Adult Health I and II

Patricia Kyriakidis, RN, PhD

Thomas Ahrens, RN, PhD, FAAN

Patricia Benner, RN, PhD, FAAN

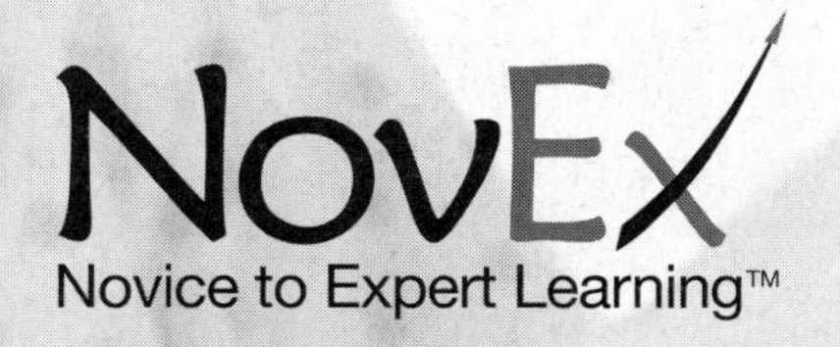

PEARSON

Boston Columbus Indianapolis New York San Francisco
Amsterdam Cape Town Dubai London Madrid Milan Munich Paris Montreal Toronto
Delhi Mexico City Sao Paulo Sydney Hong Kong Seoul Singapore Taipei Tokyo

Contributors on Adult Health 1

Thomas S. Ahrens, RN, PhD, FAAN
Patricia Ahrens, RN, BSN
Patricia E. Benner, RN, PhD, FAAN
Tammy Carroll, RN, MSN, ARNP
Kara Hanenburg, RN, MA
Halden W. Hooper, MD
Alex Johnson, RN, MSN
Kyriakos E. Kyriakidis, MD
Patricia H. Kyriakidis, RN, PhD
Jill Mallen, RN, MS, CNS
Molly McClelland, RN, PhD, CMSRN
Angela McConachie, RN, DNP, FNP-C
Nina B. Murphy, BASc
Cathy Provins-Churbock, RN, PhD, ACNP-BC
Teresa Rincon, RN, PhDc
Robert St. John, MSN, RRT
Priscilla H. Stoddard, RN, BSN, CRNA
William F. Stoddard, MD

Reviewers, Adult Health 1

Thomas Ahrens, RN, PhD, FAAN
Patricia Benner, RN, PhD, FAAN
Sarah Davis, MD
Lisa Day, RN, PhD, CNRN, CNE
Kara Hanenburg, RN, MA
Frank Hicks, RN, PhD
Halden W. Hooper, MD
Kyriakos E. Kyriakidis, MD
Patricia Kyriakidis, RN, PhD
Molly McClelland, RN, PhD, CMSRN
Angela McConachie, RN, DNP, FNP-C
Priscilla H. Stoddard, RN, BSN, CRNA
William F. Stoddard, MD

Medical Artist for Adult Health 1

George Kyriakidis, PhD

Contents

Note to Student v

Oxygenation

Module 1

Acute Bronchitis 1
Deviated Septum 10
Epistaxis 20
Allergic Rhinitis 30
Acute Rhinosinusitis 41
NovE-Cases for Module 1 51

Module 2

Airway Obstruction 52
Tracheostomy 74
Acute Lung Injury 91
NovE-Cases for Module 2 102

Module 3

COPD 103
Asthma 119
NovE-Cases for Module 3 131

Module 4

Pneumonia 132
Influenza 152
NovE-Cases for Module 4 165

Module 5

Toxic Inhalation 166
Pleural Disturbances 182
Thoracotomy 199
Pulmonary Embolism 206
Tuberculosis 225
Sleep Apnea 241
NovE-Cases for Module 5 252

Perfusion

Module 6

Acute Coronary Syndrome 253
Angina 285
NovE-Cases for Module 6 295

Module 7

Dysrhythmias 296
Electrocardiogram 326
NovE-Cases for Module 7 355

Module 8

Cardiomyopathy 356
Heart Failure 373
NovE-Cases for Module 8 400

Module 9

Hypertension 401
NovE-Cases for Module 9 419

Module 10

Endocarditis 420
Pericarditis 432
Myocarditis 443
NovE-Cases for Module 10 450

Module 11

Chronic Venous Insufficiency (CVI) 451
Arterial Vascular Diseases 464
Venous Thromboembolism (VTE) 499
Cardiac Valvular Disease 512
NovE-Cases for Module 11 525

Shock

Module 12

Overview of Shock States 526
Cardiogenic 540
Neurogenic 550
Hypovolemic 557
Anaphylactic 568
NovE-Cases for Module 12 580

Sepsis

Module 13

Sepsis 581
NovE-Cases for Module 13 600

Fluid & Electrolytes

Module 14

Fluid & Electrolyte Disturbances . . . 601
NovE-Cases for Module 14 . . . 626

Hematology/Oncology

Module 15

Platelet & Coagulation Disorders . . . 627
Anemia . . . 650
Blood Cancers . . . 677
NovE-Cases for Module 15 . . . 692

Module 16

Cancer Patient . . . 693
Treatment Toxicities . . . 728
NovE-Cases for Module 16 . . . 749

Upper Gastrointestinal

Module 17

Upper and Lower GI Bleeding . . . 750
Abdominal Pain . . . 768
Esophageal Disorders . . . 782
Peptic Ulcer Disease . . . 806
NovE-Cases for Module 17 . . . 816

Lower Gastrointestinal

Module 18

Infectious GI Disorders . . . 817
Inflammatory GI Disorders . . . 854
Structural/Obstructive GI Disorders . . . 871
NovE-Cases for Module 18 . . . 897

Hepatic Disorders

Module 19

Hepatic Disorders . . . 898
Pancreatitis . . . 926
Gallbladder Disease . . . 940
Functional GI Disorders . . . 960
NovE-Cases for Module 19 . . . 978

Renal

Module 20

Urinary Tract Disorders & CAUTI . . . 979
Ureteral Calculi or Renal Stones . . . 1004
Urinary Incontinence . . . 1020
NovE-Cases for Module 20 . . . 1038

Module 21

Acute Kidney Injury . . . 1039
Chronic Kidney Disease . . . 1064
Glomerulonephritis . . . 1085
NovE-Cases for Module 21 . . . 1099

Diabetes and Gland Disorders

Module 22

Diabetes Mellitus . . . 1100
Hyperglycemic Crisis: DKA and HHS . . . 1118
Hypoglycemia & Hyperglycemia During Hospitalization . . . 1129
Insulin . . . 1142
NovE-Cases for Module 22 . . . 1157

Module 23

Thyroid Disturbance . . . 1158
Adrenal Gland Disorders . . . 1178
Obesity . . . 1193
Pituitary Gland Disorders . . . 1207
NovE-Cases for Module 23 . . . 1217

Musculoskeletal

Module 24

Osteoarthritis & Joint Replacements . . . 1218
Fractures: Hips, Femur, Pelvis . . . 1234
NovE-Cases for Module 24 . . . 1263

Neuro

Module 25

Traumatic Brain Injury (TBI)) . . . 1264
Spinal Cord Injury . . . 1286
Neuro Inflammatory & Infectious Disease . . . 1307
NovE-Cases for Module 25 . . . 1337

Module 26

Stroke . . . 1338
Brain Tumors . . . 1373
Chronic Neurologic Conditions: Dementia and Delirium . . . 1390
Seizures . . . 1412
NovE-Cases for Module 26 . . . 1429

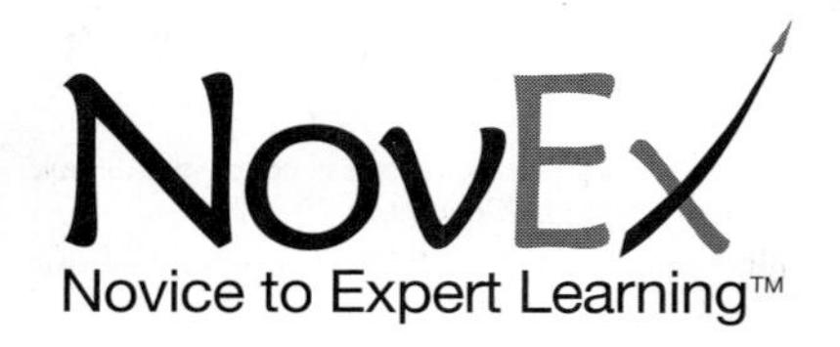

To the Student

Learning with NovEx will be different from your other nursing courses, as you will have the opportunity to practice and develop your clinical thinking and reasoning skills in a simulated clinical environment (called a NovE-case) immediately after learning the most clinically relevant content that is foundational for good patient care in each lesson (called a NovE-lesson.) It is the goal of the NovEx course to educate you to be a safer and more skillful nurse as you care for your patients. To learn more about how to maximize your learning with NovEx, read on.

About This Course

Adult Health provides the most up-to-date evidence-based practices in order to prepare you for the dynamic environment of a clinic, medical, and/or surgical unit. You will learn the most commonly diagnosed conditions and collaborative interventions in order to care for your patients with the current recommended medical standards and nursing practices.

Course Outcomes

After completing the NovE-Lessons and NovE-Cases, you should be able to:

- Recognize the clinical relevance of the most commonly diagnosed conditions and collaborative interventions that address them.
- Consider the pathophysiology, etiology, risk factors, and clinical presentation of these conditions that determine the priority patient concerns and the care that addresses them.
- Determine the most urgent and important nursing interventions and patient education required in caring for a patient with the most commonly diagnosed conditions and resulting collaborative interventions.
- Evaluate attainment of desired patient care outcomes for a patient with the most commonly diagnosed conditions and resulting collaborative interventions.

How to Prepare for Class

For each module, there are several NovE-Lessons and related NovE-Cases. The NovE-Cases solidify the knowledge acquired from the NovE-Lessons; therefore, to learn what you need to know for each patient condition in the course and be prepared for class, you will need to:

1. **Study the NovE-Lessons assigned by your instructor.** While reading, you will see:
   a. Symbols. Pay close attention as they delineate the responsibilities of the health care team. The N indicates that it is your responsibility to initiate or perform the intervention, and/or ensure the interventions is provided to the patient. The M indicates that it is the medical practitioner's or Health Care Provider's (HCP) responsibility to initiate, determine, and/or perform the interventions. When you see the "N" & "M", it is your responsibility to collaborate with the

medical practitioner or HCP in order to perform the required intervention for the patient. The (EBP) indicates research-based practices that are strongly recommended in the care of patients. These delineated interventions are central in the care and evaluation of care you provide. These essential interventions are most commonly urgent, high priority, and/or required. These interventions are fundamental to your success in this course and in clinical practice.

> **Hypokalemia**
>
> - M N — Identify and treat the underlying cause.
> - M N EBP — Provide oral potassium if patient is able to drink and hypokalemia is not severe. Should supplement with dietary intake of potassium-rich foods (Cohn, et al., 2000).
> - N — Offer a flavored beverage when administering oral potassium, for the patient to drink with or after the potassium. Oral potassium has a strong and bitter taste.
> - M N EBP — If mild to moderate (K^+ 3.0–3.4 mEq/L) and without continued potassium loss, give 10–20 mEq orally, two to four times daily (Cohn, et al., 2000).
> - M N — If severe (K^+ <2.5–3.0 mEq/L) or symptomatic (e.g., dysrhythmias, significant muscle weakness), give oral potassium 40 mEq, three to four times daily or 20 mEq IV every 2–3 hours.
> - M N EBP — If symptoms are severe and patient is unable to take orally, infuse potassium 20 mEq IV every 2–3 hours (Cohn, et al., 2000). Use of a central line is preferred due to potential phlebitis.

b. Animations and Videos. In order to adequately prepare for class and any tests administered, it is essential that you access your NovE-Lesson online so that you can view the animations and videos and learn the content you need to know in order to successfully use the practice cases. The animations and videos can assist in understanding concepts in a few short minutes that will be more easily remembered and used.

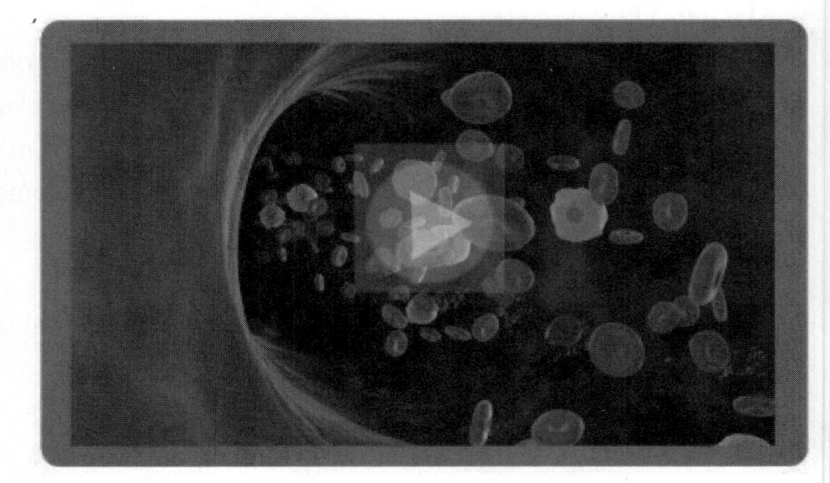

Source: © 2013 Nucleus Medical Media, All rights reserved

c. Prioritized Collaborative Interventions. Because practicing nurses must learn to prioritize the care provided to patients on a hourly basis, NovEx has carefully designed each lesson by prioritizing care to prepare you to organize, "think, and act like a nurse". Interventions are organized around urgency, safety, priority, and evidence-based. Interventions for symptom management, comfort care, and patient education that may not currently be evidence-based are presented in separate sections.

d. Treatment Algorithms. Use the summary of interventions algorithms to assist you in pulling the many detailed interventions together when caring for patients. You will find these invaluable as you problem-solve the NovE-Cases.

e. Narratives. The narratives are clinical stories of memorable situations by practicing nurses. They are incredibly interesting. These are shared with you to provide strong instances for learning. Many nurses who hear others' stories, or reflect on their own clinical situations, can learn important lessons that can forever improve their practice and make them better nurses. Some stories detail how things did not go well, which provide ways of learning that can be as rich as excellent care of patients. We believe you will find the clinical narratives engaging, worthwhile, and rich sources of knowledge you will use in your clinical practice.

f. **Concept Checks.** Use these ungraded questions to check your reading comprehension throughout the NovE-Lessons. (Place a sample callout from a lesson as an example).

Concept Check

2. Following a severe head injury, a 45-year-old male patient is in a medically-induced coma and mechanically ventilated. Which factors predispose this patient to the development of pneumonia?
   A. Age
   B. Immobilization
   C. Gender
   D. Trauma

Answer question

2. **Practice what you learned in the NovE-Lessons with the NovE-Cases when indicated in your syllabus.** Your performance will be reported to your professor and is commonly graded, so it is essential that you complete all cases assigned ***before*** class.

Class Participation

Once you have prepared for class, your professor will spend time reviewing cases and discuss the best clinical practices for your future patients using coaching cases and the practice cases that you completed before class. Coaching cases are practice cases but have real life scenarios and clinical challenges embedded as questions for the class to respond to. It is essential to your development as a clinician that you complete the assigned practice cases ***before*** class, as you may be asked to present a practice case to the class, discuss in a small group, or called upon by your instructor to answer questions based on the practice cases. Additionally, your professor will use coaching cases to discuss pathophysiological, family, psychological, spiritual, ethical, and social issues that may arise during your clinical practice.

NCLEX-Style Practice and Assessment Questions

You will have plenty of practice and test opportunities with NCLEX style questions based on the content of the NovE-Lessons and NovE-Cases. It is therefore important that you complete all NovE-lessons and NovE-Cases assigned so you will be successful.

We wish you great success, both as a student and, more importantly, as a practicing nurse.

Learning Outcomes for Acute Bronchitis

When you complete this lesson, you will be able to:

1. Recognize the clinical relevance of acute bronchitis.
2. Consider the pathophysiology, etiology, risk factors, and clinical presentation of acute bronchitis that determine the priority patient concerns.
3. Determine the most urgent and important nursing interventions and patient education required in caring for a patient with acute bronchitis.
4. Evaluate attainment of desired collaborative care outcomes for a patient with acute bronchitis.

LO1:

What Is Acute Bronchitis?

- Bronchitis occurs when the trachea (windpipe) and the large and small bronchi (airways) within the lungs become inflamed because of infection or irritation.
- Bronchitis commonly occurs after an upper respiratory infection, such as a cold or the flu, and is caused by a virus more than 90% of the time.
- This lesson focuses on acute bronchitis. Chronic bronchitis is a different, more serious condition that occurs in patients with COPD. It is manifested by prolonged cough (3 consecutive months over 2 years).

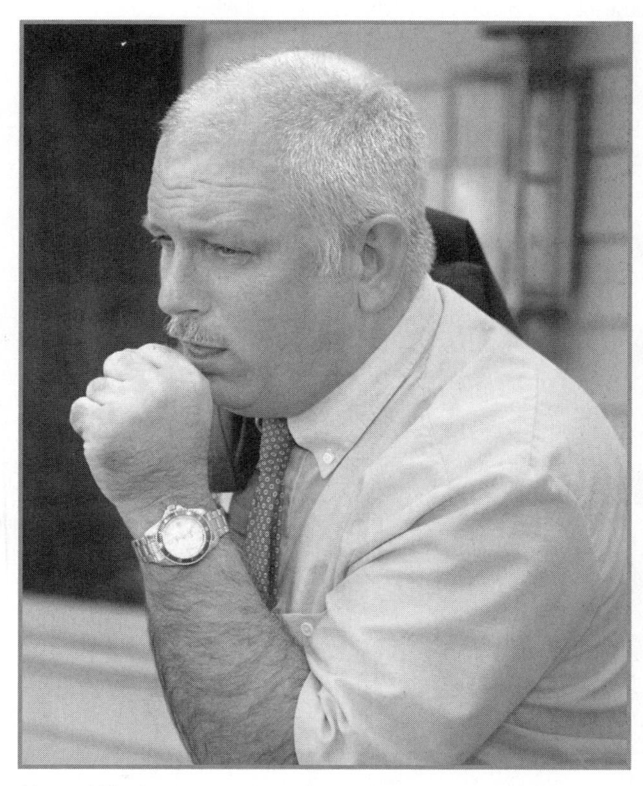

Almost 90% of acute bronchitis infections are viral, not bacterial.
Source: Lisa F. Young/Fotolia

Concept Check

1. What is the most common cause of upper respiratory infections associated with acute bronchitis?

   A. Virus

   B. Bacteria

   C. Fungus

   D. Pollutants

Answer question

LO1:

Clinical Relevance

- Acute bronchitis is among the ten top conditions that cause patients to see a health care provider.
- It is the most frequently diagnosed illness by primary care providers.
- In the United States, costs range from $200–300 million annually.
- Acute bronchitis is a common reason for antibiotic overuse and misuse (65–80% of patients with bronchitis currently receive antibiotics). Despite little evidence that supports their effectiveness, as antibiotics are active against bacteria but not viruses, antibiotics are still overprescribed. Health care providers commonly find themselves challenged by patient demands to overtreat.
- Studies show that reducing the misuse of antibiotics effectively reduces the prevalence of antibiotic-resistant bacteria.

LO2:

Pathophysiology

- Infection or irritation of the bronchial tree leads to inflammation. Inflammation can cause several problems:
  - o Edema and narrowing of the bronchioles
  - o Secretion of mucous that is usually cleared by cough
  - o Bronchospasm (contraction of the muscles lining the bronchial walls), which may manifest as wheezing
  - o More severe inflammation can cause injury and sloughing of the cells lining the bronchial tree, resulting in purulent sputum (thicker discolored sputum), but is not necessarily a sign of bacterial infection.
- Most symptoms are transient, lasting a few to 10 days, and resolve shortly after the viral infection clears. Cough, however, may persist for 2–3 weeks.
- In some patients, the inflammation can last for several months.

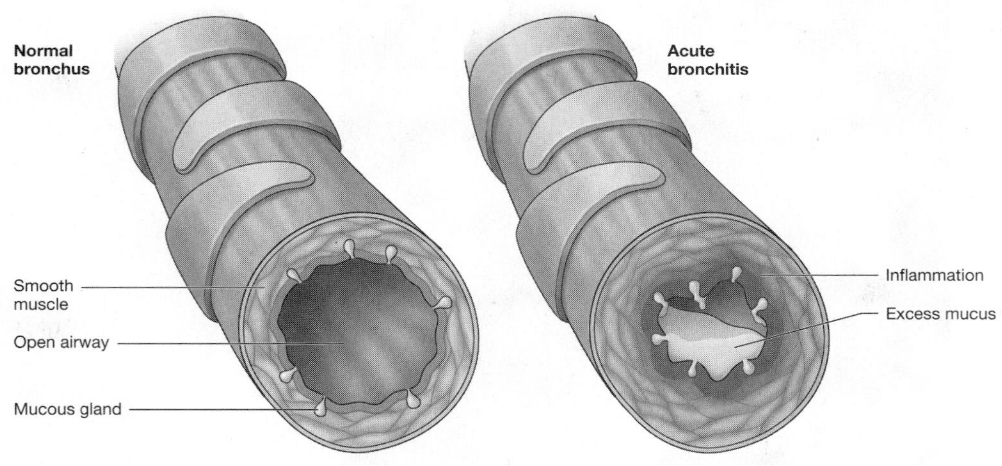

Normal versus inflamed bronchus in acute bronchitis.

Concept Check

2. Which finding indicates severe inflammation of the bronchial tree but not necessarily the presence of infection?

A. Coughing that persists beyond 1 week

B. Thick, dark sputurm

C. Wheezing that clears with coughing

D. Sudden development of sneezing

Answer question

LO2:

Risk Factors

Risk factors for acute bronchitis include:

- Smoking or exposure to secondhand smoke
- Exposure to air pollution
- Exposure to irritating vapors and chemical fumes
- Dust
- Older adults, infants, and very young children
- Pre-existing lung disease

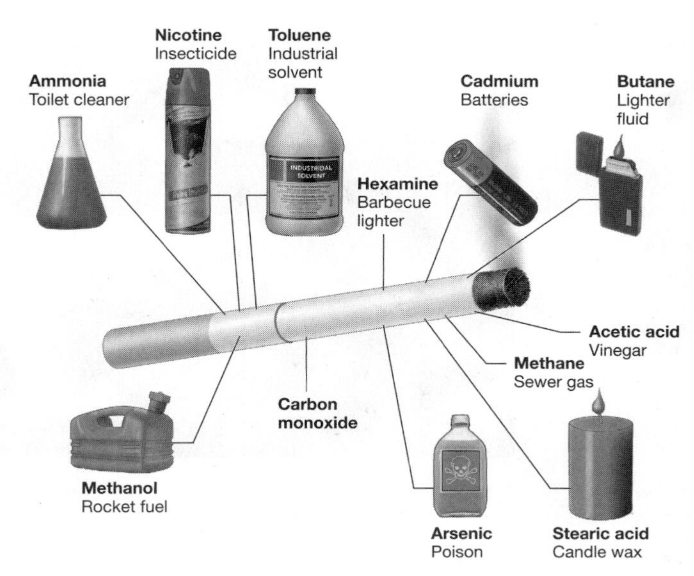

Smoking is the leading cause of preventable death in the United States. Exposure to secondhand smoke is third. Cigarettes emit multiple gases and particulates (about 4,800 gases or chemicals). Carbon monoxide, formaldehyde, nicotine, methane, toluene, carcinogenic tars, and more are breathed in as secondhand smoke.

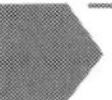

Concept Check

3. **Which situation is a risk factor for the development of acute bronchitis?**
   A. Drinking alcohol
   B. Genetic predisposition
   C. Exposure to water pollution
   D. Exposure to chemical fumes

Answer question

Causes

Acute bronchitis can develop from many conditions or factors:

- Viruses: Rhinoviruses and influenza viruses account for more than 90% of acute bronchitis.
- Bacteria (less than 10%): mycoplasma pneumoniae (most common)
- Yeast and fungi (less than 10%)
- Noninfectious triggers or irritants (less than 10%): asthma, air pollutants, ammonia, cannabis, tobacco, trace metals, others

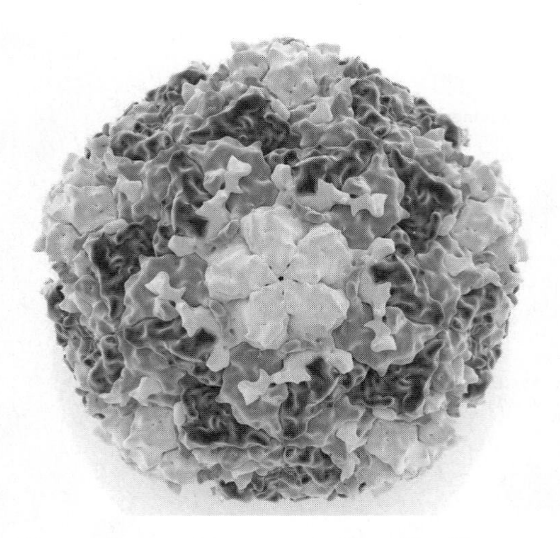

Human rhinovirus: Viruses are not living things. They are, however, highly infectious. Only 30 or so rhinoviruses (above) are sufficient to cause someone to catch a cold. Because viruses are not alive, they need a living host to reproduce. Viruses are parasites.
Source: Luk Cox/Fotolia

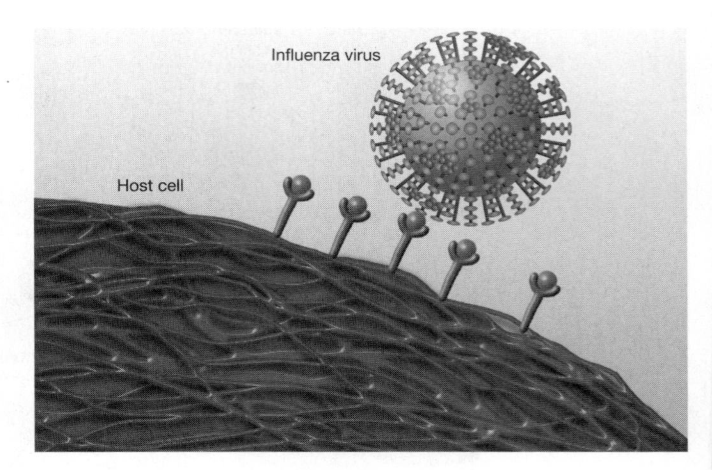

Influenza virus attaching to host cell: The influenza virus attacks by attaching itself to receptors on healthy cells in the respiratory system. The virus will pass along its genetic information into the host cell to replicate and produce more strains of the virus as well as strains with possible mutations.

LO2:

Assessment Findings

- Irritating and often persistent cough, lasting 10–21 days. Cough may be dry hacking or productive.
- Sputum production may be clear or purulent.
- Wheezing can occur in some patients.
- Low-grade fever, if any
- Chest tightness or discomfort
- Shortness of breath can be mild, even in severe cases, but uncommon.
- Hoarseness
- Malaise is not typical.
- Symptoms may all be absent in some cases.

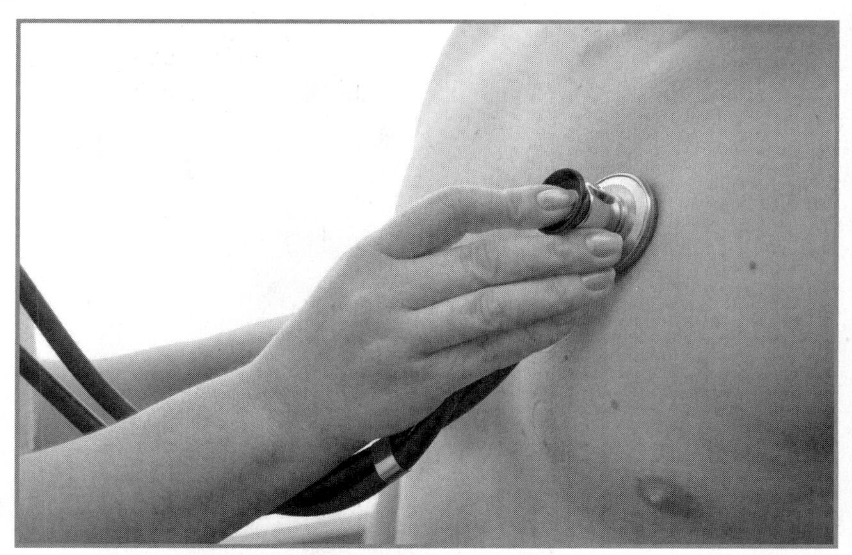

When infection causes airway irritation and inflammation or bronchitis, sputum production with a persistent cough occurs. Wheezing is frequently noted and sounds like a whistle or squeaky sound on inspiration. Chest discomfort or pain, a low-grade fever, and dyspnea may also occur.
Source: Oleg Pchelov/Shutterstock

Concept Check

4. **Which finding is least commonly associated with acute bronchitis?**
   A. Fever
   B. Chest tightness
   C. Hoarseness
   D. Shortness of breath

Answer question

Atypical Assessment Findings

Patients with acute bronchitis do not usually appear very ill. However, pneumonia can develop following bronchitis and needs to be ruled out (usually with a chest x-ray) in patients who have the following atypical symptoms:

- Fever with temperature over 101.3°F (38.5°C)
- Tachycardia: heart rate greater than 100 beats/min
- Confusion or altered level of consciousness
- Severe shortness of breath
- Hypoxemia: low pulse oximeter readings (less than or equal to 92%)
- Crackles on lung exam

If patients have these symptoms, health care providers should look for a cause other than bronchitis.

Diagnostics

- Diagnosis is clinically based on the patient's history and symptoms in the absence of other underlying diseases, such as asthma, COPD, or pneumonia.
- Chest x-ray may be needed, depending on severity and type of symptoms.
- Sputum cultures are not recommended.

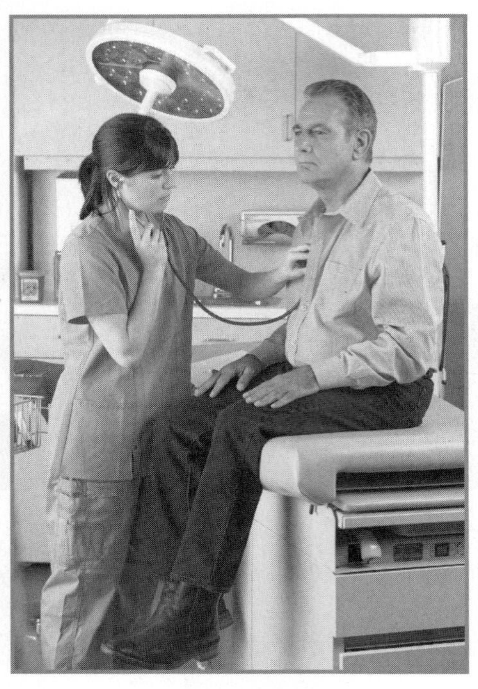

The health care provider simply uses a stethoscope to listen for wheezes in the lungs that commonly accompany bronchitis.
Source: Monkey Business/Fotolia

Concept Check

5. What is the primary diagnostic tool used to determine whether a patient with acute bronchitis has developed pneumonia?

A. Chest x-ray
B. Cardiac monitor
C. Pulse oximetry
D. Sputum culture

Answer question

Priority Patient Concerns and Desired Collaborative Care Outcomes

Prior to caring for patients with acute bronchitis, it is important to prioritize the patient's concerns that must guide the nursing care plan and interventions. Care for the patient is ordered and organized in accordance with the patient's priority and urgent needs. Desired collaborative care outcomes in patients with acute bronchitis typically include:

1. Patient will report that it is easier to expectorate mucous.
2. Patient's airways will sound clearer to auscultation.
3. Patient will report a decrease in discomfort with reduced coughing and congestion.
4. Patient will acknowledge that cough may be persistent for several weeks but should gradually become less frequent and should begin to produce clear or thin white mucous.

Considering these important care outcomes, prepare a list of the major 3–6 priority patient concerns or nursing diagnoses for patients with acute bronchitis. Be prepared to participate in a discussion of this list and/or to submit them as an assignment, as determined by your faculty. Resources you may find helpful in this assignment can include this lesson, the references, resources on nursing care plans, and standard nursing diagnoses manuals.

LO3:

Collaborative Interventions

Evidence-Based Practice

Evidence has NOT shown that antibiotics are helpful in acute bronchitis (except in pertussis, which is uncommon).

Collaborative Practice: Symptom Management

- Treatment is focused primarily on symptom relief and comfort.
- M N Administer ordered bronchodilators (albuterol/ipratropium)—normally only given if wheezing is severe and/or shortness of breath is present.
- M N Provide the most common therapy, antitussives or protussives, to relieve cough, (e.g., guaifenesin, benzonatate, chlorpheniramine and hydrocodone [Tussionex]). Recommend as an over-the-counter medication for at home use.
- N Patient Education is a major focus:
  - o Emphasize that antibiotics are almost never indicated in acute bronchitis. The only exception to this is bronchitis caused by pertussis.
  - o Encourage patient to get as much rest and hydration as possible.
  - o Teach and promote humidified air, especially while sleeping.
  - o Recommend over-the-counter analgesics for fever/pain (acetaminophen, ibuprofen).
  - o Recommend over-the-counter decongestants/antihistamines (phenylephrine, diphenhydramine) to alleviate congestion.
  - o Sitting (or elevating the head of the bed in rarely hospitalized patients) may be often more comfortable.
  - o Demonstrate and encourage effective coughing techniques, as well as turning and deep breathing.

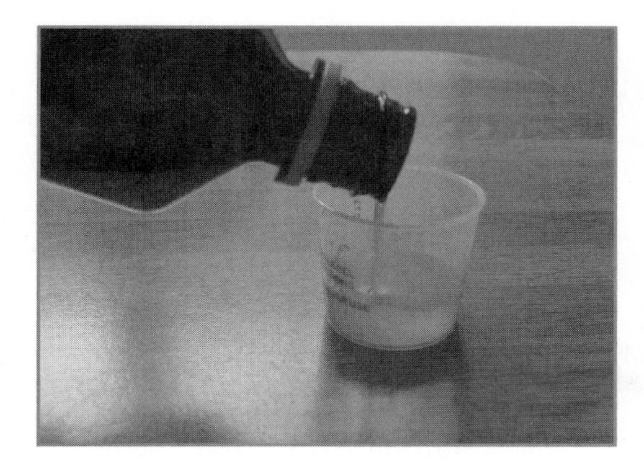

Patients often find antitussives or protussives helpful with symptom relief.

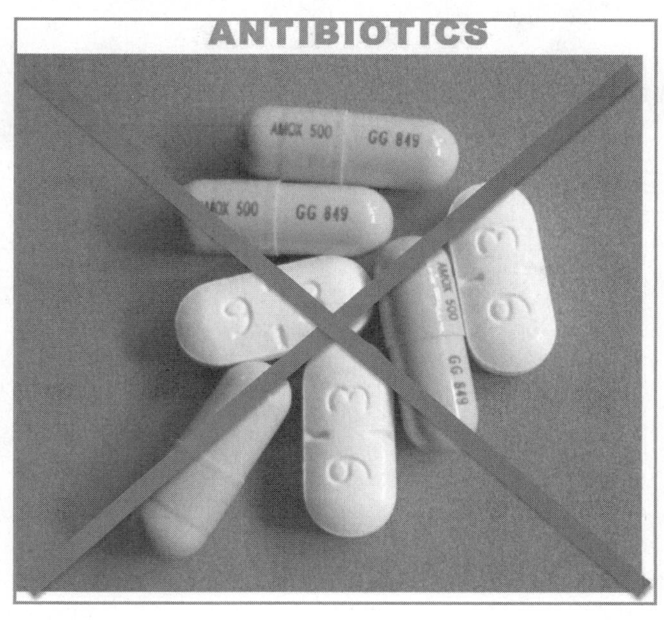

Concept Check

6. Which treatment is indicated for acute bronchitis?

A. Two-week course of antibiotics

B. Use of a dehumidifier in the bedroom

C. Prone positioning

D. Use of antitussives

Answer question

Collaborative Interventions (continued)

Nursing Support and Preventive Education

- Promote hand washing and good respiratory hygiene to prevent risk of spread of virus.
- Teach patients to avoid inhaled irritants such as smoke or chemical inhalants, (e.g., perfumes, strong odors, dust, feather pillows).
- Inform patient that cough may last for longer than 2–3 weeks, even up to 30 days.
- Encourage fluid intake of 2–3 liters per day according to patient's cardiac tolerance.
- Reinforce with family as well as patient that routine antibiotic therapy, which treats *bacterial* infections, is not helpful and not recommended with viral infections like bronchitis. Overuse and misuse of antibiotics increases the patient's and community's risk of resistant bacterial infections.

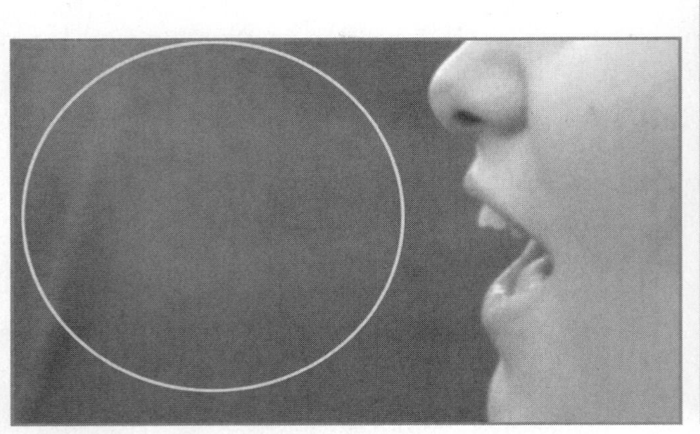

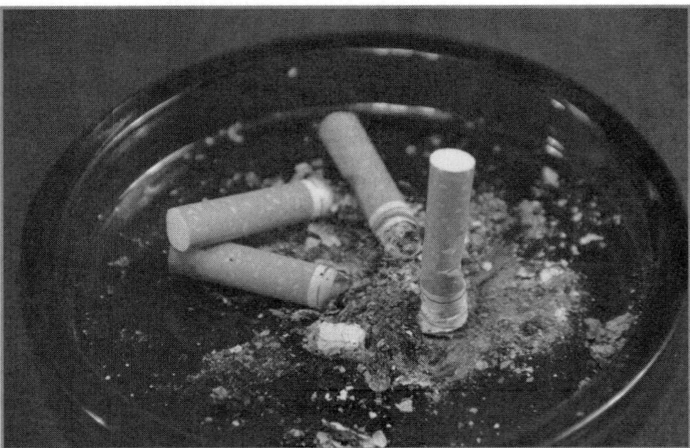

Good hygiene and smoking cessation are key patient education issues.
Sources: *(left)* Copyright © 2012, NovEx Novice to Expert Learning, LLC; *(right)* CDC/Debora Cartagena

Concept Check

7. What is a major community risk associated with inappropriate use of antibiotics?
   A. Increased cost of individual prescription drugs
   B. Increased use of emergency department services
   C. Increase in drug-resistant pathogens
   D. Increase in the number of cases of acute bronchitis

Answer question

Summary of Interventions

- Symptomatic treatments for cough and congestion include: bronchodilators (only when indicated), antitussives, rest, hydration, and antipyretics.
- Antibiotics should be considered only for those who have comorbidities that make them susceptible to pneumonia.
- Pneumonia needs to be ruled out (usually with chest x-ray) in patients who appear ill, have a rapid respiratory rate, tachycardia, crackles on lung exam, or high fever.

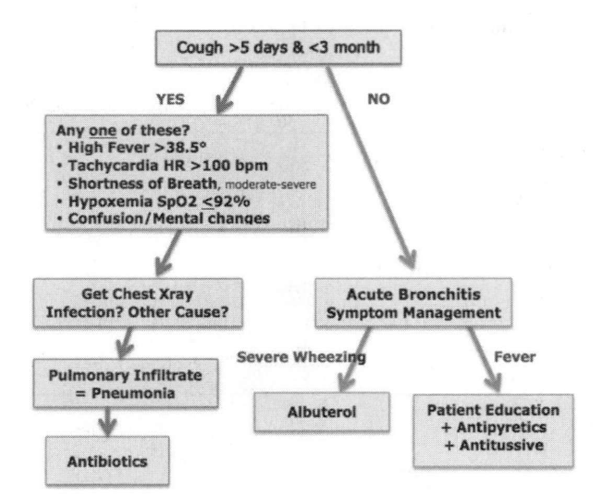

Schematic of acute bronchitis: recognition through treatment.
Source: Copyright © 2012, NovEx Novice to Expert Learning, LLC

LO4:

Evaluation of Desired Collaborative Care Outcomes

Evaluation and reassessment should reveal attainment of previously established patient outcomes. In summary:

- Patient reports that it is easier to expectorate mucous.
- Patient's airways sound clearer to auscultation.
- Patient reports a decrease in discomfort with reduced coughing and congestion.
- Cough may be persistent for several weeks but is gradually becoming less frequent and is beginning to produce clear or thin white mucous.

If the patient becomes increasingly tachypneic, tachycardic, has crackles on lung exam, or develops a high fever, additional diagnostic testing and intervention are required.

References

Blush, R.R. (2013). Acute bronchitis: evaluation and management. Nurs Practitioner: Amer J Primary Health Care, 38(10), 14-20. **www.nursingcenter.com/Inc/Static-Pages/Acute-bronchitis-Evaluation-and-management**

Ebell, M.H., Lundgren, J., & Youngpairoj, S. (2013). How long does a cough last? Comparing patients' expectations with data from a systemic review of the literature. Ann Fam Med, 11(1), 5-13. **www.annfammed.org/content/11/1/5.full**

Gonzales, R., Anderer, T., et. al. (2013). A cluster randomized trial of decision support strategies for reducing antibiotic use in acute bronchitis. *JAMA, 173*(4), 267–273. **http://www.ncbi.nlm.nih.gov/pubmed/23319069?tool=MedlinePlus**

http://www.lung.org/lung-disease/bronchitis/

http://www.aafp.org/afp/980315ap/hueston.html

http://www.crnbc.ca/Standards/CertifiedPractice/Documents/RemotePractice/740AdultAcuteBronchitisDST.pdf#search=adult%20acute%20bronchitis

Learning Outcomes for Deviated Septum

When you complete this lesson, you will be able to:

1. Recognize the clinical relevance of deviated septum.
2. Consider the pathophysiology, etiology, risk factors, and clinical presentation of deviated septum that determine the priority patient concerns.
3. Determine the most urgent and important nursing interventions and patient education required in caring for a patient with a deviated septum.
4. Evaluate attainment of desired collaborative care outcomes for a patient with a deviated septum.

LO1:

What Is a Deviated Septum?

One of the most common causes of structural nasal obstruction is acquired deviation of the septum. The septum is easily injured. Even minor blunt trauma can cause alteration in cartilage and/or septal bones.

- The patient often complains of sensation of:
  - Insufficient airflow
  - Fullness
  - Stuffiness
  - Congestion
  - Blockage within the nose
- Unilateral complaints suggest structural cause and bilateral complaints suggest mucosal cause.

LO1:

Clinical Relevance

- Obstruction to the nasal passages may make it difficult to breathe through the nose.
- Postnasal drip may result from blockage of nasal passages.
- Drying of the nasal septum may lead to nosebleeds.
- Sinus infection can occur from prolonged congestion.
- A minor annoyance can be that noisy breathing occurs during sleep.

LO2:

Pathophysiology

A deviated septum is a variation, usually significant, from the normal neutral anatomic position of the septum between the nasal passages.

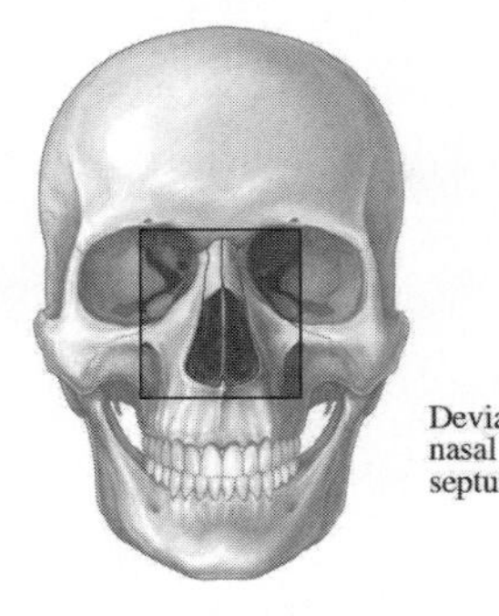

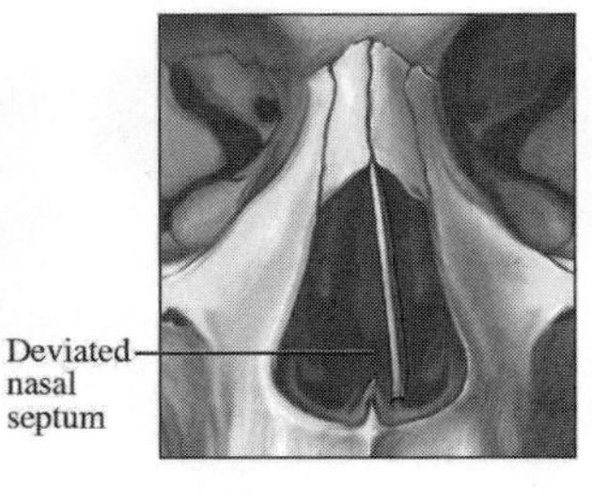

This image depicts a deviated nasal septum. The skull on the left shows where the nasal septum is normally located whereas the view on the right depicts a septum that is dislocated to the patient's left.

Risk Factors

- Normal aging does not cause septal deviation, even though symptoms from the deviation can worsen over time.
- Diseases such as allergic or chronic rhinosinusitis may potentiate obstruction caused by the septum.
- Deviated septum is often associated with nasal bone fractures, which are discussed later in this elesson.

Causes

Several causes of a deviated septum are:

- Traumatic or forceps delivery
- Sports injuries
- Motor vehicle accidents
- Traumatic events
- Idiopathic

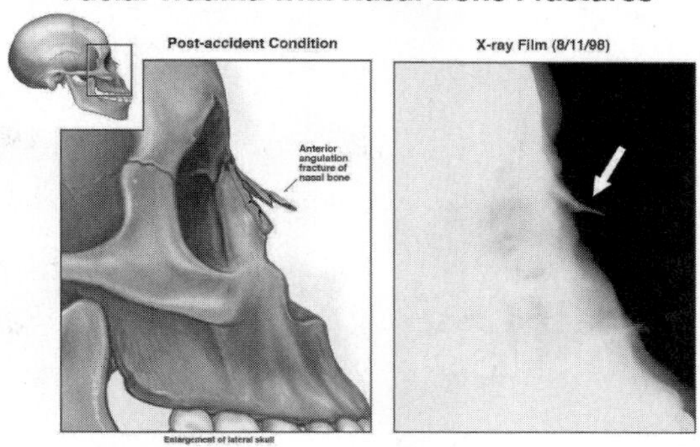

Accidents and trauma are common causes of nasal fractures, resulting in deviated septum.
Source: © 2013 Nucleus Medical Media, All rights reserved

Assessment Findings

Symptoms most often seen with a deviated septum include:

- Unilateral obstruction of nasal passage
- Frequent nasal congestion or sore throat from postnasal drip
- Facial pain or frontal headaches
- Frequent sinus infections or nosebleeds

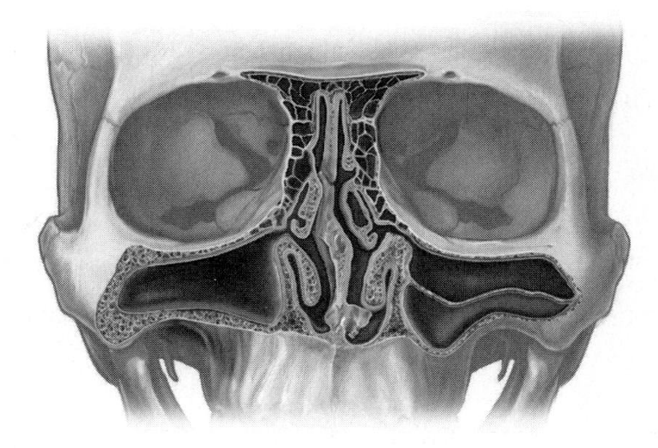

This drawing features a cutaway view of the head and the sinuses. Note the deviated septum with a narrowed passage which can cause congestion and/or obstruction.
Source: © 2013 Nucleus Medical Media, All rights reserved

Concept Check

1. **Which symptom is commonly associated with deviated septum?**
   A. Sinusitis
   B. Migraine headaches
   C. Pneumonia
   D. Choking

Answer question

Diagnostics

- Evaluation of patient with nasal symptoms should include a detailed history, physical examination, and anterior rhinoscopy with a nasal speculum or otoscope with a bright light.
- Most causes of nasal obstruction can be identified by examination of the external nose, nasal cavity, and nasopharynx.

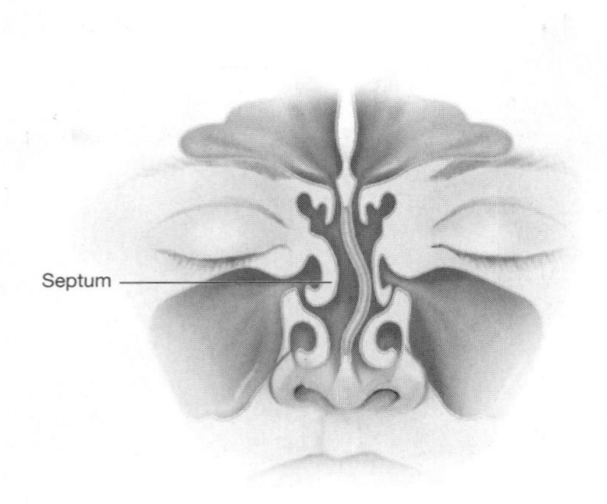

Deviated nasal septum.

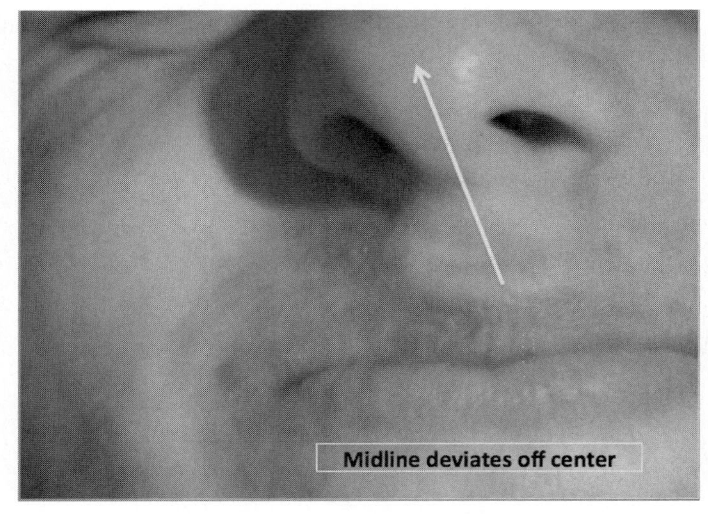

Deviated nasal septal midline.
Source: Copyright © 2012, NovEx Novice to Expert Learning, LLC

- Tests such as acoustic rhinometry, (measure of the nasal cavity using acoustic reflections) peak nasal airflow, rhinomanometry, (measure airflow and pressure in the nose during respirations) allergy testing, or mucosal biopsy may prove helpful.
- Some patients may require further evaluation:
  - o Nasal endoscopy: Used for better evaluation of internal nasal structures (normally septum should be midline)
  - o Diagnostic imaging: CT scan is helpful for assessing mucosal disorders and anatomic deformities
  - o Standard facial x-rays are usually not helpful.

Concept Check

2. **To diagnose a deviated septum caused by a mucosal abnormality, facial x-rays are considered:**
   A. necessary in the evaluation of nasal mucosa.
   B. helpful in noting anatomical disorders.
   C. useful in visualization of internal structures.
   D. not helpful when making this diagnosis.

Answer question

Priority Patient Concerns and Desired Collaborative Care Outcomes

Prior to caring for patients with a deviated septum, it is important to prioritize the patient's concerns that must guide the nursing care plan and interventions. Care for the patient is ordered and organized in accordance with the patient's priority and urgent needs. Desired collaborative care outcomes in patients with a deviated septum typically include:

1. Patient will experience less discomfort during respirations.
2. Patient will report improved ease of breathing.

Considering these important care outcomes, prepare a list of the major 3–6 priority patient concerns or nursing diagnoses for patients with a deviated septum. Be prepared to participate in a discussion of this list and/or to submit them as an assignment, as determined by your faculty. Resources you may find helpful in this assignment can include this lesson, the references, resources on nursing care plans, and standard nursing diagnoses manuals.

Concept Check

3. Which nursing diagnosis takes priority in the care of a patient with a deviated septum due to trauma?

A. Impaired airway

B. Discomfort

C. Altered Self-concept

D. Risk for injury

Answer question

LO3:

Collaborative Interventions

Collaborative Symptom Management

- Most cases of nasal obstruction due to structural cause (deviated septum) DO NOT respond to medical treatment.
- The majority of cases of nasal obstruction are effectively treated with a combination of pharmacological and surgical therapy.
- Nasal strips may be helpful in cases in which the soft tissues around the lateral external nose collapse during regular or moderate inspiration.

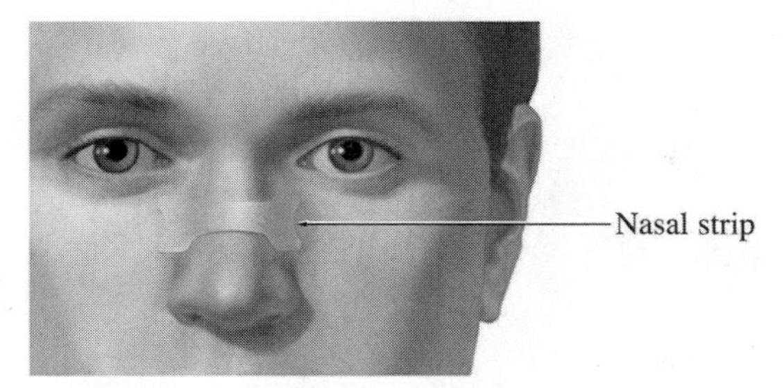

Although it is not harmful to utilize nasal strips, users must be aware that they may not improve symptoms and this treatment is not considered definitive.

Definitive Management

- In general, structural disorders, such as deviated septum, are most effectively treated with surgical intervention.
- Septoplasty is the definitive treatment. The literature suggests long-term success varies, but symptom improvement is common postsurgery.

LO4: Evaluation of Desired Collaborative Care Outcomes

Evaluation and reassessment should reveal attainment of previously established patient outcomes. In summary:

- Patient has less discomfort during respirations.
- Patient reports improved ease of breathing.

Concept Check

4. **What is the most effective treatment for a deviated septum?**
   A. Use of nasal strips
   B. Use of nasal sprays
   C. Surgical septoplasty
   D. Oral steroids

Answer question

What Is a Nasal Fracture?

- Fracture of the nasal bone and surrounding cartilage
- Usually results from blunt force trauma to the nose from a direct hit or a fall
- Can occur in isolation or associated with other facial injuries
- Associated with nasal bleeding and swelling

Fractures of Nasal Bones and Septum

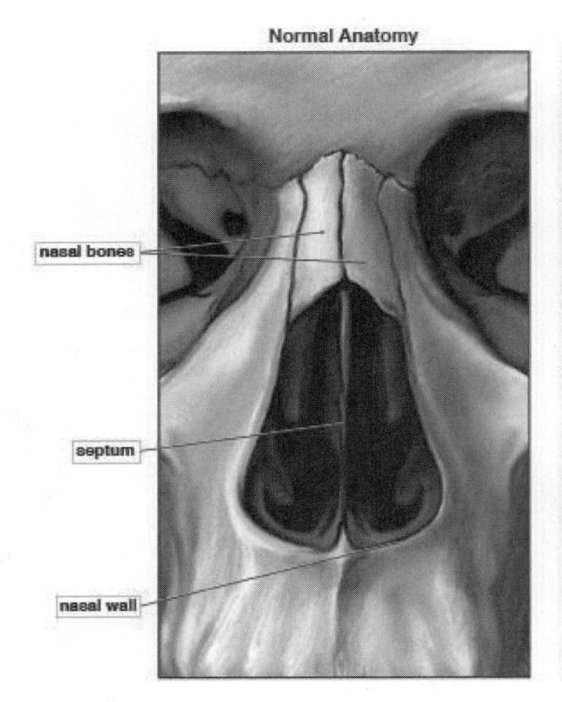

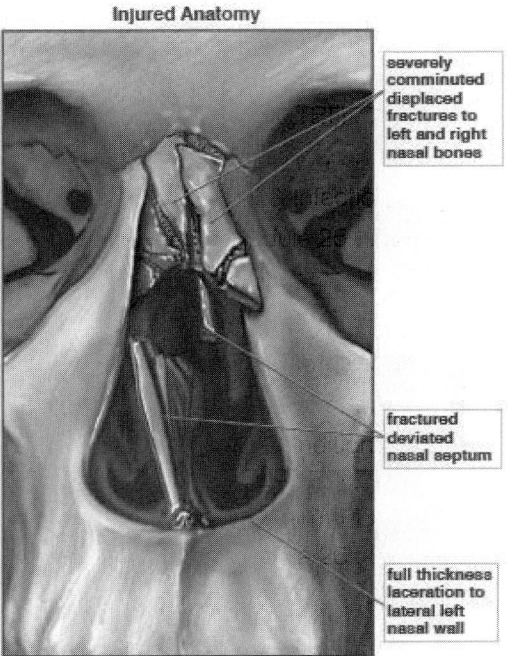

Clinical Relevance: Nasal Fractures

- Facial appearance is a serious concern of humans.
- Fractures are very common in automobile and sports injuries.
- Injury may result in both acute and chronic pain.
- Severe blood loss is not uncommon.
- The complication of nasal obstruction may result in breathing and sleeping problems.
- Self-esteem and self-image may be diminished secondary to facial scarring and disfigurement.
- In a worst-case scenario, death can occur.

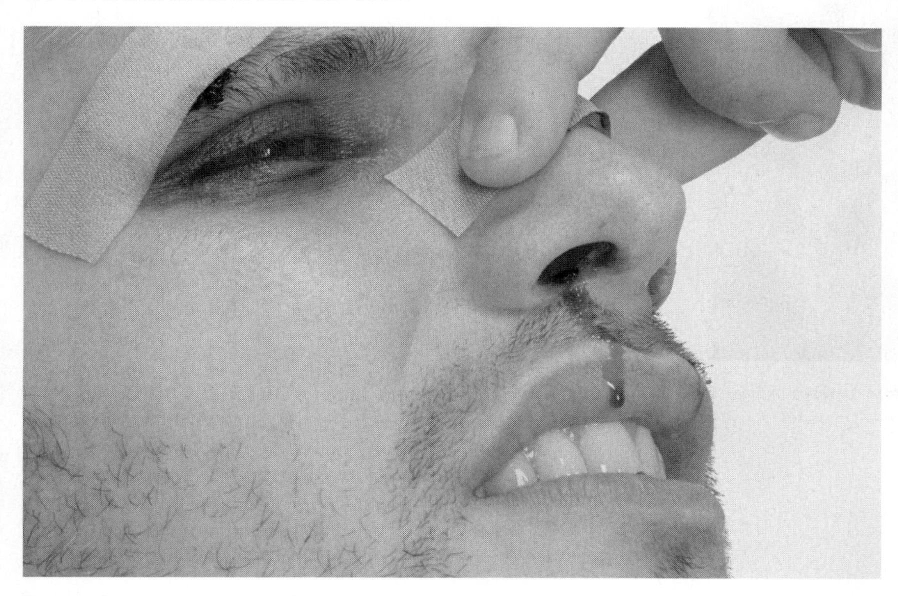

Fractured nose with epistaxis; the result of a rugby injury.
Source: Image Source Plus/Alamy

Causes and Risk Factors: Nasal Fractures

- Contact sports
- Motor vehicle accidents
- Direct blunt force trauma
- Interpersonal or domestic violence
- Falls
- Risky recreational activity

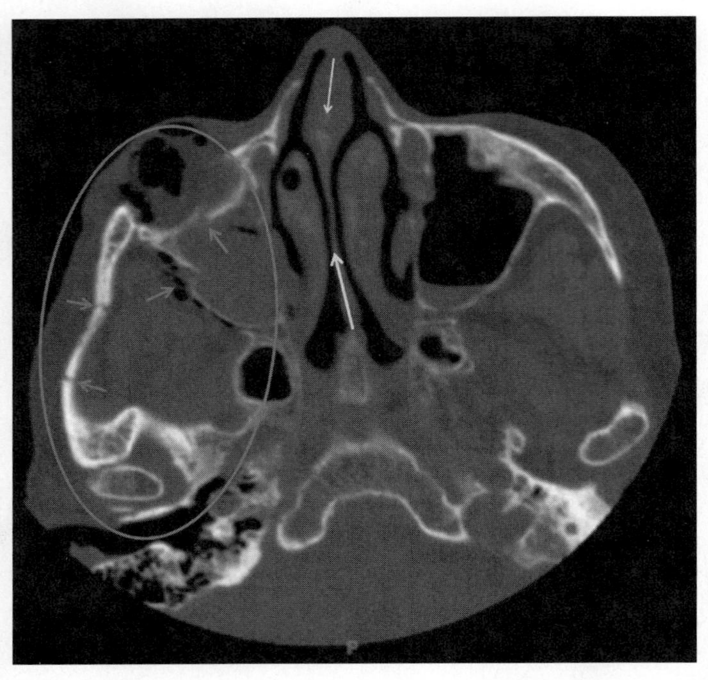

Nasal fracture (slanted yellow arrow) is not this patient's most serious injury. He also sustained extensive right facial fractures (red arrows and circle) involving the orbit of the eye and maxillary sinus.
Source: Copyright © 2012, NovEx Novice to Expert Learning, LLC

Assessment Findings: Nasal Fractures

The symptoms of nasal fracture can vary, but often include:

- Obvious swelling and pain to the nose and/or surrounding areas
- Epistaxis (nose bleeding)
- Bruising of the nose and surrounding tissues
- Lacerations and abrasions
- Inability to breathe through one or both sides of nostrils

Diagnostics: Nasal Fractures

- Focus on the basics of trauma care:
  - o Primary survey
  - o Secure airway
  - o Complete facial examination (e.g., secondary survey)
- Nasal fractures may be associated with other injuries, including orbital or facial fractures, thus a careful examination is necessary.
- Accurate diagnosis and appropriate referral to a specialist may be key to initial management of facial bone fractures.
- Fractures of the thin bones of the nasal bridge are common. Patients with a contusion or tenderness over the bridge of the nose may be assumed to have a fracture of the nasal bones.

Physical Examination

- Findings consistent with common, less severe nasal fractures include:
  - o Nosebleed
  - o Discoloration
  - o Pain and tenderness over the bridge of the nose
  - o Crepitation over the injured area
  - o Obstruction of nasal passage
  - o Displacement—the nose appears crooked
  - o Hematoma of the median septum of the nose
- Severe injuries could include a fracture of the base of the skull resulting in rhinorrhea, which is leaking of cerebrospinal fluid (CSF) from the nose. A Halo Test should be performed and if positive (the drainage forms a yellow "halo" on gauze), the drainage is probably CSF, indicating a fracture of the base of the skull.

Concept Check

5. A patient with facial trauma and possible nasal fracture has a positive halo test. What major concern should the nurse prioritize in the care of this patient?

A. Airway obstruction

B. Broken nose

C. Deviated septum

D. Cerebrospinal fluid leak

Answer question

Imaging Studies

- Nasal bone x-rays need *not* be obtained in the emergency department (ED) provided the following criteria are met:
  - o Tenderness and swelling are isolated to the bony bridge of the nose.
  - o Patient can breathe through each naris.
  - o The nose is straight (i.e., no deviation of septum).
  - o No septal hematoma is present.
- X-rays should be considered if:
  - o There is a concern that a foreign body might be present.
  - o There could be legal ramifications (e.g., alleged assault).
- Providers giving follow-up care after the injury may obtain x-rays as needed.
- CT scan is preferred for imaging nasal fractures if there is a concern about more extensive injury evidenced by severe facial trauma associated with diffuse tenderness (e.g., NOT isolated to the nasal bridge).

Priority Patient Concerns and Desired Collaborative Care Outcomes

Prior to caring for patients with nasal fractures, it is important to prioritize the patient's concerns that must guide the nursing care plan and interventions. Care for the patient is ordered and organized in accordance with the patient's priority and urgent needs. Desired corroborative care outcomes in patients with nasal fractures typically include:

1. Patient will report decrease in pain to a tolerable level.
2. Patient's airways will remain clear with no aspiration.
3. Patient will verbalize methods to avoid re-injury.
4. Patient will explain risk factors and ways of preventing further injury.
5. Patient will demonstrate acceptance of changes in appearance.

Considering these important care outcomes, prepare a list of the major 3–6 priority patient concerns or nursing diagnoses for patients with nasal fractures. Be prepared to participate in a discussion of this list and/or to submit them as an assignment, as determined by your faculty. Resources you may find helpful in this assignment can include this lesson, the references, resources on nursing care plans, and standard nursing diagnoses manuals.

Collaborative Interventions: Nasal Fractures

Evidence-Based Practice

There is no evidence-based practice (EBP) medical treatment for nasal fractures.

Collaborative Symptom Management and Comfort Care

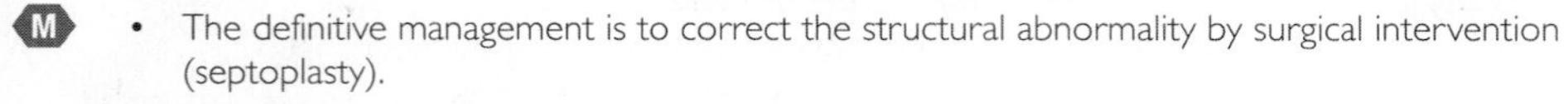

- The definitive management is to correct the structural abnormality by surgical intervention (septoplasty).
- Septoplasty is highly successful in relieving symptoms associated with nasal obstruction.
- Determine if other facial bony structures are fractured.
- Determination should be made regarding loss of consciousness with any facial injury.
- Control of bleeding is a priority with a diagnosis of deviated septum from an uncomplicated nasal fracture.
- Simple measures such as ice to the nasal area and elevating the head of the bed constrict vessels to reduce bleeding, can help relieve pressure and pain, and mitigate edema
- Symptomatic treatment for pain should be initiated. Encourage the patient to request and take pain medication as prescribed.
- Calm the patient, if needed, and teach mouth breathing to improve breathing comfort.

Patient Education

Patient education needs to be individualized, depending on the cause of the injury, but often includes:

- Teach the importance of safety measures to prevent reinjury:
  - o Appropriate use of protective sports equipment like mouth pieces and helmets, if a sports accident was the cause of injury.
  - o Importance of seatbelt use if injured in a motor vehicle accident.
  - o Environmental safety when injured in unsafe environment.
- Consider abuse as a causative factor especially in women and children. Collaborate with social worker as indicated for further intervention.
- In the elderly and very young, educate about fall precautions when appropriate.
- Educate the patient and family that facial injury and its treatment often cause significant bruising and swelling and that this condition may last for several days or weeks to transition the patient's expectations prior to seeing himself or herself. Encourage the patient to express feelings about the change in appearance. Use therapeutic communication techniques when discussing appearance or answering questions.
- Allow the patient to openly express concerns, anger, or frustration as a therapeutic intervention.

Summary of Interventions

- Septoplasty is the definitive treatment for patients with nasal obstruction due to septal deviation.
- Nasal strips can be beneficial in certain situations where the soft tissues around the lateral external nose collapse during regular or moderate respiration.
- Nasal fracture should be treated with the intent to prevent future septal deviation by returning the septum to proper alignment at the time of injury.
- Conservative treatment with ice pack may constitute the only necessary initial action.

LO4:

Evaluation of Desired Collaborative Care Outcomes

Evaluation and reassessment should reveal attainment of previously established patient outcomes. In summary:

- The patient reports a tolerable amount of discomfort.
- The patient reports reduced nasal dryness and stuffiness. Oxygen saturation levels are within the patient's normal range and no aspiration occurred.
- Patient identifies the probable cause of the injury, risk factors, and discusses methods to prevent reinjury.
- Patient discusses potential changes to appearance and verbalizes concerns.

References

http://www.mayoclinic.com/health/deviated-septum/DS00977/DSECTION=symptom

http://www.ncbi.nlm.nih.gov/pubmed/19328889

http://www.aafp.org/afp/2004/1001/p1315.html

Baring, D., Murray, C., Singh, J., Davidson, A., Syed, M. I. (2009). Prospective, blinded study of nasal injuries: comparison of doctor and nurse assessment. *J Laryngol Otol, 123*(12), 1338–1342.

Fraser, L., & Kelly, G. (2009). An evidence-based approach to the management of the adult with nasal obstruction. *Clin Otolaryngol, 34*, 151.

Learning Outcomes for Epistaxis

When you complete this lesson, you will be able to:

1. Recognize the clinical relevance of epistaxis.
2. Consider the pathophysiology, etiology, risk factors, and clinical presentation of epistaxis that determine the priority patient concerns.
3. Determine the most urgent and important nursing interventions and patient education required in caring for a patient with epistaxis.
4. Evaluate attainment of desired collaborative care outcomes for a patient with epistaxis.

LO1:

What Is Epistaxis?

- Epistaxis, commonly known as nose bleed, is a common problem, occurring in up to 60% of the general population.
- Most types of epistaxis are classified as anterior and occur in a highly vascular part of the nasal septum. Posterior epistaxis is generally a more serious type of bleed.
- Only 10% of epistaxis cases require medical attention, and surgical intervention is rarely needed.
- Most cases occur either before age 10 or between 45–65 years old.

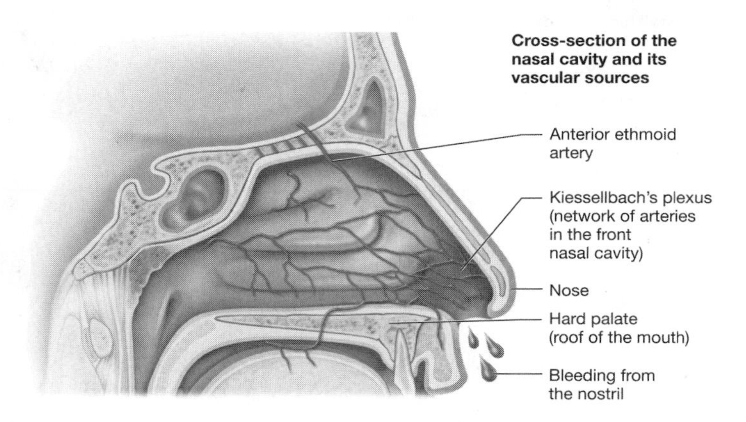

LO1:

Clinical Relevance

- Epistaxis is a common clinical condition.
- Rarely is epistaxis life threatening, unless the bleeding cannot be stopped.
- Most cases are self-limiting with basic treatment.
- Epistaxis is often frightening to the patient, as the blood loss can appear to be substantial.
- Reassurance to the patient while determining the cause and implementing treatments is an important nursing responsibility.

LO2:

Pathophysiology

- Anterior epistaxis:
  1. Usually occurs when the mucosa is eroded; blood vessels become exposed; and, subsequently, break and bleed
  2. Is of capillary origin in the majority of incidents
  3. Provides a constant ooze typical of a venous or capillary bleed
  4. May also originate anterior to the inferior turbinate
- Posterior bleeds:
  1. Develop from a ruptured blood vessel in the posterior nasal cavity
  2. Trend toward more profuse blood loss
  3. May be of arterial origin (producing a pumping of blood)
  4. Present a greater risk of airway compromise
  5. Make aspiration of blood more likely
  6. Manifest greater difficulty in controlling bleeding

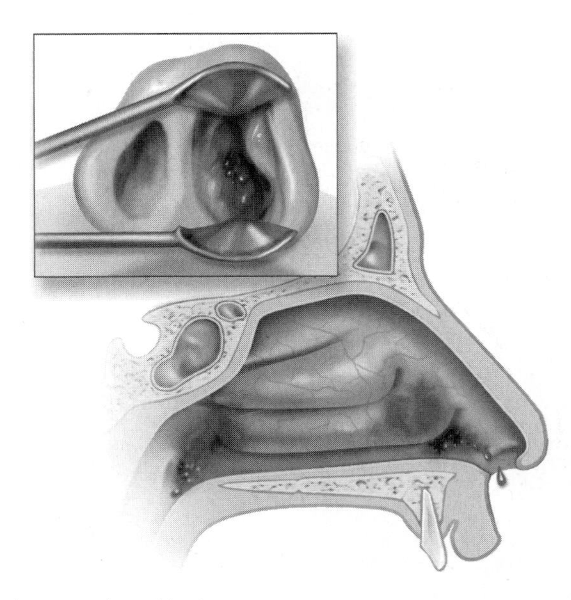

Location of nosebleed.

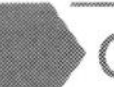

Concept Check

1. **A patient with a posterior epistaxis is at risk for what manifestation?**

   A. Aspiration

   B. Mucosal erosion

   C. Infection

   D. Hypertension

Answer question

LO2:

Risk Factors

Factors that increase the risk of epistaxis, although none are associated with high causality include:

- Male gender
- Anticoagulant use (e.g., aspirin, warfarin)
- Seasonal variation (i.e., winter months when humidity is low)
- Nose picking
- Allergic or viral rhinitis
- Foreign body or facial trauma
- Excoriation due to drug use (e.g., cocaine)
- Blood dyscrasias (e.g., hemophilia)
- Vasculopathy (e.g., vascular lesions)
- Nasal neoplasm

Causes

- Epistaxis is commonly the result of trauma. The trauma can be severe, as in the illustration, or minor, as from picking one's nose.
- However, spontaneous bleeding can occur, particularly if the patient has a coagulapathy (e.g., low blood platelets).
- Certain conditions increase the tendency to bleed (e.g., drying of the mucous membranes in patients with rhinitis).

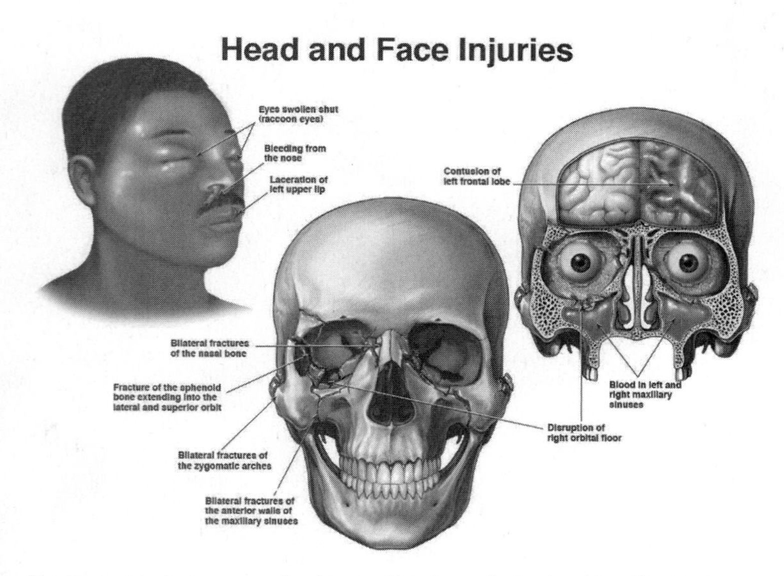

This illustration depicts external and internal injuries to the head and face. The injuries include: eyes swollen shut, bleeding from the nose, laceration of the left upper lip, contusion of the left frontal lobe of the brain, blood in the left and right maxillary sinuses, disruption of the right orbital floor, bilateral fractures of the nasal bone, the zygomatic arches and the anterior walls of the maxillary sinuses and a fracture of the sphenoid bone extending into the lateral and superior orbit.

Concept Check

2. Which test is most helpful in diagnosing the source of frequent nose bleeds?

   A. Facial x-ray

   B. Nasal endoscopy

   C. 24-hour blood pressure monitoring

   D. Complete blood count

Answer question

LO2:

Assessment Findings

- Bleeding from the nasal area presents as an ooze due to an anterior bleed or as a pumping flow due to an arterial bleed.
- Patients and families may be highly anxious due to fear and anxiety produced by the bleeding.
- Airway compromise is possible secondary to an arterial bleed.

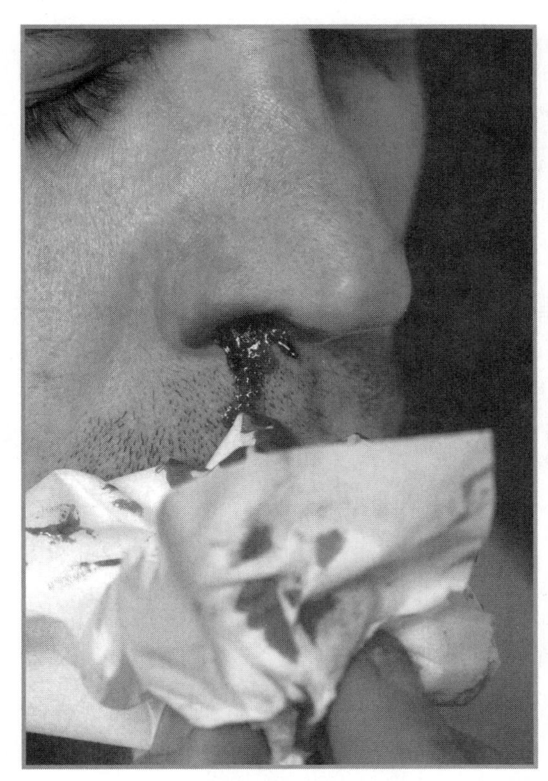

Source: The Power of Forever Photography/Getty Images

LO2:

Diagnostics

- Initial evaluation focuses on airway assessment and cardiovascular stability:
    1. Secure patent airway
    2. IV fluid resuscitation
    3. Consider emergent otolaryngologic consultation in severe cases
- Assess for symptoms related to blood loss:
    1. Chest discomfort
    2. Dyspnea
    3. Dizziness
    4. Altered mental status
    5. Tachycardia
    6. Hypotension
- Consider laboratory studies if bleeding is severe (*NOT* needed routinely):
    1. PT-INR
    2. Hemoglobin and Hematocrit
    3. Type and crossmatch

Concept Check

3. If a patient has had several hours of epistaxis, what objective data would be helpful?

A. Presence of facial bruising

B. Medication history

C. Allergy history

D. Blood pressure reading

Answer question

Detailed Evaluation of Epistaxis

- After emergency management, a more detailed examination of the nares is required.
- Preparation for the exam may include anesthetizing and vasoconstricting the nasal mucosa by topically applying agents such as lidocaine and epinephrine on saturated cotton swabs.
- Detailed examination requires a nasal speculum or otoscope speculum to look for bleeding, ulceration, or erosion. It is not uncommon to be unable to locate the source of bleeding.
- Clots can be cleared during this process with suction or by asking patient to gently blow his or her nose.

Priority Patient Concerns and Desired Collaborative Care Outcomes

Prior to caring for patients with epistaxis, it is important to prioritize the patient's concerns that must guide the nursing care plan and interventions. Care for the patient is ordered and organized in accordance with the patient's priority and urgent needs. Desired collaborative care outcomes in patients with epistaxis typically include:

1. Patient's airways will be clear and lungs will remain clear to auscultation.
2. Hemostasis will be achieved and patient will remain normovolemic as demonstrated by blood pressure, mental status, and urine output.
3. Patient will express the ability to self-manage discharge treatments with less anxiety and will exhibit a calm demeanor.
4. Patient will express knowledge of causes of epistaxis and of how to self-manage discharge treatments.

Considering these important care outcomes, prepare a list of the major 3–6 priority patient concerns or nursing diagnoses for patients with epistaxis. Be prepared to participate in a discussion of this list and/or to submit them as an assignment, as determined by your faculty. Resources you may find helpful in this assignment include this lesson, the references, resources on nursing care plans, and standard nursing diagnoses manuals.

LO3:

Collaborative Interventions

Evidence-Based Practice

- Evidence-based practice (EBP) for the treatment of epistaxis is limited.
- Treatment is designed to control blood loss.

Collaborative Symptom Management

- Controlling blood loss through pressure (tamponade) and/or cauterization is considered effective treatment even though those methods have not had randomized controlled trials and are considered limited in terms of EBP.
- For uncomplicated epistaxis, various methods can be used to control bleeding:
    - 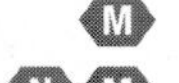 Cauterizing a bleeding vessel that can be visualized
    -  Nasal sprays to cause vasoconstriction of the nasal
    - 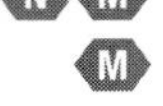 Packing the nose with various devices to tamponade the bleeding site
- 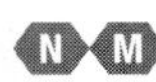 The easiest and often most effective method of managing epistaxis is application of pressure (manual tamponade) to the nasal area.
- Both patient and health care provider may need to don personal protective equipment (PPE). In addition:
    -  Teach patient to bend at the waist while sitting up to minimize swallowing of blood and risk of aspiration.
    - 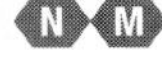 Teach patient to grasp lateral surfaces of the external nose (i.e., nasal alae) and hold firmly to the nasal septum.
    - 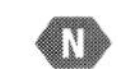 Encourage the patient NOT to check for active bleeding, but rather to hold constant pressure for a minimum of 10–15 minutes.

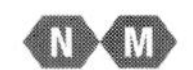 **Oxymetazoline (Afrin) to Aid Tamponade**

Many physicians recommend oxymetazoline as a treatment strategy even though little published data exists to support the practice:

- Patient blows nose to remove blood and clots so medication can absorb via nasal tissues.
- Clinician sprays nares with oxymetazoline (Afrin).
- Patient pinches lateral surfaces.

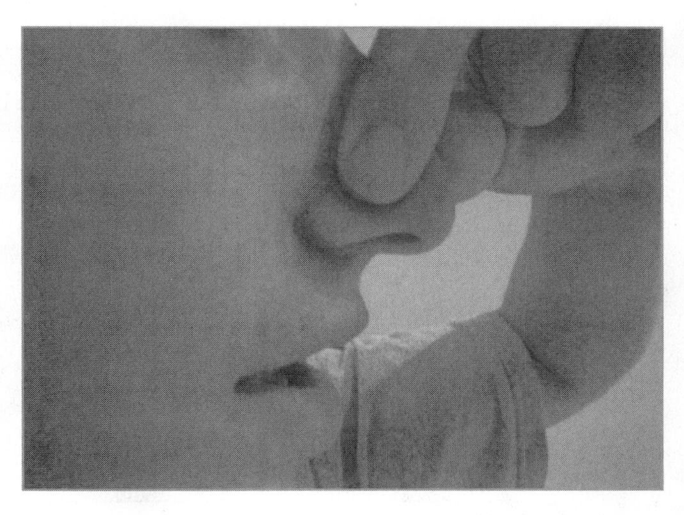

Pinch the soft part of the nose just below the bridge (the bony, hard cartilage part). Use thumb and index finger to squeeze (not too hard) for at least 10 minutes. If the nose continues to bleed, squeeze again for at least 10 minutes. While doing this, breathe through the mouth. Pinching the nose leaves little choice but to mouth breathe, but this has a positive, calming effect. If pinching the second time doesn't stop the bleeding, seek urgent medical attention.
Source: Copyright © 2012, NovEx Novice to Expert Learning, LLC

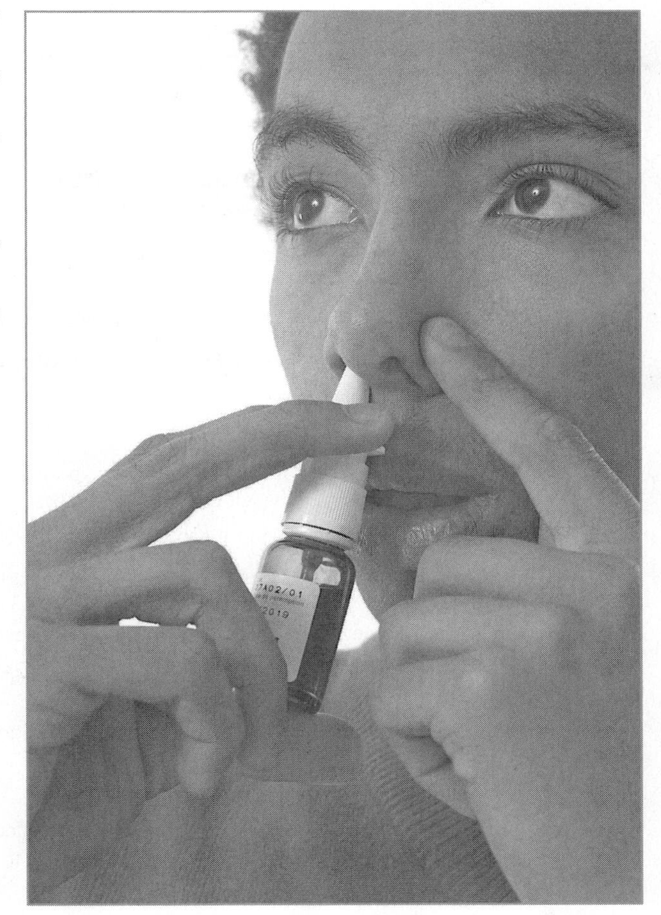

Use of nasal spray may help stop bleeding.
Source: JPC-PROD/Fotolia

Tamponade with Cotton Wool Compress

1. Have patient bend forward at waist while sitting up (to avoid aspiration or swallowing blood).
2. Place a plug of cotton wool or an absorbent compress into the bleeding nostril. Cotton will absorb drainage, providing further tamponade effect.
3. Instruct patient to expectorate further blood that accumulates in the pharynx (have emesis basin available).
4. Consider cold compress to bridge of nose.
5. Patient can perform this at home.

Management of Hypertension-Initiated Epistaxis

- Reduction of elevated BP in the setting of epistaxis has not been well studied and scientific validity of this strategy remains unclear.
- Hypertension may aggravate, but does not cause, epistaxis.
- Anxious patients may require anxiolysis with medications such as lorazepam.

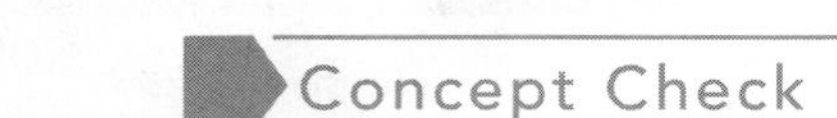

4. What is the cause of most episodes of epistaxis?
   A. Hypertension
   B. Trauma
   C. Aspirin use
   D. Allergy

Answer question

Collaborative Interventions (continued)

Source Control of Epistaxis

- If an anterior source is identified, electrical or chemical (e.g., silver nitrate) cautery may be performed.
- Analgesia and local anesthesia is very important if cautery is to be performed.

Nasal Packing May Be Chosen if Cautery Is Unsuccessful

Several packing options are available:

1. **Nasal tampons**
   a. Insert an antibiotic-coated, synthetic polymer nasal tampon (tip should be left exposed for removal).
   b. After tampon is inserted, it can be expanded by infusing saline.
2. **Nasal balloon catheters**
   a. Shown to be equally effective as packing and easier to use.
   b. Some balloons are slick after placed in water for 30 seconds and are easier to insert.
   c. Balloon catheters should not be left in place more than 3 days.
   d. Fibers in balloon may promote thrombosis.
   e. Low-pressure air balloon provides tamponade effect.
3. **Nasal packing**
   a. Use ribbon petroleum-impregnated gauze.
   b. This approach requires greater skill.
   c. Research suggests no difference in outcome between tampons versus packing.
   d. Tampons or balloon catheters suggested to be used over packing.

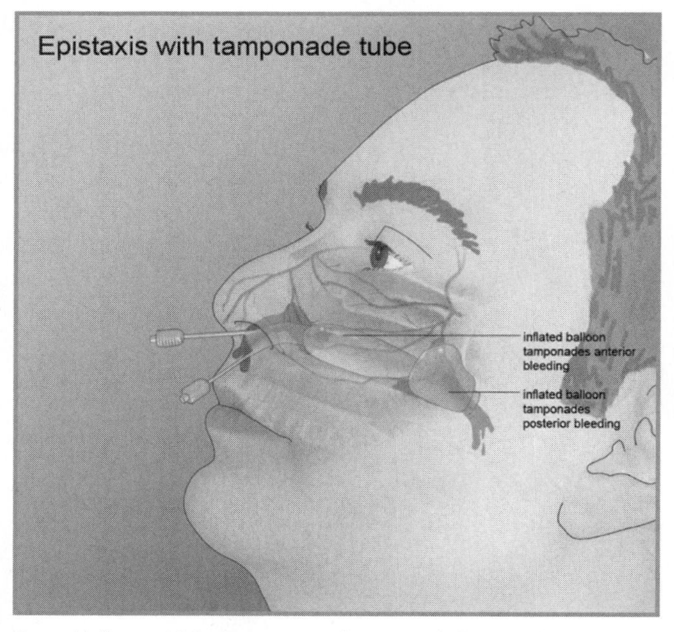

A nasal balloon with both anterior and posterior balloons is shown in place to tamponade the bleeding.
Source: Copyright © 2012, NovEx Novice to Expert Learning, LLC

Assessing for Hemostasis

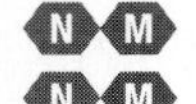

- Observe patient for 30 minutes for recurrent bleeding.
- If no anterior source is identified and bleeding has stopped, the nose should only be packed if bleeding recurs rapidly.

Persistent Bleeding and Failure to Achieve Hemostasis

- Packing is successful for anterior bleeding 90–95% of the time.
- If bilateral-nare packing fails to produce hemostasis, the odds of a more serious bleed requiring posterior packing and hospitalization increase significantly.

Support and Comfort Care

- Encourage slow controlled breathing if patient has rapid, deep, or irregular gasping respirations to reduce the possibility of aspirating blood.
- Reinforce, demonstrate, and monitor patient's ability to cooperatively follow intervention instructions, such as pinching the nares, not blowing the nose, and maintaining nasal tampon placement. Coaching and support may be needed to help patient cope with anxiety or ventilator disruption.
- Elevate the head of the bed to reduce the possibility of aspiration.
- Apply cold compress to the nose and face if bleeding is from the anterior chamber to constrict blood vessels and may help to slow bleeding.

- Explain all treatments and provide care in a calm, confident, and competent manner to increase the patient's comfort and confidence about treatment effectiveness. Support and coaching are helpful in calming the patient in the midst of large amounts of blood.

Patient Education

- Instruct the patient to return to the emergency department if bleeding recurs and cannot be stopped.
- If vital signs and respiratory function are stable after packing, patients with recurrent or severe epistaxis may be safely referred for specialist follow-up in 24–48 hours.
- Some clinicians opt for urgent otolaryngologic consultation if bilateral packing is required.
- Packing left in longer than 72 hours increases the risk of complications:
  1. Necrosis
  2. Toxic shock syndrome
  3. Sinus infections

Summary of Interventions Algorithm for Epistaxis

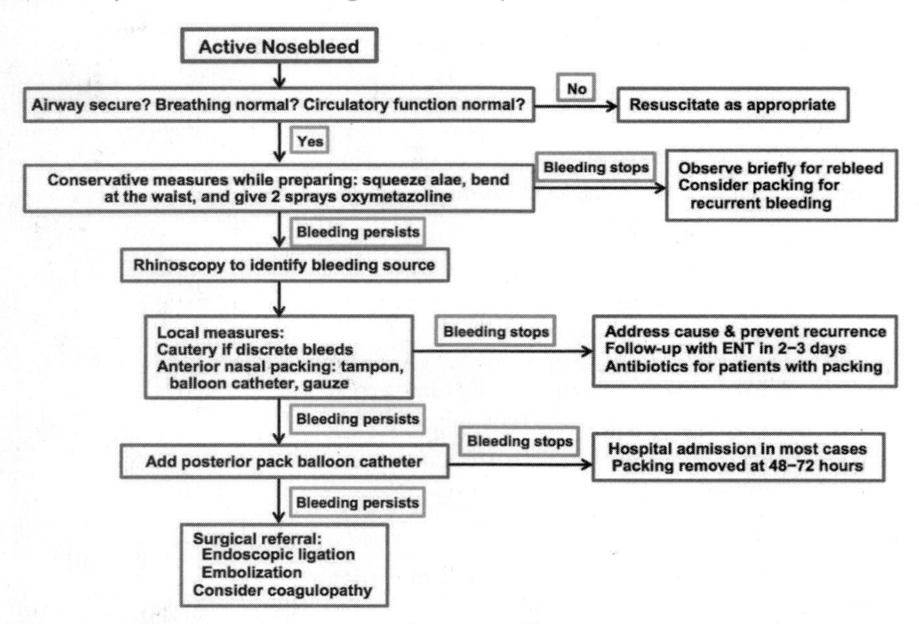

Algorithm for epistaxis management that may help guide clinical decision-making.
Source: Copyright © 2012, NovEx Novice to Expert Learning, LLC

Concept Check

5. Use of a nasal balloon catheter will require what other form of care?
   - A. Insertion of an oral airway
   - B. Administration of oxymetaxoline
   - C. Hospital admission
   - D. Manual tamponade

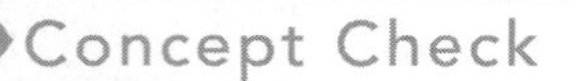

Summary of Interventions

- Epistaxis is common and rarely requires medical intervention.
- Hemostasis is often achieved by having the patient sit up, applying cool compresses to the nose, and using a manual tamponade and/or cotton wool compress.
- Oxymetazoline may be helpful.
- Patient compliance and anxiety management are key modifiable factors for minimizing bleeding.
- Nasal balloon catheters, cautery, and/or nasal packing may be needed for more severe bleeding.
- Re-bleeding, bilateral packing, or the need for posterior packing should prompt consideration for specialist referral.

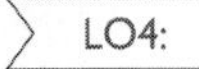

Evaluation of Desired Collaborative Care Outcomes

Evaluation and reassessment should reveal attainment of previously established patient outcomes. In summary:

- Patient's airways are clear and lungs remain clear to auscultation.
- Hemostasis is achieved. Patient remains normovolemic as evidenced by blood pressure, mental status, and urine output.
- Patient expresses the ability to self-manage discharge treatments with less anxiety and exhibits a calm demeanor.
- Patient knows the causes of epistaxis and how to self-manage discharge treatments.

References

http://emedicine.medscape.com/article/764719-overview

Douglas, R., & Wormald, P. J. (2012). Update on epistaxis. *Curr Opin Otolaryngol Head Neck Surg., 15(3)*, 180–183.

Kucik, C. J., & Clenney, T. (2005). Management of epistaxis. *Am Fam Physician, 71(2)*, 305–311.

Learning Outcomes for Allergic Rhinitis

When you complete this lesson, you will be able to:

1. Recognize the clinical relevance of allergic rhinitis.
2. Consider the pathophysiology, etiology, risk factors, and clinical presentation of allergic rhinitis that determine the priority patient concerns.
3. Determine the most urgent and important nursing interventions and patient education required in caring for a patient with allergic rhinitis.
4. Evaluate attainment of desired collaborative care outcomes for a patient with allergic rhinitis.

LO1:

What Is Allergic Rhinitis?

- Rhinitis is an inflammatory condition that affects the mucosal lining of the nose.
- Rhinitis is characterized by the presence of one or more of these symptoms: rhinorrhea, sneezing, nasal congestion, and/or itching.
- Rhinitis can either be allergic or nonallergic.

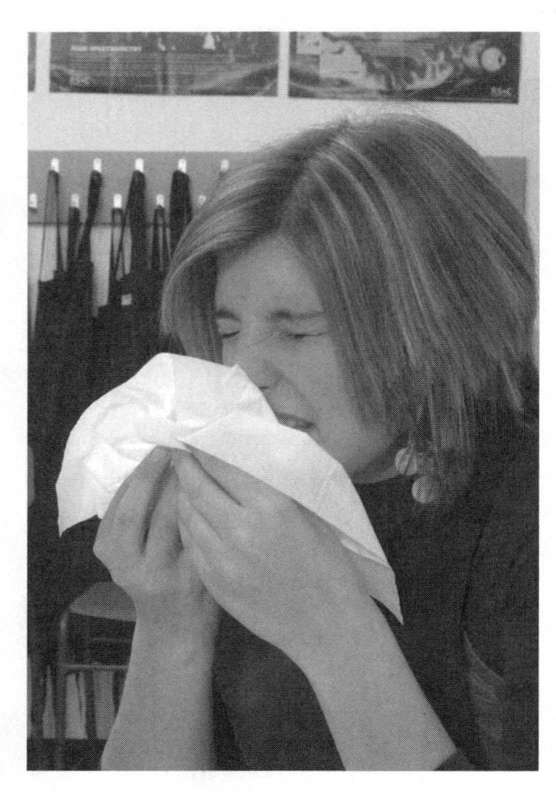

This patient shows some classic signs of rhinitis.
Source: Trevor Clifford/Pearson Education Ltd

What Are the Types of Rhinitis?

Allergic Rhinitis

This lesson focuses on allergic rhinitis as this is the more common reason for patients to seek medical care.

Nonallergic Rhinitis

- Nasal congestion and runny nose that are from no apparent cause
- Typically not harmful, but is annoying
- Commonly resolves when the cause is removed

LO1:

Clinical Relevance

- Allergic rhinitis, sometimes called "hay fever," results in lost school attendance and lost or restricted workdays. Estimated cost of decreased productivity is $2.4–4.6 billion annually.
- Up to 30% of adults and 40% of children have some degree of allergic rhinitis.
- Prevalence in industrialized world is increasing (especially urban areas) where pollution is greater.
- Rhinitis is often underdiagnosed and undertreated.
- Rhinitis accounts for at least 2.5% of clinician visits.
- Cost for over-the-counter medications and clinician visits amounts to several billion dollars each year.
- Rhinitis is frequently associated with asthma and sinusitis.
- Affected individuals suffer a decreased quality of life.

Concept Check

1. Allergic rhinitis is often associated with which two disorders?

A. Asthma and sinusitis

B. Congestive heart failure and pulmonary edema

C. Pneumonia and tuberculosis

D. Acute respiratory failure and pulmonary embolism

Answer question

Quality of Life and Cognitive Function

Allergic rhinitis is associated with a host of other problems that affect the quality of life:

- Sleep impairment
- General malaise
- Poor concentration
- Impaired athletic performance
- Anxiety
- Depression
- Impaired work performance

LO2:

Pathophysiology

- Rhinitis occurs through different mechanisms. People often have genetic or environmental predispositions to an allergen and this inherited predisposition is a major factor in the patient's response.
- Allergic rhinitis and its symptoms commonly follow a series of events that begin when atopic (predisposed, hypersensitive) patients respond to allergen exposure by producing immunoglobulin E (IgE) antibodies or allergen-specific IgE. The IgE antibodies bind to mast cells throughout the respiratory mucosa and to basophils in the blood to circulate and remove invading organisms or allergens. Patients who are hypersensitive are prone to make large amounts (10 times normal) of IgE antibodies.

Concept Check

2. A patient is referred to as "atopic." How does the nurse interpret this categorization?

A. The patient tends to exaggerate.

B. The patient has been diagnosed with multiple disease states.

C. The patient is predisposed to allergic conditions.

D. The patient has difficulty hearing due to allergic rhinitis.

Answer question

- When the same allergic "trigger" (virus, pollution, allergens, smoke) is inhaled, it attaches or binds to IgE on the mast cells. The allergen-IgE complex causes the mast cells to release inflammatory mediators (histamine, leukotrienes, and prostaglandins), initiating the hypersensitivity (overreaction) or rhinitis.

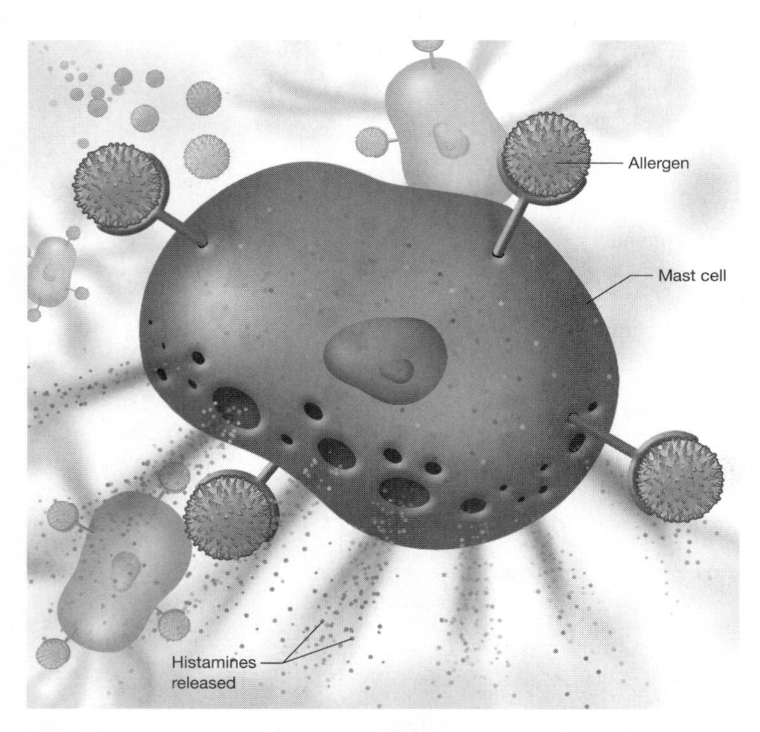

IgE antibodies (red, Y-shaped) are shown, attached to a mast cell (purple). Allergens (green) bind with the IgE, causing the mast cell to release histamines and other chemical mediators (tiny purple).

- Within minutes, after these strong and rapid-acting chemicals called inflammatory mediators (e.g., histamine) are released into the tissues, they cause inflammation by acting on the nasal mucosa, nerves, mucous glands, and blood vessels in the nasal area to produce signs and symptoms.

Sneezing, runny nose (rhinorrhea), mucosal edema, itching, and tearing ensue in response to histamine in the tissues. Similar inflammatory changes can occur in the paranasal sinus lining and cause sinusitis.

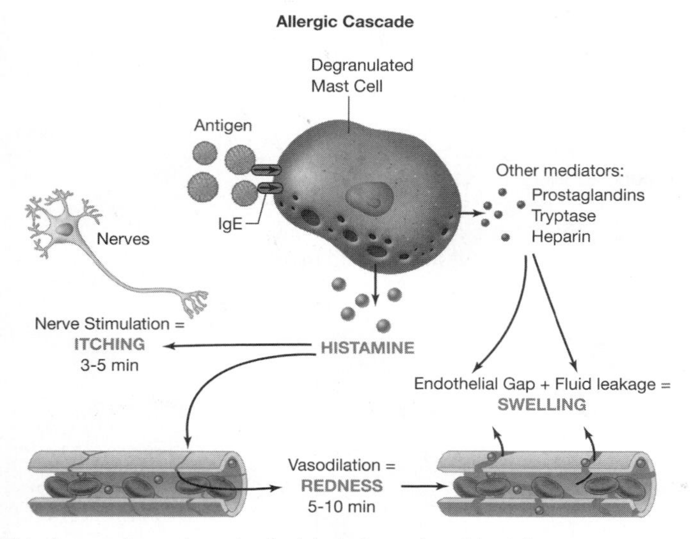

This diagram shows the pathophysiological sequelae of the inflammatory mediator effects: irritation of the nerve fibers causes itching while vasodilatory effects on blood vessels cause skin redness and swelling.

Rhinosinusitis

- Many people have an additional late reaction, within 4–15 hours, which is manifested as congestion. This reaction occurs when more and diverse inflammatory cells are recruited (e.g., macrophages, neutrophils, basophils) or triggered. The inflammatory cells also release more histamine, leukotrienes, and inflammatory chemicals. This inflammatory response affects a larger area of tissues beyond the nose, like the head and possibly other body systems as they enter the bloodstream. Thus, more systemic symptoms of inflammation (e.g., headache, fatigue) are seen.
- This pathophysiologic process is very similar to the immune response in asthma where there is a second phase of inflammatory mediators released. Again, the triggering and influx of inflammatory cells causes prolonged edema and inflammation.
- Rhinitis commonly leads to sinusitis because the nose and sinus mucosa are contiguous.
- Inflammation can also lead to obstruction of the sinus osteomeatal complex, predisposing patients to bacterial sinus infections.
- Rhinitis accounts for 30% of acute bacterial sinusitis and 80% of chronic bacterial sinusitis.

Risk Factors

- Family history (genetic predisposition)
- Male gender
- Birth during pollen season
- Firstborn status
- Early introduction of formula and food
- Maternal smoking exposure in first year of life
- Serum IgE more than 100 International Unit/mL before age 6
- Presence of allergen specific IgE
- History of eczema (atopic dermatitis)
- History of asthma

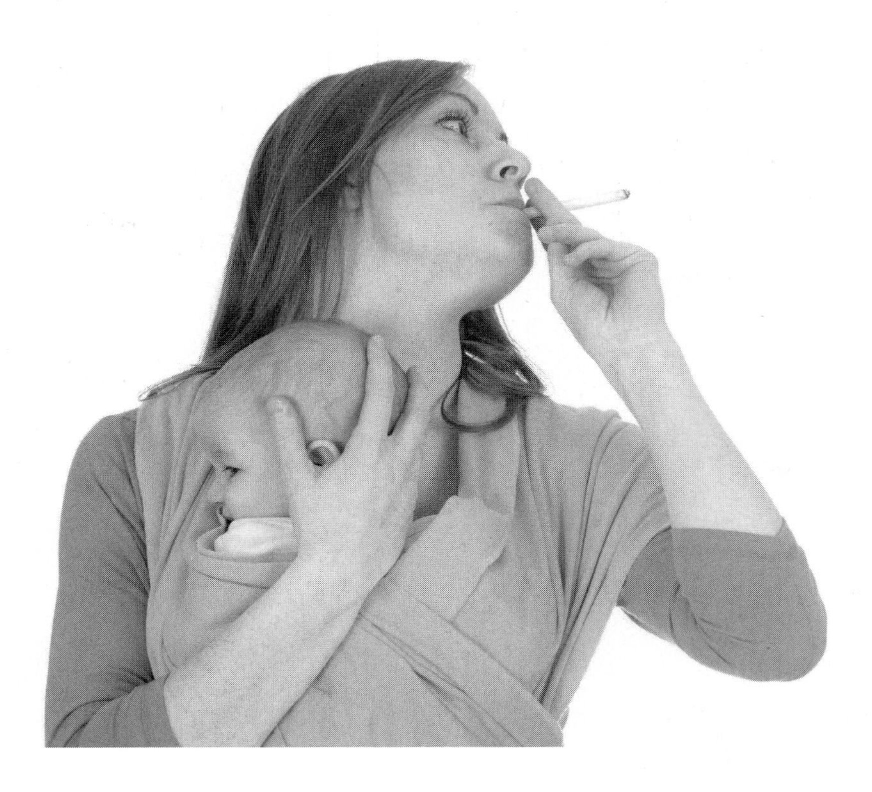

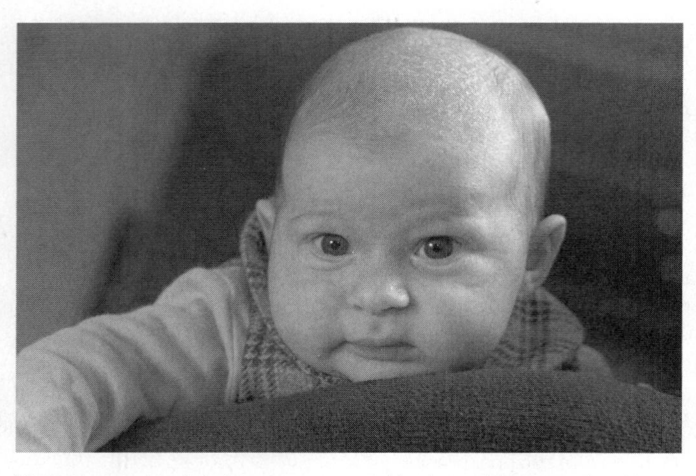

Under 1 year old, a baby's exposure to smoking (upper) increases the risk of rhinitis and sinusitis. Eczema or atopic dermatitis on the baby's face (lower) is another risk factor for rhinitis and sinusitis.
Sources: (*upper*) Marcin Sadlowski/Fotolia; (*lower*) aldegonde/Shutterstock

Concept Check

3. Which patient has the greatest risk for developing allergic rhinitis?

A. A male patient who is exposed to secondhand smoke
B. A female patient who was born in winter
C. A male patient who was exclusively breastfed until age 12 months
D. A female patient with history of colic

Answer question

Causes

- Exposure to seasonal allergens, including:
    - Trees
    - Grass
    - Weed pollens
    - Outdoor molds
- Exposure to indoor allergens that cause perennial rhinitis:
    - House dust mites
    - Cockroaches
    - Animal proteins
    - Fungi (molds)
    - Strong scents
    - Perfumes
    - Foods
- Nonallergic rhinitis:.
    - Exposure to irritants such as pollution, smoke, and cleaning solutions
    - Exposure to spicy foods
    - Some medications, e.g., for erectile dysfunction
    - Cold temperature
- Aging often offers some improvement in allergic rhinitis.

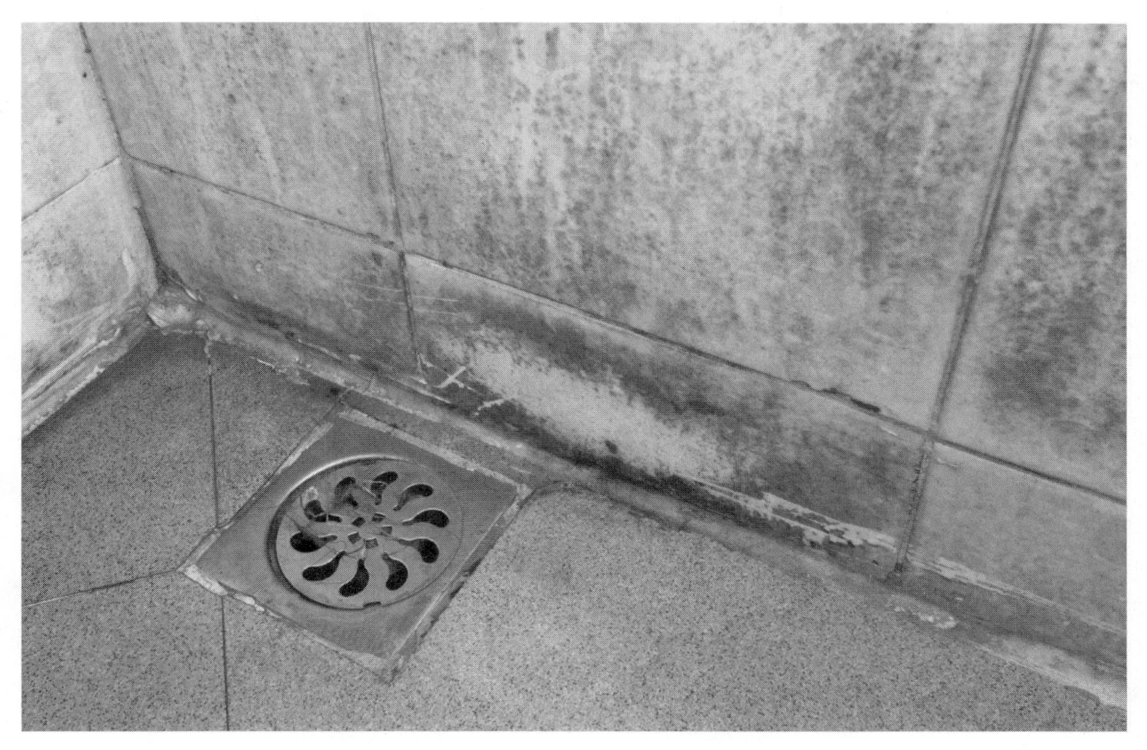

Common sources of mold may expose family members to allergens.
Source: pokko/Fotolia

Assessment Findings

- The patient usually complains of presence of one or more of the following:
    - o Nasal itching
    - o Sneezing, congestion
    - o Watery rhinorrhea
    - o Nasal congestion
    - o Postnasal drip
    - o Cough, sore throat
    - o Red, itchy, watery eyes
    - o Fatigue
- "Allergic salute" sign: pushing tip of nose upward with the hand as itching maneuver.
- Acute rhinitis is common and affects nearly everyone at some point in time.
- Most cases of rhinitis can be classified into a specific syndrome recognized primarily by patterns of symptoms and, less commonly, distinguishing physical signs.

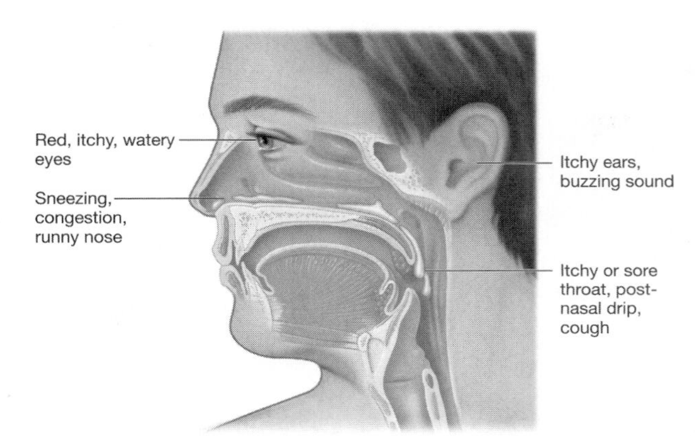

This photo provides a physical exam presentation of a patient suffering with rhinitis.

Diagnostics

Diagnosis is commonly based on the patient's history, clinical presentation, and risk factors:

- History should include:
  - o Review of symptoms
  - o Risk factors
  - o Symptoms onset with exposure to allergen
- Physical exam:
  - o Close observation of nasal mucosa, often found to be edematous with pallor or pale bluish color
  - o Speculum or otoscope exam with bright light
  - o Tenderness and/or pain to pressure over sinus cavity
  - o Clear rhinorrhea may be present anteriorly or as postnasal drip.
- Other diagnostic aids, as needed:
  - o Confirming the presence of the IgE specific to an allergen
  - o Production of symptoms with suspected allergen
  - o Topical application of steroids or antihistamines with relief of symptoms is not diagnostic.
  - o Flexible fiberoptic rhinoscopy may assist in direct observation of mucosa.

Diagnosis and Classification

- Seasonal or episodic: Symptoms occur at a particular time of year.
- Perennial or persistent: Symptoms occur all year around.
- World Health Organization (WHO) classification:
  - o Intermittent: Symptoms present less than 4 days per week or less than 4 weeks.
  - o Persistent: Symptoms persist more than 4 days per week or more than 4 weeks.
  - o Mild: Absence of symptoms seen in "moderate–severe."
  - o Moderate–Severe: One or more symptom(s) is present:
    - ■ Disturbances in sleep and rest
    - ■ Disruption in daily routines, athletic and/or leisure activities
    - ■ Interference with usual ability to function at school or work
    - ■ Worrisome symptoms

Concept Check

4. A patient diagnosed with allergic rhinitis says, "I get so stuffed up during the spring that I cannot sleep or concentrate at work. The rest of the year I am fine." Which type of allergic rhinitis does this patient probably have?

A. Episodic and mild

B. Seasonal and moderate

C. Perennial and mild

D. Persistent and intermittent

Answer question

Priority Patient Concerns and Desired Collaborative Care Outcomes

Prior to caring for patients with allergic rhinitis, it is important to prioritize the patient's concerns that must guide the nursing care plan and interventions. Care for the patient is ordered and organized in accordance with the patient's priority and urgent needs. Desired collaborative care outcomes in patients with allergic rhinitis typically include:

1. Patient will report increased comfort and reduced congestion.
2. Patient will report that breathing requires less effort.
3. Patient will remain in clinic after allergy desensitization in case emergency intervention is needed for anaphylaxis.
4. Patient will experience fewer episodes by avoiding causative allergens.
5. Patient will experience reduced severity of episodes by better controlling symptoms.

Considering these important care outcomes, prepare a list of the major 3–6 priority patient concerns or nursing diagnoses for patients with allergic rhinitis. Be prepared to participate in a discussion of this list and/or to submit them as an assignment, as determined by your faculty. Resources you may find helpful in this assignment can include this lesson, the references, resources on nursing care plans, and standard nursing diagnoses manuals.

LO3:

Collaborative Interventions

Evidence-Based Practice

Evidence-based practice (EBP) depends on the severity of disease present and focuses on symptom management:

- The most effective treatment for rhinitis that is triggered by allergens is to identify and avoid them (EBP).

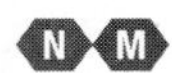

- Mild intermittent disease is treated PRN (EBP not strong):
  - o Second generation antihistamines (e.g., loratadine, Fexofenadine)
  - o Intranasal glucocorticoids
  - o Oral or nasal oxymetazoline or Azelastine: Use sparingly to avoid rebound congestion.
  - o A decongestant (e.g., ephedrine, pseudoephedrine)

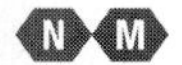

- Moderate to severe rhinitis therapy (EBP):
  - o Oral or nasal antihistamine
  - o Intranasal corticosteroid (e.g., fluticasone)
  - o Leukotriene receptor blocker (e.g., montelukast)
  - o Mucolytic (e.g., guaifenesin)

Concept Check

5. What should the patient using oxymetazoline (Afrin) for symptoms of allergic rhinitis be told?

A. Use the medication every 2 hours for the first 24 hours.

B. Reduce fluid intake while using this medication.

C. Rebound congestion is an adverse effect of this medication.

D. If you develop a headache, stop taking this medication immediately.

Answer question

Follow-Up Care

- Instruct patient in strategy of identifying and avoiding specific food and environmental allergens.
- Skin testing may be, but is not always, necessary to identify the specific allergen (EBP).
- Patients with persistent or severe symptoms or who are unresponsive to treatment:
  - may require desensitization
  - should receive a referral to an allergist
- Short-term (7 days) steroid therapy may abort a persistent allergic response.
- Safety: During and after each immunotherapy or allergy desensitization session, good patient care necessarily includes safety measures:
  - Interview patient and determine whether interfering medications (e.g., antihistamine) were taken on the day of therapy or testing that may cause interactions and alter results.
  - Monitor the patient for at least 30 minutes after injections because:
    - Severe anaphylactic response may occur as long 30 minutes after injection, although uncommon
    - Patients may experience a change in allergy symptoms as immunotherapy or allergy desensitization progresses
  - Familiarize the patient on how to recognize the potential and various adverse responses and the dangers
  - Instruct the patient to immediately report any unexpected response to therapy
  - Ensure the availability and proper functioning of resuscitation equipment before administering medications

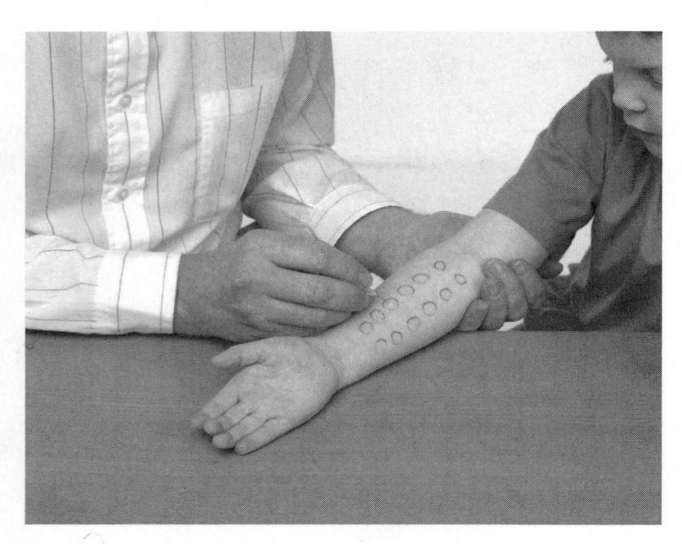

Skin testing may assist in identifying the source of recurrent allergens. Skin testing entails exposing the skin to small amounts of allergens to test for reactions.
Source: Andy Crawford/DK images

Concept Check

6. What information should be provided to a patient who will have allergy testing?

A. Do not take antihistamines the day of the test.

B. Use the steroid inhaler 1 hour before the test.

C. The test requires overnight hospitalization.

D. The test will be performed under conscious sedation.

Answer question

Collaborative Interventions (continued)

Patient Education

- Educate patient to recognize and avoid triggering allergens (e.g., dust mites, pollens, smoke, perfumes, pets, and mold) when possible.
- Educate about smoking cessation, as it can exacerbate the reaction.
- Educate patient on importance of taking prescribed medications as ordered.
- Provide available written material for patient education related to allergic rhinitis.
- Educate patient about the use of antibiotics only in situations where *bacterial* causes are suspected, as antibiotics will not eliminate a virus or allergen. Antibiotic overuse and misuse are a growing community hazard in producing drug-resistant organisms.

Concept Check

7. Which information should the nurse include in discharge planning for a patient with persistent allergic rhinitis?

A. Avoid smoking and secondhand smoke.

B. Take antibiotics on a routine schedule.

C. Have others empty cat litter boxes.

D. Avoid all citrus fruits.

Answer question

Summary of Interventions

- Instruct patient in strategy of identifying and avoiding specific food and environmental allergens.
- Skin testing may be, but is not always, necessary to identify the specific allergen.
- Patients with persistent or severe symptoms or who are unresponsive to treatment:
  - May require desensitization, followed by injection desensitization that may be given for months or years
  - Should receive a referral to an allergist
- Educate patient about smoking cessation, antihistamines, and decongestants.

LO4:

Evaluation of Desired Collaborative Care Outcomes

Evaluation and reassessment should reveal attainment of previously established patient outcomes. In summary:

- The patient experiences increased comfort with a decrease in the presenting symptoms: itching of the eyes, nose and throat, sneezing, and coughing.
- Patient reports that breathing requires less effort.
- Patient experiences fewer episodes of rhinitis by avoiding causative allergens.
- Patient has reduced severity and duration of episodes and better control of symptoms.
- Patient reports no anaphylactic reaction or readily receives emergency intervention in the clinic for anaphylaxis.

References

http://www.ncbi.nlm.nih.gov/pubmedhealth/PMH0001816/

http://onlinelibrary.wiley.com/doi/10.1111/j.1398-9995.2011.02741.x

https://www.aaaai.org/Aaaai/media/MediaLibrary/PDF%20 Documents/Practice%20and%20Parameters/rhinitis2008-diagnosis -management.pdf

http://www.aaaai.org/patients/publicedmat/tips/rhinitis.stm

http://www.aaaai.org/patients/gallery/rhinitissinusitis.asp

Crystal-Peters, J., Crown, W. H., Goetzel, R. Z., & Schutt, D. C. (2000). The cost of productivity losses associated with allergic rhinitis. *Am J Manag Care, 6*(3), 373–378.

Pearlman, A. N., & Conley, D. B. (2008). Review of current guidelines related to the diagnosis and treatment of rhinosinusitis. *Curr Opin Otolaryngol Head Neck Surg, 16*(3), 226-30.

Quillen, D., & Feller, D. (2006). Diagnosing rhinitis: Allergic vs. nonallergic. *American Family Physician, 73*, 1583–1590.

Skoner, D. P. (2001). Allergic rhinitis: Definition, epidemiology, pathophysiology, detection, and diagnosis. *J Allergy Clin Immunol, 108*(1 Suppl), S2–S8.

U.S. Department of Health and Human Services. Agency for Healthcare Research and Quality. Management of Allergic and Nonallergic rhinitis. (2002). AHQR publication 02:E023, Boston, MA. Summary, Evidence Report/Technology Assessment: No 54.

Clinical Practice Guidelines

Wallace, D. V., Dykewicz, M. S., et al. Joint Task Force on Practice, American Academy of Allergy, Asthma & Immunology, American College of Allergy, Asthma & Immunology, Joing Council of Allergy, Asthma & Immunology. (2008). The diagnosis and management of rhinitis: an updated practice parameter. *J Allergy Clin Immunol, 122*(2 Suppl), S1–S84.

Patient Education

http://www.cdc.gov/vaccines/hcp/vis/vis-statements/ppv.html

Stevens, L. M., Lynm, C., & Glass, R. M. (2001). Seasonal allergic rhinitis. *JAMA, 286*(23), 3038.

Learning Outcomes for Acute Rhinosinusitis

When you complete this lesson, you will be able to:

1. Recognize the clinical relevance of acute rhinosinusitis.
2. Consider the pathophysiology, etiology, risk factors, and clinical presentation of acute rhinosinusitis that determine the priority patient concerns.
3. Determine the most urgent and important nursing interventions and patient education required in caring for a patient with acute rhinosinusitis.
4. Evaluate attainment of desired collaborative care outcomes for the patient with acute rhinosinusitis.

LO1:

What Is Rhinosinusitis?

- Acute rhinosinusitis is inflammation of the nasal passages and sinuses that lasts less than 4 weeks.
- Although "sinusitis" is commonly used to name this illness, rhinosinusitis is preferable because the nasal mucosa is almost always involved.
- Unlike allergic rhinitis, it is usually caused by either a viral or bacterial infection.

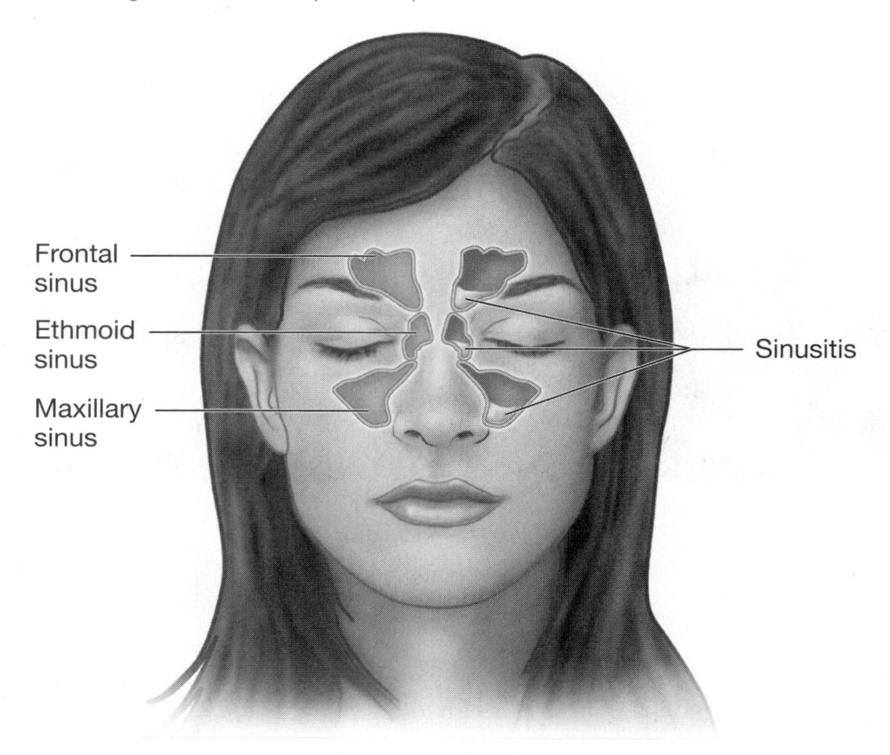

The location of sinus cavities within the skull are shown: Frontal, ethmoid, sphenoid (nasal, not shown), and maxillary sinuses.

LO1:

Clinical Relevance

- Thirty million people present each year with this illness.
- Most rhinosinusitis is caused by viral infections (see photos). However, the majority are treated with antibiotics, even though antibiotics are not effective against viruses.
- The annual health care costs are over $3,500,000,000.
- This diagnosis accounts for 20% of the prescriptions written.
- Overuse and misuse of antibiotics contributes to the growing number of antibiotic-resistant organisms that we have little means to combat.

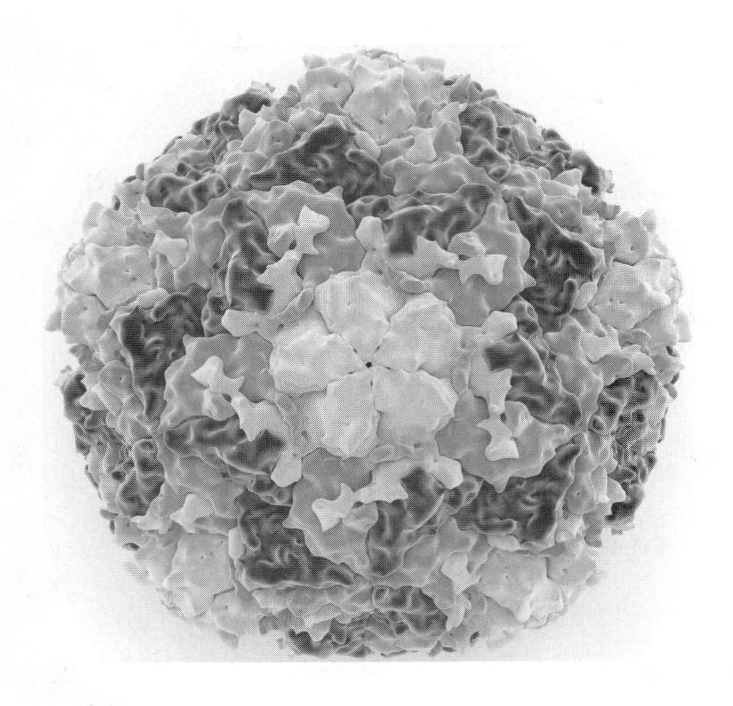

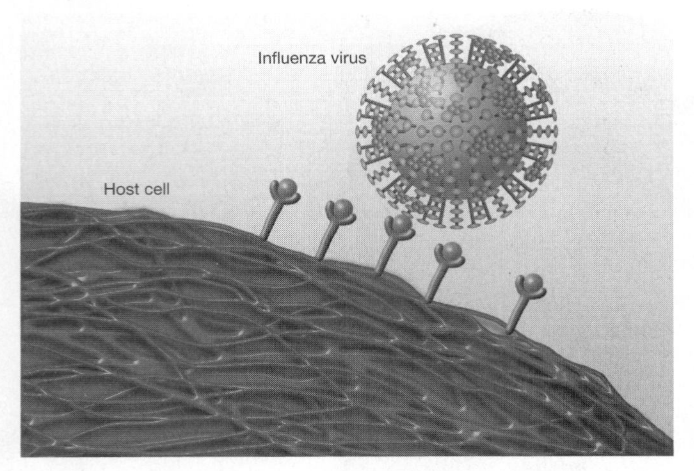

Both the rhino virus (upper) and influenza virus (lower) are commonly responsible for rhinosinusitis.
Source: (*upper*) Luk Cox/Fotolia

LO2:

Pathophysiology

Bacterial Rhinosinusitis

- Bacteria may normally reside in the nasal cavities without causing an infection.
- Mucous normally drains from the sinuses and keeps the sinuses free from bacteria. Mucous produced in the sinuses drains out the ostia (openings) into the nasal passages with the help of cilia.
- Any impairment of cilia or blockage of the ostia may result in stasis of mucous in the sinuses. Bacteria that enter through the ostia may then start to grow and cause a bacterial infection resulting in bacterial rhinosinusitis.

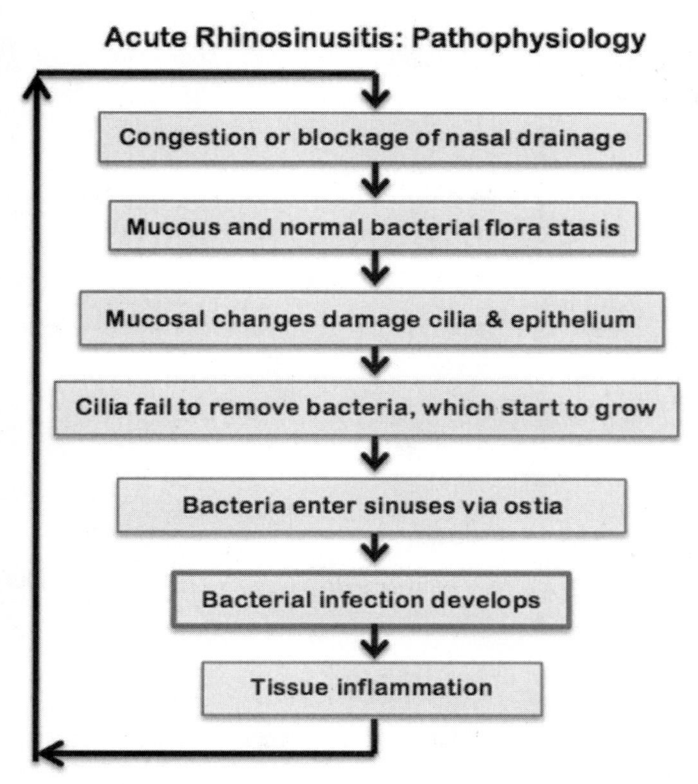
Acute Rhinosinusitis: Pathophysiology
Congestion or blockage of nasal drainage
Mucous and normal bacterial flora stasis
Mucosal changes damage cilia & epithelium
Cilia fail to remove bacteria, which start to grow
Bacteria enter sinuses via ostia
Bacterial infection develops
Tissue inflammation

Source: Copyright © 2012, NovEx Novice to Expert Learning, LLC

Viral Rhinosinusitis

- Viral infections are, by far, the most common cause of rhinosinusitis.
- Viral infections also cause inflammation of the lining of the sinuses and nasal passages as well as impairment of ciliary function.
- Patients with viral rhinosinusitis are, therefore, more predisposed to developing bacterial rhinosinusitis because the viral infection sets up the conditions for bacterial growth.
- A viral infection typically resolves without treatment within 7–10 days whereas a bacterial infection causes symptoms to persist or worsen.
- Any conditions (e.g., smoking, allergic rhinitis) that may contribute to ciliary dysfunction and compromise the ostia, predispose patients to development of bacterial rhinosinusitis.

Concept Check

1. **Which statement concerning rhinosinusitis is true?**
   - A. Viral rhinosinusitis often follows bacterial rhinosinusitis.
   - B. Viral rhinosinusitis may result in bacterial rhinosinusitis.
   - C. Bacterial rhinosinusitis is more common than viral rhinosinusitis.
   - D. There is little, if any, relationship between bacterial and viral rhinosinusitis.

Answer question

Inflammation Leading to Chronic Rhinosinusitis

- Infections of the sinus passages cause an inflammatory response. The inflammatory response produces both local and systemic effects through the release of inflammatory cytokines (damaging chemicals).
- Recurrent sinusitis with repeated inflammation of the nasal passages and sinuses leads to chronic rhinosinusitis.
- A number of changes occur including: enlargement of the mucous producing cells; fibrosis; blockage of the ostia; and presence of bacteria in mucous.

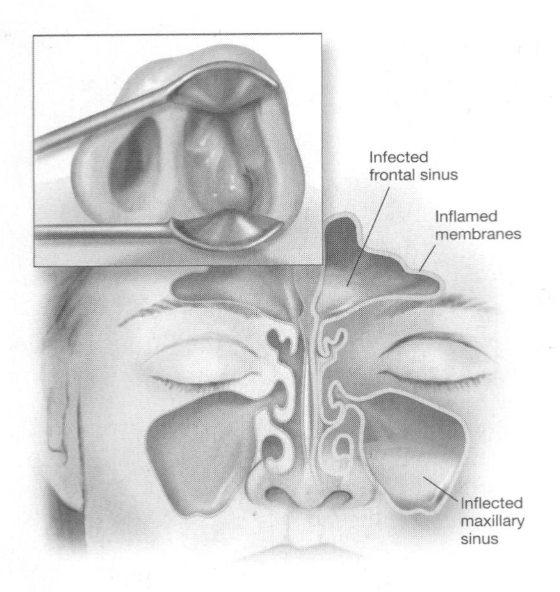

Sinusitis is an inflammation of the sinuses usually following an upper respiratory infection.

Risk Factors

- Allergic rhinitis
- Smoking
- Immunocompromised patients
- Cocaine abuse
- Nasogastric tubes
- Dental abscess

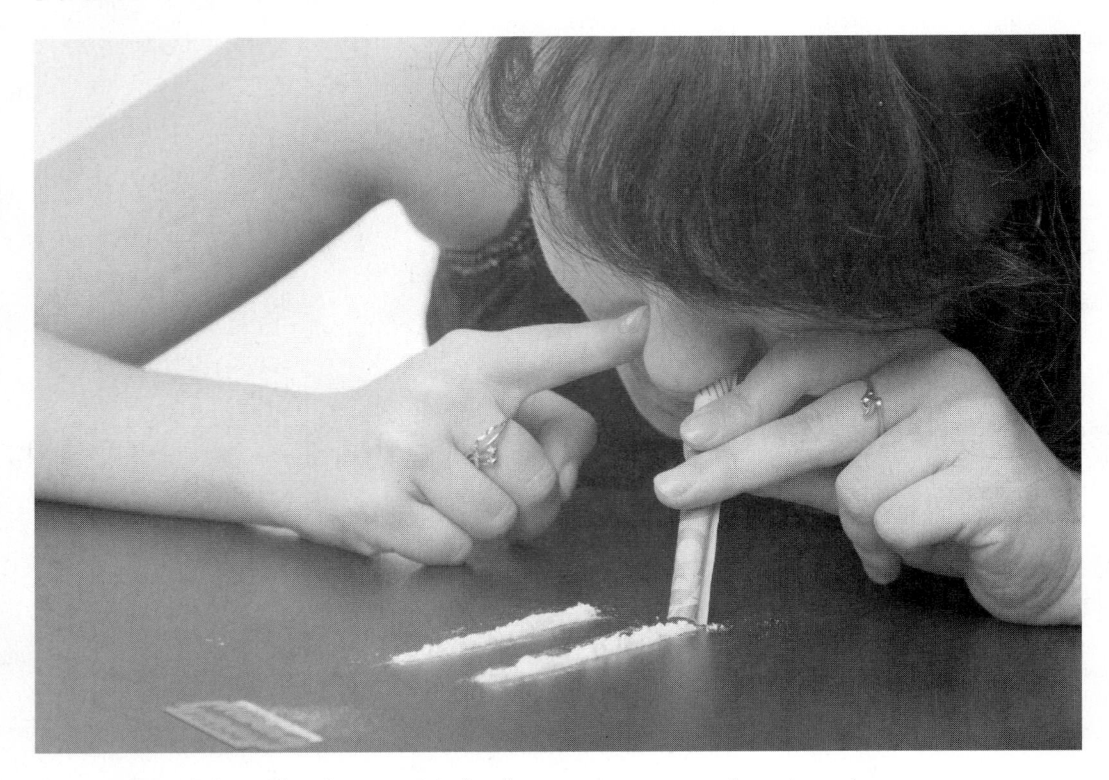

Cocaine is a risk factor for rhinosinusitis. Small amounts are not as damaging as long-term use. However, rhinitis is not the major health danger to cocaine abusers
Source: NatUlrich/Fotolia.

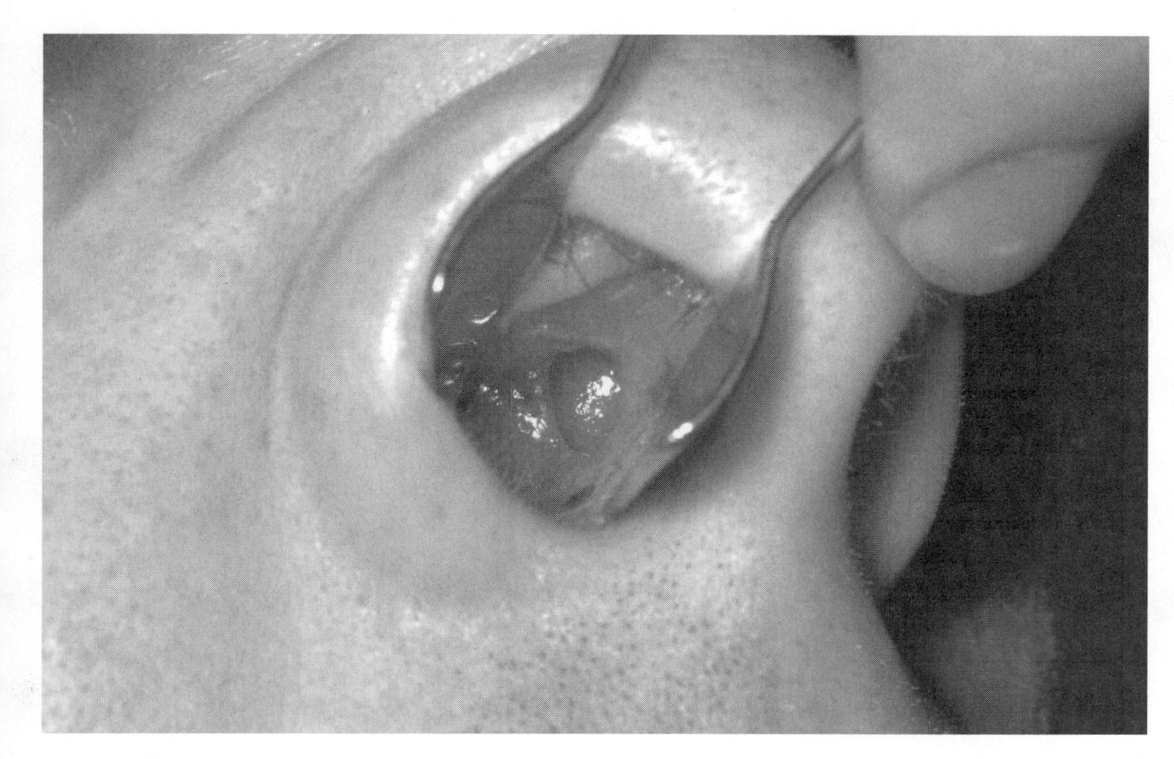

Note the destruction of the nasal septum in this patient who has been snorting cocaine. The septum can be totally destroyed due to chronic and habitual use. Always examine the nasal septum in patients with rhinosinusitis.
Source: Medical-on-Line/Alamy.

Concept Check

2. Which patients are at risk for the development of bacterial rhinosinusitis?
   A. Patients who have blockage of sinus ostia
   B. Patients with congestive heart failure
   C. Patients with a tracheostomy tube
   D. Patients who drink more than two alcoholic beverages a day

Answer question

Causes

- **Viral infections**, such as the common cold.
- **Bacterial infections**: Most common pathogens include *Streptococcus pneumoniae* and *Haemophilus influenzae*.
- Bacteria usually enter the sinuses through the ostia. Another method of **entry is through a dental abscess** in the upper molar because of the proximity to the maxillary sinuses.
- **Nosocomial infections**: Patients who are immunocompromised or who have a prolonged ICU stay are at higher risk of developing bacterial sinusitis. Pathogens are usually gram negative organisms that include pseudomonas.
- **Patients needing a nasogastric (NG) tube** are also at higher risk for bacterial sinusitis due to the mechanical damage to the nasal passage and proximity to the sinuses.
- **Fungal infections**, especially in immunocompromised patients.

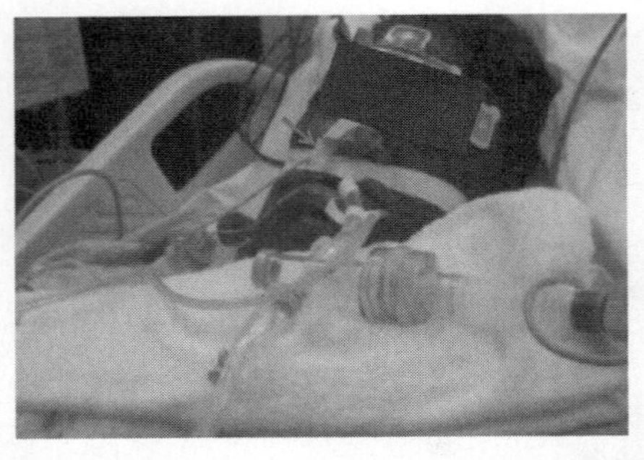

This photo shows a patient with a NG tube, which puts her at a higher risk for sinusitis.
Source: Copyright © 2012, NovEx Novice to Expert Learning, LLC

Assessment Findings

- Symptoms suggesting sinus involvement:
  1. Nasal congestion
  2. Posterior nasal drainage (often purulent)
  3. Reduced sense of smell
  4. Postnasal drip

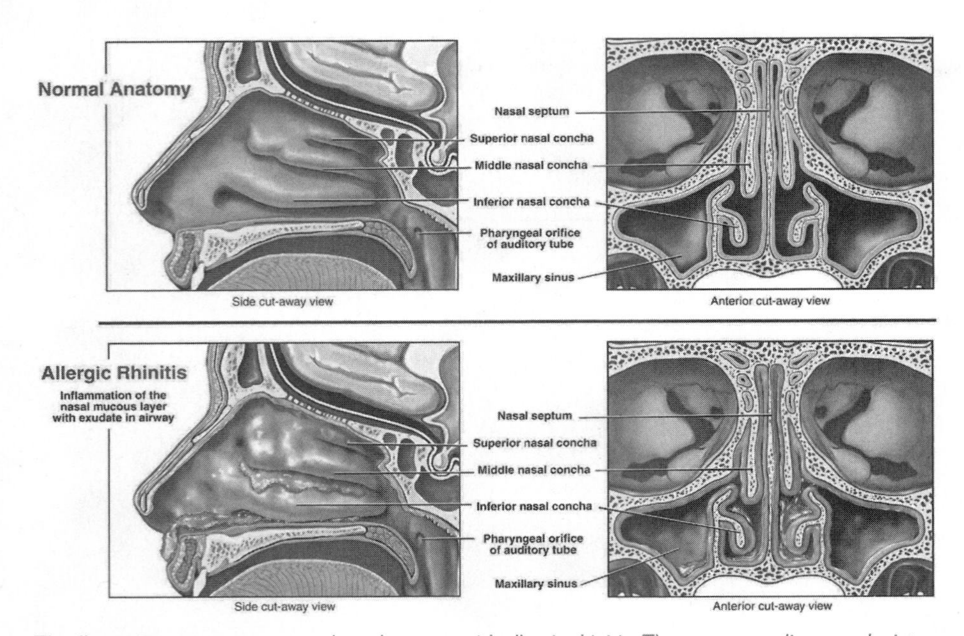

The illustrations contrast a normal nasal passage with allergic rhinitis. The two upper diagrams depict a normal nasal septum. The lower two diagrams display the same anatomy but in allergic rhinitis with mucosal inflammation and exudate.
Source: © 2013 Nucleus Medical Media, All rights reserved

- Symptoms suggesting sinus involvement (continued):
  1. Facial pressure and/or pain, including dental (see Regions of PAIN in Sinusitis figures 1–4)
  2. Headache behind forehead and/or cheekbones
  3. Cough

Regions of PAIN in Sinusitis

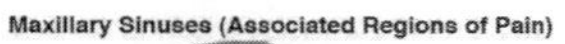

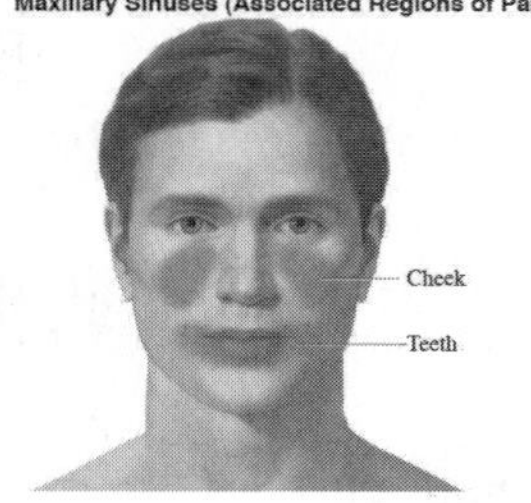

1. Maxillary Sinusitis

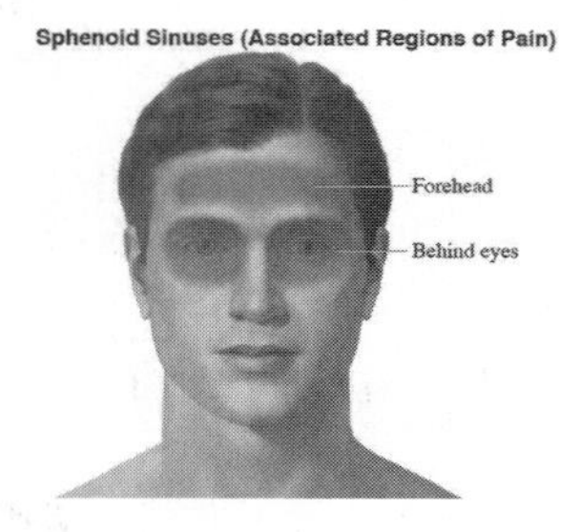

2. Sphenoid sinusitis

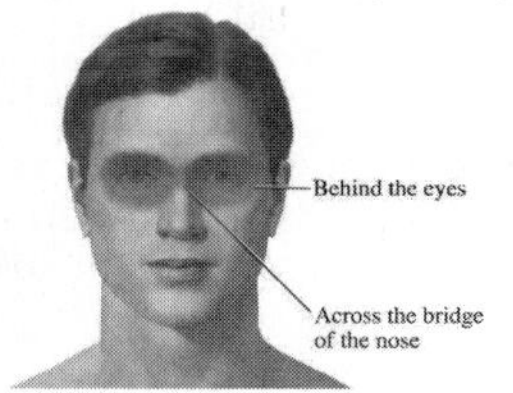

3. Ethmoid sinusitis

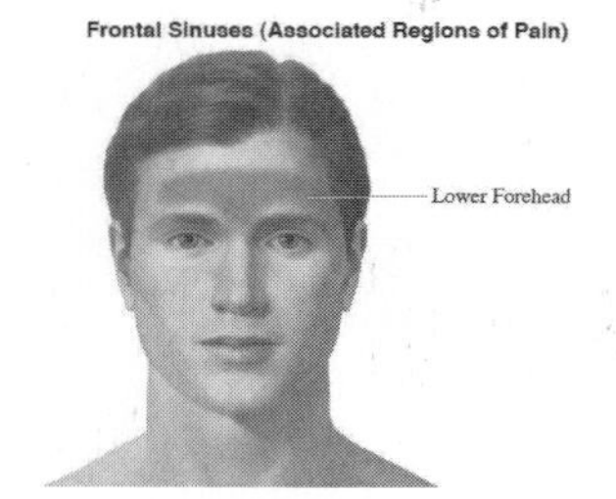

4. Frontal sinusitis

(Clockwise from top left) Maxillary sinusitis, sphenoid sinusitis, ethmoid sinusitis, frontal sinusitis.

Concept Check

3. **Which patient statement suggests that a patient's rhinosinusitis involves the ethmoid sinuses?**
   A. "I have pain in my right cheek."
   B. "My forehead hurts."
   C. "There is pain behind my eyes."
   D. "My teeth hurt."

Answer question

Bacterial versus Viral Rhinosinusitis

Symptom/Characteristic	Bacterial	Viral
Duration	>10 days	7–10 days
Fever	>102°F	<102°F
Purulent drainage	Yes	Yes
Facial pain and tenderness	More severe	Moderate
Severity	Persistent, worsens	Improves

- No single symptom has a high sensitivity or specificity in discriminating bacterial from allergic or viral sinusitis and rhinitis.
- An infection of the sinuses has the potential for causing an infection of the cerebral lining with resulting cerebral edema. The results are potentially fatal.

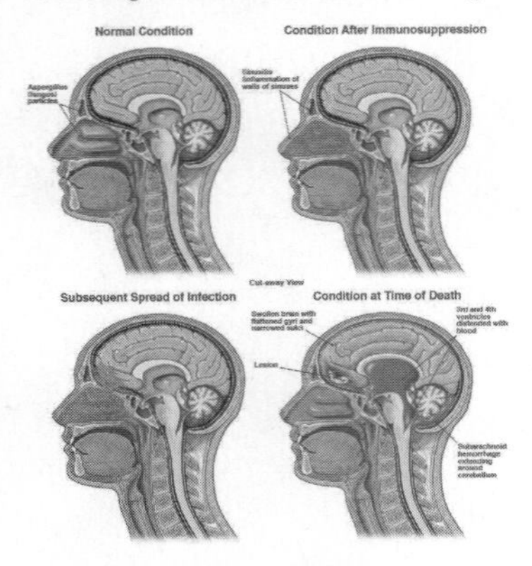

These illustrations show four progressively worsening conditions of the head and brain that begin with a sinus infection. The images include: normal sinuses, infected frontal sinuses, penetration of the infection through the thin bone layers of the skull into the brain cavity, and the final spread of infection throughout the cranium resulting in brain edema and hemorrhage.

Source: © 2013 Nucleus Medical Media, All rights reserved

Concept Check

4. Which finding suggests that the patient's rhinosinusitis is bacterial in origin rather than viral?

A. The patient's temperature is 103°F.

B. The patient has been sick for five days.

C. The patient has purulent sputum.

D. The patient denies significant facial tenderness.

Answer question

Diagnostics

CT scan is helpful in viewing the sinuses. It is usually performed in patients who are not improving with treatment.

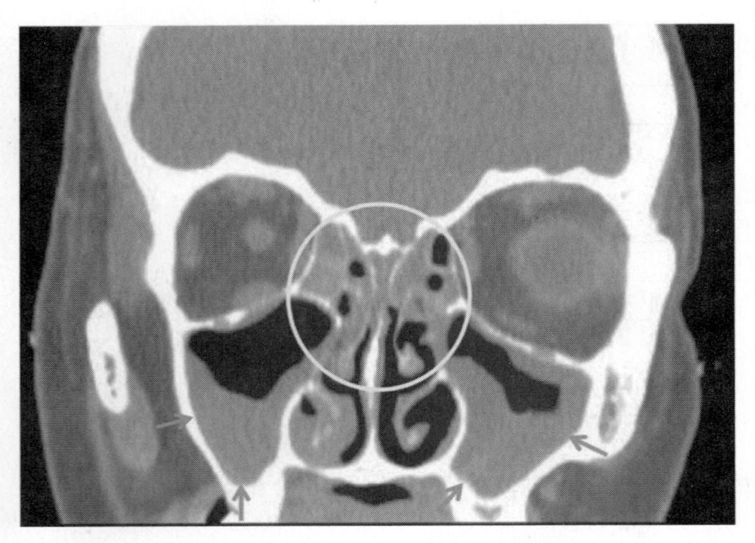

A 50-year-old man with intractable nasal congestion. This CT scan of the nasal sinuses reveals mucosal thickening of bilateral maxillary (red arrows), ethmoid, and sphenoid sinuses (circle).

Source: Courtesy of K. Kyriakidis

Priority Patient Concerns and Desired Collaborative Care Outcomes

Prior to caring for patients with acute rhinosinusitis, it is important to prioritize the patient's concerns that must guide the nursing care plan and interventions. Care for the patient is ordered and organized in accordance with the patient's priority and urgent needs. Desired collaborative care outcomes in patients with acute rhinosinusitis typically include:

1. Patient will report decreased intensity of headache and facial pain.
2. Patient will report that nasal breathing is easier and airways are clearer.
3. Patient will discuss causative factors, relate them to preventative measures, accurately discuss post discharge care, and explain why antibiotics are not indicated in a viral infection.
4. Patient will identify signs and symptoms of further infections that indicate need for follow up and treatment modification.

Considering these important care outcomes, prepare a list of the major 3–6 priority patient concerns or nursing diagnoses for patients with acute rhinosinusitis. Be prepared to participate in a discussion of this list and/or to submit them as an assignment, as determined by your faculty. Resources you may find helpful in this assignment can include this lesson, the references, resources on nursing care plans, and standard nursing diagnoses manuals.

LO3:

Collaborative Interventions

Evidence-Based Practice

Evidence-based practice (EBP) recommends ations for symptom management include:

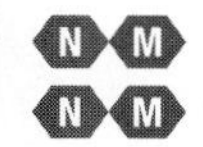

- Distinction is to be made between viral rhinosinusitis and bacterial rhinosinusitis.
- Symptomatic treatment and watchful waiting are recommended for symptoms that are indicative of viral rhinosinusitis:
    - o Symptoms lasting less than 10 days and
    - o Symptoms that show improvement after the initial 3–5 days.
    - o Second generation antihistamines (e.g., loratadine, fexofenadine)
    - o Intranasal glucocorticoids
    - o Oral or nasal oxymetazoline or azelastine: use sparingly to avoid rebound congestion
    - o Decongestant (e.g., ephedrine, pseudoephedrine)

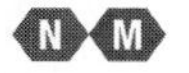

- Symptoms that the patient and/or healthcare providers may recognize, are suggestive of bacterial rhinosinusitis, and suggest the possible need for antibiotic therapy include:
    a. Symptoms that persist more than 10 days with no discernible improvement
    b. Symptoms that are worsening before 10 days, following an upper respiratory infection or if patient is immunocompromised
    c. Severe symptoms (fever more than 102° plus purulent drainage or facial pain) early, close to the time of onset

- Antibiotics are recommended, preferably amoxicillin and clavulanate as the first line drugs with doxycycline and fluoroquinolone as alternatives.

- Sinus imaging is generally not recommended except for chronic or recurrent acute rhinosinusitis.

Concept Check

5. At which point would the nurse anticipate prescription antibiotics being provided for a patient complaining of symptoms of rhinosinusitis?

A. The patient complains of purulent drainage for 8 days.

B. The patient has been sick for 7 days.

C. The patient has high fever and purulent drainage 2 days after getting sick.

D. The patient develops a cough.

Answer question

Concept Check

6. A patient has been diagnosed with rhinosinusitis. At which point would the nurse anticipate preparing this patient for sinus imaging?

A. Immediately if the patient is a child

B. Once the patient has been febrile for 4 days

C. If the condition is chronic or recurrent

D. Upon the patient's request

Answer question

Patient Education

Most of these patients must self-manage their care at home. Thus, a key intervention is patient education. Patients and/or their families should be educated about:

- Smoking cessation as it can exacerbate the process
- The importance of taking prescribed medications as ordered
- Applying warm compresses to sinus area
- Administering humidified air to keep the airway moist
- Maintaining adequate hydration to reduce the thickness of secretions
- Administering ordered analgesics, as needed
- Written material that is available to patients regarding allergic rhinitis and sinusitis
- The signs and symptoms (listed above in EBP) that indicate the need for follow-up care
- The need for influenza and pneumonia vaccinations
- The use of antibiotics only in situations where *bacterial* causes are suspected since antibiotics will not eliminate a virus or allergen. Patients should be informed that antibiotic overuse and misuse are a growing community hazard in producing drug-resistant organisms.

Concept Check

7. Which education should the nurse provide to a patient being discharged after diagnosis of viral rhinosinusitis?

A. Use cold packs over the areas of your face that are painful.

B. Take analgesics as prescribed.

C. Take your antibiotics on a regular schedule.

D. Use a humidifier at your bedside.

Answer question

Summary of Interventions

- Rhinosinusitis is commonly the result of a transient viral infection. Antibiotics should not be considered unless symptoms persist more than 10 days or they indicate a bacterial origin.
- Bacterial infection of the sinuses should be treated promptly to prevent meningeal infections.
- Symptomatic treatment for cough and congestion can include: *smoking cessation*, antihistamines, decongestants, rest, hydration, warm compresses, antipyretics, and humidified air.

LO4:

Evaluation of Desired Collaborative Care Outcomes

Evaluation and reassessment should reveal attainment of previously established patient outcomes. In summary:

- The patient has relief of or reduced severity in headache, facial pain, and coldlike symptoms. If headache or facial pain worsens or fever becomes high, additional medical attention may be necessary.
- The patient reports that nasal breathing is easier and airways are clearer.
- The patient discusses causative factors, relate them to preventative measures, accurately detail post-discharge care, and explain why antibiotics are not indicated in a viral infection.
- Patient states the signs and symptoms of worsening infection that indicate the need for follow up and treatment modifications.

References

(2007). Treatment of acute and chronic rhinosinusitis in the United States, 1999–2002. *Arch Otolaryngol Head Neck Surg, 133*(3), 260–265. doi:10.1001/archotol.133.3.260

Poole, M. D. (2004). Acute bacterial rhinosinusitis: Clinical impact of resistance and susceptibility. *The American Journal of Medicine Supplements, 117*(3), 29–38.

Scheid, D. C., & Hamm, R. M. (2004). Acute bacterial rhinosinusitis in adults: Part I. Evaluation. *Am Fam Physician, 70*(9), 1685–1692.

Sinus and Allergy Health Partnership Release: Updated Guidelines Provide Diagnosis and Treatment Recommendations for Bacterial Sinusitis.

Young, J., De Sutter, A., Merenstein, D., van Essen, G. A., Kaiser, L., Varonen, H., Williamson, I., & Bucher, H.C. (2008). Antibiotics for adults with clinically diagnosed acuterhinosinusitis: a meta-analysis of individual patient data. *Lancet, 371*(9616), 908–914.

Patient Education

Shoup, J. (2011). Management of adult rhinosinusitis. Nurs Practitioner, 36(11), 22-26. **www.nursingcenter.com/lnc/JournalArticle?Article_ID=1247571&Journal_ID=54012&Issue_ID=1247499&expiredce=1**

Vidrine, T.A. & Harrington, D. (2014). Acute rhinosinusitis in adults: Appropriate diagnosis and treatment practices in the emergency department. nurse-practitioners-and-physician-assistants.advanceweb.com/Features/Articles/Acute-Rhinosinusitis-in-Adults.aspx

http://www.cdc.gov/getsmart/program-planner/Rec-Readings.html

STOP

Go to the online course and complete the NovE-Cases assigned by your instructor for this module.

Learning Outcomes for Airway Obstruction

When you complete this lesson, you will be able to:

1. Recognize the clinical relevance of airway obstruction.
2. Consider the pathophysiology, etiology, risk factors, and clinical presentation of airway obstruction that determine the priority patient concerns.
3. Determine the most urgent and important nursing interventions and patient education required in caring for a patient with an airway obstruction.
4. Evaluate attainment of desired collaborative care outcomes for a patient with an airway obstruction.

LO1:

What Is Airway Obstruction?

- An acute airway obstruction is a complete or partial blockage of the airway. An obstruction may occur in the trachea, pharyngeal and laryngeal areas, and bronchi due to a variety of causes.

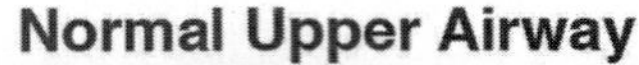

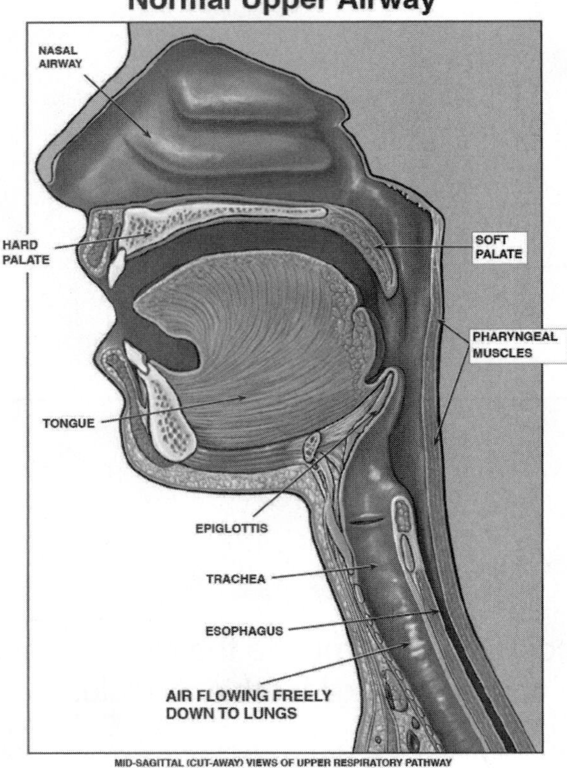

The upper respiratory system includes the hard and soft palates, pharyngeal muscles, and the trachea. Arrows show air moving normally through airway passages.

Concept Check

1. Which structures are parts of the airway?
   A. Uvula
   B. Tympanic membrane
   C. Esophagus
   D. Diaphragm

Answer question

LO1:

Clinical Relevance

- Any partial or complete airway obstruction is a medical emergency. An obstruction needs to be recognized and treated rapidly to prevent a life-altering event and/or death.
- Airway obstruction can progress rapidly, and warning signs may present for only a short period of time. Urgent intervention is essential when the airway is compromised.
- In the diagrams, the picture (right) shows airway obstruction due to a lodged bologna sandwich.
- Some of the common interventions (intubation, tracheostomy) are not life-saving, as in the situation with the bologna sandwich obstruction, because the obstruction cannot be bypassed. Instead the bologna sandwich must be urgently removed.
- The animation shows how forceps (for instance) can be used to urgently remove lodged objects.
- Protection and maintenance of the airway are the first priority.

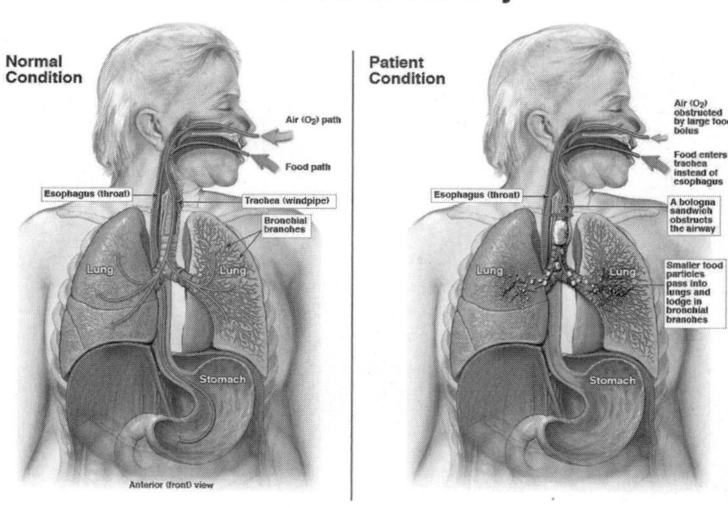

This image compares the normal, clear airway to one that is obstructed.

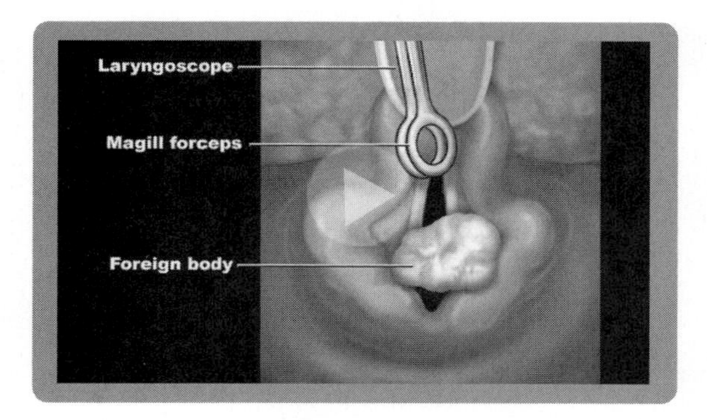

This animation show a foreign body obstructing the airway at the larynx. This object is high enough that forceps can be used to remove the object.

- About 14,000 emergency department visits each year are for airway obstruction.
- More than 34 million people are diagnosed with asthma during their lifetime, and asthma causes over 3,000 deaths per year from airway obstruction.
- Eighty-eight percent of children who choke and die from airway obstruction are 4 years of age or younger. Food items are the most common cause of choking.
- Many cases of airway obstruction or accidental strangulation, particularly in children, can be prevented by following safety recommendations.
- Angioedema may affect 10–20% of the population at some time. This rapid swelling and edema of the mucous membranes can be life-threatening.
- Alcohol is linked to 75,000 deaths per year in the United States. The airway can be obstructed by aspirated vomitus from overuse of alcohol and from the tongue falling back into the pharynx.
- Prescription opioids caused more than 11,000 people to experience respiratory depression or arrest in 2007—more than heroin and cocaine combined.

Concept Check

2. Which statement about partial airway obstruction is most accurate?

A. Because of their immature anatomy, children are unlikely to experience airway obstruction.

B. Airway obstruction typically progresses slowly.

C. Asthma can result in airway obstruction.

D. Partial airway obstructions are treated conservatively, not emergently.

Answer question

LO2:

Pathophysiology

Airway obstruction occurs when an object or other cause of occlusion of the airway is present. An obstruction prevents oxygenation.

- Obstruction can be due to edema or respiratory depression and relaxation of the airway musculature.
- Conditions that can exacerbate quickly, like the inflammation and swelling that can develop in epiglottis, can lead to severe airway obstruction in a short time even in a patient who appears relatively stable.

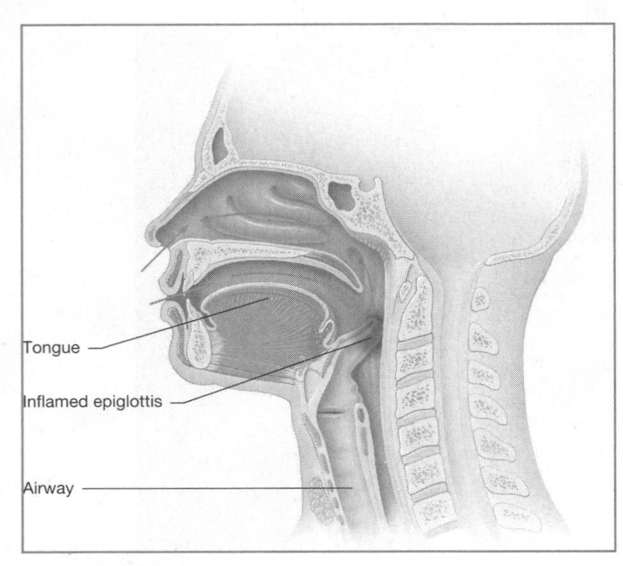

Epiglottis is caused by a pathogen and leads to inflammation and edema of the epiglottis. The swelling results in narrowing or even obstruction of the airway. Epiglottis can be life-threatening if severe.

Causes and Risk Factors

There are many causes with overlapping risk factors of airway obstruction. The most common include:

- Inflammation with edema
- Infection
- Foreign bodies
- Secretions
- Tumors
- Vocal cord paralysis
- Anatomical abnormalities
- Trauma
- Hematoma or uncontrolled bleeding
- Obstructive sleep apnea
- Overdose

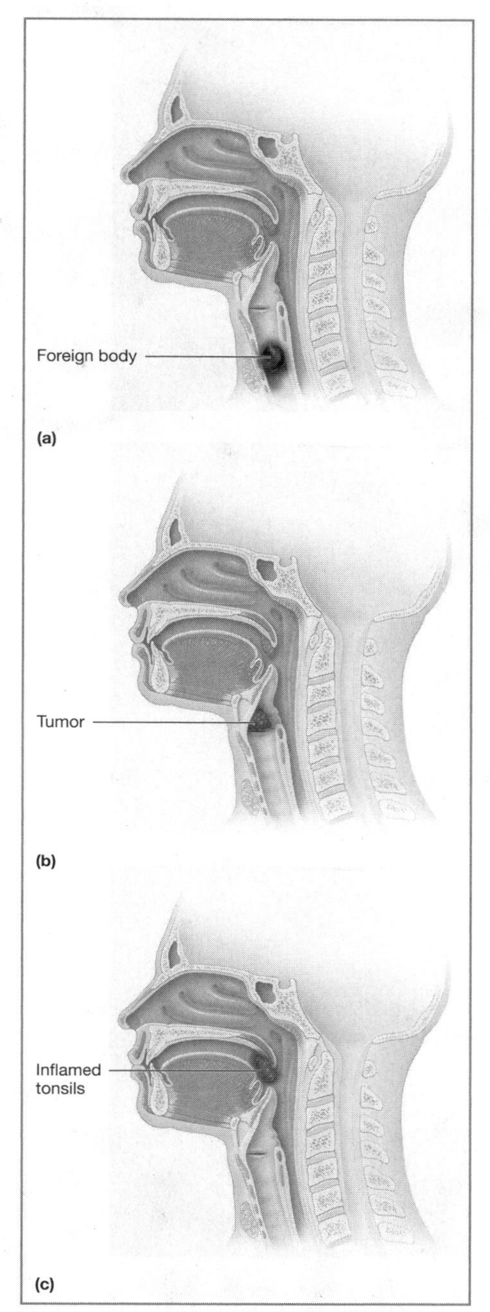

These three illustrations show common causes of airway obstruction. (a) Foreign body. (b) Tumor at the larynx. (c) Tonsillitis.

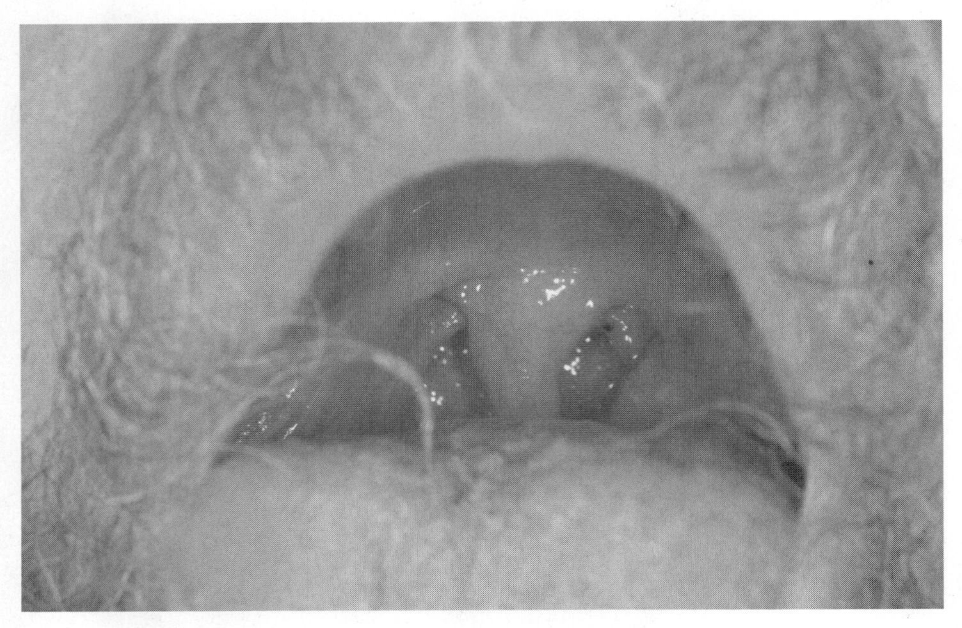

Neoplasm of the throat.
Source: Medical-on-Line/Alamy

Rapid Airway Obstruction

Some rapid onset, dangerous airway obstructive causes are due to inflammatory responses, including:

- Anaphylactic reactions
- Status asthmaticus
- Epiglottitis
- Angioedema, idiopathic, or from medications (e.g., ACE inhibitors)
- Severe laryngospasm or bronchospasm

Because these patients can rapidly digress into severe and life-threatening airway obstruction, they need to be monitored carefully and closely. Intubation or emergency tracheostomy may be needed.

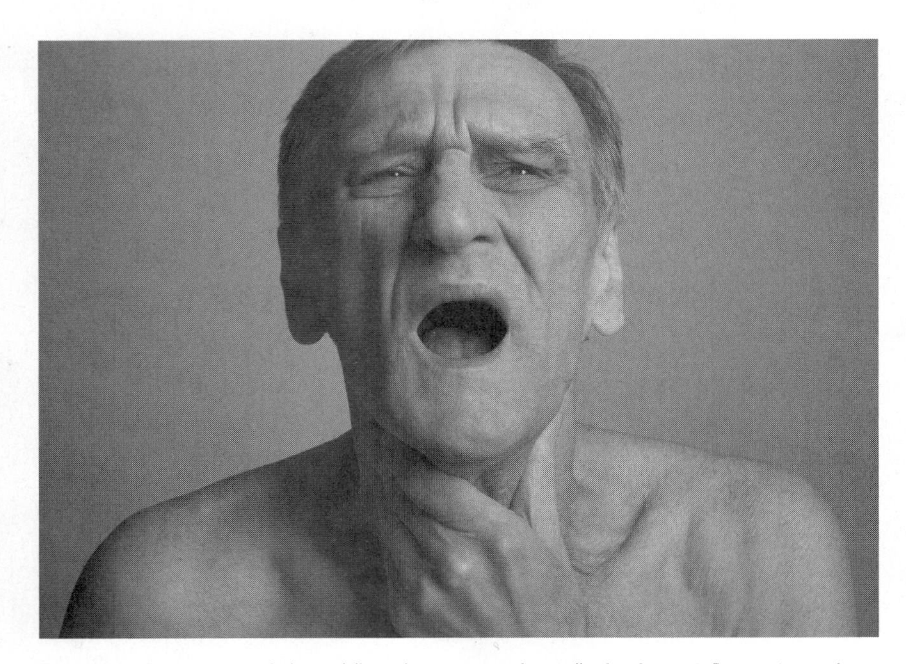

This photo depicts an anaphylactic (allergic) reaction with rapidly developing inflammation and edema in the throat. Airway occlusion can be rapid. The tongue can swell and prevent swallowing, hives can arise, and consciousness may be lost.
Source: GlebStock/Shutterstock

Infectious Airway Obstruction

Additional causes involve infections. These situations often present as less life threatening and include:

- Suppurative parotitis
- Peritonsillar abscess
- Ludwig's angina
- Epiglottitis
- Laryngitis
- Laryngotracheo bronchitis (LTB)
- Tonsillar hypertrophy
- Retropharangeal abscess

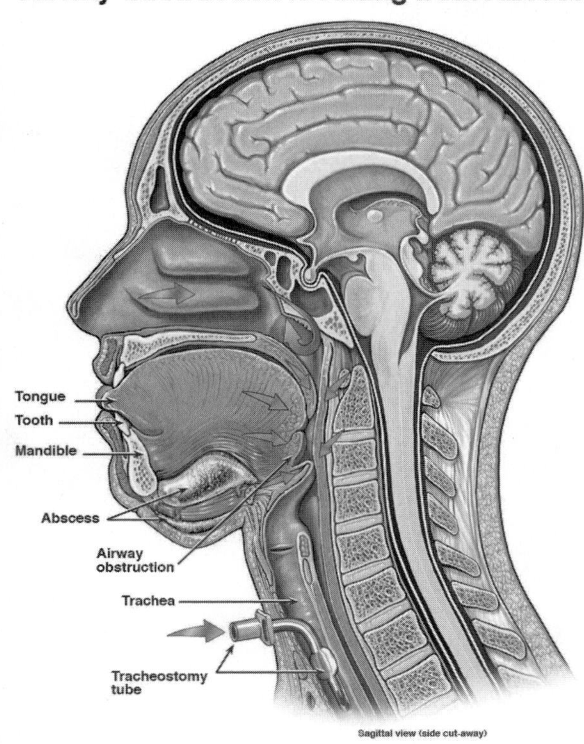

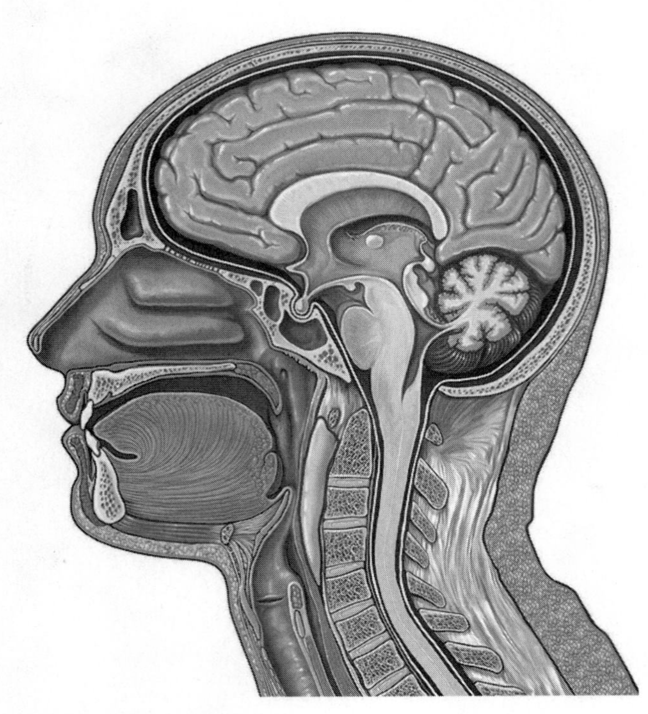

These exhibits illustrate airway obstructions resulting from abscess. Upper: The abscess under the tongue (yellow enlongated pus pocket behind the tongue and in front of the spinal cord) caused severe swelling that led to airway obstruction by pushing the tongue backwards. Lower: A retropharyngeal abscess is large and swollen into the airway.

Concept Check

3. Which source of airway obstruction is of rapid onset, therefore placing the patient in extreme danger?

A. Angioedema

B. Parotitis

C. Laryngitis

D. Tonsillar hypertrophy

Answer question

Causes and Risk Factors (continued)

Traumatic Airway Obstruction

Traumatic causes of airway obstruction include:

- Suffocation
- Strangulation
- Facial fractures
- Tracheal injury—blunt or penetrating
- Uncontrolled upper airway bleeding
- Thermal injury

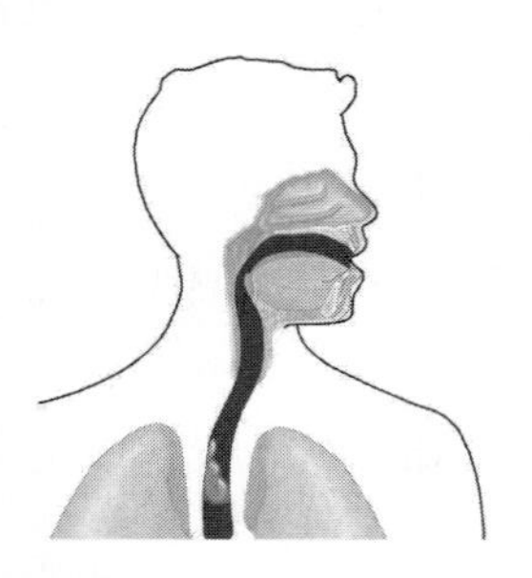

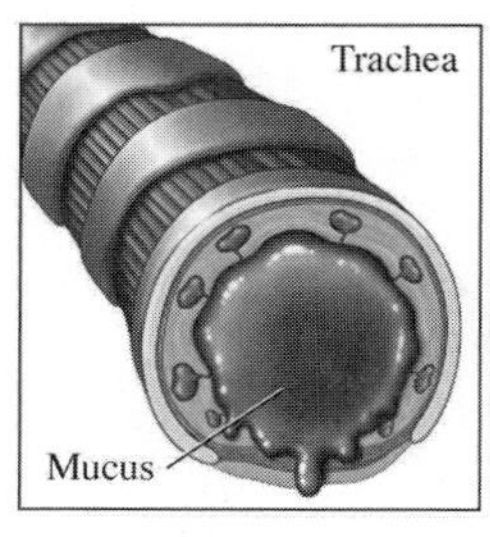

Thick, copious mucous can obstruct the airway.

Common Causes of Airway Obstruction

- Obstructive sleep apnea is a common cause of airway obstruction. In these patients, the tongue and soft tissues relax during sleep, fall back into the pharynx, and can intermittently occlude the airway.
- Aspiration of foreign bodies or fluids can also lead to airway obstruction. Important causes include food, small toys, vomitus and secretions.

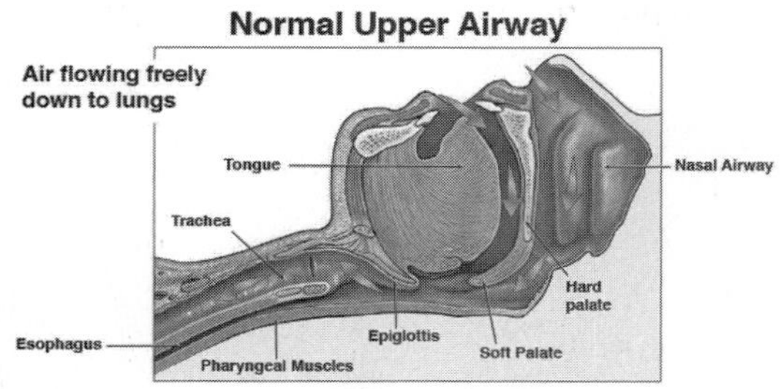

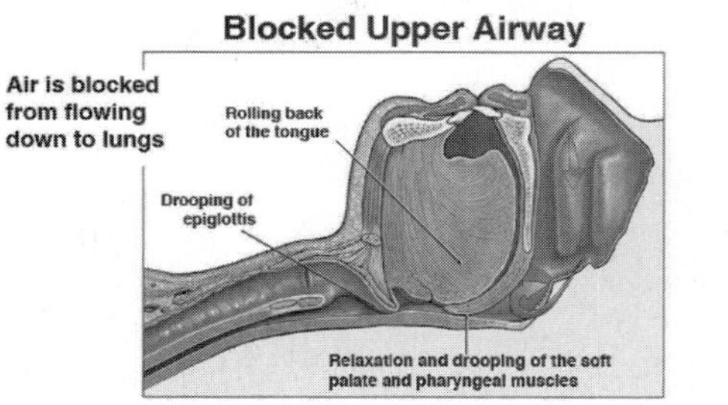

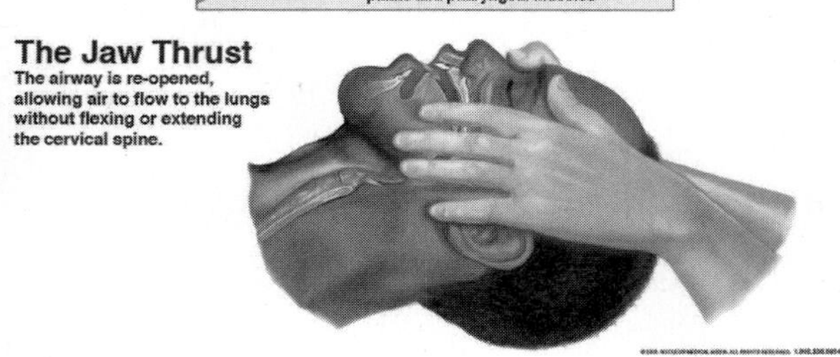

The mechanism of apnea in drug or alcohol overdose is depicted. A jaw-thrust maneuver opens the airway, but medical attention should be initiated

Drug-Related Airway Obstruction

- Drug overdose that results in central nervous system depression can result in apnea, the loss of ability to protect airway, lack of gag reflex, and relaxation of upper airway structures that block the airway.
- Examples of drug overdose include alcohol, sedatives, and narcotics. A list of culprit medications is listed in the Medication-Induced Respiratory Distress illustration.

Medication-Induced Respiratory Distress

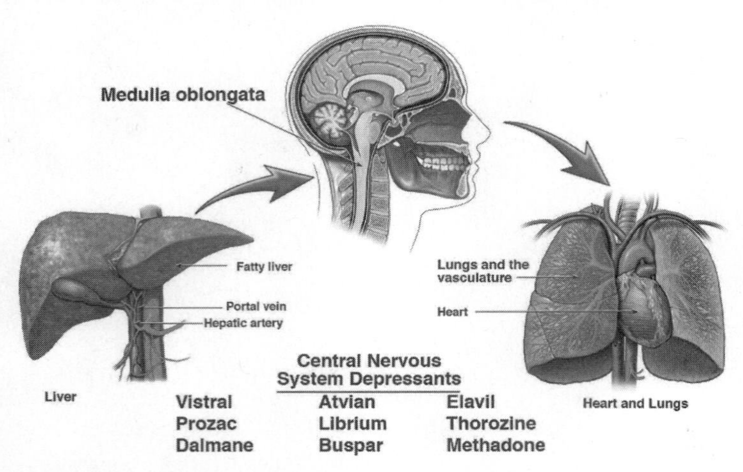

Failure in adequate metabolism of these drugs can cause CNS depression which, in turn, slows respirations and/or can lead to airway obstruction as discussed prior.

Assessment Findings

Several signs of airway obstruction can be present, including:

- Inspiratory stridor or whistling noise
- Inability to speak
- Sore throat, hoarseness
- Use of accessory muscles
- Paradoxical motion of chest wall
- Muffled or "hot potato" voice (speaking as if you have a mouth full of hot food)
- Drooling or inability to swallow, painful swallowing
- Tachypnea, dyspnea
- Tachycardia
- Nasal flaring
- Diaphoresis
- Pallor or cyanosis
- Agitation or panic
- Choking
- Confusion and loss of consciousness

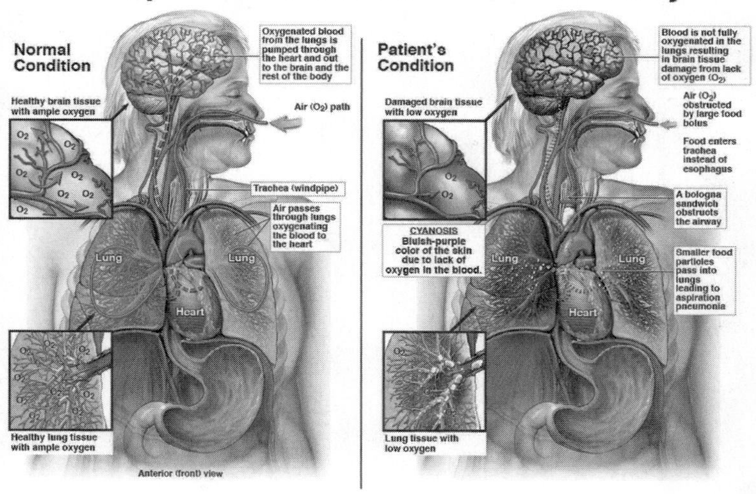

Symptoms in airway obstruction (right) are contrasted with the normal person on the left.

Clinical findings of airway obstruction include:

- Decreased breath sounds
- Low 0_2 saturation
- Tachypnea
- Tachycardia, secondary to fear and potential hypoxia
- Apnea

Diagnostics

Diagnostics will depend on the suspected cause of the airway obstruction and can include the following:

- Lab tests
  - o Toxicology screen
  - o Alcohol or drug levels
  - o Cultures—throat, abscess, and blood
    - ■ Cultures will take time to return so action is not to be delayed waiting on cultures.
  - o Arterial blood gases showing a decreased pH and rising $PaCO_2$—this situation indicates a medical emergency.
- Imaging
  - o X-ray—soft tissue
  - o CT scan to detect soft tissue swelling or abscess
  - o Fiber optic visualization

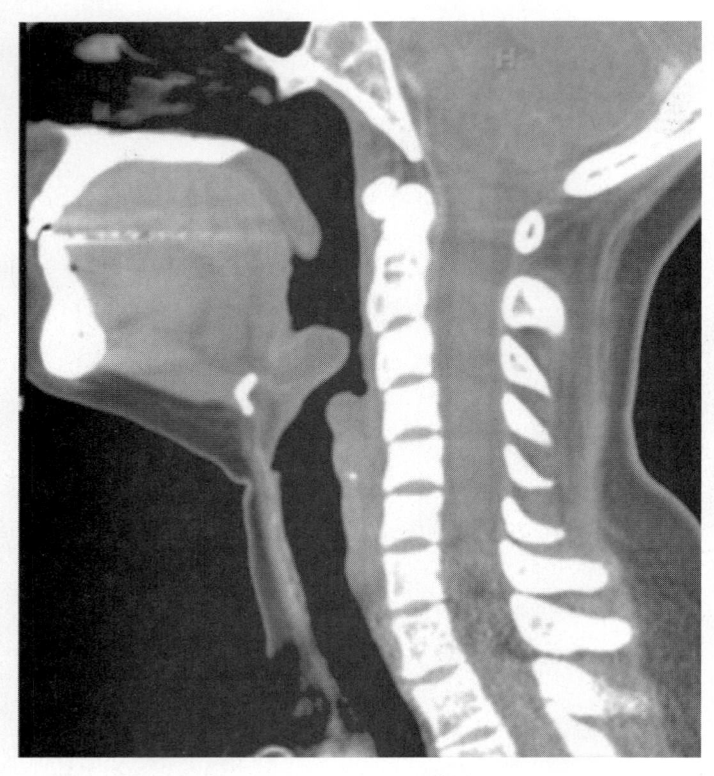

This CT scan of the neck reveals an enlarged epiglottis. The red curved line shows the location and typical size of a normal epiglottis.
Source: Courtesy of K. Kyriakidis

Priority Patient Concerns and Desired Collaborative Care Outcomes

Prior to caring for patients with an airway obstruction, it is important to prioritize the patient's concerns that must guide the nursing care plan and interventions. Care for the patient is ordered and organized in accordance with the patient's priority and urgent needs. Desired collaborative care outcomes in patients with an airway obstruction typically include:

1. Patient's lungs and airways will be clear to auscultation.
2. Patient's arterial blood gas measurements or oxygenation saturations will return to pre-incident normal.
3. Patient will experience reduced anxiety.
4. Patient will express decreased feelings of air hunger.
5. Patient will remain infection free.
6. Patient will report feeling competent to avoid situations in which airway obstruction might occur.
7. Patient will report minimal to no pain.

Considering these important care outcomes, prepare a list of the major 3–6 priority patient concerns or nursing diagnoses for patients with airway obstruction. Be prepared to participate in a discussion of this list and/or to submit them as an assignment, as determined by your faculty. Resources you may find helpful in this assignment can include this lesson, the references, resources on nursing care plans, and standard nursing diagnoses manuals.

LO3: Collaborative Interventions

An obstructed airway often presents a life-threatening situation. For patients in distress, while simultaneously assessing to pinpoint the cause, the jaw-thrust maneuver should be attempted.

Jaw Thrust

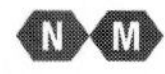

The Jaw-thrust maneuver is basic in airway management of the unconscious or airway obstructed patient (e.g., drug overdose, alcohol intoxication, anesthesia)

- It is the first, most important airway management intervention and should be performed by the first person on the scene or who confronts this kind of situation. In these individuals, the tongue tends to be displaced backwards, obstructing the airway.
- Pull the lower jaw forward to restore the patency of the airway.
- In patients with suspected neck trauma, gently pull the lower jaw forward with caution and without moving the neck.

If the jaw-thrust fails to open the airway, the urgency of the situation calls for multiple and urgent interventions.

- Many of the interventions require medications. Although medications are ordered by physicians, nurses are the key providers who:
  - o Recognize the urgency of the situation
  - o Convey the emergency
  - o Mobilize the team's response
  - o Administer the medications, provide care, and support the patient and family
  - o Monitor and evaluate the patient's responses
  - o Determine with the team if the patient is stable or requires further intervention
- There are numerous causes and therefore numerous sets of interventions in providing life-saving interventions and caring for the patient with an obstructed airway. Major causes with specific interventions include:
  - o Can't intubate, can't ventilate situations
  - o Anaphylaxis
  - o Angioedema
  - o Status Asthmaticus

Emergency Tracheostomy

A "**can't intubate, can't ventilate**" situation:

Emily Bromiley, a young British mother, was admitted for a routine surgery. Breathing problems lead to repeated failed intubation; however, the lack of clinical leadership led to her prolonged brain anoxia and death.

- Please click the video link to hear this dramatic example of how the problem of tunnel vision can lead to errors, like failure to perform a tracheotomy in a safe and timely manner in failed intubations:
  http://vimeo.com/970665
- Or click to read *The Airline Pilot who Lost his Wife:*
  http://medicalharm.org/patient-stories/martin-bromiley/

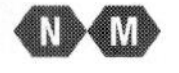

- The American Society of Anesthesiologists define "a difficult intubation" as more than three attempts at inserting an endotracheal tube. The nurse should ensure that a tracheotomy tray is at the bedside for all intubations. After 3 failed attempts, leadership is imperative to assert that a tracheostomy be performed for patient safety, in accordance with known guidelines.
  American Society of Anesthesiologists Task Force on Management of the Difficult Airway. (2003). Practice guidelines for management of the difficult airway. *Anesthesiology, 98,* 1269–1277.

Concept Check

4. The nurse is attempting to open the airway of an unconscious patient. Which action should be taken?

A. Tilt the patient's head back.

B. Pull the patient's jaw forward.

C. Use a tongue blade to depress tongue tissue.

D. Turn the patient to the left side.

Answer question

Obstruction Due to Anaphylaxis

(see Anaphylactic Shock NovE-lesson for detail)

Evidence-Based Practices (EBP) for airway obstruction due to anaphylaxis:

N M **1.** Epinephrine IM, preferably in the mid-outer thigh, urgently. Repeat in 5–15 minutes if unresolved or infuse IV fluids.

N M **2.** Rapidly infuse 1-2 liters of fluid IV to treat hypotension

N M **3.** Endotracheal intubation if needed for ventilation

Collaborative Symptom Management includes:

N M **1.** Supplemental oxygen if oxygen saturation falls below 93%

N M **2.** Corticosteroids IV (or methylprednisolone)

N M **3.** Famotidine or ranitidine IV (H2 blocker/antihistamine)

N M **4.** Diphenhydramine IV (H1 blocker/antihistamine)

Concept Check

5. **Which intervention is indicated for airway obstruction due to anaphylaxis?**
   A. Supplemental oxygen
   B. Rapid administration of antibiotics
   C. Subcutaneous epinephrine administration
   D. Slow infusion of intravenous fluids

Answer question

Obstruction Due to Angioedema

EBP for angioedema with anaphylaxis:

N M **1.** Epinephrine IM, urgently and preferably in the mid-outer thigh, for laryngeal swelling or airway obstruction. Repeat in 5–15 minutes if unresolved or infuse IV fluids.

N M **2.** Endotracheal intubation or tracheostomy if needed for ventilation.

Collaborative Symptom Management includes the major recommendations for allergic angioedema without anaphylaxis:

N M **1.** Supplemental oxygen if oxygen saturation falls below 93%

N M **2.** Corticosteroids IV, e.g., methylprednisolone for severe forms

N M **3.** Antihistamines (H1 and H2 blockers) for histamine-mediated angioedema
   - o Diphenhydramine IV (H1 blocker) or
   - o Famotidine or ranitidine IV (H2 blocker)

N M **4.** If angioedema is accelerating in severity or threatens to compromise the airway, treat as anaphylaxis.

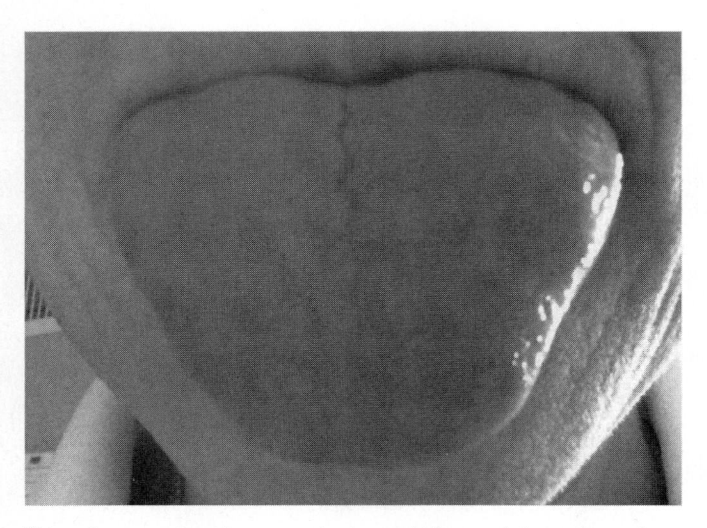

This patient experienced severe angioedema, which caused airway obstruction. He required intubation until the angioedema resolved.
Source: Copyright © 2012, NovEx Novice to Expert Learning, LLC

Obstruction Due to Status Asthmaticus

(see Asthma Nov-E lesson for details)

EBP includes:

1. Inhaled beta-2 agonists (albuterol, Xopenex) when needed as a rescue or for quick relief
2. Oxygen therapy if the patient's oxygen saturation falls below 93%.
3. Corticosteroids (methylprednisolone) when treatment for inflammation of the airways is warranted

Collaborative Symptom Management includes:

1. Parenteral bronchodilators (theophylline) if continued relaxation of the bronchiolar smooth muscle is needed
2. Magnesium sulfate intravenous if smooth muscle relaxation is needed
3. Heliox, which is a helium-oxygen mixture, if needed to reduce the work of breathing and decrease airway resistance
4. Inhaled anticholinergics (ipratropium bromide) was historically and may still be currently used, but research has not supported its continued use.

Further airway management may be necessary with endotracheal intubation, tracheostomy, or cricothyrotomy.

Obstruction Due to Peritonsillar Abscess

EBP includes:

1. Peritonsillar abscess and upper airway infections
2. Care of incision and drainage of the abscess
3. Antibiotics that should include antimicrobials effective against group A streptococcus and oral anaerobes (e.g., clindamycin, penicillin with metronidazole)—Administer IM or IV if patient is sick enough for hospitalization; orally if patient is in clinic and discharged to home.

Collaborative Symptom Management includes:

1. Steroids: may be useful in reducing symptoms
2. Position head of bed upright.
3. Humidified oxygen
4. Assist with intubation, tracheostomy, or cricothyrotomy if airway occlusion is imminent.

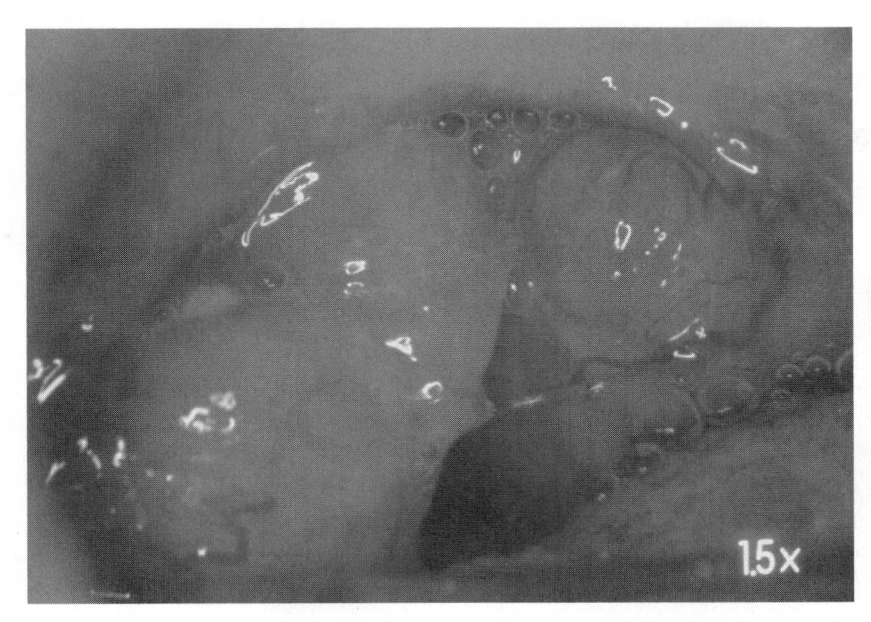

Note the huge periotonsillar abscess nearly occluding the airway. This degree of obstruction warrants emergency intervention.
Source: Science Photo Library/Custom Medical Stock

Obstruction Due to Epiglottitis

- No specific EBP is recommended.
- Treatment is focused on protection of the airway.
-  Visualization of the epiglottis should only be done in the OR with anesthesia prepared to emergently intubate or perform a tracheostomy.

Epiglottis Preventing Proper Intubation

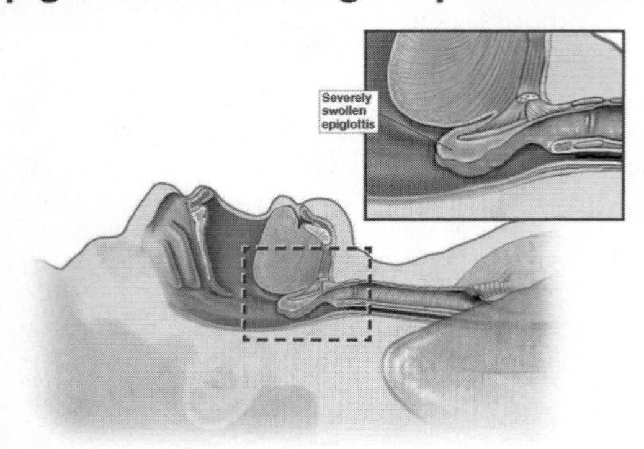

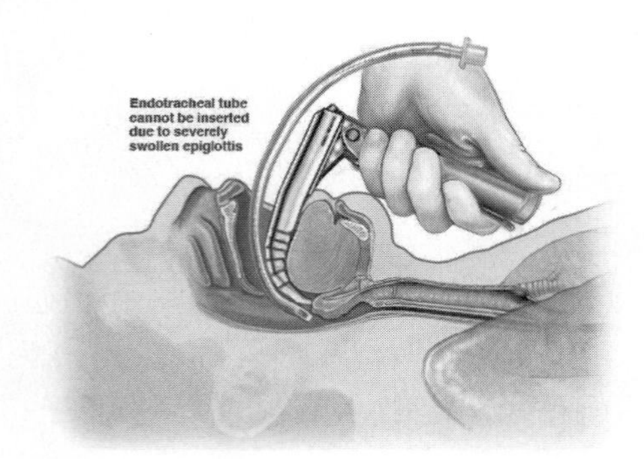

Emergency Tracheostomy Procedures

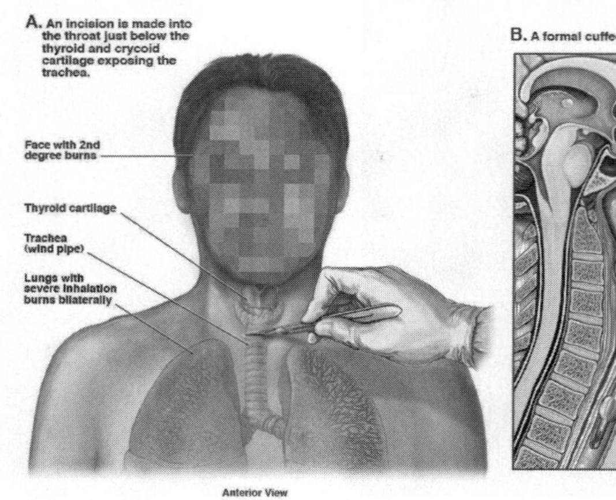

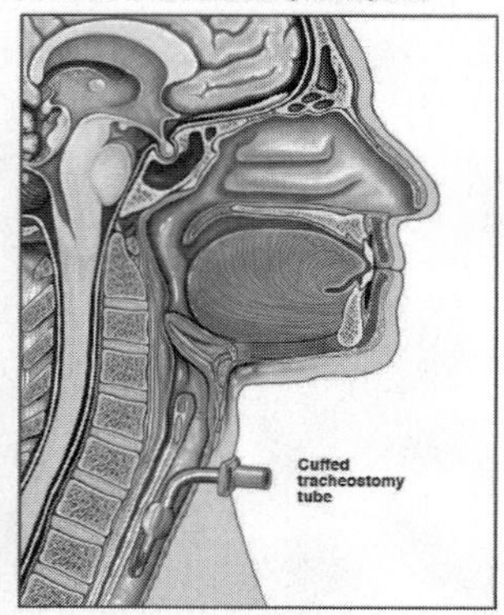

Collaborative Symptom Management includes:

M **1.** IV antibiotics, e.g., ceftriaxone, cefuroxime (effective against *H. influenzae, S. pneumoniae, Staphylococcus aureus,* and various gram-negative bacilli)

N M **2.** Steroids may be given when an anti-inflammatory medication is indicated

N **3.** Position head of bed upright

N M **4.** Bronchodilators, if wheezing is present

N **5.** Humidified oxygen

N **6.** Calm environment

M **7.** Racemic epinephrine may be attempted but has no evidence to support that it will reduce edema, especially from an abscess.

N Nursing monitoring: Patients with epiglottis require vigilant monitoring as they are vulnerable to a sudden episode of airway occlusion.

Obstruction Due to Foreign Bodies

EBP for acute aspiration of a foreign body includes:

- N M Heimlich maneuver for adults
- N M Abdominal thrusts for patients older than 1 year of age
- N M Back blows and alternating abdominal thrusts for infants younger than 1 year of age

M If the foreign body cannot be cleared, a tracheostomy may be necessary.

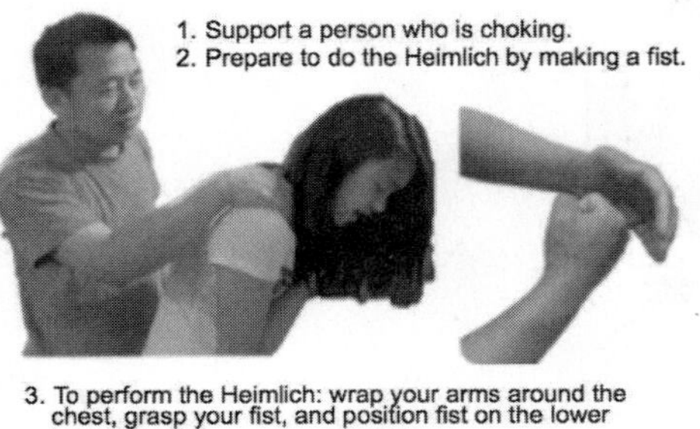

1. Support a person who is choking.
2. Prepare to do the Heimlich by making a fist.

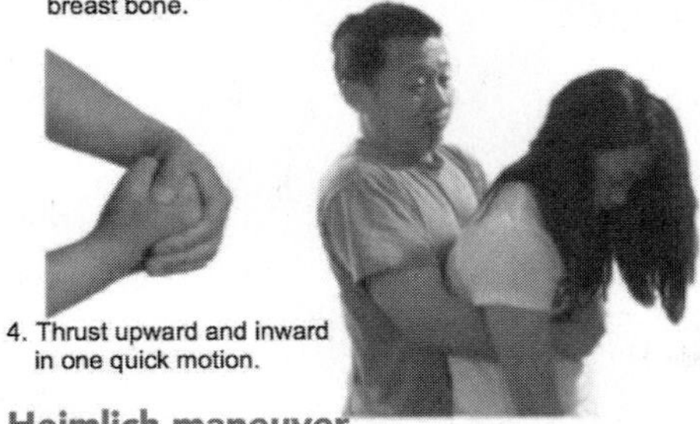

3. To perform the Heimlich: wrap your arms around the chest, grasp your fist, and position fist on the lower breast bone.
4. Thrust upward and inward in one quick motion.
Heimlich maneuver

How to perform the Heimlich maneuver for choking.
Source: Copyright © 2012, NovEx Novice to Expert Learning, LLC

Collaborative Interventions (continued)

Obstruction Due to Fluid Aspiration

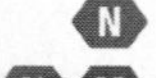

- Aspiration precautions can prevent airway obstruction.

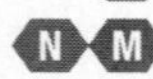

- A swallow test should be performed on all patients suspected of having swallowing difficulties. Those who are unable to pass the swallow test should be made NPO.

EBP includes:

- Antibiotics for aspiration pneumonia

Collaborative Symptom Management includes:

- Suctioning when indicated if patient is unable to clear own airway adequately

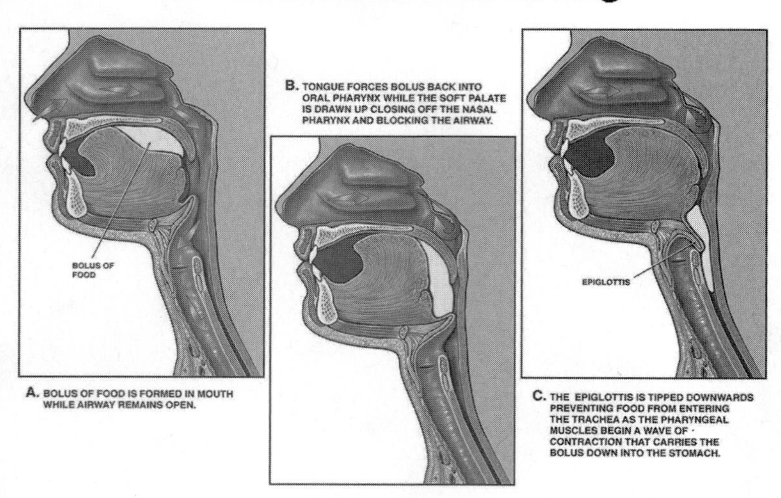

The Action of Swallowing
BOLUS OF FOOD
A. BOLUS OF FOOD IS FORMED IN MOUTH WHILE AIRWAY REMAINS OPEN.
B. TONGUE FORCES BOLUS BACK INTO ORAL PHARYNX WHILE THE SOFT PALATE IS DRAWN UP CLOSING OFF THE NASAL PHARYNX AND BLOCKING THE AIRWAY.
EPIGLOTTIS
C. THE EPIGLOTTIS IS TIPPED DOWNWARDS PREVENTING FOOD FROM ENTERING THE TRACHEA AS THE PHARYNGEAL MUSCLES BEGIN A WAVE OF CONTRACTION THAT CARRIES THE BOLUS DOWN INTO THE STOMACH.

This series of pictures illustrates and describes the mechanism of swallowing. Evaluating a patient for adequate swallowing has serious implications.

Obstruction Due to Tumors

No specific EBP exists for upper airway tumors, and management will depend on the type, location, and extent of the tumor and whether malignancy is present.

Collaborate with other members of health care team with the following as needed:

- Laser therapy
- Tracheal stenting
- Surgical intervention

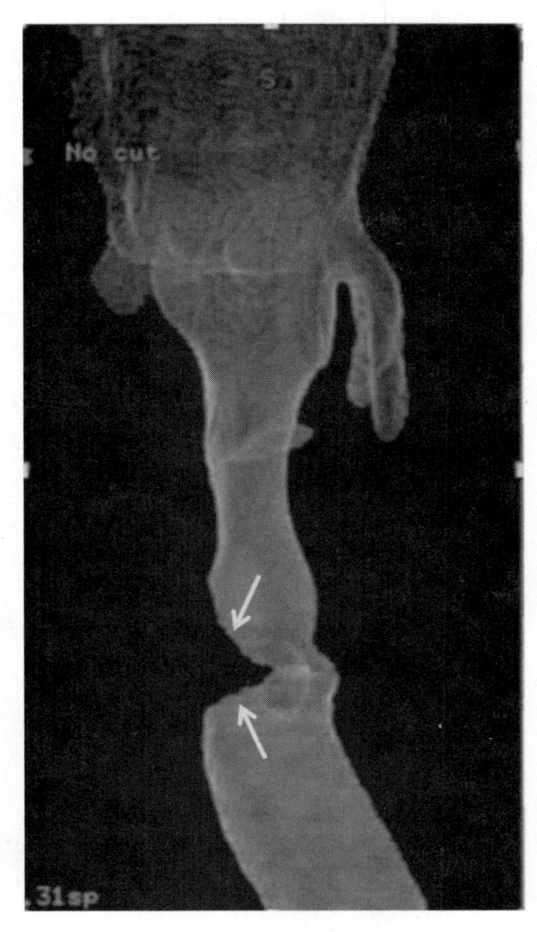

This 3D reconstruction of the patient's trachea reveals an invasion into the trachea from the left side (arrows). The thyroid cancer is not lit up, but is noticed by the obstruction it creates in the patient's trachea. The impingement on the airway requires intervention.
Source: Courtesy of K. Kyriakidis

Obstruction Due to Trauma

No specific EBP exists as patient-specific interventions are dependent on the type and extent of trauma.

N M **1.** Secure and maintain unstable airway with intubation, tracheostomy, or cricothyrotomy.

N **2.** Suction secretions from airway as often as indicated.

N M **3.** Control bleeding and swelling.

N M **4.** Supplemental oxygen if SpO_2 is less than or equal to 92%.

M **5.** Anesthetics (i.e., etomidate, ketamine) and/or paralytics (i.e., succinylcholine) for conscious patients prior to rapid sequence intubation or tracheostomy procedures.

N M **6.** Protect the cervical spine.

Penetrating Stab Wound of the Face

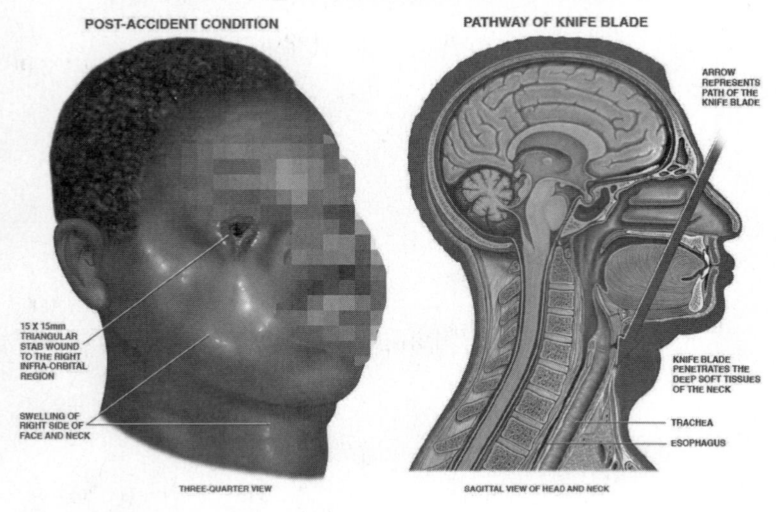

Traumatic Damage of the Trachea with Surgical Repairs

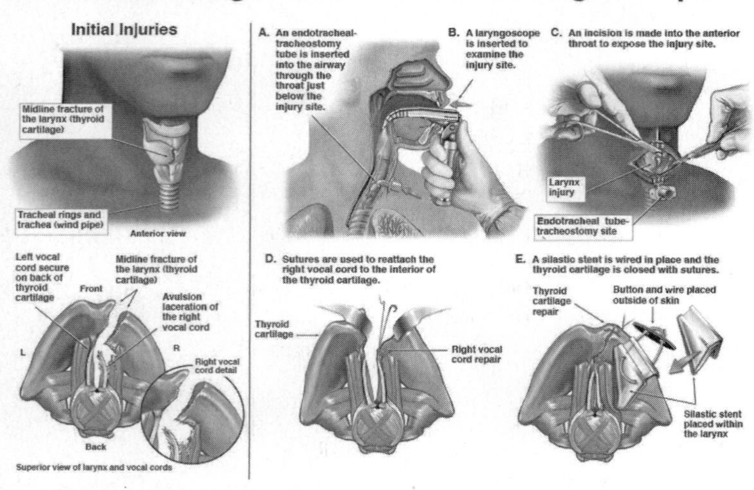

Concept Check

6. What is the best intervention for aspiration of a foreign body by a 2-year-old child?
   - A. Heimlich maneuver
   - B. Back blows
   - C. Abdominal thrusts
   - D. Back blows and alternating abdominal thrusts

Answer question

Collaborative Interventions (continued)

Obstruction Due to Drug Overdose

No specific EBP exists as patient-specific interventions are dependent on the type and extent of the substance ingested. Commonly, multiple drugs are implicated. This factor is important because multiple drugs can have a cumulative effect on respiratory depression.

N M **1.** In general, for all overdose management, the priority is airway protection and maintenance.

N M **2.** Test for gag reflex.

N M • If airway is obstructed (including intermittently), consider the jaw thrust prior to intubation.

N M • If gag reflex is absent, endotracheal intubation may be required for patients unable to protect their airway or clear secretions.

N M **3.** In addition, a general management principle is to determine from the patient and/or family what drugs have been used.

N M **4.** Follow local poison control management protocols.

N M **5.** The use of naloxone (narcotic antagonist) is a specific treatment for opiate overdose (heroin, prescription narcotics).

N M **6.** The use of flumazenil (benzodiazepine antagonist) is a specific treatment for benzodiazepines (diazepam, alprazolam) overdose.

Obstruction Due to Alcohol Intoxication

No specific EBP exists for alcohol intoxication regarding the airway. Management depends on the patient's level of sedation and the patient's ability to protect his or her airway:

N • If the airway is stable, position and keep patient on one side.

N • Give ordered anti-emetics to prevent vomiting and subsequent aspiration.

N M • Infuse IV fluids for hydration as indicated.

M • Perform drug screen to rule out other intoxicants.

N • Carefully monitor patient's condition (frequent vital signs and neuro checks).

N • If airway is obstructed (including intermittently), consider jaw thrust prior to intubation.

Obstruction Due to Obstructive Sleep Apnea

Diagnosis is made by a specialist after sleep studies are completed.

N M **1.** Use a CPAP/BiPAP machine or oral appliance

N **2.** Educate about weight loss program, if obesity is a factor

N **3.** Avoid use of alcohol 4–6 hours before bed.

N M **4.** May need to prepare patient for surgical intervention—includes revision of uvula and soft palate, craniofacial reconstruction, tracheostomy.

N M **5.** Instruct patient on pre- and postoperative teaching and care.

N **6.** Closely monitor after anesthesia.

N M **7.** Avoid benzodiazepines and narcotics if possible.

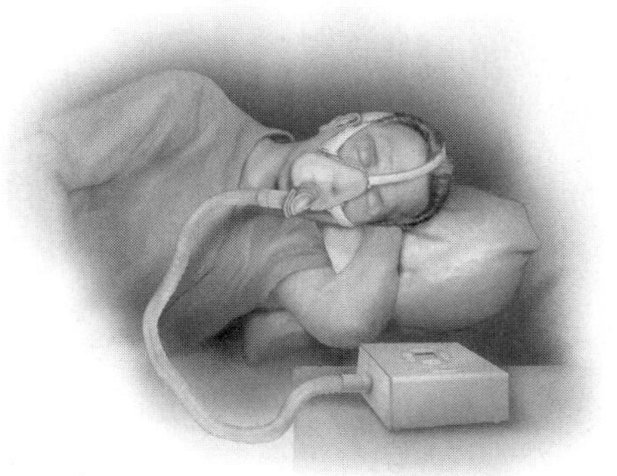

This image illustrates the use of CPAP to treat sleep apnea.

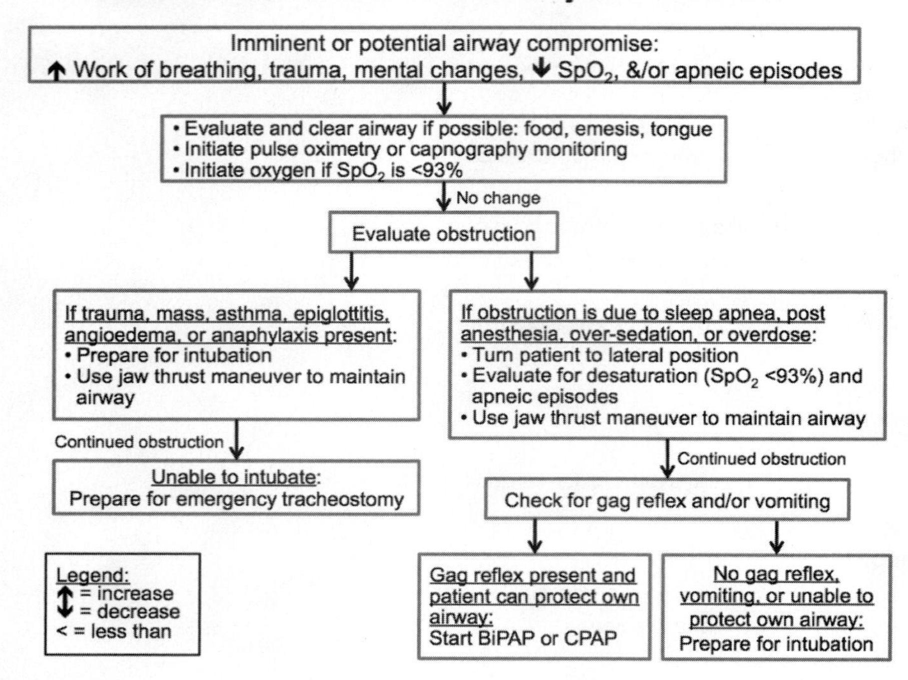

Collaborative Care: Airway Obstruction
Imminent or potential airway compromise:
↑ Work of breathing, trauma, mental changes, ↓ SpO2, &/or apneic episodes
• Evaluate and clear airway if possible: food, emesis, tongue
• Initiate pulse oximetry or capnography monitoring
• Initiate oxygen if SpO2 is <93%
No change
Evaluate obstruction
If trauma, mass, asthma, epiglottitis, angioedema, or anaphylaxis present:
• Prepare for intubation
• Use jaw thrust maneuver to maintain airway
Continued obstruction
Unable to intubate:
Prepare for emergency tracheostomy
If obstruction is due to sleep apnea, post anesthesia, over-sedation, or overdose:
• Turn patient to lateral position
• Evaluate for desaturation (SpO2 <93%) and apneic episodes
• Use jaw thrust maneuver to maintain airway
Continued obstruction
Check for gag reflex and/or vomiting
Gag reflex present and patient can protect own airway:
Start BiPAP or CPAP
No gag reflex, vomiting, or unable to protect own airway:
Prepare for intubation
Legend:
↑ = increase
↓ = decrease
< = less than

Source: Copyright © 2012, NovEx Novice to Expert Learning, LLC

Concept Check

7. Which drug would the nurse anticipate administering in an attempt to prevent an airway obstruction in a patient who has overdosed on heroin?
   A. Epinephrine
   B. Atropine
   C. Flumazenil
   D. Naloxone

Answer question

Summary of Interventions

- Control and management of the airway is the priority.
- If trauma is involved in airway obstruction, protection of the cervical spine is imperative.
- Prevention by using safety precautions, particularly in young children, can prevent death and life-altering conditions from choking on food or foreign bodies and accidental strangulation.
- Be prepared with appropriate equipment and suctioning at the bedside for the sudden deterioration of patients with infectious or inflammatory processes of the airway.
- Intervention with appropriate medications can avert airway occlusion or respiratory arrest.
- Careful and ongoing monitoring is required for any patient with the potential for airway compromise.

LO4:

Evaluation of Desired Collaborative Care Outcomes

Evaluation and reassessment should reveal attainment of previously established patient outcomes. In summary:

- The patient reports a clear airway and lungs are clear on auscultation.
- The patient has acceptable arterial blood gas levels and no evidence of hypoxemic changes to tissues.
- The patient is experiencing reduced anxiety.
- The patient reports and demonstrates comfortable respirations without air hunger.
- The patient has a normal temperature and white blood cell count.
- The patient expresses confidence in ability to avoid potential future airway obstruction.
- The patient reports being comfortable with little to no pain.

References

http://www.nlm.nih.gov/medlineplus/ency/article/000067.htm

http://www.google.com/search?client=safari&rls=en&q=airway+obstrcution&ie=UTF-8&oe=UTF-8

http://emedicine.medscape.com/article/135208-overview#a0156

http://www.aaaai.org/about-the-aaaai/newsroom/asthma-statistics.aspx

http://www.rcjournal.com/cpgs/maecpg.html

http://emedicine.medscape.com/article/764188-treatment#a1126

http://emedicine.medscape.com/article/763612-medication

http://emedicine.medscape.com/article/295807-overview

Learning Outcomes for Tracheostomy

When you complete this lesson, you will be able to:

1. Recognize the clinical relevance of a tracheostomy.
2. Consider the pathophysiology, etiology, risk factors, and clinical presentation of a patient requiring a tracheostomy that determine the priority patient concerns.
3. Determine the most urgent and important nursing interventions and patient education required in caring for a patient with a tracheostomy.
4. Evaluate attainment of desired collaborative care outcomes for a patient with a tracheostomy.

LO1:

What Is a Tracheostomy?

- A tracheostomy is an opening in the neck from the skin surface to the trachea.
- A tracheostomy is performed when breathing through the nose or mouth is not practical due to injury or disease.
- The procedure used to create the opening is called a tracheotomy.
- The tracheotomy procedure can be done surgically or percutaneously, using a bronchoscope and a series of dilators to create the opening.

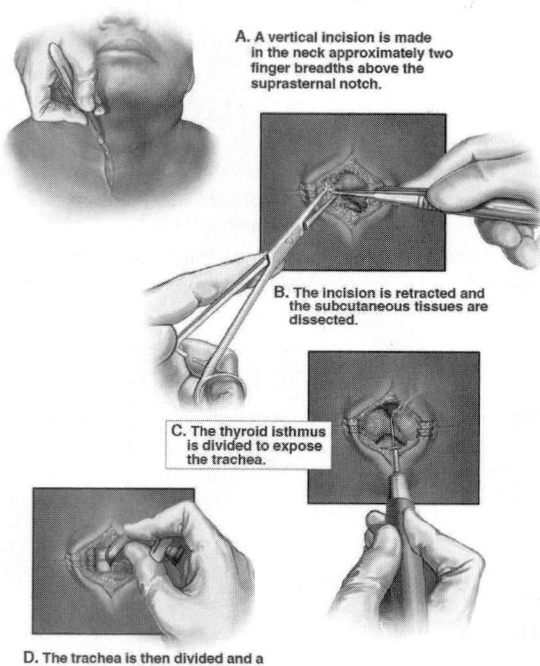

Tracheostomy Procedure
A. A vertical incision is made in the neck approximately two finger breadths above the suprasternal notch.
B. The incision is retracted and the subcutaneous tissues are dissected.
C. The thyroid isthmus is divided to expose the trachea.
D. The trachea is then divided and a tracheostomy tube is placed into the trachea.

This series of images depicts how a tracheotomy is created.
Source: © 2013 Nucleus Medical Media, All rights reserved

Tracheostomy Placement

- The placement of the tracheostomy tube is below the vocal cords.
- The markers in the illustration to the right are as follows:
  1. Vocal cords
  2. Thyroid cartilage
  3. Cricoid cartilage
  4. First tracheal ring
  5. Tracheostomy balloon cuff
- Note that the tracheal tube has a balloonlike, air-filled layer called the tracheostomy cuff, which forms a seal between the trach tube and tracheal wall to prevent aspiration and protect the airway.

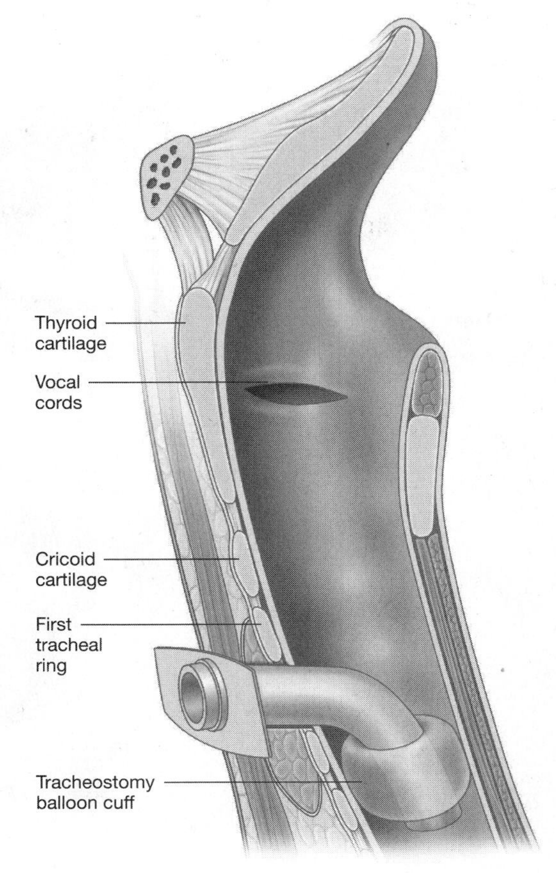

Tracheotomy (or tracheostomy) is one of the oldest known surgical procedures. It involves an incision in the neck to create an opening (stoma) directly into the airway (trachea).

LO1:

Clinical Relevance

- In most cases, tracheostomy is a life-saving procedure:
  - o To bypass an upper airway obstruction so the patient can breathe, or
  - o To provide for the safe administration of prolonged mechanical ventilation in patients with respiratory failure.
- It is also used to provide easy access to the lower airway for clearance of secretions in patients who can no longer clear and manage their own oral and lower airway secretions.

Indications

The most common indications for a tracheostomy tube are:

- Airway obstruction, which can occur from.
  - o Edema
  - o Trauma
  - o Mucous plug
  - o Severe inflammation
  - o Aspiration
  - o Tumor
- Edema of mouth and vocal cords, which require intubation or emergency tracheostomy.
- Poor airway clearance, which can be due to:
  - o Severe COPD
  - o Weak, ineffective cough from neuromuscular weakness
  - o Severe dysphasia with chronic aspiration (e.g., after a stroke, neuromuscular weakness)

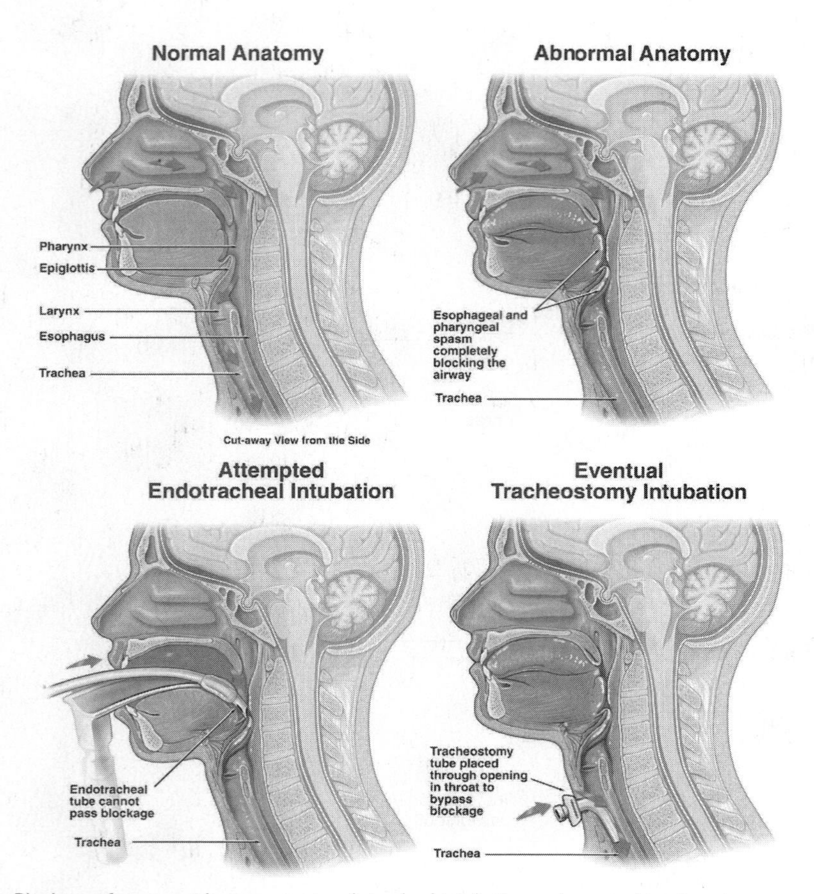

Blockage of airway with attempts at endotracheal intubation and eventual tracheostomy.

Indications (continued)

Continued from the previous page, the most common indications for a tracheostomy tube are:

- The need for long-term mechanical ventilation and:
  - o The patient will not be extubated quickly.
  - o The patient has been intubated more than 7-10 days.
  - o There is an increased need to protect the larynx, facilitate mobility, and/or enable the patient to talk.
- Patient's inability to protect his/her airway
- Endotracheal intubation not possible or desirable
- Head and neck surgery for cancer of the larynx (vocal cords) and upper airway

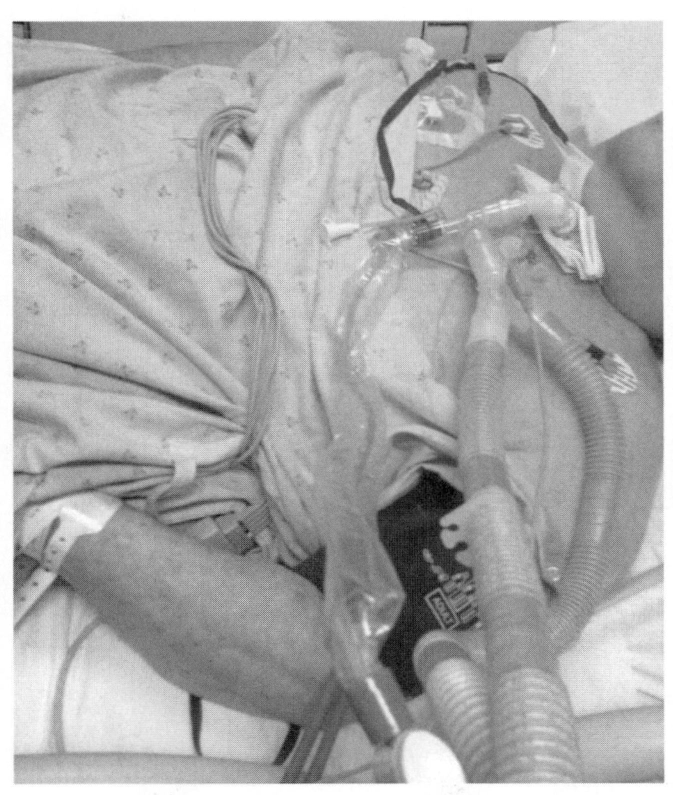

This patient required long-term mechanical ventilation following intubation. A tracheostomy was performed to avoid complications of prolonged intubation.
Source: Courtesy of K. Kyriakidis

Concept Check

1. **The nurse is planning care for a patient undergoing surgery for cancer of the larynx. The nurse should prepare to care for a patient with which type of airway?**
   A. Normal airway
   B. Endotracheal tube
   C. Tracheostomy
   D. Cricothyrotomy

Answer question

Permanent Tracheostomy

- A permanent tracheostomy (life-long dependence on a tracheal tube through which to breathe) can be performed if the original reason for the tracheostomy is considered to be permanent (e.g., head and neck cancer).
- A total laryngectomy (removal of the larygnx) creates a complete separation of the upper and lower airway. The separation prevents normal air flow to the lungs, requiring a permanent tracheostomy. For instance, in patients with head and neck cancer, total laryngectomy may be necessary. Thus, the patient must become a neck breather.

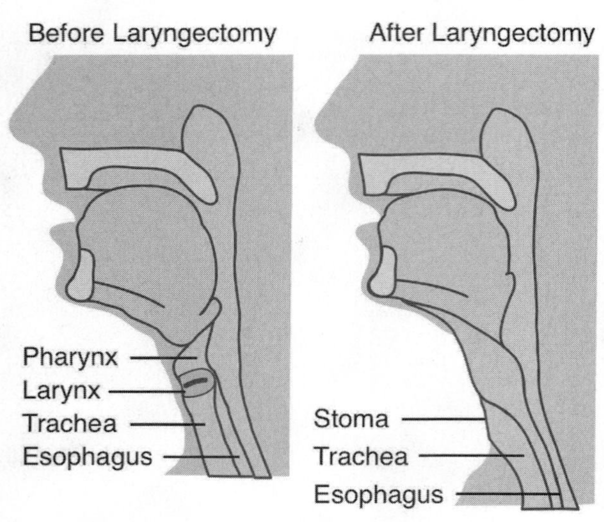

Source: Copyright © 2012, NovEx Novice to Expert Learning, LLC

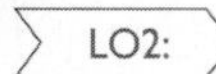

Pathophysiology

Tracheostomy Effects on Normal Physiology and Functioning

A tracheostomy bypasses upper airway function and causes the following physiologic and functional consequences:

- Loss of heat and humidification of air before it reaches the trachea as air bypasses the nasal passages and mouth
- Loss of smell as air bypasses the nose
- Lost ability to talk as air no longer passes over the vocal cords
- Increased risk of infection as air is no longer filtered by the upper airway
- Increased risk of aspiration related to increased amount of oropharyngeal secretions, the pooling of those secretions about the tracheal tube cuff, and the delayed triggers that stimulate swallowing

Assessment Findings

Warning of Partial Airway Obstruction

An airway obstruction is an emergent situation and is, therefore, a common cause for tracheostomy. Common signs of airway obstruction include:

- Increased RR; respiratory distress
- Increased work of or labored breathing
- Shortness of breath
- Use of accessory muscles
- Choking; inability to clear one's airway
- Stridor if upper airway is obstructing
- Hypoxia
- Fever and leukocytosis
- Cardiac dysrhythmias
- Pulmonary infiltrate or lobar collapse (from a mucous plug)
- Apnea

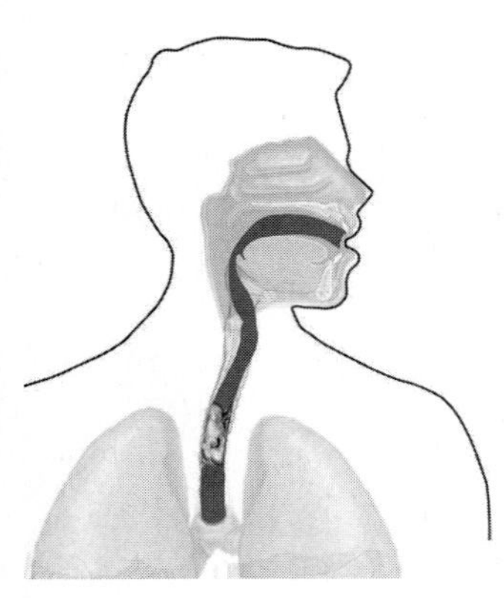

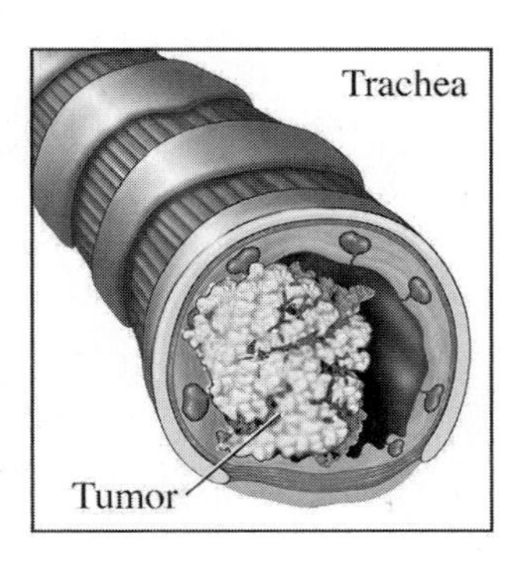

A large tumor growing is depicted in the trachea and is obstructing the trachea (yellow mass). The tumor is seen on the left and right in a cutaway view.

Concept Check

2. **Which assessment findings are common during airway obstruction?**
   A. Labored breathing
   B. Decreased respiratory rate
   C. Crackles
   D. Hot, dry skin

Answer question

Assessment Findings (continued)

Warning of Complete Airway Obstruction

- Complete airway obstruction is signaled by the lack of air movement and the ability to talk.
- Endotracheal intubation may be attempted first in controlled situations, as in the hospital environment, where there may be well-prepared and sufficient clinicians to respond to airway emergencies.
- Complete airway obstruction and the inability to intubate (pass an endotracheal tube through the obstruction) are the two major signs that a tracheostomy is required.

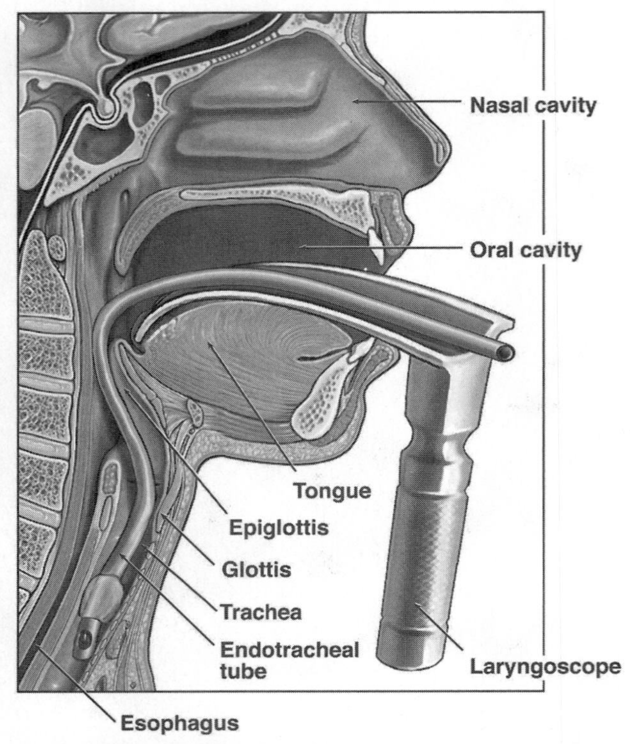

This illustration pictures endotracheal intubation with labels for anatomical parts and laryngoscope involved in insertion.
Source: © 2013 Nucleus Medical Media, All rights reserved

Emergency Tracheostomy Procedures

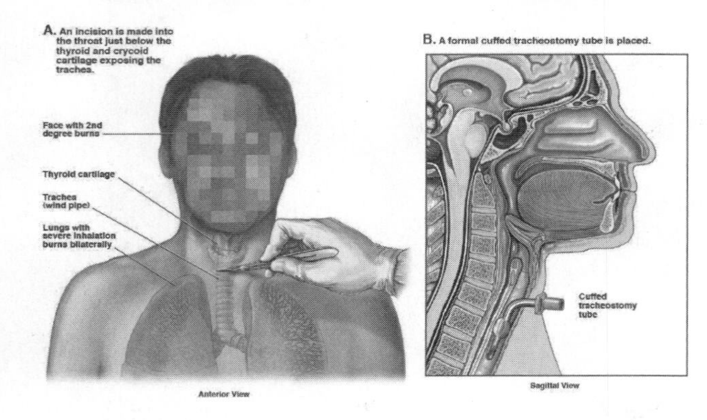

This graphic portrays the placement of a tracheostomy tube for comparison when airway obstruction precludes intubation.
Source: © 2013 Nucleus Medical Media, All rights reserved

- Complete airway obstructions, when neither intubation or tracheostomy are possible or time does not permit, are the ominous signs that an emergency cricothyrotomy may be required.
- In skilled hands, a cricothyrotomy provides rapid airway access, even in less controlled settings.
- The care of a patient with a cricothyrotomy is very similar to the care of patients with a tracheostomy.

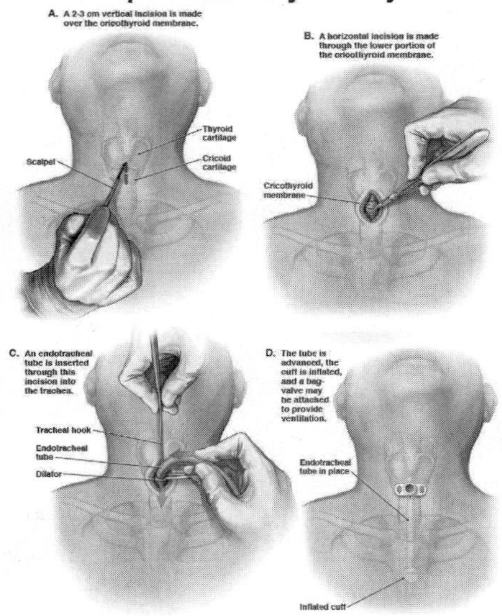

The cricothyrotomy procedure is presented.

Priority Patient Concerns and Desired Collaborative Care Outcomes

Prior to caring for patients with a tracheostomy, it is important to prioritize the patient's concerns that must guide the nursing care plan and interventions. Care for the patient is ordered and organized in accordance with the patient's priority and urgent needs. Desired collaborative care outcomes in patients with a tracheostomy typically include:

1. Patient will report decrease in discomfort.
2. Patient will be able to communicate needs.
3. Incision site will heal with no evidence of infection or excoriation.
4. Patient will manage secretions and fluids effectively, avoiding aspiration.
5. Patient will demonstrate acceptance of altered body appearance.

Considering these important care outcomes, prepare a list of the major 3–6 priority patient concerns or nursing diagnoses for patients with a tracheostomy. Be prepared to participate in a discussion of this list and/or to submit them as an assignment, as determined by your faculty. Resources you may find helpful in this assignment can include this lesson, the references, resources on nursing are plans, and standard nursing diagnoses manuals.

LO3:

Collaborative Interventions

Patients with a Tracheostomy

- A track develops over the tracheostomy in several days. However, during the first few days following a tracheostomy (trach), if the airway is lost, no track is present and the patient's airway will likely collapse. So, vigilance in preventing trach dislodgement is imperative.

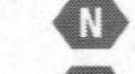

- Assess respiratory rate and breathing pattern for signs of respiratory distress.
- Monitor via oximetry to determine need for oxygen therapy.
- Use capnography to evaluate the adequacy of CO_2 clearance and to identify if the airway is lost. If the airway is lost, the capnogram ($PetCO_2$) reading is zero.
- Assess breath sounds and palpable fremitus to determine need for suctioning.
- Assess sputum for blood and plugging:
  - o Clots from blood or mucous can obstruct (plug) the tracheostomy tube. A complete obstruction will cause a medical emergency.
  - o Fortunately, suctioning can remove most clots or plugs.
  - o Keeping the humidification on the tracheostomy tube is especially important after a tracheostomy to prevent plugging.
  - o When the patient is on mechanical ventilation, a cuff must be inflated on the tracheostomy tube to prevent air loss during the ventilator-assisted breathing.

Evidence-Based Practice

- There is little evidence-based nursing for managing a patient with a tracheostomy.
- Research is needed to examine most nursing aspects in the care of patients with tracheostomies. Instead, interventions focus on comfort care, symptom relief, and prevention of complications.

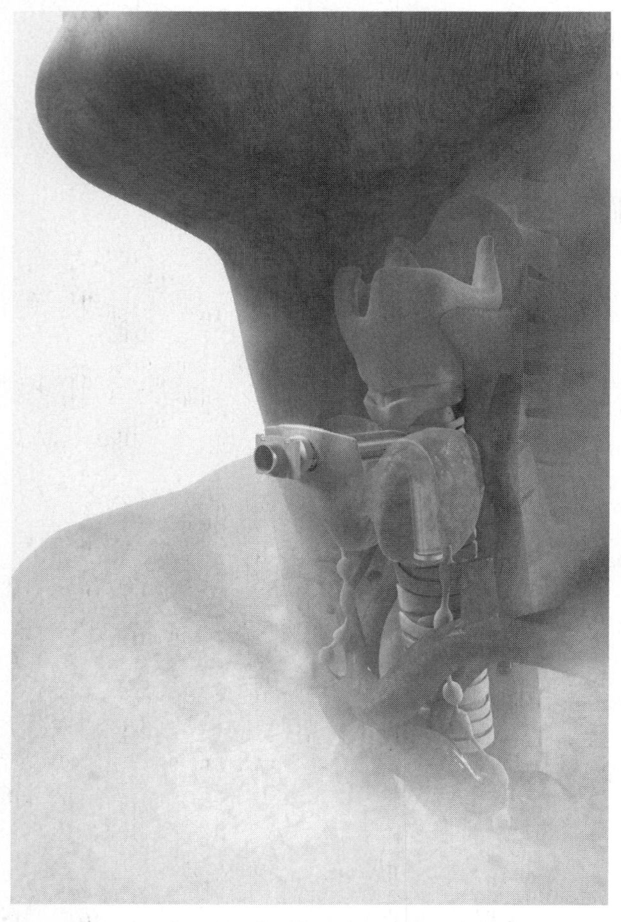

A tracheostomy tube with a fenestrated outer cannula is shown. The fenestrated holes permit air to pass through the cannula when the inner cannula is removed, allowing the patient to breathe and talk.

Source: MedicalRF.com/Alamy

- Important goals of nursing care are to prevent mucous plugging and to diagnose and treat complications as early as possible.
- Observing for signs of infection (e.g., fever, tachycardia, tachypnea, elevated WBCs) and airway obstruction are key nursing activities.
- Care requires an interdisciplinary team including patient, family, health care provider, nursing, respiratory care, speech therapy, dietician, and physical and occupational therapy.

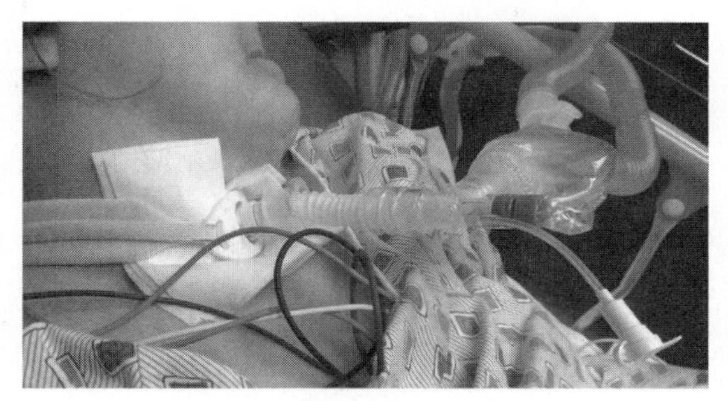

This patient, like most with tracheostomies, experiences the challenge of mucous plugs. Expectorating mucous is a greater problem when the patient's cough is not effective.
Source: Copyright © 2012, NovEx Novice to Expert Learning, LLC

Concept Check

3. What is an important goal of nursing care for patients with a newly created tracheostomy?

A. Use only evidence-based interventions.

B. Suction at least every 2 hours.

C. Prevent mucous plugging.

D. Remove both cannulas for cleaning.

Answer question

Collaborative Interventions (continued)

Postoperative Complications

Tracheostomy placement involves a surgical procedure. Observation and management, as needed, is required for symptoms of several postoperative complications, particularly:

- Bleeding around the operative site
- Pneumothorax and/or subcutaneous (sub-Q) air from a collapsed lung
- Mucous plugging, the most common complication
- Displacement of a new trach tube is, a serious complication. Most trach tubes are sutured in place for 1–2 weeks, until a track forms to prevent displacement.

Dislodged Tracheostomy Tube with Resulting Fatal Anoxic Encephalopathy

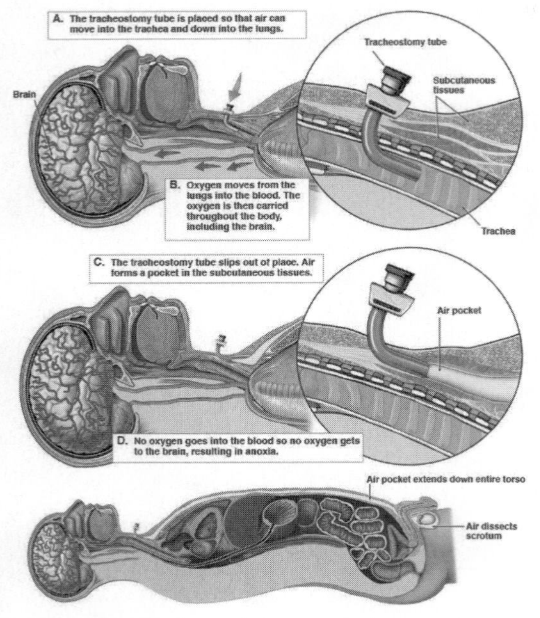

This series of images depicts the sequences of events upon dislodgement of a tracheostomy tube without effective intervention.
Source: © 2013 Nucleus Medical Media. All rights reserveda

Preventing complications in patients with a tracheostomy is essential. Avoid complications by:

- (M) Evaluating chest x-ray for correct tube placement, pneumothorax, cuff overinflation, and so forth.
- (N) Assessing sputum for blood and constantly assess for potential mucous plugging.
- (N)(M) Monitoring patient via EKG, SpO_2 and $PetCO_2$.
- (N)(M) Using high humidity trach collar (HHTC).
- (N) Cleaning or changing inner cannula every 8 hrs.
- (N) Suctioning as needed
- (N) Inflating cuff using proper technique and having respiratory therapy assist if this technique is not familiar
- (N) Preventing traction (pull caused by attachment to the ventilator tubing) on tube by using swivel adaptors and careful placement of the ventilator circuit.

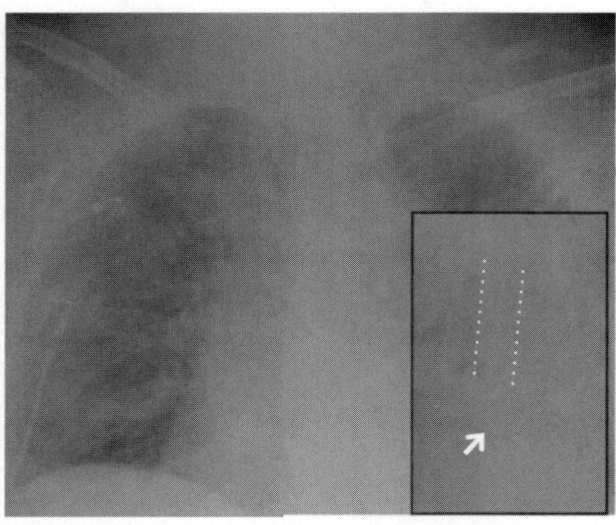

Tracheostomy and endotracheal (ET) tubes are cuffed conduits placed in the trachea either through the oropharynx or through a surgically created tracheostomy. When evaluating an ET tube (dotted line) on a chest x-ray it is important to identify the location of the tip (arrow).
Source: Courtesy of K. Kyriakidis

Concept Check

4. What is the most common complication associated with a new tracheostomy?
   A. Bleeding at the operative site
   B. Mucous plugging
   C. Pain
   D. Infection

Answer question

Tracheostomy Cuff Management

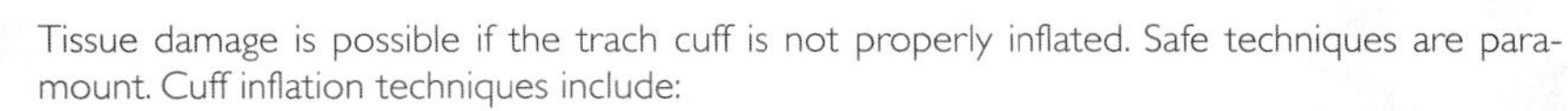

Tissue damage is possible if the trach cuff is not properly inflated. Safe techniques are paramount. Cuff inflation techniques include:

- Cuff measurement using appropriate device
- Minimal occlusive volume
- Minimal leak technique
- Cuff pressure limits that should never exceed capillary pressure, which is 24–30 cm of water pressure.
- Bivona Fome cuffs that self inflate as air should never be added to these cuffs.

Inflated Tracheostomy Cuff

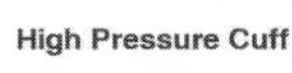
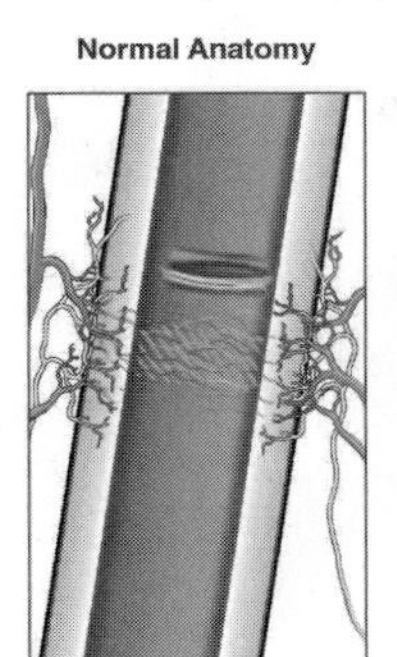
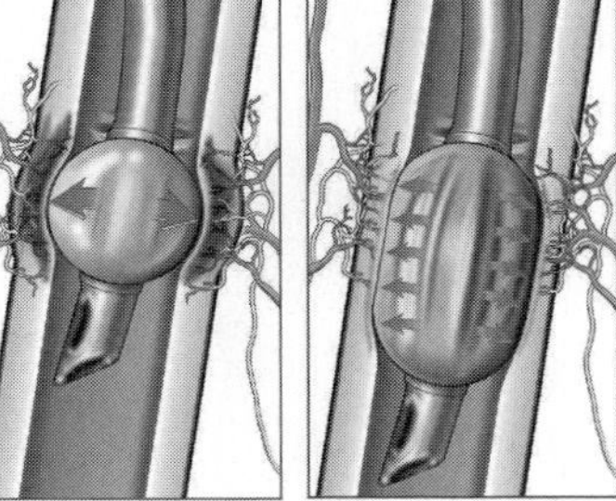
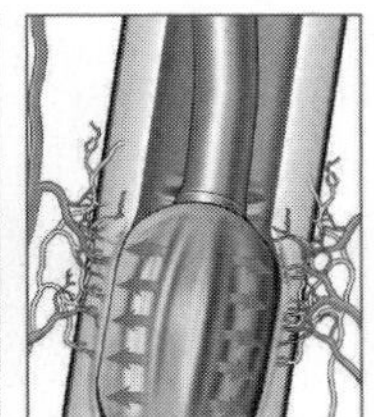

High and low pressure trach cuffs show how pressure is distributed against the tracheal wall.

Collaborative Interventions (continued)

Changing Tracheostomy Tubes

Some areas require nurses to assist with or perform tracheostomy tube changes. A review of the key points of this procedure include:

1. Check new cuff for leaks.

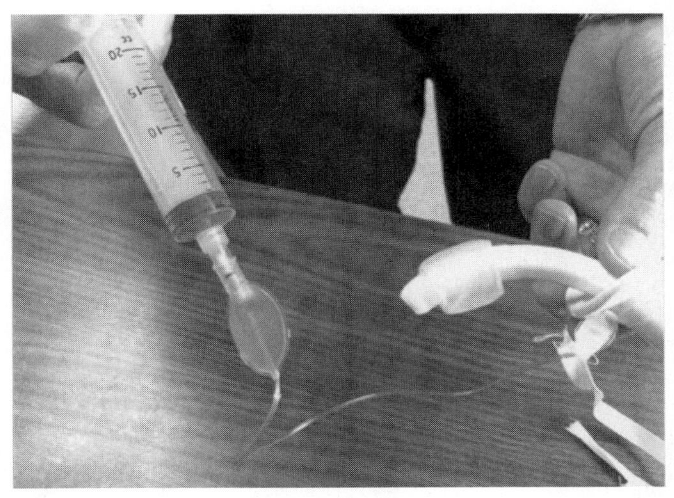

2. Deflate cuff by wrapping it around shaft.
3. Lubricate with water-soluble lubricant.
4. Apply trach ties.

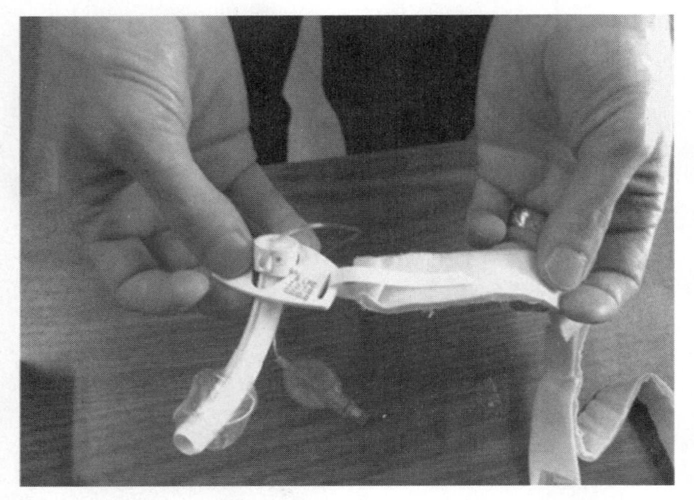

Source: Copyright © 2012, NovEx Novice to Expert Learning, LLC

5. Insert obturator in trach tube or prepare to use trach tube exchanger.
6. Position patient flat in bed with neck hyperextended on towel roll.
   - o Remove old dressing and ties. Support tube. Insert exchange device and deflate cuff.
   - o Remove old tube and insert new one over the exchange device. Remove obturator.
   - o Ensure good airflow and inflate cuff. Remove exchange device.
7. If patient is on a ventilator, give 100% O_2 for 2 min.
   - o Clean site and place dressing and holder. Replace inner cannula.

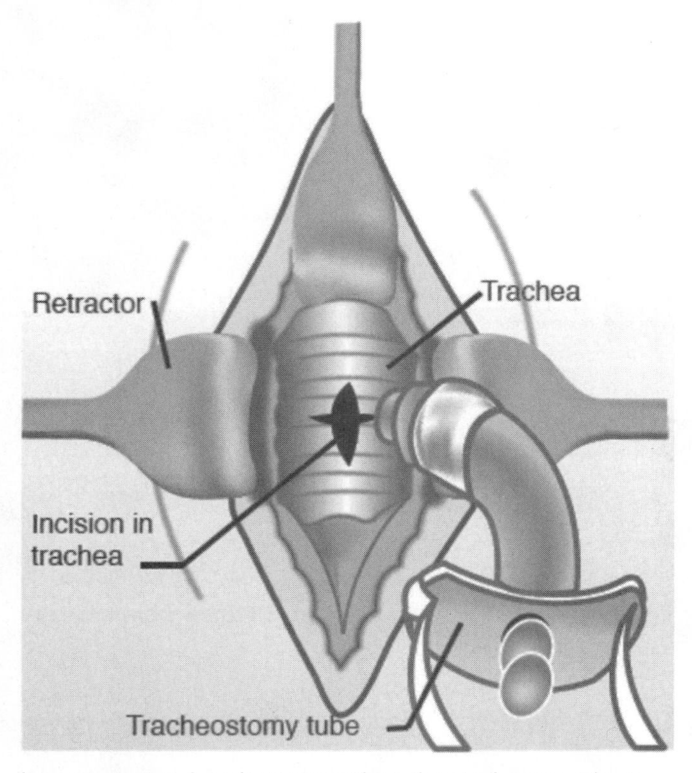

It is not uncommon during long-term ventilation that a tracheostomy tube can become disloged. Clinicians should be familiar with the tracheal structures in order to properly reinsert the tube in a ventilator-dependent patient.
Source: Copyright © 2012, NovEx Novice to Expert Learning, LLC

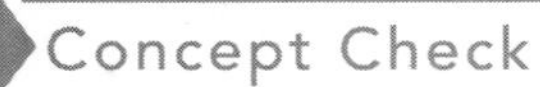

Concept Check

5. **How should the patient be positioned when it is necessary to change the tracheostomy tube?**
   A. Upright with neck extended
   B. Leaning forward with arms on the overbed table
   C. On the left side
   D. Flat in bed with neck hyperextended

Answer question

Collaborative Interventions (continued)

Airway Emergencies

Several emergencies can develop during tracheostomy use. The most dangerous are:

- Accidental decannulation in ventilator-dependent patients
- Bleeding post surgery
- Trach cuff rupture in a patient who is ventilator-dependent

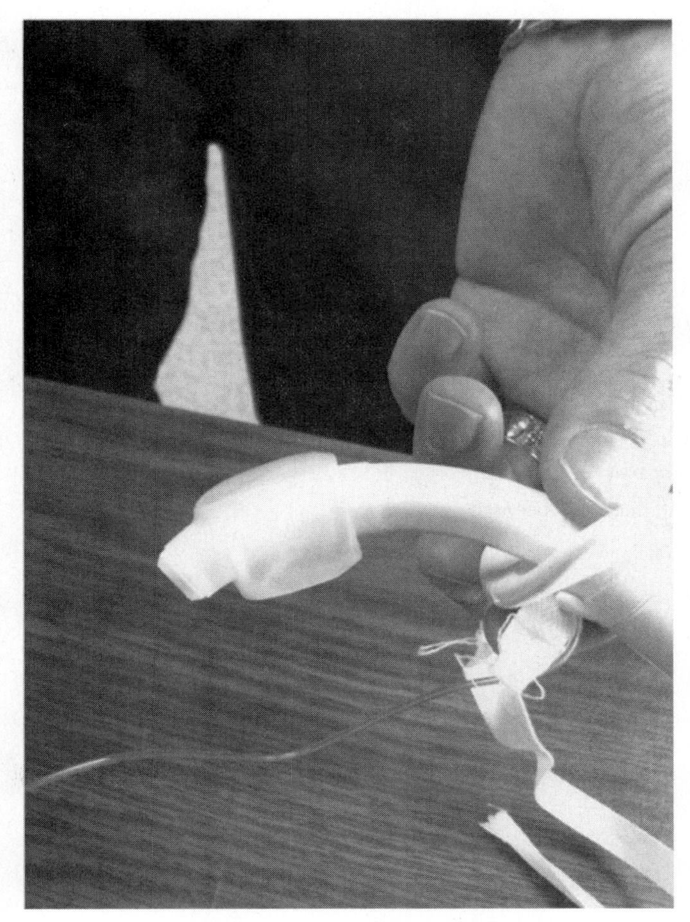

There is commonly an inflatable balloon-like cuff at the end of a tracheostomy tube. The balloon and tracheal wall interface forms a seal to prevent gas leakage around the tube, enables positive pressure ventilation, and prevents aspiration. If the balloon pressure against the trach wall is too high, serious complications like tracheal wall erosion can occur. Should the cuff rupture, ventilation can become compromised.
Source: Copyright © 2012, NovEx Novice to Expert Learning, LLC

Emergency Interventions in Case of Dislodgement

If an airway emergency develops from dislodgement of the trach tube, follow these steps:

1. Call for help: Rapid Response Team or a code.
2. Ventilate with ambu bag and oxygen over stoma, mouth and nose until a trach tube is reinserted.
3. Make one quick attempt to reinsert trach tube after laying the patient flat and hyperextending the neck back.
4. If unable to reinsert, place ET tube through upper airway if the patient had a trach to prevent longer-term complications from an ET tube.
5. If patient is a permanent neck breather and trach cannot be reinserted, ventilate over the stoma (trach site) until help arrives.

The main goal in these emergencies is to establish ventilation and oxygenation and then attempt trach reinsertion.

Concept Check

6. What nursing action is priority if a patient has accidental decannulation of the tracheostomy?

A. Have the patient hold his breath and bear down while the nurse reinserts the cannula.

B. Rinse the cannula with normal saline before attempting recannulation.

C. Call the rapid response team or a code blue.

D. Evaluate arterial blood gas measurement.

Answer question

Utilization of the Passy-Muir Speaking Valves (PMSV)

- A tracheostomy speaking valve allows the patient to talk—a critical patient need.
- Normally, a speaking valve is initiated by professional staff (e.g. speech pathologist, speech therapy) who can assess patient tolerance and respiratory status closely.
- Safest use of PMSVs is with a cuffless tube or a trach tube with a completely deflated cuff.

- If used with a cuffed tube, cuff must be completely deflated and patient must be supervised and monitored.

Concept Check

7. A patient with a cuffed tracheostomy tube is being prepared to use a PMSV. What nursing intervention is essential?

A. Completely deflate the tracheostomy cuff.

B. Completely inflate the tracheostomy cuff.

C. Remove the tracheostomy tube to fit the valve securely.

D. Replace the tracheostomy tube with the PMSV.

Answer question

Nursing Support and Patient Education

N Stoma and Mouth Care with Trach Dressing Change

Stoma and mouth care prevents dental caries and bacterial overgrowth and provides comfort.

- Should be done every 8 hr and prn.
- Keep stoma clean and dry.
- Remove old dressing. Inspect stoma.
- Clean with wound cleanser (no peroxide).
- Wipe off any mucous or blood.
- Apply pre-cut sponge to fit around the trach.
- Change trach ties that secure the trach daily. Have an assistant hold the tracheostomy securely to the neck while changing the ties to avoid inadvertent dislodgement.
- Give good mouth care using 2 min for teeth brushing and bacteriostatic mouthwash.
- Examine the mouth for mucosal inflammation or sores.
- Apply lip balm as needed for comfort.
- Every organization has a specific procedure that the nurses must follow, but generally these are the important elements.

N Aspiration Precautions

- Sit the patient with the head of the bed at 90 degrees.
- Provide thickened liquids that mitigate aspiration.
- Do not use straws.
- Purees are preferable over solids or soft foods.
- Chin tuck.
- Use Passy-Muir speaking valve (PMSV) if tolerated.
- Eat only with supervision.
- Take small sips and bites.
- Double swallow.
- If patient coughs with liquids or food, keep NPO until speech therapist can re-evaluate.
- Ensure suction setup is at the bedside and ready for use.

Summary of Interventions

- Tracheostomy is an alternative airway used for the following emergencies when endotracheal intubation is not possible:
  - o Long-term mechanical ventilation
  - o Permanent airway after head and neck surgeries for cancer or trauma
  - o For airway protection and clearance of secretions
- Patients with trachs require specific care and diligent observation to prevent occlusion and infection.
- Dislodgement or occlusion of a tracheostomy tube is a life-threatening emergency and requires immediate attention.
- Patients with a trach need careful observation for other complications such as aspiration, mucous plugging, and infection.
- Patients need evaluation for use of PMSV by speech therapy in order to allow voicing.

LO4:

Evaluation of Desired Collaborative Care Outcomes

Evaluation and reassessment reveal attainment of previously established patient outcomes. In summary:

- Patient reports reduced discomfort.
- Patient communicates needs effectively.
- Incision site is healing with no evidence of infection or excoriation.
- Patient manages secretions and fluids effectively and without aspiration.
- Patient demonstrates growing acceptance of altered body appearance.

References

http://www.passy-muir.com

http://www.mayoclinic.com/health/tracheostomy/MY00261

http://www.nhlbi.nih.gov/health/dci/Diseases/trach/trach_whatis.html

http://www.clevelandclinic.org/thoracic/Airway/Tracheostomy.htm

CARE OF PATIENTS WITH ACUTE LUNG INJURY AND ACUTE RESPIRATORY DISTRESS SYNDROME

Learning Outcomes for Acute Lung Injury and Acute Respiratory Distress Syndrome

When you complete this lesson, you will be able to:

1. Recognize the clinical relevance of acute lung injury and acute respiratory distress syndrome.
2. Consider the pathophysiology, etiology, risk factors, and clinical presentation of acute lung injury and acute respiratory distress syndrome that determine the priority patient concerns.
3. Determine the most urgent and important nursing interventions and patient education required in caring for a patient with acute lung injury or acute respiratory distress syndrome.
4. Evaluate attainment of desired collaborative care outcomes for a patient with acute lung injury or acute respiratory distress syndrome.

LO1:

What Is ALI and ARDS?

- Acute lung injury (ALI) describes the inflammatory condition that results after injury to the lung presenting with:
  - o Bilateral pulmonary opacities
  - o Hypoxemia
- Acute respiratory distress syndrome (ARDS) is the most severe form of ALI.
- ALI and ARDS are caused by a variety of conditions that result in lung injury.

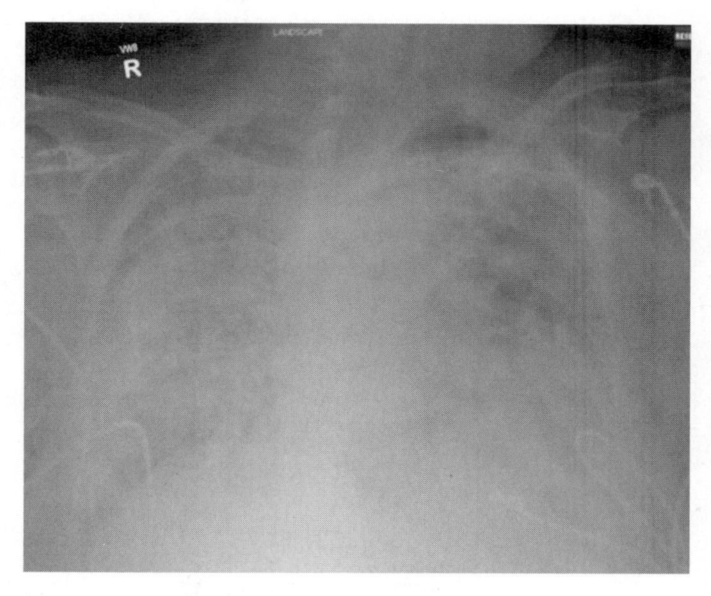

Acute respiratory distress syndrome is a situation where fluid floods the alveoli (a "white out") and interferes with gas exchange. Mortality rates with ARDS are severe and treatment is often ineffective.
Source: Copyright © 2012, NovEx Novice to Expert Learning, LLC

LO1:

Clinical Relevance

- Approximately 150,000 patients experience ARDS annually.
- Patients who develop ARDS need to be:
  1. Transferred to the intensive care unit (ICU)
  2. Intubated
  3. Supported on mechanical ventilation
     a. Early recognition of impending ARDS and intervention with ventilatory support can mitigate complicating sequelae.
- Despite aggressive treatment, the mortality in ARDS remains high (40–60%).
- The majority of ARDS survivors recover most of their lung function, but some are left with lifelong impairment.
- ARDS and sepsis are often found in combination, increasing the likelihood of multi-organ failure.
- The involvement of additional organs in the ARDS pathophysiology is an ominous sign for poor survival.

Concept Check

1. Which of the following is true regarding acute respiratory distress syndrome (ARDS)?
   A. The patient is likely to have a long history of smoking.
   B. Recovery of lung function is complete in the majority of clients.
   C. ARDS is effectively treated with steroids and fluids.
   D. Mechanical ventilation is required to effectively treat ARDS.

Answer question

LO2:

Pathophysiology

- A traumatic event that injures the lung may or may not lead to the ALI or ARDS inflammatory response.
- An inciting injury that leads to ALI or ARDS may cause injury directly to the lung (e.g., through smoke inhalation) or indirectly (e.g., through damage from sepsis).
- Damage to the alveoli results in release of inflammatory cytokines and proteases, which then cause further damage to the capillaries, tissues, and alveolar walls.
- Adverse changes occur with fluid in the alveoli:
  - o Decrease in compliance of the alveoli results in alveolar stiffness, creating greater difficulty for gas exchange in and out of the alveoli.
  - o Hypoxemia results from the worsening gas exchange.
- Alveolar compliance is diminished when:
  - o Damaged alveoli produce less surfactant, causing decreased compliance.
  - o Pressure required to inflate the alveoli increases and the alveoli collapse (atelectasis).

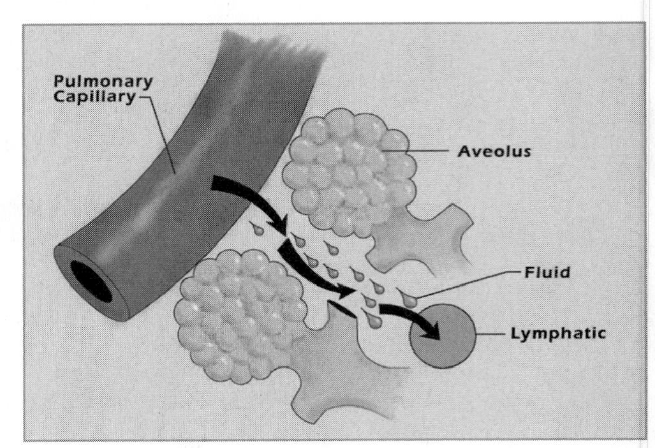

As in all inflammatory responses, the damaged capillaries dilate and leak into the interstitial spaces. Pulmonary lymphatics are overwhelmed in ALI and ARDS and unable to drain the excess fluid as quickly as it accumulates. Therefore, fluid, proteins, WBCs, and RBCs then leak into the alveoli.
Source: Copyright © 2012, NovEx Novice to Expert Learning, LLC

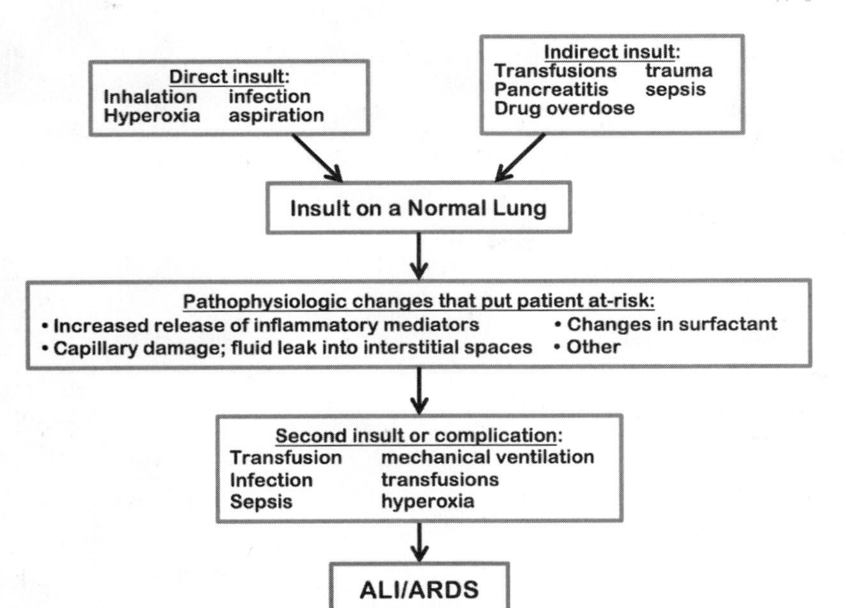

Pathophysiology of ARDS.
Source: Copyright © 2012, NovEx Novice to Expert Learning, LLC

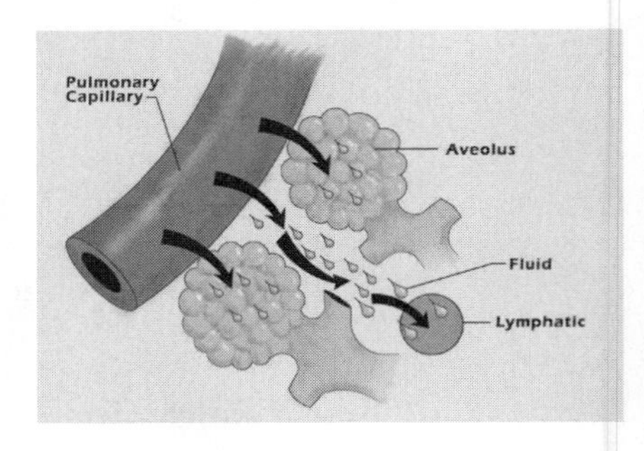

Capillary leaking into the interstitial space and alveoli in ARDS.
Source: Copyright © 2012, NovEx Novice to Expert Learning, LLC

ARDS

- In the acute phase of the syndrome (right-hand side of image below), protein rich edema fluid fills the alveolar air space, blocking O_2 delivery and resulting in damage to all normal cell components and to the alveolar wall.
- The damaged cells produce cytokines and other destructive inflammatory substances that result in: (1) loss of integrity of the alveolar wall, (2) subsequent leakage of toxic products into the interstitial space, and (3) damage to the pulmonary capillaries.
- The end result is that the patient rapidly loses the ability to maintain adequate air exchange and progresses to full-blown ARDS.

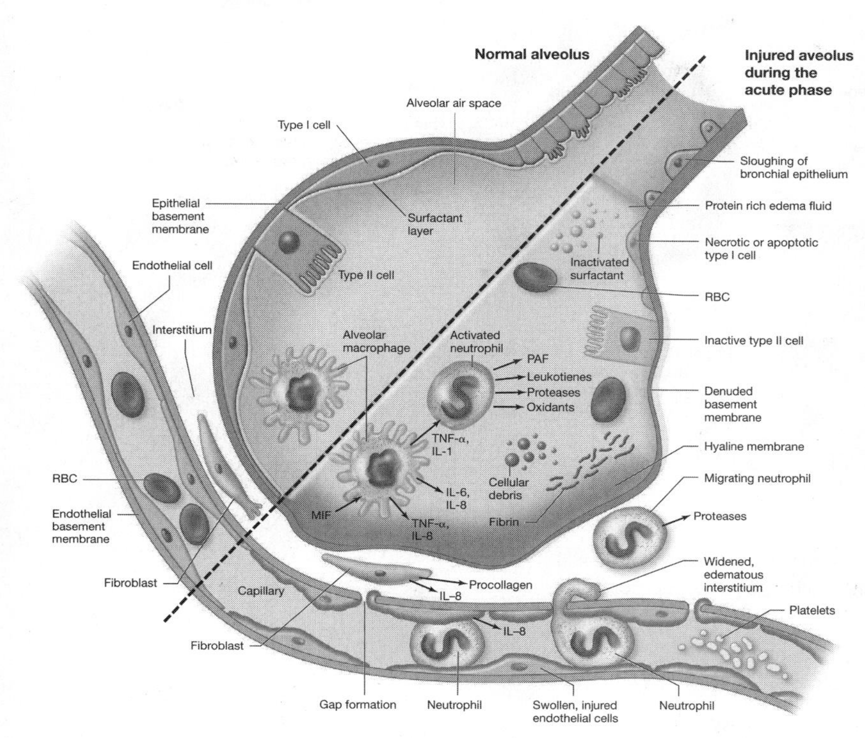

The normal alveolus (left-hand side) and the injured alveolus in the acute phase of acute lung injury and the acute respiratory distress syndrome (right-hand side).

- Collapsed fluid filled alveoli severely compromise ventilation (V) and gas exchange but continue to be perfused (Q), known as ventilation/perfusion (V/Q) mismatch. This *pulmonary shunting* produces hypoxemia.
- Hypoxemia is manifested by low PaO_2 and SpO_2 (pulse oximeter). The degree of reduction depends on the amount of oxygen administered.
- The relative degree of hypoxemia can be measured by PaO_2/FiO_2 ratio. It is obtained by dividing the arterial oxygen saturation (PaO_2 in mmHG) by the fraction of inspired oxygen (FiO_2). Example: if the PaO_2 is 80 mmHG and the FiO_2 is 40% (0.40), then the PaO_2/FiO_2 ratio is 80/0.4 = 200. The lower the ratio the worse the hypoxemia.
- CO_2 diffuses more readily and is not as affected by the fluid filled alveoli.
- The pathophysiological changes are shown in sequence in the following illustrations of the alveolar changes in ARDS.

Alveolar Changes in ARDS

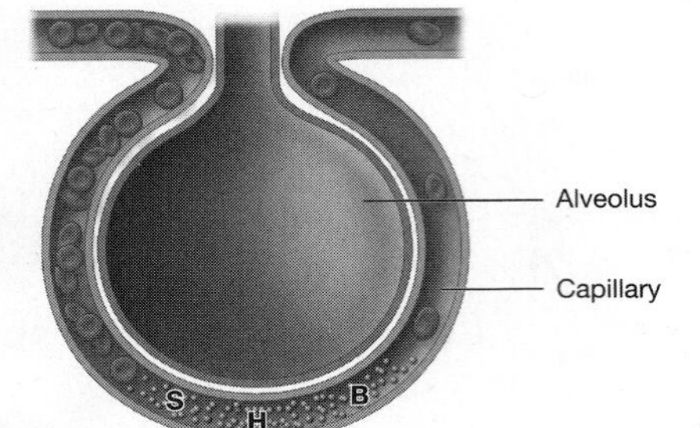

Phase 1: Injury reduces normal blood flow to the lungs. Platelets aggregate and release histamine (H), serotonin (S), and bradykinin (B).

Phase 2: Those substances, especially histamine, inflame and damage the alviolocapillary membrane, increasing capillary permeability. Fluids then shift into the interstitial space.

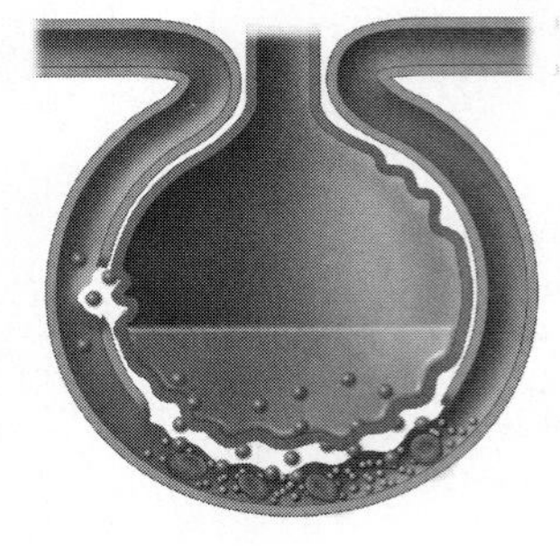

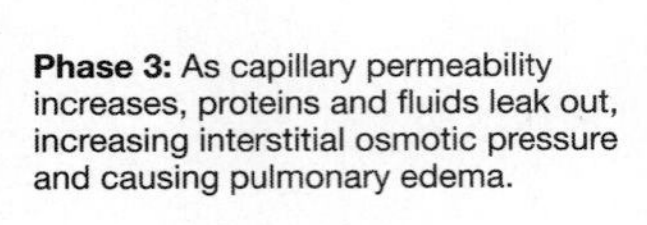

Phase 3: As capillary permeability increases, proteins and fluids leak out, increasing interstitial osmotic pressure and causing pulmonary edema.

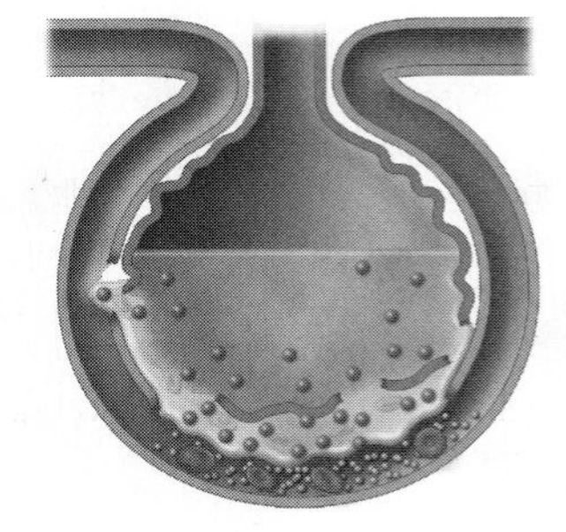

Phase 4: Decreased blood flow and fluids in the alveoli damage surfactant and impair the cell's ability to produce more. As a result, alveoli collapse, impeding gas exchange, and decreasing lung compliance.

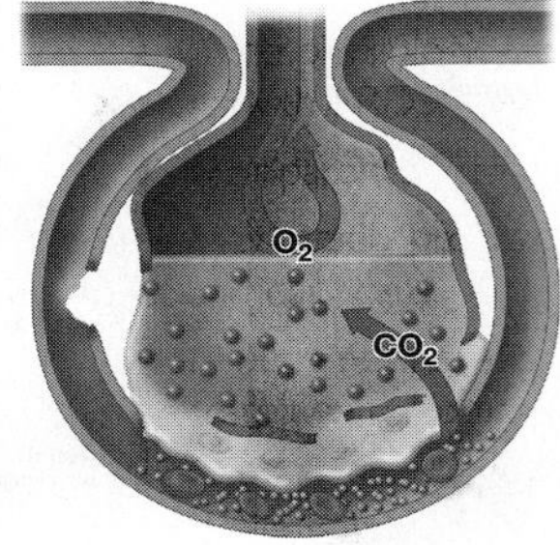

Phase 5: Sufficient oxygen cannot cross the alveolocapillary membrane, but carbon dioxide (CO_2) can and is lost with every exhalation. Oxygen (O_2) levels decrease in the blood.

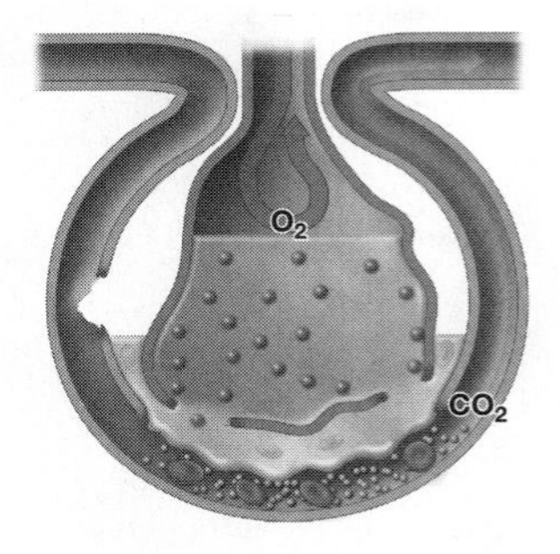

Phase 6: Pulmonary edema worsens, inflammation leads to fibrosis, and gas exchange is further impeded.

Comparing the pathological changes in the normal lung that occur in ARDS can provide a visual perception about how the lung's ability to ventilate and exchange gases deteriorates.

Causes and Risk Factors

- ALI can be caused by any condition that injures the lung either directly or indirectly.
- Direct lung injury is due to:
  - o Pneumonia
  - o Aspiration
  - o Inhalation
  - o Fat embolism
  - o Trauma (e.g., lung contusion)
  - o Near drowning
- Indirect lung injury (usually through the release of inflammatory cytokines) can be caused by:
  - o Sepsis
  - o Pancreatitis
  - o Blood transfusion
  - o Burns
  - o Cardiopulmonary bypass
- There is no evidence that ALI is more common among patients of a certain age, race, or gender.

Complications

- ALI and ARDS usually have an acute onset and resolve in about one week. Occasionally, ARDS can take several weeks to resolve.
- Patients with ARDS are commonly critically ill and require ventilation.
- Complications in ARDS patients are often due to the causes of lung injury (e.g., sepsis causing multi-organ failure).
- Barotrauma is a complication of mechanical ventilation and is more common in ARDS. Barotrauma is the damage that occurs to alveoli as a result of high pressures needed to ventilate the stiff lungs. In ARDS, air moving away from the injured parts of the lung causes over distension and higher pressures in the unaffected alveoli. The high pressures can result in pneumothoraces.
- Most other complications are related to the critical aspects of the patient's condition. Complications may include:
  - o Aspiration
  - o Malnutrition
  - o Ventilator-associated pneumonia
  - o Delirium
  - o Stress ulcers
  - o Urinary tract infections
  - o Catheter-related infections
  - o Venous thromboembolism
- Patients can have long-term consequences of a critical illness and prolonged ICU stay, not related to lung injury itself (e.g., cognitive deficits).

Concept Check

2. Which of the following puts someone at risk for development of ALI/ARDS?

A. The patient is 75 years old.

B. The patient has serious injuries from a motor vehicle crash.

C. The patient is of Asian descent.

D. The patient is male.

Answer question

Concept Check

3. The complications of ARDS most often result from which factor?

A. The original cause of the lung injury

B. The use of mechanical ventilation

C. Long term oxygen use

D. Use of steroid medications

Answer question

Assessment Findings

- Hypoxemia (low PaO_2 and SpO_2), despite oxygen therapy
- Shortness of breath
- Tachycardia, heart rate more than 100 beats per minute
- Respirations more than 20 per minute
- Anxiety
- Other signs and symptoms of ALI depend on the cause of lung injury (e.g., sepsis causing fever and hypotension).

Diagnostics

The diagnosis of ALI depends on meeting the following criteria:

- Timing: Acute
- Chest x-ray: Bilateral infiltrates that are not due to CHF
- Development of bilateral diffuse alveolar infiltrates within 4–24 hours after the injury. Chest x-ray shows widespread infiltrates that are often termed a "white out" pattern as the lungs show up white on the x-ray.

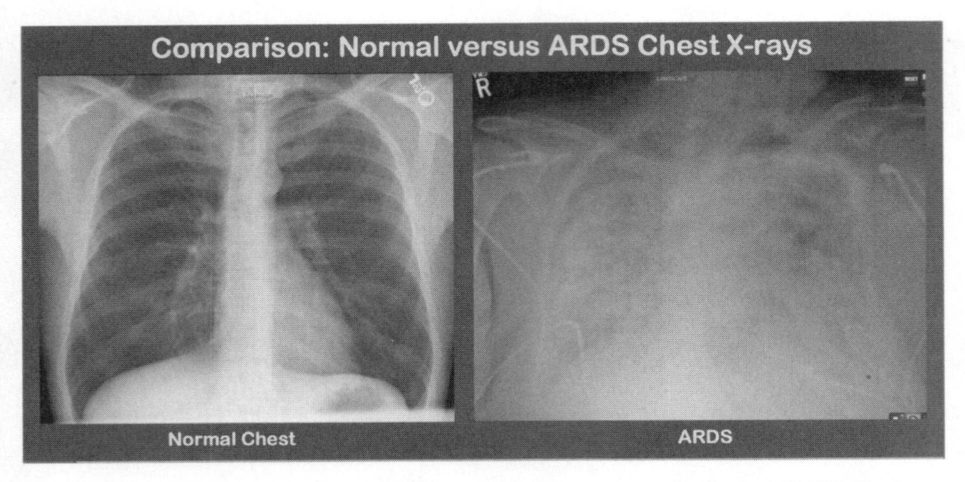

These x-rays compare the lungs of a patient with normal lungs versus one who developed ARDS. On the left, the cardiac silhouette is distinctly visible and lung fields are clear (gray with visible vasculature). On the right, note the "white out" of both lungs that is typical of the bilateral infiltrates seen in ARDS. The cardiac silhouette and mediastinum are obscured.
Source: Courtesy of K. Kyriakidis

- By definition, ALI is PaO_2 (ABG)/FiO_2) ratio is less than 300. The ratio denotes the severity of the hypoxemia.
- Older definitions stipulate that intracardiac pressures are normal or not elevated, e.g., pulmonary artery occlusion pressure (PAOP or wedge) less than 19 mmHg. However, many patients do not have cardiac pressure determinations measured by pulmonary artery catheters, so this part of the definition was eliminated.
- ARDS is the most severe form of ALI and is differentiated by the degree of hypoxemia. A patient has ARDS when the PaO_2/FiO_2 ratio is less than 200.
- Other tests that are helpful in diagnosis and treatment of ALI or ARDS are related to ruling out heart failure and evaluating the cause of ALI or ARDS.
- BNP: Levels of beta natriuretic peptide (BNP) increase with heart failure. A low BNP makes heart failure unlikely.
- Bronchoscopy is used to obtain samples of secretions from the bronchial tree for:
  - o Culture
  - o Gram stain
  - o Microscopic examination

  It is often helpful in determining the cause of lung injury and can aid in identifying an infectious organism.
- A summary of the diagnostics are provided (see the following table).

Berlin Definition of ARDS

The Berlin Definition of Acute Respiratory Distress Syndrome

		Acute Respiratory Distress Syndrome
Timing		Within 1 week of a known clinical insult or new or worsening respiratory systems
Chest imaging[a]		Bilateral opacities—not fully explained by effusions, lobar/lung collapse, or nodules
Origin of edema		Respiratory failure not fully explained by cardiac failure or fluid overload Need objective assessment (e.g., echocardiography) to exclude hydrostatic edema if no risk factor present
Oxygenation[b]	**Mild**	200 mmHg $< PaO_2/FiO_2 \leq$ 300 mmHg with PEEP or CPAP $\geq$ 5 cm H_2O[c]
	Moderate	100 mmHg $< PaO_2/FiO_2 \leq$ 200 mmHg with PEEP $\geq$ 5 cm H_2O
	Severe	$PaO_2/FiO_2 \leq$ 100 mmHg with PEEP $\geq$ 5 cm H_2O

Abbreviations:
CPAP = Continuous positive airway pressure
FiO_2 = Fraction of insired arterial oxygen
PEEP = Positive end-expiratory pressure

[a] Chest radiograph or computed tomography scan.
[b] If altitude is higher that 1000m, the correction factor should be calculated as follows: [PaO_2/FiO_2O×(barometric pressure/760)]
[c] This may be delivered noninvasively in the mild acute respiratory distress syndrome group.

Priority Patient Concerns and Desired Collaborative Care Outcomes

Prior to caring for patients with ALI or ARDS, it is important to prioritize the patient's concerns that must guide the nursing care plan and interventions. Care for the patient is ordered and organized in accordance with the patient's priority and urgent needs. Desired collaborative care outcomes in patients with ALI or ARDS typically include:

1. Patient's arterial blood gases and oxygenation saturations will approximate pre-illness level.
2. Patient will demonstrate normal lactate level and no signs of cyanosis, mental confusion, or hypoxemia.
3. Patient will remain infection free.
4. Patient's caloric intake will match energy requirements.
5. Patient will experience less fear and anxiety with support systems and comfort care so that fear and anxiety do not compromise oxygenation.

Considering these important care outcomes, prepare a list of the major 3–6 priority patient concerns or nursing diagnoses for patients with ALI or ARDS. Be prepared to participate in a discussion of this list and/or to submit them as an assignment, as determine by your faculty. Resources you may find helpful in this assignment can include this lesson, the references, resources on nursing care plans, and standard nursing diagnoses manuals.

Concept Check

4. **The widespread infiltrate often present on the chest x-ray of a patient with ARDS is often described using which term?**
   A. snow chest
   B. white out
   C. grayed
   D. fogged

Answer question

LO3:

Collaborative Interventions

Evidence-Based Practice

In managing patients with ALI and ARDS, evidence-based treatments primarily involve avoiding situations that may lead to ALI (e.g., aspiration) and therapies that prevent harm from mechanical ventilation:

- Ventilator management to prevent barotrauma:
  - N M Use the lowest effective ventilator pressures required to ventilate patients with ARDS in order to decrease the incidence of barotrauma.
  - N M Barotrauma can often be prevented by using higher respiratory rates and lower tidal volumes, while keeping the SpO_2 more than 92% and $PaCO_2$ within normal limits (35–45 mmHg).
- N M Minimizing IV fluids may enhance oxygenation by mitigating fluid leakage into the alveoli. Conservative fluid therapy also decreases both the time required for weaning the patient off the ventilator and the length of ICU stay (days in the ICU). Unfortunately, it does not decrease mortality.

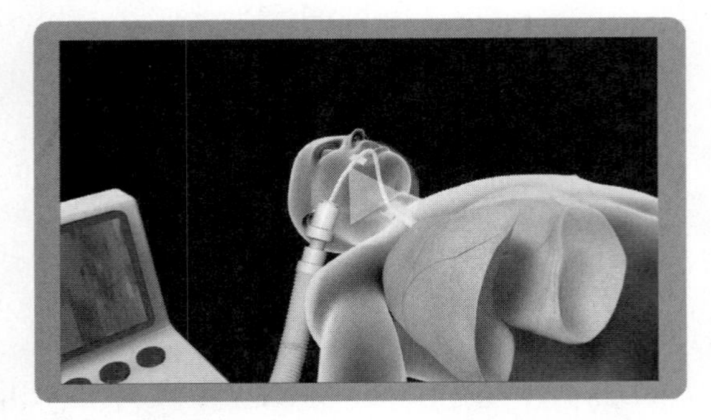

Intubation and mechanical ventilation are typically needed in severe respiratory distress. Poor oxygenation and/or gas exchange may compromise the patient's survival. These conditions threaten the vital organs, particularly the heart and brain. Intubation and mechanical ventilatory support may be lifesaving, but should be discontinued as early as possible to prevent complications. Although this animation targets patients as the audience, it is instructive to observe how and why intubation is performed.

ARDS patients commonly require intubation and mechanical ventilation. These are central to managing these patients according to EBP.

- Current mechanical ventilators are sophisticated, computer-controlled breathing machines. However, most of their basic functions are not new. Ventilators work by pushing air into the patient's lungs, exactly the opposite of normal breathing.
- A key goal in ARDS is to keep the plateau pressure (the alveolar opening pressure) less than 30 cm H_2O while keeping the SpO_2 more than 92% and $PaCO_2$ in normal limits (35–45 mmHg). This can be achieved with different modes of ventilation.
- Modes of breathing via mechanical ventilation*
  1. Intermittent mandatory ventilation (IMV) or assist-control (AC) modes are common:
     a. Ventilator delivers a preset volume.
     b. The preset volume set for delivery with each breath is called the tidal volume.
     c. The normal volume set for each breath is 6–10 mL/kg.
  2. Pressure support therapy can also be used, where pressure is the set end point instead of volume.
  3. Prevention of ventilator-associated pneumonia is paramount and requires two key nursing interventions (EBP):
     a. Raise the head of the bed to 30–45 degrees to avoid aspiration
     b. Vigilant, frequent mouth care

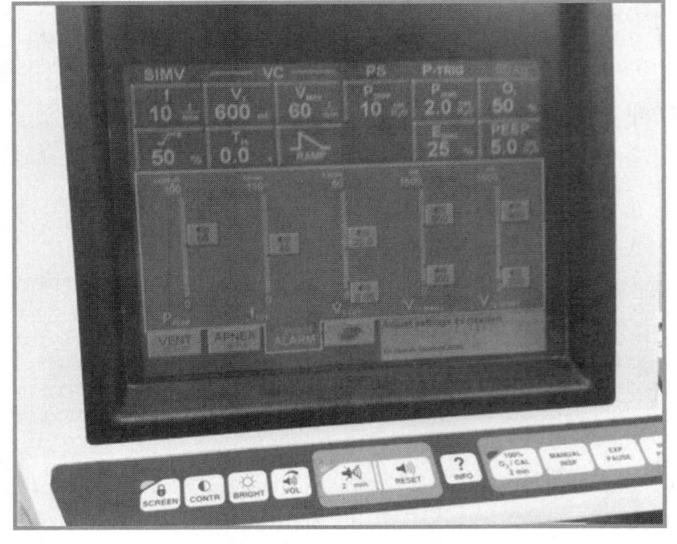

Some newer mechanical ventilators provide the operator with automated tools to obtain a static Pressure Volume (P/V) Curve in the ventilated patient. These tools provide the clinician a simple, safe, and reproducible method to assess the P/V curve for various pulmonary conditions.

*Arterial blood gases inform judgment about the adequacy of ventilation. (Ventilator adjustments are made to keep the pH and $PaCO_2$ levels normal.)

Evidence supports the removal of invasive therapies as soon as possible to prevent complications. In ALI and ARDS, weaning from the ventilator as soon as possible is of primary importance:

- Normally, this begins with a weaning trial (temporary removal of the patient from the ventilator).
- If a weaning trial is attempted, the patient may be extubated when the patient is not short of breath or tachypneic and the patient is breathing effectively (normal pH and no increase in $PaCO_2$).
- Patients are normally very happy to be off mechanical ventilation as they can return to eating and talking.
- Importantly, the patient's normal protective barriers against aspiration are restored upon removal of the ventilator and extubation.

Mechanical Ventilation Issues

- Mechanical ventilation is necessary in most patients who develop ARDS. However, it can contribute adverse effects to the very pathophysiological problems that need to be treated.
- Notice that inflammation, surfactant disruption, fibrosis, and lung compliance are potential adverse effects.
- Despite the potential adverse effects, mechanical ventilation is essential as a supportive treatment until the pathophysiological sequelae resolve.

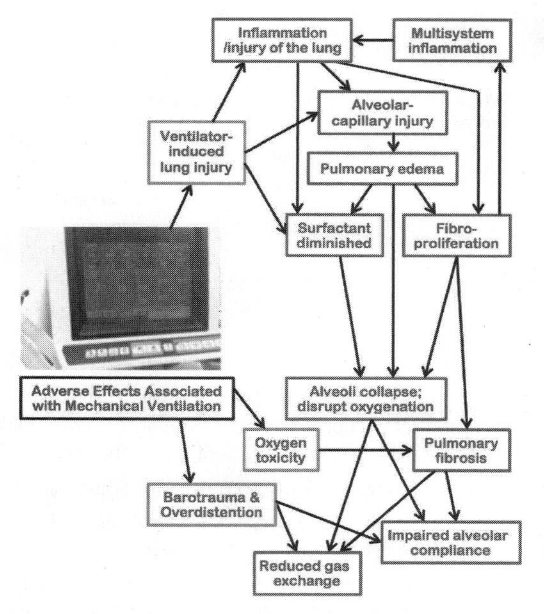

Potential adverse effects of mechanical ventilation.

Concept Check

5. What position helps to reduce risk for the development of ventilator-associated pneumonia?
   A. prone
   B. supine with head of bed at 30 degrees
   C. side-lying
   D. flat in bed

Answer question

Collaborative Interventions (continued)

Collaborative Symptom Management

- Treatment for ARDS primarily involves treating the cause of lung injury (e.g., antibiotics for sepsis). Treatment is otherwise supportive and targets prevention of ICU-related complications.
- Supporting oxygenation and ventilation.
  - o Supplemental oxygen can be used to maintain SpO_2.
  - o Mechanical ventilation is required if the patient is:
    - Hypoxemic despite supplemental oxygen
    - SOB
    - Tachypneic
    - In respiratory acidosis

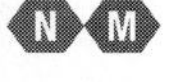

  - o Patients who are refractory to treatment require intubation or noninvasive ventilatory support with bilevel positive airway pressure (BiPAP).

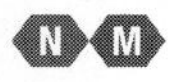

  - o Positive end expiratory pressure (PEEP) can be used to improve oxygenation.

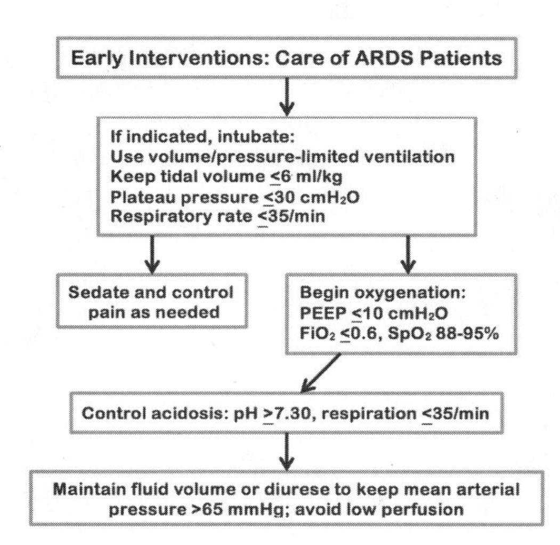

Algorithm for the initial management of ARDS: Clinical trials have provided evidence-based therapeutic goals for a stepwise approach to the early mechanical ventilation, oxygenation, and correction of acidosis and diuresis of critically ill patients with ARDS.

Concept Check

6. Which intervention is the priority for the treatment of a patient with ARDS?

A. Relieve shortness of breath

B. Treat the cause of the injury

C. Reduce metabolic alkalosis

D. Treat tachycardia

Answer question

Collaborative Comfort Care

- Nursing support of a patient on mechanical ventilation is a major factor in the patient's well-being and satisfaction. Ensuring the patient is comfortable and fostering communication are all part of nursing care of a patient on mechanical ventilation.
- N Protect the patient's airway to prevent aspiration and its complications, such as pneumonia
- N Suction, oral and endotracheal, whenever indicated to maintain a patent airway and prevent the buildup of secretions
- N M Support patient comfort with using physical, emotional, social, environmental, and pharmacologic means as indicated to improve the patient's well-being and physiologic stability. Sedation, analgesia, and communication play a heavy role in patients with ARDS.
- N M Collaborate to provide and maintain adequate nutrition via enteral or parenteral means
- N Closely monitor patient condition to identify subtle changes that may rapidly progress and that require alterations in therapy, particularly during procedures and daily care.
- N M Collaborate with team to recognize early when/if life-sustaining care becomes futile, despite excellent treatment. If futile, collaborate with patient and family to transition to compassionate and end of life care to provide a peaceful and dignified death.
- N Cluster care activities to assure frequent rest periods, as these patients have diminished respiratory reserve and may decompensate with minimal activity. Advocate for the patient's rest by collaboratively working with others to orchestrate care.
- N Explore any fear and anxiety that the patient may have. Support patients with their ways of coping with fear and anxiety and in ways that they perceive as helpful to reduce fear and anxiety. Provide explanation of equipment, environment, and interventions when elicited. Coach relaxation when the patient is receptive and it is appropriate.

N **Impact of Turning Patients**

- Blood flow goes to the dependent lung areas.
- When a patient is turned to the side, the lung that is down gets better perfusion.
- If a patient has significant injury to one lung, when turned to that side, gas exchange becomes impaired (e.g., pulse oximeter drops).
- Turning onto the side that has less lung injury allows for better gas exchange.

Additional Respiratory Therapies

With the high mortality rate, treating patients with ALI or ARDS is difficult. Additional therapies can be attempted, but all have shown limited effectiveness:

M **Nitrous Oxide** Nitric oxide is a selective pulmonary vasodilator and is used to enhance gas exchange by increasing SpO_2 and PaO_2.

A significant deterrent in using this treatment is its potential toxicity. It produces methemoglobin which cannot carry oxygen, thereby producing a "functional" anemia.

N M **Positioning** Proning (or lying face down position) may enhance gas exchange by allowing improved ventilation and perfusion to lung areas where blood flow and aeration are best.

N M **Bed Rotational Therapy** In addition to proning, bed rotational therapy techniques can be used.

- Continuous lateral rotational therapy (CLRT) and kinetic therapy (KT):
  - Each rotation is at a different angle.
  - CLRT is less than 30 degrees.
  - KT is more than 40 degrees.
- Patient tolerance may be an issue.
- Turning patients at sharp angles often requires patient sedation.

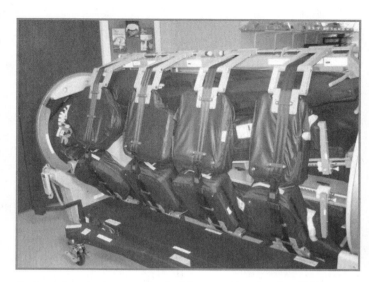

Turning patients is a key part of maintaining normal lung function. Utilizing the prone position with a rotating bed enhances the ability to turn seriously ill patients as needed. Studies continues on how often the patient should be turned. In addition, the prone (versus supine) position appears to have benefits.
Source: Copyright © 2012, NovEx Novice to Expert Learning, LLC

Evidence-Based Practice: Preventing ICU Complications

- N M Venous thromboembolism prophylaxis (e.g., with low molecular weight heparin SQ)
- N M Protocol use to decrease catheter-related infections
- N M Stress ulcer prevention in patients at high risk (e.g., with proton pump inhibitors)
- N Prevention of ventilator-associated pneumonia (e.g., keeping the head of bed at 30–45 degrees to avoid aspiration, mouth care)
- N Pressure ulcer prevention

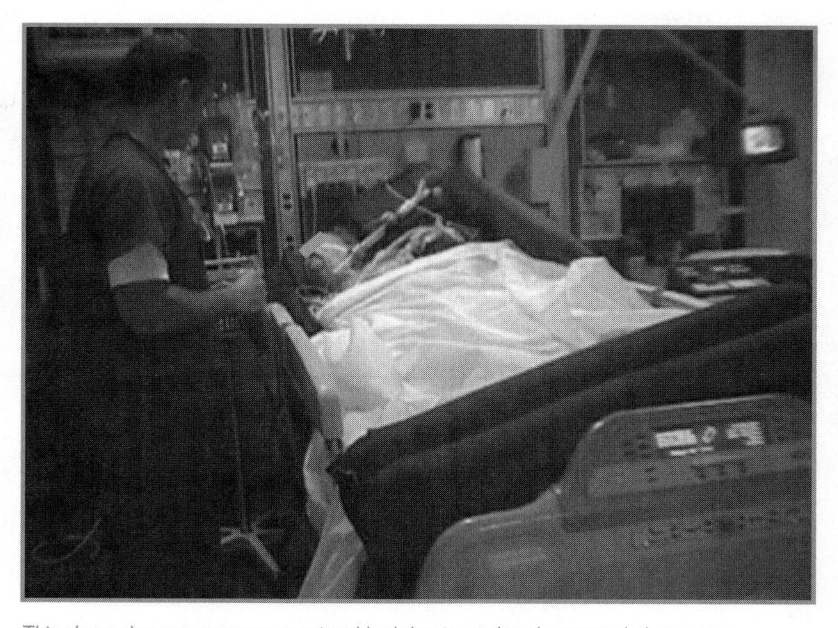

This photo shows a common rotational bed that is used as therapy to help improve ventilation and gas exchange in ALI and ARDS patients.
Source: Copyright © 2012, NovEx Novice to Expert Learning, LLC

Concept Check

7. **Which statement about positioning a patient with ALI or ARDS is true?**

   A. The proning positioning reduces risk of skin complications.

   B. Positioning the less injured lung down can improve perfusion.

   C. Positioning the less injured lung down eliminates the need for mechanical ventilation.

   D. The proning positioning prevents pneumonia in the damaged lung.

Answer question

Summary of Interventions

- Treatment of ALI is focused on:
  1. EBP:
     a. Adequate ventilation volume
     b. Optimal oxygenation
     c. Patient comfort with sedation prn
     d. Nutrition
     e. Communication with the family
  2. Treating the cause of lung injury
  3. Preventing ICU-related complications:
     a. Stress ulcer prophylaxis in patients at high risk
     b. Prevention of ventilator associated pneumonia
     c. DVT prophylaxis
     d. Using protocols to reduce incidence of catheter-related sepsis
     e. Pressure ulcer prevention

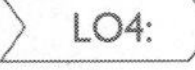

Evaluation of Desired Collaborative Care Outcomes

Evaluation and reassessment should reveal attainment of previously established patient outcomes. In summary:

- Patient's arterial blood gases and oxygen saturations approximate pre-illness level.
- Patient demonstrates normal lactate levels and no signs of cyanosis, mental confusion, or hypoxemia.
- Patient remains infection free.
- Patient's caloric intake matches energy requirements.
- Patient is experiencing less fear and anxiety with support systems and comfort care so that fear and anxiety do not compromise oxygenation.

References

http://www.ncbi.nlm.nih.gov/pubmedhealth/PMH0001164/

http://www.ards.org/learnaboutards/whatisards/brochure/

http://www.lung.org/lung-disease/acute-respiratory-distress-syndrome/

http://www.aafp.org/afp/2002/0501/p1823.html

Rubenfeld, G. D., et al. (2012). Acute Respiratory Distress Syndrome: The Berlin Definition. *JAMA, 307*(23), 2526–2533.

STOP

Go to the online course and complete the NovE-Cases assigned by your instructor for this module.

Learning Outcomes for Chronic Obstructive Pulmonary Disease

When you complete this lesson, you will be able to:

1. Recognize the clinical relevance of chronic obstructive pulmonary disease.
2. Consider the pathophysiology, etiology, risk factors, and clinical presentation of chronic obstructive pulmonary disease that determine the priority patient concerns.
3. Determine the most urgent and important nursing interventions and patient education required in caring for a patient with chronic obstructive pulmonary disease.
4. Evaluate attainment of desired collaborative care outcomes for a patient with chronic obstructive pulmonary disease.

LO1:

What Is Chronic Obstructive Pulmonary Disease?

- Conditions that are grouped as Chronic Obstructive Pulmonary Diseases (COPD) result from progressive lung diseases that cause permanent obstruction of airflow in the lungs. Exposure to pollutants and toxins, particularly from smoking, cause airway damage. The most commonly seen conditions are:
  1. Emphysema
  2. Chronic bronchitis
  3. Bronchiectasis
  4. Asthma, when no longer reversible
- Patients commonly have a combination of these diseases, although one alone can occur.

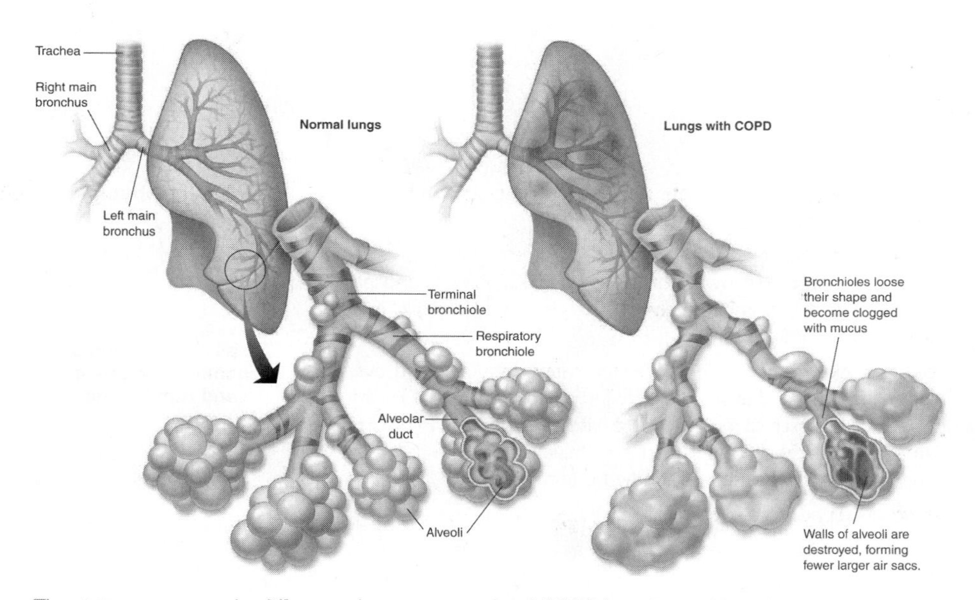

The picture compares the differences between normal and COPD lung tissues. Note the mucous, bronchioles, and alveolar changes that occur in COPD.

LO1:

Clinical Relevance

- COPD is the fourth leading cause of death in the United States and is projected to be the third leading cause of death for both males and females by 2020.
- It affects 10–24 million Americans.
- COPD costs the United States about $50 billion dollars per year.
- COPD is preventable but currently results in severe human suffering from shortness of breath, profound fatigue, severe debility, and eventual heart failure.
- Most of these costs, in suffering and resource use, are avoidable if people stopped smoking.
- Centers for Disease Control and Prevention (2010) reported that almost 20% of American adults smoke and, every day, more than 3,800 teens begin smoking.

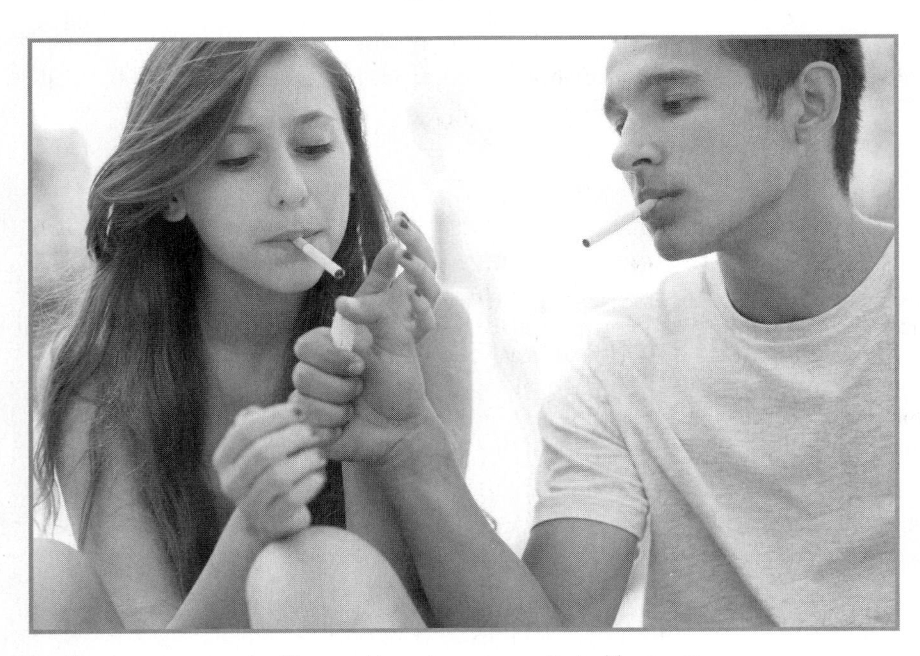

Smoking among teens under 18 years old remains a community health concern.
Source: Edyta Pawlowska/Fotolia

LO2:

Pathophysiology

- COPD develops when airflow through the lungs becomes progressively limited.
- Harmful irritants, especially and typically cigarette smoking, cause inflammation with narrowing of the bronchiolar lumens and parenchymal destruction in the alveoli with decreased alveolar elasticity and attachments.
- Toxic particles initiate the body's inflammatory response and, over many years, these changes worsen. Toxic particles attract inflammatory cells, which stimulate the release of proteases. Proteases damage alveolar walls and bronchiolar structures, which then collapse. Fibrous tissue is subsequently deposited.
- Some alveoli become hyperinflated while others are destroyed.
- Bronchial airway lumens narrow due to a number of inflammatory effects:
  1. Damage to the cilia, which interferes with clearance of mucous
  2. Damage to the endothelium (the cellular lining of the bronchial lumens)
  3. Presence of inflammatory cells in the bronchial walls
  4. Remodeling of the bronchial walls, which includes hyperplasia of smooth muscle and deposition of fibrous tissue (scarring)

Pathophysiology: Limited Airflow in COPD

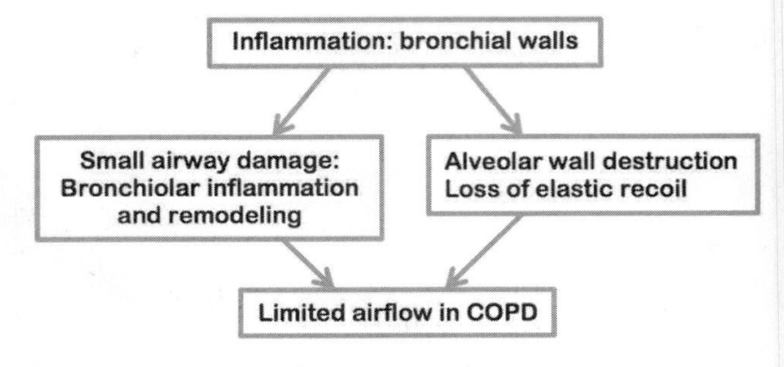

This diagram shows the relationship between inflammation and airflow limitation.
Source: Copyright © 2012, NovEx Novice to Expert Learning, LLC.

- Reduced movement of air is exacerbated by the loss of elasticity of the alveoli, so that air is increasingly trapped. Trapped air stretches and enlarges the alveoli. All increase the work of breathing and interfere with exhalation.
- Normally, during exhalation the alveoli forcefully deflate, moving air out. Destruction of alveolar tissue diminishes this elastic recoil, necessitating the use of other muscles.
- The damaging effects of chronic exposure to toxins and the resulting inflammation result in the following conditions. Most patients have a combination of these conditions rather than just one.
  - o Emphysema
  - o Chronic bronchitis
  - o Asthma
  - o Bronchiectasis

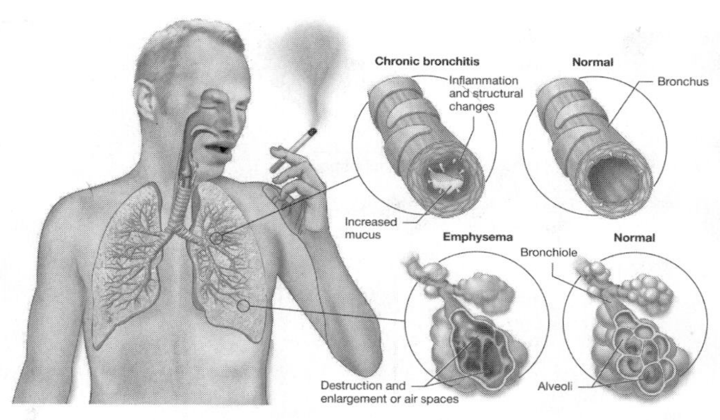

COPD is usually a combination of conditions that include bronchitis and emphysema.

Emphysema

- In emphysema, enlargement of the distal airspaces occurs through destruction of the walls between the alveoli.
- Normally there is a balance between proteases and antiproteases in tissue. It is thought that irritants such as smoke or genetic factors such as alpha1-antitrypsin deficiency results in an increase in the proteases, creating an imbalance.
- This promotes destruction of alveolar tissue, causing the walls between alveoli to be damaged and destroyed. The alveolar size becomes larger and the number of alveoli becomes smaller (see diagram), causing problems with gas exchange.
- Capillary beds lining the alveoli are also destroyed in the process, decreasing the surface area where gas can be exchanged between the capillaries and the air in the alveoli.
- The changes that occur in emphysema are irreversible.

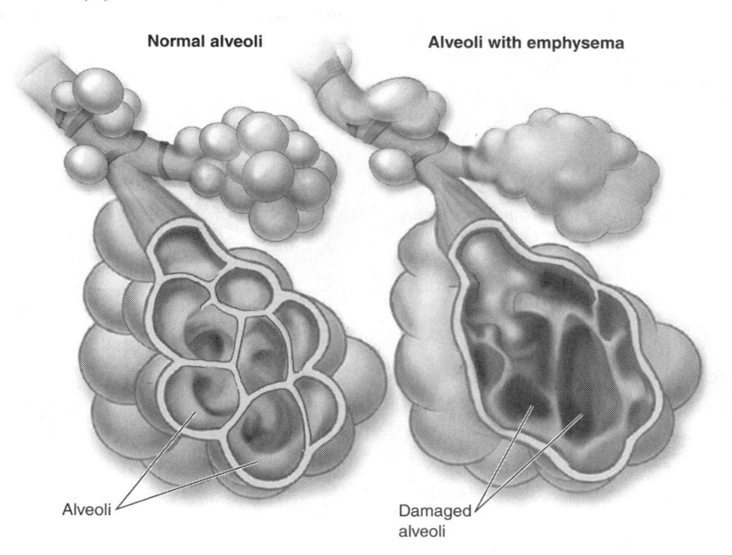

Alveolar and capillary walls breakdown in emphysema, resulting in impairment of gas exchange.

Concept Check

1. **Which situation occurs as part of emphysema?**
   A. The number of alveoli increases.
   B. Alveolar capillary beds are destroyed.
   C. There is narrowing of the bronchial lumen.
   D. Mucous production is remarkably increased.

Answer question

Chronic Bronchitis

- Chronic bronchitis is defined as a chronic cough for more than three consecutive months for two consecutive years.
- Irritants, such as tobacco smoke, cause inflammation in the bronchioles with edema, mucous overproduction, hyperplasia of the muscle walls, mucous gland enlargement, damage to the cilia, vasodilatation, bronchospasm, and congestion. Together these result in narrowing of the bronchial lumen and interference with air movement.
- Bronchitis primarily affects the airways, rather than the alveoli as in emphysema.

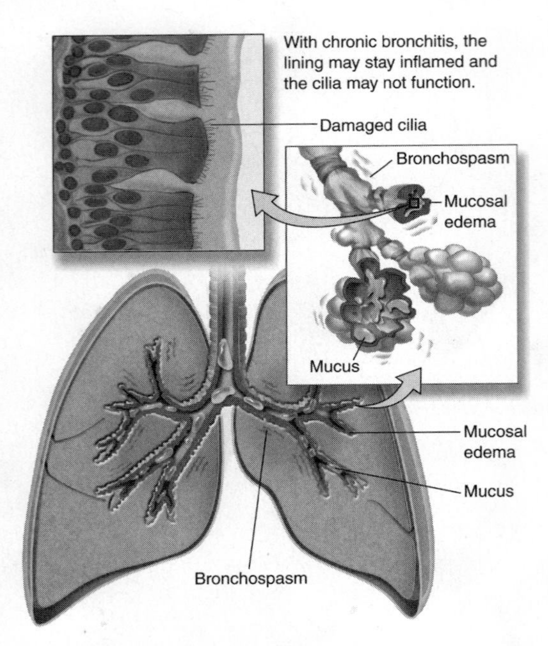

Pathophysiological changes in chronic bronchitis.

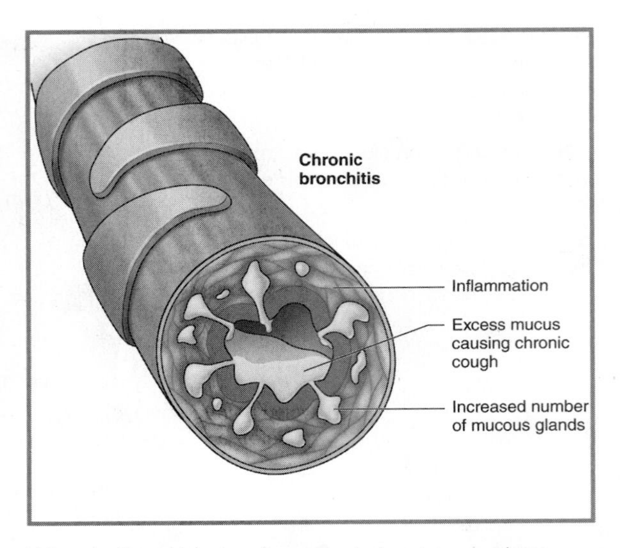

When the bronchial tubes that carry air deep into your lungs become inflamed, the inner lining swells and grows thicker, narrowing the breathing passages. These irritated membranes also secrete extra mucus, which coats and sometimes clogs the small airways. Coughing spells are the body's way of trying to clear out these secretions for easier breathing.

Concept Check

2. Which patient meets the criteria for chronic bronchitis?

A. A patient who has a 25 pack year smoking history.

B. A patient who has complained of shortness of breath for longer than 1 year.

C. A patient who has coughed for over 3 months in 2 consecutive years.

D. A patient who has been dependent on oxygen for at least a month of each of the last 4 years.

Answer question

Pathophysiology (continued)

Bronchiectasis

- Bronchiectasis is dilation of bronchioles caused by the destruction of the elastic tissue and muscles of the bronchioles by proteases released with inflammation. Mucous production is increased and tends to be thick. Despite being dilated, the bronchioles collapse easily, especially during exhalation when intrathoracic pressures increase.
- Bronchiectasis causes permanent damage to the lungs. It primarily affects air movement or ventilation.
- These patients are also susceptible to frequent bacterial infections. The reason is not clearly understood but may be related to endothelial (cells lining the airways) damage, damage to the cilia, and neutrophil dysfunction.

Concept Check

3. Which pathophysiology is associated with bronchiectasis?

A. Dilation of bronchioles

B. Reduced production of mucus

C. Airway collapse that occurs during inhalation

D. Obstruction caused by overgrowth of cilia

Answer question

Asthma

- Asthma is the reversible component of COPD. Airway inflammation causes contraction of the smooth muscles lining the bronchial walls (bronchoconstriction and bronchospasm), which is reversible with bronchodilators.

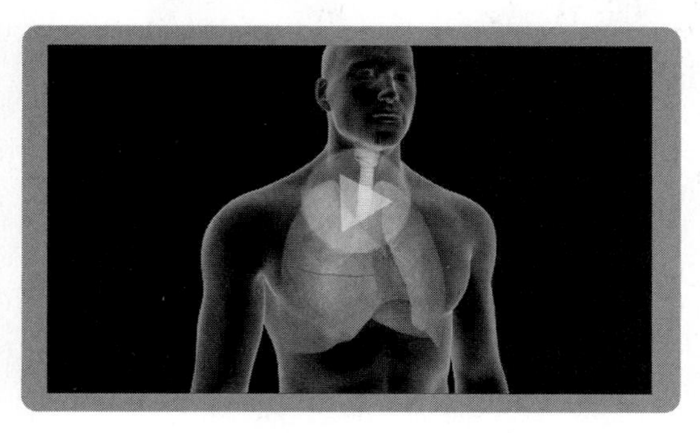

This animation provides an overview of asthma, which inflames and narrows the airways. The symptoms and triggers of asthma and medications are described.

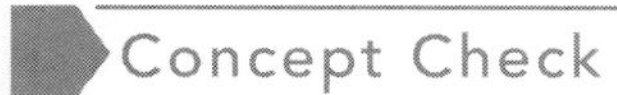

4. **Changes associated with which component of chronic obstructive pulmonary disease (COPD) are reversible?**
   A. Bronchiectasis
   B. Asthma
   C. Emphysema
   D. Chronic bronchitis

Answer question

Compensatory Mechanisms in COPD

- One may anticipate that the airway obstruction and alveolar damage would produce hypoxemia (lower PaO_2), hypercapnia (elevated $PaCO_2$) and acidosis (decreased pH). However, compensatory mechanisms initially keep these values within normal range.
- Patients compensate for airway obstruction, decreased elasticity and recoil of the lungs, and compromised gas exchange in the damaged alveoli through several mechanisms.
  1. Decreasing oxygen needs by decreasing activity.
  2. Increasing respiratory drive which is mediated by chemoreceptors in the brain and arteries that detect changes in pH and PaO_2.

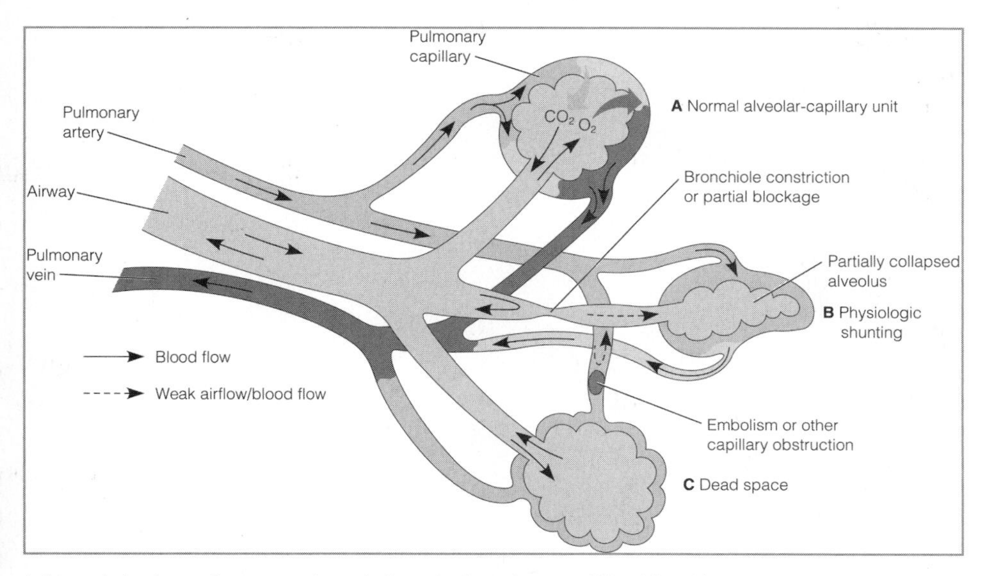

A: Normal alveolar-capillary unit with an ideal match of ventilation and blood flow. Maximum gas exchange occurs between alveolus and blood. B: Physiologic shunting: adequate perfusion but inadequate ventilation. C: Dead space: adequate ventilation but inadequate perfusion. In the latter two cases, gas exchange is impaired.

Pathophysiology (continued)

COPD Respiratory Drive

Chemoreceptors detect even small changes in pH and PaO_2. The following changes result to compensate for the worsening airflow obstruction:

1. Increasing respiratory rate
2. Forced exhalation using intercostal muscles and diaphragm
3. Use of accessory muscles, including neck and abdominal muscles, to assist exhalation
4. Pursed lip breathing, which can help prevent the collapse of the bronchioles by increasing the pressure in the airways during exhalation

Eventually, as COPD worsens, when the patient is no longer able to compensate, the PaO_2 drops and/or $PaCO_2$ increases.

An increase in $PaCO_2$ is expected to cause a drop in pH. However, when these changes occur slowly, over time, the kidneys compensate by excreting hydrogen to keep the pH near normal. Serum bicarbonate (left in the blood when hydrogen splits from it to be excreted) is reabsorbed.

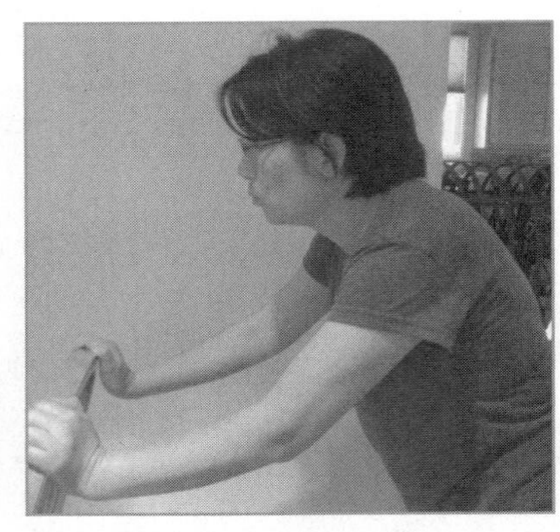

This patient shows how bending forward helps her breathe more easily during activity, but also at rest. Note that she keeps her back straight and leans forward at the waist, while leaning on a table or a chair. Pursed-lip breathing often helps. It involves inhaling through the nose but exhaling by mouth while almost closing the lips (pursing). Inhalation takes about 4 seconds and exhalation takes about 6–8 seconds.
Source: Copyright © 2012, NovEx Novice to Expert Learning, LLC

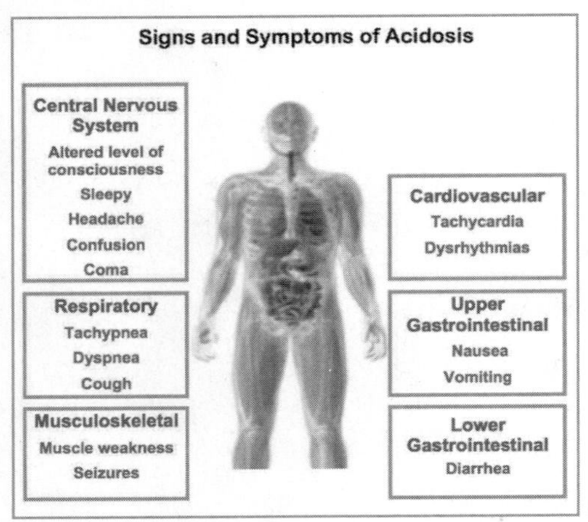

Respiratory acidosis leads to multisystem symptoms in COPD patients with advanced disease.
Source: Copyright © 2012, NovEx Novice to Expert Learning, LLC

Acute Exacerbation COPD

- Anything that worsens airway inflammation can lead to COPD exacerbation. Inflammation may increase due to infection (either bacterial or viral) or exposure to irritants (e.g., smoke). The airway lumen further narrows and mucous production increases.
- Exacerbations can lead to an acute increase in $PaCO_2$ and drop in PaO_2 if the patient can not compensate any further or quickly enough. The acute rise of $PaCO_2$ usually results in a drop in pH. A high $PaCO_2$ and low pH is therefore indicative of an acute change in respiratory status.
- Treatment with oxygen helps to correct the PaO_2 but must be used with caution in patients with chronic hypercapnia (high $PaCO_2$). Oxygen in some hypercapnic patients can suppress their respiratory drive and lead to further deterioration.

Pulmonary Hypertension in COPD

- As the arterioles and capillaries in the pulmonary vascular beds become damaged, narrowed, blocked, or destroyed, blood flow is slowed, blood backs up, and the pressure rises in the pulmonary arteries. This is called pulmonary hypertension.
- COPD induces pulmonary hypertension in two ways:
  1. Hypoxemia causes vasoconstriction that then further increases arteriolar narrowing (resistance to blood flow)
  2. Obliteration of the arteriolar and capillary vessels forces the same amount of blood to flow through fewer blood vessels
- The high pressures strain the right ventricle (RV) because it must pump against high pressures. The RV has limited capability to pump harder for an extended time without failing.

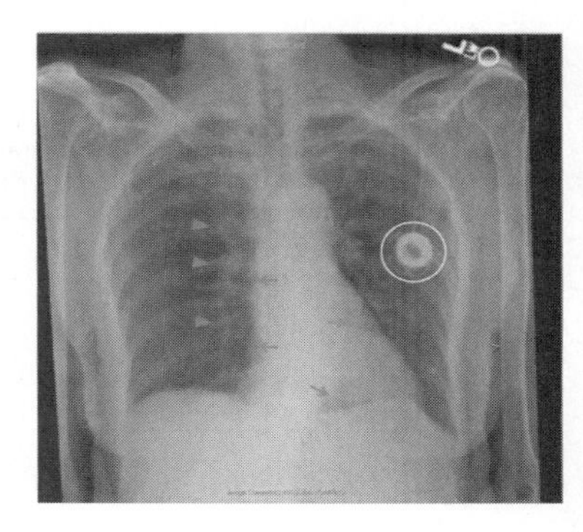

This x-ray provides a clear presentation of pulmonary hypertension and cor pulmonale (right-sided heart failure due to COPD). Note the hyperextended lung fields. The blue arrows highlight the congested, widened pulmonary vessels seen in pulmonary hypertension and the red arrows mark the outline of the right heart failure. A port-a-cath for a central line is encircled in yellow.
Source: Courtesy of Erick Kyriakidis

Cor Pulmonale

- Cor pulmonale or right-sided heart failure is often seen in COPD patients due to pulmonary hypertension. When strain is placed on the right ventricle for a long period of time, the high pressure against which the right heart must pump causes it to fail.

LO2:

Causes and Risk Factors

- Smoking is the largest risk factor for the development of COPD. Risk of developing emphysema is six times higher in smokers. Risk increases with the amount of exposure over a lifetime. The amount is sometimes quantified as pack years (packs per day × number of years smoking).
- Other inhaled irritants or pollution can increase the risk of developing COPD.
- Emphysema can be caused by genetic factors (e.g., alpha-1 antitrypsin deficiency). About 100,000 patients in the United States have this condition. These patients usually have an earlier onset (between 20–50 years old), minimal smoking history, family history of lung disease, and lower lobe prominent emphysema.

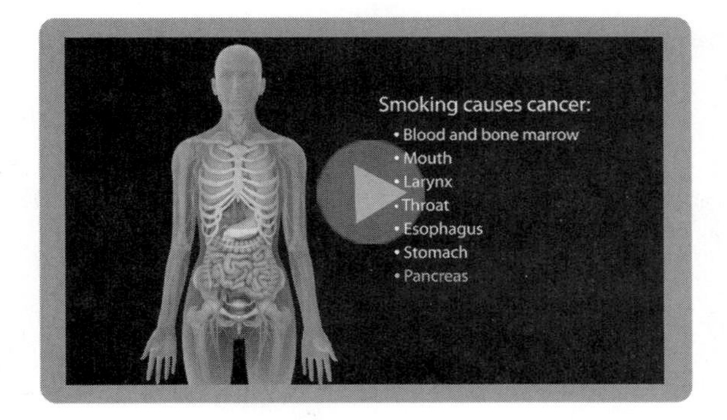

This video teaches how smoking causes multiple types of COPD. Furthermore, it examines numerous health issues that are important for teaching your COPD patients and the community about how to avoid the deadly effects of smoking.
Source: © 2013 Nucleus Medical Media, All rights reserved

Concept Check

5. A patient diagnosed with chronic obstructive pulmonary disease reports smoking two packs of cigarettes a day for the past 20 years. The nurse would record this patient's smoking history as:
   A. 10 pack years
   B. 20 pack years
   C. 30 pack years
   D. 40 pack years

Answer question

Assessment Findings

- Patients with mild COPD may not have any symptoms.
- Because few COPD patients have only bronchitis or emphysema, for instance, they tend to present with overlapping signs and symptoms.
- As the disease progresses patients sometimes decrease their activity levels to match their decreasing lung capacity.
- Common and key symptoms include chronic coughing with a large amount of sputum and dyspnea with activity. The cough is often referred to as "smoker's cough."
- Wheezing and prolonged expiration (more than 5 sec) may be present.
- Patients with more advanced disease may have dyspnea *at rest*, barrel chest, cyanosis, hypoxemia, tachycardia, weight loss, and malnutrition (see photo).
- Patients may lean forward supporting their upper body with hands on their knees or on the edge of the bed to decrease the effort necessary for breathing (see photo).
- Other patients breathe with pursed lips. This causes increased pressure in the airways to prevent collapse.
- Patients may have recurrent pulmonary infections.
- Symptoms of right heart failure may be present and should raise concern: leg edema, ascites, hepatomegaly, and jugular venous distension.

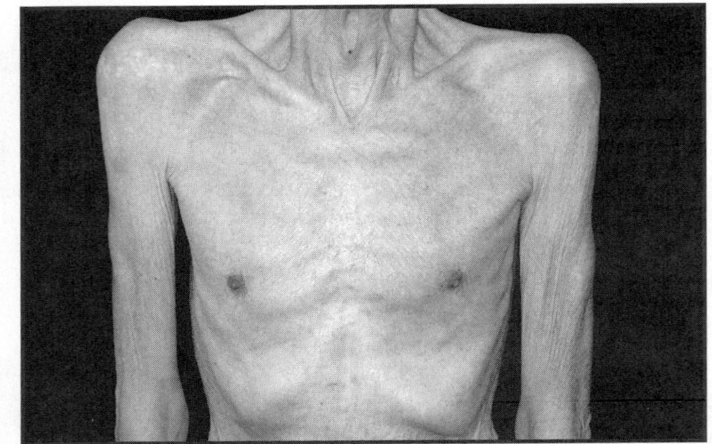

Clearly visible on this patient with COPD is the malnutrition and barrel chest.
Source: Dr. P. Marazzi/Science Source

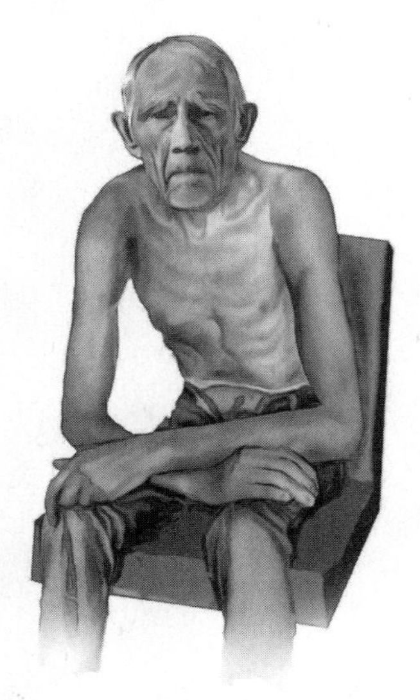

This illustration shows the common physical presentations of persons with chronic bronchitis and/or with emphysema. The barrel chest, malnutrition, fatigue, and leaning forward while breathing are typical. Most cases (80%) of COPD are due to a mixture of the two causes.

Confounding Findings from Comorbid Conditions Associated with COPD

1. **Cor pulmonale:** This is a complication caused by emphysema and presents with signs and symptoms of right heart failure and an enlarged right ventricle.
2. **Pulmonary hypertension:** An enlarged right ventricle, narrowing of the pulmonary artery, and constricted blood vessel that supply less oxygen to the body characterizes this comorbid condition.
3. **Bacterial pneumonia:** With a weakened immune system, COPD patients commonly have pneumonia, especially streptococcal, as a complication and present with cough, fever, and lung infiltrate(s).
4. **Congestive heart failure:** COPD is commonly associated with heart failure. Heart failure causes fluid overload with lower body edema and severe SOB, seen frequently in advanced stages of COPD.
5. **Pneumothorax:** An injury or weakness in lung structure allows air to escape from the lung into the chest cavity and collapses the lung, occurring more frequently with COPD because.
6. **Bronchiectasis:** Manifestations include a chronic cough with sputum production, inflammation, and infection. It may exist alone or in combination with COPD.
7. **Atelectasis:** A partial or total airway blockage results in collapse of a lung area. People with underlying lung disease are at greater risk.
8. **GERD:** The incidence is higher in COPD and doubles the risk of COPD exacerbations.
9. **Lung cancer:** Since lung cancer and COPD are both caused by smoking, it is not surprising that both conditions frequently co-exist.
10. **Heart disease:** COPD and heart disease are both strongly related to smoking and both conditions cause and are, partly, caused by decreased oxygen supply.

http://copd.about.com/od/complicationsofcopd/tp/10-Comorbid-Conditions-Associated-With-Copd.htm

LO2:

Diagnostics

- A diagnosis of COPD requires measurement of expiratory airflow limitation on pulmonary function tests (PFTs). To perform a key PFT test, called a FEV1 (forced expiratory volume in 1 second), patients are asked to take their deepest breath and exhale as fast and as completely as possible into a spirometer.
- FEV1 is the amount of air exhaled in the first second. FVC (forced vital capacity) is the total amount of air exhaled.
- The Global Initiative for Obstructive Lung Disease (GOLD) grading system defines COPD by severity. FEV1 or the GOLD spirometric criteria for COPD* are:

Stages of Severity of COPD by Global Initiative for Chronic Obstructive Lung Disease		
Stage	**FEV1: % of predicted**	**Characteristics**
Mild	≥ 80%	± Chronic symptoms (e.g., cough, sputum)
Moderate	< 80%	± Chronic cough, sputum, shortness of breath (SOB)
Severe	< 50%	Chronic cough, sputum, SOB, exacerbations
Very Severe	< 30% or <50% + respiratory failure	Severe limitations, life-threatening exacerbations, ± Cor pulmonale. If respiratory failure: PaO_2 <60 mmHg± $PaCO_2$ >50% mmHg

Pulmonary Function Tests

- The PFT results in COPD are shown below in a flow volume curve. The gold curve is normal and the pink and blue curves are obstructive conditions, showing the reduction in FVC and decrease in expiratory flow rate.
- FEV1 is a predictor of mortality and is used to assess the patient's clinical course and responsiveness to treatments.
- Other pulmonary function tests used to determine abnormalities include total lung capacity (TLC), residual volume (RV), and functional residual capacity (FRC). Abnormal increases in these PFTs are typically due to lung hyperinflation and air trapping.

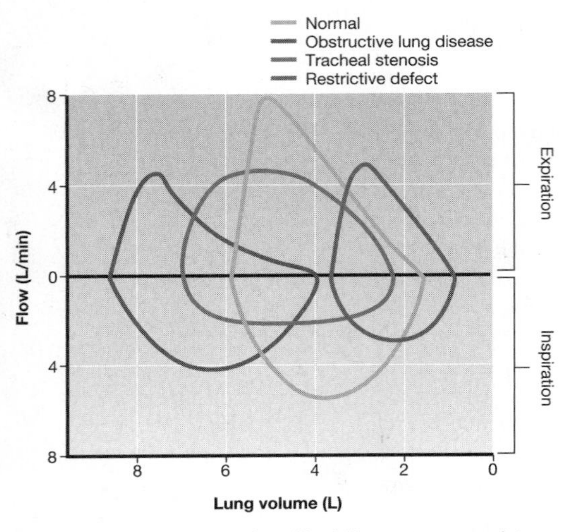

Distinctive patterns are produced by different airway conditions.

Additional Diagnostic Tests for COPD

- A chest x-ray may show overdistended lungs and flattened diaphragm as illustrated below. It may also show cardiac enlargement as the heart must increasingly work harder to pump blood forward against rising lung pressures.

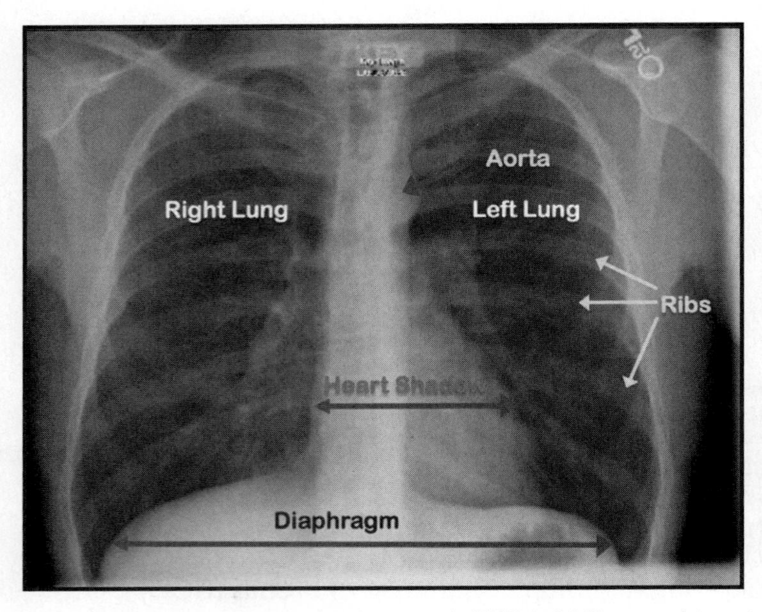

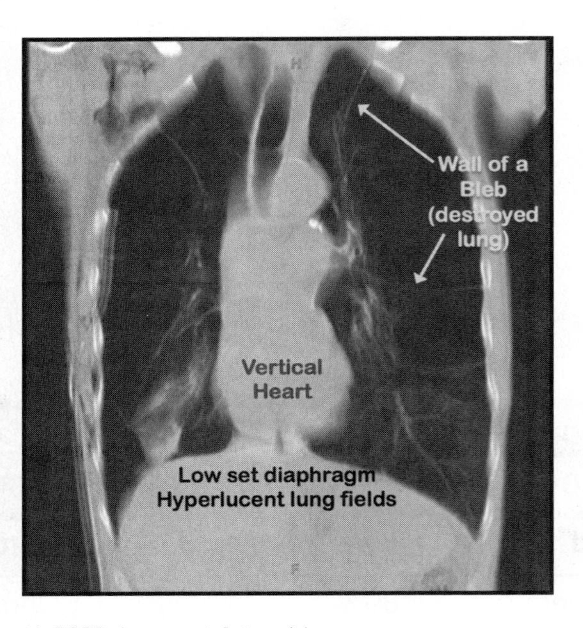

The normal chest x-ray (left) is compared to one with COPD (right). The x-ray of the patient with COPD shows overinflation of the lungs with the simultaneous pushing down (flattening) of the diaphragm.
Source: Courtesy of Erick Kyriakidis

- Arterial blood gases (ABGs) may show increased $PaCO_2$ and low PaO_2 in severe stages of COPD. Some COPD patients have a chronically elevated $PaCO_2$ (over 45 mmHg), but a normal pH (7.35–7.45) due to renal compensation with HCO_3. However, a medical emergency exists if a patient has an elevated $PaCO_2$ with a low pH. This indicates an acute ventilation problem with no time to compensate for a low pH. In this situation, a repeat blood gas should be obtained after treatment to ensure therapy has improved the pH and the $PaCO_2$.
- A chest CT may be helpful in assessing patients for lung transplantation or lung volume reduction surgery. A chest CT can also be helpful at refining a diagnosis, e.g., bronchial dilation in bronchiectasis or emphysema.

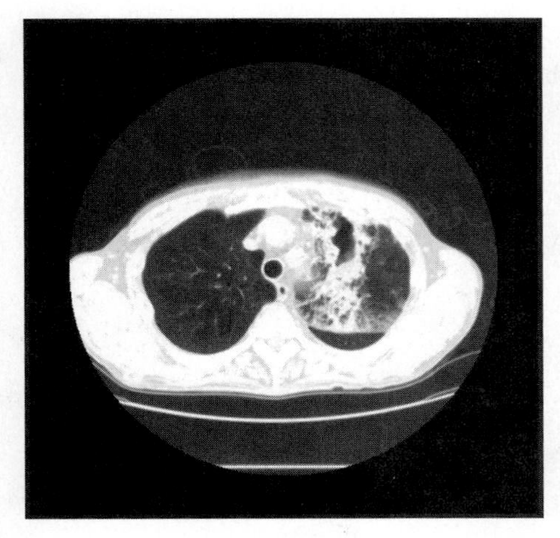

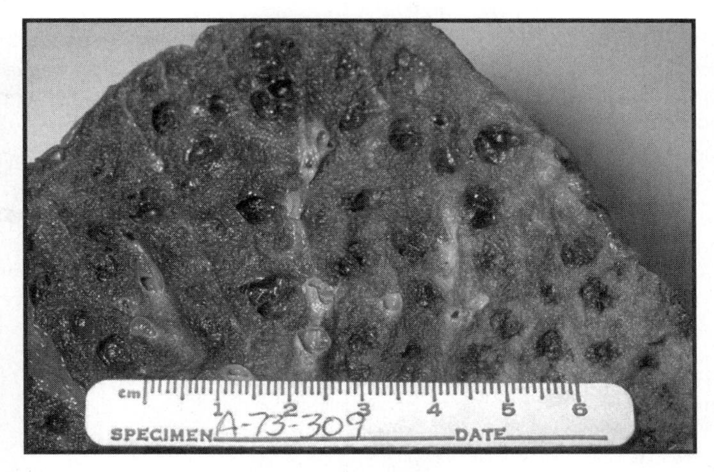

Centrilobular emphysema commonly results from smoking. The dark circular areas in both photos are irreversibly destroyed alveoli in the upper lung areas. CT scan seen on the left; Lung specimen on the right. An abscess is seen in the CT scan (large white area), likely from infection.
Sources: (*left*) Du Cane Medical Imaging Ltd./Science Source; (*right*) CDC/Dr. Edwin P. Ewing, Jr.

Priority Patient Concerns and Desired Collaborative Care Outcomes

Prior to caring for patients with COPD, it is important to prioritize the patient's concerns that must guide the nursing care plan and interventions. Care for the patient is ordered and organized in accordance with the patient's priority and urgent needs. Desired collaborative care outcomes in patients with COPD typically include:

1. Patient will report and demonstrate that respiratory effort is at usual pre-exacerbation level.
2. Pulmonary toilet will result in clearing of auscultated lung sounds.
3. Oxygen saturation values will return to patient normal levels.
4. Patient will maintain body weight appropriate for height. No additional muscle wasting will be evident.
5. Patient will identify early cues of anxiety and will verbalize methods of anxiety control. Behavioral manifestations of anxiety are absent.
6. Patient will tolerate pre-exacerbation level of activity.
7. Patient will report interest in social activities.
8. Patient will expectorate secretions effectively.

Considering these important care outcomes, prepare a list of the major 3–6 priority patient concerns or nursing diagnoses for patients with COPD. Be prepared to participate in a discussion of this list and/or to submit them as an assignment, as determined by your faculty. Resources you may find helpful in this assignment can include this lesson, the references, resources on nursing care plans, and standard nursing diagnoses manuals.

LO3:

Collaborative Interventions

Evidence-Based Practice

Evidence-based practice (EBP) for COPD is limited due to the irreversible nature of the condition. Smoking cessation and oxygen therapy to reduce pulmonary hypertension and prolong life are among the few EBP guidelines for COPD.

COPD Management

The goals of COPD treatment, outlined by GOLD guidelines, involve:

1. Symptom relief as an important focus:
   a. Smoking cessation remains the most important modality in risk reduction for treatment of COPD (EBP).
   b. Oxygen therapy (discussed in more detail below)
   c. Medications: None of the existing medications for COPD have been shown to improve the long-term decline in lung function. Medications are primarily used to control symptoms, improve function, and reduce acute exacerbations.

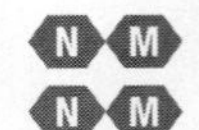

2. Improve pulmonary function: Treat the reversible part of the disease with bronchodilators.
3. Exacerbation prevention: Decrease the frequency and the severity of acute exacerbations with vaccinations (flu and pneumonia) and early treatment of infections. Proper nutrition is important.
4. Improve quality of life with: physical therapy, oxygen therapy, smoking cessation classes or support, and pulmonary rehabilitation.
5. Slow the progression of complications: oxygen therapy and rapid treatment of exacerbations. Oxygen therapy helps to reduce pulmonary hypertension.

Concept Check

6. A patient has just been diagnosed with mild chronic obstructive pulmonary disease. What is the most important information the nurse can provide?

A. How to use metered dose inhalers
B. Techniques of smoking cessation
C. Use of pulmonary function tests
D. Obesity management information

Answer question

Oxygen Therapy (EBP)

- A good guide for oxygen therapy is to keep the PaO_2 more than 55 mmHg or a pulse oximeter reading more than 93%.
- Maintaining these values helps reduce pulmonary hypertension and workload on the right heart. This is one of the only techniques that might actually improve survival rates.
- Oxygen therapy should be used with caution in patients who have chronic CO_2 retention ($PaCO_2$ levels that are elevated, but have normal pH values). The reason for this is a concern over interfering with the hypoxemic drive to breath, which relies on a lower PaO_2 level. If oxygen is given to patients with chronic CO_2 elevation, make sure to check the patient for an adverse response, i.e., a decrease in level of consciousness (a symptom of hypercapnia).
- A capnogram can be used as well, and if the $PetCO_2$ increases after oxygen is given, a fall in the pH may have occurred.
- A blood gas should be obtained if the $PetCO_2$ rises by 5–10 mmHg. If the $PaCO_2$ rises and the pH falls after oxygen therapy is given, the oxygen therapy should be reduced, or the patient may need to be placed on noninvasive positive pressure ventilation (NPPV) or intubated.

Collaborative Symptom Management and Comfort Care

COPD Pharmocologic Management: Chronic

- Short-acting bronchodilators: May be used alone or in combination, usually on an as needed basis. They include:
  - o Beta agonist (e.g., albuterol)
  - o Anticholinergic (e.g., ipratropium bromide)
- Long-acting bronchodilators are usually added if short-acting inhalers do not adequately help symptoms. They include:
  - o Beta agonists (e.g., salmeterol)
  - o Anticholinergics
- Inhaled glucocorticoids may be used if the patient has frequent COPD.

Pulmonary Hygiene

The following treatments may be helpful in a subgroup of patients who have trouble clearing their own secretions. However, there is not yet evidence that these interventions are effective:

1. Acapella is a therapeutic device for managing lung congestion. Acapella administers pressure and vibration, enabling patients to clear their congested lungs and airways.
2. Chest physiotherapy is a technique in which percussion is employed to help mobilize secretions, enabling easier clearing of secretions.
3. Vest therapy involves a vest that is worn and provides oscillation therapy to the chest, allowing mobilization of secretions and easier clearance of secretions.

COPD Acute Management

- Administer O_2 for SpO_2 less than or equal to 92%.
- If patient already has home oxygen, consider noninvasive positive pressure ventilation or intubation in patients with severe respiratory distress (i.e., labored breathing, use of accessory muscles, and altered mental status) who are not responding to oxygen therapy.
- Treat with inhaled short-acting beta 2 agonists (albuterol) and anticholinergics (e.g., ipratropium bromide).
- Systemic corticosteroids oral or IV
- Consider antibiotics for patients with moderate to severe exacerbation and purulent sputum production.

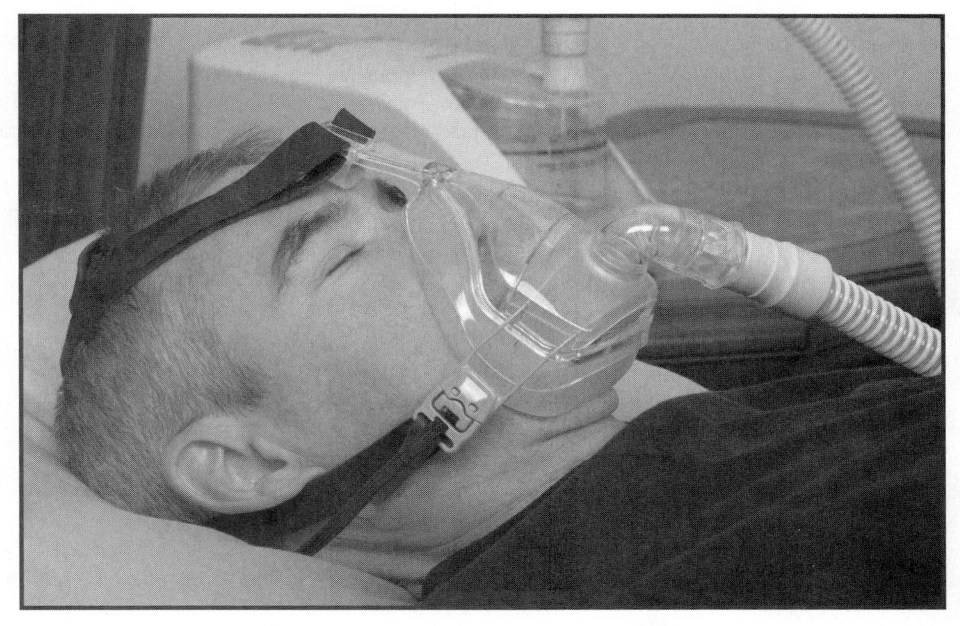

NPPV is an effective method to decrease mortality, intubation rates, and duration of hospital stay in severe exacerbations of COPD, among other conditions, and as a bridge to extubation in COPD patients.
Source: BVDC/Fotolia

Support and Comfort Care

Since COPD is a chronic condition, nurses and health care workers need to first find out what the patient's own experiential wisdom and coping strategies are, and discuss these with patients in relation to individual concerns and usual coping strategies. For example, if the patient's main concern is stigma, or visibility of illness, then coaching should address how the patient usually manages his or her concern over being stigmatized by their illness. Supportive and "helpful" coaching is aligned with the patient's own preferred ways of coping.

- Assess rate, depth, and ease of respirations at each patient encounter.
  - o Patients with COPD have little respiratory reserve and can decompensate rapidly.
  - o Be prepared to intervene quickly if changes occur.
  - o Remain cognizant that COPD respiratory drive may decrease with too much oxygen.
- Support patient's use of and/or educate about respiratory techniques. These techniques are often discovered by patients as part of their own coping with and control of their disease. Exploring the patient's own learning and effective self-management techniques supports the patient's sense of control over and coping with their disease. Techniques can include:
  - o Pursed lip breathing: increases expiratory pressure that keeps the airways open longer and reduces air trapping in collapsed alveoli.
  - o Diaphragmatic breathing: helps the patient learn to slow and control respiratory effort.
  - o Othopneic breathing positions, which are positions that improve breathing: The tripod or forward leaning position helps to increase chest expansion and relax chest muscles, thereby supporting ventilation.
- Provide hydration and humidification.
  - o Encourage at least 2 liters of fluid per day as tolerated by the patient's cardiac condition to help thin secretions for easier expectoration.
  - o Encourage use of a vaporizer or humidifier to moisten environmental air and helps to prevent uncomfortable drying of mucous membranes.

- N Provide high-calorie, high-protein foods that are easy to eat.
  - o Eating expends a great deal of energy in the dyspneic patient.
  - o Divide meals into 6 to 8 small meals throughout the day to improve meal tolerance before becoming too tired to consume sufficient calories.
  - o Large meals fill the stomach and increase pressure on the diaphragm, making respiration more difficult.
  - o Reduce or separate anxiety-producing or energy-consuming events (e.g., bathing) surrounding mealtimes which may overstress the patient's respiratory capacity and shift energy demands on breathing instead of eating. Separating mealtimes encourages better intake and more patient comfort.
- N Help patient identify factors (e.g., air hunger) that elicit anxiety or worry and discuss how the patient copes with anxiety producing events and worry:
  - o Air hunger is extremely frightening. Having a plan to avoid these occurrences and methods to regain respiratory control help to reassure the patient.
  - o Teach relaxation techniques to decrease stress and anxiety and to provide the patient with options to regain a sense of control.
- N Help patient identify a desirable level of activity and methods to attain that level.
  - o Collaborate with patient on a mild exercise plan to identify pleasurable activities that do not require physical expenditure.
  - o Encourage the patient to be as active and involved as possible to reduce anxiety and to slow physical decline.
  - o Activity goals should reflect the patient's interests and desires.
  - o Assist with dyspnea during mild exercise can increase exercise tolerance in order to avoid muscle loss and weakness.
  - o Encourage activities that do not require physical exertion and can provide engagement, diversion, and relaxation as well as comfort.
- N Monitor for any signs of infection, including changes in quality and quantity of pulmonary secretions, pain, fever, or changes in mentation.
  - o Infection can easily occur in COPD, with very rapid deterioration. Patients with COPD have difficulty recovering from severe infection.
  - o Teach patient and family to be alert for subtle signs of infection, seek health care advice early, and comply with treatment regimens to reduce the severity of infection.
  - o Avoid exposure to persons with a cold or fever.

Patient Education

- Educate patients on the proper use of inhalers is critical. There are many different types of inhalers. Educate patients on the use of the specific one(s) they use.
- Use long-acting beta agonist and steroid inhalers as directed.
- Use rescue beta agonist inhaler as needed for shortness of breath.
- Do aerobic exercise such as walking, biking, or swimming for 30 minutes daily at 80% of maximal heart rate (220 − age) × 0.8.
- Stop smoking. Assist patient to locate program or resource of choice.
- Use oxygen as prescribed.

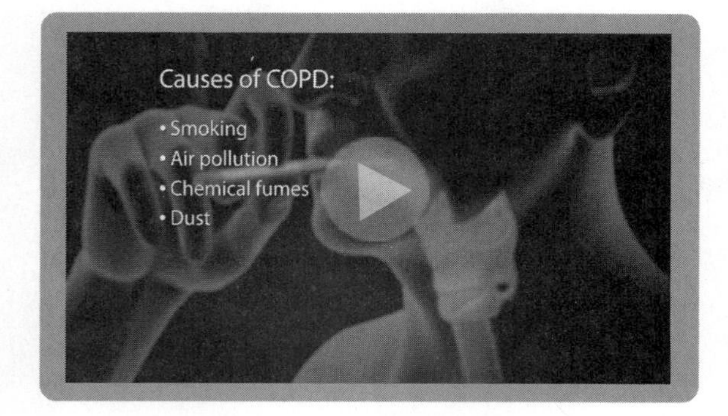

This animation shows the effect of smoking on alveolar destruction. Some aspects of COPD are not reversible (emphysema); however, smoking cessation, secretion management, exercise rehabilitation, and bronchodilator therapy can improve the quality of life of COPD patients.

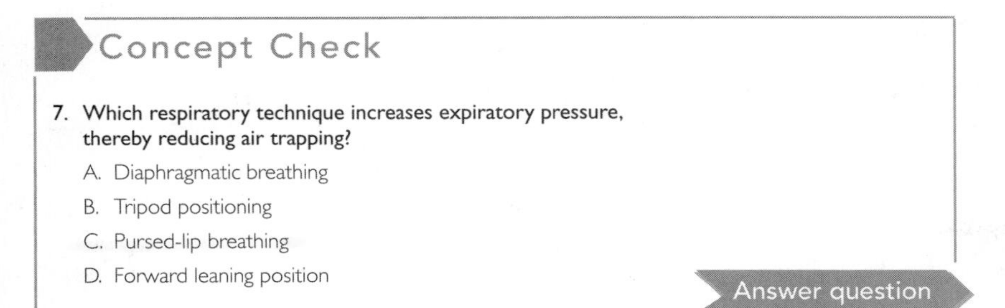

Concept Check

7. Which respiratory technique increases expiratory pressure, thereby reducing air trapping?
   A. Diaphragmatic breathing
   B. Tripod positioning
   C. Pursed-lip breathing
   D. Forward leaning position

Answer question

- Take influenza and pneumonia vaccines.
- Call primary health care provider at the first sign of an infection or exacerbation.
- Join a pulmonary rehabilitation program.
- Optimize treatment of any comorbid conditions such as sleep apnea, CHF, renal failure, sepsis, obesity, malnutrition, and diabetes.
- Advanced directives and palliative care should be discussed if respiratory failure occurs and/or intubation is needed.

Summary of Interventions

1. For treatment of acute COPD exacerbations:
   a. Administer oxygen for SpO_2 less than or equal to 92%.
   b. Bronchodilators—beta agonists and anticholinergics—if unresponsive to oxygen
   c. If unresponsive to bronchodilators, obtain ABG and consider noninvasive positive pressure ventilation or intubation.
   d. Systemic corticosteroids (glucocorticoids) if needed
   e. Antibiotics are commonly needed for patients with moderate to severe COPD exacerbation and purulent sputum production.
2. For discharge and long-term COPD treatment:
   a. Educate the patient about disease process.
   b. Educate the patient about using prescribed medications, particularly the inhalers.
   c. Improve quality of life with physical therapy, oxygen therapy, smoking cessation counseling, and pulmonary rehabilitation.
   d. Educate about when to call health care providers.
   e. Recommend influenza and pneumococcal vaccinations.

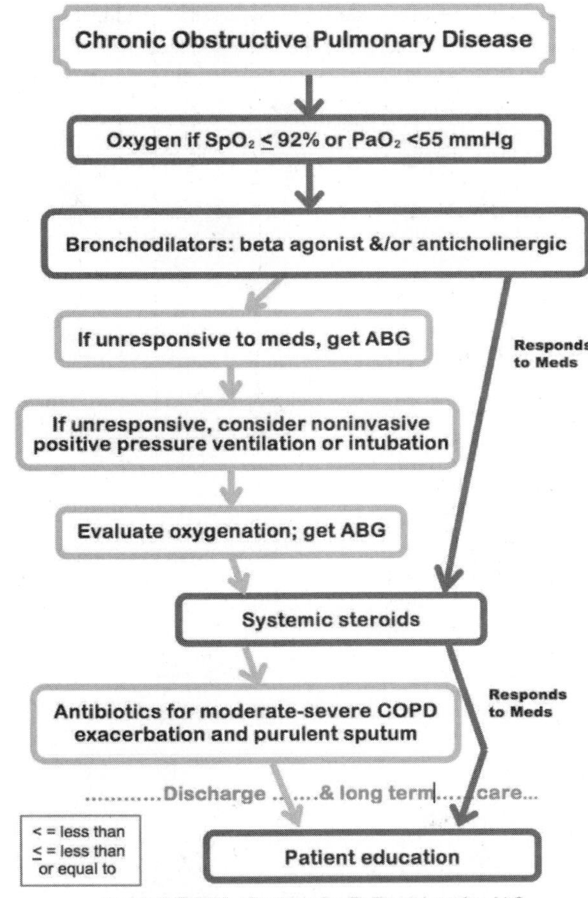
Chronic Obstructive Pulmonary Disease
Oxygen if $SpO_2 \leq 92\%$ or PaO_2 <55 mmHg
Bronchodilators: beta agonist &/or anticholinergic
If unresponsive to meds, get ABG
Responds to Meds
If unresponsive, consider noninvasive positive pressure ventilation or intubation
Evaluate oxygenation; get ABG
Systemic steroids
Responds to Meds
Antibiotics for moderate-severe COPD exacerbation and purulent sputum
...........Discharge ....& long term.....care...
< = less than
$\leq$ = less than or equal to
Patient education
Copyright © 2012, NovEx Novice To Expert Learning, LLC

Treatment guide for COPD. Note that interventions in green boxes are implemented only when needed. Interventions in blue boxes are intended to all patients.
Source: Copyright © 2012, NovEx Novice To Expert Learning, LLC

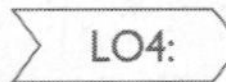

Evaluation of Desired Collaborative Care Outcomes

Evaluation and reassessment should reveal attainment of previously established patient outcomes. In summary:

- Patient reports and demonstrates that respiratory effort is at usual pre-exacerbation level.
- Pulmonary toilet produced clearing of auscultated lung sounds.
- Oxygen saturation values are at patient normal levels.
- Patient expectorates secretions effectively.
- Patient tolerates pre-exacerbation level of activity.
- Patient is maintaining body weight appropriate for height. No additional muscle wasting is evident.
- Patient identifies early cues of anxiety and verbalizes methods of anxiety control. Behavioral manifestations of anxiety are absent.
- Patient remains infection-free.

COPD is an irreversible and progressive disease. The major goal of collaborative care is to slow the decline and progression of symptoms.

References

http://www.ncbi.nlm.nih.gov/pubmedhealth/PMH0001153/

http://www.copd-international.com/library/statistics.htm

http://jama.ama-assn.org/content/301/13/1331.full

http://www.lung.org/lung-disease/copd/

http://www.cdc.gov/copd/

Practice Guidelines

Global Strategy for the Diagnosis, Management and Prevention of COPD, Global Initiative for Chronic Obstructive Lung Disease (GOLD) 2011. Available from: http://www.goldcopd.org/

Patient Education

http://www.chestnet.org/~/media/chesnetorg/Foundation/Documents/COPD/LivingWellwithCOPD2014.ashx

http://www.upmc.com/patients-visitors/education/breathing/pages/chronic-obstructive-pulmonary.aspx

Learning Outcomes for Asthma

When you complete this lesson, you will be able to:

1. Recognize the clinical relevance of asthma.
2. Consider the pathophysiology, etiology, risk factors, and clinical presentation of asthma that determine the priority patient concerns.
3. Determine the most urgent and important nursing interventions and patient education required in caring for a patient with asthma.
4. Evaluate attainment of desired collaborative care outcomes for a patient with asthma.

LO1:

What Is Asthma?

Asthma is a chronic respiratory disease, characterized by inflammation of the airways with intermittent airway obstruction. Of the Reversible Obstructive Airway Diseases (ROAD), asthma is the most common.

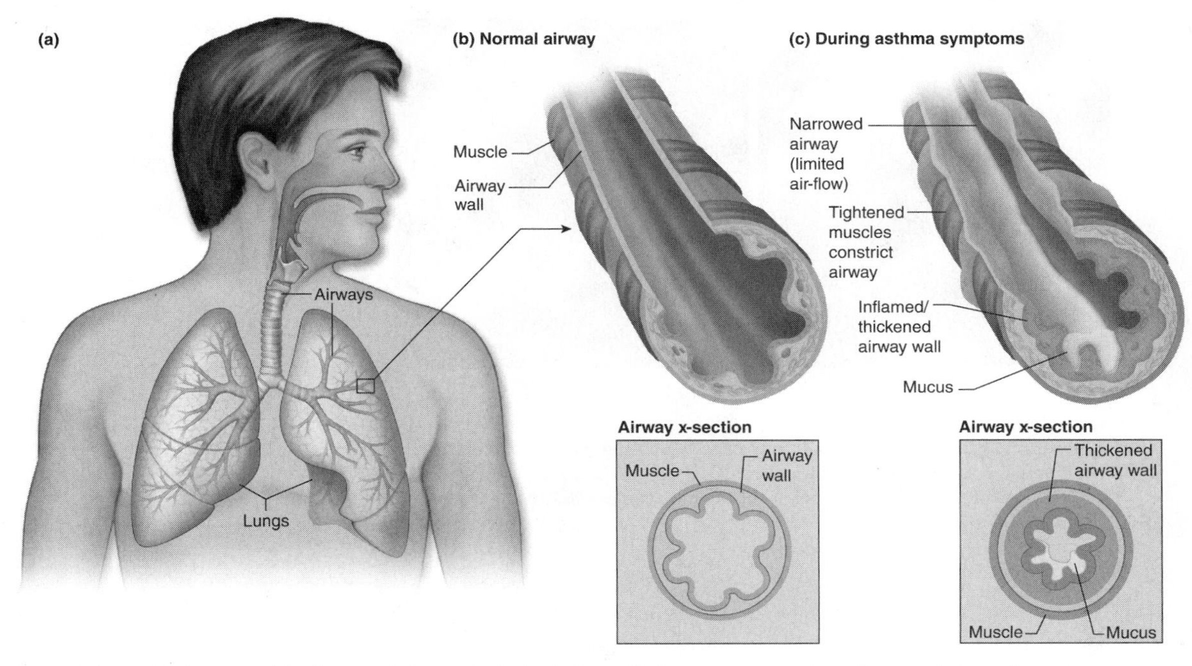

Figure A shows the location of the lungs and airways in the body. Figure B shows a cross-section of a normal airway for comparison. Figure C shows the pathophysiological consequences with narrowing airways during an asthma episode.

LO1:

Clinical Relevance

- Every nurse will care for patients with asthma, with more than 23 million people affected, 7 million of which are children. It is among the most commonly seen chronic childhood diseases.
- In the United States, asthma is responsible for approximately 11 deaths per day.
- Complications of asthma, some severe, include:
    - o Inactivity, exercise intolerance, and inability to participate in activities
    - o Lung functions can be permanently altered.
    - o Sleep loss from symptoms during the night
    - o Endotracheal intubation requiring ventilator support for respiratory failure
    - o Death
- With proper treatment and patient education, asthma is a manageable illness.
- There is no cure for asthma, although treatment can allow most people to have an active lifestyle.

Concept Check

1. **Which statement is true of patients diagnosed with asthma?**
   A. Most patients with asthma get relief from symptoms by rest.
   B. Asthma is an acute problem, so patients can be cured.
   C. Children with asthma may not be able to play sports.
   D. There is no risk of lung damage from asthma.

Answer question

LO2:

Pathophysiology

- Asthma is characterized by bronchial hyperresponsiveness that results in reversible airway obstruction.
- Triggers that cause bronchial muscle contraction include: viral infections, allergens, pollutants, exercise, and cold.

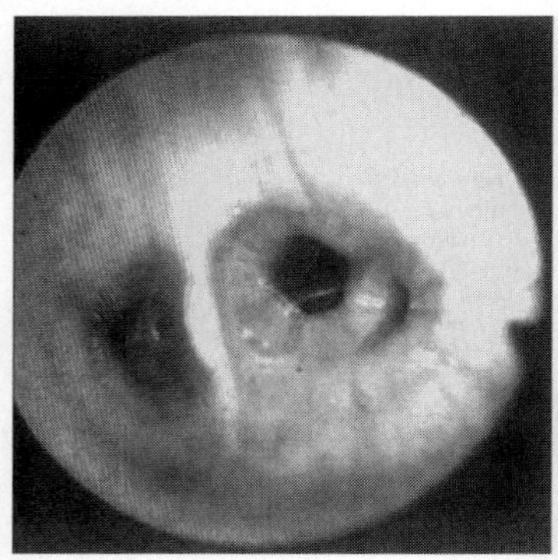

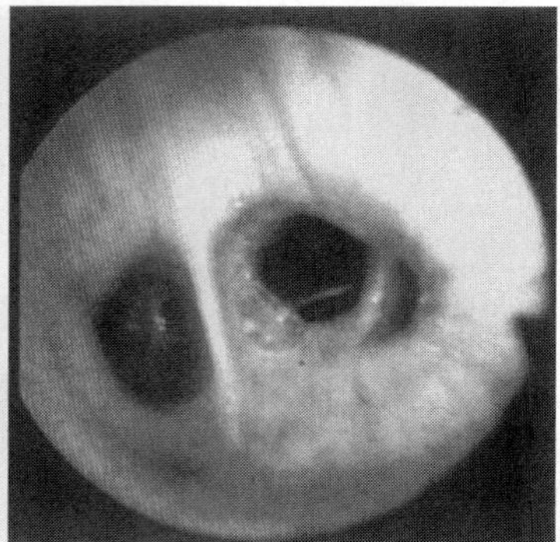

These photos, taken during bronchoscopy, reveal the pathophysiologic problem of ventilating during an asthmatic episode. *Left:* This photo shows the result of a trigger that causes severe bronchial constriction in a patient with asthma. Note that one of the airways is very tight, limiting air exchange. This exemplifies acute bronchoconstriction. *Right:* After treatment, the bronchioles relax to a more normal state with improved ventilation.
Source: CAVALLINI JAMES/BSIP SA/Alamy

- Viruses and allergens can trigger an immune response that results in release of cytokines, which:
  - o Cause inflammation and bronchiolar constriction with airway narrowing
  - o Stimulate hyper-secretion of mucous
  - o Attract more WBCs (inflammatory cells) to the bronchial tissue. The activated WBCs release more cytokines, causing a cycle of inflammation.
  - o Cause capillary leakage with mucosal edema

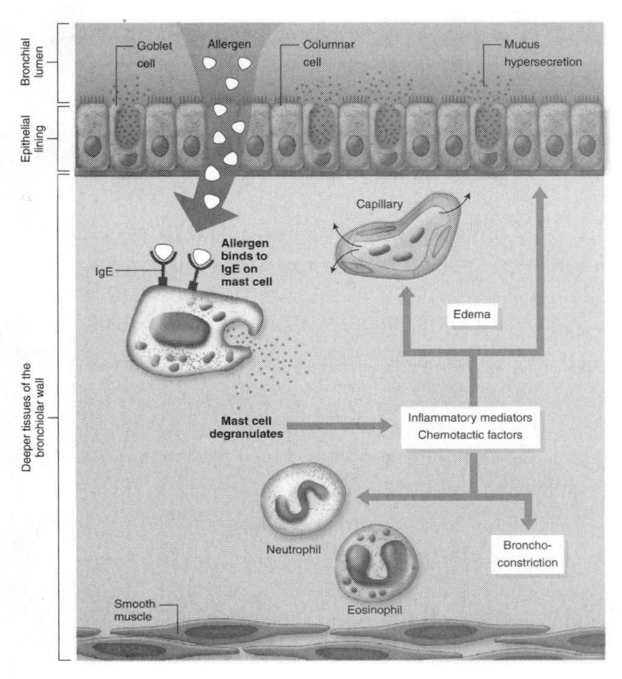

This picture depicts the pathophysiologic process by which an allergen triggers an exacerbation.

- This inflammation results in numerous changes in the airways:
  - o Dysfunction of cilia cells that help remove secretions
  - o Increased mucous production
  - o Hypertrophy and hyperreactivity of the bronchial smooth muscle, constricting the airways
  - o Thickening of the mucosa
- These changes contribute to obstruction of airflow produced and is reversible initially. However, after years of inflammation the airways may undergo permanent changes or airway remodeling, which include scarring, cellular proliferation, structural changes, and chronic nonreversible airway obstruction.
- Inflammation and bronchospasm may be triggered almost immediately and last for several hours.
- Control of inflammation is key to controlling and preventing any worsening of the asthma.

(2003). *Allergy Asthma Proc*, 24(2), 79–83

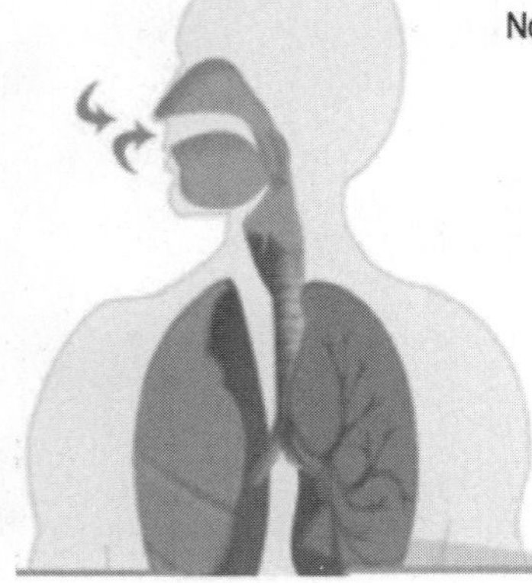

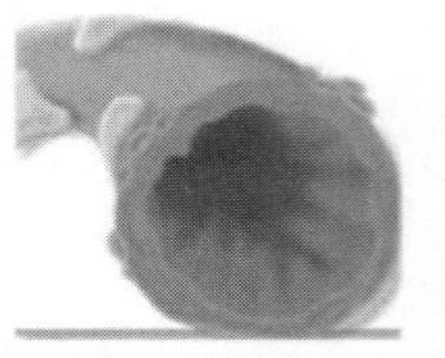

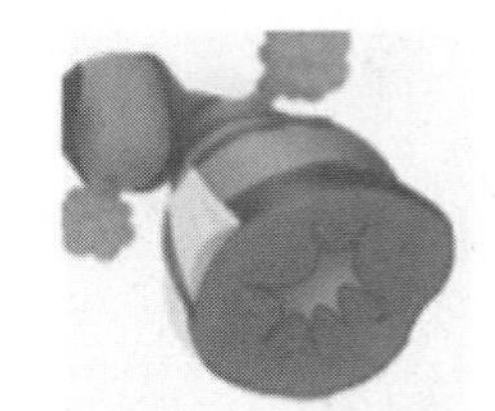

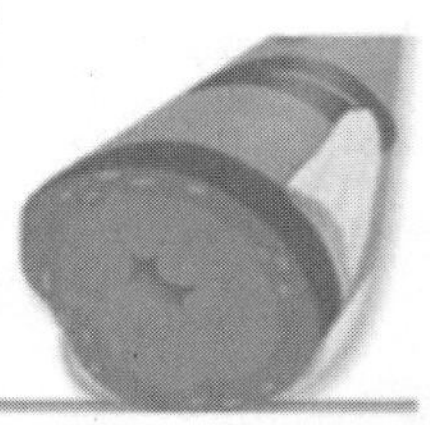

This drawing compares the airflow obstruction, bronchoconstriction, smooth muscle thickening, and mucous in normal, asthma, and severe asthma conditions.
Source: Copyright © 2012, NovEx Novice to Expert Learning, LLC

Concept Check

2. **What is a key strategy to prevent an acute asthma episode?**
   A. Control of inflammation
   B. Prevention infection
   C. Limiting exposure to toxins
   D. Use of bronchodilators

Answer question

Animated Pathophysiology

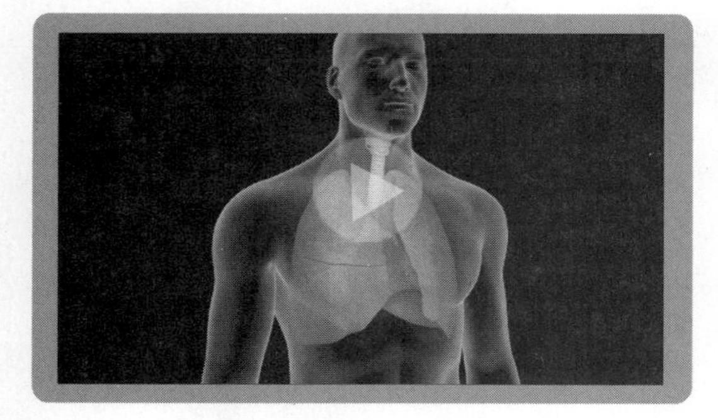

This 3D medical animation provides an overview of the upper respiratory anatomy and a lung disease that inflames and narrows the airways called asthma. The symptoms and triggers of asthma, along with various short-acting rescue and long-acting anti-inflammatory control medications are also featured in this video.
Source: © 2013 Nucleus Medical Media, All rights reserved

LO2:

Risk Factors

Risk factors for severe asthma exacerbation and prediction of poor outcomes for asthma include:

- Presence of comorbid conditions, such as COPD or heart failure
- Prior intubation for asthma exacerbation
- Frequent emergency department visits or hospitalizations for asthma

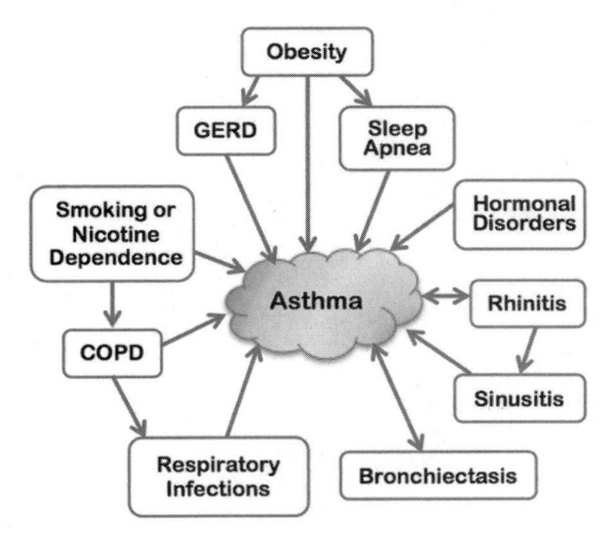

This diagram depicts the many comorbid conditions that influence asthma attacks.

Causes

- The causes of asthma are not clear. Patients who have relatives with either asthma or allergies are more likely to develop asthma. Genes related to asthma have been identified. The implications for clinical management are exciting, but not well developed yet.
- Triggers (see photo) include:
  - o Allergens: Many environmental and food allergens exist that can trigger an asthmatic episode, e.g., dust, pollen, pollution, fish, eggs, peanuts, shellfish, soy.
  - o Respiratory irritants and conditions: These may also include perfumes, strong emotions, cold air, stress, exercise, and respiratory infections.

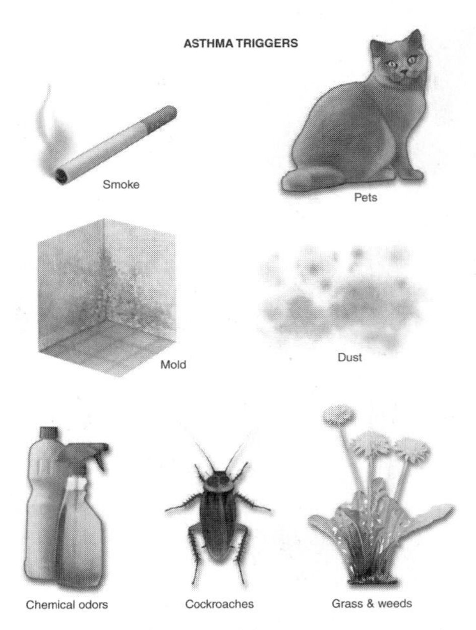

Genetic and environmental factors interact to produce asthma. These factors are targeted for treatment to help control asthma.

Concept Check

3. Which of the following is a specific asthma trigger?

A. Family history of asthma

B. Exposure to pet dander

C. History of depression

D. History of pneumonia

Answer question

Assessment Findings

Mild Asthma

- Patients with mild asthma may be asymptomatic.
- Symptoms tend to come and go and may be associated with certain triggers such as cold, certain allergens, smoke exposure, or exercise.
- Patients with mild asthma are less likely to have tachycardia and tachypnea.
- Intermittent shortness of breath may occur.
- Wheezing (high-pitched whistling sounds) on examination may be heard.

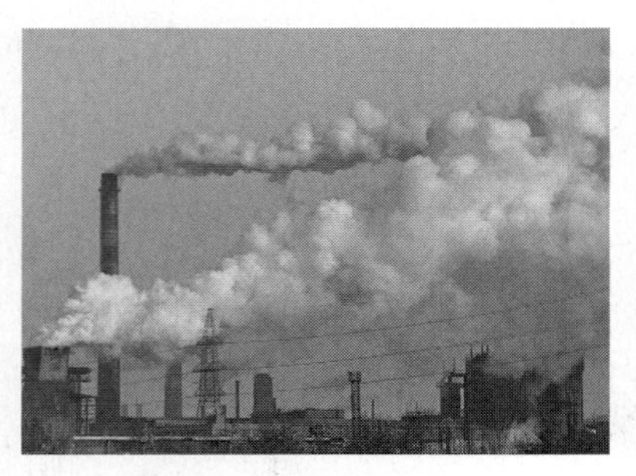

Outdoor air pollution.
Source: Nickolay Khoroshkov/Fotolia

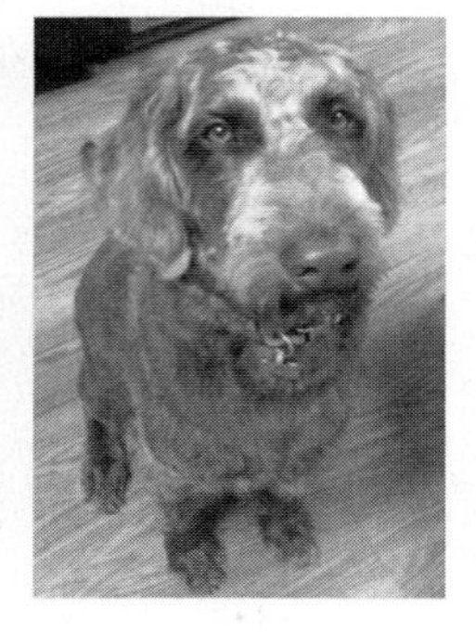

Pets.
Source: Copyright © 2012, NovEx Novice to Expert Learning, LLC

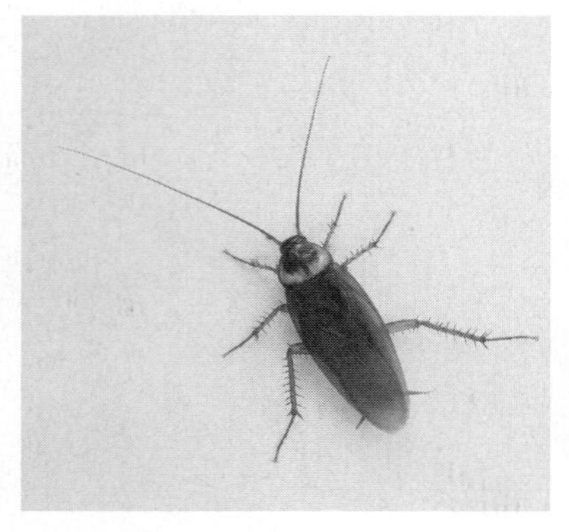

Cockroach allergen.
Source: Frank Greenaway/DK Images

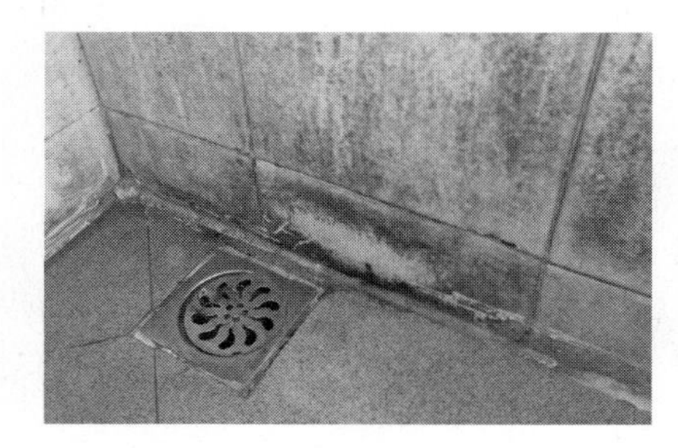

Mold.
Source: pokko/Fotolia

Moderate to Severe Asthma Exacerbation

Patients with moderate to severe asthma may experience an exacerbation of symptoms, such as:

- Tachycardia
- Tachypnea
- Use of accessory muscles, sternal retractions, cyanosis, hypoxemia
- Confusion or altered mental state
- Nocturnal waking frequently
- Diminished or absence of wheezing: When airflow is severely diminished, wheezing may not be audible because of the severely reduced airflow upon expiration.

Concept Check

4. A patient experiencing sternal retractions during an asthma exacerbation likely has what form of the disease?

A. Allergic

B. Chronic

C. Childhood

D. Severe

Answer question

Diagnostics

Diagnostic tests may include:

- Pulmonary function tests (PFT): PFTs measure reduced airflow and are usually normal unless the patient is having an exacerbation. Challenge with methacholine and exercise, which together can cause bronchospasm in asthmatics and are often used diagnostically.
- A peak flow meter (see photo) is a useful handheld device that measures the peak expiratory flow rate. This is accomplished by having the patient take a deep breath and then exhale forcefully through the meter (normal peak flow is 80–100 L/min). It is inexpensive and may be used at home or in the office. Improvement of peak flow after administration of a beta agonist is one indicator of asthma. A peak flow of less than 50% of normal indicates severe asthma.
- Chest x-ray: Typically normal but can show air trapping
- Pulse oximeter: Oxygen saturation may be abnormally low.
- ABGs: May be normal in early stage of asthma. Later, hyperventilation results in a diminished $PaCO_2$ and increased pH during an asthma exacerbation. Elevated $PaCO_2$ with a low pH is a sign of impending respiratory failure.
- Labs: Evaluate the eosinophil count (a kind of white blood cell) and IgE (an immunoglobulin)

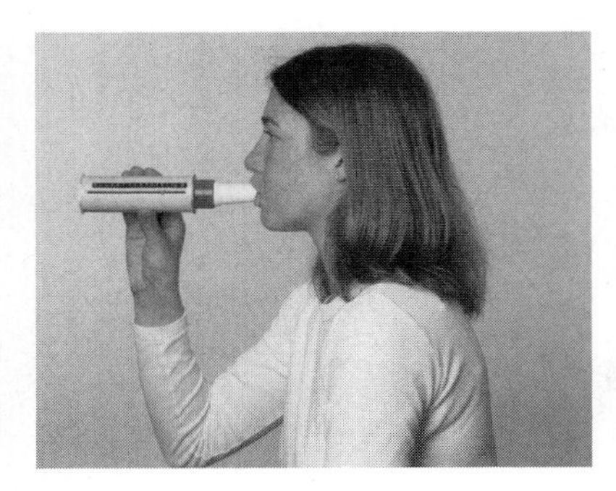

There are numerous models of peak flow meters. After taking a deep breath, one breathes out forcefully into a mouthpiece. The scale along the side of the meter measures one's airflow. Airflow diminishes with asthma

Source: Steve Gorton/Dorling Kindersley, Ltd.

Priority Patient Concerns and Desired Collaborative Care Outcomes

Prior to caring for patients with asthma, it is important to prioritize the patient's concerns that must guide the nursing care plan and interventions. Care for the patient is ordered and organized in accordance with the patient's priority and urgent needs. Desired collaborative care outcomes in patients with asthma typically include:

1. Patient will describe improvement in chest tightness and resolution of bronchospasm. If severe, arterial blood gas or pulse oximetry measures will return to the patient's pre-exacerbation level.
2. Patient will report reduced shortness of breath and breathe more comfortably. Respiratory rate and rhythm will return to the patient's normal levels.
3. Patient's lungs will sound clearer to auscultation. Peak flow levels will trend close to the patient's normal levels.
4. Activity will be tolerated close to the patient's pre-exacerbation level.
5. Patient will return to their pre-exacerbation level of work in breathing.
6. Patient will experience greater calm and will report feeling less anxious.

Considering these important care outcomes, prepare a list of the major 3–6 priority patient concerns or nursing diagnoses for patients with asthma. Be prepared to participate in a discussion of this list and/or to submit them as an assignment, as determined by your faculty. Resources you may find helpful in this assignment can include this lesson, the references, resources on nursing care plans, and standard nursing diagnoses manuals.

Concept Check

5. **A patient being evaluated for possible asthma would likely be ordered to have which test(s)?**
   A. Hemoglobin and hematocrit
   B. Urinalysis
   C. Allergy skin testing
   D. Pulmonary function test

Answer question

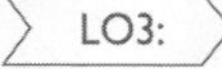

Collaborative Interventions

Evidence-Based Practice (EBP)

- There are no curative treatments for asthma. Despite substantial research, preventing and treating asthmatic episodes remain difficult. However, the research has provided some evidence-based practice in asthma.
- EBP focuses on four major types of collaborative interventions:
  1. Pharmacologic therapy
     a. Bronchodilators: Beta agonists (bronchodilators) have been shown to reduce symptoms associated with an asthmatic episode.
     b. IV or oral steroids: There is some evidence to support its use in moderate to severe asthmatic episodes.
  2. Identification of severity of asthma and evaluation of treatment effectiveness by assessing and monitoring airway obstruction
  3. Education in asthma care (e.g., proper use of inhalers, inhaled steroids, and bronchodilators for acute episodes)
  4. Control of environmental factors: Avoiding factors that precipitate an asthmatic episode have reduced the incidence and severity of episodes

Collaborative Symptom Management for Mild Asthma Exacerbations

- Pharmacologic therapy:
  - o Examples include albuterol (e.g., Proventil, Ventolin) and levalbuterol (e.g., Xopenex).
  - o Bronchodilators: Short-acting beta agonists provide quick relief of symptoms and are often referred to as "rescue" inhalers. They work by relaxing the smooth muscle of the bronchioles, cause broncho-dilation, and allow greater airflow.
  - o Beta agonists can also be used prophylactically prior to exercising to prevent asthma symptoms in patients with exercise-induced asthma.
  - o Beta agonists may be delivered in the form of metered dose inhalers (MDI) or nebulizers. These treatments are equally effective if the MDI is used properly (see illustrations). Proper use can be aided by a spacer.

Normal
Asthma Attack
After Medicine
(Muscles Spasm)
(Muscles Relaxed)

This image compares the bronchiolar state during normal breathing, during an asthmatic episode, and after successful pharmacologic intervention.
Source: Copyright © 2012, NovEx Novice to Expert Learning, LLC

- Explore potential contributing environmental factors: Evidence shows that avoiding precipitating factors that trigger an asthmatic episode can reduce the incidence and severity of asthma exacerbations (listed in "Causes").

Metered Dose Inhaler (MDI)

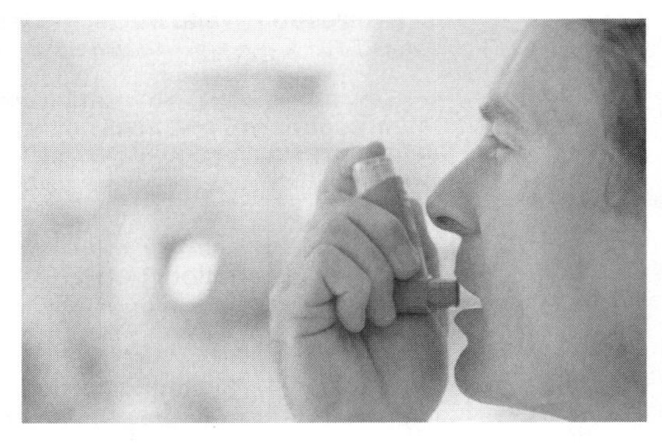

The spacer enables one to inhale the medication with ease and comfort. Two to three breaths usually delivers the full dose in adults. Slow inhalations if a whistle is heard while breathing. Spacers can be mouthpieces or masks.
Source: OJO Images Ltd/Alamy

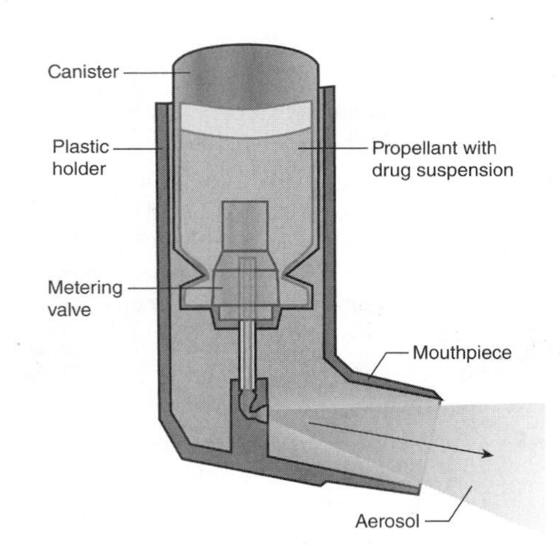

MDI's are the most common method of delivering brochodilators. Care must be taken to use a MDI properly or else medications may not be properly administered.

Nebulizer

- Nebulizers change liquid medication into inhalable aerosol mists.
- When medication is added, the mist is inhaled through a mouthpiece or by mask.
- Treatments may last 10–15 minutes, until the medication is gone.
- Nebulizer use results in higher absorption of the medication than MDI administration.
- Nebulizer are often used in the emergency department.
- Treatments can be administered in the home, workplace, or clinic.
- Specific instructions should include how to operate the machine, measure medications, add saline if indicated, and clean the machine after use.

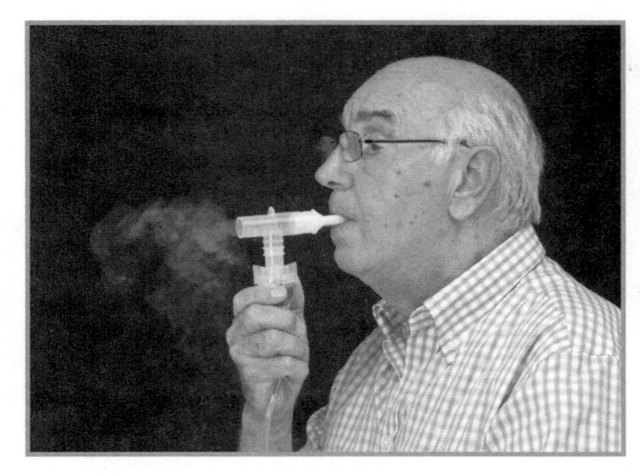

Although inhalers with a spacer may be very effective when the patient uses correct technique, many experts think that a nebulizer may be more effective, particularly in emergent situations. Instruct the patient that it is key to breath through the mouth, not the nose, in order to inhale the full dosage of the medicine
Source: Juanmonino/Getty Images.

Collaborative Symptom Management for Moderate to Severe Asthma Exacerbations

Interventions for patients with signs and symptoms of moderate to *severe* exacerbation include (see treatment schematic):

- Oxygen therapy for oxygen saturation less than or equal to 92% and/or PaO_2 more than 55 mmHg. Maintain the SpO_2 more than or equal to 93%.
- Beta agonists can be administered consecutively, up to three times every 15 minutes, until there is a response.
- In severe cases where the patient is unresponsive to initial treatment (status asthmaticus), or if the patient becomes less responsive, consider getting an arterial blood gas (ABG). This is a medical emergency situation and health care providers must act quickly.
- It is appropriate to call the rapid response team or the health care provider for help, but the nurse must act while waiting for help to arrive.
- Patients with elevated pCO_2 and low pH need BiPAP or intubation with mechanical ventilation. BiPAP should be considered before intubation since it is less invasive and prevents the hazards of intubation (e.g., ventilator associated pneumonia). Assess patient's level of consciousness before using BiPAP.
- Reassess for adequate oxygenation (PaO_2 more than 55 mmHg). If intubation is required, consider the need for sedation and paralytics.
- Corticosteroids are then recommended for patients having a moderate to severe exacerbation. Glucocorticoids (systemic corticosteroids) can be effective. The response to steroids, however, may take several hours. Both oral and intravenous corticosteroids are often effective.
- IV magnesium relaxes the smooth muscle of airways and can improve breathing.

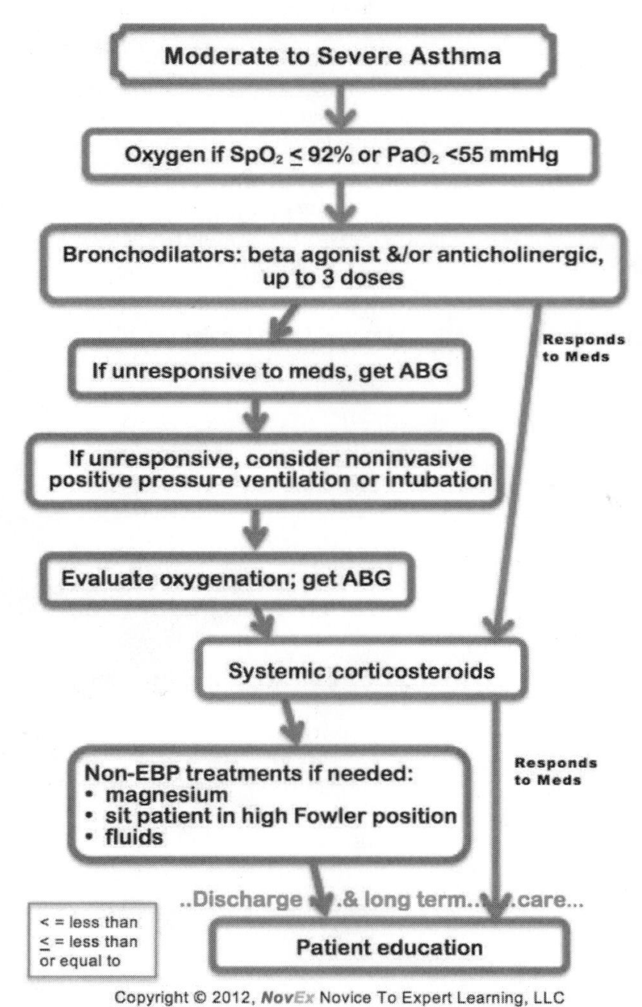

Moderate to Severe Asthma
Oxygen if $SpO_2 \le 92\%$ or $PaO_2 < 55$ mmHg
Bronchodilators: beta agonist &/or anticholinergic, up to 3 doses
Responds to Meds
If unresponsive to meds, get ABG
If unresponsive, consider noninvasive positive pressure ventilation or intubation
Evaluate oxygenation; get ABG
Systemic corticosteroids
Non-EBP treatments if needed:
• magnesium
• sit patient in high Fowler position
• fluids
Responds to Meds
..Discharge ...& long term... care...
Patient education
< = less than
≤ = less than or equal to
Copyright © 2012, NovEx Novice To Expert Learning, LLC

Source: Copyright © 2012, NovEx Novice to Expert Learning, LLC

LO3:

Monitoring Treatment Effectiveness

- Improvement in patient symptoms is the most important indication that treatments have been effective. Patients should appear more comfortable with easier breathing if they are improving. However, objective indicators can give more specific information.
- Objective measures of improvement include:
  1. Monitoring of peak flow is essential in assessing patients response to treatment:
     a. Improvement of peak flow of 10–15% of normal (or more than 200 mL), after inhaled beta agonist, indicates therapy was effective according to the American Thoracic Society.
     b. Peak flows below 50% of normal are indicative of a severe asthma attack.
     c. Following daily peak flows is an effective way to control and monitor asthma both at home and in the hospital.
  2. Repeat ABGs in acute situations, if needed, are expected to show normalization of pH (7.35–7.45) and pCO_2 (35–45 mmHg).

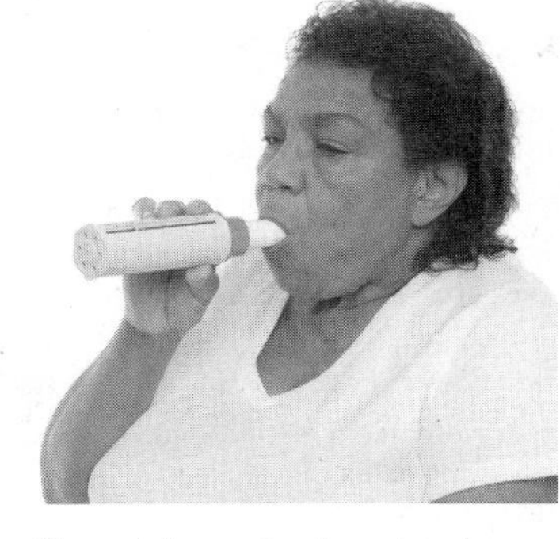

The peak flow meter shown here is a portable device used by patients at home to monitor effectiveness of therapy and provide early warning of airflow compromise.
Source: Science Photo Library/Alamy

Concept Check

6. Treatment of a patient with an asthma exacerbation is effective when:

A. oxygen is no longer required.
B. respiratory rate is less than 20 breaths per minute.
C. peak flow is less than 50% of normal.
D. the patient is more comfortable.

Answer question

Collaborative Symptom Management for Asthmatic Episodes: General Treatment

Support and Comfort Care

N M
- Treat any potential causes, such as pneumonia.

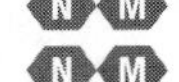

- Infuse fluids, up to 3 liters per day, to help liquefy thickened secretions that are hard to expectorate.

N
- Place patient in high Fowler position to ease respirations. They often sit without intervention because they find they breathe easier.

N
- Closely monitor patients developing respiratory fatigue. Increased $PaCO_2$ and $PetCO_2$ are dangerous signs signaling the potential requirement for intubation and mechanical ventilation.

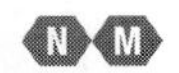

- Intubation and use of paralytics may help save the life of a patient with a severe asthmatic episode. Remember that patients receiving paralytics should first be sedated. The goal of these emergency interventions is to reduce airway resistance and improve gas exchange.

Pharmacologic Control: Chronic Asthma

- A patient with good control of the asthma should NOT be using a rescue inhaler more than twice weekly. Patients should have and know how to use the rescue inhaler, but if the frequency of use increases, medications that control airway inflammation should be added.
- Control drugs are typically taken on a daily basis and should not be skipped even when the patient is asymptomatic.
- The most commonly used control drugs are inhaled corticosteroids (ICS) such as Flovent and Azmacort. Regular use of ICS to stop the cycle of inflammation has been shown to decrease the progression of asthma, ER visits, and hospitalizations.
- Additional control drugs that may be needed can include:
  - Cromolyn sodium (Intal) or nedocromil (Tilade) are alternatives to inhaled glucocorticoids and tend to have a lower incidence of side effects.
  - Leukotriene inhibitors: Leukotriene is a cytokine that contributes to airway inflammation. These inhibitors reduce airway inflammation.
  - Omalizumab (Xolair) is used in severe asthma. It blocks a pathway in the immune systems that triggers the inflammatory response resulting in asthma symptoms.
  - Long-acting beta-agonist inhalers are often added in patients with severe asthma and are typically used in combination with an ICS.
- Effectiveness of control therapy can also be monitored with peak flows. Peak flow decreases before patients notice worsening symptoms. Changes in therapy can then be employed to prevent a severe asthma exacerbation. If peak flows begin to drop, for example, inhaled corticosteroid dose may be increased.

Patient Education

Asthma education and self-management are critical to long term control.

- Hospitals may have a nurse who specializes in asthma education. If available, consult an expert who can provide current information and support to the staff nurse.
- Asthma education should include:
  - o Disease-specific education, recognition of complications and when to call the health care provider
  - o Recognition and avoidance of asthmatic episodes and triggers; proper use of inhalers and other medications, even when stable
  - o How to use peak flow meters to evaluate treatment effectiveness: Effective use of a peak flow meter can be seen at this link: http://emedicine.medscape.com/article/1413347-overview.
  - o Exploration of the patient's self-care and coping strategies regarding repeated triggers, medication use, management of acute episodes (e.g., timing of rescue medication use), and sense of stigma of a chronic disease.
  - o Habits for healthy living: smoking cessation, healthy diet, exercise, weight management as needed, comorbid condition management, influenza, and pneumonia vaccines
  - o Having a plan in case the peak flow meter detects a change, for example: Medication changes to initiate when peak flows are decreased to 50–80% of personal best and an emergency care to be initiated when peak flows are less than 50% of baseline

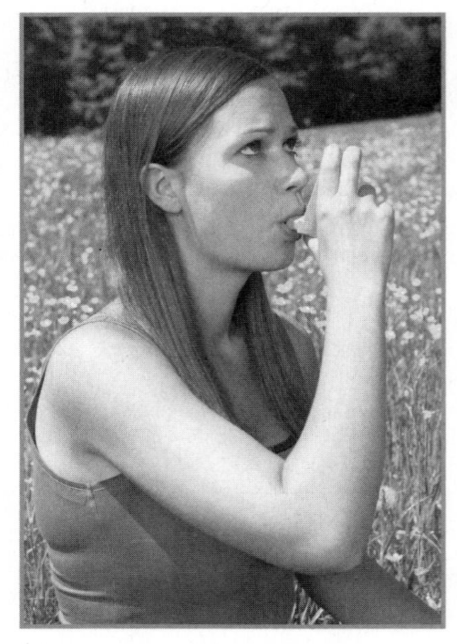

Using medications as prescribed is key to controlling asthma exacerbations.
Source: spflaum/Fotolia

Concept Check

7. Limited usage of a rescue inhaler to what determines whether or not a patient has well-controlled asthma?

A. Three times per day

B. Once or twice per week

C. Before encountering a trigger

D. After exercise

Answer question

Summary of Interventions

- Treatment of asthma exacerbations:
  - o Administer oxygen for SpO_2 less than or equal to 92%.
  - o Bronchodilators: Beta agonists, up to three doses
  - o If unresponsive to treatment, consider noninvasive positive pressure ventilation or intubation.
  - o Systemic corticosteroids (glucocorticoids) in moderate to severe exacerbations
- For discharge and chronic asthma treatment:
  - o Educate the patient about disease process.
  - o Educate the patient about using inhaled corticosteroid and rescue inhalers and other prescribed meds.
  - o Control environmental triggers of asthma.
  - o Improve quality of life with exercise, oxygen therapy, and/or smoking cessation.
  - o Explore coping and self-care.
  - o Educate the patient about when to call health care providers.
  - o Influenza and pneumococcal vaccinations

LO4:

Evaluation of Desired Collaborative Care Outcomes

Evaluation and reassessment should reveal attainment of previously established patient outcomes. In summary:

- Patient describes improvement in chest tightness and resolution of bronchospasm. If severe, arterial blood gas or pulse oximetry measures are at the patient's pre-exacerbation level.
- Patient reports reduced shortness of breath and breath more comfortably.
- Respiratory rate and rhythm approximate the patient's normal levels.
- Patient's lungs sound clearer to auscultation.
- Peak flow levels are close to the patient's normal levels.
- Activity tolerance is close to the patient's pre-exacerbation level.
- Patient is calmer and reports feeling less anxious.

Failure to attain these goals or worsening of any condition indicates that interventions are ineffective, tapered prematurely, inadequate, or a complication may be evolving. The nurse should be alert if wheezing sounds decrease without improvement of other assessment findings. This calls for good clinical judgment about impending respiratory failure. If rapid deterioration is recognized, notification of the rapid response team or initiation of code protocol may be indicated.

References

http://www.cdc.gov/nchs/data/nhsr/nhsr032.pdf

http://www.aaaai.org/media/statistics/asthma-statistics.asp

http://www.nhlbi.nih.gov/health/dci/Diseases/Asthma/Asthma_Treatments.html

http://ajrccm.atsjournals.org/content/163/2/540.full

http://emedicine.medscape.com/article/109739-overview

http://emedicine.medscape.com/article/296301-treatment

http://www.nhlbi.nih.gov/health-pro/resources/lung/naci/asthma-info/asthma-guidelines.htm

http://www.clevelandclinicmeded.com/medicalpubs/diseasemanagement/allergy/bronchial-asthma/

Becker, G., Janson-Bjerklie, S., Benner, P., Slobin, K., & Ferketich, S. (1993). The dilemma of seeking urgent care: Asthma episodes and emergency service use. *Social Science and Medicine, 37*, 305–313.

Benner, P., Janson-Bjerklie, S., Ferketich, F., & Becker, G. (1994). Moral dimensions of living with a chronic illness: Autonomy, responsibility and limits of control. In P. Benner (Ed.), *Interpretative Phenomenology: Embodiment Caring and Ethics* (pp. 225–254). Thousand Oaks, CA: Sage Publishers.

Janson-Bjerklie, S., Ferketich, S., Benner, P., & Becker, G. (1992). The clinical markers of asthma severity and risk: Importance of subjective as well as objective factors. *Heart and Lung, 21*(3), 265–272.

Lazarus, S.C. (2010). Clinical practice emergency treatment of asthma. *New England Journal of Medicine, 363*m, 755–764.

Mannam, P., & Siegel, M. D. (2010). Analytic Review: Management of lifethreatening asthma in adults. *Journal of Intensive Care Medicine, 25*(1), 3–15.

National Heart, Lung, and Blood Institute, National Asthma Education and Prevention Program, Expert Panel Report 3: Guidelines for the Diagnosis and Management of Asthma, Full Report 2007.

STOP

Go to the online course and complete the NovE-Cases assigned by your instructor for this module.

Learning Outcomes for Pneumonia

When you complete this lesson, you will be able to:

1. Recognize the clinical relevance of pneumonia.
2. Consider the pathophysiology, etiology, risk factors, and clinical presentation of pneumonia that determine the priority patient concerns.
3. Determine the most urgent and important nursing interventions and patient education required in caring for a patient with pneumonia.
4. Evaluate attainment of desired collaborative care outcomes for a patient with pneumonia.

LO1:

What Is Pneumonia?

- Pneumonia is an infection of the lung, typically caused by inhaling an organism that is pathogenic.
- In addition to inhalation, pneumonia can develop from aspiration or hematogenous spread of bacteria (see illustration).
- Many types of organisms can cause pneumonia, although most commonly the infection is caused by bacteria and viruses.

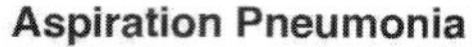

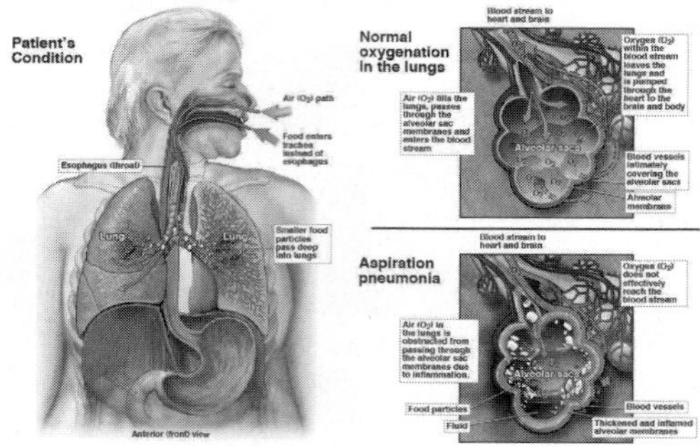

The first image (left) shows the patient condition that causes aspiration pneumonia. Food enters the trachea instead of the esophagus, and smaller food particles pass deep into the lungs. The other two images (right) compare the normal oxygenation process in the lungs with oxygenation obstructed by inflammation, fluid buildup, and a thickening of the alveolar membrane (aspiration pneumonia). Aspiration produces a pneumonia that is similar to a bacterial pneumonia.

Classification

There are several types of pneumonia based on classification:

- Community-acquired pneumonia (CAP)
- Nosocomial—three types:
  - o Hospital-acquired pneumonia (HAP)
  - o Healthcare-associated pneumonia (HCAP)
  - o Ventilator-associated pneumonia (VAP)

Classification Defined (see Assessment Findings table for distinctions):

CAP: Acquired in the community, prior to hospitalization

HAP: Occurs 48 hours or more after hospital admission

HCAP: Occurs in nonhospitalized patient with extensive health care contact:

- IV, chemo, hemodialysis, or wound care within prior 30 days
- Resident of nursing home or long term care facility
- Acute care hospitalization for 2 or more days within previous 30 days

Ventilator-Associated Pneumonia (VAP)

- In addition to the pneumonia classifications, there are two types of VAP:
  - o Early: Develops after approximately 48 hours on the ventilator
  - o Late: Develops after approximately 5 days on the ventilator
- Time of onset is important because it is related to the causing organism.
- Incidence of VAP is 9–27% of patients on mechanical ventilation.
- Mortality of VAP is high (25–50%) and is likely due to sepsis.

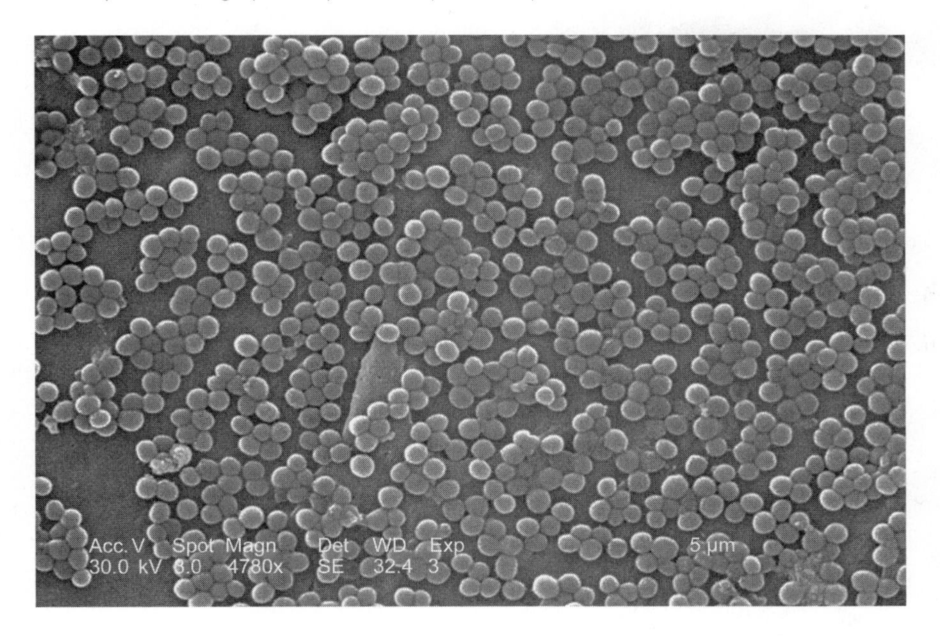

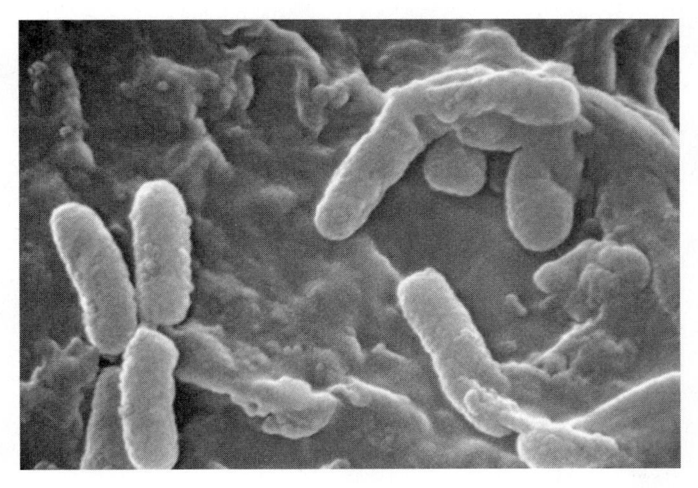

Common pathogens seen in ventilator-associated pneumonia include: methicillin-resistant *staphylococcus aureus* (upper) and *pseudomonas* (lower).
Sources: (*upper*) CDC/Janice Carr; Jeff Hageman; (*lower*) Janice Haney Carr/Center for Disease Control (CDC)—PHIL

LO1:

Clinical Relevance

- Pneumonia can be very dangerous, even fatal when sepsis develops. Pneumonia that develops into sepsis is one of the leading causes of death in the world.
- Sepsis is a systemic response to infection that can cause cell dysfunction and circulatory and coagulation problems (see Sepsis/Overview of Shock NovE-lessons).
- Most patients do not die of the pneumonia, but rather from sepsis as a complication of pneumonia.

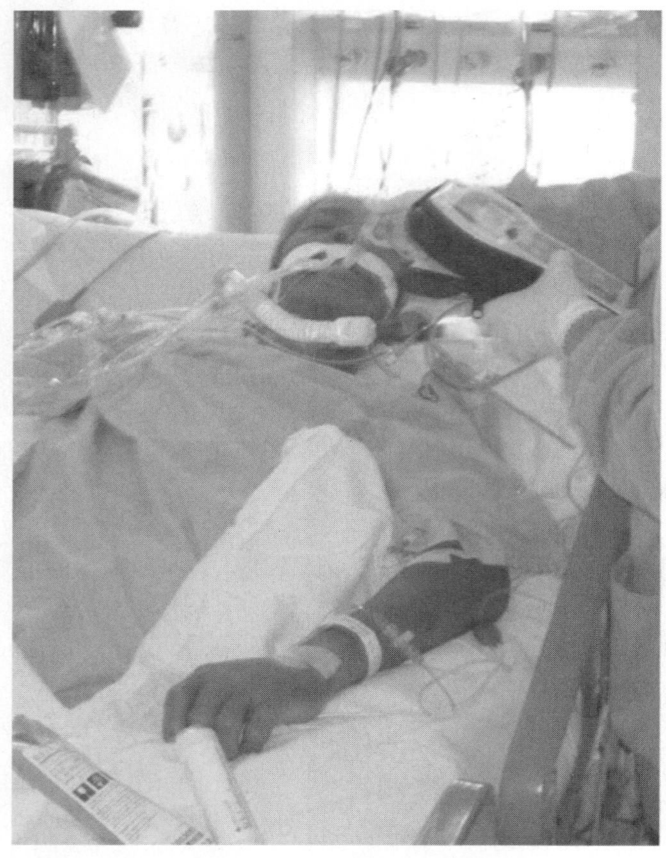

Most pneumonia patients do not require hospitalization. However, a patient is admitted for pneumonia when the pneumonia presents a serious condition that can progress to a life-threatening situation like sepsis.
Source: Copyright © 2012, NovEx Novice to Expert Learning, LLC

- Approximately 4–5 million cases of pneumonia occur in the United States per year, with 25% requiring hospitalization and with more than 55,000 deaths per year.
- The United States spends over $8 billion each year on pneumonia.
- Community-acquired pneumonia (CAP) is the most common cause of admission to hospitals for infection.
    - o Due to the enormity of resources consumed by this condition, which is heavily funded by Medicare, the Centers for Medicare & Medicaid Services (CMS) made managing CAP a "core" measure.
    - o A core measure is one that has quality measures in place to improve care and, most importantly, outcomes of patients with CAP.

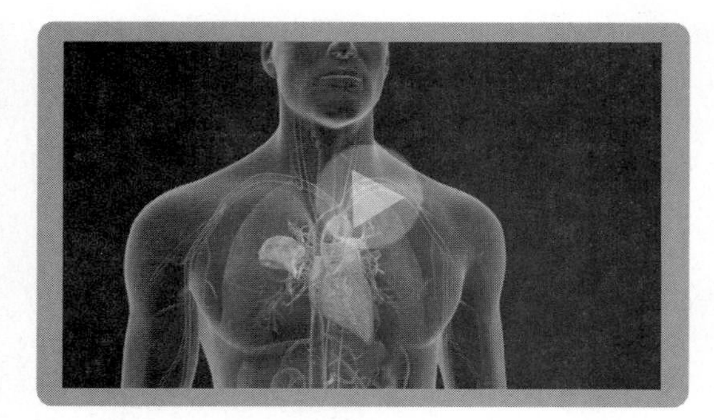

This animation features an overview of the symptoms and risk factors of pneumonia. The normal anatomy and physiology of the lungs, along with the types of pathogens that cause pneumonia, common treatment options, and ways to lower the risk for developing pneumonia are also featured.
Source: © 2013 Nucleus Medical Media, All rights reserved

Concept Check

1. **An emergency department patient who is a resident of a long-term care facility is diagnosed with pneumonia. How is this pneumonia classified?**

   A. Community-acquired pneumonia

   B. Hospital-acquired pneumonia

   C. Healthcare-associated pneumonia

Answer question

LO2:

Pathophysiology

- A pathogen enters the lungs either through inhalation, aspiration, or through the blood (hematogenous). Once a pathogen has entered, the body recognizes an invader, activating the immune system.
- The body's normal response is to contain the infection with recruitment of white blood cells (WBC) and macrophages.
- Normally, the immune response is powerful against pathogens, using neutrophils or WBCs and macrophages that reside in every body tissue to lyse (kill) most invading organisms in a period of hours to days. Thus, the immune system often prevents pathogens from spreading.

Antibody Immune System Response

- The animation provides an accurate depiction of how the immune system mounts a response to a pathogen (antigen). An antigen (bacteria) causes the body to produce antibodies against it. The antibodies then prevent harmful invaders from attaching to health body cells.
- The animation starts by depicting the flow of normal red and white blood cells through the bloodstream.
- A single pathogen (potato-looking cell) is then shown, slowly moving toward the surface of a white blood cell (WBC). The pathogen's tubular extensions are surface proteins that attach to protruding surface proteins on a WBC. More invaders then arrive and attach to the WBC, disabling it.

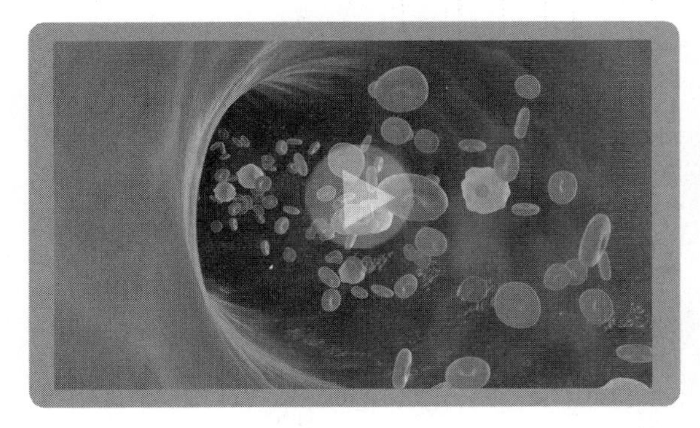

Source: © 2013 Nucleus Medical Media, All rights reserved

- Y-shaped antibodies (green) are activated by the immune system response and attack the invaders, swarming and binding to its surface proteins. The antibodies completely disable the pathogen from attaching to body cells. When antibodies attach to the antigen, it "tags" the pathogen for recognition by macrophages (whitish-gray cells with multiple arms) in the immune system. The macrophage reaches out and binds to the pathogen. It then engulfs and lyzes the pathogen.

The next animation provides a more detailed demonstration of what the macrophage does when it detects and attacks a bacterial invader:

- The animation starts with three macrophages (large brown cells) in the bloodstream, with numerous bacteria (small green rods) nearby.
- As the middle macrophage passes by, its amoeboid movement helps it navigate through the bloodstream.
- A macrophage slows down as it identifies bacteria close by and rapidly extends numerous thin, long filament-like arms or pseudopods to grab and ingest the invaders into itself.
- The macrophages then signal for and recruit more macrophages by releasing many cytokines (small blue particles) to mount a stronger response if there are too many invaders present.
- The cytokines (or pro-inflammatory cells) are chemicals that attract more macrophages and other white cells into the area.
- If the immune system becomes overwhelmed, an infection (pneumonia) develops.

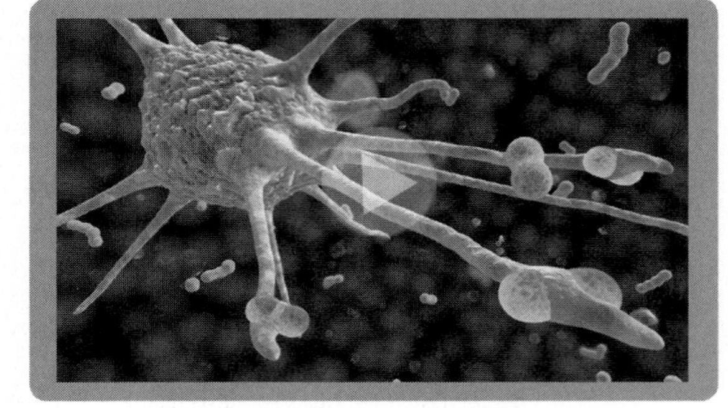

Pathophysiology (continued)

Responses to Pneumonia

When pathogens proliferate and pneumonia develops, both local and systemic responses are stimulated:

- **Local response**: Infection of the lungs (pneumonia) causes inflammation of the alveoli. The alveoli become filled with bacteria, WBCs, and fluid, forming secretions. Consolidation (large area of fluid-filled alveoli) interfere with gas exchange and can cause hypoxemia, observed as:
    - o Decreased PaO_2 (oxygen tension in arterial blood gases)
    - o Decreased SpO_2 (pulse oximeter)
- **Systemic response**:
    - o Mediators, released by the WBCs in the lung, recruit other WBCs resulting in systemic symptoms such as fever.
    - o If the infection worsens, sepsis may develop. Signs and symptoms of sepsis are the result of toxins released by the pathogens along with mediators released by WBCs. Sepsis is characterized by hypotension, metabolic acidosis (high lactate), tachycardia, and confusion.

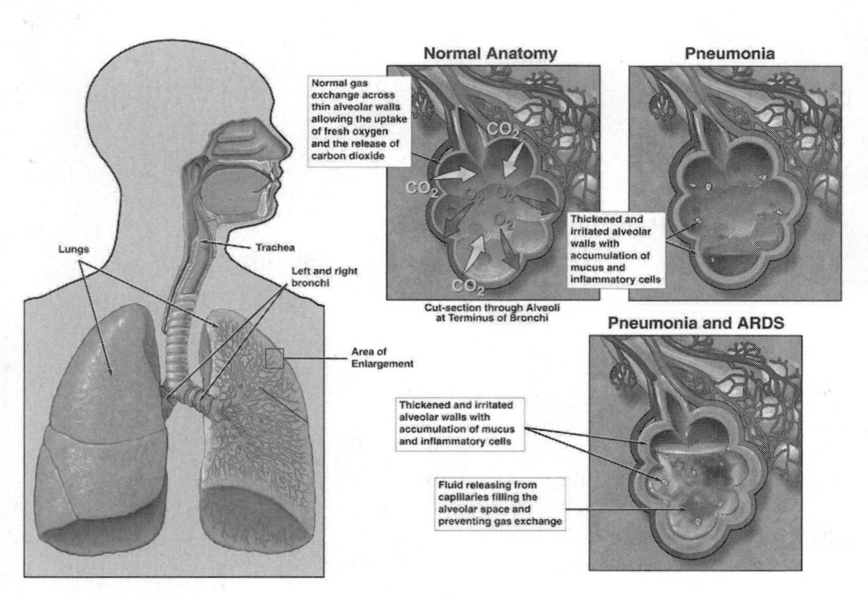

One of the dangers of pneumonia is deterioration to a worse clinical condition, such as Acute Respiratory Distress Syndrome (ARDS). While pneumonia can produce an interference in oxygen entering the blood, a condition such as ARDS produces much worse gas exchange and can be life-threatening.

- At the local alveolar level, secretions are formed and need to be cleared from the alveoli and airway to enable good gas exchange.
  - o Secretions can be different colors, depending on the infecting pathogen.
  - o Yellow or green sputum is a common sign of pneumonia.
- For most people, a strong cough effort can clear the secretions, which can then be expectorated. However, depending on the person's overall health, hydration status, cough effort, and level of consciousness, the patient may not be able to cough or cough effectively enough to clear the secretions.

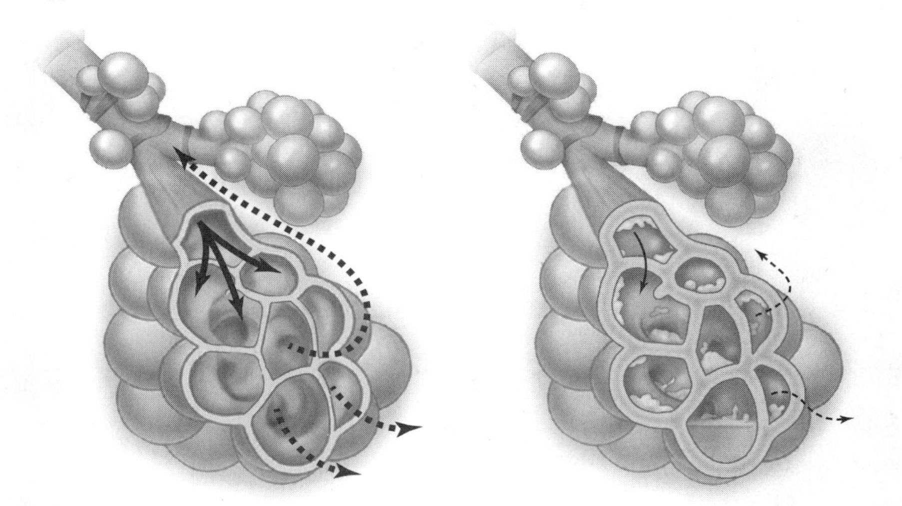

These drawings compare a normal (left) to an infection-filled (right) alveolus, impairing gas exchange.

Secretions in Pneumonia

- If the airway (or portions) cannot be cleared, obstruction for oxygen exchange can potentially further contribute to the hypoxemia, as seen in the x-ray.
- The amount of secretions produced and the patient's ability to clear the secretions should guide the clinician's vigilance in monitoring the patient to determine if further assistance is needed.

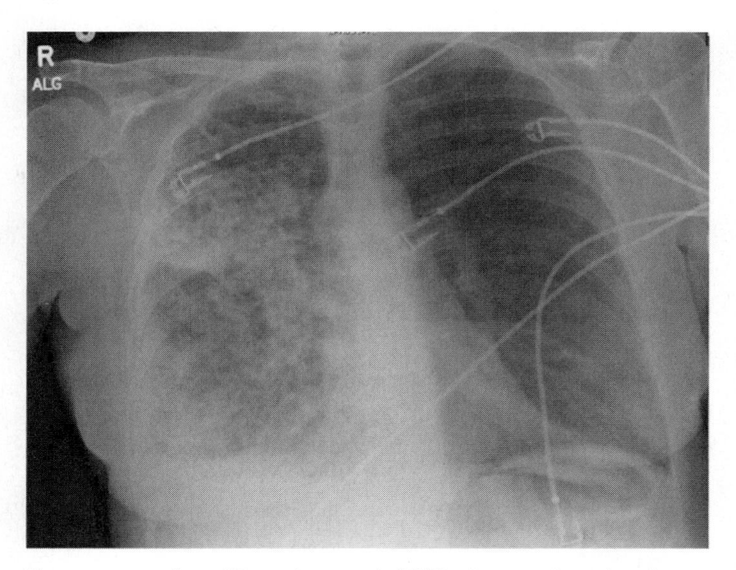

This is an x-ray of a middle-aged man with COPD who was admitted to the hospital with multiple symptoms of pneumonia. His x-ray reveals extensive right lobe infiltrates (whitish cotton appearance). His SpO_2 was abnormally low
Source: Courtesy of K. Kyriakidis

Risk Factors

Several important risk factors are present for developing pneumonia (see table for greater detail). Some of the most important are:

- Age: Very young and older patients are the most at risk.
- Comorbid states, particularly those that cause immobilization, decreased activity and inability to clear secretions (cough ineffectively)
- Institutionalization (e.g., hospital, nursing home)
- Immunosuppression, (e.g., chemotherapy, splenectomy, HIV)
- Being on a mechanical ventilator

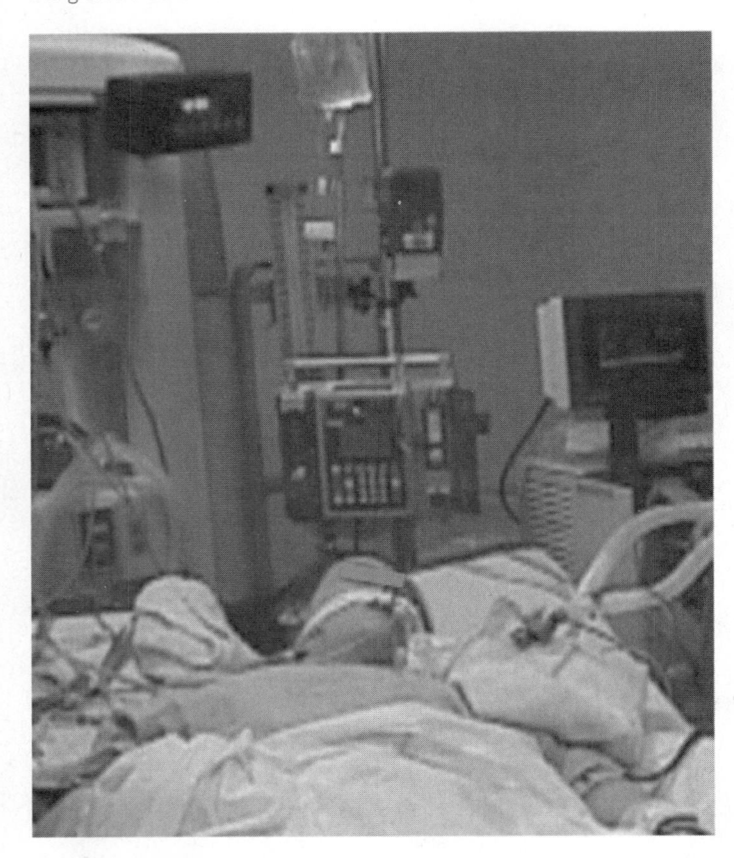

Intubation and mechanical ventilator place the patient at higher risk for pneumonia. A nurse's close observation and good clinical judgment are essential components in protecting the patient from potential hazards

Concept Check

2. **Following a severe head injury, a 45-year-old male patient is in a medically-induced coma and mechanically ventilated. Which factors predispose this patient to the development of pneumonia?**

   A. Age

   B. Immobilization

   C. Gender

   D. Trauma

Answer question

Causes

Most pneumonias are caused by exposure to and invasion by bacterial or viral infections. Immunocompromised patients, (e.g., HIV patients and patients on chemotherapy) can get unusual organisms such as fungi-causing pneumonia. Hundreds of organisms are known to cause pneumonia. Typical organisms include:

- **Bacterial**:
  - o *Streptococcus pneumoniae* is the most common and is responsible for 50% of pneumonia cases.
  - o *Haemophilus influenzae*
  - o *Chlamydia pneumoniae*
  - o *Mycoplasma pneumoniae*
  - o *Staphylococcus aureus*
  - o *Legionella*
- **Viral**: Cause almost one-third of pneumonias:
  - o Influenza virus
  - o Rhinoviruses
- **Other pathogens**:
  - o Fungal
  - o *Histoplasma*
  - o *Cryptococcus*

The most common exposure to these organisms or cause is in the community. Less common but typically more severe and devastating are the nosocomial (HAP, HCAP, VAP) causes associated with hospitalization, health care providers, and ventilator use, as more of these organisms have developed resistance to multiple antibiotics.

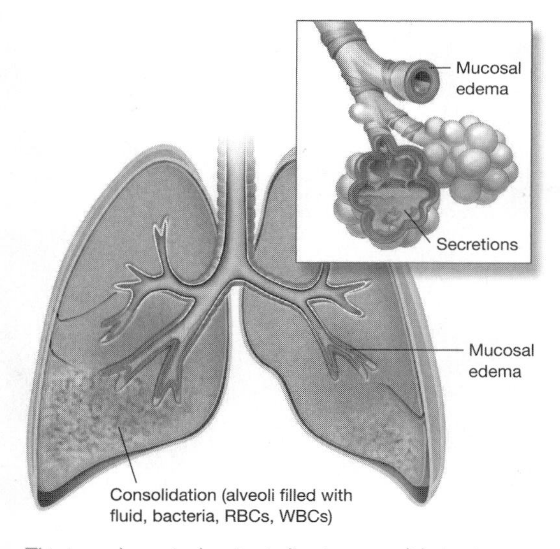

This is a schematic drawing indicating consolidation in the lower lobe of the right lung with a diagnosis of lobar pneumonia.

Comparison: Community-Acquired Pneumonia (CAP), Hospital AP (HAP) & Ventilator AP (VAP)

	CAP	HAP**	VAP
Origin	Community	In hospital or long-term care facility	On ventilator
Time of onset	Before hospitalization	≥48 hours after hospitalization	Early: ≥48 hours on ventilator Late: ≥5 days on ventilator
Incidence	Common; rising	Common; rising	9–27% on ventilators
Risk factors	Age: very young & older Comorbidities (HIV, lung, cardiac, renal) Immunosuppressed Substance abuse (drugs, alcohol, smoking) Prior antibiotics	Critically ill and in ICU Immunosuppressed Poorly controlled diabetes Aspiration Inadequate mouth care Hospitalization >2 days Invasive procedures Long-term care facility Exposure to MDR Older Alcohol abuse	**On ventilator** **On steroids** Re-intubation COPD Emergency surgery Coma Immunosuppressed Tube feedings Tracheostomy Prior antibiotics
Most common pathogens that cause pneumonia	Strep pneumoniae Myco pneumoniae H influenzae Chlamyd pneumoniae Legionella sp Respiratory viruses	ICU: S pneumoniae, S aureus, Legionella sp, Gram neg bacilli, H influenzae Multidrug resistant organisms	**Pseudomonas aerug** Gram neg bacilli MRSA Staph aureus Acinetobacter Multidrug resistant organisms
Clinical presentation (all similar)	Fever and chills Dyspnea, tachypnea Crackles & wheezes	Cough Sputum, discolored Malaise	Hemoptysis Nausea, vomiting Pleuritic pain, worsens with cough

MDR = multidrug resistance

**Healthcare-associated pneumonia (HCAP) is very similar to HAP except that patients have not been hospitalized but have had extensive health care provider exposure.

Assessment Findings

Symptoms of pneumonia can range from mild to severe. Common symptoms of the various pneumonias include:

- High fever (present in the majority of patients)
- Tachypnea and dyspnea
- Tachycardia
- Productive cough: Sputum is usually thick and yellow, green, or brown colored.
- Pleuritic chest pain (sharp pain may increase with inspiration)
- Fatigue
- Chills
- Abnormal lung sounds: crackles and, possibly, wheezing
- Headache, muscle aches, joint pains
- Nausea

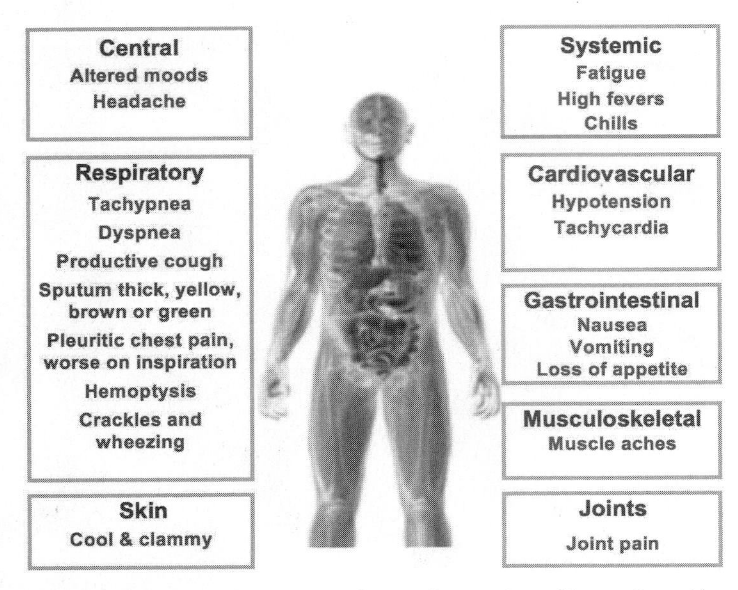

This image lists the various symptoms that may be experienced by a patient with pneumonia with lines indicating the organs and body parts affected.

Assessment Findings That Should Trigger Concerns About Sepsis

The following findings should elicit serious concern and vigilance. However, a combination of the following reveals an urgent deterioration. The clinician should alert the physician about these distinctive signs that warn of developing sepsis:

- Markedly elevated white blood cell count (15–30/mm)
- Rigors (shaking chills)
- Elevated lactate
- Hypotension (septic shock), especially when unresponsive to IV fluids
- Metabolic acidosis and/or low bicarbonate levels
- Altered mental status (from patient's baseline)

These patients need to be triaged or transferred into a more closely monitored level of care.

Geriatric Considerations

The signs and symptoms in geriatric patients may differ somewhat from a healthier or younger patient population. They may exhibit blunted responses, for instance, they:

- May not exhibit fever
- Tend to have faster respiratory rate
- Experience a higher mortality rate due to comorbid conditions
- May present with altered mental status or unexplained fall

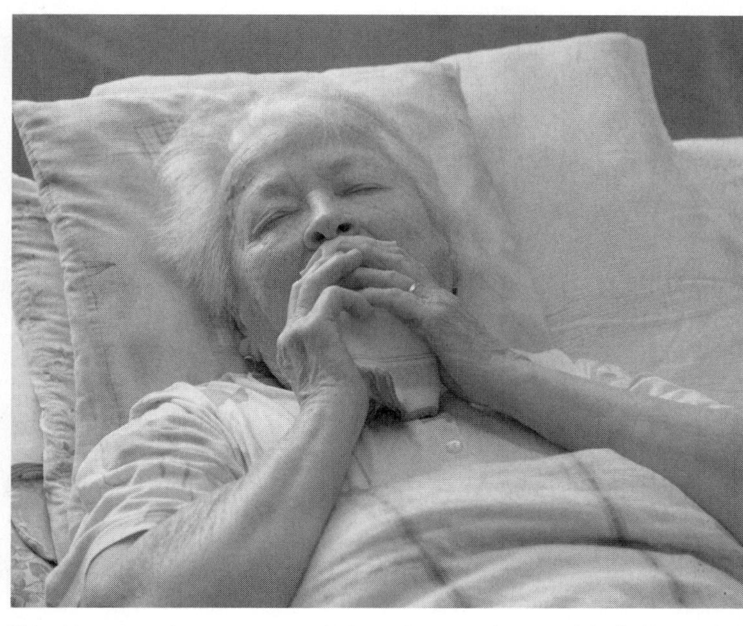

This older woman has pneumonia, which may be a complication of the flu. Pneumonia in an elder can be life threatening, from the infection itself or from the multiple organ involvement that can ensue.
Source: vbaleha/Fotolia

Diagnostics

- Clinical signs and symptoms provide the clinician with early warning signals to suspect the presence of pneumonia.
- Sputum culture—these cultures need to be obtained as soon as possible and, ideally, before beginning antibiotic therapy.
  - o Although sputum culture results take days (except for newer types of cultures), cultures should be obtained prior to antibiotic initiation in order to avoid masking the organism responsible for the pneumonia.
  - o In patients who are not improving or with unusual presentation, cultures and biopsy can be obtained with bronchoscopy (see animation).
- Blood cultures may also be obtained.
- Infiltrate on chest x-ray is the first real diagnostic criteria for a pneumonia.

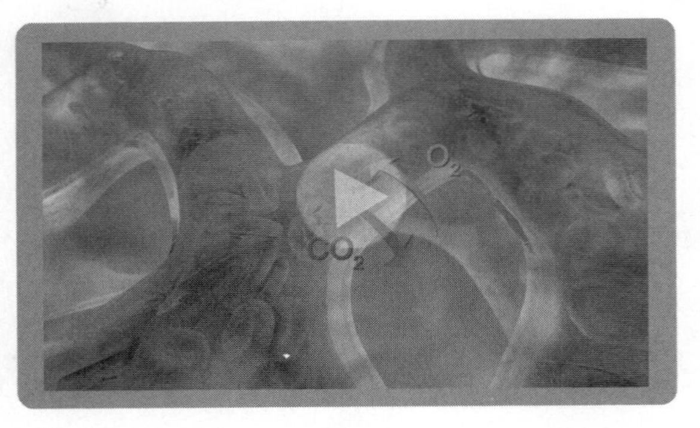

This animation explains a bronchoscopy procedure. A scope is inserted through the trachea to diagnose pulmonary problems.
Source: © 2013 Nucleus Medical Media, All rights reserved

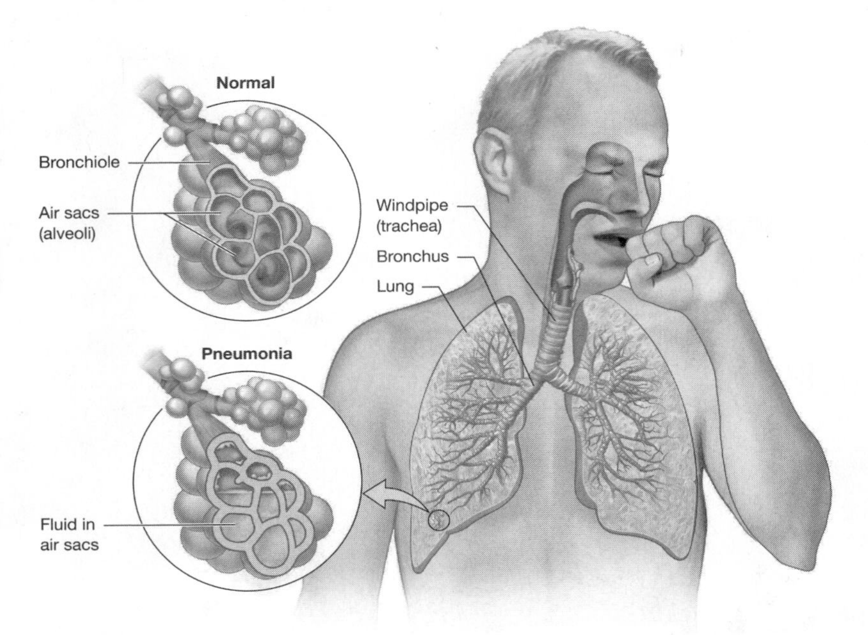

The man has pneumonia with severe coughing and fluid (pus) in his alveoli. The pus severely impairs tissue oxygenation.

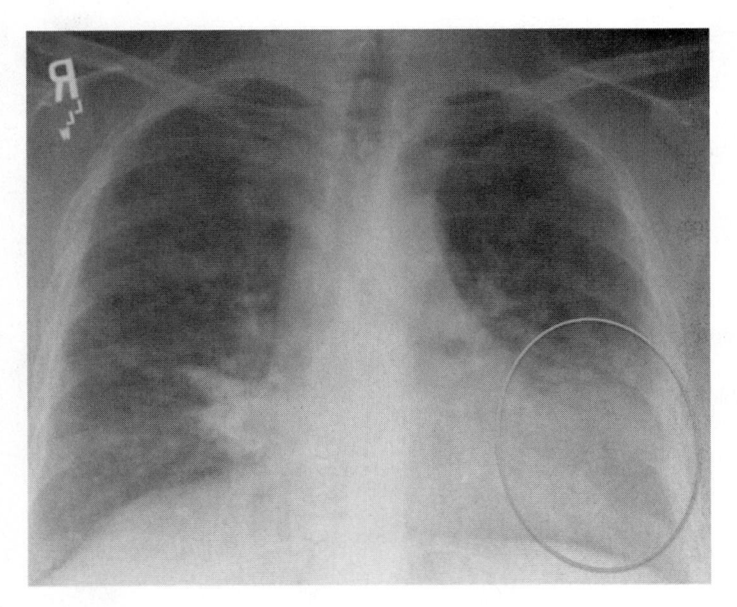

The chest x-ray shows an area of inflammation (circle) indicating the presence and location of pneumonia.
Source: Courtesy of K. Kyriakidis

Concept Check

3. Which diagnostic procedure is often indicated when a patient diagnosed with pneumonia is not showing improvement?

A. CBC

B. Dip stick of urine

C. Bronchoscopy

D. Open biopsy

Answer question

Priority Patient Concerns and Desired Collaborative Care Outcomes

Prior to caring for patients with pneumonia, it is important to prioritize the patient's concerns that must guide the nursing care plan and interventions. Care for the patient is ordered and organized in accordance with the patient's priority and urgent needs. Desired collaborative care outcomes in patients with pneumonia typically include:

1. Patient's oxygen saturation and mentation will return to pre-illness level.
2. Patient will expectorate secretions without difficulty and sound clear to auscultation.
3. Patient will tolerate usual pre-illness level of activity without distress.
4. Patient will develop no complications, have pre-illness vital signs, and sputum and blood cultures if done are pathogen free.

Considering these important care outcomes, prepare a list of the major 3–6 priority patient concerns or nursing diagnoses for patients with pneumonia. Be prepared to participate in a discussion of this list and/or to submit them as an assignment, as determined by your faculty. Resources you may find helpful in this assignment can include this lesson, the references, resources on nursing care plans, and standard nursing diagnoses manuals.

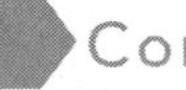

Concept Check

4. Which outcome is appropriate to guide therapy for a patient who has pneumonia?

A. The patient will tolerate the pre-illness level of activity.

B. The patient will be able to walk two blocks without shortness of breath.

C. The patient's respiratory rate will not increase with activity.

D. The patient will have clear mentation.

Answer question

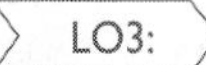

LO3:

Collaborative Interventions

Overview

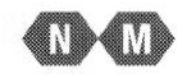

- Timely recognition of pneumonia is essential, especially in "at-risk" populations like older adults and those with comorbidities (e.g., immunosuppressed, COPD, diabetes).

- Most CAP can be treated as an outpatient with oral antibiotics. However, the patient is hospitalized if extenuating circumstances exist, for instance:
    - o Severe illness
    - o Inability for oral intake
    - o History or concern for noncompliance with meds
    - o Cognitive impairment, poor functional status, lack of support at home

CAP Performance Measures for Inpatients

- Performance measures for CAP have been derived from evidence-based practice and are required in the care of patients by the Centers for Medicare and Medicaid Services (CMS). These are often referred to as "core measures."
- Significant financial penalties and hospital reimbursement are tied to meeting these core measures in specifically named diagnoses, CAP as one.

Core measures include:

- Blood cultures: Prior to administration of antibiotics (ATB), if obtained in the ED
  - o Required for all ICU patients
  - o Optional for non ICU patients
- Antibiotic administration within 6 hours
- Empirical antibiotics according to guidelines
- Measurement of blood gases or pulse oximetry—Although this requirement has been dropped due to high compliance, it should be performed.
- Assessment or administration of pneumococcal and influenza vaccines
- Smoking cessation counseling

Evidence-Based Practices (EBP)

The main evidence-based treatment for pneumonia is antibiotics.

Although antibiotics are ordered only by health care professionals with prescriptive licenses (e.g., physicians, nurse practitioners), nurses hold responsibility for ensuring that patients receive urgent and essential treatments, like antibiotics for pneumonia. The development of advocacy and collaboration skills is essential to ensuring excellent patient care.

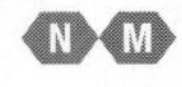

1. Mandell, L.A., Wunderink, R. G., Anzueto, A., et al. (2007). Infectious Disease Society of America/ American Thoracic Society consensus guidelines on the management of community-acquired pneumonia in adults. *Clin Infect Dis*, *44*, S27–S72.
2. Burman, M. E., & Wright, W. L. (2007). Diagnosis and Management of Community-Acquired Pneumonia: Evidence-Based Practice. *The Journal for Nurse Practitioners*, 633–649.

Evidence-Based Prevention

- Oral hygiene every 1–3 hours (discussed further)
- Vaccine for pneumonia in any patient at risk. Vaccine for influenza carries relatively equal importance because pneumonia is a common complication of influenza.

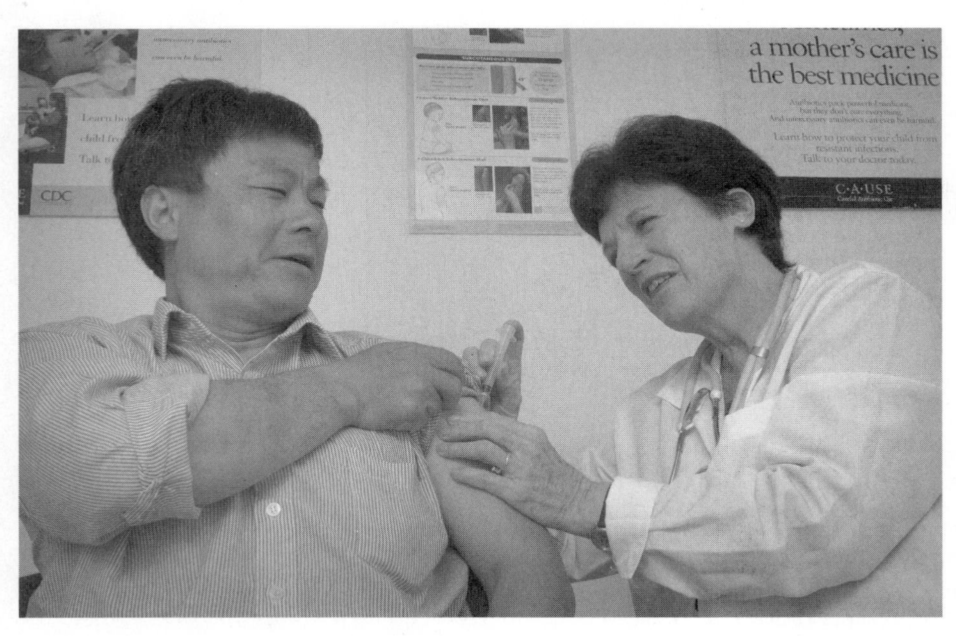

Pneumonia and flu vaccines offer greater protection against pneumonia and influenza than good hand washing, hygiene, and antiseptic technique alone can provide, particularly in infants and older adults.
Source: CDC/Judy Schmidt

Specific Antibiotics Treatment

Knowing specific antibiotics is usually not in the nurse's scope of practice. Advanced practice nurses who prescribe medications must know specific antibiotics. However, there are two key points that most nurses need to know about treatment of pneumonia and integrate into their practice:

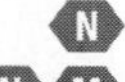

1. Patients should start on antibiotics as quickly as possible.
2. Certain patients are at higher risk for developing infection with multidrug-resistant (MDR) organisms, (e.g., pseudomonas, MRSA):
   - Patients treated with antibiotics in the past 3 months
   - Immunocompromised patients (e.g., chemotherapy, HIV, splenectomy)
   - Recent hospitalization, especially if the hospital has high MDR rates
   - Pneumonia acquired in the hospital
   - Admitted from chronic care facility
   - Critically ill patients

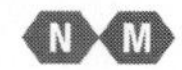

- These groups of patients usually need broader antibiotic coverage that target drug-resistant organisms such as MRSA and pseudomonas.

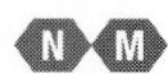

- Generally, there is a lower risk for MDR organisms in CAP unless the patient was recently on antibiotics.

Concept Check

5. **A patient admitted to the emergency department is diagnosed with community-acquired pneumonia (CAP) and will be started on antibiotic therapy once sputum specimens are obtained. Which statement in the patient's history places this patient at greatest risk for having a multiple drug resistance organism?**

A. The patient has recently traveled out of state.

B. The patient just took antibiotics for a tooth abscess.

C. The patient is vegetarian.

D. The patient lives in a large metropolitan area.

Answer question

Collaborative Interventions (continued)

Examples

Antibiotics in Hospitalized Patients for CAP

The following are examples of antibiotic treatment options. Other options may also exist as no national standard is universally accepted. While the following is a common approach to antibiotic administration, hospitals can apply their own guidelines:

Option 1—most common for community-acquired pneumonia

- Ceftriaxone—1 g IVPB q 24 hrs
- Azithromycin—500 mg IVPB q 24 hrs

Option 2—if beta lactam (ceftriaxone) allergy:

- Moxifloxacin—400 mg IVPB q 24 hrs

Option 3—if pseudomonas risk is present:

- Piperacillin/tazobactam—4.5 g IVPB PLUS
- Fluoroquinolone (e.g., ciprofloxacin)—400 mg IVPB q 8 hrs

Option 4—If methicillin-resistant staph (MRSA) is possible, then add vancomycin.

Antibiotics for *Hospital-Acquired* Pneumonia (HAP)

Treatment recommendations commonly focus on antibiotic classifications or categories. Different hospitals vary but below are examples of treatment that can be anticipated:

Option 1—most common:

- Piperacillin/tazobactam—4.5 g IVPB PLUS
- Fluoroquinolone (e.g., ciprofloxacin)—400 mg IVPB q 8 hrs
- Vancomycin

Option 2—if beta lactam allergy:

- Fluoroquinolone (e.g., ciprofloxacin)—400 mg IVPB q 8 hrs PLUS
- Vancomycin PLUS
- Aztreonam—2 g IVPB q 8 hrs

Option 3—if beta lactam allergy and suspected aspiration:

- Clindamycin—900 mg IVPB q 8 hrs OR
- Vancomycin PLUS
- Aztreonam—2 g IVPB q 8 hrs

Duration of Antibiotic Therapy

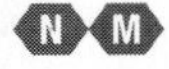

- Antibiotics should be administered for a minimum of 5 days, if afebrile for 48–72 hours, for core pathogens:
  - o Core pathogens are *H. influenzae*, *Strep pneumoniae*, *Enterobacteriaceae* and *Staph aureus*.
  - o Longer for other pathogens (e.g., multidrug-resistant organisms) or evidence of extrapulmonary infection
- M Procalcitonin can also be used to guide the length of antibiotic therapy.
  - o If the procalcitonin level has returned to normal, antibiotics can be safely discontinued.

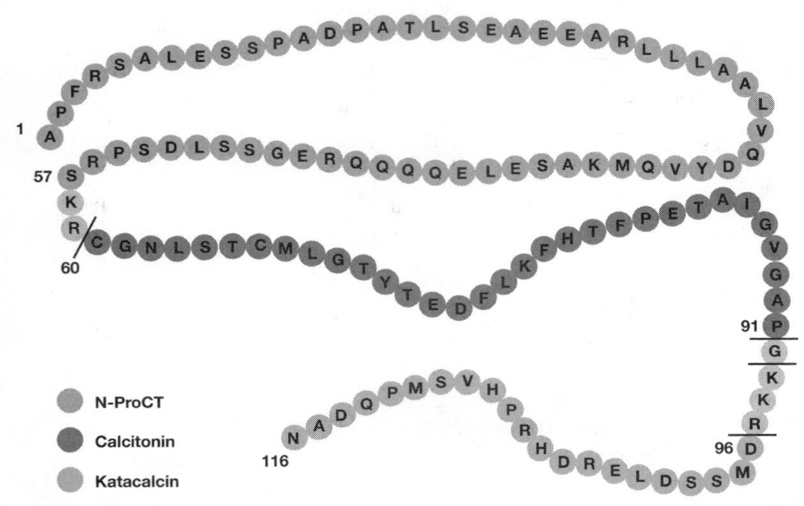

This image represents the chemical structure of procalcitonin. Procalcitonin is composed of three sections: the amino terminus (N-ProCT), immature calcitonin, and katacalcin.

Procalcitonin in Antibiotic Administration

- Procalcitonin increases in the presence of a bacterial infection.
- Normal values are less than 0.1 ng/mL.
  - o Levels less than 0.1 indicate antibiotics are not indicated or not necessary.
  - o Levels less than 0.5 ng/mL may be physiologically normal.

- The key action is to use procalcitonin in a patient with pneumonia as a guide to the timing of antibiotic withdrawal.
  - o If the procalcitonin level is decreasing, then the pneumonia is resolving.

Concept Check

6. The patient has been treated with antibiotics for community-acquired pneumonia. The nurse is aware that antibiotics can be discontinued when which condition exists?

A. The patient has been afebrile for 24 hours.

B. The patient's white blood cell count is normal.

C. The patient has been taking the antibiotics for 10 days.

D. The patient's procalcitonin level is normal.

Answer question

Transition from IV to Oral Antibiotics

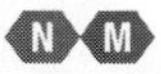

Signs of patient improvement guide the transition from an IV to an oral antibiotic. All healthcare team members should track and initiate team discussion when the majority of the following improvements are noted:

- SpO_2 greater than 92%
- Temperature less than 38°C
- Pulse less than 100 beats per min
- Respirations less than 24 per min
- Able to take oral medications
- Normal procalcitonin level

Collaborative Interventions (continued)

Vaccinations

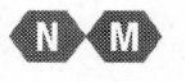

Vaccinations for pneumonia prevention are known as pneumococcal polysaccharide vaccine, PPSV23, or Pneumovax.

Vaccination for pneumonia is recommended for any person with risk factors for pneumonia, particularly:

- Patients who are immunosuppressed (low WBC, HIV infection, blood cancers, transplant patients)
- People over 65 years old
- Adults with chronic conditions, including:
  - o Heart failure
  - o COPD and asthma
  - o Diabetes mellitus
  - o Alcoholism
  - o Chronic liver disease
  - o Cigarette smoking
  - o Sickle cell disease
  - o Chronic renal failure, especially those on dialysis
- The risk is so great and the success in prevention is so strong that many hospitals initiate the vaccination prior to discharge per protocol.

Vaccine Administration

- Pneumococcal vaccine is administered intramuscularly as a 0.5 mL dose.

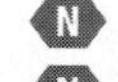

- Warning: Never administer the vaccine intradermally. It can cause severe local reactions.

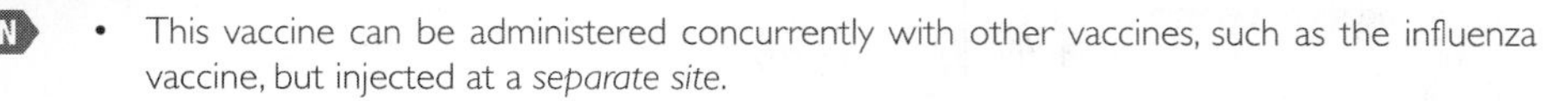

- This vaccine can be administered concurrently with other vaccines, such as the influenza vaccine, but injected at a *separate site*.

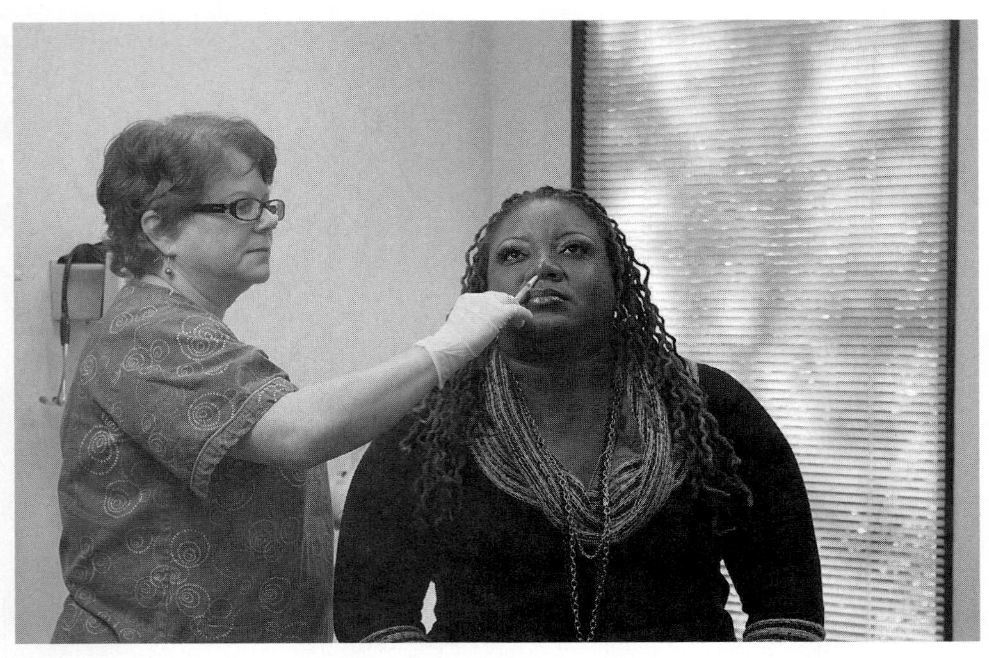

This patient is being immunized with the pneumococcal vaccine.
Source: Douglas Jordan, M.D./Center for Disease Control (CDC)–PHIL

VAP Prevention and Associated Complications

Prevention is one of the most important nursing responsibilities in a ventilated patient, as VAP is preventable. The point is emphasized by insurers who no longer reimburse hospitals when this complication occurs in patients.

N M
- The key to avoiding VAP is to avoid intubation. Use noninvasive ventilation (e.g., BiPap) if possible. If mechanical ventilation is required, progress to extubation as soon as possible.

N
- Perform or encourage oral hygiene every 1–3 hours to keep mucous membranes moist to prevent aspiration of pathogenic microorganisms.
  - **a.** Chan, E.Y., Ruest, A., Meade, M. O., & Cook, D. J. (2007). Oral decontamination for prevention of pneumonia in mechanically ventilated adults: systematic review and meta-analysis, *BMJ, 334*(7599), 889.
  - **b.** Munro, C. L, Grap, M. J., Jones, D. J., McClish, D. K., & Sessler, C. N., (2009). Chlorhexidine, toothbrushing and preventing ventilator-associated pneumonia in critically ill adults. *American Journal of Critical Care, 18(5),* 428–437.

N
- Ensure good hand hygiene and aseptic technique whenever managing the mechanical ventilator.

N
- Keep the head of bed elevated greater than 30 degrees to avoid aspiration.

N
- Mobilize the patient as early and as much as possible to prevent "never events" such as VAP spread, pressure ulcers, deep vein thrombosis, and muscle wasting. If immobile, vigilantly turn, cough, and deep breath on a schedule. Allow undisturbed rest periods throughout the day to reduce metabolic demand, promote healing, minimize sleep deprivation complications, and restore patient's energy reserves.
- Vigilance in monitoring the patient for increased work of breathing, changes in lung sounds, complaints or presence of dypsnea, and any early warning sign that may indicate impending respiratory failure. Additionally, sepsis is a common, life-threatening, and often unrecognized complication of pneumonia and carries a high mortality rate. Monitor for mental status, hemodynamic, and lactate level changes that warn of sepsis because, currently, most patients with an infection who are sick enough to be hospitalized are at risk for sepsis and life-threatening septic shock.

N
- Implement or provide leadership to implement "never event" preventive measures in all very ill patients:
  - o Initiate intermittent, sequential compression device to prevent DVT and pulmonary embolism.
  - o Remove indwelling urinary catheter at the earliest possible time. Evaluate need daily.
  - o Remove central venous catheter at the earliest possible time to prevent air embolism and vascular infections.
  - o Monitor blood sugars to maintain glycermic control.
  - o Implement fall precautions in at risk patients.
  - o Mobilize the patient early and often, as above.

Collaborative Interventions (continued)

Collaborative Symptom Management

There are numerous symptom-management interventions in patients with pneumonia that can help make them more comfortable when indicated, including:

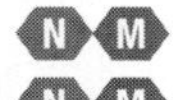

- Oxygen therapy for SpO_2 less than or equal to 92%
- Bronchodilators for wheezing
    - o Single bronchodilators or bronchodilators used in combination can help patients breathe more comfortably.
    - o Bronchodilators used in combination (DuoNeb, which is a combination of albuterol + atrovent) to keep airways open.

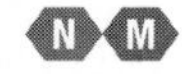

- Antipyretics (acetaminophen [Tylenol], ibuprofen [Advil]) when fever more than 101°F for patient comfort.

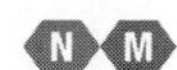

- Fluid intake to 2–3 L daily as long as heart failure is not present.

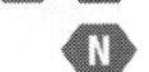

- Caution with caffeinated beverages (e.g., coffee, tea, colas) as these have diuretic effects and may enhance dehydration.

- Incentive spirometer to improve deep breathing. An incentive spirometer is a device that encourages patients to breathe deeply.

- Acapella (mucous clearance device) and/or chest vest therapy to mobilize secretion.

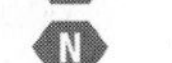

- Suctioning secretions when patients are unable to clear their airway.

Suctioning

- There are no evidence-based guidelines for suctioning a patient.
- Suctioning is designed to remove secretions that the patient cannot clear by coughing.
- One guideline is to suction the patient based on auscultation of the lungs when secretions are heard in the major airways, particularly when the inability to clear secretions increases the work of breathing.
- Suctioning is very unpleasant for most patients and should be avoided when possible.
    - o Keep in mind that suctioning cannot reach much beyond the carina. The major benefit of suctioning may be to help stimulate a cough reflex (when the catheter touches the carina).
    - o Using a suction catheter to reach the trachea is difficult, unless the patient is intubated. The catheter will have a tendency to go into the esophagus rather than the trachea.
    - o If suctioning is successful, the airways will sound clear and the pulse oximeter will increase (although initially the SpO_2 may decrease).

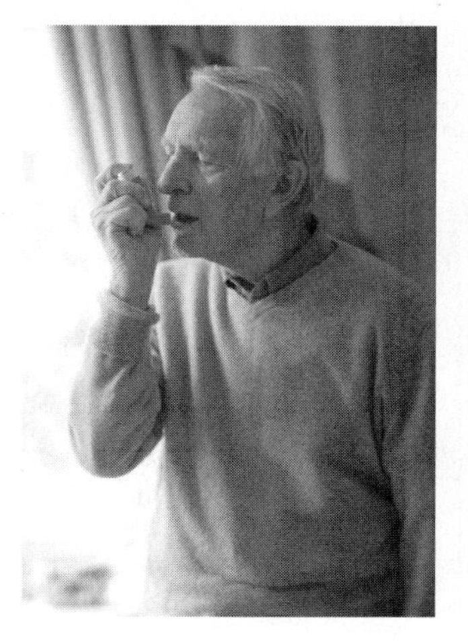

The inhaler is used to deliver a bronchodilator that can improve breathing and oxygenation. Bronchodilators also assist in expectorating secretions, reducing airway obstruction, and alleviating bronchospasm. Each improves oxygenation.
Source: Science Photo Library/Getty Images

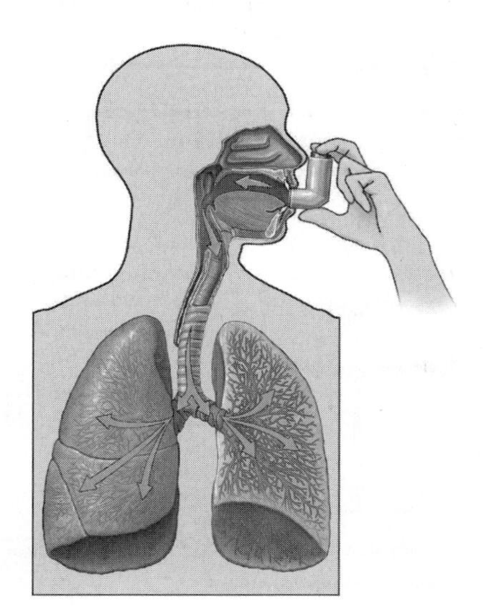

Use of an inhaler (mucous clearance device) can help mobilize secretions for the patient to clear more easily.
Source: © 2013 Nucleus Medical Media. All rights reserved

Patient Education

- Instruct patients, family members and staff to perform frequent hand washing in order to prevent spread of infection and bacteria.
- Instruct patients about the importance of compliance with prescribed medications, particularly antibiotics:
    - Take only the prescribed dose.
    - Take medication for the prescribed time period.
    - Complete the full antibiotic course unless problems arise.
    - Report problems with medications to health care provider (HCP).
- Some HCPs may continue to teach patient and families about postural drainage to utilize gravity and assist with secretion clearance if patients can tolerate it, but some contraindications and poor patient compliance have motivated alternative therapy development.
- Ambulate as often as tolerated to maintain or improve muscle compliance and functional abilities.
- Allow for periods of rest between ambulation exercises to minimize oxygen demands, fatigue and dyspnea, especially in older adults.

Concept Check

7. A nurse is providing discharge instructions to the wife of a husband diagnosed with pneumonia. The husband's treatment will occur at home. What information should be included in this teaching?

A. Allow the husband to be as active as tolerated.

B. Encourage the husband to be up in the chair at the bedside.

C. Keep the husband on bed rest until there is no fever.

Answer question

Summary of Interventions

- The key aspects of treating and preventing pneumonia include:
    - Administer the vaccine to those at risk.
    - Nursing—symptom management and comfort care such as good oral care and keeping the head of the bed at 30–45 degrees to prevent ventilator-associated pneumonia.
- Once a pneumonia is present:
    - Administer antibiotics immediately, ideally after sputum and blood cultures are obtained.
    - Cultures should be obtained as soon as possible and certainly no longer than 4 hours after admission.
    - Administer oxygen when appropriate. If unresponsive or response is inadequate, initiate BiPAP.
    - Provide symptom relief, such as the administration of bronchodilators for shortness of breath or antipyretic for fever.

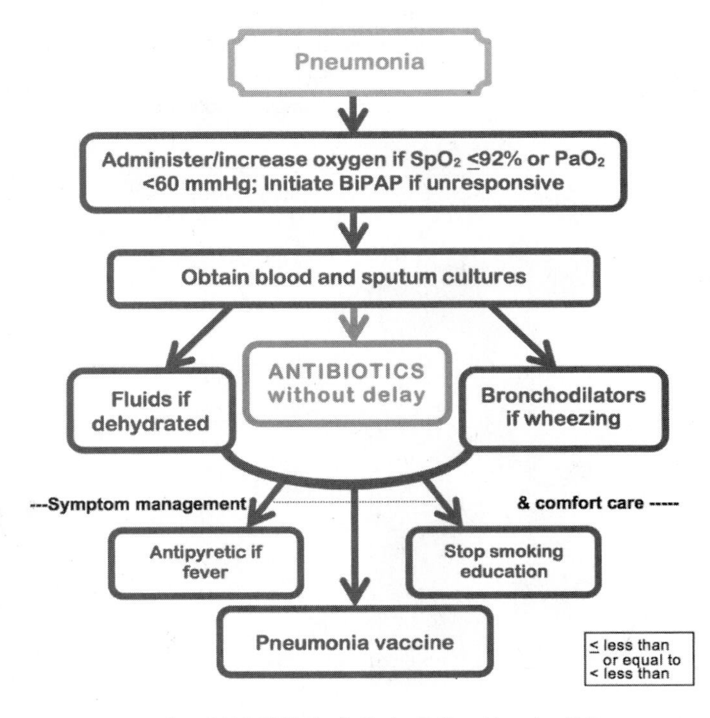
Pneumonia
Administer/increase oxygen if $SpO_2 \leq 92\%$ or PaO_2 <60 mmHg; Initiate BiPAP if unresponsive
Obtain blood and sputum cultures
Fluids if dehydrated
ANTIBIOTICS without delay
Bronchodilators if wheezing
---Symptom management
& comfort care -----
Antipyretic if fever
Stop smoking education
Pneumonia vaccine
≤ less than or equal to
< less than
Copyright © 2013, NovEx Novice To Expert Learning, LLC

Source: Copyright © 2012, NovEx Novice to Expert Learning, LLC

LO4:

Evaluation of Desired Collaborative Care Outcomes

Evaluation and reassessment should reveal attainment of previously established patient outcomes. In summary:

- The patient should exhibit no cyanosis or pallor, have a normal oxygen saturation, and mentation that is unchanged from pre-illness level.
- Patient expectorates secretions without difficulty and lungs are clear to auscultation.
- Patient tolerates usual pre-illness level of activity and has no complaint of excessive fatigue.
- The patient's vital signs and white blood cell count are at pre-illness state, there are no complications, and sputum and blood cultures are pathogen free.

References

http://www.ncbi.nlm.nih.gov/pubmed/11049791

http://journal.publications.chestnet.org/article.aspx?articleID=1081684

http://cid.oxfordjournals.org/content/31/4/1066.full

http://www.nhlbi.nih.gov/health/dci/Diseases/pnu/pnu_signsandsymptoms.html

Buckley, L. L., Schub, T., & Pravikoff D. (2013, July). Pneumonia in older adults. *Cinahl Information Systems.*

Burman, M. E., & Wright, W. L. (2007, October). Diagnosis and Management of Community-Acquired Pneumonia: Evidence-Based Practice. *The Journal for Nurse Practitioners*, 633–649.

Chan, E.Y., Ruest, A., Meade, M. O., & Cook, D. J. (2007). Oral decontamination for prevention of pneumonia in mechanically ventilated adults: systematic review and meta-analysis. *BMJ, 334* (7599), 889.

Munro, C. L., Grap, M. J., Jones, D. J., McClish, D. K., & Sessler, C. N., (2009). Chorhexidine, toothbrushing and preventing ventilator associated peneumonai in critically ill adults. *American Journal of Critical Care, 18*(5), 428–437.

Nair, G. B., & Niederman, M. S. (2001, November). Community acquired pneumonia: an unfinished battle. *Med Clin North Am, 95*(6), 1143–1161

Schuetz, P., Muller, B., Christ-Crain, M., Stolz, D., Tamm, M., Bouadma, L., Luyt, C. E., Wolff, M., Chastre, J., Tubach, F., Kristoffersen, K. B., Burkhardt, O., Welte, T., Schroeder, S., Nobre, V., Wei, L., Bhatnagar, N., Bucher, H. C., & Briel, M. (2013, July). Procalcitonin to initiate or discontinue antibiotics in acute respiratory tract infections. *Evid Based Child Health, 8*(4), 1297–1371

Practice Guidelines

American Thoracic Society. (2005, February) Infectious Diseases Society of America: Guidelines for the management of adults with hospital-acquired, ventilator-associated, and healthcare-associated pneumonia. *Am J Respir Crit Care Med, 171*, 388.

Mandell, L. A., Wunderink, R. G., Anzueto, A., et al. (2007). Infectious Disease Society of America/American Thoracic Society consensus guidelines on the management of community-acquired pneumonia in adults. *Clin Infect Dis, 44*, S27–S72.

Learning Outcomes for Influenza

When you complete this lesson, you will be able to:

1. Recognize the clinical relevance of influenza.
2. Consider the pathophysiology, etiology, risk factors, and clinical presentation of influenza that determine the priority patient concerns.
3. Determine the most urgent and important nursing interventions and patient education required in caring for a patient with influenza.
4. Evaluate attainment of desired collaborative care outcomes for a patient with influenza.

LO1:

What Is Influenza?

- Influenza is a respiratory illness caused by influenza A or B viruses that result in seasonal outbreaks worldwide.
- Responses to the infection vary from mild to severe.
- Influenza can be serious enough that it leads to hospitalization and possible death.

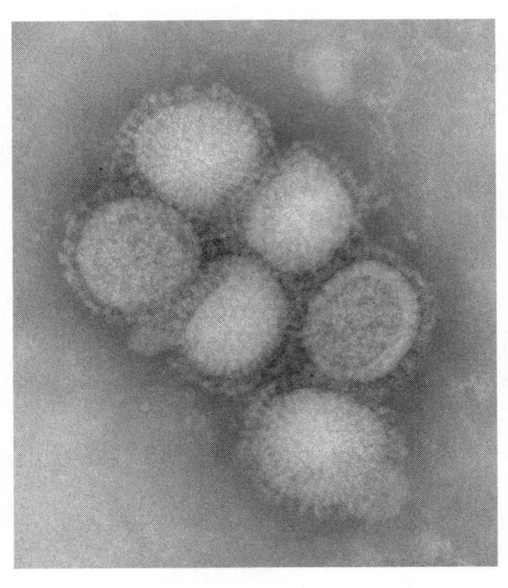

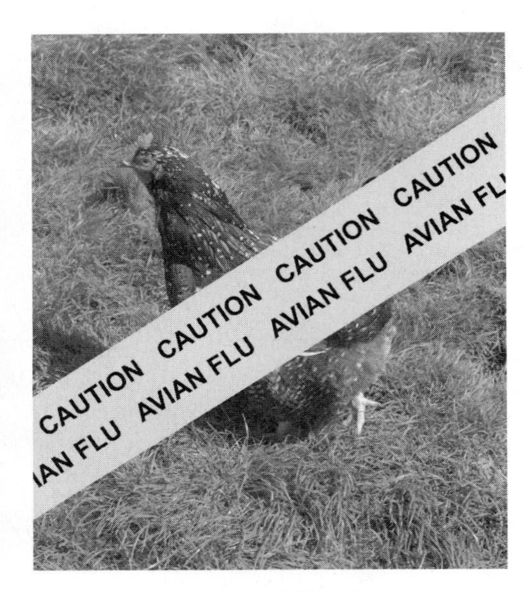

Left: The new swine flu (H1N1) influenza virus first appeared in the United States in April 2009 and became a worldwide pandemic. Viruses mutate quickly, as did this one, from a nonpathogenic strain to one that is virulent to humans. Right: Viruses have been known to mutate from pigs, birds, and other animals. Here, chickens are being destroyed after a harmful strain was discovered.
Source: (*left*) CDC/C.S. Goldsmith and A. Balish; (*right*) CS-Stock/Alamy

LO1:

Clinical Relevance

- Yearly deaths from influenza have ranged from 4,000 to 49,000.
- A large number of people are infected every year. In 2009, for example, 43–89 million people in the United States became ill with the H1N1 (swine) influenza.
- Enormous amounts of work hours are lost due to the severity of the disease and the number of people who contract it.
- It is easily preventable with vaccinations.
- The Centers for Disease Control and Prevention (CDC), along with the World Health Organization (WHO) and its reporting network, track positive test reports on influenza that occur worldwide. By monitoring disease activity, they predict target viruses for the annual influenza vaccine.
    - o Information is available at www.cdc.gov/flu/weekly/.

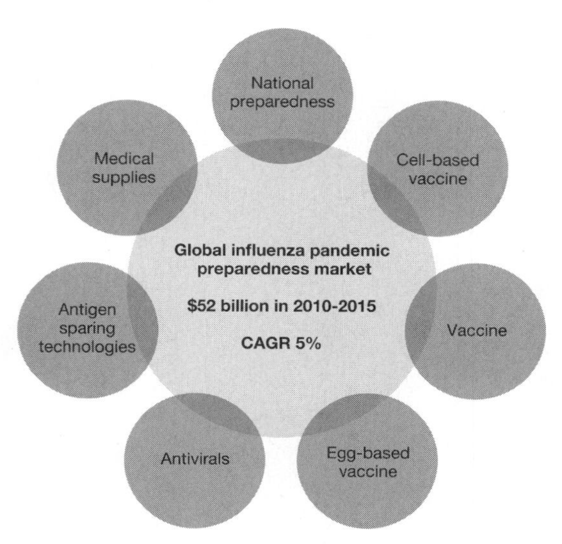

Due to recent flu outbreaks, the cost of preparedness for global influenza has tripled. Costs are expected to be about $10 billion in 2015.

LO2:

Pathophysiology

Influenza viruses infect the host by entering through the respiratory system. The viral infection causes both systemic and pulmonary effects within a short time period.

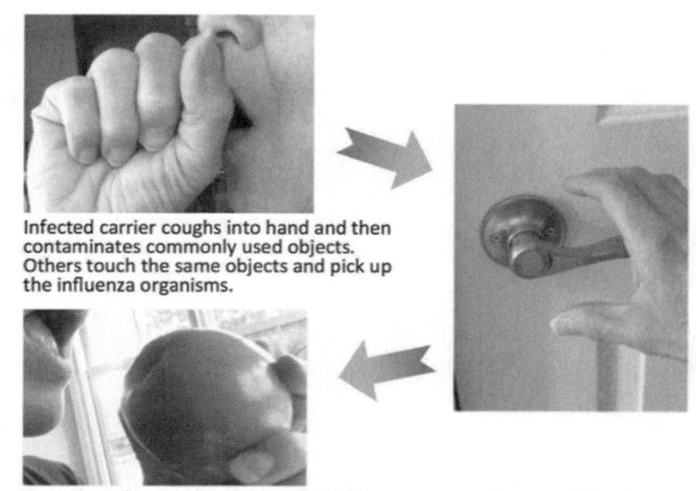

Infected carrier coughs into hand and then contaminates commonly used objects. Others touch the same objects and pick up the influenza organisms.
Once the influenza virus is transferred to an unsuspecting person hand, hand to mouth or mucous membranes inoculation is common. This is a common cycle for spread of infection.

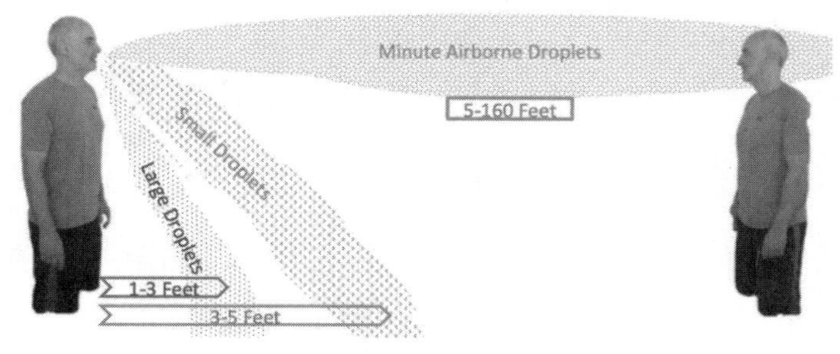

Transmission of viruses has multiple routes. Upper: Most people are familiar with direct routes (hands). Lower: Infectious droplets, however, have tremendous "reach." Covering the mouth and staying home when sick are important.

Source: (*both*) Copyright © 2012, NovEx Novice to Expert Learning, LLC

Concept Check

1. Which statement about influenza is true?

A. Influenza is a bacterial infection spread via food and water supply.

B. Influenza is a viral infection that enters the body via the respiratory system.

C. Influenza can be easily treated with antibiotics, fluids, and rest.

D. Influenza is dangerous because there are no effective methods of prevention.

Answer question

Influenza Transmission

- Large viral loads (or large numbers of the virus) of influenza are often present in respiratory secretions of infected persons. The virus can be spread in two ways:
  1. Aerosolized droplets carrying the virus are produced when an infected person coughs, expectorates, or sneezes. These droplets can then enter the respiratory track of another person.
  2. The flu can also enter a person through the mucocutaneous (e.g., eye, nose, mouth) route or by coming in contact with the virus (e.g., handshake, infected surface).
- The length of time the virus can survive on a surface varies. It can survive for 1–2 days on hard, nonporous surfaces (e.g., plastic, metal), about 15 minutes on dry paper tissues, and only 5 minutes on skin.
- Sunlight rapidly destroys the virus. For this reason, flu viruses may survive better in winter months due to the low humidity and less exposure to sunlight.
- Influenza viruses have proteins on the surface that bind to receptors in the respiratory system. These proteins determine what part of the respiratory tract they infect, as well as what species they infect (i.e., bird, pig, or human).

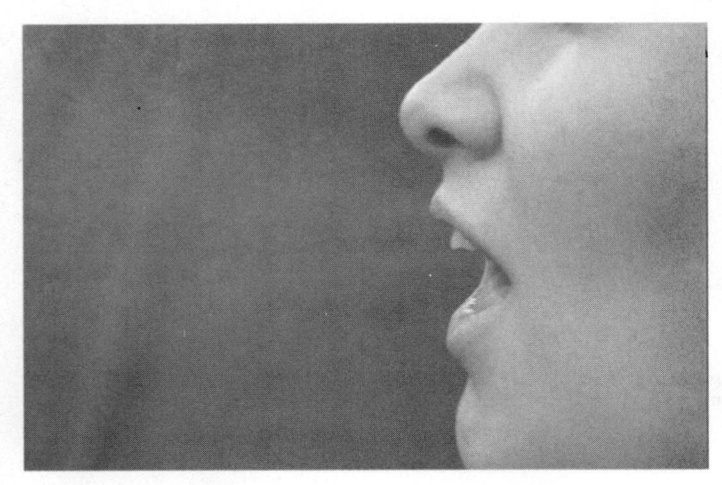

Viral transmission via cough.

Concept Check

2. What is an important measure to take to prevent the spread of influenza?

A. Opening windows to improve ventilation

B. Exposing infected patients to sunlight

C. Use of anti-inflammatory agents

D. Hand washing

Answer question

Pathophysiology (continued)

Replication

- Influenza viral proteins can mutate at times, allowing swine (pig) flu and avian (bird) flu viruses to infect humans.
- As seen in the animation, after attaching to the receptors, the virus invades the host cell and begins to replicate.
- Viruses must find a live host because they can only replicate within living tissues.
- Following replication, newly generated virus exits the host cell.
- Medications used to treat the flu attack the virus by inhibiting replication.

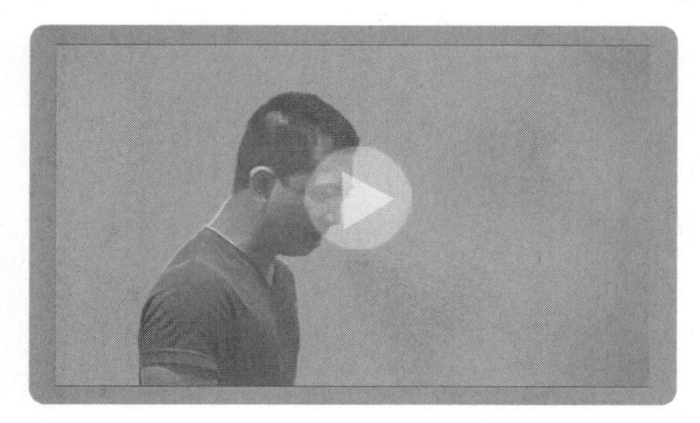

This animation describes influenza as a virus, transmission, clinical presentation, pathophysiology, treatment, and prevention.
Source: © 2013 Nucleus Medical Media, All rights reserved

- The systemic symptoms (headaches, fatigue, and fever) that are most common in influenza can result from one of two mechanisms:
  1. The body's inflammatory response and release of large amounts of chemokines and cytokines by macrophages.
  2. Viral replication is so enormous that the symptoms result from the inflammatory response to the huge amounts of cytokines produced in response to the infected cells.
- The incubation time (2–4 days) is the time between exposure and symptom development. Once infected, a person becomes infectious and begins to shed the virus 2 days before the onset of symptoms. The person usually can continue to shed the virus for one week. Immunocompromised patients may shed the virus for longer period of time (up to 3 weeks). The human body eventually produces antibodies against the proteins found on the surface of the virus that clears the infection.

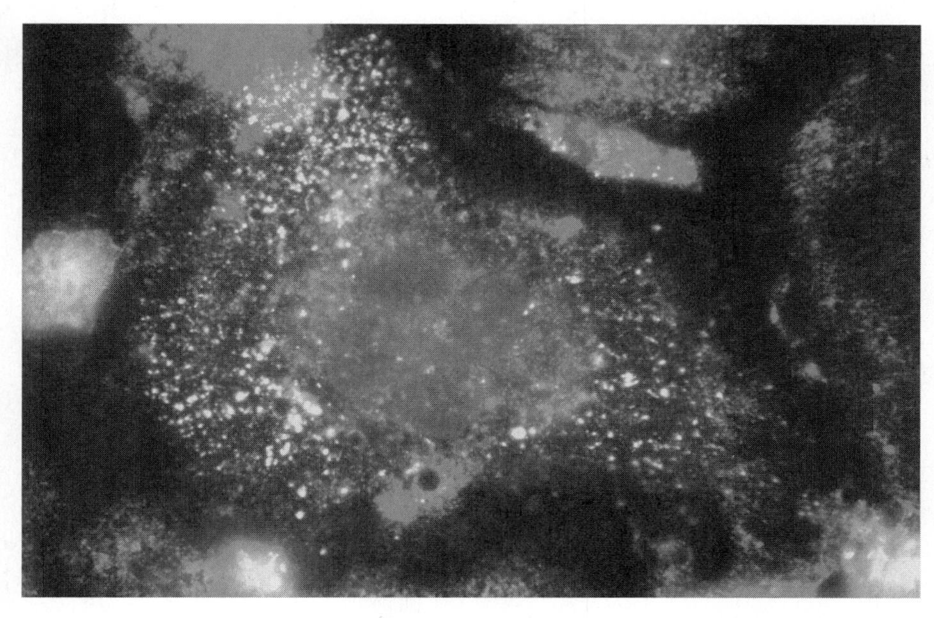

Numerous cytokines are released from the macrophage (center with 4 blue nuclei), triggering an inflammatory response after exposure to mock bacteria. The outer yellowish-green bodies arrive to bind with (yellow) and halt the overproduction of cytokines that prevent an inflammatory overresponse.
Source: Nancy Kedersha/Science Source

Concept Check

3. What is the cause of the symptoms often experienced with influenza infection, such as body aches, headache, and fatigue?

A. Inflammation

B. Fever

C. Use of non-steroidal drugs

D. The immunization

Answer question

Vaccines

- Immunity does not last long because the proteins on the surface of the virus are constantly changing. New vaccines are therefore produced each year to target the viruses that are predicted to be circulating during the flu season.
- Vaccinations become effective by causing antibodies to be produced within about two weeks. The vaccine is developed to protect against influenza A (H1N1 or swine, H3N2) viruses and influenza B viruses. There are two types of vaccines:
  1. The flu shot is a vaccine with inactivated (dead) virus.
  2. Nasal spray flu vaccine utilizes live viruses that are weakened. The nasal spray is recommended for healthy, nonpregnant people (not recommended in immunocompromised patients).
- Neither vaccine produces the flu.

Concept Check

4. The nasal spray form of the influenza vaccine could be used for which patient?

A. A 40-year-old receiving chemotherapy for cancer

B. An adolescent who is 20 weeks pregnant

C. A young adult on steroid medications with a skin rash

D. A healthy 25-year-old college student

Answer question

Complications

- Bacterial pneumonia is the most common complication in those with flu:
  - o Occurs more frequently in groups of patients with underlying chronic illness (example: COPD and heart failure).
  - o Suspicion for pneumonia increases when symptoms persist and/or suddenly worsen.
- Less commonly, complications involving the muscle and CNS also occur.
- Flu often exacerbates the patient's pre-existing condition(s). For example, the patient may also experience a heart failure exacerbation.

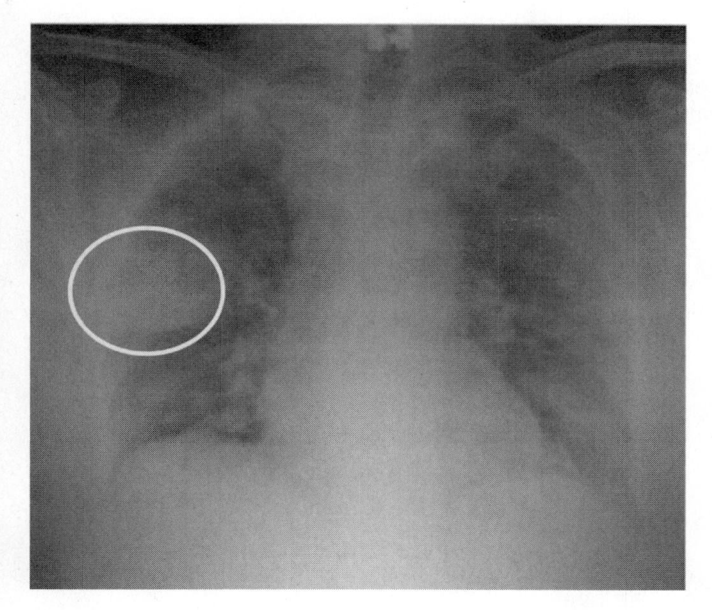

Note the patient's right upper lobe consolidation. Pneumonia is one of the most common complications of influenza.
Source: Courtesy of K. Kyriakidis

Risk Factors

Particular groups of people are at much higher risk of serious complications:

1. Age younger than 5 (especially under 2 years) or older than 65 years old
2. Comorbid conditions, especially:
   - COPD
   - Heart failure, Coronary Artery Disease (CAD)
   - Diabetes
   - Neuro and neurodevelopmental conditions
3. Immunosuppression
4. Pregnant or 2-weeks postpartum women
5. Native American and Alaskan natives
6. Morbidly obese (BMI more than 40 in adults)
7. Residents of chronic care facilities

Concept Check

5. **Which patient is most at risk for an influenza infection?**
   A. A 45-year-old healthy female
   B. A 40-year-old with well-controlled diabetes
   C. A 25-year-old who had a baby 3 months ago
   D. A 30-year-old who recently had a 50-pound weight loss

Answer question

Causes

- Influenza is an infection caused by influenza A, B, or C viruses. Generally, influenza A and B are more severe, but influenza A is the most devastating of the three on a global scale.
- H3N2 influenza A viruses (e.g., Hong Kong, Bangkok) most commonly cause the most severe conditions.
- The H1N1 (swine flu) influenza A viruses typically cause less severe illness in adults than in younger children.
- Influenza B viruses cause a moderately severe illness.
- Influenza C only causes a mild to no symptoms and does not cause the wide-spread epidemics of A or B. It is known as the "common flu."

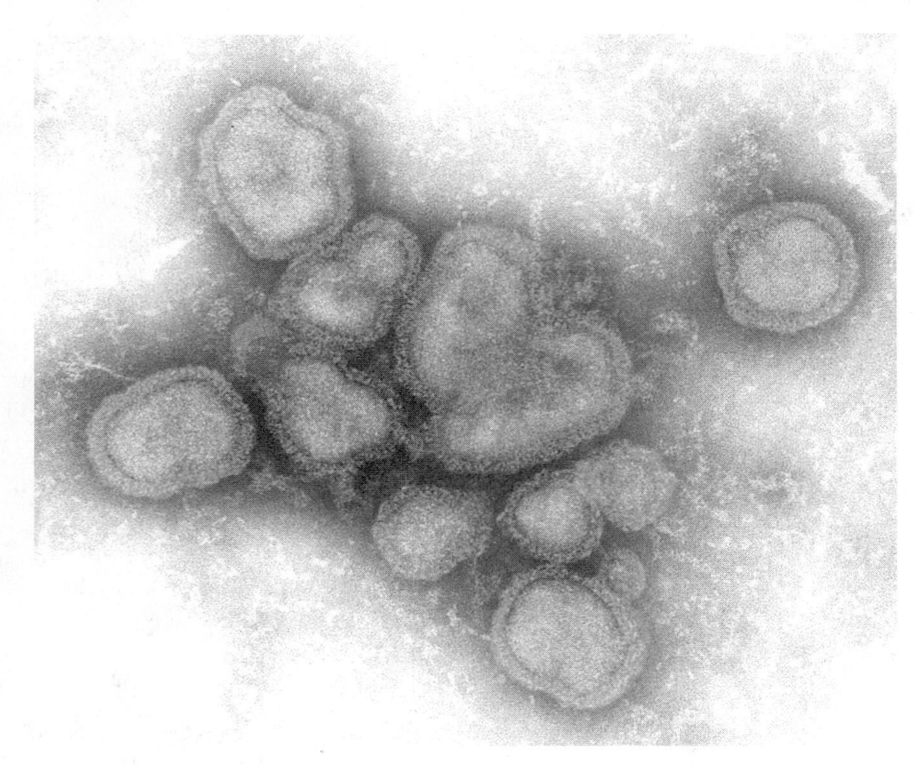

The H3N2 influenza A virus causes the most severe form of influenza. This strain had numerous hosts as genes from humans and birds were also found from mutations
Source: CDC/F.A. Murphy.

Concept Check

6. Which virus would cause the least severe influenza illness in an adult patient?

A. H1N1 virus

B. H3N2 virus

C. Hong Kong Flu virus

D. Influenza C virus

Answer question

Assessment Findings

Symptoms onset is usually abrupt:

- Fever, usually sudden
- Headache
- Myalgia
- Chills
- Malaise
- Nausea
- Vomiting
- Diarrhea
- Nonproductive cough
- Sore throat
- Nasal discharge: runny or congested nose

Systemic symptomology, abrupt onset, and increased severity are distinguishing factors for influenza over common cold.

Unfortunately, 30–50% of people who are infected are asymptomatic, making spread of the disease common.

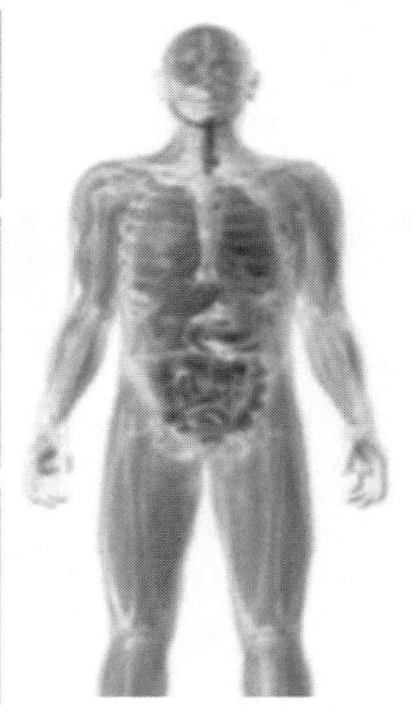

Source: Copyright © 2012, NovEx Novice to Expert Learning, LLC

Differentiating Flu Versus Cold Symptoms

Symptoms	Cold	Flu
Fever	Rare	Usual
Headache	Sometimes	Usual
Myalgias	Mild	Usual
Extreme fatigue	Never	Usual
Sinusitis	Usual	Sometimes
Sneezing	Usual	Sometimes
Sore throat	Usual	Sometimes
Chest discomfort & congestion	Mild to moderate (cough related)	Common

The key differentiating factor is that cold symptoms tend to be local whereas influenza symptoms tend to be more systemic.
Source: Copyright © 2012, NovEx Novice to Expert Learning, LLC

Concept Check

7. A patient is likely suffering from a cold rather than the flu if the patient complains of what condition?

A. Fever

B. Sudden onset of symptoms

C. Fatigue

D. Sneezing

Answer question

Diagnostics

Diagnosis is usually clinical (made via physical assessment). In the setting of an outbreak, a patient with typical symptoms is likely to have the flu without the need for further diagnostics:

- Generally few physical findings exist.
- Patient may appear hot and flushed.
- Throat is often clear, even with complaints of sore throat.
- Mild cervical lymphadenopathy may be present.
- Physical examination of chest generally unremarkable.

Laboratory testing with flu swab can confirm the diagnosis. This is sometimes helpful, for example, when a hospitalized patient presents with an acute onset of severe pulmonary disease.

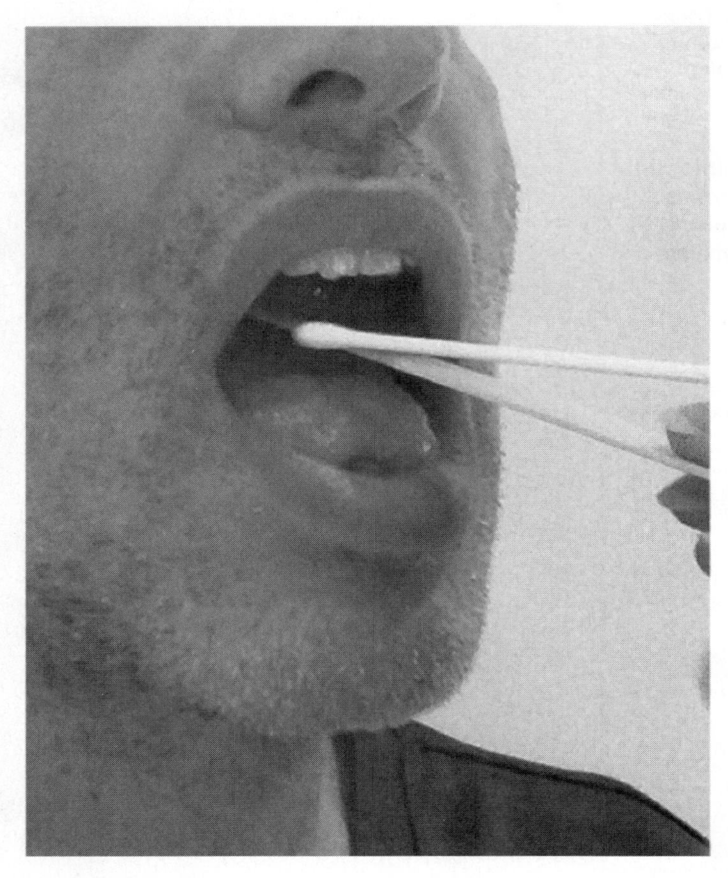

The photo displays the use of a throat swab (or can be nasal swab) to test for influenza specific organisms.

Priority Patient Concerns and Desired Collaborative Care Outcomes

Prior to caring for patients with influenza, it is important to prioritize the patient's concerns that must guide the nursing care plan and interventions. Care for the patient is ordered and organized in accordance with the patient's priority and urgent needs. Desired collaborative care outcomes in patients with influenza typically include:

1. Patient will experience reduced discomfort.
2. Patient will have restoration of body temperature within normal limits.
3. Patient will return to normal activities of daily living.
4. Patient will express normal levels of energy.

Considering these important care outcomes, prepare a list of the major 3–6 priority patient concerns or nursing diagnoses for patients with influenza. Be prepared to participate in a discussion of this list and/or to submit them as an assignment, as determined by your faculty. Resources you may find helpful in this assignment can include this lesson, the references, resources on nursing care plans, and standard nursing diagnoses manuals.

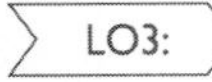

Collaborative Interventions

- Although debilitating, influenza is a self-limited infection in the general patient population (uncomplicated influenza) and does not necessarily require medical intervention. Common beneficial interventions ares:
  - o Acetaminophen or NSAIDs can be used for fever, headache, and myalgia and are self-administered by most patients.
  - o Hydration to maintain necessary fluid balance when insensible loss is higher, intake is lower, and diarrhea and vomiting may compound fluid loss.
- However, increased morbidity and mortality exist in certain high-risk patients (complicated influenza). Antivirals should be considered in these patients and issues include (EBP):
  - o Recommended for outpatients who present within 48 hours of symptom onset with confirmed or suspected influenza infection AND who are at increased risk for complications (Grade 1A evidence-based practice).
  - o Neuraminidase inhibitors (NOT a substitute for vaccination!) zanamivir and oseltamivir are active against both influenza A and B.
  - o Antivirals can also be used to prevent development of the flu, especially in patients at high risk for complications (e.g., oxygen desaturation, rapid clinical deterioration).
  - o When initiated promptly, antivirals can shorten duration of symptoms by 1 to 3 days. However, the greatest benefits are experienced when medication is given within the first 24–30 hours of onset. Limited to no benefit is observed when started 2 days or more after onset of symptoms.
- Persons at highest risk include (EBP):
  - o Patients with chronic illnesses
  - o The very young and the very old
  - o Immunocompromised patients
  - o Patients with comorbid conditions
  - o Patients in long-term care facilities
- Isolation and droplet precautions should be implemented:
  - o Wash hands with soap and water or use alcohol sanitizer before entering room and after leaving the room.
  - o Room should not be shared with other patients.
  - o Special air-handling (e.g. negative pressure) rooms are not required.
  - o Healthcare personnel should wear a mask when entering the room.
  - o Patients should wear a mask when leaving the room (e.g., being transported for tests) when still contagious.

Concept Check

8. What is the goal of using antiviral medications in a patient with the flu?

A. Reduce the duration of symptoms.

B. Interfere with the bacterial replication process.

C. Avoid the need for immunization.

D. Treat the fever.

Answer question

Collaborative Symptom Management and Comfort Care

Patients with influenza are uncomfortable, aching, and in some pain:

- Stay at home when sick or contagious to improve care of self and to reduce the rapid spread of infection
- Encourage rest to enhance recovery.
- Promote increased fluid intake due to reduced intake while sick, fever, and sometimes diarrhea.
- Administer ordered analgesics to reduce discomfort from headache, sore throat, and myalgias.
- Administer ordered antipyretics to control fever and its associated discomfort.
- Encourage patient to seek follow-up care with primary health care provider, particularly if at higher risk, to detect potential complications early.

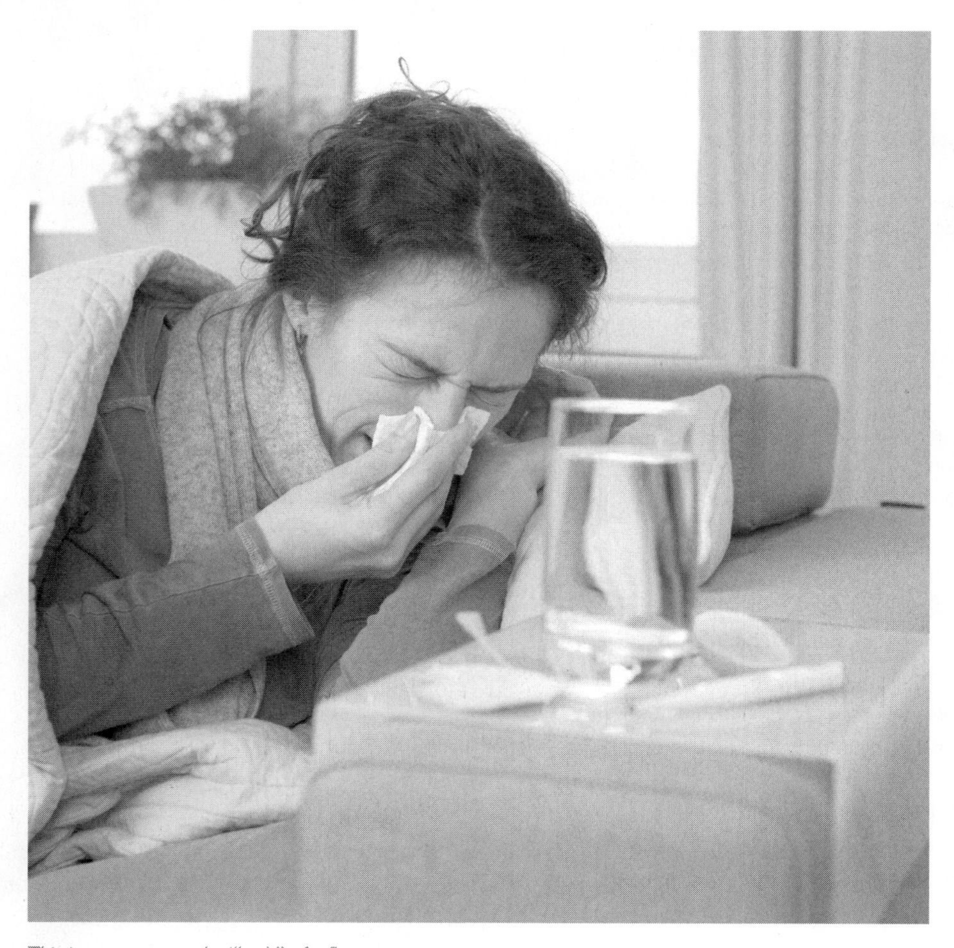

This image conveys the "look" of influenza.
Source: Subbotina Anna/Fotolia

Best Treatment Is Prevention

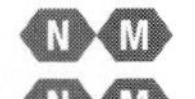

- Diligent hand hygiene practices are key in limiting the spread of influenza.
- Annual immunization is the most important preventive measure:
  - o Recommended for all individuals over six months of age in the United States (EBP).
  - o Recommended for health care providers to prevent transmission to patients (EBP).
  - o Health care organizations should offer influenza vaccines to all employees (EBP).
  - o Once infected, patients should be reminded that good hygiene is imperative to prevent transmission of the illness to others. Examples include good hand hygiene, covering the mouth when coughing and the nose when sneezing, and proper disposal of used tissue.

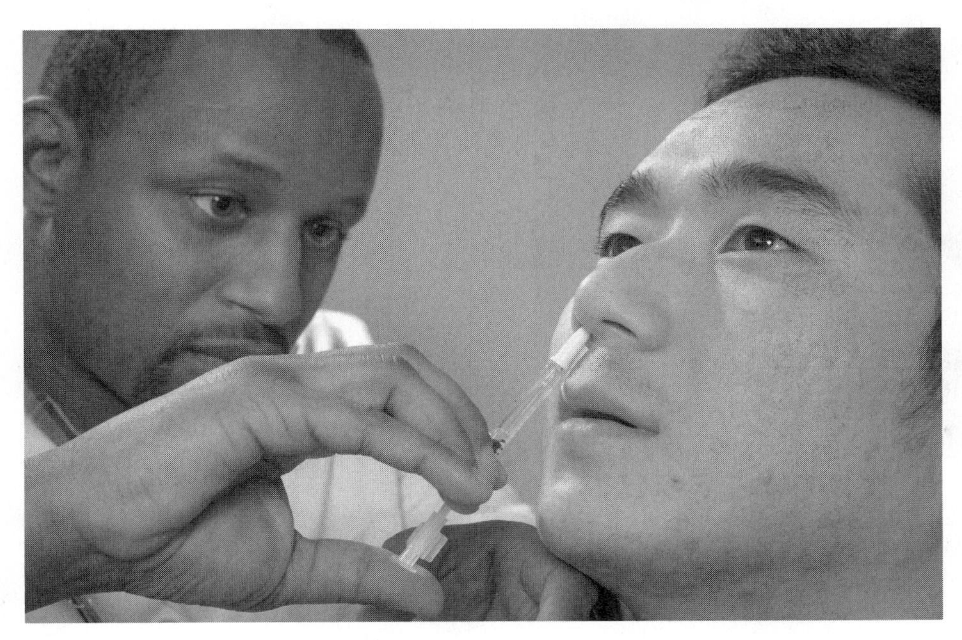

Administration of the swine flu vaccine by intranasal mist.
Source: CDC/Dr. Bill Atkinson

Collaborative Interventions (continued)

Patient Education

Patient education should inform the patient about what to expect and how to prevent the spread of the infection to others. It also needs to address and correct expectations that patients have. Educate the patient and family that:

- Uncomplicated influenza usually improves gradually over 2–5 days. However, the illness may last for one week or more.
- Patients should remain home from work, school, church, or populated environments until signs and symptoms have ceased. A general rule of thumb is to stay away from others for 24 hours after fever is gone.
- Hand hygiene with soap, water, and friction from rubbing hands together is key to prevent further transmission.
- Hand sanitizers that contain more than or equal to 60% alcohol are as, if not more, effective against viruses (and most bacteria) as hand washing.
- Antibiotics are not effective against viruses. Antibiotics are appropriate for bacterial infections (e.g., pneumonia) that typically do not develop as a complication of influenza. Taking antibiotics when not indicated and not completing the full course of antibiotic treatment when indicated have led to multidrug resistant organisms which have become individual and public health hazards.
- Follow up care is needed if their symptoms worsen as a complication as arise. Chronic health conditions place patients at higher risk for complications of influenza, especially asthma, chronic heart disease, and diabetes. These patients should be more vigilant about early follow up if symptoms persist or suddenly worsen.

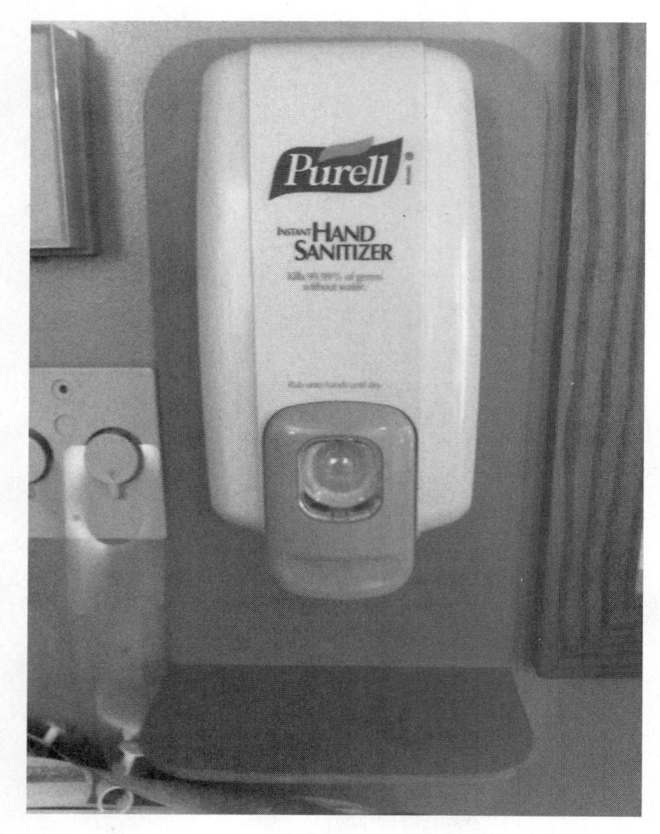

Alcohol-based hand sanitizers are an effective alternative to hand washing and critical to preventing general disease transmission, except for a few gastrointestinal organisms like *C. difficile* and norovirus.
Source: Copyright © 2012, NovEx Novice to Expert Learning, LLC

Summary of Interventions

- Influenza (type A and B) are preventable through yearly immunizations.
- Acetaminophen and NSAIDs are commonly used for symptom management and comfort.
- Antivirals can be given within 24–30 hours of symptom onset to shorten the duration of the infection.
- Careful evaluation and follow up are needed in certain populations and age groups who are at increased risk for complications from influenza.

LO4:

Evaluation of Desired Collaborative Care Outcomes

Evaluation and reassessment should reveal attainment of previously established patient outcomes. In summary:

- The patient has reduced discomfort.
- The patient body temperature is within normal limits.
- The patient is performing normal activities of daily living.
- The patient expresses the return of normal levels of energy.

References

http://www.cdc.gov/flu/about/disease/

http://www.who.int/csr/disease/influenza/en/

http://www.cdc.gov/flu/keyfacts.htm

Glezen, W. P. (2008, December). Clinical practice. Prevention and treatment of seasonal influenza. *N Engl J Med. 359*(24), 2579–2585.

Jackson, A. P., & Simenson, S. (2013, January). Management of common cold symptoms with over-the-counter medications: clearing the confusion. *Postgrad Med. 125*(1), 73–81.

Nichol, K. L. (2010, March). Pneumococcal vaccination and revaccination in the elderly population. *J Infect Dis. 201*(5), 659–661.

Clinical Practice Guidelines

Harper, S. A., Bradley, M. S, Englund, J. A., et al. (2009). Seasonal influenza in adults and children—Diagnosis, treatment, chemoprophylaxis, and institutional outbreak management: clinical practice guidelines of the Infectious Diseases Society of America. *Clin Infect Diseases, 48*, 1003–1032.

Patient Education

http://www.ucsfhealth.org/education/facts_about_the_flu/index.html

http://www.uptodate.com/contents/influenza-symptoms-and-treatment-beyond-the-basics

Butteri, M. J., Radu, C., Huq, F., Wiglesworth, A., Durso, S. C., & Bellantoni, M. (2010, September). Flu in 15: a novel 15-minute education program to promote acceptance of the influenza vaccine among health care workers. *J Am Med Dir Assoc, 11*(7), 523–537.

Chang, H. J., & Golub, R. M. (2001). Influenza. *JAMA. 306*(15), 1723.

Talbot, T. R., & Talbot, H. K. (2013, March). Influenza prevention update: examining common arguments against influenza vaccination. *JAMA, 309*(9), 881–882.

STOP

Go to the online course and complete the NovE-Cases assigned by your instructor for this module.

Learning Outcomes for Inhalation Injuries: Toxic Inhalation

When you complete this lesson, you will be able to:

1. Recognize the clinical relevance of inhalation injuries.
2. Consider the pathophysiology, etiology, risk factors, and clinical presentation of inhalation injuries that determine the priority patient concerns.
3. Determine the most urgent and important nursing interventions and patient education required in caring for a patient with inhalation injuries.
4. Evaluate attainment of desired collaborative care outcomes for a patient with inhalation injuries.

What Is Toxic Inhalation?

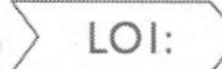

- Toxic inhalants are substances that can inflame and damage the lungs when inhaled.
- There are several different types of toxic inhalation.
  - Chemical irritants:
    a. Hydrophilic
    b. Nonhydrophilic
  - Chemical asphyxiants. Simple chemical asphyxiants are gases that displace oxygen in the air (e.g., carbon dioxide or methane):
    a. Carbon monoxide
    b. Cyanide
  - Smoke inhalation
  - Biological and chemical agents, some of which are used as weapons
- Each of the above toxins are discussed separately to provide a clearer understanding.

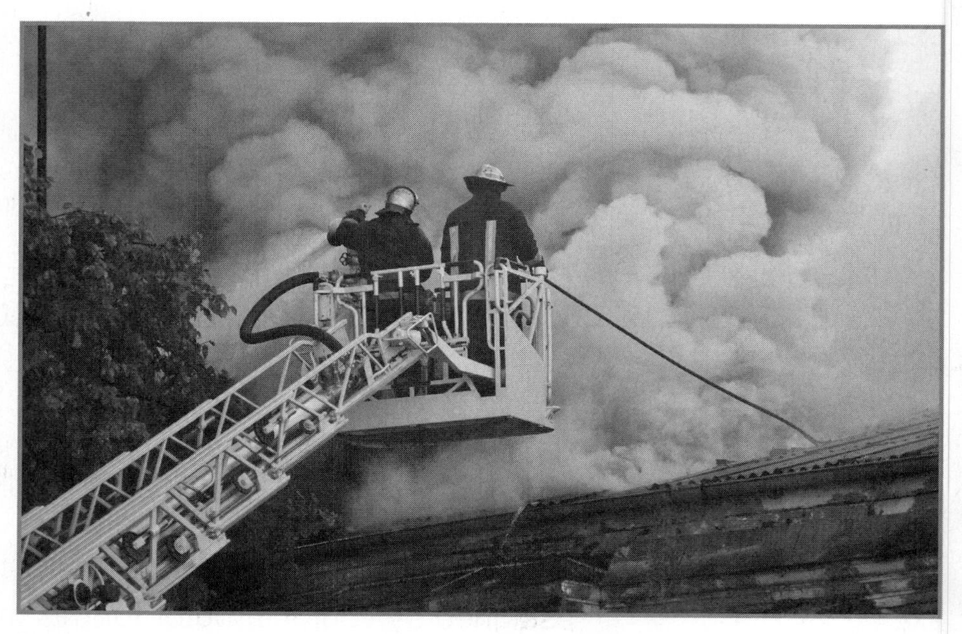

Fire deaths due to smoke inhalation outnumber fire deaths caused by burns.
Source: Ansis Klusic/Shutterstock

Clinical Relevance

LO1:

- Toxic or smoke inhalation is the leading cause of death related to fires.
- In the United States, 5,000–10,000 deaths occur from smoke inhalation each year.
- Many of these deaths are preventable through public education and safe practices.
- Toxic inhalation can pose a hazard in home, industrial, mass casualty, and military settings.
- Carbon monoxide is the leading cause of death due to poisoning in the United States.

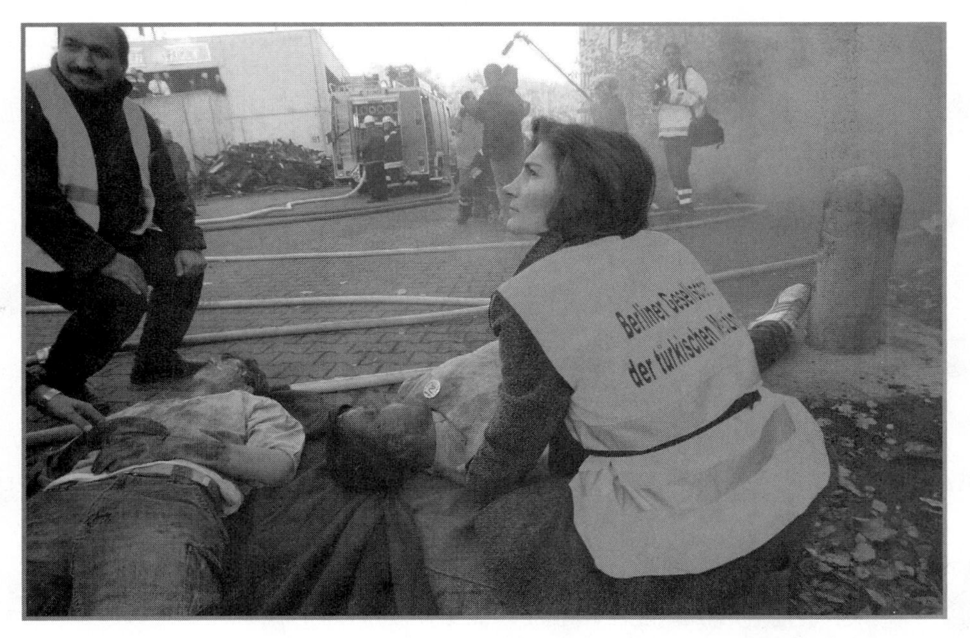

Clinicians must recognize that facial burn injuries warn of imminent inhalation injury sequelae. Early airway management can be life-saving.
Source: Caro/Alamy

LO1:

Chemical Irritants

Pathophysiology

- Chemical irritants are chemicals that irritate and can damage the lungs. Some are commonly used in household cleaning. They are inhaled and cause:
  - o Inflammation of the airways and alveoli
  - o Bronchospasm
  - o Laryngospasm
- These patients can develop acute lung injury (ALI) and acute respiratory distress syndrome (ARDS).
- The length of the exposure and the concentration of the substance are directly related to the severity of symptoms and consequences.
- Smoke damages alveoli and bronchial lining. Surfactant is inactivated and edema develops.
- Inflammatory response: Cytokines damage capillaries, edema due to leakage, hypoxemia.
- If smoke injury is severe, acute respiratory distress syndrome can develop as seen in the pathophysiologic cascade in the diagram.
- Treatment: Eventual recover from hypoxemia, lung tissue damage, and lung dysfunction.

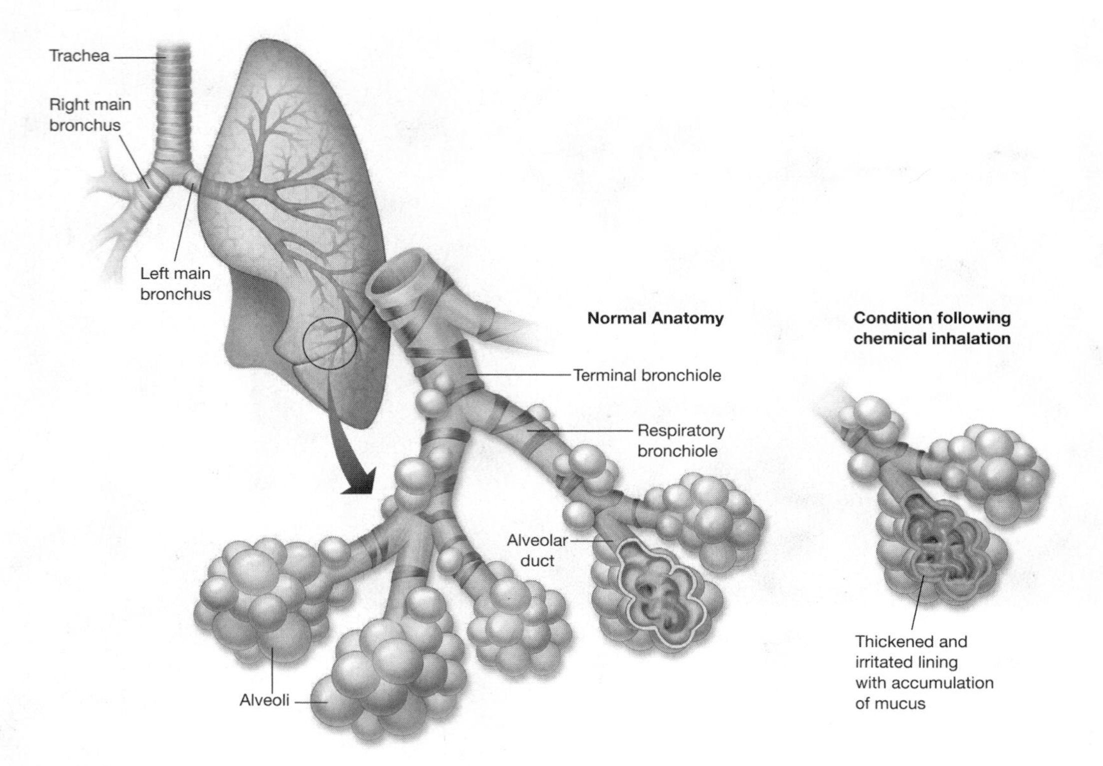

Chemical Inhalation resulting in lung damage.

LO1:

- These irritants may be divided into hydrophilic (water soluble) and nonhydrophilic.

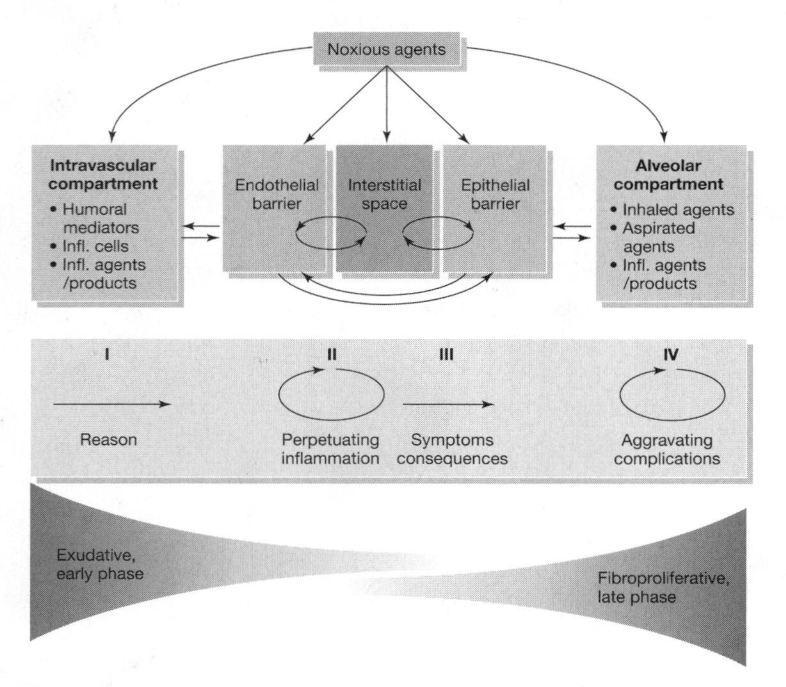

Pathophysiology of acute respiratory distress syndrome.

LO1: LO2: Chemical irritants may be divided into two categories:

- Hydrophilic (reacts with water) chemical irritants:
  - Major examples: hydrochloric acid and ammonia
  - Pathophysiological effects and symptoms are immediate and tend to affect the upper more than lower airways.
  - These chemicals often produce the warning signs of a burning sensation of the eyes and mucous membranes upon exposure.
- Nonhydrophilic:
  - Key examples: phosgene gas and nitrogen dioxide
  - Pathophysiological effects and symptoms may be delayed and may affect the entire lungs.

Causes and Risk Factors

- Exposure to cleaning solutions
- Industrial accidents

Problems with Mixing Chemicals

- Cleaning products should NEVER be mixed as the mixture can create a combination of chemicals which are volatile, flammable, and incredibly toxic. Mixing chemicals can also set off a dangerous, explosive chemical reaction.
- In particular, chlorine bleach should NEVER be mixed with ammonia (or even urine), as the chemical reaction triggered can produce poisonous fumes that can cause a severe respiratory reaction, burning in the throat and eyes, and serious lung irritation.
- In addition, chlorine can react with organic material to form trihalomethanes (e.g., chloroform), which are carcinogenic compounds.
- More than one cleanser should NEVER be poured down the toilet or used on the same cloth to avoid inadvertently mixing chemicals down the toilet or use the same cloth to apply two different cleansers.

http://www.dolceta.eu/united-kingdom/Mod3/Problems-with-mixing-chemicals.html

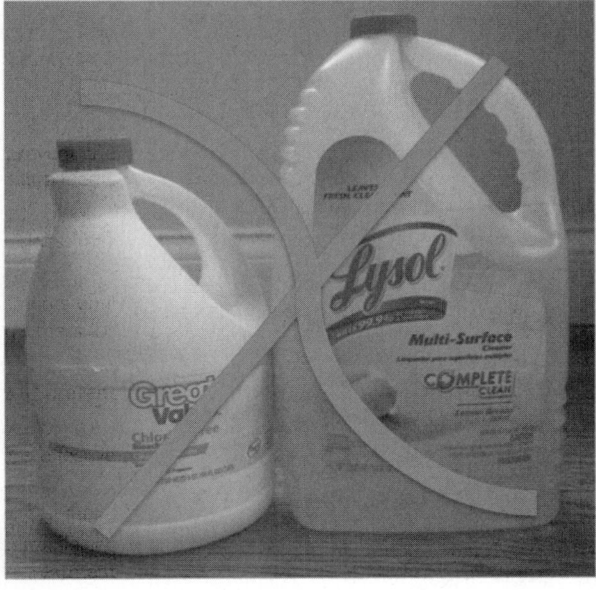

Mixing cleaning products can be dangerous.

LO2:

Chemical Irritants (continued)

Assessment Findings

- Usual symptoms are:
  - Cough
  - Wheezing
  - Shortness of breath
  - Hemoptysis
- Hydrophilic chemicals can cause:
  - Burning eyes and mouth
  - Hoarseness of the voice

LO3:

Collaborative Interventions

- Treatment is usually supportive and includes:
  - o Supplemental oxygen if SpO_2 falls below 93%
  - o Bronchodilators if required for shortness of breath or wheezing
  - o Racemic inhaled epinephrine for laryngospasm
- Patients with serious and/or prolonged exposure can develop ARDS. Patients who develop ARDS usually require intubation and mechanical ventilation.
- Patient education to prevent the dangers of chemical inhalation injury:
  - o Dangers inherent in mixing chemicals
  - o Need for adequate ventilation when using cleaners, paints, or solvents

Concept Check

1. A female patient in the emergency department complains of her throat and eyes burning and her cough developed with the past 30 minutes. She states that she has been cleaning house. She most likely has which type of chemical irritant exposure?

A. Phosgene gas and nitrogen dioxide

B. Ammonia and hydrochloric acid

C. Hydrochloric acid and phosgene gas

D. Nitrogen dioxide and ammonia

Answer question

Simple Asphyxiants: Overview

- Asphyxiants are gases, such as methane and carbon dioxide, that produce a harmful effect by displacing oxygen off the hemoglobin. Without adequate oxygen available for cells, hypoxia ensues.
- These gases have no inherent toxic effect on cells other than by causing hypoxia due to inadequate oxygen supply and hypoperfusion.
- Simple asphyxiants can produce:
  - o Hypoxia
  - o Agitation
  - o Mental status changes
  - o Cardiac arrest
- Treatment is supportive.

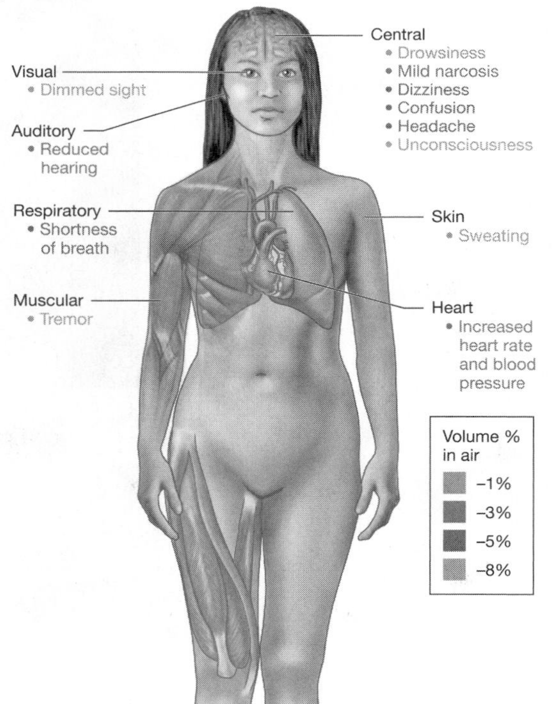

This image provides an example of the effects that a simple asphyxiant can have on multiple body systems. Carbon dioxide toxicity, common in patients with severe COPD, can be caused by other factors.

LO1:

Chemical Asphyxiants

- Chemicals can also cause asphyxiation, which causes a severe oxygen deficit, at the cellular level by vastly disrupting normal cell utilization of oxygen.
- Carbon monoxide (CO) and cyanide are the most common chemicals and are so toxic that their effects are referred to as "poisons."
- Poisoning from both chemicals occurs with smoke inhalation, so their combined asphyxiant effect can be serious.

LO1:

Carbon Monoxide (CO) Poisoning

Pathophysiology

- Carbon monoxide is an odorless, colorless, tasteless gas that is produced by incomplete burning of carbon matter, e.g., wood, gas, charcoal, even being generated by gas engines and cigarette smoking.
- Carbon monoxide diffuses rapidly into the blood stream once inhaled and interferes with the transport and utilization of oxygen.
- Interference is caused by the binding of carbon monoxide to hemoglobin and cytochromes (molecules involved in the production of energy).
- Carbon monoxide has a much higher affinity for hemoglobin (240 times higher) than does oxygen and, therefore, displaces oxygen.

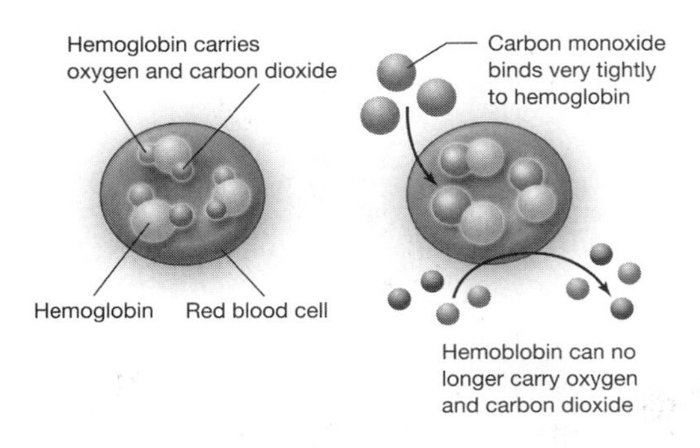

Normal oxygen and carbon dioxide are shown binding to hemoglobin. This is compared to carbon monoxide binding to hemoglobin. Without oxygen on hemoglobin to release to cells and tissues, hypoxia occurs and cellular metabolism is compromised.

Causes and Risk Factors

- House fires
- Faulty furnaces
- Portable stoves and grills used inside the house
- Car exhausts
- Intentional poisoning in suicide attempt
- Industrial chemicals that are metabolized to carbon monoxide in the liver

LO2:

Assessment Findings

- Cherry red skin
- Confusion
- Somnolence or coma
- Fatigue
- Headache
- Nausea
- Seizures
- Symptoms of cardiac ischemia (e.g., chest pain), ventricular dysrhythmias
- Pulmonary edema
- Profound lactic acidosis
- Death

Chemical Asphyxiants (continued)

Diagnostics

- Diagnosis is usually made by:
  - o History
  - o Elevated carboxyhemoglobin levels
    - a. Carboxyhemoglobin (COHb) is carbon monoxide bound to hemoglobin in the red blood cells.
    - b. COHb can be measured by determining arterial blood gas
    - c. Normal level is less than 2%.
    - d. May be slightly higher in smokers
    - e. Symptoms typically manifest between levels of 10–30%.
    - f. Severe exposure, more than 40%, can be lethal
- Low arterial pH (metabolic acidosis) may be present in more severe poisonings. Normal arterial pH is 7.40 with a normal range of 7.35 to 7.45.
- Pulse oximetry is usually normal.
- Cardiac enzymes and ECG may be ordered if the patient is having symptoms of cardiac ischemia (e.g., chest pain) and/or ventricular dysrhythmias.

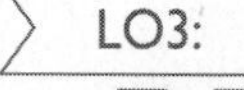

Collaborative Interventions

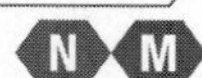

- Evidence-based practice includes high flow oxygen for carbon monoxide inhalation to improve oxygenation and to reduce the COHb level. This improves the amount of oxygen bound to hemoglobin that is then delivered to cells.

- In severe or specific cases of carbon monoxide inhalation, hyperbaric oxygen can be used. Although studies have not provided evidence for its use, hyperbaric oxygen therapy is not uncommon. Indications for use of hyperbaric oxygen include:
  - o Altered mental status or loss of consciousness
  - o Pregnancy
  - o Myocardial ischemic changes
- N Use and maintenance of smoke and CO detectors in the home should be promoted.
- N Education on not using fuel-powered devices indoors in an enclosed space and the need for proper venting should be provided.

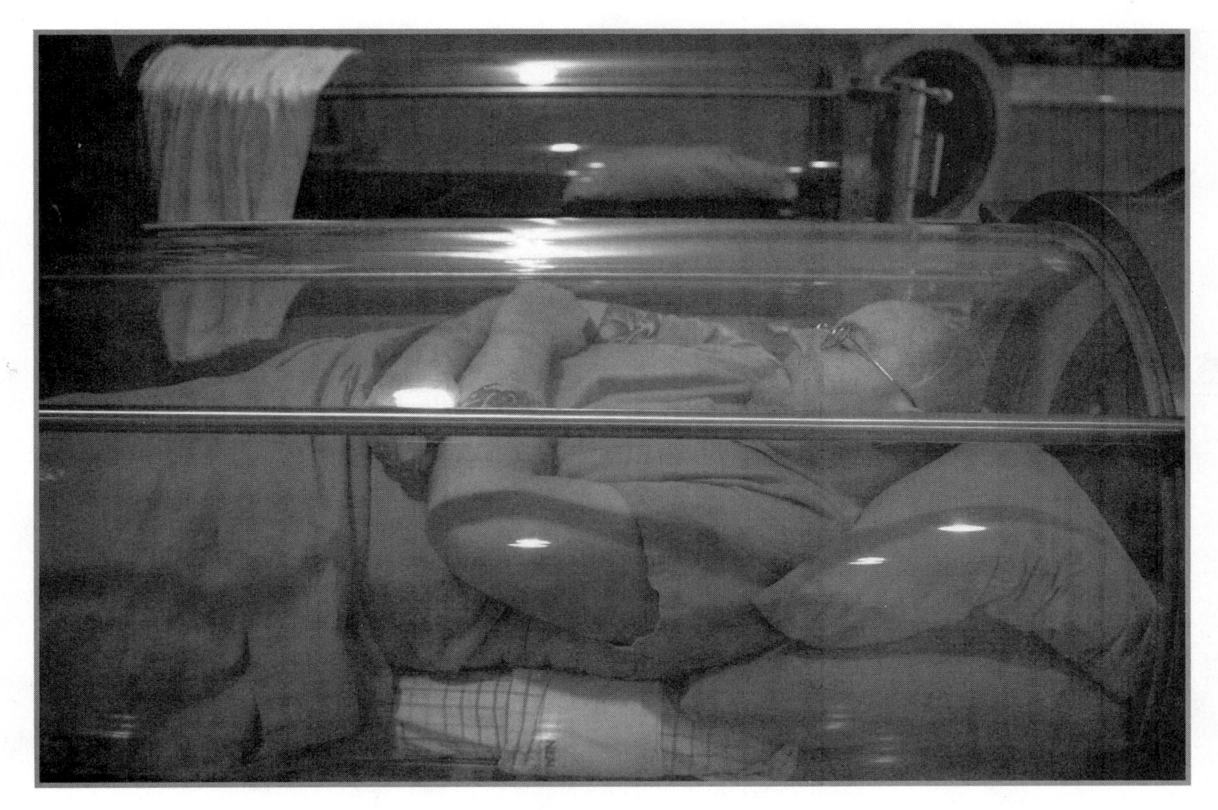

Hyperbaric therapy in patients with severe carbon monoxide poisoning may improve oxygenation.
Source: ZUMA Press, Inc/Alamy

LO3:

Long-Term Sequelae

- Neurocognitive deficits are present in about 50% of patients who had toxic levels of carboxyhemoglobin.
- The neurocognitive complications are seen as symptoms that may arise within days or as late as one year after the poisoning.
- Symptoms may include:
    - Confusion
    - Difficulty concentrating
    - Memory deficits
    - Personality changes
- The cause of these symptoms is not understood.

(2009). Complications of Carbon Monoxide Poisoning: A Case Discussion and Review of the Literature, *Prim Care Companion J Clin Psychiatry, 11*(2), 74–79.

Concept Check

2. Which finding is present in carbon monoxide poisoning?

A. Decreased pulse oximetry
B. Leukocytosis
C. Metabolic alkalosis
D. Elevated carboxyhemoglobin

Answer question

LO1:

Chemical Asphyxiants (continued)

Cyanide Inhalation

The second common type of chemical asphyxiant is the inhalation of cyanide gas, which can cause cyanide poisoning.

- The most common cause of cyanide poisoning is inhalation of fumes from a fire.
- Cyanide is produced when synthetic materials (e.g., textiles, plastics, foam, and paints) are burned.
- Cyanide binds to cytochromes (molecules that are essential in the production of energy) and block their ability to produce energy.

LO2:

Assessment Findings

- Headache
- Confusion
- Coma
- Seizures
- Hypotension
- Metabolic acidosis
- Shortness of breath
- Pulmonary edema
- Nausea and vomiting
- Hepatic failure

LO3:

Collaborative Symptom Management

- Supportive care includes:

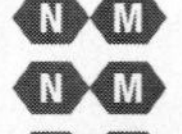

  - o Airway management
  - o Crystalloid IV solutions, e.g., Ringer's solution and 5% dextrose solution
  - o Vasopressors are titrated to manage hypotension if unresponsive to fluids
  - o Sodium bicarbonate

Antidotes that may be ordered include:

  - o Hydroxocobalamin (Cyanokit): Hydroxocobalamin combines with cyanide to form cyanocobalamin (vitamin B_{12}), which is cleared by the kidneys.
  - o Cyanide antidote kit (CAK): Amyl nitrite pearls, sodium nitrite, and sodium thiosulfate

LO2: 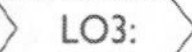

Smoke Inhalation

Pathophysiology

- Smoke often contains carbon monoxide and cyanide.
- Causes:
  1. Inhalation of hot gases may cause thermal damage to the upper airway. Blast injuries and steam inhalation may cause thermal damage to the lower respiratory tract
  2. Chemicals in smoke can damage the entire respiratory tract
  3. Systemic and multiorgan injury may be caused by toxic gases

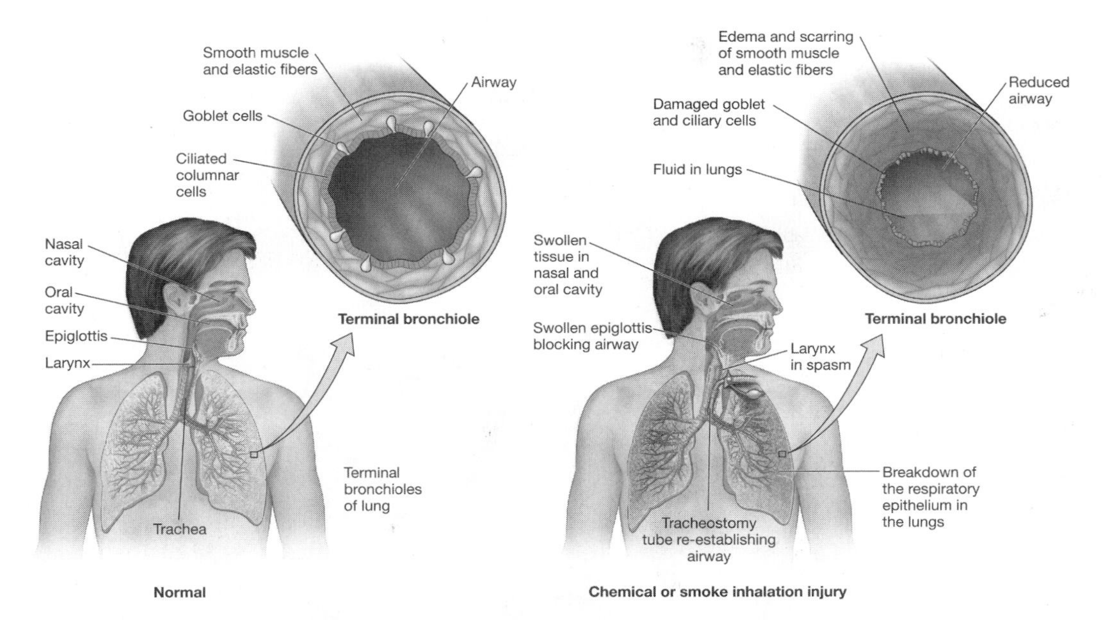

This illustration compares a normal airway to one with a severe inhalation injury from smoke or a chemical agent. The two images on the right side illustrate the damage to the bronchiole from the inhalation of a caustic agent.

Assessment Findings

LO2: LO3:

- Cough and shortness of breath are the most common signs of smoke inhalation.
- Burns and sore throat may be present.
- The severity and location of damage depends on the source of the smoke, duration of exposure, and particle size of the irritant substance.

Collaborative Symptom Management

The treatment for smoke inhalation is supportive and includes:

- N M Oxygen therapy for SpO_2 under 93%.
- N M Bronchodilators if shortness of breath is severe or wheezing arises.
- N M Intubation and mechanical ventilation if poorly responsive to less invasive interventions.

Concept Check

3. The woman (see photo) just arrived for emergency care after rescue from a house fire. In addition to what's visible in the photo, she is coughing, short of breath, and confused. She complains of nausea, sore throat, and headache. What are the most important injuries that you anticipate and need to carefully evaluate?

A. facial burns, carbon dioxide toxicity, and chloroform poisoning
B. facial burns, smoke inhalation, cyanide poisoning, and carbon monoxide poisoning
C. facial burns, smoke inhalation, ammonia toxicity, and phosgene gas toxicity
D. carbon dioxide, ammonia, phosgene gas, and cholorform poisonings

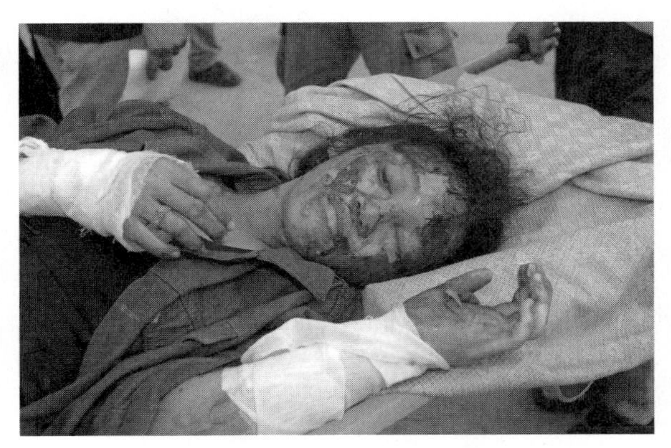

Source: DENNIS SABANGAN/EPA/Newscom

Answer question

Biological and Chemical Agents

Biological and chemical agents can cause a wide range of injuries, depending on the source, duration, and severity of exposure.

Biological Agents

- Living organisms or toxins of living organisms
- Include viruses, bacteria, fungi and their metabolites
- Anthrax and ricin are representative of the category.

Chemical Agents

- Poisonous vapors, aerosols, liquids, or solids that have toxic effects on people, animals, or plants.
- Classified as:
  - o Blister agents, e.g., nitrogen mustard
  - o Choking agents, e.g., tear gas
  - o Nerve agents, e.g., sarin, an organophosphate

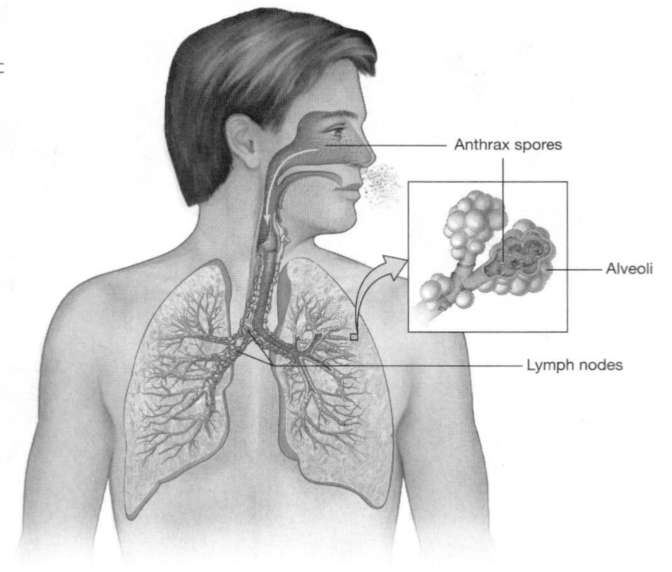

Bacillus anthracis is an infectious spore if inhaled because it releases toxins as it germinates in the moist, warm, and protected climate of the lungs. Respiratory anthrax spores can also spread into the lymph nodes, releasing toxins where they lodge.

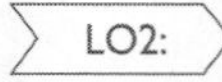

Assessment Findings

Biological Agents

Biological agents are primarily infectious agents that can cause mild to severe symptoms, which include:

- Fever, chills,
- Headache, anthralgia, myalgia, backache
- Cough, dyspnea
- Fatigue, malaise
- Hemoptysis, bleeding, petechiae, DIC
- Respiratory failure, pulmonary edema, respiratory distress
- Hypotension, shock, collapse, necrosis, multiorgan failure, death

Chemical Agents

Blister Agents

Blister agents cause intense burning on contact and may cause:

- Intense burning on contact
- Hoarseness
- Cough with copious secretions
- Necrosis of epithelial tissue
- Death occurs from pulmonary edema or mechanical asphyxia.

Choking Agents

Choking agents may cause the following symptoms:

- Cough
- Choking
- Chest pain
- Nausea and occasionally vomiting
- Headache
- Lacrimation
- Death occurs from pulmonary edema.

Chemical Nerve Agents: Organophosphate Toxicity

- Although chemical weapons with organophosphates (nerve agents) are a very real threat in this age of terrorism, they are also commonly found in insecticides that are used in agriculture, landscaping, and gardening.
- Organophosphates are also found in herbicides, solvents, and components of plastics.
- Examples are malathion, parathion, and diazinon.
- As the other chemical and biological agents are rarely seen by most health care providers, this section focuses on organophosphates.

LO2:

Assessment Findings: Organophosphate Poisoning

Organophosphates inhibit acetylcholinesterase production and can cause:

- Lacrimation (tearing of the eyes)
- Pupil constriction
- Headache
- Slurred speech
- Excessive salivation
- Chest pain
- Tachy- or bradycardia
- Hallucinations, seizures
- GI symptoms like cramping, diarrhea
- Nausea and vomiting
- Urinary incontinence
- Profuse sweating
- Respiratory issues:
  - Profuse nasal and respiratory secretions
  - Wheezing
  - Dyspnea
  - Tachypnea
  - Noncardiac pulmonary edema
- Musculoskeletal issues:
  - Weakness
  - Fasciculations
  - Paralysis
- Eventual coma and death by cardiac arrest is possible.

LO3:

Biological and Chemical Agents (continued)

Collaborative Symptom Management: Organophosphate Inhalation

N M
- Airway management and oxygenation are paramount.

N M
- Intubation and mechanical ventilatory support may be required until toxin clears.

N
- Oximetry and cardiac monitoring are indicated. Note that depending on the unit the patient is admitted to, both are automatically used.

N M
- Atropine, a powerful anticholinergic, may be administered to counter the cholinergic effects of excess acetylcholine and reactivate acetylcholinesterase, the enzyme that cleaves acetylcholine.

N M
- Diazepam is useful when convulsions or pronounced muscle fasciculations are present.

N M
- Pralidoxime (2-PAM chloride) reactivates acetylcholinesterase and is used in conjunction with atropine and diazepam.

Concept Check

4. **Which nursing intervention has priority when caring for a patient with organophosphate poisoning?**
   A. Place the patient on a cardiac monitor.
   B. Secure the patient's airway.
   C. Administer epinephrine.
   D. Obtain a baseline blood pressure reading.

Answer question

LO3:

Collaborative Interventions: Chemical and Biological Weapon Exposure to Organophosphates

- Contamination of health care providers can cripple a medical facility. Just a few micrograms (one drop!) of sarin (an organophosphate) can totally incapacitate a large medical center by inadvertent cross contamination from the patient to emergency department, radiology, lab, surgery, ICU, medical surgical, and the entire hospital.

N M
- It is extremely important to immediately isolate suspected patients.

N M
- Providers must maintain personal protection against contamination from toxic agents by using:
  - o Protective suits
  - o Masks
  - o Eye shields
  - o Gloves

N M
The proper protocol should be followed:

1. Remove all of the victim's clothing, wound dressings, and catheters (IVs, endotracheal tubes, urine catheters). Treat these as hazardous wastes.
2. Thoroughly cleanse patient with soap and water and/or decontaminate with chlorine bleach while providing basic life support.
3. Protected providers then replace dressings and catheters.

Concept Check

5. **What should the nurse do with the clothing of a patient who might have been exposed to sarin gas?**
   A. Leave it in place, covering the patient with a sterile sheet.
   B. Leave it in place while the patient is doused with copious amounts of water.
   C. Remove it and seal it in a hazardous waste bag.
   D. Remove it and send it to the hospital laundry immediately.

Answer question

Priority Patient Concerns and Desired Collaborative Care Outcomes: All Inhalation Injuries

Prior to caring for patients with toxic inhalation injury, it is important to prioritize the patient's concerns that must guide the nursing care plan and interventions. Care for the patient is ordered and organized in accordance with the patient's priority and urgent needs. Desired collaborative care outcomes in patients with toxic inhalation injury include:

1. Patient's arterial blood gases will approximate pre-exposure level.
2. Patient will demonstrate respirations and ventilation that are adequate and preclude mechanical ventilator support.
3. Patient's exposure to toxins will be minimized and no additional persons will be exposed to the poisons.
4. Patient will demonstrate adequate oxygenation to prevent hypoxemia with adequate oxygen delivery to prevent hypoxic organ damage.
5. Patient will experience minimal or no pain.

Considering these important care outcomes, prepare a list of the major 3–6 priority patient concerns or nursing diagnoses for patients with toxic inhalation injury. Be prepared to participate in a discussion of this list and/or to submit them as an assignment, as determined by your faculty. Resources you may find helpful in this assignment can include this lesson, the references, resources on nursing care plans, and standard nursing diagnoses manuals.

Collaborative Interventions

LO3:

Collaborative Symptom Management: All Toxic Inhalation Injuries

General (listed in order of priority):

1. (N)(M) Protect the rescuer from contamination.
2. (N) Remove patient from source of exposure (e.g., clothing).
3. (N)(M) Protect the patient's airway. Closely monitor patient for early warning signs of respiratory failure.
4. (N) Provide supplemental oxygen.
5. (N)(M) Identify the toxin for specific treatment or antidote through poison control agency.
6. (N)(M) Decontaminate exposed areas if appropriate to protect others from toxic injury.
7. (N)(M) Administer bronchodilators and mucolytics for symptomatic treatment.
8. No evidence-based practice (EBP) exists for most inhalation injuries other than oxygen in carbon monoxide poisoning.
9. Non-EBP includes symptomatic treatment that varies, depending on the presence of pre-existing conditions, the severity of the symptoms and the inhalant involved
10. Symptomatic management can include:
    - (N)(M) Supplemental oxygen if oxygen saturations fall below 93%
    - (N)(M) Bronchodilators if required for shortness of breath or wheezing
    - (N)(M) Anticholinergics if organophosphate poisoning is strongly suspected
    - (N)(M) Mucolytics if mucous is blocking or narrowing the airway and interfering with breathing
11. (N)(M) Intubation and mechanical ventilatory support may be required for severe inhalation injuries.

Concept Check

6. **What are the nurse's most important actions when initially caring for patients with chemical or biologic weapon exposure?**

   A. Administer bronchodilators and mucolytics.

   B. Secure intravenous access and start anticholinergics.

   C. Protect oneself from contamination and remove contaminated items from the patient.

   D. Initiate cardiac and oximetry monitoring.

Answer question

LO3: Patient Education

- Promote use and maintenance of smoke and carbon monoxide detectors in the home.
- Educate on dangers of mixing chemicals. Stress the necessity of appropriate ventilation when using cleaners, paints, or solvents.
- Instruct on the use of devices requiring fuel, the hazards of their indoor use, and the need for proper venting.
- Supply information on local poison control agency and their emergency number. For immediate help from poison control anywhere in the United States, call 1-800-222-1222.

Concept Check

7. **What topics should the nurse include in a community presentation on prevention of inhalation injury?**
   A. Working smoke detectors should be present in every home.
   B. Only mix household cleaning chemicals in small batches.
   C. Small charcoal grill use in the house if electricity or gas is lost.
   D. Carbon monoxide detectors are required only if appliances are gas.

Answer question

Summary of Interventions

- Identifying the inhaled agent is important in order to provide the most effective treatment.
- High flow oxygen is recommended for carbon monoxide (CO) poisoning. Oxygen, airway management, and intubation may be necessary.
- Supportive care is essential. May include interventions such as bronchodilators and/or mucolytics.
- Life support for airway management, cardiovascular collapse, and neurological damage or irritation may be needed.
- Decontamination is critical when indicated.
- Many inhalation injuries can be prevented through the use of CO detectors, properly working smoke detectors, and education of the public on the appropriate use and proper ventilation when using chemicals, solvents, or fueled devices.

LO4:

Evaluation of Desired Collaborative Care Outcomes

Evaluation and reassessment should reveal attainment of previously established patient outcomes. In summary:

- Patient's arterial blood gases approximate pre-exposure levels.
- Patient demonstrates respirations and ventilation that are adequate and preclude mechanical ventilator support.
- Patient's exposure to toxins is minimal and no additional persons are exposed to the poisons.
- Patient demonstrates adequate oxygenation to prevent hypoxemia with adequate oxygen delivery to prevent hypoxic organ damage.
- Patient is experiencing minimal or no pain.

References

Federation of American Scientists. (2015). Biological, chemical, and other non-nuclear threats. **http://fas.org/issues/biological-chemical-and-other-non-nuclear-threats/**

North Dakota Department of Health Emergency Preparedness & response. (2015). Bioterrorism. **http://www.ndhealth.gov/EPR/HealthTopics/Bioterrorism.asp**

Tubera, D. (2014). Management of inhalation injury in an adult burn patient. Internet J Advanced Nurs Practice, 13(1). **ispub.com/IJANP/13/1/15083**

http://www.cdc.gov/anthrax

http://emergency.cdc.gov/agent/ricin/facts.asp

http://www.jems.com/article/features/ems-responds-toxic-inhalation

http://www.fas.org/programs/bio/chemweapons/cwagents.html

http://www.bt.cdc.gov/agent/nerve/tsd.asp

http://www.osha.gov/SLTC/biologicalagents/index.html

http://en.wikipedia.org/wiki/Sarin_gas_attack_on_the_Tokyo_subway

http://www.emsworld.com/print/EMS-World/Smoke-Inhalation/1$17096

http://www.cdc.gov/mmwr/preview/mmwrhtml/mm5339a4.htm

http://www.carbonmonoxide.ie/htm/gpfactsheet-poisoning.pdf

Learning Outcomes for Pleural Disturbances

When you complete this lesson, you will be able to:

1. Recognize the clinical relevance of pleural disturbances.
2. Consider the pathophysiology, etiology, risk factors, and clinical presentation of pleural disturbances that determine the priority patient concerns.
3. Determine the most urgent and important nursing interventions and patient education required in caring for a patient with a pleural disturbance.
4. Evaluate attainment of desired collaborative care outcomes for a patient with a pleural disturbance.

LO1:

What Are Pleural Disturbances?

- Pleural disturbances involve the abnormal entry of air, blood, or fluid into the pleural space. There are three types of pleural disturbances:
  1. Fluid in the pleural space is a pleural effusion.
  2. Blood in the pleural space is a hemothorax.
  3. Air in the pleural space is a pneumothorax.
- Normally, air, blood, or other fluids are not found in the pleural space. The pleural space is a potential space between the visceral and parietal pleura. Because the pleural space cannot expand to accommodate abnormal accumulation, an effusion interferes with and compromises lung expansion and blood flow (cardiac output).
- If the air or fluid accumulation is significant, it can lead to lung collapse and the result can be fatal. Removal of the air and fluid from the pleural space is a critically important management aspect of pulmonary care.

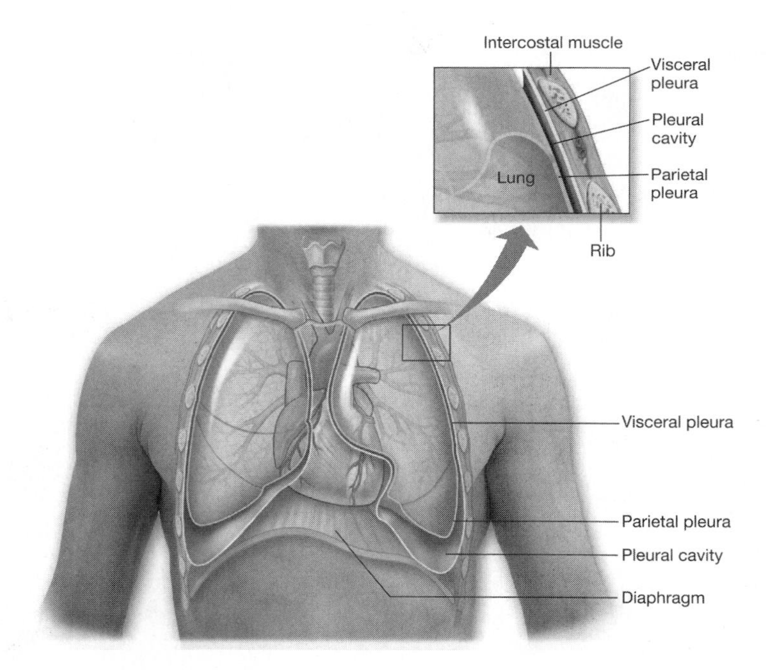

Normally, there is no air between the visceral and parietal pleura.

In this lesson, each of the pleural disturbances (pleural effusion, hemothorax, pneumothorax) is initially discussed separately followed by a discussion of a key intervention in all three disturbances—chest tubes. The many commonalities in treating pleural disturbances are discussed at the end.

LO1:

What Is a Pleural Effusion?

Pleural effusion is the presence of excessive fluid in the pleural space.

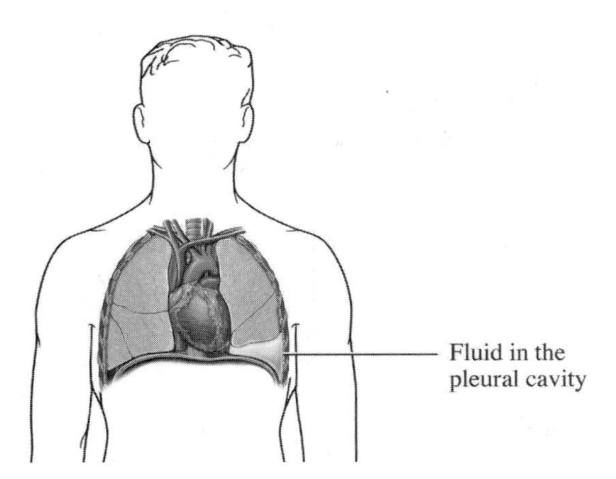

Note the effect that a small accumulation of fluid can have on lung expansion.
Source: © 2013 Nucleus Medical Media, All rights reserved

LO1:

Clinical Relevance: Pleural Effusions

- Effusions are a common problem and analysis of the fluid may suggest or confirm the underlying cause.
- Patients with large effusions can become very symptomatic, requiring intervention.
- Large effusions cause severe dyspnea (labored breathing) with increased respiratory rate and decreased volume of each breath, creating fear and anxiety in the patient.

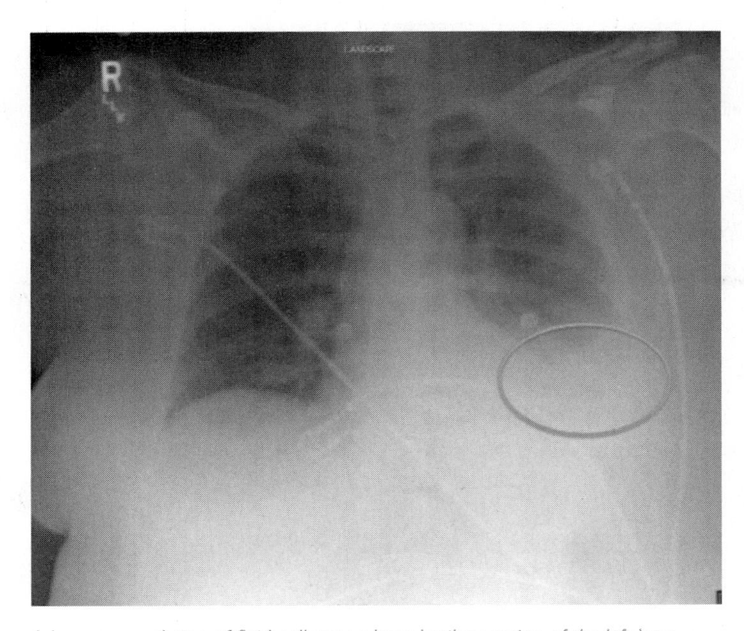

A large accumulation of fluid collapses a large basilar portion of the left lung.
Source: Courtesy of K. Kyriakidis

LO2: Pathophysiology: Pleural Effusion

- The pleural space normally contains a thin layer of fluid that acts as a lubricant, allowing the visceral pleura to slide easily against the parietal pleura during respiration.
- The small amount of normal pleural fluid (2–10 mL) is maintained by the lymphatic system of the lungs, draining away any excess fluid.
- Normally, up to 100 mL of fluid can be produced in the pleural space each hour and is drained away by the lymphatics.
- When the rate of production of fluid is greater than the capacity of the lymphatic system to drain, an effusion develops.
- Effusions cause compression of the lung and large effusions can cause dyspnea and reduction in air exchange, resulting in hypoxemia.

Causes and Risk Factors: Pleural Effusion

- Heart failure, left heart failure
  - Effusion is most commonly bilateral.
  - Occasionally only one side is involved.
- Pneumonia
  - Forty percent of pneumonias develop an associated effusion.
  - Infection of the lung causes the capillaries to leak more fluid.
  - The fluid itself may or may not be infected.
- Malignancies
  - The effusion is usually secondary to metastatic disease.
  - The effusion results from fluid production by the malignant cells.
- Malnutrition
  - Normally, the protein in blood helps keep fluid within the vascular system.
  - When protein levels in blood (e.g., albumin) drop, the result is an increased amount of fluid in the extravascular space and pleural space.

Concept Check

1. **Which statement is true regarding pleural effusion?**

   A. A pleural effusion occurs when the lymphatic system drains into the pleural space.

   B. A pleural effusion is usually the result of trauma to the chest.

   C. If a pleural effusion occurs, cancer cells must be present in the lung.

   D. Pleural effusion occurs when more fluid accumulates around the lung than the body can handle.

Answer question

Assessment Findings: Pleural Effusion

- Dullness to percussion
- Decreased breath sounds
- Pleural rub
- Large effusions may result in shortness of breath, tachypnea, hypoxemia, and tachycardia
- Many signs and symptoms depend on the cause of the effusion (e.g., fever in pneumonia or distended neck veins and leg edema in heart failure).
- The fluid level of the effusion may appear as a meniscus (U-shape of the lung edge) or as a flat opacity. Compare the right to the left inferior angles in the x-ray.

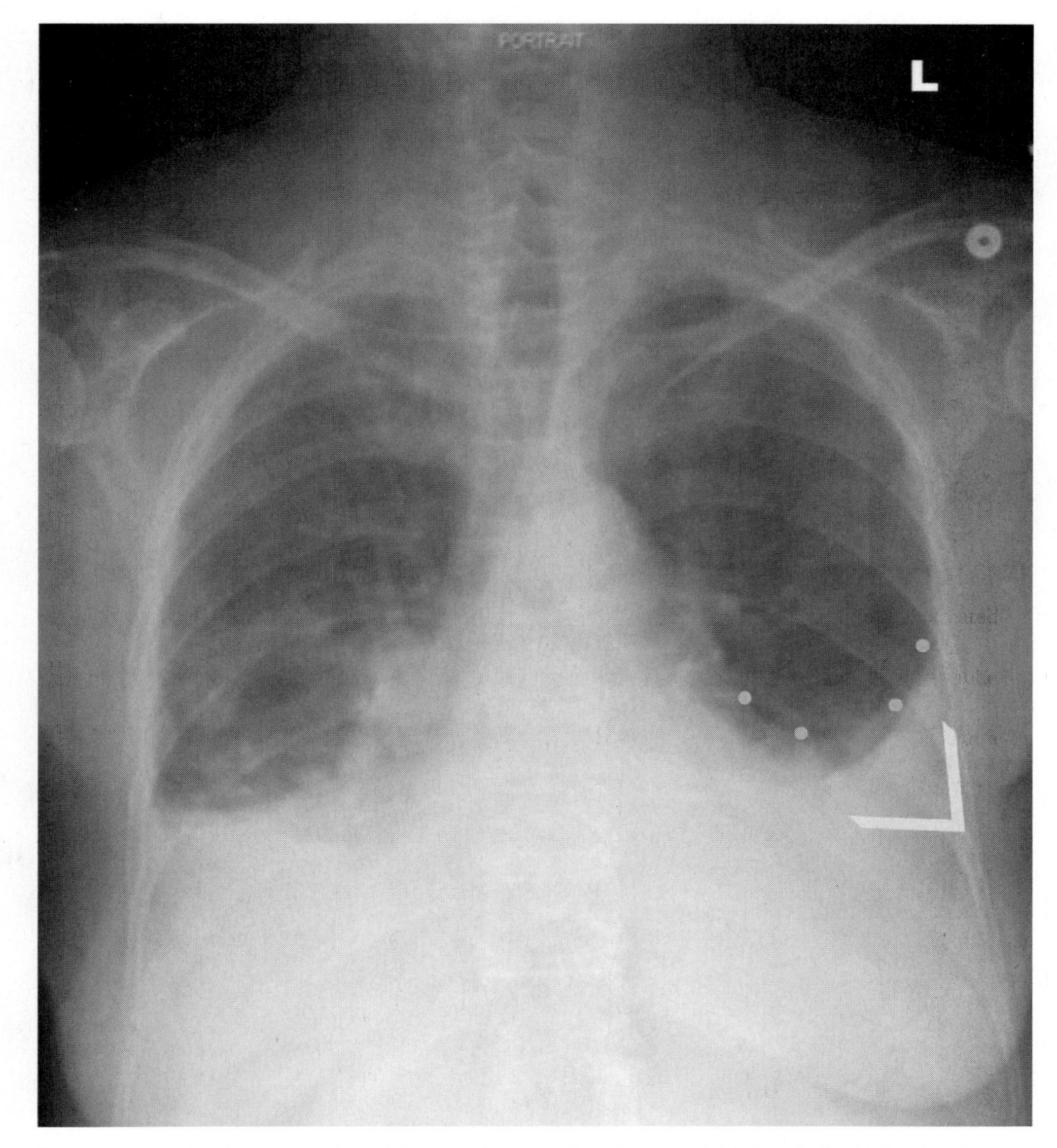

The x-ray shows the characteristic loss of the costophrenic angle in the patient's left base (yellow V shape) and a meniscus (green dots) appearance indicating the level of the effusion.
Source: Courtesy of K. Kyriakidis

Diagnostics: Pleural Effusion

- Pleural effusion is suspected on the basis of the patient's history, signs and symptoms, and physical exam.
- The diagnosis of pleural effusion is normally confirmed by x-ray. The costophrenic angle appears blunted, the lung may appear compressed, and opacity of a portion of the chest cavity is present.
- Thoracentesis is usually performed in new effusions for diagnostic purposes. The fluid is:
  - Studied microscopically
  - Cultured for organisms
  - Analyzed for levels of LDH, albumin, and protein that may assist in determining etiology

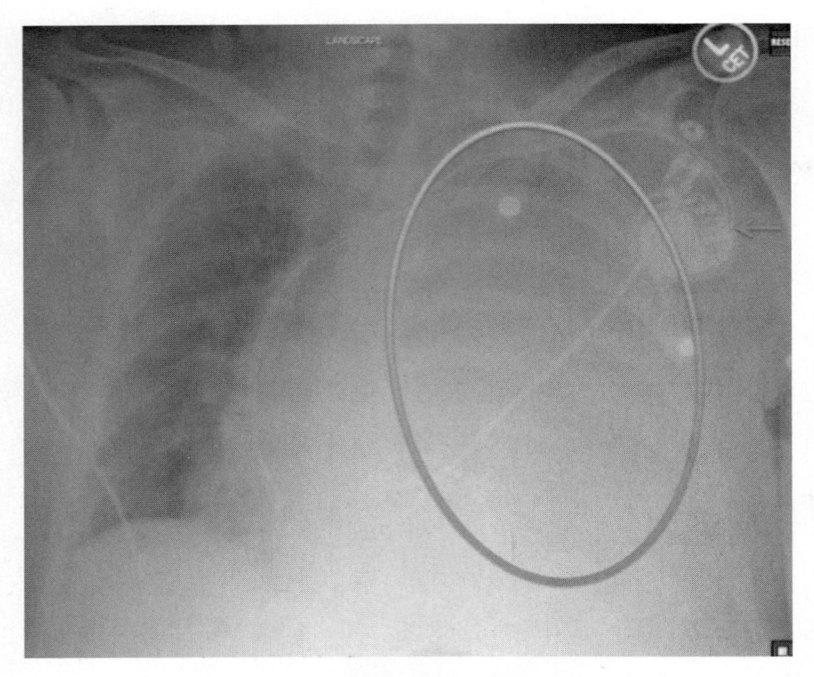

In this very sick patient, the whole left lung is affected by the large pleural effusion, seen as a white out (blue circle), and caused by a gastric ulcer perforation. A permanent pacemaker is on the patient's upper left chest. The right lung is clear.
Source: Courtesy of K. Kyriakidis

LO3:

Collaborative Interventions: Pleural Effusion

- Treatment of pleural effusion is usually targeted at the cause:
  -  Administer antibiotics for infection
  - 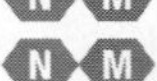 Diuresis for heart failure: Diuresis will frequently resolve an effusion caused by CHF in approximately two days. Monitor and evaluate the patient's response to diuresis.
- Large effusions, especially those causing symptoms, should be drained.
  - Drainage is accomplished by thoracentesis (aspiration of fluid through a needle inserted between the ribs into the pleural cavity).

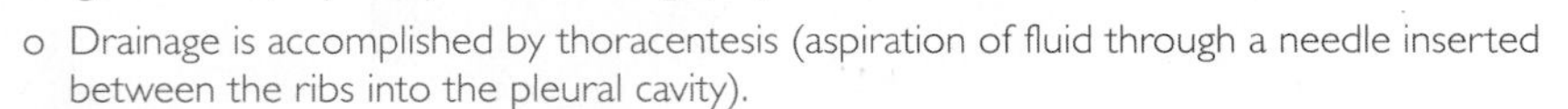

- Monitor and evaluate following thoracentesis. Effusions that rapidly re-accumulate may require placement of a chest tube or catheter positioned in the chest that allows continuous drainage.
- Pleurodesis can prevent a re-accumulation of fluid by causing the visceral and parietal pleura to adhere, thus eliminating the pleural cavity.
  - Prior to pleurodesis, the effusion is aspirated to remove all the fluid.
  - Pleurodesis is accomplished by introducing a chemical irritant into the pleural space through a chest tube. The irritant causes inflammation and scarring of the pleura, resulting in adherence.
- Infected effusions with pus (empyema) usually require a chest tube to allow drainage, in addition to intravenous antibiotics.

Concept Check

2. A patient has a recurrence of pleural effusion after being treated twice in the past few months. The nurse anticipates what intervention?

A. Aspiration and observation
B. Thorocentesis
C. Aspiration and pleurodesis
D. Chest tube placement

Answer question

Hemothorax Overview

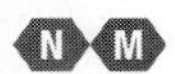

- Hemothorax is a pleural effusion that consists of blood. It usually results from trauma but can also occur spontaneously in patients taking anticoagulants.
- Patient presentation is essentially the same as the patient with any other effusion. Evidence of significant blood loss may offer a clue to the diagnosis. X-ray findings resemble those of any other pleural effusion.
- Treatment consists of the insertion of a chest tube to drain the blood from the pleural space. This procedure allows measurement of the blood loss and may tamponade (stop) the source of bleeding by reinflating the lung.

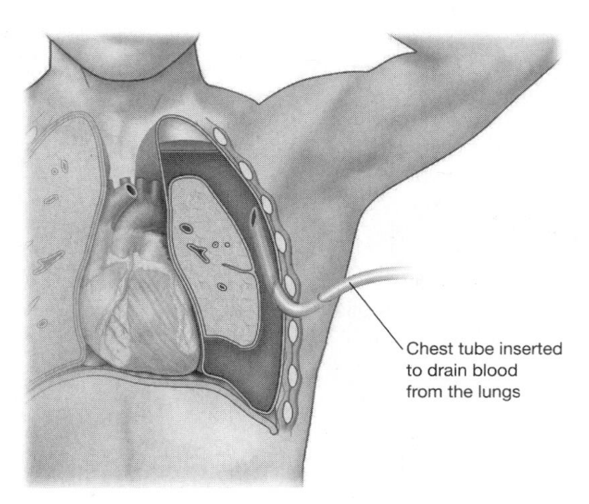

A chest tube is placed in the pleural space to drain blood that collected and allow the lung to fully expand. A chest tube drainage system is connected and suction applied. As in pneumothorax, the chest tube is removed when the lung fully re-expands.

Concept Check

3. **What is the appropriate immediate treatment for hemothorax in a symptomatic patient?**
   A. Replace lost fluids.
   B. Insert a chest tube.
   C. Institute antibiotics.
   D. Administer diuretics.

Answer question

LO1: What Is a Pneumothorax?

Air in the pleural space or the space surrounding the lung(s) is called a pneumothorax. The air exerts pressure on the collapsed lung, preventing it from re-expanding when one breathes.

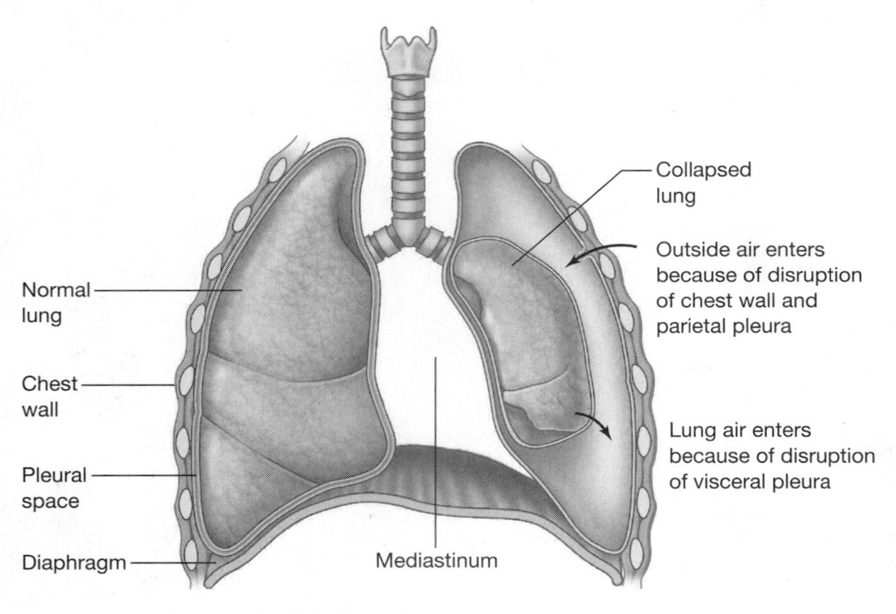

This illustration depicts a left-sided pneumothorax.

LO1: Clinical Relevance: Pneumothorax

- Pneumothorax is a common complication following invasive procedures performed in the hospital:
    - o Central line placement
    - o Thoracentesis
    - o Chest surgeries
- Tension pneumothorax (a type of pneumothorax) can cause a rapid decline in the patient and could prove fatal.
    - o Early recognition is essential for successful and urgent treatment.

LO2: Pathophysiology: Pneumothorax

- Pressure in the pleural space is normally lower than in the atmosphere.
- The pressure differential keeps the lungs expanded and the parietal and visceral pleura together.
- A defect or rent in the pleura exposes the pleural space to atmospheric air. This condition can be caused by:
    - o A penetrating knife wound
    - o Puncture of the lung by:
        - ■ Surgery
        - ■ Severe coughing
        - ■ Vehicle or other accident
- Air then moves from the higher pressure area to the lower pressure area in the pleural space.
- As air enters the space, the increased pressure causes the lung to collapse and interferes with gas exchange.

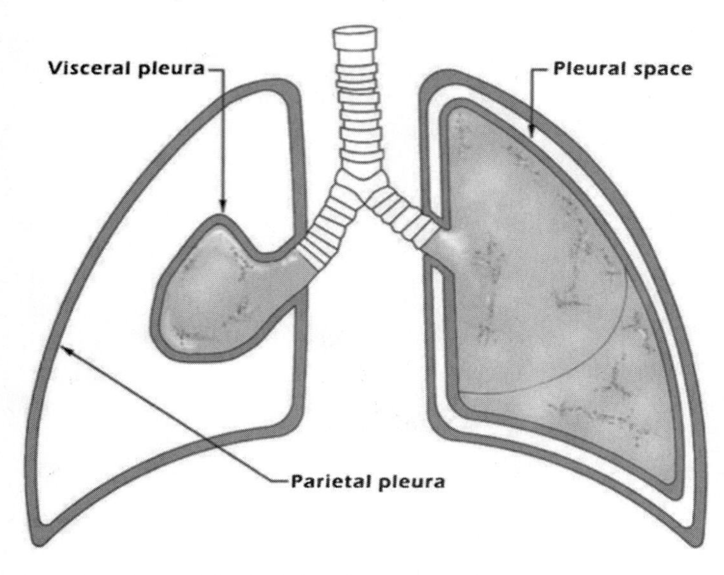

Source: Copyright © 2012, NovEx Novice to Expert Learning, LLC

Tension Pneumothorax

- Tension pneumothorax is a dangerous, often fatal event. Tension pneumothorax results when air enters the pleural space through a defect but cannot exit. A one-way valve effect occurs and the pressure in the pleural space progressively increases. This has several effects:
  - o Intrathoracic pressure increase, compressing the veins and decreasing blood returning to the heart, resulting in diminished cardiac output, which can prove fatal.
  - o The increasing pressure causes a shift of the mediastinal structures (e.g., heart and trachea) to the opposite side, causing a mediastinal shift.
- Tension pneumothorax requires immediate venting of the air from the pleural space to the atmosphere. The vent can be a chest tube or a needle inserted into the pleural space.

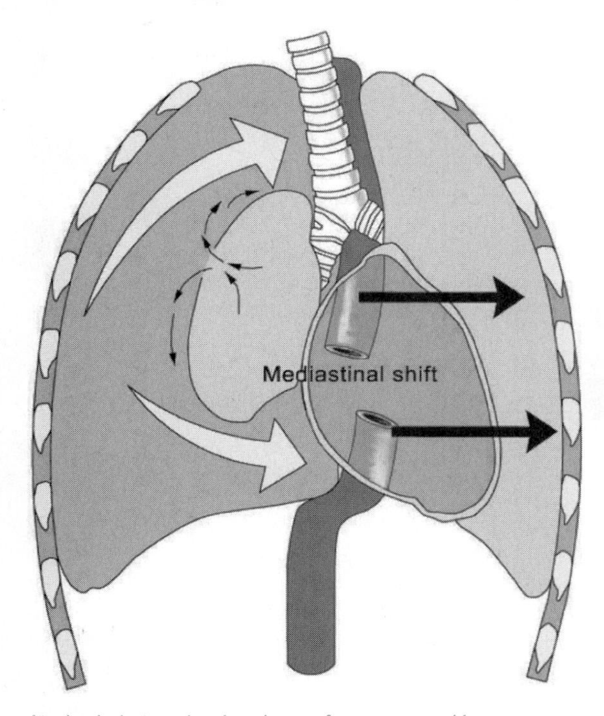

Air that leaks into the pleural space from a ruptured lung presents the danger of a tension pneumothorax. The air has no path to escape. The pressure from a tension pneumothorax compresses the lung and can also push the heart to the opposite side. The compression can severely hinder cardiac output.
Source: Copyright © 2012, NovEx Novice to Expert Learning, LLC

Causes and Risk Factors: Pneumothorax

- Spontaneous pneumothorax occurs without a known cause.
    - Primary pneumothorax occurs in patients without lung disease. Risk factors include:
        - Smoking
        - Family history
    - Secondary pneumothorax occurs in patients with lung disease. Risk factors include:
        - Emphysema
        - Pneumonia
        - Lung cancer
        - Cystic fibrosis
- Traumatic injury most commonly resulting from:
    - Blunt trauma, causing rib fracture with puncture of the lung by the sharp edge of the fractured rib.
    - Penetrating trauma, e.g., a knife or gunshot wound.
    - Barotrauma, the result of excessive pressure used to inflate the lungs when a patient is on a ventilator.

Assessment Findings: Pneumothorax

- Symptoms of patients with pneumothorax are usually related to the size of the pneumothorax and include:
    - Shortness of breath
    - Diminished breath sounds on the side of the pneumothorax
    - Dullness to percussion
    - Hypoxia
- Symptoms in tension pneumothorax can be dramatic:
    - Hypotension that develops rapidly
    - Tachycardia
    - Absent breath sounds on the side of the pneumothorax
    - Shifting of the trachea to the opposite side

Concept Check

4. Which assessment findings would make the clinician more suspicious of pleural effusion rather than a pneumothorax?

A. Shortness of breath

B. Dullness on percussion

C. Hypoxia

D. Pleural rub

Answer question

Diagnostics: Pneumothorax

- Chest x-ray discloses air around a collapsing lung.
- X-ray of a patient with tension pneumothorax exhibits a shift of the heart and trachea to the opposite side of the chest.

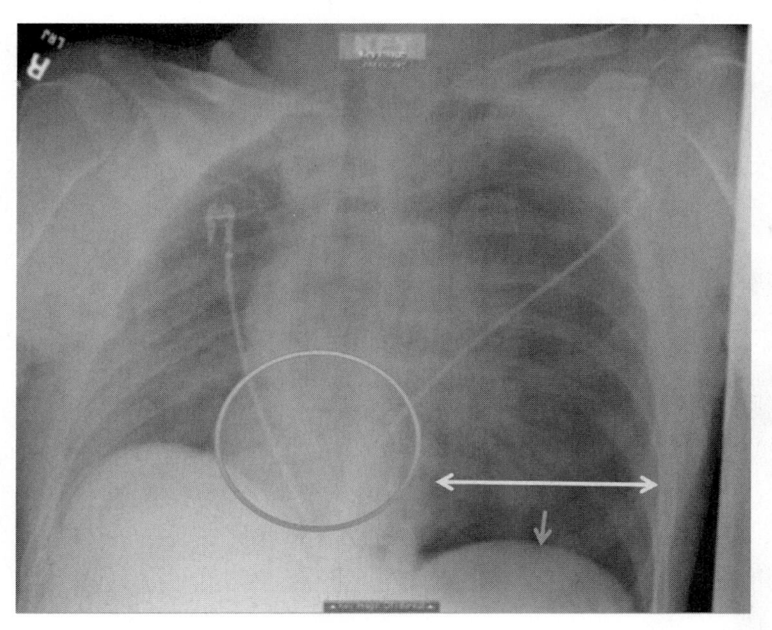

Radiographic features:

- Overexpanded hemithorax (yellow arrow)
- Shift of the mediastinum to the right side (circled)
- Depression of the hemidiaphragm (red arrow)

Source: Courtesy of K. Kyriakidis

LO3:

Collaborative Interventions: Pneumothorax

- If the pneumothorax is small and asymptomatic, the patient may be monitored and treated with supplemental oxygen (3 L/min to 100% FIO_2). These often resolve spontaneously.

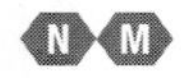

- Larger pneumothoraces usually require aspiration of air with a needle or chest tube placement.

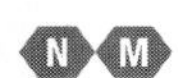

- Unstable patients, with tension pneumothorax, require immediate decompression with a needle or chest tube. Successful treatment usually results in rapid improvement.

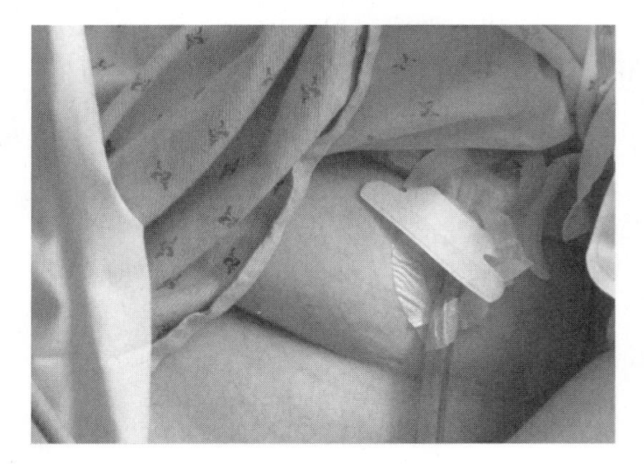

A chest tube is inserted to allow lung re-expansion.
Source: Copyright © 2012, NovEx Novice to Expert Learning, LLC

Concept Check

5. What factor determines the treatment selected for pneumothorax?
   A. Size of the pneumothorax
   B. Cause of the pneumothorax
   C. Age of the patient
   D. Presence of blood in the pleural space

Answer question

Before treatment (same patient)

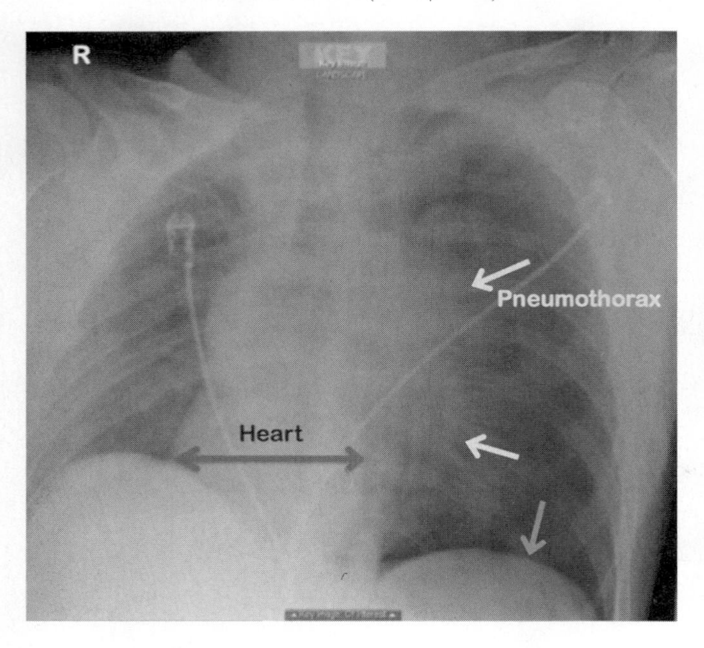

After treatment

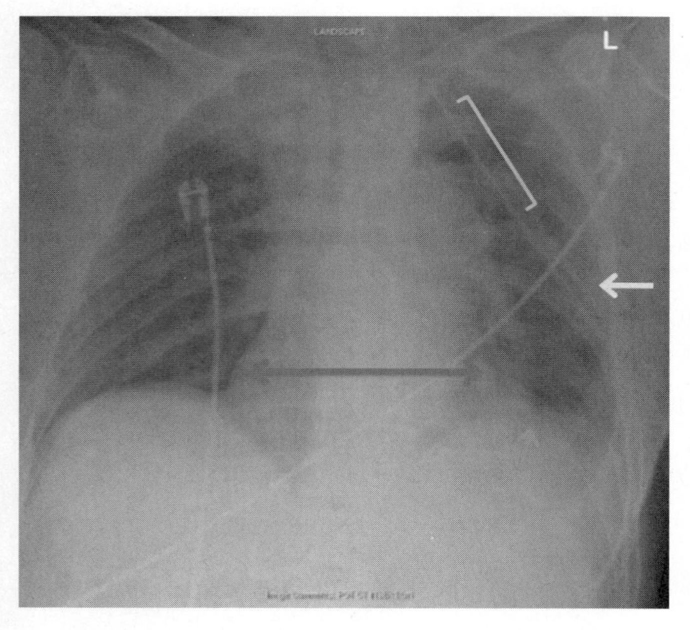

The comparison of x-rays in this patient with a tension pneumothorax (top, yellow arrows) and following treatment (bottom) highlights the re-expansion (yellow arrow) of the right lung. The dramatic shift in the heart back toward the midline is visible (blue arrows). The red arrow in the top x-ray shows how the pressure displaced the diaphragm and how treatment with a chest tube (green bracket) returns the diaphragm to normal (bottom).
Source: *(both)* Courtesy of K. Kyriakidis

Priority Patient Concerns and Desired Collaborative Care Outcomes: All Pleural Disturbances

Prior to caring for patient with pleural disturbances, it is important to prioritize the patient's concerns that must guide the nursing care plan and interventions. Care for the patient is ordered and organized in accordance with the patient's priority and urgent needs. Desired collaborative care outcomes in patients with pleural disturbances typically include:

1. Patient's respiratory effort will return to pre-incident level. Chest drainage system will remove the fluid, blood, or air from the chest cavity.
2. Patient's oxygenation saturation will return to pre-incident level.
3. Patient will report decrease in pain.
4. Patient will be infection free.
5. Patient will experience no further tissue damage.

Considering these important care outcomes, prepare a list of the major 3–6 priority patient concerns or nursing diagnoses for patients with pleural disturbances. Be prepared to participate in a discussion of this list and/or to submit them as an assignment, as determined by your faculty. Resources you may find helpful in this assignment can include this lesson, the references, resources on nursing care plans, and standard nursing diagnoses manuals.

LO3:

Collaborative Interventions: All Pleural Disturbances

Chest Tube Placement

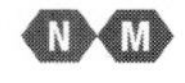

- Chest tubes are placed to help evacuate air, blood, or fluid from the thoracic cavity, and allow re-expansion of the lungs. Chest tube insertion requires assistance from the nurse. The nurse is needed to support and coach the patient through the procedure.
- (M) Chest tubes are placed into the pleural space, above the seventh intercostal space to avoid placement in organs other than the lung.
- (M) The chest tube insertion site is numbed (local anesthesia). The patient may require sedation.
- (M) An opening is made between the ribs of the chest wall (thoracostomy) through which the chest tube is placed. It is connected to a suction system for drainage.

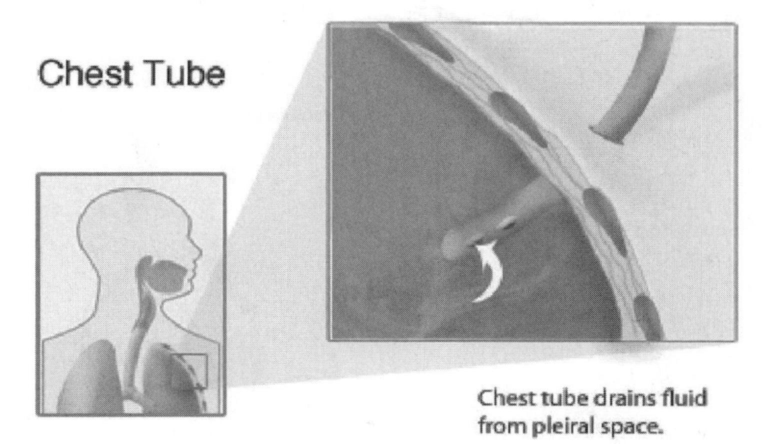

Chest Tube
Chest tube drains fluid from pleiral space.

The area for insertion is numbed (local anesthesia). The chest tube is inserted between the ribs into the pleural space and is connected to a bottle or canister that contains sterile water. Suction is attached to the system to encourage drainage. The chest tube usually remains in place until all the blood, fluid, or air has drained from the chest and the lung has fully re-expanded. When the chest tube is no longer needed, it can be easily removed.

- (M) In an emergency, a large bore needle may be used to decompress the lung and alleviate the pressure (see photo).
- (M) The chest tube is typically removed when x-rays reveal that the air, blood, or fluid is resolved, and the lung is re-expanded. The chest tube is then removed, usually without the need for sedation or an anesthetic.
- (N) Pre-medicate for pain prior to chest tube removal.

- Antibiotics may be needed if infection is a threat.

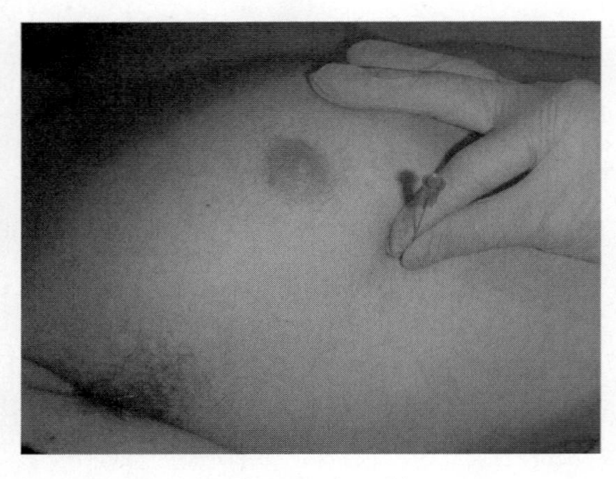

In an emergency, when the patient's vital functions are compromised and rapid deterioration ensues, needle decompression can be life-saving.
Source: Copyright © 2012, NovEx Novice to Expert Learning, LLC

Collaborative Interventions: All Pleural Disturbances (continued)

Chest Drainage System (CDS)

- The goal is to evacuate air, fluid, or blood from the pleural space.
- In order to allow air and fluid to exit without re-entering the pleural space, chest drainage systems must have a valve that allows movement in one direction only.
- CDS are designed to take advantage of gravity to achieve this.
- The devices are, therefore, always below the level of the chest.
- Commonly used CDS in today's patients have multiple features that are best understood by examining each feature additively. Each additive concept is presented below using the one, two and three chamber method, shown with the old, traditional glass bottles.

Early CDS Method

- The chest tube from the patient is connected to a valve that lets air out but not in.
    - o Balloon type valve (dry).
    - o A valve system that has an extension tube or chamber barely under the water level

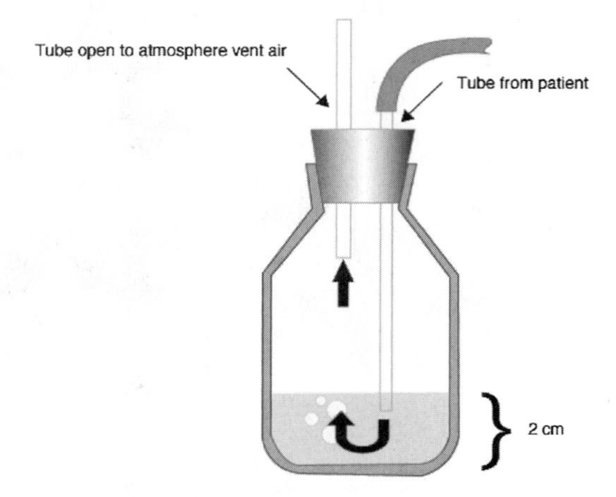

Air can push past the water to escape, but it cannot re-enter the chest.
Source: Copyright © 2012, NovEx Novice to Expert Learning, LLC

CDS with Fluid Collection Chamber

- If fluid is draining, it adds to the fluid in the water seal, and increases the resistance for air to exit the pleural space. For this reason, a second or collection chamber was added.
- The second chamber is placed in front of the valve or water seal to allow fluid to leave the pleural space without affecting the valve or depth of the water seal.

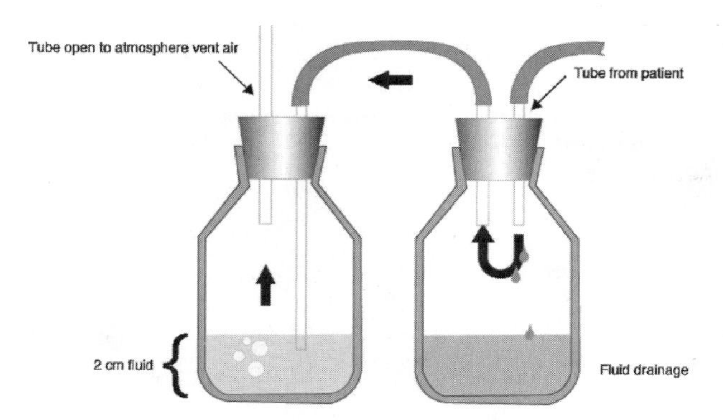

A dual-chambered drainage system encourages fluid to collect in the first bottle and allows air to escape with little resistance from the second chamber.
Source: Copyright © 2012, NovEx Novice to Expert Learning, LLC

Three Parts of a Complete CDS

Most current CDS use a three chamber system:

- Chamber 1 is the collection chamber for fluids draining from the chest.
- Chamber 2 is the water seal chamber which lets air escape from the pleural space but it cannot re-enter.
  - o Re-entry is prevented by either a valve or a water seal.
- Chamber 3 is the suction control chamber.
  - o Negative pressure in this chamber applies suction in the pleural space.
  - o The pressure in this chamber should be low, i.e., no greater than 20 cm H_2O.
  - o Many clinicians believe this chamber is not necessary and no evidence exists to support its use. However, it is still commonly applied.
  - o This chamber can be regulated by a valve, or water column.
    - ■ If water is used, one should see slight bubbling in this chamber at all times.
    - ■ If not bubbling, then the desired level of suction is not present.

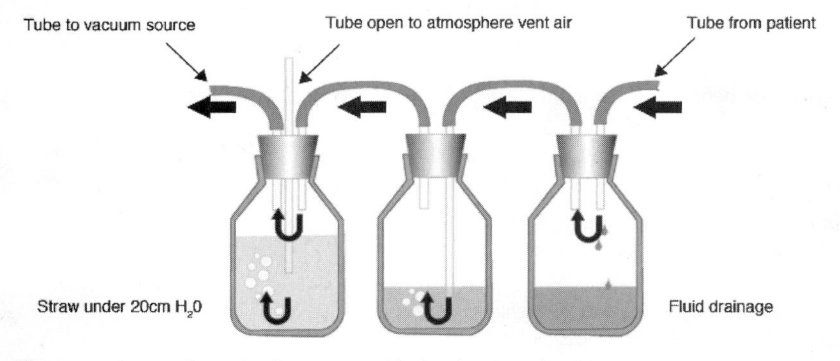

This image shows a three chamber system with chamber 1 on the right.
Source: Copyright © 2012, NovEx Novice to Expert Learning, LLC

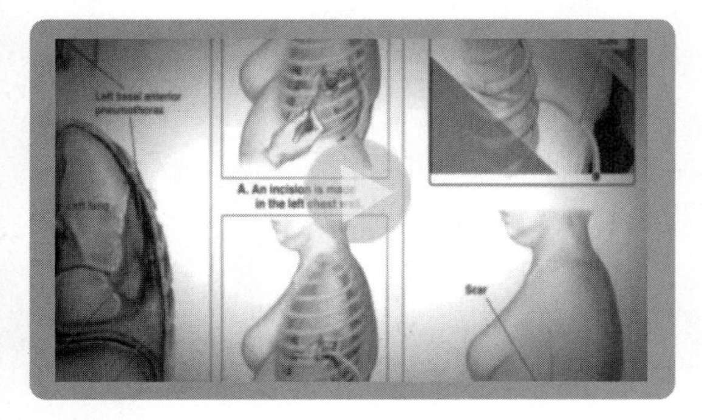

In the newer CDS, the three chambers have been combined into one collection device, as described in this video.
Source: Copyright © 2012, NovEx Novice to Expert Learning, LLC

Concept Check

6. What does bubbling in the third chamber of a three-chamber chest drainage system indicate?

A. An air leak in the system has occurred.

B. Adequate suction is in use.

C. Pleural healing is complete.

D. Pleurodesis is required.

Answer question

Suction Regulation in CDS

- *In older systems* that utilize a third chamber, fluid is placed in the third chamber.
- An open tube is placed below the water level. This tube is open at both the bottom and top.
- N As suction is applied, air is sucked into the tube and causes the water to begin to bubble.
- N M The level of negative pressure applied to the chest is determined by the water depth in the suction bottle (#3). The vacuum regulator reading does NOT determine the negative pressure transmitted to the chest.
- *Newer CDS* devices commonly utilize dry valves. However, the water seal valves are helpful since these allow observation of air that may exit from the pleural space.

Collaborative Interventions: All Pleural Disturbances (continued)

Safety and Quality Concerns

- N Observe the presence of bubbling in the water seal chamber to confirm air exiting the pleural space.
  - o *If there is bubbling, one must NOT clamp the chest tube.*
- N Do not clamp the chest tube, especially during transport. Clamping the chest tube can trap air in the pleural space and create a tension pneumothorax.
- N If there is no pleural air leak, then bubbling or tidaling (normal water level fluctuations with respirations) is no longer seen in the water seal chamber.
- N If there is no bubbling or tidaling, the chest drainage tubing may be kinked, bent, or clogged from a blood clot. Like clamping the chest tubing, kinking or bending can create a tension pneumothorax and harm the patient.
- N Always keep the CDS below the level of the patient's chest to to prevent drainage from reentering the patient's chest and to promote drainage.
- Monitor and measure chest tube drainage (amount, quality) to recognize complications early (e.g., chest tube displacement, clot preventing drainage, infection, bleeding, inadequate suction).
- N M Do not milk or strip (pull on the tubing and create suction to enhance chest tube drainage) the chest tubes to avoid generating negative pressure. Instead, move visible clots along the drainage tubing by squeezing down along the tubing.
- N Never disconnect the chest tube from the drainage tubing or reposition the chest tube. These unsafe actions can introduce infection.
- N Notify healthcare provider if excessive bleeding is noted (in cases of pleural effusion or pneumothorax) to evaluate for lung damage due to chest tube insertion.
- N Add water (depending on CDS) if low to maintain water-seal and suction levels.
- N Prior to chest tube removal, teach the patient how to do the Valsalva maneuver at maximum inspiration. Instruct the patient to Valsalva right before the healthcare provider removes the chest tube to prevent air reentry into the chest.
- N Report subcutaneous emphysema (crepitus or air bubbles under the skin around the insertion site like crackles). The majority of subQ emphysema incidences are benign and require no intervention but some situations require the need for chest tube adjustment.

Collaborative Symptom Management and Comfort Care

There are additional interventions that can provide symptom management or comfort and include:

N M • Observe and aspirate fluid, blood, or air. These simple interventions are recommended when the patient's symptoms, responses, and condition allow.

N M • Aspirate or place chest tube(s) to remove excess amounts of air or fluids when indicated.
  - o Simple aspiration is preferred in non-emergent situations.
  - o The resulting re-expansion of the lung may assist in determining the etiology of the pleural disturbance.

N • Prevent the drained air and fluid from returning into the pleural space.

N • Restore negative pressure in the pleural space to re-expand the lung. Ensure proper negative pressure and continuous drainage by preventing kinking and looping of the drainage tubing and chest tube.

N M • Provide supplemental oxygen therapy, as needed.

N • Offer reassurance, comfort measures, including family support, caring interactions, emotional support, and/or pastoral support.

N M • Provide pain management using pharmacologic and alternative therapeutic interventions.

N • Pre-medicate for pain prior to chest tube removal

N • Mobilize the patient as early as possible to prevent complications. Extra support to assist the patient may be needed. Range of motion exercises should be done until patient can be out of bed.

N • Ensure adequate periods of rest.

Patient Education: All Pleural Disturbances

N • No preventive measures are known for pneumothorax other than avoiding traumatic accidents. Emphasize to patients that seatbelts can lower their risk in case of an accident.

N • After pneumothorax, educate patient to avoid air travel and deepsea diving due to pressure changes until healthcare provider agrees it is safe.

N • Educate patient to stop smoking and provide smoking cessation information.

N • As in all conditions, educate patient about condition, medications, healthy diet, exercise, and contact healthcare provider if condition worsens.

Summary of Interventions

- Oxygen should be administered for O_2 saturations of less than or equal to 92%.
  - o Oxygen administration has been shown to increase the rate of absorption of air in a pneumothorax and should be considered even if O_2 saturation is less than or equal to 92%.
- Fluid, air, or blood can be removed from the pleural space with aspiration or by inserting a chest tube. Gas exchange is improved by re-expansion and diagnosis is made easier.
- A tension pneumothorax is a medical emergency requiring immediate decompression with insertion of a chest tube.
  - o A needle inserted into the pleural space may provide more immediate relief.

LO4: Evaluation of Desired Collaborative Care Outcomes: All Pleural Disturbances

Evaluation and reassessment should reveal attainment of previously established patient outcomes. In summary:

- The patient reports breathing is easier. Chest drainage system is operating correctly to remove fluid, blood, or air. The lung is re-expanding.
- Patient demonstrates no pallor or cyanosis. Mentation is clear.
- Patient reports pain is decreased to a tolerable level. Pain may not be totally absent due to mechanism of original injury.
- Patient is afebrile with normal white blood cell count, clear mentation, no adventitious lung sounds, and no findings associated with other organ involvement. Chest tube insertion site shows no redness, edema, or abnormal drainage.
- Patient is free from subcutaneous emphysema or other tissue involvement.

References

Pleural Effusion

Wing, S. (2004). Pleural effusion: nursing care challenge in the elderly. *Geriatr Nurs, 25*(6), 348–352.

Clinical Practice Guidelines

Hooper, C., Lee, G., & Maskell, N. (2010). Investigation of a unilateral pleural effusion in adults: British Thoracic Society pleural disease guideline 2010. *Thorax, 65*(ii), ii4–ii17.

Light, R. W. (2002). Clinical practice. Pleural effusion. *N Engl J Med, 346*, 1971–1977.

Pneumothorax

Clinical Practice Guidelines

Bethel J. (2008, July). Tension pneumothorax. *Emerg Nurse, 16*(4), 26–29.

MacDuff, A., Arnold, A., & Harvey, J. (2010). Management of spontaneous pneumothorax: British Thoracic Society pleural disease guideline 2010. *Thorax, 65*(ii), ii18–ii33.

Sharma, A., & Jindal, P. (2008). Principles of diagnosis and management of traumatic pneumothorax. *J Emerg Trauma Shock, 1*(1), 34–41.

All Pleural Disturbances

Clinical Practice Guidelines

Bauman, M. & Handley, C. (2011). Chest tube care: the more you know, the easier it gets. *American Nurse Today, 6*(9), 27–32.

Dev, S. P., Nascimiento, B., Simone, C., & Chien, V. (2007). Chest tube insertion. *N Engl J Med, 357*, e15.

Durai, R., Hoque, H., & Davies, T. W. (2010). Managing a chest tube and drainage system. *AORN J, 91*(12), 275–280.

Learning Outcomes for Thoracotomy

When you complete this lesson, you will be able to:

1. Recognize the clinical relevance of a thoracotomy.
2. Consider the pathophysiology, etiology, risk factors, and clinical presentation of a patient requiring a thoracotomy that determine the priority patient concerns.
3. Determine the most urgent and important nursing interventions and patient education required in caring for a patient with a thoracotomy.
4. Evaluate attainment of desired collaborative care outcomes for a patient with a thoracotomy.

LO1:

What Is a Thoracotomy?

- Thoracotomy is a surgical procedure used to gain access to the thoracic cavity. When performed outside the OR, it is always a resuscitative or emergency procedure to gain quick access to the heart or major vessels due to injury or trauma.
- Patients requiring emergent thoracotomy are typically in shock, tamponade, hemorrhaging, or pulseless.
- Thoracotomies are done for many nonemergent procedures such as lung resections due to cancer or types of lung disease, cardiac surgeries, infections, esophageal surgery and some endocrine resections. However, these are done in the OR.

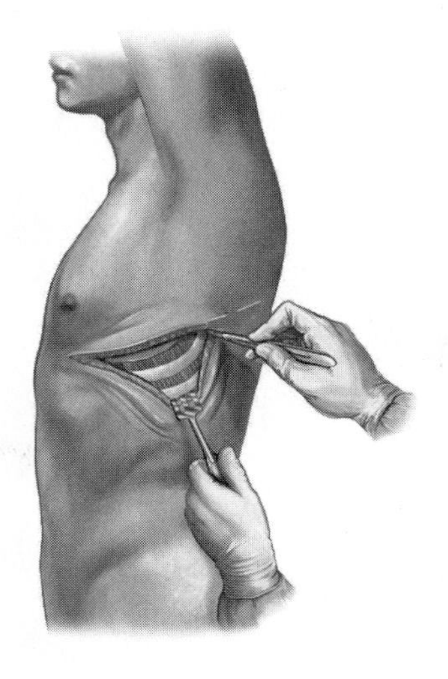

This illustrates a thoracotomy incision.

Concept Check

1. **Emergency thoracotomy is performed for which reasons?**
   A. To gain quick access to the heart
   B. To remove cancerous tissue
   C. To repair patent ductus arteriosus
   D. To access hiatal hernia

Answer question

LO1:

Clinical Relevance

Thoracotomies are important management strategies for:

- Lung resection
- Thoracic trauma
- Esophageal resection or rupture
- Cardiac surgery (on pump)

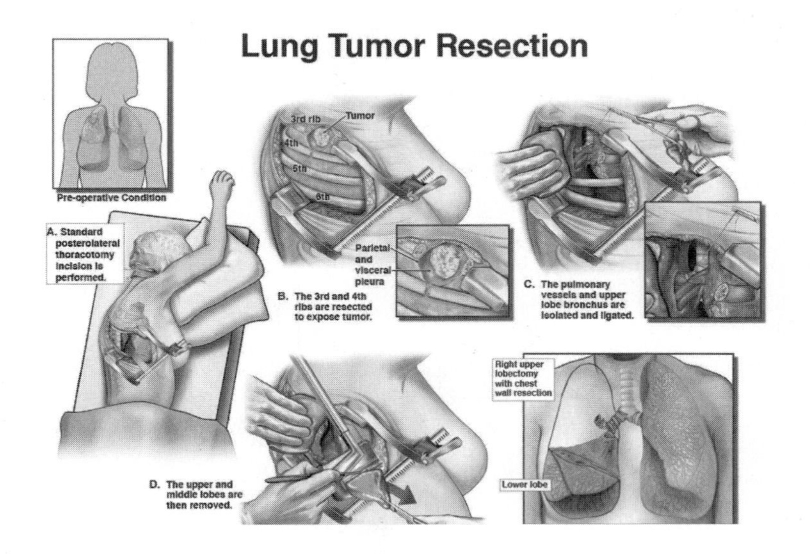
Lung Tumor Resection
Pre-operative Condition
A. Standard posterolateral thoracotomy incision is performed.
3rd rib
Tumor
4th
5th
6th
Parietal and visceral pleura
B. The 3rd and 4th ribs are resected to expose tumor.
C. The pulmonary vessels and upper lobe bronchus are isolated and ligated.
Right upper lobectomy with chest wall resection
Lower lobe
D. The upper and middle lobes are then removed.

LO2:

Types

- Thoracotomies are of three types:
  1. Posterolateral
  2. Muscle sparing
  3. Anterior approach
- The most common type is the posterolateral.
- The thoracotomy can be on the left or right side.
- Bilateral thoracotomies (transverse if connected) are sometimes needed, as in performing a lung transplant.
- For the muscle sparing thoracotomy, the latissimus dorsi is not cut but retracted, and this procedure possibly helps to decrease postoperative pain.
- The incision for the anterior thoracotomy is made on the front of the chest for procedures such as cardiac and endocrine surgery.

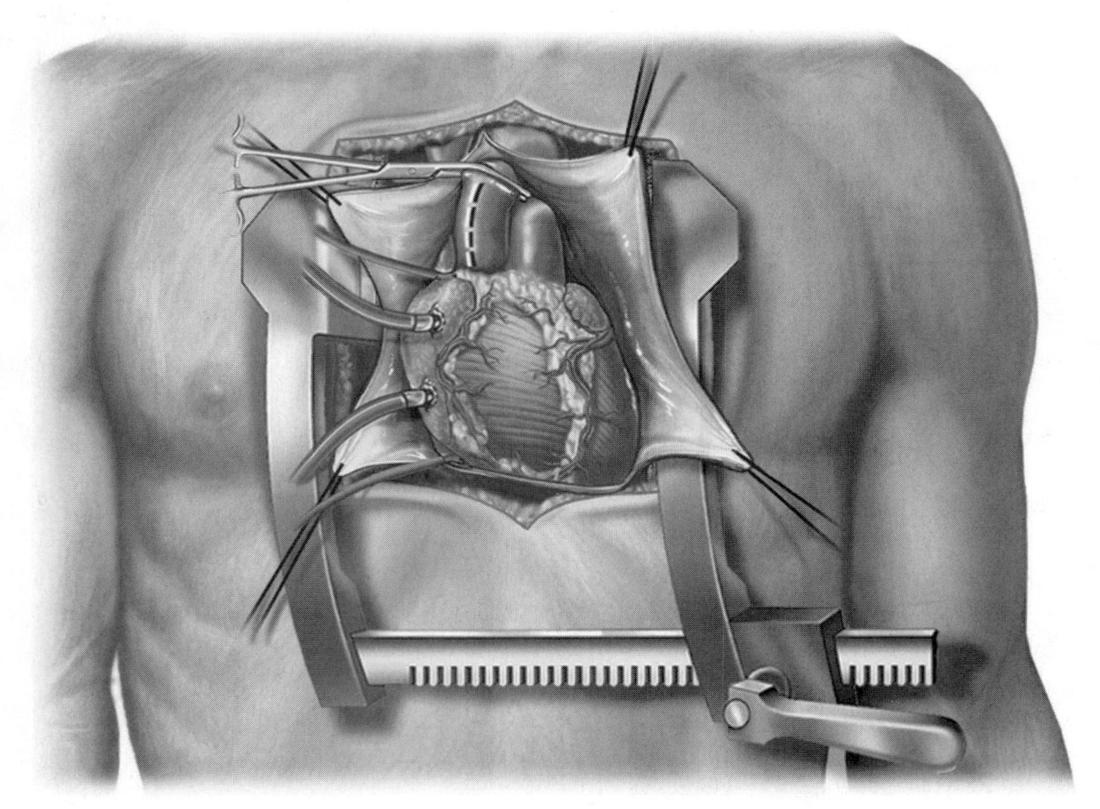

This illustration depicts a thoracotomy for an open heart surgery with retractors in place. The pericardium is open, exposing the heart, and the heart is cannulized (tubes inserted for cardiopulmonary bypass) via the right atrium and ventricle. Note how far the chest is spread open, explaining the chest pain patients have post-op.

Concept Check

2. What is the benefit of a muscle sparing thoracotomy?

A. It opens the chest more completely, allowing better visualization of structures.

B. It can result in less postoperative pain.

C. It is easier to perform than other techniques.

D. It is a faster way to gain access to chest structures.

Answer question

Concepts

- Thoracotomies present postoperatively in different patterns, depending on the type of surgery.
- Some surgeries (e.g., off pump surgery) may be relatively minor.
- Other thoracotomy surgeries involve significant postoperative management.
- One of the most common aspects of thoracotomies is the presence of chest drainage systems (CDS).

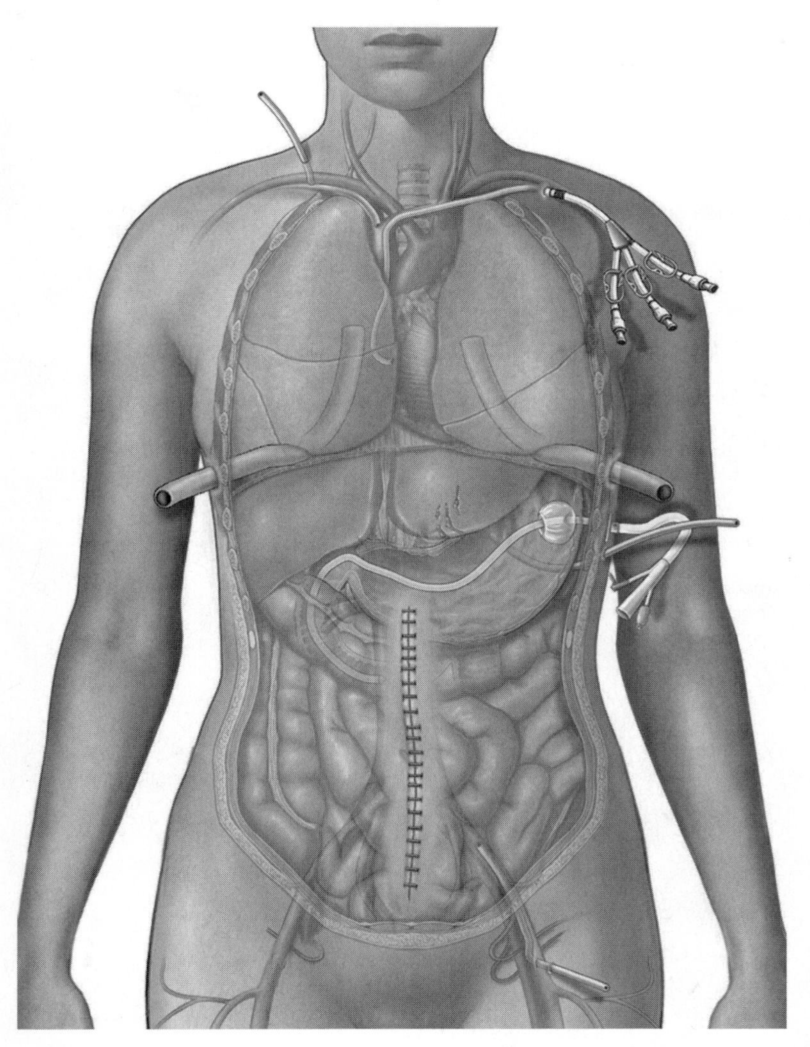

Bilateral chest tubes are shown inside the thorax and exiting the chest wall. The chest tubes are used to drain excess blood or fluid and remove air from the lung spaces.

Concept Check

3. **What equipment would be used postoperatively by a nurse caring for a patient who has had a thoracotomy?**
   A. Chest drainage unit
   B. Penrose drain into the chest cavity
   C. Tracheostomy cleaning supplies
   D. A minimum of two large-bore peripheral IVs

Answer question

Priority Patient Concerns and Desired Collaborative Care Outcomes

Prior to caring for patients with a thoracotomy, it is important to prioritize the patient's concerns that must guide the nursing care plan and interventions. Care for the patient is ordered and organized in accordance with the patient's priority and urgent needs. Desired collaborative care outcomes in patients with a thoracotomy typically include:

1. Patient will report a decrease in pain.
2. Patient's breathing pattern will return to pre-incident normal.
3. Patient's oxygen saturation will return to pre-incident normal.
4. Patient will demonstrate a progressive return to pre-surgical activities.
5. Patient will be infection free.

Considering these important care outcomes, prepare a list of the major 3–6 priority patient concerns or nursing diagnoses for patients with a thoracotomy. Be prepared to participate in a discussion of this list and/or to submit them as an assignment, as determined by your faculty. Resources you may find helpful in this assignment can include this lesson, the references, resources on nursing care plans, and standard nursing diagnoses manuals.

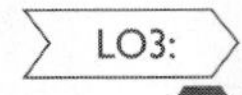

Collaborative Interventions

N

- Due to the epidural and pain medication, ongoing assessment of the thoracotomy patient involves assessment of:
  - Severity, location, quality of, and patient's responses to pain
  - Breathing rate and quality
  - Heart rate and rhythm
  - Blood pressure
- Bleeding or hemorrhage: Assess for rate of blood loss, amount, character, location, or source if visible. Depending on severity, intervention can range from using gauzex to hold pressure for mild bleeding at the surgical site to calling rapid response and the surgeon for emergency return to surgery if hemorrhaging is noted from any site.

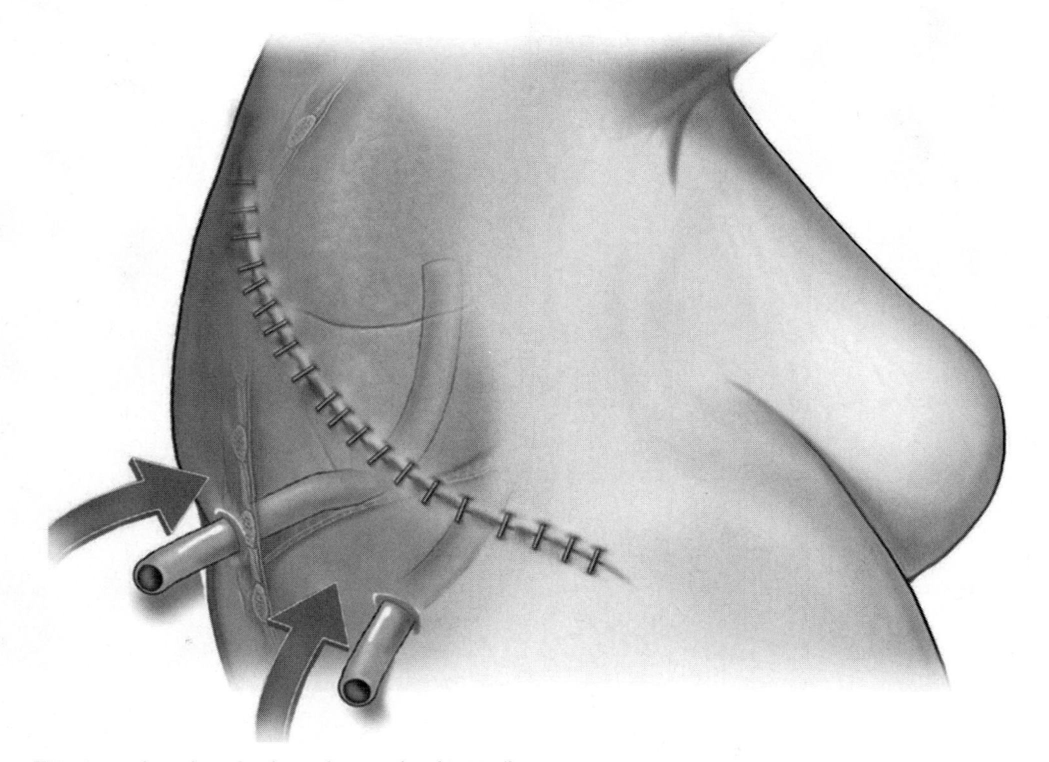

This picture shows how the chest tubes are placed internally.
Source: © 2013 Nucleus Medical Media. All rights reserved

N M

- Pain management: The thoracotomy pateint often has severe pain due to the incision and presence of chest tubes. Relief of this pain is a primary nursing responsibility:
  - o Pain after a thoracotomy can be one of the most severe that is experienced postoperatively. Administer analgesics as prescribed.
    - ■ Pain control is essential because pain can be an important cause of restricted mobilization and poor ventilation.
    - ■ Advocate for changes in the patient's pain management regimen if the patient is not getting sufficient relief.
  - o Identifying the best pain management for the patient is essential. Explore alternative modalities that may enhance pain relief, such as music, rest, family support, massage, or other methods known to the patient to be effective.

N

- Mobilization:
  - o Getting up to the bedside is important as soon as the patient is alert and oriented to prevent the multiple "never" events such as pressure ulcers, pneumonia, and deep vein thrombosis.
  - o Pre-medicate the patient for ambulation to improve the patient's willingness and ability to actively participate.
  - o Care must be taken to keep the chest drainage system below the level of the chest and protect it from disconnection or kinking.

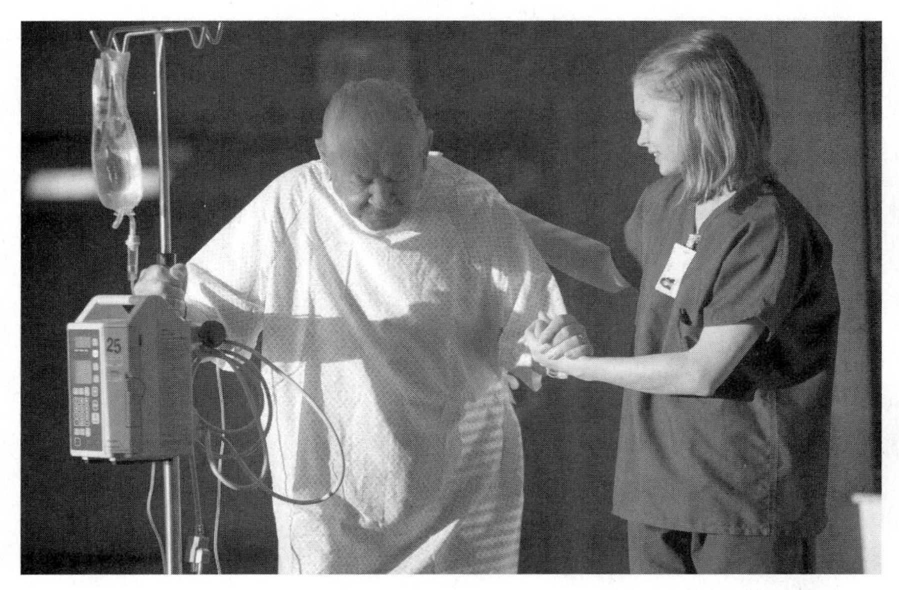

This photo represents a patient recovering from a complicated surgery which required placement of a chest tube. Despite the challenge, the patient is ambulating to prevent postoperative complications
Source: RubberBall/Alamy.

Concept Check

4. Which nursing assessment is essential following thoracotomy?

A. Pain level

B. Ability to cough

C. Return of bowel sounds

D. Neck mobility

Answer question

Concept Check

5. A patient who has a chest tube drainage system in place must be transferred to radiology. Where should the drainage system be positioned during the move?

A. On the patient's abdomen

B. On an IV standard connected to the bed

C. Below the level of the chest

D. At the foot of the bed

Answer question

Concept Check

6. How quickly after thoracotomy should the patient be gotten up to the bedside?

A. As soon as the water seal in the drainage bottle stops bubbling

B. When the patient is alert and oriented

C. The day after the procedure

D. When the affected lung is totally expanded

Answer question

- Chest tube management (see collaborative interventions regarding chest tubes, chest drainage systems, and safety concerns in the Pleural Disturbances NovE-lesson). The nurse should:
  - N o Implement care for the patient with chest tubes.
  - N o Adhere to the safety concerns.
  - N o Monitor for potential subcutaneous emphysema.

Collaborative Interventions (continued)

Subcutaneous Emphysema

- Subcutaneous emphysema or crepitus is air that can escape or leak when the pleural space connects to the subcutaneous tissue.
- N Assess for subcutaneous emphysema, which presents as a crackling or popping feel when you palpate around the chest tube insertion site or suspected area.
- N While not dangerous (since the air will be reabsorbed by the body), the cause of the air leak into the tissues should be found if moderate to extensive. Most minor leaks resolve without intervention but should be monitored closely.
- N Notify the physician if subcutaneous emphysema occurs suddenly.

Subcutaneous Emphysema

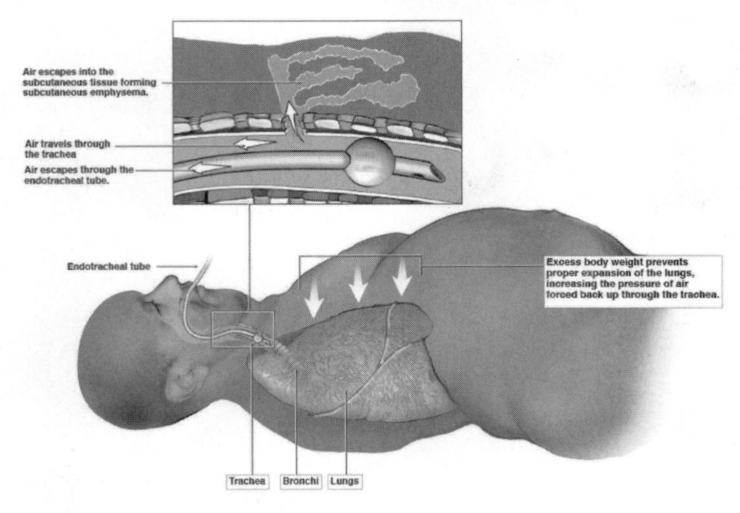
Air escapes into the subcutaneous tissue forming subcutaneous emphysema.
Air travels through the trachea
Air escapes through the endotracheal tube.
Endotracheal tube
Excess body weight prevents proper expansion of the lungs, increasing the pressure of air forced back up through the trachea.
Trachea
Bronchi
Lungs

Subcutaneous emphysema occurs when air leaks out through an unintended gap around a chest tube or, as shown here, an endotracheal tube. Air in the subcutaneous tissues signals a leak and should be investigated.

Concept Check

7. The patient has developed subcutaneous emphysema after a thoracotomy. How will the body rid itself of this air?

A. The patient will pass the air per rectum.

B. The tissues will reabsorb the air.

C. The air will be removed by insertion of a chest tube.

D. The air will be expelled through the respiratory system.

Answer question

Summary of Interventions

- Thoracotomies require careful observation for:
  - Changes in vital signs
  - Bleeding
  - Development of respiratory distress
  - Appearance of subcutaneous emphysema
- Careful attention to chest tubes is required to ensure adequate functioning.
- Pain management and comfort is important in managing patients with thoracotomies.
- Mobilization of the patient as soon as possible is important to prevent complications.

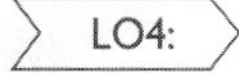

Evaluation of Desired Collaborative Care Outcomes

Evaluation and reassessment should reveal attainment of previously established patient outcomes. In summary:

- The patient reports resting comfortably and has sufficient pain relief to allow for active participation in progressive activities.
- The patient has normal respiratory rate, depth, and expansion.
- The patient's oxygen saturation levels support return to activity without supplemental oxygen
- The patient demonstrates active and progressive participation in activities of daily living and in ambulation.
- The patient has a normal white blood cell count, no fever, no purulent drainage, and clear mentation.

References

http://www.nlm.nih.gov/medlineplus/ency/article/002956.htm

http://www.ncbi.nlm.nih.gov/pmc/articles/PMC1285322/

http://journal.publications.chestnet.org/article.aspx?articleID=1054333

Gerner, P. (2008, June). Post-thoracotomy Pain Management Problems. *Anesthesiol Clin, 26*(2), 355–357. http://www.trauma.org/archive/thoracic/EDTintro.html

Learning Outcomes for Pulmonary Embolism

When you complete this lesson, you will be able to:

1. Recognize the clinical relevance of pulmonary embolism.
2. Consider the pathophysiology, etiology, risk factors, and clinical presentation of pulmonary embolism that determine the priority patient concerns.
3. Determine the most urgent and important nursing interventions and patient education required in caring for a patient with pulmonary embolism.
4. Evaluate attainment of desired collaborative care outcomes for a patient with pulmonary embolism.

LO1:

What Is a Pulmonary Embolism (PE)?

- Pulmonary thromboembolism ("emboli," if plural) occurs when a thrombus (blood clot) travels into the pulmonary arterial tree, obstructs blood flow through the lungs, and interferes with blood return to the heart.
- Air, fat, tumor, or other mass can also embolize or cause pulmonary arterial blockage in the lungs.
- The vast majority of PEs are thrombus related, so this lesson focuses on thromboembolism. Air, fat, and amniotic fat embolism are discussed briefly at the end of the lesson.

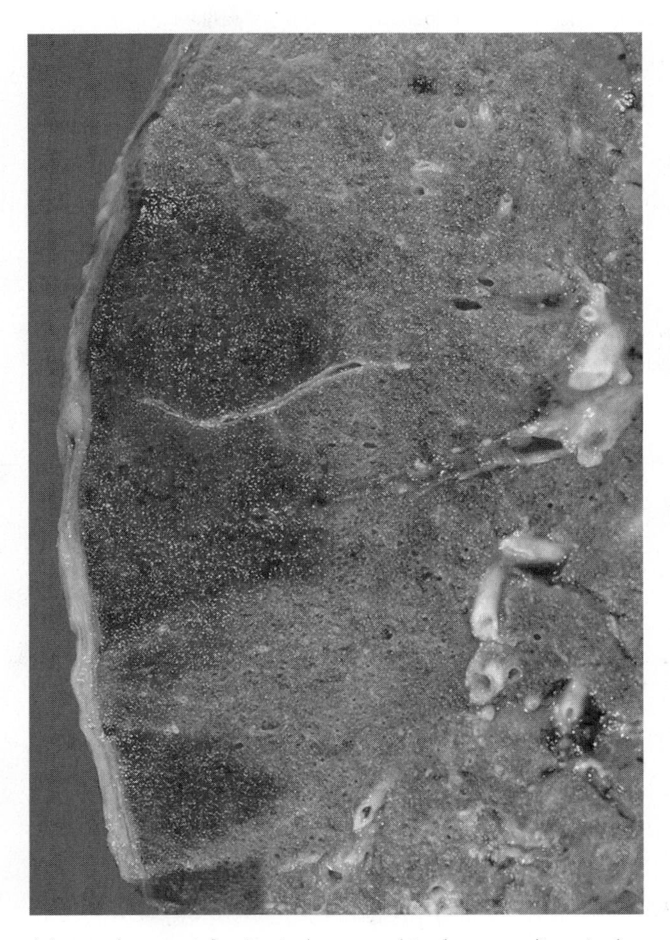

A large pulmonary infarction is shown, resulting from a medium-sized thromboembolus. This infarction has begun to organize at the margins.
Source: Yale Rosen/Custom Medical Stock Photo—All rights reserved

LO1:

Clinical Relevance

- Pulmonary emboli (PE) are potentially lethal events. PE results in approximately 200,000 deaths per year.
- The most common, yet preventable, cause of death in U.S. hospitals is PE.
- Prevention of deep vein thrombosis (DVT) is an important nursing role.

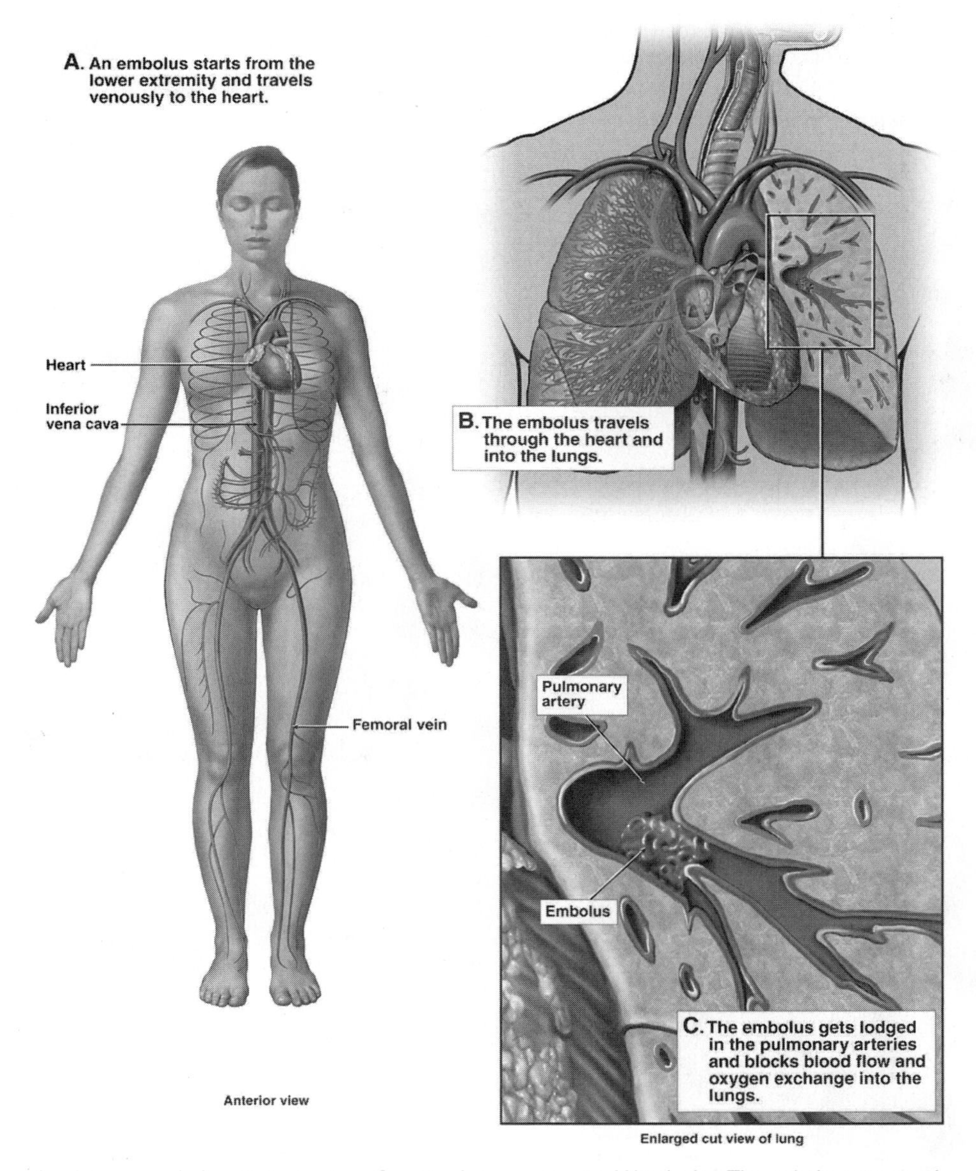

A. An embolus starts from the lower extremity and travels venously to the heart.
Heart
Inferior vena cava
Femoral vein
Anterior view
B. The embolus travels through the heart and into the lungs.
Pulmonary artery
Embolus
C. The embolus gets lodged in the pulmonary arteries and blocks blood flow and oxygen exchange into the lungs.
Enlarged cut view of lung

A pulmonary embolus starts in a vein, often in a deep venous vessel like the leg. The embolism can travel up the vein into the lung and become wedged in the pulmonary artery. This blocks blood flow into that part of the lung producing symptoms of shortness of breath and right-sided heart failure. A pulmonary embolism can be fatal if it is large enough.
Source: Nucleus Medical Art Inc/Alamy

LO2:

Pathophysiology

- A blood clot is most commonly formed in the deep veins (DVT). Some people are predisposed to clot formation because of a hypercoagulable state, venous stasis, or damage.
- The blood clot breaks away and travels from the venous system, through the right heart, and into the lungs.
- Usually within seconds, the embolus lodges in a blood vessel when the vessel becomes too small to permit passage.
- If the embolism is large and lodges in a main pulmonary artery, death can occur quickly. A saddle embolus is the largest type of embolus, which bridges across and occludes both right and left pulmonary arteries. Mortality is almost 100%.
- If the clot occludes in a small pulmonary artery, symptoms may not even be present.
- Multiple pulmonary emboli may occur simultaneously or over time.

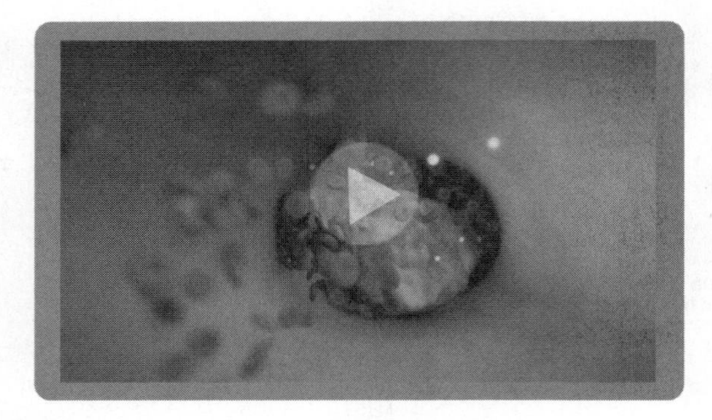

This animation illustrates the formation of a deep vein thrombosis: blood cell accumulation on the venous valves, a clot, venous blockage, and embolization.

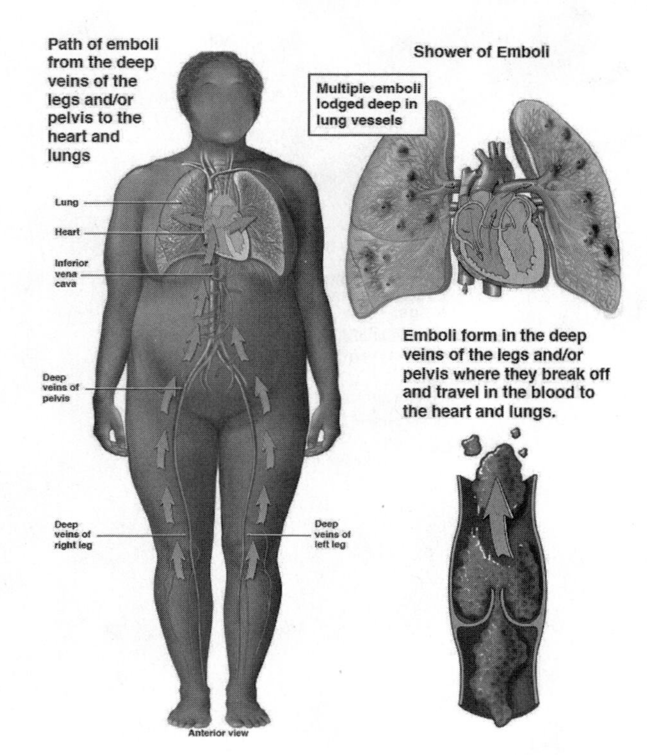

A close look shows a clot forming on a valve and that travel to the lungs if it breaks off.

Concept Check

1. **A patient is suspected of having a saddle embolus. What is the probable result of this occurrence?**

   A. The patient will likely experience additional emboli within 24 hours.

   B. The patient will experience minimal shortness of breath.

   C. The patient will have ischemia in both legs.

   D. The patient will die.

Answer question

- When a pulmonary embolism occurs, blood flow is impeded by the embolism and is diverted into other arteries. The result is increased blood pressure in the remaining pulmonary vascular beds, known as pulmonary hypertension.

Three major problems can result from embolism:

1. **Right ventricular overload:** With the sudden pulmonary hypertension, the right ventricle is unable to effectively pump against the increased pressure load, resulting in dysfunction of the right ventricle.
2. **Compromised perfusion to vital organs:** Reduced blood flow through the lungs results in far less blood return to the left ventricle. This reduces cardiac output and, potentially, produces a significant and even fatal hypoperfusion to vital organs.
3. **Impaired gas exchange:** A ventilation/perfusion mismatch occurs in the lung resulting in diminished gas exchange.

Concept Check

2. **What is the pathophysiologic reason for the development of pulmonary hypertension as a result of pulmonary embolism?**

   A. Diversion of blood into the pulmonary vascular bed.

   B. Epinephrine release due to anxiety and shortness of breath.

   C. Cytokine release from injured tissue.

   D. Airway compromise from pressure on the airway.

Answer question

Pathophysiology (continued)

Ventilation/Perfusion (V/Q) Mismatch

- A ventilation/perfusion mismatch is an imbalance between ventilation and perfusion.
- Normally, perfusion and ventilation occur throughout the lungs. A pulmonary embolus decreases perfusion into an area where ventilation continues, causing a mismatch. The mismatch can be seen on a V/Q scan.
- An increase in physiologic dead space results. Physiologic dead space occurs when alveoli and airways are unable to participate in gas exchange due to lack of perfusion.

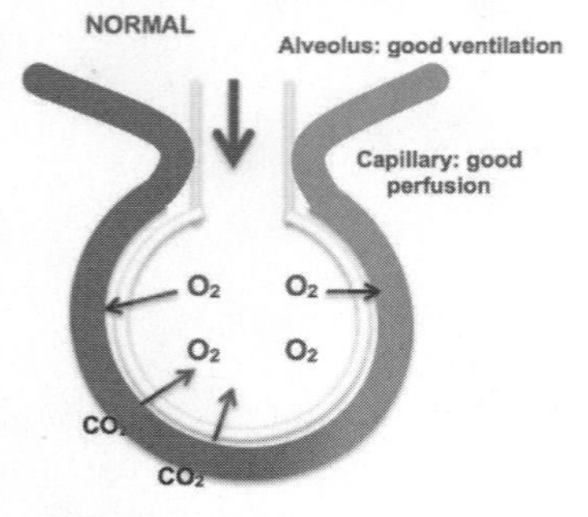

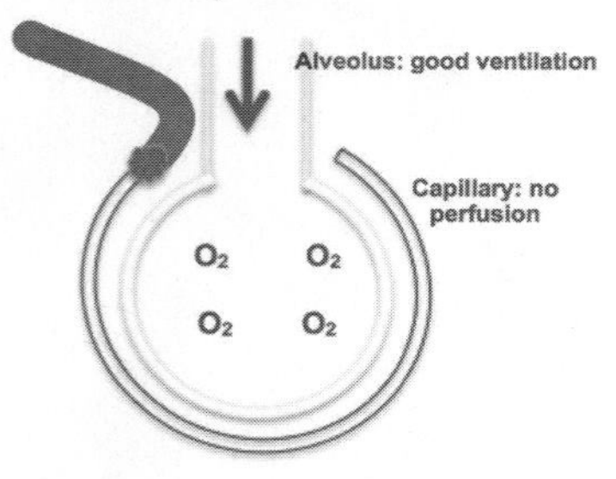

Normal ventilation (upper) of the alveolus is matched by normal perfusion via the capillary to produce good gas exchange. A pulmonary embolus (lower) blocks perfusion so that no gas exchange occurs, despite good ventilation of the alveolus, resulting in hypoxemia.
needed, (b) no transition to. NovEx Novice to Expert Learning, LLC

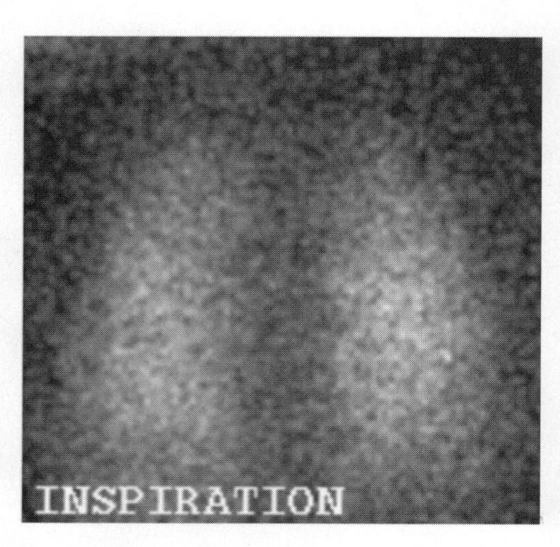

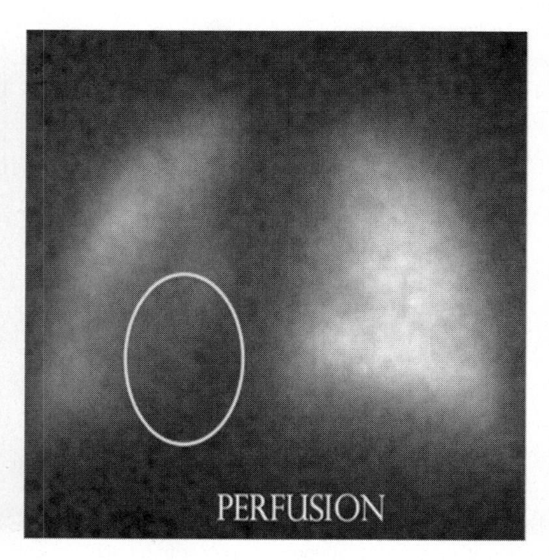

Note that the ventilation in the ventilation/perfusion scan is normal, with homogenous symmetric uptake and no defects. The perfusion scan shows decreased blood flow in the right lower lung (circle).
Source: (*left*) Copyright © 2012, NovEx Novice to Expert Learning, LLC; (*right*) Courtesy of K. Kyriakidis

Concept Check

3. The ventilation/perfusion mismatch associated with pulmonary embolism is due to which factor?
   A. Decreased capillary perfusion
   B. Decreased alveolar ventilation
   C. Increased capillary perfusion
   D. Increased alveolar ventilation

Answer question

- Increased dead space causes a reduction in exhaled carbon dioxide ($PetCO_2$), detectable by capnography. A sudden or significant drop in capnography readings can help with diagnosis, if needed.
- V/Q mismatch can also result in hypoxemia.
- Some effects on blood gases may occur but are often subtle and not easily detectable. Respiratory alkalosis (decrease in $PaCO_2$) develops due to tachypnea. The overventilation acts as a compensation mechanism.

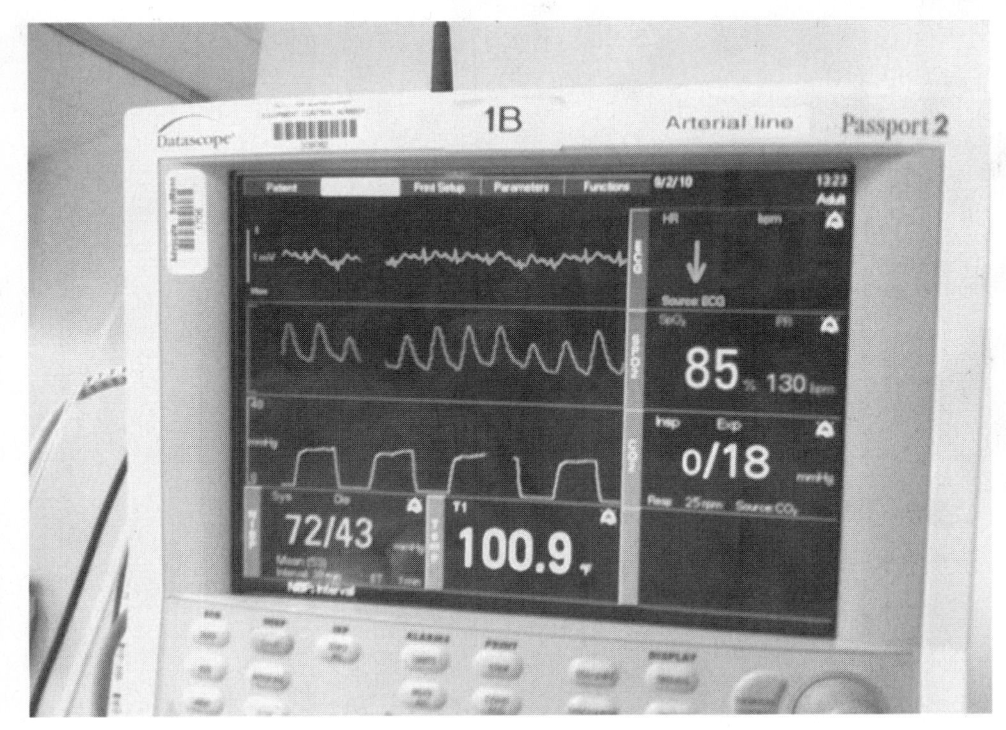

Because capnography can immediately detect and warn of low exhaled CO_2 levels, current guidelines for Advanced Cardiac Life Support and by the British and Irish Anaesthetist Association include the use capnography during a code. It can assist in the rapid diagnosis of pulmonary embolism.

Risk Factors

Predisposing factors for thromboembolism include:

- Family history of hypercoagulable conditions (PE, DVT)
- Surgery within prior 3 months
- Venous insufficiency
- Leg or pelvic trauma
- Prolonged bed rest
- Prolonged travel
- Contraceptives
- Cancer
- Dehydration
- Smoking
- Obesity

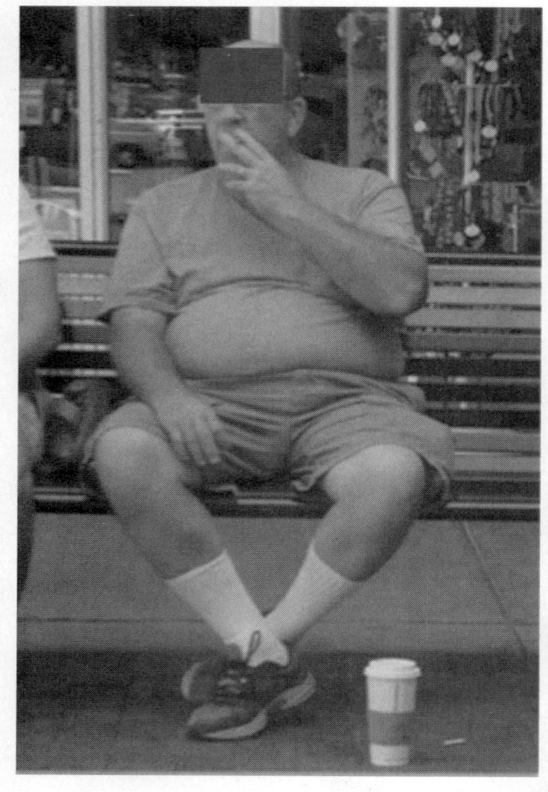

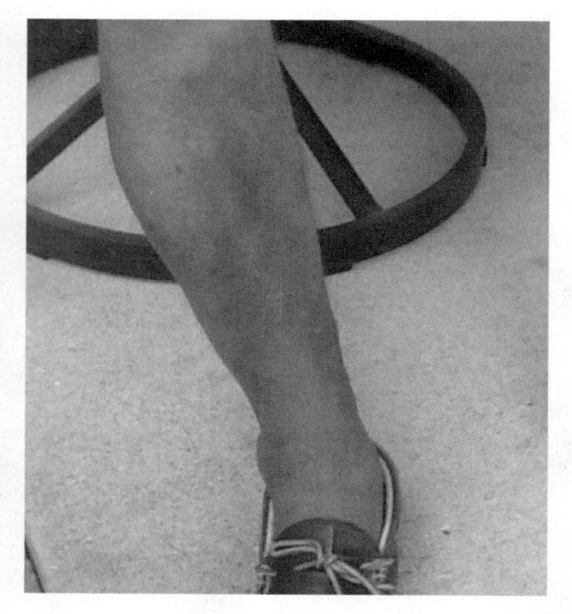

Smoking (left) and chronic venous insufficiency (right) are only two of the key risk factors for DVT leading to pulmonary embolism.
Source: *(both)* Copyright © 2012, NovEx Novice to Expert Learning, LLC

Causes

- Hypercoagulable state:
  - o Inherited. For example, patients with factor V Leiden have five times the risk of pulmonary embolism.
  - o Acquired. For example, malignancy and oral contraceptives are but two of many.
- Venous endothelial injury or stasis (e.g., chronic venous insufficiency or recent hip or knee surgery)
- Three additional causes of PE are not common but are briefly described: air, fat, and amniotic fluid.

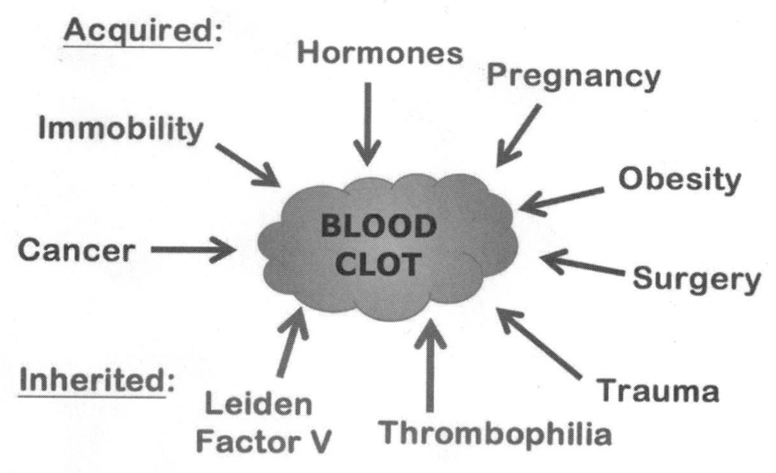

Factor V is a protein that helps blood to clot normally. Factor V Leiden, first identified in 1994, is a genetic mutation that is found in 5–8% of people of European descent. It increases the risk of abnormal venous blood clotting and thromboembolism but does not cause increased risk of bleeding.
Source: Copyright © 2012, NovEx Novice to Expert Learning, LLC

Air

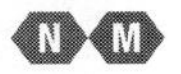

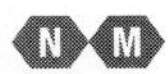

- **Pathophysiology:** An air embolism can occur when air enters the blood stream through an open venous access (e.g., IV disconnection, insertion), particularly a central line when the patient is in the supine or sitting position. If large enough, it can be fatal.
- **Treatment:** Trendelenburg position. Unless it is a large air embolism, treatment is generally supportive and based on symptoms.
- **Prevention:** Central lines should be placed, changed, or opened with the patient in Trendelenberg position.

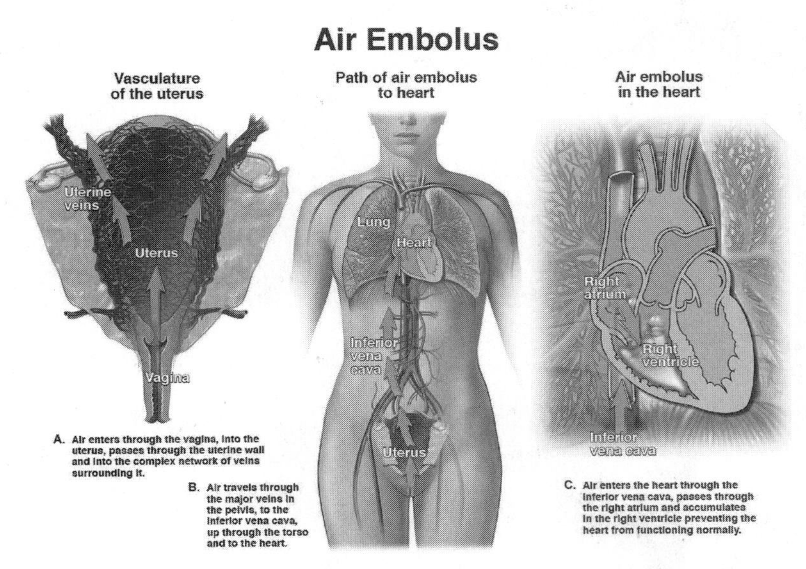
Air Embolus
Vasculature of the uterus
Path of air embolus to heart
Air embolus in the heart
Uterine veins
Uterus
Vagina
Lung
Heart
Inferior vena cava
Uterus
Right atrium
Right ventricle
Inferior vena cava
A. Air enters through the vagina, into the uterus, passes through the uterine wall and into the complex network of veins surrounding it.
B. Air travels through the major veins in the pelvis, to the inferior vena cava, up through the torso and to the heart.
C. Air enters the heart through the inferior vena cava, passes through the right atrium and accumulates in the right ventricle preventing the heart from functioning normally.

If an air embolism travels into the right ventricle and obstructs blood flow, it can produce severe hypovolemia and even death.
Source: © 2013 Nucleus Medical Media, All rights reserved

Causes (continued)

Fat

- Fat emboli are mutliple small fat globules entering the bloodstream and may have widespread effects. They are related to:
  - Traumatic injury (90% in severe skeletal injuries) and more commonly after pelvic and long bone fracture, e.g., femur or tibia
  - Orthopedic surgeries
  - Soft tissue damage and burns
  - Nontraumatic situations: post-CPR, pancreatitis, lipid infusions, liposuction
- Manifests 12–72 hours after injury
- **Treatment:** Usually supportive but fat embolism may be difficult.

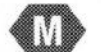

- **Prevention:** Early surgical fixation of fractures reduces risk of fat embolism.

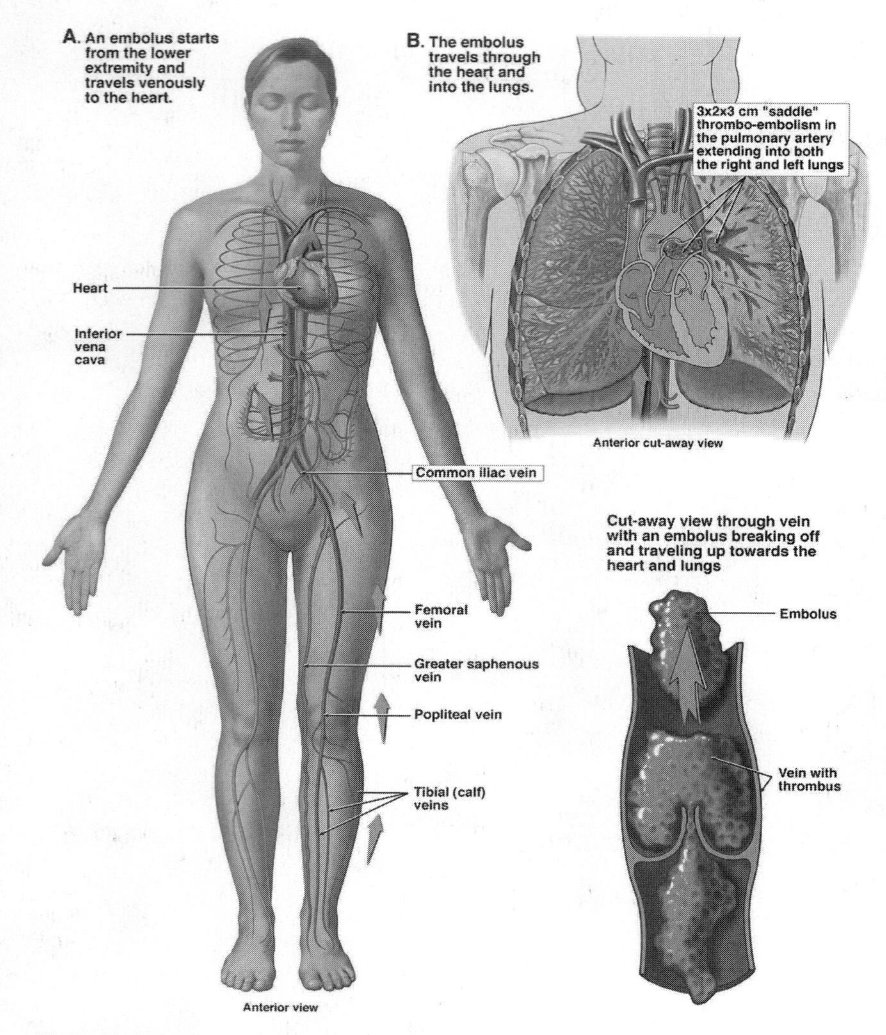

A. An embolus starts from the lower extremity and travels venously to the heart.
B. The embolus travels through the heart and into the lungs.
3x2x3 cm "saddle" thrombo-embolism in the pulmonary artery extending into both the right and left lungs
Heart
Inferior vena cava
Anterior cut-away view
Common iliac vein
Cut-away view through vein with an embolus breaking off and traveling up towards the heart and lungs
Embolus
Femoral vein
Greater saphenous vein
Popliteal vein
Vein with thrombus
Tibial (calf) veins
Anterior view

The mechanism of injury from fat embolism is the same as an air or blood clot embolism.
Source: Nucleus Medical Art Inc/Alamy

Concept Check

4. Development of fat embolism is often related to which condition?
   A. Traumatic injury
   B. Dehydration
   C. Placement of a central line
   D. Complications during labor and delivery

Answer question

Causes (continued)

Amniotic Fluid

- Amniotic fluid embolism (AFE) is amniotic fluid that enters the maternal circulation. Although uncommon, AFEs have mortality rates of 80–90%. It causes a massive anaphylactoid reaction. There is an 80% chance of maternal cardiopulmonary arrest.
- **Presentation:** AFE is unpredictable with no definitive warnings or clues. Unlike other emboli, it does not occur in an artery.
- **Treatment:** Generally supportive and based on symptoms that present, but treatment differs from thromboembolism and may be very difficult.

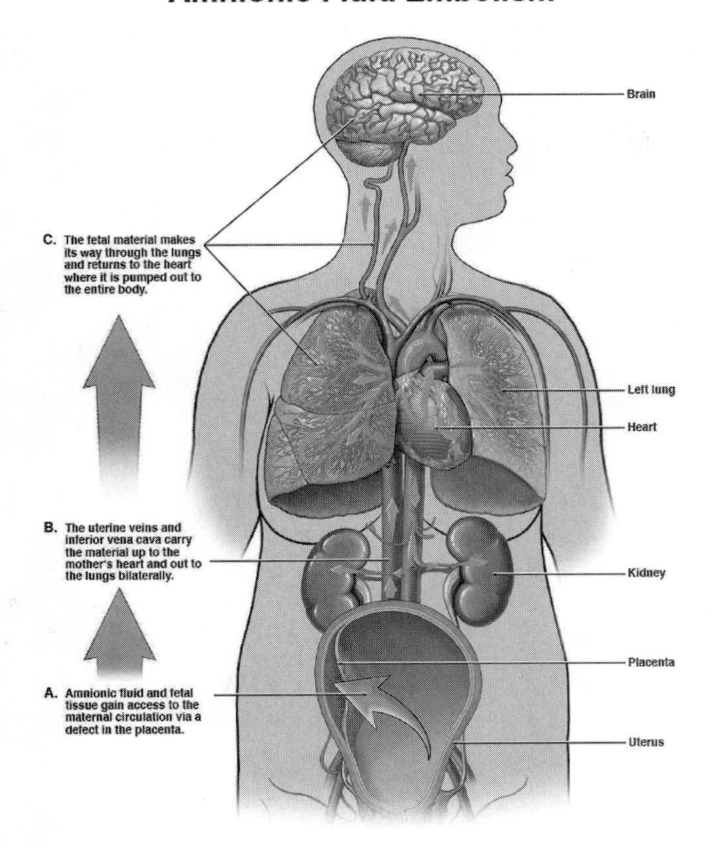
Amnionic Fluid Embolism
Brain
C. The fetal material makes its way through the lungs and returns to the heart where it is pumped out to the entire body.
Left lung
Heart
B. The uterine veins and inferior vena cava carry the material up to the mother's heart and out to the lungs bilaterally.
Kidney
Placenta
A. Amnionic fluid and fetal tissue gain access to the maternal circulation via a defect in the placenta.
Uterus

Amniotic fluid embolism is an unusual event that can occur when pregnant. Ruptured membrane or veins allow entry of fetal cells and tissue, with amniotic fluid and other debris, into maternal circulation. A subsequent allergic reaction can lead to cardiac and respiratory collapse and even death.
Source: © 2013 Nucleus Medical Media, All rights reserved

Assessment Findings

Symptoms of pulmonary embolism can be subtle or dramatic. There are classic patterns of signs and symptoms that strongly suggest a PE:

- Dyspnea, sudden difficulty breathing
- Tachypnea with respirations over 20
- Tachycardia or heart rate over 100
- Chest pain (often pleuritic)
- Hypoxemia

There are additional commonly accompanying signs and symptoms:

- Pleural rub
- Anxiety
- Feeling of impending doom
- Hemoptysis
- Clammy or bluish-colored skin
- A sudden decrease in the $PetCO_2$ value, resulting from areas of ventilation without perfusion (a high V/Q situation)
- Syncope
- Cardiopulmonary arrest
- Sudden death

Isolated Symptoms That Should Trigger Suspicion of a PE

Symptoms of PE can be vague and may not present in a typical pattern. Strongly consider the possibility of a PE when the following present as an isolated symptom, especially in high-risk patients (e.g., family history, recent hip or knee surgery, immobility):

- Unexplained tachycardia
- Hypoxemia
- Feeling of impending doom with a sudden onset

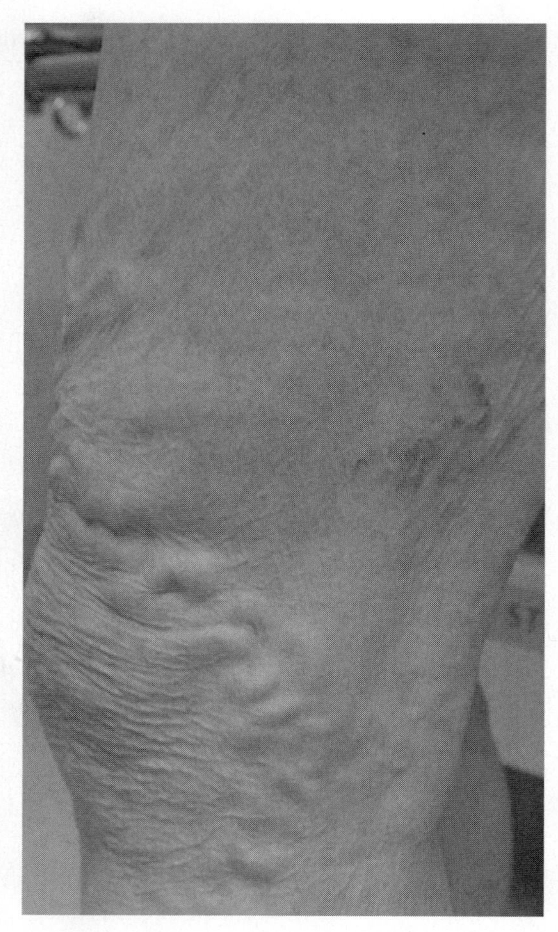

Clinicians' level of surveillance should be heightened when patients with severe varicose veins are taken for joint surgery.

Deep Vein Thrombosis (DVT)

Deep Vein Thrombosis (DVT) is responsible for a majority of pulmonary emboli. Recognizing signs and symptoms of DVT can therefore be helpful but are not always reliable:

- Calf pain
- Calf and leg edema
- Palpable popliteal cord
- Erythema of the calf, sometimes confused with cellulitis

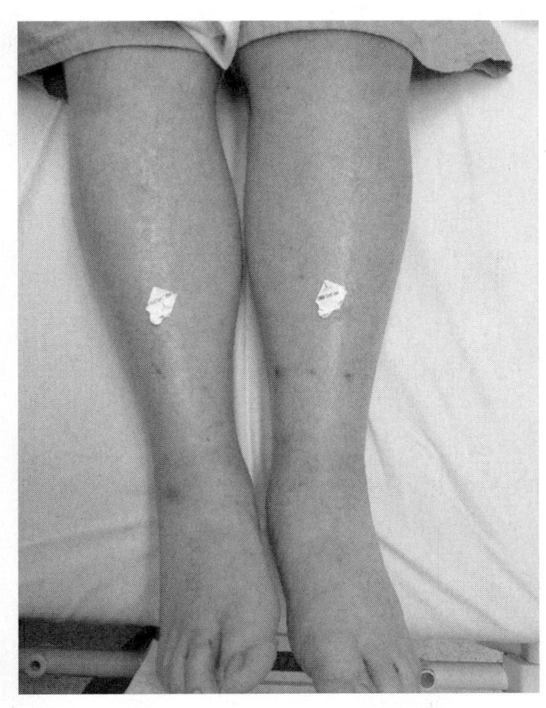

This patient developed subtle but definite swelling in her left calf and pain in the back of her knee, which worsens when walking. This early warning stage should elicit concern from clinicians. Ultrasound confirmed DVT.
Source: Courtesy of K. Kyriakidis

Diagnostics

- Pulmonary angiography is the most definitive test but is also the most invasive.
- Chest CT with contrast picks up clinically significant or larger pulmonary emboli and is the most common method currently used for diagnosis.
- D-dimer increases when there is thrombosis. D-dimer is a fibrin degradation product seen in the blood after a blood clot is lysed by fibrinolysis. D-dimer, however, has low specificity in diagnosing pulmonary emboli since it is present in many other conditions. Normal value is 0.5 mcg/mL.
- Chest x-ray is of limited value but may show dilated pulmonary artery or pleural effusion. It can be helpful in evaluating shortness of breath from causes other than PE.
- V/Q lung scan shows a ventilation–perfusion mismatch in the area of the clot(s) but often provides inconclusive results.
- Arterial Blood Gases (ABGs) may show decreased O_2 and CO_2, depending on the size of the clot.
- Venous duplex ultrasound scanning can be used to evaluate for DVT. A patient with DVT and signs or symptoms suggestive of PE is likely to have a PE.
- Echocardiogram may show pulmonary hypertension.

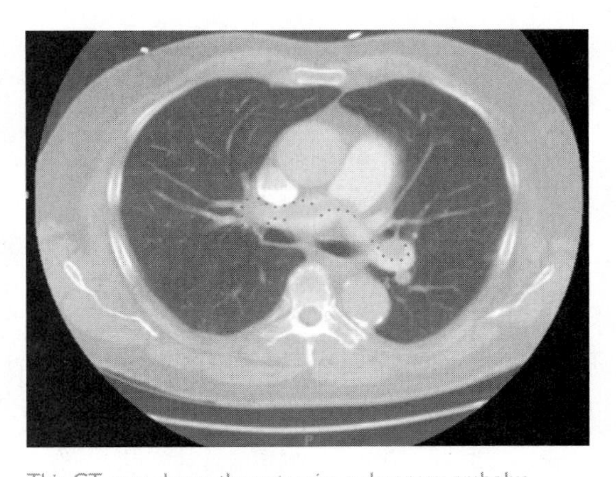

This CT scan shows the extensive pulmonary embolus (partially outlined in red) that blocks the main pulmonary artery, straddles both main branches, and therefore causes obstruction to blood flow to both left and right pulmonary arteries. This is known as a saddle embolus.
Source: Courtesy of K. Kyriakidis

Capnography

- Capnography is used to measure exhaled CO_2 which is the end-tidal CO_2 volume. If the $PetCO_2$ value suddenly decreases, the reason is either hyperventilation or a regional loss of pulmonary blood flow.
- Typically, hyperventilation does not produce a rapid sudden drop in $PetCO_2$ like a pulmonary embolism.

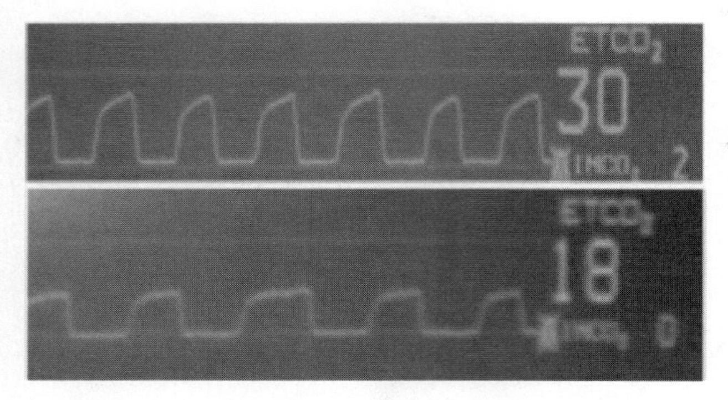

Upper: The top capnogram is normal. Lower: When a pulmonary embolism occurs, it produces an increase in physiologic dead space. This increased dead space produces a decrease of exhaled CO_2 since air reaching the lungs does not have carbon dioxide added. Thus, when exhaled, it has less carbon dioxide than normal.
Source: Copyright © 2012, NovEx Novice to Expert Learning, LLC

Priority Patient Concerns and Desired Collaborative Care Outcomes

Prior to caring for patients with a pulmonary embolism, it is important to prioritize the patient's concerns that must guide the nursing care plan and interventions. Care for the patient is ordered and organized in accordance with the patient's priority and urgent needs. Desired collaborative care outcomes in patients with a pulmonary embolism typically include:

1. Patient will report decrease in shortness of breath.
2. Patient's ventilation/perfusion ration will normalize.
3. Patient will have improved oxygen saturation or arterial blood gases.
4. Patient will report feeling calmer and less anxious.
5. Patient will demonstrate knowledge of prevention and management strategies.

Considering these important care outcomes, prepare a list of the major 3–6 priority patient concerns or nursing diagnoses for patients with a pulmonary embolism. Be prepared to participate in a discussion of this list and/or to submit them as an assignment, as determined by your faculty. Resources you may find helpful in this assignment can include this lesson, the references, resources on nursing care plans, and standard nursing diagnoses manuals.

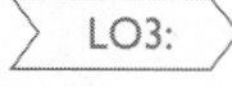

Collaborative Interventions

Evidence-Based Practices

The focus of treatment for pulmonary embolism centers on blood clots or thrombi.

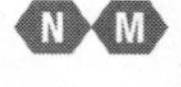

- Administration of anticoagulants, usually agents such as heparin for immediate anticoagulation and oral warfarin (Coumadin) for long-term anticoagulation.

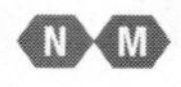

- Rivaroxaban (oral factor Xa inhibitor) is now FDA approved for treatment of acute PE. The advantages are significant: (a) no laboratory monitoring is needed, (b) no transition to warfarin is required, and (c) the dosage is fixed and oral. Patients with kidney dysfunction (creatinine clearance < 30 mL/min) should not be treated with this drug.
- Ventilator support (such as mechanical ventilation or BiPap) if a threat to breathing is present.

- Anticoagulants should be started immediately.
- Anticoagulants and particularly thrombolytics place patients at increased risk of bleeding and adverse reactions. Close observation is needed to detect early warning signs.

Concept Check

5. A patient is diagnosed with pulmonary embolism from a deep vein thrombosis. Which medication does the nurse anticipate administering immediately?
   A. Antibiotic
   B. Ace inhibitor
   C. Anticoagulant
   D. Cardiac glycoside

Answer question

Anticoagulation for Thrombotic PE

- Adequate anticoagulation prevents further clot formation but does not help lyse the current clot.
- N M Unfractionated IV heparin or low molecular subQ heparin is the treatment of choice for acute management. Close observation is needed to detect early warning signs of adverse patient responses.
  - M o Unfractionated heparin requires titration and the monitoring of partial thromboplastin time (PTT). Goal is to maintain the activated partial thromboplastin time (APTT) = 46–70 seconds (1.5–2.3 times control).
- Long-term management is with warfarin.
  - M o INR (International Normalized Ratio) goal is usually 2.0–3.0. Warfarin usually requires several days to take effect. Therefore, treatment is usually started in conjunction with heparin, which works immediately. Heparin is later discontinued after INR is therapeutic.

Collaborative Interventions (continued)

Collaborative Symptom Management and Comfort Care

- M Pulmonary embolectomy is the placement of a catheter in a major blood vessel in an attempt to remove the embolism in patients who are hemodynamically unstable and/or fail routine therapy. This is sometimes performed by thoracotomy.
- N M Administer ordered thromboytics, including drugs such as urokinase and alteplase, to enhance breakdown of existing clot, including drugs such as urokinase and alteplase. Thrombolytics are not recommended for most patients but can be used for patients who are hemodynamically unstable and/or fail routine therapy.
- M Inferior vena cava (IVC) filter placement can be used in patients who cannot be anticoagulated.
- N M Administer ordered analgesics for pain control and to decrease myocardial oxygen demand. Agents such as fentanyl or morphine are commonly used.
- N M Give supplemental O_2 for SpO_2 levels less than 92%.
- N High Fowler's position (sitting up) may help reduce shortness of breath.

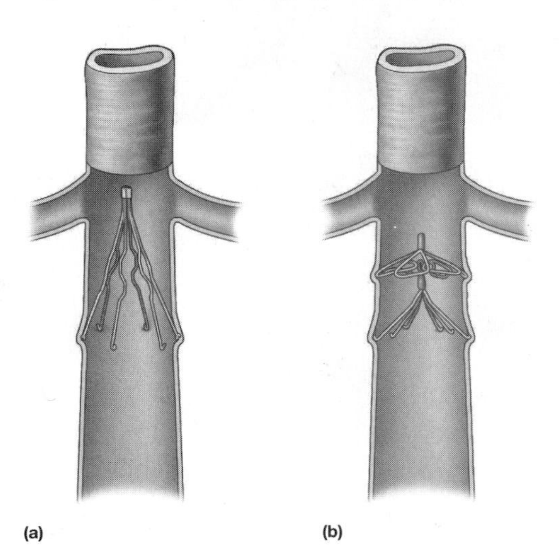

This illustration demonstrates how the inserted filters into the vena cava help to reduce the incidence of recurrent blood clots moving to and blocking the pulmonary circulation.

Prevention

- N — Low molecular weight heparin or unfractionated subcutaneous heparin is the mainstay of venous thromboembolism prophylaxis during hospitalization..
- N M — In patients who are at high risk for bleeding, intermittent pneumatic compression devices may be used.
- N M — High-risk patients who cannot be anticoagulated may have placement of IVC filter.
- N — There is little evidence that graduated compression stockings are effective although often recommended.
- N M — In low-risk patients, maintaining activity is good preventive therapy.
    - Early postoperative ambulation is encouraged.

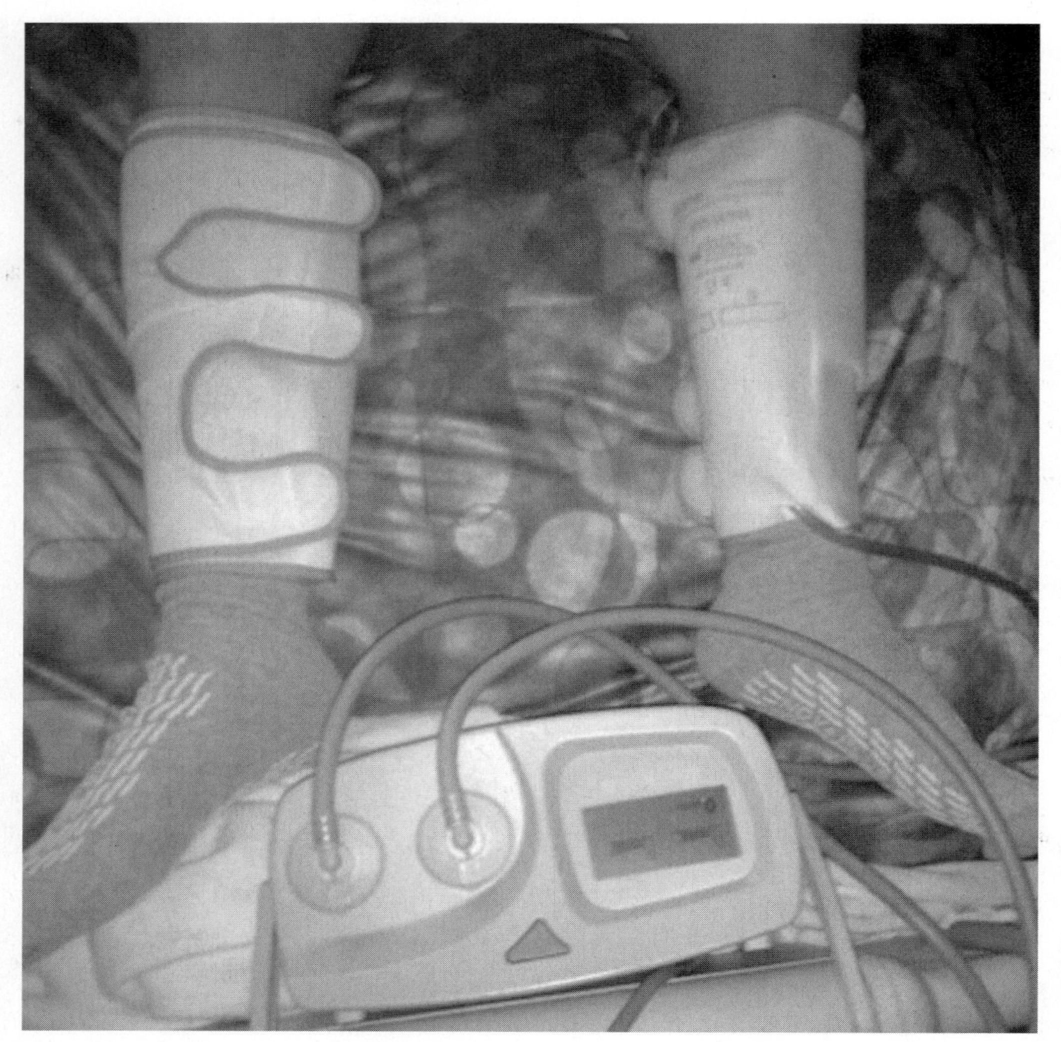

The patient who is at high risk for DVT is shown with the intermittent, sequential compression device in place.
Source: Courtesy of K. Kyriakidis

IVC Filters

Placement of a filter in the IVC is sometimes performed to prevent clots from moving from the lower extremities to the heart. It is usually inserted percutaneously via the femoral vein in the groin.

- Indications include:
  - o Absolute contraindication to or complication of anticoagulation (e.g., active or severe bleeding)
  - o Recurrent PE despite adequate anticoagulant therapy
  - o Hemodynamic or respiratory compromise that is severe enough for another PE to be lethal

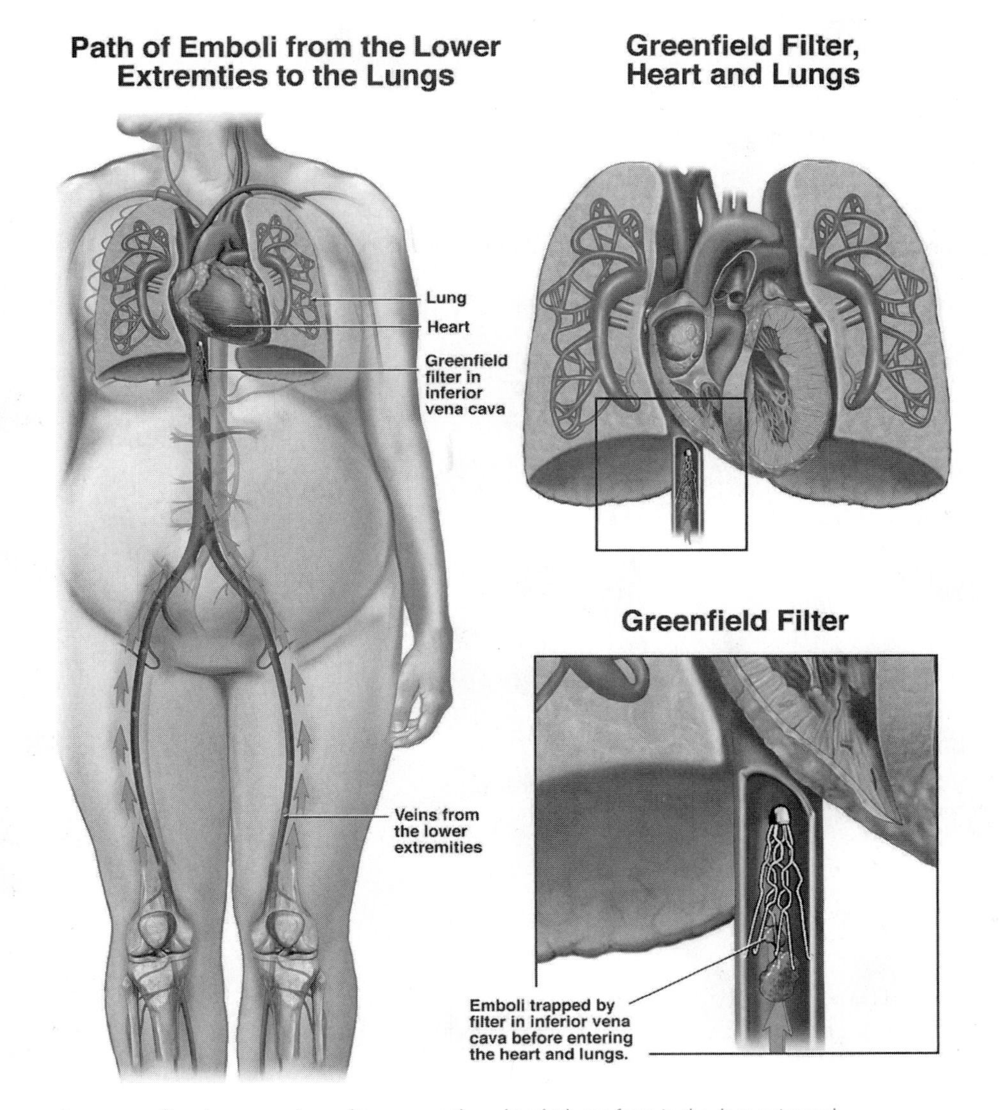

A vena cava filter is commonly used to prevent thrombi, which can form in the deep veins and embolize, from reaching the lungs. This image depicts the placement of a Greenfield filter in the inferior vena cava.

Collaborative Interventions (continued)

Collaborative Support and Patient Education

Prevention

- Maintain activity:
    - o Early postoperative ambulation
    - o Lower extremity exercise
- Low molecular weight heparin or unfractionated heparin, both subcutaneous during hospitalization. Educate the patient about anticoagulants used and the transition to their post-discharge meds.
- Intermittent pneumatic compression devices may be used when patients cannot be anticoagulated. Graduated compression stockings, although commonly recommended, have not been shown to reduce the incidence of PE or DVT.
- Central venous line: Before central lines are placed or the line is opened, either raise the patient's legs or place the patient in a Trendelenburg position to prevent accidental air embolism.

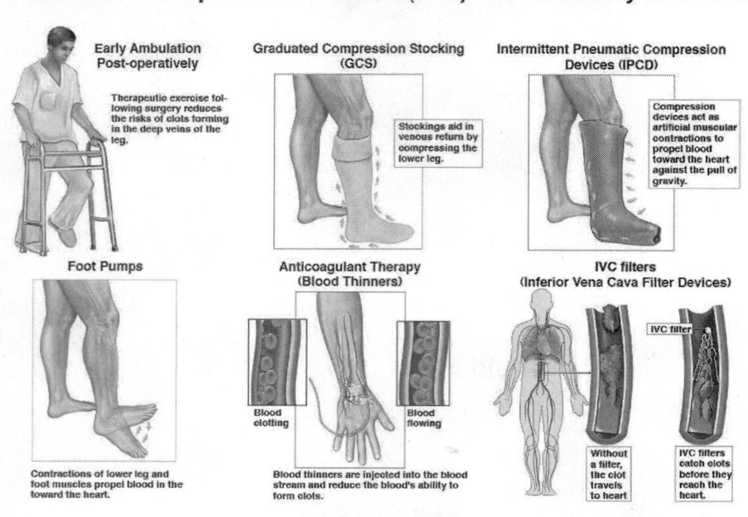

Nursing support of the patient in terms of preventing an emboli from forming include early postoperative ambulation, compression stockings, lower extremity exercise, and administration of anticoagulants.

Concept Check

6. **Which patient situation would indicate that use of an inferior vena cava filter should be considered?**

    A. The patient had surgery 6 months prior to the pulmonary embolism.

    B. The patient has had multiple pulmonary emboli.

    C. The patient had few symptoms when the pulmonary emboli occurred.

    D. The patient is young.

Answer question

Summary of Interventions

Treatment focuses on prevention of new thrombus formation:

- Treatment is usually with anticoagulation.
- Treatment is started immediately.
- Prevention with low molecular weight or unfractionated heparin.

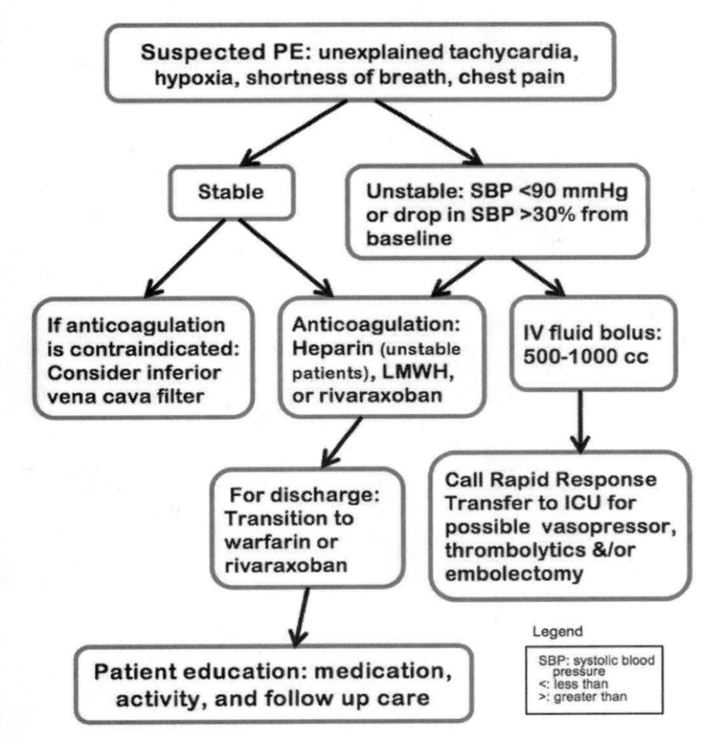

Concept Check

7. Which nursing intervention will help to prevent the development of deep vein thrombosis and pulmonary embolism?
   A. Early postoperative ambulation
   B. Use of graduated compression stockings
   C. Maintenance of an intermittent infusion port
   D. Administration of a prophylactic antithrombotic

Answer question

LO4: Evaluation of Desired Collaborative Care Outcomes

Evaluation and reassessment should reveal attainment of previously established patient outcomes. In summary:

- The patient's respirations are regular and unlabored.
- The patient's ventilation/perfusion ratio is within normal limits.
- The patient's skin is warm and dry, and color is appropriate for race.
- The patient is calm.
- The patient accurately describes a plan for preventing recurrence and for managing treatment plan.

References

Penaloza, A., Roy, P. M., & Kline, J. (2012, August). Risk stratification and treatment strategy of pulmonary embolism. *Curr Opin Crit Care, 18*(4), 318–325.

Vacca, V. M., & Jehle, J. (2013, March). Acute pulmonary embolism. *Nursing, 43*(3), 25–26.

Clinical Practice Guidelines

Hirsh, J., Guyatt, G., Albers, G. W., Harrington, R., Schünemann, H. J., & American College of Chest Physician. (2008, June). Antithrombotic and thrombolytic therapy: American College of Chest Physicians Evidence-Based Clinical Practice Guidelines (8th Edition). *Chest, 133*(6 Suppl), 110S–112S.

Patient Education

Merrigan, J. M., Piazza, G., & Lynm, C . (2013). Pulmonary Embolism. *JAMA* , *309*(5), 504.

Learning Outcomes for Tuberculosis

When you complete this lesson, you will be able to:

1. Recognize the clinical relevance of tuberculosis.
2. Consider the pathophysiology, etiology, risk factors, and clinical presentation of tuberculosis that determine the priority patient concerns.
3. Determine the most urgent and important nursing interventions and patient education required in caring for a patient with tuberculosis.
4. Evaluate attainment of desired collaborative care outcomes for a patient with tuberculosis.

LO1:

What Is Tuberculosis?

- Tuberculosis (TB) is an infection caused by *Mycobacterium tuberculosis.*
- For much of modern history, tuberculosis was a major cause of death.
- The French physician Laennec, credited with developing the modern stethoscope in the early 19th century, identified the terms we use for lung sounds primarily by the sounds tuberculosis made. Laennec died of TB at the age of 44.

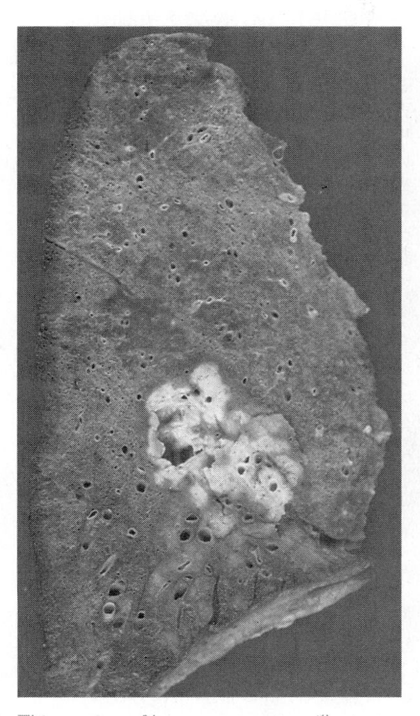

This section of lung post-mortem illustrates a caseous (cheese-like) tuberculoma with cavitation. A tuberculoma is a tumor-like, non-cancerous mass that is caused by tuberculosis.
Source: Yale Rosen, MD/Custom Medical Stock Photo—All rights reserved

LO1:

Clinical Relevance

- *Mycobacterium tuberculosis* (TB) is second only to human immunodeficiency virus (HIV) as the leading cause of death worldwide from a single infectious agent.
- Tuberculosis experienced a resurgence in the late 1980s and early 1990s.
- Multiple factors contributed to the increased incidence:
  - o Deterioration of public health infrastructure
  - o HIV epidemic, resulting in compromised immunity
  - o Multidrug-resistant (MDR) tuberculosis
  - o Homelessness, war, famine, crowded conditions
  - o Inadequate infection control measures in health care facilities
- Worldwide incidence peaked in 2003 and has since declined. The 2004 rate was the lowest recorded rate in the United States since national reporting began in 1953.

LO2:

Pathophysiology

- TB is classified as:
  - o Primary active infection
  - o Dormant
  - o Reactivation tuberculosis: TB recurs. Reactivation tuberculosis results from a previously dormant focus seeded at the time of primary infection.
- Lungs are the major site for infection, though seeding to any organ in the body is possible. Generally, the *Mycobacterium* is initially contained by host's defense (immune) systems, and the infection becomes latent or dormant.
- The apical–posterior segments of the upper lobes of the lung are frequently involved.
- Someone with latent or dormant TB may never have any clinical symptoms. However, if the patient's immune system becomes compromised, the disease can become active.

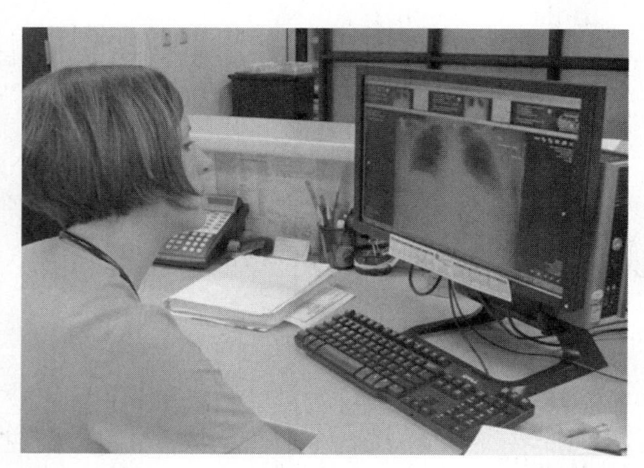

Mycobacterium invade the lungs as the major target of infection. The apices are the most commonly-affected area in pulmonary TB. TB can remain dormant in the lungs before reactivation.

- TB is caused by the tubercle bacillus. This bacillus establishes an infection in the lungs after it is inhaled in small 5–10 micron droplets. For face masks to protect against TB, they must filter particles this small.
- These small droplets reach the alveoli of the lungs, where they start to multiply, enabling the infection to spread.
- The immune system responds by: 1) attempting to kill the bacilli and 2) walling it off within a nodular granulomatous structure called the tubercle.
- Most granulomas resolve so TB does not spread. However, when the granulomas are not resolved, they may reactivate and spread the infection.

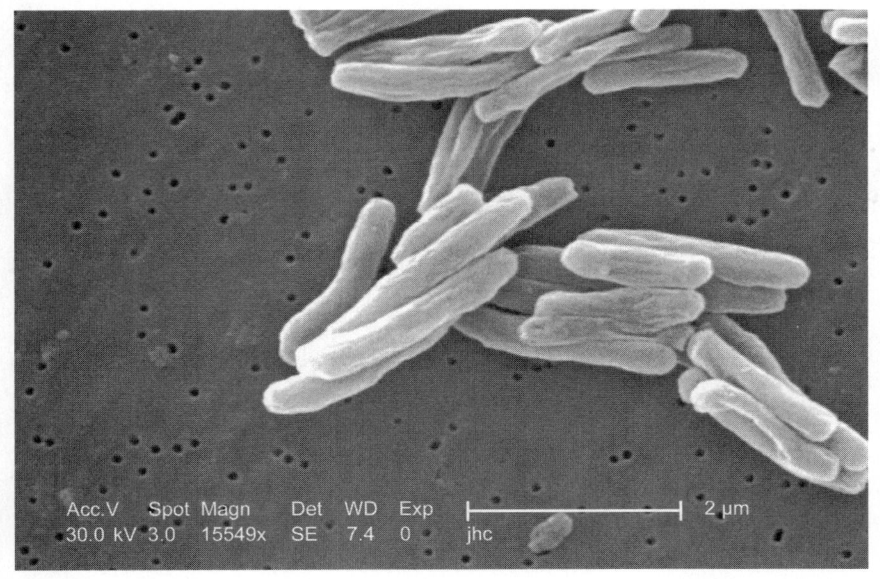

Under high magnification the acid-fast mycobacteria can be seen growing end-to-end in a culture. The way they grow creates a cordlike appearance.
Source: Centers for Disease Control and Prevention (CDC)

Pathophysiology (continued)

- When the bacterial replication is not controlled, the tubercle enlarges, and infection may spread through the lymph system. The lymph nodes then become infected, resulting in lymphadenopathy.
- Bacteremia may accompany the initial infection. Without an effective immune response, progressive destruction of the lung occurs. Destroyed lung areas result in cavities (cavitation), most commonly in the apices.
- Continued growth of the bacilli allows them to spread to other organs, producing a myriad of lesions resembling millet seeds, thus termed miliary TB.
- Spread of TB to organs other than the lungs can manifest in many ways, among them
  - o Neuro: cranial nerve deficits
  - o Cardiac: pericarditis
  - o Skeletal: osteomyelitis (e.g., knee, spine, hip)
  - o Genital tract: endometritis, salpingitis, infertility

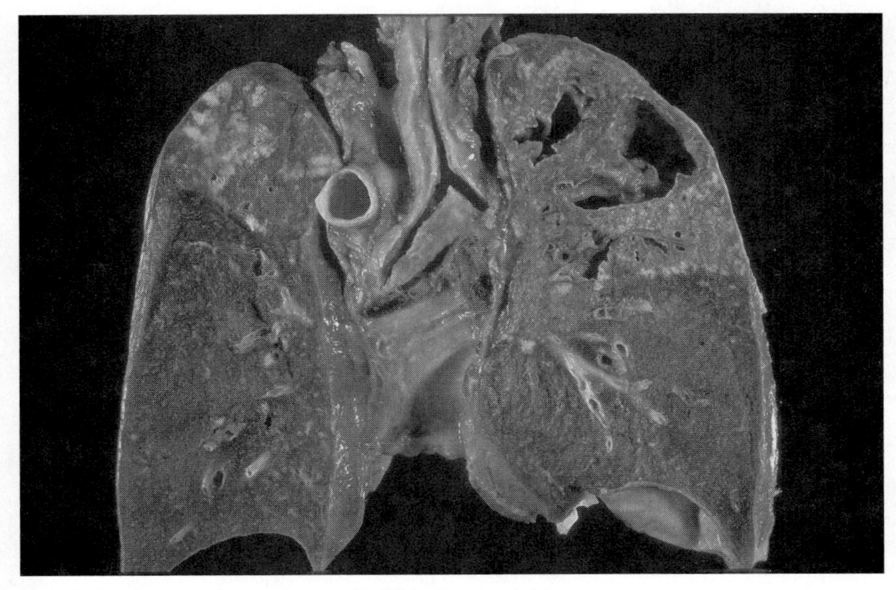

Note the huge cavities of tissue destroyed by TB in the upper-left lung.
Source: Yale Rosen/Custom Medical Stock

Concept Check

1. **Which statement is accurate for a patient with miliary tuberculosis?**
   A. Miliary tuberculosis is resistant to antimicrobial treatment.
   B. Miliary tuberculosis is located in organs outside of the lung.
   C. The miliary tuberculosis will be contained by the immune response.
   D. This type of tuberculosis will have minimal impact on lung tissue.

Answer question

- Fortunately, most people have successful isolation of the TB infection with the tubercle formation in the lungs. However, as stated, the disease can recur. Reactivation TB often occurs with immunosuppression, but can occur in 5–10% of cases without immunosuppression.
- The disease process in reactivation TB tends to be localized with less lung injury. The lesion typically occurs at the lung apices. Disseminated disease is unusual, unless the host is severely immunosuppressed.
- One benefit of latent TB is the likelihood of protection against subsequent TB exposure.
- Treatment often cures the patient, as seen in the before and after x-rays. With a growing number of patients infected by drug-resistant strains of TB, cure can be a serious challenge.

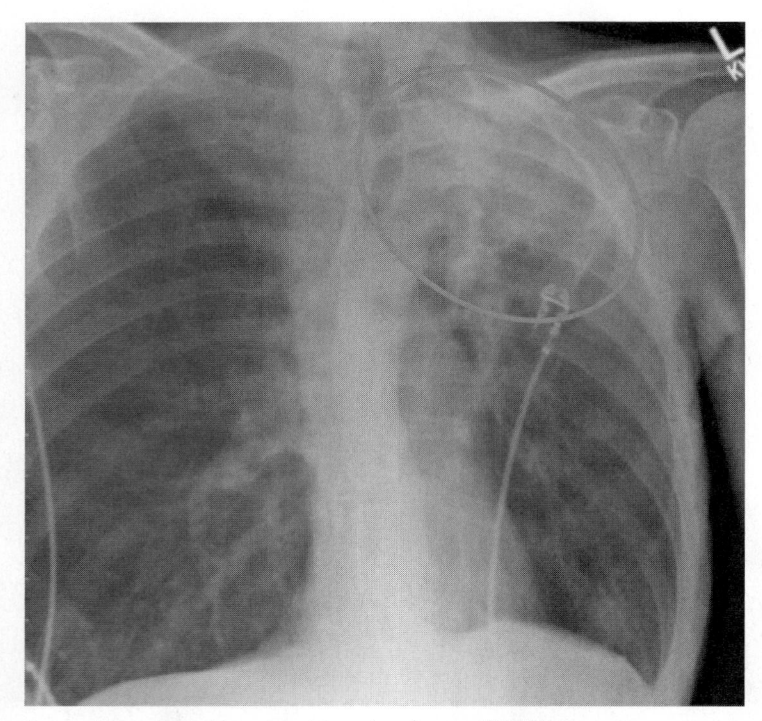

A man who smokes and has severe bilateral emphysema (COPD) developed cough, sputum production, and blood-tinged sputum. Sputum staining showed tubercle bacilli or tuberculosis. His chest x-ray showed left apical consolidation (circle) with a central cavity-like lesion (arrow).
Source: Courtesy of Erick Kyriakidis

Concept Check

2. **A recurrent infection of tuberculosis is likely if the infected person:**
   A. fails to take medications as prescribed.
   B. receives live vaccines.
   C. undergoes chemotherapy for cancer.
   D. has surgery.

Answer question

Complications

- Primary active TB may result in multisystem organ failure, septic shock, and Acute Respiratory Distress Syndrome (ARDS).
- Subacute or chronic forms may result in failure to thrive; hence the past reference to TB as "consumption."
- Complications of endobronchial TB include:
  - Airway obstruction
  - Impingement of perihilar lymph nodes
  - Endobronchial ulceration or perforation
  - Atelectasis
  - Bronchiectasis
  - Tracheal or bronchial stenosis

Microbiology

- The *Mycobacterium* genus includes more than 50 other species.
- Staining characteristics: The cell wall of the TB bacillus stains positive with Gram stain. The bacillus structure resists distaining by acid alcohol, leading to the term acid-fast bacillus (AFB).
- Tuberculosis is caused not only by *M. tuberculosis* but also occasionally by *M. bovis* and rarely by *M. africanum*, *M. microti*, *M. canetti*, *M. caprae*, and *M. penepedii.*

Risk Factors

- Increased risk of new TB infection exists in these situations:
  - Close contact with persons with active pulmonary TB
  - Casual contact with persons with highly contagious and active TB
  - Health care workers and those in other occupations exposed to patients with untreated, contagious, and active TB (e.g., prison facilities, homeless shelters, immigrants from areas with high incidence of TB.)
- High risk of reactivation exists in persons with:
  - HIV infection
  - Transplant, chemotherapy, or other major immunocompromising condition
  - Lymphoma, leukemia, head and neck cancer
  - Abnormal chest x-ray with apical fibronodular changes typical of healed TB
  - Silicosis
  - Renal failure (requiring dialysis)
  - Treatment with TNF-alpha inhibitors, commonly used to treat inflammatory conditions

TB Transmission

- Infection is person to person via airborne infectious aerosol that is produced when a person:
  - Coughs
  - Sneezes
  - Talks
  - Produces sputum
- Becoming infected is influenced by:
  - Duration of exposure
  - Ventilation in infected environment
- Be aware that suspended airborne particles are infectious even after the TB infected person leaves the room.
- Fortunately, extrapulmonary TB is NOT contagious.
- Not everyone who is exposed to TB acquires the disease. Approximately 10% of chronically exposed people with normal immune systems will develop TB.
- Those who develop the disease will not always show symptoms until later:
  - 50% in first 2–3 years following exposure
  - 50% in the remote future

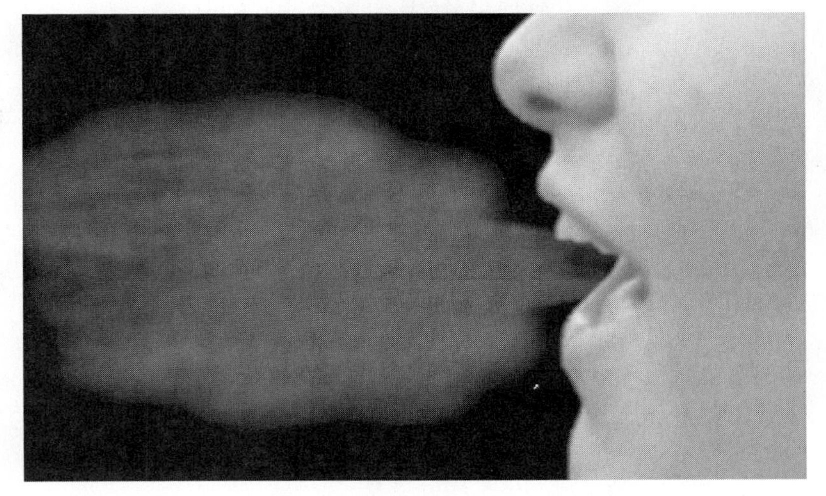

Coughing or talking causes organisms from an infected person to become aerosolized, making disease transmission a risk. TB *Mycobacterium* remains suspended in air for several hours, which is the reason for isolation in preventing transmission.
Source: Copyright © 2012, NovEx Novice to Expert Learning, LLC

Types of TB Infections

- Primary tuberculosis:
  - o Fever—70% (duration 2–10 weeks)
  - o Chest pain—25%
  - o Pleuritic chest pain
  - o Coughing, may have bloody sputum
  - o Erythema nodosum (red to violet subcutaneous nodules) on pretibial areas of lower extremities (women more than men)
- Reactivation tuberculosis:
  - o Accounts for 90% of adult non-HIV TB
  - o Result of a previously dormant infection
  - o Most common location is apical posterior segment of the lung

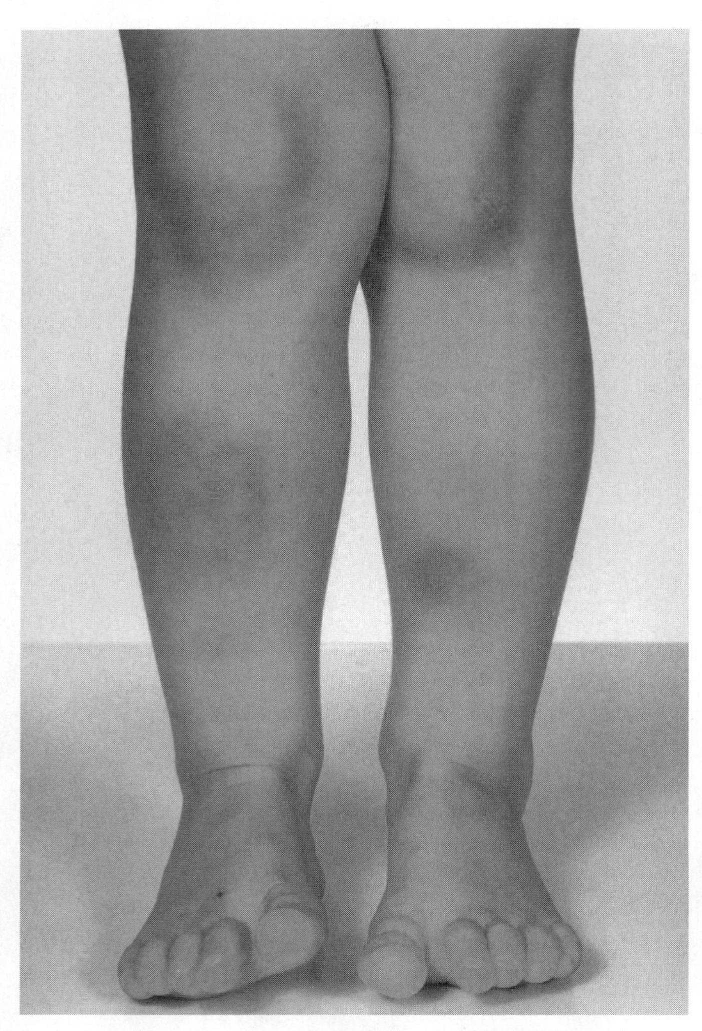

Erythema nodosum is a subcutaneous manifestation where red lumps form over the pre-tibial areas of the lower leg.
Source: Medical-on-Line/Alamy

Non-Pulmonary Forms of TB

- Gastrointestinal involvement:
    - o Abdominal pain, nausea, vomiting, or diarrhea may be present. Hepatomegaly or cholestatic jaundice may also be observed.
    - o Liver function test abnormalities are common, with elevated aspartate aminotransferase (AST) and alanine aminotransferase (ALT).
- Skin involvement:
    - o Cutaneous involvement is relatively uncommon.
    - o Cutaneous tuberculosis may manifest as 5–10 mm macules (see top photo), papules, or as a generalized rash. Advanced HIV infection is also a predisposition to TB skin manifestations.
- Central nervous system (CNS) involvement:
    - o Spread to the CNS presents as meningitis
    - o MRI can detect tuberculomas in the CNS

Concept Check

3. Cutaneous tuberculosis is associated with which problem?

A. Liver failure

B. HIV infection

C. Meningitis

D. Hearing impairment

Answer question

- Cardiovascular involvement: Cardiovascular manifestations of TB are usually clinically silent. The most common CV manifestation is pericarditis, sometimes resulting in aortic aneurysm. Pericarditis is inflammation of the outer sac of tissue enclosing the heart.
- Adrenal involvement: Adrenal insufficiency associated with infection of the adrenals has been reported.
- Other organ involvement: Tuberculosis has presented in nearly every area and organ in the body, including bone (osteomyelitis), eyes, larynx, middle ear (otitis media), and the thyroid.

Assessment Findings

- The earliest description of tuberculosis symptoms was written during 668–626 B.C.: "The patient coughs frequently, his sputum is thick and sometimes contains blood. His breathing is like a flute, his skin is cold but his feet are hot. He sweats greatly and his heart is much disturbed."
- These symptoms are still found today in patients with active tuberculosis infection.
- Physical examination may be normal.
- Signs and symptoms often begin insidiously and include:
    - o Fever
    - o Pleuritic chest pain
    - o Fatigue
    - o Weight loss
    - o Night sweats
    - o Cough (nonproductive early, progressing to productive with yellow or yellow-green sputum, rarely foul-smelling)
    - o Arthralgias (joint aches and pain)
    - o Pharyngitis
    - o Hemoptysis (presents later in disease process, due to sloughing or endobronchial erosion)
    - o Hypoxemia (abnormally low concentration of blood oxygen)
    - o Signs of pleural effusion

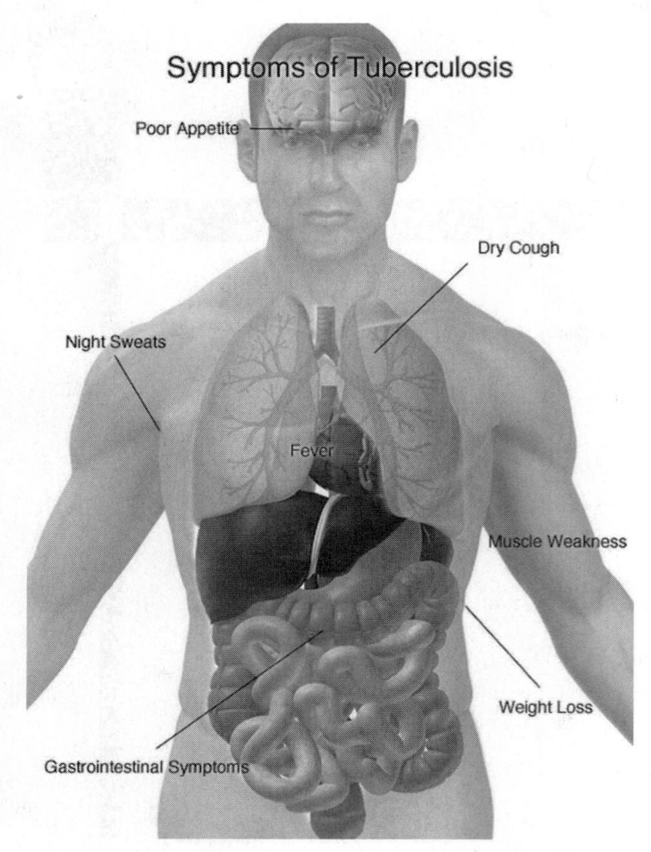

TB can infect and interfere with the function of almost every organ in the body.
Source: Copyright © 2012, NovEx Novice to Expert Learning, LLC

Physical Assessment

- TB symptoms are often nonspecific or absent in mild to moderate disease.
- Dullness with decreased tactile fremitus (vibration caused by speaking felt on the chest wall) may indicate pleural thickening or effusion.
- Clubbing of the nail beds occurs only when persistent hypoxemia is present.
- Crackles on inspiration may be present.
- Tubular breath sounds, diminished breath sounds, pleural rub, or wheezing may be heard with a stethoscope.
- Distant hollow breath sounds over cavities may be heard. This is also called "amphoric," due to the sound made by blowing across the mouth of an antique jar.

Concept Check

4. Which finding indicates TB has progressed to a late stage?

A. Non-productive cough
B. Fever
C. Hemoptysis
D. Night sweats

Answer question

Diagnostics

- Sputum culture: Positive AFB smear is confirming of TB diagnosis (see photo).
- Bronchoscopy may aid diagnosis: Brushings of the lesions and additional cultures can be obtained during the bronchoscopy.
- Purified Protein Derivative (PPD)–TB skin test
- Chest x-ray
- Interferon-Gamma Release Assays (IGRAs) are whole-blood tests that can aid in diagnosing *Mycobacterium tuberculosis* infection, including both latent tuberculosis infection (LTBI) and active tuberculosis (TB) disease.
- There are 2 IGRAs approved by the U.S. Food and Drug Administration (FDA) and are commercially available in the United States:
    - QuantiFERON®-TB Gold In-Tube test (QFT-GIT)
    - T-SPOT® TB test (T-Spot)

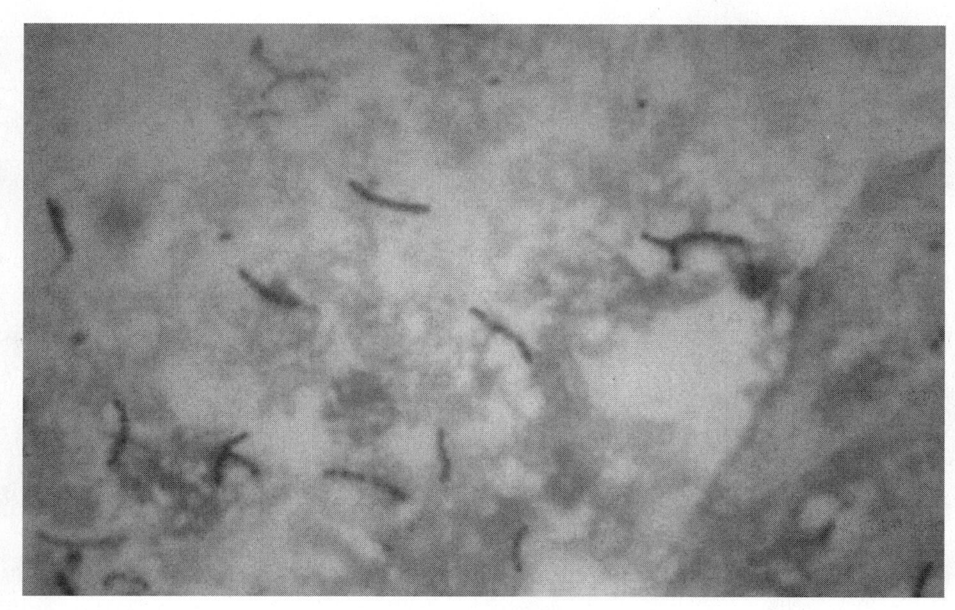

The photo is taken from a sputum culture. As is common, an acid-fast smear was used.
Source: George P. Kubica/Center for Disease Control (CDC)—PHIL

Laboratory Findings

- Lab findings may be normal in early pulmonary TB.
- Findings late in the disease may include:
    - Anemia
    - Leukocytosis
    - Thrombocytopenia
    - Elevated sedimentation rate
    - Hypoalbuminemia
    - Hyponatremia from SIADH (Syndrome of Inappropriate Antidiuretic Hormone secretion) may be noted.
- Positive blood cultures are rare except in HIV-infected patients. However, mycobacterial blood cultures are a rapid method of diagnosis.

Diagnostics (continued)

Radiologic Abnormalities

- Hilar adenopathy
  - o May be complicated by right middle lobe collapse.
- Pleural effusion
- Pulmonary infiltrates:
  - o Most often located in perihilar region and on right side.
  - o Commonly, ipsilateral hilar enlargement is found.
- Radiographic findings generally resolve slowly, often requiring more than 1 year.
- Some forms of TB may present with normal radiographs.
- CT scan is more sensitive than chest radiograph for diagnosis.

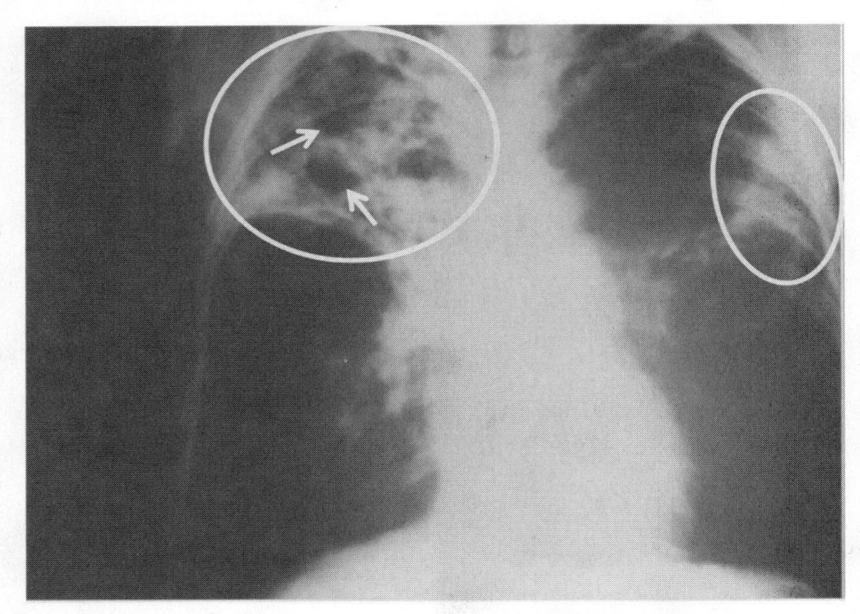

This x-ray reveals bilateral pulmonary tuberculosis. The advanced stage TB also shows cavities from lung destruction.

PPD

- PPD is *the* tuberculin skin test that identifies individuals who have been infected with *Mycobacterium tuberculosis*. It does not differentiate between old and new infection.
- Test procedure:
  1. Dose of Tuberculin = 5 tuberculin units (TU)
  2. Injection is intradermally on the dorsal side of forearm
  3. Inflammatory reaction noted in 24–72 hours
  4. Interpret test at 48–72 hours

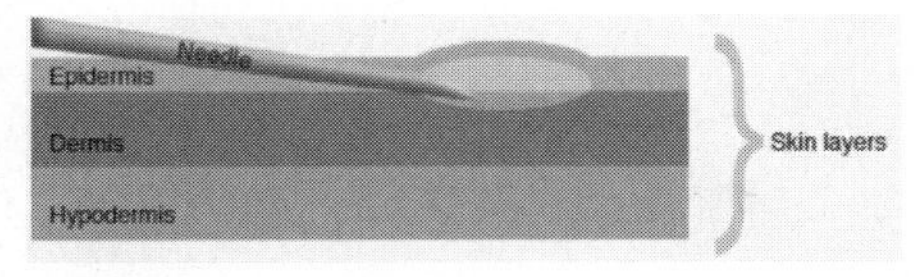

This illustration shows that the needle is inserted in the intradermal space and the bevel of the needle is aimed upward during injection.

Diagnostics (continued)

PPD Evaluation

- Diameter of induration is the determinant of test result.
- The induration is the raised, palpable, hardened area. Erythema or redness is not measured.
- Technique: Use a pen and begin measurement 1–2 cm away from margin of test.
- Mark when pen reaches the margin and resistance is felt. Repeat from opposite side. The distance between lines equals diameter.

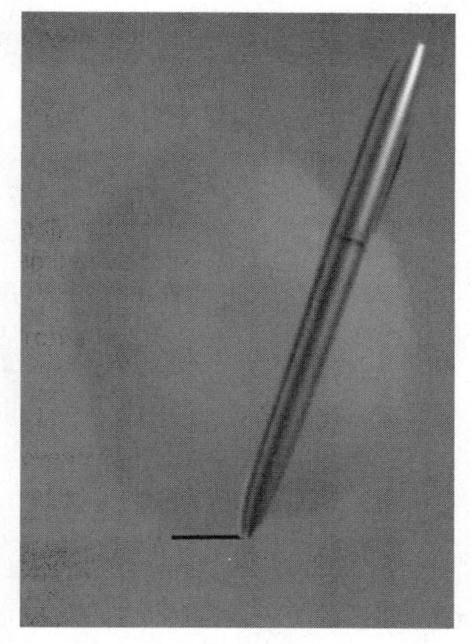

This photo illustrates how to correctly mark an induration with a pen for measurement. A normal PPD skin reaction or test is less than 15 mm or less than 1.5 cm of induration.
Source: Copyright © 2012, NovEx Novice to Expert Learning, LLC

Measuring PPD Reaction

- Read reaction 48–72 hours after injection.
- Measure only induration.
- Record reaction in millimeters.
- Fifteen mm or greater is considered positive. One inch = 25.4 mm.
- Note that the mm scale is on the right side of the ruler at right.
- The photo below reflects a positive reading at almost 50 mm. The skin reaction is called a wheal.

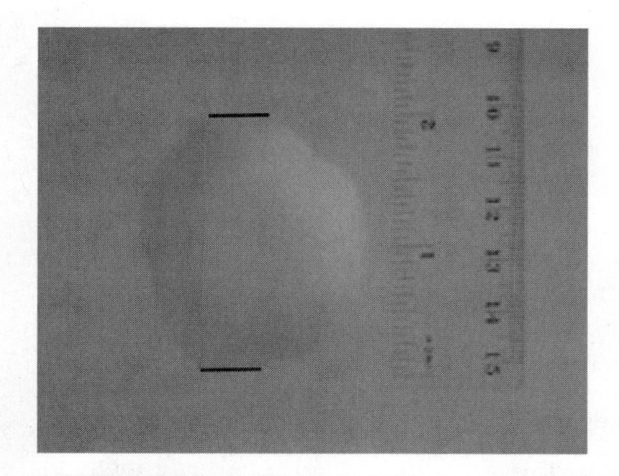

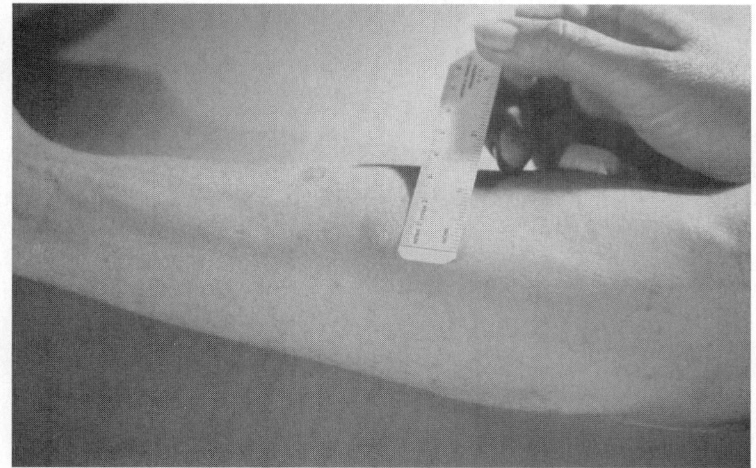

Upper: The PPD reaction is read at 72 hours. The induration is measured at approximately 50 mm and is, therefore, positive for TB. Lower: The photo compares correct and incorrect readings of the PPD positive skin test.
Sources: *(upper)* Copyright © 2012, NovEx Novice to Expert Learning, LLC; *(lower)* CDC/Donald Kopanoff

Priority Patient Concerns and Desired Collaborative Care Outcomes

Prior to caring for patients with tuberculosis, it is important to prioritize the patient's concerns that must guide the nursing care plan and interventions. Care for the patient is ordered and organized in accordance with the patient's priority and urgent needs. Desired collaborative care outcomes in patients with tuberculosis typically include:

1. Patient will be able to expectorate respiratory secretions to clear airways.
2. Patient's oxygen saturation levels will be within normal limits.
3. Patient will maintain weight appropriate for height and body build.
4. Patient will be able to complete activities of daily living without dyspnea or fatigue.
5. Patient will engage in social interaction.
6. Patient will accurately discuss treatment regimens.
7. Patient will outline methods to prevent transmission of disease to others.

Considering these important care outcomes, prepare a list of the major 3–6 priority patient concerns or nursing diagnoses for patients with tuberculosis. Be prepared to participate in a discussion of this list and/or to submit them as an assignment, as determined by your faculty. Resources you may find helpful in this assignment can include this lesson, the references, resources on nursing care plans, and standard nursing diagnoses manuals.

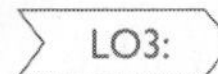

Collaborative Interventions

Evidence-Based Practice

- Evidence-based practice for the management of TB involves two key factors:
  1. Isolating the patient or having the patient wear a mask to prevent exposing others while waiting for a room
  2. Initiation of appropriate antibiotic therapy
- Treatment of the tuberculosis patient involves isolation until the infection is controlled and the rapid administration of antituberculosis agents. If a patient has a new positive PPD, prophylactic antibiotics (e.g., rifampicin, isoniazid, pyrazinamide, or Rifater) are likely to be initiated.
- In the past, a four-drug regimen was given, lasting over 6 months:
  1. Isoniazid (INH)–isonicotinylhydrazine
  2. Rifampin–rifampicin
  3. Pyrazinamide–pyrazinamide
  4. Ethambutol-ethambutol
- Newer drugs, like Rifater, combine drugs in an attempt to improve compliance. Rifater, for example, includes INH, rifampin, and pyrazinamide.
- Second-line drugs or resectional surgery may be necessary.
- Dilation, endobronchial stents, and resection have been used in the management of small airway stenosis.

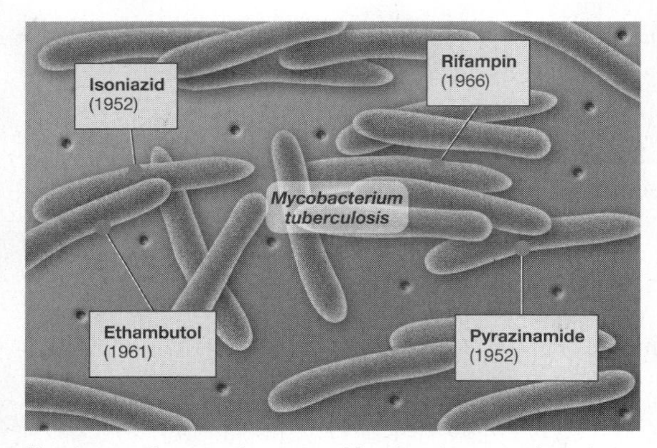

The drawing illustrates the action of first-line drugs on tubercular bacteria.

Isolation Practice

- Airborne isolation rooms (previously called negative pressure isolation) required:
  1. Any hospitalized patient suspected of having active pulmonary or laryngeal TB should be placed immediately in airborne isolation. Patients with suspected infection and those who have confirmed TB remain in isolation until they are not contagious.
  2. The door should be kept closed and negative pressure verified daily.
  3. If the patient is coughing, or a negative pressure room is not available, place a simple N95 face mask on the patient. This helps contain airborne particles.
  4. However, health care personnel should still use a N95 respirator mask (close fit, effective filtration of organisms) when caring for the patient. Appropriate respirator masks (e.g., N95) should be worn by all personnel entering the patient's room or coming into contact with the patient who has suspected tuberculosis. If in doubt about the patient's infectious status, wear a mask.
- Appropriate respiratory hygiene and cough etiquette:
  - o Cover mouth when coughing.
  - o Wear a face mask if around others.
  - o Dispose of used paper tissues only in appropriate disposal container.
- Strict adherence to facility isolation policy, especially during procedures associated with increased risk of transmission:
  - o Endotracheal intubation
  - o Bronchoscopy
  - o Sputum induction
  - o Aerosol treatments

Concept Check

5. If it is necessary for a patient suspected of having pulmonary tuberculosis to leave isolation, what is the best course of action?

A. Place a mask on the patient during transport and testing.

B. Reschedule the procedure until diagnosis is confirmed.

C. Inform all personnel who with be in contact with the patient of the diagnosis.

D. Give the patient a dose of anti-microbial agents prior to the test.

Answer question

Collaborative Interventions (continued)

Supportive Care

- Obtain ABGs and x-rays as ordered to monitor gas exchange status.
- Schedule activities gradually increasing in duration as tolerated.

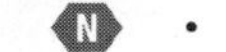

- Consult nutritionist to assist patient avoid weight loss.
- Collaborate with social services to assist with:
  - o Housing issues
  - o Treatment incentives for smoking cessation
  - o Drug abuse cessation programs, as indicated

Multidrug-Resistant (MDR) TB

- Strains of TB have developed resistance to several of the most effective first-line drugs.

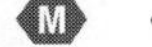

- Cure requires combinations of antibiotics that alone are not effective.
- Treatment of MDR TB is not only longer, but far more costly.

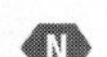

- Patient education is critical as patients must take the medications as prescribed and for the full length of time prescribed to prevent development of MDR TB.

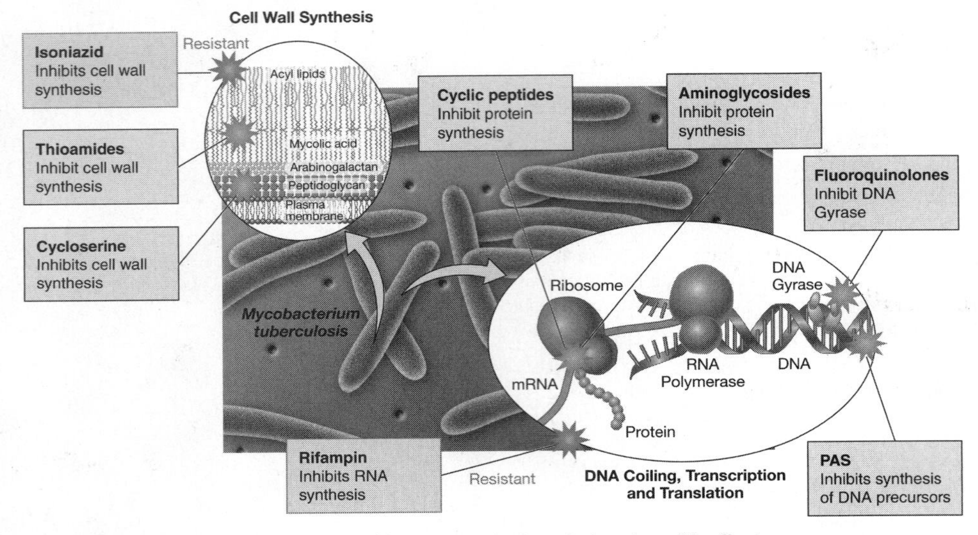

This drawing illustrates multidrug-resistant (X = resistance) tuberculosis and possible effective treatments.

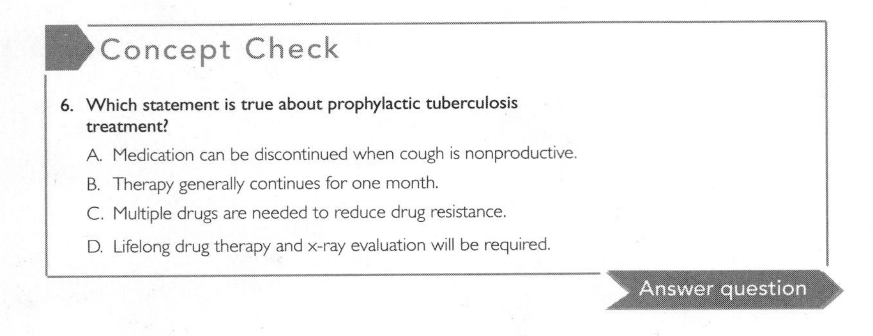

Concept Check

6. Which statement is true about prophylactic tuberculosis treatment?

   A. Medication can be discontinued when cough is nonproductive.

   B. Therapy generally continues for one month.

   C. Multiple drugs are needed to reduce drug resistance.

   D. Lifelong drug therapy and x-ray evaluation will be required.

Answer question

Collaborative Interventions (continued)

MDR Tuberculosis Treatment

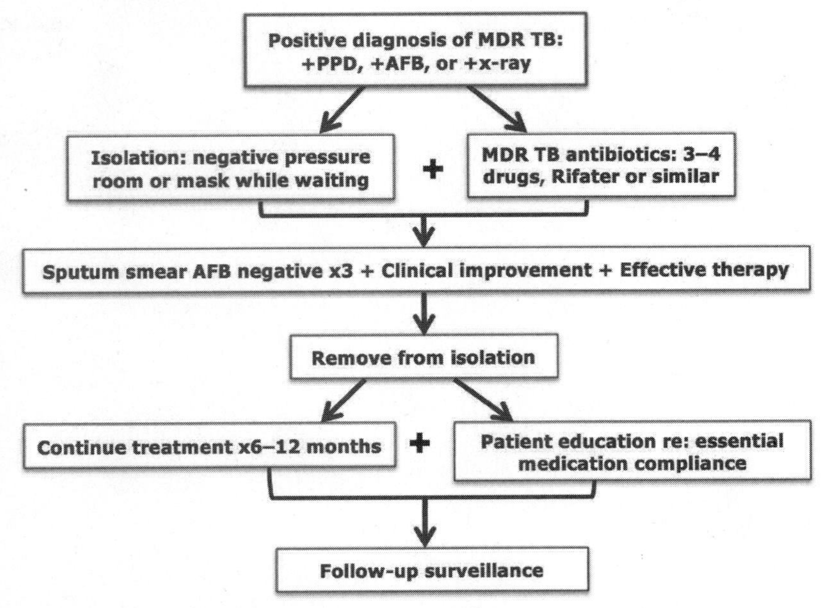

Discontinuation of Airborne Isolation

- Patient may be transferred to conventional hospital room once the diagnosis of TB has been ruled out, or when the patient is being treated and meets ALL of the following criteria:
  - o Patient is on effective therapy.
  - o Patient is improving clinically.
  - o Three consecutive sputum samples, obtained on different days, are smear-negative for AFB.

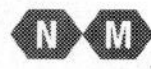

- Modifications to the isolation protocol may be made by the health care provider for patients with positive AFB smears or MDR tuberculosis.

Patient Education

Patient education is extensive:

- Teach appropriate measures to prevent the spread of the disease (i.e., isolation rooms with negative ventilation, face masks, appropriate disposition of tissues.)
- Educate patient on the critical nature of medication regimen adherence to all medications for the full duration of the prescription. Avoiding MDR TB is essential.
- Educate patient on side effects of TB medications, such as hepatotoxicity and symptoms to watch for.
- Educate the patient about potential complications and provide instructions about when to call the health care provider.
- Teach appropriate coughing and airway clearance techniques (i.e., incentive spirometry, abdominal splinting, coughing, and deep breathing techniques)
- Encourage appropriate food choices and consumption to meet metabolic requirements, such as high quality proteins and foods rich in antioxidants.

Strategies and Targets for Control

- The five-component Directly Observed Therapy, Short-course (DOTS) strategy was developed in the mid-1990s by the World Health Organization (WHO) as a response to increased global attention to tuberculosis.
- The five elements are:
  1. Government commitment to TB control
  2. Case detection among symptomatic patients
  3. Standardized drug therapy for all sputum smear-positive cases under proper case management conditions
  4. Regular drug supply
  5. Monitoring system for program supervision and evaluation.
- The DOTS model was subsequently implemented in 184 countries, which vastly improved quality and outcomes.

Summary of Interventions

- Early diagnosis and aggressive treatment
- Prevent the spread of TB by strict adherence to airborne isolation procedures and the use of N95 face masks.
- Treatment should consist of antituberculosis multidrug therapy preferably contained in one pill (i.e., Rifater) to improve compliance.
- Worldwide strategies are in place to:
  1. Improve government commitment.
  2. Increase early recognition.
  3. Pursue aggressive treatment.
  4. Provide adequate supplies of drugs.
  5. Monitor for the spread of TB.

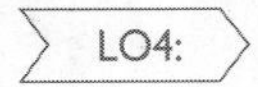

Evaluation of Desired Collaborative Care Outcomes

Evaluation and reassessment should reveal attainment of previously established patient outcomes. In summary:

- Patient demonstrates effective coughing technique and disposes of tissues appropriately. Lungs are progressively clearer to auscultation.
- Patient's skin is warm, dry, with no cyanosis. Mentation is clear.
- Patient exhibits no findings of muscle wasting. Body weight returns to patient's desired level.
- Patient maintains a daily activity schedule with no reports of excessive fatigue.
- Patient reports participation in social activities.
- Patient describes personal plan for adhering to medication schedule, identifies normal and adverse reactions to medications, and discusses findings that indicate need to contact the health care provider.
- Patient discusses ways to prevent transmission of TB to others in the community.

References

Horsburgh, C. R. Jr., Goldberg, S., Bethel, J., Chen, S., Colson, P. W., Hirsch-Moverman, Y., Hughes, S., Shrestha-Kuwahara, R., Sterling, T. R., Wall, K., & Weinfurter, P. (2010, February). Latent TB infection treatment acceptance and completion in the United States and Canada. Tuberculosis Epidemiologic Studies Consortium. *Chest, 137*(2), 401–409.

Kessenich, C. R., & Cronin, K. (2013, March). Screening options for tuberculosis. *Nurse Pract. 38*(3), 16–18.

York, N. L., & Kane, C. (2013). Caring for the critically ill patient with tuberculosis. *Dimens Crit Care Nurs. 32*(1), 6–11

Clinical Practice Guidelines

Treatment of Tuberculosis: Guidelines. 4th edition. Geneva: World Health Organization; 2010. Full free text version

Tuberculosis and Air Travel: Guidelines for Prevention and Control. 3rd edition. Geneva: World Health Organization; 2008

Patient Education

Punnoose, A. R., Lynm, C., & Golub, R. M. (2013). Tuberculosis. *JAMA. 309*(9). 938.

Learning Outcomes for Sleep Apnea

When you complete this lesson, you will be able to:

1. Recognize the clinical relevance of sleep apnea.
2. Consider the pathophysiology, etiology, risk factors, and clinical presentation of sleep apnea that determine the priority patient concerns.
3. Determine the most urgent and important nursing interventions and patient education required in caring for a patient with sleep apnea.
4. Evaluate attainment of desired collaborative care outcomes for a patient with sleep apnea.

LO1:

What Is Obstructive Sleep Apnea?

- Apnea is a period of time during which breathing stops or is markedly reduced while one is sleeping. While no exact definition is present, an apnea episode can be said to occur when a person stops breathing for 10 seconds or more.
- Obstructive sleep apnea (OSA) or obstructive sleep apnea syndrome results from recurrent episodes of apnea during sleep.
- Episodes of apnea can occur as much as 800 times per night.
- The repeated disruption from a deep sleep to a lighter sleep prevents restful and restorative sleep.

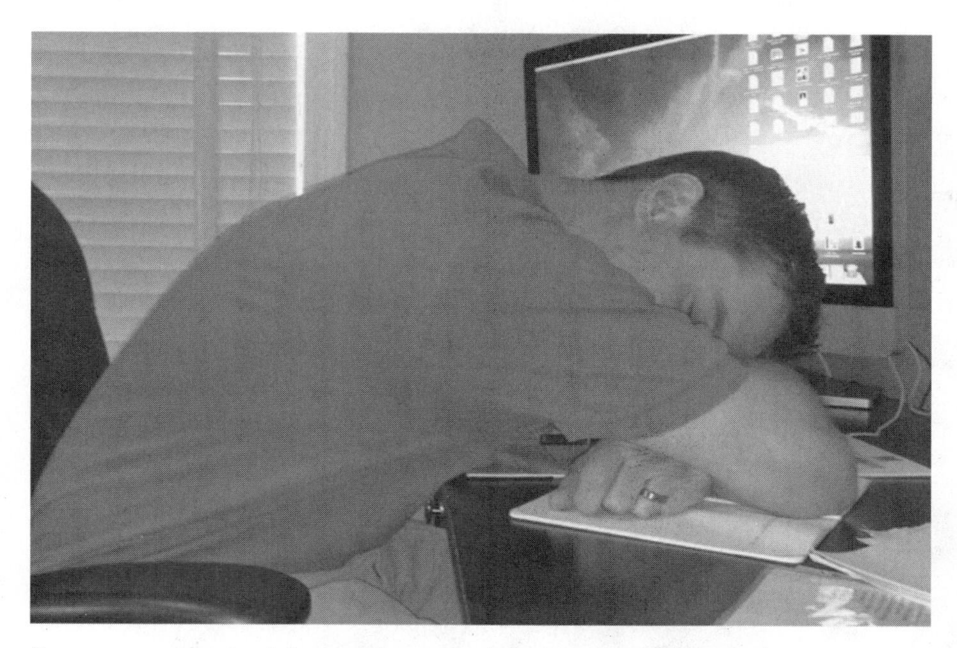

Sleep apnea creates major challenges with concentration and productivity during the day.

LO1:

Clinical Relevance

OSA Effects

The major impact of OSA on individuals is sleep deprivation resulting in:

- Daytime fatigue from repeated nocturnal awakenings
- Severe daytime drowsiness and irritability
- Falling asleep while at work, watching TV, driving, or performing other activities that require attention
- Difficulty concentrating

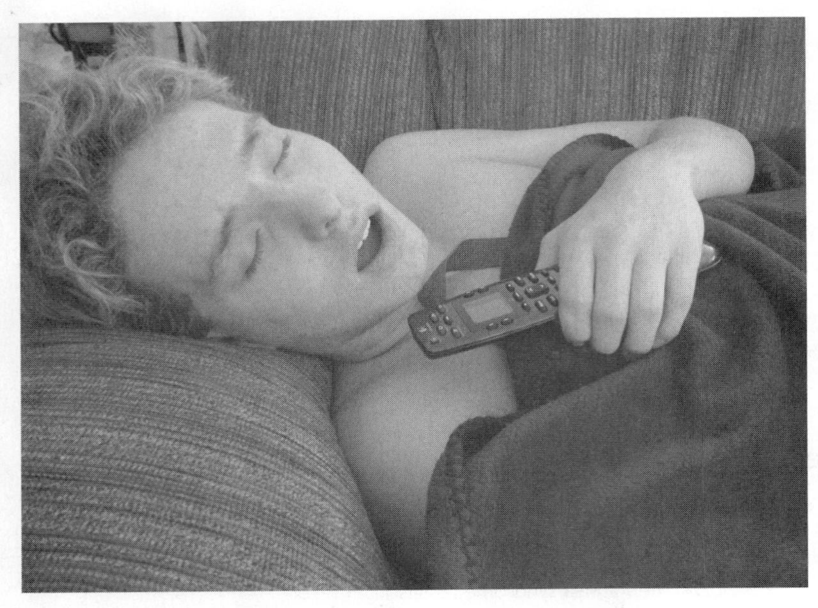

Falling asleep while watching TV, driving, and working disturb normal daily function and can be dangerous in some instances.
Source: Copyright © 2012, NovEx Novice to Expert Learning, LLC

- OSA is a significant factor in motor vehicle accidents, including fatalities.
- It affects more than 12 million people according to the National Heart, Lung, and Blood Institute.
- It increases the risk for:
  - Cardiovascular events
  - Sudden death
  - Cardiac dysrhythmias
  - Stroke
  - Right heart failure
  - Hypertension
  - Hyperglycemia
- Obesity is the best documented risk factor for OSA, with a high correlation for patients with both conditions.
- One in 25 middle-aged men and one in 50 middle-aged women have sleep apnea.

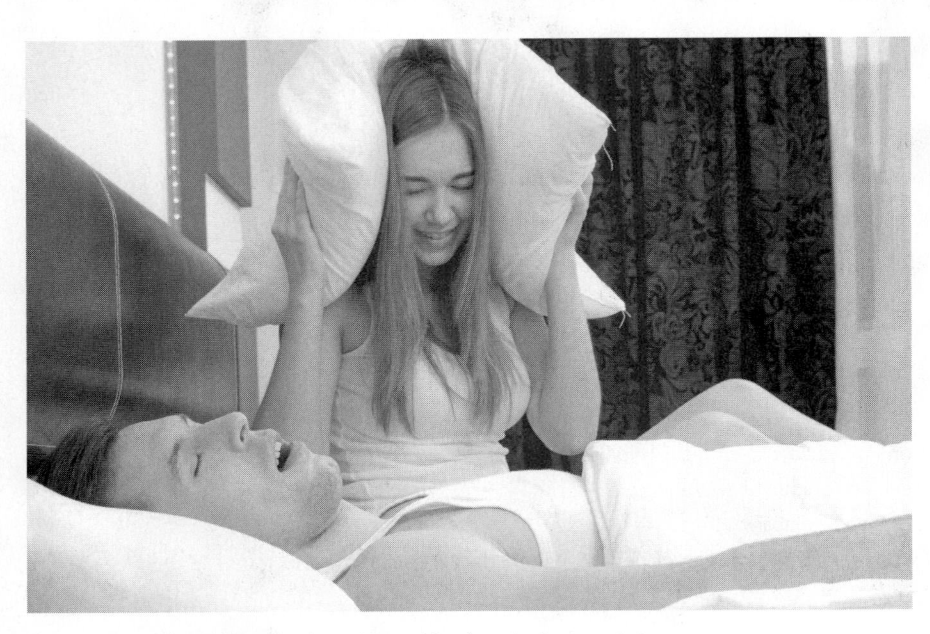

Sleep apnea can disrupt sleep for the patient and for those in close proximity.
Source: Georgerudy/Fotolia

Concept Check

1. Which patient is most at risk for obstructive sleep apnea?

A. A 45-year-old female with hypertension

B. An infant delivered at 28 weeks' gestation

C. A 25-year-old male with diabetes

D. A 55-year-old female with a BMI of 32

Answer question

LO2:

Pathophysiology

Types of Sleep Apnea

- There are two types of sleep apnea:
  1. Obstructive sleep apnea (OSA)
  2. Central sleep apnea (CSA)
- OSA is caused by a mechanical obstruction (complete or partial blockage) in the upper airway when breathing during sleep. For example, mechanical obstruction, such as when oropharyngeal area muscles relax and allow the airway to collapse, can cause blockage of the airway.
- CSA is caused when there is a disturbance in how the ventral lateral surface of the medulla in the brain responds to changes in carbon dioxide concentration. This results in disturbance of the automatic signals to breathe, producing periods of apnea. CSA is most often found in premature infants and adult patients with heart failure.
- OSA is the most common type of sleep apnea, with 90% of sleep apnea patients having this type.

Mechanics

- During a sleep apneic episode, the diaphragm and chest muscles work harder to open the obstructed airway. Breathing usually resumes with a loud gasp, snort, or body jerk as the person gasps for air. This loud gasping is known as a "resuscitative snort" as the airway is forced open.
- These episodes can interfere with sound sleep.

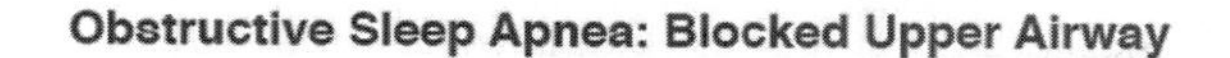

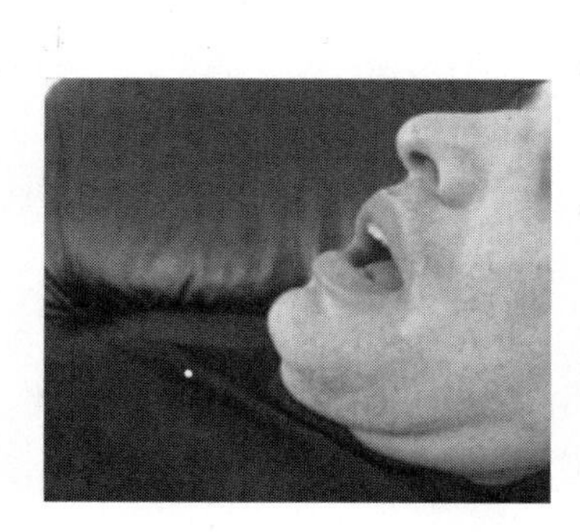

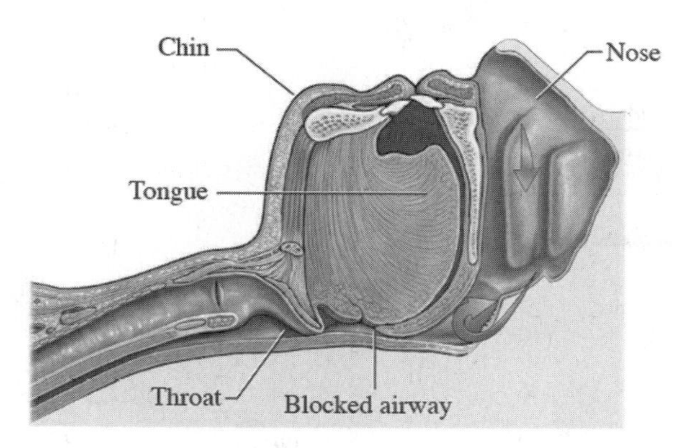

Left: The back position during sleep allows the airway to collapse when the muscles and supporting structures relax. Right: The illustration depicts relaxation of the tongue and surrounding soft tissues, which causes blockage of the upper airway. The blockage causes obstructive apnea during sleep while lying down.

Sources: *(left)* Copyright © 2012, NovEx Novice to Expert Learning, LLC; *(right)* © 2013 Nucleus Medical Media, All rights reserved

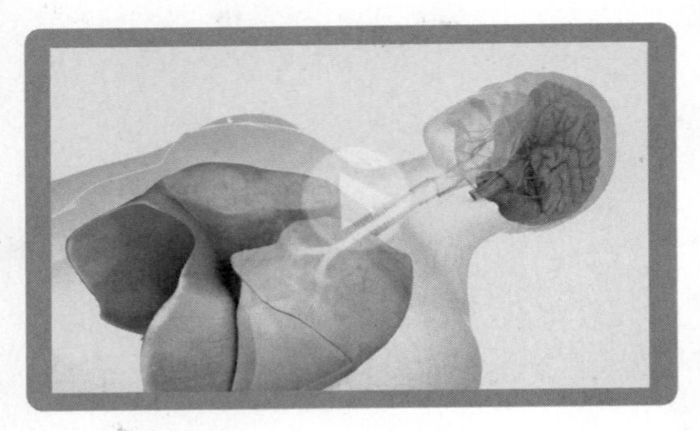

This non-narrated 3D animation shows what happens during normal breathing, snoring and sleep apnea. Snoring is due to the vibrating of respiratory structures and is demonstrated here with the vibrated uvula. Sleep apnea occurs when a person has pauses in their breathing or shallow breaths while sleeping because the pharynx collapses and air cannot pass through to the lungs. The brain suffers from lack of oxygen (brain turns blue), sends out a signal to breathing (yellow waves), and the patient wakes enough to breathe again.

- The cycle of sleep apnea is seen in the diagram.
- Apneic episodes can also reduce the flow of oxygen to vital organs. The episodic but repeated hypoxemia places patients at higher risk for cognitive disorders and other medical conditions.

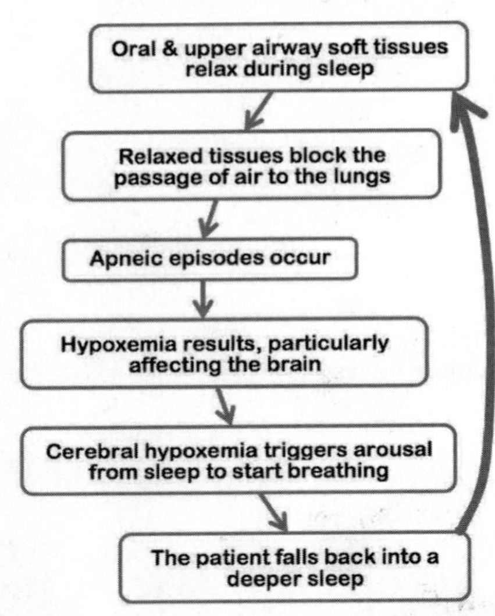

This diagram depicts the pathophysiological mechanisms that occur in sleep apnea.

Pathophysiology (continued)

Morbidity and Mortality

- Cardiovascular changes occur with decreases in blood oxygen concentrations during episodes of sleep apnea. Over time, these changes can result in chronically elevated blood pressure.
- Many people with obstructive sleep apnea develop hypertension or experience difficulty in controlling pre-existing hypertension.
- Dysrhythmias, such as atrial fibrillation, tachycardia, and bradycardia, are more likely to develop in people with OSA.
- Pulmonary hypertension and right heart failure may develop.
- Heart failure, especially right-sided heart failure with pulmonary hypertension, is a late finding indicative of advanced disease.
- Recurrent, multiple episodes of low blood oxygen concentration secondary to OSA can lead to sudden death from a cardiac event, particularly in those people with concomitant cardiac disease.

Concept Check

2. Which statement is correct regarding sleep apnea?

A. Central sleep apnea is due to lack of muscle tone in the diaphragm and intercostals.

B. Obstructive sleep apnea is the result of low levels of oxygen in the blood.

C. Central sleep apnea is the more common form of the problem.

D. Obstructive sleep apnea can result in cardiac disturbances.

Answer question

Risk Factors

- Risk factors for OSA include:
  - Obesity
  - Thick neck
  - Enlarged tonsils and adenoids
  - Narrow throat with low-lying palate
  - History of a stroke
  - Diabetes
  - Hypertension
  - Cigarette smoking

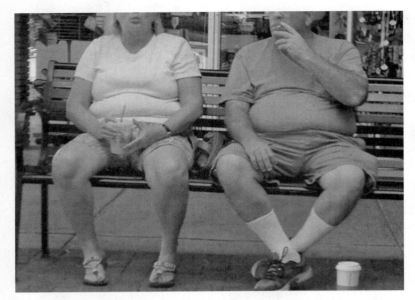

Obesity and smoking are strongly linked to obstructive sleep apnea. Further, the increased fatty tissue that accompanies obesity also surrounds the throat, increasing the weight on the airway in a supine position.
Source: Copyright © 2012, NovEx Novice to Expert Learning, LLC

Numerous questionnaires and scoring systems have been developed to assess a patient's risk for OSA, particularly before surgery. An example is the STOP-BANG score, which has been found to be very sensitive. The STOP-BANG score is a short series of questions that is reliable in predicting one's susceptibility to sleep apnea.

STOP-BANG Score

Assign one point for each positive response. Patients with a score of 5–8 are at high risk for moderate to severe sleep apnea. Do you:

- Snore loudly
- Often feel tired during daytime
- Have a history of observed apnea
- Have a history of high blood pressure or are you being treated for hypertension
- Have a BMI greater than 35
- Have an age of 50 or older
- Have a neck circumference more than 40 cm
- Belong to the male gender

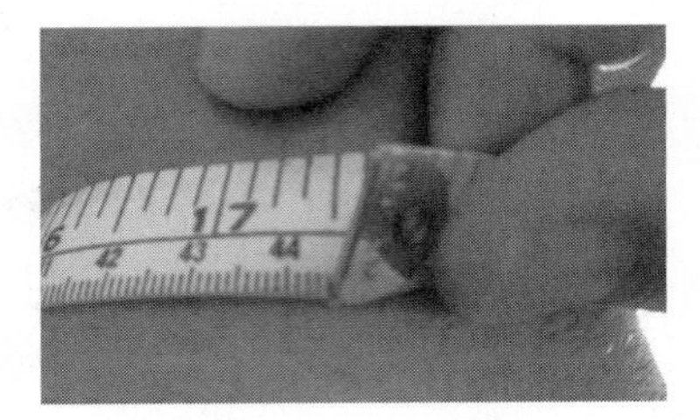

This patient has a neck circumference at 44.5 cm, increasing his risk for apnea.
Source: Copyright © 2012, NovEx Novice to Expert Learning, LLC

Concept Check

3. Which of the following are considered modifiable risk factors for sleep apnea?

A. Basal metabolic rate (BMI) of 25
B. Blood pressure of 170/95
C. Male gender
D. History of tonsillectomy at age 10

Answer question

Causes

Several characteristics of patients who develop OSA include:

- Low-lying palate with a narrow throat opening
- Enlarged tonsils and adenoids
- Obese neck
- Obese abdomen
- Relaxation of the muscles causing collapse in the oropharyngeal area blocking the airway

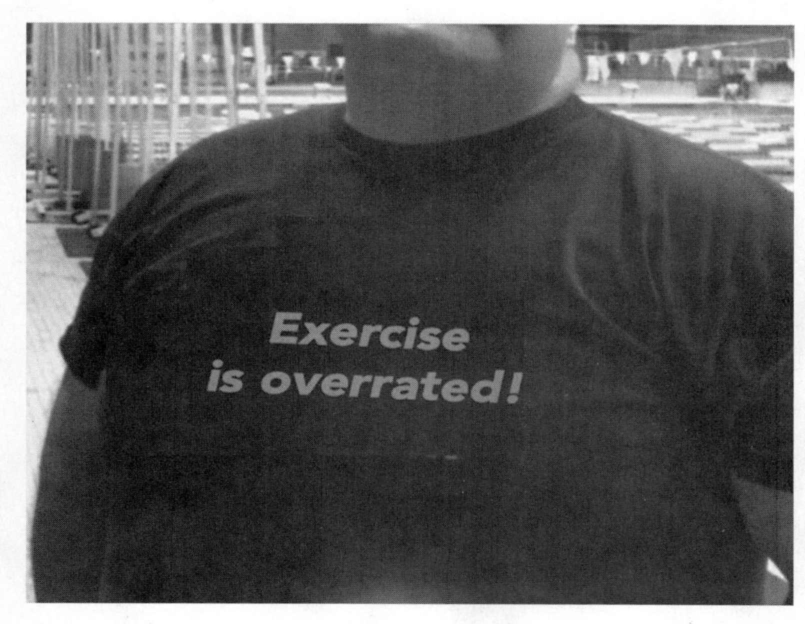

Obesity is closely associated with OSA.

Assessment Findings

- Daytime sleepiness and fatigue
- Dry mouth or sore throat upon awakening
- Morning headaches
- Difficulty concentrating, forgetfulness, depression, or irritability
- Night sweats
- Loud resuscitative snorting that ends the apneic episode
- Restlessness during sleep
- Sexual dysfunction
- Snoring that disturbs others in the home
- Sudden awakening with a sensation of gasping or choking
- Difficulty getting up in the morning
- Partner may notice periods of apnea

Diagnostics

Polysomnogram (PSD)

- The polysomnogram is used to diagnose OSA. It is performed in a sleep lab and is supervised by a trained technologist.
- The test measures:
  - o Air flow
  - o Blood oxygen levels
  - o Breathing patterns
  - o Electrical activity of the brain
  - o Eye movements
  - o Heart rate
  - o Muscle activity

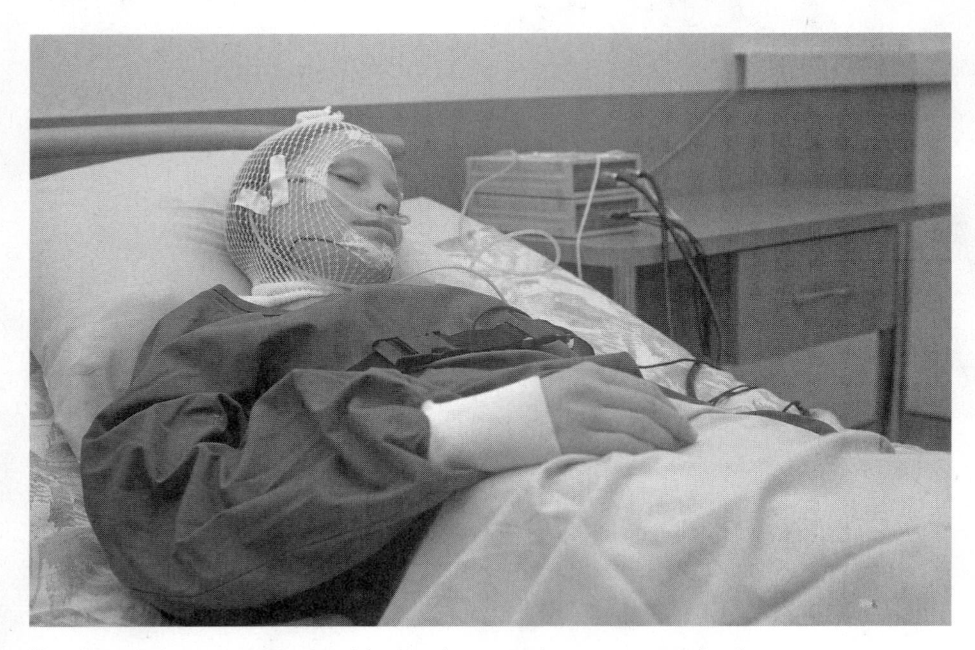

This photo shows a patient in a sleep lab who is having a polysomnogram test for sleep apnea.
Source: SEGUIN TEDDY/BSIP/BSIP SA/Alamy

Priority Patient Concerns and Desired Collaborative Care Outcomes

Prior to caring for patients with sleep apnea, it is important to prioritize the patient's concerns that must guide the nursing care plan and interventions. Care for the patient is ordered and organized in accordance with the patient's priority and urgent needs. Desired collaborative care outcomes in patients with sleep apnea typically include:

1. Patient will establish a pattern of regular respiration.
2. Patient's airway will be clear.
3. Patient will verbalize fewer feelings of fatigue.
4. Patient will report sleeping through the night.
5. Patient will discuss accurate management techniques.

Considering these important care outcomes, prepare a list of the major 3–6 priority patient concerns or nursing diagnoses for patients with sleep apnea. Be prepared to participate in a discussion of this list and/or to submit them as an assignment, as determined by your faculty. Resources you may find helpful in this assignment can include this lesson, the references, resources on nursing are plans, and standard nursing diagnoses manuals.

LO3:

Collaborative Interventions

Mild OSA

Conservative treatment in mild cases of sleep apnea include:

- N M Weight loss: As little as a 10% weight loss can reduce the number of sleep apnea events for most patients.
- N Avoid the use of alcohol and sleeping pills, which relax the airway and exacerbate OSA.
- N Sleep in side position and avoid sleeping on back.
- N M Use nasal sprays to reduce snoring and improve airflow for sinus problems.
- N Avoid sleep deprivation.

Moderate to Severe OSA: Evidence-Based Practice

- Evidenced-based treatments focus on:
  - o N M Weight loss
  - o N M The use of positive pressure during sleep. Use of CPAP should be based upon the recommendation of a board certified sleep medicine specialist.
- Nocturnal Continuous Positive Airway Pressure (NCPAP or CPAP) is the mainstay of therapy for moderate to severe OSA:
  1. Is a type of noninvasive positive pressure ventilation (NIPPV).
  2. Pressure is used to assist breathing.
  3. An air blower forces air through the nose and/or mouth.
  4. The air pressure is adjusted to prevent upper airway collapse during sleep.
  5. The pressure is constant and continuous.
- Bilevel positive airway pressure (BiPAP) is a type of NIPPV and is used if CPAP is ineffective.
- Educate patient as in mild OSA. Patients should be instructed that apneic episodes return when CPAP is stopped or it is used improperly.
- N M Coaching and informational support are helpful in a patient's adjustment when using a continuous positive airway pressure mask.
- N Research has shown that success in the first week of CPAP use increases the likelihood of long-term use.

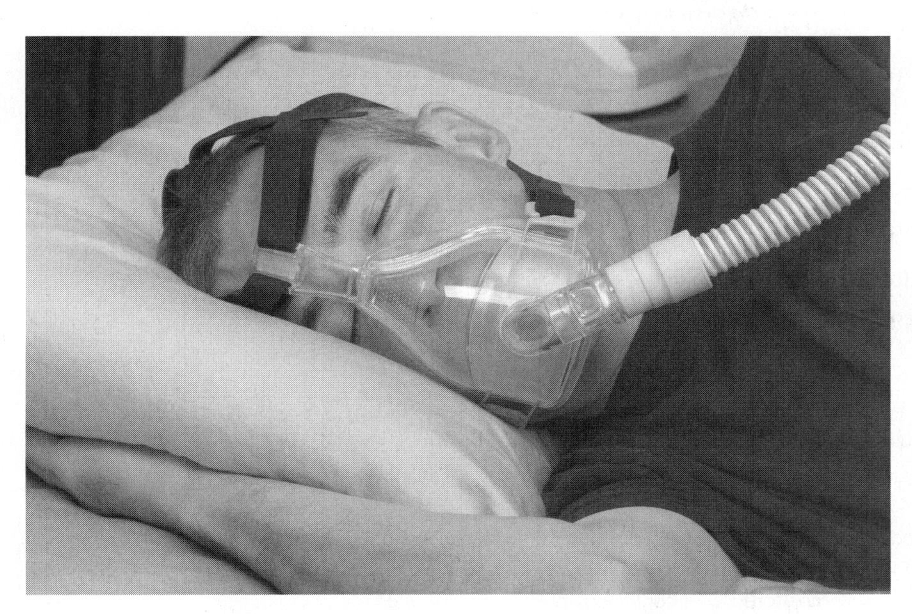

A CPAP device is shown delivering air pressure to maintain an open airway during sleep. It enables sound, restful, and uninterrupted sleep.
Source: BVDC/Fotolia

Concept Check

4. If periods of sleep apnea continue after the initiation of CPAP, the problem may be associated with what factor?

A. The patient's BMI

B. Frequency of CPAP use

C. Patient's blood pressure

D. Use of sleep medications

Answer question

Collaborative Interventions (continued)

Additional OSA Treatment Options

N M
- Oral appliances may help some patients with mild OSA keep the airway open by positioning the jaw forward.

M
- Surgery to remove upper airway obstruction may be effective in certain patients (e.g., patients with large tonsils or adenoids).

N M
- Tracheostomy is done if OSA is severe and patient fails CPAP. This is usually considered in the setting of severe respiratory and cardiac failure.

N
- Positional therapy, (i.e., avoid sleeping on one's back) may be beneficial.

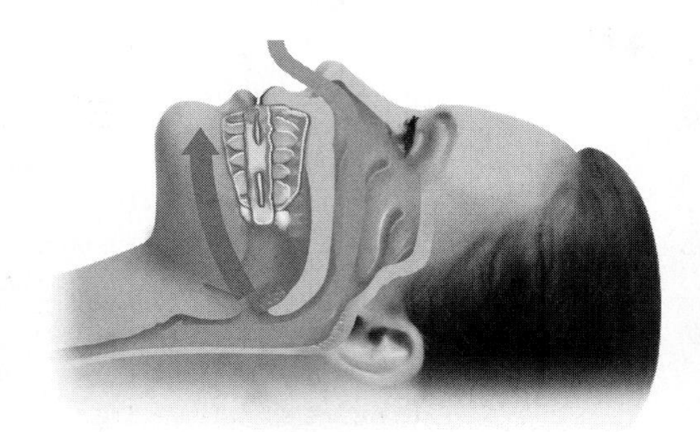

Use of an oral device can assist in moving oral and upper airway structures to prevent obstruction of the airway. Opening the airway allows more normal respirations.

Concept Check

5. In what manner should a patient with obstructive sleep apnea be instructed to sleep if not using CPAP?

A. In a cool, dark room

B. Positioned on the side

C. Flat in a recliner upright

D. Without a pillow

Answer question

OSA as a Complication After Surgery

- Patients with diagnosed or undiagnosed sleep apnea are at higher risk of postoperative respiratory and cardiovascular complications. If unattended to, the first warning of complications can be respiratory arrest.

N M
- If the patient has known OSA, ask the patient to bring CPAP to the hospital.
- Risk for sleep apnea should be assessed (e.g., use STOP-BANG score) before surgery.

N M
- Attentiveness to sleep apnea during minor procedures with conscious sedation is also essential.

N M
- Capnography is advocated as an essential monitoring device in high-risk patients because it alarms when a patient stops breathing.

N
- Patients should be more closely monitored with continuous pulse oximetry after surgery, particularly if capnography is not used. However, the pulse oximeter will not alarm as early as capnography.

N M
- Opiates (narcotics), benzodiazepines, and hypnotics should be used with caution, only when needed, and as little as possible. Avoid sedatives. Use nonsteroidal anti-inflammatory drugs.

N M
- Patients who are not on CPAP should be positioned laterally or upright during postoperative recovery because the supine position predisposes to apneic events.

N M
- Patients on CPAP or BiPAP should continue its use after surgery.

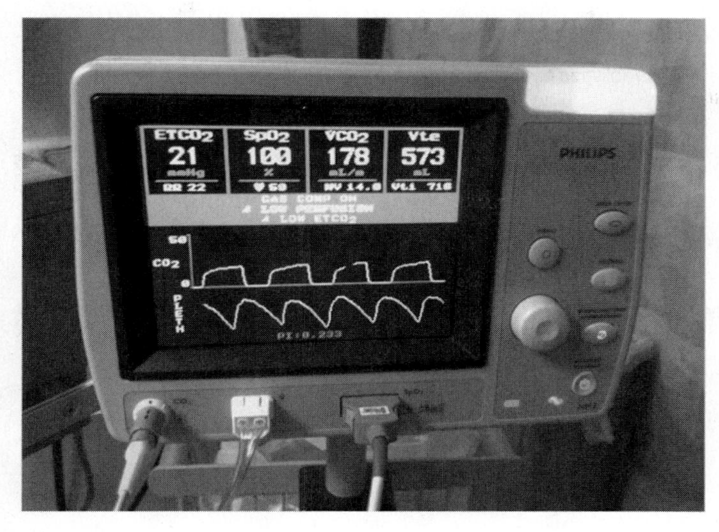

Monitoring via capnography (seen here) can provide a life saving alert for patients with sleep apnea, particularly those who have not been diagnosed. Unlike oximetry that only alarms after the patient has dangerously low oxygen sats, capnography alarms immediately when the patient stops breathing.
Source: Copyright © 2012, NovEx Novice to Expert Learning, LLC

Patient Education

Patient education should emphasize:

- Weight loss
- Exercising 30 minutes per day on most days
- Avoidance of alcohol
- Avoidance of sedating drugs such as tranquilizers and sleeping pills
- Sleeping on the side or abdomen rather than on the back
- Smoking cessation
- Proper use of adjunctive equipment such as mouthpieces or CPAP

Summary of Interventions

- Diagnosis should be made by a board certified sleep medicine specialist after a formal sleep study (PSD).
- Educate the patient: weight management, alcohol and sleeping pill use, sleeping positions, and sleep deprivation.
- Some cases of OSA can be modified by lifestyle changes and appropriate use of an appliance.
- CPAP is the treatment of choice for moderate–severe OSA.

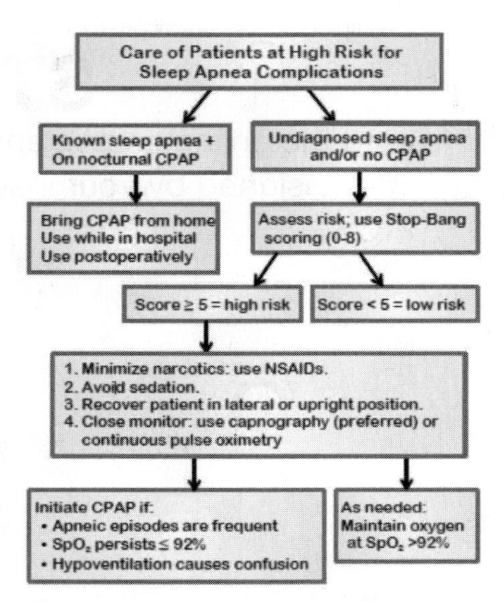

Source: Copyright © 2012, NovEx Novice to Expert Learning, LLC

LO4:

Evaluation of Desired Collaborative Care Outcomes

Evaluation and reassessment should reveal attainment of previously established patient outcomes. In summary:

- Patient's respirations during sleep are even and equal in depth with no periods of apnea.
- Patient has reduced or absent snoring.
- Patient reports less daytime drowsiness with sufficient energy to achieve daily goals.
- Patient reports sleeping through the night, and this information is validated by partner.
- Patient reports efforts at risk factor control.
- Patient uses CPAP or other adjunctive equipment correctly and routinely.

References

Chai, C. L., Pathinathan, A., & Smith, B. (2006, October). Continuous positive airway pressure delivery interfaces for obstructive sleep apnea. *Cochrane Database Syst Rev, 18*(4), CD005308.

Chung, S. A., Yuan, H., & Chung, F. (2008, November). A systemic review of obstructive sleep apnea and its implications for anesthesiologists. *Anesth Analg, 107*(5), 1543–1563.

Ye, L., Pack, A. I., Maislin, G., Dinges, D., Hurley, S., McCloskey, S., & Weaver, T. E. (2012, August). Predictors of continuous positive airway pressure use during the first week of treatment. *J Sleep Res, 21*(4), 419–426.

Clinical Practice Guidelines

Morgenthaler, T. I., Aurora, R. N., Brown, T., et al. (2008). Practice parameters for the use of autotitrating continuous positive airway pressure devices for titrating pressures and treating adult patients with obstructive sleep apnea syndrome: An update for 2007. *Sleep, 31*(1), 141–147.

Strohl, K. P., Brown, D. B., Collop, N., et al. (2013). An official American Thoracic Society clinical practice guideline: Sleep apnea, sleepiness, and driving risk in noncommercial drivers. *Amer J Resp Crit Care Med, 187*(11), 1259–1266.

Patient Education

http://www.aasmnet.org

http://www.sleepfoundation.org

http://www.nhlbi.nih.gov

STOP

Go to the online course and complete the NovE-Cases assigned by your instructor for this module.

Learning Outcomes for Acute Coronary Syndrome

When you complete this lesson, you will be able to:

1. Recognize the clinical relevance of acute coronary syndrome.
2. Consider the pathophysiology, etiology, risk factors, and clinical presentation of acute coronary syndrome that determine the priority patient concerns.
3. Determine the most urgent and important nursing interventions and patient education required in caring for a patient with acute coronary syndrome.
4. Evaluate attainment of desired collaborative care outcomes for a patient with acute coronary syndrome.

LO1:

What Is Acute Coronary Syndrome?

Acute coronary syndrome is the general term given to the various occlusive coronary conditions.

- Acute Coronary Syndrome (ACS) occurs when blockage of a coronary artery results from thrombus formation that partially or completely occludes the lumen.
- Partial occlusion (typically >70%) causes myocardial ischemia while total occlusion results in infarction (death) of the muscle supplied by the artery.
- The severity of ischemia depends on the degree and duration of the occlusion to the coronary artery.

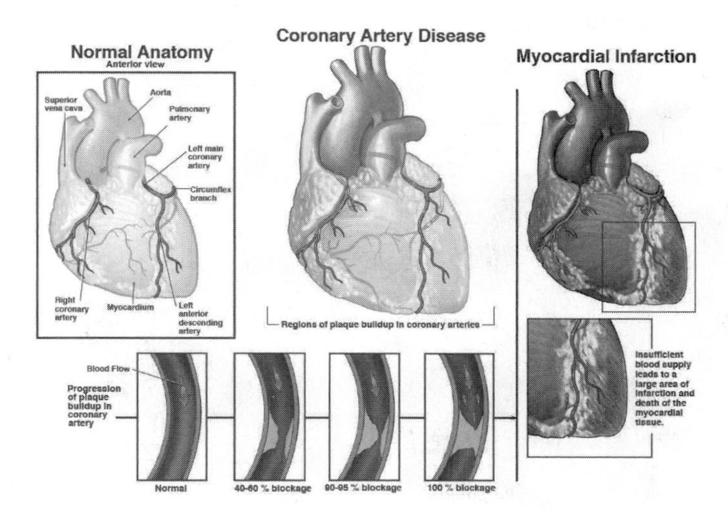

This illustration features the normal anatomy of the heart, coronary disease, and myocardial infarction. The first graphic labels the main arteries of the heart. Enlargements of arterial walls show normal, 40–60% blockage, and 90–95% blockage due to plaque buildup. The last graphic shows a large area of myocardial infarction.

Coronary Artery Circulation

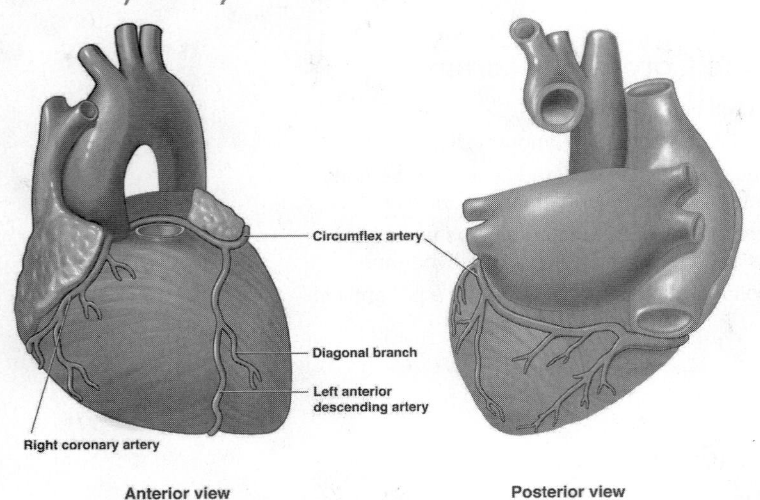

This drawing shows the coronary artery supply to muscle areas of the heart. Understanding which arteries supply the various parts of the heart can assist in better anticipating the needs of and caring for patients with ACS.

Normal Anatomy of the Heart

Right subclavian artery
Left common carotid artery
Left subclavian artery
Superior vena cava
Aortic arch
Left pulmonary artery
Left main coronary artery
Right coronary artery
Pulmonary trunk
Circumflex artery
Right atrium
Left atrium
Anterior inter-ventricular artery
Marginal artery
Cardiac muscle
Right ventricle
Left ventricle
Pulmonary semilunar valve
Atrioventricular (tricuspid) valve
Inferior vena cava
Descending aorta
Apex of heart
Aortic semilunar valve
Left pulmonary veins
Bicuspid (mitral) valve
Septum
Chordae tendineae
Papillary muscles

This drawing depicts a cutaway view of the heart's anatomy, revealing the internal heart structures. Understanding the anatomic locations of the arteries in relation to the structures provides a clearer idea about what damage occurs where with an infarction.

LO1:

Clinical Relevance

- Cardiovascular disease is listed as the leading cause of death in the United States.
- Coronary heart disease accounts for roughly 1 out of 6 deaths in the United States.
- Every 25 seconds, someone has a coronary event and, about every minute, someone dies.
- Every year close to 935,000 people have a heart attack with two-third of them experiencing their first attack.
- Almost $109 billion is spent on ACS yearly in the United States.
- Treatment and recognition have improved, but risk factors continue to persist (e.g., smoking, obesity, and other detrimental lifestyle choices).

Women and Heart Disease

- One-third of all deaths worldwide among women are attributed to heart disease.
- Almost twice as many women die from heart attacks in the first year after the attack (42%) as compared to men (24%).
- Women under the age of 50 are twice as likely to die from a heart attack as men in that age group.
- The majority of women experiencing a heart attack have atypical or no pain, but instead experience vague chest discomfort, heartburn, or flu-like symptoms.
- Diabetes doubles the risk for heart attack for women.
- Prognosis is worsened for women who are experiencing marital difficulties.
- Women are included as participants in only 24% of heart disease studies.

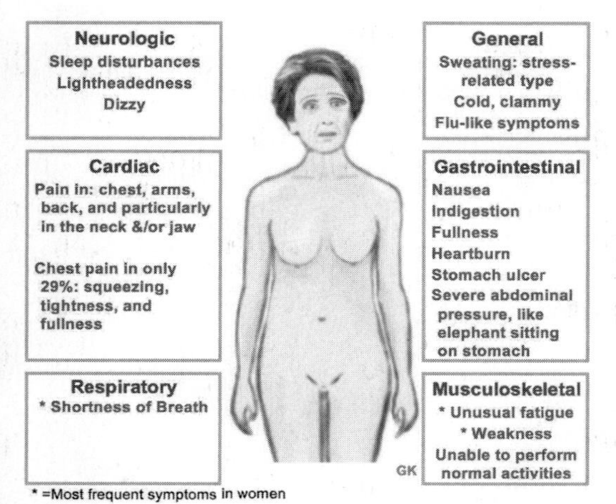

This image shows the primary symptoms associated with a heart attack.

Source: Courtesy of George Kyriakidis/Santa Ana, CA

Concept Check

1. **Which statement regarding coronary disease is accurate?**

   A. Cardiovascular disease is the second leading cause of death in the United States behind cancer.

   B. Women tend to have more severe chest pain than do men.

   C. Studies reveal that heart disease affects men and women equally.

   D. More women than men die in the first year after having a myocardial infarction.

Answer question

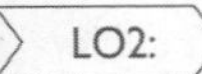

LO2: Pathophysiology

Forms of Acute Coronary Syndrome (ACS)

- Myocardial infarction (MI) is also known as a heart attack. Angina is another name for ischemia.
- There are three forms of ACS:
  1. **ST**-**E**levation **M**yocardial **I**nfarction (STEMI), meaning the MI caused ST segment elevation on the 12-lead EKG
  2. **N**on–**ST-E**levation **M**yocardial **I**nfarction (NSTEMI), meaning there was no ST segment elevation on EKG
  3. Unstable Angina (UA)
- Stable angina is more easily treated but often results in hospitalization and management issues. This stable form of angina is detailed in the Angina NovE-lesson.
- The extent of damage from ACS is influenced by the extent to which the smaller surrounding collateral vessels enlarge. Collateral circulation can supply blood flow to the affected area, reducing potential infarct size.

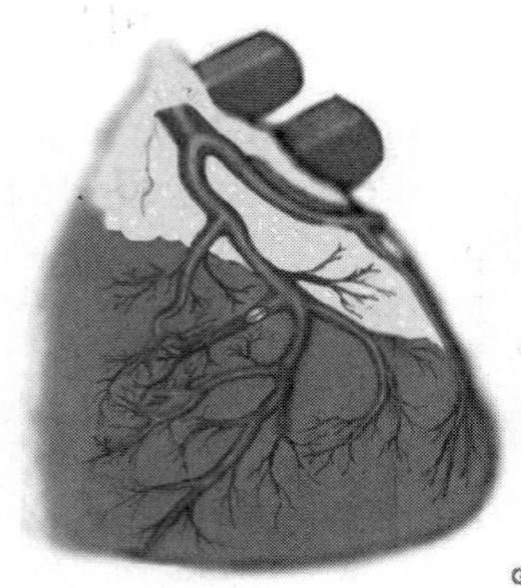

This picture depicts an occlusion in an artery (brown), cutting off blood flow and oxygen to a segment of the heart. Surrounding and infiltrating that segment are small collateral vessels (dense vessels) that can enlarge to supply blood flow and oxygen, rendering the myocardium viable after the occlusion.
Source: Courtesy of George Kyriakidis/Santa Ana, CA

Atherosclerosis in ACS

- Atherosclerosis is a process consisting of multiple stages, resulting in disruption of the arterial walls from plaque buildup. Plaque forms from cholesterol and other substances that cause progressive obstruction of the coronary arteries and, ultimately, result in thrombosis and myocardial infarction.
- The process includes:
  - o Injury to the endothelium
  - o Fatty streak formation (see photo)
  - o Inflammatory fibrous cap atheroma formation
  - o Thrombus formation

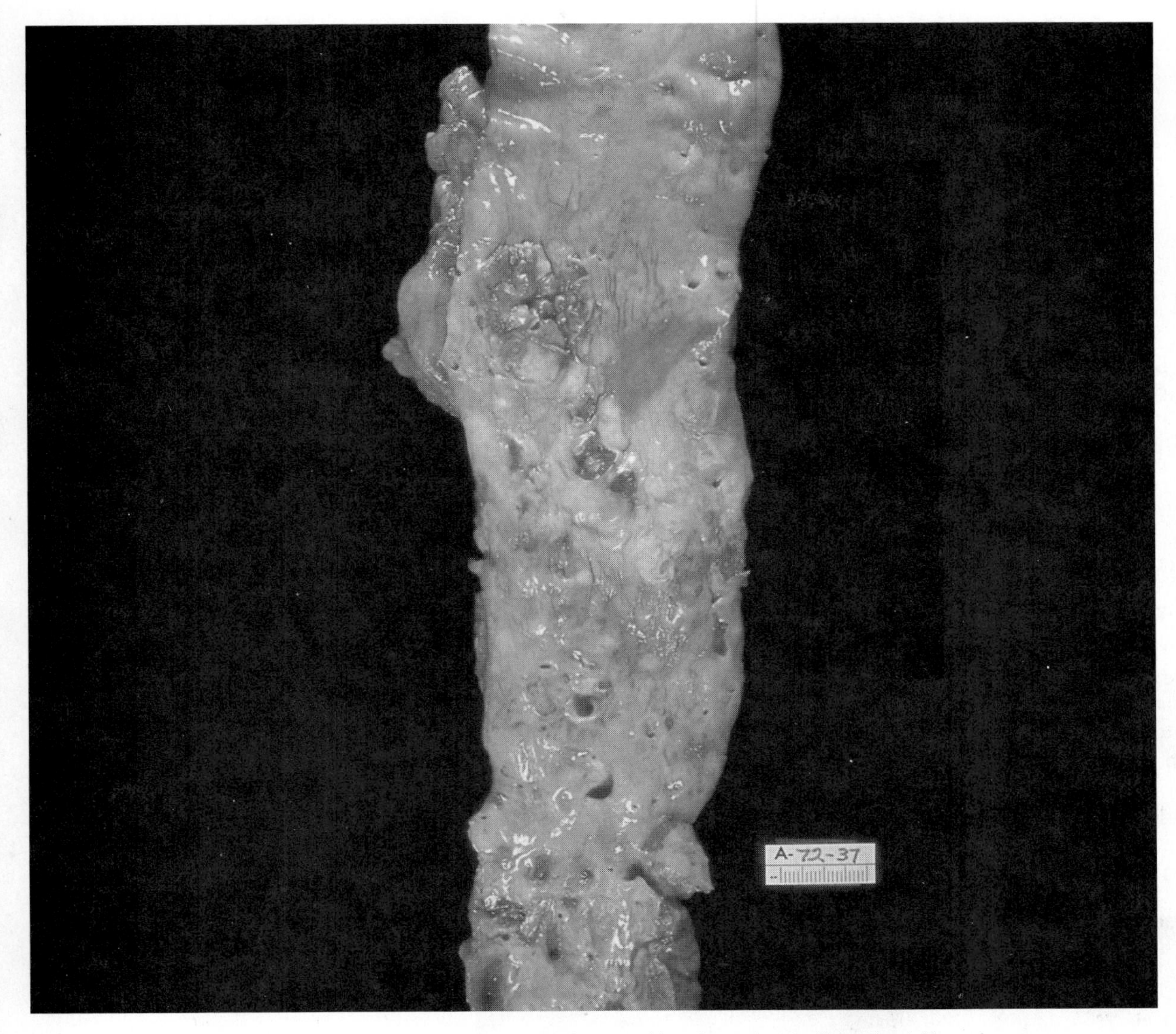

The photo shows the yellow dots and streaks known as fatty streaks created by atherosclerosis. Plaque has infiltrated and lines this arterial wall.
Source: CDC.gov/Dr. Edwin P. Ewing, Jr.

Injury to the Endothelium

- Injury is likely the result of multiple factors that include hypertension and hyperlipidemia.
- Inflammatory mediators released by the injured endothelium attract monocytes, which migrate into the tunica intima of the artery.

Fatty Streak Formation

- Monocytes transform into macrophages and ingest oxidized LDL cholesterol, leading to foam cell formation.
- These macrophages are also very active in producing multiple inflammatory mediators, some of which promote clotting.
- Deposition of cholesterol in the arterial walls results in fatty streaks.

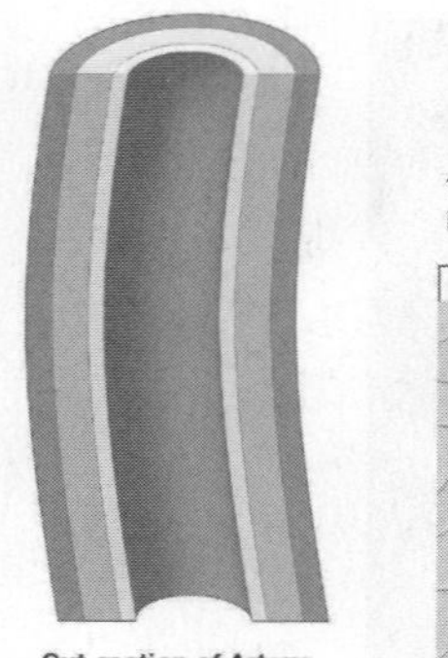

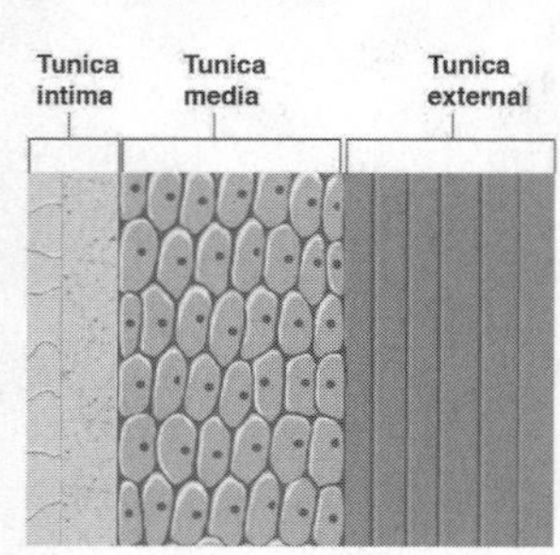

The Layers of an Artery: Tunica intima lines the lumen of the artery with endothelial cells. Tunica media contains smooth muscle cells. Tunica externa is the outermost layer of a blood vessel and primarily contains collagen.
Source: © 2013 Nucleus Medical Media, All rights reserved

Pathophysiology (continued)

Inflammation in ACS

Formation of inflammatory fibrous cap atheroma:

- Smooth muscle cells migrate from the tunica media into the intima, where they proliferate. Collagen produced by the smooth muscle cells is deposited along the lumen, forming a fibrous cap.
- Macrophages produce proteases, which release the lining endothelial cells into the blood. This disruption of the endothelium predisposes the artery to clot formation.
- In advanced lesions, smooth muscle cells and macrophages may die, forming a central necrotic area.
- These inflammatory plaques are unstable and may rupture.

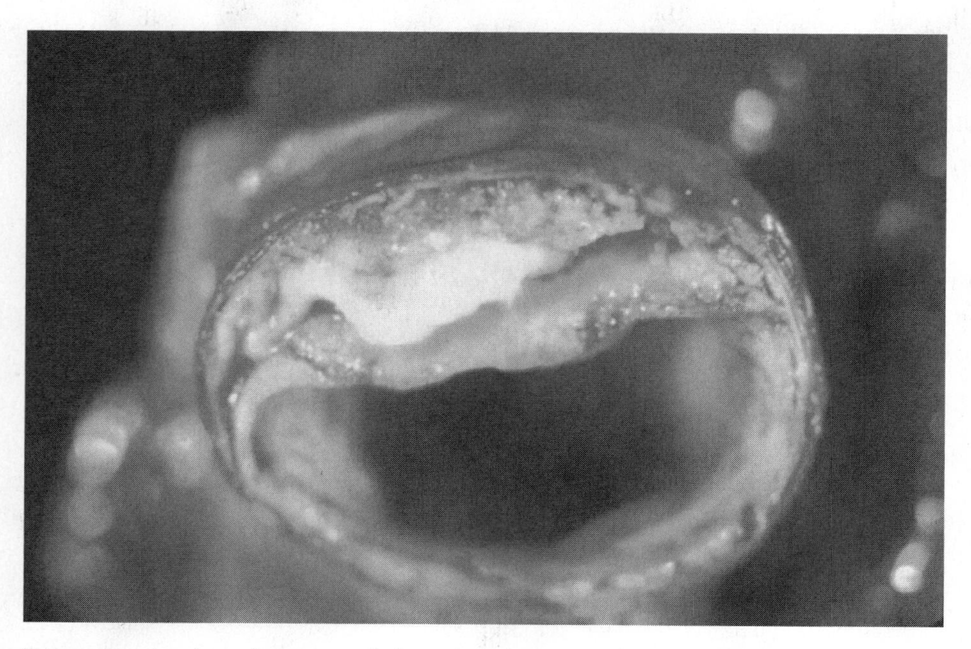

This cross section shows the anatomy of a large plaque in an artery. Smooth muscle cells (pinkish red) above a cholesterol core (light yellow) are proliferating in the intima. These cells are covered by a collagen plaque.
Source: VEM/BSIP/Alamy

Thrombosis

All forms of ACS involve thrombosis. This occurs as a result of two processes:

- The endothelium (covering the plaque) becomes compromised. These areas are prone to thrombus formation.
- Rupture of the plaque, exposing the cholesterol core, results in thrombus formation within the plaque, sometimes extending into the coronary lumen. Thrombus formation within the plaque results in enlargement of the plaque. Thrombus formation in the lumen can occlude the artery.

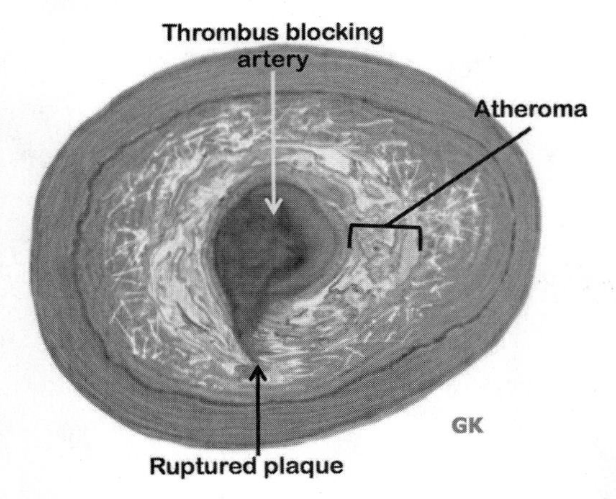

In this image, the pathologic regions are depicted with the tear in the arterial wall, the ruptured cholesterol plaque, and the thrombus occluding the artery.
Source: Courtesy of George Kyriakidis/Santa Ana, CA

Pathophysiology (continued)

Unstable Angina

- Thrombus formed in a coronary artery that does not completely block the lumen results in unstable angina.
- Thrombus formation may also stimulate temporary vasoconstriction.
- Blood flow is interrupted and ischemia that results can cause chest pain and other symptoms.
- The thrombus may spontaneously resolve or progress to completely occlude the lumen resulting in a myocardial infarction.
- The changing size of the thrombus and vasoconstriction can produce fluctuating symptoms.

Myocardial Infarction

- Bits of thrombus may embolize over time affecting numerous small arterioles. Small areas of myocardium may be affected. Lack of blood flow results in myocardial cell death in these patchy areas.
- Sudden development of a thrombosis occluding the entire lumen produces an ST elevation myocardial infarction. Myocardial cell death occurs in the area supplied by that vessel and usually involves the entire thickness of that part of the heart (known as a transmural MI).

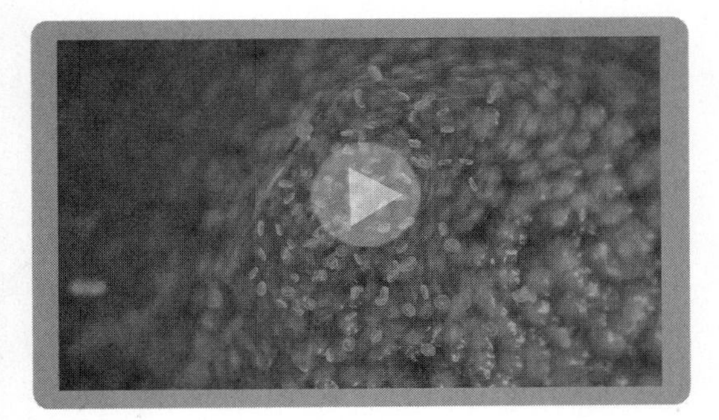

This animation demonstrates the pathophysiologic development of a myocardial infarction due to atherosclerosis, which causes chronic inflammation and subsequent damage of the blood vessels. The atherosclerotic plaque grows and can rupture, resulting in blockage of the vessel or an MI.
Source: © 2013 Nucleus Medical Media, All rights reserved

- Myocardial cell death occurs in myocardial infarction, releasing proteins into the blood that can be measured. These include myoglobin and troponin.
- Myocardial cell damage can have several effects:
  - o Function of the heart may be affected if a large area is involved. A large portion of the heart may lose its contractile force (systolic function) as well as the ability to relax and fill with blood (diastolic dysfunction).
  - o The heart becomes predisposed to deadly ventricular dysrhythmias, including ventricular fibrillation.
  - o Valves may be affected if the papillary muscles are attached to the infarcted region. If the coronary vessel supplying the papillary muscle is occluded, it can rupture with sudden, severe heart failure.
  - o A small myocardial area of infarction may not cause perceptible problems, unless the patient experiences multiple small MIs.
  - o However, larger areas of infarction may cause the patient functional limitations due to the heart's reduced systolic function and, therefore, cardiac output.
  - o Multiple MIs reduce the heart's capability to the point that it begins to fail. See the Heart Failure NovE-Lesson for a detailed understanding.
  - o An MI that causes extensive damage to a large portion of the ventricle and/or involves valvular dysfunction commonly results in either sudden death or rapid onset of severe heart failure and cardiogenic shock.

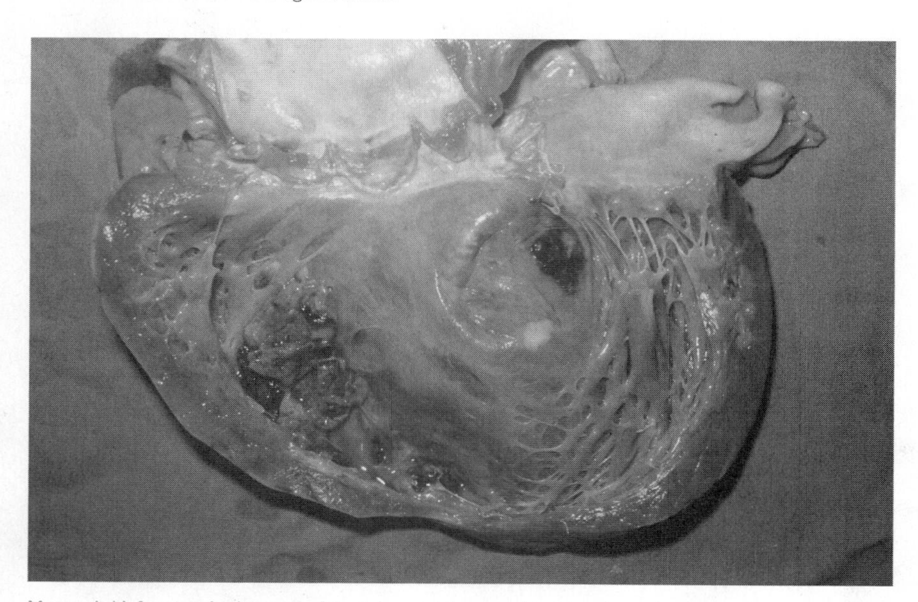

Myocardial Infarction: In this view of the left ventricle, note the extensive and transmural necrosis indicated by the dramatic wall thinning (apex or lower edge) and darkened discoloration that extends from the apex upward to the middle of the ventricle. This infarct is approximately 8–24 hours old.
Source: Biophoto Associates/Photo Researchers, Inc/Science Source

Concept Check

2. Unstable angina is the result of which pathophysiologic process?

A. Total occlusion of a coronary artery by a blood clot

B. Temporary vasoconstriction

C. Collapse of a coronary artery

D. Rupture of a coronary artery

Answer question

Concept Check

3. As a result of a myocardial infarction, a patient's heart has decreased ability to contract. Which function has been affected?

A. Papillary

B. Systolic

C. Diastolic

D. Thrombotic

Answer question

Causes and Risk Factors

- There are several fixed risk factors that increase the risk of ACS, but are difficult or impossible to modify. These include:
  - o Family history of CAD
  - o Gender: male
  - o Ethnicity: increase in African American and Caucasians
  - o Age: increase with age
- Fortunately, there are some modifiable risk factors. The nurse should address these in discharge planning:
  - o Smoking
  - o Obesity
  - o Hypertension
  - o Diabetes: type 2
  - o High cholesterol
  - o Medical noncompliance
  - o Sedentary lifestyle
  - o Stress

Assessment Findings

ST elevation myocardial infarction (STEMI) classic symptoms include:

- Chest pain: although chest pain is considered "the" classic symptom of ACS, not all patients with ACS present with chest pain.
- As many as one-third or more patients have no pain at all.
- The classic symptoms of chest pain can include a pain worse than anything the patient has ever felt.
- There may be a feeling of impending doom.
- Unbearable chest pain (like an elephant sitting on their chest) is often described by patients.

Chest pain associated with heart attack

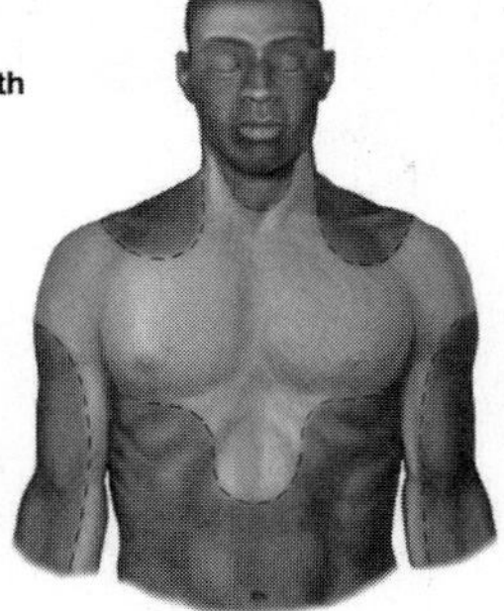

This image highlights areas that are commonly referred to when a patient is describing chest pain symptoms (angina pectoris) associated with a heart attack, or myocardial infarction.

- Patients with acute myocardial infarction who do NOT experience chest pain have a higher mortality rate, delay essential treatment, and are therefore less likely to:
  - Be diagnosed
  - Get thrombolytics
  - Receive percutaneous coronary intervention (PCI)
  - Be prescribed a drug regimen

  than are those patients with MI presenting with chest pain.
- These patients are more commonly older, more commonly women, and have a history of diabetes or heart failure.
- Pain symptoms may be located in the arm (more commonly the left), back, shoulder, neck, throat, and jaw.
- Stress symptoms may be present and include sweating, shortness of breath, nausea and vomiting, indigestion, palpitations, dread, and anxiety.
- Patients may present with very vague symptoms. Older patients may present with altered mental status.
- The clinical manifestations of an MI are similar to those of angina.

Neurologic
Altered mental status
Anxiety
Lightheadedness
Dizzy

General
Sweating
Cold, clammy
Dread; feeling of doom
Sudden death
Flu-like

Cardiac
Pain in: chest, arms, shoulder, back, neck, throat, &/or jaw
Chest pain: Crushing, heaviness, burning, fullness, pressure, tightness, squeezing, aching
Palpitations
Hypo- or hypertension
Dysrhythmias

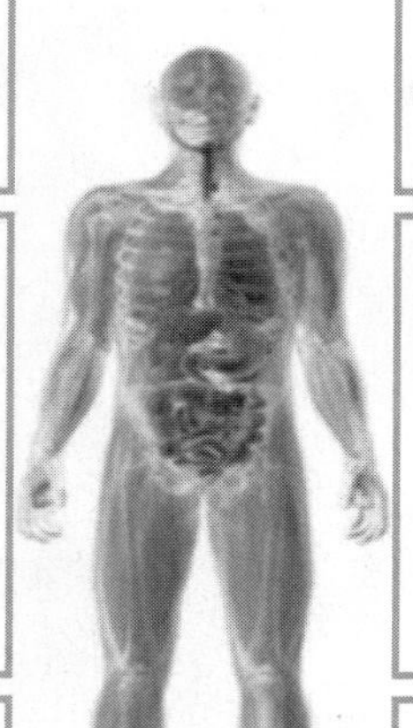

Respiratory
Shortness of Breath
↓ Oxygen saturation
Dyspnea

Gastrointestinal
Nausea, vomiting
Indigestion
Fullness

Musculoskeletal
Fatigue
Unable to perform normal activities

This picture illustrates the most common areas of pain experienced during an attack of angina or MI with reddened regions representing the painful areas. Symptoms of ACS vary. Possible areas of pain delineate where the pain or discomfort commonly radiate to beyond the chest.
Source: Copyright © 2013, NovEx Novice to Expert Learning, LLC

Assessment Findings (continued)

Unstable Angina

- Unstable angina (UA) usually presents with chest pain similar to acute myocardial infarction.
- Symptoms however do not tend to be as severe.
- UA is differentiated from stable angina in one or several of the following:
  - It is new in onset.
  - It occurs with less exertion or at rest.
  - It occurs with increased frequency.
- Patient with stable angina have symptoms of chest pain that are more stable and predictable in terms of what triggers an episode.

Differentiating Unstable Angina versus NSTEMI

Unstable Angina (UA)	VS	NSTEMI
*Angina when at rest >20 minutes. *New onset severe angina less than 2 months. *More frequent angina attacks with increasing duration and intensity.	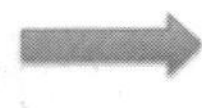	Symptoms similar to that of UA but pain presents with ***more severe and prolonged*** pain than UA.
Symptoms can include shortness of breath, tachycardia, hypo- or hypertension, decreased 02 sat., rhythm disturbances.		Symptoms can include shortness of breath, tachycardia, hypo- or hypertension, decreased 02 sat., rhythm disturbances.
EKG - ST-segment depression or T-wave inversion.		EKG - ST-segment depression or T-wave inversion.
Cardiac biomarkers are ***not*** elevated.	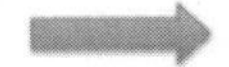	Cardiac biomarkers ***will be elevated in NSTEMI.***

Unstable angina presents with similar symptoms to acute myocardial infarction but are shorter in duration and typically less severe.

Diagnostics

- When diagnosing ACS, specifically a myocardial infarction, three common assessments are made:
  - o Patient symptoms
  - o 12-lead EKG
  - o Laboratory data
    - ■ Cardiac biomarkers (release of proteins into the blood that are measured when there is myocardial cell death).
- If any two of the three are suggestive of a myocardial infarction, immediate transport to a cardiac catheterization lab without delay is the treatment of choice.
- Patient symptoms have been discussed. Biomarkers and 12-lead EKG are the next two diagnostics for ACS.

Concept Check

4. **What assessment is most commonly used to diagnose myocardial infarction?**
   A. Blood urea nitrogen level (BUN)
   B. Patient history
   C. Patient symptoms
   D. CT scan

Answer question

Diagnostics (continued)

Troponin: A Good Cardiac Biomarker

- A biomarker is a biological marker or measure that indicates, in this case, the presence and severity of a disease state.
- Enzymes like troponin (cTnI) are located primarily in the cardiac cells and give specific information regarding cardiac damage.
- When cell death occurs, contents of the cell, including enzymes such as troponin, are released into the extracellular fluid. The enzymes may then leak into the bloodstream, allowing diagnostic measurement.
- Troponin is the most sensitive and specific marker for cardiac muscle damage and therefore considered the gold standard.
- The detection of troponin in the blood is therefore a good and reliable biomarker for cardiac injury and infarction.

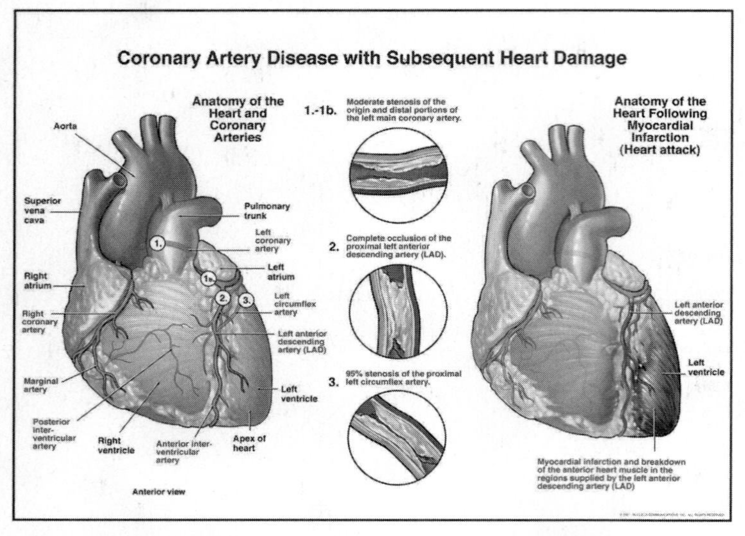

Coronary artery disease with subsequent heart attack. This is a clear depiction showing blocked coronary arteries, including the left main coronary, left anterior descending (LAD), and the left circumflex. Each artery shows evidence of severe occlusion and stenosis. Due to extensive muscle damage, the resulting myocardial infarction, or heart attack, is fatal.

Obtaining Cardiac Enzymes (Biomarkers)

- Chest pain centers are dedicated to rapid intervention and treatment of ACS, in particular STEMI/NSTEMI.
- Point-of-care testing devices have become the rapid way to aid in the diagnosis and treatment of ACS.
- Cardiac biomarkers can be obtained at the bedside and within minutes of arrival. A normal venous blood draw provides the blood sample needed for point-of-care testing.
- Results from a point-of-care device can be available in 10 minutes. However, if the patient has clear symptoms of a myocardial infarction and the EKG shows signs of an MI, transport to the catheterization lab should occur without waiting for the results of the troponin to become available.
- Troponin is the most common cardiac biomarker used in the assessment of ACS.
- Troponin is one of several types of proteins located in the heart. The troponin complex is located on the thin filament of striated and cardiac muscle and regulates the movement of calcium between actin and myosin.
- After a period of hours following cardiac damage, these enzymes appear in the blood. This leaking of troponin occurs only when there has been irreparable damage or cell death. It is therefore a good indicator of the severity of cardiac damage.

Actin Myosin Cross-Bridging

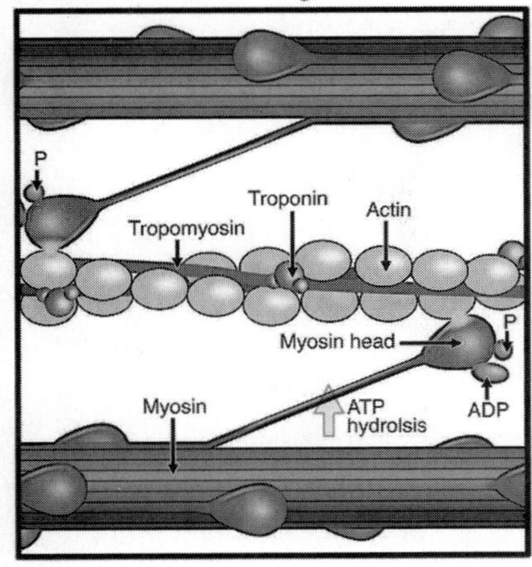

ATP = Adenosine triphosphate
ADP = Adenosine diphosphate
P = Phosphate

This image shows the cross-bridge cycle. Actin (A) bridging with myosin (M) and ATP to produce contraction. When the myocyte is damaged, the troponin (seen in the middle) is released and can be measured.

- Cardiac troponin has three components: T, C, and I. Cardiac troponin I is often referred to as cTnI. cTnI is a highly sensitive test for myocardial injury, but, like any test, the cTnI is not perfect.
- Other cardiac markers exist, for example, (creatine phosphokinase-MB CPK-MB), but are not as accurate as cTnI at identifying myocardial injury.
- Though highly accurate, an elevation in CPK is not always specific to an acute injury as in myocardial infarction.

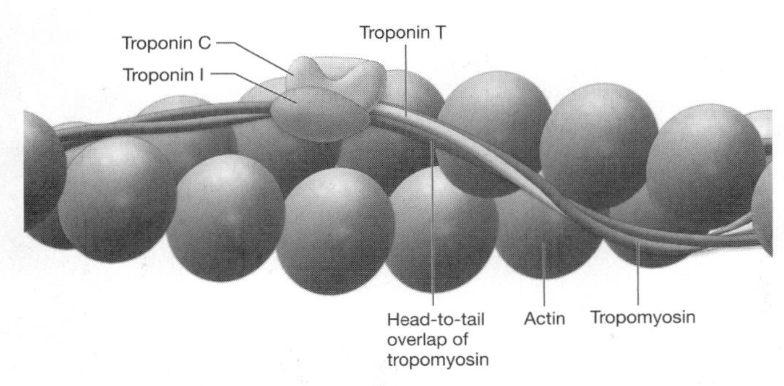

This model shows how troponin I, T, and C interrelate with actin and myosin.

- Most healthy individuals have undetectable cTnI (Troponin) of less than 0.01 ng/mL with 99th percentile value of 0.4 ng/mL.
- Therefore, any level above 0.4 ng/mL is considered to be an elevation and indicative of myocardial injury. Grossly elevated cTnI values, such as more than 2 ng/mL, are associated with myocardial infarction.
- Pattern of cTnI release is biphasic:
  1. Detectable in the blood in 2–4 hr.
  2. Peaks in 12–38 hr.
  3. Remains elevated for 5–10 days but should be steadily declining.

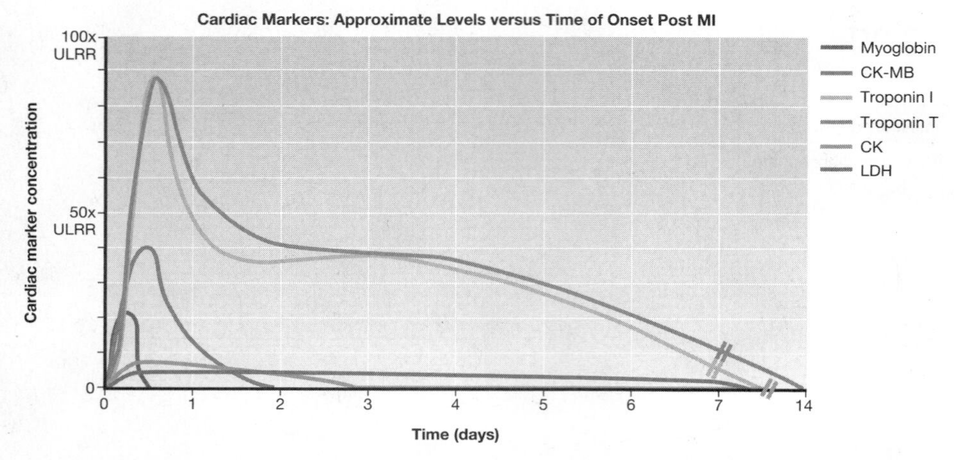

This graph depicts the relative concentrations and duration of the cardiac biomarkers upon cardiac muscle damage. Note that the troponin peaks higher and lasts longer than the CPK-MB or other biomarkers.

- Indications for the evaluation of cTnI include any symptoms that are suspicious of ACS. Elevated cTnI alone, with the absence of other signs of ACS, is not enough to make the diagnosis of myocardial infarction.
- Measurement of cTnI, when evaluating chest pain and other ACS symptoms, is often a serial measurement. cTnI may not appear in the blood for 2–4 hr following the onset of symptoms of a myocardial infarction (MI).
- For that reason, one single negative result is insufficient to rule out an MI. Serial sampling is recommended. Commonly, if symptoms are suspicious of ACS, the test is repeated in 90 min, then in 6 hr, and finally at the 12-hr mark from the original test.

Diagnostics (continued)

Limitations of Biomarkers

- The most frequent reasons that enzymes are elevated, other than from acute myocardial infarction, are:
  - o Blunt chest trauma
  - o Myocarditis
  - o Congestive heart failure
  - o Left ventricular hypertrophy
- In some cases, other enzyme tests, such as CPK-MB, may be helpful in determining the acuity of myocardial damage.
- CPK-MB typically increases in 2–4 hr and decreases in 24–48 hr, returning to normal much faster than cTnI.

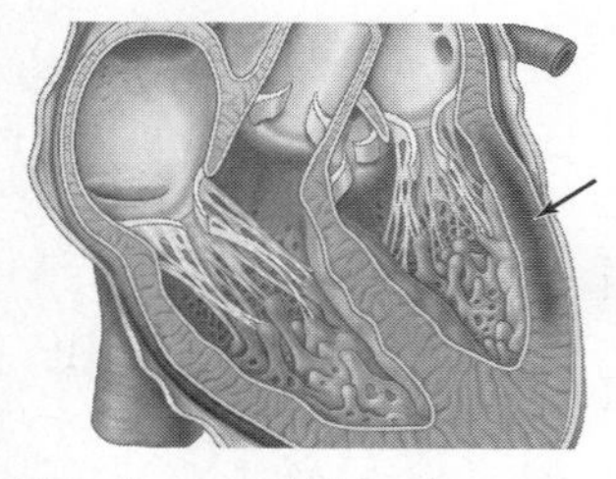

(a) Acute myocardial infarction

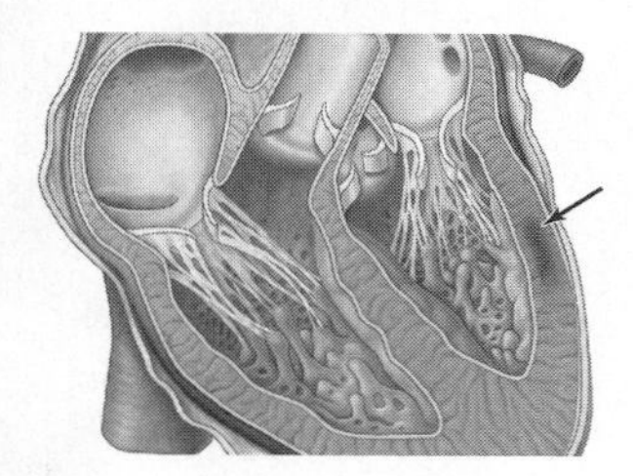

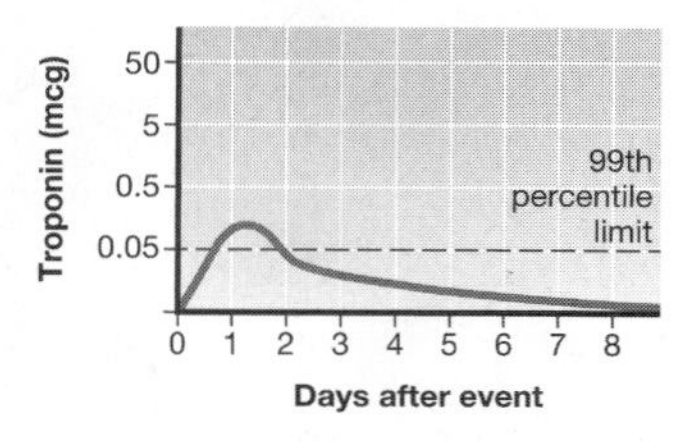

(b) Minor myocardial injury

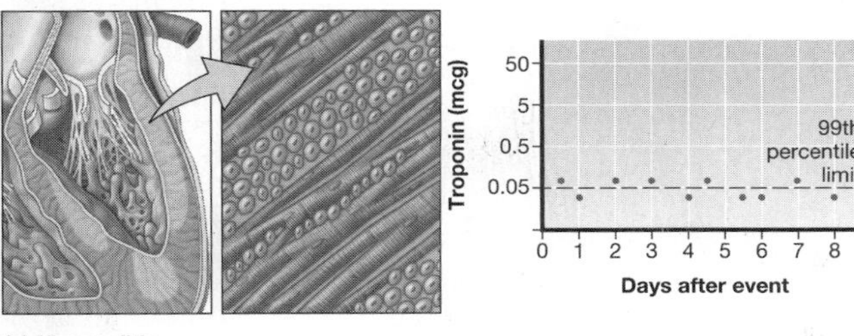

(c) Myocarditis

The pattern of troponin release is depicted for (a) acute myocardial infarction, (b) minor myocardial injury, and (c) myocarditis. In acute myocardial infarction, troponin increases significantly within hours of symptom onset and then gradually decreases over several days. Minor myocardial injury leads to troponin concentrations only slightly above the decision limit (dotted line) for a shorter period. In myocarditis, troponin concentrations remain at or slightly above the decision limit for days to weeks. Pattern differences can assist in recognizing or ruling out certain diagnoses.

Diagnostics (continued)

Electrocardiogram and Acute Coronary Syndrome

Cardiac ischemia produces changes that can be recognized on EKG (see Electrocardiogram NovE-lesson for more information). STEMI produces characteristic ST segment elevation, but other changes, such as ST depression and T wave changes, can be seen in unstable angina and non-ST elevation MI.

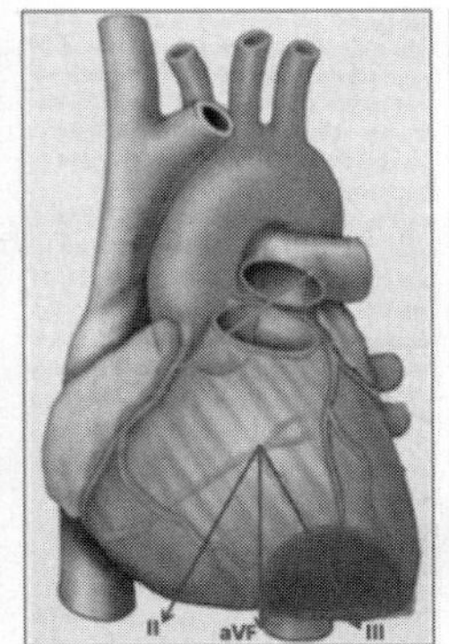

Inferior MI shows EKG changes in leads II, III, and aVF.

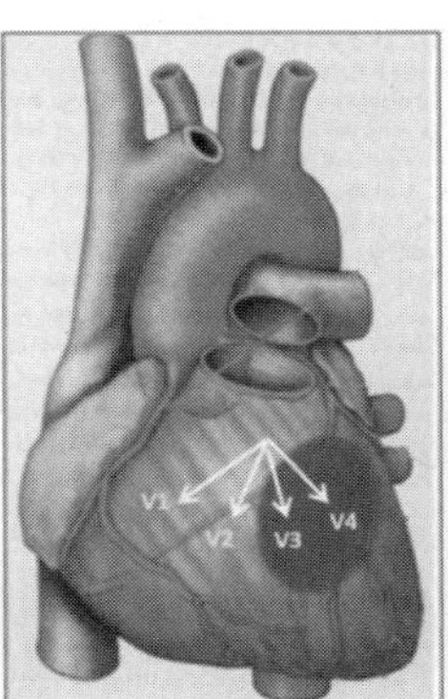

Anterior MI produces EKG changes in leads V1-V4.

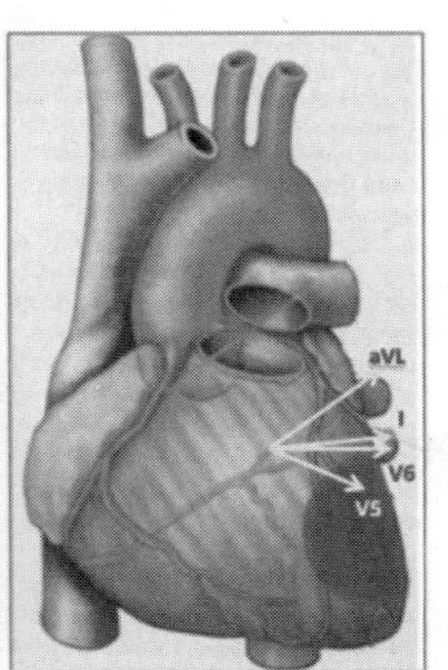

Lateral MI shows EKG changes in leads I, aVL, and V5-V6.

This image shows three different types of STEMIs and the leads that typically reflect EKG changes.

Source: Adapted from Osborn, Medical Surgical Nursing, p. 1054, fig 37-4.

Electrocardiogram and ST-Elevation Myocardial Infarction (STEMI)

- When identifying a myocardial infarction, the 12-lead EKG can be used.
- ST elevation, indicating myocardial injury, is the most common EKG finding used in identifying myocardial infarctions.
- If two contiguous leads show ST elevation, a myocardial infarction should be suspected, for example, ST elevation in V1 and V2, or Lead II and III.
- STEMI signifies complete blockage of the coronary artery and myocardial death.
- Q wave formation (negative inflection prior to the R wave) is an indication of myocardial death.
    - o Q wave formation does not occur for about 24 hr.
    - o An early MI does not have Q wave formation, but does have ST elevation.

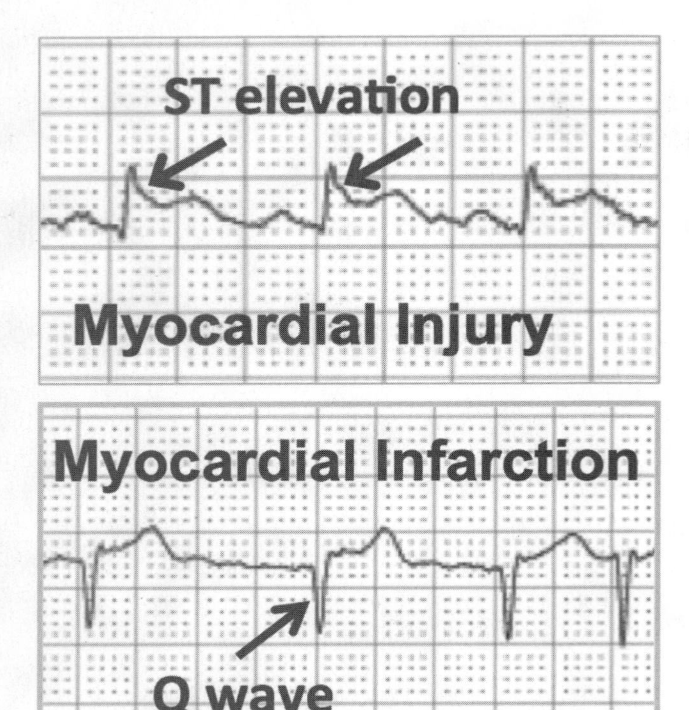

Upper: ST segment elevation indicates acute myocardial injury, resulting in STEMI or ST Elevation MI. Lower: Deep Q waves with ST elevation are seen in both V2 & V3 leads indicating an anterior infarction.
Source: *(both)* Courtesy of K. Kyriakidis

- Understanding the EKG leads that reflect specific areas of the heart enables the health care provider to determine the location of a myocardial infarction or injury.
- Specific MIs are associated with particular complications. By recognizing the location of the infarction, the health care provider can anticipate and be prepared for early warning signs of those complications.
- The table below shows the specific EKG leads associated with particular types of MIs and the associated coronary artery.
- Depending on the extent of damage, there may be more or fewer leads involved.

Localizing the MI:

Location of Infarction	ST-Elevations	Reciprocal ST-Depressions	Affected Coronary Artery
Inferior or inferolateral MI*	II, III, AVF	I, aVL	RCA (90%), left circumflex (10%)*
Extensive anterior MI	V1–V6, I, aVL	None	LAD (proximal)
Septal MI	V1–V2	None	LAD
Apical anterior MI*	V1–V2 to V3–V6	None	LAD (mid)
Mid-anterior MI*	aVL, I, V2–V3	--	LAD
Lateral MI*	I, aVL, V6,	II, III, aVF, RS in V1–V2	Left circumflex
Right ventricular MI	V1, V3R–V6R	I, aVL	Right coronary
Posterior MI	V7–V9	V1–V3	RCA or LCX
* Changes from traditional understandings			

Based on autopsy or cardiovascular MRI comparisons to EKG findings, this is a summary of the classification system that correlates Q waves and/or ST-T abnormalities with myocardial ischemic and infarct locations. LAD = left anterior descending

The table shows the EKG leads associated with each type of myocardial infarction and the associated coronary artery involved. Understanding which EKG leads reflect certain areas of the heart enables the clinician to determine where a myocardial infarction is located.
Source: Copyright © 2013, NovEx Novice to Expert Learning, LLC

Ex. 1: what type of ACS problem is this patient experiencing and in what location(s)?

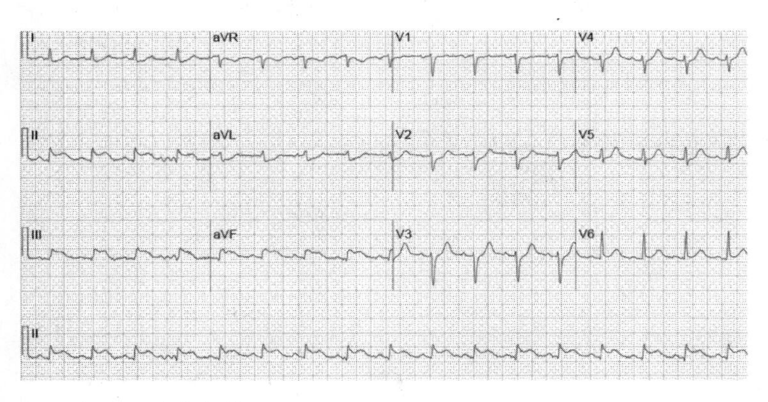

Source: Courtesy of K. Kyriakidis

Answer: ST segment elevation in leads II, III, and aVF indicate acute inferior wall MI.

Ex. 2: Identify the ACS problem in this patient and name the location(s) involved.

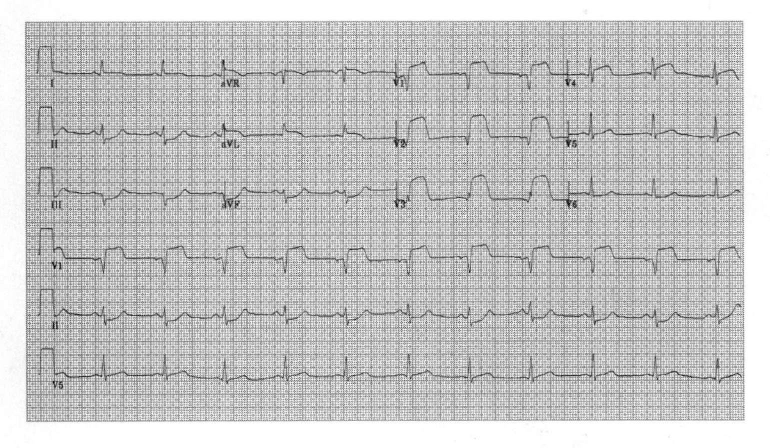

Answer: ST segment elevation in leads I, aVL, and V1–V4, with reciprocal ST changes in II, III, and aVF, are consistent with indicate an acute anterior and septal wall MI. Urgent reperfusion is needed!

Ex. 3: What problem is this patient experiencing and what does it mean for the patient?

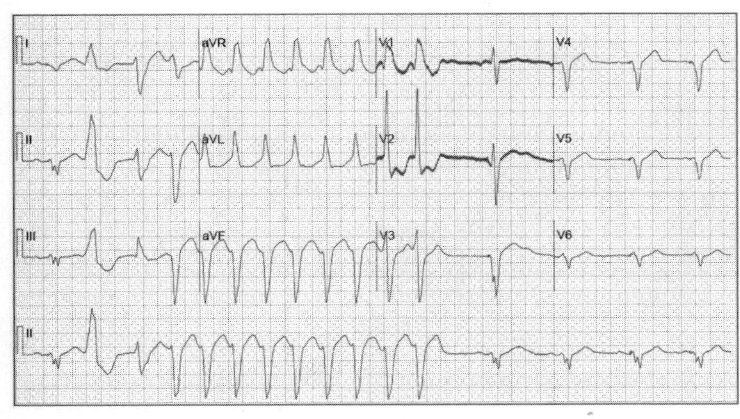

Source: Courtesy of K. Kyriakidis

Answer: The ventricular paced rhythm is interrupted by a rapid, wide complex, regular rhythm. The patient's BP falls and he feels faint. The run of ventricular tachycardia forewarns of further, potentially life-threatening dysrhythmias.

Diagnostics (continued)

Conduction Defects in ACS

- Development of conduction defects like a left bundle branch block (LBBB) is serious since the defects indicate a loss of electrical conduction fibers and the crucial surrounding myocardium.
- The development of LBBB is particularly worrisome since the left bundle is large and difficult to block without substantial loss of myocardium.
- The LBBB is characterized by a wide QRS complex (greater than 0.12 sec) and a QS wave in V1.
- Abnormal depolarization of the heart due to the conduction defect leads to less coordinated and less effective ventricular contraction.

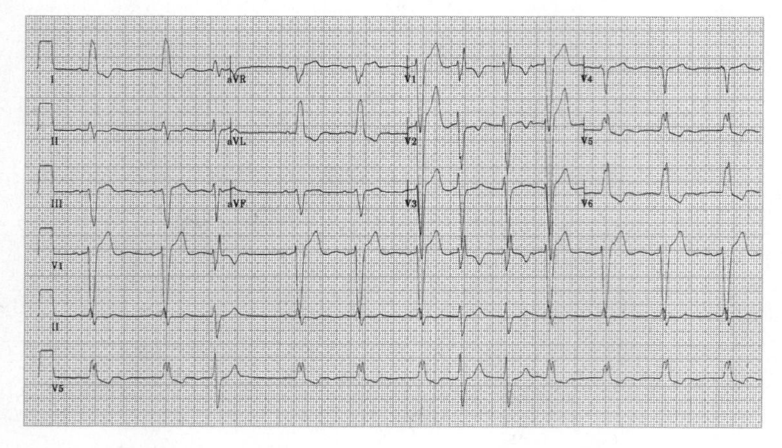

This EKG shows the classic findings of a patient with LBBB: (1) QRS > 0.12 sec with mid-slurring. (2) Frontal plane QRS vector variable. (3) V1 rS with upright T wave. (4) V5 and V6 predominantly upright with inverted T. (5). Lead I predominantly upright with inverted T.

Non-ST Elevation Myocardial Infarction (NSTEMI)

- NSTEMI occurs when there is sufficient coronary artery obstruction to cause myocardial damage and with subsequent elevation of cardiac enzymes but not enough to produce ST elevation.
- EKG often shows ischemic changes such as ST-segment depression or T-wave inversion.

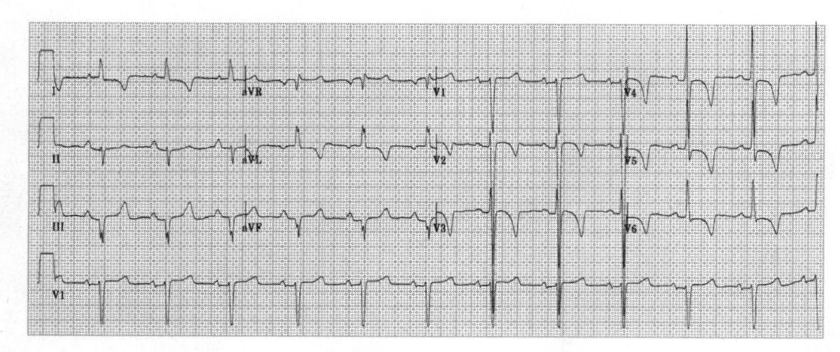

EKG showing NSTEMI key findings: Marked ST segment depression and T-wave inversion in the lateral precordial leads (V5, V6), consistent with subendocardial injury.

Priority Patient Concerns and Desired Collaborative Care Outcomes

Prior to caring for patients with acute coronary syndrome, it is important to prioritize the patient's concerns that must guide the nursing care plan and interventions. Care for the patient is ordered and organized in accordance with the patient's priority and urgent needs. Desired collaborative care outcomes in patients with acute coronary syndrome typically include:

1. Patient will receive supportive and therapeutic interventions to minimize further deterioration of cardiac tissue perfusion, as needed.
2. Patient's cardiac output will stabilize and/or be maximized to the degree possible with treatment and in accordance with the patient's wishes.
3. Patient will experience minimal to no pulmonary edema.
4. Patient's chest pain will dissipate and/or be controlled therapeutically as indicated.
5. Patient will exhibit a calmer demeanor and rest more peacefully after discussion of treatment plan, probable outcomes, and reassurance that care providers are vigilantly watching over the patient and know how to care for them if problems arise.
6. Patient will tolerate gradual increases in daily activity level without fatigue.

Considering these important care outcomes, prepare a list of the major 3–6 priority patient concerns or nursing diagnoses for patients with acute coronary syndrome. Be prepared to participate in a discussion of this list and/or to submit them as an assignment, as determined by your faculty. Resources you may find helpful in this assignment can include this lesson, the references, resources on nursing care plans, and standard nursing diagnoses manuals.

LO3:

Collaborative Interventions

Evidence-Based Practice (EBP)

Emergency Transport and Treatment

The American Heart Association (AHA) recommends that evidence–based practices (EBP) be used in the care of patients with acute coronary syndrome. The recommendations are numerous and detailed. Because almost every nurse will care for these patients, given the extensive prevalence of ACS, those details are specified in the remainder of this lesson. An overview of ACS is provided in a schematic.

- Emergency medical services (EMS) are aware of the AHA guidelines. They are instructed (1) to transport patients to the nearest appropriate facility and (2) to initiate prehospital treatment in patients with signs of STEMI/ACS.
- Progressive critical care transport, like Fletcher Allen's fleet in Vermont, for possible STEMI patients can include:
  - o Assessing patients using 12-lead EKG in the ambulance to activate treatment early
  - o Making a diagnosis with the Emergency physician before ever arriving at the hospital
  - o Determining whether to transport the nearest Emergency Department or instead to the primary angioplasty center to access the most appropriate treatment
- According to the current American College of Cardiology (ACC)/AHA guidelines, the strongest recommendation for patients with a STEMI is to get prompt Percutaneous Coronary Intervention (PCI) **in less than 90 min of symptom onset**. Obtaining diagnostic tests beyond the EKG should NOT delay transport to cardiac catheterization:
  - o Once at the emergency department, "**Door-to-PCI" time should be less than 30 min** in order to restore myocardial perfusion and limit myocardial loss. Percutaneous coronary intervention is the highest priority.

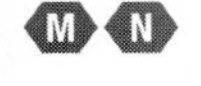

  - o Administration of medications, although important, should NOT delay transport to cardiac catheterization.

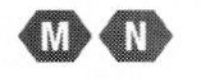

- If cardiac catheterization cannot be accomplished within 90 min, a thrombolytic agent should be administered.
  - o "Door-to-drug" time should be less than **30 min**.

Concept Check

5. Which EKG finding is most commonly used to identify myocardial ischemia?

A. Q wave formation

B. Flattening of the R-wave

C. ST elevation

D. Peaking of the T-wave

Answer question

Collaborative Interventions (continued)

Cardiac Catheterization and PCI

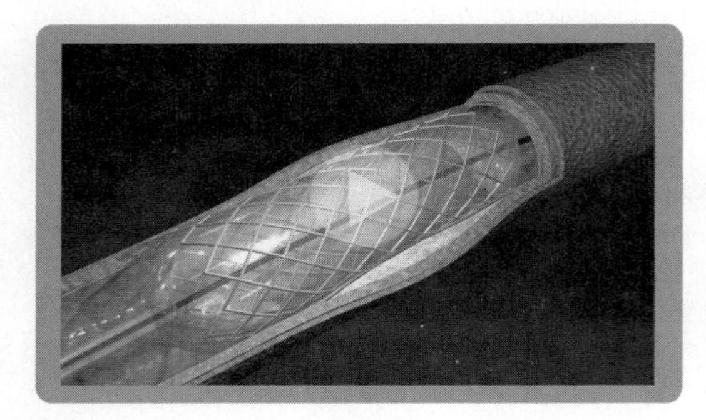

This animation depicts a coronary angiography or catheterization procedure. It begins by showing the buildup of plaque in an artery wall of the heart, blocking the flow of blood. Afterward, contrast dye is injected into the coronary arteries, illuminating the location of the blockage. A guide wire with balloon is then inserted and positioned at the diseased section. The balloon inflates to widen the lumen, the metal stent is then placed, and the lumen of the artery is opened.

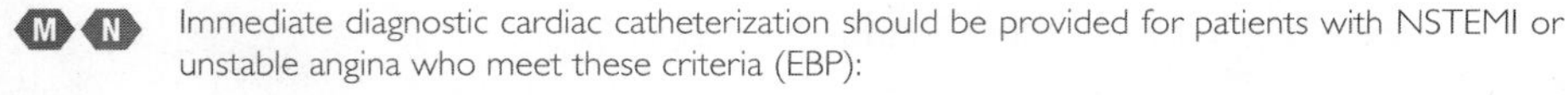

Immediate diagnostic cardiac catheterization should be provided for patients with NSTEMI or unstable angina who meet these criteria (EBP):

- Cardiogenic shock
- Heart failure
- Sustained ventricular tachycardia
- Recurrent angina at rest despite treatment

The remaining patients may undergo cardiac catheterization under less emergent circumstances.

Post-PCI Care

Following PCI, which may be the first time one meets the ACS patient, immediate patient care includes the following:

- The femoral artery sheath, used during cardiac cath, commonly remains in place for 1–2 hr postprocedure for emergency access. Coagulation studies are performed prior to sheath removal to ensure the patient is not at excessive risk of bleeding.
- Observe puncture site frequently for bleeding or hematoma: Assess neurovascular status distal to puncture site in the limb by checking pulses and sensation distal to the sheath (e.g., popliteal, pedal, dorsalis, tibial).
- Obtain vital signs every 15 min for the first hour, every 30 min for an hour, and preferably every hour for 2 hr, followed per facility protocol or if symptoms arise. Vitals also include O_2 sats.

- Removal of sheath is usually done by specially trained nursing staff. Pressure is applied for 20 min (minimum) or more after removal of sheath to prevent bleeding.
- Obtain an EKG upon return from procedure and repeat for any onset of chest pain. Monitor for any signs of reperfusion dysrhythmias such as bradycardias or ventricular irritability.
- Monitor for any signs of chest pain, back pain, or leg pain.
- Bed rest (supine) for 2–6 hr to prevent site clot from dislodging or hematoma formation. Progress to sitting position when site is stabilized per medical protocol. Pain relief to promote rest period.
- Ensure that sterile dressing is intact over puncture site.
- Pressure over the site if the patient has bleeding. May need to notify physician, depending on extent of bleeding.
- Adequate hydration and urinary output monitored to clear radiographic IV dye used in procedure.
- Oral antiplatelet medications may be given prior to procedure. The patient is discharged on this medication and continues it for up to 12 months if stenting is used. Most patients remain on aspirin therapy for life.
- Pain control as needed for post-PCI discomfort.

Concept Check

6. Which pulse should the nurse monitor in a patient after standard percutaneous coronary intervention?

A. Tibial

B. Radial

C. Carotid

D. Brachial

Answer question

Evidence-Based Thrombolytics

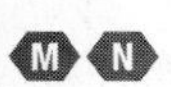

If PCI is not available, thrombolytics are the next most important intervention. Thrombolytics are:

- A group of medications that dissolve blood clots (thrombolysis) by converting plasminogen to plasmin, which is generally responsible for clot breakdown
- Recommended for STEMI within 12 hours of symptom onset but is most effective within the first 2 hr.
- Given when arriving at an emergency department (ED). The door-to-drug time should be less than 30 min per AHA guidelines if PCI is not available. Door refers to entry at the ED. *Drug* refers to administration of the thrombolytic
- Used primarily if PCI is not available or is delayed
- Are NOT recommended for unstable angina or for NSTEMI.

Thrombolytics are tissue plasminogen activators (tPA) and include:

- Alteplase (tPA): First recombinant tissue-type plasminogen activator
- Reteplase (rPA): Second generation thrombolytic with a more rapid onset and lower bleeding risk
- Tenecteplase: Similar to alteplase and approved in 2000
- Urokinase: most often used for thrombolysis of peripheral intravascular thrombus or for occluded catheters. It cannot be administered repeatedly without antigenic problems.
- Streptokinase: inexpensive but has a high incidence of side effects (febrile or allergic reactions) as it is produced from streptococcal bacteria. The antigenic problems prevent its use more than once in a 6-month period.
- Anistreplase: a streptokinase activator complex with side effects similar to streptokinase.

Collaborative Interventions (continued)

Overview: Care of ACS Patients

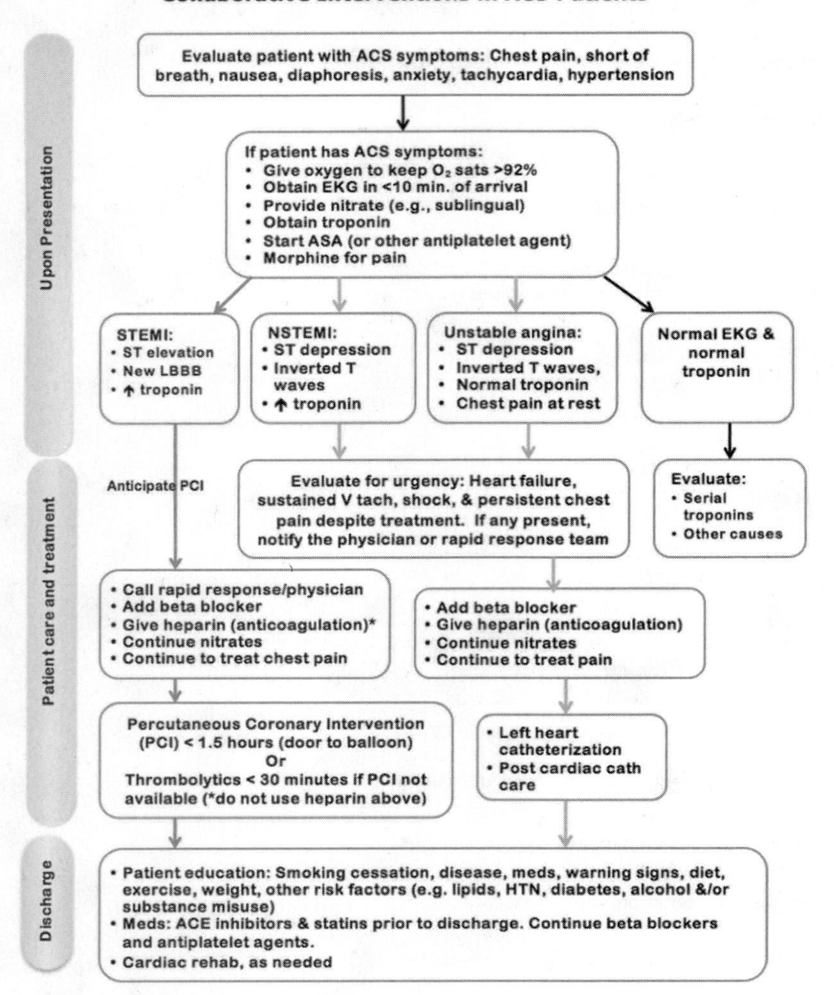

Collaborative Interventions in ACS Patients
Upon Presentation
Patient care and treatment
Discharge
Evaluate patient with ACS symptoms: Chest pain, short of breath, nausea, diaphoresis, anxiety, tachycardia, hypertension
If patient has ACS symptoms:
• Give oxygen to keep O_2 sats >92%
• Obtain EKG in <10 min. of arrival
• Provide nitrate (e.g., sublingual)
• Obtain troponin
• Start ASA (or other antiplatelet agent)
• Morphine for pain
STEMI:
• ST elevation
• New LBBB
• ↑ troponin
NSTEMI:
• ST depression
• Inverted T waves
• ↑ troponin
Unstable angina:
• ST depression
• Inverted T waves,
• Normal troponin
• Chest pain at rest
Normal EKG & normal troponin
Anticipate PCI
Evaluate for urgency: Heart failure, sustained V tach, shock, & persistent chest pain despite treatment. If any present, notify the physician or rapid response team
Evaluate:
• Serial troponins
• Other causes
• Call rapid response/physician
• Add beta blocker
• Give heparin (anticoagulation)*
• Continue nitrates
• Continue to treat chest pain
• Add beta blocker
• Give heparin (anticoagulation)
• Continue nitrates
• Continue to treat pain
Percutaneous Coronary Intervention (PCI) < 1.5 hours (door to balloon) Or Thrombolytics < 30 minutes if PCI not available (*do not use heparin above)
• Left heart catheterization
• Post cardiac cath care
• Patient education: Smoking cessation, disease, meds, warning signs, diet, exercise, weight, other risk factors (e.g. lipids, HTN, diabetes, alcohol &/or substance misuse)
• Meds: ACE inhibitors & statins prior to discharge. Continue beta blockers and antiplatelet agents.
• Cardiac rehab, as needed

This schematic provides an overview of the care of patients with acute ACS. Included are the evidence-based practices as well as essential supportive, comfort, and non-EBP interventions needed to provide excellent care. The interventions are organized and ordered by urgency and priorities. The overview is not all-inclusive but points out the most essential interventions in all patients. All early and essential care can be provided pre-hospitalization. Depending on the circumstances, some interventions are initiated earlier when possible.

M N

- The overview schematic is intended to provide a general understanding about all the important interventions that are needed in the care of an ACS patient.
- However, patients may call 911, present in the emergency department, or health care provider's office, with different entry points along the schematic. A schematic cannot account for every entry point, but can provide an overview of the care that most ACS patients need.

M N

- The most urgent priorities when the patient first presents are:
  1. To gather info about the patient's symptoms, get an EKG, and obtain lab information.
  2. If any two of these three are suggestive of myocardial infarction, immediate transport for PCI is warranted.
  3. If PCI is unavailable or delayed, thrombolytics should be administered within 30 min.
- Following the most urgent priorities, the overview schematics can help guide subsequent care of the patient with STEMI, NSTEMI, or unstable angina.

Initial Priorities in ACS

M N markers: N

Oxygen, per protocol:

- Immediately administer 2–4 LPM via nasal cannula to maintain O_2 sat greater than 92%. (If the patient has first had PCI, the patient may already be on oxygen.)
- If the O_2 sat is less than or equal to 92%, continue to increase the oxygen.
- While oxygen administration has not been studied, it is a universally expected standard of practice.
- While oxygen therapy does not have a major impact on coronary perfusion, it might slightly improve oxygen delivery to the heart.

M N

Nitrates (e.g., nitroglycerin):

- Part of the initial therapy in ACS management
- The goal is to reduce preload through vasodilation plus improve myocardial blood flow.

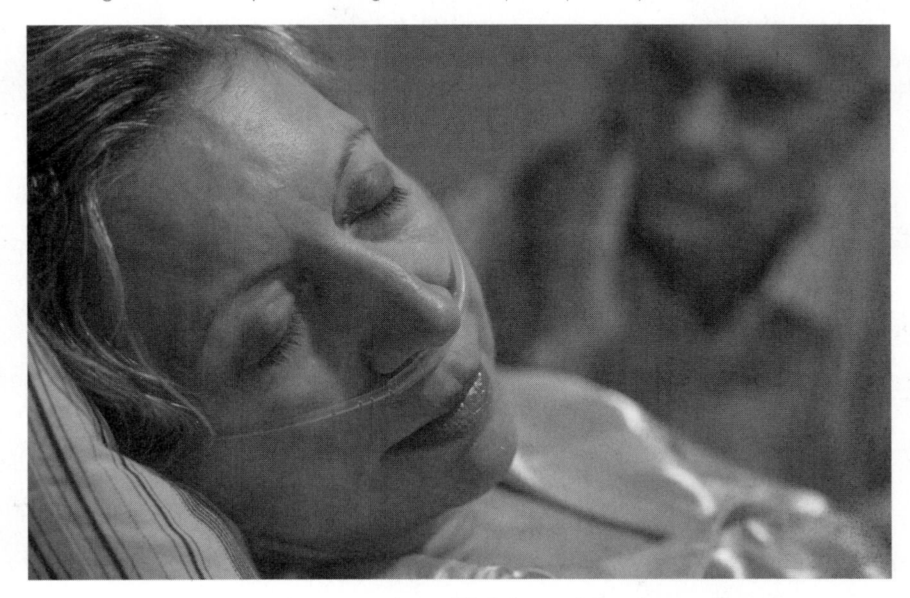

This photo shows a patient needing oxygen after an MI. Oxygen is delivered via nasal cannula.
Source: CandyBox Images/Fotolia

Collaborative Interventions (continued)

Evidence-Based Medications: Nitrates

Nitroglycerin is commonly used for ACS to control pain and lower blood pressure. Nitrates dilate coronary arteries, improving collateral blood flow to the myocardium and lower blood pressure due to vasodilation effect. It can also be given by oral spray or transdermal.

- It is often given prior to arrival by EMS and continued in the department emergency for symptomatic relief of chest pain.
- It is usually given sublingual every 5 min, up to three doses.
- Nitroglycerin in a paste may be added to provide sustained relief of pain.
- If pain is not relieved, an IV infusion may be initiated and titrated for pain. IV use may cause hypotension, particularly if the patient is dehydrated, and often causes headache.

Evidence-Based Medication Priorities

M N

- Antiplatelet administration is a key initial treatment for ACS.
  - o Aspirin should be given immediately upon suspicion of STEMI.
  - o Clopidogrel (Plavix) should be given when possible, often after cardiac catheterization.
  - o IIb/IIIa inhibitor (e.g., abciximab [ReoPro])
  - o The goal of antiplatelets is to prevent further clot formation.

M N

- Anticoagulant should be administered as soon as possible.
  - o Dose-based heparin
  - o The goal of anticoagulants is to prevent further clot formation.

M N

- Beta blockers are started prior to cardiac catheterization if possible (if the patient is not hypotensive or bradycardic).
  - o May be started IV initially, but converted to oral as soon as possible, for example, metoprolol (Lopressor, Toprol-XL)

- o The goal of the beta blocker is to reduce myocardial oxygen consumption.

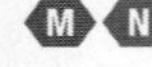

- ACE inhibitors are important in patients with elevated blood pressure.
  - o Examples of ACE inhibitors: captopril (Capoten)
  - o The goal is to reduce myocardial work by reducing systemic vascular resistance via blood pressure reduction.

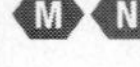

- Pain relief with vasodilation or opioids are essential for is patient comfort.
  - o Nitrates and narcotics (e.g., morphine) are drugs of choice.
  - o The goal is to improve the patient's comfort and improve myocardial blood flow through vasodilation.

- HMG-CoA reductase inhibitors (statins) are used post cardiac catheterization. AHA/ACC recommend that all patients with ACS receive high-dose statin therapy prior to discharge, regardless of their baseline low-density lipoprotein (LDL) level:
  - o Prior to discharge, initiation of statins is part of home management (e.g., lovastatin [Mevacor]).
  - o The goal is to reduce future incidents of ACS by reducing the formation of cholesterol and other lipids, thereby decreasing inflammation in the plaques and stabilizing them.

Concept Check

7. The nurse would evaluate for relief of chest pain after which drug is administered?

A. Aspirin

B. Nitroglycerin

C. Lovastatin

D. Clopidogrel

Answer question

Collaborative Interventions (continued)

Evidence-Based Medications: Antiplatelets

- Antiplatelet drugs are one of the first agents given in ACS. Antiplatelet agents prevent the formation of blood clots by interfering with the clumping or aggregation of platelets.
- There are three types of antiplatelet agents:
  - o Aspirin blocks the production of thromboxane A_2 that causes platelets to clump; 162–325 mg is given ASAP when symptoms present. It is often given prior to arrival by EMS or is given on arrival in the emergency department.
  - o Thienopyridines block adenosine diphosphate receptors on the surface of the platelets preventing aggregation or clumping. This can be given prior to PCI and continued for 1–9 months or longer if stenting is done.
    - a. Clopidogrel (Plavix): loading dose of 300 mg orally; maintenance dose of 75 mg daily.
    - b. Ticlopidine: loading dose of 500 mg orally; maintenance dose of 250 mg twice daily.
  - o Glycoprotein IIb/IIIa inhibitors are given intravenously. They can be used as an adjunct to PCI with or without stent placement. They inhibit the receptor on the surface of platelets (glycoprotein IIb/IIIa) to prevent clumping of platelets. The drugs in this category are the most potent antiplatelet drugs:
    - a. Abciximab: Loading dose of 0.25 mg/kg IV bolus. Maintenance of 0.125 mcg/kg/min (max 10 mcg/min).
    - b. Eptifibatide: IV bolus of 180 mcg/kg. Maintenance dose of 2.0 mcg/kg/min for with normal creatinine clearance.
    - c. Tirofiban: Loading dose of 0.4 mcg/kg/min over 30 min. Maintenance dose of 0.1 mcg/kg/min for normal creatinine clearance.

Evidence-Based Medications: Anticoagulants

- Anticoagulants are started prior to PCI to prevent further clots from forming.
- Heparin (unfractionated) is used to prevent the formation of clots or extension of existing clots by binding to enzyme inhibitor, antithrombin III, which inactivates several clotting factors.
- It does not cause thrombolysis.
  - o Loading dose of 60 mg/kg (max 4,000 units) as IV bolus.
  - o Maintenance of 12 units/kg/hr (max to 1,000 units/hr).

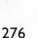

The Effect of Heparin on the Blood Vessels

Initial Condition

Large amounts of clotting agents move through the bloodstream. Blood begins to leak through a small defect in the vessel wall.

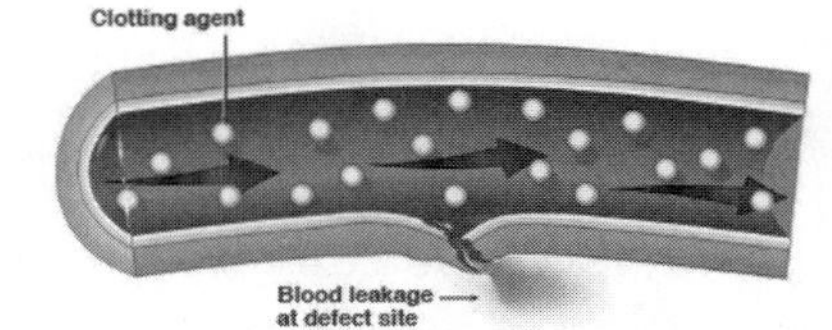

Effective Clotting

Clotting agents collect at the defect site, effectively stopping the leakage of blood.

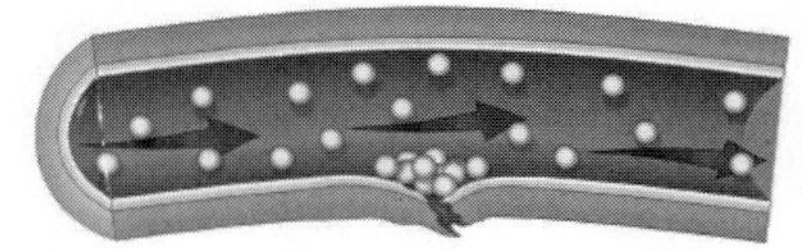

Thrombus Formation

When too many clotting agents accumulate, a thrombus forms, partially blocking blood flow.

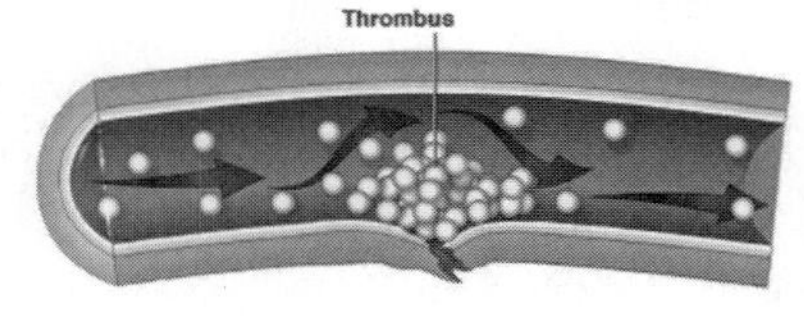

Low Dose Heparin

Low doses of heparin clear the thrombus yet leave enough of the clotting agents for the effective closure of the vessel wall defect.

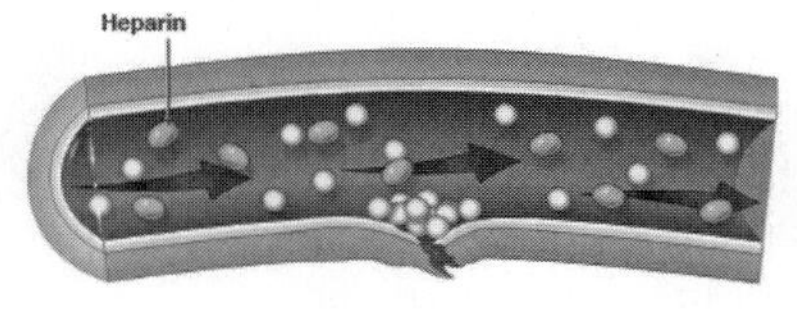

High Dose Heparin

High doses of heparin completely eliminate clotting agents. This leads to uncontrolled hemorrhage through the vessel wall defect.

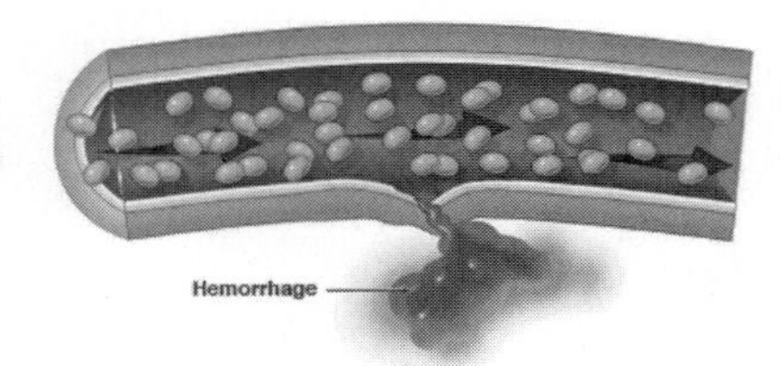

This series describes the effect of heparin on the blood vessels. It includes three illustrations describing the normal anatomy and physiology involved in the clotting. Two additional illustrations compare the effects of a low and a high dose of heparin on the blood vessels.

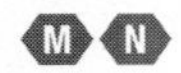

- Enoxaparin is a low molecular weight heparin with similar action to that of unfractionated heparin and can be used as an alternative to unfractionated heparin for STEMI.
  - o The loading dose is 30 mg IV bolus.
  - o Maintenance dose is 1 mg/kg subcutaneous every 12 hr.

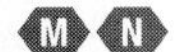

- Bilvalirudin provides anticoagulation by thrombin inhibition.
  - o The loading dose by IV bolus is 0.1 mg/kg.
  - o The maintenance dose is 0.25 mg/kg/hr by infusion.

Collaborative Interventions (continued)

Patient Education: Anticoagulant and Antithrombotic Drugs

Patient education is necessary following initiation of anticoagulant/antithrombotic therapy of any type and should include:

- Patients need to understand that antithrombotic therapy can make it easier to bleed, even from a minor injury.
- Patients should also be cautioned to observe for signs of unusual bleeding while using these medications.
- Patients should be taught to seek emergency medical attention if they have bleeding that will not stop, bloody stool, or coffee ground emesis.
- Alcohol moderation is important as alcohol may increase the risk of gastrointestinal bleeding with medications such as clopidogrel.
- If any surgery is planned for the patient, including dental surgery, the patient should notify the caregiver about anticoagulant use.
- Patients who have a certain type of stent (drug eluting) should not stop their antiplatelet agent for at least one year.
- Patients should be cautioned that other agents can increase bleeding, such as aspirin or NSAIDs (nonsteroidal anti-inflammatory drugs). Over-the-counter medications should be used only after consulting with one's caregiver.

Priorities Evidence-Based Medications: Beta Blockers

- Beta blockers block stimulation of beta 1 and 2 adrenergic receptors that results in lowered blood pressure and heart rate as well as provides vasodilation.
- Beta blockers have been shown to reduce infarct size and to reduce short-term and long-term mortality.

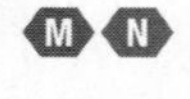

- They can be given PO or IV in ACS prior to PCI if the patient is not hypotensive and their heart rate is greater than 60 beats/min.

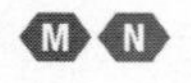

- The beta blockers are:
  - o Metoprolol: PO or IV
  - o Labetalol: PO or IV
  - o Carvedilol: PO
  - o Propranolol: PO or IV
  - o Timolol: PO
  - o Sotalol: PO

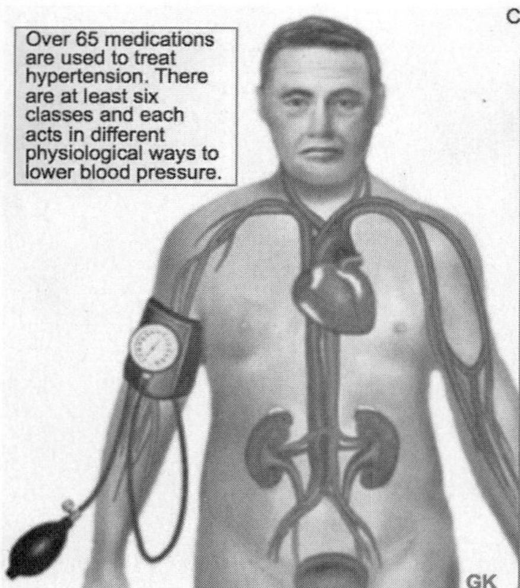

Over 65 medications are used to treat hypertension. There are at least six classes and each acts in different physiological ways to lower blood pressure.
GK
Commonly used antihypertensive drugs and how they work
ACE Inhibitors:
Cause vasodilatation by interfering with angiotensin II production. Lowering angiotensin II reduces vasoconstriction.
Angiotensin II Receptor Blockers:
Block the action of angiotensin II, thereby relaxing the vessels.
Diuretics:
Renal excretion of sodium and water lower blood volume and pressure.
Calcium Channel Blockers: Cause vascular relaxation.
Adrenergic Inhibitors:
Includes alpha & beta blockers. Alpha blockers dilate blood vessels while beta blockers lower heart rate and contractility.
Vasodilators:
Cause arterial and venous dilation.

This image depicts the treatments for high blood pressure (hypertension), listing the six most common antihypertensives. These include adrenergic inhibitors (alpha blockers and beta blockers), calcium blockers, ACE inhibitors, angiotensin II receptor blockers, vasodilators, and diuretics.

Source: Courtesy of George Kyriakidis/Santa Ana, CA

Evidence-Based Medications: ACE Inhibitors and ARBs

- Angiotensin Converting Enzyme (ACE) inhibitors block the conversion of angiotensin I to the potent vasoconstrictor angiotensin II.
- Similarly, angiotensin receptor blockers (ARBs) block angiotensin II receptors, preventing their vasconstrictive action.
- Both types of medications dilate both arteries and veins to reduce preload, afterload, and blood pressure.
- Both medication types reduce ventricular remodeling that contributes to left ventricular dysfunction and heart failure. Research has also shown a decreased risk of death in ACS patients, particularly in patients with low EF or heart failure.
- ACE inhibitors are typically preferred over ARBs because there is more supporting evidence of the efficacy.
- M ARBs are recommended when ACE inhibitors are poorly tolerated.
- M N An ACE inhibitor is usually started or continued within 24 hr (early is better) of admission and is continued at discharge unless contraindicated.
- M N The ACE inhibitors are all given orally: lisinopril, captopril, enalapril, quinapril, and ramipril. Hypotension is possible, so BP should be monitored.
- ARBs include candesartan and valsartan that are preferred based on clinical trial evidence; other ARBs are eprosartan, irbesartan, losartan, olmesartan, and telmisartan.

Collaborative Interventions (continued)

Comfort Medications: Pain Management

- M N Pain control with analgesics may be necessary if nitrates, oxygen, and other urgent interventions do not relieve pain.
- N Pain relief is a priority and should not be delayed.
- Morphine is the most common opiate used for pain relief. It is an essential therapy for those patients with severe chest pain as it is typically effective and rapid acting.
- N Clinicians must monitor the potential side effects of morphine that causes CNS and respiratory depression. Further, morphine can cause hypotension. The patient must be monitored closely when morphine is given together with beta blockers, ACE inhibitors, and/or nitrates, which can all act synergistically to cause hypotension.

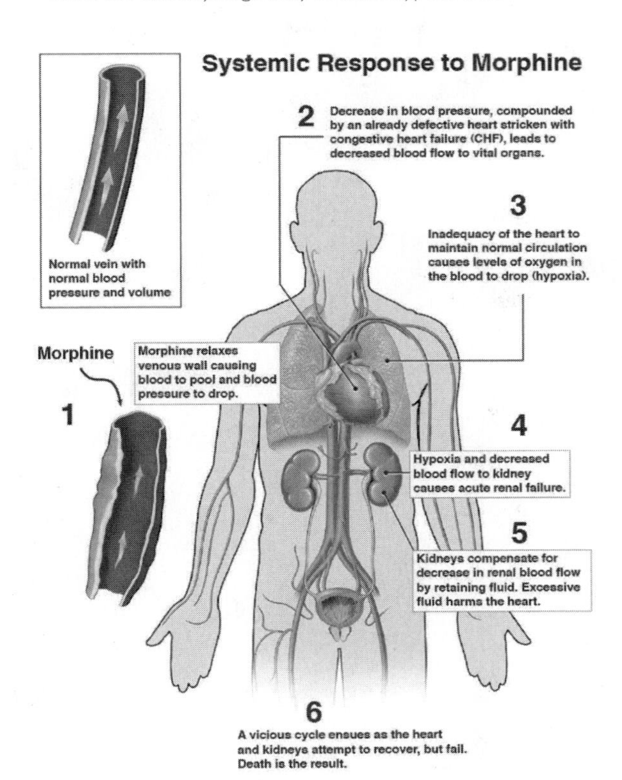
Systemic Response to Morphine
Normal vein with normal blood pressure and volume
2 Decrease in blood pressure, compounded by an already defective heart stricken with congestive heart failure (CHF), leads to decreased blood flow to vital organs.
3 Inadequacy of the heart to maintain normal circulation causes levels of oxygen in the blood to drop (hypoxia).
Morphine
1
Morphine relaxes venous wall causing blood to pool and blood pressure to drop.
4 Hypoxia and decreased blood flow to kidney causes acute renal failure.
5 Kidneys compensate for decrease in renal blood flow by retaining fluid. Excessive fluid harms the heart.
6 A vicious cycle ensues as the heart and kidneys attempt to recover, but fail. Death is the result.

This image depicts the potential risks of administering morphine with vigilant monitoring afterwards or administering too much.

Evidence-Based Medications: Statins

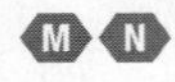

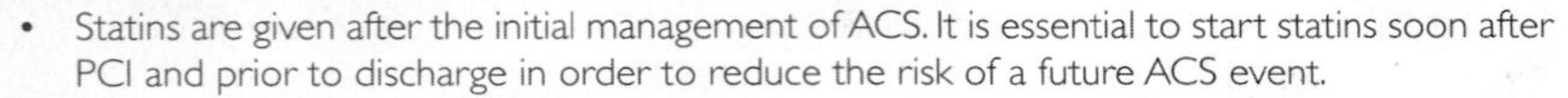

- Statins are given after the initial management of ACS. It is essential to start statins soon after PCI and prior to discharge in order to reduce the risk of a future ACS event.

- Statins are a class of HMG-CoA reductase inhibitor medications. Statins work by slowing the production of cholesterol in the body. Normally, statins are prescribed for patients who have an LDL cholesterol above 100 mg/dL and also have risk factors for coronary artery disease (such as a previous ACS event).
- When given (orally) during hospitalization after a PCI and then continued at discharge, statins have been shown to reduce the risk of another MI.
- The statin drugs include:
  - o Lovastatin
  - o Pravastatin
  - o Rosuvastatin

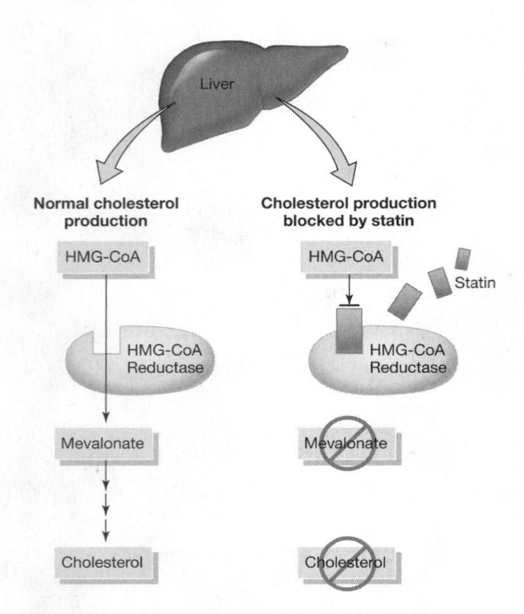

This simplified illustration shows how cholesterol synthesis is blocked by a statin or HMG-CoA Reductase Inhibitor to lower blood cholesterol and its damage effects throughout the body.

- Treatment with statins and a low-saturated fat diet also result in some regression of the size of atheromas or fatty plaque formations.
- In addition, inflammation within the atheroma decreases, and the plaque becomes more stable. The plaque becomes less thrombophilic (promotes less clotting) and is less likely to rupture.

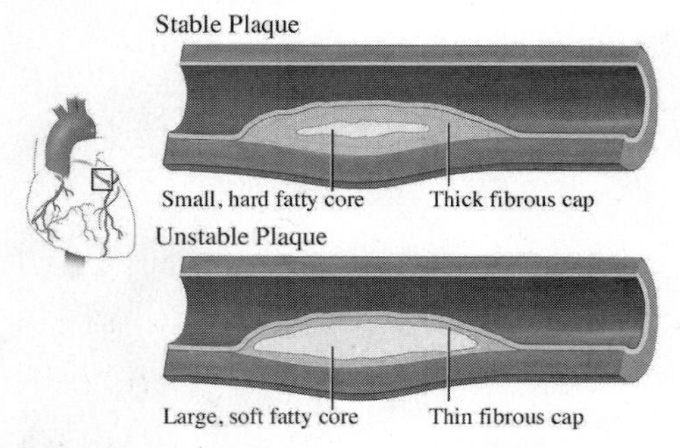

These illustrations compare a stable to an unstable plaque formation in the coronary arteries. Note the hard, fatty core and thick fibrous cap of the stable plaque, making it unlikely to rupture. In contrast, the unstable plaque core has liquefied, the fatty core enlarged and the fibrous cap thinner, making it vulnerable to rupture.

Collaborative Interventions (continued)

Patient Education and Rehabilitation

Education of patients with ACS conditions is extensive because these patients commonly have comorbid conditions that exacerbate the development of ACS. In addition, recovery from ACS is progressive, extended, and minimally includes:

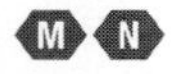

- Patients need substantial education regarding disease process, complications, medications, exercise, diet, smoking cessation, alcohol and/or substance misuse, and modifiable risk factor management. This includes dietary consultation, particularly if comorbid factors, such as diabetes, hypercholesterolemia, and hypertension, are present.
- **Cardiac rehabilitation** is an integral part of post-ACS management. While cardiac rehabilitation has limited evidence on improving survival following an event, it has been shown to improve the quality of life.
  - o Cardiac rehabilitation is more than just improving exercise habits. A change in exercise habits has the potential to act as a stimulus for improving additional aspects of rehabilitation, for example, lifestyle changes and optimization of psychosocial support.
  - o The outcome measures of cardiac rehabilitation include improvement in quality of life (QOL), for example, the patient's perception of physical improvement; satisfaction with risk factor alteration; psychosocial adjustments in interpersonal roles; and the potential for returning to a pre-ACS lifestyle.
  - o For the majority of patients the best predictors of rehabilitation outcome are psychosocial, not physiological. Psychological findings about adjustment to MI and lifestyle change must be integrated with routine care.
  - o Referral to a cardiac rehabilitation program post discharge is an important part of patient education and management of post-ACS quality of life.
  - o Family members, especially the partner, should be included in the rehabilitation process.

- **Medications:** Adhering to medications and developing a routine for taking medications are essential for slowing the progress of disease. If, for any reason, medications are not tolerated, patients should be educated to contact the primary care provider so that medication adjustment can be considered.
- **Diet:** A heart healthy diet is encouraged. A nutritionist should provide the patient and family with detailed nutritional plans that are tailored for the patient. More importantly, a diet that takes the particular patient's needs into consideration can improve the patient's adherence to change. With all the best intentions in the past, simply informing the patient what to eat has had little impact.

Collaborative Interventions (continued)

Cardiac Revascularization in ACS

- Cardiac revascularization is considered in many ACS patients, depending on the severity, location, and extent of their disease.
- Although patients who have coronary artery bypass grafting (CABG) surgery go to the ICU post-op, medical–surgical nurses often prep patients for surgery or receive them post-ICU stay.
- An overview is provided to familiarize nurses who care for these patients before and/or after surgery.
- In ACS patients, particularly those with unstable angina, there are a host of reasons why medical management may not be the best option. For instance, despite maximum therapy, a patient with UA may continue to become less stable.
  - o Or, cardiac catheterization and stenting may be unsuccessful at re-establishing perfusion of the heart. Additionally, for some patients, balloon angioplasty and stenting are not recommended. Those patients may require coronary artery bypass grafting (CABG) (see animation).
  - o CABG is briefly discussed as most of those patients receive care in specialty units.
  - o Nursing care for a patient having CABG surgery is primarily delivered in the intensive care unit.

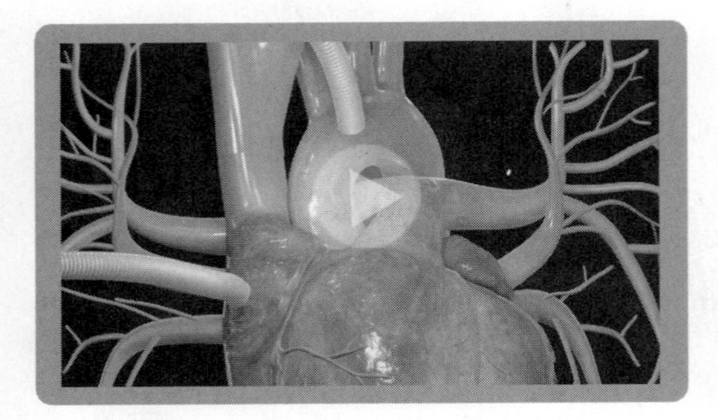

This shows a CABG procedure. It reviews the midline sternal incision, connection to a perfusion machine, and two grafts for bypass. After the procedure, the heart is restarted and a drainage tube is placed to remove excess fluid. Postoperative care is also included.

Source: © 2013 Nucleus Medical Media, All rights reserved

Postoperative Care

- Post-CABG, the patient is intubated for a short time (less than 24 hr), but may be extubated prior to leaving the operating room.
- Following the ICU stay (usually 24–48 hr), the patient is transferred to a cardiac step-down area for discharge preparation.
- The patient is monitored (cardiac) but is unlikely to still be hemodynamically monitored.
- Chest tubes may remain in place if still draining.
- A cardiac pacemaker (temporary) and pacing wires are in place until just prior to discharge.
- Early mobilization and patient education are central nursing goals.

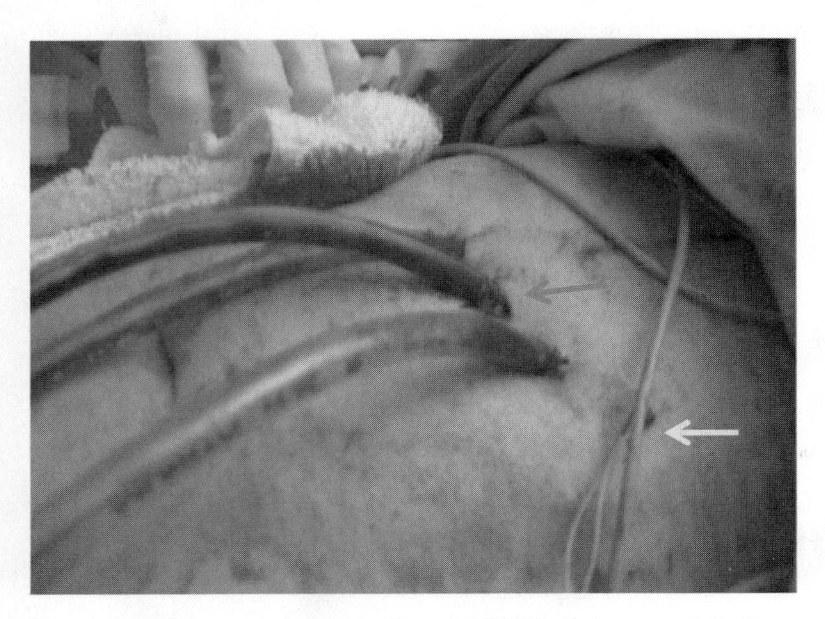

The thin pacing wires are seen (yellow arrow) in a post-CABG patient as surgery is finishing. Additionally, the patient has chest tubes (red arrow) exiting the skin substernally to remove any blood from pooling around the heart. Both sites are covered with sterile dressings and safety precautions are paramount.

Source: Copyright © 2013, NovEx Novice to Expert Learning, LLC

- Monitoring and care of the patient by nurses involves:
  - o Managing the patient's pain while increasing mobilization
  - o Observing for signs of infection (primarily in the sternal wound or groin areas if the saphenous vein is used)
    - ■ Look for redness, swelling, pain, or purulent drainage along the wound

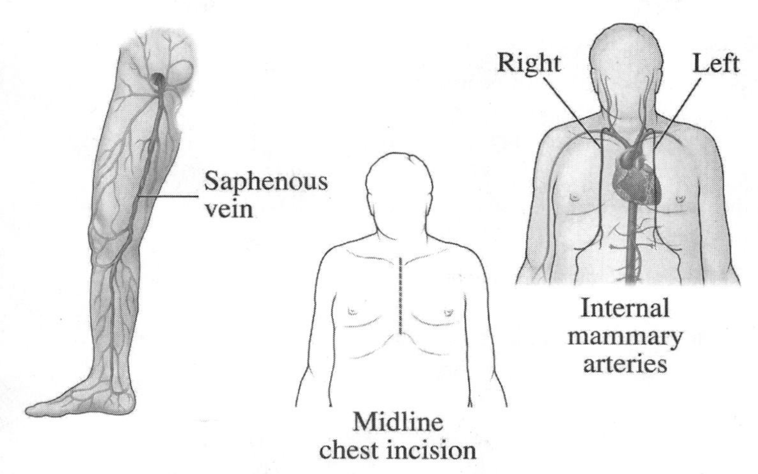

This drawing points out potential incision sites a patient may have after CABG surgery. The midline sternal wound may be seen along with other various donor graft sites. The saphenous vein and the internal mammary artery are commonly used.

- o Monitoring for excessive bleeding into the mediastinal tube which may indicate cardiac graft bleeding
  - ■ Small amounts of blood loss are normal (e.g., less than 100 mL/8 hr).
- o Managing wounds of both the surgery and the donor vein site
- o Encouraging early ambulation, which, like any surgery, is a key to helping rapid patient recovery
- o Progressing toward extubation from mechanical ventilation when the patient can eat again. A sore throat is common after intubation, but usually is a temporary condition.
- o Educating the patient for discharge, healthy living, and risk modification

- Nurses and various team members should collaborate with the patient and family to plan ways that the patient can follow the many recommended and important activities known to reduce the risk of additional coronary events and improve the quality of life, including:
  - o Cardiac rehabilitation
  - o Reduce modifiable risk factors
  - o Adhere to their medication regime
  - o Understand the signs of ACS and know what to do if needed
  - o Engage in a healthier lifestyle around diet, exercise, weight management, management of comorbid conditions (e.g., HTN, diabetes), stress reduction, smoking cessation, and substance misuse.

Summary of Interventions

- CAD is the leading cause of death in the United States. Early recognition and rapid intervention saves lives. In ACS, "time is muscle" saved. ACC/AHA guidelines provide excellent recommendations on how to intervene in a timely way.
- The goal for ACS is to restore myocardial perfusion and to limit myocardial damage. Intervention priorities include:
  - o Antiplatelets and EKG within 10 min of arrival
  - o For STEMI: Door-to-PCI less than 90 min. If PCI unavailable, then door-to-drug (thrombolytics) less than 30 min
  - o ACS medications within guideline time/frame with diagnostic troponin levels
  - o EBP indicates patients should receive:
    - ■ Antiplatelets, anticoagulation, beta blockers, ACE inhibitors, and nitrates as part of their initial treatment
    - ■ Statin therapy prior to discharge
  - o Obvious and important therapies that have not been researched include pain relief and oxygen therapy for SpO_2 values less than or equal to 92%. Prior to discharge, patient education should be initiated and cardiac rehabilitation should be advised when indicated.
    - ■ Educate patient about reduction in variable risk factors and medical compliance can decrease the incidence of ACS and reduce the risk of death.
    - ■ Cardiac revascularization for patient who do not respond to medical management or require surgical intervention.

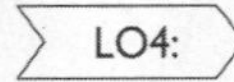

Evaluation of Desired Collaborative Care Outcomes

Evaluation and reassessment should reveal attainment of previously established patient outcomes. In summary:

- Patient has no further cardiac compromise, as seen by an improving EKG, a stable and acceptable rhythm, and resolving cardiac enzymes.
- Patient's hemodynamics are within normal limits, mentation is clear, and chest pain is absent.
- Patient reports no chest pain.
- Patient confidently discusses plan of care, reports feeling more comfortable with health situation, and reflects a calmer demeanor.
- Patient tolerates gradual increases in daily activities with no chest pain or excessive fatigue.

References

Braunwald, E., Antman, E., Beasley, J., et al. (2000). ACC/AHA guidelines for the management of patients with unstable angina and non-ST-segment elevation myocardial infarction: Executive summary and recommendations. *Circulation, 102*, 1193–1209.

Davies, M. J. (2000). Coronary Disease: The pathophysiology of acute coronary syndromes. *Heart, 83*, 361–366.

Munro, N. (2009). Acute coronary syndromes. In K. Carlson (Ed.), AACN Advanced Critical Care Nursing (pp. 207–236). St. Louis, MO: Saunders Elsevier.

Kirkwood, P. (2009). Heart disease in women. In K. Carlson (Ed.), AACN Advanced Critical Care Nursing (pp. 276–296). St. Louis, MO: Saunders Elsevier.

O'Connor, R. E., Brady, W., Brooks, S., et al. (2010). 2010 American Heart Association guidelines for cardiopulmonary resuscitation and emergency cardiovascular care science: Part 10: Acute coronary syndromes. *Circulation, 122*, S787–S817.

O'Gara, P., Kushner, F., Ascheim, D., et al. (2013). 2013 ACCF/AHA guideline for the management of ST-elevation myocardial infarction: Executive summary. *Circulation, 127*, 529–555.

Overbaugh, K. (2009). Acute coronary syndrome. *American Journal of Nursing, 109*(5), 42–52. Clinical Practice Guidelines

Patient Education

American Heart Association

Women's Heart Foundation. Improved Survival, Prevention, Early Intervention, and Gender Care. **www.womensheart.org**

Learning Outcomes for Angina

When you complete this lesson, you will be able to:

1. Recognize the clinical relevance of angina.
2. Consider the pathophysiology, etiology, risk factors, and clinical presentation of angina that determine the priority patient concerns.
3. Determine the most urgent and important nursing interventions and patient education required in caring for a patient with angina.
4. Evaluate attainment of desired collaborative care outcomes for a patient with angina.

LO1:

What Is Angina?

- Angina is not itself a disease. Instead, it is the symptom of underlying coronary heart disease.
- **Angina** is defined as chest discomfort or pain that results when heart muscle fails to get sufficient oxygen.
- Angina is best understood as the symptoms a person may experience when coronary artery disease (CAD) is present. It is a warning sign for myocardial ischemia.

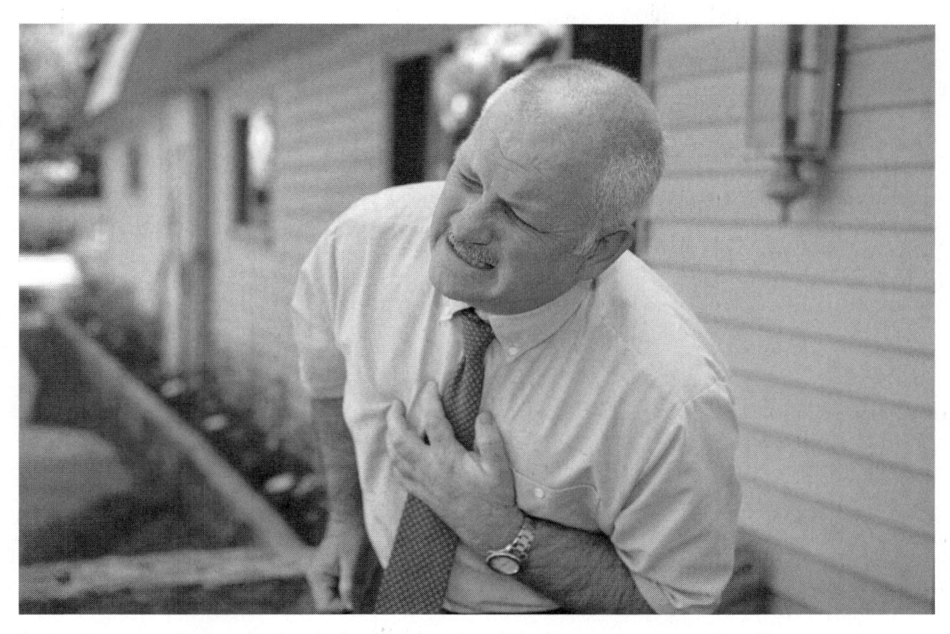

Angina is commonly described as feeling like there's an "elephant sitting on my chest."
Source: Lisa F. Young/Fotolia

LO1:

Clinical Relevance

- Almost 9.8 million Americans have angina yearly.
- Worsening angina (known as "unstable") can be a warning sign of both impending myocardial infarction (MI) and the potential for sudden death.
- While angina can be mild to severe, it poses a significant challenge regarding quality of life. The pain of angina can be disabling by either limiting normal daily activities or paralyzing the patient with fear of pain episodes that limit involvement in daily activities.
- Angina can be a risk factor for developing further myocardial disease, particularly MI and heart failure.
- Early recognition of angina symptoms allows one to promptly evaluate and treat the patient for heart disease.

Concept Check

1. What is the best definition of angina?

A. A disease of the heart muscle
B. Chest pain resulting from ischemia
C. Myocardial infarction
D. A warning that death is imminent

Answer question

LO2:

Pathophysiology

- Angina is a symptom of cardiac ischemia or insufficient oxygen supply to meet cardiac demands.
- Angina can be stable or unstable. Stable angina occurs during exertion or while under stress, whereas unstable angina occurs at rest, without an attributable reason. This lesson focuses on stable angina.
- Angina or cardiac ischemia occurs when: Oxygen demand > Oxygen delivery
- Exertion or exercise increases heart rate, contractility, and work of the ventricles, all of which increase oxygen demand.
- When oxygen demand exceeds supply, metabolism switches from aerobic to anaerobic, creating potential metabolic, electrical, and mechanical dysfunctions of the heart. Angina (pain) results from the chemical stimulation of the nerve signals to the brain, initiated by the oxygen imbalance.
- Angina or ischemia, however, almost always occurs in the setting of atherosclerosis and narrowing of one or more coronary arteries by greater than 70%. (The development of atherosclerosis is discussed in more detail in the Care of Patients with Acute Coronary Syndrome NovE-lesson.)
- As an overview, atherosclerosis occurs when plaque forms within the walls of the arteries and arterioles. The arterial walls become inflamed and damaged as fatty tissue, cholesterol, and cellular debris build up, bulge into the vessel lumen, and impinge on blood flow. Plaque additionally causes the arterial walls to thicken and harden. Hence the term *hardening of the arteries* evolved in reference to *arterio*sclerosis, a term used almost interchangeably with atherosclerosis.
- Healthy coronary arteries are capable of increasing blood flow up to 6-fold compared to resting blood flow. Oxygen extraction (the percentage of oxygen in the blood used by cells or tissues) by the cardiac muscle cells also improves while exercising.

Concept Check

2. Which term is often used to describe atherosclerosis?

A. Unstable angina
B. Stable angina
C. Hardening of the arteries
D. Myocardial infarction

Answer question

- In atherosclerotic (partially blocked) arteries, blood flow is impaired by narrowing of the blood vessels and the ability of the vessel to vasodilate is impaired. Usually patients are asymptomatic even with exertion until narrowing of an artery approaches 70%.
- Ischemia tends to occur first in areas of the heart that are supplied by the most narrowed arteries.
- Chronically ischemic areas of the heart can develop collateral circulation in order to compensate for the compromised blood supply. Collateral blood vessels are vessels that develop and supply the ischemic area of the heart by increasing in size over time to provide more blood flow.
- A less common type of angina, Prinzmetal or variant angina, is due to coronary spasm (temporary stenosis of the artery due to vasoconstriction) rather than atherosclerosis.

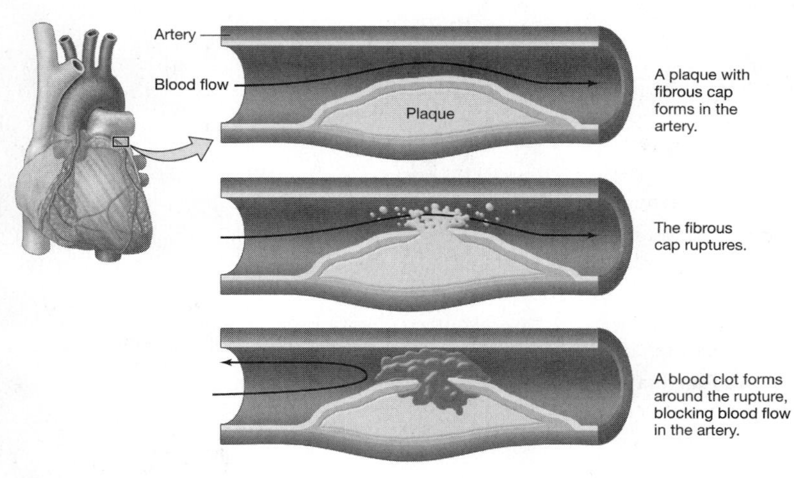
Artery
Blood flow
Plaque
A plaque with fibrous cap forms in the artery.
The fibrous cap ruptures.
A blood clot forms around the rupture, blocking blood flow in the artery.

This pathology in this disease involves a decrease in supply of coronary blood flow and resulting decrease of oxygen delivery to a level below the required baseline metabolic needs of the myocardium. Coronary blood flow is interrupted by fibrin and platelet plugs developing on a fissured or ruptured atherosclerotic plaque in most cases. Recent research reveals that coronary vasospasm plays a role in some patients.

Concept Check

3. Which type of angina is thought to be caused by vasoconstriction?
   A. Stable
   B. Unstable
   C. Infarction
   D. Prinzmetal

Answer question

Risk Factors

The risk factors for developing angina are the same as those for atherosclerosis.

- Hypertension
- Hypercholesterolemia
- Diabetes
- Smoking
- Family history
- Age
- Obesity and/or sedentary lifestyle
- Unhealthy diet
- Renal disease

Causes

- Arterosclerosis, the major cause
- Smoking
- Hyperlipidemia
- Hypercholesteremia
- Hypertension
- Diabetes
- In patients with atherosclerosis, there are factors that trigger angina due to the oxygen imbalance:
  - o Increased demand of the heart through exertion (e.g., climbing stairs)
  - o Decreased oxygen carrying capacity as occurs with anemia
  - o Hypoxemia (e.g., lung disease, pneumonia, high altitudes)
  - o Decreased cardiac output (e.g., heart failure)

Assessment Findings

- Stable angina is a clinical syndrome characterized by discomfort or pain in the chest, jaw, teeth, shoulders, neck, back, or arms.
- Angina pain is commonly described as "an elephant sitting on one's chest," squeezing, pressure, and tightness.
- Occasionally, discomfort or indigestion may occur in the epigastric area (referred to as pain).
- Chest pain may be accompanied by shortness of breath, nausea and vomiting, diaphoresis, weakness, to name a few.
- The pain is typically elicited by exertion or emotional stress and relieved by rest and/or nitroglycerin.
- Angina can present with sudden onset, with or without risk factors for cardiac disease.
- The pain is unlike acute coronary syndrome (ACS) pain, in that **the pain of angina is relieved by rest and/or with nitroglycerin**.
- If patients experience symptoms of chest pain, they should rest to see if the pain goes away. If the pain has not diminished after 20 min, help should be sought in the nearest emergency facility.

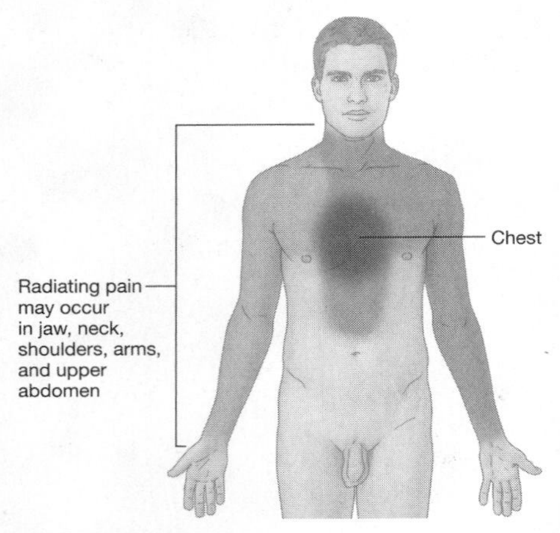
Chest
Radiating pain may occur in jaw, neck, shoulders, arms, and upper abdomen

Signs and symptoms of angina.

Concept Check

4. Which symptoms are often present during stable anginal episodes?

A. Hot, dry skin

B. Headache

C. Pain unrelieved by rest

D. Shortness of breath

Answer question

Atypical Assessment Findings

- Women and patients with diabetes are more likely than men to have atypical angina symptoms.
- Patients who present with atypical symptoms are therefore at risk for delay in recognition and treatment. These symptoms include:
  - o Shortness of breath without pain
  - o Epigastric or throat discomfort
  - o Pain may be burning or sharp
  - o Jaw pain or ache
  - o Dizziness, weakness, and confusion

Classification of Angina

- Classification of angina according to the Canadian Cardiovascular Society:

  Grade I: Pain occurs only with strenuous or prolonged exertion.

  Grade II: Pain occurs with activities, such as quickly climbing stairs, exertion (e.g., rapid walking) after eating, activity in the cold when under stress, or shortly after waking up in the morning.

  Grade III: Pain occurs when walking one to two blocks on level ground or climbing a flight of steps at a normal pace.

  Grade IV: Unable to perform any physical activity without pain, and experiencing pain at rest (unstable angina)

Angina Requiring Medical Attention

Signs and symptoms of angina that are concerning and require medical attention:

- Increased frequency or duration of angina episodes
- Angina at rest
- New onset of angina

These can be signs that angina is becoming unstable and/or of an impending MI. These patients require immediate evaluation and treatment at the earliest possible time (see Care of Patients with Acute Coronary Syndrome NovE-lesson for further discussion).

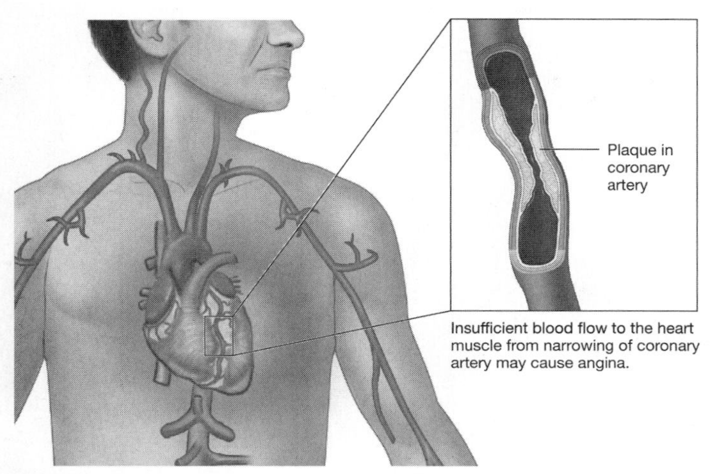

Plaque in coronary artery
Insufficient blood flow to the heart muscle from narrowing of coronary artery may cause angina.

Stable angina is a specific type of pain in the chest caused by inadequate blood flow through the blood vessels (coronary arteries) of the heart muscle (myocardium).

Diagnostics

- Patients who present with angina symptoms require a diagnositc workup, which initially includes a complete physical examination and blood work.
- This evaluation reveals information about the cardiac risk factors discussed earlier and can support one's suspicions and concerns.
- Cardiac biomarkers can be obtained, specifically, troponin I. These markers are typically normal in angina, unlike an ST elevation myocardial infarction (STEMI) or non-ST elevation myocardial infarction (NSTEMI), where the biomarkers are elevated.
- They are evaluated to determine their risk and the extent of their disease using a variety of diagnostic tests that includes:
  - o Electrocardiogram (EKG)
  - o Exercise stress test
  - o Echocardiography

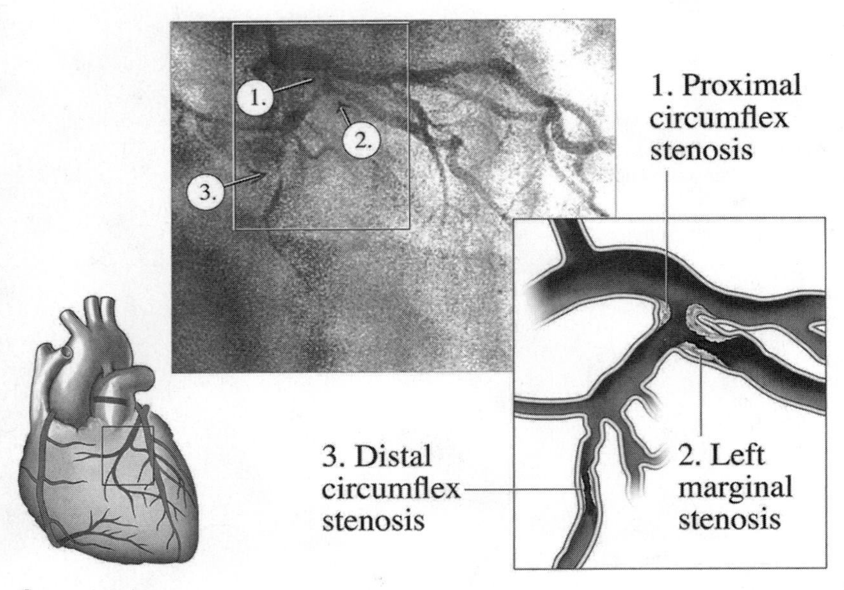

Coronary angiogram.

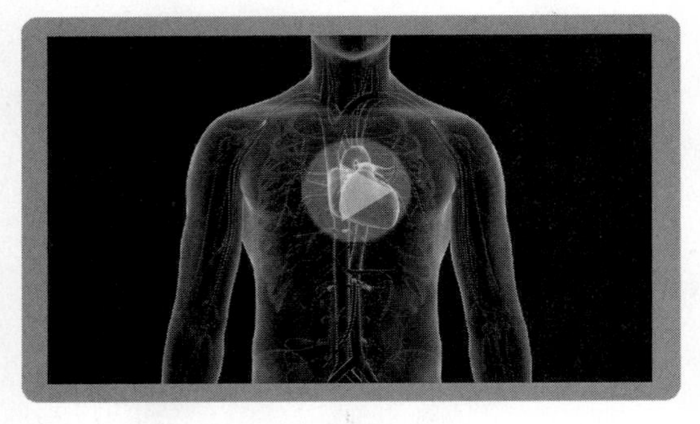

This animation depicts a coronary angiography (cardiac catheterization) procedure. It begins by showing the buildup of plaque in an artery wall of the heart, slowing the flow of blood and shows the heart valves pumping. Afterwards, the patient lies on a testing table while contrast dye is injected into the arteries of the heart, showing the location of the blockage.

- EKG can be performed when the patient has symptoms or during a stress test (see EKG). Patients with angina may have ST depression, as opposed to the ST elevation seen in myocardial injury during symptoms or during a stress test. Patients with angina are expected to have:
  - o ST depression in more than one contiguous lead.
  - o ST depression greater than or equal to 1 mm.

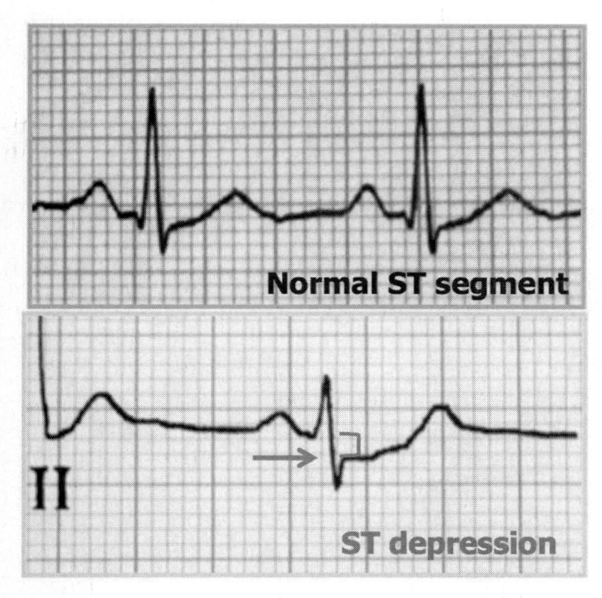

Upper: A patient complaining of chest pain shows a normal EKG with no ST segment changes during stress test. Lower: In comparison, another patient shows 2 mm (0.02 mV) of horizontal ST segment depression during an exercise stress test, indicating a positive test for ischemia.

- A resting EKG in an asymptomatic patient is often normal.
- A stress test involves evaluation of the patient during exercise under controlled circumstances, usually on a treadmill or bike. EKG is monitored simultaneously, looking for changes that occur with ischemia.
- An echocardiogram can also be used in addition to an EKG during stress testing.
  - o While the echocardiogram is more accurate, it is also more costly.
- Cardiac catheterization may be indicated if further or more specific evaluation is needed.

Priority Patient Concerns and Desired Collaborative Care Outcomes

Prior to caring for patients with angina, it is important to prioritize the patient's concerns that must guide the nursing care plan and interventions. Care for the patient is ordered and organized in accordance with the patient's priority and urgent needs. Desired collaborative care outcomes in patients with angina typically include:

1. Patient will report no further chest pain or chest pain that is unrelieved by minimal intervention.
2. Patient will receive supportive and therapeutic interventions to minimize further deterioration of cardiac tissue perfusion, as needed.
3. Patient will exhibit a calmer demeanor and rest more peacefully after discussion of the treatment plan, probable outcomes, and reassurance that care providers are vigilantly watching over and treating the cause of the pain.
4. Patient will tolerate return to daily activity level with no new chest pain or fatigue.

Considering these important care outcomes, prepare a list of the major 3–6 priority patient concerns or nursing diagnoses for patients with angina. Be prepared to participate in a discussion of this list and/or to submit them as an assignment, as determined by your faculty. Resources you may find helpful in this assignment can include this lesson, the references, resources on nursing care plans, and standard nursing diagnoses manuals.

LO3:

Collaborative Interventions

Evidence-Based Practice

- Three evidence-based practice (EBP) treatments of angina are proposed:

M N 1. Nitrates are the most effective intervention for managing acute symptoms.
   - Nitroglycerin sublingually is the most common method of administration.
   - IV nitroglycerin can also be used when pain is unrelieved by sublingual or requires immediate relief.
   - Patients can develop a tolerance to nitrates, requiring increasing doses over time.
   - Long-acting nitrates (e.g., isosorbide dinitrate) may help prevent anginal episodes but are not used during an acute episode.

M N 2. Beta blockers are commonly administered to help reduce myocardial oxygen consumption by lowering heart rate and contractility. Commonly used beta blockers include:
   - Metoprolol, atenolol, and bisoprolol

M N 3. Calcium channel blockers (CCBs) provide benefits similar to beta blockers and can be used in place of beta blockers. Long-acting CCBs include:
   - Nifedipine, felodipine, verapamil, and diltiazem

M N
- In addition, aspirin should be given at a dose of 81–325 mg daily to patients with angina.
  - o Less evidence is available for other antiplatelets such as clopidogrel.

Acute Anginal Episode

Patients who experience an acute episode of angina may be at home, work, or in the hospital. The following interventions are needed and, depending on where the patient is, the patient or health care provider may administer the following interventions, as needed:

- N The first most important intervention is to stop activity and rest. Fortunately, patients commonly do this without prompting or thinking.
- N If the patient has been previously treated for angina, administration of a sublingual (SL) nitroglycerin for pain or symptom relief per protocol is appropriate.
- N For unrelieved pain, patients can repeat nitroglycerin SL up to 3 times, each time waiting only 5 min before taking another nitroglycerin.
- If pain is unrelieved by rest and three doses of nitroglycerin, the patient should call 911 if not in a health care facility.
- N Educate patients to see or talk to their physician or health care provider (HCP) if the angina is new in onset or if there are changes in its presentation or duration.
- N Administer ordered nitroglycerin (NTG)
- N Administer ordered analgesics for pain per protocol as needed.
- N Educate patients on risk reduction (i.e., smoking cessation programs, weight reduction strategies).
- M N Collaborate or consult with other members of the health care team to assist with risk reduction (i.e., nutritionist, social work, trainer).
- N Instruct patient on side effects and proper use of NTG.
- N Implement relaxation strategies (i.e., dim lights, soothing music).
- N Educate patient on activity levels and monitoring for chest discomfort.

Concept Check

5. What is the rationale for administering atenolol to a patient having angina?

A. It slows the heart rate.

B. It dilates vessels.

C. It prevents clotting.

D. It increases blood pressure.

Answer question

Collaborative Interventions (continued)

Patient Education

Education of each patient and/or family needs to be adapted to each specific situation, depending on the patient's risk factors, condition, and complications. However, details that should generally be included with both the patient and family involve:

- M N Angina means that:
  - There is underlying coronary heart disease.
  - Patients are at an increased risk of heart attack compared with those who have no symptoms of cardiovascular disease.
  - One episode of angina is not a signal of an impending heart attack.
- N A person with angina should learn the pattern of his or her angina—what triggers an angina attack, what it feels like, how long episodes usually last, and how much medication relieves the pain. If the pattern changes sharply—if episodes exacerbate (e.g., become more frequent, last longer, occur without exercise)—or if the symptoms are those of a heart attack, seek medical help immediately, perhaps best done by seeking an evaluation at a nearby hospital emergency department.
- N When the pattern of angina changes, the risk of heart attack in subsequent days or weeks is much higher.

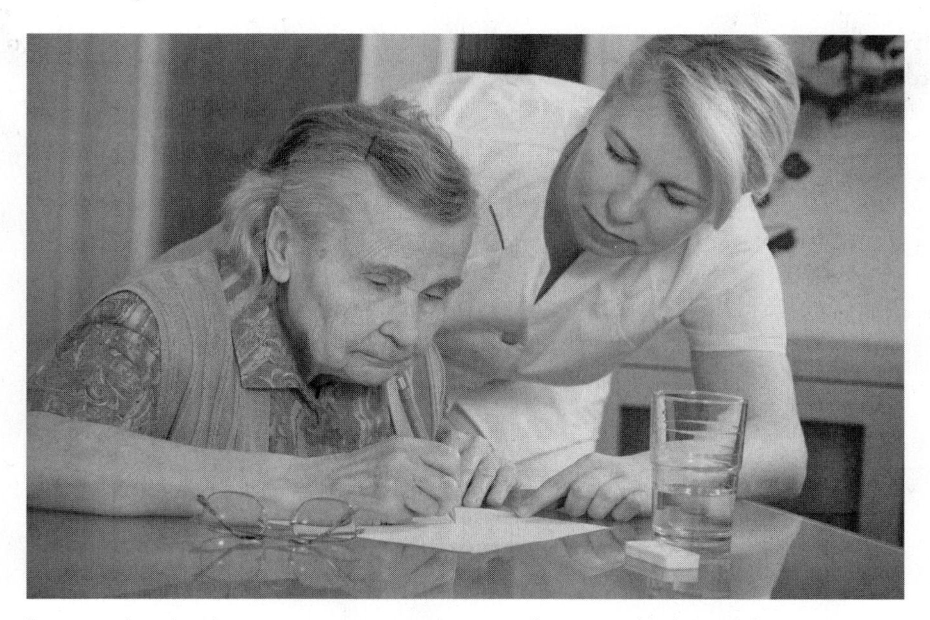

Patients with cardiac disease require extensive education to learn to modify their risk factors.
Source: Alexander Raths/Fotolia

N

- Patients with angina should be educated about how to prevent further episodes by modifying their risk factors for cardiac disease whenever possible.

N

- Discharge instructions that encourage interactive learning, allowing the patient and family to be involved together in the learning process, results in better retention of information. Key areas to address include:
  - o Symptom recognition, disease process, complications—if symptoms return or increase in frequency, immediate medical attention should be sought.
  - o If chest discomfort occurs, first stop and rest.
  - o If angina does not dissipate immediately with rest, attempt up to three doses of SL nitroglycerin, 5 min apart.
  - o If discomfort is not relieved, call 911 for immediate help.
  - o Cardiac rehabilitation may be beneficial.
  - o Exercise, as suggested by the health care provider, should be encouraged.
  - o Patients should be educated to identify when and what triggers their symptoms in order that they cease that activity before reaching that point.
  - o Activities that trigger symptoms, including sex, should be modified to prevent the onset of symptoms.
  - o Activity tolerance may be improved by medications.
  - o Medication compliance can control and prevent symptoms.
  - o Smoking cessation and dietary considerations can improve long-term results.
  - o Management of comorbid conditions and lifestyle changes can reduce symptoms and improve quality of life.
  - o Weight management will reduce the cardiac workload.

Concept Check

6. What is the benefit of weight management for the patient with stable angina?

A. It improves the patient's self-image.

B. It reduces cardiac workload.

C. It reverses cardiac damage.

D. It eliminates need for exercise.

Answer question

Summary of Interventions

- Discomfort with angina is usually transient and responds to rest and/or nitroglycerin.
- The primary treatment for angina involves reducing risk factors for CAD and symptom relief:
  - o Nitroglycerin for immediate symptom relief
  - o Beta or CCBs to reduce myocardial oxygen consumption
  - o Aspirin for antiplatelet benefits

Concept Check

7. The nurse would evaluate that nitroglycerin has had its intended effect if which situation occurs?

A. The patient is less short of breath.

B. The patient had a headache.

C. The patient's chest pain resolves.

D. The patient's respiratory rate slows.

Answer question

LO4: Evaluation of Desired Collaborative Care Outcomes

Evaluation and reassessment should reveal attainment of previously established patient outcomes. In summary:

- The patient has no chest pain but has explained what he will do to intervene should chest pain reoccur.
- Patient's hemodynamics are within normal limits, mentation is clear, and chest pain is absent.
- The patient is working on control of his risk factors for angina and reports feeling less anxious about health status.
- The patient performs normal activities of daily living and has no chest pain.

References

Conway, B., & Fuat, A. (2007). Recent advances in angina management: implications for nurses. *Nurs Stand, 21*(38), 49–56.

Leeper, B., Cyr, A. M., Lambert, C., & Martin, K. (2011). Acute coronary syndrome. *Crit Care Nurs Clin North Am, 23*(4), 547–557.

Clinical Practice Guidelines

Jneid, H., Anderson, J. L., Wright, R. S., et al. (2012). 2012 ACCF/AHA Focused Update of the Guideline for the Management of Patients With Unstable Angina/Non–ST-Elevation Myocardial Infarction (Updating the 2007 Guideline and Replacing the 2011 Focused Update). *Circulation, 126,* 875–910.

The Task Force on the Management of Stable Angina Pectoris of the European Society of Cardiology. (2006). Guidelines on the management of stable angina pectoris. *European Heart Journal, 10,* 1–63

Patient Education

American Heart Association. What is Angina? **www.heart.org/idc/groups/heart-public/@wcm/@hcm/documents/downloadable/ucm_300287.pdf**

Hildreth, C. J., Burke, A. E., & Glass, R. M. (2009). Chest pain. *JAMA, 301*(14), 1498. doi:10.1001/jama.301.14.1498

National Heart, Lung, and Blood Institute. Living with Angina. **http://www.nhlbi.nih.gov/health/health-topics/topics/angina/livingwith.html**

STOP

Go to the online course and complete the NovE-Cases assigned by your instructor for this module.

Learning Outcomes for Dysrhythmias*

After completion of the EKG NovE-lesson, followed by this lesson, you will be able to:

1. Recognize the clinical relevance of dysrhythmias.
2. Consider the pathophysiology, etiology, risk factors, and clinical presentation of dysrhythmias that determine the priority patient concerns.
3. Determine the most urgent and important nursing interventions and patient education required in caring for a patient with dysrhythmias.
4. Evaluate attainment of desired collaborative care outcomes for a patient with dysrhythmias.

*This NovE-Lesson is not a comprehensive Dysrhythmias course, but is instead a overview of key dysrhythmias and interventions that most nurses should understand.

LO1:

What Are Dysrhythmias?

Dysrhythmia means abnormal rhythm. A dysrhythmia is a disturbance in the heart's normal rhythm and/or rate and represents a defect in the normal sequence and/or rate of electrical activation (depolarization) of the cardiac muscle cells.

- The heart has a natural pacemaker and a normal sequence of depolarization that follows the cardiac conduction system. Any additional impulse or conduction out of sequence is considered a dysrhythmia.
- Dysrhythmias present with the heart beating either irregularly (premature or abnormal contractions), too fast (**tachycardias**), or too slow (**bradycardias**).
- The term **arrhythmia** is often used, but technically arrhythmia means the absence of a rhythm. There is only one arrhythmia, an asystole, but many dysrhythmias.
- Dysrhythmias are concerning because they can reduce stroke volume and cardiac output, slightly or completely. Dysrhythmias range from benign to lethal.

Concept Check

1. **What is a major concern regarding dysrhythmias?**
   A. They are the predominant cause of pulmonary embolism.
   B. They can reduce stroke volume.
   C. They often reduce preload.
   D. They increase systemic vascular resistance.

Answer question

LO1:

Clinical Relevance

- Many patients with heart disease develop dysrhythmias that interfere with daily living.
- Depending on the type of dysrhythmia, it also causes distress, creates discomfort, and can be anxiety provoking.
- Dysrhythmias are a significant cause of death following a myocardial infarction. Many can be prevented or effectively treated if detected early.
- Approximately 500,000 people in the United States die each year from heart disease. Lethal dysrhythmias are thought to be a common cause of death.
- Cardiovascular disease is a frequent comorbid condition in patients being treated for other conditions. Because all nurses care for these patients and urgent situations arise, understanding basic dysrhythmias and interventions is essential.
- Dysrhythmias occur frequently following cardiac injury. Because some conduction defects can serve as an early warning before a clinically dangerous event, clinicians can detect and prevent many life-threatening dysrhythmias.

Electrophysiology

A Review of the Normal Cardiac Conduction and the EKG

- This lesson is intended to follow the Electrocardiogram NovE-lesson. Please complete the Electrocardiogram lesson first in order to gain the foundation necessary for this one, as a brief overview is provided here.
- The top image shows how the conduction system of the heart is situated anatomically. The lower image shows an EKG of normal conduction.
- The sinoatrial (SA) node is the natural pacemaker of the heart. When it spontaneously depolarizes, it sends a depolarization wave throughout the atria. This depolarization creates the P wave on EKG, followed by atrial contraction.
- The depolarization then passes through the atrioventricular (AV) node and bundle of His, between the atria and the ventricles. This produces the PR interval.
- The depolarization wave continues through the Purkinje fibers, depolarizing the ventricles. This produces a QRS complex on EKG and ventricular contraction follows.
- Cells immediately repolarize (resulting in the T wave formation) and the cycle repeats itself as the SA node automatically depolarizes again.

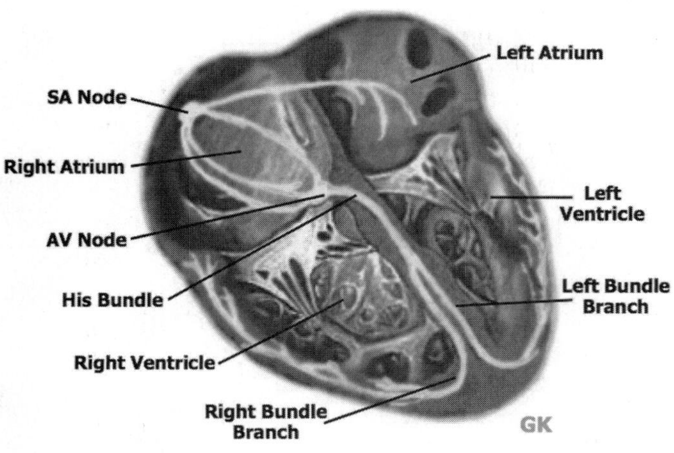

This diagram shows the cardiac conduction system as it is anatomically situated. All major conduction system structures are labeled.
Source: Courtesy of George Kyriakidis/Santa Ana, CA

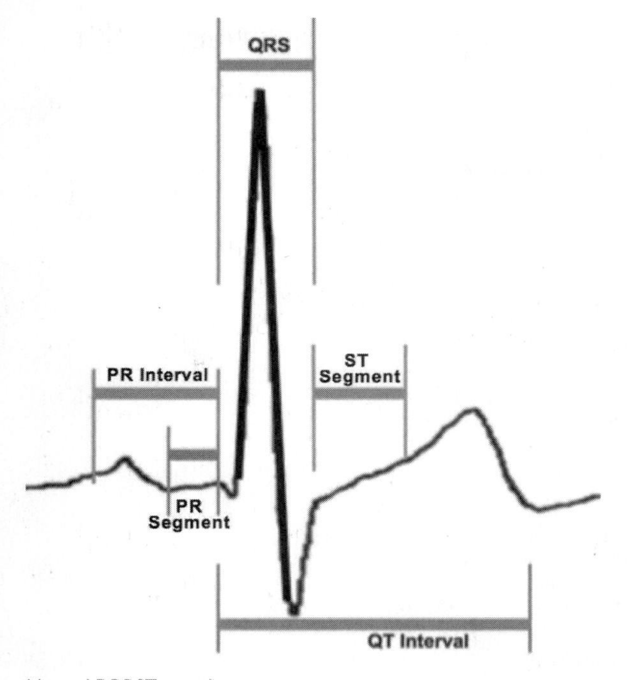

Normal PQRST complex.
Source: Courtesy of George Kyriakidis/Santa Ana, CA

Concept Check

2. What occurs in response to the electrical activity that produces QRS complex?

A. Contraction of the atria

B. Filling of the ventricles

C. Contraction of the ventricles

D. Resting of both the atria and the ventricles

Answer question

- When the SA node automatically fires regularly and the conduction system conducts every impulse at a constant speed in synchrony with the SA node, a sinus rhythm is produced.
- If normal conduction occurs at a heart rate between 60–100 beats per minute (bpm), the rhythm is referred to as normal sinus rhythm or NSR.

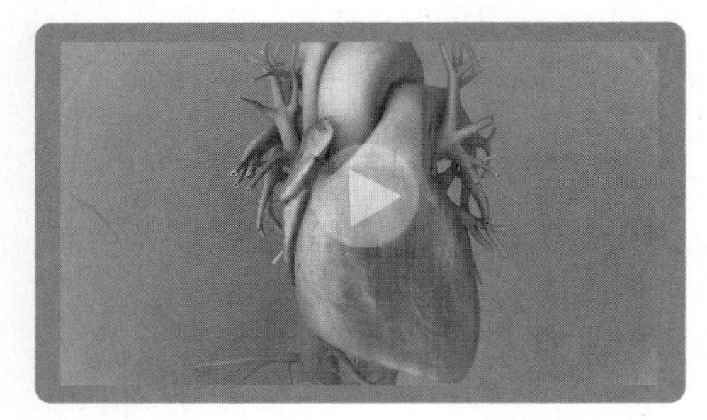

This animation provides an anatomical overview of the cardiac conduction system of the heart, depicting the sequence of events producing a heartbeat.

Source: © 2013 Nucleus Medical Media, All rights reserved

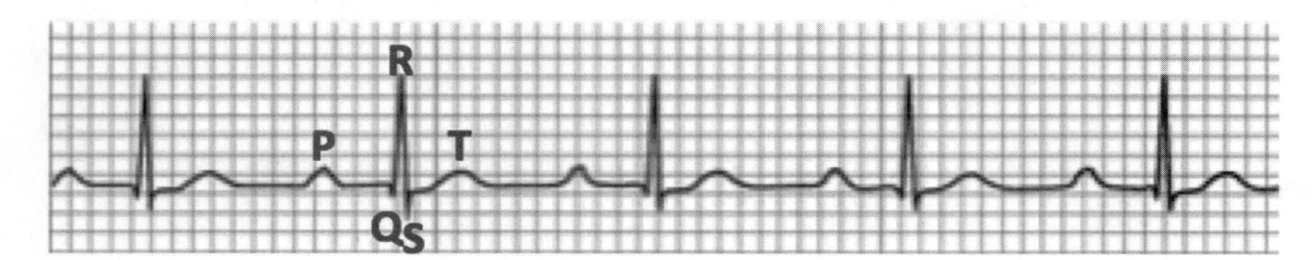

EKG showing normal sinus rhythm.

Source: Courtesy of K. Kyriakidis

Electrophysiology (continued)

Dysrhythmia Pathogenesis

- Dysrhythmias may be the result of:
  - o Faulty initiation of impulses
  - o Abnormal conduction
  - o Both

A 31-year-old female presented with fatigue, shortness of breath, and syncope. While gardening, she experienced shortness of breath and dizziness. She went to talk to her husband and "passed out." She was not responsive to her name when he shook her. She regained consciousness in 5 minutes, but is still short of breath, tired, and dizzy. Her review of systems is grossly normal. Her vitals are: temperature, 96.4°F; heart rate varying 30–110 bpm; respirations, 18–20 per minute, blood pressure, 88/42 mmHg; and oxygen saturation of 94% on room air. Her physical examination: An EKG confirms atrioventricular block, brachycardia, and multiple macular erythematous lesions with central pallor on both thighs.

This patient was diagnosed with Lyme Disease that commonly causes myocarditis (infection of the heart muscle) and conduction defects. The patient required temporary pacing until the Lyme disease resolved after treatment.

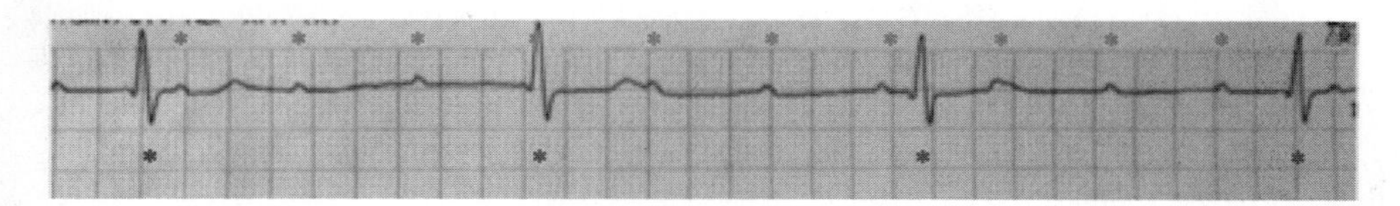

The rhythm demonstrates atrioventrricular (AV) block with two independent rhythms: a junctional rhythm that is conducting at a rate of 32 bpm (blue asterisks) and a sinus tachycardia at 109 bpm (red asterisks). In this case, the AV node fails to conduct the sinus impulses, so the AV node (or junction) takes over pacing the heart, but at a much slower rate.
Source: Courtesy of K. Kyriakidis

Initiation of Impulses

- Cardiac muscle throughout the heart has the ability to spontaneously initiate an impulse.
- This characteristic is called **automaticity** and is responsible for the generation of impulses by the SA node.
- An increased rate of automaticity within or outside the SA node can cause tachycardias.
- A decreased rate of automaticity causes bradycardias.
- Impulses can also arise in areas other than the SA node (ectopic foci) resulting in:
  - Atrial dysrhythmias (e.g., premature atrial contractions, atrial flutter)
  - Ventricular dysrhythmias (e.g., premature ventricular contractions)

Abnormal Electrical Impulse Initiation and Conduction due to Ventricular Ectopy

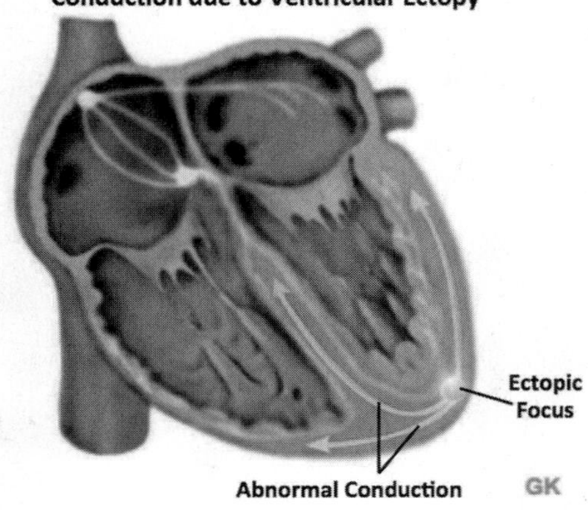

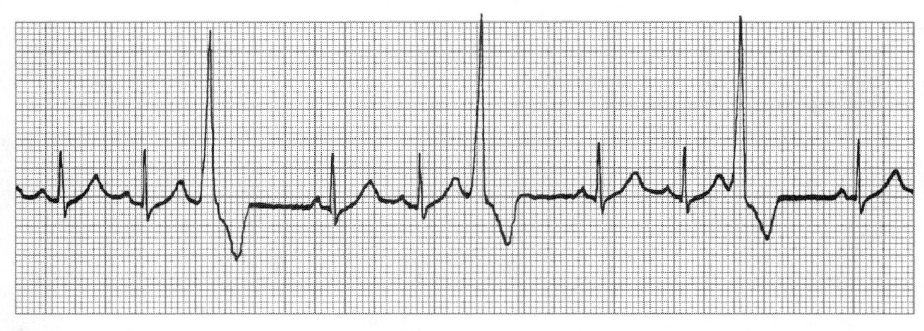

Upper: Note the ectopic focus site originating in the ventricles. The spread of depolarization cannot follow the normal, fast conduction pathway and takes longer to spread throughout the heart.
Lower: The EKG shows normal sinus rhythm (NSR) with early, wide, bizarre QRS complexes, premature ventricular contractions (PVCs). The wide QRS reflects ventricular origin due to the prolonged length of time needed for depolarization. PVCs occur in patients with heart disease and can warn of more serious disease or lethal dysrhythmias or can be benign. PVCs are also common in healthy people due to stress, too much caffeine, anxiety, or medications and are typically benign.
Source: (*upper*) Courtesy of George Kyriakidis/Santa Ana, CA

Conduction Abnormalities

- Delay in the conduction of impulses results in either prolonged conduction intervals (widened QRS) or in heart block (e.g., 2nd° AV block).
- Presence of an accessory (alternative, additional) pathway results in an impulse circling back and prematurely reentering parts of the heart, known as reentry dysrhythmias. This early reactivation causes fast dysrhythmias. Impulses can travel through AV node down toward the ventricle and reenter the atria through the accessory pathway. In A, the impulse first travels down the AV node and reenters the atria through the accessory pathway. In B, the impulses travel down the accessory pathway and return up the AV node to the atria. These are almost always tachydysrhythmias.

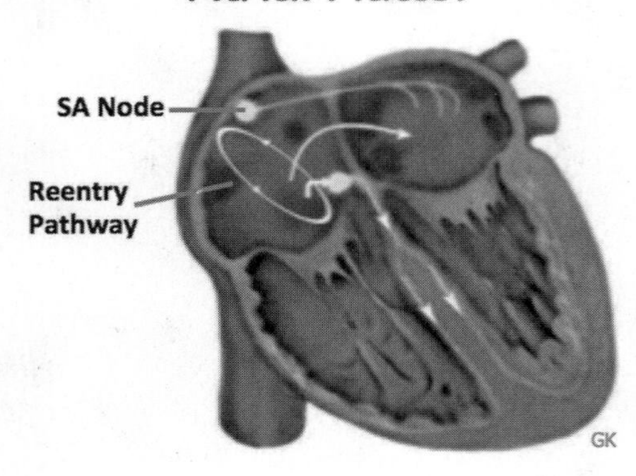

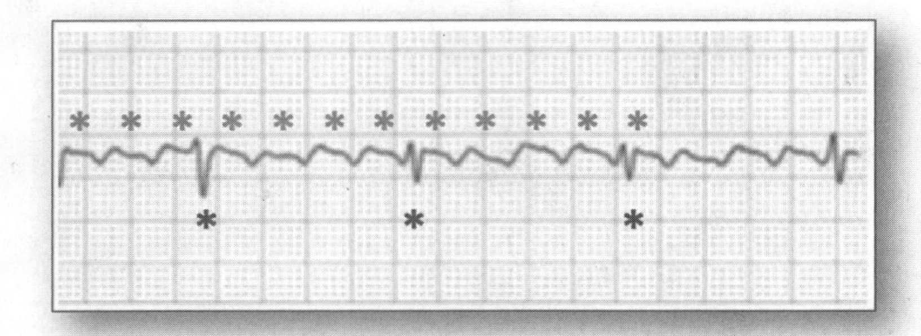

Upper: The image depicts the circular and rapid path of the impulse as it reenters the atria repeatedly, causing the rapid reentrant dysrhythmia known as atrial flutter. The rate of the reentrant impulses exceeds the number of impulses that the AV node can conduct, so many are blocked.
Lower: Atrial flutter is seen as an example of reentry, with its rapid circular conduction (red asterisks). The AV node is blocking three of every four impulses and keeps the ventricular rate (blue asterisks) controlled or below 100 beats per minute.
Sources: (*upper*) Courtesy of George Kyriakidis/Santa Ana, CA; (*lower*) Courtesy of K. Kyriakidis

LO2:

Pathophysiology

- Dysrhythmias can compromise hemodynamics, particularly at very fast and very slow heart rates. When dysrhythmias occur, the heart cannot pump blood efficiently and, if sufficiently compromised, cardiac output and tissue perfusion drop.
- Tachycardias do not allow adequate diastolic filling of the heart prior to contraction, so arterial pressure and output immediately fall (see example). Tachycardias also increase the oxygen demand on the heart and may cause ischemia.
- Similarly, bradycardias can compromise perfusion when there are too few contractions per minute.
- Some dysrhythmias, such as ventricular fibrillation, result in no stroke volume.

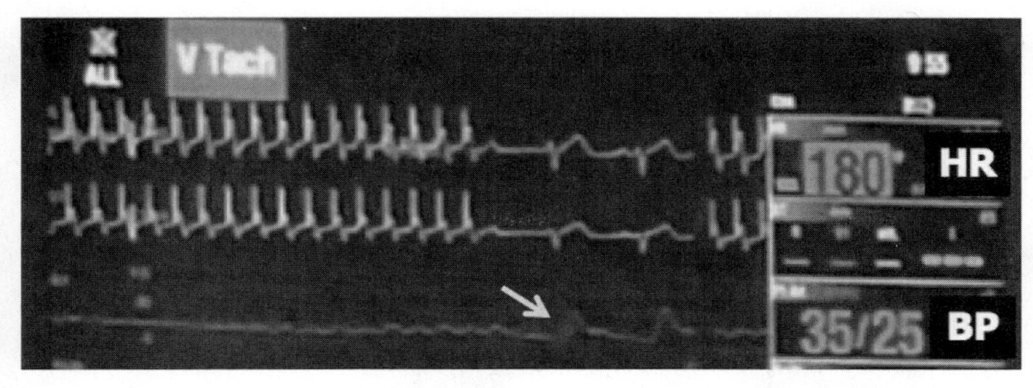

This EKG strip shows V tach (green) with spontaneous conversion to sinus rhythm. Note the dramatic increase in arterial pressure (red) from 32/25 to 88/35, which coincides with the conversion to sinus rhythm. This image illustrates the effect that dysrhythmias can have on cardiac output and stroke volume.
Source: Courtesy of Dr. Jaime Sosa/Medellin, Colombia

Causes and Risk Factors

Dysrhythmias can be caused by a variety of factors including hypoxia, disturbances in electrolytes (particularly potassium, possibly magnesium), and structural abnormalities of the heart. Other common causes include:

- Coronary artery disease
- Heart failure
- Cardiomyopathy
- Thyroid problems
- Fluid and electrolyte imbalances
- Valvular disease
- Congenital defects
- Inflammatory processes
- Autonomic dysfunction
- Medications
- Drugs and alcohol use (caffeine)
- Myocardial infections

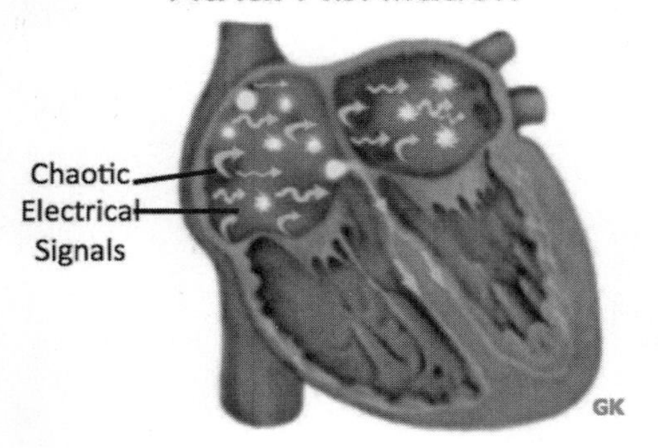

Atrial fibrillation is a common dysrhythmia with many causes. The image shows multiple, simultaneous electrical impulses firing throughout the atria. The chaotic impulses bombard the AV node, which allows few impulses to conduct into the ventricles.
Source: Courtesy of George Kyriakidis/Santa Ana, CA

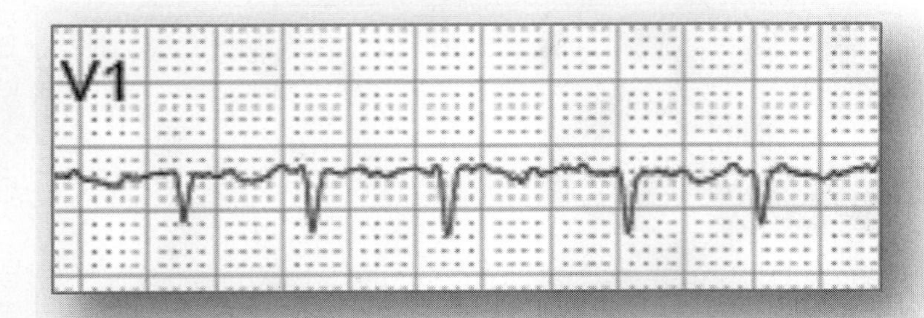

The story of a 53-year-old man illustrates how dysrhythmias and their cause can manifest. The patient presented in good health with new onset tachycardia, weight loss, exhaustion, dyspnea, and palpitations. Atrial fibrillation was noted on EKG. Hyperthyroidism was diagnosed as the cause and treated.
Source: Courtesy of K. Kyriakidis

Assessment Findings

The physical signs of dysrhythmias range from asymptomatic to dramatic:

- Light-headedness, dizziness
- Palpitations, tachycardia, bradycardia
- Shortness of breath, tachypnea
- Hypotension
- Pulse may be regular or irregular
- Pulse may be thready or absent
- Syncope, loss of consciousness
- Chest pain or discomfort

Diagnostics

Electrophysiologic Diagnostic Tools

- A 12-lead EKG is the most commonly used method to diagnose a dysrhythmia:

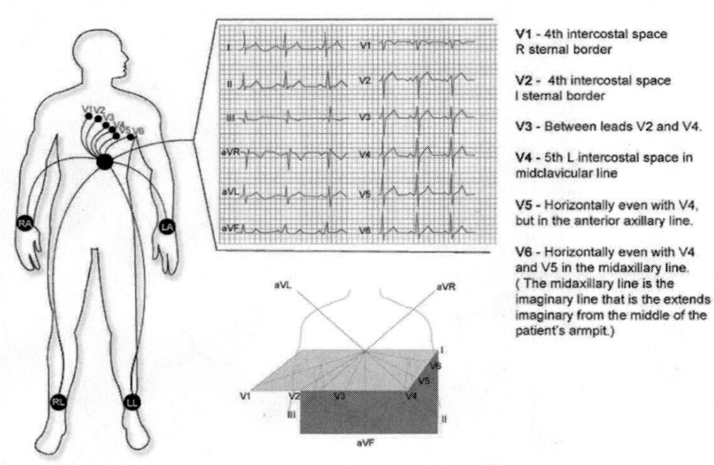

V1 - 4th intercostal space
R sternal border
V2 - 4th intercostal space
l sternal border
V3 - Between leads V2 and V4.
V4 - 5th L intercostal space in
midclavicular line
V5 - Horizontally even with V4,
but in the anterior axillary line.
V6 - Horizontally even with V4
and V5 in the midaxillary line.
(The midaxillary line is the
imaginary line that is the extends
imaginary from the middle of the
patient's armpit.)
RA
LA
RL
LL
aVL
aVR
aVF

This image depicts how an EKG is obtained and an example of the information that it provides. It also shows how electrical impulses traveling in multiple directions are recorded.
Source: Copyright © 2013, NovEx Novice to Expert Learning, LLC

- Nurses in hospitals and outpatient settings often monitor patients by using a few chest leads (3 or 5) to assess a patient's heart rhythm. It is important to verify a dysrhythmia by assuring that the monitor is functioning and leads are properly placed prior to assessment. Monitor artifacts or disconnection can mimic lethal dysrhythmias.
- A variation of monitoring is a 24-hr rhythm exam, often called a Holter exam.

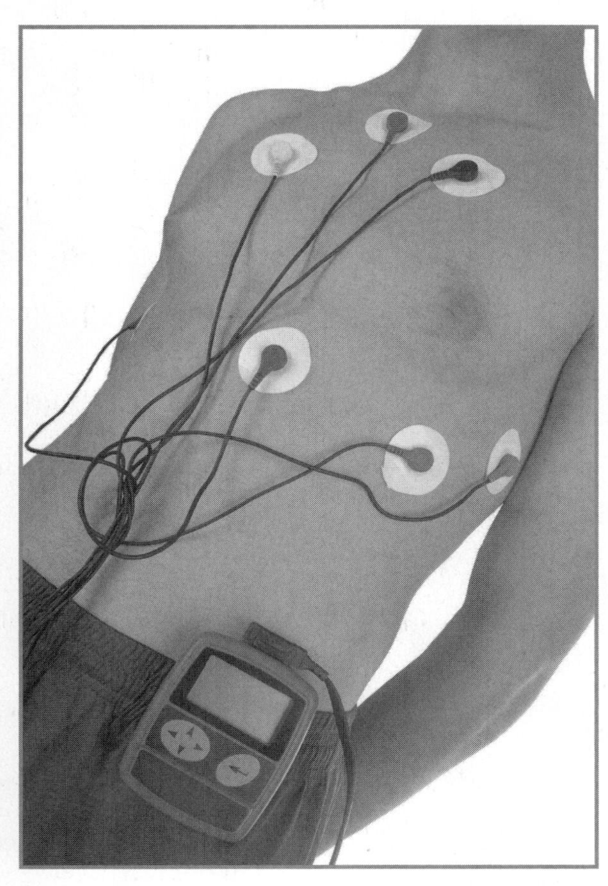

Patient with Holter monitor.
Source: papa1266/Fotolia

- o The Holter monitor records cardiac rhythm for a designated amount of time (usually 24 hours) to capture any irregularities.
- o A 12-lead EKG is more specific in identifying some types of dysrhythmias.
- Electrophysiological studies is another precise way to identify the type and origin of dysrhythmias.

Assessing the Rhythm

Accurate rhythm interpretation is predicated on accurate and thorough assessment of the complexes and intervals. The development of a systematic assessment is the basis of an accurate interpretation as it sets up one's ability to reason accurately. Steps should include:

- P waves:
  - o Normal (upward), abnormal, or absent? All look the same?
  - o P-P intervals, regular or irregular?
  - o Atrial rate normal, fast, or slow?
- PR interval:
  - o Normal, short, prolonged, or absent?
  - o Are PR intervals the same (constant)? If no, is there a pattern of variation?
- QRS complexes:
  - o Normal (for the lead), abnormally wide, or absent? Constant?
  - o QRS width, normal, prolonged, variable with pattern or variable with no pattern?
  - o R-R intervals, regular or irregular?
  - o Ventricular rate, normal, fast, or slow?
- P-P = R-R (to define the relationship between the atria and ventricles)? Is there a P wave in front of every QRS?
- ST segment, elevation or depression—this is only interpreted on a 12-lead EKG
- QT interval, normal, short, or prolonged? Constant?

Each component above must be assessed to accurately interpret dysrhythmias, unless they are lethal. This method provides the information needed to determine if the rhythm is normal or abnormal.

Diagnostics (continued)

Differentiating Normal Versus Abnormal Rhythms

Listed below are the expected normals for each EKG component in order to determine the presence of a dysrhythmia.

Rate	60 – 100 bpm (atrial & ventricular)
Rhythm	P - P intervals are consistent & regular throughout R - R intervals are consistent & regular throughout P-P equals R-R
P Waves	Positive (upright in Lead II), monomorphic
PQRST	One P wave precedes every QRS
PR Interval	0.12 - 0.20 seconds, constant
QRS	≤ 0.12 seconds
QT interval	≤ 0.44 seconds

Dysrhythmia Interpretation

Once the diagnostic results are obtained, the challenge is determining whether or not a dysrhythmia is present. If so, one must then interpret what kind of dysrhythmia before appropriate interventions can be implemented. The most common dysrhythmias that require diagnosis include:

- **Sinus Dysrhythmias**
  - Normal Sinus Rhythm
  - Normal Sinus Rhythm with Interference
  - Pulseless Electrical Activity
  - Sinus Tachycardia
  - Sinus bradycardia
  - Asystole (no rhythm)
- **Atrial Dysrhythmias**
  - Premature Atrial Contraction (PAC)
  - Atrial Tachycardia
  - Atrial Flutter
  - Atrial Fibrillation
  - Paroxysmal Supraventricular Tachycardia
- **AV Nodal Heart Blocks**
  - 1st degree AV block
  - 2nd degree AV block, Mobitz type I (Wenckebach)
  - 2nd degree AV block, Mobitz type II
  - 3rd degree AV block
  - Paced Rhythm (treatment for AV block)
- **Ventricular**
  - Premature Ventricular Contractions (PVC)
  - Ventricular tachycardia
  - Ventricular fibrillation

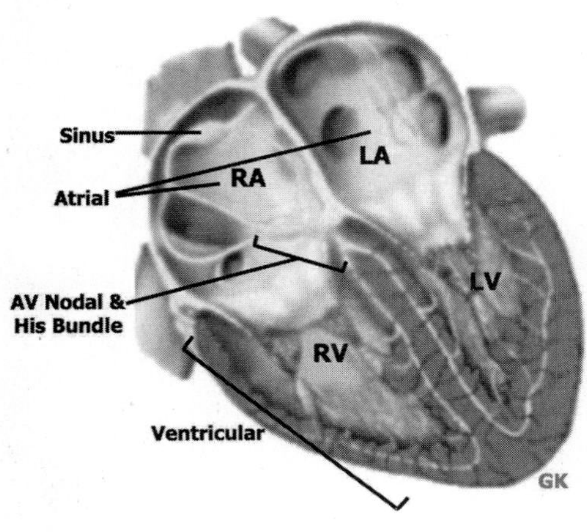

The diagram depicts the general locations of the dysrhythmia origins within the cardiac conduction system.
Source: Courtesy of George Kyriakidis/Santa Ana, CA

Concept Check

3. What is the normal length of the PR interval?
   A. 0.60–1.0 seconds
   B. 0.12–0.20 seconds
   C. 0.05–0.12 seconds
   D. 0.14–0.44 seconds

Answer question

Concept Check

4. Which monitor type provides the most specific information about dysrhythmias?
   A. 3-lead
   B. 5-lead
   C. Holter
   D. 12-lead

Answer question

Priority Patient Concerns and Desired Collaborative Care Outcomes

Prior to caring for patients with dysrhythmias, it is important to prioritize the patient's concerns that must guide the nursing care plan and interventions. Care for the patient is ordered and organized in accordance with the patient's priority and urgent needs. Desired collaborative care outcomes in patients with dysrhythmias typically include:

1. Patient will have no further decrease in cardiac output.
2. Patient will have no evidence of myocardial damage.
3. Patient will have no evidence of stroke.
4. Patient's peripheral tissues will remain intake with no damage.
5. Patient's demeanor will be calm.
6. Patient will report no chest pain.

Considering these important care outcomes, prepare a list of the major 3–6 priority patient concerns or nursing diagnoses for patients with dysrhythmias. Be prepared to participate in a discussion of this list and/or to submit them as an assignment, as determined by your faculty. Resources you may find helpful in this assignment can include this lesson, the references, resources on nursing care plans, and standard nursing diagnoses manuals.

Interpreting Sinus Dysrhythmias

Normal Sinus Rhythm

Normal Sinus Rhythm (NSR) occurs when the heart's natural pacemaker is automatically initiating normal impulses and controls the heart's rate and rhythm. Any rhythm that does not meet the criteria for NSR is considered a dysrhythmia. Below are examples of NSR configurations.

Criteria and Example

- P-P: regular, rate 60–100 bpm, upright and monomorphic (same shape) P waves
- PR: normal (0.12–0.20 sec); constant
- QRS: normal <0.12 sec
- R-R: regular, rate 60–100 bpm
- ST segment: this must be interpreted from a 12-lead EKG
- QT: normal and <0.44 sec
- P-P = R-R: yes, meaning that one P wave is always present prior to a QRS complex and that this is a constant relationship

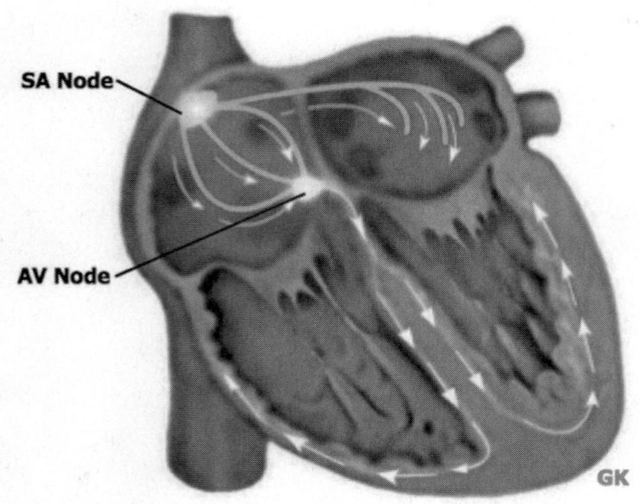

The SA node is depicted as initiating the electrical impulse, which then depolarizes both atria toward the AV node.
Source: Courtesy of George Kyriakidis/Santa Ana, CA

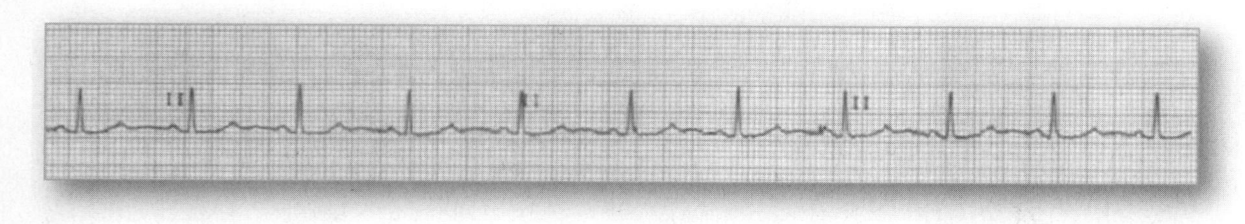

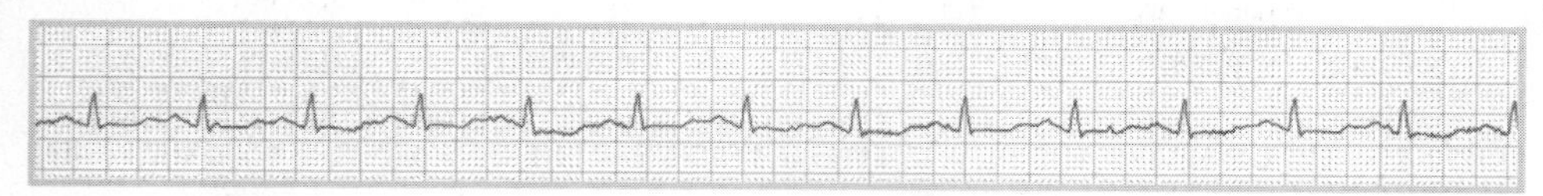

Upper: NSR: P waves upright and monomorphic, atrial & ventricular rate = 78, PR = 0.14, P-P = R-R, QRS = 0.08, QT = 0.40
Lower: NSR: P waves upright and monomorphic, atrial & ventricular rates = 88, PR = 0.18, P-P = R-R, QRS = 0.11, QT = 0.41
Source: (*both*) Courtesy of K. Kyriakidis

Normal Sinus Rhythm with Interference

- **Normal Sinus Rhythm** (NSR) with interference occurs when extraneous electrical or muscular activity is produced or an EKG electrode/lead comes loose.
- With a loose electrode, the baseline is extremely erratic, but QRSs can be seen and remain regular.
- The electrical waves with tremors and interference are too rapid and narrow to reflect actual cardiac activity. Most striking is that the R-Rs can be "marched through" or measured at a constant interval through the interference.
- Although each of these EKG patterns are bizarre and can appear problematic, accurate assessment would discount a real dysrhythmia.
- N Treatment: Troubleshoot the cause to correct the problem so that the patient may be adequately monitored and cared for.

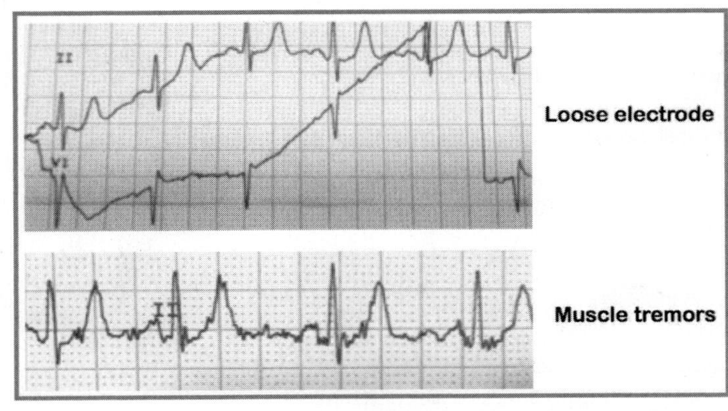

Normal sinus rhythm is seen with (1) a loose electrode causing an erratic baseline and (2) muscle tremor interference mimicking an atrial fibrillation-like baseline except that the P waves and QRS complexes are easily seen. NSR can been seen and the PQRST can be "marched through" the interference.
Source: Courtesy of K. Kyriakidis

Pulseless Electrical Activity

Pulseless Electrical Activity (PEA) occurs when the heart's electrical activity continues even in normal sinus rhythm, but the patient has no pulse.

- One must always be aware that the monitor does not reveal the patient's hemodynamic state or cardiac output. Most of the time, if there is normal electrical activity, the patient has the expected mechanical contraction of the heart. But touching the patient, talking to him or her, and ensuring there is a pulse is at the heart of good care.
- M N Treatment: If there is no pulse, immediately initiate basic life support and call a code for help.

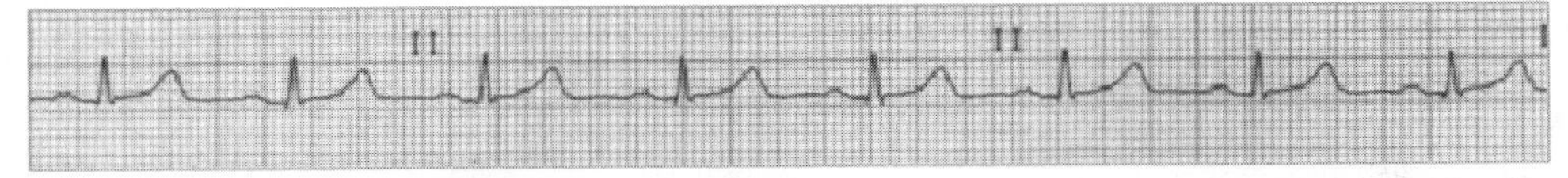

This sinus rhythm + No pulse = Pulseless Electrical Activity = No Cardiac Output
Source: Courtesy of K. Kyriakidis

Interpreting Sinus Dysrhythmias (continued)

Sinus Tachycardia

Sinus tachycardia is diagnosed when the HR is >100 bpm but the rhythm is constant and originates in the SA node.

Criteria (same as NSR except rate) and Example:

- P-P: regular, rate >100 bpm, upright and monomorphic
- PR: normal (0.12–0.20 sec); constant
- QRS: normal <0.12 sec
- R-R: regular, rate >100 bpm
- ST segment: this must be interpreted from a 12-lead EKG
- QT: normal <0.44 sec.
- P-P = R-R: yes, with 1:1 and constant P:QRS relationship
- This rhythm is not lethal and often noted with physical activity, fever, fight and flight responses, and hypovolemia. It is commonly seen as a compensatory mechanism for other disturbances.

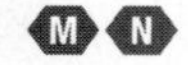

- Treatment is usually related to removing or correcting the cause (e.g., infection, dehydration, shock, compromised cardiac output). Treating the tachycardia itself may worsen or mask the condition. Treat the underlying cause, if needed.

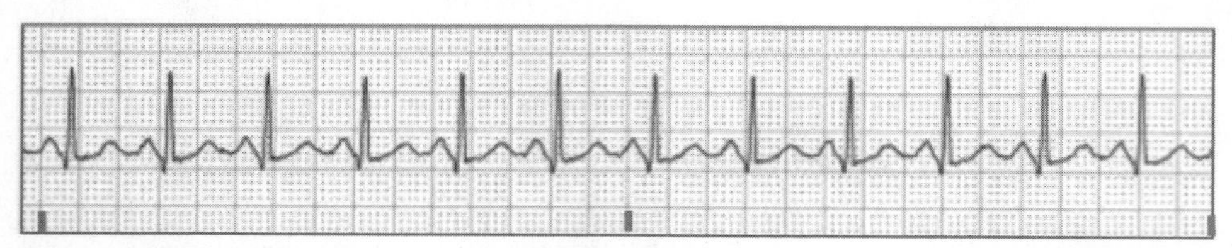

Note the example of sinus tachycardia. In this 6-second strip (red marker at bottom = 3 sec intervals), the rate is approximately 120–130.

Source: Courtesy of K. Kyriakidis

Sinus Bradycardia

Sinus bradycardia is a result of decreased rate of impulse generation by the SA node. Sinus bradycardia is diagnosed when the HR is less than 60 bpm and a regular rhythm including constant P-P and P-R intervals.

Criteria (same as NSR except rate) and Example:

- P-P: regular, rate >60 bpm, upright in lead II and monomorphic
- PR: normal (0.12–0.20 sec); constant
- QRS: normal <0.12 sec
- R-R: regular, <60 bpm
- P-P = R-R: yes, with 1:1 and constant P:QRS relationship

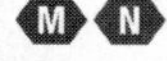

Treatment: For many patients who are healthy and exercise, their resting pulse may be less than 60 bpm. No treatment is indicated. Unless the patient is symptomatic, most bradycardias are not treated but watched.

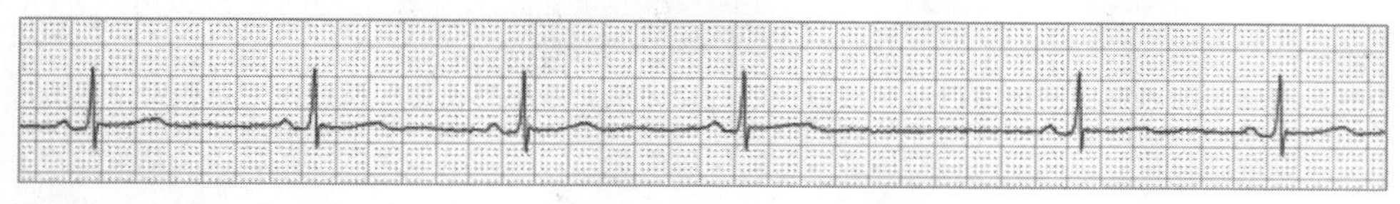

This is an example of sinus bradycardia with a heart rate of about 46 beats per minute. This particular rhythm additionally has a sinus arrhythmia or slightly irregular firing of the SA node so the the P-P is not consistently regular.

Source: Courtesy of K. Kyriakidis

Asystole

Asystole occurs when all electrical activity in the heart fails, no pacemaker cells fire, and therefore no cardiac contractions are produced. There is simply a flatline. It is the only true arrhythmia.

- P-P: absent
- PR: absent
- QRS: absent

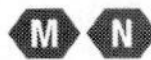

- Treatment: Asystole is the most lethal dysrhythmia. Immediate, aggressive CPR and medical interventions are required to save the patient's life.

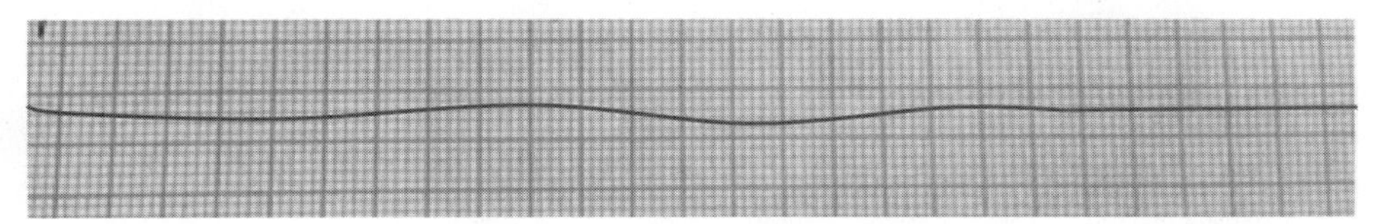

Asystole.
Source: Courtesy of K. Kyriakidis

Treatment for Asystole and PEA:

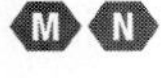

- When a clinician identifies a patient in asystole, basic and advanced cardiac life support (BCLS and ACLS) must be initiated immediately. Call for rapid response team and/or health care provider as assistance is urgently needed.

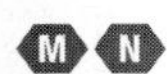

- Following the treatment guidelines, once an IV line is established, epinephrine 1 mg every 3–5 minutes should be given per protocol. Vasopressin can be administered instead. Other medications (atropine) and pacing have not proven to be effective.

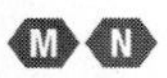

- The most important treatment is to find the underlying cause and treat it. This may include: hypoxia, hyper/hypokalemia, hypothermia, drug overdose, myocardial infarction, hypovolemia, pulmonary embolism, cardiac tamponade, tension pneumothorax, hypoglycemia, and acidosis. The cause should urgently be identified and corrected.

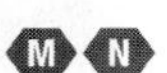

- Health care providers should know or collaborate with the patient and/or family to determine the patient's code preference, particularly in patients who are at high risk for life-threatening events.
- Despite immediate and excellent care, outcomes for patients experiencing asystole are very poor. Asystole, following defibrillation, has even worse outcomes.

Interpreting Atrial Dysrhythmias

Premature Atrial Contractions

Premature atrial contractions (PACs) are impulses that arise from an ectopic focus (outside of the SA node) within the atria. The P wave shape or morphology appears different than the SA nodal P waves and present early.

Criteria and Example:

- P-P: regular, except the early ectopic beat, P wave morphology (shape) differs, earlier than P-P of NSR
- PR: varies from, often longer than, the regular PR interval.
- QRS: normal <0.12 sec
- R-R: shorter R-R with ectopic beat followed by a longer R-R (known as a compensatory pause for longer repolarization, R-R regular for NSR)
- P-P = R-R: yes, with 1:1 and constant P:QRS relationship

If the PAC is very early, the AV node may not conduct it (not yet repolarized), so no QRS follows. This is a benign dysrhythmia and the patient tends to be asymptomatic.

- Treatment: Usually, no treatment is indicated. With frequent, multifocal (multiple origins) PACs, identify and treat the underlying cause when indicated.

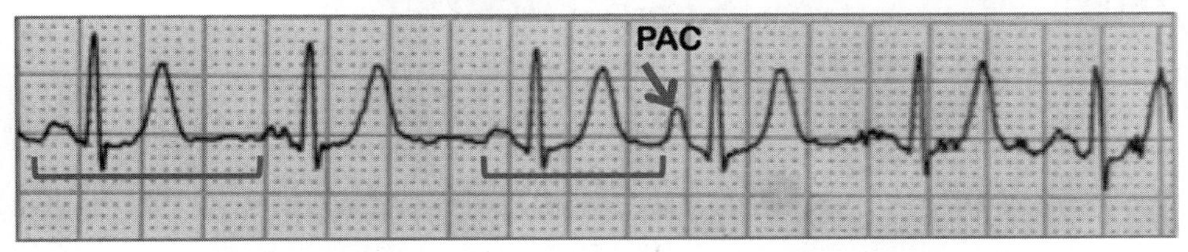

This EKG shows normal sinus rhythm with premature atrial contractions. Notice the peaked and early P wave with QRS. The timing and morphology of the early P wave signals that its origin differs from the SA nodal P wave. Also characteristic is the shortened P-P and R-R interval in the PAC.
Source: Courtesy of K. Kyriakidis

Atrial Tachycardia

Atrial tachycardia is a type of supraventricular tachycardia that originates from an ectopic atrial focus, outside the SA node. It is typically not lethal. However, it may require nursing interventions, depending on symptoms.

Criteria and Example:

- P-P: regular if visible, P wave morphology differs from NSR; rate 140–220 bpm, upright, may gradually accelerate at onset
- PR: constant, may vary from regular PR
- QRS: normal <0.12 sec
- R-R: constant, rate same as atria
- P-P = R-R: yes, with 1:1 and constant P:QRS relationship
- Treatment:
  1. Vagal or valsalva maneuvers, such as coughing or bearing down to mimic a bowel movement, may be attempted as they have the least potentially harmful consequences.
  2. A certified health care provider may attempt carotid massage, a vagal maneuver that carries a higher risk.
  3. Adenosine 6 mg IV may be given. If unresponsive, Adenosine 12 mg may be given. If the patient is still unresponsive, collaborate with physician about whether Adenosine 12 mg is again administered or a different intervention is preferred.
  4. Synchronized cardioversion is initiated at any point if the patient becomes unstable.

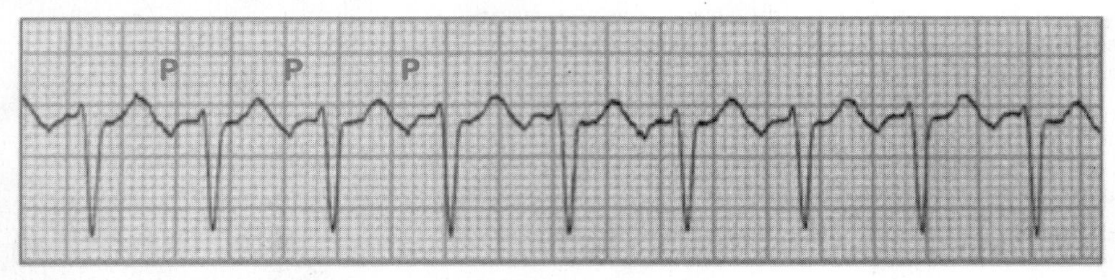

In this V1 lead, the visible, regular P waves, although inverted, indicate an atrial tachycardia with normal conduction through the ventricles (QRS <0.10). Heart rate is 140 bpm.

Atrial Flutter

Atrial flutter is a rapid but regular dysrhythmia that originates from an atrial ectopic focus and continues in a self-sustaining loop. The rate is fast (>100 bpm) and typically has a block (not all the impulse pass through the AV node to the ventricles) associated with the rhythm producing a sawtooth pattern in the EKG. The faster the heart rate, the greater the patient's hemodynamic compromise.

Criteria and Examples:

- P-P: P waves absent; regular flutter waves often discernable, "sawtooth" pattern morphology, rate typically 300 (range 240–340)
- PR: AV node block 1–4 flutter waves for each one that conducts
- QRS: usually normal <0.12 sec
- R-R: typically 2:1 conduction pattern; usually regular
- P-P does not equal R-R: is a ratio of the flutter waves (2:1, 3:1, 4:1)

Treatment: If patient is stable, antiarrhythmic medications can be used to slow the rate or return it to NSR. If unstable, cardiovert starting at low energy.

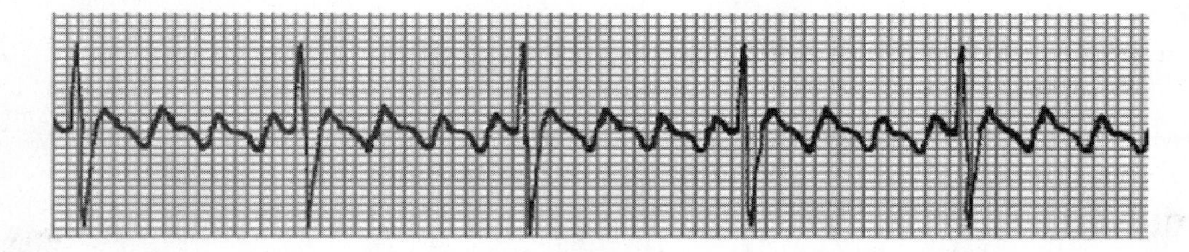

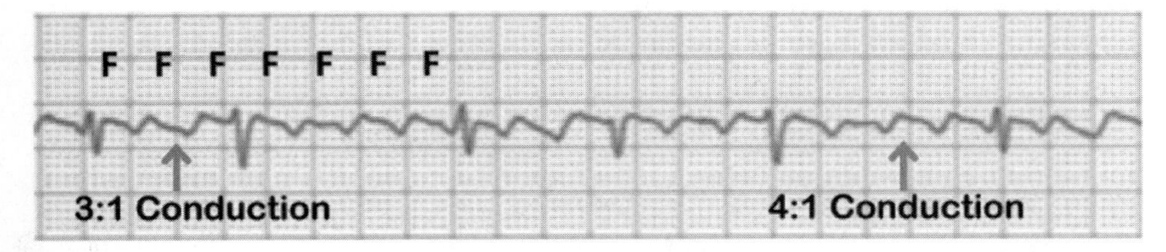

Upper: Atrial flutter with a 4:1 conduction (i.e., only one out of every four flutter waves conducts through the AV node). Lower: Atrial flutter with variable degrees of conduction. 3:1 conduction means one atrial flutter impulse of three is conducted through the AV node into the ventricles.
Source: (*lower*) Courtesy of K. Kyriakidis

Interpreting Atrial Dysrhythmias (continued)

Atrial Fibrillation

Atrial fibrillation (A-fib) is one of the most common of the atrial tachycardias. Normally the rhythm is not lethal but can produce severe symptoms that include exercise limitations, shortness of breath (SOB), syncope, and stroke when thrombi are present. A-fib is often associated with cardiac pathology.

- The rhythm is characteristically irregular (R-R intervals occur randomly and variably). QRS duration is usually normal.

Criteria and Example:

- P-P: no P waves, chaotic baseline of rapid atrial activation, rate is 300–600 bpm, coarse A-fib can appear similar to flutter, but is irregular
- PR: none
- QRS: normal <0.12 sec
- R-R: irregularly irregular, rate often 90–170 bpm
- P-P does not equal R-R: no relationship

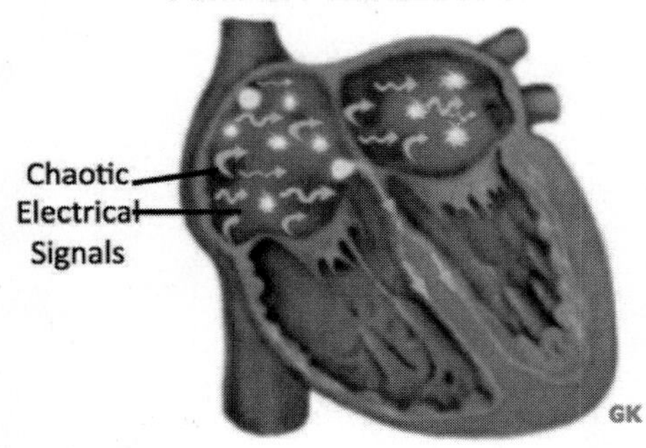

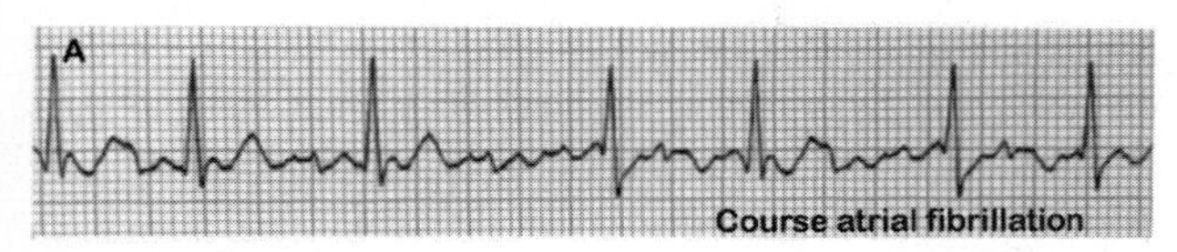

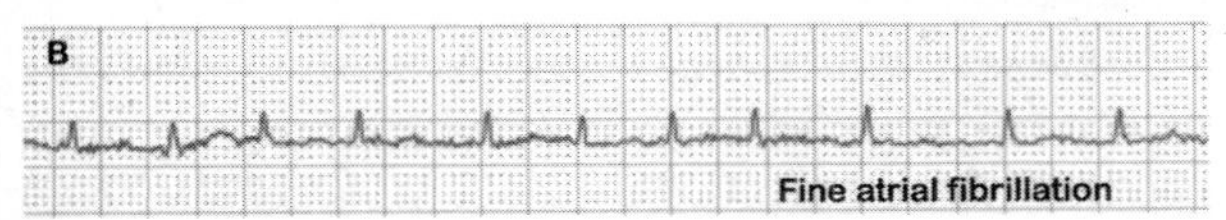

Upper: The image depicts the mechanism of atrial fibrillation. Middle: In this EKG showing course A-fib, the baseline is coursely fluctuating and irratic. Lower: In contrast, this EKG demonstrates a finely fluctuating baseline. In both dysrhythmias, P waves are absent and the R-Rs are irregular.
Sources: (*upper*) George Kyriakidis/Santa Ana, CA; (*lower*) Courtesy of K. Kyriakidis

- In A-fib, atrial contraction, which normally contributes 15% of diastolic filling for stroke volume, is lost. This is referred to as losing the "atrial kick." Cardiac output is further compromised due to the decreased ventricular filling time with the rapid heart rate that often accompanies A-fib.

Treatment:

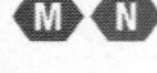

- Because blood passively flows through the quivering atria in A-fib, blood easily pools, predisposing to clot formation. Anticoagulation is needed to prevent potential emboli to the lungs and brain.

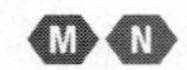

- A-fib can be treated with antiarrhythmic drugs, medications to reduce heart rate, and if unstable, synchronized cardioversion. Medications that reduce heart rate include beta blockers and calcium channel blockers (e.g., verapamil, diltiazem).

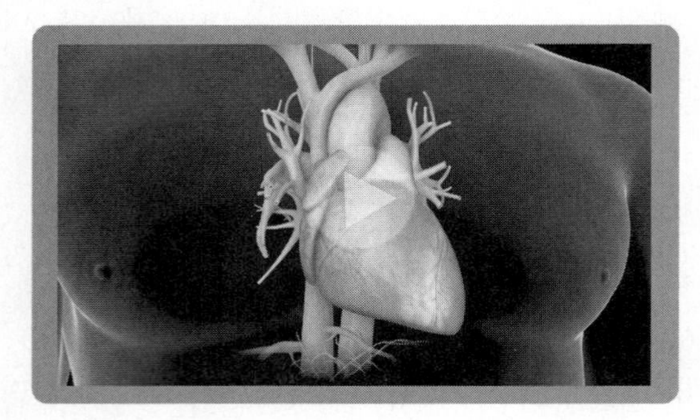

This animation shows what happens during A-fib, the risks associated with having A-fib and the common treatments for A-fib. A-fib is an abnormality in the pace or force of your heartbeat. In A-fib, the heart's upper chambers contract in a fast, twitching fashion, resulting in an irregular, uncoordinated heartbeat.

- Prevention of complications due to A-Fib
  - o A-fib is the most common dysrhythmia encountered. Clot formed in the atria can dislodge and embolize to the brain and cause a stroke.

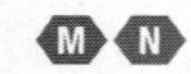

  - o To prevent emboli, patients are usually anticoagulated with either warfarin or thrombin inhibitors. The advantage of thrombin inhibitors is that INR does not need to be monitored.

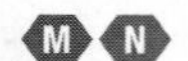

  - o Patients at high risk for falls and bleeding are sometimes treated with aspirin instead.

Interpreting Atrial Dysrhythmias (continued)

Paroxysmal Supraventricular Tachycardia (PSVT)

PSVT is an extremely fast reentrant tachycardia. Paroxysmal means intermittent, with an abrupt onset and stop. Supraventricular refers to the ectopic focus being above the ventricles, noted by the narrow QRS, but is often unidentifiable. Reentrant refers to the dual pathway in its pathogenesis.

SVT is a rapid, narrow complex tachycardia that meets the same criteria but either does not have an abrupt onset or endpoint or where the onset or endpoint are not observed is known as a supraventricular tachycardia (SVT).

Criteria and Example:

- P-P: usually hidden in T waves of the preceding beats, regular if visible, rate 150–250 bpm; P-P is not discernible in SVT
- PR: constant if measurable
- QRS: typically normal <0.12 sec
- R-R: usually regular, rate same as atria
- P-P = R-R: yes, with 1:1 and constant P:QRS relationship

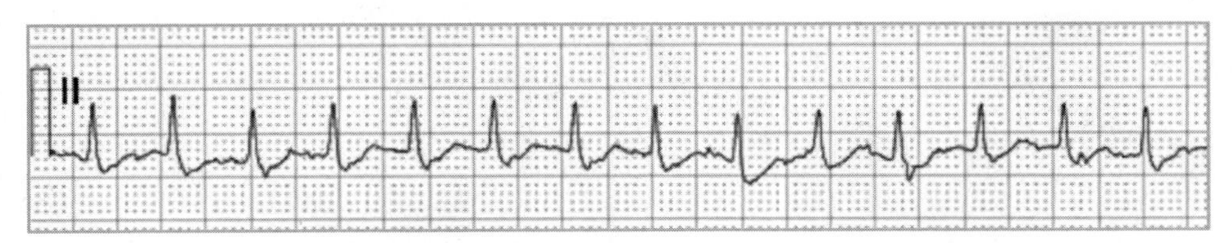

This rhythm is considered to be a SVT rather than PSVT because the onset or endpoints were not observed. The rhythm has a narrow QRS, which indicates that the initiating focus is above the ventricles (supraventricular). The heart rate is about 167 bpm, making it a tachycardia. Upon close examination of the baseline, there is no consistent hint of a P wave which differentiates this dysrhythmia from an atrial tachycardia.

Source: Courtesy of K. Kyriakidis

Concept Check

5. **What is a common feature of atrial fibrillation?**
   A. Irregular rhythm
   B. Shortened QRS duration
   C. Inverted P wave
   D. Peaked T wave

Answer question

Rapid heart rate in PSVT often causes dizziness and shortness of breath.

- Treatment for PSVT and SVT:

M N 1. Vagal or valsalva maneuvers, such as coughing or bearing down to mimic a bowel movement, may be attempted as they have the least potentially harmful consequences.

M N 2. A certified health care provider may attempt carotid massage, a vagal maneuver that carries a higher risk.

M N 3. Adenosine 6 mg IV may be given. If unresponsive, Adenosine 12 mg may be given. If the patient is still unresponsive, collaborate with physician about whether Adenosine 12 mg is again administered or a different intervention is preferred.

M N 4. Synchronized cardioversion is initiated at any point if the patient becomes unstable.

Interpreting AV Heart Blocks

Classification of AV Heart Blocks

- An AV nodal heart block occurs when there is a delay, block, or dissociation in the AV nodal area of the conduction pathways of the heart.
- Some of the heart blocks are relatively benign, while others require rapid interventions.
- There are four categories of AV heart blocks:
  - o 1st° AV block
  - o 2nd° AV block, Mobitz Type I or Wenckebach
  - o 2nd° AV block, Mobitz Type II
  - o 3rd° AV block or complete AV block

1st° AV Block

1st° AV block occurs when there is a delay in conduction through the AV node. It is defined by a prolonged PR interval. It is fairly common and benign. 1st° AV block is diagnosed when the P-R interval is constant but >0.20 sec.

Criteria (same as NSR except the PR interval) and Example:

- P-P: regular, upright, and monomorphic
- PR: prolonged >0.20 sec; constant
- QRS: normal <0.12 sec
- R-R: regular
- P-P = R-R: yes, with 1:1 and constant P:QRS relationship
- N Treatment consists of monitoring for symptoms and for progression to second and third degree blocks.

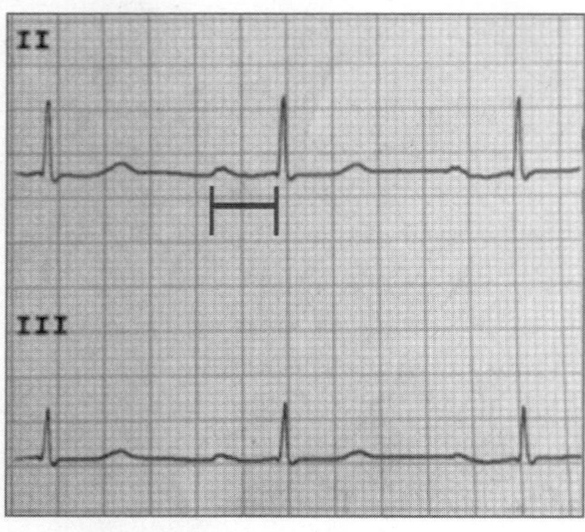

In this rhythm, note the prolonged, but constant length of the PR interval. What is the measurement of the PR interval? What is (please calculate) the heart rate? This rhythm demonstrates how two abnormalities can occur together. What do you call this rhythm? (Answer below)
Source: Courtesy of K. Kyriakidis

Answer: The PR interval is .28 sec, making this a 1st° AV block. The heart rate is 58 bpm, categorizing this as a sinus bradycardia. The correct name for this dysrhythmia is a sinus bradycardia with a 1st° AV block.

2nd° AV Block, Mobitz Type I or Wenckebach

2nd° AV block Mobitz Type I occurs when AV nodal conduction progressively takes longer and longer (seen as the P-R interval progressively lengthening) until an impulse is blocked (seen as a QRS complex is dropped). This rhythm is sometimes called Wenckebach. Wenckebach does not typically digress into a complete heart block.

Criteria (same as NSR except rate) and Example:

- P-P: regular, rate 60–100 bpm, upright and monomorphic (same shape) P wave
- PR: progressively lengthens until a QRS fails to follow a P wave
- QRS: normal <0.12 sec
- R-R: progressive shortening in each cycle until the dropped QRS
- P-P does not equal R-R
- Treatment: A Wenckebach block is typically benign and resolves without treatment. The patient should be monitored for any deterioration in the rhythm.

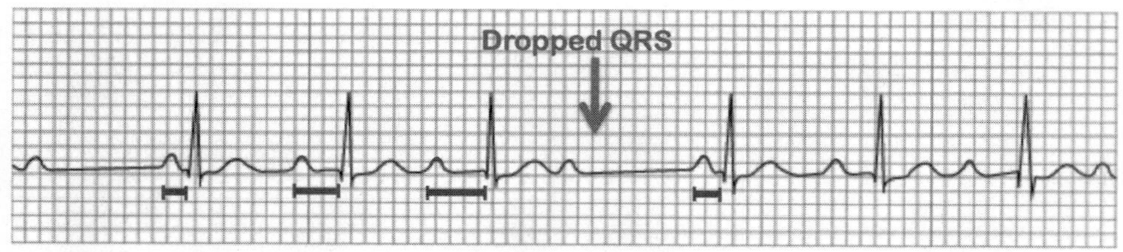

This EKG shows 2nd° AV block Mobitz Type I with the hallmark prolongation of the PR interval until a QRS is suddenly dropped (a P wave seen with the impulse not conducted into the ventricles). During the long pause, the AV node recovers, which allows conduction of the next impulse, and the PR interval shortens again.
Source: Copyright © 2013, NovEx Novice to Expert Learning, LLC

2nd° AV Block, Mobitz Type II

2nd° AV block Mobitz Type II arises from underlying bundle of His disease. Unlike Mobitz I, Mobitz Type II is dangerous due to the risk of progressing to a complete heart block (3rd° AV block). It can be diagnosed when P waves occur without the presence of QRSs—often more than one. Unlike Wenckebach, the PR interval remains constant.

Criteria and Examples:

- P-P: regular, upright and monomorphic
- PR: constant whether normal or prolonged
- QRS: normal <0.12 sec or wide
- R-R: regular until a dropped QRS
- P-P does not equal R-R: constant 1:1 P:QRS relationship until a dropped QRS complex
- There may be only brief warning before digressing into complete AV block.

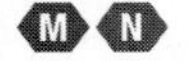

- Treatment commonly requires a pacemaker.

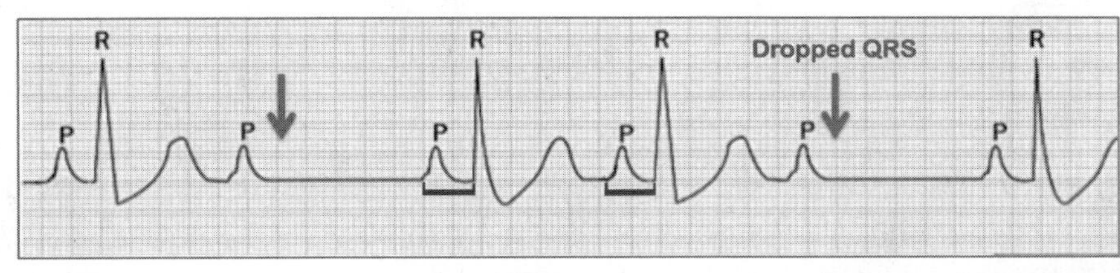

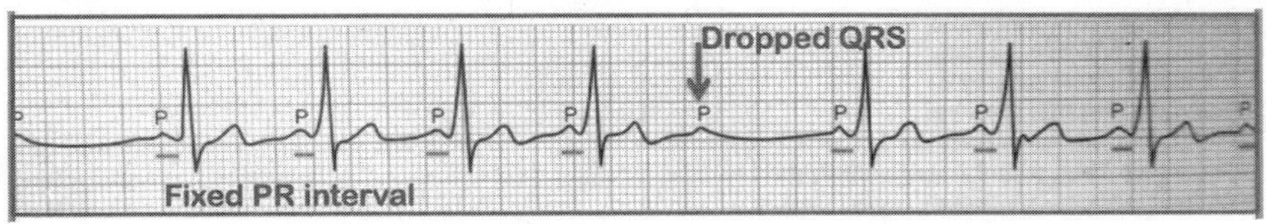

Both EKGs show 2nd° AV block Mobitz Type II with fixed PR intervals and 1:1 P:QRS ratios until the suddenly dropped QRS complex(es), signaling the potential for complete block and cardiac arrest. The upper EKG shows normal ventricular conduction (narrow QRS at 0.10 sec) whereas the lower EKG shows slowed ventricular conduction system (wide QRS at 0.14 sec).

3rd° AV Heart Block

In 3rd° AV block there is no conduction through the AV node/His bundle. If a pacemaker below the atria fires, an AV junctional (narrow QRS) or ventricular escape rhythm (wide QRS) may take over. 3rd° AV block is diagnosed when there is no association between the P waves and the QRS waves. The P waves and QRS complexes occur at constant intervals, but they are not in sync with each other. Without mechanical (pumping) coordination of the atrial and ventricular contractions, cardiac output drops. The ventricular rate often determines the patient's temporary hemodynamic stability. 3rd° AV block is an emergency situation requiring immediate and invasive intervention.

Criteria and Example:

- P-P: regular, rate usually 60–100 bpm, upright and monomorphic
- PR: all variable
- QRS: may be normal or wide, usually monomorphic if present
- R-R: usually constant, rate <60 bpm
- P-P does not equal R-R: P waves have no relationship to QRSs (AV dissociation)

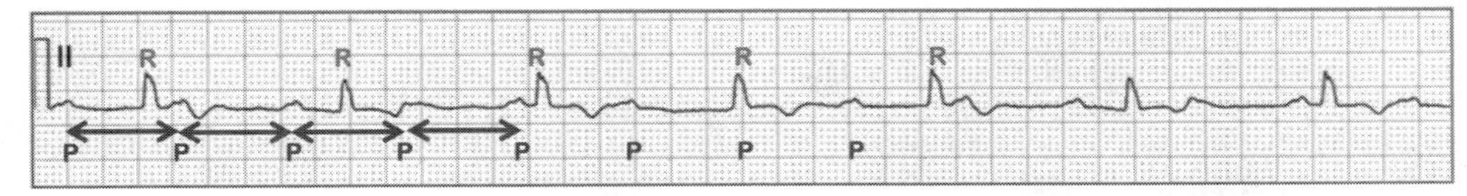

Note that the P-P intervals (blue arrows) and the R-R intervals (red arrows) are constant but different instead of equal. The atrial and ventricular rates are unrelated, with both internally but independently paced (dissociated). the effective heart rate is 53 bpm.

Source: Courtesy of K. Kyriakidis

Interpreting AV Heart Blocks (continued)

Heart Block Treatments

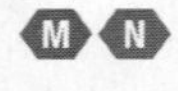

- Patients in 2nd° (Mobitz Type II) and 3rd° AV block urgently need external (transcutaneous) or transvenous pacing until a permanent pacemaker can be inserted. Patients with 3rd° AV block commonly present with dizziness and lightheadedness due to a slow heart rate.

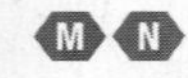

- Emergency medications: During the delay of preparing for pacemaker insertion, epinephrine is the drug of choice for symptomatic and hemodynamically unstable patients with heart block. Levophed and dopamine can be used, when needed, to improve hemodynamic stability.

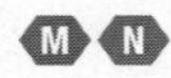

- Review the patient's medications for drugs that can slow conduction through the AV node. These include digoxin, beta blockers, and some calcium channel blockers (e.g., verapamil, diltiazem). Heart blocks are commonly related to myocardial damage so the condition is most often irreversible.

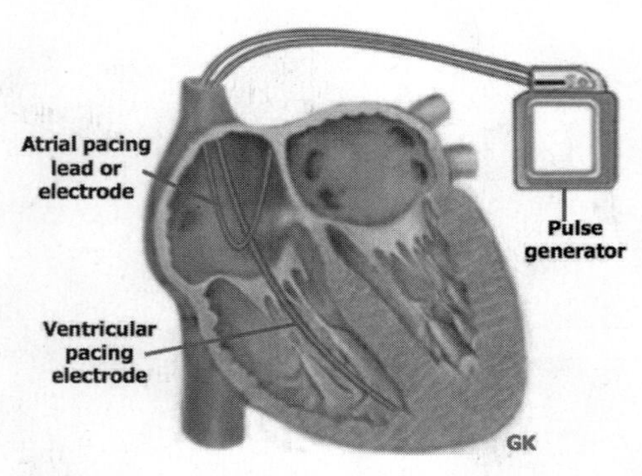

This drawing depicts a permanent pacemaker with pacing wires in both atrium and ventricle. Dual heart chamber pacing provide synchronous pacing to maximize stroke volume.

Source: Courtesy of George Kyriakidis/Santa Ana, CA

Paced Rhythm

A **paced rhythm** is produced by an artificial pacemaker, which generates impulses (seen as spikes) at a specified rate. Using a single chamber (ventricular) pacemaker, the QRSs immediately follow when "capture" occurs, meaning that the ventricles conduct the impulses. However, dual chamber atrioventricular (AV) pacemakers are now common and can produce one, two, or no pacing spikes with accompanying atrial and/or ventricular responses, depending on the ability of the patient's heart to function.

- When the pacemaker does not capture, the EKG then shows only spikes.
- P waves may or may not appear. If the heart initiates its own rhythm and it is faster than the pacemaker, the EKG shows the switch (back and forth) with the patient's own heart taking over temporarily.
- Paced rhythms cause wide, bizarre QRSs because the electrical impulse is initiated in the right ventricular and does not depolarize the ventricles along the normal electrical pathways. At first glance, a paced rhythm can be misinterpreted as V-tach. It is critical to note that the heart rate is <100 bpm and the patient is responsive with a pulse.

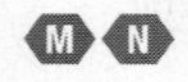

- When a ventricular pacer takes over, atrial kick (15% of the stroke volume) is lost. For borderline heart failure patients, the reduction in cardiac output when pacing is just enough to tip them into heart failure. They need dual atrial ventricular pacing.

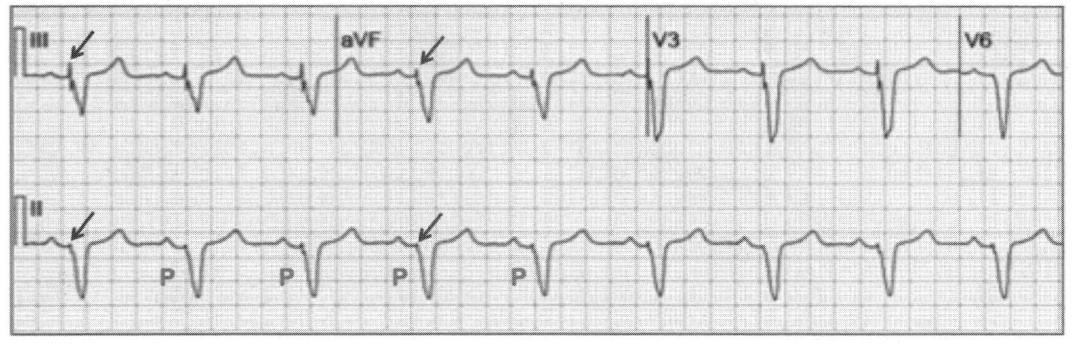

This EKG (4 leads) shows a patient with an AV pacemaker. Atrial pacing spikes are not present because the SA node is firing normally, indicated by the normal, regular P waves. However, very narrow, sharp, short pacing spikes (blue arrows) follow each P wave when the atrial impulse is blocked in the AV node. Ventricular pacing is required so a wide, bizarre QRS follows each pacing spike and reflects "ventricular capture." This EKG shows 1:1 capture, meaning every QRS is initiated by the pacemaker and effectively conducts. The very tall narrow rods, just to the left of the letters aVF, V3, and V6, are simply lead separators on the EKG.

Source: Courtesy of K. Kyriakidis

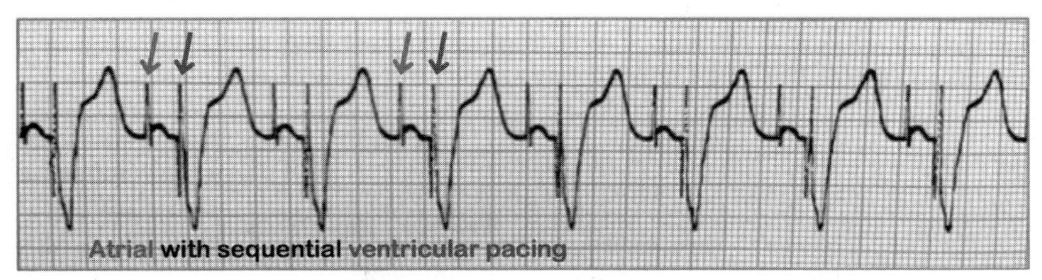

An AV sequential pacing rhythm is noted by the synchronized atrial (red arrows) and ventricular (blue arrows) pacing to maximize cardiac output.

Interpreting Ventricular Dysrhythmias

Premature Ventricular Contractions

Premature ventricular contractions (PVCs) develop from foci in the ventricles rather than in the sinoatrial node. The QRS is widened, and occurs early (prior to the expected QRS). Generally, PVCs are benign and will resolve without incident. These are sometimes experienced by the patient as a sudden pounding in the chest.

Criteria and Examples:

- P-P: regular if visible, upright and monomorphic for underlying NSR; none with PVC
- PR: constant for underlying rhythm, none for PVC
- QRS: normal <0.12 sec for NSR; ectopic PVCs are wide, bizarre and variable >0.12 sec
- R-R: constant for NSR; underlying rate same as atria; shortened with PVC followed by prolonged compensatory pause due to abnormal delayed activation
- P-P = R-R for underlying NSR
- Treatment: There is typically no treatment needed for PVCs as they are not usually harmful.

  - o If PVCs are bothersome, instruct the patient to avoid common triggers, such as caffeine and smoking.
  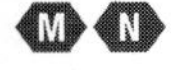
  - o If PVCs compromise cardiac function and/or oxygen delivery, consider medications such as beta blockers, calcium channel blockers, or anti-dysrhythmic drugs.

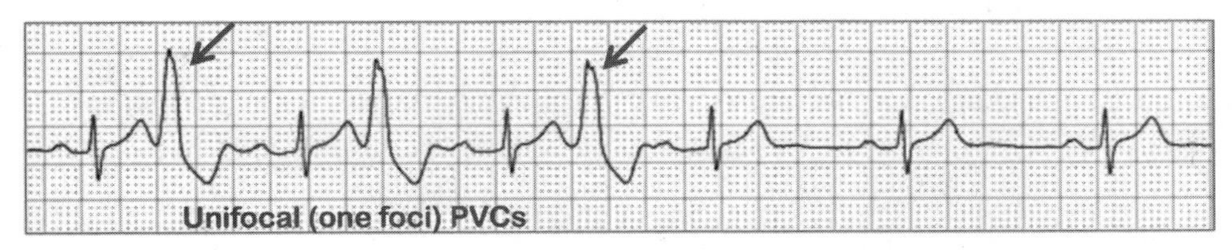

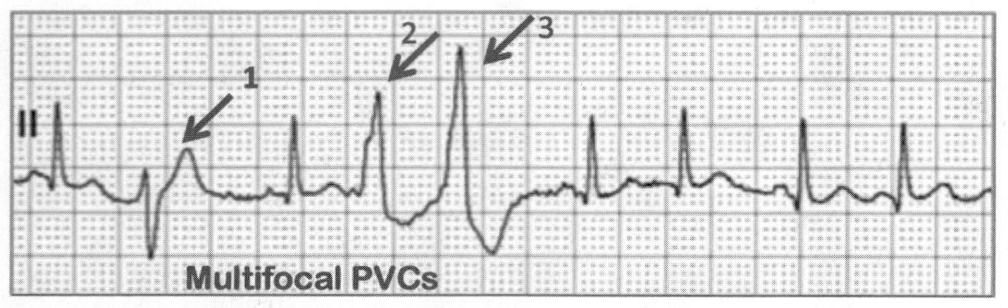

Upper: NSR with Premature Ventricular Contractions that are unifocal or initiated by one ectopic focus. Lower: Sinus tachycardia with multifocal PVCs, originating from three separate locations.
Source: (*both*) Courtesy of K. Kyriakidis

Lethal Ventricular Rhythms

- Two of the most dangerous dysrhythmias are:
  - o Ventricular Tachycardia (V-tach)
  - o Ventricular Fibrillation (V-fib)

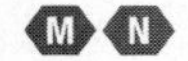

- These rhythms can result in sudden cardiac death and are almost always symptomatic because there is essentially little to no blood pumped from the heart. Ventricular fibrillation and pulseless V-tach result in loss of consciousness and require immediate cardioversion or defibrillation. The rapid response or code team is called and typically needed for assistance.

Ventricular Tachycardia

Ventricular Tachycardia (VT) is a lethal dysrhythmia where the heart is contracting and the cardiac output plummets. The rhythm is typically regular in monomorphic V-tach and irregular in polymorphic (multishaped) V-tach. Patients may have short bursts (nonsustained) or long, sustained V-tach.

Criteria and Examples:

- P-P: none typically visible, AV dissociation if present
- PR: none
- QRS: wide, bizarre, >0.12 sec; mono- or polymorphic
- R-R: can be constant; typically >150 bpm

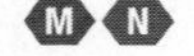

- Treatment: In pulseless V-tach, cardioversion is the highest priority. CPR is started if there is a delay. Additional treatment following ACLS guidelines is often needed to prevent recurrence.

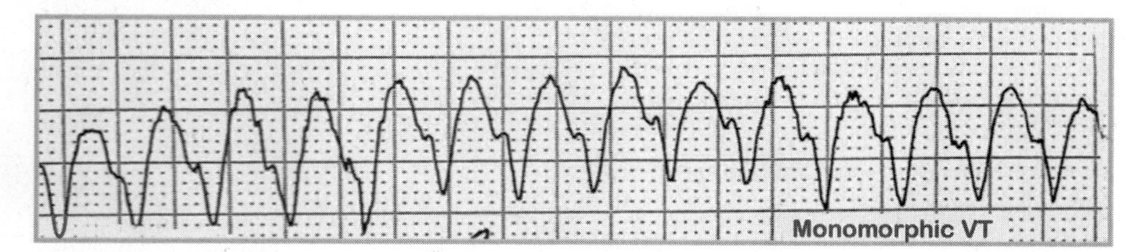

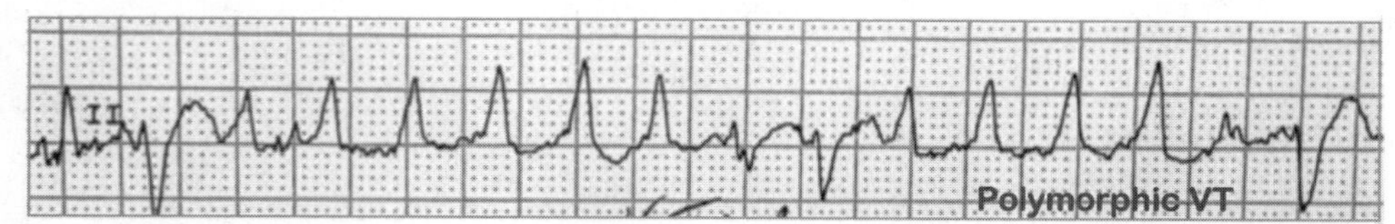

Upper: The EKG shows monomorphic V-tach at a rate of 214 bpm. All QRS complexes look very similar and all are pointed in the same direction. Although this patient was awake during the first 15 seconds of the V tach, he lost consciousness as his BP fell. Lower: EKG shows polymorphic V-tach where the QRS complexes are constantly twisting and pointing in changing directions. Rate is 200–205 bpm.
Source: (*both*) Courtesy of K. Kyriakidis

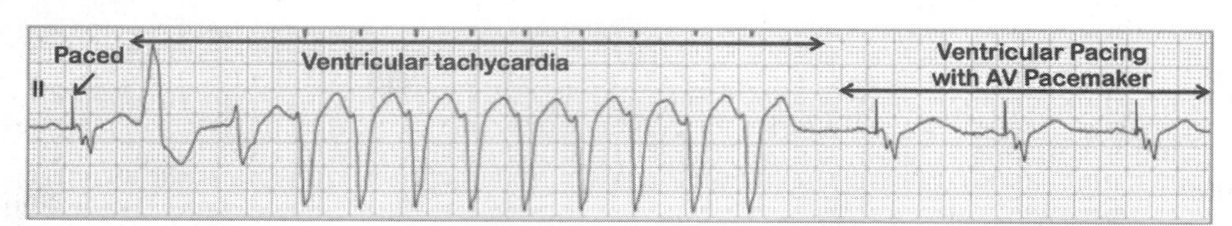

A patient has an underlying paced rhythm but suddenly has a burst of V tach. The ventricular electrode of his newly placed AV pacemaker became dislodged, began flopping inside the ventricle and causing irritability, and caused a burst of unsustained V tach.
Source: Courtesy of K. Kyriakidis

Ventricular Fibrillation

Ventricular fibrillation (V-fib) is a lethal, pulseless dysrhythmia requiring rapid CPR, defibrillation, and advanced cardiac life support (ACLS) interventions by the team. In V-fib, the heart has hundreds of simultaneous but ineffective impulses, which cause the heart to quiver in chaotic motion without contracting. Because there is no real ventricular contraction in V-fib, there is no cardiac output so the patient loses consciousness quickly and asystole ensues without successful intervention.

Criteria and Example:

- P-P: no discernible P waves
- PR: no PR intervals
- QRS: erratic or fibrillatory waves, may be coarse (large) or fine (small)
- R-R: no QRS to measure

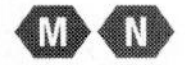

- Treatment: In pulseless V-fib, defibrillation is the highest priority. CPR is started if there is a delay. Additional treatment following ACLS guidelines is commonly needed to treat and/or prevent recurrence.

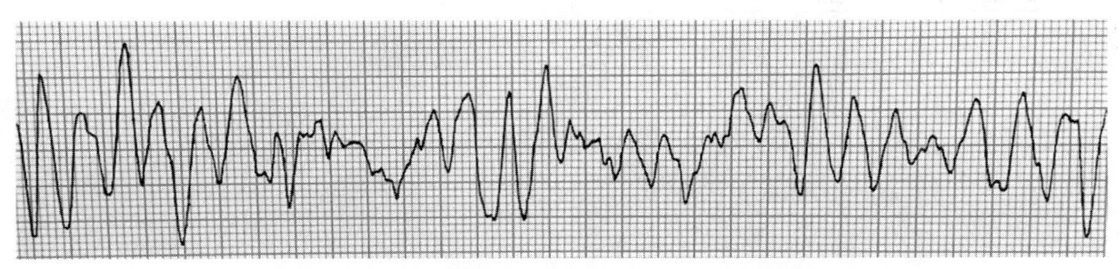

This EKG shows the erratic, rapid, disorganized "rhythm" of coarse ventricular fibrillation.

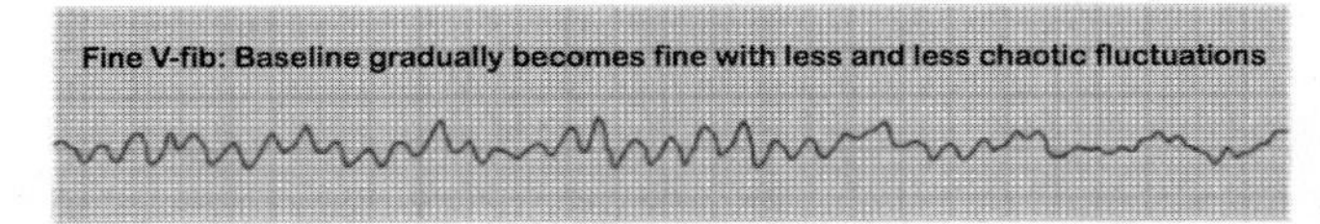
Fine V-fib: Baseline gradually becomes fine with less and less chaotic fluctuations

This ventricular fibrillation has finer or smaller fluctuations and is termed "fine" V-fib.

LO3:

Collaborative Interventions

Overview of Basic Guidelines

The American Heart Association (AHA) has been the leader in defining Basic and Advanced Cardiac Life Support (BLS & ACLS) guidelines for the treatment of dysrhythmias. Early and basic interventions are based on the 2010–2015 ACLS & BLS Guidelines. The full guidelines are most appropriate for cardiac and critical care specialties. Basics when an abnormal rhythm is detected include:

- Assess ABCs (airway, breathing, circulation) and treat. Start O_2 for hypoxia or SpO_2 <92%. Place patient on monitor/telemetry.
- Determine if patient is stable, unstable, or pulseless. Initiate urgent treatment in pulseless and unstable patients. If pulseless, begin CPR according to BLS standards (30 compressions/2 breaths). Call rapid response team.
- Identify the general type of dysrhythmia: Tachycardia (rate >100 bpm) or normal/bradycardia (rate <100 bpm)
- Is the QRS wide or narrow? P waves present?
- Look for causes of the dysrhythmia and treat causes if identifiable.
- Treat the dysrhythmia and hemodynamic instability. Prevent complication.
- Educate the patient about the dysrhythmia and any ongoing treatment.

Assess Circulation, Airway, and Breathing (CAB)

A guide is offered to assist in clinical reasoning, judgment, and interventions for dysrhythmias. Because there are many and some complex guides, the Dysrhythmia Reasoning Guide Overview is provided to help prioritize and focus on the most clinically relevant interventions. It includes:

- Evaluate the patient's consciousness and mental status. If unconscious, call Rapid Response or Code to get help.
- Check pulse, airway, and breathing.
- If there is no pulse, start CPR (30 compressions/2 breaths). If there is a pulse but no breathing, support ventilation and oxygenation.
- If breathing, check O_2 saturation. If SpO_2 <92%, start nasal oxygen.
- Check blood pressure.
- Place on monitor if dysrhythmia is noticed without a monitor.

Dysrhythmias Reasoning Guide: Overview

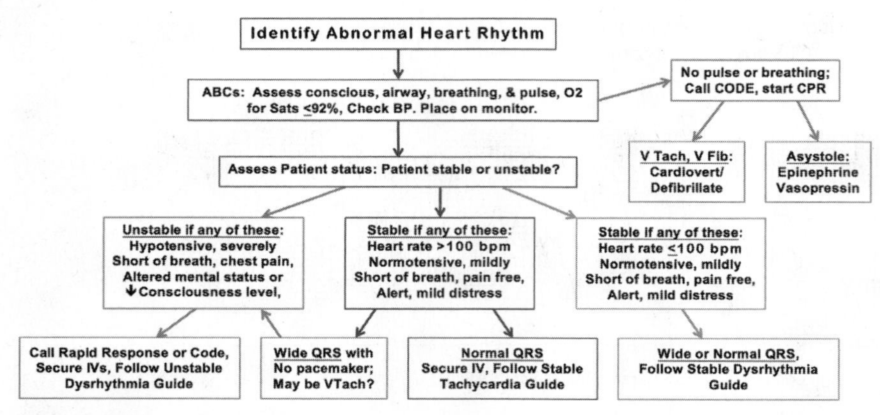

This guide may be useful in assisting a clinician to determine how to approach dysrhythmias.

Collaborative Interventions (continued)

Patients with Unstable Dysrhythmias

The Dysrhythmia Reasoning Guide has multiple pathways that end by pointing to three continued paths. Each path is discussed and another detailed guide provided for each. They are color coded for easier recognition.

- Patients with some or all of the following are **unstable (red) and require emergent treatment:**
  - o Altered level of consciousness or mental status from baseline
  - o Chest pain
  - o Severe shortness of breath
  - o Hypotension
- **If unstable, follow the Unstable Dysrhythmias Reasoning Guide:**

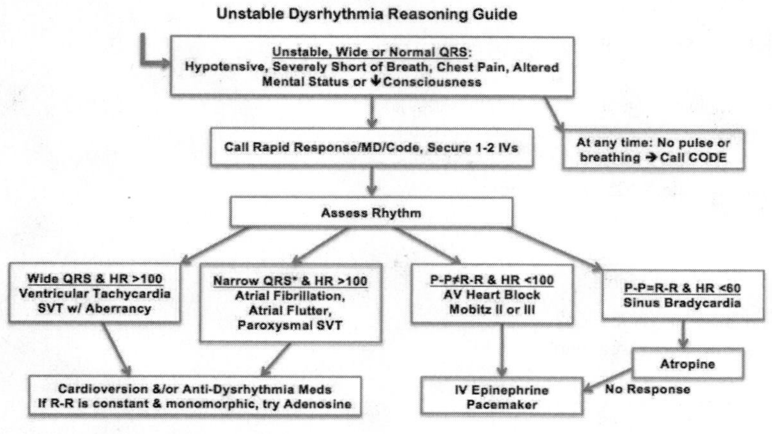

This guide may be useful in assisting the nurse to determine how to approach dysrhythmias.

Concept Check:

6. A patient is given atropine for sinus bradycardia. Which response indicates that the expected outcome of this medication has been achieved?
   A. Heart rate 85
   B. Widened QRS
   C. Regulation of R-R
   D. Development of Mobitz Type II

Answer question

Unstable Dysrhythmias

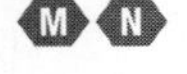

- Call Rapid Response Team, health care provider, or Code because all these situations are urgent and help is needed. Secure 1–2 IVs.
- Is the heart rate (HR) >100 or <100 bpm?
- Is the QRS wide or narrow?

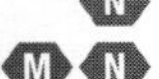

  - A wide complex tachycardia is likely to be a ventricular tachycardia and requires urgent treatment: cardioversion and/or antiarrhythmic medications.

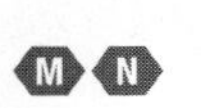

  - Narrow QRS complex tachycardias are commonly due to paroxysmal supraventricular tachycardia (PSVT), A-fib, and atrial flutter. When the patient is very unstable with a fast HR, cardioversion is the intervention of choice to prevent complications. With milder symptoms, medication may be administered to slow the HR.

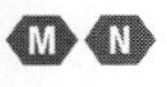

  - If the tachycardia is regular with monomorphic QRSs (QRSs all look the same) and may be due to PSVT, adenosine may be administered.

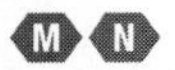

  - Patients with HR <100 bpm in 2nd° AV block type II and 3rd° AV block urgently require a pacemaker (e.g., transvenous or transcutaneous) (see animation).

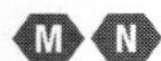

  - Unstable bradycardic patients may respond to atropine or may need a pacemaker.

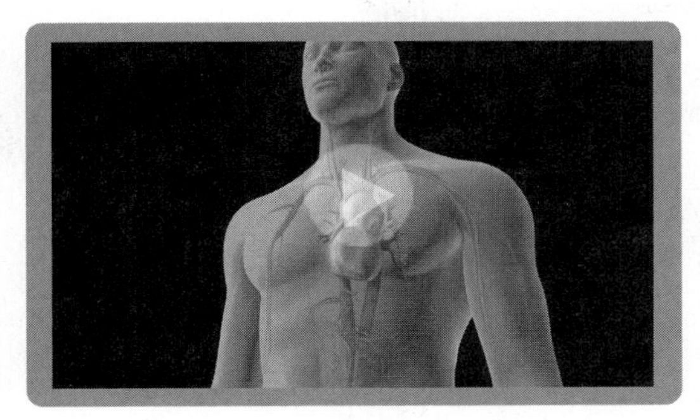

This animation depicts an abnormal heart rhythm, and how normal heart rhythm can be restored with electrical cardioversion. A heart with abnormal signals and atrial fibrillation is shown forming a blood clot which results in a stroke. Next, the steps of the cardioversion procedure are illustrated: the placement of EKG electrodes, the placement of cardioversion paddles, the delivery of shock to the chest and heart, and the restoration of normal electrical signals within the heart.

Collaborative Interventions (continued)

Stable Patients with Tachycardias

- A second path from the Dysrhythmia Reasoning Guide leads to stable patients with tachycardias. Patients with **HR >100 bpm** who also have some or all of the following are **considered stable (blue), but require urgent intervention:**
  - Normotensive
  - Same baseline level of consciousness/mental status
  - Mild to no shortness of breath
  - Free of chest pain
  - May experience mild distress
- **If stable, follow the Stable Tachycardia Reasoning Guide:**

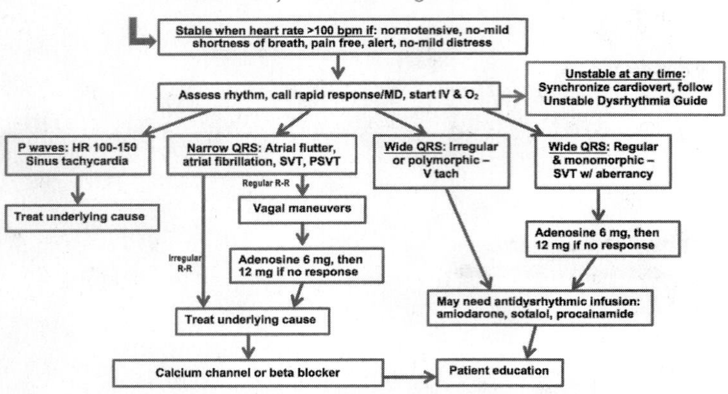

This guide may be useful in assisting the nurse to determine how to approach dysrhythmia.

Source: Copyright © 2012, NovEx Novice to Expert Learning, LLC

- Interventions such as carotid massage or valsalva maneuvers can cause vagal blocking of the AV node and interrupt the dysrhythmia.
- Adenosine, 6 mg IV, followed by a saline flush is the first line medication used to convert SVT in a stable or unstable but conscious patient, according to AHA guidelines. Adenosine works by temporarily blocking the AV node. If SVT persists, an additional two doses of 12 mg (each followed by saline flush) can be attempted. Patients may feel the brief and transient arterial hypotension, accompanied by a short or breathtakingly long sinus pause.
- If three doses of adenosine fail, diltiazem (a calcium channel blocker) can be administered.
- If SVT persists or the patient is unstable (hypotension, altered mental status), synchronized cardioversion may be required. AHA recommends cardioversion in all unstable patients with tachycardia as the first intervention except in SVT. Good clinical judgment is required in each patient situation to determine the significance and effect of the hypotension. With the overarching guide of "do no harm," adenosine is the first treatment of choice, with fewer potential harmful effects than cardioversion.
- Cardioversion can be used to restore normal sinus rhythm in many dyshythmias. These include V-tach, V-fib, PSVT, A-fib, and atrial flutter.
- Long-term treatment includes radiofrequency ablation in which the abnormal tissue or accessory pathway in the heart is then identified and destroyed. This is usually accomplished with heart catheterization. It has been used in treatment of atrial flutter, A-fib, V-fib, V-tach, and PSVT.
- Treatment for tachydysrhythmias can require medications. These include:
    - o Antiarrhythmics: These medications may be used for wide QRS complex tachycardias. Antiarrhythmics include amiodarone, sotalol, and rhythmol. These medications affect the ion channels so they may also cause other dysrhythmias. Prolongation of QT intervals often must be monitored in patients undergoing treatment.
    - o Calcium channel blockers: May be given for HR control. A-fib and atrial flutter are often treated without restoring normal sinus rhythm. Verapamil 2.5–10 mg IV can be administered over 2 minutes and 5–10 mg can be repeated after 15–30 min. Similarly, diltiazem 20 mg (0.25 mg/kg) may be given directly into the IV over 2 minutes and it can be repeated in 15 min, 25 mg (0.35 mg/kg) IV.
    - o Beta blockers: May help by decreasing automaticity of the atrial cells as well as slowing conduction through the AV node. Propranolol is a commonly used medication and 1–3 mg is given IV at 1 mg/min. May repeat every 2–5 min for total of 5 mg.

  These medications can also be given orally for home use.

Concept Check

7. **What is the purpose of carotid massage for a patient with stable tachycardia?**

   A. Increasing blood flow to the brain
   B. Blocking the AV node to interrupt the rhythm
   C. Preventing clot migration through the carotids
   D. Stimulating baroreceptors to stabilize blood pressure

Answer question

Collaborative Interventions (continued)

Stable Patients with Dysrhythmias

N • A third path from the Dysrhythmia Reasoning Guide leads to Stable Patients with dysrhythmias. Patients with **HR ≤100 bpm** who also have some or all of the following are **considered stable (green), but require further evaluation and potential treatment:**
  - o Normotensive
  - o Same baseline level of consciousness or mental status
  - o Mild to no shortness of breath
  - o Free of chest pain
  - o May experience mild distress

N • **If stable, follow the Stable Dysrhythmias Reasoning Guide:**

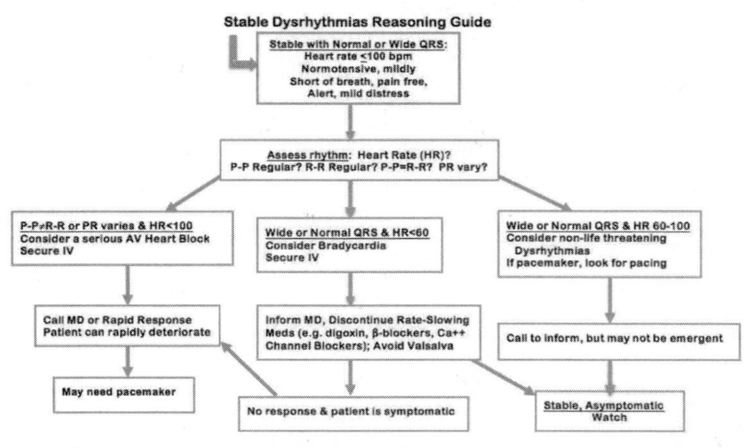

Stable Dysrhythmias Reasoning Guide
Stable with Normal or Wide QRS: Heart rate ≤100 bpm Normotensive, mildly Short of breath, pain free, Alert, mild distress
Assess rhythm: Heart Rate (HR)? P-P Regular? R-R Regular? P-P=R-R? PR vary?
P-P≠R-R or PR varies & HR<100 Consider a serious AV Heart Block Secure IV
Wide or Normal QRS & HR<60 Consider Bradycardia Secure IV
Wide or Normal QRS & HR 60-100 Consider non-life threatening Dysrhythmias If pacemaker, look for pacing
Call MD or Rapid Response Patient can rapidly deteriorate
Inform MD, Discontinue Rate-Slowing Meds (e.g. digoxin, β-blockers, Ca++ Channel Blockers); Avoid Valsalva
Call to inform, but may not be emergent
May need pacemaker
No response & patient is symptomatic
Stable, Asymptomatic Watch
** The guide is not exact and may have overlapping categories, but the clinician should collaborate with a skilled dysrhythmia interpreter for greater accuracy. This overview guide cannot account for every scenario but can assist to provide safe care.

This guide may be useful in assisting the nurse to determine how to approach dysrhythmias.

Source: Copyright © 2012, NovEx Novice to Expert Learning, LLC

M N • Call Rapid Response Team, health care provider, or Code because all these situations are urgent and help is needed. Secure 1–2 IVs.

N • Is the HR >100 or <100 bpm?

N • Is the QRS wide or narrow?

M N o A wide complex tachycardia is likely to be a ventricular tachycardia and requires urgent treatment: cardioversion and/or antiarrhythmic medications.

M N o Narrow QRS complex tachycardias are commonly due to paroxysmal supraventricular tachycardia (PSVT), A-fib, and atrial flutter. When the patient is very unstable with a fast heart rate, cardioversion is the intervention of choice to prevent complications. With milder symptoms, medication may be administered to slow the heart rate.

M N o If the tachycardia is regular with monomorphic QRSs (QRSs all look the same) and may be due to PSVT, adenosine may be administered.

M N o Patients with HR <100 bpm in 2nd° AV block type II and 3rd° AV block urgently require a pacemaker (e.g., transvenous or transcutaneous) (see animation).

M N o Unstable bradycardic patients may respond to atropine or may need a pacemaker.

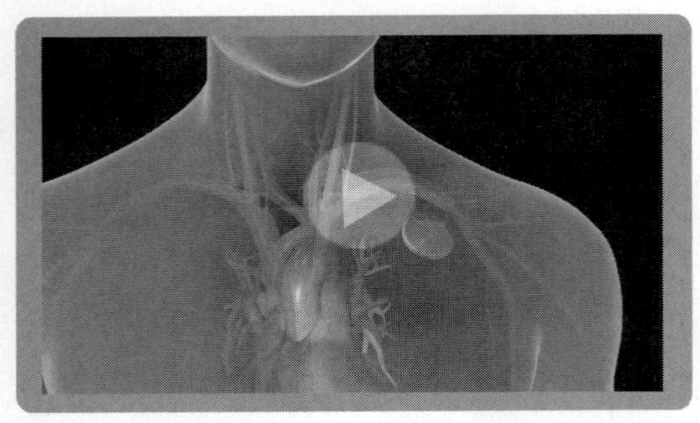

A pacemaker is a small, battery-powered device made up of two parts, a pulse generator and the leads. This animation demonstrates the steps involved in placing a pacemaker. The pulse generator of the pacemaker gives off impulses that cause the atria and/or ventricles to contract. It is positioned under the skin, below the collarbone on either side of the chest. The leads carry signals between the pulse generator and the heart in both directions. The surgeon makes a small incision beneath your collarbone. The pacemaker's leads are inserted into the subclavian vein and then threaded toward the right side of your heart. Your surgeon views x-ray images on a video screen to position the leads correctly.

Collaborative Interventions (continued)

Patient Education

- Educate regarding dysrhythmia and treatment:

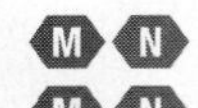

  - o Dysrhythmia involved

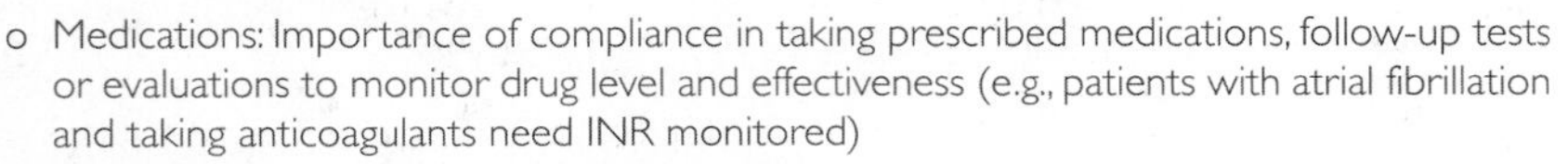

  - o Medications: Importance of compliance in taking prescribed medications, follow-up tests or evaluations to monitor drug level and effectiveness (e.g., patients with atrial fibrillation and taking anticoagulants need INR monitored)

  - o Symptoms indicating dysrhythmia onset and what to do

  - o Complications and what to do if needed
  - o When to call the health care provider or seek treatment

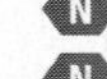

  - o Risk factor modification (e.g., smoking cessation)

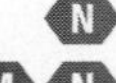

- Monitoring: Patients need to understand that they are at increased risk for stroke if not taking their medication properly.

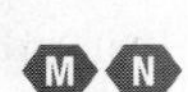

- Education about tests and treatment options, such as Holter monitoring or ablation, when appropriate.

Summary of Interventions

- Management of dysrhythmias varies and can include physical maneuvers, medication, electrical shock, surgical intervention with or without implanted devices to control heart rate.
- When a life-threatening dysrhythmia does not allow time for diagnosis using a 12-lead EKG, it is important to verify the dysrhythmia by checking that the monitor is functioning and leads are properly placed prior to treatment. Monitor artifact or disconnection can mimic lethal dysrhythmias.
- Assess the stability of the patient. Patients who have a tachydysrhythmia and are unstable usually require immediate cardioversion. Unstable patients with bradycardia and/or heart block may require pacing.
- Treat the cause of the dysrhythmia. Dysrhythmias are precipitated by numerous causes including cardiac ischemia, pulmonary embolus, infection/sepsis, electrolyte abnormalities, hypoxia, endocrine problems (e.g., hypothyroidism), trauma, or drugs.
- Successful treatment of the patient requires recognition and treatment of the underlying problem. A dysrhythmia may be the first sign of a more serious problem, such as cardiac ischemia or pulmonary embolus.

LO4:

Evaluation of Desired Collaborative Care Outcomes

Evaluation and reassessment should reveal attainment of previously established patient outcomes. In summary:

- Patient's hemodynamic measurements (if available) reveal that cardiac output is stable. Patient's heart rate is within normal limits, heart rhythm is stable, mentation returns to pre-illness state, and urine output is within the patient's normal volume
- Patient's EKG reveals no further cardiac damage caused by the dysrhythmia.
- Patient's mentation is clear or at the patient's pre-illness level.
- Patient's skin is warm and dry and pulses are as strong as pre-illness state.
- Patient calmly discusses treatment regimen and personal perceptions of illness.
- Patient denies chest pain and demonstrates no signs of pain.

References

American Heart Association. Arrhythmias. **watchlearnlive.heart.org/CVML_Player.php?moduleSelect=arrhyt** [These are animated dysrhythmias]

Beasley, B. (2010). Understanding EKGs: A practical approach. Upper Saddle River, NJ: Pearson Education.

Chulay, M.A. & Burns, S. (2010). AACN essentials of progressive care nursing, 2nd edition. New York, NY: The McGraw-Hill Companies.

Dubin, D. (2000). Rapid interpretation of EKG's (6th edition). Tampa, FL: COVER Publishing CO.

Sinz, E., Navarro, K., & Soderberg, E. (Eds). (2013). Advanced Cardiovascular Life Support: Provider Manual. Dallas, TX: American Heart Association.

Walraven, G. (2011). Basic arrhythmias, 7th edition. Boston, MA: Brady.

Clinical Practice Guidelines

Incorporated American Heart Association. (2011). Advanced cardiovascular life support (ACLS) provider manual. Dallas, TX: American Heart Association.

Patient Education

Heart arrhythmias: Mayo Clinic (2013). Lifestlye and home remedies. **http://www.mayoclinic.org/diseases-conditions/heart-arrhythmia/basics/lifestyle-home-remedies/con-20027707**

National Heart, Lung, and Blood Institute. Living with an Arrhythmia. **http://www.nhlbi.nih.gov/health/health-topics/topics/arr/livingwith.html**

Texas Cardiac Arrhythmia. Patient Education. **http://tcaheart.com/patient-education**

Learning Outcomes for Electrocardiograms

When you complete this lesson, you will be able to:

1. Recognize the clinical relevance of an electrocardiogram.
2. Consider the physiology and techniques associated with electrocardiograms that determine the priority patient concerns.
3. Determine the most urgent and important nursing interventions and patient education required in caring for a patient having an electrocardiogram.
4. Evaluate attainment of desired collaborative care outcomes for a patient requiring an electrocardiogram.

LO1:

What Is an Electrocardiogram?

- An electrocardiogram (EKG) is a noninvasive test that reflects the electrical activity of the heart.
- For the heart muscle to contract and pump blood, an electrical stimulation is needed. The stimulus rapidly passes through the atria and ventricle, the muscles contract, and that stimulus or impulse is recorded via EKG.
- The electrical impulses are recorded using 12 electrodes or leads (typically 12) that are placed on the skin around the heart. Each electrode records the impulse from a different "viewpoint." The 12 different recordings produce what is known as the 12-lead EKG.
- The EKG is recorded on special graph paper and printed at an exact speed so that accurate measurements can be obtained about impulse speed, location, path of movement (depolarization), or direction. This information allows a knowledgeable clinician to better understand how the patient's heart is functioning.

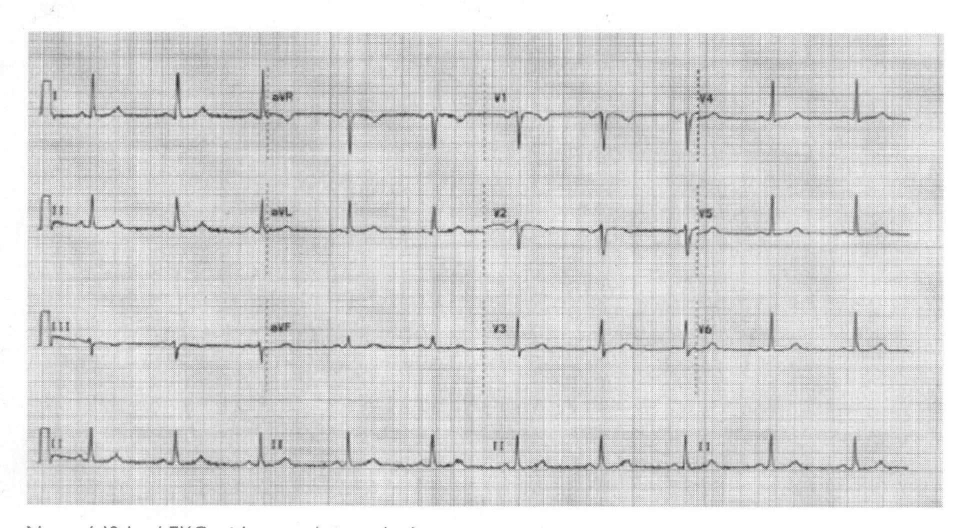

Normal 12-lead EKG with normal sinus rhythm.
Source: Courtesy of K. Kyriakidis

LO1:

Clinical Relevance

- The EKG is an important diagnostic tool. The 12-lead EKG is useful in determining the presence of cardiac ischemia, injury, cardiac infarction, conduction disturbances, drug toxicity, and electrolyte imbalance.
- The 12-lead EKG is also useful in reflecting the size of the heart chambers and the electrical impulse axis. The axis shows the common direction of cardiac electrical activity.
- An EKG is one of the most common, noninvasive and nonpainful diagnostic tests performed.

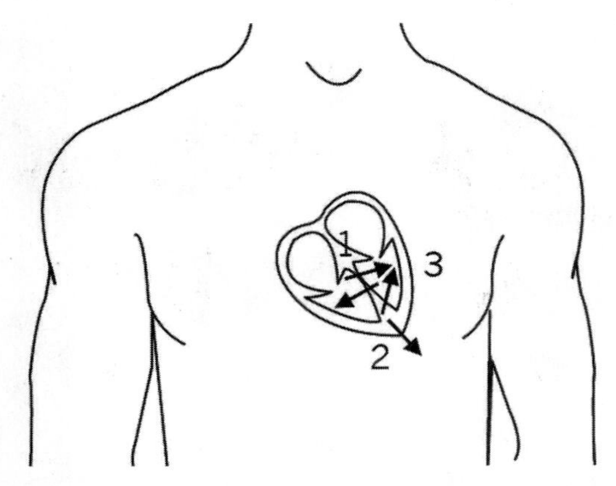

This image shows the phases (1–3) of depolarization (electrical movement) through the heart. The arrows indicate the changing direction that the impulse is moving through the heart over time. The EKG, which reflects the impulse movement, can therefore reveal normal and abnormal cardiac electrical activity, depending on the EKG lead.

Source: Copyright © 2013, NovEx Novice to Expert Learning, LLC

Concept Check

1. **Which information can the 12-lead EKG help to determine?**
   A. Presence of cardiac murmur
   B. Size of heart chambers
   C. Presence of air around the heart
   D. Amount of plaque in vessels

Answer question

Components of a Cardiac Cycle

Cardiac Muscle Depolarization and the EKG

- Cardiac muscle cells maintain a voltage difference between the inside of the cell and the outside.
- For cardiac muscle to contract, it first requires an electrical stimulus or impulse resulting from depolarization.
- Depolarization (phase 0) occurs when there is rapid movement of ions through channels causing a rapid change in the voltage across the cell membrane.
- With repolarization (phase 3), the voltage gradient returns back to baseline. As groups of myocytes depolarize, EKG is able to record changes in voltages.

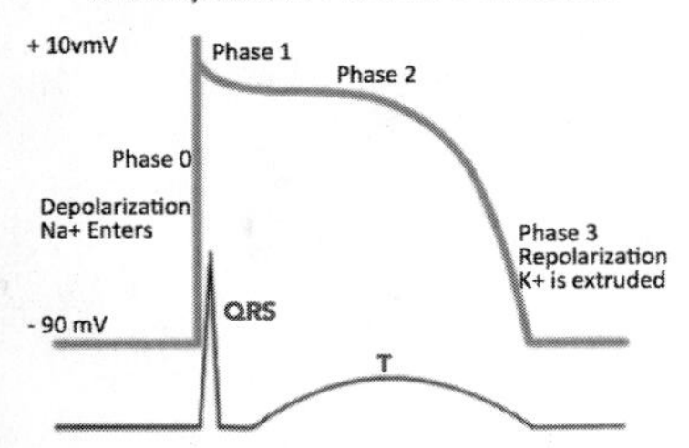

This image shows the action potential in a heart muscle cell along with the movement of ions.

Source: Courtesy of George Kyriakidis/Santa Ana, CA

Components of a Cardiac Cycle (continued)

Normal Cardiac Conduction System and the EKG

Depolarization cycle of the heart muscle

- The sinus (SA) node is the natural pacemaker of the heart as it is made up of spontaneous pacemaker cells. When it spontaneously depolarizes, it sends a depolarization wave through the atrium. This depolarization creates the **P wave**, which is followed by atrial chamber contraction.

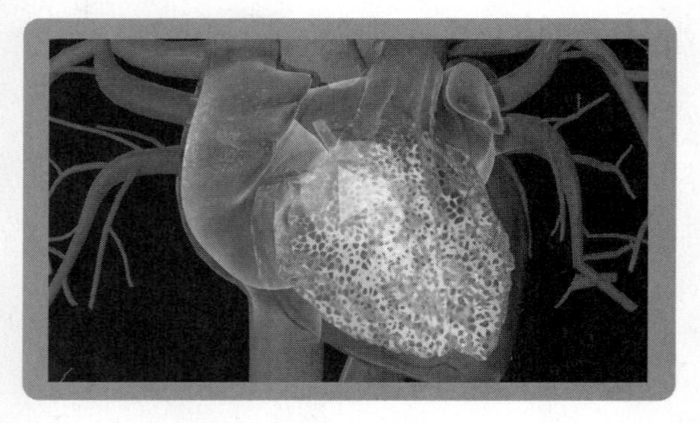

This animation provides an anatomical overview of the cardiac conduction system of the heart, depicting the mechanical and electrical sequence of events producing a heartbeat.

Source: © 2013 Nucleus Medical Media, All rights reserved

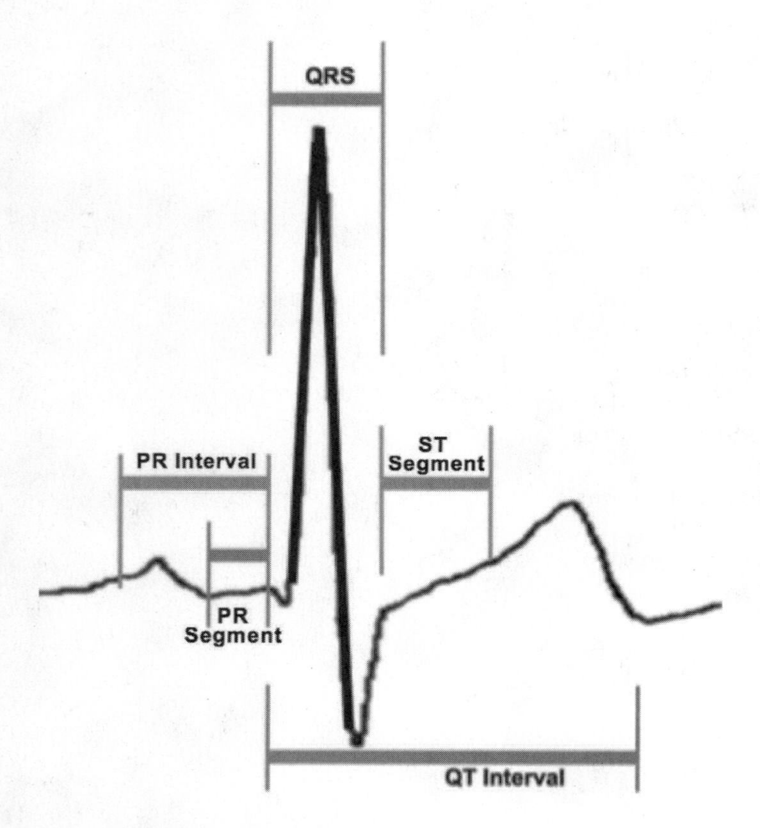

The PQRST complex intervals are delineated to show how to precisely measure the various cardiac intervals. These are important for dysrhythmia interpretation.

Source: Courtesy of George Kyriakidis/Santa Ana, CA

- The depolarization or impulse then passes through the atrioventricular (AV) node, between the atria and the ventricles. This produces the **PR segment**.
- Of greater interest than the PR segment is the **PR interval**, which represents atrial and AV nodal depolarization.
- The depolarization wave continues through the bundle of His in the ventricles before dividing into three bundle branches (one right, two left). The bundle branches rapidly spread the impulse into the vast Purkinje fiber system, which then causes depolarization of the ventricles. The **QRS complex** represents the impulse through the ventricles. Ventricular contraction follows.
- Repolarization occurs (resulting in the T wave formation). The cycle repeats itself as the SA node automatically depolarizes again.

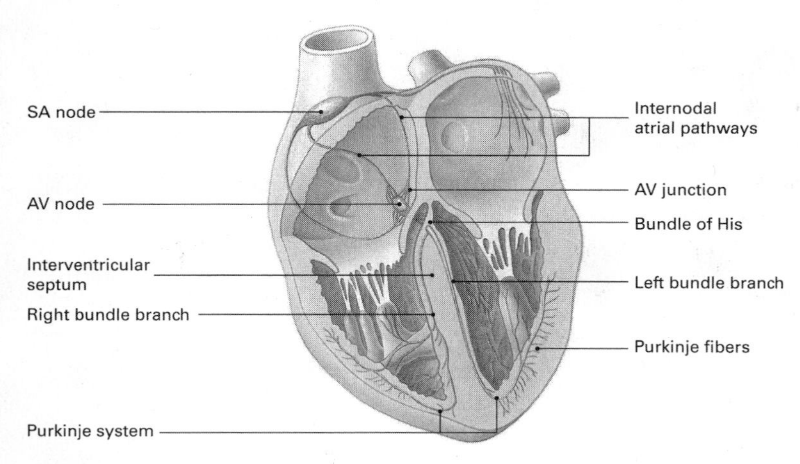

The anatomical location of the normal conduction system is shown.

When the electrical system of the heart is healthy and functioning normally, a normal sinus rhythm (NSR) is produced.

Components of a Cardiac Cycle (continued)

Normal Sinus Rhythm (NSR)

These are examples of NSR at differing heart rates:

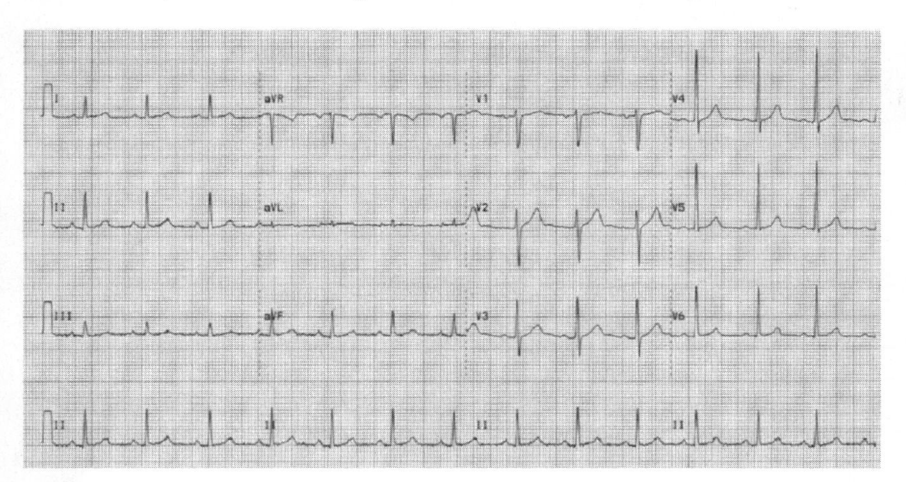

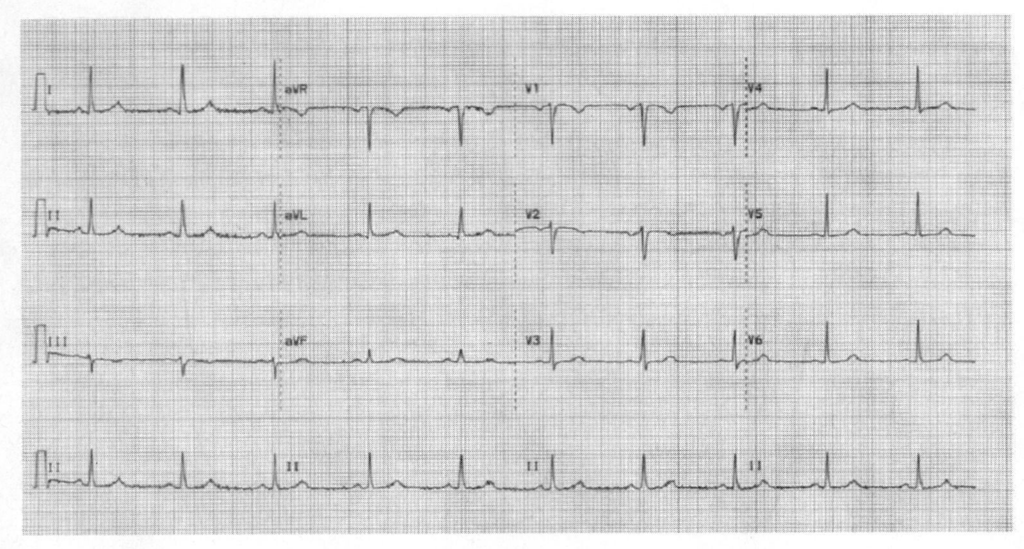

The EKGs are examples of NSR. Notice in the upper EKG that the heart rate is faster, at 79 bpm. The lower EKG shows a slower but normal heart rate at 60 bpm.
Source: (*both*) Courtesy of K. Kyriakidis

Interpreting the Normal EKG

EKG Paper

- The EKG paper is a grid of horizontal and vertical lines creating small squares. Each square measures 1 × 1 mm.
- Horizontal lines on the graph paper reflect the electrical energy or voltage.
- Vertical lines on the graph paper reflect time. Each 1 mm box equals 0.04 sec.
- The example (see drawing) reveals how rapidly the impulse travels through the heart, in 0.32 sec (8 mm) from the beginning of the P wave through the end of the QRS.

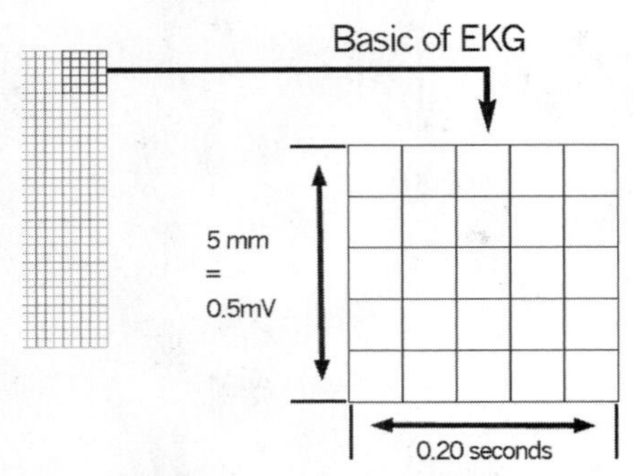

This image illustrates the standards used for measurement in EKG interpretations. Exact measurement of PQRST complexes and intervals is the basis for good and accurate interpretations.
Source: Copyright © 2013, NovEx Novice to Expert Learning, LLC

Concept Check

2. Each small box on EKG paper is equivalent to how many seconds?
   A. 0.04 seconds
   B. 0.20 seconds
   C. 1 second
   D. 0.08 seconds

Answer question

- Analysis of the monitor strip (from a single lead) is made after examination of each wave in relation to the electrical activity in the three prominent deflections of the cardiac cycle.
- These three deflections consist of a P, QRS, and T wave formation.
- Unlike a monitor strip of one lead, a 12-lead EKG has six limb leads involving the arms and legs, II, III, aVF, I, aVR, aVL, and six precordial (chest) leads, V1–V6.
- Dysrhythmias can be interpreted from a monitor lead or 12-lead EKG, but myocardial ischemia, injury, and infarction must be interpreted from a 12-lead EKG.

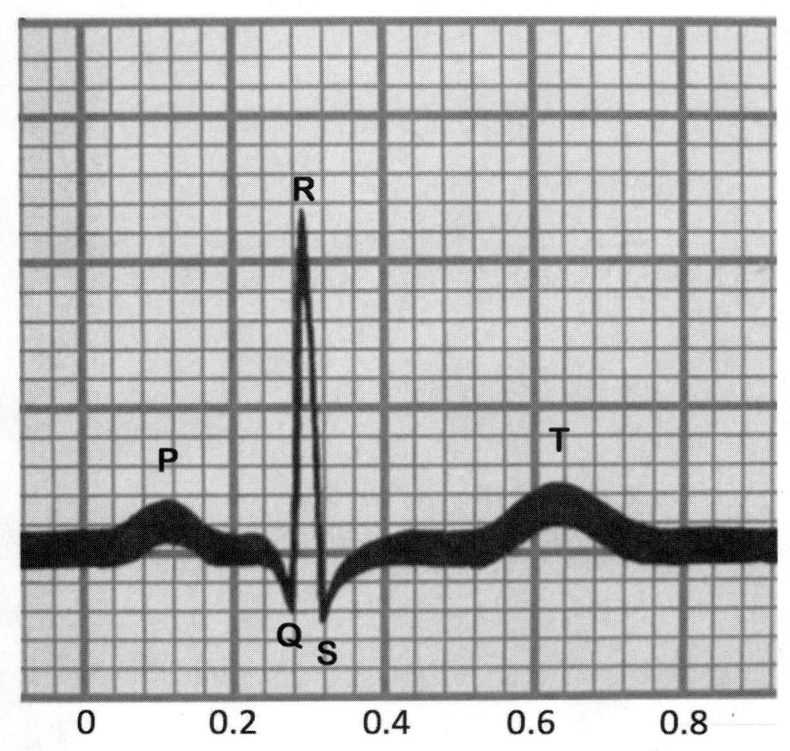

Time factors into EKG analysis. This image illustrates the amount of time involved in one cardiac cycle. This example shows that the electrical cycle in the heart took approximately 0.6 seconds. Intervals on the EKG graph paper denote time in seconds.

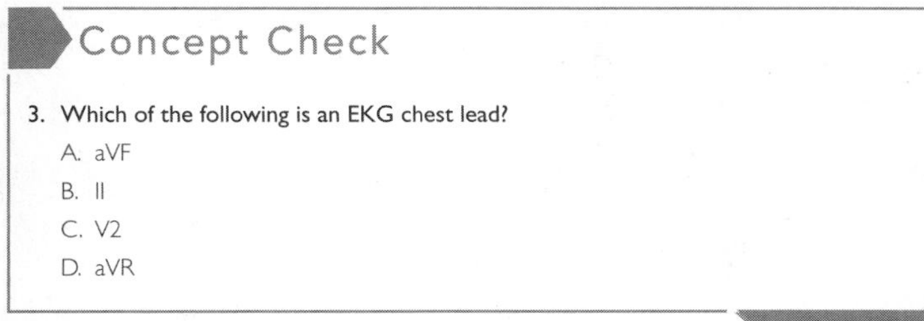

Concept Check

3. Which of the following is an EKG chest lead?
   A. aVF
   B. II
   C. V2
   D. aVR

Answer question

Components of a Cardiac Cycle (continued)

P Wave

- Atrial depolarization normally originates in the SA node.
- The P wave is produced by the atrial depolarization. Atrial contraction takes place immediately after depolarization (<1 sec).
- P waves are normally small (<3 mm), upright, and appear uniform.
- Unusual appearing P waves (e.g., downward) may originate from a place other than the SA node (ectopic focus).

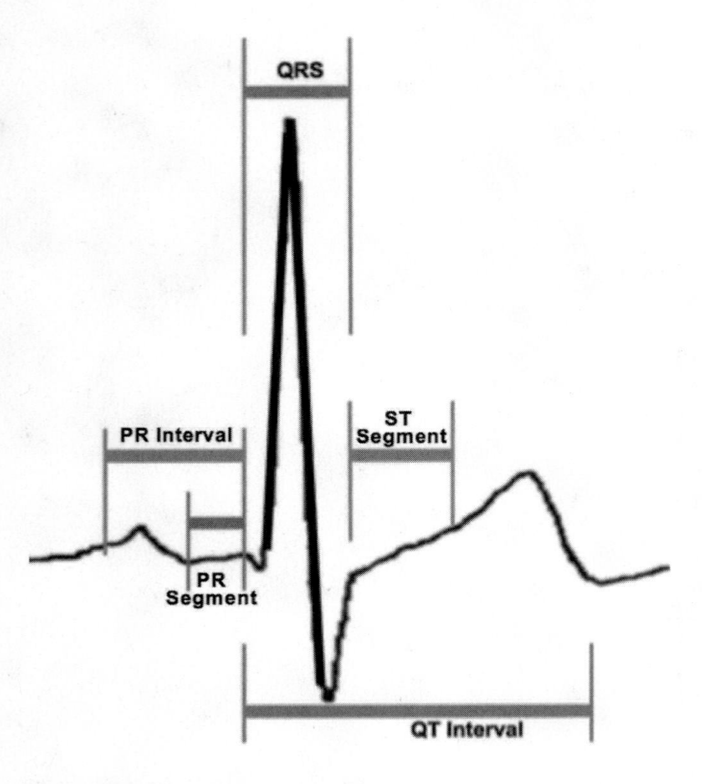

This image represents the PQRST intervals and how to measure each. The intervals have exact points for measurement with normals and abnormals for each. Incorrect measurements can lead to erroneous understandings of the patients conditions.
Source: Courtesy of George Kyriakidis/Santa Ana, CA

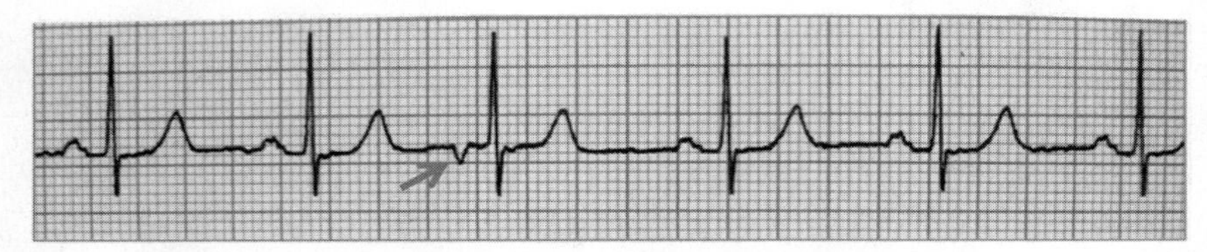

This image shows the P wave is downward (red arrow) compared to the normal appearing P wave. This suggests that the early PQRST with an inverted P wave originates from an ectopic (abnormal) focus.

PR Interval

The PR interval is the measurement of time between atrial depolarization (beginning of the P wave) and ventricular depolarization (beginning of the QRS complex).

- This is the time it takes for the electrical impulse to move through the atrium and AV node and the bundle of His.
- A normal PR interval measures 0.12 to 0.20 sec.
- A longer PR interval (greater than 0.20 sec) indicates an AV block (1st° block) or delayed conduction through the AV node, producing a delay of the electrical impulse to the ventricle.

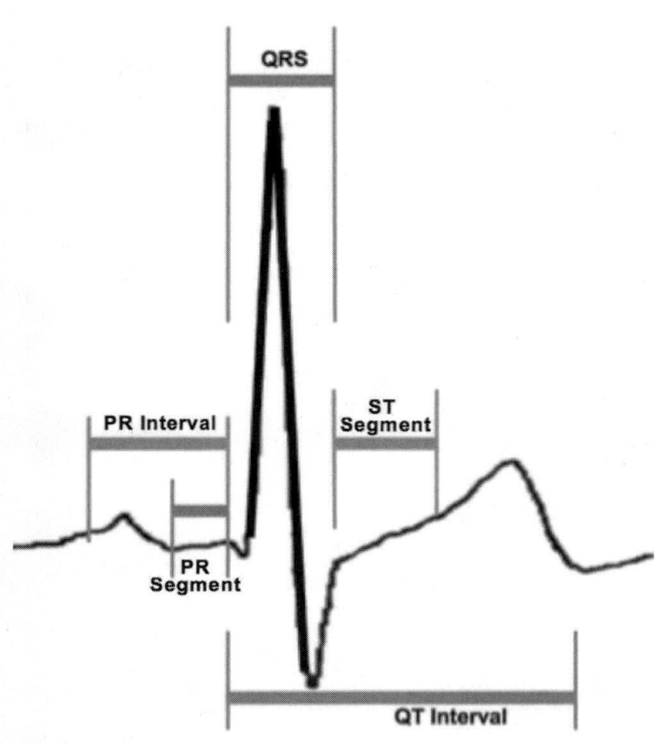

PQRST intervals.
Source: Courtesy of George Kyriakidis/Santa Ana, CA

What is the PR interval measurement? Is it normal or abnormal?

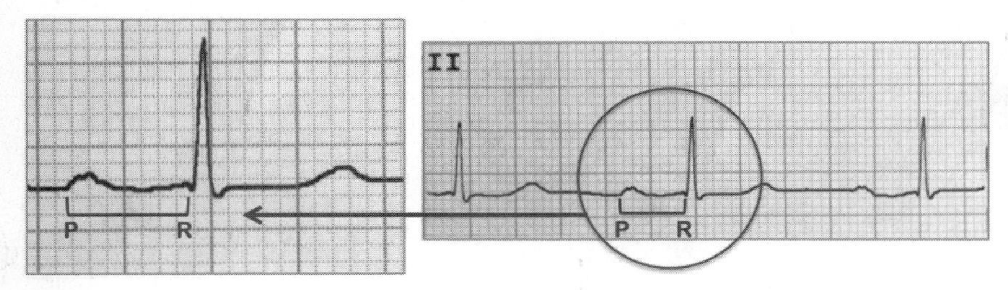

Source: Courtesy of K. Kyriakidis

Answer: The PR interval = 7 boxes. 7 × 0.4 = 0.28 sec: Abnormally long. This is 1st° AV block.

Components of a Cardiac Cycle (continued)

PR Segment

The PR segment reflects the time (prolonged, compared to other structures) it takes for the electrical impulse to pass through the AV node into the ventricle.

- During the time it takes the electrical impulse to travel through the AV node, it does not produce any muscle contraction. This segment is normally flat or isoelectric (zero electric potential).
- The PR segment is measured from the end of the P wave to the beginning of the QRS complex.
- The PR segment is not considered clinically relevant.

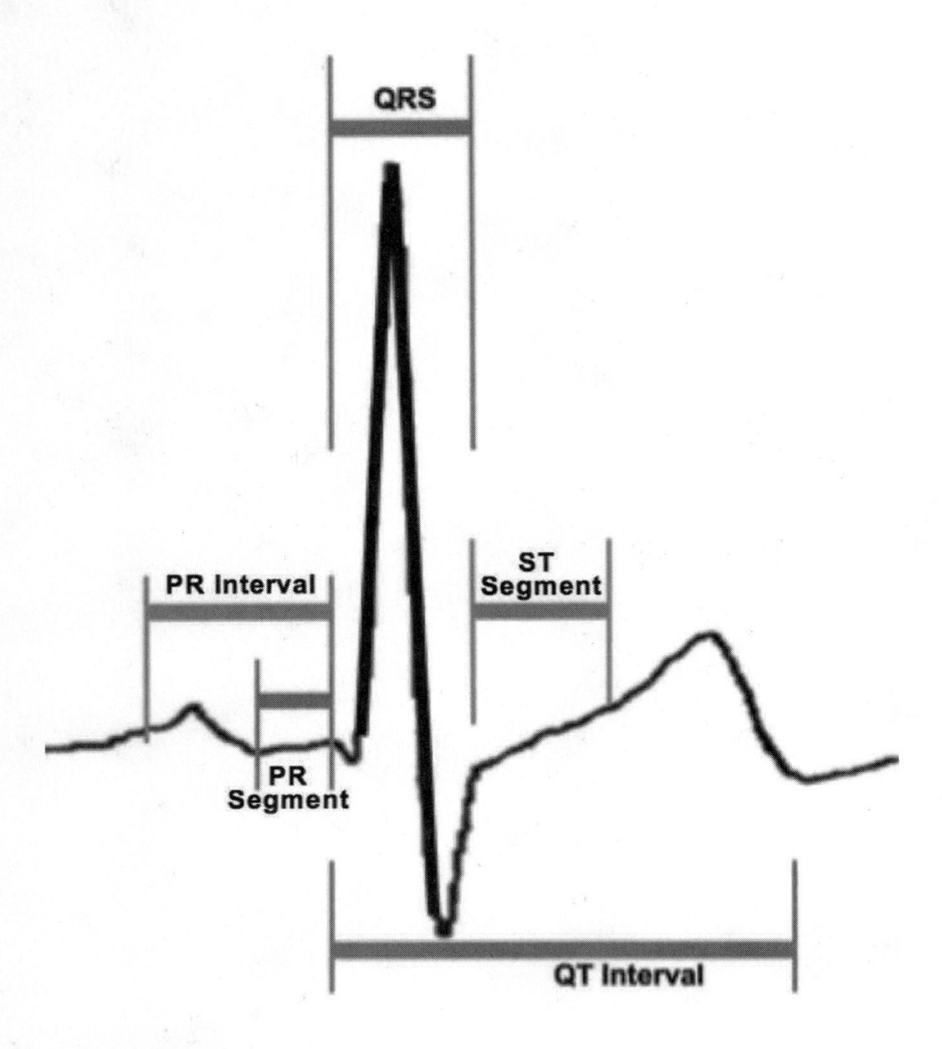

PQRST intervals.
Source: Courtesy of George Kyriakidis/Santa Ana, CA

QRS Complex—The Q wave

There are three consecutive waves that form the QRS complex. The QRS complex reflects the electrical activity, with ventricular depolarization followed immediately by ventricular contraction.

- The first downward wave (deflection) in this complex is the **Q wave**. The Q wave can be absent, small, or, large.
- Large Q waves are a sign of a prior myocardial infarction. The scar tissue from a previous injury does not conduct electrical impulses, which creates the pathologic Q wave. If the QRS has only one negative deflection, it is referred to as a QS wave.
- Pathologic Q waves are commonly 0.04 sec wide and greater than one-third in depth of the height of the R wave.

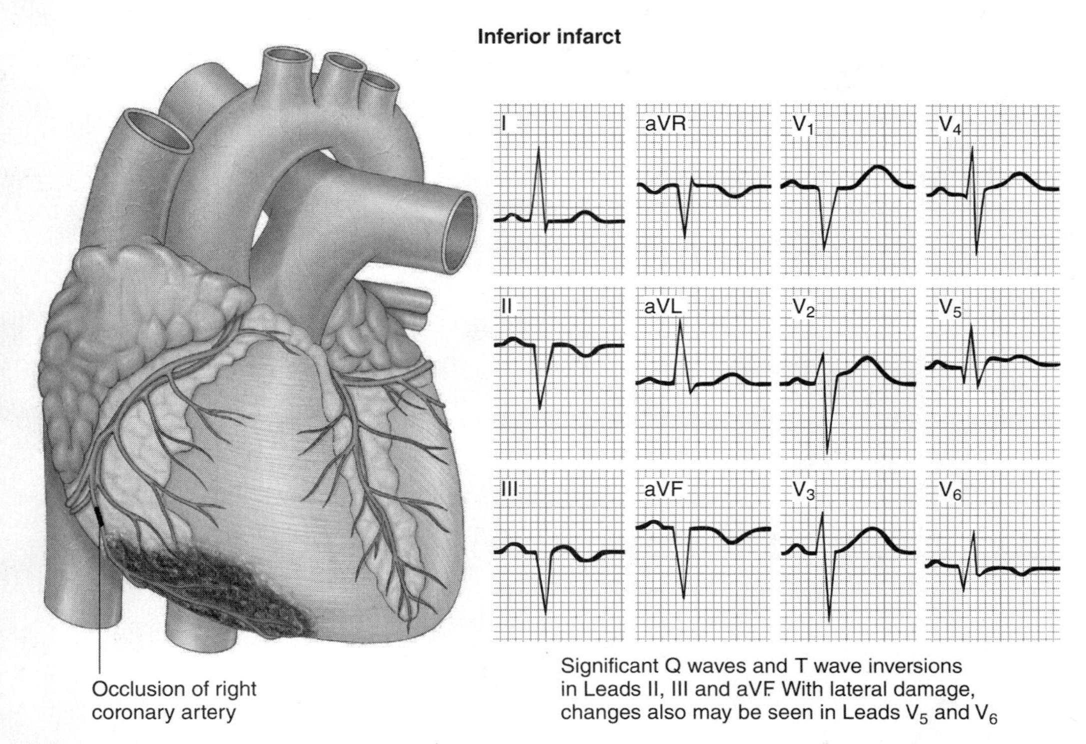

The image of the heart illustrates an inferior wall MI, caused by occlusion of the right coronary artery. The EKG that accompanies this infarction reveals deep and distinct Q waves in the inferior leads (II, III, and aVF). The infarction extends into the lateral wall, reflected by the smaller Q waves in V5–V6.

QRS Complex—The R wave

The **R wave** is the first upward deflection in the QRS complex after the P wave.

- The R wave is large and easy to see when looking at an EKG in most leads.
- The R wave signifies early ventricular depolarization prior to contraction.
- The R wave is most prominent in leads I, II, III, aVL, aVF, V5, V6, and less prominent in leads V1, V2, aVR.

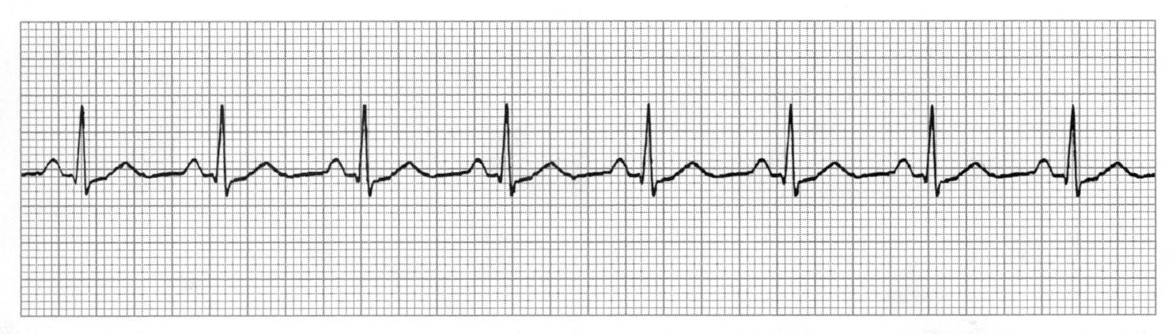

This is a normal sinus rhythm. Notice the very small and nonpathologic Q wave and the tall prominent R wave in leads I, II, III, and aVF. In many EKGs, a small S wave in the QRS complex can be observed.

Components of a Cardiac Cycle (continued)

QRS Complex—The S Wave

The S wave is seen as the first downward deflection following the upward R wave.

- It signifies late repolarization of the ventricles.
- The S wave appears more prominent in V1, V2, aVR, and less prominent in leads I, II, III, aVL, aVF, V5, V6.
- Many patients are monitored in a modified V1 (MVL1) lead (see rhythm example).

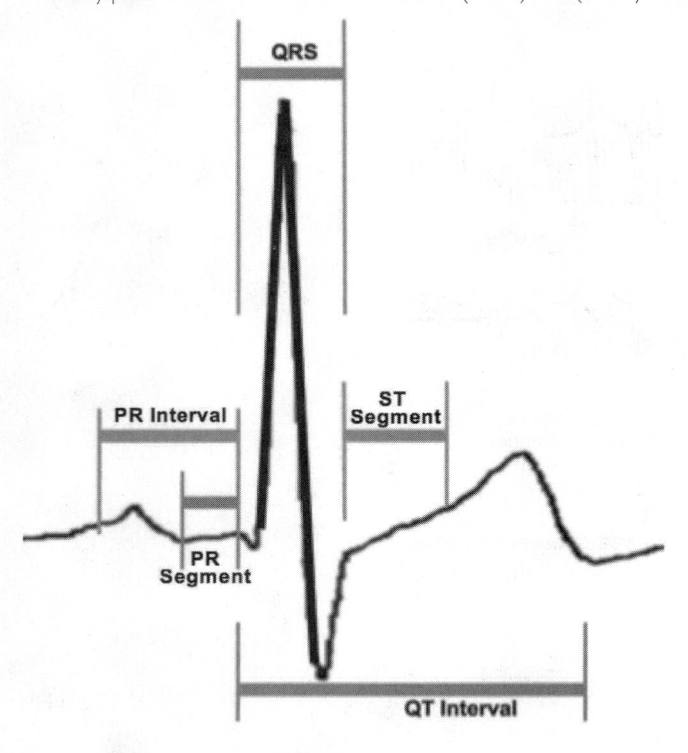

PQRST intervals.
Source: Courtesy of George Kyriakidis/Santa Ana, CA

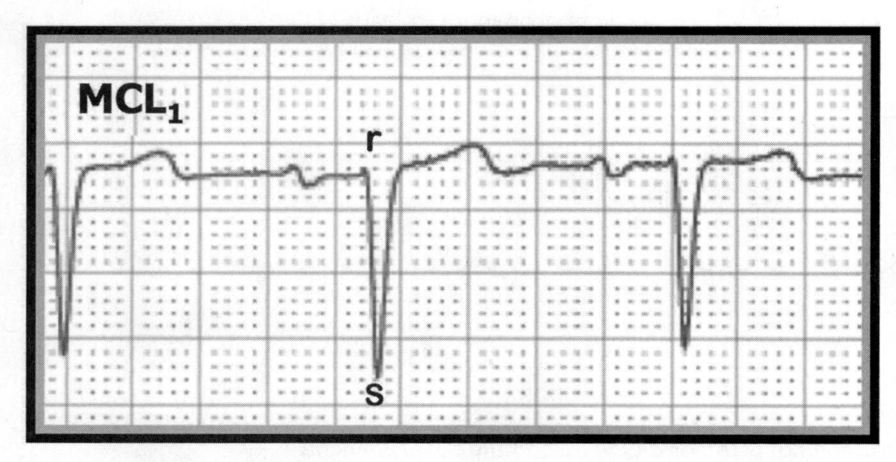

In this MCL1 lead, notice there is no Q wave (normal), the first upward R wave is very small, and the next downward deflection (S wave) is large. The lower case "r" and upper case "S" denote their relative size. This is a normal sinus rhythm using an MCL1 lead placement.
Source: Courtesy of K. Kyriakidis

PP Interval

The time between the beginning of one P wave and the beginning of the next P wave. This interval signifies the atrial (usually SA node) rate.

RR Interval

The time between the peak of one QRS complex and the peak of the next QRS complex. This is helpful in determining the ventricular rate.

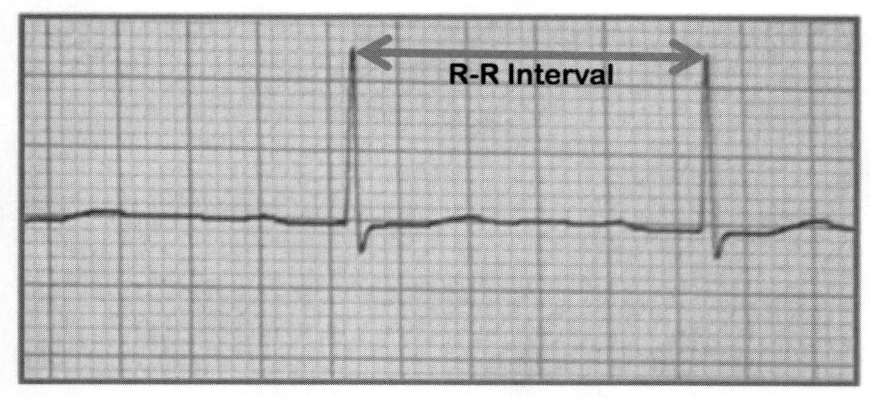

This image illustrates the correct measurement of the R-R interval. In addition to providing the basis for calculating the ventricular heart rate, its measurement for consistency informs about the regularity of the impulse initiation and conduction.
Source: Courtesy of K. Kyriakidis

T Wave

The T wave is the third prominent deflection in the EKG, follows the QRS, and signifies ventricular repolarization.

- The T wave normally appears as an upward deflection, rounded, and slightly asymmetrical.
- The morphology of the T wave can change in the presence of ischemia, ventricular hypertrophy, bundle branch blocks, and electrolyte imbalances. These can cause a flattened, biphasic, or inverted (upside down) T wave. Changes can also be benign.
- Hyperkalemia can give the T wave a tall and peaked appearance.

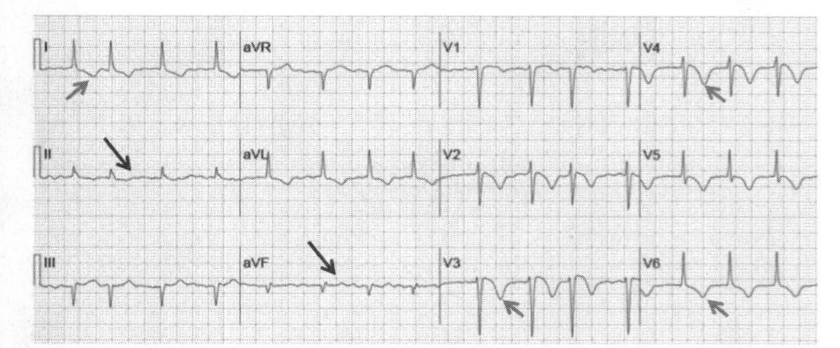

This EKG reveals an underlying atrial fibrillation as the rhythm, so the P waves are missing. Note the red arrows that point out the abnormally inverted T waves in leads I, aVL, and V2-V6. Blue arrows highlight the flattened T waves in leads II and aVF.
Source: Courtesy of K. Kyriakidis

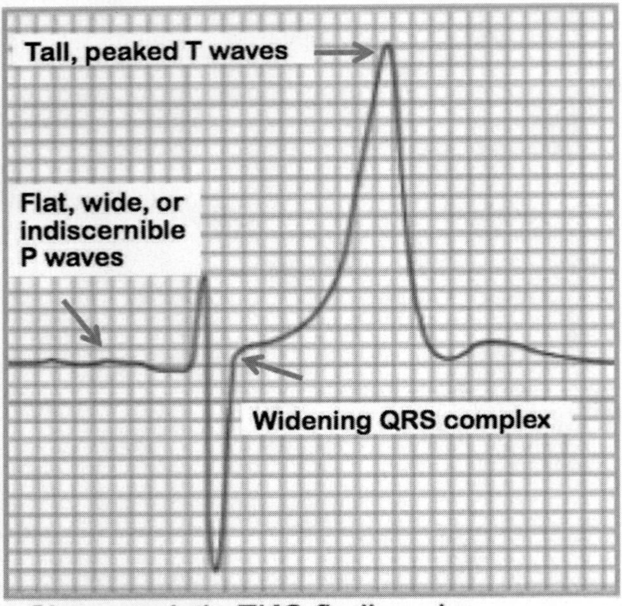

Characteristic EKG findings in hyperkalemia: tall, peaked T waves

T waves can be large in various cardiac conditions, but the T waves in this example are very peaked and tall. The "peaked" T waves warn of hyperkalemia which can be dangerous.
Source: Copyright © 2013, NovEx Novice to Expert Learning, LLC

Components of a Cardiac Cycle (continued)

ST Segment

The ST segment is the period immediately following ventricular depolarization. Since it reflects time when there is no electrical activity, a normal ST segment is flat or isoelectric.

- The ST segment is measured from the end of the QRS complex to the beginning of the T wave. The junction of the QRS and T waves is known as the J point.
- The ST segment is an important diagnostic finding in acute myocardial ischemia and infarction. **When acute myocardial injury occurs, the ST segment may be elevated.** This is referred to as ST segment myocardial infarction (STEMI).
- ST segment depression can indicate myocardial ischemia. It can be observed in NSTEMI and unstable angina.

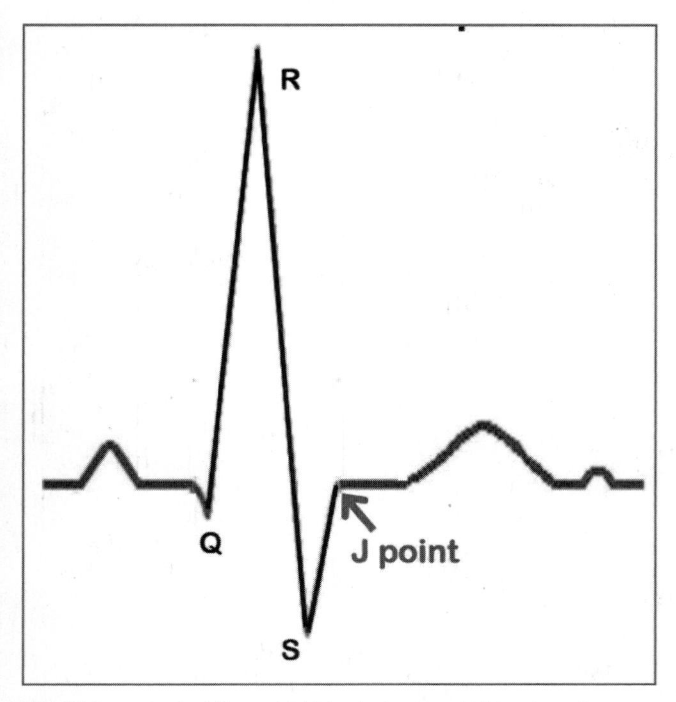

This QRS complex and T wave highlight the J point, which is where the beginning of the ST segment is measured.
Source: Courtesy of George Kyriakidis/Santa Ana, CA

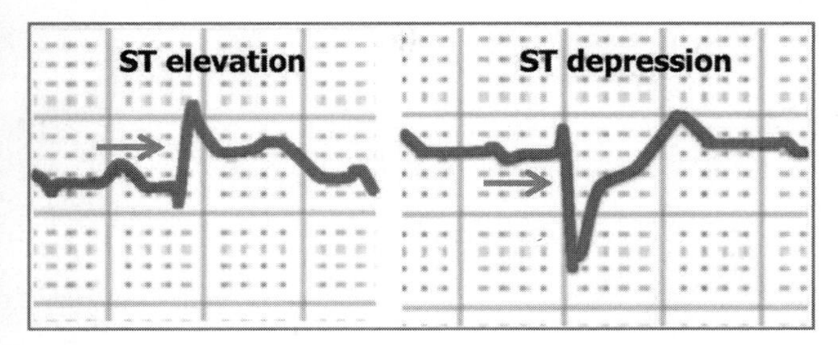

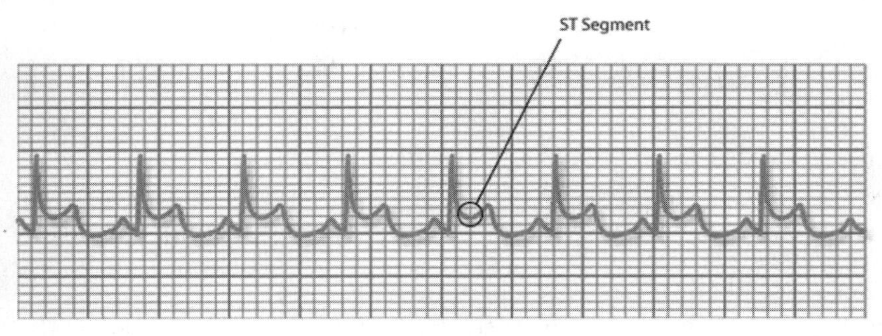

Upper: Note comparison of ST segments: ST elevation, which commonly indicates myocardial injury compared to ST depression, which can indicate myocardial ischemia. Lower: The EKG rhythm strip depicts a sinus tachycardia with ST elevation.
Sources: *(upper)* Courtesy of K. Kyriakidis; *(lower)* Copyright © 2013, NovEx Novice to Expert Learning, LLC

QT Interval and U Wave

The QT interval is the time it takes for ventricular depolarization and repolarization.

- The QT interval is measured from the beginning of the QRS complex to the end of the T wave. The time interval is normally < 0.40 sec.
- Normal factors that can influence the QT interval include heart rate, age, and gender. Medications and genetic abnormalities can prolong the QT and predispose a patient to lethal dysrhythmias (see examples below).

Occasionally, an additional wave may appear after the T wave called a **U wave**.

- A U wave is seen as a small (0.5 mm) upward deflection occurring right after the T wave.
- The **U wave** may reflect repolarization of the Purkinje fibers or can be present with electrolyte disturbances (hypokalemia).

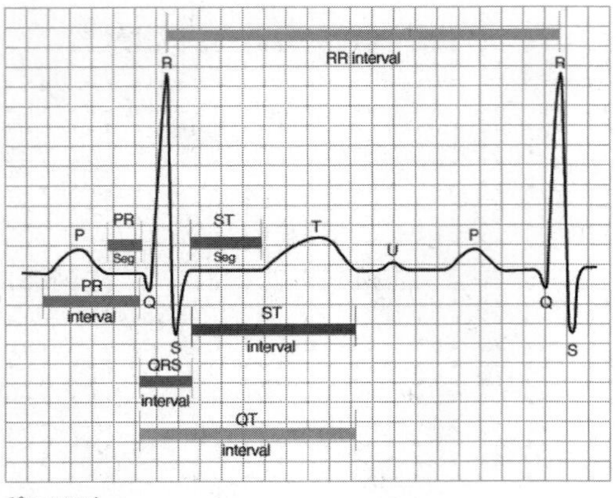

QT interval and U wave.

Source: Copyright © 2013, NovEx Novice to Expert Learning, LLC

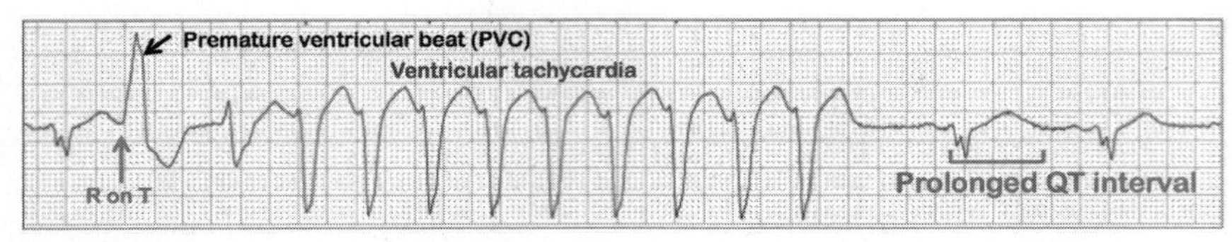

This EKG strip shows a life-threatening rhythm, V tach, that can occur when the QT interval is prolonged. This QT interval (above) is 0.64 sec, making the patient vulnerable to the ectopic ventricular impulse that initiated V tach. The V tach spontaneously resolved but intervention was necessary to prevent recurrence.

Source: Courtesy of K. Kyriakidis

Concept Check

4. What is the normal configuration of a T wave?
   A. Slightly asymmetrical
   B. Biphasic
   C. Inverted
   D. Peaked

Answer question

LO2:

Calculating Rate

Accurate Method

- Normal atrial (P-P interval) and ventricular (R-R interval) heart rates are 60–100 beats/min. For the rhythm to be normal, the atrial rate must equal the ventricular rate (P-P = R-R).
- Less than 60 is termed **bradycardia**.
- Greater than 100 is termed **tachycardia**.

Rate can be calculated by counting the number of small boxes contained in the RR interval (peak of one QRS to peak of the next).

Small boxes × 0.4 sec = time elapsed.

Rate = 60/(the time elapsed during RR interval) = **60/(number of boxes × 0.04)**

Example: 60/(**17** × 0.04) = **88** bpm

Example: 60/(17 x 0.04) = 88 beats/minute

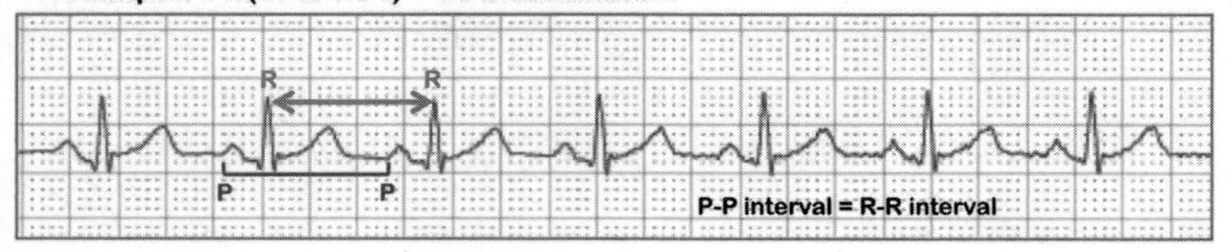

This example shows how to measure the appropriate intervals to calculate the heart rate.

Source: Courtesy of K. Kyriakidis

The "6 Seconds" Method

- The "6 Seconds" method uses 6 seconds as marked by notches on the EKG paper.
- This method is quick but not very accurate. It can give a rapid idea about the patient's heart rate but should not be used when documenting or obtaining accurate information.
- This method is useful with irregular rhythms when calculations are also inaccurate or hard to determine.
- To calculate the rate, first count the number of QRSs in 6 seconds, then, multiply the number of QRS's by 10 to get the estimated heart rate.
- 6 Seconds example: **9** QRSs × 10 = **90** bpm
- Now, calculate the heart rate using the prior method.

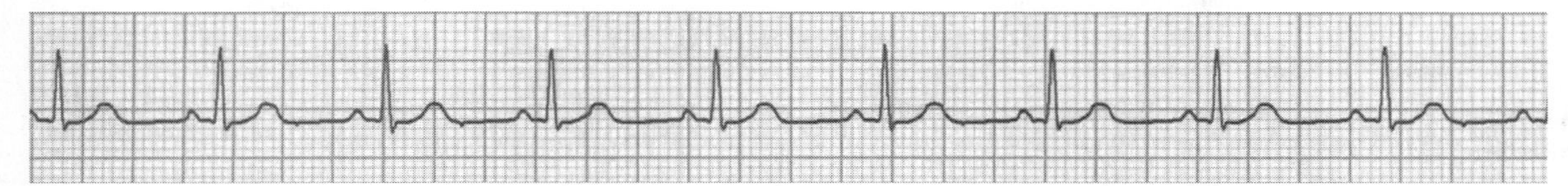

Answer: 60/ (19 × 0.04 sec) = 88 bpm

The "Quick Look" Method

- The "quick look" method of *estimating* the rate is counting the number of large boxes (5 small boxes in each) between two QRS complexes.
- This is only an estimated rate, not a reliable or an accurate one, but in an urgent situation, it provides a ballpark idea about the patient's situation.
- The estimation is derived from dividing 300 by the number of large boxes between the R-R. Example: 2 boxes within an R-R interval = 300/2 = HR 150.

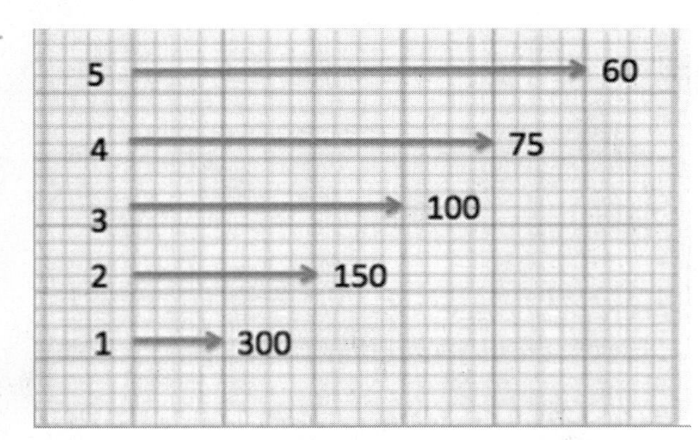

Quick look rate calculator; Heart Rates Estimations by Large Boxes

- Quick look example: Almost **4** large boxes between R-R = 300/**4** = **HR 75**
- To be more accurate, **What is the calculated rate?**

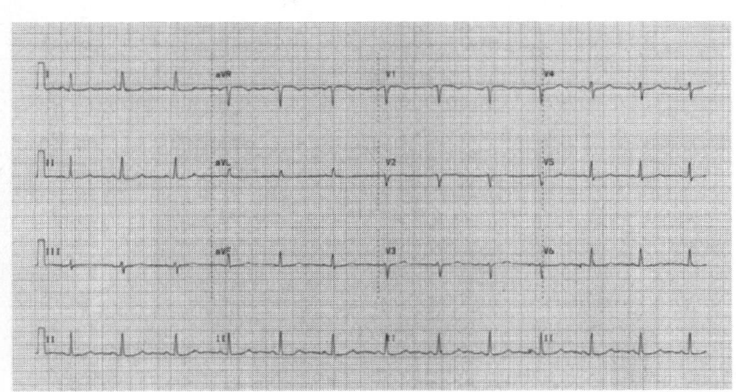

Source: Courtesy of K. Kyriakidis

Answer: 60/(19 × 0.04) = 79 bpm

Assessing Rhythm

Accurate rhythm interpretation is predicated on accurate and thorough assessment of the complexes and intervals. The development of a systematic assessment is the basis of an accurate interpretation. Steps should include:

1. P waves:
   - o Normal (upward), abnormal, or absent? All look the same?
   - o P-P intervals regular or irregular?
   - o Atrial rate normal, fast, or slow?
2. PR interval:
   - o Normal, short, prolonged, or absent?
   - o Are PR intervals the same (constant)? If not, is there a pattern of variation?
3. QRS complexes:
   - o Normal (for the lead), abnormally wide, or absent? Constant?
   - o QRS width normal, prolonged, variable with a pattern or variable with no pattern?
   - o R-R intervals regular or irregular?
   - o Ventricular rate normal, fast, or slow?
4. P-P = R-R (to define the relationship between the atria and ventricles)? Is there a P wave for every QRS?
5. ST segment elevation or depression: this is only interpreted on a 12-lead EKG.
6. QT interval: normal, short, or prolonged? constant?

Use of this method informs one if the rhythm is normal or abnormal.

- Clinicians who care for cardiac or monitored patients, with any frequency, find calipers indispensible (see top photo).
- Calipers are metal tools for accurately measuring EKG intervals, segments, and rates.
- Calipers can be used to more easily and accurately measure intervals on graph paper with the very small boxes as seen in the lower photo.
- This tool is especially helpful in assessing whether intervals are equal and constant.

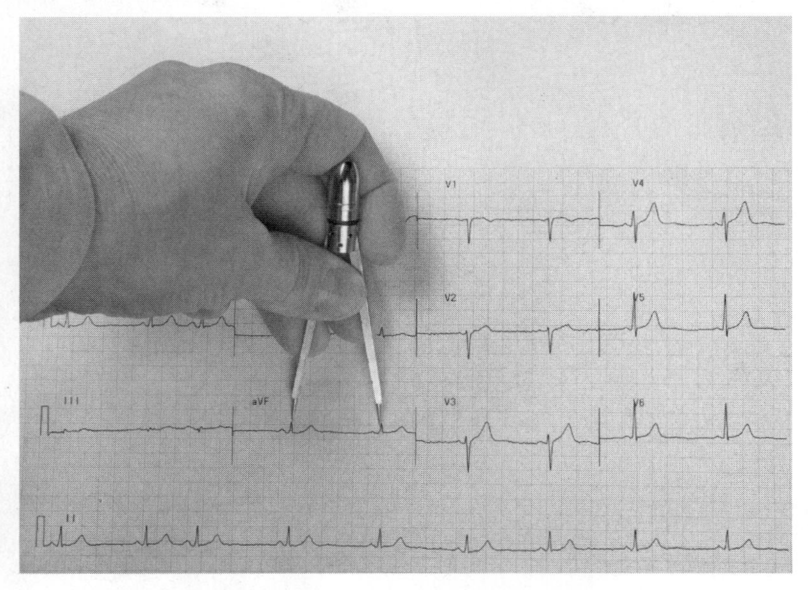

Photo shows the use of calipers in the measurement of the R-R interval.
Source: Howard/Fotolia

Example 1: Complete an assessment of the rhythm

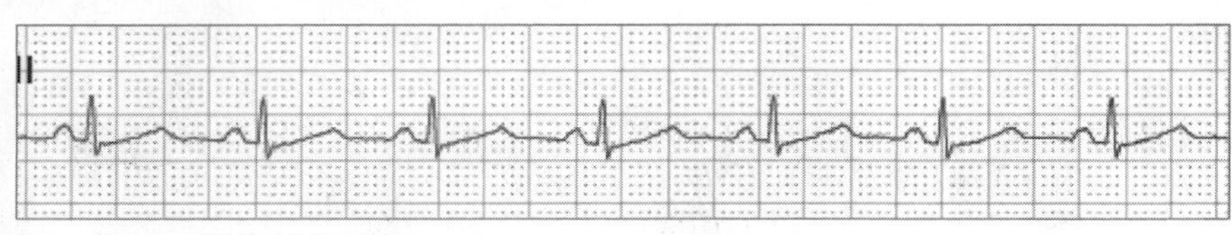

Source: Courtesy of K. Kyriakidis

Ex. 1—Rhythm Assessment:
P-P: normal, constant, rate 83 bpm
PR: 0.14 sec, constant
QRS: 0.08 sec, constant, R-R regular, rate 83 bpm
P-P = R-R: sinus and fast = **Normal sinus rhythm**
QT: 0.40 sec (normal)

Example 2: Complete an assessment of the rhythm

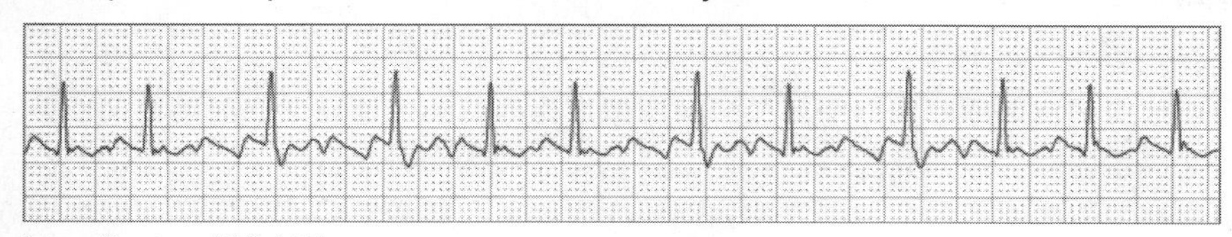

Source: Courtesy of K. Kyriakidis

Ex. 2—Rhythm Assessment:
P-P: absent, erratic baseline
PR: absent
QRS: 0.08 sec, constant, R-R irregular, cannot calculate—estimated rate 103–115 bpm
P-P ≠ R-R: not sinus, **abnormal, or dysrhythmia** (atrial fibrillation)
QT: about 0.28 sec (normal) but not clearly discernible

12-Lead EKG

Lead Placement Summary

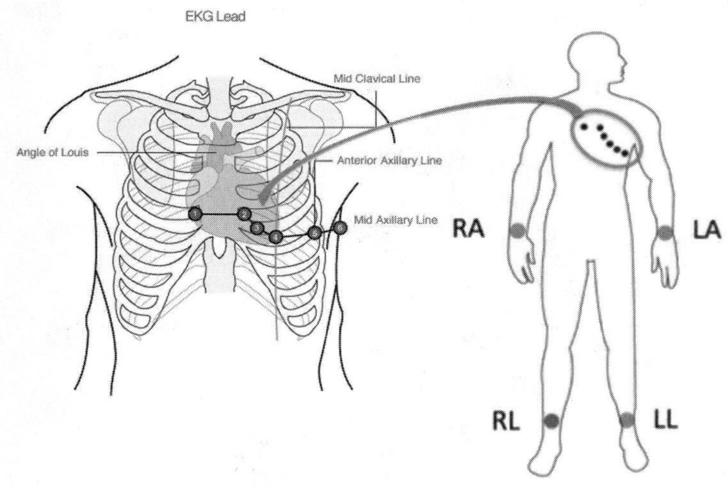

Left: Proper placement of six chest or V leads. Right: Proper placement of four limb electrodes to produce the three augmented and three standard limb leads in the 12-lead EKG.
Source: *(both)* Copyright © 2013, NovEx Novice to Expert Learning, LLC

Three Standard Limb Leads

Lead I

Measures the voltage from the right arm to the left arm and observes electrical activity moving to the left.

Lead II

Measures the voltage from the right arm to the left leg and observes electrical activity moving toward the left and downward.

Lead III

Measures voltage from the left arm to the left leg and observes electrical activity moving toward the right and downward.

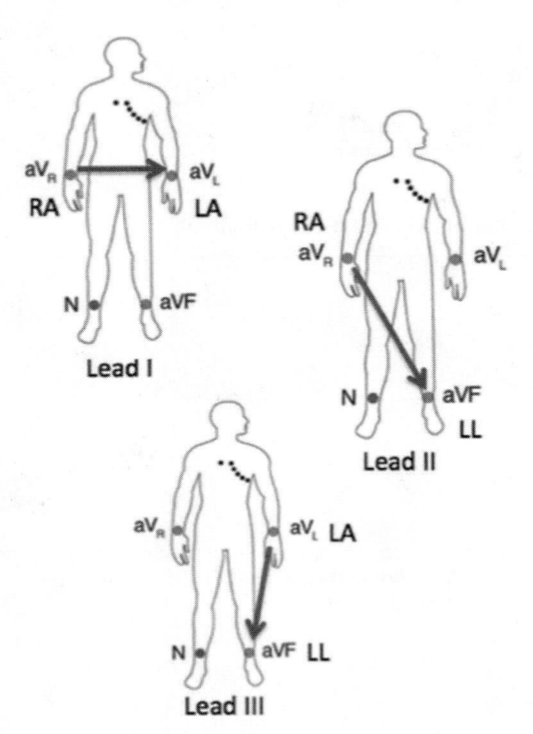

Three standard limb leads.
Source: Copyright © 2013, NovEx Novice to Expert Learning, LLC

Three Augmented Leads

The augmented leads are created by using combinations of electrodes. Two electrodes are combined to form an average and then compared to a third positive electrode. The right leg serves as a ground.

aVF

Two arm leads are averaged, with left foot as the positive electrode.

aVL

Right arm and left foot are averaged, with left arm as the positive electrode.

aVR

Left foot and left arm are averaged, with right arm as the positive electrode.

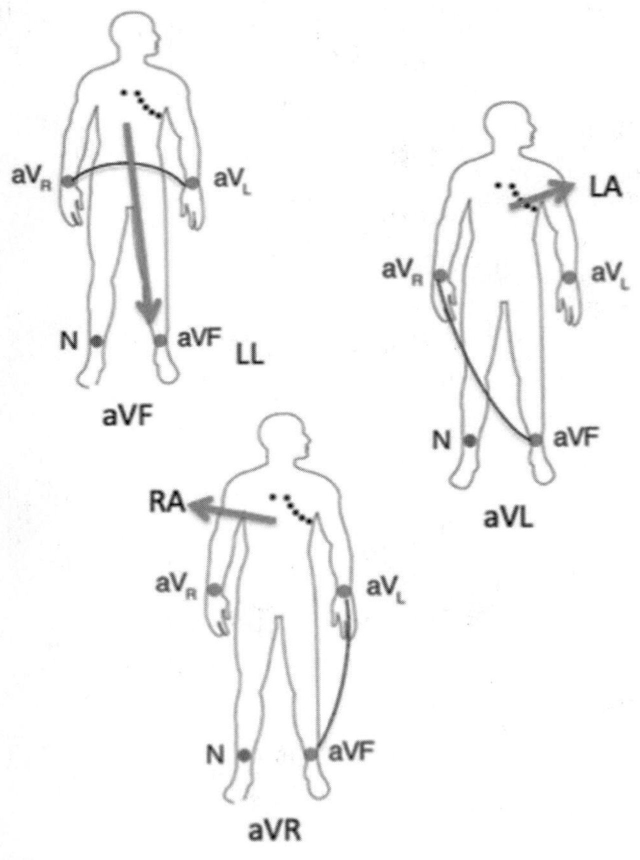

Three augmented leads.
Source: Copyright © 2013, NovEx Novice to Expert Learning, LLC

Six Chest Leads

There are six chest (precordial) leads V1–V6.

- V1: 4th intercostal space (ICS), to the right of the sternal border
- V2: 4th ICS, left of the sternal border
- V3: exactly between V2 and V4
- V4: 5th ICS, midclavicular line
- V5: 5th ICS, anterior axillary line
- V6: 5th ICS, midaxillary line

Correct lead placement is important for accuracy and validity.

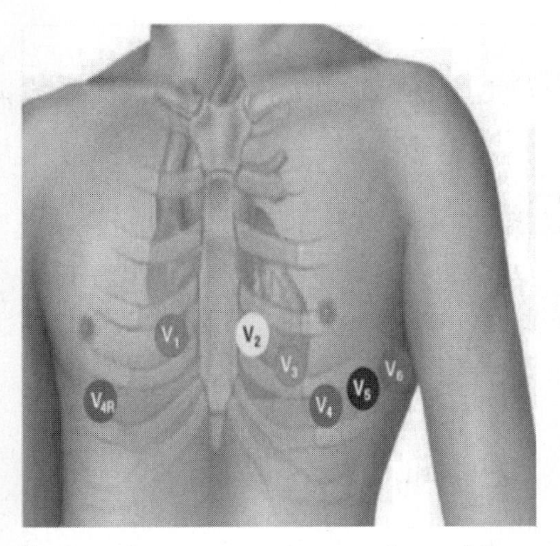
Illustration depicting proper placement of precordial or chest EKG leads.
Source: Copyright © 2013, NovEx Novice to Expert Learning, LLC

LO3:

What Can an EKG Represent?

EKG is a central tool in diagnostics as it can provide significant amounts and types of information that saves heart muscle and lives. Accurate and rapid interpretation is critical in guiding correct treatment. This lesson details the most salient information in the care of most patients who require a 12-lead EKG or cardiac monitoring. Two primary functions include:

1. **Dysrhythmia Detection:** Dysrhythmias are abnormal heart rhythms and rhythm disturbances. These can be interpreted from a monitor strip using a single lead (two in some situations). A 12-lead EKG can also be used for dysrhythmia interpretation but is a less convenient or efficient method when dysrhythmias are the focus.
2. **Injury Patterns of Ischemia and Infarction:** A 12-lead EKG is necessary to interpret patterns of ischemia and infarction that occur in acute coronary syndrome (ACS) conditions. Infarctions (STEMI or NSTEMI) manifest different patterns than ischemia. Further, multiple leads are commonly needed to understand the meaning and location of ischemia (stable or unstable) and infarction patterns.

Dysrhythmias

Dysrhythmias represent a defect in the electrical conduction system of the heart affecting the heart rate, regularity, speed, reliability, or sequence of the electrical activity of the heart.

- Dysrhythmias can be fast or slow, regular, or irregular, or chaotic.
- Dysrhythmias can range from benign to life threatening.
- Heart blocks can affect the capacity and speed of conduction.
- Normal EKG morphology is commonly altered by conduction abnormalities.

Due to the importance and detail necessary to understand Dysrhythmias, please refer to the NovE-Lesson on Dysrhythmias for a more in-depth look at specific dysrhythmias and interpretation.

Injury Patterns

Ischemia and Infarction

The most common injury patterns in ACS involve ischemia, NSTEMI, and STEMI.

- Each ACS condition manifests different EKG patterns. The most important information to obtain from the EKG includes the **type** of injury and its **location**.
- The type of injury is obtained by interpreting ST segment and T wave changes and/or Q waves. The location of the changes on the 12-lead EKG generally reflects the specific coronary artery involved and the myocardial area where damage occurred.
- The diagram points out the changes that can occur. Each is discussed as follows:
  1. Q waves
  2. ST segment elevation
  3. ST segment depression
  4. T wave changes (hyperacute peaking, inversion, flattening)

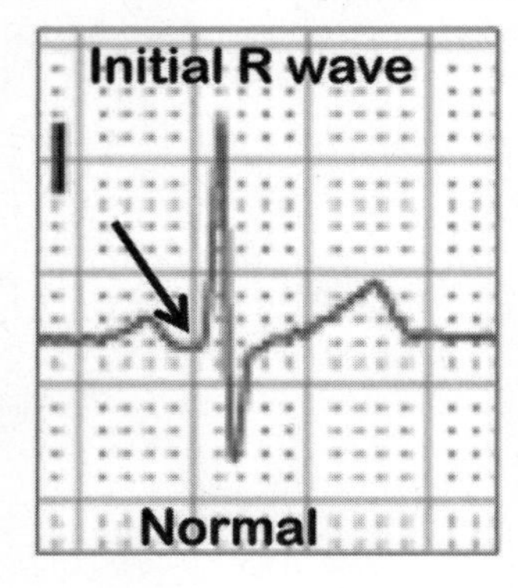

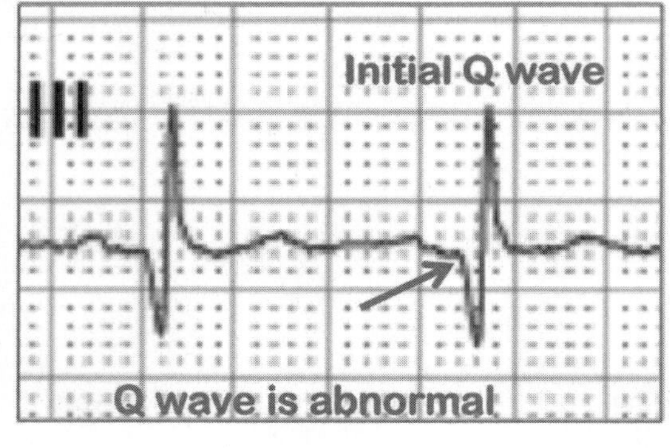

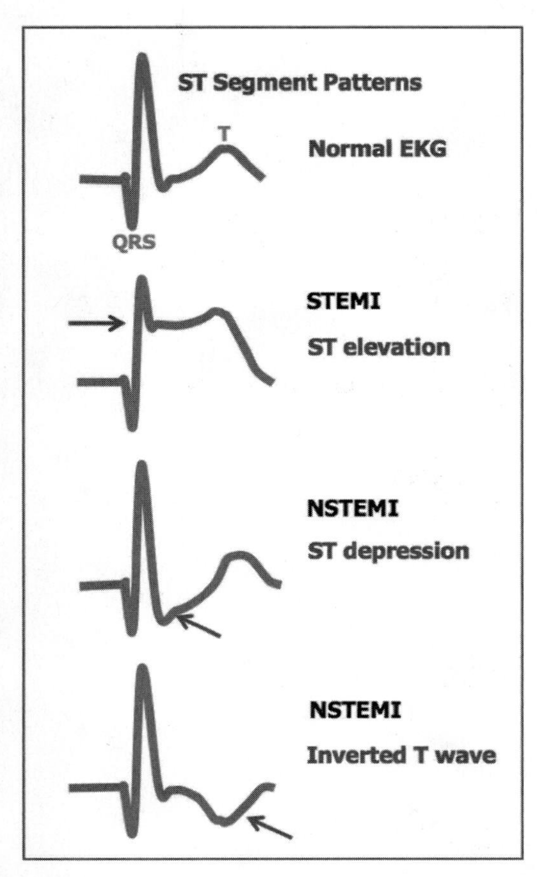

Upper: Q wave. Lower: This diagram allows comparison of the ST-T wave changes that occur in STEMI versus NSTEMI. Note that ST elevation occurs only in a STEMI.

Sources: (*upper*) Courtesy of K. Kyriakidis; (*lower*) Copyright © 2013, NovEx Novice to Expert Learning, LLC

What Can an EKG Represent? (continued)

T Wave Changes

T wave abnormalities, specific to ACS, can indicate cardiac ischemia and can occur prior to ST segment changes.

- Hyperacute T waves (see V2–V3) are tall, peaked, wide, symmetrical changes that accompany acute injury. They are the first EKG change noted in STEMI or can coincide with ST elevation, and Q waves, as seen in the EKG example.
    - Inverted T waves can be pathologic for cardiac ischemia, particularly if in a pattern (see lower EKG, leads II, III, and aVF). These point out inferior wall ischemia.
    - There are frequent instances of diffuse T wave changes or with no pattern. These may or may not reflect cardiac ischemia.
- A key finding is NEW T wave inversion, as those more commonly reveal an important or impending condition.
- Symmetrically inverted T waves are strongly correlated with ischemia.

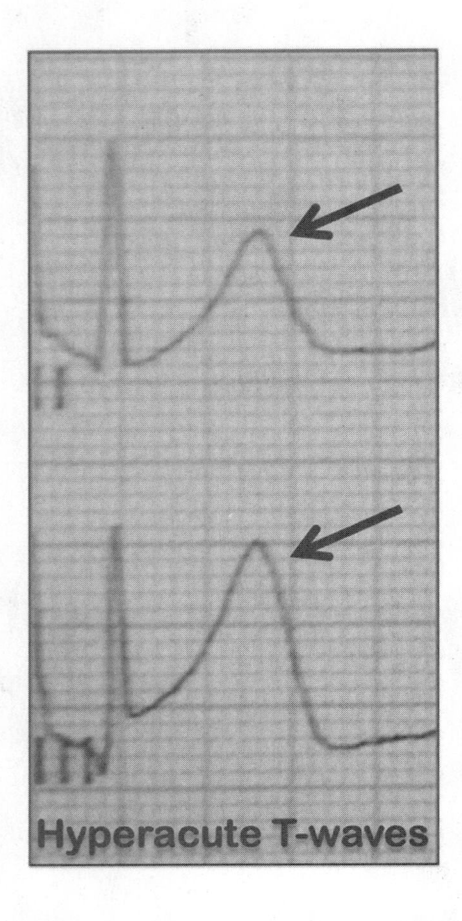

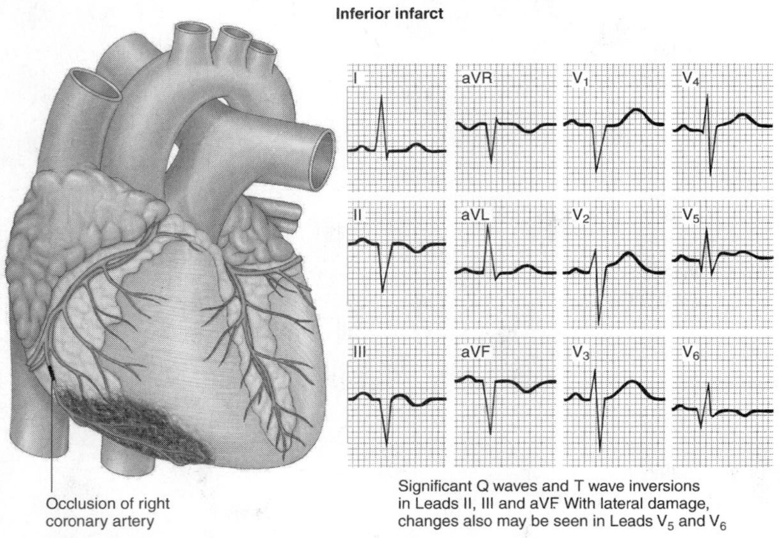

Upper: Hyperacute or large and wide T waves are commonly seen with STEMI along with the ST elevation and Q waves. Lower: Inverted T waves may indicate ACS, but are associated with a wide range of conditions. However, in this EKG, the pattern of T wave changes along with the deep Q wave in Leads II, III, and aVF point at inferior wall ischemia.

What Can an EKG Represent? (continued)

ST Depression

Like T wave changes, ST depression can indicate cardiac ischemia.

- Ischemia-related ST depression is typically localized to reflect the affected myocardial region but can present diffusely across leads.
- ST depression must meet criteria to have significance.
- Horizontal and downsloping ST depression is most highly correlated with ischemia.
- Reciprocal (mirror image) ST depression can be seen in leads opposite STE after STEMI.

Types of ST Depression

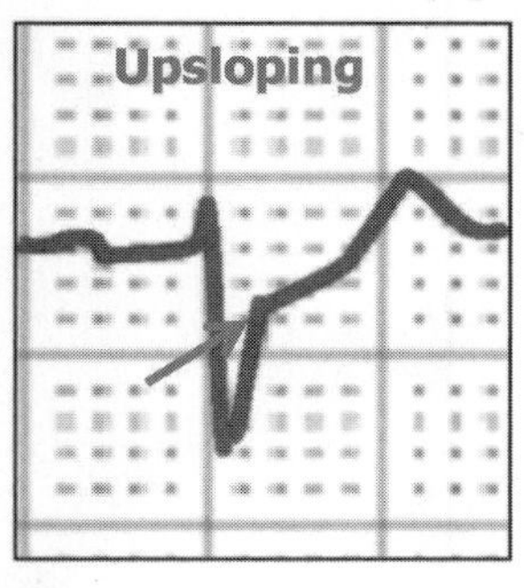

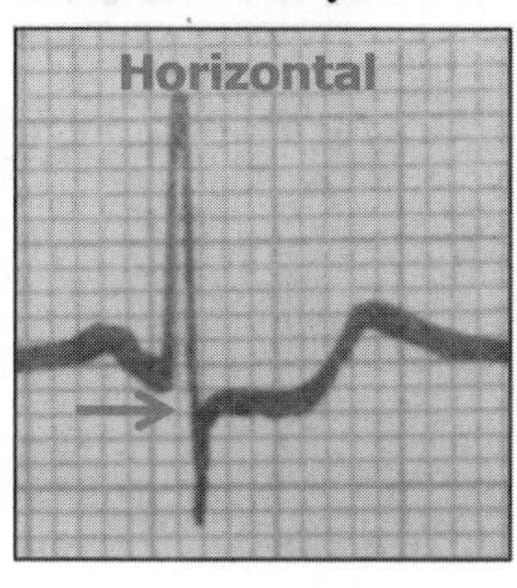

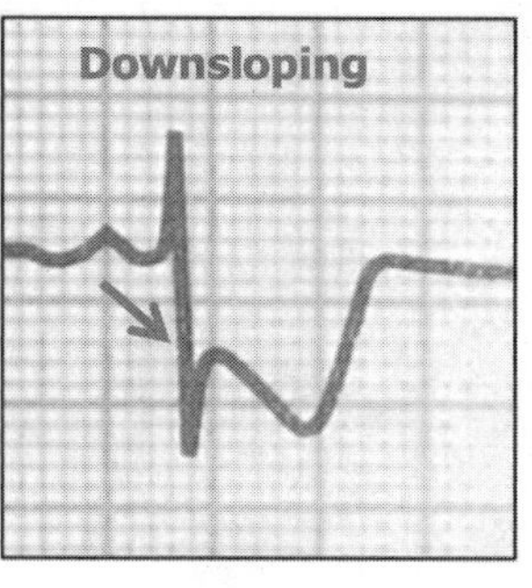

This diagram details the three types of ST Depression. ST depression is a key EKG finding in a patient with NSTEMI.
Source: (*left*) Courtesy of K. Kyriakidis

- ST depression with or without T wave inversion in at least two leads is common in non–Q wave NSTEMI.
- NSTEMI must be diagnosed along with other information such as clinical presentation and biomarkers as the EKG is not specific for a firm diagnosis.

Concept Check

5. **What is the typical first step in the interpretation of EKG rhythm?**
   A. Measure QRS duration
   B. Determine P wave and R wave relationship
   C. Assess P wave
   D. Evaluate T wave configuration

Answer question

What Can an EKG Represent? (continued)

Infarction

ST Segment Elevation

STE is another early EKG change during a myocardial infarction (MI). **It is a serious sign of myocardial injury or STEMI.**

- ECG criteria were defined by the joint ESC/ACCF/AHA/WHF* committee for STEMI (see left illustration). Criteria refer to the number of mV (0.1 mV = 1 mm = 1 small box) of elevation to qualify as a positive finding.
- The EKG (picture to right) provides examples in V1–V3 of varying degrees of STE, indicating a STEMI. The example also meets all criteria as the STE occurs in two or more leads in the same region (septal wall).

*Joint Task Force of the European Society of Cardiology, American College of Cardiology Foundation, the American Heart Association, and the World Health Federation

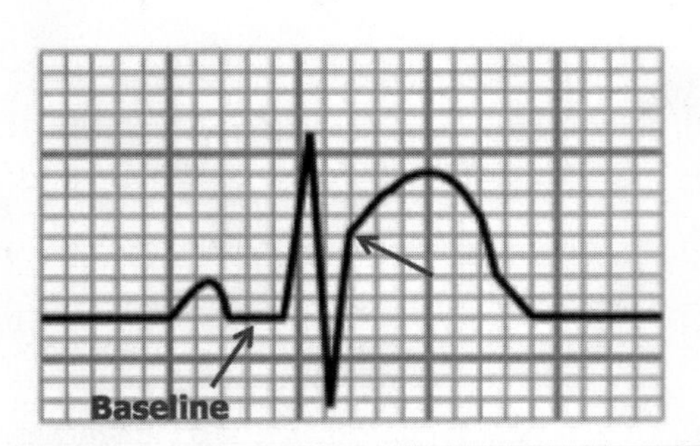

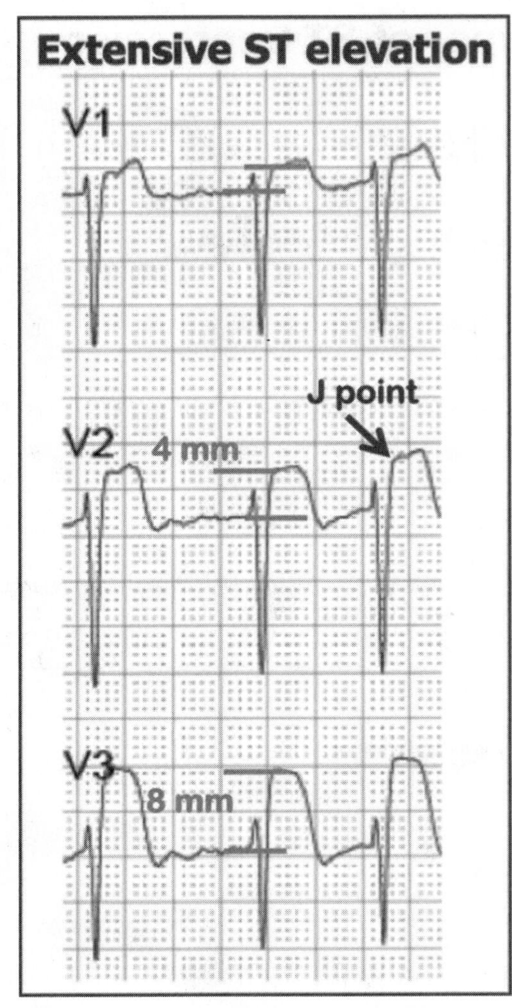

Left: The QRS complex is used to show the ST segment elevation seen in STEMI. The EKG criteria for ST elevation are listed. Right: Leads V1–V3 in this EKG demonstrate the EKG criteria for ST elevation in a STEMI regarding degree of elevation and presence in multiple leads in the same region.
Source: (*right*) Courtesy of K. Kyriakidis

- The ST segment elevation present on specific EKG leads provides information about the likely coronary artery or arteries involved.
- STE can be transient in transmural ischemia and then resolve or disappear when the ischemia is treated. This type of STE seen on the EKG commonly reflects location of the ischemia (see localization chart for EKG patterns).
- It is important to note that there are a small but significant number of patients who will have a normal EKG or nonspecific EKG changes in the presence of an MI. The EKG should be viewed in conjunction with the clinical presentation, biomarkers, and other tests to determine if myocardial damage has occurred.
- **Identification of STE in STEMI is an important guide to treatment** (see EKG). These patients should be immediately transported for percutaneous coronary intervention (PCI). The EKG example shows STE greater than 0.1 mV in III, aVF, and V1–V6, >0.2 mV in V2–V3, and Q waves in II and aVF, which are compelling evidence for urgent PCI.

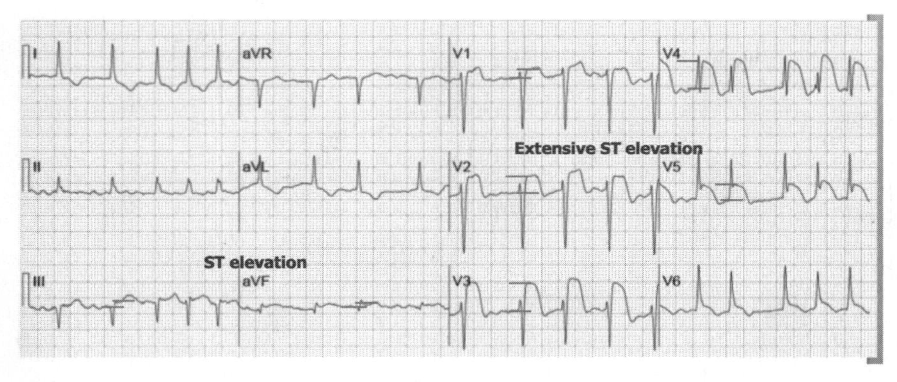

EKG: Acute inferior-septal STEMI. The extensive ST elevation is noted in the inferior (III and aVF) and septal (V1–V5) leads.
Source: Courtesy of K. Kyriakidis

What Can an EKG Represent? (continued)

The Q Wave

Q wave is the first downward deflection after the P wave and is normally small.

- A Q wave commonly appears post-STEMI (after 24 hours).
- Q waves are not always present following MI, depending on the duration of the occlusion, the extent of the myocardial damage, and the collateral blood flow to the damaged area.
- For Q waves to be diagnostic of MI (see top EKG), they must be greater than or equal to 0.04 sec wide, one-third the height of the R wave, and occur in greater than or equal to two or more contiguous or adjacent leads.
- Examine the lower EKG to find the location and extent of the pathologic Q waves. What do these mean?

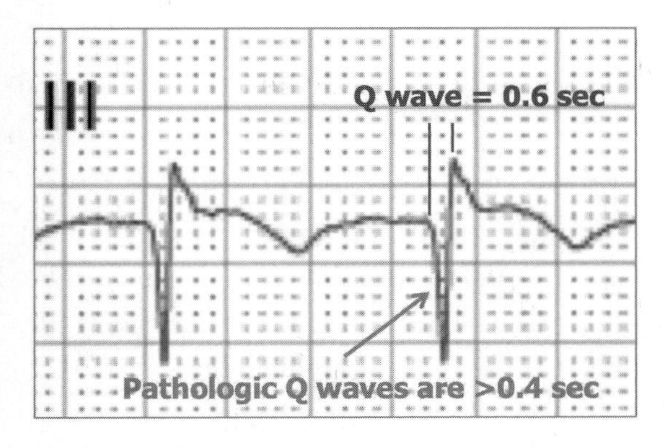

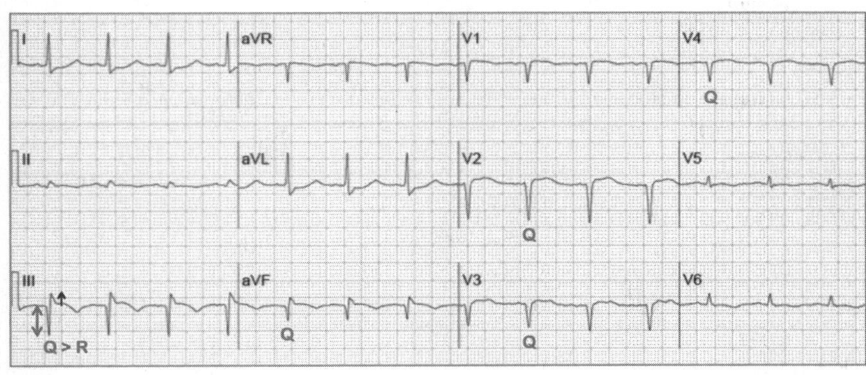

Upper: This example of a Q wave meets the criteria of being greater than 0.4 sec wide with the Q wave greater than 1/3 the height of the R wave. Lower: Notice the Q waves in contiguous leads III and aVF, which suggest inferior wall infarction. Additionally, the deep Q or QS waves in contiguous leads V2–V4 suggest an anteroseptal MI. Without acute ST elevation, the MIs are of indeterminant age.
Source: *(both)* Courtesy of K. Kyriakidis

- Identification of Q waves is important in guiding clinical judgment and determining the course of treatment. An MI that is at least a day old will *not* respond to thrombolytic therapy. Early interventional treatments are no longer useful.
- What pathologic Q waves do you find below? What do these mean?

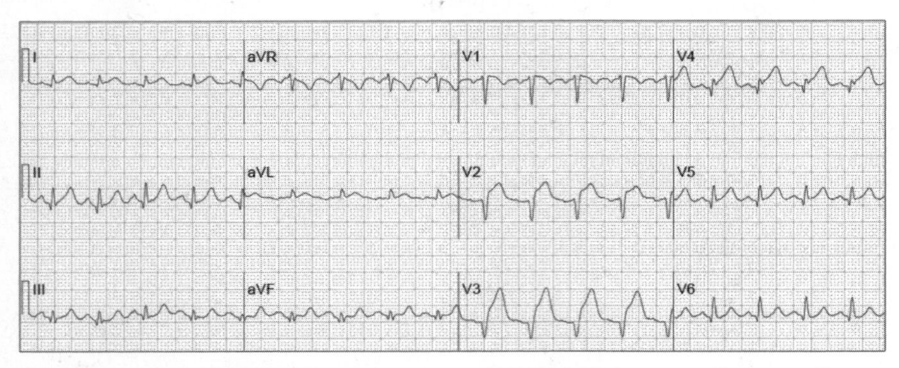

The Q waves in leads V2–V4 reveal an acute anteroseptal MI. With ST elevation and hyperacute T waves in the same leads, the STEMI is thought to be acute. Q waves are also visible in the inferior leads (II, III, and aVF) without ST segment changes, indicating that the MI may be old.
Source: Courtesy of K. Kyriakidis

- The EKG can reflect injury patterns that correspond to the affected coronary arteries.

EKG Q Wave and ST-T Abnormalities Suggest Location of Myocardial Injury, Infarction, or Transmural Ischemia

EKG Lead	Myocardium Affected	Coronary Artery
II, III, AVF	Inferior or Inferolateral Wall*	Right Coronary (90%), Left circumflex (10%)*
V1-V6, I, aVL	Extensive Anterior Wall	LAD (proximal)
V1-V2	Septal Wall	LAD
V1-V2 to **V3-V6**	Apical Anterior Wall*	LAD (mid)
aVL, I, V2-V3	Mid-Anterior Wall*	LAD
I, aVL, V6, **RS in V1-V2**	Lateral Wall*	Left Circumflex
V1, V3R-V6R	Right Ventricular Wall	Right Coronary
V7-V9	Posterior Wall	Posterior Descending?
aVR ST ↑ >V1; ST in ≥ 7 leads	"Widow Maker"; Sudden Death*	Left Main Coronary
* Changes from traditional understandings		

*Based on autopsy or cardiovascular MRI comparisons to EKG findings, LAD = Left anterior descending
Source: Copyright © 2013, NovEx Novice to Expert Learning, LLC

- Based on autopsy and/or cardiovascular MRI comparisons to EKG findings, this is a summary of the classification system that correlates Q waves and/or ST-T abnormalities with myocardial ischemic, injury, and infarct locations. The table lists the most current evidence regarding EKG findings and related myocardial regions with the associated coronary arteries.
- An **extensive anterior MI** that involves the left main coronary artery, above the left anterior descending (LAD) and circumflex arteries, is often called the "widow maker" because most patients die suddenly.
- **Anterior MIs** are the most lethal because of the amount of muscle damage and the injury to the ventricular conduction system. The occlusion occurs at the LAD artery.
- **Lateral MIs** involve occlusion of the left circumflex artery. Seeing the location of the arteries helps one understand how various MIs got their labels.
- **Inferior MIs** are the second most lethal because they often produce dysrhythmias, such as 2nd degree heart block. Inferior MIs involve occlusion of the right coronary artery (RCA).

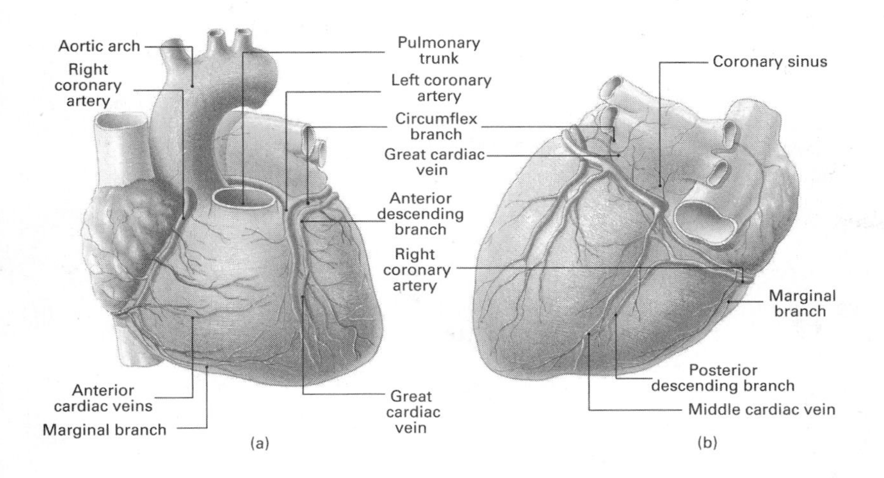

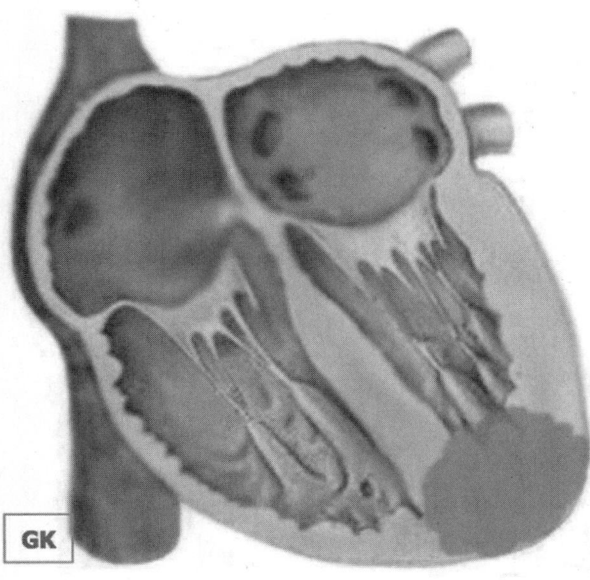

Upper: This picture shows the location of the coronary arteries to provide a visual understanding about what myocaridal area is affected by each type of MI. Lower: The MI is located in the anterior and septal areas of the heart. One may expect to see ST elevation in leads V2–V4.
Source: (*lower*) Courtesy of George Kyriakidis/Santa Ana, CA

Concept Check

6. Q wave and ST-T abnormalities only in V1 through V2 most likely indicate ischemia in which area of the heart?

A. Posterior wall

B. Septal wall

C. Anterior wall

D. Lateral wall

Answer question

Concept Check

7. Which myocardial infarction is most lethal?

A. Anterior

B. Inferior

C. Lateral

D. Posterior

Answer question

Priority Patient Concerns and Desired Collaborative Care Outcomes

Prior to caring for patients having an EKG, it is important to prioritize the patient's concerns that must guide the nursing care plan and interventions. Care for the patient is ordered and organized in accordance with the patient's priority and urgent needs. Desired collaborative care outcomes in patients having an EKG typically include:

1. Patient will be calm during the procedure.
2. Patient will demonstrate understanding of the procedure.

Considering these important care outcomes, prepare a list of the major 3–6 priority patient concerns or nursing diagnoses for patients having an EKG. Be prepared to participate in a discussion of this list and/or to submit them as an assignment, as determined by your faculty. Resources you may find helpful in this assignment can include this lesson, the references, resources on nursing care plans, and standard nursing diagnoses manuals.

Summary

- EKG is one of the most common and useful diagnostic tools used in medicine.
- This NovE-Lesson is meant to provide a basic understanding of what an EKG is, what it represents, and how it is used in the care of patients.
- An EKG reflects information about the electrical condition of the heart, electrolyte imbalances, dysrhythmias (both lethal and nonlethal), drug toxicities, and myocardial ischemia and damage.
- It is important to be familiar with the normal configuration of an EKG and to be aware of acute injury patterns in order to provide excellent care of patients and maximize their outcomes.
- Accurate lead placement is imperative to obtain accurate information from an EKG.
- An EKG alone is not diagnostic in the absence of a thorough history and physical assessment.
- EKG rhythm is an **electrical** representation but does not verify **mechanical activity** of the heart, that is, the actual contraction to produce stroke volume. Remember that there are situations when the EKG can show a normal rhythm but the heart is not pumping at all. One must always verify by physical exam that the patient's clinical presentation is consistent with the EKG representation.

LO4:

Evaluation of Desired Collaborative Care Outcomes

Evaluation and reassessment should reveal attainment of previously established patient outcomes. In summary:

- Patient lies quietly and calmly during procedure.
- Patient accurately describes the purpose of the procedure, his role in accurate testing, and any follow-up required.

References

Ahrens, T. S., Prentice, D., & Kleinpell, R. (2010). *Critical Care Nursing Certification: Preparation, Review and Practice Exams* (6th ed.).

Dubin, D. (2000). *Rapid interpretation of EKG's: An interactive course.* Tampa, FL: COVER Publishing Co.

Thygesen, K., Alpert, J. S., Jaffe, A.S., Simoons, M. L., Chaitman, B. R., White, H. D., ... Mendis, S. (2012). Third universal definition of myocardial infarction. *Circulation*, 126, 2020-2035 (Criteria for diagnosis of acute MI).

Clinical Practice Guidelines

ACC/AHA guidelines for the management of patients with ST-elevation myocardial infarction: A report of the American College of Cardiology/American Heart Association Task Force on Practice Guidelines (Committee to Revise the 1999 Guidelines for the Management of Patients with Acute Myocardial Infarction). Antman, E. M., Anbe, D. T., Armstrong, P.W., Bates, E. R., Green, L. A., Hand, M., ... Jacobs, A. K. (2004). American College of Cardiology, American Heart Association Task Force on Practice Guidelines, Canadian Cardiovascular Society. *Circulation*, 110(9), e82.

ACC/AHA Guidelines update in 2007: www.acc.org/qualityandscience/clinical/statements.htm (Accessed on September 18, 2007).

STOP

Go to the online course and complete the NovE-Cases assigned by your instructor for this module.

Learning Outcomes for Cardiomyopathy

When you complete this lesson, you will be able to:

1. Recognize the clinical significance of cardiomyopathy.
2. Consider the pathophysiology, etiology, risk factors, and clinical presentation of cardiomyopathy that determine the priority patient concerns.
3. Determine the most urgent and important nursing interventions and patient education required in caring for a patient with cardiomyopathy.
4. Evaluate attainment of desired collaborative care outcomes for a patient with cardiomyopathy.

LO1:

What Is Cardiomyopathy?

- Cardiomyopathy (CM) refers to diseases of the heart muscle.
- There are different types of cardiomyopathies, each with their different causes, signs, symptoms, and treatment.
- Cardiomyopathy is a primary disturbance in the cardiac muscle. Generally, in CM, the heart muscle becomes enlarged, thick, or rigid, resulting in failure of the muscle (myocytes) to function properly:
  - o Myocyte dysfunction weakens the heart's ability to pump.
  - o Abnormal muscle tissue can disrupt fibers in the electrical conduction system and lead to dysrhythmia.
- The ventricular chamber of the heart may become dilated, but often the ventricular muscle mass thickens so the heart appears enlarged.
- As myopathy worsens, one of two things usually happens:
  1. The heart becomes weaker and is less able to pump blood through the body. Heart failure is then likely.
  2. Rhythm disturbances develop, with potentially fatal rhythms such as ventricular fibrillation or tachycardia.
- Ischemic heart disease is considered, at least in the United States, as the leading cause of some cardiomyopathies. However, there is some controversy regarding this statement.
- The American Heart Association's (AHA) scientific statement on cardiomyopathies does not include ischemic origins. Their definition essentially states:

  "Cardiomyopathies are a group of diseases of the myocardium associated with mechanical and/or electrical dysfunction that usually (but not invariably) exhibit inappropriate ventricular hypertrophy or dilatation and are due to a variety of causes that, frequently, are genetic."
- AHA then goes further to state:

  "Cardiomyopathies are categorized into two groups: (1) primary cardiomyopathies (predominantly involving the heart) and (2) secondary cardiomyopathies (accompanied by other organ system involvement)."
  - o Primary cardiomyopathies are subdivided into those which are genetic, mixed (predominantly nongenetic but, less commonly, genetic), or acquired. The genetic cardiomyopathies include hypertrophic obstructive cardiomyopathy (HCM) and arrthymogenic right ventricular dysplasia (ARVD).
  - o Mixed cardiomyopathies include dilated cardiomyopathy (DCM) and restrictive cardiomyopathy (RCM).
  - o Acquired cardiomyopathies include myocarditis, stress-induced (Takotsubo), peripartum, tachycardia-induced, and infants of insulin-dependent diabetic mothers.

Concept Check

1. **Which cardiomyopathy has a strong genetic link?**

   A. Hypertrophic obstructive cardiomyopathy

   B. Dilated cardiomyopathy

   C. Restrictive cardiomyopathy

   D. Myocarditis

Answer question

LO1:

Clinical Relevance

- Cardiomyopathies can result in sudden cardiac death, often without prior symptoms.
- For example, HCM is the leading cause of sudden cardiac death in people under 24 years of age, affecting 1 in 500 people.
- Cardiomyopathies are responsible for more than 10,000 deaths per year if ischemic heart disease is included in the definition.

Types of Cardiomyopathy

There are four main types of cardiomyopathy:

1. Dilated cardiomyopathy (DCM)
2. Hypertrophic obstructive cardiomyopathy (HCM)
3. Restrictive cardiomyopathy (RCM)
4. Arrhythmogenic right ventricular cardiomyopathy (ARVC) or arrhythmogenic right ventricular dysplasia (ARVD)

Each type of cardiomyopathy is discussed.

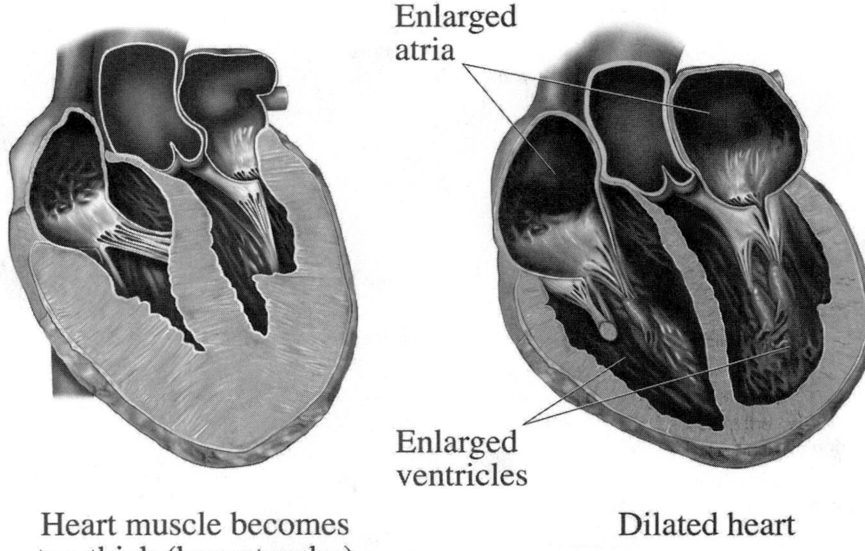

This illustration shows cardiomyopathies: one with hypertrophy (thickened walls) (left) and one that has thin, dilated walls (right).
Source: Nucleus Medical Art Inc/Alamy

LO1:

What Is Dilated Cardiomyopathy?

- Dilated cardiomyopathy (DCM) is the most common type of cardiomyopathy and is the most likely type seen in the hospitalized patient. It has also been referred to as congestive cardiomyopathy.
- While more common in African Americans, it can occur in any group of patients. It can affect individuals at any age, but the majority of patients diagnosed are middle-aged or young adults.
- In the majority of patients (about 80%), the precise cause of the cardiomyopathy cannot be determined.
- DCM is characterized by dilatation (enlarging and thinning) and weakness. Both ventricles can be affected.

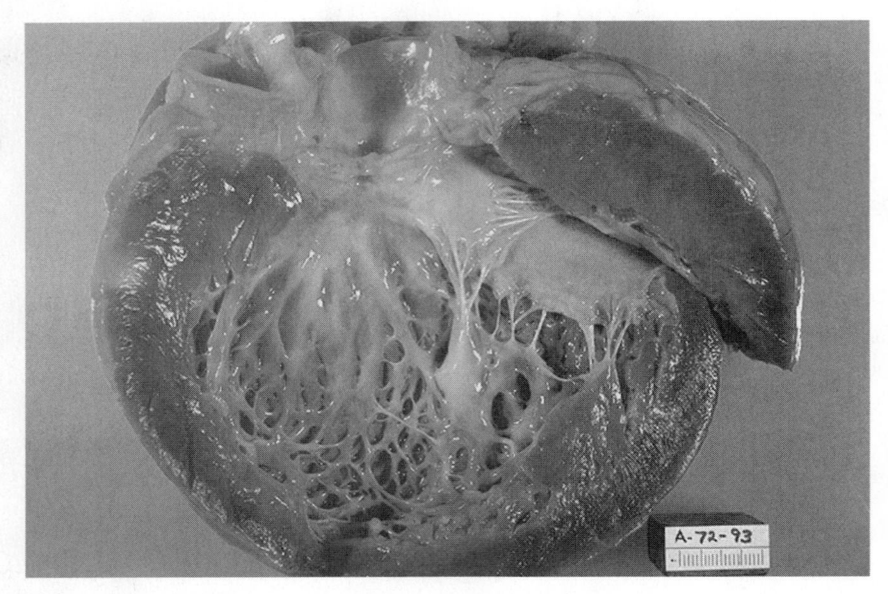
A-72-93

An autopsy, the heart of a patient who died from idiopathic cardiomyopathy, shows the abnormal thick, dilated left ventricular walls. Note the abnormally increased fibrosis (whitish color) of the endocardium. By comparison, the heart with dilated cardiomyopathy is similarly dilated, but the ventricular walls are much thinner than normal. Both causes of cardiomyopathy can lead to heart failure and death.
Source: CDC/Dr. Edwin P. Ewing, Jr.

LO2:

Pathophysiology: DCM

- In DCM, the heart muscle becomes dysfunctional resulting in both weakening of the heart and a tendency for fast rate dysrhythmias.
- As the heart weakens, it becomes enlarged in size, and its walls tend to thin (thus the term *dilated*).
- In DCM, the enlargement of the ventricles results in decreased performance in the heart's ability to pump or eject blood during systole. The weakening of the heart produces reduced stroke volume and lower ejection fractions.
- The abnormal muscle allows electrical impulses to be conducted outside the normal pathways, resulting in dangerous and potentially fatal ventricular dysrhythmias.

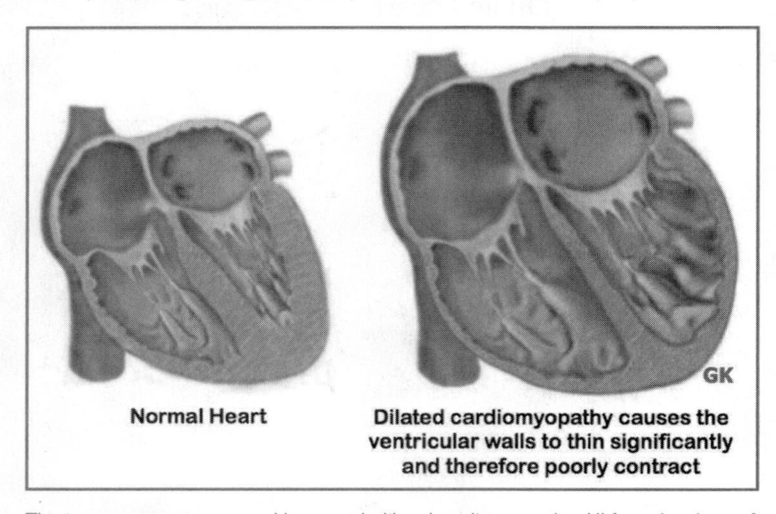
GK
Normal Heart
Dilated cardiomyopathy causes the ventricular walls to thin significantly and therefore poorly contract

This image contrasts a normal heart with dilated cardiomyopathy. All four chambers of the heart with DCM are dilated. The ventricular walls are especially thinned. There is no evidence of scarring.
Source: Courtesy of George Kyriakidis/Santa Ana, CA

Risk Factors: DCM

Factors that can lead to DCM include:

- Viral infections
- Alcohol and drug abuse
- Sustained or severe stressors on the heart
- Chemotherapy
- Nutritional and vitamin deficiencies
- Family history

Causes: DCM

- Alcohol (alcoholic cardiomyopathy) or cocaine abuse
- Ischemic heart disease
- Infections: Viral are the most common (e.g., myocarditis).
- Stressors on the heart, such as:
  - o Tachycardias, usually atrial, which persist for prolonged periods of time
  - o Apical ballooning syndrome, also called Takotsubo cardiomyopathy (named after the Japanese scientist who discovered it), results from emotional stress and is also called broken heart syndrome
  - o Pheochromocytomas that release cardiac stimulants that is catecholamines
  - o Vitamin deficiencies (e.g., thiamine, calcium, magnesium)
  - o Genetic disorders (e.g., muscular dystrophy [MD])
  - o Chronic renal failure
  - o Cardiac muscle infections (e.g., Lyme disease)
  - o Chemotherapy
  - o Pregnancy (e.g., peripartum cardiomyopathy)
- Idiopathic: Fifty percent of with unknown cause of DCM have a genetic history in one or both parents with DCM

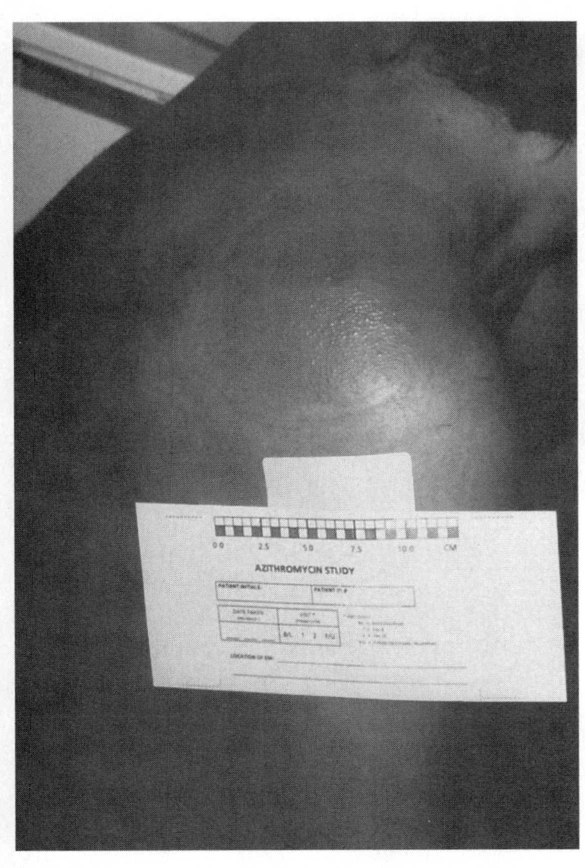

A tick bite is seen on this patient's shoulder, which caused the characteristic rash of erythema migrans. The patient was diagnosed with Lyme disease. The bacteria can migrate to the heart and other organs if left untreated.
Source: CDC

Concept Check

2. **What pathophysiology is associated with dilated cardiomyopathy?**
   A. Increased stroke volume
   B. High ejection fractions
   C. Ventricular dysrhythmias
   D. Very slow heart rate

Answer question

Assessment Findings: DCM

- Patients with DCM have systolic dysfunction.
- Atrial and/or ventricular dysrhythmias can occur and cause sudden cardiac arrest and death.
- Clinically, the most common symptoms are related to systolic heart failure, such as:
  - Dyspnea, orthopnea, and cough
  - Dependent or pitting edema (see photo)
  - Fatigue and/or shortness of breath
  - Cardiogenic shock in severe cases
  - Weight gain
  - Syncope (caused by abnormal heart rhythms)

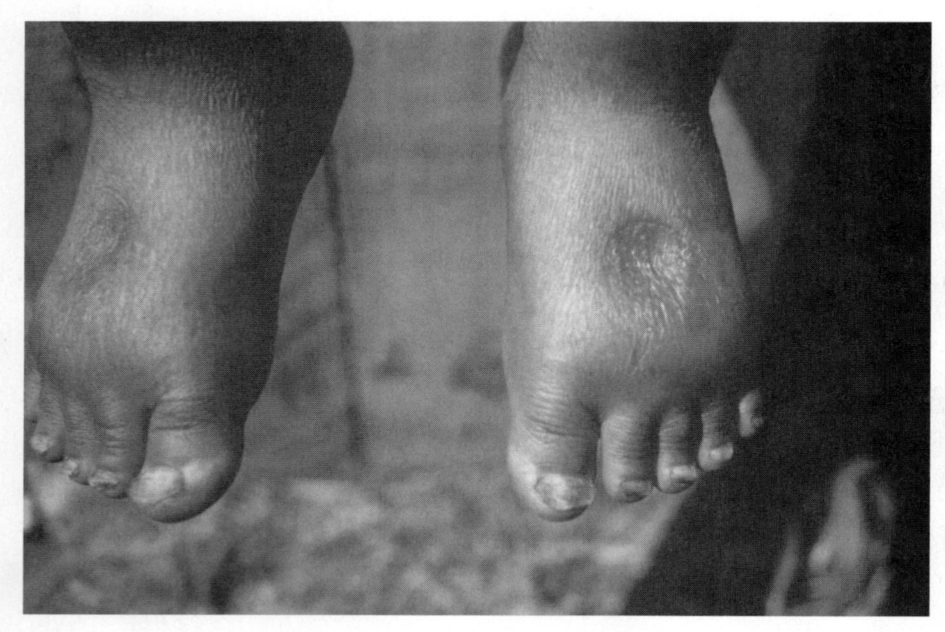

A patient with dilated cardiomyopathy presents much like a patient with heart failure . . . with pitting edema.
Source: CDC/Dr. Lyle Conrad

Diagnostics: DCM

- DCM is seen best on an echocardiogram (EKG).
- EKG may show disturbances related to conduction (e.g., left bundle branch block) or high voltages.
- Chest x-ray may show an enlarged heart.

Priority Patient Concerns and Desired Collaborative Care Outcomes: DCM

Prior to caring for patients with dilated cardiomyopathy, it is important to prioritize the patient's concerns that must guide the nursing care plan and interventions. Care for the patient is ordered and organized in accordance with the patient's priority and urgent needs. Desired collaborative care outcomes in patients with dilated cardiomyopathy typically include:

1. Patient's cardiac output will return to optimal personal level.
2. Patient will evidence as few findings associated with ineffective cerebral tissue perfusion as possible.
3. Patient will evidence as few findings associated with ineffective cardiac tissue perfusion as possible.
4. Patient's oxygen saturations levels will return to optimal personal level.
5. Patient will be normovolemic.
6. Patient will return to activities of daily living with as little dyspnea or fatigue as possible.
7. Patient will report being less anxious.

Considering these important care outcomes, prepare a list of the major 3–6 priority patient concerns or nursing diagnoses for patients with dilated cardiomyopathy. Be prepared to participate in a discussion of this list and/or to submit them as an assignment, as determined by your faculty. Resources you may find helpful in this assignment can include this lesson, the references, resources on nursing care plans, and standard nursing diagnoses manuals.

LO3:

Collaborative Interventions: DCM

Evidence-Based Practice

Evidence-based practice (EBP) treatment is limited, with the primary treatments focused on relieving heart failure:

N M
- Preload reducers: diuretics (e.g., furosemide)

  AND

N M
- Afterload reducers
  - o ACE inhibitors (e.g., captopril)
  - o Beta blockers (e.g., metoprolol)
  - o Angiotensin receptor blockers (e.g., losartan)

N M
- Implantation of a pacemaker or defibrillator may be considered, especially if the myopathy is producing significant cardiac symptoms, dysrhythmias, and/or the ejection fraction is low (e.g., less than 35%).

Patient Education: DCM

N M
- Educate patient about the condition, medications, complications, when to call the health care provider, smoking cessation, and weight management.

N M
- Educate patient about safe and preferred types of exercise:
  - o Unless the patient has ARVC, noncompetitive aerobic exercise is the general recommendation (Cleveland Clinic).
  - o Aerobic exercise can include such activities as biking, cross-country skiing, rollerblading, swimming, and walking.
  - o Heavy weight lifting is discouraged in anyone with any form of cardiomyopathy (Cleveland Clinic).
  - o A good reference is www.livestrong.com/article/327324-can-you-exercise-with-an-enlarged-heart/#ixzz2AheOBaZd.

N
- A low-sodium, healthy diet is encouraged.

N
- Fluid retention is a good warning sign of complications. Weighing daily can provide a clue to fluid retention.

N
- Take medication as prescribed.

Concept Check

3. Which forms of exercise are appropriate for a patient with dilated cardiomyopathy?

A. Volleyball

B. Swimming

C. Weight-lifting

D. Basketball

Answer question

LO4:

Evaluation of Desired Collaborative Care Outcomes: DCM

Evaluation and reassessment should reveal attainment of previously established outcomes. In summary:

- Patient's skin is warm and dry, mentation is clear, and urine output is adequate.
- Patient is awake and alert and has experienced no mentation changes.
- Patient has experienced no chest pain.
- Patient's oxygen saturation levels are within patient's normal parameters.
- Patient's blood pressure is stable and urine output is adequate.
- Patient reports tolerating return to normal range of daily activities without dyspnea or fatigue.
- Patient discusses disorder calmly and reports no excessive anxiety.

LO1:

What Is Hypertrophic Obstructive Cardiomyopathy?

- Hypertrophic obstructive cardiomyopathy (HOCM) or hypertrophic cardiomyopathy (HCM) can present almost any time after age 12 and is the leading cause of sudden cardiac deaths in young people.
- The intraventricular septum enlarges in this condition and can obstruct blood flow out of the left ventricle into the aorta.
- However, the enlarged and thickened tissue is also prone to electrical disturbances, making fatal dysrhythmias a possibility.

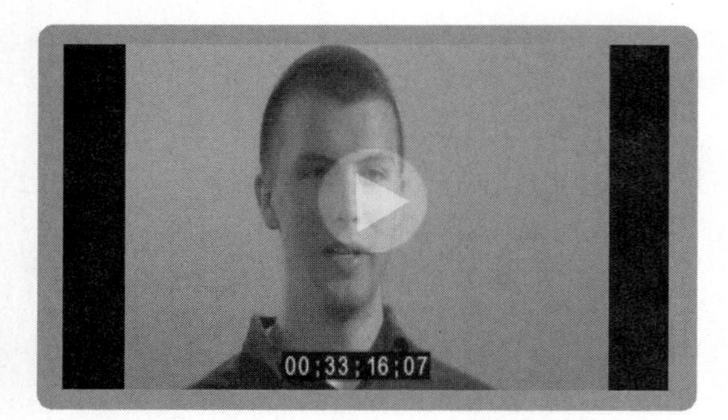

This is a video of a young man, Nick, who was diagnosed with HCM and he relates his story, his experience of living with HCM. It contributes knowledge that is rarely shared with learners and shapes the way one uses knowledge and cares for a person. Nick's story should help you better connect to the feelings and experience from the patient's viewpoint. Expert clinicians have shown that this is a very important aspect of being an excellent clinician.

Source: Copyright © 2013, NovEx Novice to Expert Learning, LLC

LO2:

Pathophysiology: HCM

- The muscle of the heart, particularly the intraventricular septum, enlarges. This can produce three problems:
  - o The enlarged muscle can obstruct blood flow into the aorta.
  - o The reduction in coronary artery blood flow can cause myocardial ischemia.
  - o The enlarged muscle conducts impulses abnormally, resulting in potentially fatal dysrhythmias.
- The muscle hypertrophy is both excessive and abnormal (in disarray). Electrical impulses are not conducted normally in the enlarged portion of the heart.
- While the septum is most noticeably enlarged, other parts of the heart can hypertrophy as well, such as the left ventricle. HCM is distinguished from an enlarged athlete's heart, which can also have a thicker septum and LV wall, but unlike HCM, the athlete's myocardial hypertrophy is symmetrical and the wall is generally less than or equal to 12 mm in thickness.

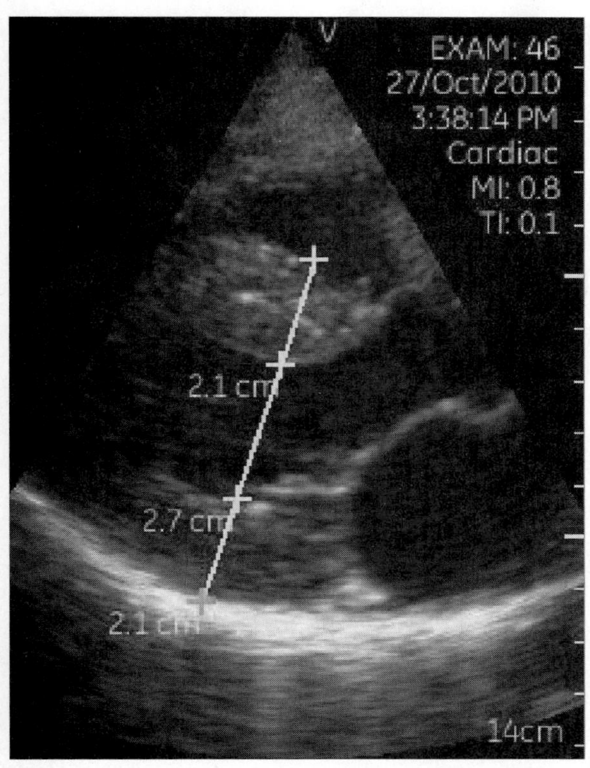

An echocardiogram showing septal hypertrophy between the LV (left ventricle) and RV (right ventricle).

Source: Copyright © 2013, NovEx Novice to Expert Learning, LLC

Causes and Risk Factors: HCM

- HCM is a genetic condition, affecting 1 in 500 people.

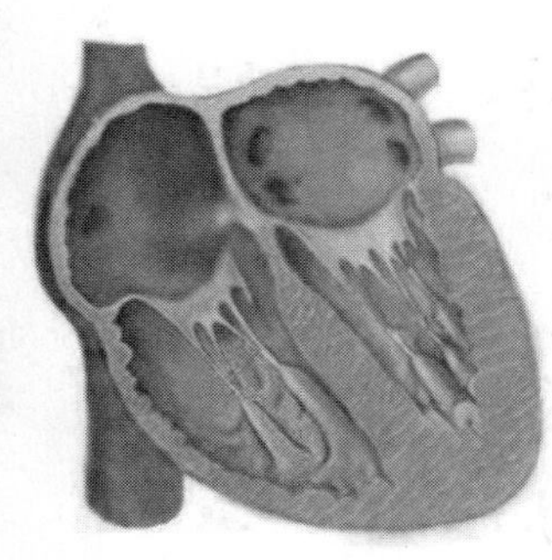

Although HCM typically compromises the left ventricle (the main pumping chamber), it can involve both lower chambers of the heart. The muscle fibers of the heart thicken, making it harder for the heart to relax and allow adequate diastolic filling for the next contraction. Notice the striking thickness of the interventricular septum, between the two ventricles, which causes significant cardiac output problems.

Source: Courtesy of George Kyriakidis/Santa Ana, CA

Assessment Findings: HCM

Key symptoms include:

- Palpitations
- Syncope, particularly with exercise
- Fatigue
- Shortness of breath with exertion (90%)
- Chest pain (75%)
- Sudden cardiac arrest or death (see video)
- Fainting

Diagnostics: HCM

- The clinical diagnosing of HCM is best accomplished with an echocardiogram (echo). The intraventricular septum is disproportionately large. A portable handheld ultrasound can now be used to accurately recognize HCM and does not require the expense of hospital or clinical-based equipment.
- An EKG can detect the enlarged heart in many cases, with as many as 90% of cases of HCM being diagnosed on the EKG. However, the EKG can give false positives, leading to echocardiograms which were not necessary.
- Genetic testing can confirm the diagnosis of HCM.
- Cardiovascular MRI (CMR) has shown diagnostic advantages over 2-D echo as echo at times underestimates or misses areas of ventricular wall thickening. Images of the heart's edges and LV outflow tract obstruction may be clearer.

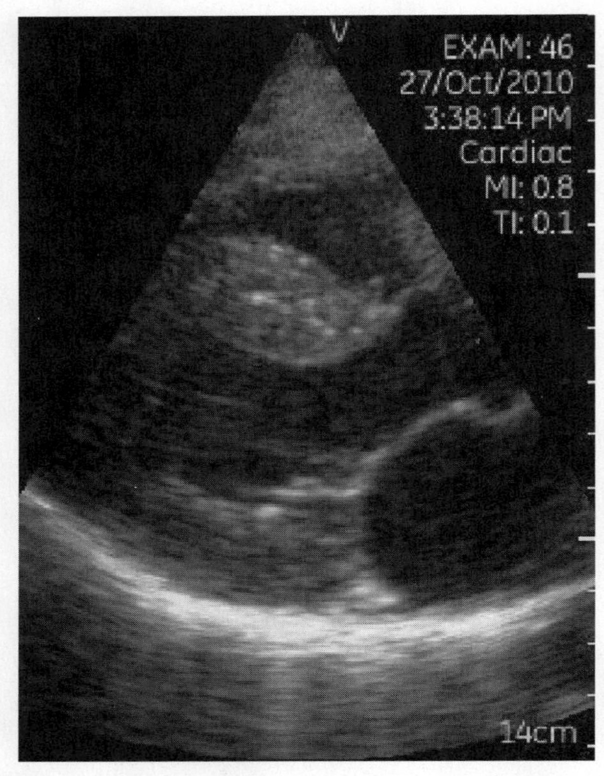

This echocardiogram reveals some key features noted in patients with HCM: asymmetric hypertrophy of the ventricular septum, systolic anterior motion of the mitral valve, and partial closure of the aortic valve during early systole.
Source: Copyright © 2013, NovEx Novice to Expert Learning, LLC

Priority Patient Concerns and Desired Collaborative Care Outcomes: HCM

Prior to caring for patients with hypertrophic cardiomyopathy, it is important to prioritize the patient's concerns that must guide the nursing care plan and interventions. Care for the patient is ordered and organized in accordance with the patient's priority and urgent needs. Desired collaborative care outcomes in patients with hypertrophic cardiomyopathy typically include:

1. Patient's cardiac output will not decrease.
2. Patient will tolerate normal levels of activity.
3. Patient will not experience trauma.
4. Patient will take measures to prevent exacerbations of disorder.
5. Patient will discuss feelings associated with diagnosis and will feel in control of health outcomes.

Considering these important care outcomes, prepare a list of the major 3–6 priority patient concerns or nursing diagnoses for patients with hypertrophic cardiomyopathy. Be prepared to participate in a discussion of this list and/or to submit them as an assignment, as determined by your faculty. Resources you may find helpful in this assignment can include this lesson, the references, resources on nursing care plans, and standard nursing diagnoses manuals.

LO3:

Collaborative Interventions: HCM

Evidenced-Based Practice

EBP management of HCM is limited. Most treatments are not yet supported by research and focus on relieving and preventing symptoms:

- M N Medications for HCM include beta blockers (e.g., metoprolol). Calcium channel blockers (e.g., diltiazem) are given if beta blockers are not tolerated.
- M N Strenuous exercise is usually discouraged, although this is not an evidence-based recommendation.
- M N Noncontact mild exercise is usually allowed, particularly if an implantable cardioverter defibrillator (ICD) is in place.
- M Myectomies (removal of a portion of the intraventricular septum) and alcohol ablation (small septal MI induced by alcohol that results in septal wall thinning) are also therapies that can be used in this condition.
- M N An implantable defibrillator or pacemaker is often used if a lethal dysrhythmia develops.
    - o Patient education following placement of an implantable defibrillator is essential.
    - o Patients may need lifestyle modifications that require education.

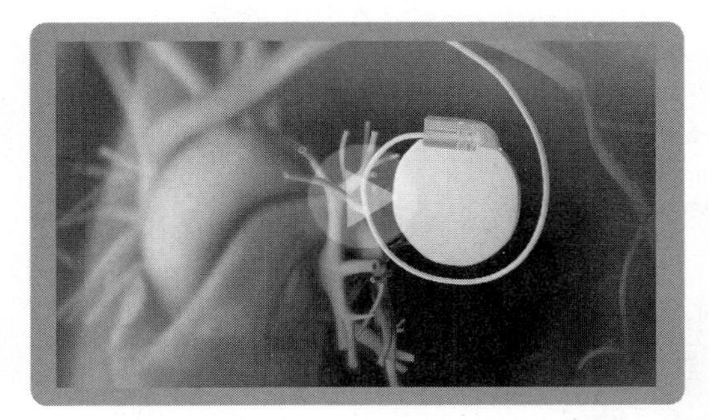

This animation explains how an ICD is implanted to restore the heart's normal rhythm and prevent sudden cardiac death. A lead wire is threaded through the subclavian vein until it reaches the right ventricle. If the heart experiences dysrhythmia, the Automatic Implantable Cardioverter Defibrillator device can send electrical shocks through the wire to reset the heartbeat back to normal.

Collaborative Interventions: HCM (continued)

Patient Education

Patient and parent education should include:

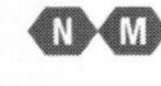

- There is a 50/50 chance of passing on the disorder to children. Screening family members with echocardiograms is, therefore, important.

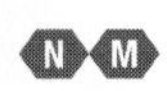

- Avoid participation in competitive sports and strenuous exercise but maintain an active, healthy lifestyle that includes exercise and a healthy diet.

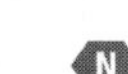

- Take medications as prescribed by the health care provider.

- Keep regular visits to cardiologist for evaluation.

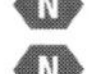

- Pay attention to the following:
    - o Notify health care provider if there is a change in your symptoms; especially, if you feel that you nearly pass out, do pass out, have increased or new chest discomfort, increased or new palpitations, increased fatigue.
    - o Manage other conditions that contribute to worsening of HCM: hypertension, diabetes, obesity, and hyperlipidemia. Follow treatment based on relevant existing guidelines.
    - o Lifestyle recommendations: no smoking, maintain normal weight, avoid use of alcohol and illegal drugs, get sufficient sleep and rest, and reduce unnecessary stress.

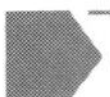

Concept Check

4. Which condition may lead to worsening of hypertrophic cardiomyopathy?

A. Alzheimer's disease

B. Hypertension

C. Gastric cancer

D. Pancreatitis

Answer question

LO4:

Evaluation of Desired Collaborative Care Outcomes: HCM

Evaluation and reassessment should reveal attainment of previously established outcomes. In summary:

- Patient's skin is warm and dry, mentation is clear, and urine output is adequate.
- Patient reports being able to return to activities of daily living without dyspnea or fatigue.
- Patient has not experienced trauma.
- Patient accurately relates measures to prevent trauma.
- Patient is able to discuss diagnosis and treatment modalities without anxiety.
- Patient relates a plan to help manage personal health.

LO1:

What Is Restrictive Cardiomyopathy?

- Restrictive Cardiomyopathy (RCM) is an uncommon myocardial disease.
- While it is the least common of the cardiomyopathies, RCM presents with a different dysfunction—diastolic dysfunction.
- The ventricle is too stiff to fully and rapidly dilate during diastolic filling, so it fails to fill with a normal volume. Stroke volume and cardiac output are compromised.

Viral Myocarditis (Inflammation of the Cardiac / Heart Muscle)

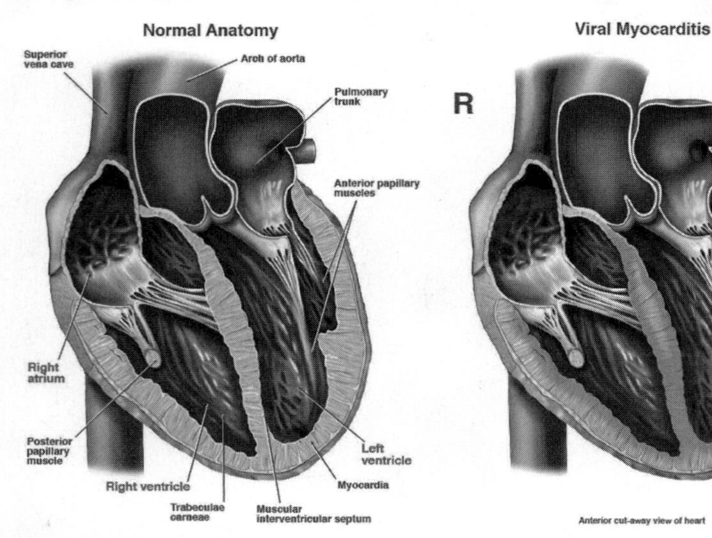

Cardiomyopathies can be the result of infections or chemo toxic agents. These myopathies tend to produce a rigid heart or a restrictive cardiomyopathy

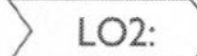

Pathophysiology: RCM

- RCM is different from the other myopathies in that the myocyte contractile strength is normal, wall thickness is normal, but the ventricular muscle is stiff and noncompliant.
- The stiff ventricular chamber does not allow blood to enter as easily and the chamber has limited volume capacity to accommodate blood.
- The result is a drop in stroke volume and a rise in cardiac pressures.
- RCM is an example of diastolic dysfunction, whereas most other myopathies are characterized by systolic dysfunction.
- RCM is also called infiltrative cardiomyopathy.

Concept Check

5. Which cardiomyopathy has primarily diastolic effects?

A. Dilated cardiomyopathy
B. Restrictive cardiomyopathy
C. Hypertrophic obstructive cardiomyopathy
D. Alcoholic cardiomyopathy

Answer question

Risk Factors: RCM

Several risk factors for RCM include:

- Diabetes
- Infiltrative disorders (e.g., amyloidosis, endomyocardial fibrosis)
- Advanced age
- Noninfiltrative disorders (e.g., scleroderma)
- Radiation
- Chemotherapy

Causes: RCM

Several types of RCM are present:

- Idiopathic, or no known cause
- Infiltrative (e.g., amyloidosis, sarcoidosis)
- Treatment-induced (e.g., chemotherapy)
- Malignancy, from a myocardial cancer or metastasis
- Noninfiltrative, (e.g., familial [genetic], scleroderma, diabetic)

Assessment Findings: RCM

Symptoms of RCM appear late in the course of the disease, and, when symptoms occur, they are typically those of heart failure:

- Dyspnea, orthopnea
- Fatigue
- Paroxysmal nocturnal dyspnea
- Ascites and dependent edema
- Chest pain
- Palpitations

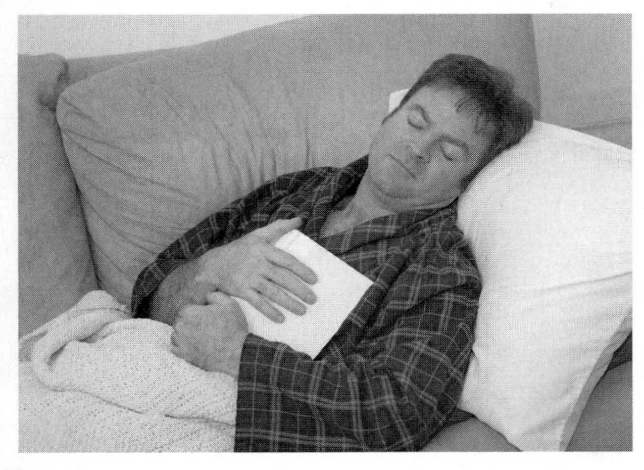

People with RCM are typically orthopneic and have trouble breathing when they are lying down. In fact, they cannot sleep unless their head is elevated like the man in this photo. Orthopnea is a hallmark sign of heart failure.

Source: Lisa F. Young/Fotolia

Diagnostics: RCM

- An echocardiogram is the best way to detect RCM; however, it is not as easily diagnosed as other cardiomyopathies. Echocardiogram features include:
  - o A nondilated or even small left ventricular size
  - o Impaired left ventricular filling that results in low or normal diastolic volumes
  - o No muscular hypertrophy, but infiltrates may cause increased LV wall thickness
  - o Systolic ejection typically remains normal in the early stage.
  - o Normal to slightly low ejection fraction
  - o Atrial enlargement

Priority Patient Concerns and Desired Collaborative Care Outcomes: RCM

Prior to caring for patients with restrictive cardiomyopathy, it is important to prioritize the patient's concerns that must guide the nursing care plan and interventions. Care for the patient is ordered and organized in accordance with the patient's priority and urgent needs. Desired collaborative care outcomes in patients with restrictive cardiomyopathy typically include:

1. Patient will maintain or improve ability to manage activities of daily living.
2. Patient will remain infection free.
3. Patient will demonstrate understanding of medical regimen and activity restrictions.
4. Patient will express confidence in ability to manage changes associated with illness.

Considering these important care outcomes, prepare a list of the major 3–6 priority patient concerns or nursing diagnoses for patients with restrictive cardiomyopathy. Be prepared to participate in a discussion of this list and/or to submit them as an assignment, as determined by your faculty. Resources you may find helpful in this assignment can include this lesson, the references, resources on nursing care plans, and standard nursing diagnoses manuals.

LO3:

Collaborative Interventions: RCM

Evidence-Based Practice

Evidence-based practice for RCM is primarily symptomatic. Treatment is very similar to the treatment for heart failure:

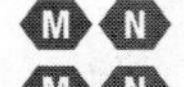

- Diuretics such as furosemide (Lasix)
- Antiarrhythmics:
  - o For atrial dysrhythmias, diltiazem
  - o For ventricular dysrhythmias, amiodarone

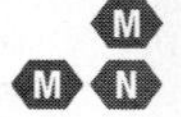

- Implantable pacemaker or defibrillator
- Anticoagulant therapy if atrial fibrillation is present (e.g., heparin for short term, warfarin for long term)

- Transplantation can be considered in some forms of restrictive cardiomyopathy

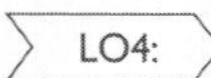

Evaluation of Desired Collaborative Care Outcomes: RCM

Evaluation and reassessment should reveal attainment of previously established outcomes. In summary:

- Hemodynamic measurements reveal that patient's cardiac output has stabilized.
- Patient expresses acceptance of the unknown nature of this disorder and confidence in own ability to manage symptoms.
- Patient accurately describes the basic pathophysiology, treatments, and potential complications associated with the disorder.

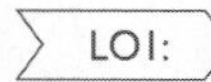

What Is Arrhythmogenic Right Ventricular Cardiomyopathy?

- In this myopathy, the right ventricle is the chamber of the heart that is centrally affected. ARVC is a specific type of cardiomyopathy.
- Arrhythmogenic right ventricular cardiomyopathy or dysplasia (also called ARVC, ARVD, and ARVC/D) is a genetic disorder that is uncommon (ranges 1 in 1,500 to 1 in 5,000) and results in a dysplasia of the muscle (abnormality in muscle structure).
- The muscle atrophies and is replaced by fat and fibrosis, leading to abnormal heart rhythms. Additionally, the right ventricle contracts poorly and abnormally. Because the RV dilates and is dysfunctional, heart failure results.
- The abnormality of the right ventricle that occurs in ARVC is prone to dysrhythmias that are potentially dangerous, even fatal.
- ARVC is 3 times more common in men than women.
- Despite being uncommon, ARVC accounts for 20% of sudden cardiac death in people under 35 years of age.

LO2:

Pathophysiology: ARVC/D

- In ARVC, the right ventricle can have limited or general thinning and dilatation. The condition often occurs in segments of the ventricle, occasionally extending to the left ventricle.
- The normal muscle of the myocardium is replaced by fibrous tissue and fat.
- This abnormal tissue does not contract normally and predisposes to electrical disturbances, producing dysrhythmias. Potentially fatal dysrhythmias, for example, ventricular tachycardia or fibrillation, can occur without symptoms.

Causes and Risk Factors: ARVC/D

- ARVC is primarily a genetically transmitted condition, with higher occurrence in certain regions of Greece and Italy.
- However, the understanding of ARVC is still developing since it is likely underdiagnosed and incompletely understood.

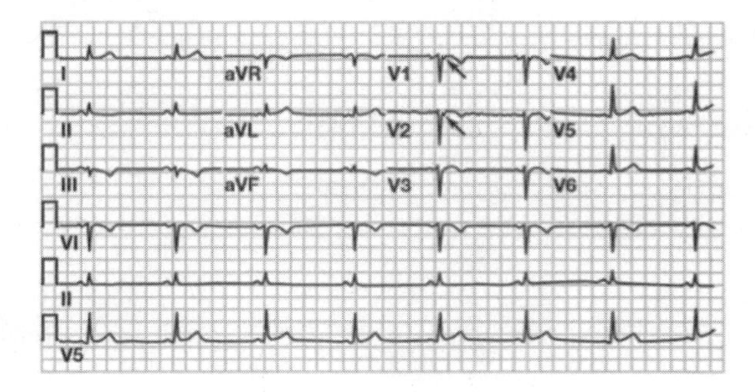

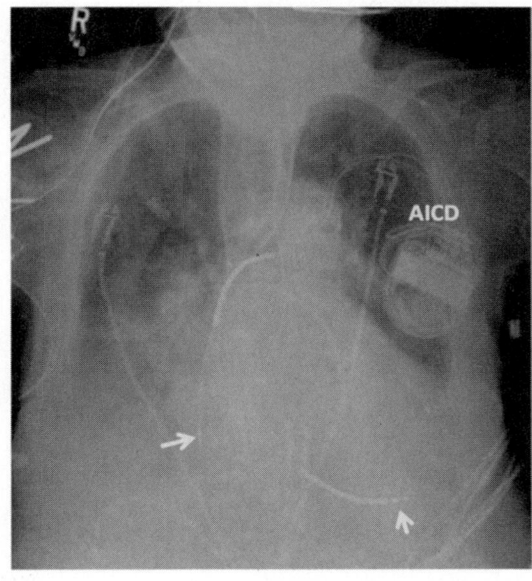

Upper: EKG with typical signs for ARVC; negative T waves and epsilon waves in the precordial or V leads (arrow). Lower: Chest x-ray after AICD with pacemaker implantation. Both the atrial and ventricular leads are visible (arrows).
Source: (*lower*) Courtesy of K. Kyriakidis

Assessment Findings: ARVC/D

- Most affected people do not know they have ARVC. The first symptom may be a dysrhythmia or sudden death.
- The most common symptom is palpitations, which feels like fluttering in the chest.
- Symptoms vary depending on the type, significance, and duration of the dysrhythmia. All the major symptoms are produced from a fast dysrhythmia, ventricular in nature.
- The event may be self-terminating, and the patient may not notice significant symptoms or think anything of it. If the rhythm disturbance is prolonged, the patient may feel faint or dizzy.
- Less commonly, patients with ARVC develop symptoms of heart failure: dependent edema, shortness of breath with activity, inability to comfortably perform daily activities, orthopnea, and easy fatigue with exercise.
- Other vague symptoms can present as well, including lightheadedness.

Diagnostics: ARVC/D

- ARVC is difficult to diagnose due to vague or absent symptoms. No one test can definitively diagnose ARVC.
- Patient history may help. If the patient has complaints of syncope, easy fatigue, family history of sudden cardiac death not due to ischemic heart disease, suspicion should be aroused.
- Electrocardiogram, an exercise stress test, an echocardiogram, cardiac MRI, and a 24-hr Holter monitor are the most common tests to evaluate the patient for dysrhythmias or abnormal muscle structure.
- An electrophysiology study (EP study), right ventriculogram, and biopsy may be recommended to completely evaluate ARVC. Due to the incomplete infiltrative pattern of the disease, biopsies may miss the affected part of the heart.

Priority Patient Concerns and Desired Collaborative Care Outcomes: ARVC/D

Prior to caring for patients with ARVC/D, it is important to prioritize the patient's concerns that must guide the nursing care plan and interventions. Care for the patient is ordered and organized in accordance with the patient's priority and urgent needs. Desired collaborative care outcomes in patients with ARVC/D typically include:

1. Patient's cardiac output will stabilize or improve from baseline.
2. Patient will discuss feelings associated with having a potentially lethal and unpredictable disorder.
3. Patient will demonstrate increased knowledge of disorder and treatment modalities.

Considering these important care outcomes, prepare a list of the major 3–6 priority patient concerns or nursing diagnoses for patients with ARVC/D. Be prepared to participate in a discussion of this list and/or to submit them as an assignment, as determined by your faculty. Resources you may find helpful in this assignment can include this lesson, the references, resources on nursing care plans, and standard nursing diagnoses manuals.

Concept Check

6. What is the most common symptom of ARVC/D?

A. Headache
B. Chest pain
C. Palpitation
D. Edema

Answer question

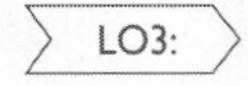

Collaborative Interventions: ARVC/D

Evidence-Based Practice

- Evidence-based practice for ARVC is limited. Therapy is instead focused on relieving symptoms of heart failure or preventing an episode of a lethal dysrhythmia.
  - o Many patients with ARVC are prescribed antiarrhythmic medications such as beta blockers, ACE-inhibitors or amiodarone that can lessen the frequency and severity of dysrhythmias.
  - o Use of an ICD is a common therapy to prevent sudden cardiac death.
  - o If the area of the dysrhythmia can be identified, the area might be treated with alcohol ablation. However, because ARVC is a progressive disease, the dysrhythmias are not permanently cured by this procedure.
  - o If heart failure is present, standard heart failure therapy should be utilized (e.g., preload and afterload reduction). Patients with ARVC heart failure are often prescribed an ACE inhibitor.
  - o Rarely, heart transplantation could be considered if all the above therapies are unsuccessful.

Patient Education: ARVC/D

Education of patients with ARVC/D includes routine instructions but also should include instruction some specialized issues:

- ARVC/D is a genetically inherited condition so siblings and children of the patient should strongly consider screening.
- Avoid strenuous exercise: Although there is not clarity about the relationship between ARVD and exercise, exercise is a cause of dysrhythmia in many, particularly in very young athletes and males. As in HCM, sudden death may occur. Patients with ARVC are advised to avoid vigorous exercise but maintain an active, healthy lifestyle and a healthy diet. Discuss details with the physician.
- Avoid stimulants of all types as they increase the risk of dysrhythmias. This includes, but is not limited to: caffeine, nicotine, chocolate, and pharmacologic stimulants like pseudoephedrine (Sudafed) and stimulant-containing cold or flu mediations. Consulting a pharmacist prior to purchasing over-the-counter drugs can assist the patient from inadvertent intake of unfamiliar stimulants.
- Avoid alcohol consumption, a known cause of dysrhythmia (EBP).
- Take medications as prescribed by the physician.
- Keep regular visits to cardiologist for evaluation. Siblings and children who do not yet have indications of ARVC/D should follow up every 2–5 years because the problem can develop over time.
- Pay attention to the following:
  - o Notify MD if there's a change in your symptoms; especially, if you feel that you nearly pass out, do pass out, have increased/new chest discomfort, increased/new palpitations and increased fatigue.
  - o Manage comorbid conditions that may contribute to ARVC/D worsening.
  - o Lifestyle recommendations: no smoking, maintain normal weight, avoid use illegal drugs, get sufficient sleep and rest, and reduce unnecessary stress.
- Pregnancy: Women can experience uncomplicated pregnancy. If on medication or with an AICD, a physician may need to modify medication regimen. A cardiologist should be involved in the care of a mother during pregnancy.
- Illnesses that cause fever, fluid or electrolyte imbalances such as a GI virus, or decreased absorption of medication predispose to dysrhythmic events.
- Inform family about learning to perform CPR in an emergency.

Summary of Interventions

- Treatments vary, depending on the type of cardiomyopathy diagnosed. Primary treatment centers around management of heart failure.
- The implantation of a pacemaker, defibrillator, or an ICD is a common treatment.
- Most common medications include diuretics and afterload reducers (e.g., ACE inhibitors).

Concept Check

7. Which patient outcome is assessed to determine successful treatment of cardiomyopathy?

A. Patient no longer eats meat.

B. Patient no longer reports early morning headaches.

C. Patient joins a competitive softball league.

D. Patient has regular heart rate and rhythm.

Answer question

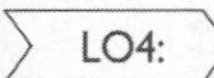

Evaluation of Desired Collaborative Care Outcomes: ARVC/D

Evaluation and reassessment should reveal attainment of previously established outcomes. In summary:

- Decreased CO: Patient's skin is warm and dry, mentation is clear, and urine output is adequate.
- Powerlessness: Patient is able to discuss improved control over ARVC/D events by adhering to recommendations on medication, exercise, and substance use.
- Knowledge: Patient is able to discuss diagnosis, treatments, and key patient education information for home care.

References

Hickey, K.T., & Rezzadeh, K. (2013). Hypertrophic cardiomyopathy: a clinical and genetic update. *Nurse Pract, 38*(5), 22–31.

Smith, K. M., & Squiers, J. (2013). Hypertrophic cardiomyopathy: an overview. *Crit Care Nurs Clin North Am. 25*(2), 263–272.

Clinical Practice Guidelines

Gersh, B. J., Maron, B. J., Bonow, R. O., et al. (2011). 2011 ACCF/AHA Guideline for the Diagnosis and Treatment of Hypertrophic Cardiomyopathy: A Report of the American College of Cardiology Foundation/American Heart Association Task Force on Practice Guidelines. *Circulation, 124*, 2761–2796.

Patient Education

Chang, J. H., Lynm, C., & Glass, R. M. (2009). Hypertrophic Cardiomyopathy. *JAMA, 302*(15), 1720.

Hypertrophic Cardiomyopathy Foundation. Patient Education Topics. **www.4hcm.org**

Johns Hopkins Medicine. ARVD/C Questions and Answers. **www.hopkinsmedicine.org/heart_vascular_institute/clinical_services/centers_excellence/arvd/patient_resources**

Learning Outcomes for Heart Failure

When you complete this lesson, you will be able to:

1. Recognize the clinical relevance of heart failure.
2. Consider the pathophysiology, etiology, risk factors, and clinical presentation of heart failure that determine the priority patient concerns.
3. Determine the most urgent and important nursing interventions and patient education required in caring for a patient with heart failure.
4. Evaluate attainment of desired collaborative care outcomes for a patient with heart failure.

LO1:

What Is Heart Failure?

- The Heart Failure Society of America (HFSA) defines heart failure as "a syndrome characterized by elevated cardiac filling pressure or inadequate peripheral oxygen delivery, at rest or during stress, caused by cardiac dysfunction" (Heart Failure Society of America, 2011).
- In broader terms, heart failure (HF) is a complicated disease process characterized by a set of typical symptoms that results from abnormal function of the heart.
- Diseases (e.g., myocardial infarction, cardiomyopathy, valvular diseases) that damage or place increased demand on the heart can lead to heart failure. Heart failure leads to a reduced stroke volume and cardiac output, producing many symptoms.
- There are several subsets of heart failure (e.g., left-sided, systolic) and each subset can be acute or chronic.

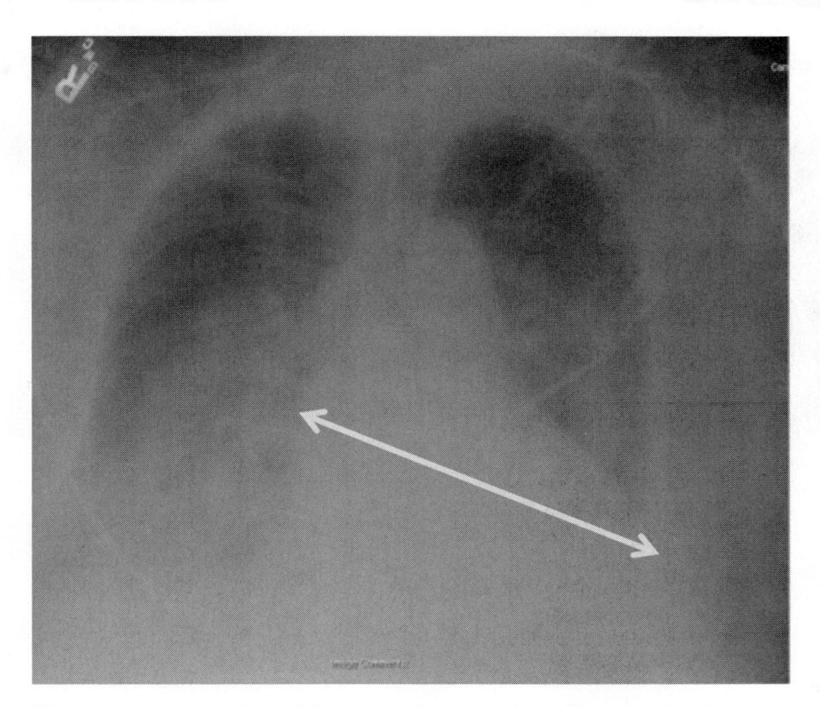

This patient is in severe heart failure with pulmonary edema. The patient's enlarged heart (arrow) far exceeds its normal size and is contracting so poorly that fluid is backed up into the lungs bilaterally. Pulmonary congestion is noted by the cotton ball-appearing, whitish markings on the x-ray.
Source: Courtesy of K. Kyriakidis

LO1:

Clinical Relevance

- The effect of heart failure on patient care is hard to overestimate. Heart failure is the leading cause of morbidity and mortality in the United States, with 5 million cases currently.
- There are approximately 550,000 new cases of HF every year (Weintraub et al., 2010).
- Heart failure utilizes more Medicare dollars than any other diagnosis. The current cost of heart failure is estimated at $37 billion dollars annually.
- The increasing costs are related to an aging population, increased survival from cardiac conditions, and improvement in management of sudden cardiac death.
- Almost every clinician frequently cares for patients for or with heart failure.
- Heart failure is more common in women. Although it occurs in all age groups, it is predominantly seen in older adults.
- Heart failure is a chronic condition and is not curable with present treatment, but can be managed.
- Depending on the severity of failure, many patients with heart failure can lead productive lives with optimal medical support.
- Heart failure is a progressive condition and eventually leads to a decline in functional abilities due to weakening of the heart.

Concept Check

1. **Which types of interventions have been shown to cure heart failure?**
   A. Use of medications
   B. Lifestyle modifications
   C. Electrophysiological procedures
   D. Heart failure is not currently considered curable.

Answer question

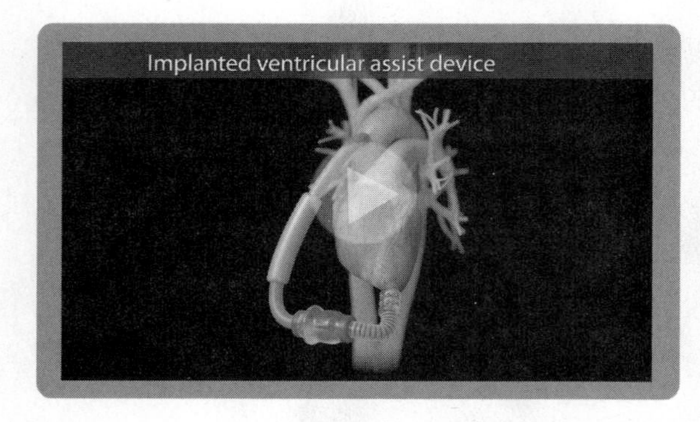

This animation provides an overview of heart failure, from clinical presentation through treatments.

LO2:

Pathophysiology

Heart failure is characterized by:

- Reduced stroke volume (SV; the amount of blood pumped by a single contraction, or beat, of the ventricles). Normal stroke volume is 50–100 mL/beat. Clinical signs and symptoms of HF are in response to a decreased SV. Stroke Index (SI) is a better indicator as it accounts for differing body sizes. Normal SI is 33–47 mL.
- Decreased cardiac output (CO; the total amount of blood pumped by the heart over a period of *a minute*). Measured in liters per minute (L/min). Normal CO is 4–8 L/min.
  - o CO has two determining factors: heart rate (HR) and SV. Normal HR is 60–100 bpm.

    CO = SV x HR
  - o Cardiac Index (CI) is a better indicator of CO since it accounts for body size. Normal CI is 2.5–4 L/m^2/min.

There are four factors that determine stroke volume and cardiac output:

1. Preload: The ventricular volume or pressure at the *end of diastole* that stretches the heart. The pressure in the ventricle is influenced by venous return to the heart.
2. Afterload: The resistance to ventricular ejection. The higher the afterload, the harder the heart has to work to contract and pump blood to the body.
3. Contractility: The capability of the myocardium to contract and eject blood from the heart.
4. Heart rate: Number of ventricular contractions (heart beats) per minute. The heart rate may increase to compensate for increased preload, increased afterload, and/or decreased contractility.

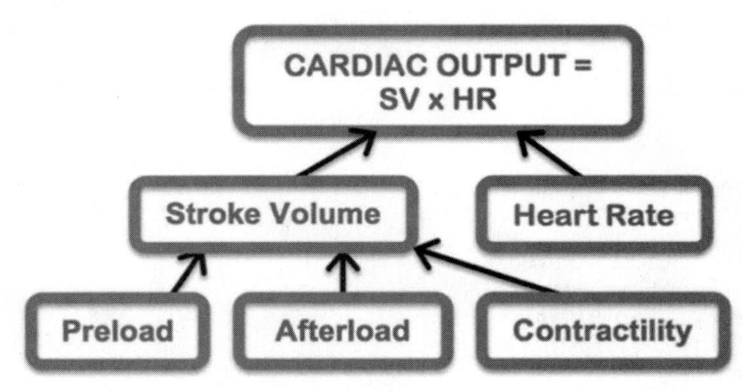

Determinants of cardiac output.
Source: Copyright © 2013, NovEx Novice to Expert Learning, LLC

Preload

- Preload is the blood volume in the ventricle during relaxation (end-diastolic volume). Fluid retention results in increased blood volume, increased venous return, and therefore increased preload. Changes in preload have two effects.
  1. Positive effect of increasing preload: The higher the preload, the more forceful the contraction of the ventricle to empty and the higher the CO, to a point. This principle is known as the Frank–Starling law (see diagram). Increasing contractile force is how the heart compensates for a weakening heart and heart failure. However, when preload is too high, the negative effects begin to compromise SV and CO.

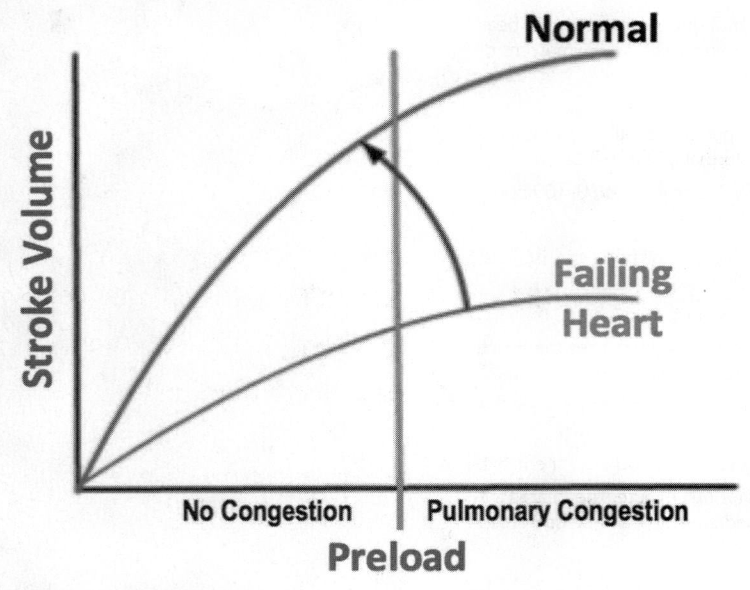

The Frank–Starling law shows that the higher the preload (to a point prior to congestion), the higher the stroke volume or cardiac output. Some interventions, such as medications, can strengthen contractility and enable the heart to increase stroke volume with the same preload. Improvement in contractility is depicted on the graph by the shift to a higher curve (arrow).

Source: Copyright © 2013, NovEx Novice to Expert Learning, LLC

2. Negative effect of increasing preload: When increases in preload overstretch the heart muscle, the result is minimal or no improvement in the force of contraction (see the peak and right side of the Frank–Starling curve in the diagram). When the end-diastolic volume/pressures are too high, the heart cannot adequately empty, causing blood to backup in the venous systems of the lungs or periphery. Abnormally high venous pressures can then lead to pulmonary and/or systemic edema. In patients with acute heart failure high pulmonary pressure is a more important factor.

- Several medications (e.g., diuretics, nitrates) used to treat heart failure lower or help control preload. They work primarily by decreasing the pressures and/or volume in the venous system. Nitrates lower preload by causing venodilation.

Afterload

- Afterload is the pressure the heart must overcome to eject blood into the high pressure within the aorta. The higher the afterload, the more work the heart must do.
- Increased afterload and work on the heart eventually causes hypertrophy and/or dilation of the ventricle.
- When afterload is too high and sustained, it contributes to what is called a "downward spiral into irreversible heart failure" if there is no effective intervention.
- Vasodilators (e.g., ACE inhibitors and angiotensin receptor blockers [ARBs]) can decrease the work required to eject blood by decreasing the pressure against which the heart has to pump.

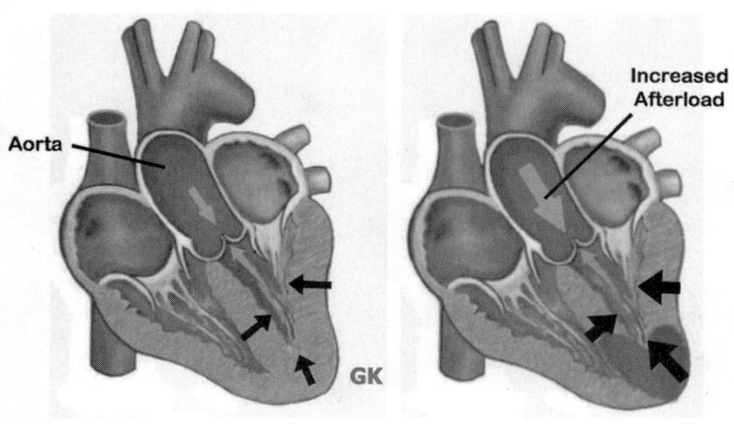

Left: During systole, the left ventricle (LV) must generate enough force to pump against the aortic pressure. Right: With increased afterload and myocardial damage from various causes, the LV must work harder, despite the damage, but cannot sustain adequate cardiac output. Heart failure ensues.
Source: Courtesy of George Kyriakidis/Santa Ana, CA

Pathophysiology (continued)

Contractility

- Contractility is the force with which the myocardium contracts to eject blood with each beat.
- A measure of the heart's contractility is ejection fraction (EF). EF is the percentage of blood in the ventricle that is "ejected" with each beat.

  $$EF = (SV/\text{end-diastolic volume}) \times 100\%$$

  A normal EF is 55–70%.
- EF is commonly measured with an echocardiogram.
- An EF of less than 55% may indicate ventricular weakening; however, a much lower EF (e.g., <40%) is usually required to provoke symptoms, such as fatigue and shortness of breath in the patient. Heart failure caused by a diminished EF or a dysfunction in contractility is called **systolic heart failure**.
- Medications such as digoxin, dobutamine, and milrinone are used to increase contractility, except in diastolic heart failure.
- Heart failure can also be caused by a stiff (noncompliant) ventricle, meaning that the heart is unable to relax and fill normally. Unable to adequately fill, SV and CO are compromised. Heart failure due to abnormal ventricular filling, with a normal or high ejection fraction, is called **diastolic heart failure (DHF)**.
- DHF is commonly due to hypertension, which results in hypertrophy of the heart muscle and a stiff, noncompliant ventricle. Ischemia of the heart can also cause stiffening of the ventricle. A stiff, noncompliant ventricle is one that does not easily expand as blood flows into it. In DHF, ventricular filling is the main problem.

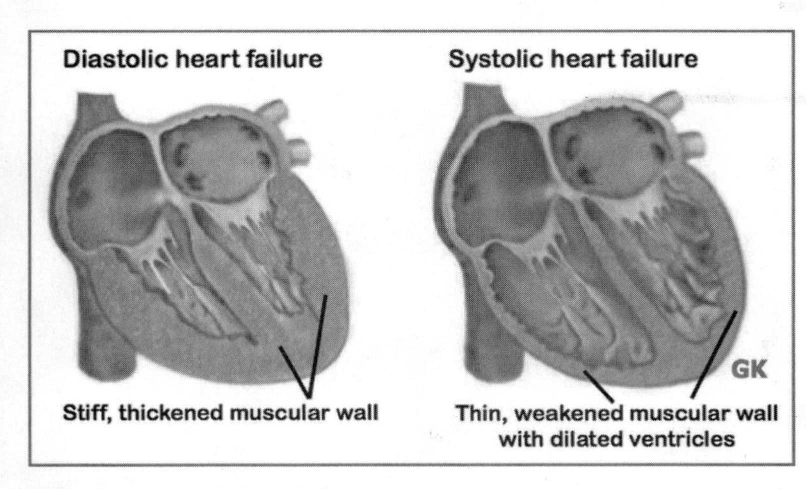

Diastolic versus systolic heart failure.
Source: Courtesy of George Kyriakidis/Santa Ana, CA

- An analogy to the heart normally filling with blood is inflating a new balloon. The effect of systolic failure on the heart is therefore like a used, overstretched balloon that has been repeatedly overinflated. The overstretched balloon inflates easily, but does not deflate efficiently or fully. Systolic failure therefore is from a loss in contractility.
- DHF, on the other hand, is best compared to multiple balloons layered together. The balloons deflate easily but are difficult to inflate due to the thickened wall.
- It is possible to have both diastolic and systolic heart failure together. In combined failure, the heart neither fills properly (diastolic failure), nor empties forcefully (systolic failure). When this occurs, the ejection fraction is low and the ventricle is stiff.
- The end result of diastolic and systolic heart failure is that stroke volume decreases. Symptoms of diastolic and systolic heart failure are therefore very similar and overlapping, particularly when the patient has both types of HF.

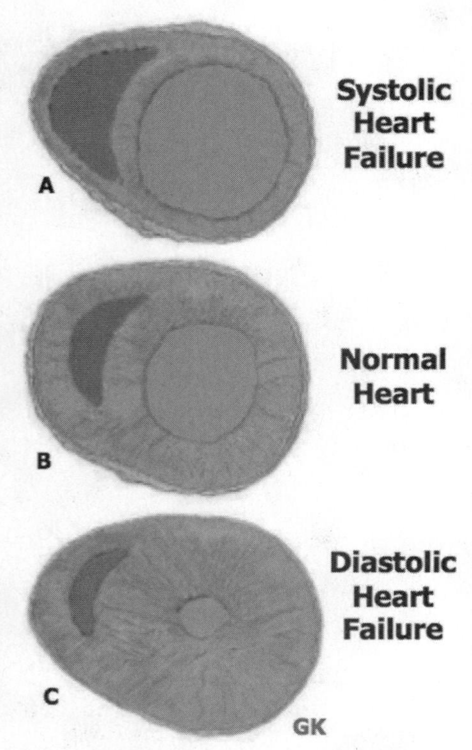

Dilated systolic failure versus normal heart versus hypertrophied diastolic heart failure.
Source: Courtesy of George Kyriakidis/Santa Ana, CA

Heart Rate (HR)

- Increasing HR can initially compensate for a decreased stroke volume (SV). At first, cardiac output (CO) is maintained.

$$\downarrow SV \times \uparrow HR = \text{Stable CO}$$

- As heart failure progresses, the CO eventually falls as the heart progressively ejects less blood, despite the tachycardia.
- Tachycardia also fails as a compensatory mechanism when the HR is too high because there is too little time for the ventricles to adequately fill.

Pathophysiology (continued)

Ventricular Remodeling

- Heart failure is usually a chronic condition that develops over several years. The changes that result to the structure and functioning of the heart is called "remodeling." These changes occur at many levels: structural (e.g., dilation of heart), cellular changes, and hormonal changes. Early remodeling changes occur to compensate for decreasing stroke volume and perfusion.
- Unfortunately, the same mechanisms, particularly neurohormonal ones, that compensate for heart failure become deleterious to the heart over the long term by causing ventricular remodeling. Long-term remodeling causes global ventricular dilation that worsens contractility, distortion of the ventricle's shape and ability to function normally, and hypertrophy that hinders contractile function. Without treatment, remodeling leads to death.
- Treatments for chronic heart failure work by targeting these remodeling changes to prevent further deterioration.

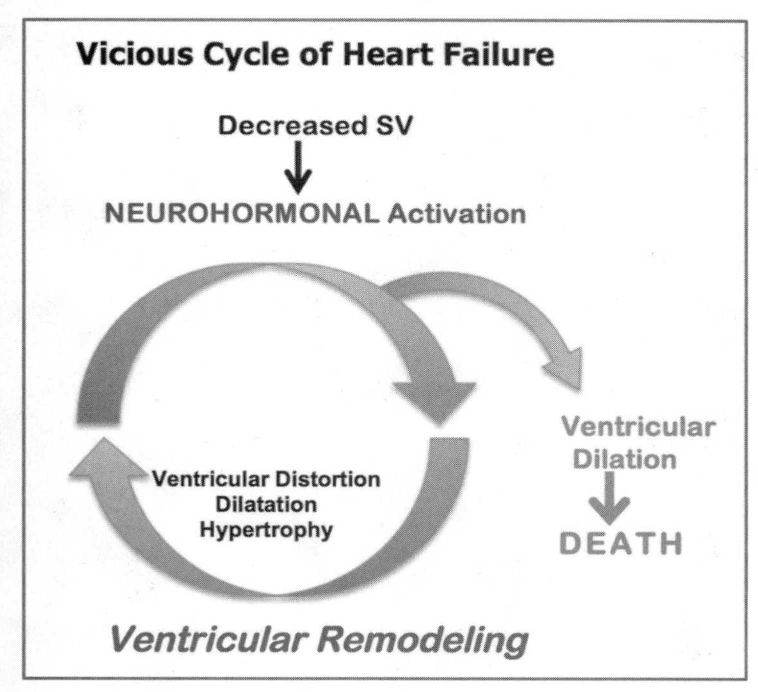

Ventricular remodeling begins shortly after an acute myocardial injury. Without treatment, chronic heart failure often develops and spirals downward over time with continued remodeling.
Source: Copyright © 2013, NovEx Novice to Expert Learning, LLC

Heart Failure Compensatory Mechanisms

- When the heart weakens and stroke volume falls, blood flow and oxygen delivery to the organs are compromised. Several neurohumoral (combined nervous system and hormones) compensatory mechanisms are activated in an attempt to maintain cardiac output:
  - Sympathetic nervous or vascular response: increased heart rate, contractility and vasoconstriction to maintain blood pressure and flow
  - Antidiuretic hormone (ADH): large increase in ADH promotes water retention to improve cardiac output
  - Renin-angiotensin activation: fluid retention by kidneys to increase blood volume and improve cardiac output
  - Additional neurohumoral substances: increased release of other substances (e.g., atrial and brain natriuretic peptides, endothelin) contribute to improving cardiac output
- Initially, these compensatory mechanisms are helpful, but over time, these same mechanisms contribute to ventricular remodeling, resulting in the vicious cycle leading to decompensated heart failure.
- Heart failure is usually a chronic condition that develops over several years. These numerous hormonal mechanisms cause deleterious changes that usually worsen heart failure over time.

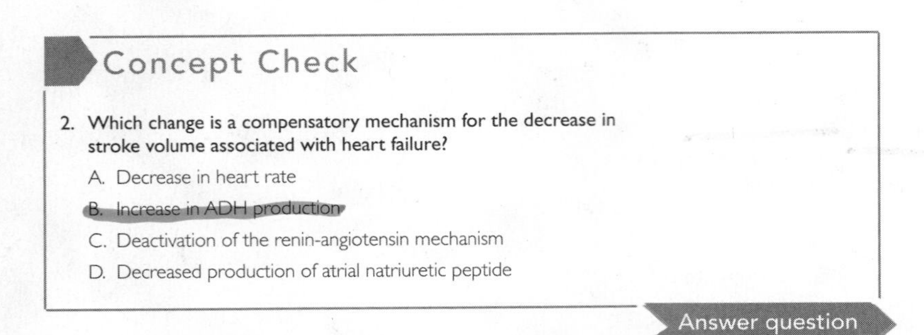
Concept Check

2. Which change is a compensatory mechanism for the decrease in stroke volume associated with heart failure?
   A. Decrease in heart rate
   B. Increase in ADH production
   C. Deactivation of the renin-angiotensin mechanism
   D. Decreased production of atrial natriuretic peptide

Answer question

- Despite initially improving cardiac output, these compensatory mechanisms inevitably fail. Treatments work by targeting these changes to prevent further deterioration.
- Unless a disease condition severely damages portions of the myocardium, the total amount of blood pumped by the heart (CO) is *initially* maintained by the compensatory increase in HR. Increased HR enables adequate perfusion of the organs (e.g., kidneys, brain).
- When SV falls to below 50 mL and compensatory mechanisms fail, CO and CI drop (CI to less than 2.2 mL/m^2/min). Perfusion then falls, prompting the downward spiral into irreversible heart failure.
- Decreased CO and SV result in several changes (see the Compensated Heart Failure schematic):
  1. Decreased renal perfusion is sensed as hypovolemia resulting in fluid retention. Excess fluid, which the heart cannot manage, causes weight gain, dependent edema, and venous engorgement.
  2. The drop in CO triggers vasoconstriction to maintain blood flow and perfusion. However, vasoconstriction increases the afterload (pressure the heart must pump against) and places further strain on the weakened ventricle. Unable to adequately eject blood, the ventricle distends and preload increases, causing pulmonary and/or venous congestion. As fluid load further increases, both ventricles can decompensate and biventricular failure can ensue.
  3. Coronary perfusion falls. Myocardial ischemia ensues and ejection fraction drops, further hindering SV and CO.
  4. Reduced SV results in higher end-diastolic volume and pressure, additively increasing preload.
  5. The downward spiral eventually causes biventricular failure and a vicious cycle of failure or cardiogenic shock.

Pathophysiology Schematic: Compensated Heart Failure

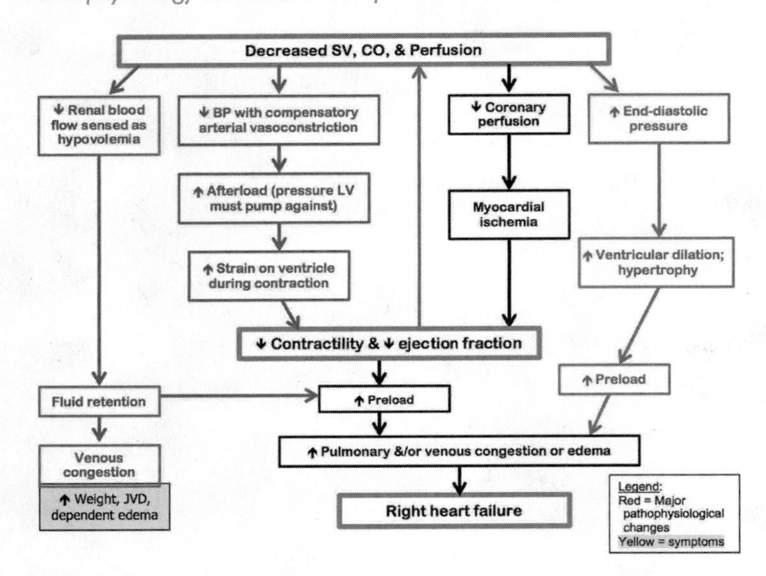

This schematic shows the numerous pathophysiologic mechanisms that compensate for early left heart failure to support cardiac output. However, the physiologic alterations contribute to the development of right heart failure. Left untreated, heart failure deteriorates. Note the limited symptoms that warn clinicians of heart failure in its compensated phase.

Pathophysiology (continued)

Pathophysiology by Heart Failure Subset

There are several clinical subsets of heart failure, and combinations of the subsets, that determine the clinical manifestations (signs and symptoms) and most appropriate interventions:

1. Acuity: Acute, chronic, or acute on chronic (chronic with an acute episode)
2. Location: The side(s) of the heart that is involved: right-sided, left-sided, or both (biventricular)
3. Functional impairment: The principal functional impairment: systolic dysfunction, diastolic dysfunction, or systolic and diastolic dysfunction
4. Severity: The New York Heart Association (NYHA) classification system (I–IV)
   - Left ventricular systolic failure is the most common type of HF, occurring in almost 60% of cases.
   - An understanding of each individual subset, the similarities and differences, contributes to a clearer understanding for each patient with heart failure.

Acute vs. Chronic HF

Heart failure can be acute or chronic

- **Acute heart failure** (decompensated)* is a sudden worsening of heart failure with new and/or rapid onset of symptoms. Acute HF often results from a change in medical condition (e.g., change in medications). Some changes are life threatening (e.g., myocardial infarction, ventricular tachycardia) and require emergency treatment. Patients who present in the emergency department or hospital are typically in acute, rather than chronic, heart failure. Treatment of acute heart failure is focused on symptom relief, restoration of oxygenation, and perfusion. Most patients present to the emergency department or the health care provider's office with new onset HF or an acute exacerbation of their chronic HF.
- **Chronic heart failure** (compensated)* is a long-term condition that develops over time. Symptoms gradually worsen and tend to be stable. The deterioration that occurs is in large part due to the compensating mechanisms themselves. Treatment of chronic heart failure focuses on preventing remodeling and decreasing mortality.
- **Acute or chronic heart failure is an acute exacerbation of heart failure in a patient who already has chronic HF.** A person can have acute or chronic heart failure when an acute exacerbation occurs (e.g. myocardial infarction, dysrhythmia) in a patient with stable chronic heart failure.

*Acute and chronic heart failure may be due to either systolic, diastolic, left heart, and/or right heart dysfunction (e.g., left systolic and diastolic failure).

Left Heart Failure

- Left heart failure (LHF) is the most common type of failure and presents with pulmonary symptoms.
- Pulmonary symptoms dominate since there are increased left ventricular (LV) and atrial pressures, causing increase pressures in the pulmonary vasculature. The increased pressure results in increased extravascular lung water, interfering in gas exchange (especially of oxygen) and manifested by:
  - o Low pulse oximeter readings
  - o Shortness of breath, orthopnea
  - o Crackles in dependent regions of the lungs, cough
- However, the most dangerous effects of left-sided heart failure are loss of stroke volume and cardiac output. These lead to tissue hypoxia. Severe LHF (see Severe Heart Failure schematic) can be manifested by hypotension and life-threatening loss of perfusion (cardiogenic shock). Symptoms include:
  - o Weak pulses
  - o Confusion and decreased level of consciousness
  - o Low urine output
  - o Cool, clammy skin

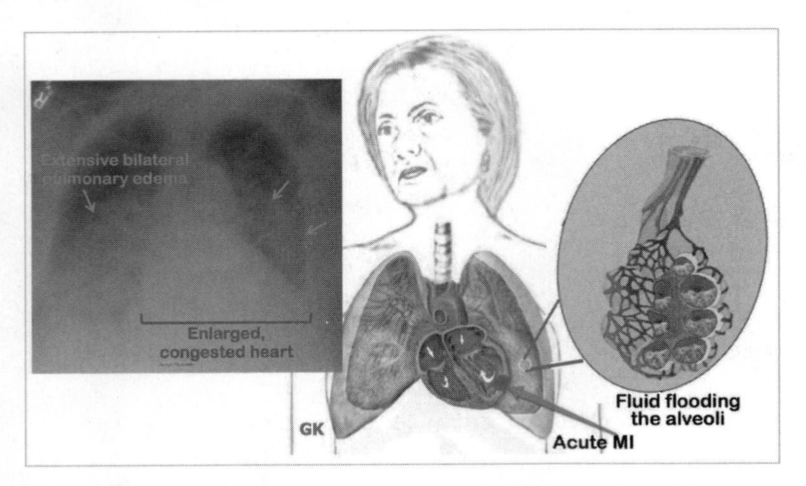

Following MI or other significant myocardial damage (middle image), heart failure leads to pulmonary congestion (x-ray on left). When the pulmonary vasculature is congested, fluid leaks into the alveoli (right image) and hinders gas exchange.
Sources: (*left*) Courtesy of K. Kyriakidis; (*middle/right*) Courtesy of George Kyriakidis/Santa Ana, CA

Pathophysiology Schematic: Severe Heart Failure

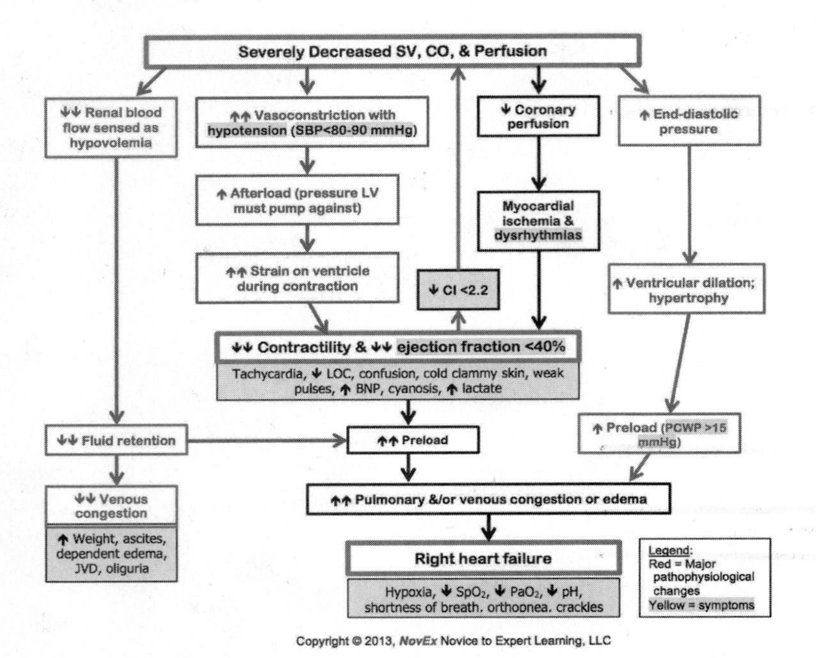

This schematic shows how the compensatory mechanisms eventually fail in left heart failure and contribute to the worsening of both left and right heart failure. The biventricular failure inevitably leads to cardiogenic shock.
Source: Copyright © 2013, NovEx Novice to Expert Learning, LLC

Right Heart Failure

The pathophysiology of right heart failure is typically related to pulmonary hypertension (most commonly from left heart failure) or right heart damage. Despite the cause, stroke volume is diminished.

Chronic Right Heart Failure

- Left heart failure is the most common cause of right heart failure that develops over time. Left heart failure, leads to pulmonary hypertension. The high pulmonary pressure increases the pressure against which the right ventricle (RV) must pump (the afterload on the RV).
- Afterload places undue strain on the RV that normally pumps against low pressures (see the RV Failure schematic). Sustained increases in pulmonary pressure eventually cause right ventricular hypertrophy or dilation. Without much contractile reserve, the RV is unable to adapt to the high afterload and fails.
- Right heart failure develops over time into chronic right HF.
- However, depending on how acute and how high the afterload is, the RV can exhaust rapidly and, without medical intervention, it can suddenly and irreversibly fail.

Schematic: Pathophysiology of Right Ventricular Failure

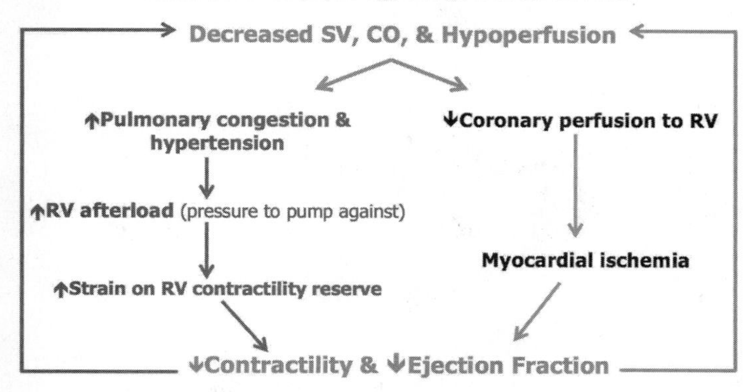

- When right heart failure is caused by pulmonary hypertension (arterial vasoconstriction) due to lung diseases (e.g., COPD, hypoxemia from sleep apnea) or conditions (e.g., pulmonary embolism), it is called **cor pulmonale**.
- A consequence of right heart failure is the systemic backup of venous blood returning to the RV, reflected as an elevated central venous pressure (CVP). Normal CVP is 2–6 mmHg, whereas a CVP greater than or equal to 10 mmHg is considered elevated. The increased CVP causes extensive venous congestion (e.g., seen as peripheral edema, jugular distension, hepatic distention, and ascites). In most conditions, given this pathophysiology, RV failure can be identified if the CVP is markedly elevated without pulmonary congestion.
- The elevated CVP and preload on the RV can lead to an adaptive RV dilation, up to a point. Continued high preload eventually contributes to RV failure, as occurs in left heart failure.

Acute Development of Right Heart Failure

- Acute development of right heart failure (e.g., damage to the right ventricle from myocardial infarction) can be devastating if significant in size. There can be a sudden drop of blood flow (or CO) from the RV through the lungs. This diminishes blood return to the LV and systemic hypotension ensues. The hemodynamic deterioration is compounded when the CO drops the aortic pressure as a key determinant of coronary blood flow drops, and causes inadequate coronary perfusion. Inadequate coronary blood flow leads to RV ischemia, which then exacerbates the decline in contractility.
- Initially increasing the preload or end-diastolic volume with intravenous fluids can be helpful temporarily, because there is a rapid compensatory increase in contractility (Frank–Starling curve). However, the contractile reserves in the RV are limited as it is a much thinner muscle than the LV and is made to pump against low pressures. When the RV can no longer compensate, there can be a sudden hemodynamic collapse, further reducing CO. Unless medical intervention such as tissue plasminogen activator (TPA) or angioplasty occurs, this catastrophic deterioration is likely to spiral into irreversible RV failure.
- Early recognition of acute RV failure, alone or in combination with left-sided failure, is important because of its inherent instability and the propensity to abruptly and irreversibly decompensate.

Pathophysiology (continued)

Systolic Versus Diastolic HF

- **Systolic heart failure** is a clinical syndrome with symptoms of congestion and low cardiac output caused by impaired ventricular ejection function. The major hemodynamic alterations include:
  - o Reduced ejection fraction leading to reduced SV and CO
  - o Depressed contractility
  - o Increased afterload and LV wall stress
  - o Increased ventricular volume and abnormal diastolic filling with LV dilation
  - o Increased LV diastolic pressure, increased pulmonary hypertension
  - o Increased LV diastolic pressure, increased pulmonary hypertension

  *More common in men
- **Diastolic heart failure** is HF with normal or near-normal ejection fraction. The major hemodynamic derangements include:
  - o Normal or near-normal ejection fraction
  - o Decreased LV relaxation resulting in high LV diastolic pressure
  - o LV wall stiffness
  - o Resultant pulmonary and RV alterations

  *More common in women

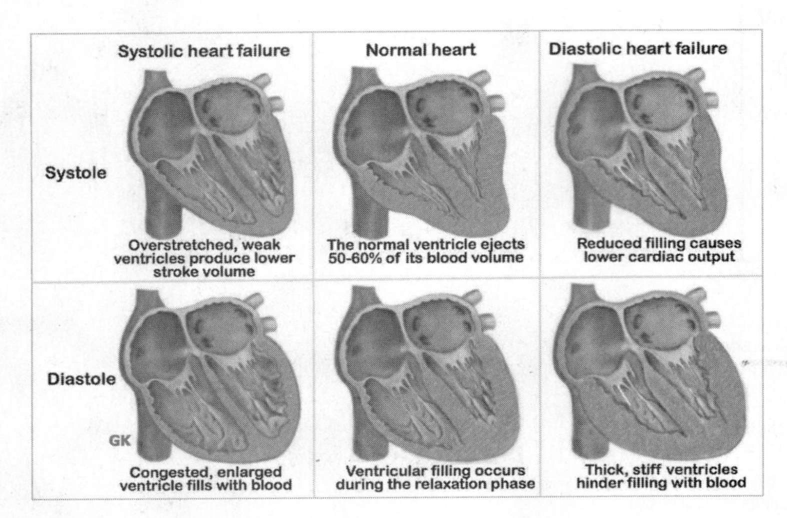

Systolic versus diastolic heart failure during systole and diastole.
Source: Courtesy of George Kyriakidis/Santa Ana, CA

- Systolic and diastolic HF share similar characteristics (signs and symptoms, some hemodynamics), but have dissimilarities in their pathogenesis (mechanism that caused the disease).
- Distinguishing between systolic and diastolic failure is important therapeutically because studies have not yet shown that patients with diastolic failure respond as well to the same therapies used in patients with systolic failure. Despite the few studies in diastolic HF, health care providers continue to treat patients similarly because of the clinical responses.
- Important exceptions:
  1. Contractility agents, such as digoxin, should not be used in diastolic HF.
  2. Patients with diastolic HF may be more sensitive to volume changes due to ventricular stiffness, so fluids should be titrated with greater care.

New York Heart Association Classification in Patients with Cardiac Disease

Class	Severity	Functional Capacity during Activity
I	Mild	Experiences no limitation in normal daily activity
II	Mild	Experiences minor limitations in functional daily activities but comfortable when inactive
III	Moderate	Experiences moderate and restricting limitations during physical activity but comfortable when inactive
IV	Severe	Experiences discomfort in most, if not all, physical activities, to the point of discomfort at rest

HF patients are often classified according to functional capacity to help guide treatment and patient education.

Risk Factors

- Hypertension
- Coronary artery disease
- Valvular diseases
- Obesity
- Diabetes
- Kidney disease
- Aging
- Smoking

Concept Check

3. **Which patient is at highest risk for developing heart failure?**
   A. A patient with diabetes mellitus
   B. A patient who smokes
   C. A patient with hypertension
   D. A patient with cancer

Answer question

Causes

Each of the following conditions has its own prognosis and treatment. **Chronic conditions** associated with heart failure include:

- Hypertension: single largest risk factor!
- Cardiac valve disease (e.g., aortic stenosis)
- Coronary artery disease: cause of 2/3 of systolic HF cases
- Infections (e.g., myocarditis)
- Left to right heart shunts (e.g., septal defects)
- Cardiomyopathies (e.g., hypertrophic, alcoholic): diseases of the heart muscle with unknown causes.

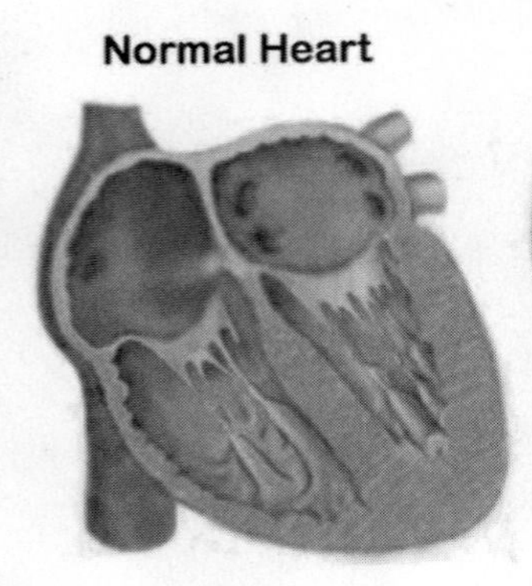

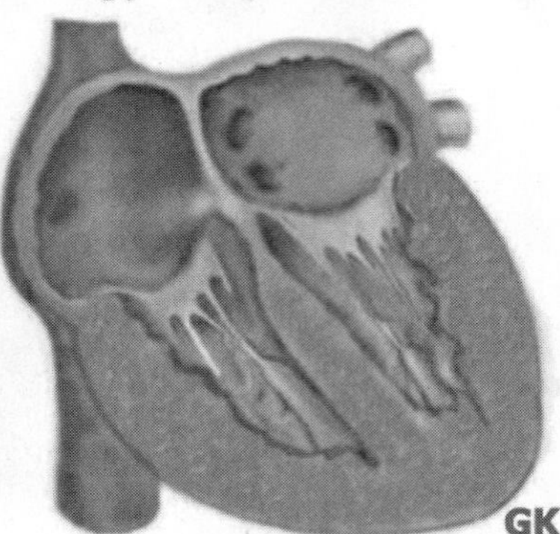

The hypertrophied heart (right) is contrasted to a normal heart. It makes visible why hypertension is the biggest risk factor for heart failure. A hypertrophied heart can be twice the size of a normal one.
Source: Courtesy of George Kyriakidis/Santa Ana, CA

- Coarctation (narrowing) of the aorta
- Prolonged tachydysrhythmias
- Toxins such as cocaine, alcohol, chemotherapy, or medications causing cardiac depression
- Ventricular filling disorders that prevent adequate blood flow into the ventricles during diastole, such as mitral or tricuspid stenosis, cardiac tamponade, restrictive pericarditis, or restrictive cardiomyopathy
- Less common conditions that produce increased metabolic demand may cause heart failure (e.g., anemia, thyrotoxicosis, fever, arteriovenous fistulas).

Specific Causes

Cardiomyopathies

Cardiomyopathies are diseases of the heart muscle with unknown causes. There are four main categories of cardiomyopathy which cause heart failure:

1. Dilated Cardiomyopathy: A loss of contractility results in the heart being overstretched, dilated or enlarged, and weakened. This is the most common of the cardiomyopathies.
2. Hypertrophic Cardiomyopathy: This hereditary condition causes the development of ventricular wall thickening and stiffness that leads to compromise in ventricular filling.
3. Arrythmogenic Right Ventricular Dysplasia: This genetic disorder allows fatty and fibrous tissue to progressively replace myocardial tissue, primarily in the right ventricle.
4. Restrictive Cardiomyopathy or Diastolic Dysfunction: The development of stiff, noncompliant ventricular walls results in restrictive contraction, similar to the pathophysiologic effects in hypertrophic cardiomyopathy. Unlike dilated cardiomyopathy, the ventricle is typically not enlarged.

Right Heart Failure

- Left heart failure
- Cor pulmonale: right heart failure caused by pulmonary hypertension resulting from lung diseases (e.g., sleep apnea, COPD)
- Pulmonary embolism
- Posterior myocardial infarction

Concept Check

4 What is cor pulmonale?

A. Right heart failure caused by lung disease
B. Left heart failure
C. A type of myocardial infarction
D. Pulmonary hypotension

Answer question

Assessment Findings

General Assessment Findings

Understanding the signs and symptoms of heart failure is enhanced by considering the type of heart failure present:

- **Left-Sided and/or Systolic Heart Failure**
  - o The most common side of the heart to fail is the left side.
  - o Systolic failure accounts for 67% of patients in heart failure.
  - o Left systolic HF accounts for 60% of patients in heart failure.
  - o Patient with left and systolic failure present with primarily *pulmonary symptoms*, such as pulmonary congestion, edema, difficulty breathing, and difficulty oxygenating. The increased left ventricular and atrial pressures cause pulmonary vascular overload, leakage, and poor gas exchange (e.g., arterial blood gas abnormalities). The ability to rapidly and accurately recognize the predominance of the symptoms as pulmonary prepares one to make better clinical judgments.
- **Right-Sided Heart Failure**
  - o The most common reason for right heart failure is left heart failure.
  - o Right heart failure that is caused by lung disease (e.g., COPD, sleep apnea) and pulmonary hypertension is called cor pulmonale.
  - o Patients with right heart failure present primarily with *systemic symptoms*, such as dependent edema, venous distention, hepatic congestion, jugular venous distention, ascites, and weight gain because systemic venous congestion. Noticing the predominance of systemic symptoms can assist in quickly identifying the nature of the problem and intervening appropriately.
- **Biventricular Heart Failure**
  - o Many patients with chronic left heart failure eventually develop biventricular failure.
  - o Patients with right and left heart failure predictably present with both pulmonary and systemic manifestations.
- **Combinations of Severe Heart Failure or Severe Left and/or Systolic Heart Failure**
  - o Severe heart failure results in rapidly deteriorating stroke volume and cardiac output and leads to tissue hypoxia.
  - o Symptoms of shock caused by life-threatening hypoperfusion and hypotenison across organ systems are notable.

When patients have combinations of right, left, systolic, and/or diastolic heart failure, the signs and symptoms cross subsets:

Typical symptoms of LEFT heart failure include:

1. Shortness of breath, cannot lie flat
2. Orthopnea
3. Paroxysmal nocturnal dyspnea
4. Cough (frothy, blood-tinged)
5. Peripheral edema and weight gain
6. Tachycardia, often irregular
7. Crackles
8. Fatigue, weakness
9. Low urine output
10. Loss of appetite or sleep
11. Palpitations (heart pounding)
12. S3 and/or S4 gallop, murmur
13. Pulsus alternans, weak pulses
14. Cool, clammy skin
15. Pleural effusion

Typical symptoms of RIGHT heart failure include:

1. Dependent edema
2. Nocturia
3. Jugular venous distention or CVP ≥ 10 mmHg
4. Tachycardia, often irregular
5. Fatigue, weakness
6. Palpitations (heart pounding)
7. Enlarged liver with hepatojugular reflux
8. Ascites
9. Weight gain
10. Shortness of breath, often due to pulmonary disease

Typical symptoms of SYSTOLIC heart failure include:

1. Tachycardia, dysrhythmias
2. Fatigue, reduced functioning
3. Shortness of breath
4. Orthopnea
5. Crackles
6. Cough
7. S3 and/or S4 gallop, murmur
8. Peripheral edema
9. Loss of appetite or sleep
10. Palpitations
11. Pulsus alternans
12. Pleural effusion
13. Ventricular dysrhythmias

Typical symptoms of DIASTOLIC heart failure include:

1. **Flash, or sudden, pulmonary edema (unlike most HF)
2. **Normal or near-normal ejection fraction
3. **Loud S4 gallop
4. Shortness of breath, tachypnea (particularly on exertion)
5. Orthopnea
6. Jugular venous distention
7. Crackles
8. Peripheral edema
9. Tachycardia, especially atrial fibrillation
10. Cough
11. Fatigue

**** Key Distinctions**

New York Heart Association Classification in Patients with Cardiac Disease

Class	Severity	Signs & Symptoms during Activity
I	Mild	Asymptomatic or almost no symptoms
II	Mild	No notable signs at rest. Experiences dyspnea, fatigue and palpitations during daily activities.
III	Moderate	No notable signs at rest. Experiences dyspnea, fatigue and palpitations while attempting to do some daily activities
IV	Severe	Symptomatic at rest with any with any slight activity.

Diagnostics

B-Type Natriuretic Peptide

1. B-Type Natriuretic Peptide (BNP) is a hormone secreted by the heart. BNP levels increase in response to wall tension of the ventricles.
2. BNP increases as the heart decompensates in heart failure.
3. As a routine, guideline-recommended test, the BNP should be obtained to evaluate dyspnea and chest pain.
4. BNP readings indicate:
   - o Less than 100 pg/mL — No heart failure
   - o 100–300 pg/mL — Presence of heart failure
   - o Greater than 300 pg/mL — Mild heart failure
   - o Greater than 600 pg/mL — Moderate heart failure
   - o Greater than 900 pg/mL — Severe heart failure

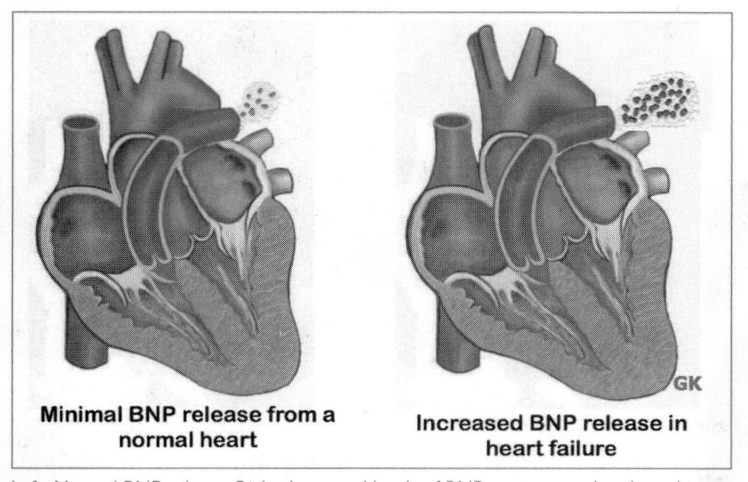

Left: Normal BNP release. Right: Increased levels of BNP are commonly released in heart failure.
Source: Courtesy of George Kyriakidis/Santa Ana, CA

BNP Levels in Evaluating Shortness of Breath

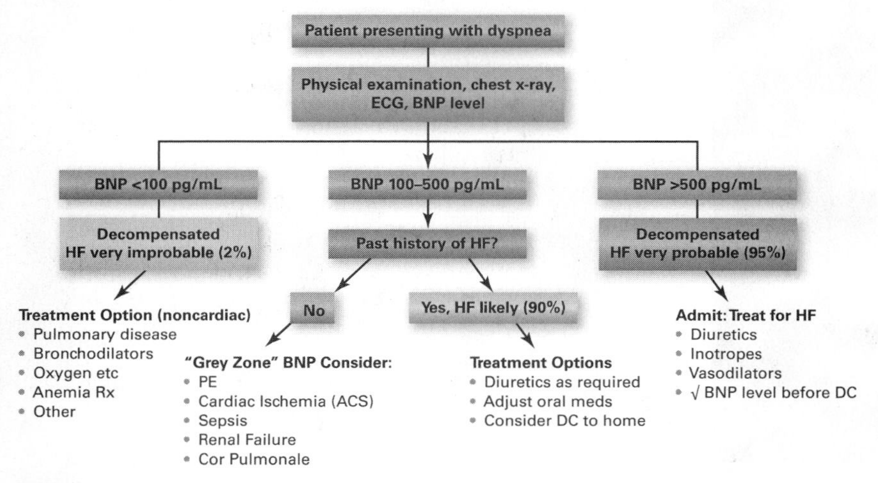

This diagram presents a chart that shows management of a patient in heart failure. Specifically the heart failure is guided by the patient's BNP level. This illustration is a very helpful summary of management of heart failure.
Source: Adapted from Maisel A. *Rev Cardiovasc Med.* 2002;3(Suppl 4):S10-S17. Mueller C et al. *N Engl J Med.* 2004;350:647-54.

- When the cause of shortness of breath (SOB) in a patient is unclear, obtaining a BNP level may help differentiate cardiac from non cardiac causes.
- BNP levels less than 100 pg/mL suggests a cardiac cause with heart failure as the probable reason. The higher the level, the more likely heart failure is the cause of SOB. For example, levels greater than 400 pg/mL are highly suggestive of heart failure.
- If BNP is low normal, the cause of SOB is likely to be noncardiac.

Diagnostics (continued)

Evaluation and Treatment of P atients Presenting with Acute Dyspnea

Evaluate **EF: Echocardiogram** may reveal a decreased ejection fraction, LV hypertrophy, valvular heart disease, or pericardial effusion.

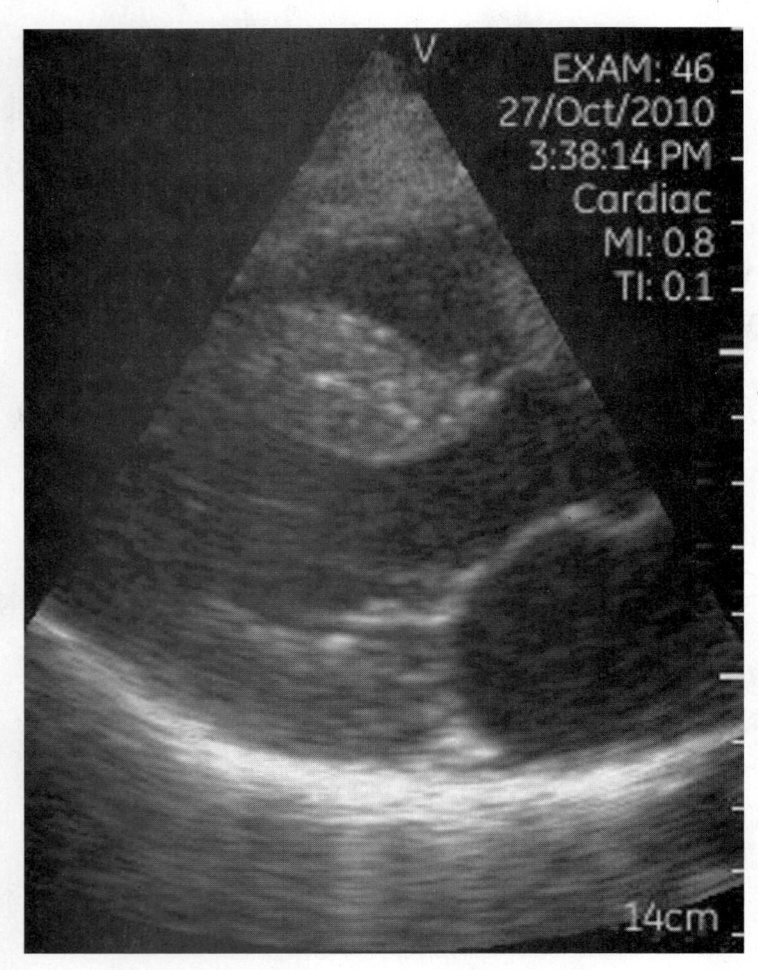

This is an example of an echocardiogram, which is an ultrasound test that often helps diagnose heart failure. This ultrasound view is called a long axis parasternal view and shows the left atrium, a closed mitral valve, and a contracting left ventricle. There are many causes of heart failure. Echocardiogram can often help differentiate the type of heart failure.

Source: Copyright © 2013, NovEx Novice to Expert Learning, LLC

Chest x-ray: Patients with left heart failure may have pulmonary edema, pleural effusions, and enlarged heart.

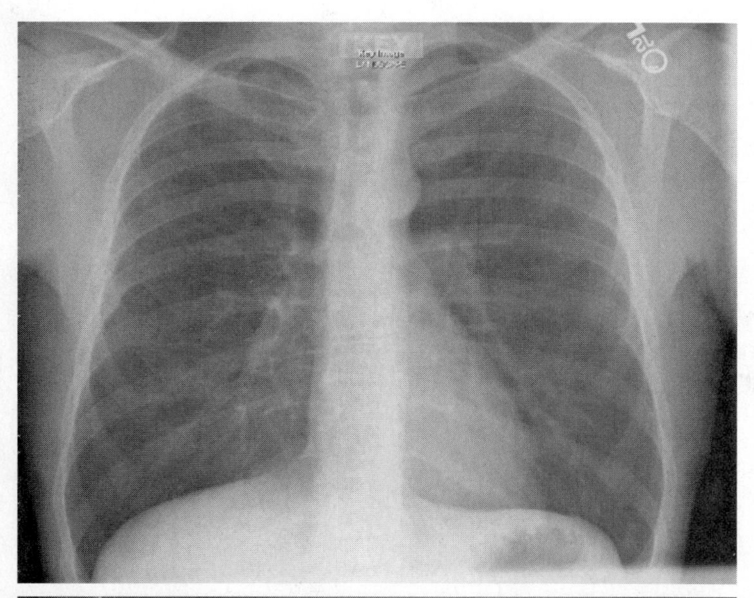

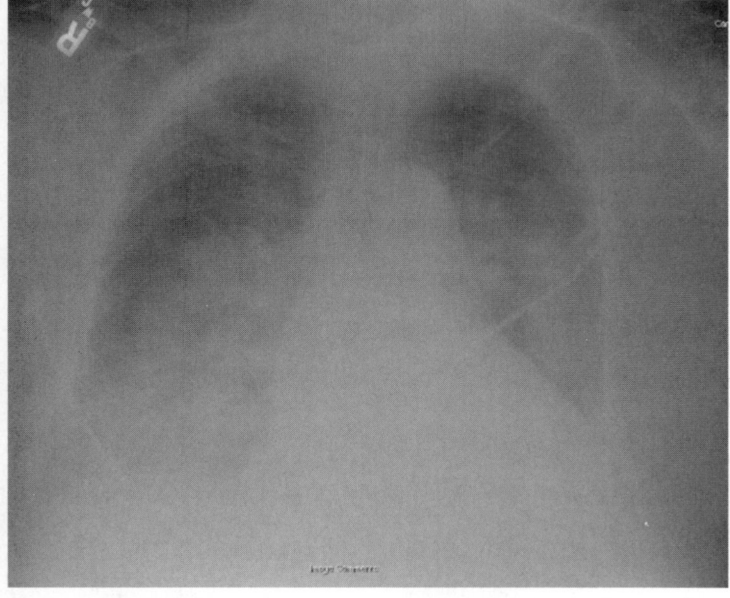

X-rays comparing normal heart (upper) versus heart failure. Lower: Pulmonary congestion is noted bilaterally (whitish shadows) with an enlarged heart.
Source: (*both*) Courtesy of K. Kyriakidis

Pulmonary artery catheterization is an invasive procedure that allows measurement of CO, SV, peripheral vascular resistance, and preload (wedge pressure).

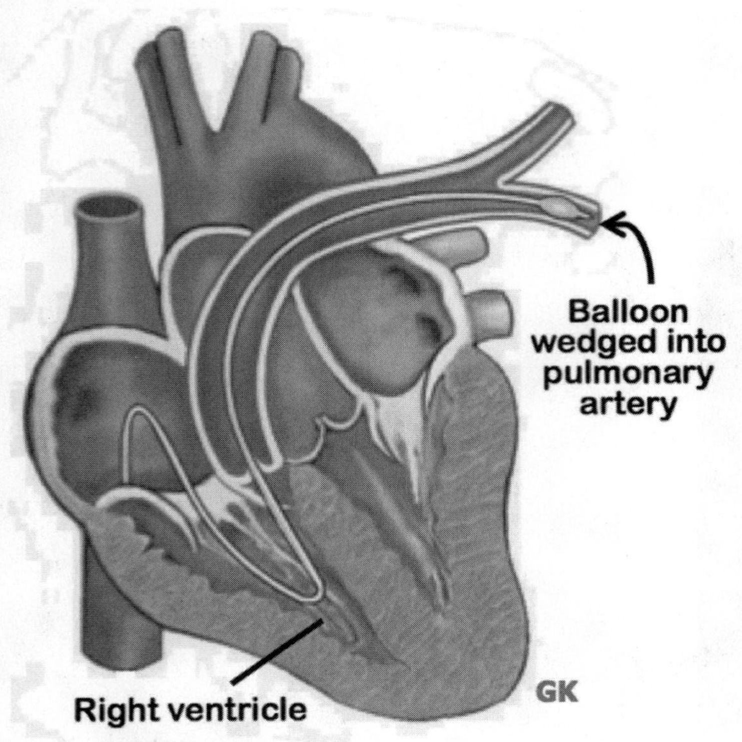

Balloon-tipped, pulmonary artery catheters can be used to measure pulmonary capillary wedge pressure (PCWP), which reflects preload, to evaluate the degree of heart failure.
Source: Courtesy of George Kyriakidis/Santa Ana, CA

Additional testing may help diagnose causes of heart failure:

- CBC to evaluate for anemia.
- Thyroid function tests to rule out thyroid disease.
- Left heart catheterization to evaluate for cardiac ischemia.

Priority Patient Concerns and Desired Collaborative Care Outcomes

Prior to caring for patients with heart failure, it is important to prioritize the patient's concerns that must guide the nursing care plan and interventions. Care for the patient is ordered and organized in accordance with the patient's priority and urgent needs. Desired collaborative care outcomes in patients with heart failure typically include:

1. Patient will be as normovolemic as possible to achieve hemodynamic stability.
2. Patient will tolerate prehospitalized activities with minimal dyspnea and/or fatigue.
3. Patient will have oxygen saturation levels with personal acceptable levels.
4. Patient's cardiac output will return to personal normal.
5. Patient will evidence increased knowledge of disease management and therapeutic modalities.
6. Patient will have no reduced anxiety or anxiety that they are able to comfortably cope with.

Considering these important care outcomes, prepare a list of the major 3–6 priority patient concerns or nursing diagnoses for patients with heart failure. Be prepared to participate in a discussion of this list and/or to submit them as an assignment, as determined by your faculty. Resources you may find helpful in this assignment can include this lesson, the references, resources on nursing care plans, and standard nursing diagnoses manuals.

LO3:

Collaborative Interventions

Management of Heart Failure

Goals in the treatment of heart failure:

- To correct the underlying problem
- Improve the quality of life by controlling and reducing symptoms
- Slow the progression of the disease
- Reduce the need for emergency department visits or hospitalization
- Increase survival

Evidence-Based Guidelines for Comprehensive Heart Failure Management

- The Heart Failure Society of America has evidence-based guidelines for heart failure management. The 2010 guidelines follow fairly simple recommendations:
  - o Level A is for treatments that have a randomized controlled trial (RCT) supporting use. Level A is the highest recommendation level.
  - o Level B is for treatments that have research, but not as rigorous as an RCT.
  - o Level C is for treatments with less research, and is more of an expert opinion.
- The level of support for therapies will be listed for each of the treatments presented here.
- In heart failure, there are several types of clinical presentations, acute and chronic management. Treatments are similar, but specific actions may be slightly altered depending on the patient symptoms. The following is a guide to managing each type of heart failure. However, for more comprehensive review, additional reading is encouraged.
- (http://www.heartfailureguideline.org/)

Collaborative Interventions (continued)

Evidence-Based Guidelines for Chronic Heart Failure Management

In chronic heart failure management (see Chronic Systolic Heart Failure schematic), actions include:

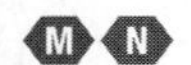

1. Afterload reduction: Level A
   - o ACE inhibitors (e.g., captopril) are the most common treatment for chronic heart failure and first line therapy. ACE inhibitors improve survival as well as symptoms, and are not typically withdrawn if symptoms improve. Major side effects that may warrant discontinuation include: hypotension, hyperkalemia, persistent cough, acute renal failure, anaphylactic reaction, angioedema.
   - o Recommendations include other afterload therapies (e.g., Angiotensin Receptor blockers such as losartan) for patients who are allergic to, or unable to tolerate, ACE inhibitors. These patients may or may not have symptomatic HF but do have LV ejection fractions less than 40%.

2. Beta-adrenergic receptor blockade with beta blockers (e.g., metoprolol, carvedilol): Level A
   - o Beta blockers are negative inotropes (decrease contractility) and chronotropes (decrease heart rate). Paradoxically, beta blockers improve symptoms, survival, need for hospitalization in chronic heart failure patients. Beta blockers are used in stable patients, who are symptomatic and/or with low ejection fractions (less than 40%). Use may be limited, or even withheld in patients with low cardiac output, a significant bradycardia or reactive airways disease (e.g., asthma).

*Evidence shows that either beta blockers or ACE inhibitors can be used initially, adding the other as indicated.
**A few randomized clinical trials using the above treatments in diastolic heart failure show insufficient evidence of reduced morbidity or mortality. They have demonstrated effectiveness in systolic heart failure.

3. Diuretics (e.g., furosemide) are used to achieve normal volume status: Level A.

   Other diuretics can be employed as well:
   - o If potassium sparing is desired, then a diuretic-like aldosterone (spironolactone) can be used. Spironolactone has been shown to improve survival in a select group of patients with CHF.
   - o Hydrochlorothiazide (a thiazide diuretic) is also a common therapy.

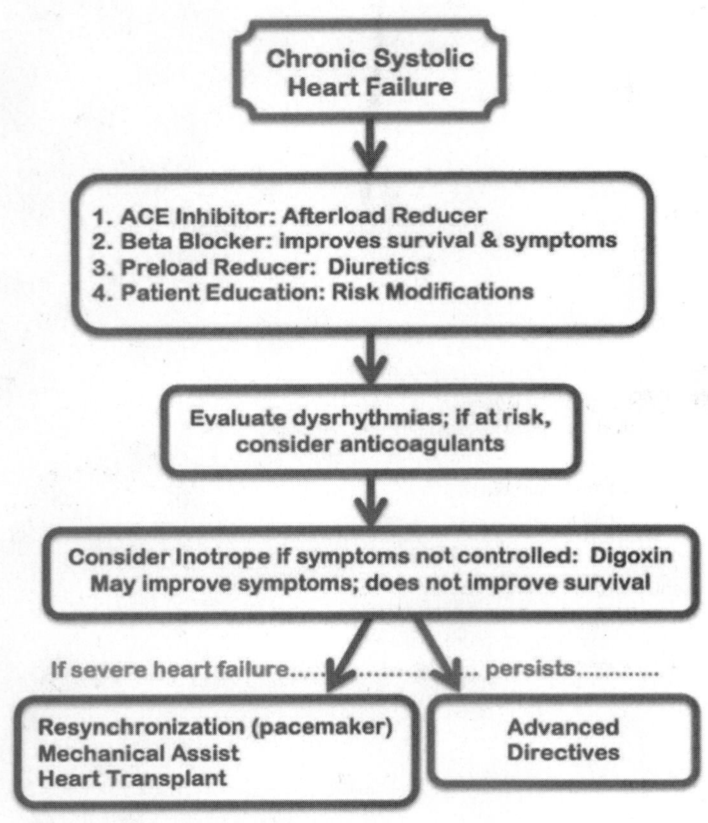

M N **4.** Improving contractility: Level B

- o The only long-term contractility agent is digitalis (digoxin is the most commonly used). Due to the toxicity of digitalis preparations, close monitoring is required for any patient receiving digitalis preparations. Contractility agents should not be used in diastolic heart failure.

N **5.** Managing modifiable risks: Patient education should begin as early as possible and plays a key role in managing patients with heart failure. These include:

- o Medications, dosages, and necessity to take them as ordered
- o When to call your health care provider
- o Daily monitoring of weight at home. An increase in weight may alert the health care provider and patient of a possible worsening of the patient's condition before symptoms develop.
- o Sodium reduction (usually to 2 grams daily) helps decrease fluid retention. Restrict fluid if the patient has hyponatremia.
- o Diet modifications, such as a low-cholesterol diet, may be helpful in patients with coronary artery disease.
- o Smoking cessation
- o Vaccination: influenza and pneumococcal
- o Weight loss in obese patients
- o Alcohol reduction
- o Exercise rehabilitation

N **6.** Dysrhythmias that compromise cardiac output (uncontrolled atrial fibrillation, life-threatening ventricular dysrhythmias) should be evaluated for treatment. Clinically, this intervention should take precedence prior to adding an inotrope for continued and unresponsive heart failure.

N **7.** Anticoagulants may need to be considered in patients with dysrhythmias (e.g., atrial fib) that increase the risk for blood clots.

M N **8.** Advanced treatment through devices such as intra-aortic balloon pumps, left ventricular assist devices (LVAD), cardiac resynchronization therapy (atrial-ventricular or biventricular synchronous contraction via pacemaker) and heart transplant may be used when other therapies are failing.

9. The benefit of these devices in diastolic HF is unproven.

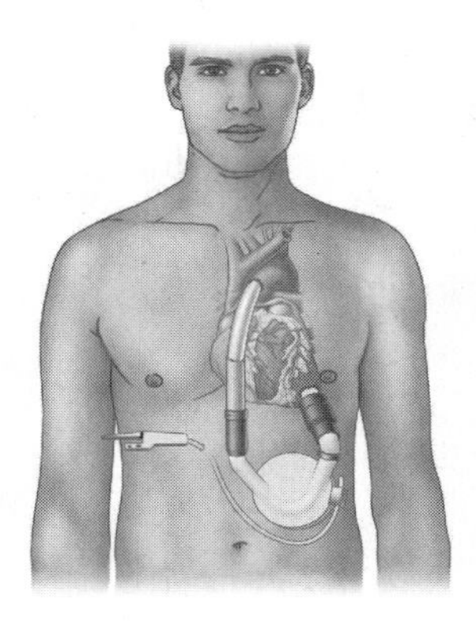

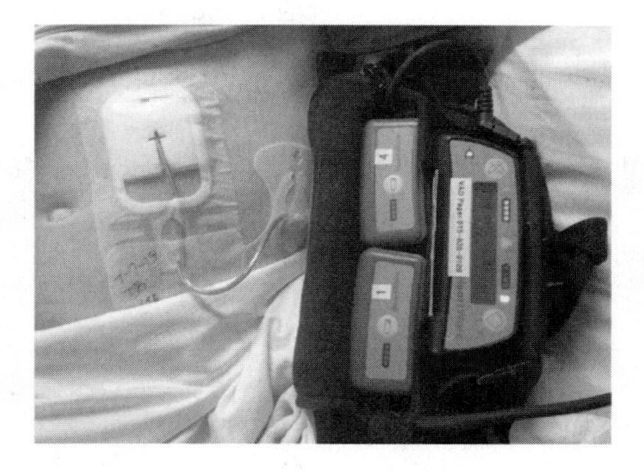

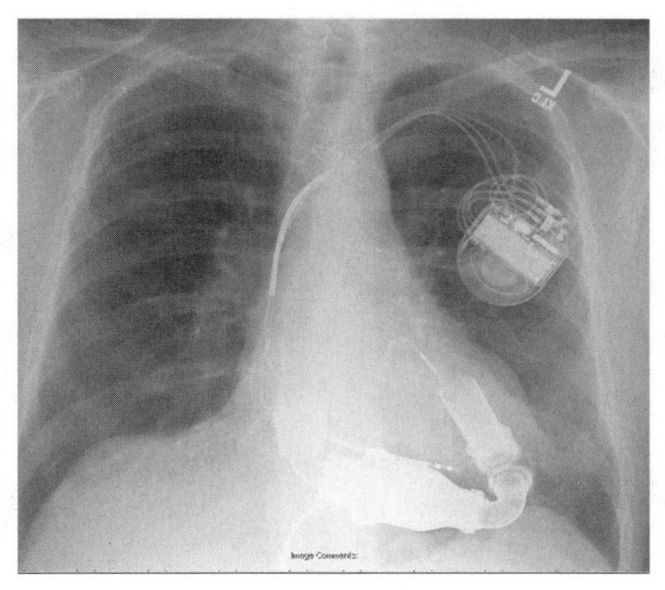

Upper left: One of the many models of the internally implanted LVAD is represented here. The newest models tend to be lighter and smaller. Upper right: This photo shows an LVAD in place in a patient who is awaiting heart transplantation. Visible are the connection line, the control unit, and battery pack that make mobility possible. Lower: The x-ray shows an implanted LVAD in the heart with an AV pacemaker visible above the heart.
Source: (*upper right*) Courtesy of Sarah Dresen; (*lower*) Courtesy of K. Kyriakidis

Collaborative Interventions (continued)

M N **Advance Directives**

- Discussion of advance directives is especially important in heart failure patients. As nurses begin to educate patients and their families about the progressive, manageable, but non reversible issues of heart failure, they should begin discussions about the importance of advanced directives in the early education sessions, just after heart failure is diagnosed.
- Nurses can educate patients about how decisions they make regarding their advanced directives can provide guidance for and comfort to family members in carrying out their wishes. Nurses should reassure patients that conscientious symptom management typically improves longevity, but for most heart failure patients, it is heart failure rather than other diseases that they succumb to at the end of life.
- Nurses can make patients and their families aware that they share responsibility in assisting the patient explore symptom management options for the future time, when those symptoms become very difficult to alleviate. Decisions do not need to be made immediately. Early discussion, however, provides the patient and family with the time to consider what is best for the patient.

Racial Considerations

- African Americans comprise about one third of all heart failure patients.
- According to research, African American patients who are treated with isosorbide dinitrate (a vasodilator and preload reducer), in addition to hydralazine (vasodilator), have improved survival rates. African Americans have a poorer response to nitrates alone, when compared to other groups, but hydralazine has been shown to enhance the efficacy of nitrates.
- African Americans have a 3.0–4.5 higher associated risk of angioedema with the use of ACE inhibitors. Angioedema is caused by vascular leakage and swelling of deep dermis or subcutaneous tissue. The edema is commonly seen in the facial area and can be problematic if the edema threatens the airway.

Concept Check

5. Which medication is given to reduce afterload in a patient with chronic heart failure?

A. ACE inhibitor

B. Beta blocker

C. Diuretic

D. Anticoagulant

Answer question

Concept Check

6. In which instance would the nurse question use of digoxin for a patient with heart failure?

A. Systolic heart failure is present.

B. The patient is African-American.

C. Diastolic heart failure is present.

D. The patient is over age 65.

Answer question

Collaborative Interventions (continued)

Evidence-Based Guidelines for Acute Heart Failure Management

In acute heart failure, the emphasis is on immediate symptom relief. These actions for acute management are generally Level C. Key actions include (see Acute Heart Failure schematic):

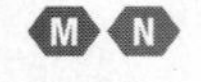

1. Treatment of fluid overload (preload reduction) is most often achieved with diuretics. The goal of diuretic therapy is to reduce lung congestion (pulmonary capillary wedge pressure <15 mmHg or CVP >10 mmHg).
   - o Furosemide (Lasix) is the most common treatment.
   - o Critical intervention is slowing IV fluid intake to a minimum.
   - o Nitrates can also be helpful. If possible, measure stroke volume to evaluate preload reduction. Symptom relief is another important although more subjective, indication of the effectiveness of therapy. Urine output may improve with diuretic use, but may not be a reliable indication of improved stroke volume.

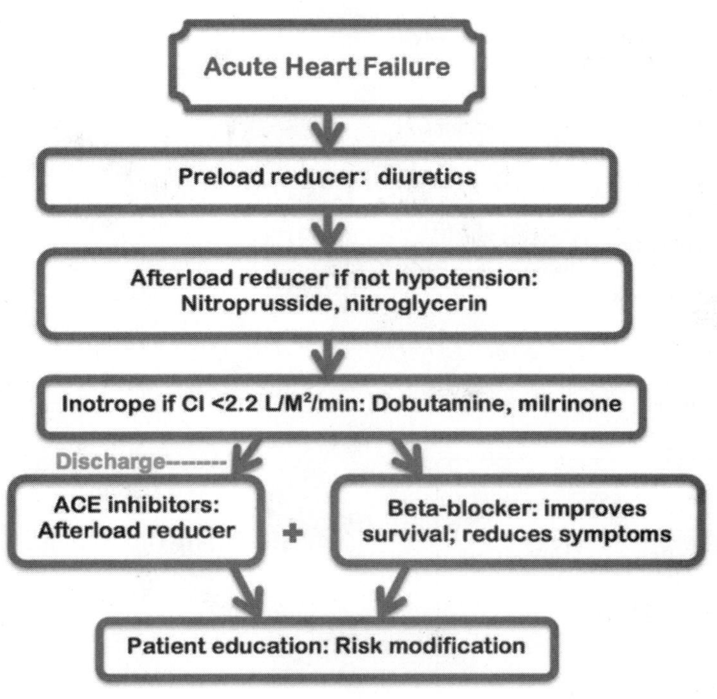

Inotrope if CI <2.2 L/M²/min: Dobutamine, milrinone

Beta-blocker: improves survival; reduces symptoms

Source: Copyright © 2013. NovEx Novice to Expert Learning, LLC

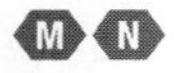

2. If the blood pressure is very high, immediate relief (afterload reduction) is a key strategy for improving stroke volume and can be obtained via medications, such as (Level C). First-line afterload reduction medication:
   - o Nitroprusside is the most rapid acting afterload reducer, but can only be given for a short time due to the production of thiocyanide (cyanide poisoning can develop)
   - o Nitroglycerin
   - o Escalation of dosages is a common practice for both preload and afterload reducers if symptom relief is not achieved.
   - o Additional afterload reducers, such as ACE inhibitors are ideal for long term management if the patient is not hypotensive, but may not act rapidly enough for symptom relief in an acute exacerbation of heart failure.

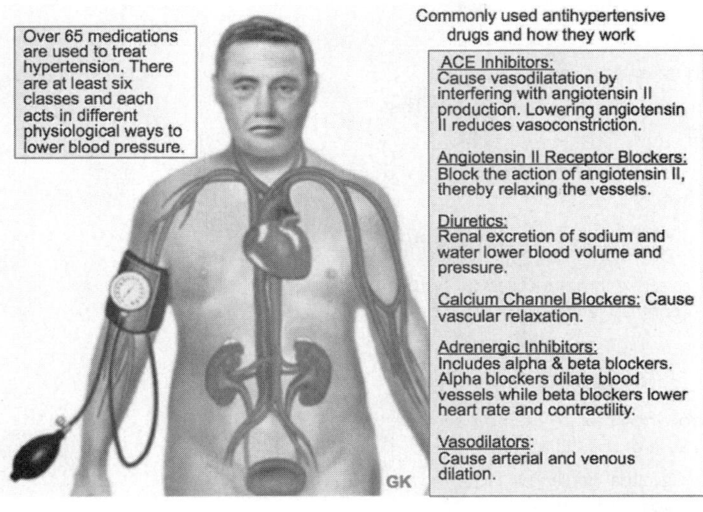

Over 65 medications are used to treat hypertension. There are at least six classes and each acts in different physiological ways to lower blood pressure.
Commonly used antihypertensive drugs and how they work
ACE Inhibitors: Cause vasodilatation by interfering with angiotensin II production. Lowering angiotensin II reduces vasoconstriction.
Angiotensin II Receptor Blockers: Block the action of angiotensin II, thereby relaxing the vessels.
Diuretics: Renal excretion of sodium and water lower blood volume and pressure.
Calcium Channel Blockers: Cause vascular relaxation.
Adrenergic Inhibitors: Includes alpha & beta blockers. Alpha blockers dilate blood vessels while beta blockers lower heart rate and contractility.
Vasodilators: Cause arterial and venous dilation.
GK

Hypertension management is a key to successfully treating heart failure. This illustration demonstrates the common treatments for hypertension management.
Source: Courtesy of George Kyriakidis/Santa Ana, CA

M N **3.** If afterload reduction therapy and diuretics are ineffective or if hypotension prohibits their use, then inotropic agents can be employed to directly increase the heart's contractility:

- o The most common inotrope used in acute situations is dobutamine.
- o Milrinone can also be used (digitalis preparations are not usually used in acute heart failure management)
- o Inotropes can directly improve stroke volume to increase end-organ perfusion and tissue oxygenation ($ScvO_2$, StO_2). Normal $ScvO_2$ and StO_2 are 70–80%.
- o While potentially increasing strength, inotropic agents can have contradictory effects because they also increase myocardial oxygen consumption (MvO_2). The increase in MvO_2 has the potential of worsening the heart failure over time. However, in short-term situations, inotropes can be helpful.

M N **4.** For chronic heart failure patients with an acute exacerbation, evidence-based therapy (e.g., ACE inhibitors, beta blockers) should be reviewed and maximized prior to discharge to manage symptoms, provide comfort, and prevent readmissions.

Concept Check

7. Which medication is the first-line treatment for a patient in heart failure who is also very hypertensive?

A. Nitroprusside

B. Furosemide

C. Dobutamine

D. Milrinone

Answer question

Collaborative Interventions (continued)

M N Management of Acute Heart Failure

- Tachycardia should not be treated in acute heart failure since this is a compensatory mechanism for a low stroke volume. A rapid heart rate in HF is a symptom and not a goal of treatment. Focus on the cause of the tachycardia.
- Oxygen therapy should be used for SpO_2 values less than or equal to 92%.
- Heart failure patients are at high risk of venous thromboembolism and should be placed on prophylaxis (e.g., with low molecular weight heparin) when hospitalized.
- Nitrates should be avoided in patients taking erectile dysfunction drugs due to the possibility of a dangerous drop in blood pressure.
- For all heart failure patients, but especially for those in acute decompensated HF, nurses need to carefully monitor total IV fluids to prevent overload and exacerbation of HF.
- It is important to observe electrolytes, especially sodium and potassium, in heart failure. This is particularly important after diuretics are administered.
  - o Sodium levels may decrease due to fluid overload and diuretic therapy.
  - o Potassium levels may decrease due to loop diuretic therapy.

M N Management of Diastolic Heart Failure

Evidence for treating diastolic heart failure (DHF) is limited, as research has focused on systolic heart failure. Treatment is primarily empiric and focuses on controlling stressors that worsen diastolic failure:

1. Control hypertension, both systolic and diastolic.
2. Diuretics to manage pulmonary and peripheral edema. Care is used in excessively reducing preload with venodilators or diuretics. Patients with diastolic heart failure are more sensitive to blood pressure and intravascular volume changes because of the stiff ventricle.
3. Control dysrhythmias that cause hemodynamic stress (e.g., atrial fibrillation, tachycardias). Patients with diastolic failure are more sensitive to sinus tachycardia and tachydysrythmias (e.g., atrial fibrillation) because filling of the ventricle is more time dependent.
4. Treat myocardial ischemia if present.
5. Contractility agents, such as digoxin, may worsen diastolic failure.
6. Beta blockers may have several beneficial effects. They help relax the ventricle and slow the heart rate to allow more time for filling.

Summary of Interventions

- Afterload reduction achieved usually with ACE inhibitors (e.g., captopril), but also angiotension receptor blockers (e.g., losartan) in chronic heart failure. These are to be used cautiously in patients with acute heart failure and may need to be discontinued if the patient is hypotensive.
- Treatment with beta blockers helps reduce re-hospitalizations, emergency department visits, and symptoms in chronic heart failure patients. These are to be used cautiously in patients with acute heart failure and may need to be discontinued if the patient is hypotensive.
- Diuresis may be prescribed to maintain normal volume. Usually achieved with loop diuretics, such as furosemide, in both acute and chronic heart failure to alleviate congestion.
- Drugs that improve contractility are often prescribed. Dobutamine is the most common inotrope used in acute heart failure with hypotension and/or shock. In chronic heart failure, some health care providers still use digoxin. These treatments do not improve survival but help with symptoms.
- Combination drug therapy is common but warrants more vigilant monitoring.
- Patient education and close monitoring of patients plays a key role in the long-term management of heart failure patients.

Summary of Heart Failure

- Heart failure is a progressive and incurable condition.
- Heart failure affects 5 million people in the United States and is the leading cause of morbidity and mortality.
- Heart failure must be well managed or recurrence is common.
- Heart failure is categorized in four stages from mild to severe, and can also be categorized as: acute (sudden onset) and chronic (long-term management); systolic (impaired contraction or ejection) and diastolic (impaired ventricular relaxation and filling).
- The left ventricle fails most often, producing pulmonary symptoms (e.g., shortness of breath, pulmonary crackles, low SpO_2 values). Right ventricular failure, which is often the result of left ventricular failure or pulmonary disease, produces signs of venous congestion (e.g., dependent edema).
- Most patients who go to the emergency department or hospital for treatment present in a new or evolving acute heart failure, rather than chronic.
- The goal of management of acute heart failure consists of treating the underlying problem, reducing preload, reducing afterload, and improving contractility.
- The goal of managing chronic heart failure is reducing mortality by targeting the maladaptive compensatory mechanisms. Key medications are beta blockers and ACE inhibitors.
- Risk factor modifications are essential to avoid exacerbations of acute HF: diet, when to call the health care provider, medications, smoking cessation, exercise, weight control.
- Treat comorbid conditions: diabetes, high cholesterol, hypertension.

LO4: Evaluation of Desired Collaborative Care Outcomes

Evaluation and reassessment should reveal attainment of previously established patient outcomes. In summary:

- Patient is hemodynamically stable with mininal to no peripheral edema and lungs are clear to auscultation.
- Patient has been able to return to prehospitalized daily activities and reports minimal to no dyspnea or increased fatigue.
- Patient's oxygen saturation levels are at personal normal level.
- Patient has warm, dry skin, mentation is clear, vital signs are normal, and urine output is balanced with intake.
- Patient accurately describes home management of this disorder including findings that indicate need to return for care and plans for future testing.
- Patient appears calm with no physiological expressions of anxiety or is able to calmly and comfortably cope with low levels of anxiety.

References

Moser, D., Riegel, B., Paul, S., et al. (2009). Heart failure. In K. Carlson (Ed.), *AACN Advanced Critical Care Nursing (pp. 237–275)*. St. Louis, MO: Saunders Elsevier.

Riegel, B., & Moser, D. (2013). 20 things you didn't know about heart failure. *Journal of Cardiovascular Nursing, 28*(2), 109–110.

Hamdani, N., & Paulus, W. (2011). Treatment of heart failure with normal ejection fraction. *Curr Treat Options Cardiovasc Med, 13*(1), 26–34.

Heart Failure Society of America. (2011). **http://www.hfsa.org/hfsa-wp/wp/about-hfsa/quick-heart-failure-facts/**

Clinical Practice Guidelines

Yancy, C., Jessup, M., Bozkurt, B., et al. (2013). 2013 ACCF/AHA guideline for the management of heart failure: Executive summary. *Circulation, 128*, 1810–1852.

Jessup, M., Abraham, W., Casey, D., Feldman, A., Francis, G., Ganiats, T., Konstam, M., Mancini, D., Rahko, P., Silver, M., Stevenson, L., & Yancy, C. (2009). 2009 Focused Update: ACCF/AHA guidelines for the diagnosis and management of heart failure in adults: A report of the American College of Cardiology Foundation/American Heart Association Task Force on Practice Guidelines: developed in collaboration with the International Society for Heart and Lung Transplantation. *Circulation, 119*, 1977–2016.

Weintraub, N., Collins, S., Pang, P., Levy, P., Anderson, A., Arslanian-Engoren, C., Gibler, B., McCord, J., Parshall, M., Francis, G., & Gheorghiade, M. (2010). Acute Heart Failure Syndromes: Emergency Department Presentation, Treatment, and Disposition: Current Approaches and Future Aims- A Scientific Statement From the American Heart Association. *Circulation, 122*(19).

Patient Education

American Association of Heart Failure Nurses. Patient Education. **www.aahfnpatienteducation.com**

Torpy, J. M., Lynm, C., & Golub, R. M. (2011). Heart failure. *JAMA, 306*(19), 2175.

STOP

Go to the online course and complete the NovE-Cases assigned by your instructor for this module.

Learning Outcomes for Hypertension

When you complete this lesson, you will be able to:

1. Recognize the clinical relevance of hypertension.
2. Consider the pathophysiology, etiology, risk factors, and clinical presentation of hypertension that determine the priority patient concerns.
3. Determine the most urgent and important nursing interventions and patient education required in caring for a patient with hypertension.
4. Evaluate attainment of desired collaborative care outcomes for a patient with hypertension.

LO1:

What Is Hypertension?

- Hypertension (HTN) is generally defined as a systolic blood pressure (SBP) greater than 140 mmHg and/or a diastolic blood pressure (DBP) greater than 90 mmHg.
- However, some evidence suggests that certain at-risk patient populations may benefit from lower blood pressure goals for optimal risk factor modification (e.g., diabetics).
- Systolic blood pressure, diastolic blood pressure, or both systolic and diastolic pressures may be elevated.
- Systolic pressure is a more important indicator of risk in adults, particularly in those who are over 50 years of age.

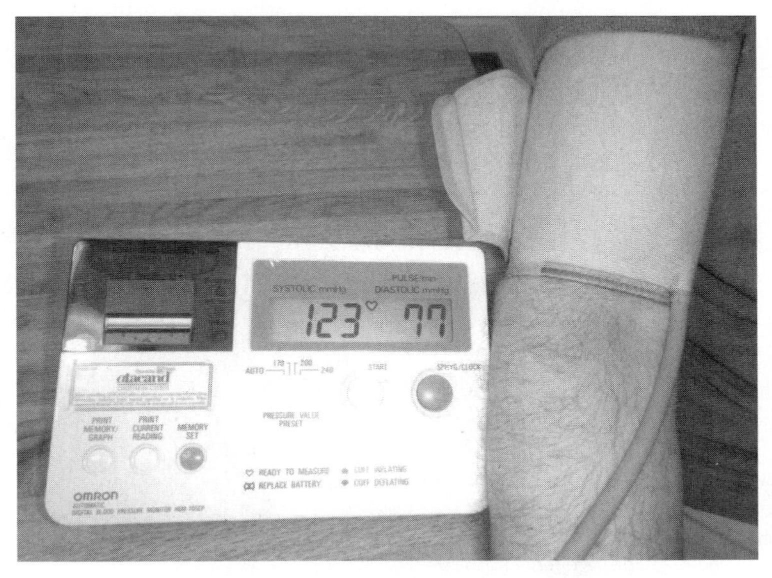

This photo depicts a patient with a sphygmomanometer wrapped around his arm. A sphygmomanometer is a device used to measure blood pressure.
Source: Courtesy of K. Kyriakidis

JNC 7 Hypertension Definitions

The seventh report of the Joint National Committee (JNC 7) revised definitions of hypertension in 2003 based upon blood pressure that is persistently elevated after three to six visits over a several-month period.

Blood Pressure Classification	Systolic BP mm/Hg		Diastolic BP mm/Hg
Normal	<120	AND	<80
PreHypertension	120-139	OR	80-89
Stage 1 Hypertension	140-159	OR	90-100
Stage 2 Hypertension	≥160	OR	≥100

This table presents the systolic and diastolic blood pressure parameters for hypertension that were defined by the JNC 7's seventh report of the JNC on prevention, detection, evaluation, and treatment for patients with high blood pressure. The Department of Health and Human Services, the National Institutes of Health, and the National Heart, Lung, and Blood Institutes collaborated on this project.

The above definitions of hypertension refer to chronic hypertension and are valid in people without a current illness and for people who are not being treated with hypertension medications.

Concept Check

1. **In patients over 50 years of age, which blood pressure is most important?**
   A. Systolic
   B. Diastolic
   C. Neither are more important.
   D. Difference between systolic and diastolic

Answer question

What Are Acute Hypertensive Events?

Blood pressure can rise rapidly and to severe levels in a short period of time. Two types of critical situations need immediate attention:

- **Hypertensive urgency** occurs when the SBP is greater than 180 mmHg and/or DBP is greater than 110 mmHg and there is no end-organ damage (end organ refers to any organ that can be harmed by hypertension, e.g., kidneys, heart, brain).
- **Hypertensive emergency** occurs when the SBP is greater than 220 mmHg and/or DBP is greater than 140 mmHg or there is evidence of organ dysfunction:
  - o Renal effects: acute renal failure (e.g., elevated creatinine, BUN compared to baseline)
  - o Cardiac effects: Pulmonary edema, heart Failure, unstable angina
  - o Neurologic effects: headache, encephalopathy (e.g., mental status changes, seizures)
  - o Retinal effects: Papilledema, exudates, hemorrhages

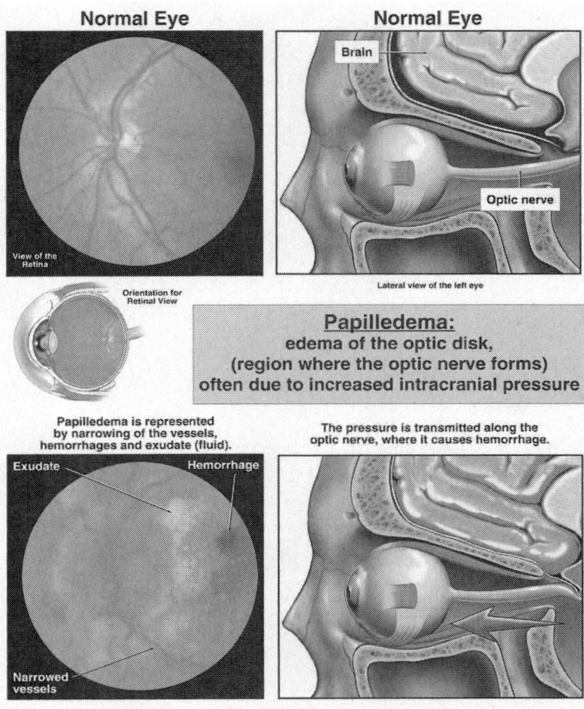

Normal eye anatomy, compared with papilledema (edema or swelling of the optic nerve or disc), shows normal retina and optic nerve. On papilledema images, the retina shows narrowed blood vessels, presence of exudate, and hemorrhage (bleeding). The cutaway view shows how increased intracranial pressure is transmitted down the optic nerve where it causes hemorrhage to the retina.
Source: Nucleus Medical Art Inc/Alamy

LO1:

Clinical Relevance

- Complications of hypertension can be devastating and include renal failure, MI, stroke, dementia, heart failure.
- The economic effects of hypertension are staggering. It is one of the most costly of all clinical conditions:
  - o The actual costs are difficult to quantify, since they include both medical costs and income lost from time off work.
  - o Some studies suggest the cost is as high as 12% of the total health care budget.
  - o Regardless of the actual cost, hypertension is one of the most important public health issues.

Total Costs = $73.4B; Direct Costs = $54.2B

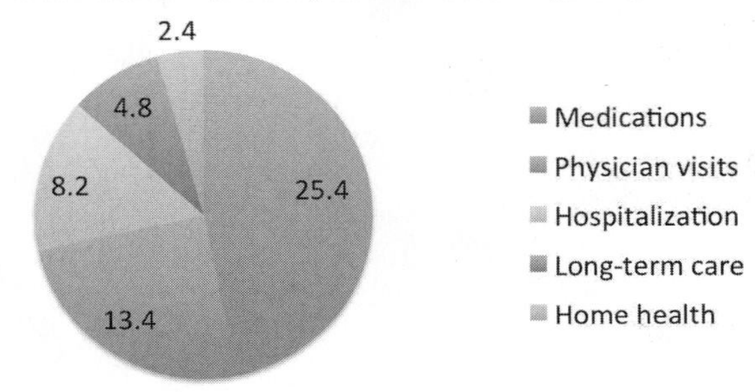

The latest projections by the American Heart Association Health Disease and Stroke Statistics estimated (for 2009) that hypertension would cost $73.4 billion (B), with $19.2 B in costs due to lost productivity. The diagram shows the breakdown in direct costs.
Source: Copyright © 2013, NovEx Novice to Expert Learning, LLC

Epidemiology

- Hypertension is the most common reason for office visits of nonpregnant adults to health care providers in the United States and accounts for the greatest use of prescription drugs.
- U.S. prevalence is approximately 29–31% of those 18 years old or older:
  1. Incidence is increasing based on census bureau data.
  2. Further increases are expected with aging population.
  3. Hypertension is found in over half of patients over 65 years of age.
  4. It is concomitant with the rise in obesity rates.

LO2:

Pathophysiology

- Blood pressure remains stable with the help of baroreceptors. These are receptors that sense pressure and are located in the arterial walls of the carotid sinuses, aortic arch, and carotid arteries. Even small changes are sensed. If blood pressure begins to drop, reflex responses by the baroreceptors result in tachycardia and vasoconstriction. The baroreceptors are reset to a higher blood pressure in patients with hypertension.
- Development of hypertension is a complex process that involves genetics, damage to blood vessel walls, change in hormone balance (e.g., renin, angiotensin), and, eventually, damage to the perfused organs (e.g., brain, heart, kidneys). This is referred to as end-organ damage.
- High blood pressure exerts increased pressure on the blood vessel walls that, over time, damages the arterial walls. Initially, there is intimal thickening; eventually, plaque forms, and the arterial walls become stiffer. This process is called **atherosclerosis**.
- Mediators are normally released from the blood vessel walls that cause vasoconstriction as well as vasodilation. As the blood vessel wall is damaged the balance shifts towards vasoconstriction.
- With mild to moderate hypertension, perfusion of organs is autoregulated and remains relatively constant. This occurs because increases in blood pressure are counteracted by vasoconstriction. Damage of the end organs takes place over years.
- With more severe hypertension, autoregulation is lost, and organs may be affected rapidly by increasing pressure in the capillaries and increased perfusion. For example, the brain can develop edema, which manifests as confusion (encephalopathy) and headache. Acute renal failure and heart failure can also develop.

Chronic Hypertension

Chronic hypertension is the chronic elevation of blood pressure. It often results in the development of atherosclerosis and heart failure. The higher the blood pressure, the greater the risk of developing these serious problems:

- Stroke
- MI and/or CAD
- Renal failure
- Peripheral arterial disease
- Heart failure

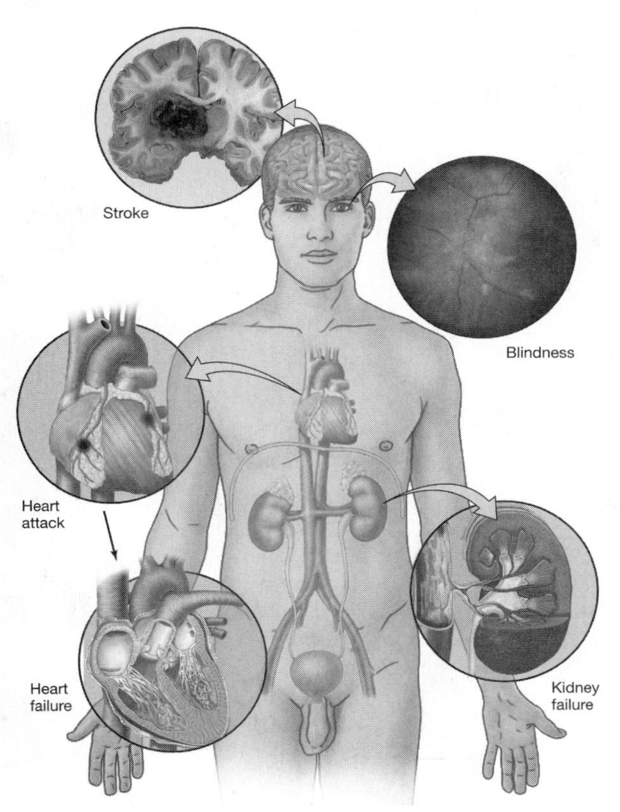

Hypertension can affect multiple organs.

Acute Hypertension

Acute hypertension is the sudden, severe rise in blood pressure that can result in acute end-organ damage over a short period of time. End-organ damage often presents as:

- Confusion (encephalopathy)
- Renal failure
- Pulmonary edema or heart failure
- Intracerebral hemorrhage
- Aortic dissection

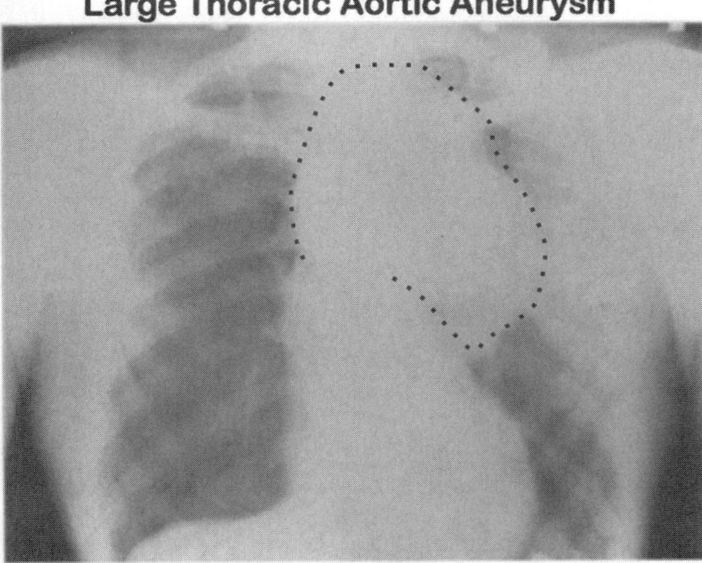

This x-ray features a large thoracic aortic aneurysm that involves the aortic arch. Note the enormous size of the aneurysm, just above the heart that expands across the upper and middle chest area. Hypertension increases the risk of dissection, a life-threatening situation.
Source: CDC

Risk Factors

Incidence tends to be more common (and severe) in the following population subsets:

- African American
- Those with:
  - o Family history (e.g., genetics)
  - o Increased sodium intake
  - o Excess alcohol intake
  - o Obesity
  - o Sedentary lifestyle
  - o Dyslipidemia
  - o Certain personality traits (e.g., hostile attitude, impatience)
- Metabolic syndrome

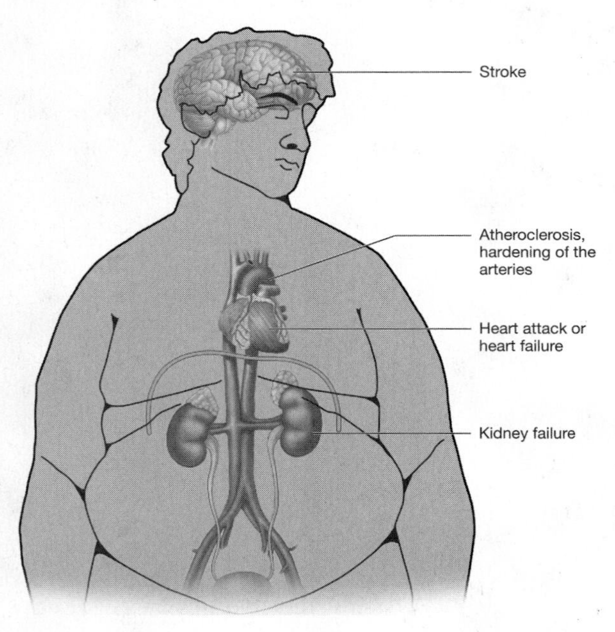

Obesity is an important risk factor for hypertension, but both conditions are very closely associated with numerous cardiovascular diseases, as shown in the image.

Concept Check

2. Which ethnic group is at the highest risk for primary hypertension?

A. Caucasians

B. Asians

C. African Americans

D. Hispanics

Answer question

Metabolic syndrome is a group of traits that are strongly associated with hypertension and are commonly seen together. If one is present, the others are likely to develop:

- Hypertension
- Hypertriglyceridemia
- Central obesity
- Hyperglycemia or diabetes
- Elevated uric acid or gout

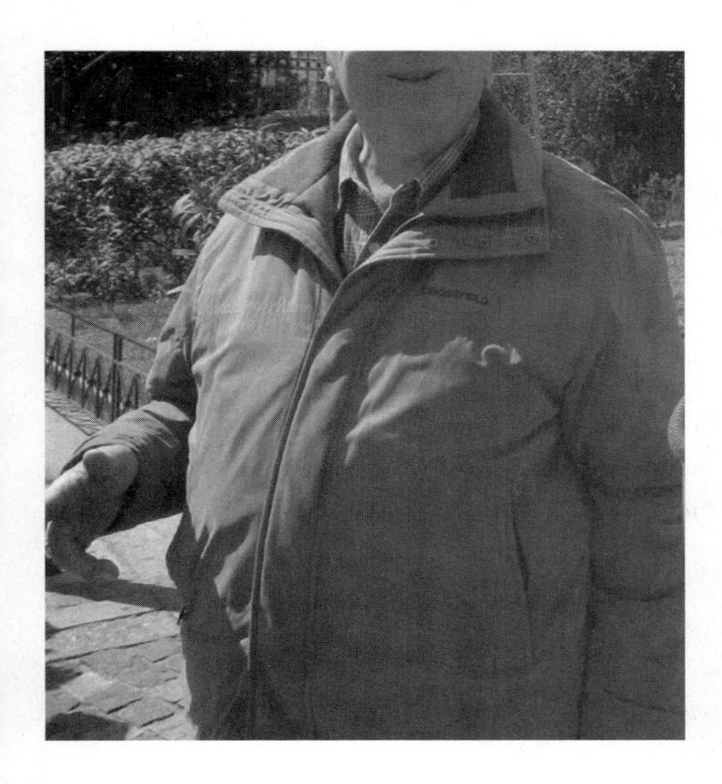

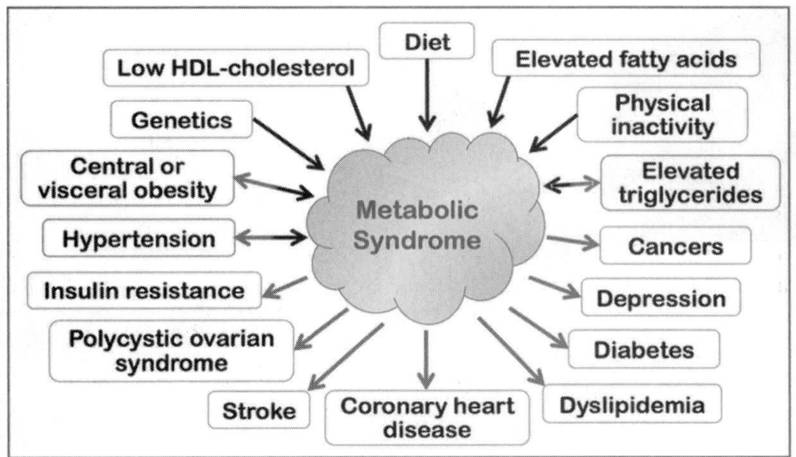

Upper: This photo reveals the typical habitus of a person with metabolic syndrome who is at high risk for hypertension. Lower: This diagram details the major causes and health consequences of metabolic syndrome. Metabolic syndrome has a significant role in health and wellness.

Sources: (*upper*) Courtesy of K. Kyriakidis; (*lower*) Copyright © 2013, NovEx Novice to Expert Learning, LLC

Causes

In Primary Hypertension

- Primary hypertension (formerly called essential hypertension) is hypertension with no known cause. It is the most common type of HTN (95%).
- Primary hypertension may be due to several factors, including:
  - Genetics: Hypertension is much more common in people who have hypertensive parents. Understanding of the role of genetics in hypertension is evolving, and it may prove to be a definitive cause of hypertension.
  - Increased sympathetic (beta adrenergic) activity (the most common current thought on the etiology of hypertension)
  - Greater than normal angiotensin II stimulation

In Secondary Hypertension

Secondary hypertension is hypertension with a known cause:

- Acute and chronic renal failure
- Renal artery stenosis
- Obstructive sleep apnea
- Certain medication (e.g., oral contraceptives, chronic NSAID use, some antidepressants)
- Adrenal dysfunction
    - o Pheochromocytoma
    - o Primary aldosteronism
- Other endocrine disorder (e.g., hypothyroidism, hyperthyroidism, hyperparathyroidism)
- "White-coat" hypertension. This is a mild, isolated hypertension noted when blood pressure is usually normal but increased when taken by a health care provider.

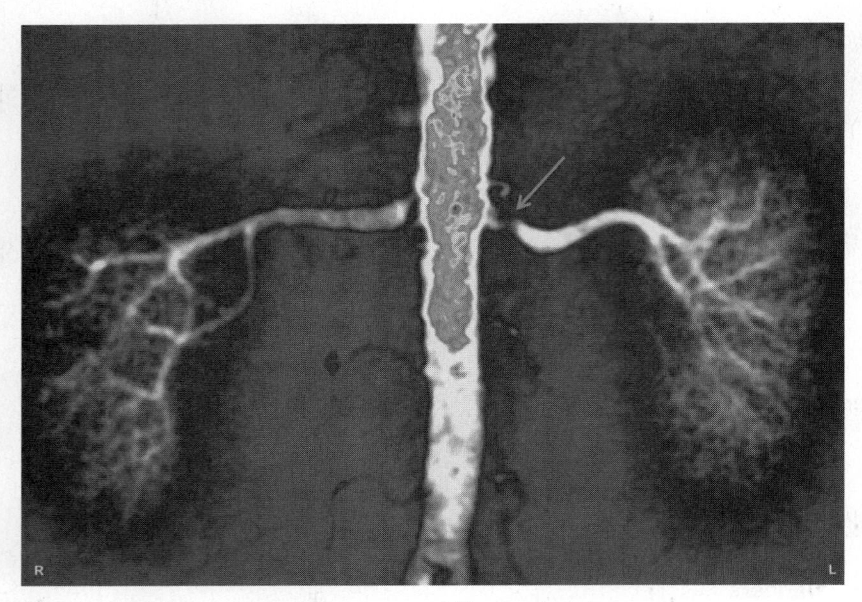

A narrowing of the artery that supplies oxygen-rich blood to the kidneys.
Source: BSIP SA/Alamy

Concept Check

3. Which situation is a cause of primary hypertension?

A. Increase in beta adrenergic activity
B. Hypothyroidism
C. Acute or chronic renal failure
D. Obstructive sleep apnea

Answer question

Assessment Findings

- Hypertension is asymptomatic until there is end-organ damage. It is therefore known as the *silent killer*.

Symptomatic patients present, as seen in the following table.

Parameter	Hypertensive Urgency Asymptomatic	Hypertensive Urgency Symptomatic	Hypertensive Emergency
Blood pressure	≥ 180/100	≥ 180/100	Commonly > 220/140
Symptoms	Headache, anxiety but often no symptoms	Severe headache, shortness of breath (SOB)	SOB, chest pain, nocturia, weakness, altered mental status
Physical findings	No end-organ damage or dysfunction, no clinical cardiovascular disease	End-organ damage with cardiovascular disease present, stable	Encephalopathy, papilledema, visual loss, pulmonary edema, renal failure, CVA, cardiac ischemia, nausea or vomiting
Treatment	Observe 1–3hr, initiate or resume medication, adjust dose of inadequate medication	Observe 3–6 hr, lower BP with short-acting oral medication or adjust current medications	Establish IV line, baseline labs, cardiac and blood pressure monitoring, start parenteral antihypertensive therapy
Follow-up (F/U) plan	F/U within 1–2 days with primary health care provider or clinic	F/U within 1–2 days with primary health care provider or clinic	Admission to the ICU, treat to initial goal blood pressure (lowering by 25% over several hours within the first 24–48 hr), additional diagnostics

This table lists the symptoms of hypertensive conditions, along with findings and treatment. Current follow-up recommendations are now within 1–2 days.

Table 2 from www.clevelandclinicneded.com/medicalpubs/diseasemanagement/nephrology/hypertensive-crises/

Diagnostics

History and Physical Examination

- When interviewing the patient, seek information that might reveal the presence of chronic hypertension:
  - o History of renal disease
  - o History of familial hypertension
  - o Use of NSAIDS, contraceptives, or other HTN-related medications
  - o Heart failure
  - o Trauma to the kidneys
- On physical exam, look for signs of end-organ damage that may be due to hypertension. Examples include:
  - o Venous engorgement from heart failure (e.g., pitting edema of the feet)
  - o Retinopathy, retinal hemorrhage
  - o CNS involvement (e.g., headache, changes in behavior)
  - o Chest pain

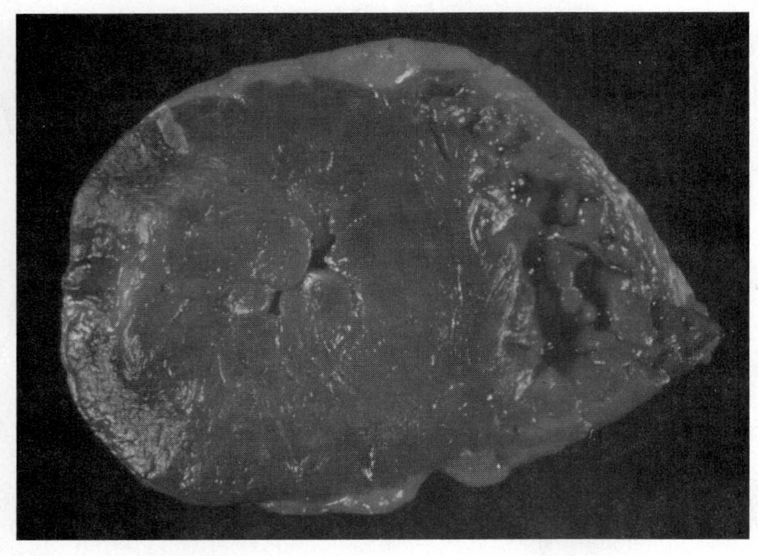

Over time, hypertension is associated with enlargement of the left ventricle. This photo reveals an extremely enlarged and hypertrophied ventricle (3/4 of the heart's mass—middle and left), which would be noticeable on physical examination. Left ventricular hypertrophy may be suspected if the apical impulse is >3 cm and/or displaced to the left.

Diagnostics (continued)

Measuring Blood Pressure and Screening for Hypertension

- Measurement of blood pressure is a key nursing activity. Use of proper measurement and technique is essential for maximum accuracy of interpretation, diagnosis, and management.
- It is important to verify the blood pressure by taking it at intervals. Provide a calm environment for the patient. Check the pressures in both arms. Verify the condition of the equipment if you are using an automatic blood pressure device. Checking a manual blood pressure may be necessary to confirm accuracy.
- Screening for hypertension. The 2007 United States Preventive Services Task Force (USPSTF) Guidelines on screening for hypertension recommend screening:
  - o Every two years for patients with BP <120/80 mmHg.
  - o Yearly for patients with systolic pressure 120–139 mmHg or a diastolic pressure of 80–89 mmHg (or prehypertension in JNC 7).

Once sustained hypertension has been identified and confirmed, the work-up should ascertain:

- The extent of any target organ (i.e., end-organ) damage.
- The patient's cardiovascular risk status.
- Any identifiable (and often curable) causes of hypertension.
- Most patients with essential hypertension undergo limited work-up due to the limited usefulness of extensive laboratory testing.
- It is important to be aware of clinical cues suggesting the presence of one of the causes of secondary hypertension (an indication for a more extensive evaluation).
- Many causes of secondary hypertension can be cured, resulting in partially or completely normal blood pressure. However, it is not cost effective to perform a complete evaluation in every hypertensive patient.

Testing for hypertension primarily centers on examining potential causes or the effects of hypertension. For example:

- Echocardiography is the most sensitive method to detect left ventricular hypertrophy (better than the EKG) due to hypertension. Left ventricular hypertrophy in hypertension may be a worse prognostic sign since it indicates the heart has enlarged over time to adapt to the high blood pressure.
- Electrocardiogram to look for hypertrophy.

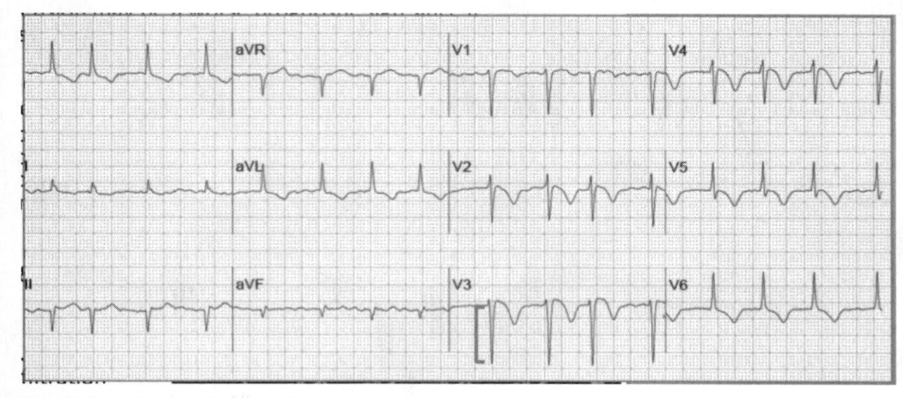

The EKG may be an indicator of hypertension. Left ventricular hypertrophy commonly accompanies hypertension, as seen here in the EKG. Note the voltage (vertical height or depth) in V1–V6 and in aVL.
Source: Courtesy of K. Kyriakidis

- Useful lab tests include:
  - o Electrolytes or blood chemistries, especially sodium (Na)—low sodium levels can indicate volume overload and a source of hypertension
  - o Fasting lipids that include HDL, LDL, triglycerides, and total
  - o Urinalysis
  - o Hematocrit
- Renal function tests (e.g., estimated glomerular filtration rate)

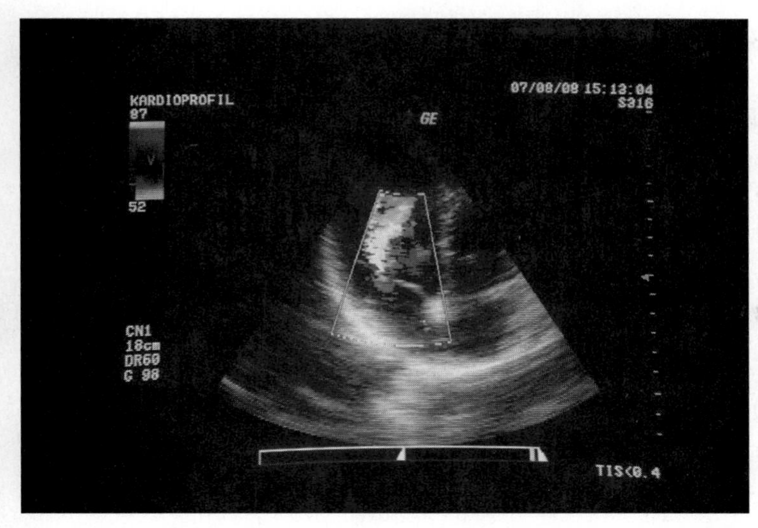

Doppler echocardiogram of the heart.
Source: StockLite/Shutterstock

Priority Patient Concerns and Desired Collaborative Care Outcomes

Prior to caring for patients with hypertension, it is important to prioritize the patient's concerns that must guide the nursing care plan and interventions. Care for the patient is ordered and organized in accordance with the patient's priority and urgent needs. Desired collaborative care outcomes in patients with hypertension typically include:

1. Patient will manifest no findings of decreased cerebral tissue perfusion.
2. Patient will manifest no findings of decreased renal perfusion.
3. Patient will manifest no findings of decreased peripheral tissue perfusion.
4. Patient will manage health more effectively.
5. Patient will demonstrate knowledge of disease process and management.
6. Patient will comply with therapeutic regimen.

Considering these important care outcomes, prepare a list of the major 3–6 priority patient concerns or nursing diagnoses for patients with hypertension. Be prepared to participate in a discussion of this list and/or to submit them as an assignment, as determined by your faculty. Resources you may find helpful in this assignment can include this lesson, the references, resources on nursing care plans, and standard nursing diagnoses manuals.

Concept Check

4. How often should a person have blood pressure screening if today's reading is 118/72 mmHg?

A. Every 6 months

B. Every 1 year

C. Every 2 years

D. Every 5 years

Answer question

LO3:

Collaborative Interventions

Evidence-Based Practices (EBP)

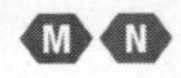

- The guidelines for hypertension management come from the National Heart, Lung, and Blood Institute (NHLBI). New guidelines are being developed at this time. The following algorithm includes the EBP for hypertension.
    1. Lifestyle modifications for prehypertension (<140/<90 mmHg), as a part of all hypertension management
    2. Thiazide diuretics for initial BP management
    3. A second drug, an Angiotensin Conversion Enzyme Inhibitor (ACE inhibitor), Angiotensin Receptor Blocker (ARB), Beta Blocker (BB), or Calcium Channel Blocker (CCB), may be needed in addition to a thiazide to keep BP in target range.
- No uniform agreement exists regarding the choice of a second drug class to be prescribed for initial therapy.
- Wide variability exists among patients regarding their response to the second drug used in their treatment regimen.
- A second medication may be chosen based on comorbid conditions (e.g., ACE inhibitor in patients with diabetes). Closer monitoring may be required until stabilized.

Patients require regular monitoring of BP to evaluate the patient's progress in meeting BP goals. BP monitoring is particular important in patients receiving any pharmacologic treatment.

Concept Check

5. Which drug class is commonly used for initial hypertension management?

A. ACE inhibitors

B. Thiazide diuretics

C. ARBs

D. Beta blockers

Answer question

Antihypertensive Medications

Initial Management

- Antihypertensive medications should generally be initiated if the systolic pressure is ≥140 mmHg and/or the diastolic pressure is persistently ≥90 mmHg, despite optimized nonpharmacologic therapy.
- Starting with two drugs may be considered in patients with blood pressures above 160/100 mmHg. This approach may improve the likelihood that target blood pressures are achieved within a reasonable time frame. However, patients need to be educated and cautioned due to increased risk of orthostatic hypotension.
- Lower blood pressure goals (≤130/80 mmHg) should be considered in patients with established diseases, such as:
    - o Cardiovascular disease
    - o Diabetes
    - o Chronic kidney disease complicated by proteinuria

Common oral agents for treatment of hypertensive urgencies:

Oral Antihypertensive	Dose	Onset of action and Duration	Cautions
Captopril (ACE Inhibitor)	25 mg orally	15-30 minute onset 2-6 hours duration	Hypotension, renal failure
Clonidine (alpha agonist)	0.1-0.2 mg orally	30-60 minute onset 8-12 hours duration	Hypotension, drowsiness
Labetalol (BB)	200-400 mg orally	1-2 hours onset 2-12 hour duration	Bronchospasm, orthostatic hypotension
Amlodipine (CCB)	2.5-5 mg orally	1-2 hours onset 12-18 hour duration	Tachycardia, hypotension

Antihypertensive medications that are needed in emergency situations are listed above. Clinically salient information that a nurse must know is included.

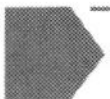

Concept Check

6. What is the onset of action of oral captopril?
   A. 1–2 hours
   B. 30–60 minutes
   C. 15–30 minutes
   D. 1–2 minutes

Answer question

Collaborative Interventions (continued)

Collaborative Supportive Care and Symptom Management

- Closely monitor patient's blood pressure, fluid status, and hemodynamic responses to pharmacologic agents, particularly if polypharmacologic treatment is implemented.
- Avoid orthostasis and injury by slowing getting a patient out of bed. Allow time to adjust when moving from lying down to sitting and then to standing.

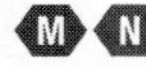

- Monitor ongoing diagnostic test results to recognize any early warning signs of problems.

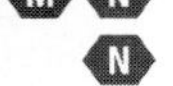

- One of the most important nursing interventions is to assist the patient with lifestyle modification. This is not easy for many patients, since these changes directly alter the patient's daily preferences and lifestyle (including areas where they may obtain much of the joy in their life). Some key areas to help manage hypertension include:
  - o Smoking cessation
  - o Exercise programs: Participate in at least 30 min of aerobic activity daily (EBP). Dynamic resistance exercise is a reasonable form of exercise for lowering BP (EBP).
  - o Salt restriction: While a controversial recent study suggested this might not be as important, all major guidelines still suggest limiting sodium intake by up to 50% of normal (e.g., to 100 meq per day [approximately 2.3 g sodium]).
  - o The Dietary Approaches to Stop Hypertension (DASH) diet combines salt restriction with increased consumption of fruits and vegetables and low-fat dairy products.
  - o Weight management programs to progress toward the patient's acceptable to ideal body weight
  - o Stress reduction: Alternative methods that are evidence-based and may be reasonable to employ are transcendental meditation, biofeedback, and device-guided breathing. Yoga, other cognitive and behavioral relaxation techniques, and acupuncture were not found to be effective in lowering BP.
  - o Alternative approaches may be added to lifestyle modifications and/or medications to to lower medication use and optimize efficacy. Health care providers will find the American Heart Association's evidence-based algorithm for implementing alternative approaches a reliable guide for clinical judgment and practice. (http://hyper.ahajournals.org/content/early/2013/04/22/HYP.0b013e318293645f)
  - o Limiting use of alcohol, particularly in those who consume more than two drinks per day

- Consult nutritionist as indicated.

Chronic Hypertension

- Most patients present with a slow or progressive (chronic) development of HTN.
- Studies show antihypertensive therapy compared to placebo has been associated with 20–25% reduction in the incidence of major cardiovascular events (e.g., stroke, heart failure, myocardial infarction).
- JNC 7 includes recommendations for risk stratification and treatment. All patients should undergo appropriate nonpharmacologic (lifestyle) modification. Decisions regarding antihypertensive medication generally should not be made until after an adequate trial of nonpharmacologic therapy.

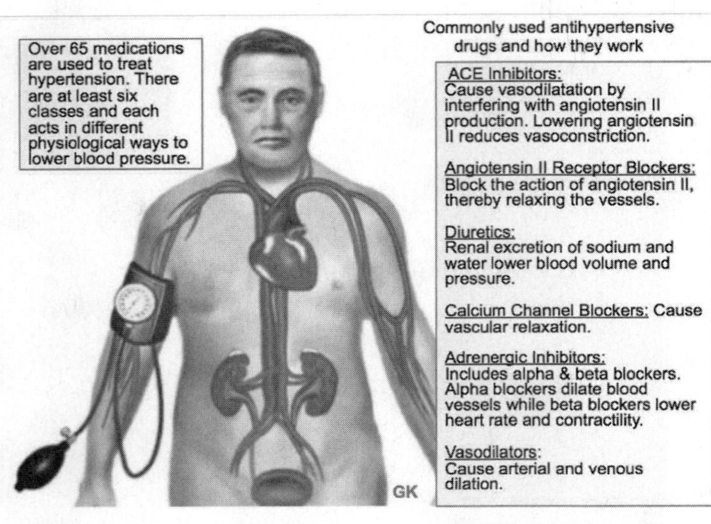

Over 65 medications are used to treat hypertension. There are at least six classes and each acts in different physiological ways to lower blood pressure.
Commonly used antihypertensive drugs and how they work
ACE Inhibitors:
Cause vasodilatation by interfering with angiotensin II production. Lowering angiotensin II reduces vasoconstriction.
Angiotensin II Receptor Blockers:
Block the action of angiotensin II, thereby relaxing the vessels.
Diuretics:
Renal excretion of sodium and water lower blood volume and pressure.
Calcium Channel Blockers: Cause vascular relaxation.
Adrenergic Inhibitors:
Includes alpha & beta blockers. Alpha blockers dilate blood vessels while beta blockers lower heart rate and contractility.
Vasodilators:
Cause arterial and venous dilation.
GK

This illustration graphically represents the treatments for high blood pressure (hypertension), listing the six most common drug types used to treat the disease. These include adrenergic inhibitors (alpha blockers and beta blockers), calcium blockers, ACE inhibitors, Angiotensin II receptor blockers, vasodilators, and diuretics.

Source: Courtesy of George Kyriakidis/Santa Ana, CA

Noncompliance

- Because hypertension is asymptomatic until there is end-organ damage and medications often have side effects, compliance is a major problem. Factors contributing to noncompliance that need to be explored and evaluated include:
  - o Poor access to health care and medications
  - o Lack of education regarding implications of organ dysfunction
  - o Unwillingness to modify secondary risk factors

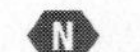

- Collaborate with the patient to modify behaviors and habits:
  - o Individualize diet modifications when affected by cultural or other differences.
  - o Consult social services when patient cannot access needed therapies or community resources that support improved lifestyle management (e.g., support groups, walking or activity groups).
  - o Collaborate with family regarding family lifestyle modifications.
  - o Collaborate with patient regarding the patient's commitment and individualized needs to improve compliance.

Collaborative Interventions (continued)

Hypertensive Urgencies and Emergencies

- A number of both parenteral and oral antihypertensive drugs may be used in the management of hypertension. Oral agents are primarily used in asymptomatic patients.
- IV agents are primarily used for emergency situations. Due to the rapid and potent effects of IV agents, patients initially require constant monitoring and possible titration of the medications until stabilized.
- Other nuances in hypertension management exist.
  - o Initial choice for oral agents could be clonidine or captopril (ACE inhibitor).
  - o However, clonidine may be preferred if the patient has ACE inhibitor allergy. These agents lower blood pressure more slowly than parenteral agents and have a more limited ability to control degree of BP reduction. Captopril has more evidence to support its initial use.
- Monitor and evaluate the degree of blood pressure reduction, which is the major determinant of reduction in cardiovascular risk in patients with hypertension, NOT the choice of the antihypertensive drug itself.
- The fundamental determination in the treatment of a hypertensive emergency is not the absolute blood pressure but the degree of and/or progression of end-organ damage. Therefore, one should monitor and track development or progression of:
  - o Heart failure or pulmonary edema
  - o Unstable angina
  - o Cerebral infarction or hemorrhage
  - o Acute renal failure
  - o Retinopathy
  - o Hypertensive encephalopathy
- Evaluate and collaborate regarding the type of hypertensive emergency and the clinical status of the patient as these influence the choice of the antihypertensive agent.
- **Recognize hypertensive urgencies:** A systolic pressure greater than 180 or a diastolic pressure greater than 110 mmHg *and* no end-organ damage. Urgencies do not commonly require admission to the hospital. The goal of treatment for hypertensive urgencies is the gradual reduction of blood pressure within 24 hours. These patients can be placed on mono or combination therapy based on their history and risk factors. Close outpatient follow up by a primary health care provider or clinic is warranted to frequently monitor BP and the patient's response to medications. Additionally, a follow up allows for the considerable patient education that is initially needed.
- **Swiftly recognize and intervene in hypertensive emergencies:** Also called **Malignant hypertension**, with a systolic blood pressure >220 mmHg or a diastolic value >140 mmHg and/or evidence of end-organ damage. Emergencies require immediate hospitalization.
  - o While immediate treatment to lower the blood pressure is required due to evidence of end-organ damage, **the goal is a gradual decrease in the mean arterial pressure (25%) over a period of 24 hours.** These patients often have impaired blood pressure autoregulation and a rapid reduction or normalization of blood pressure can lead to organ hypoperfusion.
- For hypertensive emergencies and urgencies, an INITIAL goal is recommended to reduce blood pressure to **less than or equal to 160/100 mmHg over several days**.

Intravenous Agents

Common IV or parenteral drugs for treatment of hypertensive emergencies include:

- Nitroprusside is generally considered the most effective parenteral drug.
- Nitroglycerin is similar in action, but not as potent as nitroprusside, and produces more venous dilation than arterial dilation. It should be considered for patients with heart failure or symptomatic coronary disease.
- Optimal choice of agent may vary according to underlying causes of hypertensive emergency.

Drug	Dose	Onset/duration (after stopping infusion)	Caution
Sodium nitroprusside	0.25-10 mcg/kg/min IV infusion	Onset: immediate Duration: 2-3 min	Nausea, vomiting, thiocyanate intoxication
Nitroglycerin	5-10 mcg/min IV infusion	Onset: 2-5 min Duration: 5-10 min	Headache, tachycardia, vomiting, flushing
Hydralazine	5-20 mg as IV bolus	Onset: 10 min Duration: 20-30 min	Tachycardia, headache, vomiting, aggravation of angina
Labetalol	20-40 mg IV bolus every 10 min or infusion of 2 mg/min	Onset: 5-10 min Duration: 15-30 min	Bronchospasm, heart block, bradycardia
Esmolol	500 mcg/kg bolus or 50-100 mcg/kg/min IV infusion	Onset: 1-5 min Duration: 15-30 min	1st AV block, asthma, heart failure
Phentolamine (usually reserved for hypertensive crisis due to pheochromocytoma)	5-10 mg IV bolus	Onset: 1-2 min Duration: 10-30 min	Tachycardia, orthostatic hypotension

Some of the key antihypertensive medications that every nurse will administer in an urgent situation are listed above. Clinically salient information that a nurse must know is included.
Source: Copyright © 2013, NovEx Novice to Expert Learning, LLC

Permissive Hypertension

- There are situations, most commonly in ischemic stroke, where maintaining the elevated blood pressure is beneficial. After an ischemic stroke, it is recommended that blood pressure be kept higher than normal to prevent vasospasm and to improve perfusion of the affected area of the brain.
- The American Stroke Association has a consensus recommendation that the blood pressure not be lowered following acute ischemic stroke unless:
  - o There is evidence of hypertensive end-organ damage (e.g., pulmonary edema) or
  - o Systolic BP >220 mmHg or diastolic BP >120 mmHg.

Collaborative Interventions (continued)

Summary of Hypertensive Emergencies and Urgencies

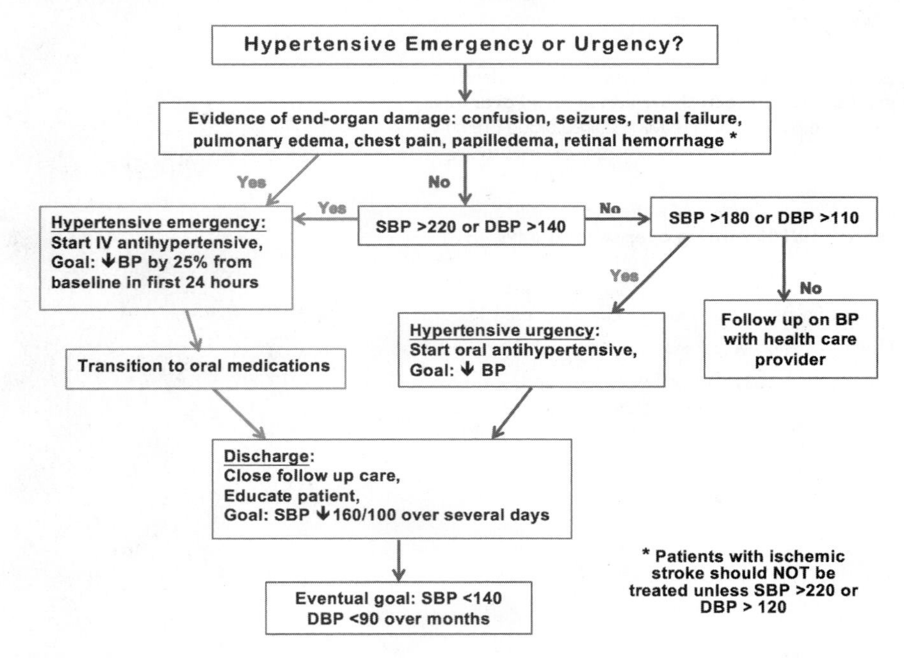

This algorithm summarizes the key collaborative interventions that are generally needed to care for patients who have a hypertensive emergency or urgency.
Source: Copyright © 2013, NovEx Novice to Expert Learning, LLC

Patient Education

- N Educate patient about dietary modifications. For most patients, a moderate reduction of sodium is needed and the DASH diet offers helpful guidance. Individualize dietary planning to account for culturally significant factors. Interestingly, evidence does not support improvement in overall cardiovascular health by significantly lowering fat intake.
- N Assist patient to understand a good personal body weight.
- N Educate about the evidence-based role of daily aerobic activity (at least 30 minutes) in lowering BP.
- N Minimize alcohol use and avoid substance abuse.
- N Smoking cessation can improve hypertension as well as multiple other medical illnesses.
- N Participate in stress reduction activities.
- N Educate the patient regarding the disease, when to contact the health care provider, when to seek immediate care, routine BP monitoring, symptoms of complications, taking prescribed medications, and follow-up care.
- N Prepare the patient on how to avoid dizziness, fainting, falls, or injury from orthostatic hypotension by gradually moving from lying down, to sitting, to standing.
- N Ensure patients understand the importance of adhering to their therapeutic regime and this cannot be overemphasized. The difficult part of ensuring compliance in a hypertensive patient is that the symptoms of hypertension are often so subtle as to be unrecognized by the patient. Significant end-organ damage is often present before the patient realizes anything is wrong or has a sense of not being completely healthy.
- N Ensure family members are also taught (or significant others) to help encourage and support patient compliance. Share handouts, web sites, and other informational sites that are available for the patient. However, the patient must be motivated to adhere to the treatment program; otherwise, the information provided may not be followed.
- M N As importantly, community education on prevention of hypertension, involving the lifestyle and risk factor modifications detailed above, are essential in reducing the individual and national burden of hypertension.

Summary of Interventions

- Evidence-based intervention for chronic HTN includes:
  - o Thiazide diuretics
  - o Afterload reducers (e.g., ACE inhibitors, angiotensin receptor blocker)
- Acute management for urgency or emergency:
  - o Oral antihypertensive for asymptomatic patients
  - o IV medication in symptomatic patients
- Nonpharmacologic in all patients: Risk factor modification (e.g., weight reduction), dietary modification, exercise program

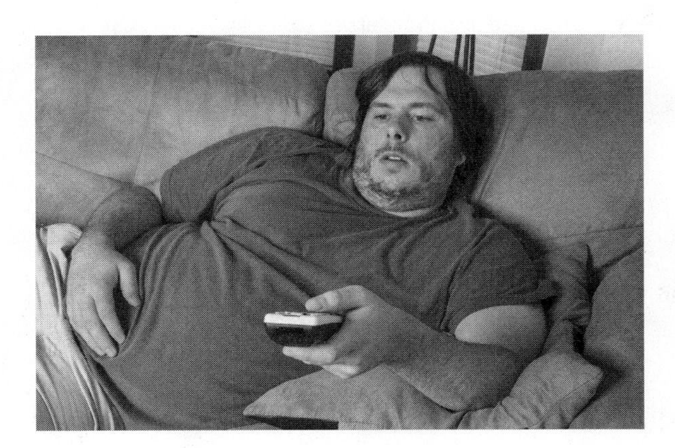

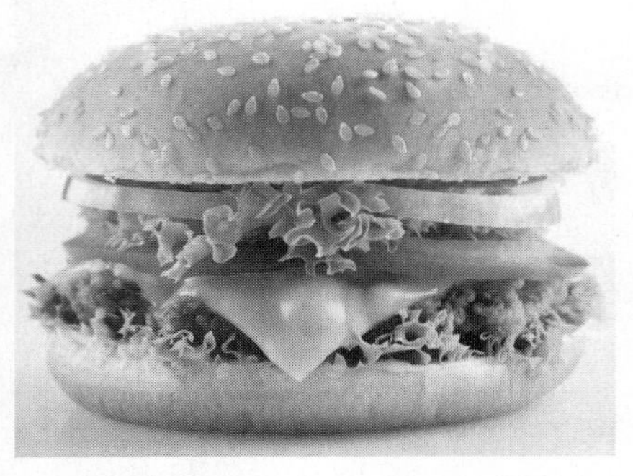
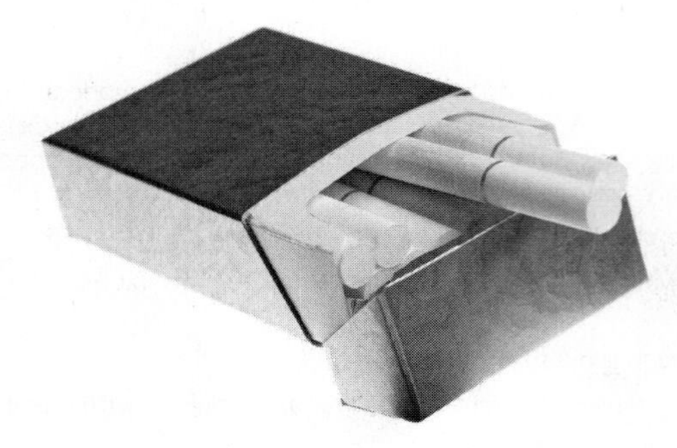

For many, hypertension is a wake-up call. Educating patients on the hazards of unhealthy eating, smoking, and obesity are key interventions for every patient.

Sources: (*upper*) © txking/Shutterstock.com; (*lower left*) volff/Fotolia; (*lower right*) Roman Sigaev/Fotolia

Concept Check

7. Which treatment is generally appropriate for a patient with hypertensive urgency?

A. Admission and treatment in an intensive care unit

B. Admission to a general treatment area, but not ICU

C. Measures to rapidly reduce blood pressure to normal range

D. Close follow-up by personal health care provider

Answer question

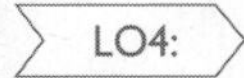

LO4:

Evaluation of Desired Collaborative Care Outcomes

Evaluation and reassessment should reveal attainment of previously established outcomes. In summary:

- Patient has clear mentation and manifests no findings of stroke.
- Patient's urine is clear and electrolytes are balanced.
- Patient's skin and peripheral tissues are warm, dry, and intact.
- Patient blood pressure has decreased to desired range.
- Patient accurately describes measures needed to decrease blood pressure.
- Patient takes medications as prescribed and is following the recommended diet and exercise program.

References

Aggarwal, M., & Khan, I. (2006). Hypertensive crisis: Hypertensive emergencies and urgencies. *Cariology Clinics, 24*, 135–146. www.ncbi.nlm.nih.gov/pubmed/12243377

Clark, C. E., Smith, L. F., Taylor, R. S., & Campbell, J. L. (2010). Nurse led interventions to improve control of blood pressure in people with hypertension: Systematic review and meta-analysis. *Brit Med J, 341*, c3995.

Hill, M. N., Miller, N. H., Degeest, S., et al. (2011). Adherence and persistence with taking medication to control high blood pressure. *J Am Soc Hypertens, 5*(1), 56–63.

Jamerson, K., Weber, M. A., Bakris, G. L., Dahlof, B., Pitt, B., Shiv, V., ... Velazquez, E. J., the ACCOMPLISH Trial Investigators. (2008). Benazepril plus amlodipine or hydrochlorothiazide for hypertension in high-risk patients. *N Engl J Med, 359*, 2417–2428

Smithburger, P. L., Kane-Gill, S. L., Nestor, B. L., & Seybert, A. L. (2010). Recent advances in the treatment of hypertensive emergencies. *Crit Care Nurse, 30*(5), 24–30.

Clinical Practice Guidelines

Brook, R. D., Appel, L. J., Rubenfire, M., et al. (2013). Beyond medications and diet: Alternative approaches to lowering blood pressure: A scientific statement from the American Heart Association. *Hypertension, 61*(6), 1360–1383.

Chobanian, A. V., Bakris, G. L., Black, H. R., Cushman, W. C., Green, L. A., Izzo, J. L. ... Roccella, E. J. (2003). The Seventh Report of the Joint National Committee on Prevention, Detection, Evaluation, and Treatment of High Blood Pressure: The JNC 7 report. *JAMA, 289*, 2560.

Patient Education

Torpy, J. M., Lynm, C., & Glass, R. M. (2010). Hypertension. *JAMA, 303*(20), 2098.

STOP

Go to the online course and complete the NovE-Cases assigned by your instructor for this module.

Learning Outcomes for Inflammation of the Heart: Endocarditis

When you complete this lesson, you will be able to:

1. Recognize the clinical relevance of endocarditis.
2. Consider the pathophysiology, etiology, risk factors, and clinical presentation of endocarditis that determine the priority patient concerns.
3. Determine the most urgent and important nursing interventions and patient education required in caring for a patient with endocarditis.
4. Evaluate attainment of desired collaborative care outcomes for a patient with endocarditis.

LO1:

What Is Endocarditis?

- Endocarditis is an inflammation of the inner lining of the heart, primarily affecting the heart valves, and is typically the result of an infection.
- Infections causing endocarditis are most commonly bacterial in origin.

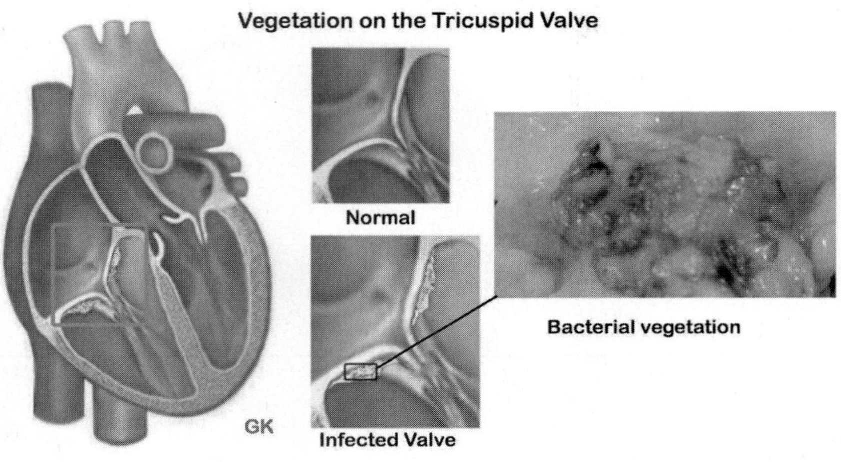

This picture portrays an aortic valve infection. The first image (left) displays the entire heart with a small window making the valve visible. The second image displays normal and healthy heart and valves. The third image shows the same valve with bacterial growth on the ventricular side of its cusps.
Source: Courtesy of George Kyriakidis/Santa Ana, CA

Concept Check

1. The infection causing infectious endocarditis is most likely caused by which organism?
   - A. Bacteria
   - B. Virus
   - C. Fungus
   - D. Prion

Answer question

LO1:

Clinical Relevance

- Although endocarditis can present initially with few symptoms, complications from endocarditis can be catastrophic if not treated early.
- Nurses need to be aware of complications of endocarditis such as heart failure, irregular heart rhythms or murmurs, and septic embolism to any organ.

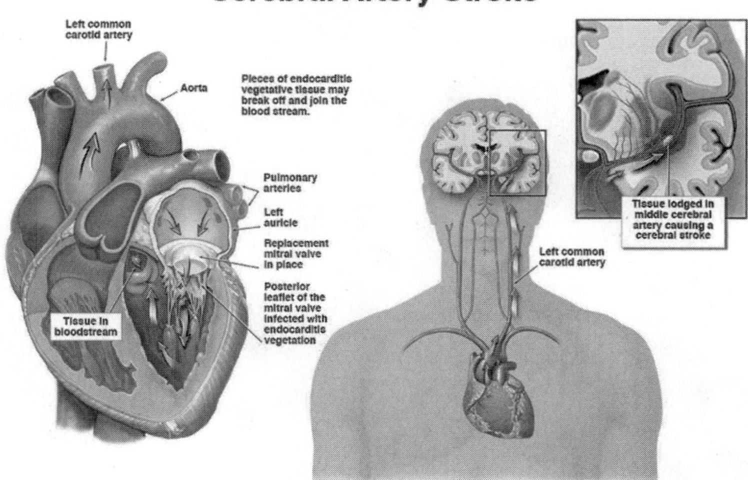

This exhibit depicts a heart with a leaflet of the mitral valve infected with endocarditis vegetation, a pre-existing prosthesis of the mitral valve in place, and a piece of tissue breaking off from the infected area and flowing away in the bloodstream. Then you see the tissue path up to the middle cerebral artery, where the piece of tissue lodges, causing a cerebral stroke.

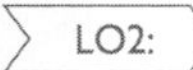

Pathophysiology

- Endocarditis most often occurs in people who already have a heart valve abnormality, heart valve replacement, or abuse IV drugs.
- The usual etiology of endocarditis is seeding of the heart valve by bacteria that are in the bloodstream (bacteremia).
- The source of bacteremia may be from an infection (e.g., cellulitis), an invasive procedure (e.g., central line, pacemaker, bronchial biopsy), or something as simple as tooth brushing that allows bacteria to enter the bloodstream.
- The microorganisms that typically cause endocarditis are *S. aureus; Streptococcus viridans;* group A, C, and G streptococci; and enterococci. Fungal infections may also occur.
- Bacteria (or other causative organisms) adhere to the valve surface and eventually invade and damage the valvular leaflets.
- The infected valve causes persistent bacteremia.
- Damage to the valves causes deformities that can prevent normal closure and result in regurgitation. The regurgitant murmur is usually audible with a stethoscope.

The mitral regurgitation that develops from a deformed valve from endocarditis can be heard in this audio clip.

Aortic Valve Deformity and Surgical Replacement

Normal Anatomy

Posterior noncoronary cusp
Right coronary cusp
Left coronary cusp
Aorta
Superior view of aortic valve
Aortic valve
Left ventricle
Anterior cut-away view of heart

Aortic Valve Deformity
Bacterial endocarditis
Fused right and left coronary cusps

Surgical Replacement
Aortic valve replaced with #23 Carbomedics prosthetic valve

This exhibit illustrates an aortic valve deformity and replacement. First, the normal anatomy of the valve is shown. Next, deformity caused by bacterial endocarditis is depicted where the right and left valve cusps are fused. Finally, the surgical replacement can be seen.

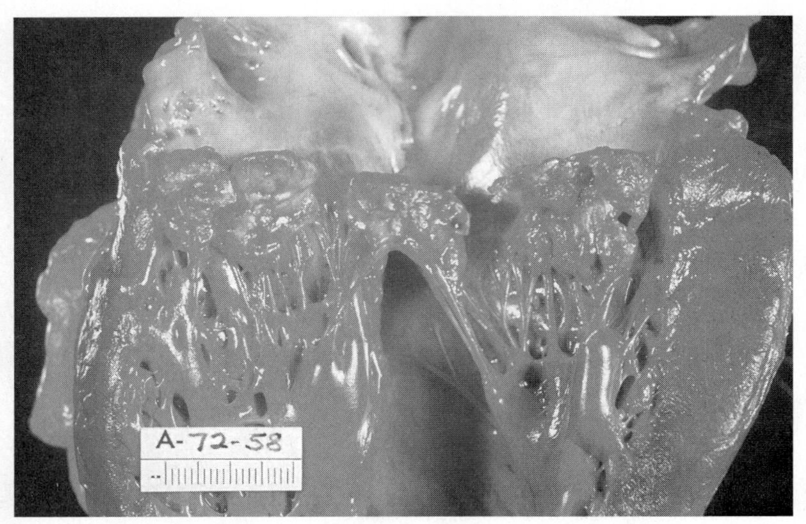

This photo at autopsy shows the extensive and devastating infective vegetations invading the mitral valve due to *Haemophilur parainfluenzae* infection.
Source: CDC/Dr. Edwin P. Ewing, Jr.

- A thrombus may form on the damaged surface of the valve. When the thrombus becomes infected, it forms a vegetation consisting of platelets, fibrin, inflammatory cells, and bacteria.
- Pieces of the brittle vegetation may break off (septic emboli) of the constantly moving valve leaflet and migrate to other organs causing complications, like infective occlusions, vessel aneurysm (called a mycotic aneurysm), and possible aneurysm rupture.
- Aortic and mitral valve endocarditis (from the left heart) can result in septic emboli to the brain, gastrointestinal (GI) tract, kidneys, and extremities.
- Tricuspid and pulmonic valve endocarditis (right heart) can "flick" septic emboli to the lungs.

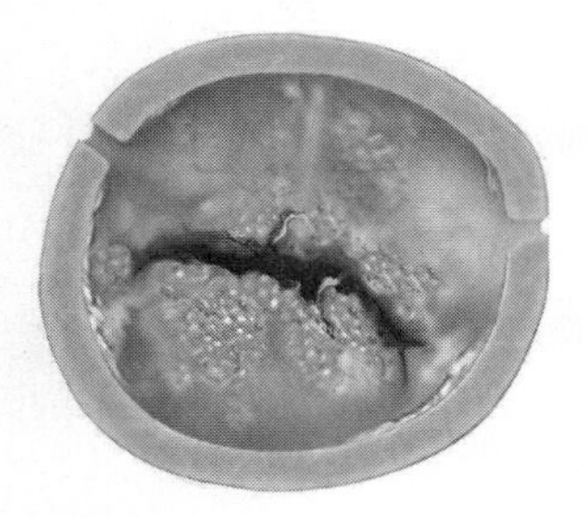

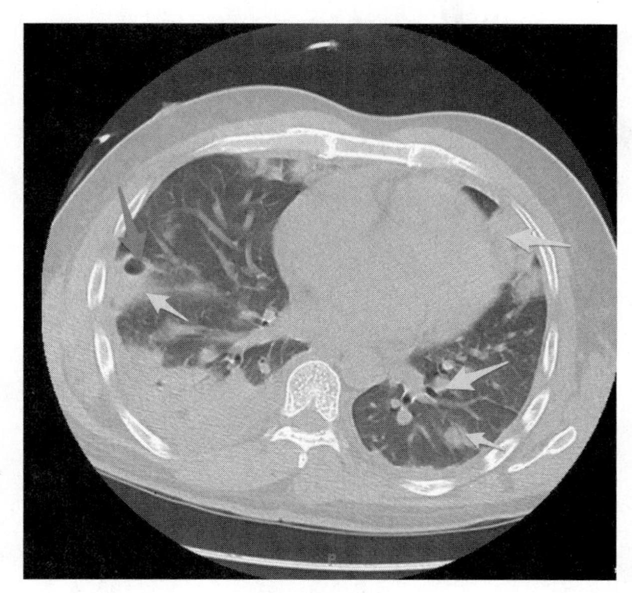

Upper: This drawing shows the pathology of an infected aortic valve. Bacterial colonies invaded the right and left aortic cusps which fused. Lower: Multiple septic emboli are seen in the lungs of a young IV drug user. Brittle vegetations on his tricuspid valve broke off. Emboli can travel to any organ, depending on the valve of origin.
Sources: (*upper*) © 2013 Nucleus Medical Media, All rights reserved; (*lower*) Courtesy of K. Kyriakidis

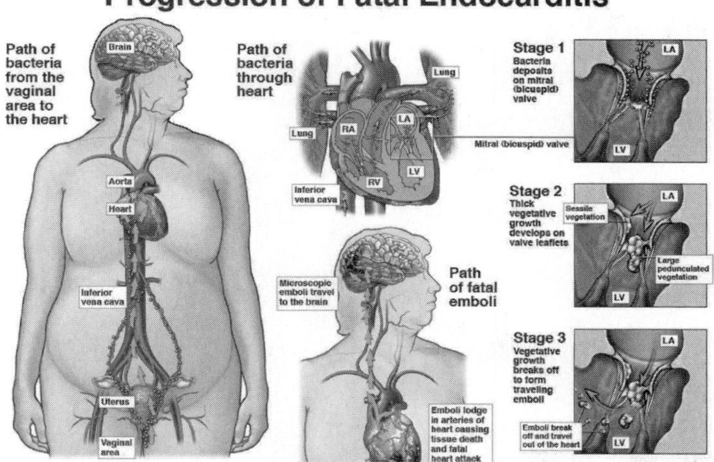

This stock medical exhibit shows multiple views of the heart and circulatory system describing the progression of fatal endocarditis. The following views are illustrated: (1) normal anatomy of the heart and bicuspid (aortic) valve, (2) pathway showing the spread of bacteria from the vaginal area to the heart, (3) bacteria collecting on leaflets of the bicuspid valve, (4) early stages of endocarditis with vegetative growth on the valve leaflets, (5) advanced endocarditis with vegetative emboli breaking off and entering the blood flow, and (6) pathway showing the emboli traveling in the blood flow from the heart to the brain.
Source: © 2013 Nucleus Medical Media, All rights reserved

LO1:

Pathophysiology (continued)

Incidence of Cardiac Valve Involvement

Infective endocarditis (IE) most commonly affects the valves in this order of frequency:

1. Mitral valve
2. Aortic valve
3. Combined mitral/aortic valve
4. Tricuspid valve
5. Pulmonic valve (rare)

In addition to infecting natural valves, equal rates of infection occur in mechanical and bioprosthetic valves.

Aortic Endocarditis

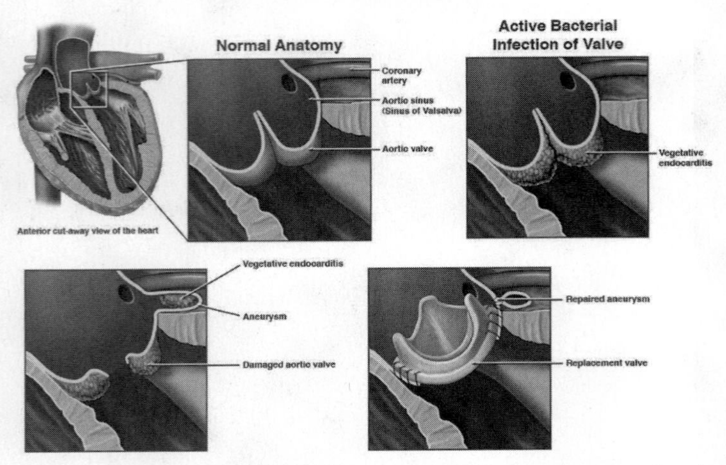

This series of illustrations depicts a normal aortic valve that then becomes infected, developing vegetative endocarditis and an associated aneurysm. This condition is treated surgically with repair of the aneurysm and a replacement artificial aortic valve.

Concept Check

2. The valve vegetations associated with infective endocarditis are composed of which material?
   A. Platelets
   B. Red blood cells
   C. Cholesterol
   D. Potassium

Answer question

Concept Check

3. What valve is most commonly affected by infective endocarditis?
   A. Aortic
   B. Tricuspid
   C. Mitral
   D. Pulmonic

Answer question

Causes and Risk Factors

- Central venous access lines, pacemaker catheters
- Prior valve surgeries
- Valvular abnormalities (e.g., mitral valve regurgitation, mitral valve prolapse, rheumatic heart disease)
- Existing artificial heart valves
- Congenital heart defects or diseases
- IV drug abuse: 75% of cases occur without underlying valve disease; 50% of these cases involve the tricuspid valve; most common infective organism is *Staphylococcus aureus.*
- Invasive procedures (such as urethral catheterization, cystoscopy, rigid bronchoscopy, or implanted cardiac devices) in patients with valvular disease

Assessment Findings

Symptoms of endocarditis are often vague but can progress rapidly or more insidiously over a prolonged time. Symptoms are caused by the immune response to infection, toxins produced by the microorganism, and valvular insufficiency. Symptoms from septic emboli depend on which side of the heart is infected:

- Fatigue, generalized muscle aches
- Fevers, chills, diaphoresis
- Dyspnea, hypoxia from heart failure or from septic emboli to the lung
- New or changing heart murmur

BACTERIAL ENDOCARDITIS FROM THE INJURY WITH DAMAGE TO THE AORTIC VALVE

NORMAL AND UNDAMAGED HEART

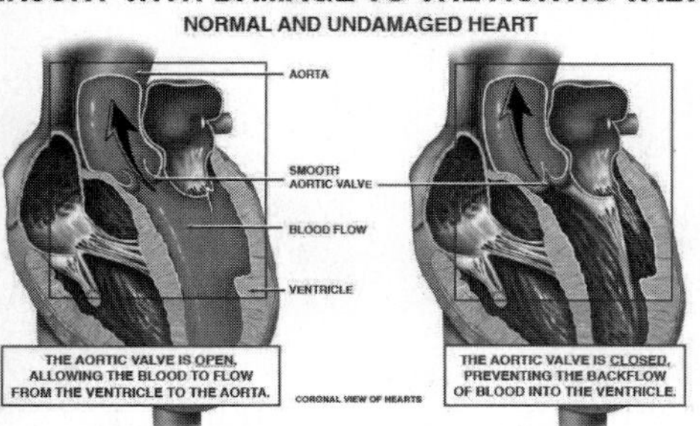

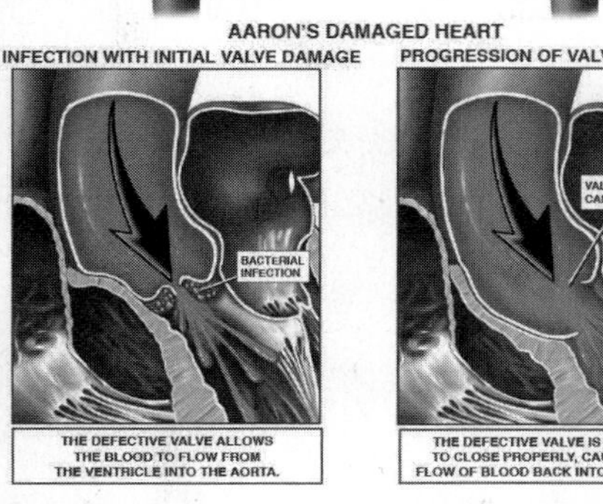

This series of pictures illustrates how a bacterial infection infects the aortic valve, damages it, and causes regurgitant flow back into the ventricle during diastole. This is how heart failure can occur.

Source:

- Weight loss
- Abdominal pain can be caused by septic emboli to GI tract
- Skin changes:
    - o Splinter hemorrhages under nails from vasculitis
    - o Petechiae, usually of the extremities and mouth
    - o Red, painful nodes on the pads of the fingers and toes (Osler nodes) result from immune deposits in the subcutaneous tissue.
    - o Painless, red to reddish-purple spots on the palms and soles (Janeway lesions) are the result of septic emboli.

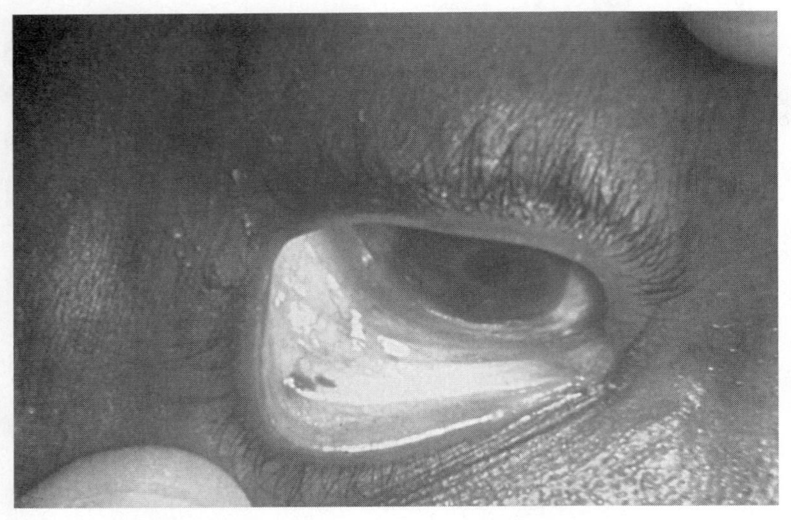

Petechial hemorrhages in the conjunctiva also signal septic emboli.
Source: CDC/Dr. Thomas F. Sellers/Emory University

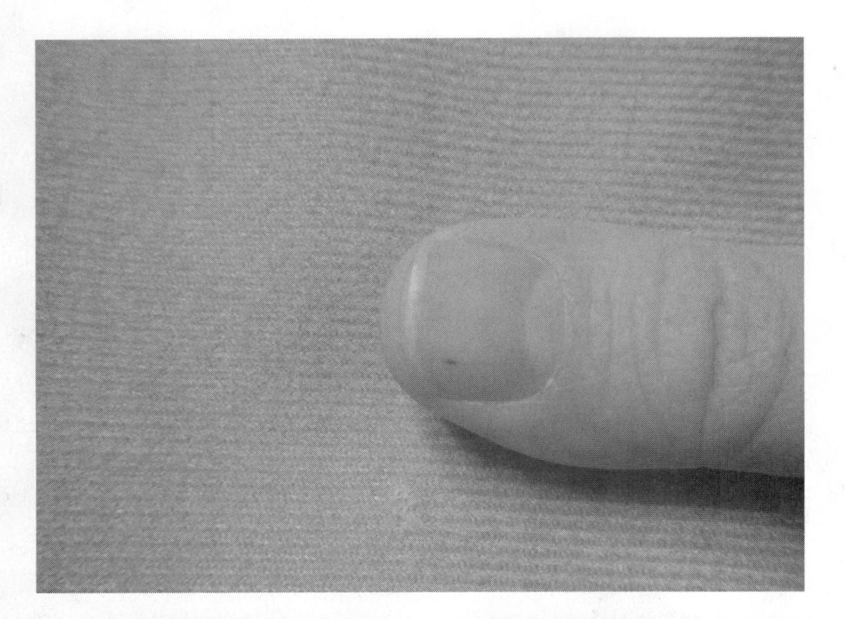

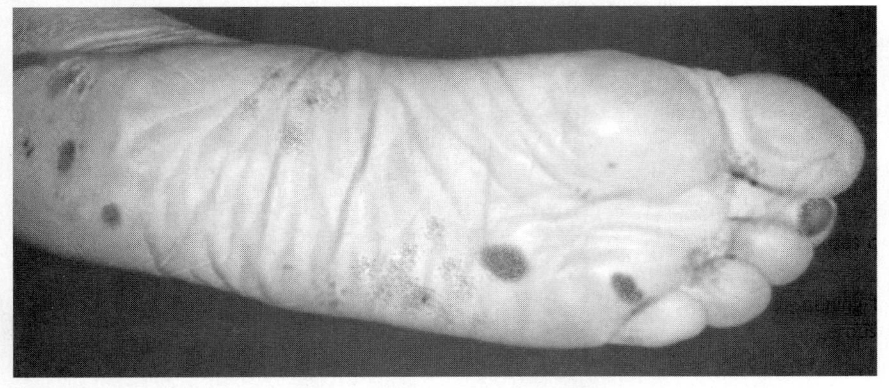

Upper: On close inspection, hemorrhages that appear like splinters (splinter hemorrhages) are seen in the nail beds. Lower: Note the deep purple spots on the patient's feet, known as Janeway lesions.
Sources: *(both)* Copyright © 2013, NovEx Novice to Expert Learning, LLC

Concept Check

4. Where are the splinter hemorrhages that are common to infective endocarditis found?

A. Soles of the feet

B. Warm areas such as axilla and groin

C. Pads of the fingers

D. Under nails

Answer question

Diagnostics

- Blood cultures: Cultures can be diagnostic and commonly identify the organism. Meticulous cleansing, allowing the decontaminant to dry, and preventing contamination during the blood draw are paramount. Obtain 3 sets of blood cultures over time (e.g., 10 minutes apart if different peripheral sites, about 60 minutes apart if at the same site), preferably before antibiotics are started. If the patient is critically ill or the disease is progressing rapidly, cultures should be obtained over a short period of time (less than 1 hr) so that antibiotics can quickly be started.
- Echocardiogram
  - Valvular dysfunction is best identified with an echocardiogram.
  - Infectious vegetations can be detected on echo. Transesophageal echocardiogram is more sensitive than transthoracic echocardiogram for viewing vegetations.
- Other tests that can be helpful include:
  - EKG: To look for conduction abnormalities (e.g., heart block) that can be caused by endocarditis.
  - Erythrocyte sedimentation rate (ESR): Inflammatory indicator
  - C-reactive protein (CRP): Inflammatory indicator
  - Coagulation tests
  - Lactate level: Tissue hypoxia indicator

Priority Patient Concerns and Desired Collaborative Care Outcomes

Prior to caring for patients with endocarditis, it is important to prioritize the patient's concerns that must guide the nursing care plan and interventions. Care for the patient is ordered and organized in accordance with the patient's priority and urgent needs. Desired collaborative care outcomes in patients with endocarditis typically include:

1. Patient will have no findings associated with decreased cerebral tissue perfusion or stroke.
2. Patient will have no findings associated with decreased peripheral tissue perfusion.
3. Patient will report decreased fatigue and increased ability to participate in routine daily activities.
4. Patient's body temperature will be within normally expected range.
5. Patient will report being pain free.
6. Patient will report feeling calmer regarding health status.

Considering these important care outcomes, prepare a list of the major 3–6 priority patient concerns or nursing diagnoses for patients with endocarditis. Be prepared to participate in a discussion of this list and/or to submit them as an assignment, as determined by your faculty. Resources you may find helpful in this assignment can include this lesson, the references, resources on nursing care plans, and standard nursing diagnoses manuals.

LO3:

Collaborative Interventions

Goals for treatment include:

M N **1.** Early diagnosis of IE

M N **2.** Identification of the infective organism and sensitivity testing for the organism

M N **3.** Prolonged administration of intravenous antibiotics, 4–6 weeks; discharge to home care is possible even with prolonged antibiotic therapy

M N **4.** Careful monitoring of toxic side effects of the antibiotics

M N **5.** Early identification of complications

M **6.** Aggressive surgical intervention as needed

Evidence-Based Practice

M N Evidence-based practice data-limited in endocarditis. Treatment of endocarditis can be difficult. Due to the absence of blood flow in the valve leaflets, antibiotics typically have little impact. Though difficult to treat, **antibiotics are the mainstay of therapy** for Infectious Endocarditis (IE). Because the pathogens that cause endocarditis are many and virulent, the American Heart Association (AHA) recommends at least nine different antimicrobial treatment regimens for the various infective pathogens. (See AHA Guidelines for details.)

- Antibiotic therapy is typically effective with 4–6 weeks duration in natural valves.
- Only bactericidal (and no longer bacteristatic) antibiotics have proven effective against endocarditis currently.
- Treatment is prolonged in patient with resistant organisms, highly virulent pathogens, or complications.
- Most patients become afebrile within 3–7 days, depending on the organisms.
- Embolic complications are most common during the first two weeks of treatment.
- Prior to discharge, ensure that the patient is fully compliant with all interventions and demonstrates the ability to manage their care and antibiotic.
- Follow-up blood cultures are important to confirm antibiotic effectiveness.

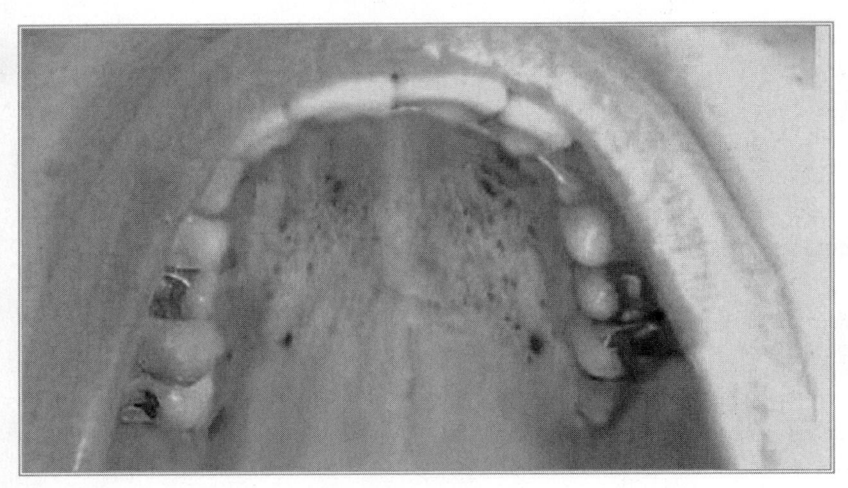

Petechiae can signal early microvascular complications of endocarditis to other organs. Early detection can lead to further intervention.

Source: Copyright © 2013, NovEx Novice to Expert Learning, LLC

Concept Check

5. What is the primary treatment for infective endocarditis?

A. Anticoagulation with aspirin

B. Prolonged administration of IV antibiotics

C. Short course of oral antibiotics

D. Placement of a dual-chamber pacemaker

Answer question

Collaborative Symptom Management

- Administer ordered antibiotic therapy. Empiric IV antimicrobial coverage is initiated to cover all likely pathogens, until the specific pathogen can be identified. Some of the antibiotics commonly used are penicillin G, oxacillin, ceftriaxone, vancomycin, Gentamicin, Unasyn, cefepime, ciprofloxacin, doxycycline, and Zosyn.
- Monitor labs to evaluate effectiveness of antibiotic therapy.
- Monitor heart sounds, report new murmurs or changes to health care provider.
- Assess for septic emboli: pulmonary infarction if tricuspid or pulmonary valves (e.g., decreasing SpO_2, dyspnea); cerebral/GI/GU/peripheral emboli if mitral or aortic valves (e.g., dysrhythmias, heart failure, decreased urine output, stroke, bowel infarction, cold, or pulseless limb).

Mitral Valve Endocarditis with Resulting Cerebral Embolus

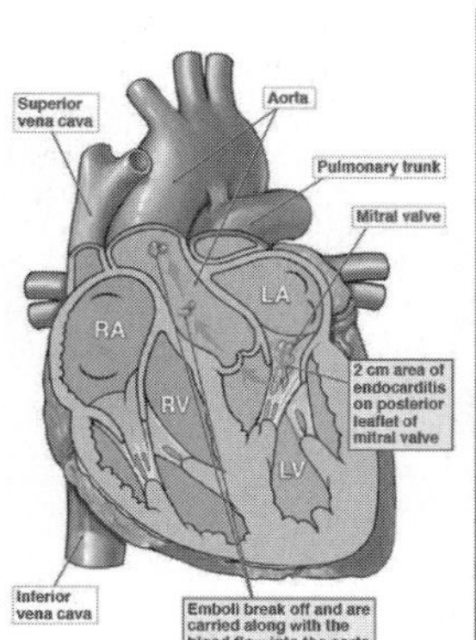

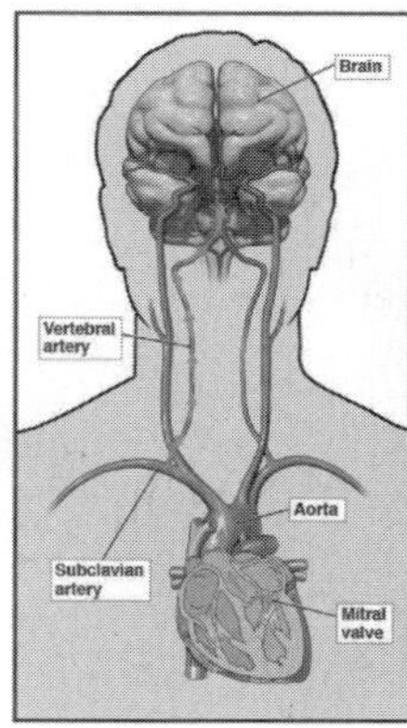

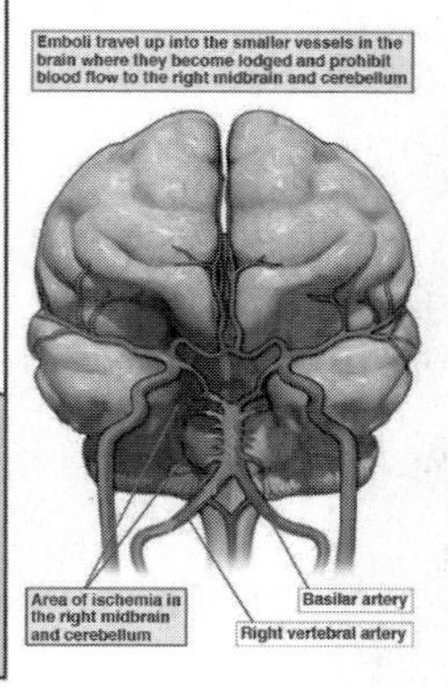

Endocarditis is depicted on the posterior mitral valve leaflet. Emboli break off, travel through the aorta (shown by arrows), through the subclavian and vertebral arteries, and embolize in the brain. In the last image, the darkened area in the brain represents ischemia or stroke.

Concept Check

6. A patient is more likely to have a bowel infarction from infective endocarditis if the disorder affects which valve?
   A. Tricuspid
   B. Pulmonary
   C. Aortic
   D. Pyloric

Answer question

- Administer ordered antipyretics for fever.

- Administer ordered analgesics for discomfort and reduction of inflammation.
- Offer reassurance and comfort measures to reduce anxiety.
- Educate patient on disease process and potential need for surgical intervention to replace damaged and infected valve.

Collaborative Interventions (continued)

Valve Replacement

A small number of patients require valve replacement surgery if one the following conditions exists:

- Heart failure occurs due to mitral or aortic valve damage.
- New septic emboli despite treatment
- Not responding to antibiotic therapy

Post-op measures for aortic or mitral valve replacement includes observing for dysrhythmias, hemorrhage, pulmonary effusion, infection, and stroke.

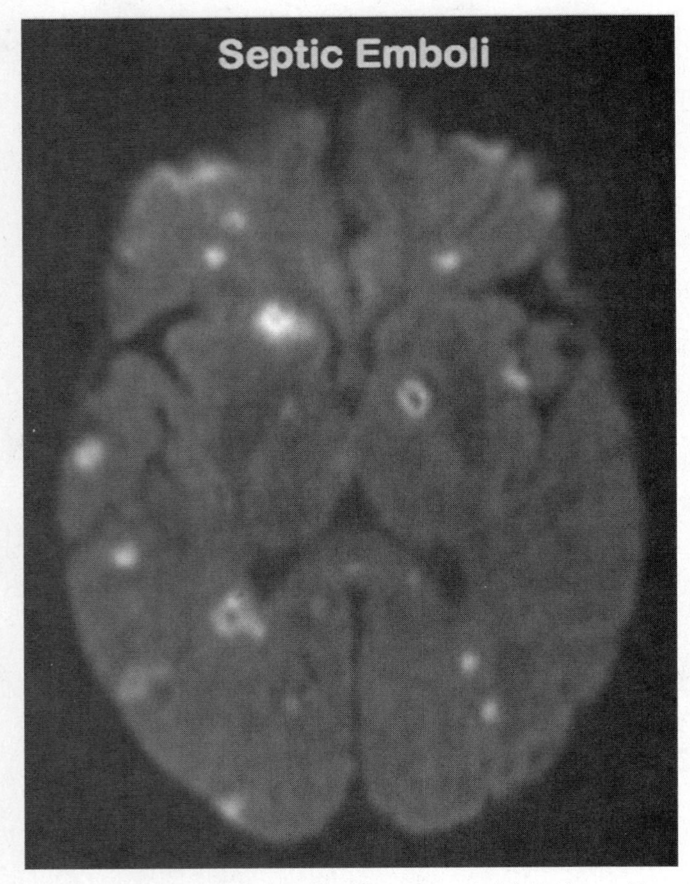

This MRI scan shows numerous infected or septic emboli (whitish spots) have showered the brain, affecting all lobes and areas. The patient has infective endocarditis and, tragically, the brittle edges of the friable valve are breaking off, embolizing, and infecting the brain.
Source: Courtesy of K. Kyriakidis

Concept Check

7. In which case is valve replacement necessary in the treatment of endocarditis?

A. Dysrhythmias occur.
B. The patient is allergic to latex.
C. Septic emboli develop following conservative treatment.
D. The infection has not cleared after 2 weeks of medication treatment.

Answer question

Patient Education

- N • Educate patient about endocarditis, symptoms of complications, follow up care, when to contact health care provider, medication adherence, and adverse medication effects or toxicity.
- N • Avoid the use of illicit IV drugs, the dangers of dirty needle use, and assist with drug rehabilitation referral if desired and indicated.
- N • Educate about the necessity of good dental care and oral hygiene.
- N • Educate about prevention, recognition, and management of heart failure, when indicated. Heart failure has the greatest impact on the patient's prognosis. (EBP)
- N • Discuss the potential of valve replacement in patients with moderate and severe valvular damage or destruction.
- N • Educate the patient and family in the administration and/or care required for long-term home IV antibiotic therapy.

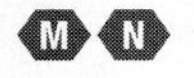

Endocarditis Prophylaxis

- There are no studies that show the benefit of prophylaxis for endocarditis. However, the American Heart Association (AHA) guidelines recommend that patients at highest risk for endocarditis receive antibiotic prophylaxis for procedures that cause significant bacteremia.
- Procedures that put patients at higher risk primarily include dental procedures that involve manipulation of the gums.
- Specific invasive procedures (e.g., urethral catheterization, cystoscopy, rigid bronchoscopy, implanted cardiac devices) may also put these patients at risk.
- IV drug users are at high risk for endocarditis. The greatest chance of protection is prevention by either using clean needles with sterile hygiene or discontinuing IV drug use.

AHA Prophylaxis Guidelines

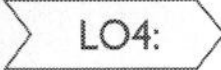

The American Heart Association has issued these guidelines. Patients with the following conditions should receive antibiotic prophylaxis:

- Prosthetic heart valve
- A history of infective endocarditis
- Unrepaired cyanotic congenital heart disease
- Repaired congenital heart defects with prosthetic material during the first six months after the procedure
- Repaired congenital heart disease with residual defects
- Heart transplant with significant valvular regurgitation
- Patients with more common valvular abnormalities and diseases no longer need to receive prophylaxis (e.g., aortic stenosis, mitral prolapse, mitral regurgitation, atrial or ventricular septal defect, hypertrophic cardiomyopathy).

Summary of Interventions

- A new murmur with fever should immediately point to endocarditis.
- The recommended treatment, though problematic, is the administration of a prolonged course (4–6 weeks) of intravenous antibiotics.
- Surgical replacement of an affected valve may be necessary.
- Close monitoring for vascular complications from endocarditis is important.

LO4:

Evaluation of Desired Collaborative Care Outcomes

Evaluation and reassessment should reveal attainment of previously established patient outcomes. In summary:

- Patient has clear mentation and expected sensation and movement of all muscle groups.
- Patient's skin and peripheral tissues are warm, dry, and intact.
- Patient has returned to normal daily activities and reports no unusual fatigue.
- Patient has no fever.
- Patient reports having no illness-associated pain.
- Patient calmly expresses understanding of illness and treatment plan.

References

Reimer-Kent, J. (2007). Infective endocarditis: A review and update of a clinical enigma. *Can J Cardiovasc Nurs, 17*(3), 5–12.

Smith, M. A., Smith, T. L., & Davidson, B. T. (2007). Managing the infected heart. *Crit Care Nurs Clinics North Amer, 19*(1), 99–106.

Practice Guidelines:

DeSimone, D. C., Tleyjeh, I. M., Correa de Sa, D. D., et al. (2012). Incidence of infective endocarditis caused by viridans group streptococci before and after publication of the 2007 American Heart Association's endocarditis prevention guidelines. *Circulation, 126*, 60–64.

Wilson, W., Taubert, K. A., Gewitz, M., Lockhart, P. B., Baddour, L. M., Levison, M., ... Quality of Care and Outcomes Research Interdisciplinary Working Group. (2007). Prevention of infective endocarditis: guidelines from the American Heart Association Rheumatic Fever, Endocarditis, and Kawasaki Disease Committee, Council on Cardiovascular Disease in the Young, and the Council on Clinical Cardiology, Council on Cardiovascular Surgery and Anesthesia, and the Quality of Care and Outcomes Research Interdisciplinary Working Group. *Circulation, 116*, 1736–1754. doi: 10.1161/ CIRCULATIONAHA.106.183095.

Patient Education

Infective endocarditis. Cleveland Clinic. **my.clevelandclinic.org/heart/disorders/valve/sbe.aspx**

Infective endocarditis. Patient.co.uk **www.patient.co.uk/health/infective-endocarditis-leaflet#**

Learning Outcomes for Inflammation of the Heart: Pericarditis

When you complete this lesson, you will be able to:

1. Recognize the clinical relevance of pericarditis.
2. Consider the pathophysiology, etiology, risk factors, and clinical presentation of pericarditis that determine the priority patient concerns.
3. Determine the most urgent and important nursing interventions and patient education required in caring for a patient with pericarditis.
4. Evaluate attainment of desired collaborative care outcomes for a patient with pericarditis.

LO1:

What Is Pericarditis?

- Pericarditis is an inflammation of the pericardial sac or the sac around the heart.
- Pericarditis can occur acutely (rapidly) or chronically over time.
- Pericarditis can occur in isolation or be a manifestation of systemic disease (e.g., systemic lupus).

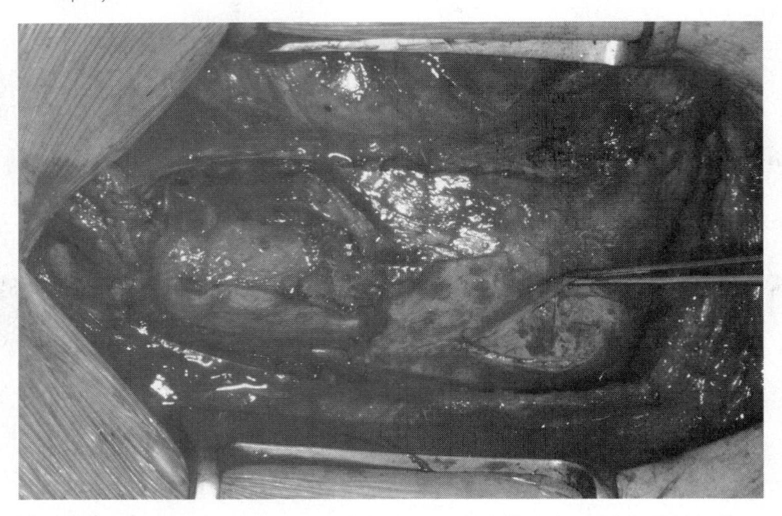

This photo shows constrictive pericarditis where a thick fibrin layer of the pericardium constricts normal contraction and heart movement. Without effective intervention, cardiac output can become severely limited.
Source: MICHAEL ENGLISH, M.D. Custom Medical Stock Photo/Newscom

Concept Check

1. **Which statement regarding pericarditis is accurate?**
   A. Pericarditis can have an acute onset.
   B. Pericarditis always indicates an underlying pathology.
   C. Pericarditis is not treatable.
   D. Pericarditis is inflammation of the heart wall.

Answer question

LO1:

Clinical Relevance

- Pericarditis can be asymptomatic but commonly causes chest pain and EKG changes that can be confused with acute coronary syndrome.
- While most forms of pericarditis are not life threatening, the most urgent and serious side effect of pericarditis is pericardial tamponade, a dangerous condition that can lead to death in the absence of immediate attention.

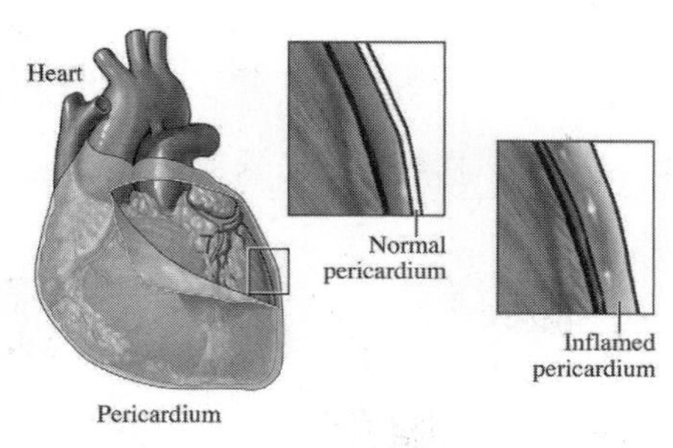

This series of pictures depicts a normal heart with a normal pericardium. The picture points out the change in appearance with inflammation in acute pericarditis.
Source: © 2013 Nucleus Medical Media, All rights reserved

LO2:

Pathophysiology

- Pericarditis is an inflammation of the pericardial lining that causes thickening of the two pericardial sac layers. This inflamed, thick lining can cause chest pain, changes in cardiac performance, and, possibly, the development of increased fluid in the pericardial sac.
- An effusion, which is an accumulation of fluid in the pericardial space, can accompany pericarditis. While some fluid is normally present in the pericardial space, too much fluid produces a constrictive effect on heart movement, known as cardiac tamponade.
- In a few situations, an infection (e.g., tuberculosis) or metastatic tumor in the pericardium can lead to bleeding into the pericaridal space or a hemorrhagic type of effusion. This is referred to as hemorrhagic pericarditis.

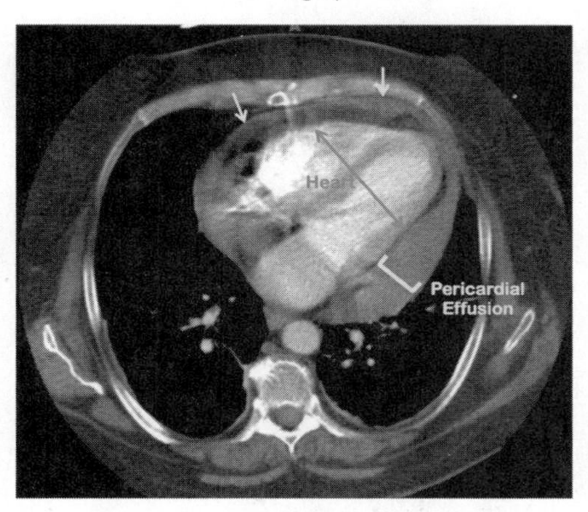

This CT scan demonstrates a significant pericardial effusion (yellow arrows and bracket) that compromises both cardiac output and pulmonary function.
Source: Courtesy of K. Kyriakidis

Pericarditis with Pericardial Tamponade

- Cardiac tamponade, with its constrictive effect around the heart, can produce a condition where the heart cannot relax and fill with blood.
- The effect of tamponade is noticed more on inspiration, where the increased venous return produces a more distended ventricle. This produces an increase in pressure in the pericardial sac. The increased pressure constricts the movement of the ventricles and drops stroke volume. The decrease in stroke volume will eventually produce a drop in blood pressure during inspiration.
- If the tamponade worsens and severely constricts ventricular filling, the deleterious drop in stroke volume causes severe hypotension and can lead to death.
- As the most dangerous complication of pericarditis, cardiac tamponade requires immediate intervention, such as a pericardiocentesis.

Concept Check

2. When are the effects of cardiac tamponade most noticeable?

A. Early in the morning

B. When the patient breathes in

C. When the patient is in the prone position

D. When dysrhythmia is present

Answer question

Constrictive Pericarditis

- The majority of patients present with acute pericarditis. However, chronic pericarditis can develop.
- In chronic pericarditis, the pericardium develops scarring and can become calcified, consequently, losing its elasticity and its ability to expand as the heart dilates during diastole.
- The ventricles, therefore, cannot expand within the constricted space in order to adequately fill and, therefore, stroke volume becomes fixed or unable to vary as needed. Diastolic dysfunction evolves and, eventually, cardiac output decreases.
- This creates a situation similar to cardiac tamponade.

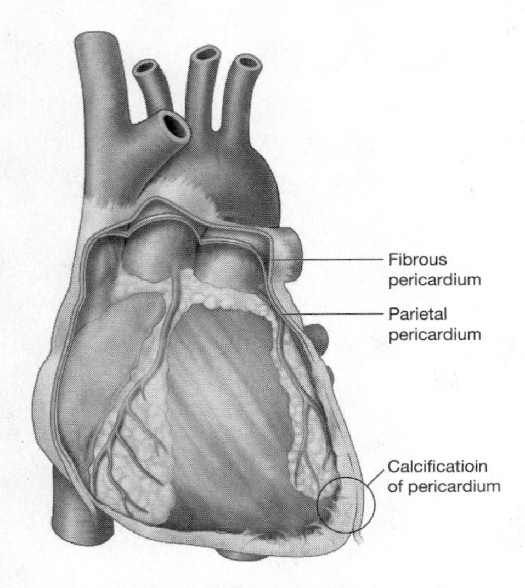

A hallmark of constrictive pericarditis is massive calcification of the pericardium. In constrictive pericarditis, the massive amount of calcified pericardium (yellowish white outer layer) causes limited stroke volume.

Causes and Risk Factors

Systemic

- Viral infections are the most common cause (see animation), but periocarditis can also result from any type of infection, including viral, bacterial, fungal, parasitic, TB, and HIV.
- Connective tissues disorders (e.g., rheumatic fever and lupus).
- Adverse effects of certain medications, such as procainamide, minoxidil, bleomycin, and methyldopa.
- Malignancy
- Renal failure has been associated with pericarditis, possibly related to an influx of proteins into the pericardial space. However, the exact pathophysiology is not well understood.

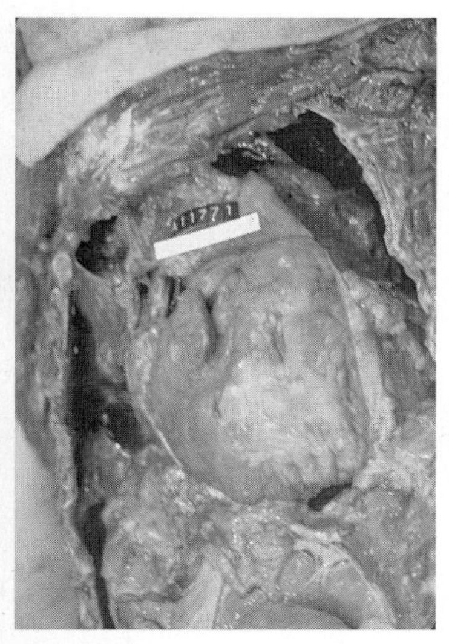

This is an autopsy specimen of a person who died with constrictive pericarditis.

Isolated Causes

- Myocardial infarction (MI) is a common cause.
- Cardiac surgery
- Post-irradiation to the chest for malignancy (cancer)
- Traumatic injury to the chest or heart

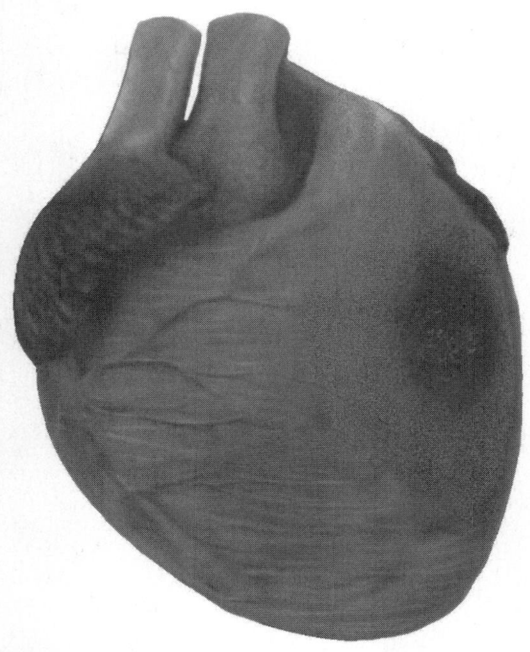

This photo shows the fibrinous pericarditis (deep reddened area) that developed following an anterior MI.
Source: Courtesy of George Kyriakidis/Santa Ana, CA

Concept Check

3. What is the most common etiology of pericarditis?

A. Connective tissue disorders
B. Medication
C. Malignancy
D. Viral infection

Answer question

Assessment Findings

- Fever is commonly present because of the infectious or inflammatory process.
- The most common symptom is chest or precordial pain.The pain may be similar to an acute MI, angina, or pleurisy (sharp and stabbing).
  - o Chest pain may be mild to severe, occur slowly or suddenly, and can radiate.
  - o Pain usually worsens with deep inspiration and when the patient, is lying supine.
  - o Pain is often positional: sitting up and leaning forward usually diminishes the pain.
- A "friction rub" often accompanies pericarditis. A friction rub is a scratchy sound (like walking in snow) heard when listening to the heart over the lower sternal border, best heard when leaning forward. It can be so loud that it blocks out other heart sounds.
- Signs and symptoms that are also common include difficulty breathing, palpitations, and elevated jugular venous pressure (distended jugular neck veins).
- A syndrome of hypotension, distended neck veins and muffled heart sounds (called Beck's triad) has traditionally been used to describe cardiac tampanade.
- A pericardial effusion (excessive fluid in the pericardial space) can be present without producing a tamponade. In this case, careful monitoring of the effusion is necessary to detect and prevent a tamponade from developing. A pocket-sized ultrasound technique (such as a Vscan) is the easiest, most accurate method to monitor for this dangerous complication.
- To monitor for tamponade, exam techniques such as auscultation for muffled heart sounds with a stethoscope are limited in protecting the patient. However, if a pocket-sized ultrasound or common echocardiogram is not available, use of the stethoscope to detect distant heart sounds is necessary.

Assessment Findings for Pericardial Tamponade

- Pericardial tamponade is a rare but life-threatening complication of pericarditis. Pressure from the fluid buildup compresses the myocardium, which causes impaired ventricular filling and results in hemodynamic compromise.
- As the condition worsens, hypotension, mental status changes, cyanosis (bluish color of mucous membranes), loss of peripheral pulses, lethal dysrhythmias (especially pulseless electrical activity), and death can occur.
- **Pulsus paradoxus** (a drop of 10 mmHg in systolic blood pressure with inspiration) **can be present with tamponade** and is a warning sign.
- Venous engorgement may also become apparent, such as jugular venous distention (JVD).
- If the patient has a decreased stroke volume from a tamponade, the fluid can be removed by a pericardiocentesis (drain the fluid from the sac).
- Pulsus paradoxus is more easily noticed when the patient has an arterial line and pressure tracing visible. However, the fading in and out of the audible systolic pressure sounds when using a sphygmomanometer are readily detectable if the blood pressure is not done rapidly. When suspected, one can slow or stop cuff pressure release when the first sound is audible to determine whether it is fading in and out with respirations.

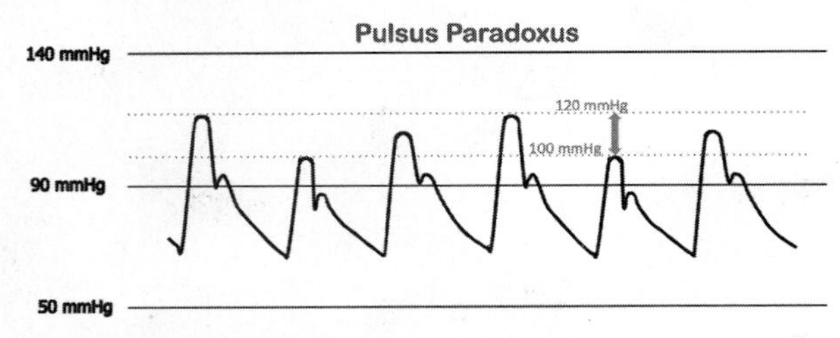

This tracing shows pulsus paradoxus with a 20 mmHg drop in systolic BP during inspiration. The systolic sound can be heard fading in and out.

Diagnostics

- EKG: ST-segment elevation in all leads except aVR is very suggestive of a general inflammation of the heart (e.g., pericarditis).
- Echocardiogram: Best and preferred test to confirm pericardial effusion or tamponade, as the fluid in the pericardial sac can be visualized, but will not likely detect a pericarditis.
- Radiology tests that may be ordered to detect complications of pericarditis, but not for pericarditis, itself, include:
  - o Chest x-ray: May detect an effusion and enlargement but not pericarditis.
  - o CT scan: Good detail but may need intravenous contrast for clear distinction. It is an accurate test for effusions or tamponade, but not for pericarditis.
  - o MRI: Will provide a detailed soft tissue view without exposing the patient to radiation or contrast dyes, but will not likely be ordered for pericarditis.
- Cardiac enzymes (troponin I) may be elevated. White blood cell count might also be elevated, but is not diagnostic for pericarditis.

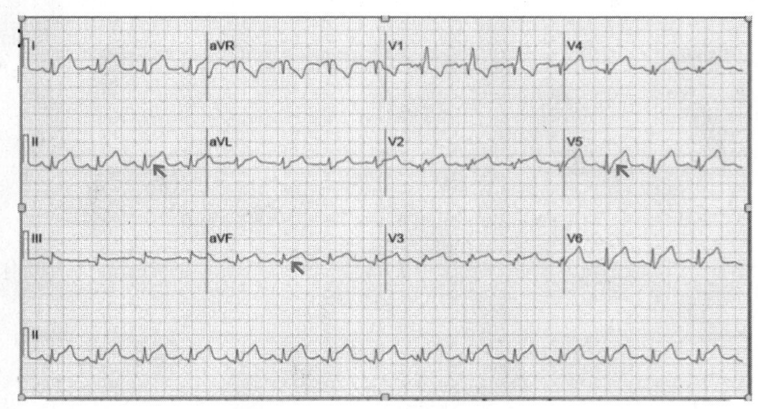

Note the ST segment elevation throughout the 12 leads.
Source: Courtesy of K. Kyriakidis

Concept Check

4. **Which diagnostic tool is the easiest, most accurate method of monitoring a pleural effusion?**
   A. EKG
   B. Troponin
   C. Handheld ultrasound
   D. Chest x-ray

Answer question

Priority Patient Concerns and Desired Collaborative Care Outcomes

Prior to caring for patients with pericarditis, it is important to prioritize the patient's concerns that must guide the nursing care plan and interventions. Care for the patient is ordered and organized in accordance with the patient's priority and urgent needs. Desired collaborative care outcomes in patients with pericarditis typically include:

1. Patient will be pain free.
2. Patient will have no findings associated with decreased cardiac output.
3. Patient will tolerate daily activities.
4. Patient will be calm.

Considering these important care outcomes, prepare a list of the major 3–6 priority patient concerns or nursing diagnoses for patients with pericarditis. Be prepared to participate in a discussion of this list and/or to submit them as an assignment, as determined by your faculty. Resources you may find helpful in this assignment can include this lesson, the references, resources on nursing care plans, and standard nursing diagnoses manuals.

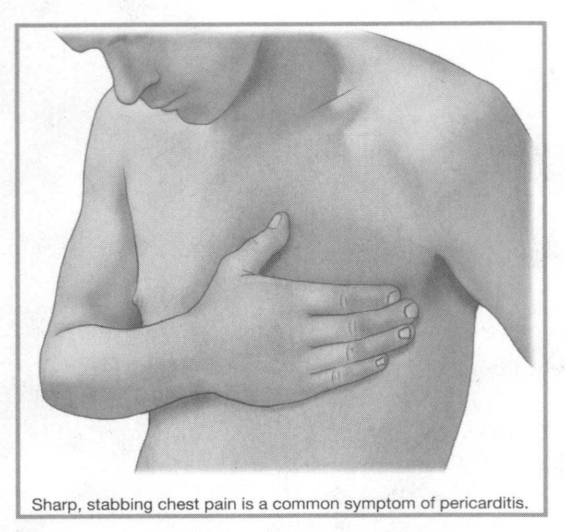

Sharp, stabbing chest pain is a common symptom of pericarditis.

Patients with acute pericarditis commonly have sharp, stabbing chest pain. It typically presents without warning and is located in the substernal or left chest area. One or both shoulders may be involved. Sitting up and leaning forward often eases pericardial pain, whereas lying down and deep breathing exacerbates it.

LO3:

Collaborative Interventions

Evidence-Based Practice (EBP)

M N
- Evidence-based treatment for pericarditis suggests that anti inflammatory, particularly non-steroidal anti-inflammatory (NSAIDs) medications (e.g., aspirin [ASA], ibuprofen, naproxen, ketorolac, indomethacin, and colchicine), are the *mainstay of treatment.*

M N
- Aspirin is the best choice if the pericarditis is a result of a myocardial infarction because other NSAIDs, like ibuprofen, can interfere with healing of the infarction site.

M N
- If a source is known, it needs to be treated or removed. For example, a bacterial infection should be treated with antibiotics.

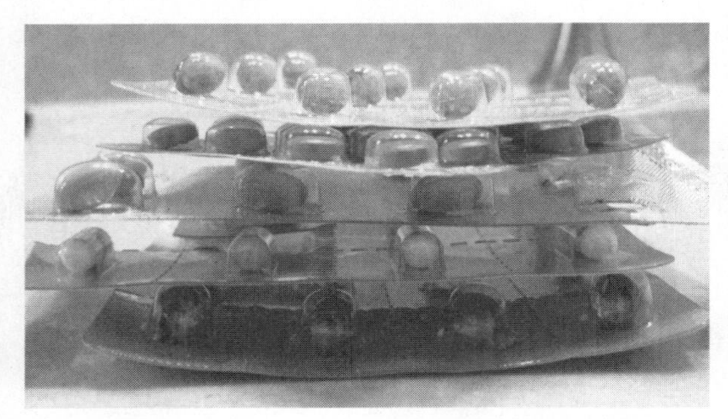

NSAIDs are commonly used to treat pericarditis, as well as other types of pain, fever, and inflammation. They are typically safe in most patients without having the mild side effects or additive problems of opioids and steroids.
Source: Copyright © 2013, NovEx Novice to Expert Learning, LLC

Collaborative Symptom Management and Comfort Care

Interventions that have not yet been sufficiently studied, but effective, include:

M N
- Corticosteroids (e.g., methylprednisolone or prednisone) may be tried, but are not used as first-line treatment.

M N
- Antipyretic agents (e.g., acetaminophen) will control the fever if the patient is uncomfortable. NSAIDs are also effective antipyretics.

M N
- Managing the patient's pain is an essential part of helping the patient with pericarditis. A limited course of narcotic pain medication (e.g., fentanyl, morphine, or hydromorphone) can be used to alleviate severe pain in addition to the NSAID treatment.

M N
- While on NSAID treatment, patients who have or are at risk for gastrointestinal disorders may require concurrent gastrointestinal protection by taking a daily proton pump inhibitor (PPI) (e.g., omeprazole, pantoprazole, esomeprazole).
- Administer anti-inflammatories with food to avoid gastrointestinal complications or discomfort.
- Elevate the head of the bed (HOB) to at least 45°.
- Encourage patient to lean forward, using the bedside table as support, to alleviate chest pain or discomfort.
- Maintain bed rest as indicated.
- Be prepared for pericardiocentesis. Have pericardiocentesis tray on hand. Review the procedure if unfamiliar.
- Monitor vital signs and heart sounds frequently.
- Report symptoms of decreased cardiac output findings to health care providers ASAP (e.g., dyspnea, peripheral edema, fatigue, hypotension, jugular venous distention [JVD]).

Interventions that have not yet been sufficiently studied but are effective for early detection or prevention of serious complications include:

M N
- Anticoagulants are contraindicated in order to prevent an increase in pericardial fluid or pericardial tamponade. Collaboration with the team is important to ensure this safety precaution.

N
- Report symptoms of decreased cardiac output findings or pulsus paradoxus to health care providers ASAP (e.g., dyspnea, hypotension, onset of fatigue, jugular venous distention, peripheral edema).

M N
- Perform continuous EKG monitoring to detect dysrhythmias that may indicate the development of cardiac tamponade. The most dangerous dysrhythmia is electromechanical dissociation (EMD), which is described as the presence of a cardiac rhythm without a pulse, also referred to as pulseless electrical activity (PEA).

M N
- Monitoring with ultrasound (pocket-sized or common echocardiography) is more sensitive to early changes of pericardial effusion.

M N
- Pulse oximetry should be used to monitor for hypoxemia if heart failure develops.

N
- Signs of development of a pericardial tamponade such as increased chest pain, shortness of breath, neck vein distention, or hemodynamic instability warrant a call for the Rapid Response Team for any patient who is not in an intensive care setting. This situation can rapidly become an emergency. Pericardiocentisis is imperative, as CPR is not likely to be effective.

Concept Check

5. Which medication is contraindicated in the treatment of pericarditis?
   - A. NSAIDs
   - B. Anticoagulants
   - C. Opioid pain relievers
   - D. Proton pump inhibitors

Answer question

Collaborative Interventions (contiued)

Cardiac Tamponade: Emergent Complication of Pericarditis

- The objective of treatment is to relieve the tamponade by inserting a needle into the pericardial fluid and aspirating or draining the fluid.
- M N Treatment of cardiac tamponade requires removing fluid from the pericardial sac, a procedure known as pericardiocentesis. An emergency pericardiocentesis tray is typically available.
- M A pericardial window (or surgical removal of a small section of pericardium drain that is left in place) may also be performed if there is a possibility of tamponade developing or if it recurs. A pericardial window is surgically created by removing a small section of the pericardium and leaving a drain in place until the effusion subsides. The window prevents tamponade.

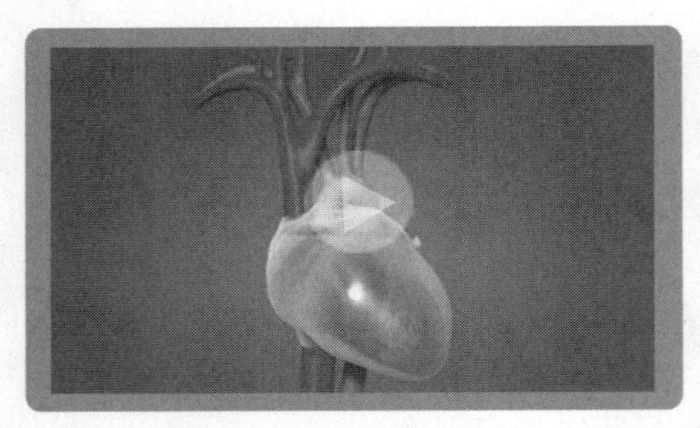

This animation demonstrates the treatment of cardiac tamponade by illustrating the fluid buildup in the pericardium and the needle aspiration procedure (pericardiocentesis) used to remove the fluid.

- M N Educate the patient about pericarditis and the interventions that are needed. Instruct the patient about any needed cooperation during the procedure as indicated.
- M N Local anesthesia is provided.
- N The patient is placed supine with the head elevated at a 45° angle.
- M N Insertion of the needle into the pericardium can be guided by an echocardiogram or by an EKG lead attached to the needle. It can be done blindly in life-threatening situations.
- M N If an EKG lead attached to the needed is used to guide needle insertion, the nurse vigilantly monitors the EKG for sudden ST elevation. ST elevation signals myocardial injury and indicates that the needle is in the pericardial space.
- M The needle is inserted at a 45° angle, lateral to the left side of the xiphoid, 1 to 2 cm inferior to the left of the xiphochondral junction. Blood is aspirated during introduction of the needle. Pericardial blood should not clot. Rapid clotting of pericardial blood can mean the pericardial needle has entered the heart and has been inserted too far.
- M N Usually, some immediate improvement in cardiac performance is noted upon aspiration of fluid from the pericardial sac. Post pericardiocentesis, the nurse should monitor for signs of bleeding in the pericardial space. Symptoms could include decreased heart sounds or evidence of pericardial tamponade.

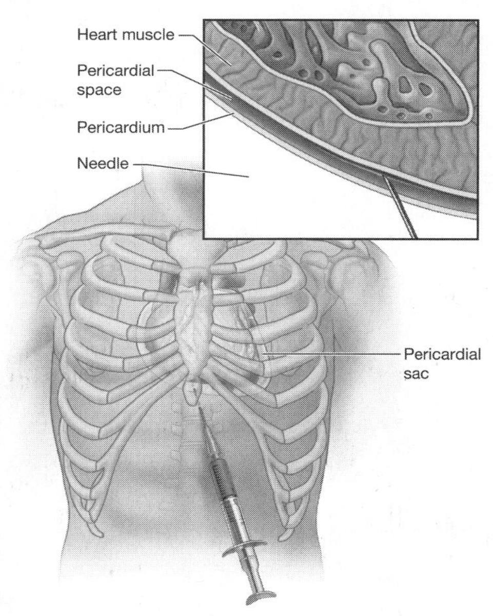

Pericardiocentesis may be required in patients with pericarditis to remove fluid from the pericardium. In addition to the emergent situations already described, when pericarditis arises from unknown origins, the fluid may be analyzed by the laboratory for infectious or malignant causes.

Concept Check

6. During pericardiocentesis, what EKG change signals that the needle is in the pericardial space?

A. Q waves

B. T wave inversion

C. ST elevation

D. Prolonged QRS interval

Answer question

Patient Education

For patients with acute pericarditis, educational needs are limited because the condition typically resolves without further problem within 2 weeks. For patients with recurrent pericarditis, the educational focus is on treating and managing the underlying chronic problem that is causing the pericarditis. Education can include:

- N If on corticosteroids, instruct the patient to not stop taking these medications without the health care provider's instructions.
- N Educate about symptoms of recurrence, when to seek medical attention, and follow-up visits.
- N Continue medication and rest for pain relief and recovery as instructed.
- N Prevention of pericarditis is almost impossible other than recommending good hygiene.

Concept Check

7. Where is the needle placed during pericardiocentesis?

A. In the right ventricle

B. In the left ventricle

C. In the space between the pericardium and the heart

D. Slightly into the heart muscle at the apex

Answer question

Summary of Interventions

- Pericarditis is managed by pain relief, primarily **anti-inflammatory agents**.
- A pericardiocentesis may be needed if an effusion develops. The most dangerous effusions lead to a tamponade, a potentially life-threatening event.
- The key nursing roles are:
  - o Closely monitor the patient.
  - o Manage pain.
  - o Detect early development and effects of a pericardial tamponade.
  - o Educate the patient about the condition.

LO4:

Evaluation of Desired Collaborative Care Outcomes

Evaluation and reassessment should reveal attainment of previously established patient outcomes. In summary:

- Patient has no chest pain.
- Patient's skin is warm and dry, mentation is clear, and urine output is balanced with intake.
- Patient reports returning to daily activities without pain or dyspnea.
- Patient calmly discusses disorder, treatment modalities, and treatment plan.

References

Gaudino, M., Anselmi, A., Pavone, N., & Massetti, M. (2013). Constrictive pericarditis after cardiac surgery. *Ann Thorac Surg, 95*(2), 731–736.

Htwe, T. H. & Khardori, N. M. (2012). Cardiac emergencies: infective endocarditis, pericarditis, and myocarditis. *Med Clin North Am, 96*(6), 1149–1169.

Humphreys, M. (2006). Pericardial conditions: signs, symptoms and electrocardiogram changes. *Emerg Nurse, 14*(1), 30–36.

Clinical Practice Guidelines:

Khandaker, M. H., Espinosa, R. E., Nishimura, R. A., Sinak, L. J., Hayes, S. N., Melduni, R. M., & Oh, J. K. (2010). Pericardial disease: Diagnosis and management. *Mayo Clinic Proceedings, 85*(6), 572–593.

Patient Education

American Heart Association

Harvard Medical School, Patient Education Center: **Patienteducationcenter.org/articles/pericarditis**

UpToDate. Pericarditis in Adults. **http://www.uptodate.com/contents/pericarditis-in-adults-thebasics?source=see_link**

Learning Outcomes for Inflammation of the Heart: Myocarditis

When you complete this lesson, you will be able to:

1. Recognize the clinical significance of myocarditis.
2. Consider the pathophysiology, etiology, risk factors, and clinical presentation of myocarditis that determine the priority patient concerns.
3. Determine the most urgent and important nursing interventions and patient education required in caring for a patient with myocarditis.
4. Evaluate attainment of desired collaborative care outcomes for a patient with myocarditis.

LO1:

What Is Myocarditis?

- Myocarditis is an inflammation of the heart muscle.
- It typically involves:
    - o An infection of the heart
    - o The infiltration of inflammatory cells into the myocardium
    - o Cardiac myocyte damage or necrosis
- It does not involve blockage of the coronary arteries.
- It can affect all ages.

Viral Myocarditis (Inflammation of the Cardiac / Heart Muscle)

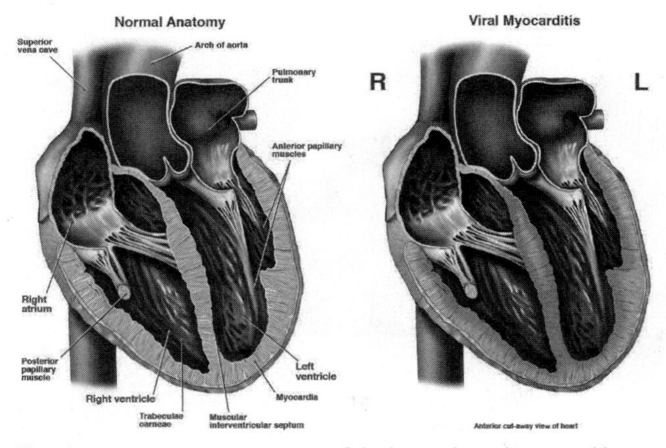

The above anterior cutaway views of the heart show the normal heart on the left and a heart infected with viral myocarditis on the right, the reddened areas indicating the affected cardiac myocytes.

Concept Check

1. **Which statement about myocarditis is accurate?**
    A. It is slowly progressive, so it occurs primarily in adulthood.
    B. It results from blockage of the coronary arteries.
    C. It is an infiltration of the heart muscle.
    D. It involves infection of the valve leaflets.

Answer question

LO1:

Clinical Relevance

- Myocarditis can be benign, or it can lead to death from heart failure and/or ventricular dysrhythmias.
- Since there are many causes of myocarditis, nursing attention to the individual patient should be attuned to:
  - o Signs of heart failure
  - o Irregular heart rhythms
  - o Abnormal heart sounds
- Patients with inflammatory conditions of the heart can present with few symptoms or can have catastrophic presentations. The nurse should be prepared to manage each of the inflammatory conditions.
- Myocarditis is thought to be the culprit in up to 20% of all cases of sudden death in young adults (Myocarditis Foundation).

LO2:

Pathophysiology

- Patients may present with small to large areas of inflammation of the cardiac muscle.
- One, two, or all three of the following mechanisms may result in inflammation:
  - o The infection infiltrates the myocardial tissue, resulting in dysfunction of the affected myocytes. If myocyte damage is extensive, heart failure can develop.
  - o The immune system is activated locally and/or systemically with macrophages and/or inflammatory cells invading the cardiac muscle, resulting in immune-mediated myocardial injury.
  - o Cellular and humoral mechanisms, in conjunction with the immune system, may activate cells that produce or contribute to cardiac muscle inflammation, ventricular dysfunction, and necrosis.

Concept Check

2. Which mechanisms cause myocarditis?

A. Decreased hormone production

B. Activation of the immune system

C. Damage to vessels

D. Damage to alveoli

Answer question

- Myocarditis may injure the cardiac myocytes sufficiently to diminish the heart's ability to contract, resulting in cardiomyopathy, a condition of extreme heart weakness.
- Dysrhythmias can develop due to alteration or damage in the normal electrical conduction system. As seen in the 12-lead EKG, the patient suffered diffuse damage to the electrical conduction system throughout the heart.

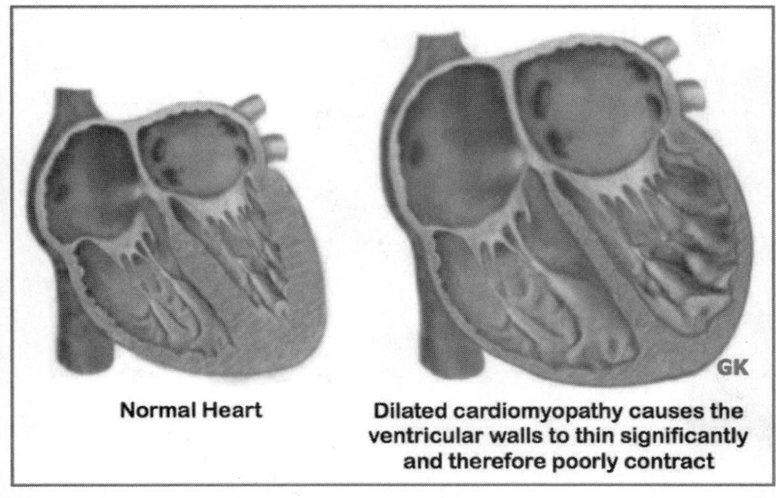

GK
Normal Heart
Dilated cardiomyopathy causes the ventricular walls to thin significantly and therefore poorly contract

As myocarditis damages the myocytes and the heart dilates, the conduction system is disruptive and dysrhythmias are common.

Source: Courtesy of George Kyriakidis/Santa Ana, CA

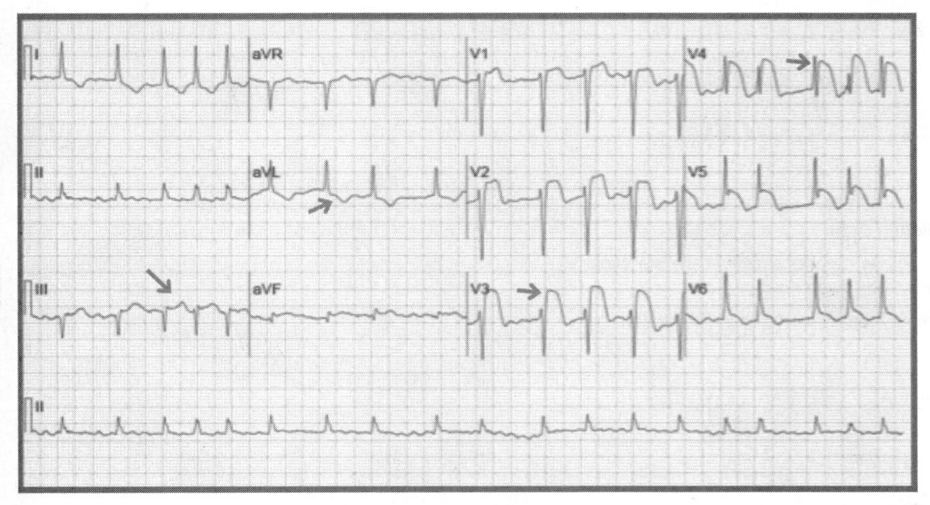

This EKG reveals the diffuse and multiple abnormal changes that can be found in patients with myocarditis. Red arrows point out the ST segment elevations in III, aVF, and V1–V6; ST depression with inverted T waves in I and aVL; and atrial fibrillation.

Source: Courtesy of K. Kyriakidis

Causes and Risk Factors

- Causes of myocarditis may be categorized as:
  - Infectious
  - Toxic, primarily chemical in origin
  - Immunologic (e.g., Kawasaki disease) occurring as an autoimmune reaction
- Acute viral myocarditis is by far the most common infectious etiology. A complication of upper respiratory infection (URI)—influenza, common cold—can include myocarditis.
- Other infections such as GI infections, Lyme disease, and Chagas disease are among other causes of myocarditis.
- Toxic causes of myocarditis include medications, particularly alcohol and chemotherapeutic drugs.
- Myocarditis can also be caused by radiation therapy.

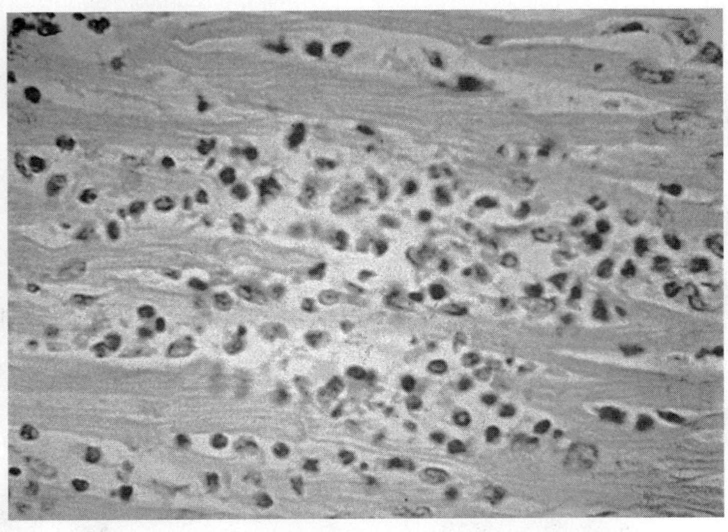

The interstitial lymphocytic infiltrates (dark dots) shown here are characteristic for myocarditis. Many myocarditis cases are probably subclinical. Some may be a cause for sudden death in young persons from lethal dysrhythmias. There is usually little necrosis. The most common viral agent is Coxsackie B.
Source: CDC/Armed Forces Institute of Pathology, Charles N. Farmer

Assessment Findings

Myocarditis can present as very mild and asymptomatic or so severe that a heart transplant may be indicated.

- Dysrhythmias may be the first recognizable sign. Dysrhythmias vary from fast to fatal.
  - o Ventricular fibrillation can occur but present as sudden death.
- Chest pain is a commonly reported symptom. The pain is described as a sharp, stabbing, precordial pain. The pain may mimic an ischemic episode or myocardial infarction.
- Symptoms of heart failure are typically present if cardiomyopathy with a heart failure pattern has developed.

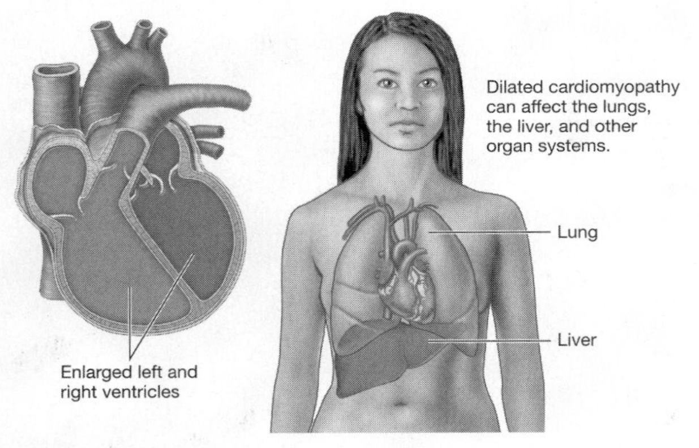

Dilated cardiomyopathy can affect the lungs, the liver, and other organ systems.
Lung
Liver
Enlarged left and right ventricles

Dilated cardiomyopathy involves enlargement of the heart muscle and is the most common type of cardiomyopathy. The heart muscle is weakened and cannot pump blood efficiently. Decreased heart function affects the lungs, liver, and other body systems.

- Systemic symptoms include:
  - o Fever
  - o Skeletal myalgia
  - o Malaise
  - o Anorexia (loss of appetite)
  - o Joint pain
  - o Leg and joint swelling
- Myocarditis symptoms usually develop 1–2 weeks after an upper respiratory viral illness. Some patients present acutely with fulminant congestive heart failure (CHF) secondary to widespread myocardial involvement and damage.
- Sudden death occasionally occurs.

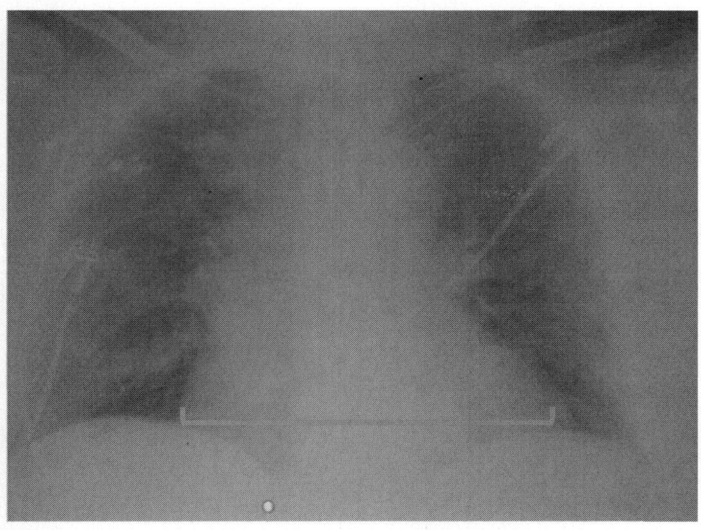

This patient was seen in the ED with an acute onset of respiratory distress and found to have congestive heart failure. The patient's huge heart size is depicted by the red bracket. Viral myocarditis, based on additionally findings, was suspected and confirmed.
Source: Courtesy of K. Kyriakidis

Concept Check

3. Which substance is particularly implicated in the development of toxic myocarditis?

A. Dietary cholesterol
B. Alcohol
C. Vitamin A
D. Aspirin

Answer question

Concept Check

4. What descriptor is often used in reporting chest pain from myocarditis?

A. Dull
B. Epigastric
C. Sharp
D. Tearing

Answer question

Diagnostics

- Troponin I elevation, suggesting general myocardial muscle injury, may prove beneficial when considering a possible myocarditis diagnosis.
- Echocardiogram—myocarditis could be suggested by a weakened ventricular contraction (with low ejection fraction), decreased wall motion, an enlarged heart, and suggestion of possible valve problems.
- The patient's history may reveal potential risk factors (e.g., recent upper respiratory infection) that are suggestive of myocarditis.
- Biopsy of the endocardium and myocardium should reveal edema with inflammatory infiltrates and myocardial cell necrosis.

Priority Patient Concerns and Desired Collaborative Care Outcomes

Prior to caring for patients with myocarditis, it is important to prioritize the patient's concerns that must guide the nursing care plan and interventions. Care for the patient is ordered and organized in accordance with the patient's priority and urgent needs. Desired collaborative care outcomes in patients with myocarditis typically include:

1. Patient will have no unanticipated findings associated with decreased cardiac output at their specific stage of recovery.
2. Patient will not experience any continued decrease in cardiac tissue perfusion.
3. Patient will be pain free.
4. Patient will be normovolemic.
5. Patient will balance rest with gradually increasing activities of daily living to return to a personal normal.
6. Patient will calmly discuss health status.

Considering these important care outcomes, prepare a list of the major 3–6 priority patient concerns or nursing diagnoses for patients with myocarditis. Be prepared to participate in a discussion of this list and/or to submit them as an assignment, as determined by your faculty. Resources you may find helpful in this assignment can include this lesson, the references, resources on nursing care plans, and standard nursing diagnoses manuals.

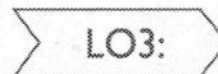

Collaborative Interventions

Evidence-based treatments for myocarditis are limited.

Collaborative Symptom Management

- Treatment is mostly based on interventions that provide the best observed outcomes but have not been sufficiently studied. Interventions are primarily targeted at symptomatic management of heart failure.
- Heart failure is managed with:
  - Preload reducers, primarily diuretics (e.g., furosemide)
  - Afterload reducers, primarily ACE inhibitors (e.g., captopril, lisinopril)
  - Possibly digitalis (e.g., digoxin) for inotropic support
- Other treatment of myocarditis involves managing complications:
  - Dysrhythmias
    - Atrial
    - Ventricular
    - Heart block, possibly requiring the use of a pacemaker
  - Thromboembolism
- Systemic immune suppression is not recommended when infection is the suspected cause.

Concept Check

5. Pharmacotherapy for myocarditis is focused on which outcome?

A. Increasing afterload
B. Increasing preload
C. Control of dysrhythmias
D. Immune suppression

Answer question

- Some of the following interventions may be useful based on diagnosis:
  - A primary intervention for myocarditis is rest (e.g., bed rest, decreasing environmental stimuli, balancing nursing interventions to allow for rest). And as healing occurs, gradual return to activities starting with ROM exercises while observing tolerance. Teaching also focuses on identifying and treating symptomology as return to daily activities occurs.
  - Monitor for signs and symptoms of heart failure:
    - Dyspnea
    - Peripheral edema
    - Jugular venous distention

- Monitor cardiac rhythms.
- Administer ordered preload and/or afterload reducers:
  - Diuretics
  - ACE inhibitors
- Monitor lung or pulmonary status, reporting new lung sounds, (e.g., wheezes, rhonchi).
- Auscultate lungs and monitor breath sounds.
- Obtain history, especially details relating to recent infections and/or radiation therapy.
- Administer ordered pain medications when needed.
- Provide comfort and reassurance to patient and family.
- Monitor for signs and symptoms of infection (e.g., fever, increased WBC) and notify health care provider if identified.

Concept Check

6. Which intervention is essential in the treatment of myocarditis?

A. Monitoring body temperature

B. Keeping the patient psychologically stimulated

C. Encouraging ambulation and activity

D. Keeping the patient sedated

Answer question

Patient Education

Education of patients can vary, depending on the degree of damage and long-term problems that are expected. When applicable, the health care provider may want to include:

- Education about rest as a primary intervention

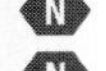

- Continuing gradual activity and exercise

- Educate about disease, symptoms that warrant seeking care, complications, adherence to medications, smoking cessation, weight management, and a healthy diet.

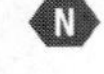

- Refer to patient education for heart failure as patients with long-term problems from myocarditis commonly have heart failure.

- Educate the patient about the potential for cardiac transplant.
- Educate the patient and family about advanced directives.

Summary of Interventions

- Evaluate cardiac status for signs and symptoms of dysrhythmias, cardiomyopathy, and heart failure.
- Institute treatment for cardiomyopathy and heart failure:
  - Preload reducers
  - Afterload reducers
  - Digitalis
- Comfort and reassure patient and patient's family.
- Appropriate therapy for any treatable etiology:
  - Toxic myocarditis: remove toxin, withhold offending medication.
  - Bacterial etiology: treat with appropriate antibiotic
- Educate the patient regarding issues of heart failure, its prevention, detection, lifestyle modifications to minimize exacerbations, long-term potential medical interventions, and advanced directives.

Concept Check

7. What therapy is appropriate for myocarditis that is caused by a specific medication?

A. Discontinue the medication

B. Half the dose of the medication

C. Administer antibiotics

D. Administer radiation therapy

Answer question

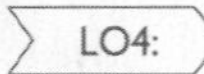

Evaluation of Desired Collaborative Care Outcomes

Evaluation and reassessment should reveal attainment of previously established patient outcomes. In summary:

- Patient is warm and dry, has clear mentation, and cardiac output hemodynamics have returned to pre-illness or optimally expected levels for their given stage of recovery.
- Patient's EKG reveals no continued cardiac damage and a normal sinus or stable rhythm.
- Patient reports no pain associated with this disease.
- Patient's blood pressure is stable and intake and output are balanced.
- Patient reports balancing rest with gradually increasing activities of daily living to return to a personal normal without dyspnea, chest pain, or excessive fatigue.
- Patient calmly discusses the disease process and treatment modalities.

References

Ginsberg, F. & Parrillo, J. E. (2013). Fulminant myocarditis. *Crit Care Clin, 29*(3), 465–483.

Khandaker, M. H., Espinosa, R. E., Nishimura, R. A., Sinak, L. J., Hayes, S. N., Melduni, R. M. & Oh, J. K. (2010). Pericardial disease: Diagnosis and management. *Mayo Clin Proceedings, 85*(6), 572–593.

Shammas, N. W., Padaria, R. F., & Coyne, E. P. (2013). Pericarditis, myocarditis, and other cardiomyopathies. *Prim Care, 40*(1), 213–236.

Shauer, A., Gotsman, I., Keren, A., Zwas, D. R., Hellman, Y., Durst, R., & Admon, D. (2013). Acute viral myocarditis: Current concepts in diagnosis and treatment. *Isr Med Assoc J, 15*(3), 180–185.

Simmons-Holcomb, S. (2006). Recognizing and managing different types of carditis. *Nursing, 36 Suppl Cardiac*, 4–9.

Clinical Practice Guidelines

Heart Failure Society of America, Lindenfeld, J., Albert, N. M., Boehmer, J. P. et al. (2010). Myocarditis: current treatment: HFSA 2010 comprehensive heart failure practice guideline. *J Care Fail, 16*(6), e176–e179.

Patient Education

Myocarditis Foundation. Discover Myocarditis Causes, Symptoms, Diagnosis, and Treatment. **www.myocarditisfoundation.org/about-myocarditis/**

STOP

Go to the online course and complete the NovE-Cases assigned by your instructor for this module.

Learning Outcomes for Vascular Diseases: Chronic Venous Insufficiency

When you complete this lesson, you will be able to:

1. Recognize the clinical relevance of chronic venous insufficiency.
2. Consider the pathophysiology, etiology, risk factors, and clinical presentation of chronic venous insufficiency that determine the priority patient concerns.
3. Determine the most urgent and important nursing interventions and patient education required in caring for a patient with chronic venous insufficiency.
4. Evaluate attainment of desired collaborative care outcomes for a patient with chronic venous insufficiency.

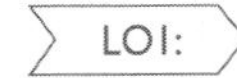

What Is Vascular Disease?

Vascular diseases involve any condition that affects the blood vessels and result in damage that reduces or blocks blood flow. These can be divided into arterial and venous diseases:

1. Arterial Diseases (see Arterial Disease NovE-lesson):
   - Peripheral Arterial Disease (PAD), also widely known as Peripheral Vascular Disease (PVD)
   - Carotid Artery Disease
   - Renal Artery Disease
   - Aortic Disease: Aneurysms
   - Cardiac Valvular Disorders (see CVD NovE-lesson)
2. Venous Diseases:
   - Venous Thromboembolism (VTE) (see VTE NovE-lesson)
   - Chronic Venous Insufficiency (CVI)

This NovE-lesson focuses on Chronic Venous Insufficiency.

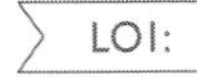

What Is Chronic Venous Insufficiency?

- Chronic venous insufficiency (CVI) occurs when the deep veins and the venous valves in the extremities (predominantly in the legs) no longer return blood effectively to the heart. The sluggish blood return creates pooling of blood, known as stasis.
- Typically, this results from chronic conditions that cause damage to the veins and valves.
- CVI is also called venous insufficiency, chronic peripheral venous insufficiency, and chronic venous disease (CVD).
- Peripheral vascular disease refers to vascular (*arterial*) conditions and is not used for venous-related conditions.

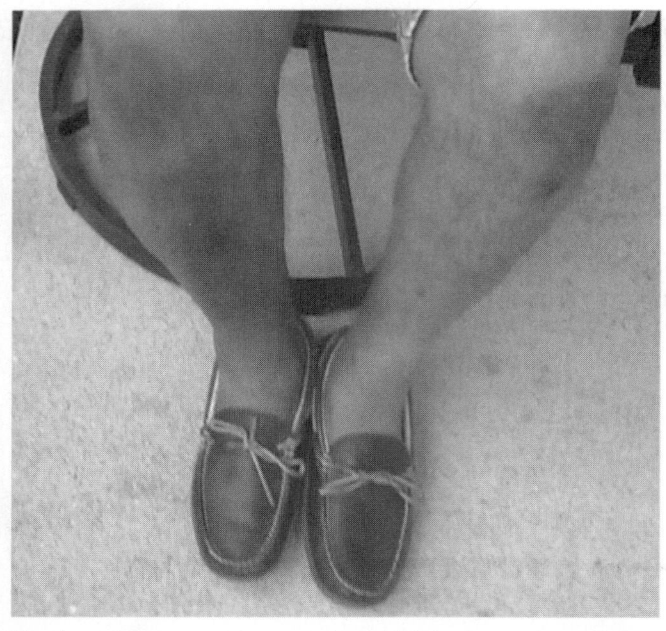

This photo shows a common presentation of CVI: hardening of the skin; constant lower limb swelling; and dark, bluish pigmentation (patient's left leg).
Source: Copyright © 2013, NovEx Novice to Expert Learning, LLC

LO1:

Clinical Relevance

- Vascular diseases are common. Venous disease is responsible for 30% of all vascular disease spending, projected to be $3 billion per year for CVI in the United States alone.
- Almost 24 million patients in the United States suffer from varicose veins and a half million from venous stasis–related ulcers.
- CVI affects quality of life, causing leg edema, pain, chronic ulceration, and infection. CVI also increases the risk for of deep vein thrombosis (DVT) and pulmonary embolism (PE).

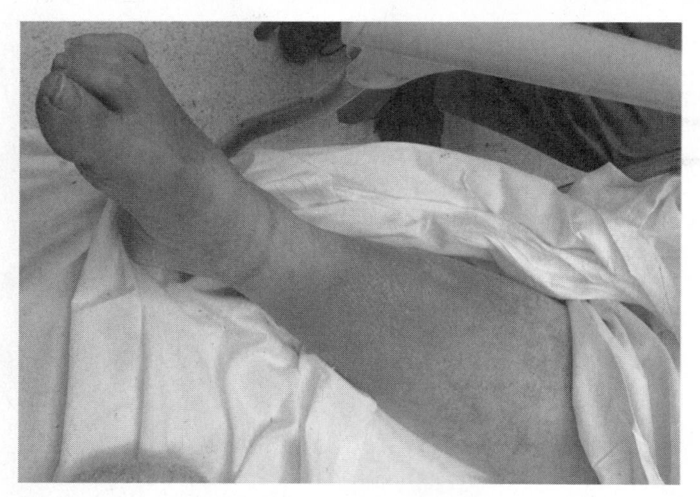

Chronic venous stasis is commonly accompanied by swelling, sensation changes, and painful ulcers that are difficult to heal. The poorly healing ulcers place the patient at high risk for infection, immobility, and reduced quality of life. This photo illustrates the progressive problems. Note the healing ulcer above the ankle.
Source: Courtesy of K. Kyriakidis

Concept Check

1. **What is the best description of chronic venous insufficiency?**
   A. Lack of blood flow to the legs
   B. Pooling of blood in the extremities
   C. Clotting of blood in the veins
   D. Peripheral vascular disease

Answer question

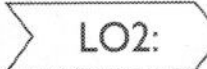

Pathophysiology

- Veins are thin-walled vessels. Pressure exerted by blood within the veins is low compared to the arteries.
- Blood returns to the heart through the veins and a series of one-way valves that allow blood to flow only toward the heart.
- Calf and leg muscle contractions that occur through activity provide the force to push the blood forward.
- When the valves are damaged, gravity plays a more significant role by impairing the return of blood and raising hydrostatic pressure. Slowing of blood flow causes venous stasis or blood pooling in dependent areas such as the legs.
- The increased hydrostatic pressure results in numerous significant pathophysiologic changes.

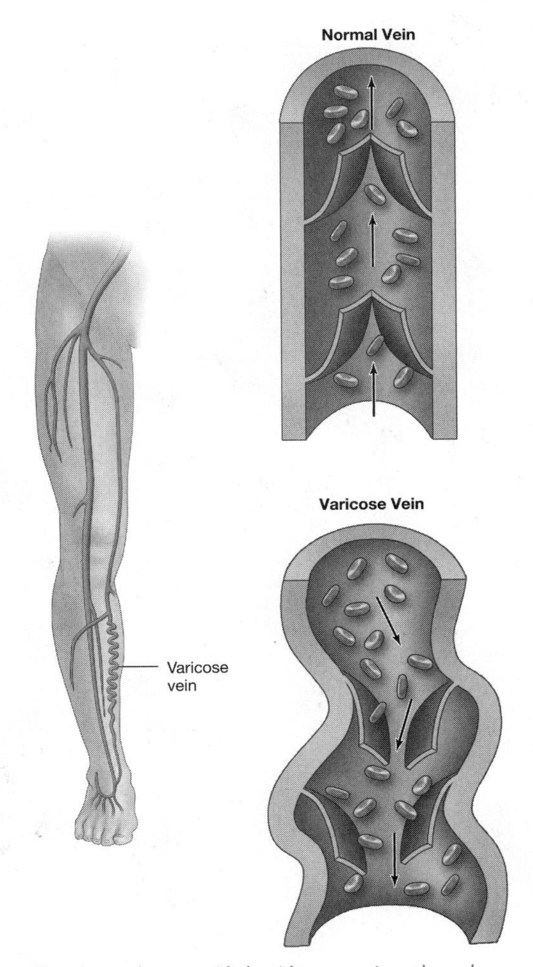

The picture features side by side cut sections through venous valves. The upper image demonstrates elements of normal venous function and blood flow. The lower image reveals faulty or incompetent valves resulting in venous insufficiency, bulging veins, and backflow of blood.

- Venous stasis from CVI can lead to deep vein thrombosis (DVT) but, conversely, a DVT can be the cause of CVI.
- When a DVT develops and blocks a large vein, it places pressure on venous walls and valves, damaging them over time. The valves no longer function to prevent backward blood flow through the veins. Varicose veins can be one result.

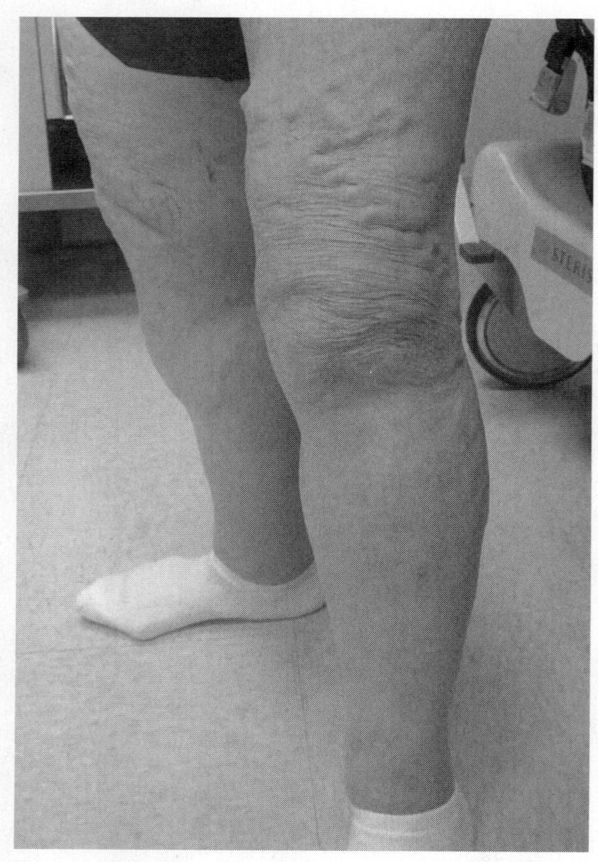

The patient has severe varicose veins that are most prominent in her left leg, particularly above the knee. The patient has disseminated telangiectasis or purplish spider veins on both legs, but they are most visible on the right inner thigh.

Source: Copyright © 2013, NovEx Novice to Expert Learning, LLC

Pathophysiology (continued)

The major pathophysiological changes that occur include:

- Telangiectasias are very small cutaneous venules that dilate and appear as short purplish spider web lines or webs on the skin.
- Varicosities are superficial veins that become distended and tortuous, and can be painful.
- Increased hydrostatic pressure in the capillaries causes leakage of fluid and RBCs into the tissue.
- Leg edema is caused by leakage of fluid from the capillaries into the surrounding tissue. Eventually, the lymphatic system becomes overwhelmed and cannot remove or alleviate the edema buildup.

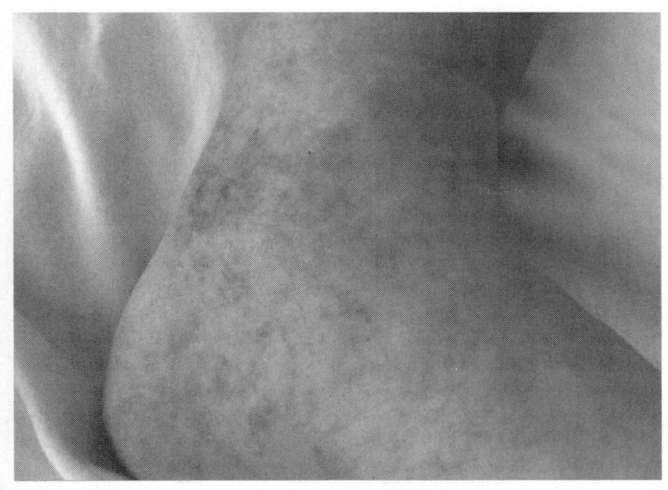

A close-up view of an ankle in a patient with CVI reveals spider veins or telangiectasias. These develop in affect many areas but often occur on the lower extremities. These small widened blood vessels are not typically painful even though they are disfiguring.

- Leakage of RBCs from the damaged capillaries results in hemosiderin deposition in the skin, resulting in a brownish blue hyperpigmentation.
- Stasis dermatitis can also develop, characterized by erythema, dry skin, pruritus, and crusting and is sometimes confused with cellulitis.
- Ulcerations commonly occur on the medial side of the ankle or over a vein.
- Lipodermatosclerosis is the development of inflammation of the subcutaneous fat.
- Patients with CVI become prone to development of cellulitis.

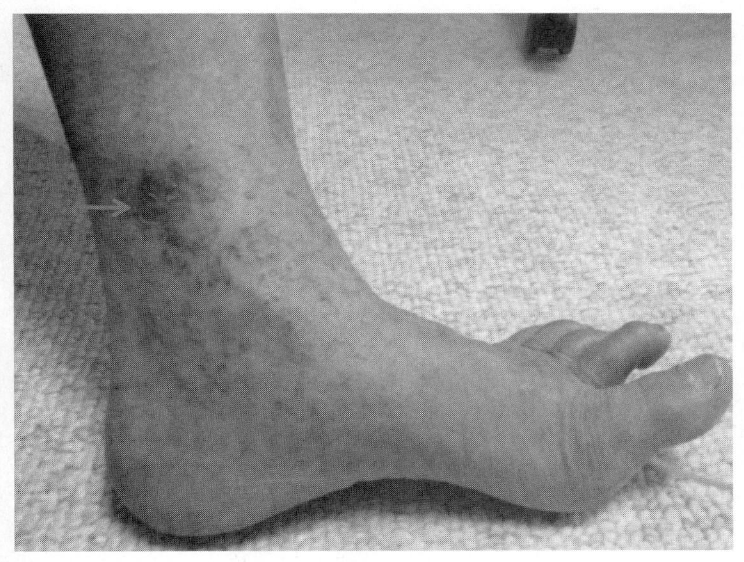

A patient with CVI shows signs of developing a venous stasis ulcer above the inner ankle. Some ulcers can be more severe.

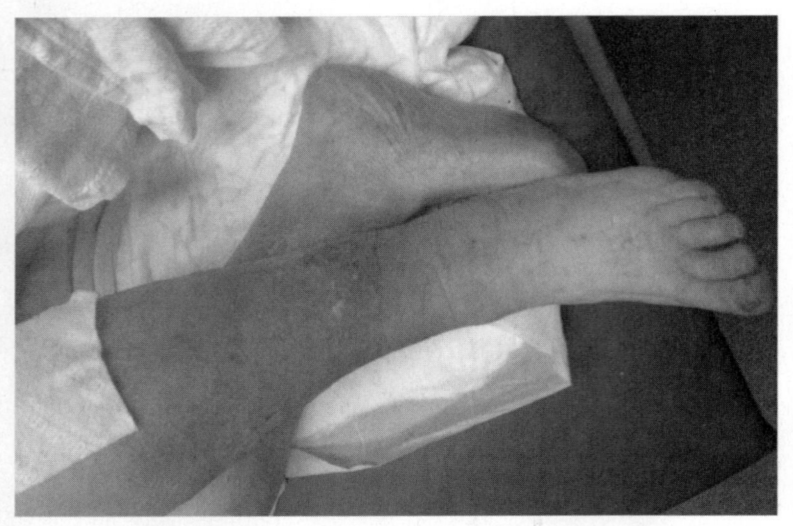

CVI is more severe in this patient's legs. The photo illuminates a cellulitis, which is a common complication.
Source: Courtesy of K. Kyriakidis

Concept Check

2. What findings are common with varicosities?

A. They are deep veins.
B. They are distended.
C. They look like spider webs.
D. They are short, thin lines.

Answer question

Concept Check

3. Where are telangiectasias most commonly located?

A. Lower extremities
B. Abdomen
C. Upper extremities
D. Neck

Answer question

Risk Factors

- Age greater than 50
- History of DVT
- Female gender, due to the close association with pregnancy
- Obesity
- Pregnancy
- Smoking
- Genetic predisposition
- Standing or sitting for long periods without activity

Concept Check

4. Which patients are at higher risk for chronic venous insufficiency?

A. Males
B. People who are obese
C. People who drink alcohol
D. People who are over 35

Answer question

Causes

- Deep venous thrombosis is the most common cause of severe CVI.
- Congenitally weak vein walls or abnormal or absent valves
- Pregnancy
- Trauma

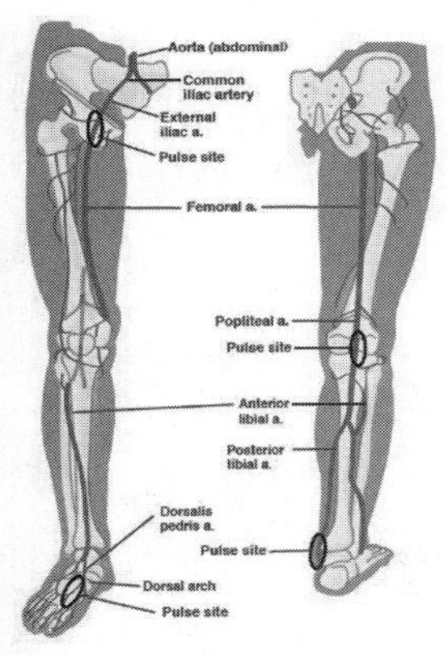

The illustrations depict the names of the veins and the locations in the lower extremity that is most often involved in the formation of deep vein thromboses.
Source: Copyright © 2013, NovEx Novice to Expert Learning, LLC

Assessment Findings

- Aching, burning, cramping, or throbbing pain
- Telangiectasias and/or varicose veins
- Skin changes can include:
  - o Brownish blue hyperpigmentation
  - o Stasis dermatitis (e.g., erythema, pruritus, crusting)
  - o Ulcerations, commonly on the medial side of ankle or over a vein
  - o Ulcers usually pink or red with irregular borders
  - o Lipodermatosclerosis—thickened and hardened skin
  - o Cellulitis (e.g., erythema, induration, fever)

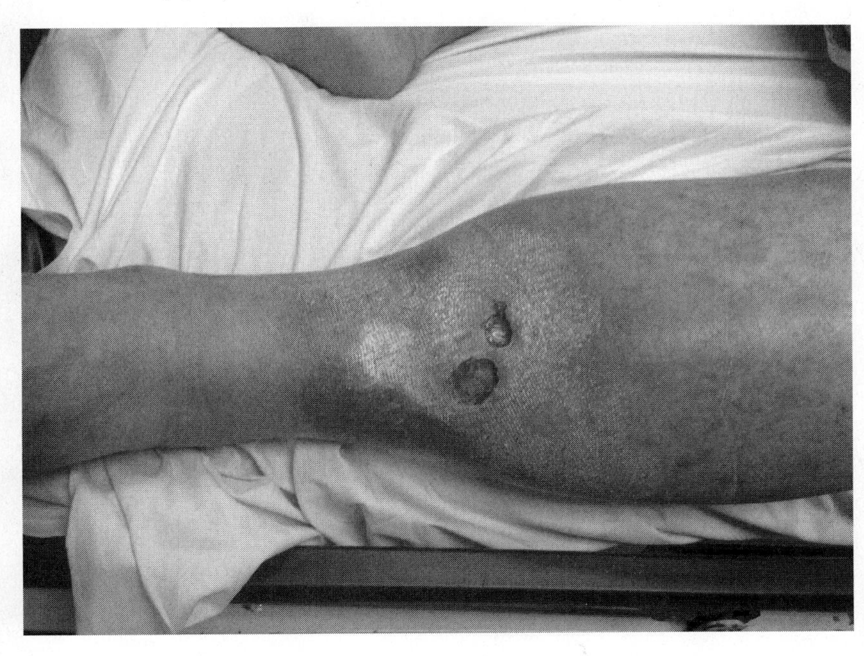

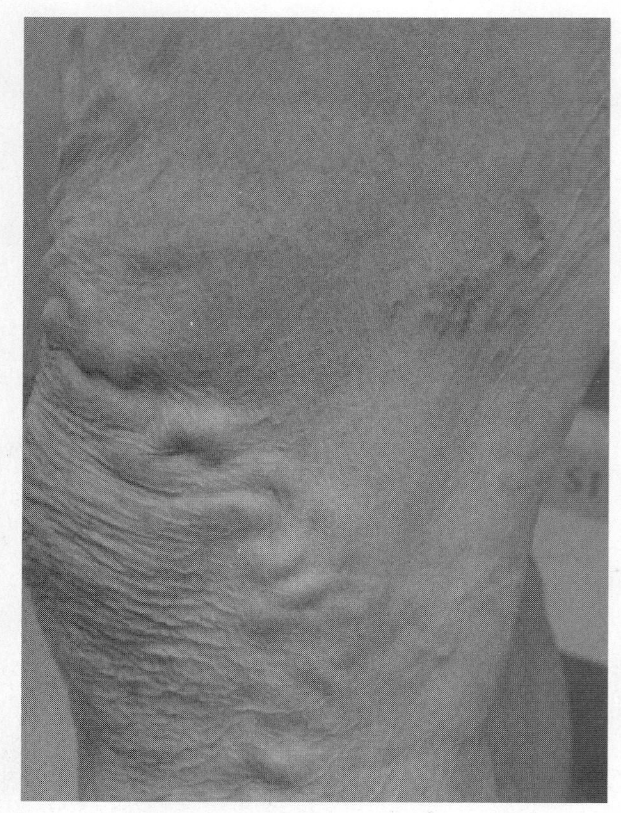

Upper: This photo reveals an ulceration and cellulitis. Note that this patient demonstrates every skin change listed above. Leg edema can also be observed. Lower: A close-up photo of severe varicose veins makes the venous pooling in the tortuous, distended veins visible.
Source: (*upper*) Courtesy of K. Kyriakidis; (*lower*) Copyright © 2013, NovEx Novice to Expert Learning, LLC

- Leg edema may be accompanied by fluid leaking from the skin (weeping). This can happen in one or both legs.
- Heaviness or leg fatigue
- Pulses, unless associated with PAD, as pulses help differentiate CVI from PAD
- Restless legs
- Pain of CVI is often relieved by walking, elevating the legs, or the use of compression stockings (opposite of PAD).

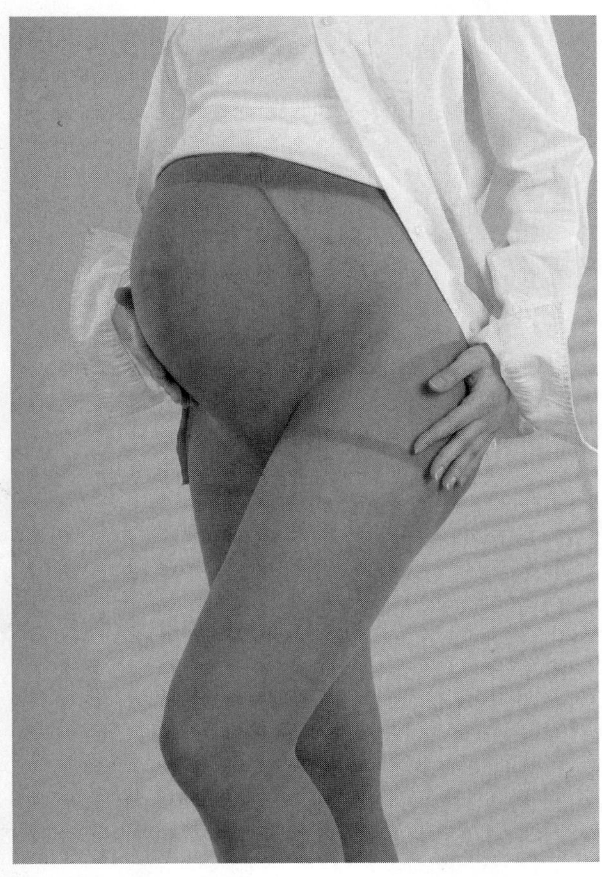

The elastic components of this maternity elastic stocking produces graduated pressure that increases distally so that the greatest compression occurs in the feet and lower part of the extremity, less on the thigh, and still less on the lower abdomen.
Source: Fotoskat/Fotolia

Concept Check

5. A patient has lipodermatosclerosis by history. Which finding will be present on exam?
   A. Ulcers with red or pink borders
   B. Hardened skin
   C. Blue hyperpigmentation
   D. Crusting on the skin

Answer question

Diagnostics

- Diagnosis of CVI is primarily based on signs and symptoms found on physical examination.
- CVI may be confirmed through imaging: Venous duplex ultrasound (see upper photo) may reveal evidence of previous or acute deep venous thrombosis and incompetence of the venous valves.

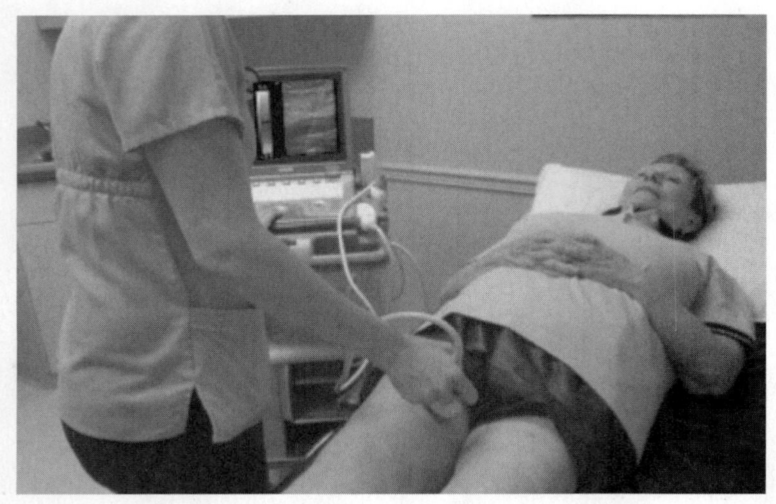

Ultrasound imaging is commonly performed using venous duplex to noninvasively diagnose thombotic occlusions from CVI.

Priority Patient Concerns and Desired Collaborative Care Outcomes

Prior to caring for patients with chronic venous insufficiency, it is important to prioritize the patient's concerns that must guide the nursing care plan and interventions. Care for the patient is ordered and organized in accordance with the patient's priority and urgent needs. Desired collaborative care outcomes in patients with chronic venous insufficiency typically include:

1. Patient will have gradual, progressive healing toward intact skin.
2. Patient will have minimal edema with gradual but progressive healing and intact tissues.
3. Patient will accurately discuss prevention of further breakdown and treatment modalities.
4. Patient will report decreased pain.
5. Patient will demonstrate care of their body to remain infection-free.

Considering these important care outcomes, prepare a list of the major 3–6 priority patient concerns or nursing diagnoses for patients with chronic venous insufficiency. Be prepared to participate in a discussion of this list and/or to submit them as an assignment, as determined by your faculty. Resources you may find helpful in this assignment can include this lesson, the references, resources on nursing care plans, and standard nursing diagnoses manuals.

Concept Check

6. Which intervention may relieve leg pain associated with CVI?

A. Placing the legs in a dependent position
B. Assisting the patient to ambulate
C. Removing constrictive stockings
D. Applying hot compresses

Answer question

LO3:

Collaborative Interventions

Evidence-Based Practice

The goal of treatment for CVI focuses on decreasing lower extremity edema, alleviating symptoms, and healing ulcers. The following measures are beneficial:

- Increasing activity and performing ankle flexion exercises

- Use of graduated compression stockings helps with edema. These should be put on in the morning before edema worsens.

- Frequent leg elevation, movement, and sleeping with legs slightly elevated help reduce edema and promote ulcer healing.
- Treatment of stasis dermatitis with topical agents helps alleviate dry skin and pruritus.
- Treatment of cellulitis with antibiotics and leg elevation is beneficial. EBP does not support the use of compression in patients with cellulitis.
- Ulceration is commonly difficult to treat because the ulcerated areas require circulation for healing. Patients are commonly treated in the clinic setting. Although evidence is not strong and effective treatment depends on the type, size, and location of the ulcer, current recommendations include:
  - Collaborate with a wound specialist to help evaluate and individualize care.
  - Wound debridement is essential when indicated.
  - Elevate the legs above the heart level at least 30 minutes 3–4 times a day.
  - Simple exercise like walking or ankle flexion can improve extremity hemodynamics.
  - Consider administration of aspirin which has been shown to accelerate healing.
  - Culture the ulcer and administer antibiotics as indicated.
  - Cleanse and dress the wound. Medicated compression bandaging may be indicated.
  - Continuous compression therapy when pulses are present. Research shows it has improved healing by 97%.
  - Consider intermittent pneumatic compression with resistant edema and nonhealing ulcers.
  - Apply barrier cream, escin (horse chestnut seed extract), or topical corticosteroid with venous stasis dermatitis.
- Monitor patients with cellulitis and ulceration carefully for any signs of sepsis. They are at increased risk for systemic inflammatory response.
- Pentoxifylline and aspirin help with microcirculation and healing of leg ulcers.
- Additional therapies are implemented but, to date, research has shown them to be ineffective: hyperbaric oxygen therapy, therapeutic ultrasound, and electromagnetic therapy.

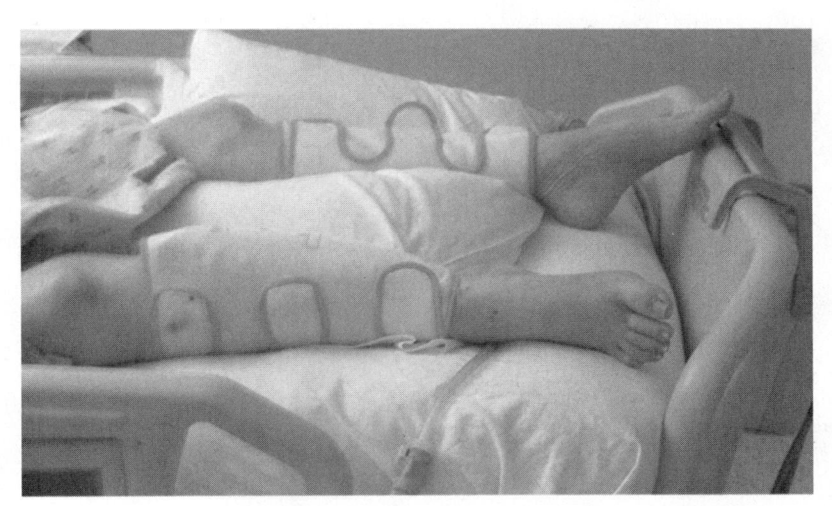

This photo demonstrates a patient whose lower extremities have bilateral compression devices applied.
Source: Courtesy of K. Kyriakidis

Concept Check

7. **Which standard treatment is used for cellulitis resulting from chronic venous insufficiency?**
   A. Antibiotics
   B. Strict bed rest
   C. Head of bed elevation
   D. Compression

Answer question

Collaborative Interventions (continued)

Surgical Management

- Surgery for superficial veins consists primarily of ablation and helps with cosmetic appearance and pain.
- Deep venous insufficiency has no clearly effective treatment. Valvuloplasty may be attempted, but is associated with a high incidence of postoperative deep venous thrombosis (DVT). Venous bypass surgery may be attempted as well, but is not considered to be standard of care.
- Postoperative (postop) care includes the interventions that all postop patients receive (e.g., fluid and electrolye balance, pulmonary support, vital signs monitoring, nausea and vomiting management, bowel and bladder management, prevention of never events, emotional support, infection control measures). Care of patients after vascular surgery includes:
  - o Collaborate with patient to manage pain.
  - o Wound care at multiple sites to prevent infection, careful inspection of wounds to detect poor wound healing or infection early
  - o Apply pressure dressings. Educate patient and family about how to apply the pressure dressings in those who must have them for 6 weeks postop.
  - o Elevate affected extremity to minimize postop edema.
  - o Gradually begin and increase mobility and ambulation.
  - o Avoid long periods of standing or sitting with legs dependent.

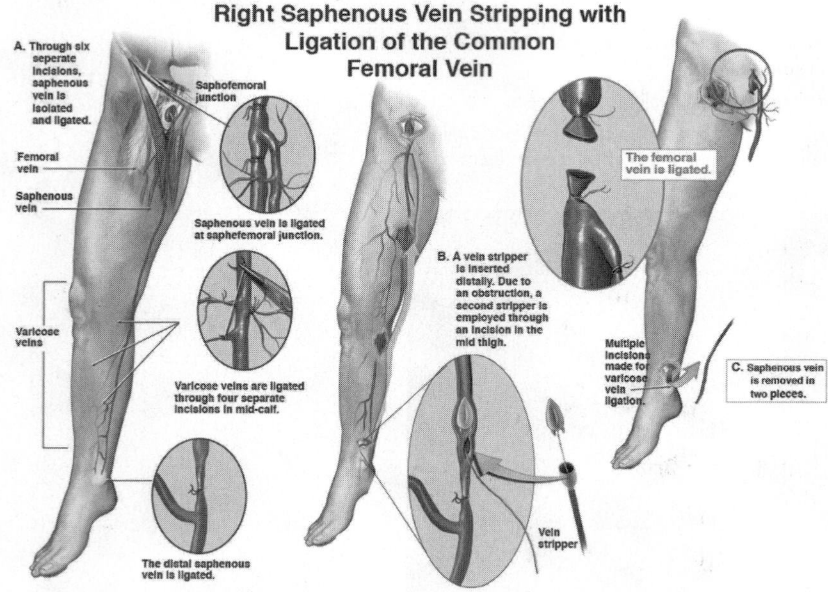

Varicose veins of the lower extremity are treated with surgical isolation and ligation of the femoral vein followed by insertion of a stripper device and stripping or removing the veins in the lower leg.

Patient Education

- Instruct patients that compression stockings may reduce swelling, if severe. These do not include the antiembolism knee or thigh high stockings used in the hospital to prevent DVT, which are ineffective in CVI. Effective stockings must exert at least 20–30 mmHg pressure at the ankle. Specific instructions are provided when purchased regarding care of the extremity, care of the stockings, application, avoidance of wrinkles, and maintenance.
- Collaborate with physician and wound care specialist to educate the patient regarding the specific care prescribed (e.g., skin care, emollients, barrier creams, topical corticosteroids, dressings).
- Elevate the legs higher than the heart level for at least 30 minutes 3–4 times per pay.
- Avoid sitting or standing for long periods. During travel, stop and take a walk every hour.
- Walk daily and/or perform ankle flexion exercises to improve circulation. Over 35% of patients with CVI do not walk 10 minutes once a week.

- Avoid wearing restrictive clothing that hinders blood flow from any part of the lower body or an extremity.
- Smoking cessation can improve overall health in addition to circulation
- Replace meals with a healthier diet.
- Attaining a healthy body weight can improve cardiovascular performance.
- Collaborate with health care provider to carefully manage comorbid conditions that can exacerbate CVI and its complications.
- Instruct about good foot and leg care: keep clean and dry, use warm water and mild soap, pat skin dry, use moisturizer, wear comfortable shoes and cotton socks, prevent accidental foot and leg injuries, and inspect feet and legs daily.
- Avoid sitting with crossed legs or legs in a dependent position. Change positions often to avoid blood pooling in the extremities.
- Adherence to the full antibiotic course should be emphasized when treating for cellulitis.

Summary of Interventions

- Reduce leg edema.
- Reduce sitting or standing.
- Elevate legs.
- Wear compression stockings when prescribed.
- Increase activity.
- Treat ulcers and cellulitis with topical agents and antibiotics when indicated.
- Utilize intermittent pneumatic compression in severe CVI
- Stripping of varicose veins, if needed
- Educate the patient regarding disease, lifestyle modifications, wound and leg care, and prevention measures.

LO4:

Evaluation of Desired Collaborative Care Outcomes

Evaluation and reassessment should reveal attainment of previously established patient outcomes. In summary:

- Patient has progressively healing wounds or intact skin over both lower extremities.
- Patient's tissues are progressively healing, less edematous, or are intact.
- Patient actively participates in treatment and describes taking preventative measures such as elevating feet, eating a more healthy diet, avoiding constrictive clothing, and participating in an exercise routine.
- Patient reports that pain in extremities has decreased.
- Patient or family demonstrates care of the patient's body, knows signs of infection, and has no untreated signs of infection.

References

Allen, L. (2009). Assessment and management of patients with varicose veins. *Nurs Stand, 23*(23), 49–57.

González-Consuegra, R. V., & Verdú, J. (2011). Quality of life in people with venous leg ulcers: an integrative review. *J Adv Nurs, 67*(5), 926–944.

Huang, T. W., Chen, S. L., Bai, C. H., Wu, C. H., & Tam, K. W. (2013). The optimal duration of compression therapy following varicose vein surgery: a meta-analysis of randomized controlled trials. *Eur J Vasc Endovasc Surg, 45*(4), 397–402.

Menon, J. (2012). Managing exudate associated with venous leg ulceration. *Br J Community Nurs, 17*(Suppl 4), S6–S16.

O'Meara, S., Cullum, N., Nelson, E. A., & Dumville, J. C. (2012). Compression for venous leg ulcers. *Cochrane Database Syst Rev, 11*, CD000265.

Sadick, N. S. (2005). Advances in the treatment of varicose veins: ambulatory phlebectomy, foam sclerotherapy, endovascular laser, and radiofrequency closure. *Dermatol Clin, 23*(3), 443–55, vi.

Simms, K. W., & Ennen, K. (2011). Lower extremity ulcer management: best practice algorithm. *J Clin Nurs, 20*(1–2), 86–93.

Clinical Practice Guidelines

Herschthal, J., & Kirsner, R. S. (2008). Current management of venous ulcers: an evidence-based review. *Surg Technol Int, 17*, 77.

Nicolaides, A. N., Allegra, C., Bergan, J., Bradbury, A., Cairols, M., Carpentier, P., et al. (2008). Management of chronic venous disorders of the lower limbs: Guidelines according to scientific evidence. *International Angiology, 27*(1), 1–59.

Patient Education

Medline Plus. Varicose Veins. **http://www.nlm.nih.gov/medlineplus/varicoseveins.html**

Merrigan, J. M., Hamdan, A., Lynm, C., & Livingston, E. H. (2012). Varicose veins. *JAMA, 308*(24), 2638.

Learning Outcomes for Vascular Diseases: Arterial Vascular Diseases

When you complete this lesson, you will be able to:

1. Recognize the clinical relevance of arterial vascular diseases.
2. Consider the pathophysiology, etiology, risk factors, and clinical presentation of arterial vascular diseases that determine the priority patient concerns.
3. Determine the most urgent and important nursing interventions and patient education required in caring for a patient with arterial vascular diseases.
4. Evaluate attainment of desired collaborative care outcomes for a patient with arterial vascular diseases.

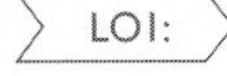

What Is Vascular Disease?

Vascular diseases involve any condition that affects the blood vessels and result in damage that reduces or blocks blood flow. These can be divided into arterial and venous diseases:

1. Arterial Diseases:
   - Peripheral Arterial Disease (PAD), also widely known as Peripheral Vascular Disease (PVD)
   - Carotid Artery Disease
   - Renal Artery Disease
   - Aortic Disease: Aneurysms
   - Cardiac Valvular Disorders (see CVD NovE-lesson)
2. Venous Diseases (see VTE and CVI NovE-lessons):
   - Venous Thromboembolism (VTE)
   - Chronic Venous Insufficiency (CVI)

This NovE-lesson focuses on Arterial Vascular Diseases.

What Are Arterial Diseases?

- Unlike venous diseases, the arterial diseases share many commonalities and can be understood as a group.
- The most common cause of all arterial diseases is atherosclerosis.
- Therefore, the pathophysiology, causes, and risk factors for peripheral arterial disease, carotid artery disease, renal artery disease, and aneurysms are similar. Treatment is usually related to risk factor modifications and achieving reperfusion.

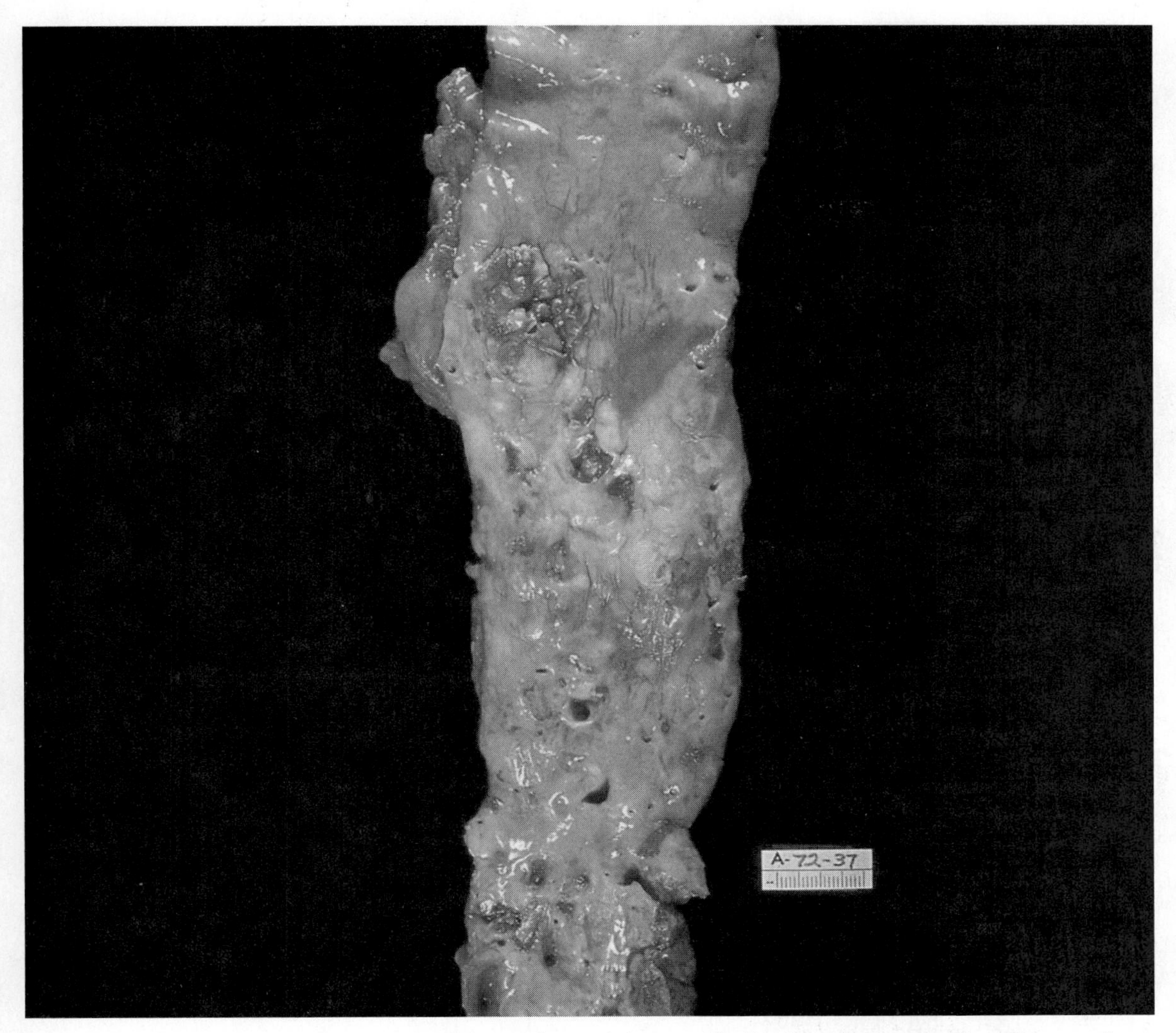

This is an autopsy specimen displaying severe atherosclerotic changes in the aorta. The blood vessel wall is normally reddish, not yellow.
Source: CDC.gov/Dr. Edwin P. Ewing, Jr.

What Is Peripheral Arterial Disease?

Peripheral arterial diseases (PAD) are the diseases that result in narrowing or occlusion of the peripheral arteries.

PAD is also commonly known as peripheral vascular disease (PVD) and peripheral arterial occlusive disease (PAOD).

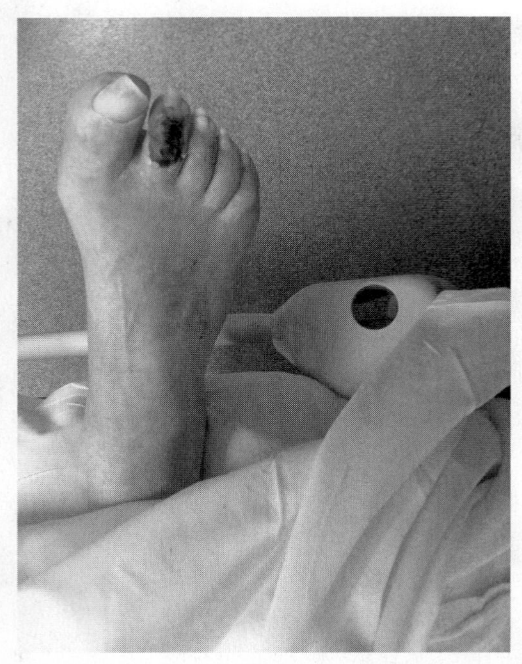

This patient has an infected and necrotic lesion on the second toe caused by PAD. This condition results from inadequate blood flow through the leg. The underlying cause is often narrowing of blood vessels due to fatty deposits (atherosclerosis), although other conditions can produce similar symptoms. Lack of blood produces pain or aching after walking, and encourages the development of leg ulcers. Without effective and immediate intervention, the gangrene in this patient's toe can spread to the foot and results in high risk for sepsis.
Source: Courtesy of K. Kyriakidis

Concept Check

1. **What is the most common cause of arterial vascular disease?**
   - A. Trauma
   - B. Atherosclerosis
   - C. Illegal drug use
   - D. Hypotension

Answer question

LO1:

Clinical Relevance: PAD

- Symptoms of PAD can significantly affect quality of life by interfering with the capacity to walk.
- PAD has numerous complications, including poor wound healing and development of gangrene that can result in limb amputations.
- The presence of PAD is closely correlated with other vascular diseases such as coronary artery disease, hypertension, ischemic stroke, and renal artery stenosis. This places PAD in the highest health risk category.
- A total of $4.5 billion per year is spent on PAD-related treatment in the United States. ([2008]. *Vasc Med, 13*(3), 209–215.)
- Prevalence of PAD/PVD affects 8 million people in the United States.

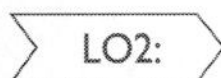

Pathophysiology: PAD

- PAD is primarily the result of atherosclerosis (see animation).
- An *atheroma* is a plaque that builds up inside the vessel wall and consists of a core of cholesterol covered by proteins with a fibrous intravascular outer layer. This buildup leads to narrowing of the arteries and eventually results in ischemia of the involved extremity or affected area (see illustration).
- When activity occurs, the increased demand for blood flow to the muscles cannot be met due to impaired arterial flow, causing pain and cramping. Once activity stops, the pain slowly resolves as the muscular metabolic demands drop. This is known as intermittent claudication.

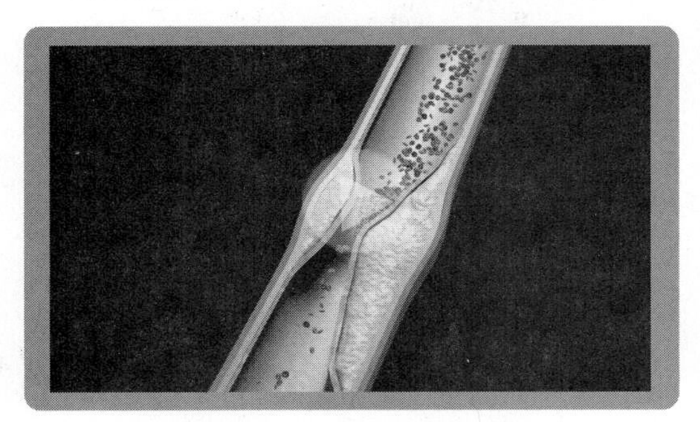

This 3D medical animation depicts an artery blocked by atherosclerotic plaque, occurring over time.

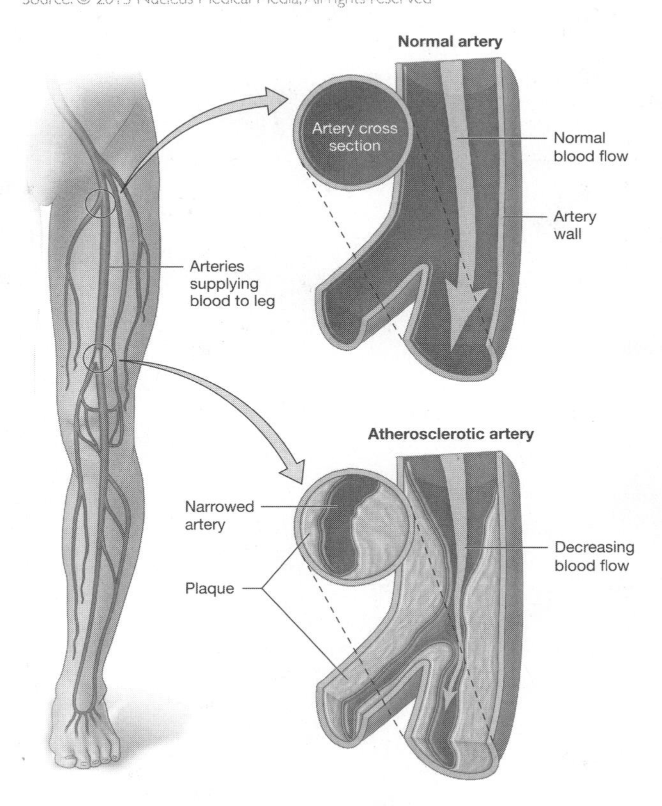

This is an illustration of a normal artery and an atherosclerotic artery with decreased blood flow.

- Severe vascular occlusion may eventually progress to the point that ischemia is present at rest.
- Further narrowing can eventually lead to complete occlusion of medium and large arteries. When this occurs gradually, collateral (extra) blood vessels can develop to supply blood to compromised areas.
- Atherosclerosis usually progresses over a prolonged period of time; however, formation of clot or embolism in a peripheral artery may cause a sudden occlusion.

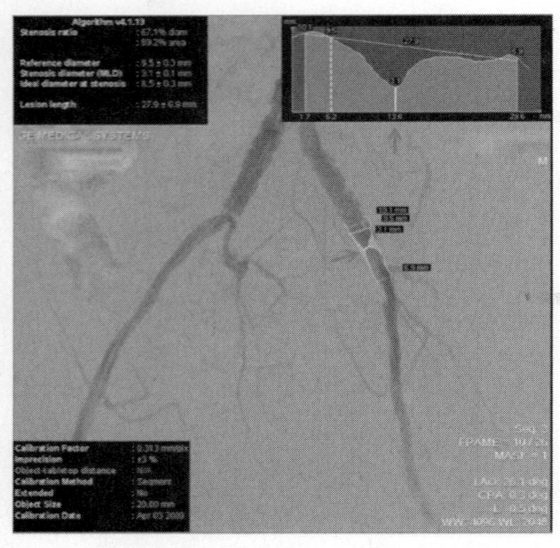

An occlusion can be seen in the popliteal artery, and the blood flow to the lower leg is obstructed. An inset also appears showing the site of the occlusion in greater detail.
Source: Courtesy of K. Kyriakidis

Acute Arterial Occlusion

- Acute occlusion can occur when a thrombus, an embolus, or an acute trauma jeopardizes perfusion. Predisposing factors for thrombus formation include sepsis, hypotension, and low cardiac output.
- An embolism may originate in the heart, aorta, or peripheral artery and lodges in an artery. Emboli are most often from a cardiac origin (80%) and tend to lodge at artery bifurcations where the vessels narrow.
- An embolus is the most common cause of sudden ischemia and is a medical emergency since it may result in development of tissue necrosis (gangrene).
- The site of the occlusion, presence of collateral circulation, and type of occlusion (thrombus or emboli) determine the severity of the acute event.

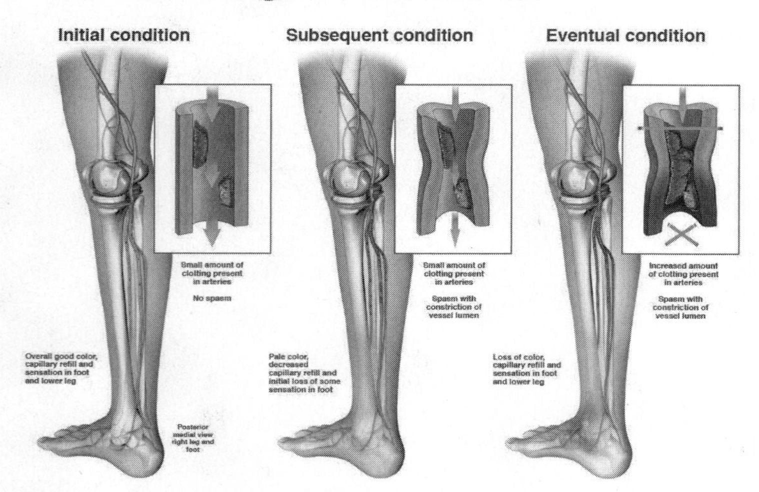

This series of images show how clotting and vasospasms can cause a gradual worsening of condition over time. The overall views allow us to show color changes to the foot with text noting the slowing of capillary refill and loss of sensation. The enlarged cutaway views reveal the actual areas of thrombosis within the arteries and the spasm with constriction of the muscular walls.
Source: © 2013 Nucleus Medical Media, All rights reserved

Risk Factors: PAD

Risk factors are similar to those associated with the development of CAD, cerebrovascular disease, renal artery disease, and aneurysms:

- High blood cholesterol levels
- Diabetes
- Insulin resistance
- Smoking
- Hypertension
- Obesity
- Inactivity
- Age
- Family history
- Sleep apnea
- Alcohol

Emerging risk factors:

- High levels of C-reactive protein (CRP)
- Elevated triglycerides (fats)

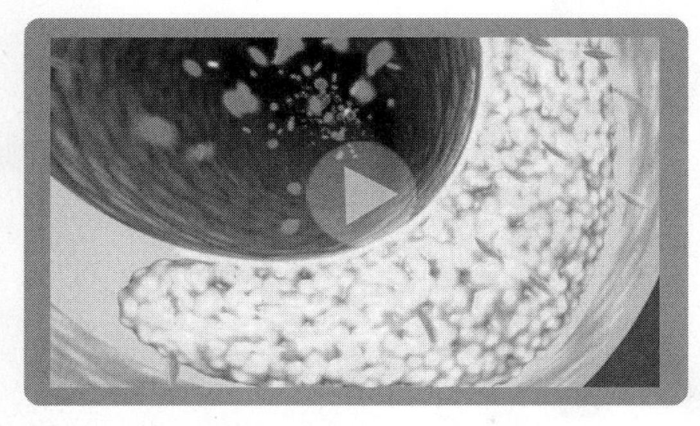

This animation demonstrates buildup of plaque in an arterial wall, eventually blocking the blood flow. Cholesterol is seen entering the arterial wall. Monocytes then enter and form foam cells. Smooth muscle cells then migrate into the atheromatous plaque.
Source: © 2013 Nucleus Medical Media. All rights reserved

Causes: PAD

Atherosclerosis (atherosclerotic plaques or atheromas) is the most common cause of peripheral vascular disease.

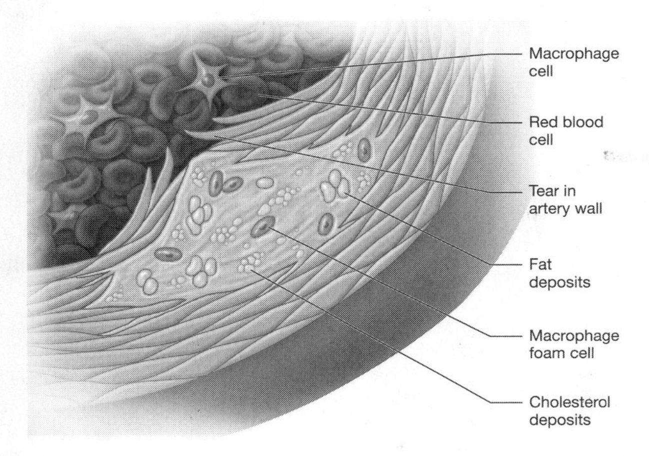

A blood clot begins to form after the fibrous cap on the fatty plaque ruptures.

Other causes of PAD/PVD include:

- Raynaud's phenomenon or disease: Spasms of the small arteries of the hands and feet precipitated by exposure to cold, causing paresthesias, numbness, and pain in the fingers or toes, which may also be cold and white.
- Buerger's disease: Inflammation and thrombosis affect the medium-sized arteries, veins, and nerves. The progressive blockage causes pain and ischemia to the hands and feet. This disease has a strong association with tobacco use.
- Other vascular inflammatory disorders, such as giant cell arteritis.

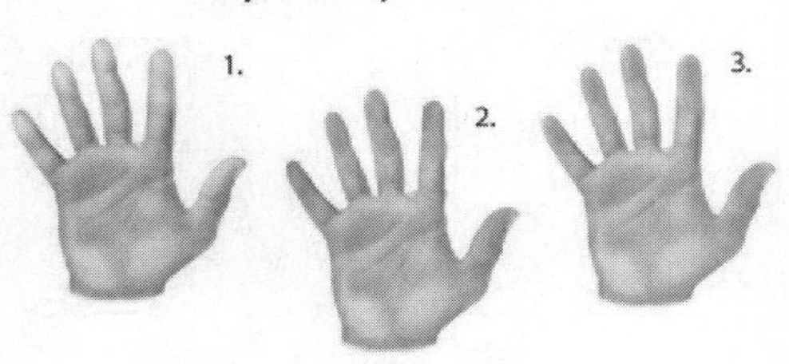
Raynaud's phenomenon
1.
2.
3.
Fingers become white due to the lack of blood flow, then blue as vessels dilate to keep blood in tissues, finally red as blood flow returns

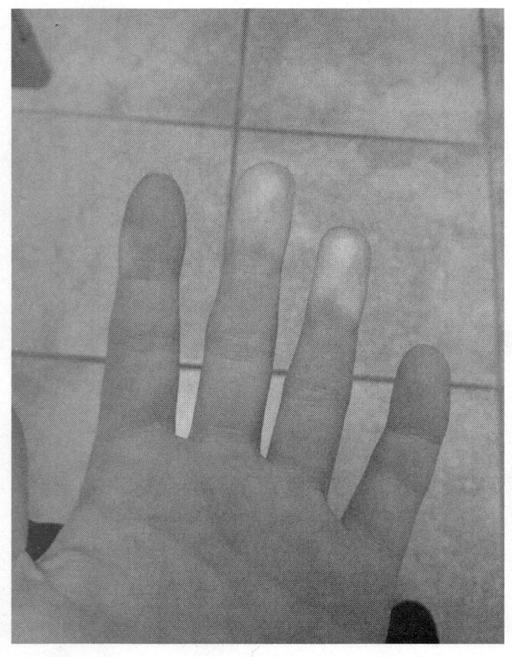

Left: Vasospasm of Raynaud's disease causes such strong vasoconstriction that it cuts off blood flow. The finger tips turn pale, cold, and some pain is experienced. Patients can learn to avoid precipitating factors. Right: Physical exam findings are demonstrated in Raynaud's disease.

Concept Check

2. What area of the body does Raynaud's phenomenon typically affect?

A. Trunk

B. Ears

C. Legs

D. Feet

Answer question

Assessment Findings: PAD

Signs and symptoms are related to decreased perfusion of the limbs. The severity depends on the extent of occlusion of the blood vessels.

- Claudication or intermittent claudication is the development of pain or cramping in the extremities with ambulation, resulting from limb ischemia. It starts upon ambulation and does not improve until the patient stops walking.
- Ischemic rest pain: Pain from ischemia at rest occurs from progressive occlusion of the peripheral artery.
- Nail and skin changes
- Decreased pulses
- Bruits
- Cool extremities
- Limb pallor or cyanosis
- Numbness
- Possibly asymptomatic in the early stages

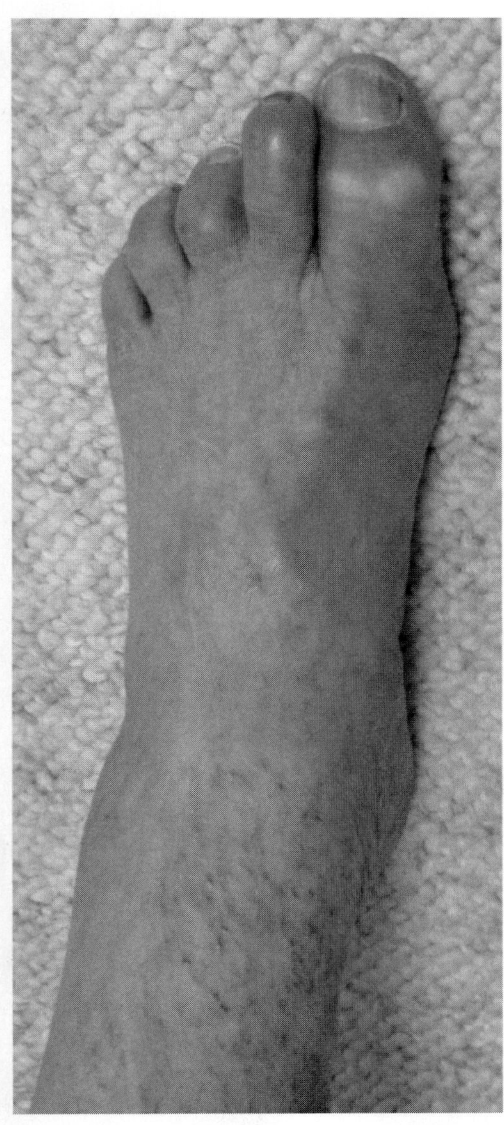

The effects of arterial disease are noted in the patient's thick and brittle nails, shiny skin, areas of pallor, and cyanosis (purplish hue) of the toes. Most striking is the reddish discoloration (rubor) that indicates significant hypoperfusion and hypoxemia when the legs are dependent. This patient also has signs of chronic venous insufficiency as a complicating factor.

As the PAD worsens, more serious signs and symptoms develop:

- Poor wound healing
- Paresthesias: abnormal sensation (e.g., burning, itching, tingling, prickling)
- Ulceration: This typically occurs on the feet: tips of the toes, between toes, bony protuberances, and heals of the foot.
- Pulseless extremity
- Gangrene: Necrotic tissue that develops from persistent ischemia. It is commonly seen in the distal toes but can affect an entire limb.

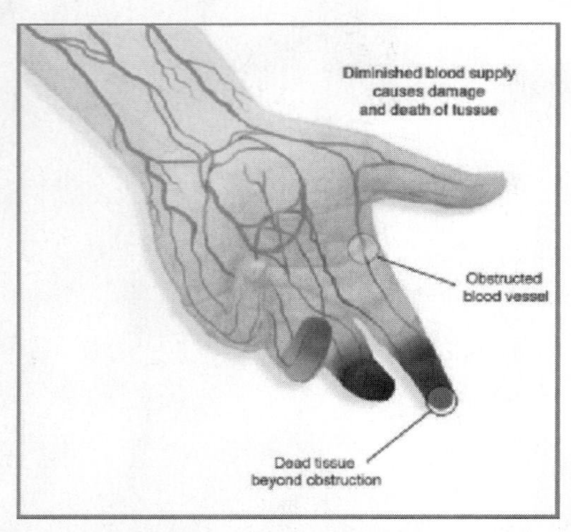
Diminished blood supply
causes damage
and death of tissue
Obstructed
blood vessel
Dead tissue
beyond obstruction

Arterial occlusion can occur in the fingers or hand, causing patients to lose their digits to gangrene and amputation.
Source: Copyright © 2013, NovEx Novice to Expert Learning, LLC

Amputation Procedure for Gangrene of Distal Left Foot

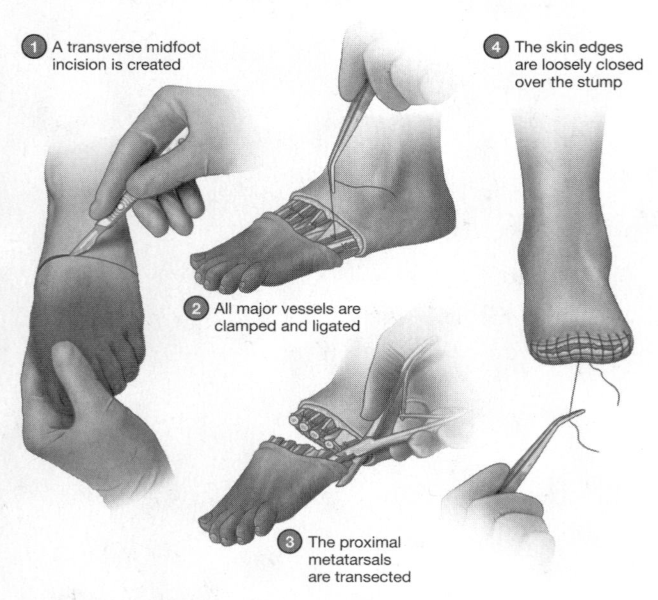
1 A transverse midfoot incision is created
2 All major vessels are clamped and ligated
3 The proximal metatarsals are transected
4 The skin edges are loosely closed over the stump

This series of illustrations shows gangrene in the distal portion of the foot with a midfoot amputation. It is hoped that circulation to the midfoot area is sufficient for the wound to heal without the need for further amputation.

Concept Check

3. What assessment finding is associated with intermittent claudication?
   A. Pain with ambulation
   B. Cramping during rest
   C. Hypertension with activity
   D. Palpitations with activity

Answer question

Acute Arterial Occlusion

Symptoms are known as the five "Ps":

- Pulseless extremity
- Pain
- Pallor and cold extremity
- Paresthesias and numbness
- Paralysis of the extremity

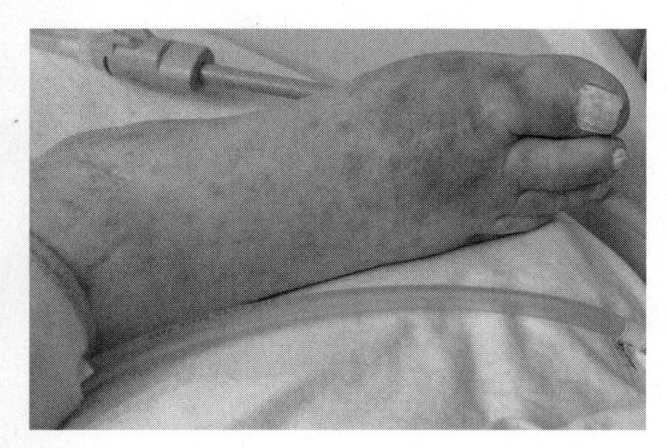

Pallor, cyanosis, and a very weak pulse in an elevated foot reveal significant peripheral arterial disease.
Source: Courtesy of K. Kyriakidis

Diagnostics: PAD

- Ankle-Brachial Index (ABI): Ratio based on comparison of systolic BP (SBP) in the ankle to the SBP in the arm (brachial artery). If the pressure is lower in the legs than arms, this could indicate PAD. ABI is strongly recommended as the first noninvasive test that should be performed (EBP). Most health care organizations have delineated a specific procedure to follow when measuring ABI. However, the American Heart Association has made evidence-based recommendations for measurement and interpretations that all clinicians should know and these include:
  1. A Doppler with gel should be used to measure SBP in both arms and both ankles.
  2. Accuracy depends on an appropriate cuff size (width over 40% of limb circumference). Ankle cuff placement must have lower cuff edge 2 cm above the superior aspect of the medial malleolus.
  3. Do not apply cuff over distal bypass or ulcers. Avoid contaminating any wound.
  4. ABI is measured after patient has rested 5–10 min in supine position and has relaxed in a comfortable room.
  5. No smoking for >2 hrs prior to ABI measurement.
  6. Accuracy depends on no patient movement during measurement.
  7. Use Doppler probe to find the clearest signal.
  8. Inflate cuff to about 20 mmHg above the last audible signal. Deflate slowly to detect signal reappearance.
  9. Follow a set sequence to obtain SBP in all four limbs, ending with repeat measurement of the first. Discard first SBP in first arm if SBP difference is >10 mmHg.
  10. Calculation: $\frac{\text{Highest ankle SBP}}{\text{Highest brachial SBP}}$
  11. Outpatient prognostic indicator: $\frac{\text{Lowest ankle SBP}}{\text{Higher brachial SBP}}$
- Arterial doppler studies: Ultrasound measures blood flow through the arteries and can identify the significance of an obstruction to guide therapy.

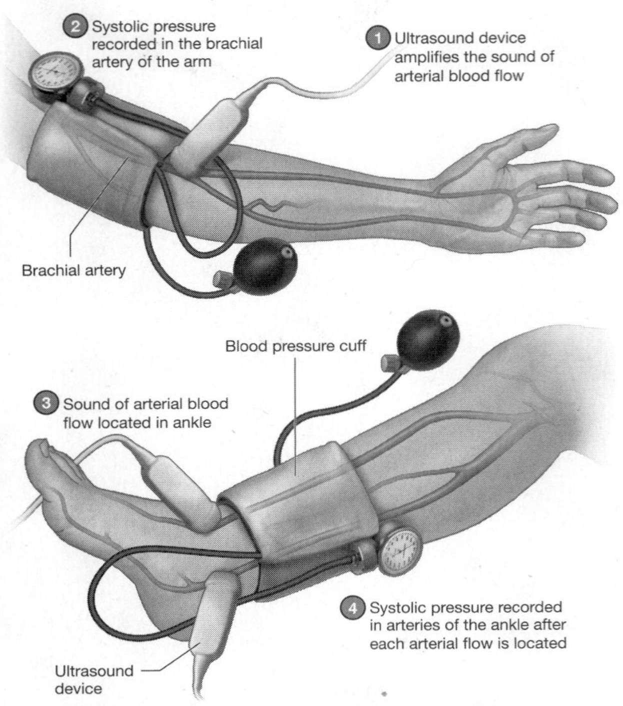
2 Systolic pressure recorded in the brachial artery of the arm
1 Ultrasound device amplifies the sound of arterial blood flow
Brachial artery
Blood pressure cuff
3 Sound of arterial blood flow located in ankle
4 Systolic pressure recorded in arteries of the ankle after each arterial flow is located
Ultrasound device

This image shows the locations and some of the details in how to obtain accurate systolic BPs in ABI measurement.

ABI ratio	Interpretation	Action
≥ 0.9	Within normal	Follow; prevent progression
0.8-0.9	Mild PAD	Aggressive risk factor control
0.5-0.8	Moderate PAD	Consult vascular specialist
≤ 0.4	Severe PAD	Consult vascular specialist. Consider revascularization for non-healing wound

This table provides interpretation of ABI measurements and the appropriate actions needed in the patient's care.

Source: Copyright © 2013, NovEx Novice to Expert Learning, LLC

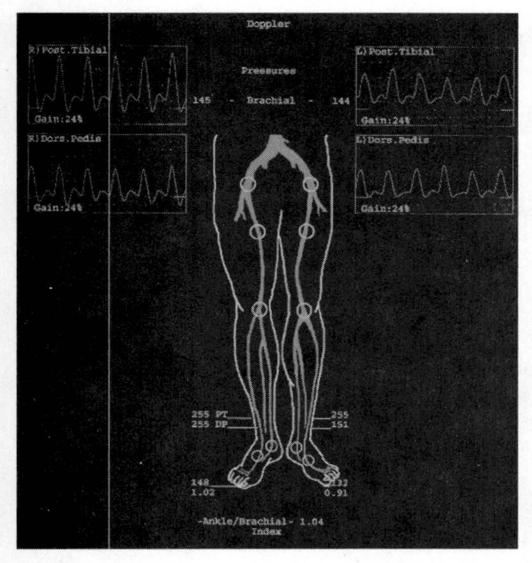

This image shows a bilateral arterial duplex doppler result of the legs using the ABI technique. Understanding the results helps guide care of the patient in their daily activities. This patient has bilateral vascular disease. Given the patient's history of renal failure, an infected foot, and four gangrenous toes, this diagnosis was anticipated.
Source: Courtesy of K. Kyriakidis

- CTA: Computerized tomographic angiography
- Angiography: Invasive, but most accurate

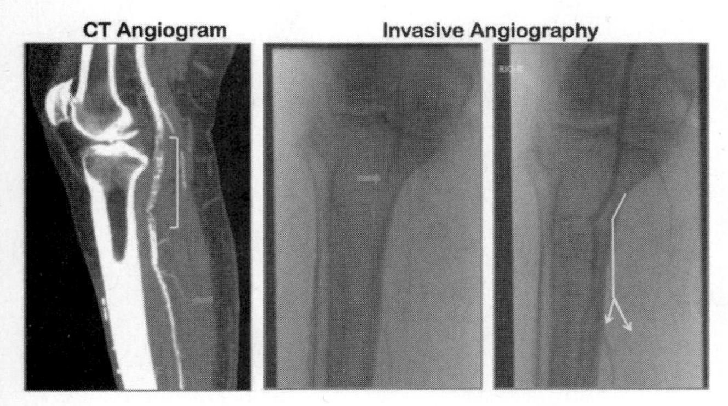

Three images examine the same patient's popliteal artery status. Left: In a CTA, the extensive and severe blockage (bracket) from PAD is seen behind the knee. In the mid-calf, complete occlusion (arrow) is present. Middle: An invasive angiogram (dye injected to visualize actual blood flow) reveals that the blockage completely occludes the popliteal artery (arrow). Right: Urgent thromboembolectomy resulted in the return of blood flow (yellow arrows). This series of photos assist in understanding the information that various diagnostic tests may offer.
Source: Courtesy of K. Kyriakidis

Priority Patient Concerns and Desired Collaborative Care Outcomes: PAD

Prior to caring for patients with PAD, it is important to prioritize the patient's concerns that must guide the nursing care plan and interventions. Care for the patient is ordered and organized in accordance with the patient's priority and urgent needs. Desired collaborative care outcomes in patients with PAD typically include:

1. Patient will have sufficient tissue perfusion to peripheral tissues with pulses present, even if weak.
2. Patient will be pain-free at rest and with low level or necessary activities.
3. Patient will tolerate usual (or at least necessary) activities of daily living.
4. Patient will describe strategies she or he is using for prevention and treatment modalities.

Considering these important care outcomes, prepare a list of the major 3-6 priority patient concerns or nursing diagnoses for patients with PAD. Be prepared to participate in a discussion of this list and/or to submit them as an assignment, as determined by your faculty. Resources you may find helpful in this assignment can include this lesson, the references, resources on nursing care plans, and standard nursing diagnoses manuals.

Concept Check

4. What is the ankle-brachial index?

A. A graph of dial and pedal pulses
B. A comparison of skin temperature at the foot and the wrist
C. A comparison of arm and leg blood pressures
D. A chart comparing coloration differences between the arm and the leg

Answer question

Concept Check

5. What diagnostic test for peripheral artery disease is most accurate?

A. ABI
B. Doppler studies
C. CTA
D. Angiography

Answer question

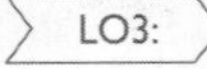

Collaborative Interventions: PAD

Evidence-Based Practices

The primary goal of therapy is to improve circulation to extremities, reduce symptoms, and minimize tissue loss or limit the degree of amputation:

- Antiplatelet agents (e.g., aspirin or clopidogrel) are effective in decreasing the risk of stroke and MI in patients with PAD. Anticoagulation with warfarin has not been effective in improving outcomes in PAD.
- Statins can reduce progression of atherosclerosis and intermittent claudication.
- Medications that can improve symptoms of intermittent claudication include cilostazol and pentoxifylline.
- Control of comorbid diseases, such as hypertension and diabetes, is essential in PAD management.
- Nonpharmacological treatment is effective and includes educating the patient to avoid disease progression: healthy diet, risk factor modification, smoking cessation, and exercise.
- Surgical intervention with revascularization (bypass or angioplasty) is indicated when medical therapy either fails or is insufficient.

Alternate Treatment Options for Acute Arterial Occlusion

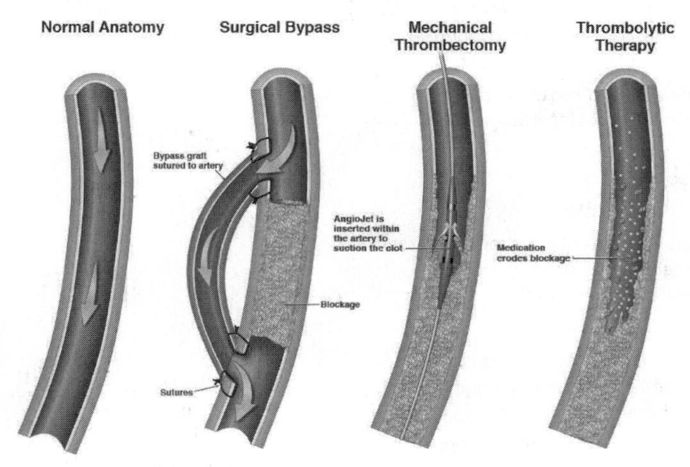

The series of illustrations compares various treatment options if medical therapy fails. First, is a normal artery that is clean and patent. Second, an arterial bypass surgically performed around an isolated blockage in an artery. The bypass graft channels blood flow around the blockage. A third option is a thrombectomy using a catheter to spray saline, break up, and suction the clot particles away. Lastly, thrombolytic therapy can be used to "bust" the clots.

Source:

EBP Surgical Intervention

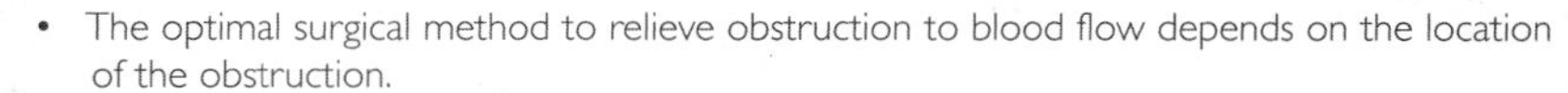

- The optimal surgical method to relieve obstruction to blood flow depends on the location of the obstruction.

- Endovascular therapies (balloon angioplasties, atherectomy, and laser angioplasties, stents) can provide effective symptom relief in patients with peripheral vascular disease.

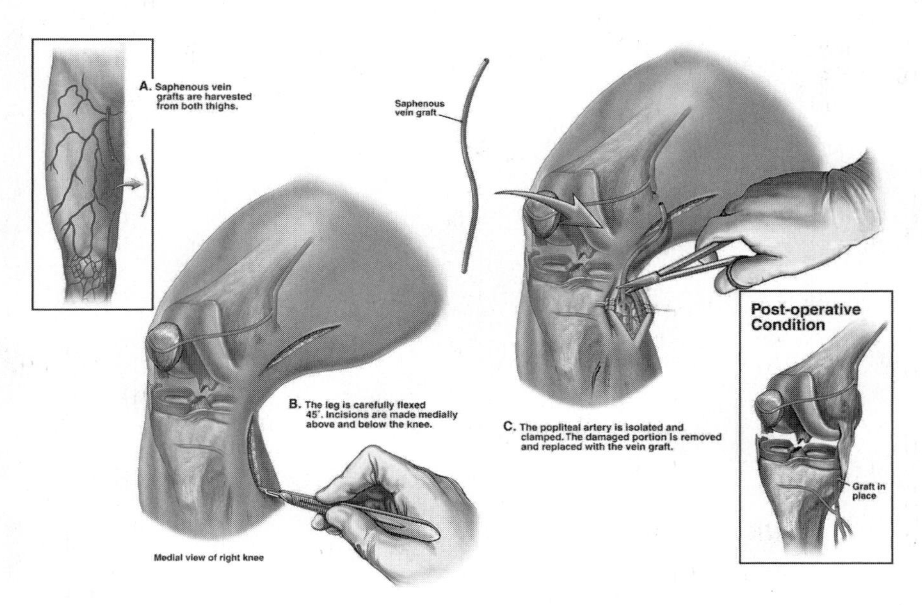

This series of illustrations depicts a femoral popliteal bypass procedure. First, a saphenous vein graft is harvested from the thigh. After the knee is incised above and below the joint, the popliteal artery is isolated and clamped. The damaged portion is removed and replaced with the vein graft.

Source: Nucleus Medical Art Inc/Alamy

Postoperative Considerations

- Routine assessment of blood flow is an important nursing measure both pre- and postoperatively. Blood flow assessment should be done often post op (e.g., every hour). Frequency of assessment can be diminished over time if graft patency is present.
- Blood flow assessment includes pulse quality, strength, capillary refill, and sensation. Blood flow is a central in ongoing assessement of PAD patients, preoperatively, postoperatively, and in follow-up visits.
- Pulse presence does not necessarily mean that the graft has good patency.
  - o Doppler assessment is a better parameter to measure flow than palpation.
- Loss of blood flow following surgery can be due to bypass graft failure or obstruction as a result of clot formation. If a clot forms, there is a danger of potential embolization. Emboli can obstruct an artery beyond the site of surgery and may result in partial loss of the involved extremity. Immediate evaluation by the team is needed.
- Assist with early mobilization and ambulation.
- Prevent never events such as DVT, IV catheter-related infections, catheter-associated urinary infections, possible blood incompatibility, pressure ulcer, fall, or surgical site infections.
- Postoperative bleeding might be manifested by discoloration and bruising in any area, but particularly around the surgical site. Evaluate to determine the need for further intervention or observation.
- Pain is usually not severe but may need management with opioids.
- Long-term follow-up care should include ABI measurements, which provides a prognostic indicator for PAD progression (EBP).

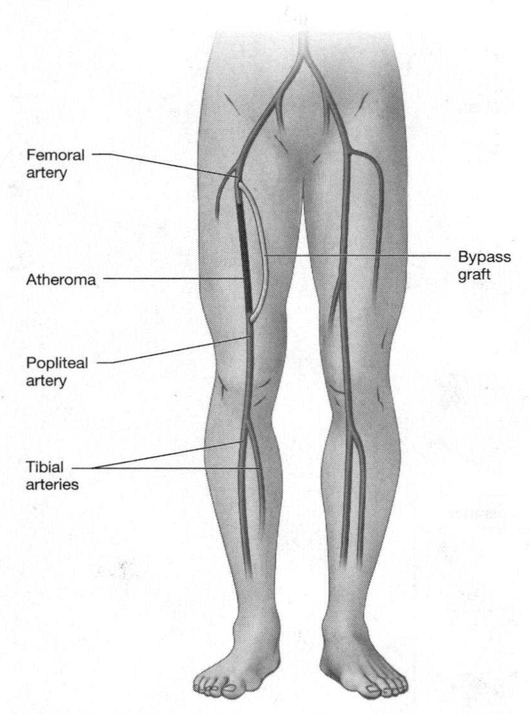

A bypass graft is shown connecting the popliteal to the femoral artery, thus bypassing an atheromatous plaque in the upper popliteal artery.
Source: Copyright © 2013, NovEx Novice to Expert Learning, LLC

Collaborative Interventions: PAD (continued)

Acute Arterial Occlusions

- Acute arterial thrombosis or embolization is a medical emergency.
- An arterial obstruction is identified through ultrasound flow studies.
- Clinically, the patient typically presents with pain, often severe, in the affected area.
- Assessment for pulses most commonly reveals that pulses are diminished or absent distal to the area of obstruction.
- Immediate anticoagulation with IV unfractionated heparin is indicated.
- Pain management is essential until definitive therapy, such as thrombolysis or surgery, can be performed.
- Emergency procedures include urgently mobilizing the team and preoperative or preparation (e.g., IVs, NPO, antibiotics) for catheter-based thrombolysis, embolectomy, or bypass surgery for viable limbs.

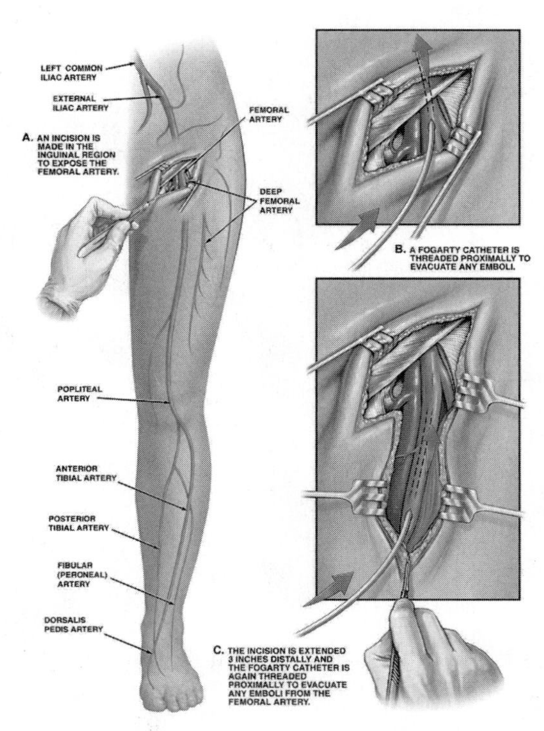
LEFT COMMON ILIAC ARTERY
EXTERNAL ILIAC ARTERY
FEMORAL ARTERY
A. AN INCISION IS MADE IN THE INGUINAL REGION TO EXPOSE THE FEMORAL ARTERY.
DEEP FEMORAL ARTERY
B. A FOGARTY CATHETER IS THREADED PROXIMALLY TO EVACUATE ANY EMBOLI.
POPLITEAL ARTERY
ANTERIOR TIBIAL ARTERY
POSTERIOR TIBIAL ARTERY
FIBULAR (PERONEAL) ARTERY
DORSALIS PEDIS ARTERY
C. THE INCISION IS EXTENDED 3 INCHES DISTALLY AND THE FOGARTY CATHETER IS AGAIN THREADED PROXIMALLY TO EVACUATE ANY EMBOLI FROM THE FEMORAL ARTERY.

Surgical embolectomy procedure. Accurately depicts surgery to remove embolism (embolus) from the femoral artery in the leg.

Source: Nucleus Medical Art Inc/Alamy

Patient Education

Patients have a central role in collaboratively managing their PAD as an outpatient. Patient education is targeted at comfort care, safety, and prevention of disease progression with the hope of avoiding surgery. Issues include:

N • Instruct patient to walk for exercise and to prevent progression of PAD. Walk until pain occurs, rest until pain is gone, and then continue walking. Development of collateral circulation over time can improve the patient's exercise duration.

N • Avoidance of trauma, tissue damage, or injury which can lead to prolonged wounds and infection. These can result in amputation. Wear sturdy, protective, and comfortable shoes. Avoid tissue damage or injury. Infections can lead to amputations.

N • Instruct about good foot, nail, and leg care: Keep clean and dry, use warm water and mild soap, pat skin dry, use moisturizer, wear comfortable shoes and cotton socks, prevent accidental foot and leg injuries, and inspect feet and legs daily. Keep nails cut straight across and filed.

M N • Aggressive wound care in patients with non-healing wounds can prevent surgery in up to two thirds of patients. Collaborate with a wound specialist and health care provider on interventions and with the patient regarding strict compliance to prevent gangrene.

N • Avoid prolonged exposure to the cold, caffeine, emotional stress and nicotine due to vasoconstriction, which can reduce blood flow to affected extremities.

N • Avoid sitting or standing for long periods. During travel, stop and take a walk every hour.

N • Avoid wearing constrictive clothing that hinders blood flow from any part of the lower body or an extremity.

N • Smoking cessation can improve overall health in addition to circulation.

N • Risk factor modifications should include a healthier diet and attaining a healthy body weight.

N • Educate about disease, symptoms that trigger seeking medical care, complications, medications and adherence to prescribed regimen, follow-up visits, and management of comorbid conditions, especially hypertension and diabetes.

Concept Check

6. Which assessment is most strongly recommended to predict the progression of peripheral arterial disease?

A. Presence of a pulse in the extremity

B. Ankle-brachial index

C. Capillary refill time

D. Decrease in pain in the extremity

Answer question

Concept Check

7. Which medication is recommended for immediate use when an acute arterial occlusion occurs?

A. Warfarin

B. Heparin

C. Aspirin

D. Vitamin K

Answer question

Summary of Interventions: PAD

Peripheral Disease:

- Antiplatelet agents (aspirin, clopidogrel) can decrease the risk of thrombi and emboli.
- Statins can reduce progression of atherosclerosis.
- Good management of comorbid conditions is essential.
- Nonpharmacological treatments include diet modification, smoking cessation, and exercise.
- Medications (cilostazol, pentoxifylline) can relieve claudication symptoms.
- Surgical intervention if medical therapy either fails or is insufficient.

Acute Arterial Occlusion:

- Anticoagulants and invasive intervention is indicated in the medical emergency of acute arterial occlusion.

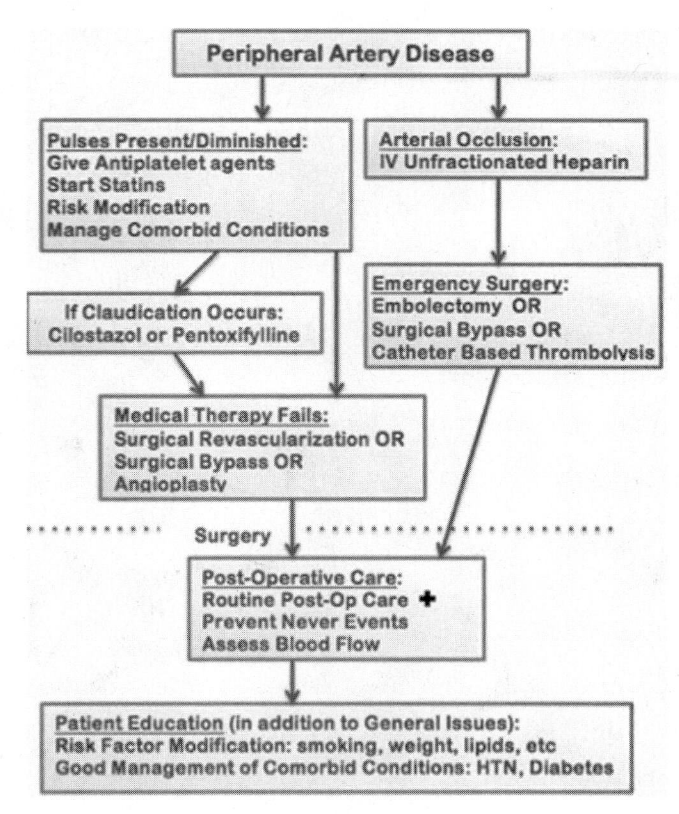

Source: Copyright © 2013, NovEx Novice to Expert Learning, LLC

LO4:

Evaluation of Desired Collaborative Care Outcomes: PAD

Evaluation and reassessment should reveal attainment of previously established outcomes. In summary:

- Patient's peripheral tissues are no colder and not more pale than prior to acute event. Pulses are present, even if weak.
- Patient experiences fewer episodes or reduced duration of intermittent claudication.
- Patient is able to participate in normal (or at least necessary) daily activities without pain and demonstrates walking to claudication.
- Patient demonstrates adherence to preventative strategies and accurately explains treatment modalities.

LO1:

What Is Carotid Artery Disease?

- Carotid artery disease is the narrowing of the carotid arteries that supply blood to the brain.
- The most common cause is atherosclerosis.
- The pathophysiology and risk factors are the same as that for PAD.

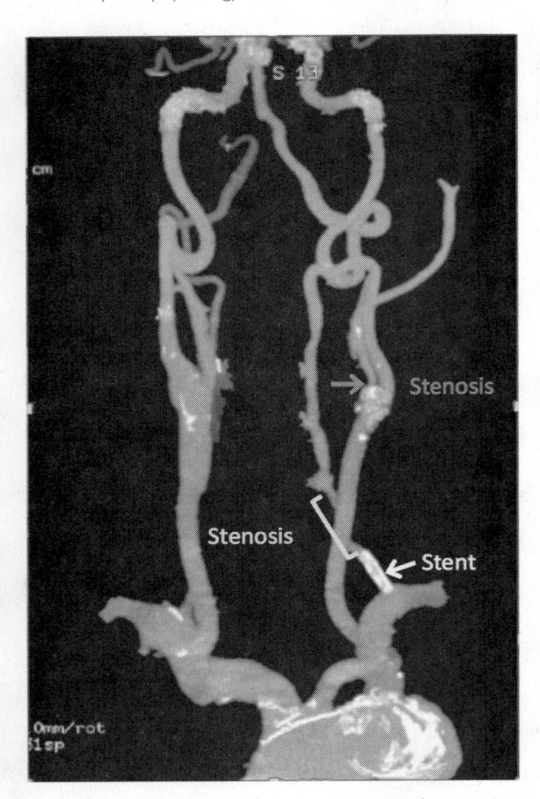

In this 3D reconstruction, there are two severely stenotic arteries. The vertebral artery, stented prior (white arrow), now shows severe narrowing (yellow bracket) above the stent. The internal carotid (red arrow) points at a small but severely occluded area at its bifurcation.

Source: Courtesy of K. Kyriakidis

LO2:

Pathophysiology: Carotid Artery Disease

- Carotid artery disease is also known as carotid artery stenosis. Carotid artery disease also occurs as the result of plaque or atheroma formation on the carotid arteries located on each side of the neck.
- The internal carotid arteries supply oxygen-rich blood to the brain. The external carotid arteries supply oxygen-rich blood to the face, scalp, and neck.
- The plaque buildup hardens and narrows the lumen of the artery restricting blood flow to the brain. If a piece of the atheroma or plaque breaks off, a thrombotic stroke can occur.

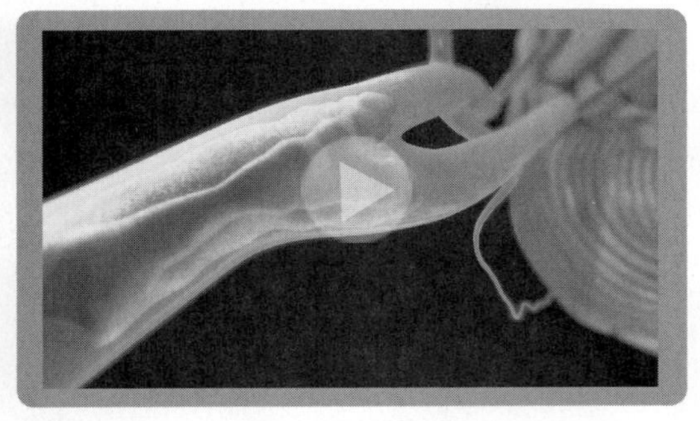

This animation demonstrates the development of carotid artery disease and shows common consequences.

Source: © 2013 Nucleus Medical Media. All rights reserved

Assessment Findings: Carotid Artery Disease

- Stroke:
  - o Sudden unilateral weakness or paralysis
  - o Loss of function of face or limbs
  - o Difficulty speaking
  - o Visual disturbances
  - o Dizziness
  - o Confusion
  - o Loss of balance or coordination
- Transient Ischemic Attack (TIA): Same symptoms as a stroke but lasts less than 24 hours

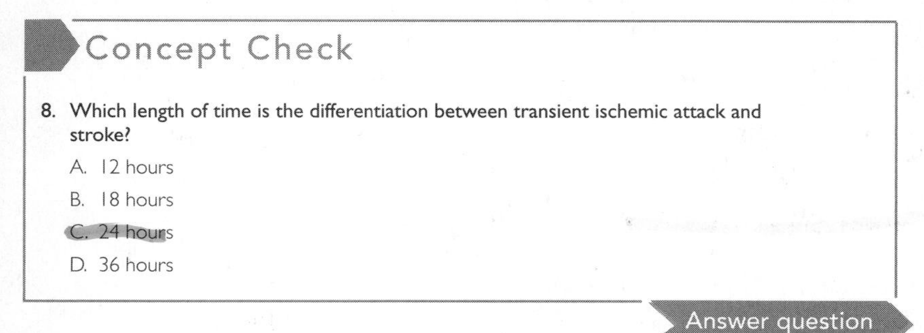

Concept Check

8. **Which length of time is the differentiation between transient ischemic attack and stroke?**

   A. 12 hours

   B. 18 hours

   C. 24 hours

   D. 36 hours

Answer question

Diagnostics: Carotid Artery Disease

- Physical Exam: A bruit
- Carotid Doppler
- Computer tomographic angiography
- Magnetic resonance angiography
- Carotid angiography, usually done with cerebral angiography

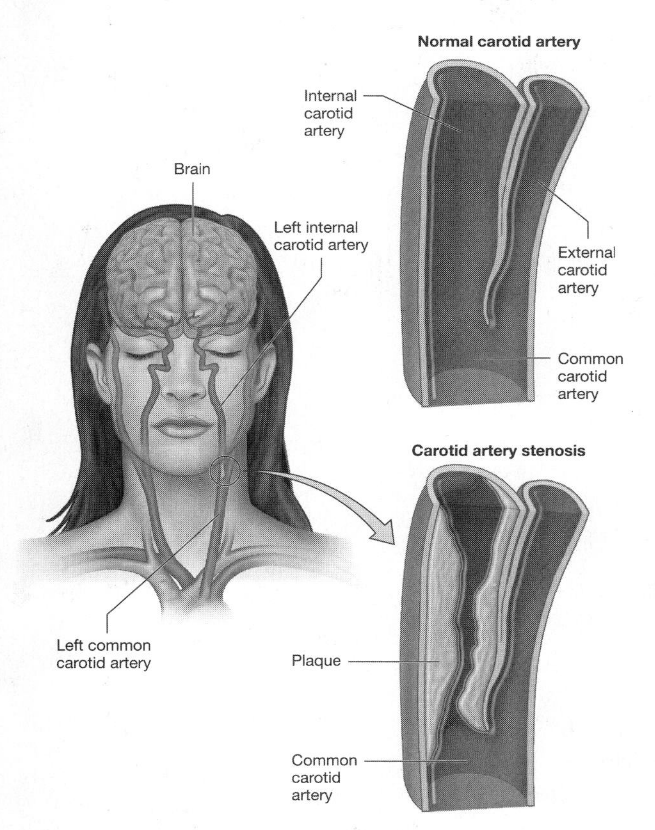

This exhibit portrays carotid artery stenosis with Doppler imaging. It consists of an orientation view to demonstrate where the carotid artery is. It also includes a visual comparison between a normal carotid vessel and one with stenosis.

Priority Patient Concerns and Desired Collaborative Care Outcomes: Carotid Artery Disease

Prior to caring for patients with carotid artery disease, it is important to prioritize the patient's concerns that must guide the nursing care plan and interventions. Care for the patient is ordered and organized in accordance with the patient's priority and urgent needs. Desired collaborative care outcomes in patients with carotid artery disease typically include:

1. Patient will have effective cerebral tissue perfusion.
2. Patient will demonstrate increased knowledge of treatment modalities for disorder.
3. Patient will have decreased anxiety associated with disorder.

Considering these important care outcomes, prepare a list of the major 3–6 priority patient concerns or nursing diagnoses for patients with carotid artery disease. Be prepared to participate in a discussion of this list and/or to submit them as an assignment, as determined by your faculty. Resources you may find helpful in this assignment can include this lesson, the references, resources on nursing care plans, and standard nursing diagnoses manuals.

LO3:

Collaborative Interventions: Carotid Artery Disease

Evidence-Based Practices

Treatment goal is to prevent carotid disease from worsening and to prevent stroke.

M N
- Antiplatelet agents including ASA and clopidogrel

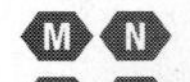

- Risk factor modification: Controlling hypertension, dyslipidemia, diabetes, smoking cessation, exercise, and weight management

- Carotid endarterectomy or carotid stenting
- If the patient has atrial fibrillation, anticoagulants should be used for prevention of stroke.
- Plaque removal

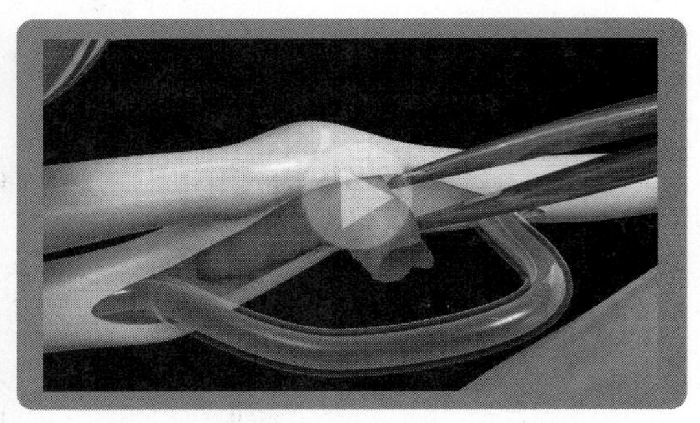

This animation briefly repeats the development of carotid artery disease, but goes on to review preparation for and care following carotid endarterectomy. The carotid endarterectomy procedure is depicted from incision, to clamping and use of a shunt, to plaque removal.

Collaborative Support Care

N
- Postoperative complications are low. The most common complication is bleeding at the site. The nurse should be aware of discomfort, site discoloration, edema at the site, and expansion or bleeding at the site. Some patients need wound exploration for bleeding. However, an emergency airway for insertion should be at the bedside in case of airway obstruction.

N
- Monitor for cranial nerve damage (e.g., impaired speech, dysphagia, gag reflex). Swallowing may be impaired if damage to cranial nerve is present.

N
- Post endarterectomy or postoperatively, monitor the patient carefully for any neurological alterations warning of embolization, cerebral ischemia (e.g., slurred speech, confusion, agitation, visual changes, paresthesias, paralysis).

Patient Education

N
- Patient education should include:
  - o Management of comorbid conditions, particularly hypertension and diabetes
  - o Instruction about medications, particularly statins in patients with hypercholesterolemia or coronary heart disease
  - o Wound care instructions as indicated

o Routine education about disease, symptoms warranting follow-up, complications, healthy diet, smoking cessation, healthy weight, exercise, and risk factor modification.

LO4:

Evaluation of Desired Collaborative Care Outcomes: Carotid Artery Disease

Evaluation and reassessment should reveal attainment of previously established patient outcomes. In summary:

- Patient has no disruption of motor, sensory, or cognitive function.
- Patient accurately discusses treatment.
- Patient identifies anxiety and openly discusses potential treatment and outcomes.

LO1, 2, 3, 4:

Brief Overview: Renal Artery Stenosis

- Renal artery stenosis is another but less common arterial disease. It reduces or occludes blood flow to the kidneys.
- Like most arterial diseases, it commonly results from atherosclerosis.
- It may cause:
  - o Diminished kidney function
  - o Hypertension that suddenly worsens
- Diagnostics includes renal arteriography.
- Treatment includes:

  - o Educate the patient regarding risk factor modification
  - o Revascularization with angioplasty or surgery

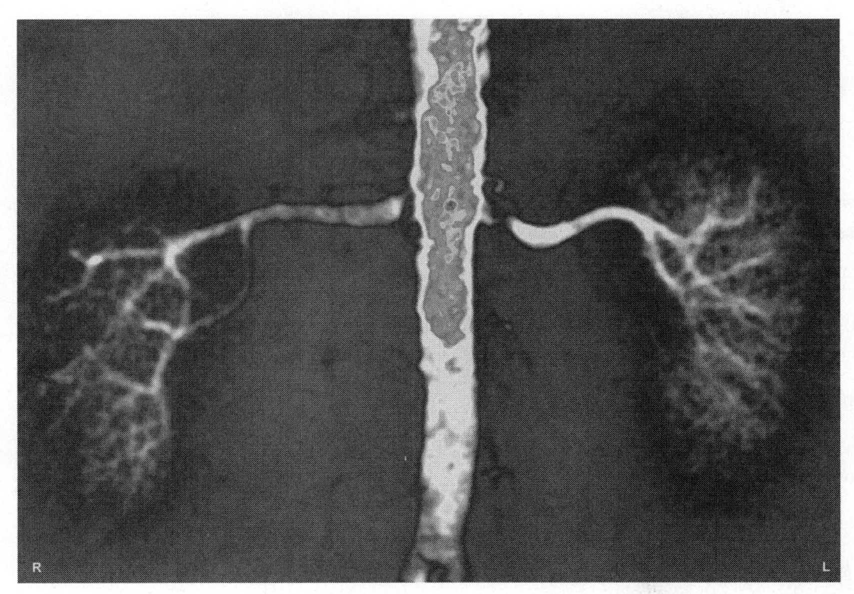

The kidneys are represented as oval clusters of blood vessels on either side of the central aorta (bright yellow). Note two major findings: Large atheromatous plaque (long brownish discoloration) in the upper half of the aorta and the thread-like stenotic left renal artery (red arrow). The left renal artery has severe narrowing.
Source: BSIP SA/Alamy

Concept Check

9. What is the most common complication associated with carotid endarterectomy?

A. Worsening hypertension
B. Edema at the incision site
C. Bleeding
D. Impaired swallowing

Answer question

LO1:

What Is an Aneurysm?

- An aneurysm is a bulging (resembling a balloon) of an arterial wall. It may occur in any blood vessel (e.g., brain, aorta).
- It may go unnoticed until quite enlarged.
- It may remain unknown for years until it ruptures. The larger an aneurysm becomes, the greater the chance it will rupture.

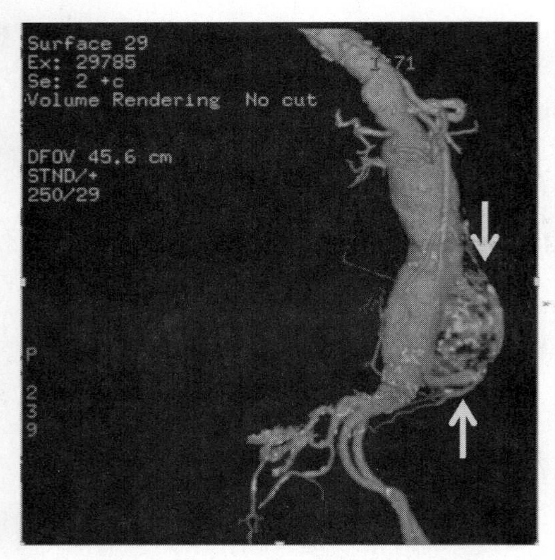

This 3D image is computer generated from a real patient's abdominal aortic aneurysm. The large, solid, pinkish-red vessel is the aorta while the transparent bulge (arrow) is the aneurysm.
Source: Courtesy of K. Kyriakidis

What Is an Aortic Aneurysm?

- Aortic aneurysms may be divided into thoracic and abdominal types.
- Abdominal aortic aneurysms (AAA) are more common (65% of aneurysms) than thoracic aneurysms.
- Aneurysms can typically take on one of two patterns:
  - o Weakness and bulging of the entire vessel wall or
  - o Weakness within the vessel wall with intimal wall tear, called dissection.

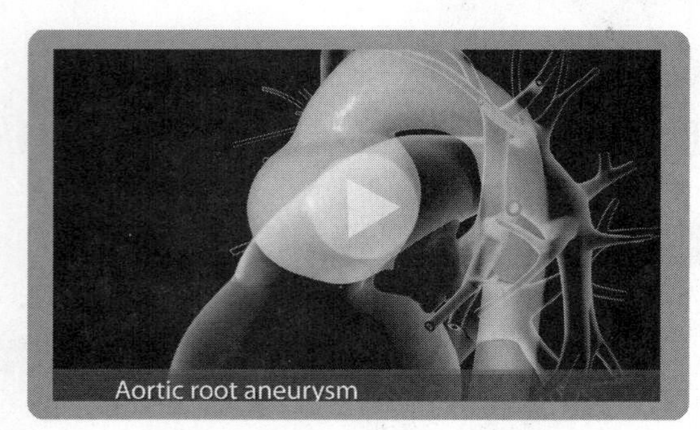

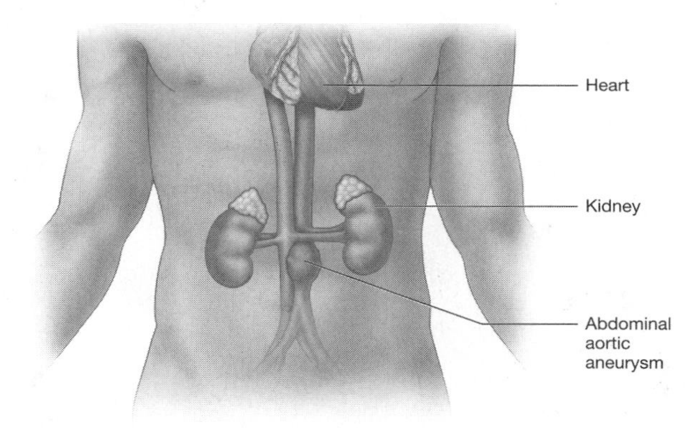

Upper: This animation shows how an aneurysm develops. Stable versus unstable symptoms are described. Lower: This image pictures an abdominal aortic aneurysm below the level of the renal artery and above the femoral arteries. Further dissection can cause serious renal damage.

Concept Check

10. Which type of aortic aneurysm is the most common?
    - A. Abdominal
    - B. Thoracic
    - C. Aortic root
    - D. Renal

Answer question

LO1:

Clinical Relevance: Aneurysms

- Aortic dissection is a life-threatening complication of aneurysm. Because of the rapid progression of shock due to loss of vascular volume, immediate surgical treatment is necessary. Aortic dissection may also occur without the presence of an aneurysm.
- At least 50% of patients who experience a ruptured abdominal aortic aneurysm (AAA) die before reaching the hospital. Mortality is commonly the result of a delay in surgical intervention.
- Survival after a ruptured AAA is less than 20%.

Aortic Dissection with Pericardial Tamponade

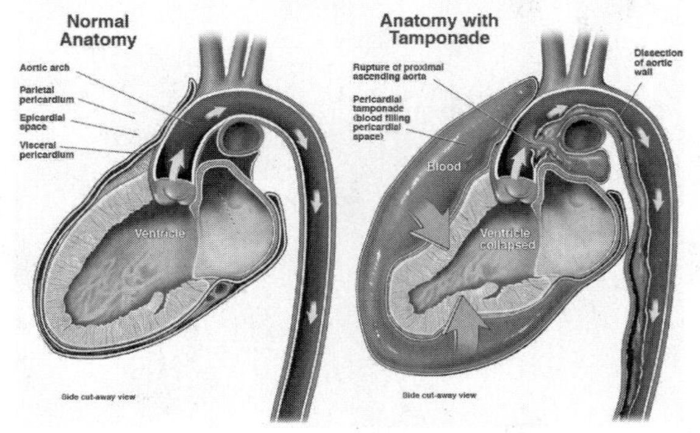

This illustration compares a normal heart with aortic dissection and resulting cardiac tamponade.

LO2:

Pathophysiology: Aneurysms

- An aneurysm forms when part of the vessel wall is damaged or weakened. The weakening may occur as a result of atherosclerosis, inflammatory disease, connective tissue disease, or infection. As pressure increases within the vessel, the vessel balloons out at its weakest point.
- The swelling can be small or large. If the pressure becomes great enough or is sustained long enough, there is the risk of rupture, which can lead to hemorrhage, loss of perfusion, and sudden death.

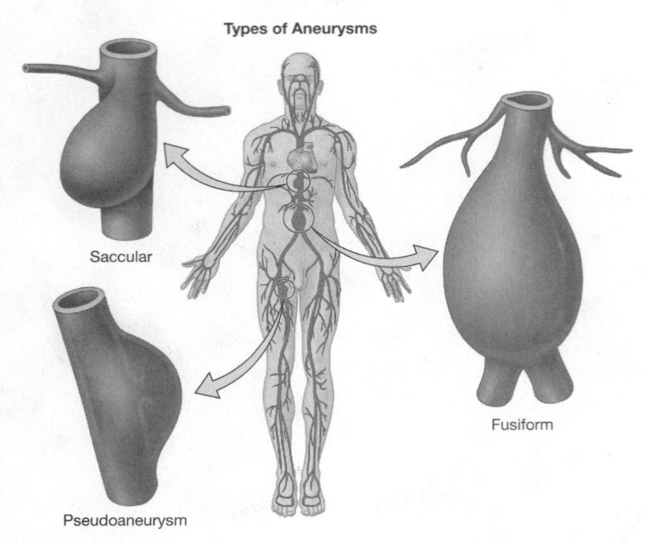

Aneurysms have different shapes: fusiform or saccular. Shape assists in identifying true aneurysms, which involves all three layers of the arterial wall. A fusiform aneurysm is shaped like a ball and bulges out circularly around the aorta, whereas a saccular-shaped aneurysm is more one-sided. The fusiform shape more commonly occurs.

- Rupture of an aneurysm or dissection results in rapid progression of shock, loss of vascular volume and perfusion, potential bleeding into the pericardial sac (with resultant tamponade), and disruption of the aortic valve with resultant left ventricle (LV) failure.
- Dissection affecting vital organs or organ arteries can cause concurrent complications, such as myocardial infarction, renal failure, and stroke.

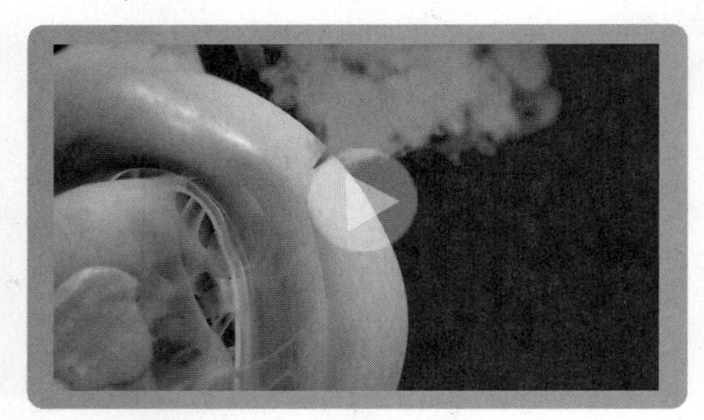

This animation reviews thoracic aortic dissection. Thoracic versus abdominal dissection symptoms are differentiated.

Risk Factors: Aneurysms

- Hypertension
- Smoking
- Atherosclerosis
- Hypercholesteremia
- Age (greater than 60 years old)
- Male gender
- Drug abuse (especially cocaine)
- Heavy alcohol use
- Lower estrogen levels after menopause
- Genetic connective tissue disorders (e.g., Marfan syndrome, Loeys-Dietz syndrome, Ehlers-Danlos syndrome, Turner syndrome)
- Infections or vasculitis
- Congenital arteriovenous malformation
- Polycystic disease
- Coarctation of the aorta
- Family history
- Previous aneurysm
- Trauma

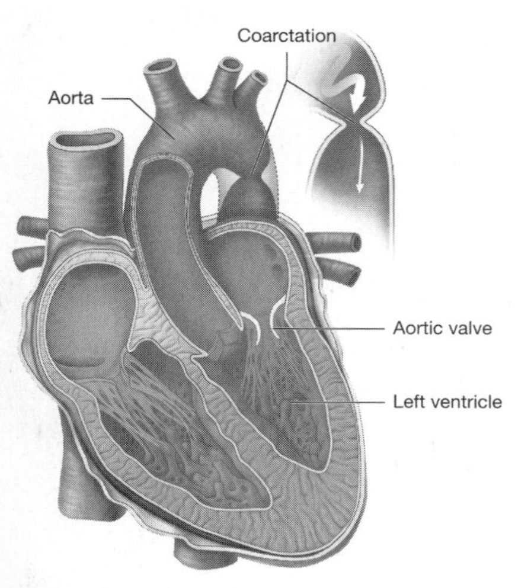

Coarctation of the aorta is a narrowing, or constriction, in a portion of the aorta. The condition forces the heart to pump harder to get blood through the aorta and to the rest of the body. This condition puts a person at higher risk for aneurysm.

Concept Check

11. What is a risk factor for the development of aneurysm?
    A. High estrogen levels
    B. Congenital vessel disorders
    C. Moderate alcohol consumption
    D. Hypotension

Answer question

Causes: Aneurysms

- Atherosclerosis
- Hypertension
- Uncontrolled diabetes
- Trauma or injury
- Vasculitis

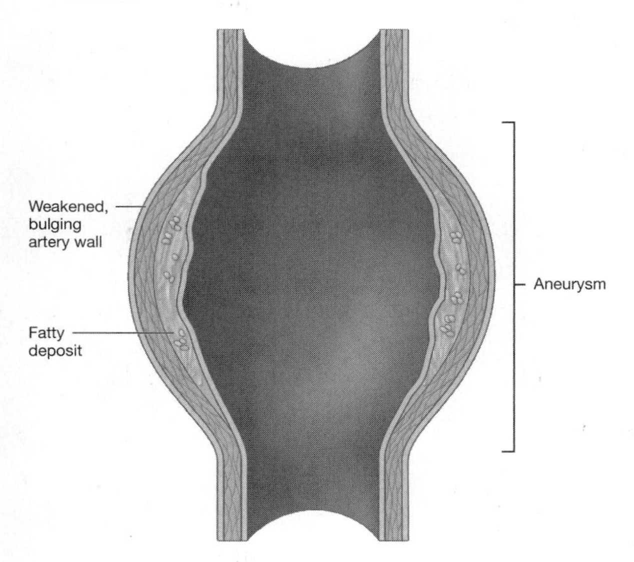

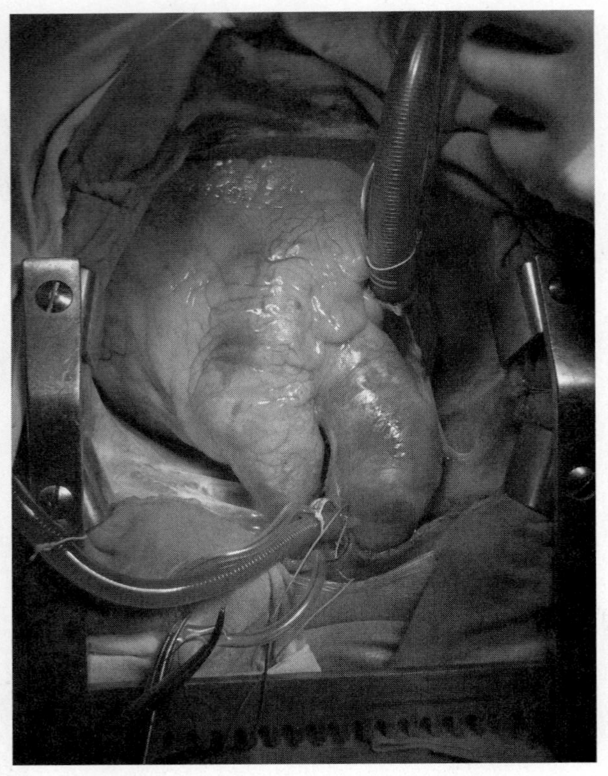

Upper: Hypertension is a frequent cause of aneurysms. The cerebral, coronary, and lower limb arteries and aorta are most commonly affected. Lower: This photo shows a large ascending aortic aneurysm (between the two cannula), which is bulging near the aortic arch. An aneurysm of this size is prone to rupture. Unlike a large abdominal aneurysm that may be palpable on physical examination, this one is in the thoracic cavity and cannot be palpated. The aneurysm is located deep in the chest, making surgical resection challenging. Here, the chest is open and the heart (left upper organ covered in a yellow fat layer) is visible in the left upper area.

Source: (*lower*) Stockphoto/Thinkstock

Assessment Findings: Aneurysms

Aneurysm Dissection or Rupture

Thoracic Aneurysm

- Sudden, severe, and unrelenting back pain or pain between shoulder blades
- Rapid and uneven radial or carotid pulses
- Sudden hypotension; shock
- Shortness of breath

Abdominal Aortic Aneurysm (AAA)

- Severe, sudden, and constant abdominal or flank pain
- Abdominal distension
- Sudden hypotension; shock
- Palpable pulsating mass

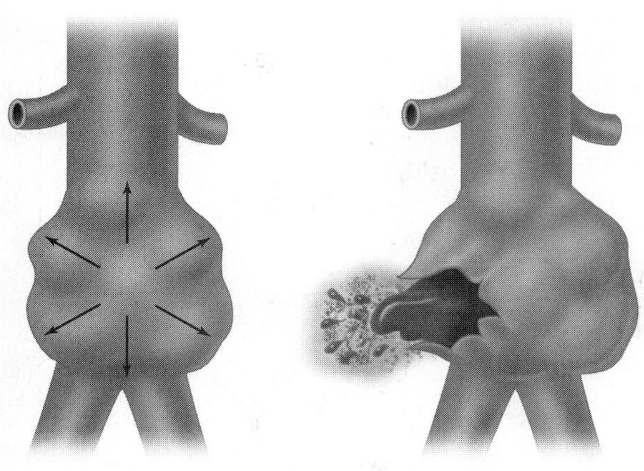

AAAs typically form slowly over several years without any symptoms. The risk for rupture with lethal outcomes heightens after the diameter exceeds 5 cm or about 2 in. as the aortic wall is thin. Rupture rapidly leads to hemorrhage, hypotension, and then shock. Mortality following rupture is very high (about 80%).

Diagnostics: Aneurysms

- Use of computed tomography (CT) and magnetic resonance imaging (MRI) to identify abdominal and thoracic vascular structures is common practice.
- Routine chest and abdominal x-rays and ultrasound may detect the aneurysm, although not sensitive.
- Angiography

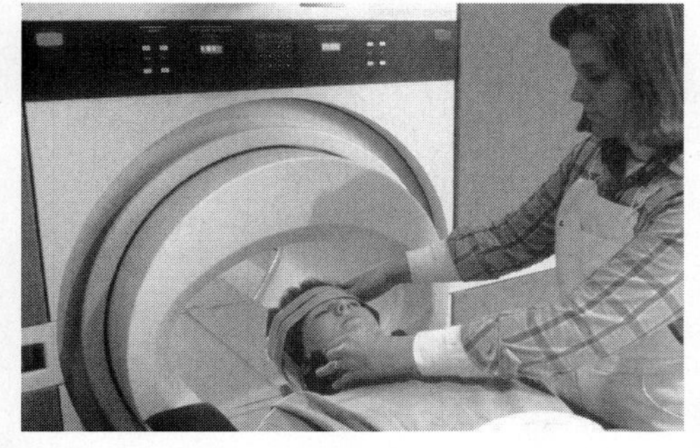

This patient is being prepared for an MRI scan. Patients pass through the MRI, which can assist in illuminating problems like an aneurysm. CT and MRI provide excellent data for diagnosis.
Source: National Cancer Institute

Priority Patient Concerns and Desired Collaborative Care Outcomes: Aneurysms

Prior to caring for patients with aneurysms, it is important to prioritize the patient's concerns that must guide the nursing care plan and interventions. Care for the patient is ordered and organized in accordance with the patient's priority and urgent needs. Desired collaborative care outcomes in patients with aneurysms typically include:

1. Patient will avoid shock state.
2. Patient will report being less fearful.
3. Patient will report decrease in pain.

Considering these important care outcomes, prepare a list of the major 3–6 priority patient concerns or nursing diagnoses for patients with aneurysms. Be prepared to participate in a discussion of this list and/or to submit them as an assignment, as determined by your faculty. Resources you may find helpful in this assignment can include this lesson, the references, resources on nursing care plans, and standard nursing diagnoses manuals.

* These nursing diagnoses are applicable for patients with an aneurysm prior to rupture. However, if or when the aneurysm ruptures, the risk for shock changes to an actual complication.

LO3:

Collaborative Interventions: Aneurysms

Care of patients with aneurysm is determined by two key factors:

1. Stability of the patient's condition
2. Severity, size, and extent of the aneurysm

These key factors influence clinical reasoning and determine treatment approaches:

1. Aneurysm is stable.
2. Aneurysm is dissecting, creating instability.
3. Aneurysm has ruptured.

Evidence-Based Practice: Aneurysms in Stable Patients

- Small, stable aneurysms in the descending or abdominal aorta are commonly asymptomatic and sometimes found while the patient is undergoing a study for a different problem. Small aneurysms are treated conservatively and watched. Treatments include:

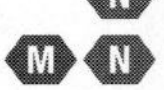

  - o Risk factor modification

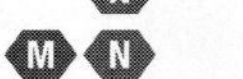

  - o Hypertension control (beta blockers are drugs of choice; calcium channel blockers are used if beta blockers are contraindicated): Strongly recommended

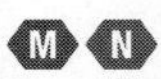

  - o Treatment of hyperlipidemia: May be helpful

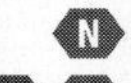

  - o Smoking cessation: Strongly recommended

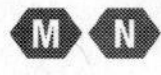

  - o Screening for abdominal aortic aneurysm in first-degree relatives: Strong

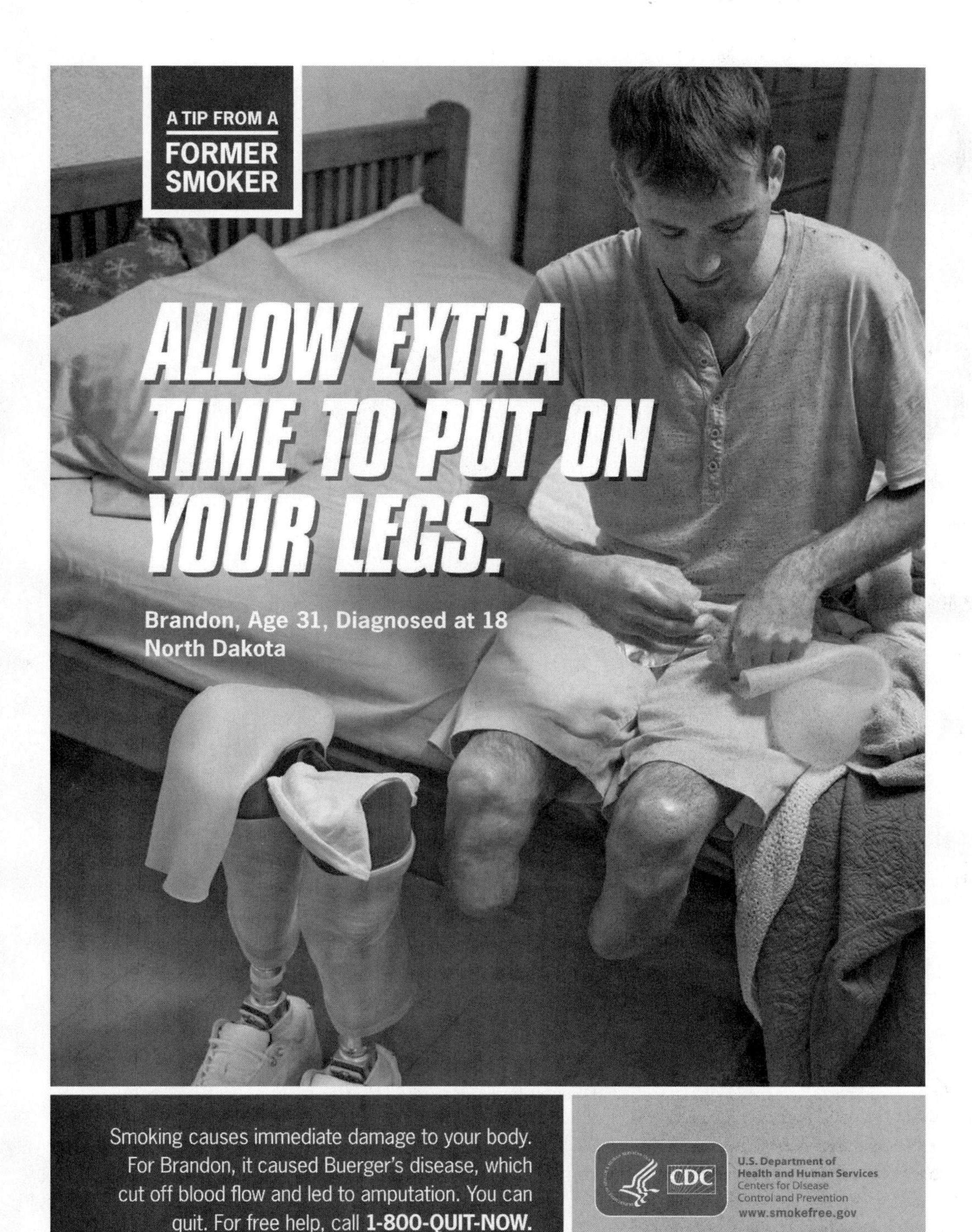
A TIP FROM A
FORMER SMOKER
ALLOW EXTRA TIME TO PUT ON YOUR LEGS.
Brandon, Age 31, Diagnosed at 18
North Dakota
Smoking causes immediate damage to your body. For Brandon, it caused Buerger's disease, which cut off blood flow and led to amputation. You can quit. For free help, call 1-800-QUIT-NOW.
CDC
U.S. Department of Health and Human Services
Centers for Disease Control and Prevention
www.smokefree.gov

From the Antismoking campaign, sponsored by the Centers for Disease Control and Prevention.
Source: Office on Smoking and Health, National Center for Chronic Disease Prevention and Health Promotion, Centers for Disease Control and Prevention

- Larger (greater than 4.5 cm) or rapidly enlarging aneurysms usually require surgery to avert rupture:
  - o Replacement with a graft is the most common surgical intervention for repair. The closer the aneurysm is to the heart, the more difficult the surgery. Thoracic aneurysms of the descending and abdominal aorta offer the surgeon a better operative field and reduce postoperative complications.
  - o Endovascular surgical grafting techniques are more commonplace. When effective, this approach eliminates the need for cross-clamping of the aorta and therefore decreases most of the complications of major aortic surgery.

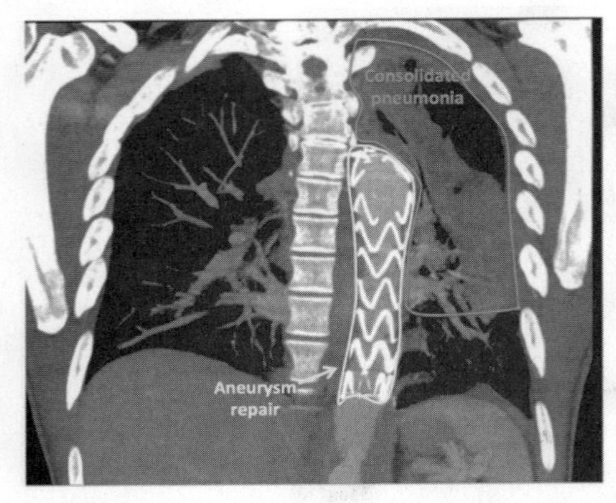

The CT scan of the chest reveals a very sick patient who has had a thoracic aortic aneurysm repair. The graft (outlined in yellow) is prominent. the patient unfortunately developed necrotizing pneumonia, seen on this CT, with consolidation in the left upper lung.
Source: Courtesy of K. Kyriakidis

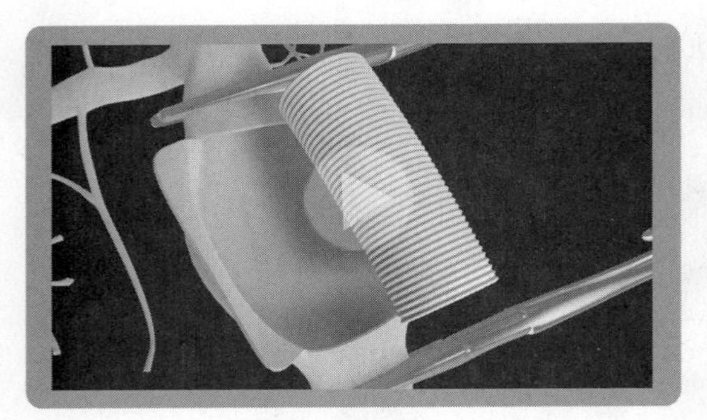

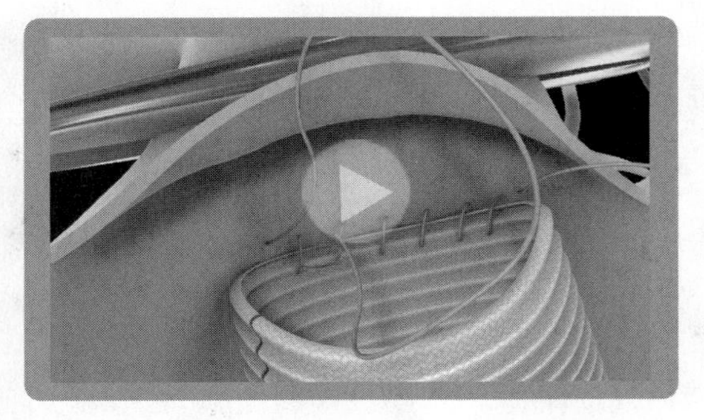

The 3D animations depict types of surgical repairs. Left: An open repair procedure for an abdominal aortic aneurysm is shown. Right: This is an endovascular or less invasive approach to an aneurysm repair.
Source: (*both*)

Unstable Patients with Dissecting Aneurysm

Aortic dissection is an unstable, life-threatening situation that commonly leads to rupture. Although very experienced clinicians may vary somewhat in their practice, recommended priorities and/or simultaneous interventions include:

- Help is needed, so call the Rapid Response team immediately.

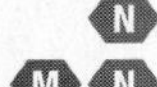

- When dissection or rupture is suspected or imminent, anticipate and prepare for the massive infusion of fluid and blood products perioperatively:
    - o Insert two large-bore IVs (size 14).
    - o Type and crossmatch for packed red cells and fresh frozen plasma.
- Stabilize the patient as much as possible while preparing for surgery:
    - o Begin volume infusion, or volume resuscitation, with IV fluids when indicated.

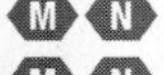

    - o Immediate surgical preparation and treatment are critical. Alert the vascular operating room team.

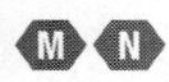

    - o When patients with dissection present with hypertension, urgent treatment and strict control are critical. These take priority as soon as the IV access is available because of the high risk for progressive aortic dissection or aneurysm rupture. Close monitoring and rapid intervention are imperative. **Evidence-based practice:** IV beta blockers and IV nitroprusside, if needed, are employed to rapidly control hypertension. Care is taken not to administer oral or long-acting antihypertensives in case of rupture and ensuing hypotension.

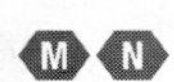

- Relief of severe, unremitting chest and/or abdominal pain with analgesics is an important intervention while diagnostic or surgical or medical interventions progress. Treatment of hypertension can sometimes also relieve pain. Avoid analgesics if rupture has occurred as they may harm the patient by exacerbating hypotension.

Patient with Ruptured Aortic Aneurysm

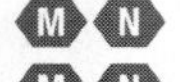

- Rupture is an emergency situation, and surgery without delay is the only lifesaving intervention.

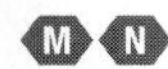

- Help is needed. The Code or Rapid Response teams are called urgently for resuscitation on the way to surgery.
- Rapid and severe hypotension and shock ensue.
- Morbidity and mortality are very high and are complicated by the comorbid conditions (often multiple) that most aneurysm patients have.
- Ensure large bore IV access is present before surgery in the event that large amounts of blood and fluid become necessary for resuscitation.
- In both dissection and rupture, the patient may be aware and scared. Emotional support and a moment for family are critical for the patient's well-being. Talk to the patient about what is being done to help them in a positive manner. Because this is a crisis situation, the family should be strongly supported during this brief visit that urgent care is ongoing. Pastoral care can be helpful to many families.

Abdominal Aortic Aneurysm

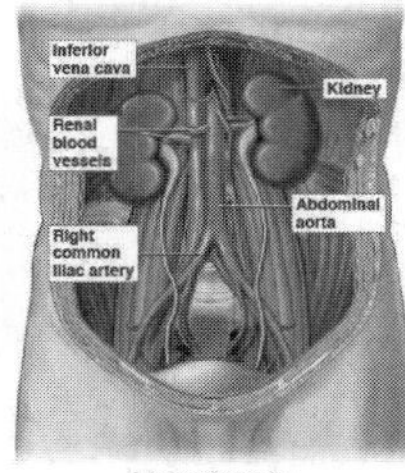

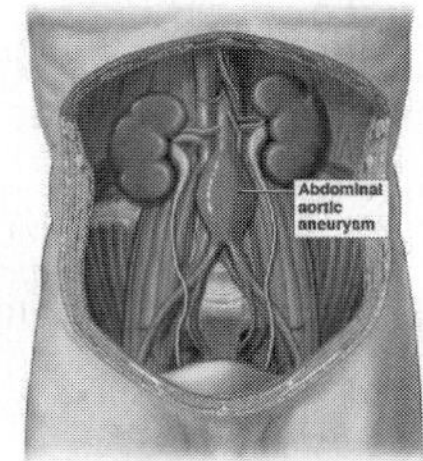

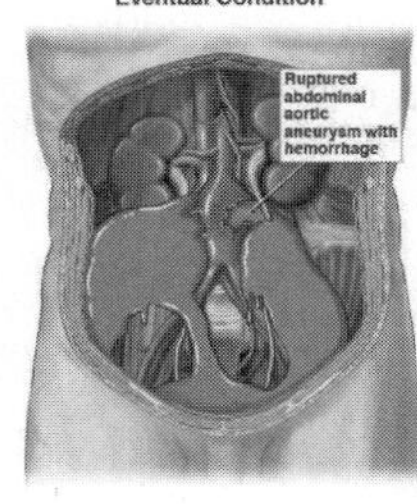

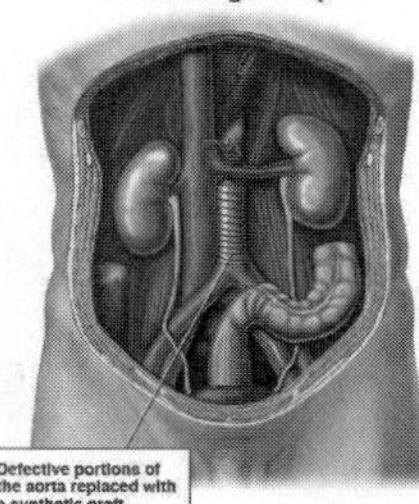

A diagram of the normal aorta is compared to the second illustration of an abdominal aortic aneurysm. The third picture depicts an aortic rupture with hemorrhage. The last illustration shows surgical repair.

Concept Check

12. What is the drug of choice for controlling hypertension in patients who are being medically managed for a small, stable aneurysm?

    A. Calcium channel blocker

    B. Diuretic

    C. Beta blocker

    D. Angiotension receptor blocker

Answer question

Collaborative Interventions: Aneurysms (continued)

Postoperative Complications

- Complications with the repair of a ruptured abdominal aortic aneurysm (AAA) are the same as with elective AAA repair, but more frequent. After rupture of AAA, patients have:
  - o 50% chance of renal failure
  - o 20% chance of MI
  - o Longer period requiring ventilator support
  - o Increased risk of colon ischemia

M N
- The most serious complication following aortic surgery is MI, accounting for almost half of the postoperative mortality. Monitoring cardiovascular performance such as troponin level and stroke volume is important.

M N
- The second most common complication from aneurysm repair is bleeding, which results from injury or coagulopathies. The nurse must be aware of hypovolemia symptoms as indicating a potential bleed.

M N
- Frequent assessment for strong femoral pulses, which indicate patency of the aorta.

M N
- Acute kidney injury, the third complication, is especially high in patients with pre-existing kidney disease. Acute kidney injury is usually caused by prolonged ischemia from extended aortic cross-clamping above the renal arteries, hypotensive episodes, and/or atheroembolization to the renal arteries. Renal function is assessed by measuring urine volume (fluid intake and urine output), electrolytes, and serum and urine creatinine.

M N
- Evidence-based practice: Postoperative antibiotics for prophylaxis should not be continued past 24 hours.

M N
- Prevent "never events" (e.g., DVT, catheter-related [IV and urinary] infections).

Postoperative Considerations

M N
- Acute limb ischemia is most commonly the result of atheroembolism and can occur in one or both legs. It is important to recognize significant cutaneous ischemia since it may occur despite maintenance of palpable pedal pulses (blue-toe syndrome or "trash foot").

N
- Assessment of pulses, skin color, temperature, movement, and sensation should be completed hourly. Pain in an extremity can be a significant indicator of acute ischemia.

N
- Bowel and spinal cord ischemia are less common complications but are associated with a high incidence of morbidity and mortality. Early recognition of any abnormal return of neuro or bowel function should trigger collaborative evaluation.

M N
- Respiratory complications may be avoided through routine postoperative therapy (e.g., incentive spirometry, early ambulation, and, if necessary, postural drainage and percussion).

M N
- Central IV and urinary catheter should be discontinued as soon as feasible.

N
- Prevention of never events is critical in these high-risk patients (e.g., DVT, catheter-associated urinary tract infections, pressure ulcers, falls, ventilator-acquired pneumonia, surgical site infection, air embolism, blood incompatibility, glycermic events, objects left in surgery).

M N
- Assist patient to mobilize and/or ambulate at the earliest possible time.

Concept Check

13. What is the most serious complication following aortic surgery?

A. Myocardial infarction

B. Bleeding

C. Acute kidney damage

D. Infection

Answer question

Concept Check

14. Which finding is a significant indication of acute extremity ischemia?

A. Pain in the extremity

B. Flushed skin

C. Bogginess of tissues in the area

D. Induration of the skin

Answer question

Summary of Interventions: Aneurysms

- Small and stable aneurysms: Watch or treat using risk factor modification, hypertension and lipid control, smoking cessation, and screen first-degree relatives.
- Larger or enlarging aneurysms: Surgical repair should be strongly considered.
- Aneurysm dissection: Get help, anticipate and prepare for urgent surgical repair and massive fluid and blood replacement, strict and immediate control of hypertension, mobilize vascular team, and pain control.
- Aneurysm rupture: Emergency surgery is the only life-saving intervention. Repeat interventions for dissection.

Dissection, Leak, or Rupture

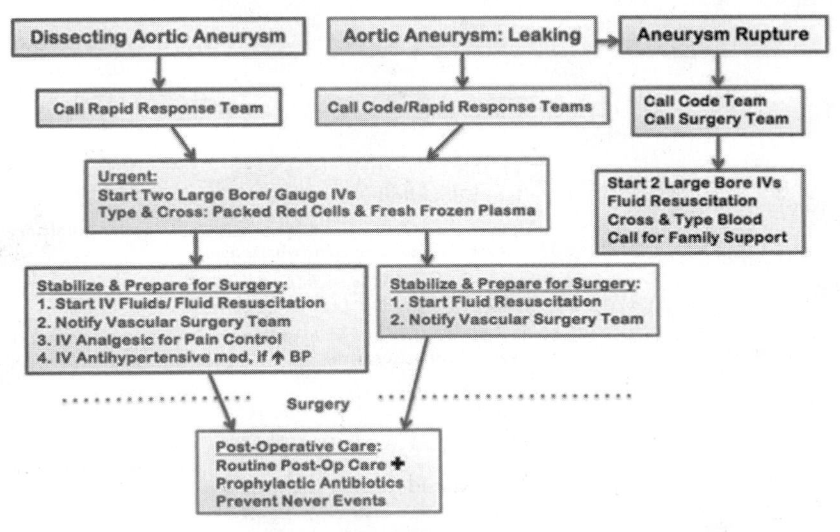

Source: Copyright © 2013, NovEx Novice to Expert Learning, LLC

LO4:

Evaluation of Desired Collaborative Care Outcomes: Aneurysms

Evaluation and reassessment should reveal attainment of previously established patient outcomes. In summary:

- Patient has clear mentation, skin is warm and dry, hemodynamic measurements are within expected levels, and urine output balances fluid intake.
- Patient identifies cause of fear and reports that fearful feelings have decreased.
- Patient reports reduction in pain.

References

(August 2008). National health care costs of peripheral arterial dease in the Medicare population. *Vascular Medicine, 13*(3), 209–215.

Bonham, P. A., & Kelechi, T. (2008). Evaluation of lower extremity arterial circulation and implications for nursing practice. *J Cardiovasc Nurs, 23*(2), 144–152.

Chaikof, E. L., Brewster, D. C., Dalman, R. L., Makaroun, M. S., Illig, K. A., Sicard, G. A., et al. (2009). Care of patients with abdominal aortic aneurysm: The Society for Vascular Surgery Practice Guidelines. *Journal of Vascular Surgery, 50*(8S), 1–48.

Dolinger, C., & Strider, D.V. (2010). Endovascular interventions for descending thoracic aortic aneurysms: The pivotal role of the clinical nurse in postoperative care. *J Vasc Nurs, 28*(4), 147–153.

Oran, N.T., & Oran, I. (2010). Carotid angioplasty and stenting in carotid artery stenosis: neuroscience nursing implications. *J Neurosci Nurs, 42*(1), 3–11.

Smith, L. (2012). Identifying and managing peripheral arterial disease. *Nurs Times, 108*(43), 12–14.

Stordahl, N. J., & Back, M. R. (2000). The efficacy of carotid endarterectomy: a vascular surgery perspective reducing hospital stay. *Medsurg Nurs, 9*(3), 113-121.

Tinkham, M. R. (2009). The endovascular approach to abdominal aortic aneurysm repair. *AORN J, 89*(2), 289–302.

White, A., Broder, J., Mando-Vandrick, J., Wendell, J., & Crowe, J. (2013). Acute aortic emergencies—part 2: aortic dissections. *Adv Emerg Nurs J, 35*(1), 28–52.

Clinical Practice Guidelines

Aboyans, V., Criqui, M., Abraham, P. et al. (2012). Measurement and interpretation of the ankle-brachial index: A scientific statement from the American Heart Association. *Circulation, 126*, 2890–2909. doi: 10.1161/CIR.0b013e318276fbcb

2011 Writing Group Members, 2005 Writing Committee Members, ACCF/AHA Task Force Members. (2011). 2011 ACCF/AHA Focused Update of the Guideline for the Management of patient with peripheral artery disease: A report of the American College of Cardiology Foundation/American Heart Association Task Force on practice guidelines. *Circulation, 124*, 2040.

Olin, J. W., Allie, D. E., Belkin, M., Bonow, R. O., Casey, D. E., Creager, M. A., Gerber, T. C., Hirsch, A. T., Jaff, M. R., Kaufman, J. A., Lewis, C. A., Martin, E. T., Martin, L. G., Sheehan, P., Stewart, K. J., Treat-Jacobson, D., White, C. J., Zheng, Z. J.; American Association of Cardiovascular and Pulmonary Rehabilitation; American Diabetes Association; Society for Atherosclerosis Imaging and Prevention; Society for Cardiovascular Magnetic Resonance; Society of Cardiovascular Computed Tomography; PAD Coalition; American Academy of Podiatric Practice Management; ACCF/AHA Task Force on Performance Measures, Masoud, F. A., Bonow, R. O., DeLong, E., Erwin, J. P. 3rd, Goff, D. C. Jr, et al. (2010). ACCF/AHA/ACR/SCAI/SIR/SVM/SVN/SVS 2010 performance measures for adults with peripheral artery disease. A Report of the American College of Cardiology Foundation/American Heart Association Task Force on Performance Measures, the American College of Radiology, the Society for Cardiac Angiography and Interventions, the Society for Interventional Radiology, the Society for Vascular Medicine, the Society for Vascular Nursing, and the Society for Vascular Surgery (Writing Committee to Develop Clinical Performance Measures for Peripheral Artery Disease). *Vasc Med, 15*(6), 481–512.

Patient Education

Cleveland Clinic. Diseases & Conditions. **http://my.clevelandclinic.org/heart/disorders/vascular/whatis.aspx**

Hamdan, A., Livingston, E. H., & Lynm, C. (2013). Treatment of varicose veins. *JAMA, 309*(12), 1306.

Medline Plus. Vascular Diseases. **http://www.nlm.nih.gov/medlineplus/vasculardiseases.html**

Medscape. Venous Insufficiency Clinical Presentation. **http://emedicine.medscape.com/article/1085412-clinical**

National Heart, Lung, and Blood Institute. What Are the Signs and Symptoms of Carotid Artery Disease? **http://www.nhlbi.nih.gov/health/health-topics/topics/catd/signs.html**

National Heart, Lung, and Blood Institute. What Is Carotid Artery Disease? **http://www.nhlbi.nih.gov/health/health-topics/topics/catd/**

Sugerman, D.T. (2013). Vascular screening. *JAMA, 310*(12), 1302.

Texas Heart Institute. Peripheral Vascular Disease. **http://www.texasheartinstitute.org/HIC/Topics/Cond/pvd.cfm**

Torpy, J. M., Lynm, C., & Glass, R. M. (2007). Transient neurological attack. *JAMA, 298*:(24), 2978.

Zeller, J. L., Burke, A. E., & Glass, R. M. (2009). Aortic aneurysms. *JAMA, 302*(18), 2050.

Learning Outcomes for Vascular Diseases: Venous Thromboembolism (VTE)

When you complete this lesson, you will be able to:

1. Recognize the clinical relevance of venous thromboembolism.
2. Consider the pathophysiology, etiology, risk factors, and clinical presentation of venous thromboembolism that determine the priority patient concerns.
3. Determine the most urgent and important nursing interventions and patient education required in caring for a patient with venous thromboembolism.
4. Evaluate attainment of desired collaborative care outcomes for a patient with venous thromboembolism.

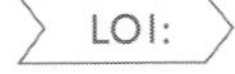

What Is Vascular Disease?

Vascular diseases involve any condition that affects the blood vessels and result in damage that reduces or blocks blood flow. These can be divided into arterial and venous diseases:

1. Arterial Diseases (see Arterial Disease NovE-lesson):
   - Peripheral Arterial Disease (PAD), also widely known as Peripheral Vascular Disease (PVD)
   - Carotid Artery Disease
   - Renal Artery Disease
   - Aortic Disease: Aneurysms
   - Cardiac Valvular Disorders (see CVD NovE-lesson)
2. Venous Diseases:
   - Venous Thromboembolism (VTE)
   - Chronic Venous Insufficiency (CVI) (see CVI NovE-lesson)

This NovE-lesson focuses on Venous Thromboembolism.

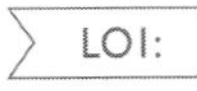

What Is Venous Thromboembolic Disease?

- Venous thromboembolism (VTE) refers to clots (thrombi) that form in the deep veins. Because a VTE has the potential of dislodging, or a piece breaking off and traveling towards the heart (embolism), it needs to be treated immediately.
- VTE includes problems of both thrombosis and embolism. A deep vein thrombosis (DVT) is a thrombosis that may embolize.

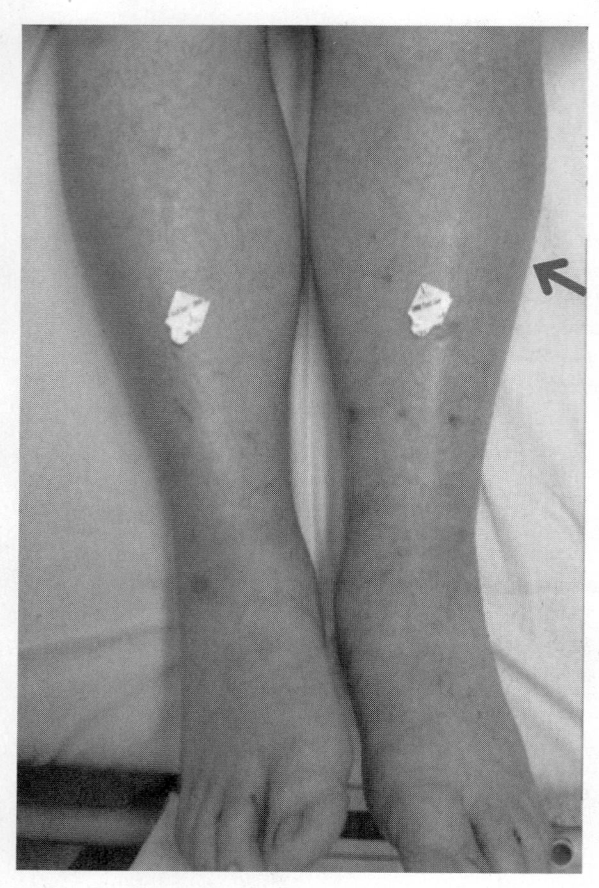

This photo shows a patient with a DVT (arrow) who complained of leg pain. Although her calf is only subtly enlarged, her foot shows swelling from the occlusion, preventing venous return.
Source: Courtesy of K. Kyriakidis

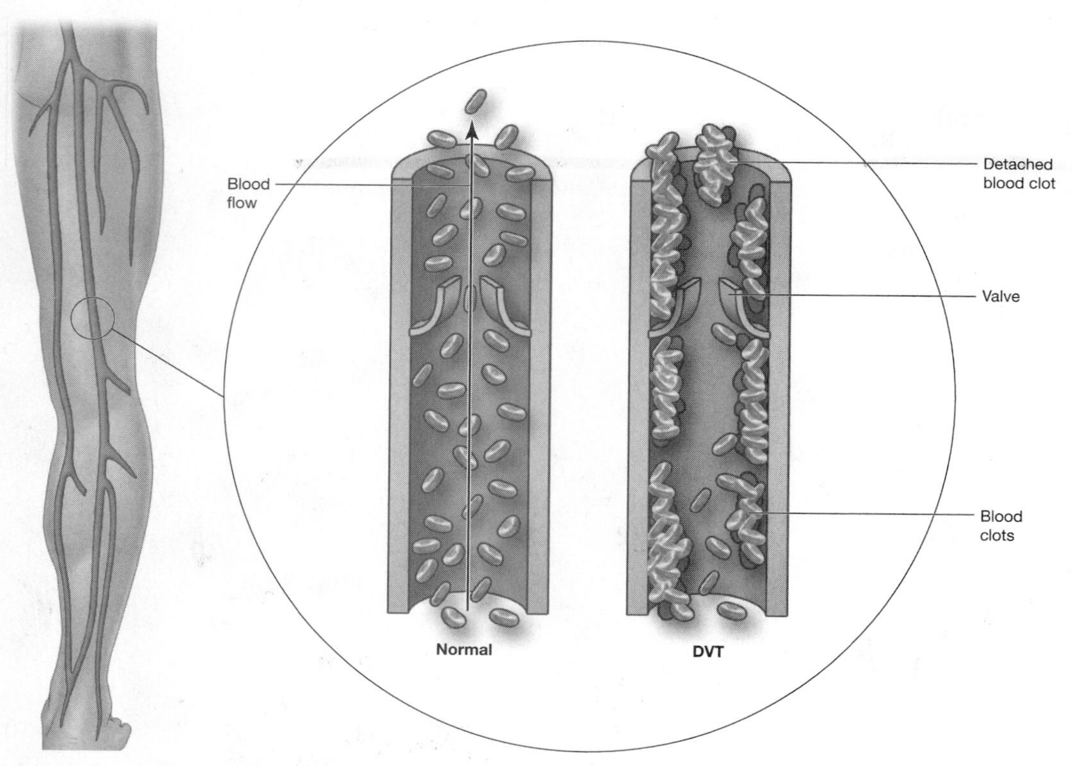

This illustration shows DVT formation.

Concept Check

1. A blood clot that dislodges from a deep vein and travels toward the heart is called a(n):

   A. Thrombus

   B. Embolism or embolus

   C. DVT

   D. PE

Answer question

LO1:

Clinical Relevance

- Pulmonary embolism (PE) is a complication of DVT, which is potentially fatal. PE results in approximately 200,000 deaths per year.
- Both DVT and PE are *preventable*.
- Post-thrombotic syndrome (PTS), the name given to chronic venous insufficiency (CVI) caused by a DVT, is a common debilitating complication (50% prevalence) resulting in edema, pain, and chronic ulceration.

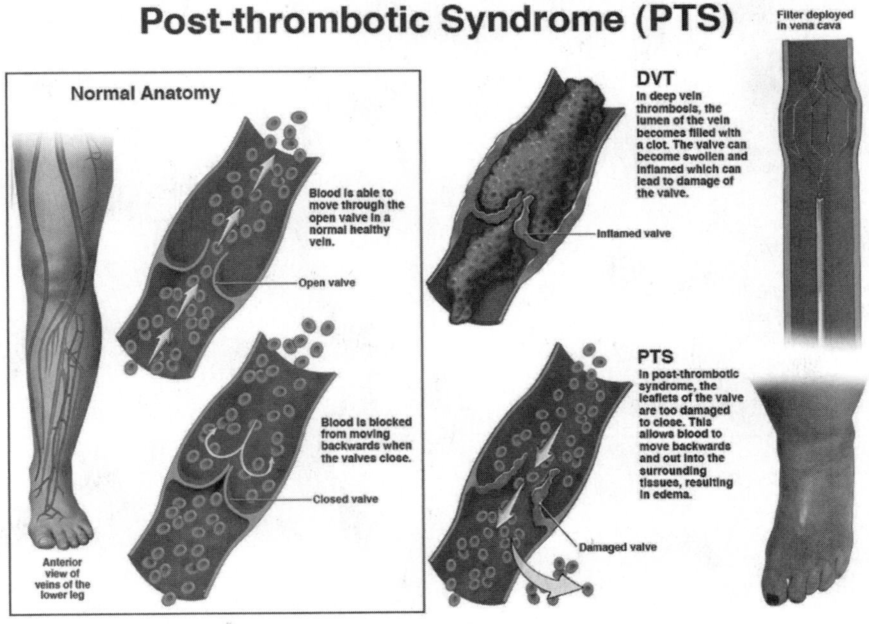

This medical exhibit features PTS with seven images. The first image portrays an anterior view of the veins of the lower leg. The second image shows a cutaway view of a vein with an open valve. The third image is a cutaway view of a vein with a closed valve. The fourth image pictures a cutaway view of a vein with a large clot. The fifth image shows a cutaway view of a vein that has been treated for a DVT and the valve is damaged. The sixth image features a filter deployed in a vena cava, and the seventh image illustrates a swollen foot suffering from PTS.

LO2:

Pathophysiology

- Clots are most commonly formed in the deep veins. Some people are predisposed to clot formation because of a hypercoagulable state (e.g., factor V Leiden), venous stasis, or venous damage.
- Fibrin binds red or white blood cells with platelets to form small or large clots.
- Thrombi form where vessels are damaged and/or blood flow is stagnant, particularly around valve "pockets," as seen in the illustration.
- Venous clots also damage the walls and valves in the veins, causing chronic venous insufficiency (post-thrombotic syndrome).
- The immediate danger that clots pose is in potentially embolizing from the venous system through the right heart and lodging in the lungs.

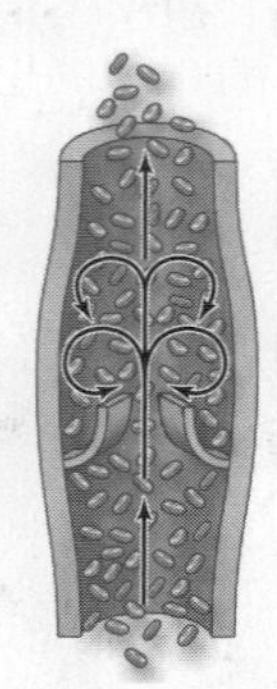

Normal blood flow through a vein

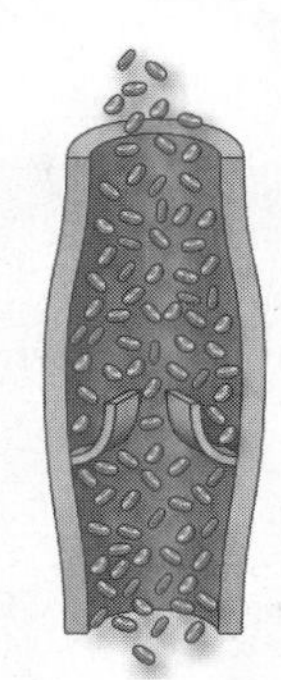

Early development of a thrombus

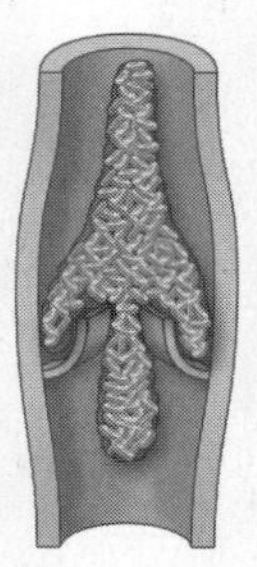

Continued development of a thrombus

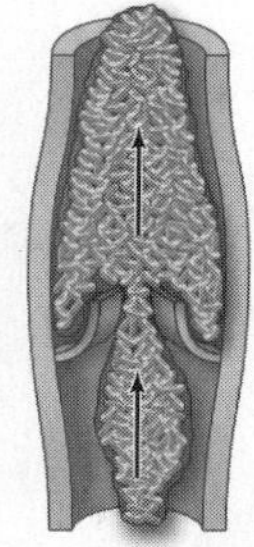

Final development of a thrombus

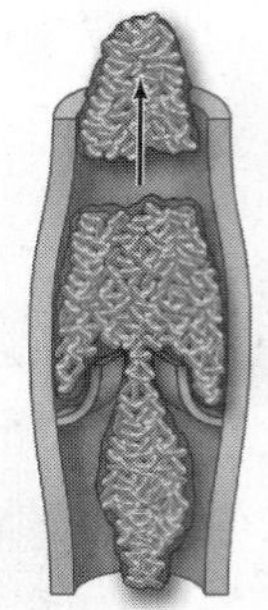

Development of an embolus

This series of illustrations depict the pathophysiological process of venous thromboembolism. The upper images show an early accumulation (right) of red cells behind the valves and along the vessel wall near the valves as compared to the normal vein. However, the lower images depict the gradual, but continued clot formation and growth until the thrombus occludes the vein. Some thrombi will have fragments (lower right) dislodge and embolize; hence, the term thromboembolism.

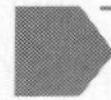

Concept Check

2. Where are clots most commonly formed?

A. In deep veins
B. In deep arteries
C. In superficial veins
D. In superficial arteries

Answer question

Concept Check

3. A clot that forms in a vein deep in the leg has the highest potential to lodge in which organ?

A. Brain
B. Lung
C. Kidney
D. Intestine

Answer question

Venous thromboembolism (VTE) basically results in two major clinical presentations:

1. Deep vein thrombosis (DVT) typically forms in the deep veins of the legs and grows or extends upward. DVT is the most common manifestation of VTE.
2. Pulmonary embolism (PE) occurs in 50–60% of patients with DVT but only about 30% are symptomatic. PE is the most serious of the two clinical presentations of VTE.

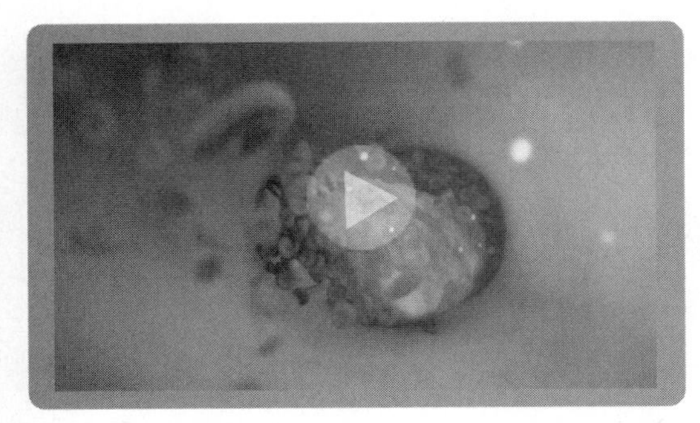

This animated depiction of DVT shows how a blood clot forms during poor blood flow, blood cells accumulate to form a thrombus, and the thrombus dislodges. When the thrombus breaks loose, it migrates to the lungs, causing a PE.

Risk Factors

- Hospitalization, immobility
- Central venous lines (catheters, pacemaker wires)
- Major surgery or trauma
- Chronic medical conditions (cancer, heart failure, pulmonary disease, inflammatory bowel syndrome)
- Hormones, oral contraceptives, pregnancy
- Obesity
- Genetic predisposition (e.g., factor V Leiden, deficiency of Protein C or S, high levels of factor VIII)
- Family history
- Smoking
- Prolonged travel, sitting, standing
- Pregnancy

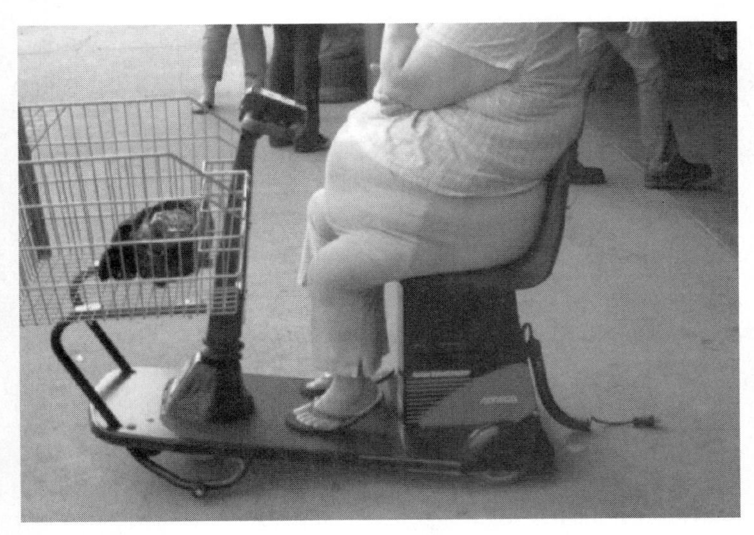

Circulation published a study that showed that body weight, waist and hip circumference, body mass index, and total body fat are predictors of VTE risk. Women with a greater hip circumference were at greater risk of VTE, while men with a higher waist circumference had more VTEs.

Concept Check

4. **Which genetic condition may be implicated in an increase in coagulability?**
   A. Hemophilia
   B. Factor V Leiden
   C. Down syndrome
   D. Low levels of factor VIII

Answer question

Causes

- Hypercoagulable states:
  - o Inherited (e.g., patients with factor V Leiden have five times the risk of pulmonary embolism)
  - o Acquired (e.g., malignancy, oral contraceptives)
- Venous endothelial injury or stasis (e.g., CVI or recent hip or knee surgery)
- Traumatic injury
- Malignancy: DVT may be the first presenting symptom.

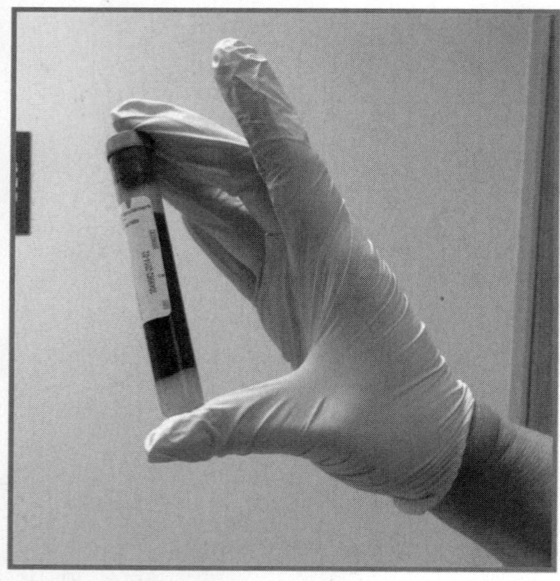

A common genetic problem that increases the risk of VTE is factor V Leiden. Although the majority of patients with factor V Leiden do not develop VTE, it can have critical consequences or be life threatening for those who do. Women are more likely than men to have this genetic abnormality.

Assessment Findings

1. DVT is responsible for a majority of pulmonary emboli. Recognizing signs and symptoms of DVT can therefore be helpful, although they are not always reliable:
   - Calf pain
   - Calf and leg edema
   - Palpable popliteal cord
   - Erythema of the calf, sometimes confused with cellulitis
   - Homan's sign is a patient's increased resistance when the foot is dorsally flexed without accompanying pain. It is used but not reliable and is not considered dangerous.
2. If a pulmonary embolus develops, the patient may show sudden shortness of breath, chest pain, hypoxemia, cough, clammy bluish or purplish skin, tachycardia, fainting, and great anxiety. Unfortunately, some PEs are subclinical and the patient might not show any symptoms. If the embolus is large, circulation to both lungs may be obstructed and sudden death can occur.

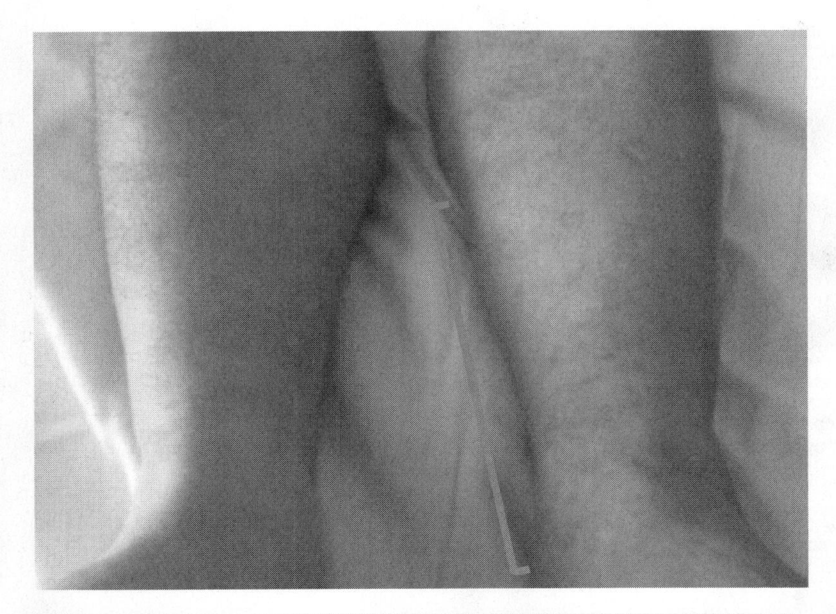

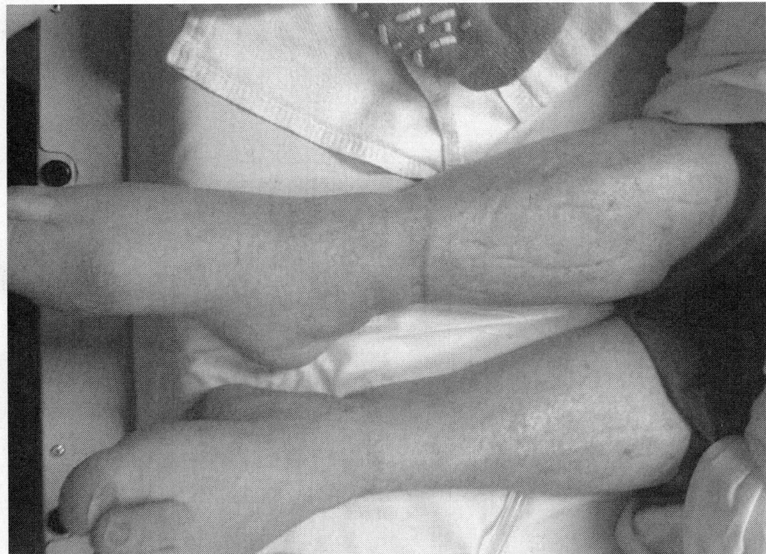

These photos illustrate the clinical presentation of DVT. Upper: The patient's left lower leg, just below the calf, is slightly enlarged, the foot and ankle are swollen, and the leg is more reddened and purplish as compared to the normal right leg, indicating possible DVT. Lower: DVT effects in this patient's lower right leg are more subtle. This calf is not discernibly red or swollen, but calf pain and the very swollen foot and ankle raise suspicion and warrant further study.
Source: (*upper*) Copyright © 2013, NovEx Novice to Expert Learning, LLC; (*lower*) Courtesy of K. Kyriadkidis

Diagnostics

- Diagnostic studies are particularly important in DVT since the signs and symptoms upon physical exam are commonly nonspecific or unreliable. Venous duplex can be used to evaluate DVT. It is the most common test employed to diagnose DVT.
- Contrast venography is invasive but the most reliable test. It can help visualize the presence of thrombus formation.
- Elevated D-dimer suggests there is thrombosis. D-dimer is a fibrin degradation product seen in the blood after a blood clot is lysed by fibrinolysis. D-dimer, however, has low specificity in diagnosing pulmonary emboli since it is present in many other conditions. Normal value is 0.5 mcg/mL.

Normal vein collapses when compressed | **Vein with a DVT cannot be compressed**

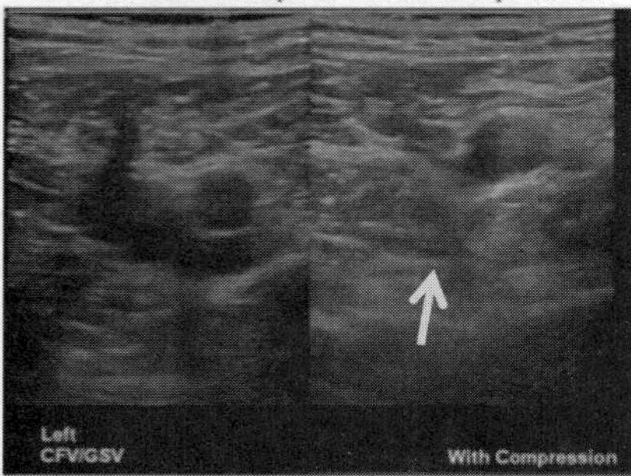

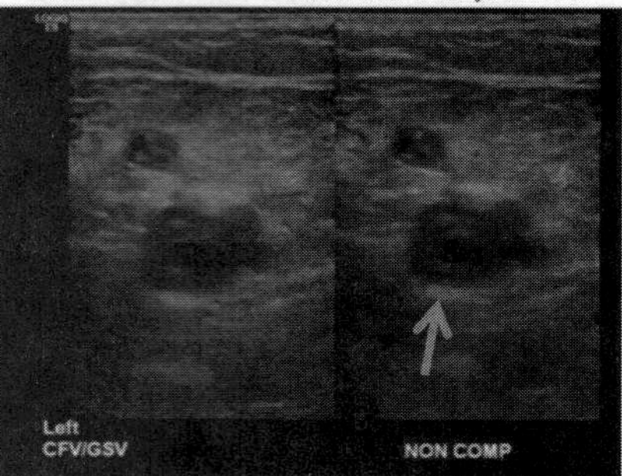

These four venous duplex images, two normal on the left and two showing a DVT on the right, demonstrate how to identify a DVT. On the left, the normal vein is shown first. The yellow arrow points to the collapsed or compressed vein when external pressure is applied. Nothing is occupying the venous space to prevent it from compressing. On the right, a DVT occupies the venous space. When external pressure is applied, the DVT prevents the vein from compressing (red arrow).

Normal vein with blood flow | **DVT obstructing blood flow**

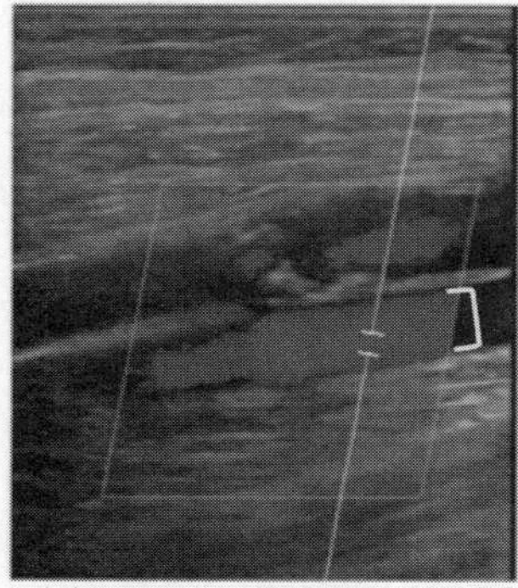

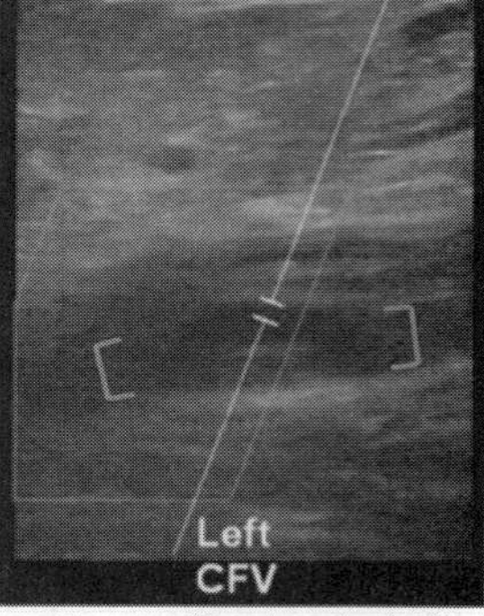

Although less accurate, duplex ultrasound is more common and less invasive in diagnosing a VTE. The two images allow comparison between normal and abnormal venous studies. Left: Normal blood flow (navy blue demarcated by a yellow bracket) appears in the ultrasound. Right: A DVT occluding the vein is seen between the red brackets.

Source: (*all*) Courtesy of K. Kyriakidis

Priority Patient Concerns and Desired Collaborative Care Outcomes

Prior to caring for patients with VTE, it is important to prioritize the patient's concerns that must guide the nursing care plan and interventions. Care for the patient is ordered and organized in accordance with the patient's priority and urgent needs. Desired collaborative care outcomes in patients with VTE typically include:

1. Patient will have no increased impairment of peripheral tissue perfusion than prior to the VTE.
2. Patient's arterial blood gases or oxygen saturation level will resolve toward normal as oxygen support is gradually reduced and discontinued.
3. Patient will report reduction of pain.
4. Patient will remain normovolemic.

Considering these important care outcomes, prepare a list of the major 3–6 priority patient concerns or nursing diagnoses for patients with VTE. Be prepared to participate in a discussion of this list and/or to submit them as an assignment, as determined by your faculty. Resources you may find helpful in this assignment can include this lesson, the references, resources on nursing care plans, and standard nursing diagnoses manuals.

Concept Check

5. Which test is the most accurate in the diagnosis of deep vein thrombosis?

A. D-dimer

B. Venous duplex

C. PT/PTT

D. Troponin

Answer question

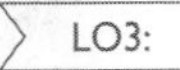

Collaborative Interventions

Evidence-Based Practice

The focus of treatment for DVT centers on the prevention and treatment of blood clots:

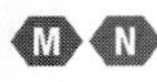

- Anticoagulation prevents further clot formation, but does not help lyse the current clot. Activated PTT (APTT) tests the same effects of heparin but activators are added to the blood sample. Activators shorten the clotting time required for the test. Treatment for specific types of DVTs include:
  - o Anticoagulants should be started immediately if the thrombus affects the deep veins in the upper leg (popliteal, femoral, or iliac veins). DVTs in this location are at highest risk for causing PE. Oral warfarin (Coumadin) is used for long-term anticoagulation
  - o Calf vein thrombosis is less likely to result in PE but is often treated with anticoagulation to prevent propagation to the upper leg and to help prevent post-thrombotic syndrome.
  - o Anticoagulants and, particularly, thrombolytics place patients at increased risk of bleeding and adverse reactions. For this reason, thrombolytics that lyse clots are rarely considered unless symptoms are severe and onset is recent.
- Acute management is to give unfractionated IV heparin or low-molecular subQ heparin as the treatment of choice:
  - o Unfractionated heparin requires titration and the monitoring of partial thromboplastin time (PTT), which is the time it takes for a clot to form, helps track the effects of the heparin.
  - o Goal is to maintain the APTT = 46–70 sec (1.5 to 2.3 times control).
- Long-term management is daily oral warfarin.
  - o INR goal is usually 2.0–3.0. Warfarin usually requires several days to take effect. Therefore, treatment is usually started in conjunction with heparin, which works immediately. Heparin is discontinued after the INR is within therapeutic range.

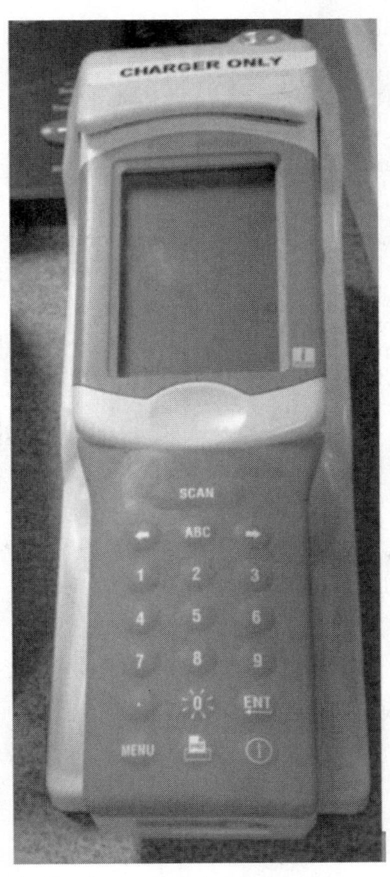

Small analysers, this being an example, very quickly and accurately determine the PT and INR values of a patient on warfarin sodium and guide the dosage determination with predetermined guidelines.
Source: Courtesy of K. Kyriakidis

Concept Check

6. What is the advantage of APTT testing over PTT testing?

A. APTT testing is much less expensive.

B. APTT testing is more accurate.

~~C. APTT testing is quicker.~~

D. APTT testing is noninvasive.

Answer question

Prevention

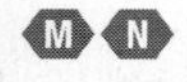

- As stated, low-molecular-weight heparin or unfractionated subQ heparin is the mainstay of VTE prophylaxis. Patients requiring longer-term anticoagulation (e.g., patients after hip replacement) are sometimes treated with warfarin for prevention.

- An (inferior vena cava) IVC filter may be placed in high-risk patients who cannot be anticoagulated (see illustration). The IVC filter does not prevent thromboembolism but instead filters out the embolus from reaching the lung.

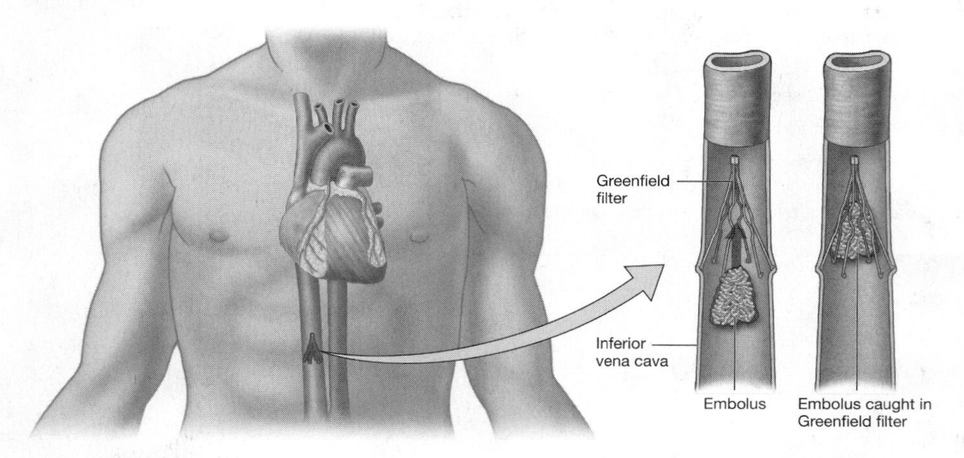

This illustration shows the placement of an IVC filter to protect the lungs from VTE. It can be inserted percutaneously to mitigate complications.

- Identify patients at high risk for close observation and/or prophylaxis: general and abdominal-pelvic surgical patients with Caprini scores greater than or equal to 5 (physicians score patients according to risk factors); patients having hip or knee arthoroplasty; colorectal, pelvic, hip fracture, spinal cord, cancer, bariatric, or trauma surgery; and obese patients.
- Instruct the patient to do leg exercises every 2 hours while at bedrest. Leg exercises involve flexion, extension, and rotation of feet, particularly against a footboard or hard surface.
- Avoid crossing legs while lying or sitting as this promotes venous stasis.
- Early and frequent ambulation or mobilization can help prevent thrombus formation.
- Encourage hydration if not prohibiting cardiac problems. Avoid caffeine which acts as a diuretic.
- In patients who are at high risk for bleeding, intermittent pneumatic compression devices may be used.
- There is little evidence that graduated compression stockings are effective, although often recommended.
- In low-risk patients, maintaining activity is a good preventative therapy. Early postoperative ambulation is strongly encouraged.

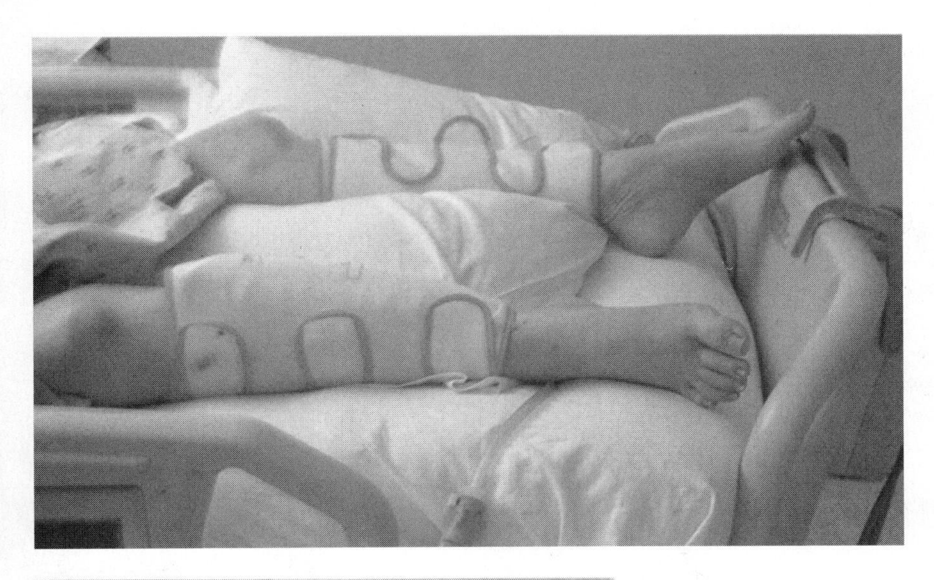

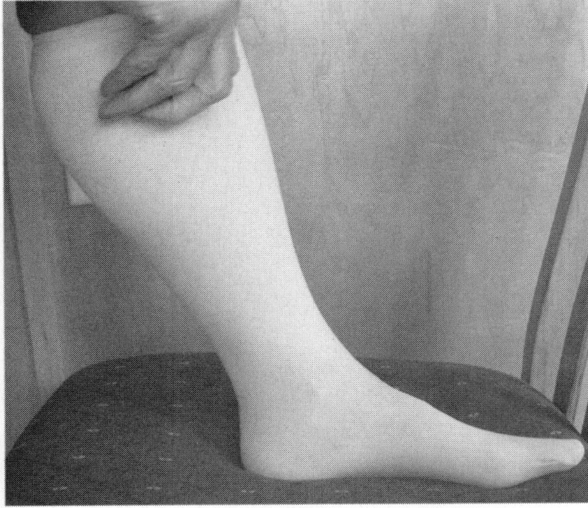

Upper: This is one example of the intermittent pneumatic compression or sequential compression devices used to prevent thromboembolism in at-risk patients.
Lower: At discharge, this patient is utilizing compression stockings.
Source: (*upper*) Courtesy of K. Kyriakidis; (*lower*) Copyright © 2013, NovEx Novice to Expert Learning, LLC

Concept Check

7. **Which statement regarding graduated compression stockings is accurate?**
   A. There is abundant evidence that they reduce venous thromboembolism.
   B. They are dangerous and should not be used.
   C. They are superior to Intermittent pneumatic devices in protecting against VTE.
   D. They are often prescribed despite evidence regarding their effectiveness.

Answer question

Collaborative Interventions (continued)

Patient Education

Educate the patient for prevention of VTE:

- N Maintain activity:
  - o Early ambulation, especially, postoperatively
  - o Exercise lower extremities by performing ankle flexion exercises.
- M N Rest is indicated in the acute phase of a VTE until anticoagulation is achieved. Then regular activity is important to avoid further coagulation disturbances.
- N In the acute phase, do not massage the area due to the danger of dislodging a thrombus and causing an embolus.
- M N Low-molecular-weight heparin or unfractionated heparin, both are subcutaneous.
- M N Intermittent pneumatic compression devices when patients cannot be anticoagulated.
- N Smoking cessation is important to avoid or prevent further damage from vascular disease and vasoconstriction.
- N Avoid caffeine and alcohol which can cause diuresis.
- N Transform meals to healthier diet.
- N Avoid sitting with legs in a dependent position or standing for long periods. During travel, stop and take a walk every hour. Change positions often to avoid blood pooling in the extremities.
- N Avoid wearing restrictive clothing that hinders blood flow from any part of the lower body or an extremity.
- N Collaborate with health care provider to carefully manage comorbid conditions that can exacerbate CVI and its complications.
- N Inform health care providers and dentist about taking anticoagulants due to increased risk of bleeding.
- N Birth control pills should be evaluated since they may promote hypercoagulability.
- N Weight management and exercise programs are important to help avoid venous stasis and vascular disease.

(Graduated compression stockings, although commonly recommended, have not been shown to reduce the incidence of PE or DVT.)

Summary of Interventions

Treatment focuses on prevention of new thrombus formation:

- Treatment is usually with anticoagulation.
- Treatment is started immediately.
- Aim for prevention with low-molecular-weight or unfractionated heparin.
- Educate the patient for prevention.

LO4: Evaluation of Desired Collaborative Care Outcomes

Evaluation and reassessment should reveal attainment of previously established patient outcomes. In summary:

- Patient's skin is as warm, mentation is as clear, and tissues are as intact as prehospital or prior condition allows.
- Patient has no findings of respiratory distress and arterial blood gases/oxygen saturation levels trend toward normal for patient.
- Patient states that pain-relief measures are adequate.
- Patient's blood pressure is stable, mentation is back to pre-illness state, and urine output is balanced with fluid intake.

References

Abad Rico, J. I., Llau Pitarch, J.V., & Rocha, E. (2010). Overview of venous thromboembolism. *Drugs, 70*(Suppl 2), 3–10.

Arabi, Y. M., Khedr, M., Dara, S. I., Dhar, G. S., Bhat, S. A., Tamin, H. M., Afesh, L.Y. (2013). Use of intermittent pneumatic compression and not graduated compression stockings is associated with lower incident VTE in critically ill patients: a multiple propensity scores adjusted analysis. *Chest, 144*(1), 152–159.

Chapman, N. H., Brighton, T., Harris, M. F., Caplan, G. A., Braithwaite, J., & Chong, B. H. (2009). Venous thromboembolism—management in general practice. *Aust Fam Physician, 38*(1-2), 36–40.

Duffin, C. (2012). Professions team up in a bid to eradicate hospital acquired VTE. *Nurs Stand, 27*(4), 11

Greig, M. F., Rochow, S. B., Crilly, M. A., & Mangoni, A. A. (2013). Routine pharmacological venous thromboembolism prophylaxis in frail older hospitalised patients: where is the evidence? *Age Ageing, 42*(4), 428–434.

Ryan, K. & Johnson, S. (2008). Preventing DVT: a perioperative perspective. *J Perioper Pract, 19*(2), 55–59.

Pebanco, G. D., Kaiser, S. A., Haines, S. T. (2013). New pharmacologic methods to prevent venous thromboembolism in older adults: a meta-analysis. *Ann Pharmacother, 47*(5), 605–616.

Smith, K. (2011). Preventing venous thromboembolism. *Nurs Manag (Harrow), 18*(3), 12–17.

Walker, L. & Lamont, S. (2008). Graduated compression stockings to prevent deep vein thrombosis. *Nurs Stand, 22*(40), 35–38.

Welle, M. K. (2012). Understanding the new emerging oral anticoagulants for venous thromboembolism prophylaxis. *Orthop Nurs, 31*(5), 265–278.

Clinical Practice Guidelines

Guyatt, G. H., Eikelboom, J. W., Gould, M. K., Garcia, D. A., Crowther, M., Murad, M. H., Kahn, S. R., Falck-Ytter, Y., Francis, C. W., Lansberg, M. G., Akl, E. A. & Hirsh, J., American College of Chest Physicians. Approach to outcome measurement in the prevention of thrombosis in surgical and medical patients: Antithrombotic Therapy and Prevention of Thrombosis, 9th ed: American College of Chest Physicians Evidence-Based Clinical Practice Guidelines. *Chest, 141*(2 Suppl), e185S–e194S.

Meissner, M. H., Gloviczki, P., Comerota, A. J., Dalsing, M. C., Eklof, B. G., Gillespie, D. L., Lohr, J. M., McLafferty, R. B., Murad, M. H., Padberg, F., Pappas, P., Raffetto, J. D., Wakefield, T. W., Society for Vascular Surgery, & American Venous Forum. Early thrombus removal strategies for acute deep venous thrombosis: clinical practice guidelines of the Society for Vascular Surgery and the American Venous Forum. *J Vasc Surg, 55*(5), 1449–1462.

Patient Education

http://www.nhlbi.nih.gov/health/health-topics/topics/dvt/

http://www.cdc.gov/ncbddd/dvt/facts.html

http://ajrccm.atsjournals.org/content/159/1/1.long

Sugerman, H. J., Eklöf, B. G., Toff, W. D., Burke, A. E., & Livingston, E. H. (2012). Air travel related deep vein thrombosis and pulmonary embolism. *JAMA, 308*(23), 2531.

Torpy, J. M., Burke, A. E., & Golub, R. M. (2011). Thrombophlebitis. *JAMA, 305*(13), 1372.

Learning Outcomes for Vascular Diseases: Cardiac Valvular Disorders

When you complete this lesson, you will be able to:

1. Recognize the clinical relevance of cardiac valvular disorders.
2. Consider the pathophysiology, etiology, risk factors, and clinical presentation of cardiac valvular disorders that determine the priority patient concerns.
3. Determine the most urgent and important nursing interventions and patient education required in caring for a patient with cardiac valvular disorders.
4. Evaluate attainment of desired collaborative care outcomes for a patient with cardiac valvular disorders.

What Is Vascular Disease?

Vascular diseases involve any condition that affects the blood vessels and result in damage that reduces or blocks blood flow. These can be divided into arterial and venous diseases:

1. Arterial Diseases (see Arterial Disease NovE-lesson):
    - Peripheral Arterial Disease (PAD), also widely known as Peripheral Vascular Disease (PVD)
    - Carotid Artery Disease
    - Renal Artery Disease
    - Aortic Disease: Aneurysms
    - Cardiac Valvular Disorders
2. Venous Diseases (see VTE and CVI NovE-lessons):
    - Venous Thromboembolism (VTE)
    - Chronic Venous Insufficiency (CVI)

This NovE-lesson focuses on Cardiac Valvular Disorders.

LO1:

What Is Cardiac Valvular Disease?

- Cardiac valvular disease occurs when there is damage or structural change to the four valves controlling the normal unidirectional blood flow through the heart.

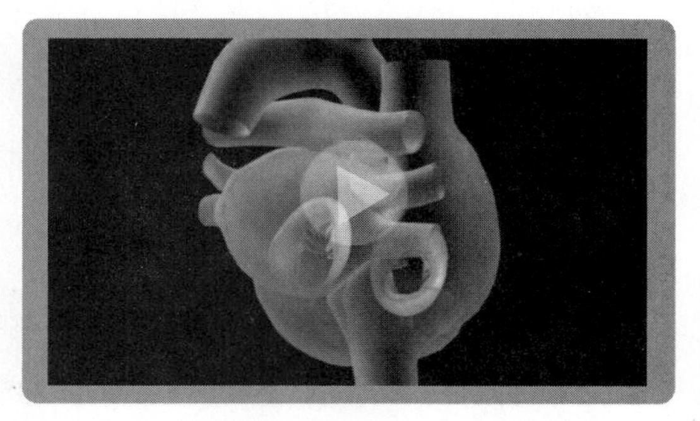

This animation demonstrates the normal functioning (opening and closing) of all four heart valves.
Source: © 2013 Nucleus Medical Media, All rights reserved

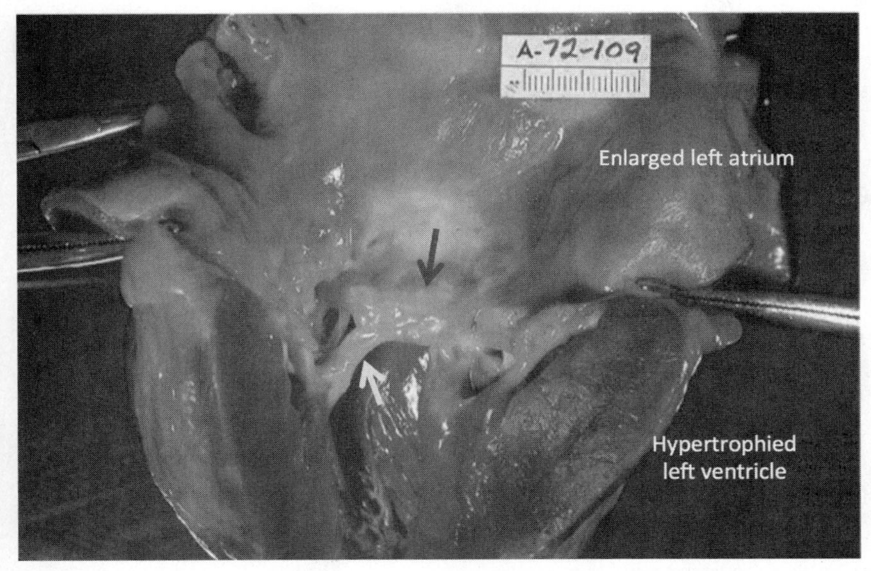

Rheumatic heart disease caused thickening of the mitral valve (blue arrow) and the chordae tendinae (yellow arrow), resulting in stenosis. The left atrium enlarged over time as blood flow diminished and backed up. Note the left ventricular hypertrophy that evolved from working to sustain cardiac output.
Source: CDC/Dr. Edwin P. Ewing, Jr.

- There are four cardiac valves—aortic, pulmonic, tricuspid, and mitral. Each of the four valves can best be heard over certain anatomical positions on the anterior chest:
    1. Aortic: 2nd intercostal space right of sternum
    2. Pulmonic: 2nd intercostal space left of sternum (Pulmonary)
    3. Tricuspid: Left lower sternal border (LLSB)
    4. Mitral: 5th intercostal space midclavicular line
- Each valve can be either stenosed or regurgitant, or both.
- Due to frequency of occurrence, only the mitral and aortic valve disorders are highlighted in this module.

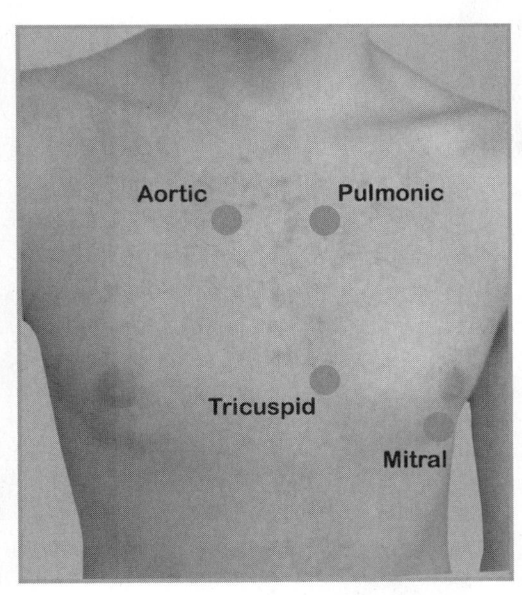

This illustration indicates the proper locations for auscultation of heart sounds made by the four cardiac valves.
Source: Copyright © 2013, NovEx Novice to Expert Learning, LLC

Concept Check

1. **Which terms are used to describe diseased valves? (Select all that apply.)**
   A. Regurgitant
   B. Bifurcated
   C. Dysrhythmic
   D. Stenotic
   E. Incompetent

Answer question

LO1:

Clinical Relevance

- Approximately 5 million people are diagnosed with heart valve disease each year.
- Valvular disease increases the risk for other medical problems, such as dysrhythmias and heart failure. For example, if a patient has mitral regurgitation (insufficiency or prolapse), blood is pumped back into the atrium during systole, decreasing stroke volume. The heart has to work harder to maintain cardiac output.
- If the patient has aortic stenosis (AS), the heart has to pump against a higher resistance, creating left ventricular hypertrophy and eventual heart failure.

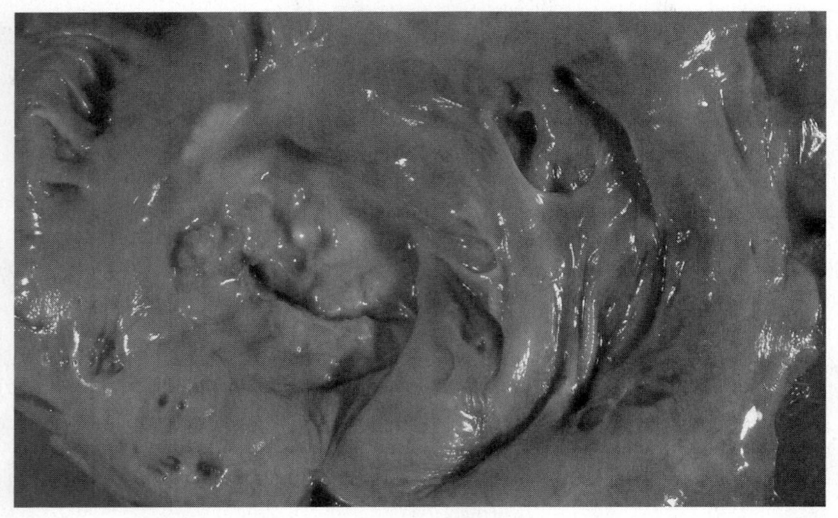

Mitral valve is stenosed and regurgitant, preventing normal forward blood flow and creating backward flow. Without timely and appropriate intervention, the combination of the two problems creates such a heavy workload on the heart that it is not sustainable.
Source: Yale Rosen/Custom Medical Stock Photo—

Concept Check

2. **Where is the mitral valve best auscultated?**
   A. 2nd intercostal space right of the sternum
   B. 2nd intercostal space left of the sternum
   C. Left lower sternal border
   D. 5th intercostal space at the midclavicular line

Answer question

LO2:

Pathophysiology

Cardiac valves are designed to permit blood flow in one direction. They normally channel blood flow in a single pathway through the four chambers of the heart during the cardiac cycle.

Valvular disorders arise when one or more heart valves is or becomes damaged and dysfunctional. Dysfunction can involve restriction of forward blood flow and/or backward flow. These two fundamental dysfunctional problems compromise stroke volume and cardiac output. The two types of valvular disease can involve four valves:

1. Regurgitation or insufficiency: Valve leaflets do not fully seal when closed, allowing blood to flow back into the preceding heart chamber. Regurgitant flow causes volume overload with dilation of the chamber.
    a. Mitral and tricuspid regurgitation increases the work on the ventricles. Systolic murmurs are present as a portion of blood flow reverses its normal path. Over time, the increased workload on the heart causes heart failure.
    b. Aortic or pulmonary regurgitation is less dangerous but can, also, interfere with cardiac ejection and stroke volume, as blood returns into the heart during diastole due to the incompetent valve. Heart failure, hypertension, and dysrhythmias may ensue.

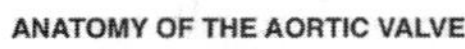

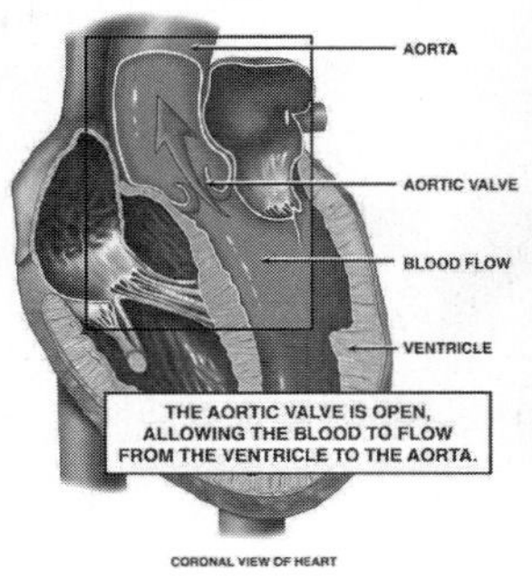

ANATOMY OF THE AORTIC VALVE

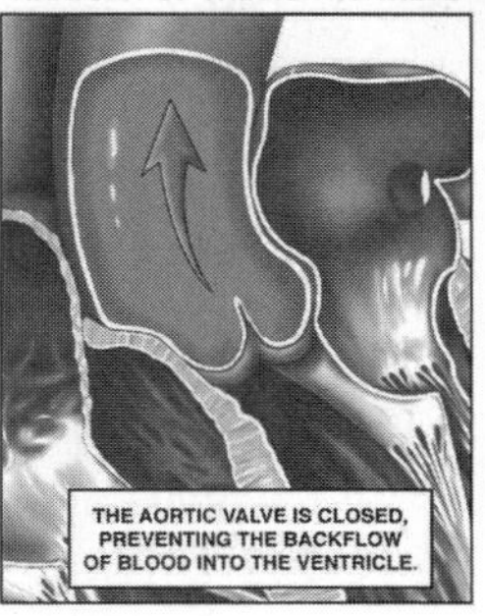

THE AORTIC VALVE IS CLOSED, PREVENTING THE BACKFLOW OF BLOOD INTO THE VENTRICLE.

FUNCTION OF DEFECTIVE VALVE

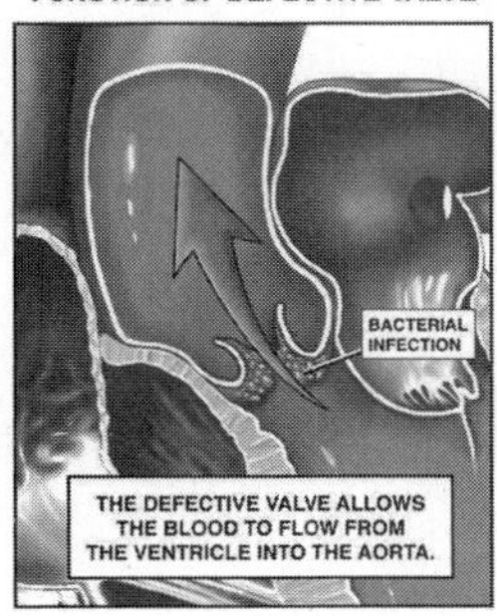

BACTERIAL INFECTION
THE DEFECTIVE VALVE ALLOWS THE BLOOD TO FLOW FROM THE VENTRICLE INTO THE AORTA.

FUNCTION OF DEFECTIVE VALVE

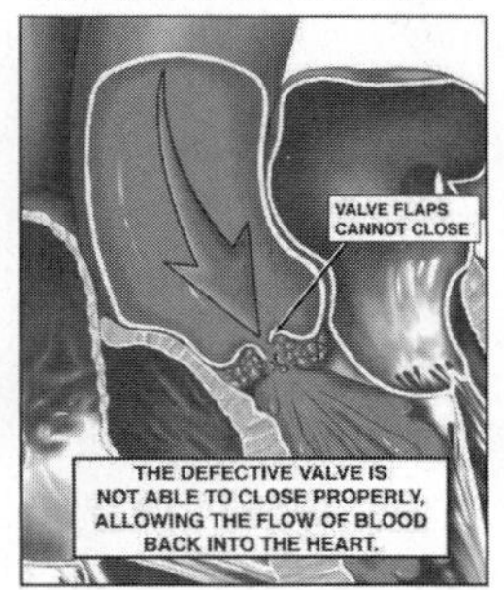

This comparison shows a striking difference between healthy and defective aortic valves.

2. Stenosis: Thickening or stiffness of the valve leaflets with calcification does not allow the valve to open fully during ejection. The partially closed valve then creates resistance to flow and a high pressure gradient across the valve. The higher pressure causes an elevated afterload (the heart's work to contract against an increased pressure load), eventually resulting in both atrial and ventricular hypertrophy.
    a. Mitral and tricuspid stenosis increases the workload on the atria. Diastolic murmurs are present when the atria contracts during ventricular filling, as blood cannot easily pass through the valves.
    b. Aortic or pulmonary stenosis creates increased workload on the heart as the ventricle must contract harder to force blood through a partially closed valve, leading to ventricular hypertrophy, dysrhythmias, and heart failure.

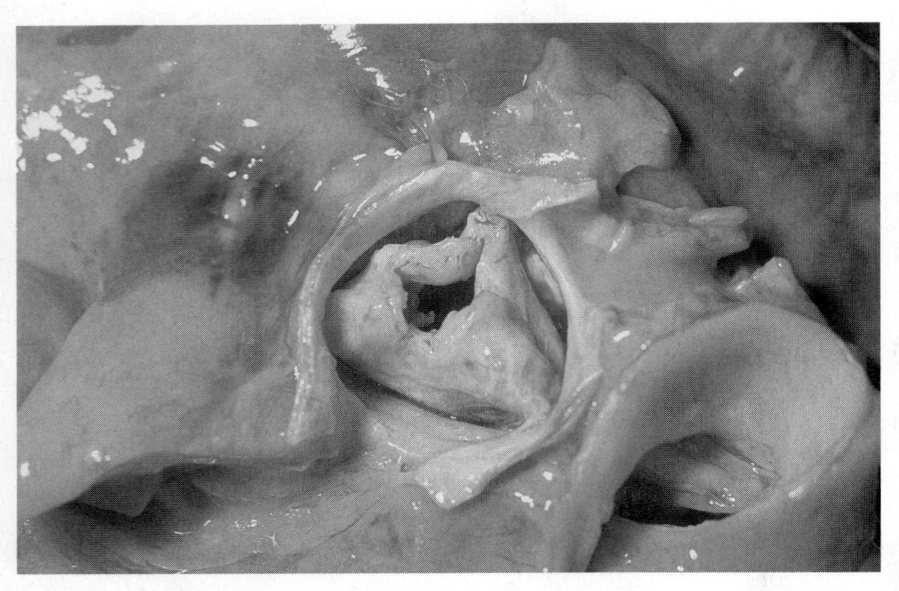

Note the thickened and fused stenotic cardiac valve leaflets that prevent the aortic valve from opening normally during systole. This photo assists in understanding how hard the heart must work to eject blood forward against the partially closed valve. The development of heart failure is inevitable.
Source: CDC/Dr. Edwin P. Ewing, Jr.

Risk Factors

The most common general risk factors for the development of cardiac valvular disease include:

- Aging
- Hypertension
- Coronary artery disease
- Smoking
- Myocardial infarction
- Infections
- Genetics (e.g., family history of valve disease)

Additional risk factors include:

- Diabetes
- Inactivity
- Radiation exposure (e.g., cancer therapy)
- Connective tissue diseases
- Obesity
- IV drug abuse

Causes

Causes of valvular disease can include:

- Rheumatic fever, which is the primary cause of acquired valvular disease
- Degenerative changes (from atherosclerosis)
- Congenital defects (mitral valve prolapse) (see diagram)
- Infections (infective endocarditis)
- Papillary muscle rupture from MI (see photo)
- Trauma
- Systemic diseases (Lupus)
- Congenital disorders (Marfan syndrome)

The mitral and aortic valves are more frequently affected by acquired valvular heart disease than either the pulmonic or tricuspid valves.

However, mitral regurgitation progresses slowly, and patients are often asymptomatic for years without knowing the disorder exists.

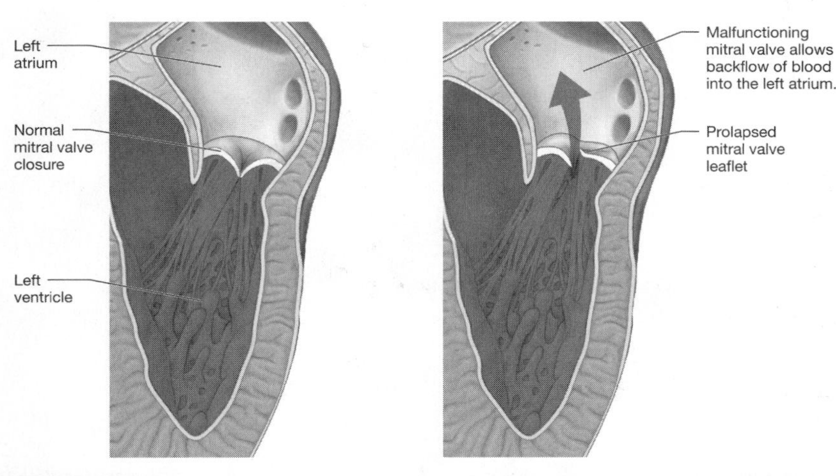

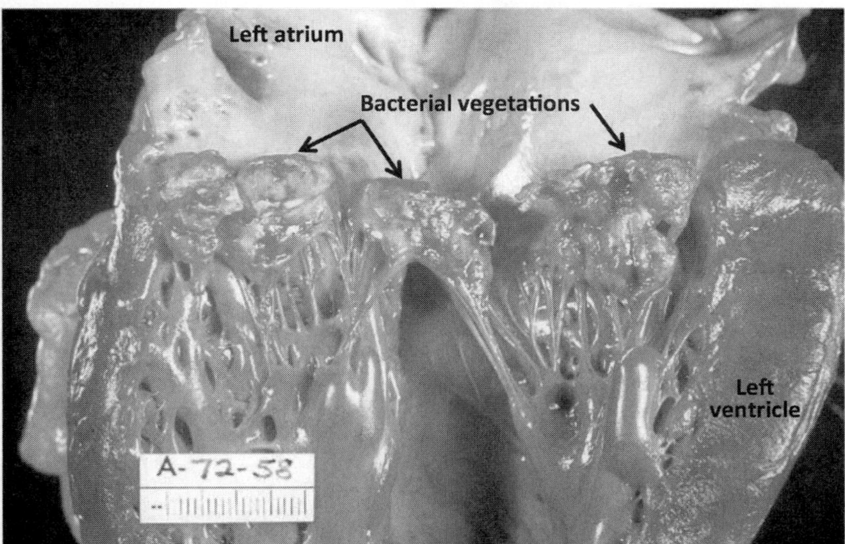

Upper: Mitral valve prolapse is a common cause of valvular disease that allows backflow of blood or regurgitation into the left atrium. Lower: Bacteria have invaded the thin, flexible leaflets of the mitral valve and caused thickening and destruction (arrows). With the huge vegetations, there is little movement of the valve due to both stenosis and regurgitation.
Source: (*lower*) CDC/Dr. Edwin P. Ewing, Jr.

Concept Check

3. What is the primary cause of acquired valvular disease?

A. Atherosclerosis
B. Myocardial infarction
C. Rheumatic fever
D. Trauma

Answer question

Assessment Findings

Aortic Insufficiency or Regurgitation

Aortic insufficiency (AI) leads to left ventricular overload, which eventually results in left ventricle (LV) hypertrophy and dilation. The clinical presentation of AI includes:

- Dyspnea, orthopnea, and paroxysmal nocturnal dyspnea (shortness of breath at night)
- Fatigue
- Widened pulse pressure
- Angina (if coronary artery disease is present)
- Abnormal heart sounds, including S3 and holodiastolic (throughout diastole) murmur heard best in aortic area (2nd intercostal space just right of the sternum)
- Sinus tachycardia, to compensate for a drop in stroke volume
- Elevated left ventricular filling pressures

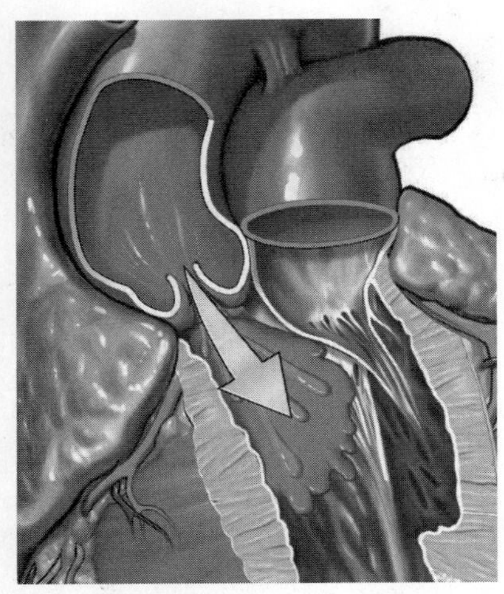
This drawing depicts blood flow back into the left ventricle during diastole due to aortic regurgitation. The abnormal volume that regurgitant blood adds to the normal filling volume and pressure causes heart failure over time.

Aortic Stenosis

Aortic stenosis (AS) causes narrowing of the valve, which obstructs blood flow during systole from the left ventricle into the systemic circulation. AS symptoms include:

- Syncope and fatigue, both due to a loss of stroke volume and cardiac output
- Palpitations, if supraventricular dysrhythmias develop
- Systolic murmur
- Angina, if coronary artery disease is present
- As the stenosis worsens and the valve narrows, symptoms of left ventricle failure are present.

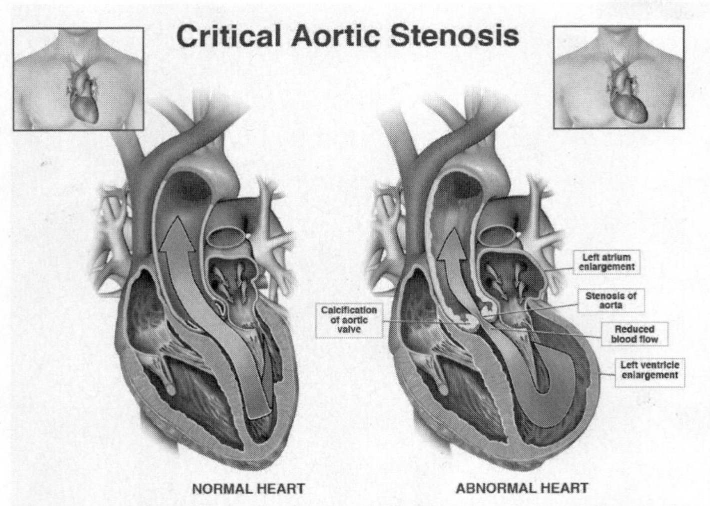

The diagrams compare blood flow from left atria to left ventricle and through the aortic valve. A normal heart shows normal flow, whereas severe calcification of the aortic valve causes critical AS, which limits blood from being ejected from the heart.

Assessment Findings (continued)

Mitral Insufficiency or Regurgitation

- **Mitral insufficiency** allows blood to be ejected back into the left atrium. Patients are commonly without symptoms. They may even be surprised to know they have a valve disturbance (this is common with all valve disturbances). However, if the insufficiency is significant, symptoms will begin to present, including:
  - o Dyspnea, orthopnea, and paroxysmal nocturnal dyspnea
  - o Elevated atrial and ventricular pressures, particularly as the heart fails
  - o Pulmonary hypertension
  - o Pulmonary crackles as heart failure develops
  - o Atrial fibrillation as the left atrium distends
  - o Holosystolic murmur heard best at the apex and lying on left side (left 5th intercostal space at the midclavicular line)
  - o The third heart sound (S3), also called ventricular gallop, produces a lub, dub, dub sound.

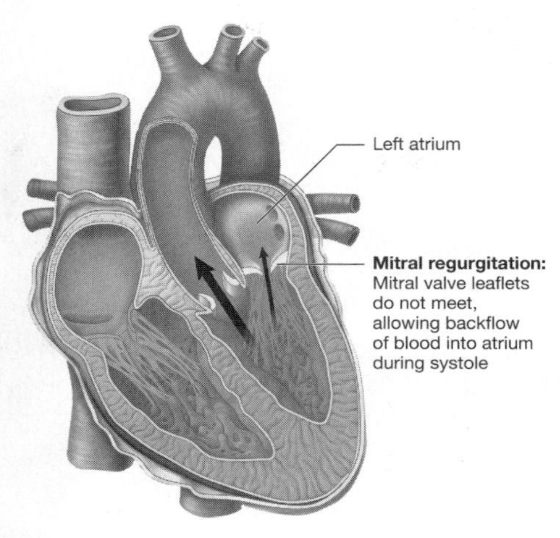

Left atrium
Mitral regurgitation:
Mitral valve leaflets
do not meet,
allowing backflow
of blood into atrium
during systole

Mitral regurgitation may be caused by either an abnormality of the mitral valve (degenerative mitral valve disease) or by weakness of the heart muscle that is not strong enough to adequately close the valve (functional mitral regurgitation).

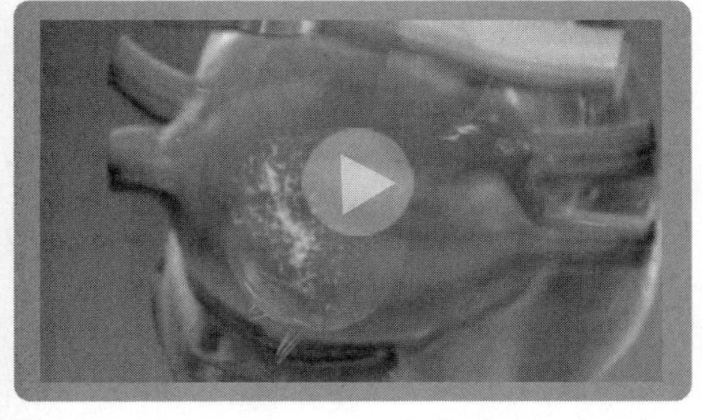

This animation demonstrates normal valve function (systole and diastole). It shows normal mitral valve function compared to mitral valve regurgitation, which occurs due to incomplete closure of the mitral valve.

Mitral Stenosis

Rheumatic fever is responsible for **mitral stenosis** in many patients. As the opening of the valve progressively narrows, the symptoms become more pronounced. The symptoms include:

- Dyspnea on exertion (DOE)
- Cough, due to pulmonary congestion. Hemoptysis occurs if pulmonary congestion is severe.
- Progressive fatigue
- Increased pulmonary and right ventricular pressures
- Atrial fibrillation
- Diastolic murmur, best heard at the apex of heart
- Peripheral edema
- Development of an emboli secondary to clot formation around the valve—this symptom can be severe if an emboli occurs in the cerebral circulation.
- Eventual right-sided heart failure, as pulmonary congestion begins to interfere with right heart function.

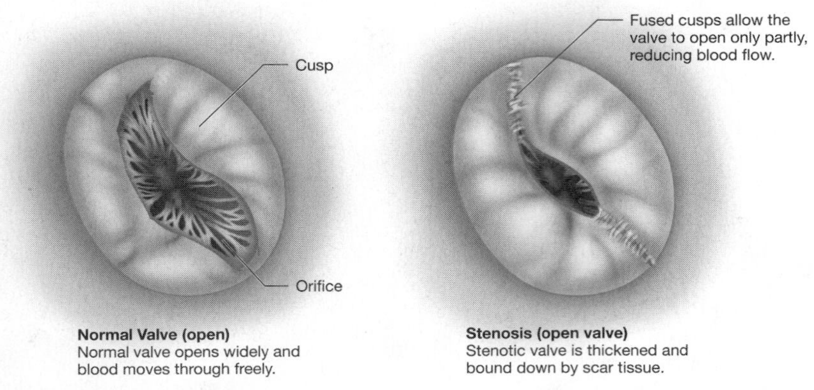
Cusp
Orifice
Normal Valve (open)
Normal valve opens widely and blood moves through freely.
Fused cusps allow the valve to open only partly, reducing blood flow.
Stenosis (open valve)
Stenotic valve is thickened and bound down by scar tissue.

This image helps to compare a normal mitral valve to a stenosed or narrowed valve.

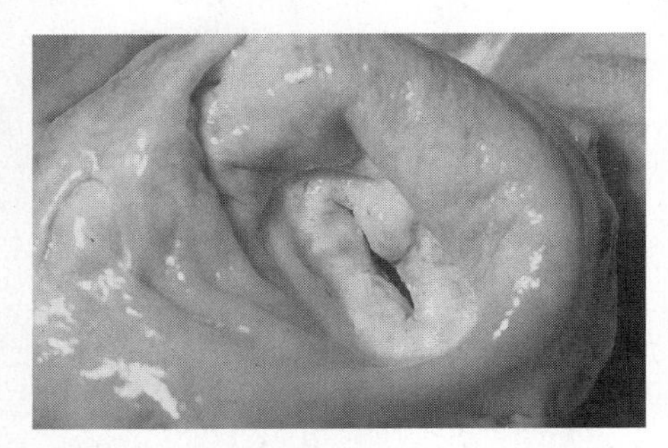

This photo shows an actual stenotic mitral valve. The stenosis is so severe that the valve leaflets have fused together, leaving a very small and insufficient opening for blood to be ejected from the ventricle. A valve that is this severely stenotic must be replaced or surgically repaired for the heart to effectively pump.

Source: CDC/Dr. Edwin P. Ewing, Jr.

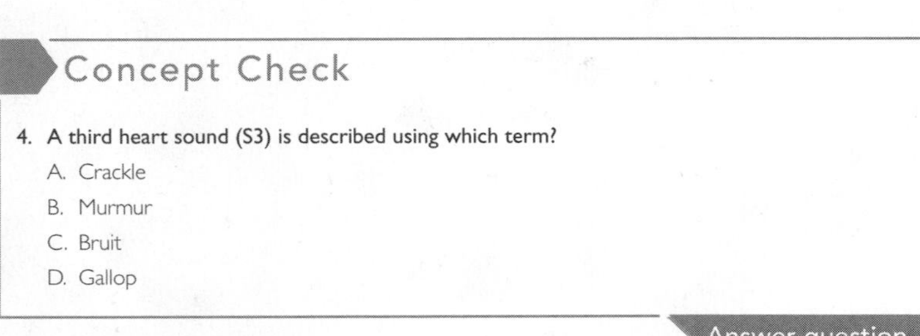

Concept Check

4. A third heart sound (S3) is described using which term?
   A. Crackle
   B. Murmur
   C. Bruit
   D. Gallop

Answer question

Diagnostics

Diagnosis of cardiac valve disease is made by:

- Physical exam: Presence of murmurs, evidence of enlarged heart, or fluid in the lungs
- EKG: Recording of electrical activity of the heart can detect left ventricular hypertrophy, myocardial ischemia, myocardial damage, and rhythm disturbances.
- Imaging: Echocardiogram can detect blood flow through the valves and pressures within the heart chambers (see animation).
- Transesophageal echocardiogram (TEE): Similar to echocardiogram but gives a clearer picture of the valves
- Cardiac catheterization: Using dye and x-rays to examine more details of coronary vessels, valves, and heart chambers
- Other tests can be used (e.g., exercise stress echocardiogram, radionuclide scans, magnetic resonance imaging [MRI]).

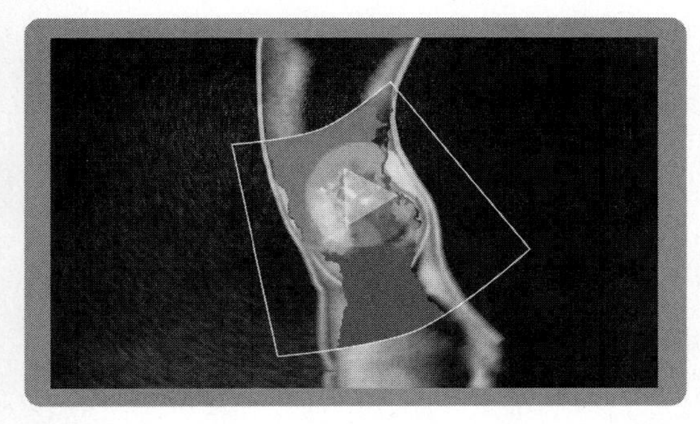

This medical animation depicts four different types of echocardiograms; transthoracic, Doppler, stress, and TEE. An echocardiogram is a test that uses sound waves to create a moving picture of the heart.

Priority Patient Concerns and Desired Collaborative Care Outcomes

Prior to caring for patients with cardiac valvular disease, it is important to prioritize the patient's concerns that must guide the nursing care plan and interventions. Care for the patient is ordered and organized in accordance with the patient's priority and urgent needs. Desired collaborative care outcomes in patients with cardiac valvular disease typically include:

1. Patient's skin is warm and dry, mentation is clear, and there are minimal to no findings indicating inadequate cardiac output or heart failure that is not being appropriately treated.
2. Patient's lungs are clear to auscultation or have greatly reduced crackles and urine output is balanced with fluid intake.
3. Patient reports return to individualized levels of daily activities with minimal to no dyspnea, chest pain, or excessive fatigue.
4. Patient verbalizes understanding of treatment plan, disease process, and interventions to prevent complications.

Considering these important care outcomes, prepare a list of the major 3–6 priority patient concerns or nursing diagnoses for patients with cardiac valvular disease. Be prepared to participate in a discussion of this list and/or to submit them as an assignment, as determined by your faculty. Resources you may find helpful in this assignment can include this lesson, the references, resources on nursing care plans, and standard nursing diagnoses manuals.

Concept Check

5. Which diagnostic test gives the clearest picture of valvular damage?

A. Electrocardiogram
B. Echocardiogram
C. Transesophageal echocardiogram
D. Exercise stress echocardiogram

Answer question

LO3:

Collaborative Interventions

Evidence-Based Guidelines: Management of Cardiac Valvular Disease

M N • Evidence-based treatments for valve disturbances vary depending on disease severity. For example, most valve disturbances are treated medically, if possible. The valve that is commonly replaced surgically is the aortic valve. Mitral valve replacement is the next most common surgery. Medical therapy is attempted prior to surgery, unless symptoms are severe and unlikely to resolve with medical management.

M N • For mild heart valve disease, no intervention may be needed. If the patient is asymptomatic and has no evidence of hypertrophy or other cardiac dysfunction, the patient may need only periodic monitoring by a health care provider or an advanced practice nurse.

- However, as the valve dysfunction worsens, ACC/AHA clinical practice recommendations include:
  - M N o Diuretics for heart failure
  - M N o Antidysrhythmic agents for treatment of atrial tachycardias and fibrillation
  - M N o ACE inhibitors for afterload reduction in heart failure
  - M N o Beta blockers for rate control and heart failure
  - M N o Patients with severe aortic stenosis are very sensitive to medications that cause even small changes in preload and afterload. Thus, medications should be used with caution and monitored closely.
  - M N o Anticoagulants when an embolic event has occurred or the patient is at risk
    - ■ In 2006, the ACC/AHA valvular disease guidelines were published that recommended long-term oral anticoagulation (target INR 2.5, range 2.0 to 3.0) in patients with mitral stenosis who have a prior embolic event, left atrial thrombus, or paroxysmal, persistent, or permanent AF, since all forms of AF carry a similar risk for thromboembolism.
    - ■ In 2008, the ACCP consensus conference suggested the addition of low-dose aspirin (50 to 100 mg/day) in patients who have an embolic event or who have left atrial thrombus despite oral anticoagulation at a therapeutic INR.

Concept Check

6. Which valve is most often replaced surgically?

A. Aortic

B. Pulmonic

C. Tricuspid

D. Mitral

Answer question

M

Surgical Treatments

- Severe heart valve disease often requires valve repair or replacement, particularly for aortic disease.
  - o Valve replacement has become common, even in octogenarians, or persons in their 80s, with good functional outcomes.
  - o All valves can be replaced, with aortic and mitral valves being the most likely.
- Minimally invasive surgery can be utilized for some valve repairs. This type of surgery is easier for the patient and shortens recovery time. However, its use is limited to uncomplicated valve replacement.
- Medical therapy is still necessary for heart failure, angina, and dysrhythmias.

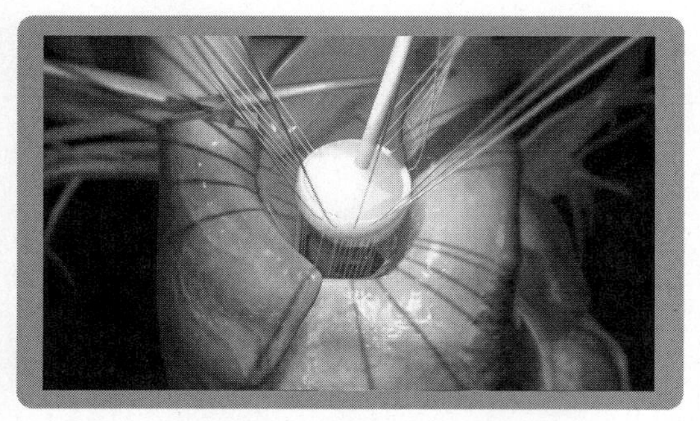

This animation demonstrates valve damage, the hemodynamic consequences of the damage, and surgical replacement of the valve.

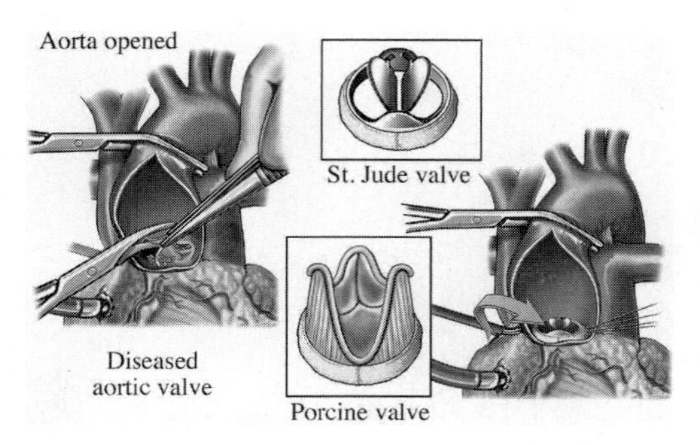

Comparison of two types of heart valve replacement, an artificial version and a donor version from a pig.

Collaborative Interventions (continued)

Postoperative Collaborative Interventions

Valve replacement care postoperatively is similar to most surgical care, once the patient is transferred from ICU. Care includes:

- M N Early weaning and extubation from mechanical ventilation
- M N Early removal of most catheters, tubes, and lines (e.g., urinary, NG, central)
- N Incision care
- N Electrical safety precautions are necessary to when handling the external pacemaker or pacing wires. Follow hospital safety protocol to prevent microshock. Collaborate with surgeon to remove the pacing wires in the absence of dysrhythmias.
- N Early mobilization and ambulation
- M N DVT and pressure wound prophylaxis
- M N Minimize the use of blood products and follow safety precautions prior to infusions. Monitor the patient vigilantly for adverse reactions.
- N Avoiding straining during bowel movement (may require a stool softener) and if overweight, attempting a diet
- M N Exercise rehabilitation for improvement in quality of life

M N Medications used preoperatively may be removed because the valve has been repaired or replaced. New medications are prescribed and may be lifelong, requiring thorough patient education.

Patient Education

Depending on the type of cardiac valve disorder and/or medical management versus surgical replacement, patient education varies.

- Issues that may need to be addressed in patients being medically managed can include:
  - o Educate the patient about their disease, symptoms that require seeking medical care, follow-up visits, likely complications when appropriate, smoking cessation, weight management, alcohol and substance avoidance, healthy diet, and light exercise.
  - o Educate thoroughly about the complex medications that may be needed to maintain stability and prevent heart failure (e.g., afterload reducers, diurectics, antidysrhythmics, anticoagulants).
  - o Educate about heart failure and prevention.
  - o Educate about prophylactic antimicrobial therapy for prevention of endocarditis.
  - o Instruct to avoid competitive sports if valvular dysfunction is moderate to severe.
  - o Assist patient to identify and educate patient about risk factor modification.
  - o Educate about valve replacement in patients likely to need surgery.
  - o Educate about advanced directives.

- After prosthetic valve replacement, the major educational issues for continued care and patient education are:
  - o Educate the patient about how important adherence to antithrombotic medications and routine monitoring is in preventing valve thrombosis and thromboembolism. Thromboembolism and anticoagulation are the most common causes of complications (EBP).
  - o Instruct the patient about the need for follow-up visits within a month postoperatively and the routinely for annual visits for evaluation of valve function (EBP).
  - o Educate about antimicrobial prophylaxis for bacterial endocarditis prior to invasive procedures that can cause bacteremia. Post-valve replacement patients are at high risk for endocarditis (EBP).
  - o Educate about the need for regular but moderate exercise. Evidence-based guidelines and recommendations are available regarding participation in competitive sports but evaluation is required (EBP).
  - o Instruct patients who may become or plan to become pregnant that antithrombotic therapy requires adjustment to prevent potential fetal harm. Discussions and planning with their health care provider is imperative.

Concept Check

7. What is the most common cause of complications after prosthetic valve replacement?

A. Pneumonia

B. Bowel infarction

C. Valve thrombosis

D. Surgical site infection

Answer question

Summary of Interventions

- Interventions for valve disturbances aim to resolve the symptoms produced by each valve dysfunction:
  - o Diuretics for heart failure
  - o Antidysrhythmic agents for development of atrial tachycardias and fibrillation
  - o Afterload reduction with agents such as ACE inhibitors
  - o Beta blockers for rate control and heart failure
  - o Anticoagulants when an embolic event has occurred or the patient is at risk
- Surgery is the corrective treatment, where the valve is replaced or repaired.
- Educate the patient regarding infective endocarditis prophylaxis.
- Educate the patient for health maintenance, risk factor modification, medication management, follow-up care, and advanced directives.

LO4: Evaluation of Desired Collaborative Care Outcomes

Evaluation and reassessment should reveal attainment of previously established patient outcomes. In summary:

- Patient's skin is warm and dry, mentation is clear, and there are minimal to no findings of inadquate cardiac output or heart failure that are not being appropriately treated.
- Patient's lungs are clear to auscultation or have greatly reduced crackles, and urine output is balanced with fluid intake.
- Patient reports return to personal level of daily activities with minimal or no dyspnea, chest pain, or excessive fatigue.
- Patient verbalizes understanding of treatment plan, disease process, and interventions to prevent complications.

References

Dirks, J. & Howland-Gradman, J. (2009). Valvular disease and surgery. In K. Carlson (Ed.), *AACN Advanced Critical Care Nursing* (pp. 322–346). St. Louis, MO: Saunders Elsevier.

Fuster, V., Ryden, L. E., Cannom, D. S., Crijns, H. J., Curtis, A. B., Ellenbogen, K. A., ... Wann, L. S. (2006). ACC/AHA/ESC 2006 Guidelines for the Management of Patients with Atrial Fibrillation: A Report of the American College of Cardiology/American Heart Association Task Force on Practice Guidelines and the European Society of Cardiology Committee for Practice Guidelines (Writing Committee to Revise the 2001 Guidelines for the Management of Patients with Atrial Fibrillation). Journal of American College of Cardiology, 48, e149.

Lauck, S., Mackay, M., Galte, C., & Wilson, M. (2008). A new option for the treatment of aortic stenosis: Percutaneous aortic valve replacement. *Critical Care Nurse, 28*, 40–51

Leeper, B. (2009). Valvular disease and surgery. In K. Carlson (Ed.), *AACN Advanced Critical Care Nursing* (pp. 322–346). St. Louis, MO: Saunders Elsevier.

Leung Wai Sang, S., Chaturvedi, R. K., Iqbal, S., Lachapelle, K., & de Varennes, B. (July 2012). Functional quality of life following open valve surgery in high-risk octogenarians. *Journal of Cardiac Surgery, 27*(4), 408–414.

Lynn-McHale Wiegand, D. (2003). Advances in cardiac surgery: Valve repair. *Critical Care Nurse, 23*, 72–90.

Nugteren, L. B., & Sandau, K. E. (2010). Critical review of health-related quality of life studies of patients with aortic stenosis. *Journal of Cardiovascular Nursing, 25*(1), 25–39.

Rosborough, D. (2006). Cardiac surgery in elderly patients: Strategies to optimize outcomes. *Critical Care Nurse, 26*, 24–31.

Clinical Practice Guidelines

Bonow, R. O., Carabello, B. A., Chatterjee, K., et al. (2008). 2008 Focused update incorporated into the ACC/AHA 2006 guidelines for the management of patients with valvular heart diseease: a report of the American College of Cardiology/American Heart Association Task Force on Practice Guidelines (Writing committee to Develop Guidelines for the Management of Patient with Valvular Heart Disease). *Circulation, 118*, e523–e661.

Vahanian, A., Baumgartner, H., Bax, J., Butchart, E., Dion, R., Filippatos, G., ... ESC Committee for Practice Guidelines. (2007). Guidelines on the management of valvular heart disease: The Task Force on the Management of Valvular Heart Disease of the European Society of Cardiology. *European Heart Journal, 28*, 230.

Patient Education

American Heart Association website: Learn about heart valve problems, signs and symptoms, and more.

www.heart.org/HEARTORG/Conditions/More/HeartValveProblemsandDisease/Heart-Valve-Problems-and-Disease_UCM_450280_SubHomePage.jsp

STOP

Go to the online course and complete the NovE-Cases assigned by your instructor for this module.

Learning Outcomes for Shock States: Overview

When you complete this lesson, you will be able to:

1. Recognize the clinical relevance of shock.
2. Consider the pathophysiology, etiology, risk factors, and clinical presentation of shock that determine the priority patient concerns.
3. Determine the most urgent and important nursing interventions and patient education required in caring for a patient with shock.
4. Evaluate attainment of desired collaborative care outcomes for a patient with shock.

LO1:

What Is Shock?

- Shock is a condition in which there is inadequate oxygen delivery or utilization for the cells to function.
- Shock states present as life-threatening situations and are among the most dangerous conditions a patient, or health care provider, can face. Shock is dangerous because it can cause multiorgan damage, failure, and death.
- Depending on the type of shock, symptoms can vary. There are three common shock states:
  - o Hypovolemic
  - o Cardiogenic
  - o Septic: **Sepsis, including septic shock, is a significant and under-diagnosed clinical problem. It is among the highest health care cost burdens** and it is included as a separate chapter NovE-Lesson under "Care of Patients with Sepsis."
- Additional, less common, but no less dangerous, shock states include:
  - o Neurogenic shock
  - o Anaphylactic shock

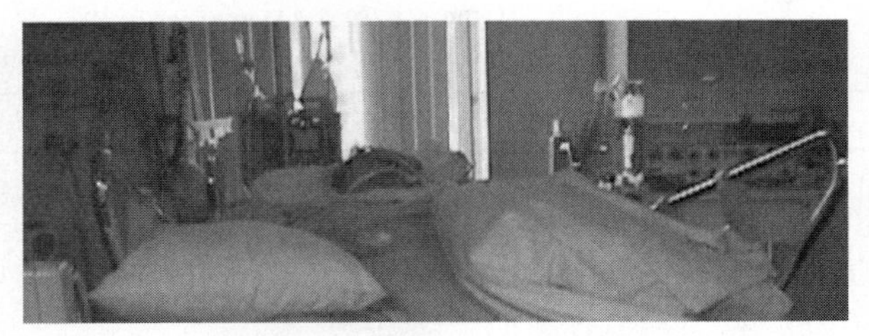

Patients in shock are usually transferred to the ICU, but all nurses are likely to see patients who are anywhere in the hospital and develop shock or who present in the emergency department.

Concept Check

1. Which shock state is most common?

A. Anaphylactic

B. Hypovolemic

C. Neurogenic

D. Irreversible

Answer question

LO1:

Clinical Relevance

- Shock states are a leading cause of death; yet, they are often missed until the late stages.
- Shock states are often the terminal event for many clinical conditions. For example, patients with most clinical conditions (e.g., MI, trauma) are unlikely to die until they reach the shock phase.
- Early recognition of shock states can be lifesaving.
- Urgent treatment is needed to prevent irreversible organ damage.
- Mortality is very high; 50–80% of patients die, often after extensive treatment and suffering.

LO2:

Pathophysiology

- Shock is the result of the loss of blood flow (oxygen delivery) to the tissues. Inadequate blood flow to tissues can ultimately cause life-threatening cellular dysfunction and death.
- The loss of blood flow in shock results from two major pathophysiological mechanisms:
  - o **Loss of macrocirculation**, which leads to a decrease in stroke volume and cardiac output. Conditions manifesting this situation include:
    - a. Hypovolemic shock (reduced circulating volume)
    - b. Cardiogenic shock (impaired cardiac function)
    - c. Early sepsis (caused by infection)
  - o **Loss of vascular tone and increased capillary permeability** (distributive shock) includes:
    - d. Septic shock (late sepsis)
    - e. Anaphylactic shock (associated with allergic reactions)
    - f. Neurogenic shock (caused by nervous system injury)
- All forms of shock, whatever the mechanism, interfere with the delivery of adequate amounts of blood flow and oxygen to the tissues.

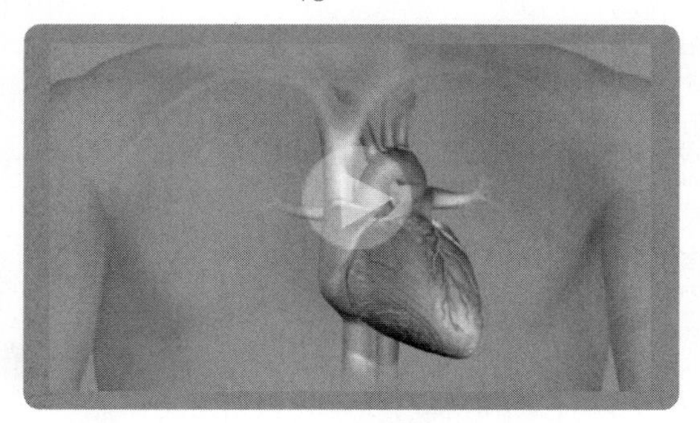

This animation addresses compensated and uncompensated shock.

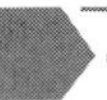

Concept Check

2. **Loss of macrocirculation is manifested in which shock state?**

   A. Late stage septic
   B. Neurogenic
   C. Anaphylactic
   D. Cardiogenic

Answer question

Macrocirculatory Shock

- Macrocirculation refers to blood flow in the heart and the large blood vessels (arteries, veins). Microcirculation refers to the smallest blood vessels (arterioles, venules, capillaries) within the organs and the periphery.
- Blood flow is evaluated from a macro perspective by measuring stroke volume and cardiac output. It is the most important component of oxygen delivery.
- Loss of other components required for oxygen delivery (e.g., hemoglobin or arterial saturation) can be compensated for by increasing cardiac output (e.g., increase in heart rate) to a point.
- The compensatory increase in heart rate and vasoconstriction shunts blood flow to the vital organs, away from, and at the expense of, nonvital organs (e.g., gut, kidneys, limbs) and the periphery.
- Once cardiac output can no longer be increased or sustained (compensatory mechanisms fail), the only method the body has to compensate for a decreasing cardiac output is to increase the extraction of oxygen from the hemoglobin. Increased oxygen extraction results in decreased tissue and venous levels of oxygen as reflected in the oxygen saturation of venous blood, such as SvO_2, $ScvO_2$, or StO_2 levels. Normal saturation levels for venous blood are greater than 70%.
- Preferential shunting of blood flow to vital organs compromises microcirculation and tissue (end organ) oxygenation, creates a maldistribution of blood flow, and if prolonged, leads to metabolic acidosis, severe vasodilation, and circulatory collapse.
- A low cardiac output, therefore, threatens the patient's survival and needs to be immediately addressed. Recognition of early warning signals is a key nursing role.

Microcirculatory Shock (also called Distributive Shock)

- Distributive shock refers to the impaired distribution of blood flow due to severe vasodilation that causes widespread tissue hypoxia. It is also referred to as microcirculatory shock because the microcirculation is most affected by inadequate blood flow, oxygen delivery, and tissue oxygenation. In this type of shock, the cascade of harmful sequelae primarily occurs in the microvasculature.
- Shock can be present due to microcirculatory loss of blood flow, even if macrocirculation (stroke volume and cardiac output) is normal.
- Vascular changes, such as severe vasodilation, loss of vasomotor tone, and increased capillary permeability, can cause loss of blood flow to tissues with significant pooling of blood in the venous and capillary vasculature. These changes are commonly sudden, severe, and demand urgent interventions.
- Compensatory mechanisms (vasoconstriction, increased heart rate) increase cardiac output, but preferentially shunt blood to the vital organs, essentially bypassing the periphery. The shunting results in slow or sluggish microcirculation.
- Despite the body's attempt to compensate by increasing cardiac output to offset the vascular changes, threats to tissue perfusion in the microcirculation can rapidly develop.
- If blood cannot reach tissues, such as occurs with microcapillary obstruction in sepsis, or if the cells cannot use oxygen (cellular dysoxia), the shock state worsens as cellular dysfunction leads to death of those cells. When enough cells die, the organ begins to fail.

Concept Check

3. Which pathophysiological factor is present in microcirculatory shock?

A. Decreased cardiac pumping strength

B. Decreased circulating blood volume

C. Severe vasodilation

D. Increased vasomotor tone

Answer question

Pathophysiology (continued)

Normal Tissue Oxygenation

- Understanding oxygenation is essential in understanding shock. Oxygenation starts in the lungs, but is dependent on a functioning cardiovascular system and hemoglobin to deliver oxygen to the tissues.
- Normal oxygenation occurs when arterial blood (oxygenated blood from the lungs) delivers oxygen bound to hemoglobin in the form of oxyhemoglobin (SaO_2) to the tissues.
- The tissues remove only some of the oxygen from the hemoglobin and return the remaining 75% as oxyhemoglobin back to the lungs. This oxyhemoglobin is the only oxygen reserve in the body.
- A decrease in the amount of oxygen returning to the heart, e.g., SO_2 <70%, represents a potential threat to oxygenation.

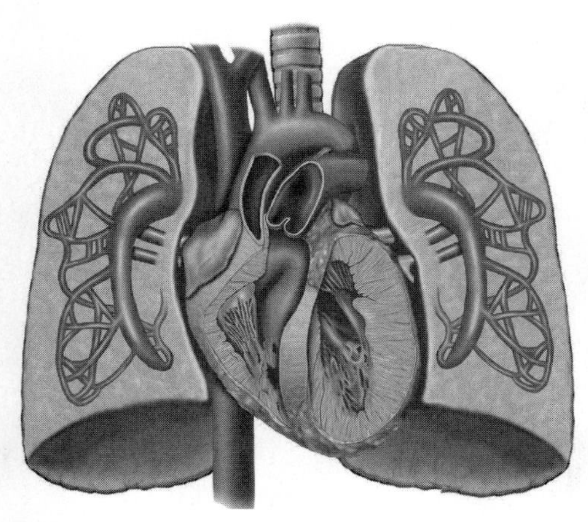

Oxygenation is normally well protected for tissue delivery. A reserve of oxygen exists in the venous blood as long as cardiac output is adequate.
Source: © 2013 Nucleus Medical Media, All rights reserved

Impaired Tissue Oxygenation

- Tissue oxygenation can be impaired by a few key factors, all of which occur in shock states:
  - o A loss of blood flow to the tissues: This occurs in hypovolemic shock (loss of circulating volume), cardiogenic shock (impaired cardiac function), and early sepsis.
  - o Maldistribution of blood: In later stages of sepsis, septic shock develops and results in a maldistribution of blood flow that may interfere with oxygen delivery. This also occurs in neurogenic, anaphylactic, and hemorrhagic shock.
  - o Cellular utilization of oxygen may be directly impaired.
    1. The cells' inability to use oxygen is common in sepsis, predisposing them to cell stunning (reversible cell dysfunction) and apoptosis (programmed cell death), both of which are likely to occur.
    2. Oxygen deprivation can also occur from an impairment in hemoglobin, for instance, from a toxin.
    3. Oxygen is not available for use when hemoglobin is unable to bind with and carry it, which occurs, for example, in carbon monoxide and cyanide poisoning. Even with normal blood flow, these conditions prevent oxygen from reaching the tissues.

Concept Check

4. What is the meaning of the term apoptosis?

A. Stunning of a cell
B. Programmed death of a cell
C. Neurogenic dysfunction at a cellular level
D. Presence of toxins at the cellular level

Answer question

- In distributive shock, blood flow is typically shunted away from the periphery in favor of the vital and central organs. Thus, microvascular blood flow is compromised. Sluggish or even lack of blood flow allows cells to aggregate, causing **microcapillary obstruction**. Oxygenated blood is then unable to reach tissues.
- Unoxygenated tissues can go into a hibernation or a stunned state where they do not function. Stunned tissues can recover and function, but stunning can also be the precursor to **apoptosis** (preprogrammed cell death).
- In both conditions, oxygen is not delivered for tissue consumption.
- If poor blood flow persists, delayed return of blood flow (reperfusion) may not reverse the hypoxic cell injury.

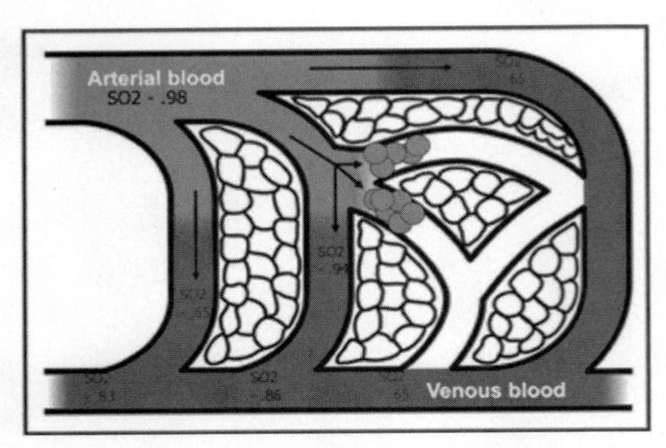

Some types of shock present with microcapillary obstruction and interfere with blood flow to tissues beyond the obstruction.
Source: Copyright © 2013, NovEx Novice to Expert Learning, LLC

Pathophysiology (continued)

Measuring Tissue Oxygenation

Blood Lactate

Recognition of the presence and severity of tissue hypoxia is critical. The only practical measure of tissue hypoxia is **blood lactate**.

- Normally, the Krebs cycle produces over 95% of the energy in humans but requires oxygen to function.
- Carbohydrate (glucose) breakdown does not need oxygen and can generate a small amount of energy (adenosine triphosphate) without oxygen (**anaerobic metabolism**). So, when the supply of oxygen for energy production does not meet the demand, **anaerobic metabolism takes place (Cori cycle)** and produces lactate.
- **Without oxygen, lactate generation is the only way to produce more energy.** However, anaerobic metabolism is inefficient and unsustainable.
- Without oxygen, hydrogen ions (H^+) are produced along with lactate. Prolonged production of H^+ can create a dangerous metabolic acidosis.
- Normal lactate values are 1–2 mmol. **Lactate levels greater than 4 mmol** are considered to be a highly dangerous indicator of **tissue hypoxia**.
- A rise in lactate may signal the depletion of oxygen and tissue hypoxia.

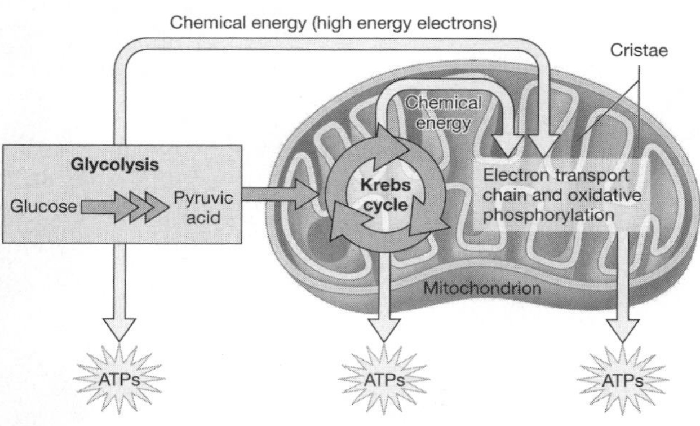

The Krebs cycle (**aerobic** metabolism) is at the center of energy generation. Lactate, via the Cori cycle, is produced with adenosine triphosphate (ATP) as an alternative source of energy if the Krebs cycle has inadequate oxygen available.

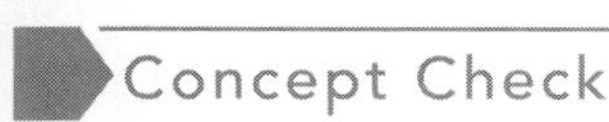

Concept Check

5. What is the normal level of serum lactate?
   A. 1–2 mmol
   B. 4–6 mmol
   C. 8–10 mmol
   D. 12–14 mmol

Answer question

Venous Oxyhemoglobin SvO_2

- Normally, about 25% of the oxygen carried by the hemoglobin is removed by the tissues from arterial blood. As previously stated, the remaining 75% is transported as oxyhemoglobin and returns unused to the lungs.
- Therefore, another indicator of a threat to tissue oxygenation is venous oxyhemoglobin (SvO_2), which acts as the only reserve of oxygen in the body. Normal is 60–80%.
- Humans rarely dip into this reserve of oxygen. Typical venous oxygen levels can be obtained from the blood returning to the heart from the right atrium and pulmonary artery:
  1. Blood from the right atrium allows measurement of oxygen saturation of central venous oxygen ($ScvO_2$). Normal is 70–75%.
  2. Blood from the pulmonary artery allows measurement of oxygen saturation of the mean pulmonary artery (SvO_2). Normal is 60–80%.
- Newer technology (StO_2 device) allows oxyhemoglobin to be measured noninvasively. StO_2 measures tissue oxygen. The device is laid on the thenar aspect of the thumb and measures oxyhemoglobin in the muscle. This measurement provides an early sign of an increase in oxygen extraction, representing a threat to tissue oxygenation (StO_2). Normal is 70–75%.

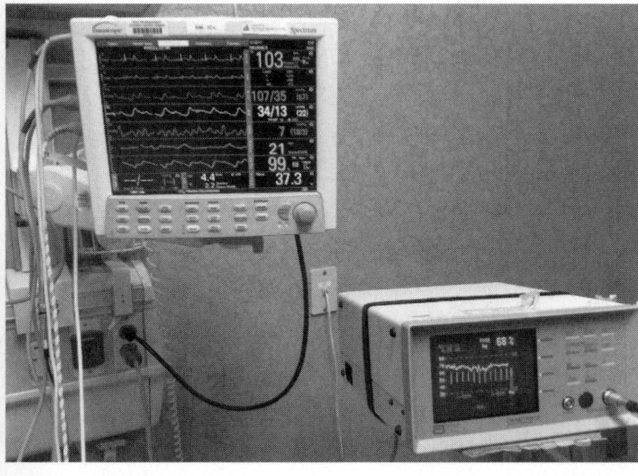

StO_2 measuring device.

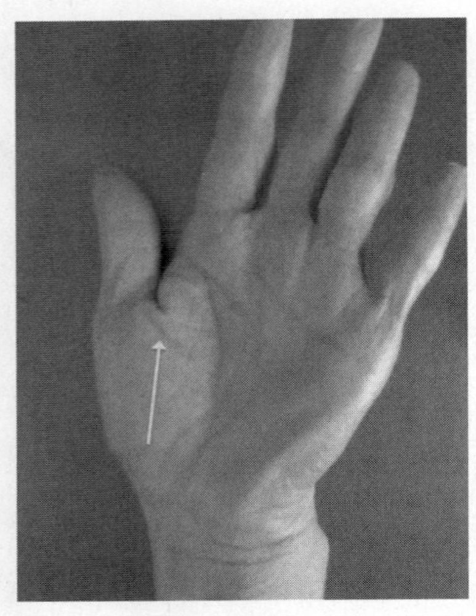

Thenar is the muscle pad at the base of the thumb.

Pathophysiology (continued)

Abnormally Low SvO_2 Levels

- While not easy to obtain from the right atrium, central venous oxyhemoglobin levels are good warning signs of increased oxygen extraction by the tissues. So, whenever venous oxyhemoglobin decreases, a threat to tissue oxygenation exists.
- The main reason the SvO_2 levels decrease is a low cardiac output. A loss of blood flow means hemoglobin—more specifically, oxyhemoglobin—cannot reach the tissues.
- Improving cardiac output usually improves SvO_2 levels.
- Other causes, such as a loss of hemoglobin or oxyhemoglobin (as measured by a pulse oximeter, providing a SpO_2 reading), may cause a decrease in SvO_2 levels, but only if the cardiac output fails to increase to offset the loss.

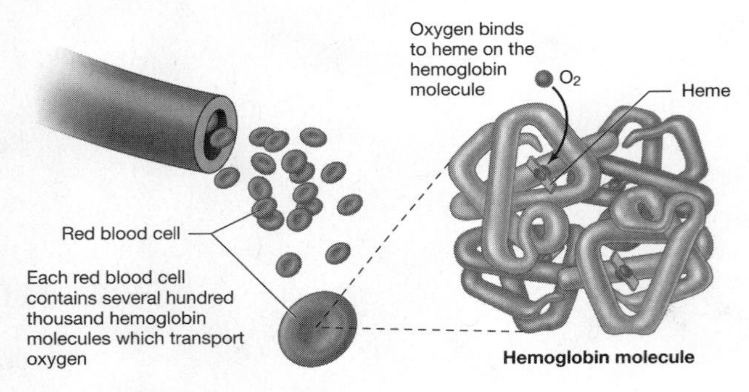

Hemoglobin transports oxygen.

Stages of Shock

Shock is commonly thought to evolve in three stages (see shock schematic):

- Stage 1 is known as the compensatory or early, reversible stage of shock when multiple systems respond to maintain perfusion, oxygenation, and fluid volume, which prevents cellular damage. At this stage, symptoms are barely perceptible. However, the compensatory mechanisms are unable to sustain the body and soon begin to fail.
- Stage 2 is the progressive or intermediate stage of shock that evolves when the compensatory mechanisms begin to fail to perfuse and oxygenate body organs and tissues. During this stage, cells are damaged and begin to dysfunction, creating more extensive cellular damage.
- Stage 3 is the irreversible or refractory stage of shock when cellular damage, anoxia, and death become extensive enough to prevent recovery. With widespread cellular death, multiple organ dysfunction syndrome (MODS) develops, the organs stop functioning and death ensues.

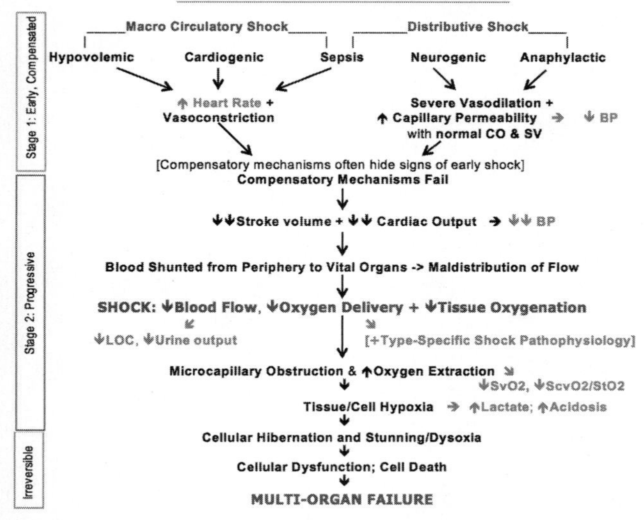

This schematic provides an overview of the pathophysiology of all shock states. It may assist in visualizing how the various deleterious processes evolve and relate. These eventually result in shock and death, if not treated effectively and in a timely manner.

Assessment Findings

Early Signs: Cardiac Output, Stroke Volume, and Heart Rate

- Cardiac Output (CO) is comprised of two components:
  1. Stroke volume or how much blood the heart pumps with each beat. Normal is 60–100 mL/beat. Stroke volume index is a better indicator as it accounts for body size. Normal is 33–47 mL/m^2/beat.
  2. Heart rate (HR)
- The earliest sign to change when the heart begins to fail (either from heart failure, hypovolemia, or sepsis) is stroke volume. As such, stroke volume is an incredibly important parameter to measure and evaluate.
- Heart rate will increase to compensate for a low stroke volume. Tachycardias, though, are nonspecific and can change for reasons other than a decrease in stroke volume. An increase in heart rate is an important clinical sign to evaluate, but it is not as accurate as stroke volume measurement.

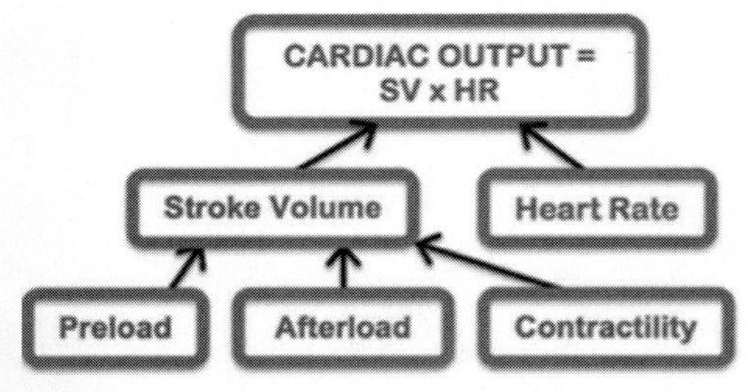

Determinants of cardiac output.

Blood Pressure in Shock

- Blood pressure is commonly but erroneously depended upon in clinical practice as an early warning sign of hemodynamic instability. However, this diagram reflects how the compensatory mechanisms (increased heart rate and vasoconstriction) often mask early signs of shock. Increased vasoconstriction is closely associated with increased systemic vascular resistance (SVR), which results in a deceivingly normal blood pressure. So, a fall in blood pressure is actually a later indicator of shock, when the compensatory mechanisms begin to fail.

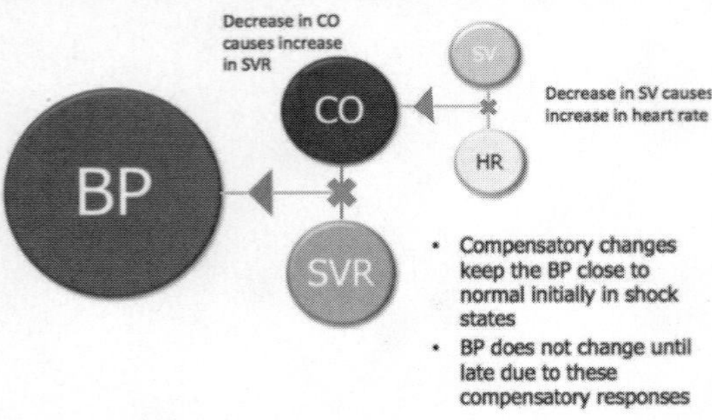

Diagram of blood pressure in shock.
Source: Copyright © 2013, NovEx Novice to Expert Learning, LLC

Progressive to Irreversible Shock

The different shock states can present with some similar physical signs and symptoms. Signs and symptoms that are specific to particular types of shock are detailed in additional NovE-Lessons. Similarities include:

- Tachycardia, as a compensatory mechanism for both reduced stroke volume and loss of vascular tone
- Changes in level of consciousness
- Hypotension, MAP less than 65 mmHg
- Oliguria (low urine output)
- Cold, clammy skin

Unfortunately, these physical findings are often inconsistent, late, and do not assist in differentiating the type of shock. These symptoms do, however, stress the likelihood of shock.

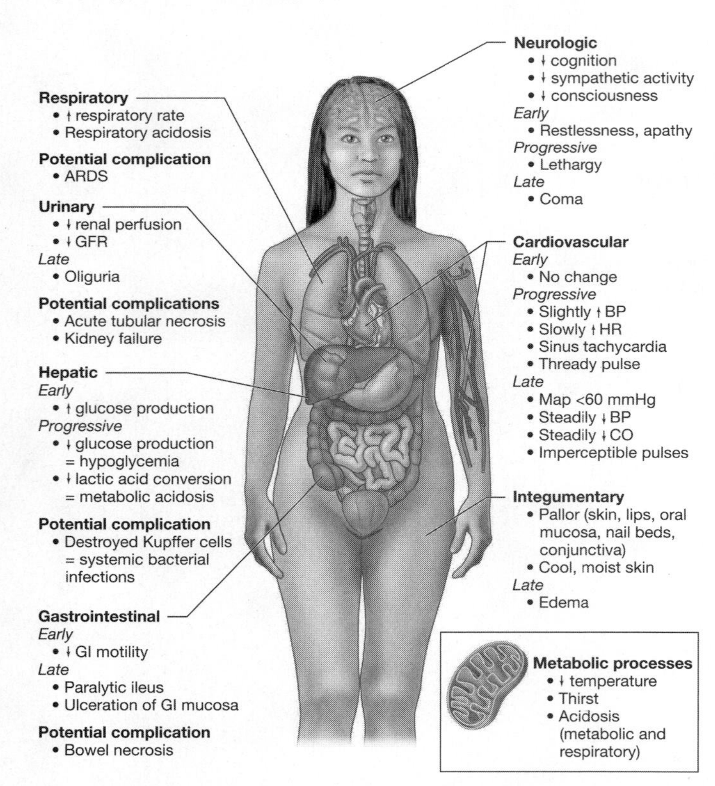

Shock is a multisystem catastrophe for the entire body of the victim. The effects on the individual body systems are listed on this illustration.

Diagnostics

The primary diagnosis of shock can be made by evaluating impaired tissue oxygenation. This can be determined by:

- History: Reported fluid or blood losses, trauma, history of current anticoagulant therapy or bleeding disorders, eating disorders, cardiac disease, diabetes. History can help identify the type of shock state and, therefore, a potential treatable cause.
- Hypotension, with a MAP <65 mmHg
- Measuring blood lactate levels: Lactate values >4 mmol/L, along with a metabolic acidosis, suggests tissue hypoxia and shock.
- Low cardiac output (or cardiac index) and stroke volume:
    - o Measures of CO and SV need to be performed (normal CI >2.5 L/min/m^2; SV 50–100 mL).
    - o Echocardiogram can be performed to evaluate SV, CO, and ejection fraction.
- 12-lead EKG may assist in recognition of cardiac ischemia or damage.
- Low venous oxyhemoglobin values (e.g., <50%)
- Chest x-ray or CT scan may be helpful.

Priority Patient Concerns and Desired Collaborative Care Outcomes

Prior to caring for patients with shock, it is important to prioritize the patient's concerns that must guide the nursing care plan and interventions. Care for the patient is ordered and organized in accordance with the patient's priority and urgent needs. Desired collaborative care outcomes in patients with shock typically include:

1. Patient will have normal lactate levels and return to normal tissue oxygenation evaluated by StO_2.
2. Patient will maintain strong and equal pulses, MAP >65 mmHg, and heart rate within normal.

Considering these important care outcomes, prepare a list of the major 3–6 priority patient concerns or nursing diagnoses for patients with shock. Be prepared to participate in a discussion of this list and/or to submit them as an assignment, as determined by your faculty. Resources you may find helpful in this assignment can include this lesson, the references, resources on nursing care plans, and standard nursing diagnoses manuals.

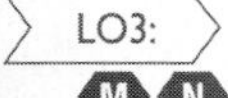

Collaborative Interventions

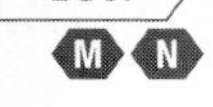

- Evidence-based practice treatments are designed to address the problem causing the shock state. Despite extensive research in shock management, treatment is not limited to the shock state, but rather to addressing the cause of shock. Examples of causes are blood transfusions in anaphylaxis and infections in sepsis. Treating shock without treating its cause typically results in poor or fatal outcomes.
- Generally, all shock treatment has the same goal. However, the specific treatments utilized to achieve the goals are a function of the type of shock.

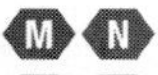

- The goals are to improve stroke volume (>50 mL) and tissue oxygen levels (SvO_2 >70%).

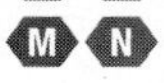

- If stroke volume measurements and SvO_2 levels are not available, reestablishing mean arterial pressure >65 mmHg is a common target.

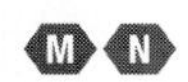

- In all types of shock, if the level of consciousness is decreased and respiratory effort is threatened, be prepared to either place the patient on bilevel positive airway pressure (BiPAP) or to intubate the patient. Airway protection is an essential part of managing shock.

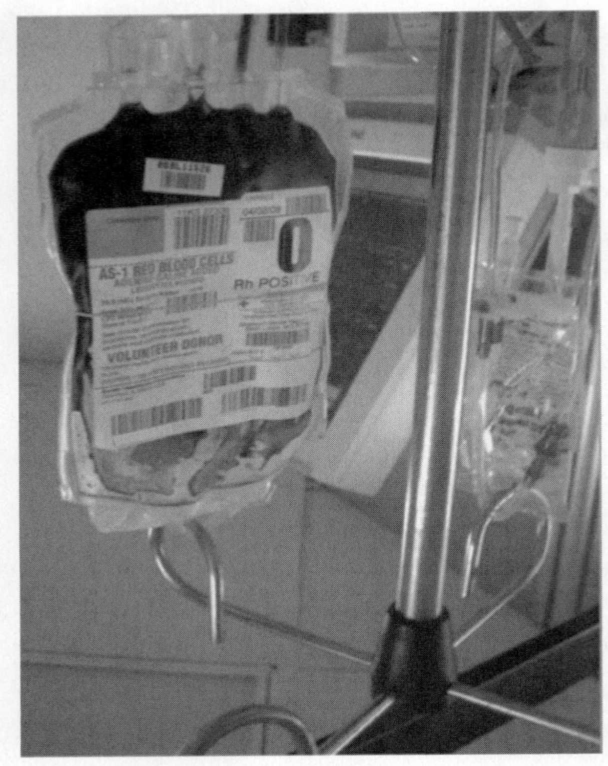

The use of blood transfusions should be performed with caution due to potential side effects, like anaphylactic shock. However, blood products are commonly used in patients with shock due to the ability to both provide rapid volume expansion and improve oxygen delivery.

Source: Copyright © 2013, NovEx Novice to Expert Learning, LLC

Concept Check

6. **Which finding indicates impending shock?**
   A. Decreased heart rate
   B. Decreased cardiac output
   C. Decreased blood pressure
   D. Decreased respiratory rate

Answer question

Collaborative Support and Comfort Care

Because patients in shock are critically ill, nursing care is necessarily focused on urgent, life-saving, and life-sustaining interventions. Patients in shock require that the health care providers draw from multiple areas of knowledge in an integrated way. What all patients in shock need is:

- Continuous monitoring, evaluation, and documentation of their ever-changing physiological status:
  - o Assessment of all body systems, particularly cardiovascular, respiratory, neurological, renal, and gastrointestinal
  - o Hemodynamic monitoring, when available and indicated: central venous pressure, arterial pressure, cardiac output, stroke volume
  - o Multiple medication and fluid administration that must be titrated to the patient's responses and tolerance
  - o Trends in diagnostic tests (e.g., labs, scans)

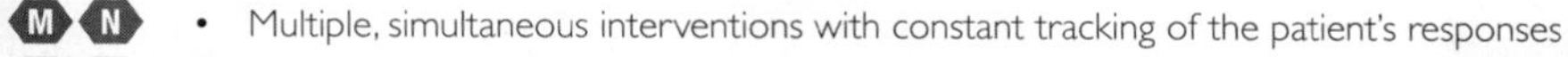

- Multiple, simultaneous interventions with constant tracking of the patient's responses

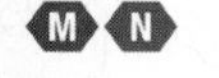

- Pain management is a challenge in the acute phase if the patient is hemodynamically unstable because sedatives and analgesics can contribute to or complicate the instability.
- Prevention of the many never events, which patients in shock are very susceptible to (e.g., pressure ulcers, catheter-associated urinary tract infections, venous catheter-related infections, deep vein thrombosis, ventilator-associated pneumonia)
- Emotional, spiritual, and psychosocial support that can involve family, clergy when desired, health care providers, and health team members
- Provide needed periods of uninterrupted sleep to minimize the impact of sleep deprivation, stress, and continuous activity. Cluster care and patient involvements (e.g., visitors, hygiene care) that are planned with the team and family.
- Frequent but realistic and honest encouragement with information to patients about their status and care being provided
- Nutritional support must be started at the earliest possible time, as soon as the patient can tolerate feedings or an infusion.

Patient Education

- In patients with shock, the mortality rate is extremely high. Emergent and lifesaving interventions are implemented unless the patient and/or family determine these are not the patient's preference or not in the patient's best interest.
- For patients who are in irreversible shock, extensive and extraordinary care can create needless pain and suffering.
- Communication with the family about possible outcomes is an important responsibility of the clinical team. The health care provider may initiate discussion or assist the team to ensure that communication is complete, understood, and realistic.
- Understanding patient's wishes is just as important as initiating therapy, since the patient's wishes may not include aggressive resuscitation or the potential pain and suffering that extensive, heroic care may create:
  - o For example, an 89-year-old patient with a history of dementia, incontinence, and tube feedings may not wish aggressive therapy to be instituted.
  - o For example, a 39-year-old woman with three young children is in the end stage of breast cancer. Heroic measures are anticipated but are not expected to improve her condition.
  - o Communication prior to shock state development is far more beneficial than trying to communicate after shock has developed.
- Educate patients and/or family about living wills and advanced directives. A living will and advanced directives are ways of communicating the patient's preferences for treatment in end-of-life conditions and guiding health care providers in their care of the patient. These legals documents allow the patient's voice to be heard when patients cannot speak for themselves. Specific treatments and care can be detailed (e.g., mechanical ventilation, feeding tube).
- Collaborate with the patient's health care proxy if one has been empowered with power of attorney to make the patient's medical decisions.
- Collaborate with patient and/or family to provide pastoral and social services support.
- Provide loved ones open access and privacy to be with and support the patient, based on the patient's preferences, tolerance, and responsiveness.

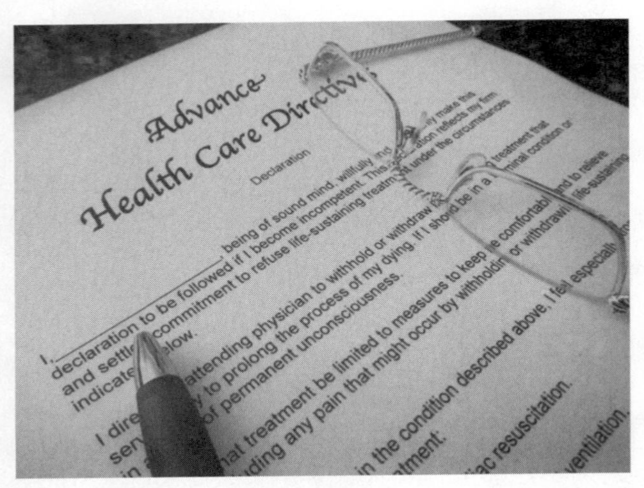

A living will is intended to provide health care providers with specific directives about treatments that comply with the patient's wishes. It designates the use or refusal of various kinds of burdensome and/or invasive medical care. It may further detail the patient's wishes about the administration or withholding of food and water by any means. The living will is implemented when the patient becomes too ill to refuse care or to give informed consent. An example: "If I suffer an irreversible, incurable disease or illness and my physician's judgment is that my condition is terminal, I direct that any life-prolonging or life-sustaining interventions that would delay my death be withheld or withdrawn."

Concept Check

7. When are living wills implemented?

A. When a patient reaches age 85

B. When a patient is too ill to refuse care

C. When a patient becomes terminally ill

D. When a patient requires tube feeding

Answer question

Summary of Interventions

The goals for managing any shock state are to rapidly restore blood flow and tissue perfusion.

- Treatment of each type of shock, as well as condition-specific differences, are detailed in additional NovE-Lessons. Key interventions will include:
  - o Treatment for hypovolemic shock is fluid resuscitation, but all shock states may use vasopressors if the initial treatment does not restore MAP to >65 mmHg.
  - o Treatment of cardiogenic shock is primarily inotropes and could even involve mechanical aids such as intra-aortic balloon pumping.
  - o Treatment for septic shock initially includes antibiotics and fluids.
  - o Neurogenic shock treatment depends on the type of shock, but primarily involves removing any aggravating factors (such as distended bladder), but also volume resuscitation and vasopressors if needed.
  - o Anaphylactic shock treatment includes epinephrine and antihistamines.

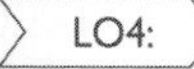

Evaluation of Desired Collaborative Care Outcomes

Evaluation and reassessment should reveal attainment of previously established patient outcomes. In summary:

- Patient has normal lactate levels and normal tissue oxygenation evaluated by StO_2.
- Patient has strong and equal pulses, MAP >65 mmHg, and heart rate within normal.

References

Ahrens, T. (2010). Stroke volume optimization versus central venous pressure in fluid management. *Critical Care Nurse* 30(2), 71–2.

Agency for Healthcare Research and Technology (2007). AHRQ Technology Assessment Review—Esophageal doppler ultrasound-based cardiac output monitoring for real-time therapeutic management of hospitalized patients. Rockville, MD: Agency for Healthcare Research and Quality.

Angus, D. C., & van der Poll, T. (2013). Severe sepsis and septic shock. *N Engl J Med, 369*, 840–851. DOI: 10.1056/NEJMra1208623.

Ekbal, N. J., Dyson, A., Black, C., & Singer, M. (2013). Monitoring tissue perfusion, oxygenation, and metabolism in critically ill patients. *Chest, 143*(6), 1799–1808.

Kleinpell, R. M., & Burns, S. (2010). Multisystem problems. In M. Chulay & S. Burns (Eds.), *AACN's essentials of Progressive care nursing (2nd ed., pp. 247–253)*. New York, NY: The McGraw-Hill Companies.

Thiel, S. W., Kolleff, M. H., & Isakow, W. (2009). Non-invasive stroke volume measurement and passive leg raising predict volume responsiveness in medical ICU patients: An observational cohort study. *Critical Care*, 13, R111 doi:10.1186/cc7955

Vincent, J. L., & DeBacker, D. (2013). Circulatory shock. *N Engl J Med, 369*, 1726–1734. DOI: 10.1056/NEJMra1208943.

Clinical Practice Guidelines (depend on type of shock)

Patient Education

www.nlm.nih.gov/medlineplus/ency/article/000039.htm

Learning Outcomes for Cardiogenic Shock

When you complete this lesson, you will be able to:

1. Recognize the clinical relevance of cardiogenic shock.
2. Consider the pathophysiology, etiology, risk factors, and clinical presentation of cardiogenic shock that determine the priority patient concerns.
3. Determine the most urgent and important nursing interventions and patient education required in caring for a patient with cardiogenic shock.
4. Evaluate attainment of desired collaborative care outcomes for a patient with cardiogenic shock.

LO1:

What Is Cardiogenic Shock?

Cardiogenic shock occurs as the result of impaired cardiac output. This shock state is typified by clinical signs of tissue hypoxia, which occurs in conjunction with insufficient intravascular volume.

Cardiogenic shock primarily involves failure of the **left ventricle**. Myocardial damage (left picture) can cause permanent impairment and shock. A few conditions, such as tamponade (right picture), may cause shock but the shock conditions can be very limited if treatment is quickly implemented and successful.

Normal Diastole

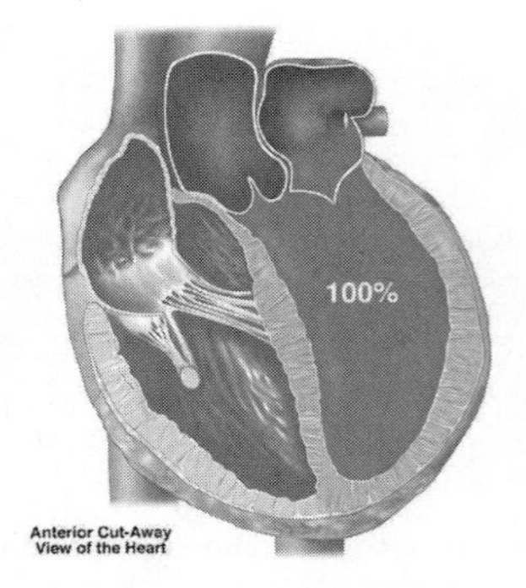

Normal Systole
Normal Ejection Fraction Approximately 0.55

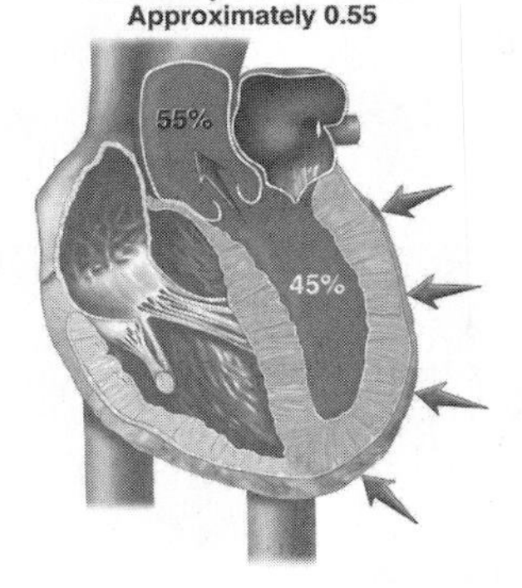

Initial Systolic Condition
Ejection Fraction 0.25

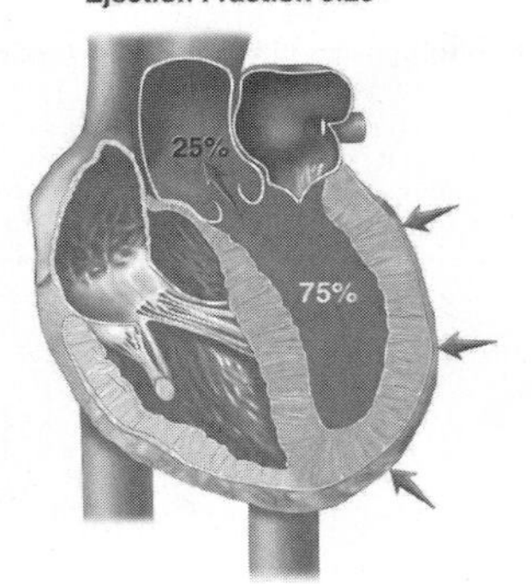

Subsequent Systolic Condition
Ejection Fraction 0.47

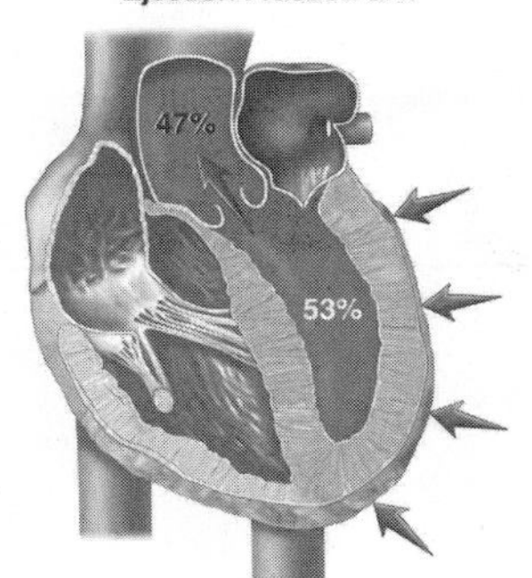

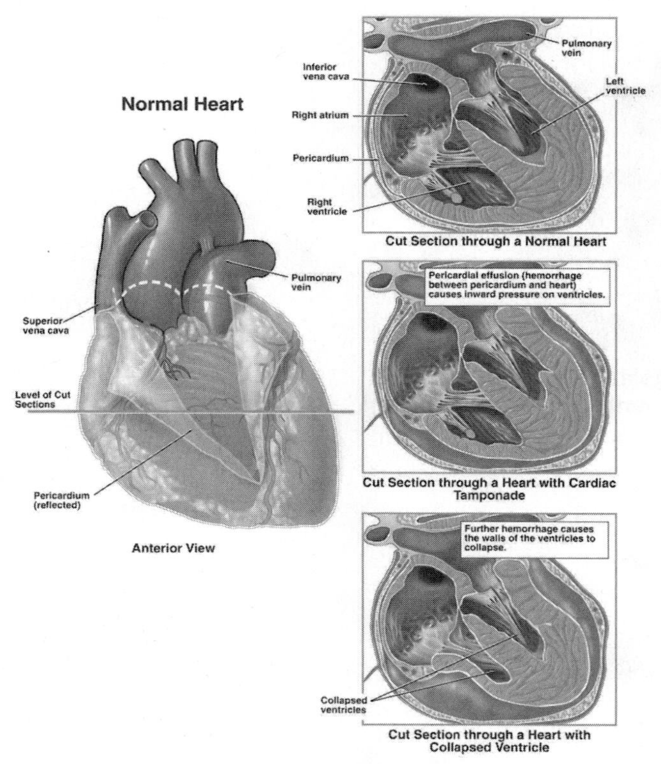

Upper: Heart attack with subsequent heart failure is a leading cause of cardiogenic shock.
Lower: Cardiac tamponade (hemorrhage or fluid within the pericardium) can cause subsequent ventricular collapse. Fluid or blood can accumulate between the heart wall and the pericardial sac, impede ventricular filling during diastole, and eventually cause the collapse of the ventricles, stopping the heart from beating.
Source: (*both*) Nucleus Medical Art Inc/Alamy

Concept Check

1. **Failure of which heart chamber is the primary cause of cardiogenic shock?**
   A. Right atrium
   B. Right ventricle
   C. Left atrium
   D. Left ventricle

Answer question

LO1:

Clinical Relevance

- Cardiogenic shock is the major cause of death following myocardial injury or dysfunction, particularly when heart failure ensues.
- Mortality ranges 50–80% despite treatment.
- Development of cardiogenic shock is the terminal event in many causes of death.
- Every nurse should understand the basics of cardiogenic shock management because almost all nurses will see this type of shock during their career. Early recognition is critical in order to transfer these patients to critical care for intensive intervention and care. The prognosis is dire, despite the best care available, so early detection is the best prevention.

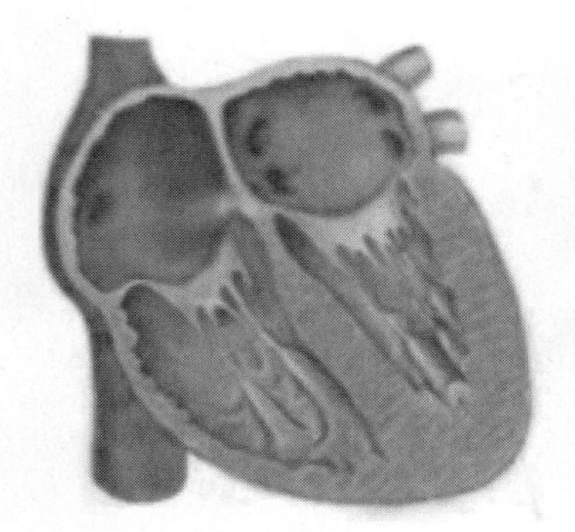

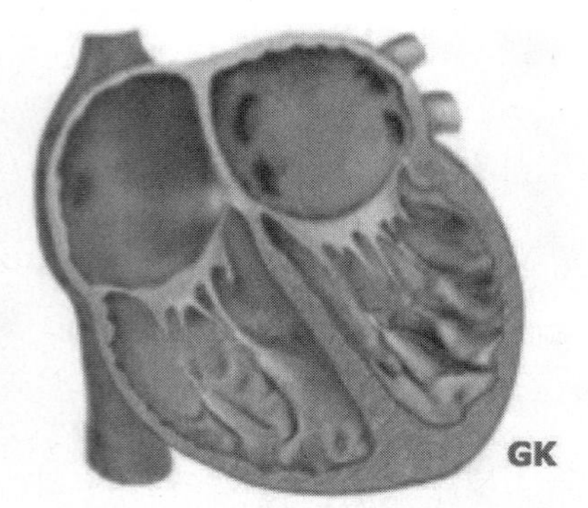

Heart enlargement, dysfunction, and failure are major causes of cardiogenic shock. This picture compares a normal (left) with an enlarged heart (right).
Source: Courtesy of George Kyriakidis/Santa Ana, CA

Concept Check

2. What is the most critical aspect of care for a patient who may develop cardiogenic shock?
   A. Early detection of developing shock
   B. Initiation of hemodynamic monitoring
   C. Transfer of patient to a high-level care unit
   D. Administration of medication to increase heart rate

Answer question

LO2:

Pathophysiology

- Cardiogenic shock results from a decrease in stroke volume, followed by a decrease in cardiac output.
- The decrease in stroke volume can be due to a weakened heart (low ejection fraction) as seen in myocardial infarctions and heart failure:
  - A decrease in stroke volume can also be due to trauma and blood loss from the ventricles.
  - Tamponade (fluid in the pericardial sac) can also restrict heart contraction and reduce stroke volume.
- The vascular system will respond to a decrease in cardiac output by vasoconstriction:
  - Systemic vascular resistance (SVR) is a term used to describe the vascular resistance to blood flow.
    - A high SVR impedes blood flow.
    - A low SVR offers less resistance to blood flow.
  - The vasoconstriction causes a rise in SVR. This rise will keep the blood pressure close to normal.
  - However, tissue perfusion may be threatened, even with a normal blood pressure, if the resistance is too high.
  - Measures of tissue oxygenation are essential in shock to measure the adequacy of tissue oxygenation.
    - Lactate
    - $ScvO_2$
    - StO_2

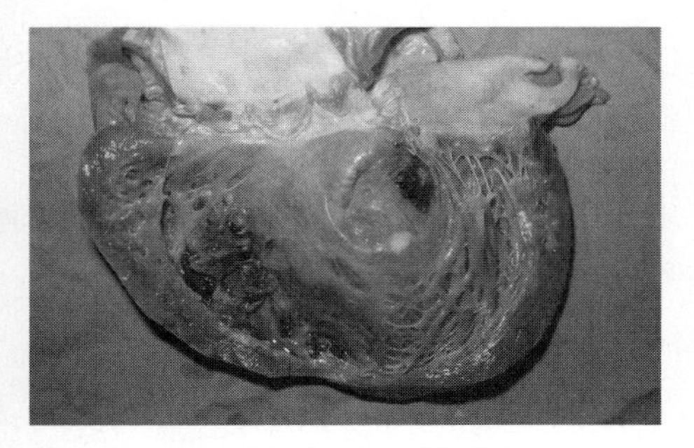

A massive myocardial infarction of the left ventricle (darker, thinner areas) in the lower third of the ventricle, severely compromises cardiac output. Heart failure and cardiogenic shock rapidly ensue. A massive MI with cardiogenic shock is commonly fatal.
Source: Biophoto Associates/Photo Researchers, Inc/Science Source

- Cardiogenic shock is the result of a drop in left ventricular stroke volume.
- Right ventricular failure can also produce cardiogenic shock by failing to deliver blood to the left ventricle.
    - o Technically, this produces left ventricular hypovolemia, but is the result of right ventricular failure.

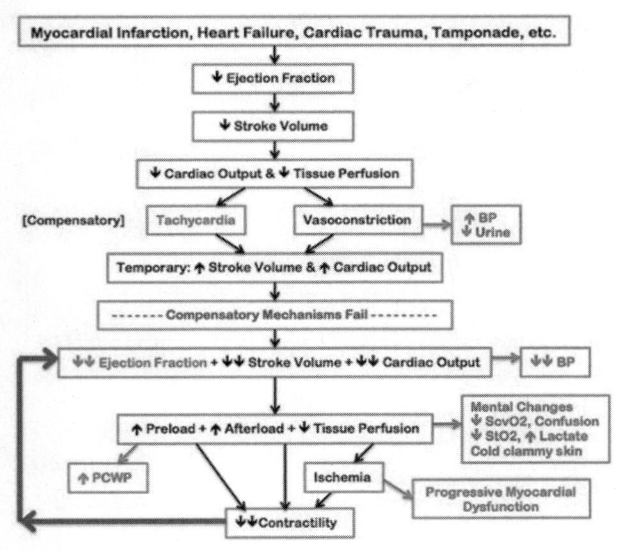

Pathophysiology of cardiogenic shock. **Bold** = refractory shock phase; red = signs and symptoms.
Source: Copyright © 2013, NovEx Novice to Expert Learning, LLC

Risk Factors

- Coronary artery disease
- Cardiac trauma

Causes

Cardiogenic shock can be produced by any of the following:

- Myocardial infarction
- Heart failure secondary to underlying conditions, such as hypertension
- Cardiomyopathies
- Infections such as sepsis, myocarditis, or endocarditis
- Obstructive disorders, such as massive pulmonary embolism or pulmonary hypertension
- Cardiac tamponade
- Aortic dissection
- Life-threatening dysrhythmias (e.g., ventricular fibrillation, pulseless ventricular tachycardia, heart blocks)
- Cardiac valvular disease
- Myocardial contusion
- Ventricular wall rupture
- Right ventricular pump failure

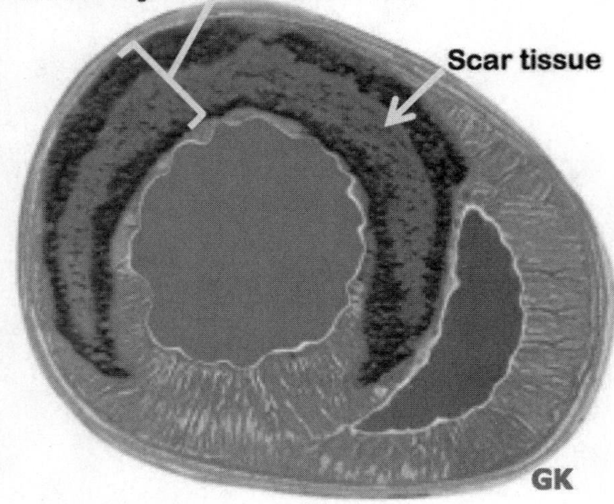

This patient's heart reveals an extensive myocardial infarction. The scar tissue indicates that the infarction occurred at least a few days to a week ago. With this degree of myocardial damage and dysfunction, heart failure and shock are expected.
Source: Courtesy of George Kyriakidis/Santa Ana, CA

Concept Check

3. Which dysrhythmia puts the patient at risk for cardiogenic shock?

A. Ventricular fibrillation
B. Isolated premature ventricular contractions
C. Supraventricular tachycardia
D. Sinus arrhythmia

Answer question

Assessment Findings

- All shock states can present with very similar physical symptoms: **tachycardia, hypotension, altered mental status, decrease in urine output, and cool, clammy skin.**
- Hemodynamic definition: *Persistent* systolic pressure of less than 90 mmHg for more than 30 minutes; pulmonary wedge pressure greater than 15 mmHg and cardiac index less than 2.2 $L/min/m^2$
- Cardiac output is reduced and vascular resistance is increased. The increased vascular resistance results from vasoconstriction that shunts blood flow away from the skin, producing a typical cold, clammy skin.
- In addition, cardiogenic shock presents with the symptoms of **heart failure**. The patient may have pulmonary symptoms, such as crackles in both lungs and poor gas exchange as manifested by a decreased pulse oximeter value. Severe heart failure essentially deteriorates into cardiogenic shock.
- The patient may be very anxious if still awake, may be extremely short of breath, and may have a sense of impending doom.

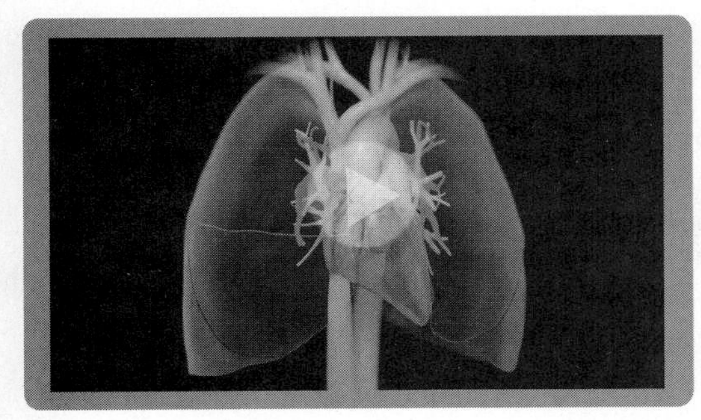

This animation provides a brief review of heart failure which leads to cardiogenic shock when unsuccessfully treated or in its end stage.

Cardiogenic Shock

- Right heart failure might be present with symptoms of venous engorgement. However, the main symptoms of **cardiogenic shock** are the result of **left ventricular failure**.
- Distinctions between shock types:
  - o Cardiogenic shock is characterized by pulmonary congestion and high CVP.
  - o Septic, neurogenic, and anaphylactic shock can present with **warm skin**.
  - o Neurogenic shock can present with **bradycardia**.
- Unfortunately, these physical signs are often inconsistent, late, and do not help differentiate the type of shock.
- Unlike neurogenic shock, severe bradycardia can be a late and ominous sign in all types of shock or, less frequently, a presenting sign. In cardiogenic shock, severe bradycardia can either be a major contributing factor in the progression of shock or it may reflect the late hemodynamic collapse.
- If the patient has the above symptoms, a shock state is likely present. However, shock states can occur much earlier than the physical symptoms reflect, due to the body's ability to initially compensate for shock.

Concept Check

4. What finding is associated with cardiogenic shock?

A. Low CVP
B. Hypertension
C. Hot, dry skin
D. Pulmonary congestion

Answer question

Diagnostics

When acute MI or heart failure are known or strongly suspected, the patient's clinical presentation provides the foundation for the diagnosis. When physical findings point at cardiogenic shock, immediate tests to confirm or disconfirm the diagnosis include:

- Electrocardiogram: To detect myocardial ischemia, injury, and/or infarction presence, location, and size
- Echocardiogram: Can evaluate and confirm the severe reduction in ventricular function and cardiac output and possible cause.
- Angiography: Emergent angiographic evaluation can assist in identifying patients who may benefit from revascularization.

Priority Patient Concerns and Desired Collaborative Care Outcomes

Prior to caring for patients with cardiogenic shock, it is important to prioritize the patient's concerns that must guide the nursing care plan and interventions. Care for the patient is ordered and organized in accordance with the patient's priority and urgent needs. Desired collaborative care outcomes in patients with cardiogenic shock typically include:

1. Patient's cardiac output will improve and stabilize.
2. Patient's peripheral tissue perfusion will return to a sustainable level, on treatment if needed, to prevent abnormal pH, lactate, StO_2, and $ScvO_2$ levels prior to discharge.
3. Patient will be normovolemic or maintained near normal with ongoing therapy.
4. Patient will convey being less anxious and/or participate when possible and appropriate in end-of-life decisions.

Considering these important care outcomes, prepare a list of the major 3–6 priority patient concerns or nursing diagnoses for patients with cardiogenic shock. Be prepared to participate in a discussion of this list and/or to submit them as an assignment, as determined by your faculty. Resources you may find helpful in this assignment can include this lesson, the references, resources on nursing care plans, and standard nursing diagnoses manuals.

LO3:

Collaborative Interventions

Evidence-Based Practice

M N

- Remove the cause: Evidence-based treatment for cardiogenic shock centers on removing the cause, whenever possible, and strengthening the heart. For example, if pericardial tamponade (fluid buildup around the heart) is the cause, it can be treated with a pericardiocentesis so that heart function can rapidly return to normal.

M N

- Managing cardiogenic shock is similar to treating heart failure because, if severe heart failure worsens, cardiogenic shock is the consequence:
  - o Preload reducers: When preload is very high, preload reducers, such as diuretics, can be given but with caution, since these agents can also reduce the blood pressure even further
  - o Inotropes: Dobutamine or milrinone can increase contractility and improve stroke volume.

M N

- Vasopressors: If there is evidence of volume overload and dobutamine has not increased stroke volume, cardiac output, and MAP, vasopressors can be added.

M N

  - o Norepinephrine and dopamine are both first-line vasopressor choices; however, evidence supports the preferred use of norepinephrine over dopamine due to the increased rate of adverse events with dopamine (e.g., twice the incidence of dysrhythmias). Administer the lowest possible dose needed for hemodynamic support, as higher doses are associated with higher mortality. In severe hypotension, norepinephrine is the recommended medication.

M N

- The American Heart Association recommends atropine as the first-line drug in the treatment of *severe bradycardia*, except for 3rd degree and 2nd degree type II AV (shown here) heart blocks. If inadequate or no response to atropine, prepare for immediate transcutaneous pacing. Epinephrine or dopamine may be used while awaiting a pacemaker if transcutaneous pacing fails.

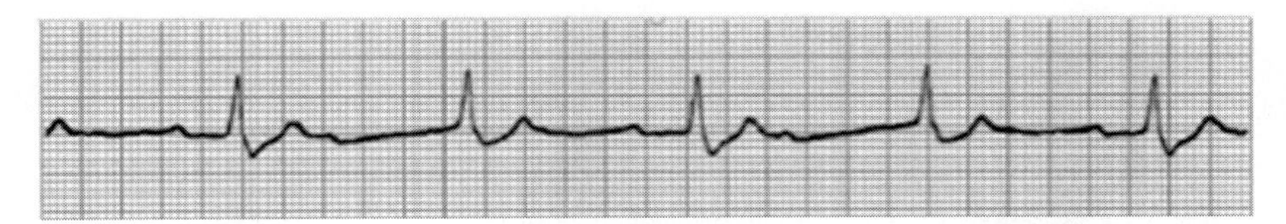

Severe bradycardia may be a source of cardiogenic shock.

Concept Check

5. Which medication is used as a preload reducer in cardiogenic shock?

A. A diuretic
B. An inotrope
C. An antithrombotic
D. A vasopressor

Answer question

Concept Check

6. In which instance would atropine be indicated for a patient in cardiogenic shock?

A. Third-degree heart block
B. Severe bradycardia
C. Second-degree heart block
D. Atrial fibrillation

Answer question

Symptom Management and Comfort Care

Many patients develop cardiogenic shock as a result of myocardial infarction (MI). In patients with an MI, particularly those manifesting early warning signs of shock, nursing interventions include:

N
- Place patient at rest to minimize cardiac workload. Once in shock, which by definition includes hypotension, elevating the head of the bed is ill advised.

N
- Call for the Rapid Response Team if available or other team members.

N
- Initiate oxygen per nasal cannula if the SpO_2 <93%.

M N
- Patients in cardiogenic shock do not always complain of pain unless they are having an acute MI or unstable angina. If they are infarcting, pain relief is essential. Morphine IV is a preferred medication but caution is needed as it is likely to exacerbate the hypotension.

M N
- Fluid therapy may be initiated if the patient is hypovolemic. Conversely, a diuretic may be given if the patient is fluid overloaded.

N
- Prepare the patient for immediate transfer to either the ED if in an outpatient setting or to ICU if already in the hospital, as the hypotension reveals that the compensatory mechanisms are failing.

N
- Provide emotional support and visitation as much as the patient tolerates. Offer the spiritual support of clergy as the patient and family desire. Provide ongoing communication about the multiple and often frightening interventions to tame the technological and crisis environment to the degree possible. Avoid eliciting any more communication from the patient than is essential to provide uninterrupted rest. There is often a delicate balance between too much and too little and is patient-specific. When in doubt, ask the patient to indicate how much is preferred.

Collaborative Support Interventions

M N
- The aortic counterpulsation balloon or the intra-aortic balloon pump (IABP) may be used in cardiogenic shock.
- The IABP reduces afterload of the left ventricle and increases blood flow into the coronary arteries, making it useful in treating refractory heart failure and cardiogenic shock.

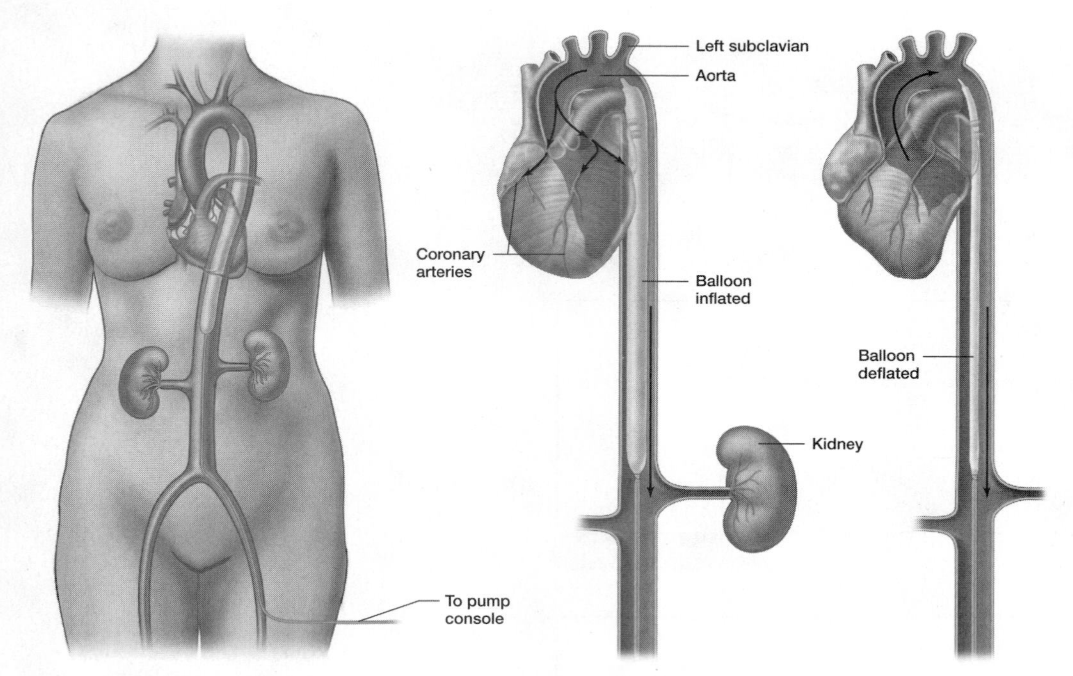

The images show how the IABP functions to decrease afterload (and, therefore, cardiac workload) and improve myocardial blood flow. The balloon inflates during diastole which assists coronary artery perfusion and deflates during systole to reduce resistance against which the left ventricular must pump.

- The IABP may be used as an adjunct to medical treatment for cardiogenic shock or as a cardiac augmentation mechanism when surgery is imminent.
- However, a recent study has indicated that IABP does not improve outcomes in cardiogenic shock. Physicians may still be using this device despite the new evidence. Reference: http://www.nejm.org/doi/full/10.1056/NEJMoa1208410?query=featured_home

Concept Check

7. What is one benefit of using intraaortic balloon pump (IABP) in the treatment of cardiogenic shock?

A. Left ventricular afterload is increased.

B. Blood flow through the coronary arteries is increased.

C. Heart rhythm can be controlled.

D. Left ventricular preload is increased.

Answer question

Summary of Interventions

- Cardiogenic shock is a medical emergency requiring immediate treatment.
- Management of cardiogenic shock centers on strengthening the heart or removing the cause (if possible) of the cardiogenic shock.
  - o Diuretics can reduce preload or fluid overload.
  - o Inotropes can improve contractility.
  - o Vasopressors, in extreme cases, can maintain MAP and blood flow.
- Mechanical assist devices, such as intra-aortic balloon pumps (IABP) can be used if the patient fails to respond to the first- and second-line therapies.

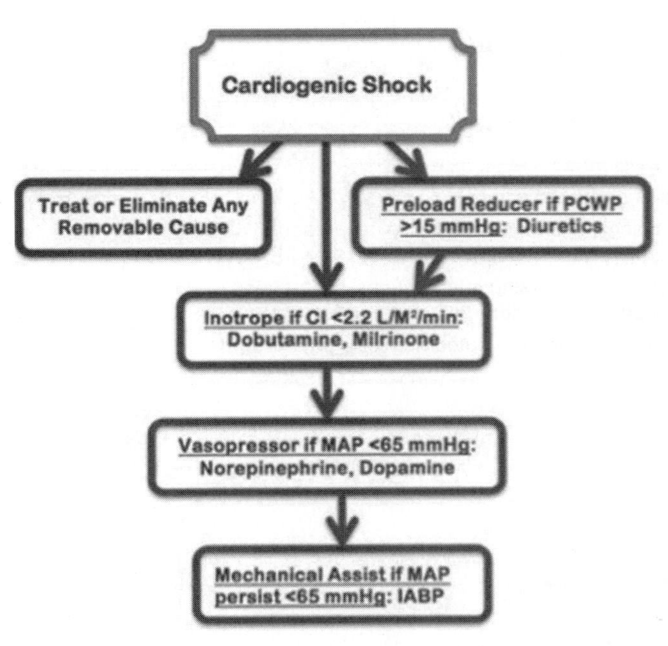

LO4: Evaluation of Desired Collaborative Care Outcomes

Evaluation and reassessment should reveal attainment of previously established patient outcomes. In summary:

- Patient has clear mentation and strong and regular pulses.
- Patient's peripheral tissues are perfused sufficiently to prevent abnormal pH, lactate, StO_2, and $ScvO_2$ levels.
- Patient's fluid intake and urine output are balanced, with treatment as needed.
- Patient participates in end-of-life decisions and reports feeling less anxious or scared and appears calmer.

References

Barata, I. A. (2013). Cardiac emergencies. *Emerg Med Clin North Am, 31*(3), 677–704.

Chulay, M., & Burns, S. (2010). *AACN essentials of critical care nursing (2nd edition)*. New York, NY: The McGraw-Hill Companies.

Josephson, L. (2008). Cardiogenic shock. *Dimensions in Crit Care Nurs, 27*(4), 160–170.

Klein, T., & Ramani, G. V. (2012). Assessment and management of cardiogenic shock in the emergency department. *Cardiol Clin, 30*(4), 651–664.

O'Connor, C. M., & Rogers, J. G. (2012). Evidence for overturning the guidelines in cardiogenic shock. *N Engl J Med, 367*, 1349–1350.

Clinical Practice Guidelines:

Antman, E. M., Anbe, D. T., Armstrong, P. W., et al. (2004). ACC/AHA guidelines for the management of patients with ST-elevation myocardial infarction: executive summary: a report of the American College of Cardiology/American Heart Association Task Force on Practice Guidelines. *Circulation, 110*, 588–636.

Patient Education:

Mayo Clinic Staff. (2011). Cardiogenic shock. Mayoclinic.com website

National Heart, Lung, and Blood Institute. (2011). What is cardiogenic shock? **http://www.nhlbi.nih.gov/health/health-topics/topics/shock/**

Learning Outcomes for Neurogenic Shock

When you complete this lesson, you will be able to:

1. Recognize the clinical relevance of neurogenic shock.
2. Consider the pathophysiology, etiology, risk factors, and clinical presentation of neurogenic shock that determine the priority patient concerns.
3. Determine the most urgent and important nursing interventions and patient education required in caring for a patient with neurogenic shock.
4. Evaluate attainment of desired collaborative care outcomes for a patient with neurogenic shock.

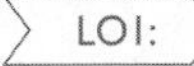

What Is Neurogenic (or Spinal) Shock?

- Neurogenic or spinal shock is the result of an injury to the spinal cord.
- While it is not a common form of shock, any injury to the spine should be a warning that neurogenic shock can subsequently occur.
- The symptoms of this shock are much the same as any shock state, with a few notable exceptions, primarily the presence of a bradycardia.
- Neurogenic shock most commonly occurs in spinal cord injuries above T6 level.
- The development of neurogenic shock can occur immediately or within hours and can last for several weeks.

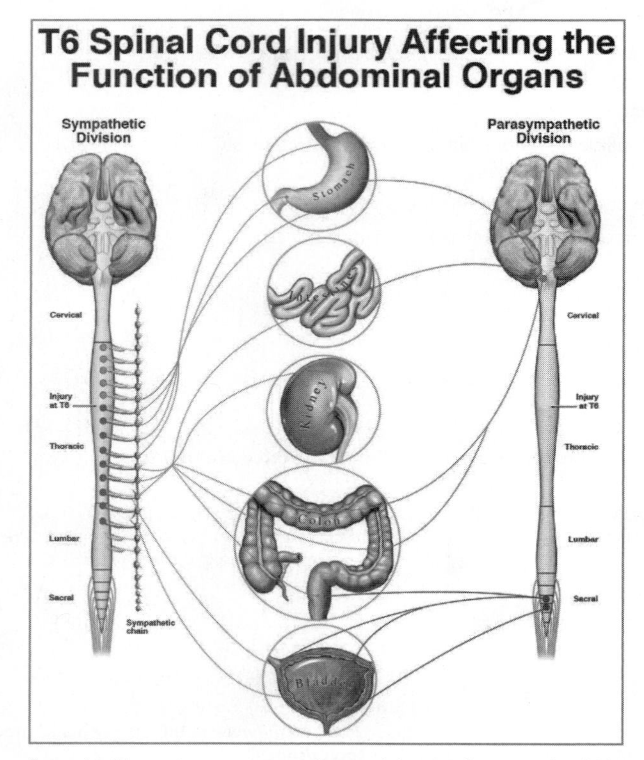

From this illustration, one can see how an injury to the cervical or high thoracic spinal cord (above T6) results in damage to the autonomic nervous system, affects important abdominal organs, and can cause neurogenic shock.

Concept Check

1. **Neurogenic shock most often occurs when the patient has an injury in which part of the spine?**
   A. Sacral
   B. Below L2
   C. Between T6 and L1
   D. Above T6

Answer question

LO2:

Pathophysiology

- Neurogenic or spinal shock results from the loss (often temporary) of sympathetic vascular tone and reduced autonomic function leading to widespread arterial and venous vasodilation as a result of an injury to the spinal cord or brain.
- This loss of vascular tone and autonomic dysfunction occurs below the level of injury. Blood pooling in areas below the level of injury decreases blood return to the heart, causing a significant reduction in the cardiac output and resultant hypotension.
- The mechanisms of neurogenic shock are unclear. It may be related to ion change within the damaged cells, particularly the loss of intracellular potassium and subsequent accumulation of potassium outside the cells. This ion change alters impulse transmission, resulting in the symptoms associated with neurogenic shock.
- Over time, this process can correct itself. The electrolytes (e.g., potassium) can return to normal with subsequent return of function.
- Depending on the severity of injury, the patient may return to normal or can have residual symptoms.
- The prior condition of the patient (e.g., young, healthy) influences how likely the patient is to have complete recovery and return to normal daily activities.

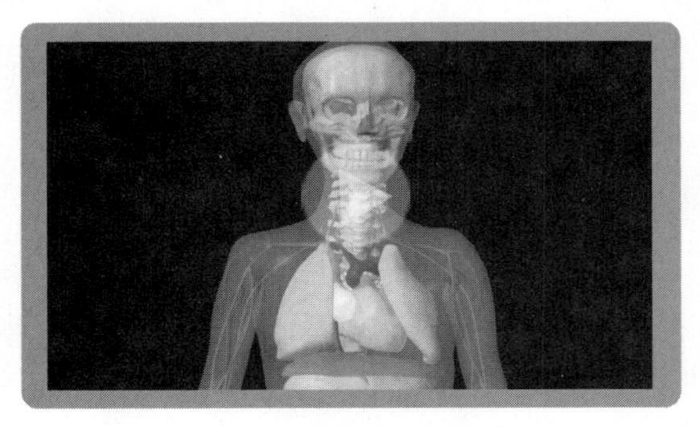

The short animation gives a brief overview of neurogenic shock.

Concept Check

2. **Which pathophysiology is present in neurogenic shock?**
   A. Increased blood return to the heart
   B. Hypertension
   C. Loss of vascular tone below the injury
   D. Venous vasoconstriction

Answer question

Causes and Risk Factors

- Cervical or high thoracic spinal cord injury: Accidents and violence account for the vast majority of spinal cord injuries. Those most at risk are young men, average age of 38. Alcohol is a contributing risk factor.
- **In a hypotensive trauma patient with no bleeding and bradycardia, consider neurogenic shock**.
- Traumatic brain injury
- General or spinal anesthesia
- Drugs (e.g., barbiturates)

Cervical Injury

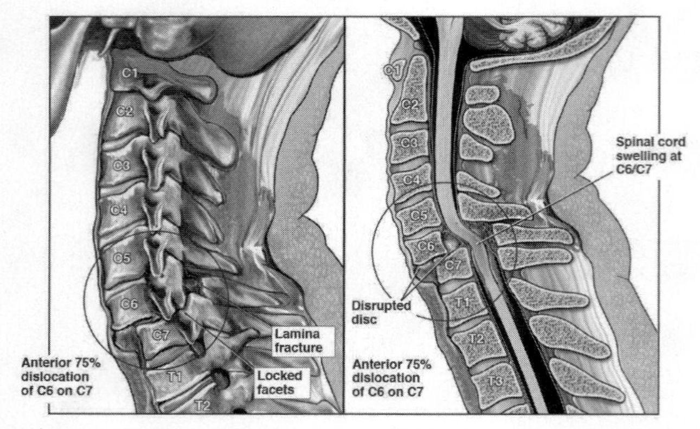

This medical exhibit features two view of 75% dislocation of C6/C7 and spinal cord injury.

Assessment Findings

- Neurogenic shock is characterized by:
  - o Bradycardia (more common with injury above T3): This sign differs from other manifestations that are typical in shock.
  - o Hypotension (mean arterial pressure [MAP] less than 65 mmHg)
- In addition, there are traditional signs of shock:
  - o Reduced urine output
  - o Low stroke volume and cardiac output
  - o Change in level of consciousness (which could also be due to head injury in this type of shock)
  - o Hypothermia
  - o Malaise
- Due to the loss of sympathetic vascular tone, most commonly with an injury above the level of T6, additional signs from spinal injury include:
  - o Areflexia below level of injury
  - o Skin is warm and dry (unlike other shock states)
  - o Inability to perspire below level of injury

C5, 6,7 Quadriplegic Spinal Cord Injury

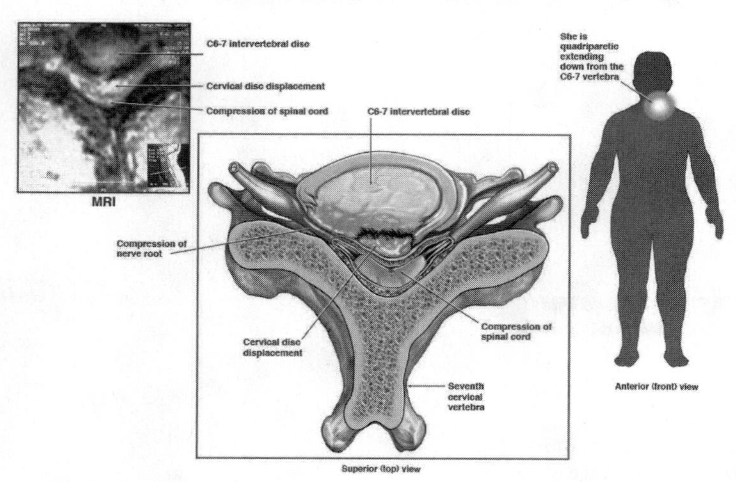

This exhibit portrays a C5–7 quadriplegic spinal cord injury. The MRI of the injured area in the neck shows the C6–7 intervertebral disc, cervical disc displacement, and compression of the spinal cord. The middle drawing helps clarify the cervical disc displacement and compression of the spinal cord. The third illustration shows how much of the body is affected by the injury.

Concept Check

3. What is a major difference in assessment findings between neurogenic shock and other shock states?

A. Presence of MAP below 65 mmHg

B. Reduction of urine output

C. Bradycardia

D. Presence of hyperthermia

Answer question

Diagnostics

- Neurogenic shock does not have a definitive diagnostic test.
- If shock is present and the patient has suffered a spinal cord or head injury, be suspicious of neurogenic shock. The key differentiating clinical sign in shock is the presence of *bradycardia*. Rarely do other types of shock present with bradycardia. Instead, most present with tachycardia.

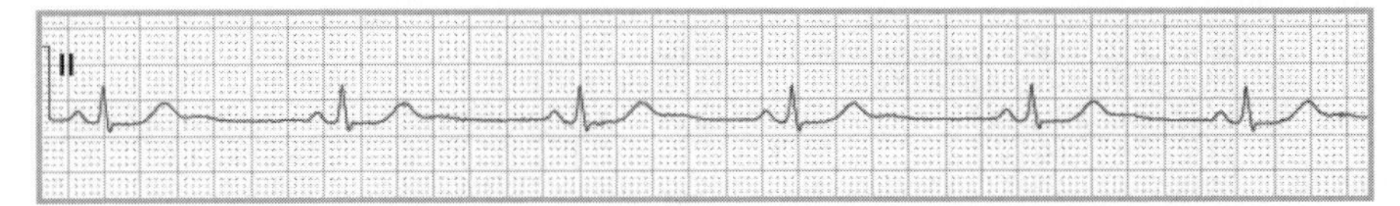

A bradycardia with a heart rate of 44 beats per minute is observed in a patient with neurogenic shock.
Source: Courtesy of K. Kyriakidis

Priority Patient Concerns and Desired Collaborative Care Outcomes

Prior to caring for patients with neurogenic shock, it is important to prioritize the patient's concerns that must guide the nursing care plan and interventions. Care for the patient is ordered and organized in accordance with the patient's priority and urgent needs. Desired collaborative care outcomes in patients with neurogenic shock typically include:

1. Patient will have effective tissue perfusion.
2. Patient's cardiac output will return to normal pre-illness level.

Considering these important care outcomes, prepare a list of the major 3–6 priority patient concerns or nursing diagnoses for patients with neurogenic shock. Be prepared to participate in a discussion of this list and/or to submit them as an assignment, as determined by your faculty. Resources you may find helpful in this assignment can include this lesson, the references, resources on nursing care plans, and standard nursing diagnoses manuals.

LO3:

Collaborative Interventions

Evidence-Based Practice

- Evidence-based treatments for neurogenic shock include life-support treatments:
  - N — Help is needed. Call Rapid Response Team.
  - M N — Airway management (care must be taken to protect the spinal cord) and tissue oxygenation: Maintain tissue oxygenation by supporting cardiac output if needed.
  - Hemodynamic support
    - M N — A mean arterial pressure **(MAP) goal of 85–90 mmHg is desirable to support spine perfusion**, but a MAP of at least 65 mmHg or greater should be maintained. **Vasopressors (e.g., norepinephrine [Levophed]) may be used if fluids alone are not effective.**
    - M N — Large amounts of fluid may be required. Depending on the degree of vasodilitation and the severity of blood pooling, several liters of fluids may be rapidly infused to support the MAP. Normally crystalloid agents are used (e.g., normal saline) but the health care provider might request a non-sodium based solution like D5W.
    - M N — **Atropine** to treat bradycardia. If unresponsive to atropine, an external cardiac pacemaker may be required.
- M N — Less evidence is present to support the administration of **high dose steroids**, such as hydrocortisone.

Concept Check

4. When are vasopressors used in the treatment of neurogenic shock?

A. If atropine is not effective

B. If fluid resuscitation is not effective

C. If high dose steroids are not effective

D. If external pacing is not effective

Answer question

Supportive and Comfort Care

- Immobilize the cervical spine until diagnostics confirm or disconfirm a dangerous injury. A cervical (C) collar, a head immobilzer, and logrolling are among the precautionary methods.
- Large amounts of fluids are administered to maintain tissue perfusion and blood pressure. Fluids along with electrolytes and urine output must be monitored closely to detect early warnings of cord swelling or increased damage due to excess fluid (e.g., decreasing motor movement, abnormal reflexes).
- Monitor closely for respiratory complications.
- Continuously monitor for hypothermia secondary to severe vasodilation and excessive heat loss. Treatment of the primary problem is the goal; however, external warming and managing heat loss by reducing skin exposure may be indicated.
- Pain control if shock is due to injury.
- Once stabilized, attentive care must be provided to prevent the many hazards of immobility and multiple invasive devices (e.g., DVT, pneumonia, infections, pressure ulcers, malnutrition, bowel dysfunction). (See Spinal Cord Injury NovE-Lesson in Neuro, if applicable.)
- Emotional and spiritual support should be offered and guided by the patient and family preferences.

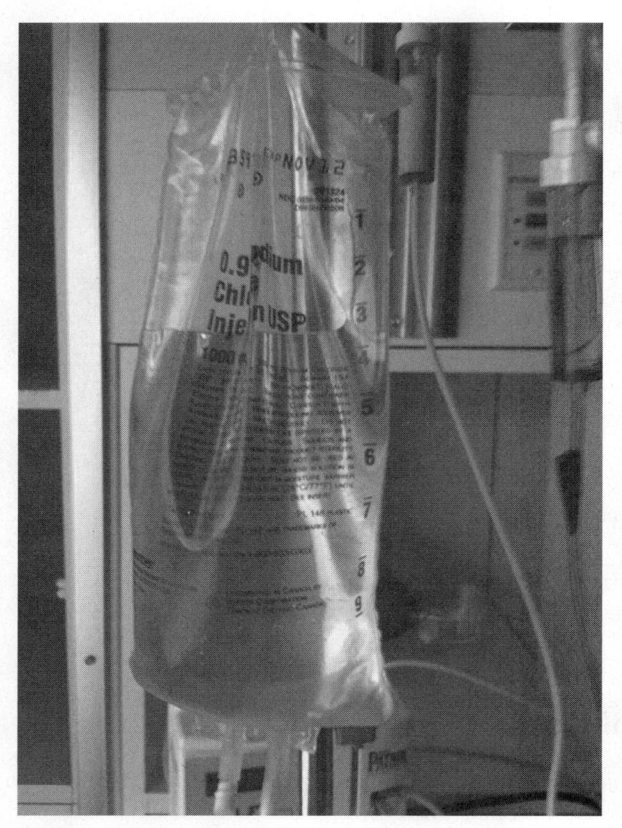

Preparation for large volume infusions requires a number of intravenous (IV) pumps. Vasopressors may also be needed.

Source: Copyright © 2013, NovEx Novice to Expert Learning, LLC

Concept Check

5. Rapid fluid administration may be decreased if the patient in neurogenic shock develops which finding?

A. Decreased urine output

B. Hypothermia

C. Respiratory crackles

D. Pain

Answer question

Concept Check

6. At which point can a patient fully immobilized for possible neck injury be taken out of immobilization?

A. After x-rays are completed

B. If the patient complains of discomfort

C. When injury is disconfirmed

D. When a neurosurgeon is present

Answer question

Summary of Interventions

- Management of neurogenic shock is similar to other forms of shock:
  - o Help is needed. Call Rapid Response Team
  - o Airway support, if needed
  - o Hemodynamic support
    - Fluids
    - Vasopressors
    - The key difference would be to administer an agent, such as atropine, to increase the heart rate if bradycardia is present.

Concept Check

7. Which nursing strategy is indicated for a patient in neurogenic shock?

A. Avoid administering pain medication to prevent the masking of symptoms.

B. Place the patient in left side-lying or recovery position.

C. Keep the patient fully exposed to allow for easy monitoring of injuries.

D. Monitor for the development of pressure ulcers.

Answer question

LO4:

Evaluation of Desired Collaborative Care Outcomes

Evaluation and reassessment should reveal attainment of previously established patient outcomes. In summary:

- Patient's skin is warm and dry, mentation is clear, and urine output is adequate.
- Patient's heart rate and blood pressure are normal and pulses are regular and easily palpable.

References

Casha S., & Christie S. (2011). A systematic review of intensive cardiopulmonary management after spinal cord injury. *Journal of Neurotrauma, 28*(8), 1479–1495.

Dooney N., & Dagai A. (2011). Anesthetic considerations in acute spinal cord trauma. *International Journal of Critical Illness and Injury Science, 1*(1), 36–43.

Hickey, J.V. (2009). The clinical practice of neurological and neurosurgical nursing. 6th ed. Philadelphia, PA: Lippincott Williams & Wilkins.

King, K., & Olson, D. (2007). What you should know about neurogenic shock. *American Nurs Today, 2*(2), 36, 38.

Wuermser, L.A., Ho, C. H., Chiodo, A. E., Kirshblum, S. C., & Scelza, W. M. (2007). 1. Spinal cord injury medicine. 2. Acute care management of traumatic and nontraumatic injury. *Archives of Physical Medicine and Rehabilitation, 99*(3 Suppl 1), S55–S61.

Patient Education

Chen, D. (2011-2015). Experts\ Spinal cord injury: video series. **www.facingdisability.com/expert-topics/spinal-cord-injury-101**

National Institutes of Health. (2014). Spinal cord injury. **www.nlm.nih.gov/medlineplus/spinalcordinjuries.html**

www.ninds.nih.gov

Learning Outcomes for Hypovolemic Shock

When you complete this lesson, you will be able to:

1. Recognize the clinical relevance of hypovolemic shock.
2. Consider the pathophysiology, etiology, risk factors, and clinical presentation of hypovolemic shock that determine the priority patient concerns.
3. Determine the most urgent and important nursing interventions and patient education required in caring for a patient with hypovolemic shock.
4. Evaluate attainment of desired collaborative care outcomes for a patient with hypovolemic shock.

LO1:

What Is Hypovolemic Shock?

- Hypovolemic shock is a macrocirculatory type of shock and is produced by the loss of circulating or intravascular blood volume, resulting in inadequate delivery of key nutrients, primarily oxygen.
- It is typically an emergency situation in which rapid and severe blood loss leads to multiorgan failure and death.
- Losing close to 20% of one's normal blood volume results in hypovolemic shock.

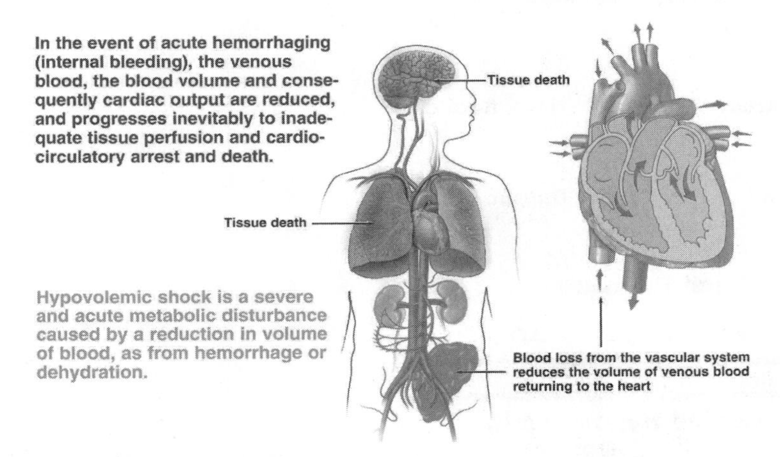

In the event of acute hemorrhaging (internal bleeding), the venous blood, the blood volume and consequently cardiac output are reduced, and progresses inevitably to inadequate tissue perfusion and cardiocirculatory arrest and death.
Tissue death
Tissue death
Hypovolemic shock is a severe and acute metabolic disturbance caused by a reduction in volume of blood, as from hemorrhage or dehydration.
Blood loss from the vascular system reduces the volume of venous blood returning to the heart

This exhibit depicts the sequence of events leading to death in hypovolemic (low blood volume) shock.
Source: Nucleus Medical Art Inc/Alamy

LO1:

Clinical Relevance

Hemorrhage is preventable but remains a leading cause of hypovolemic shock and death.

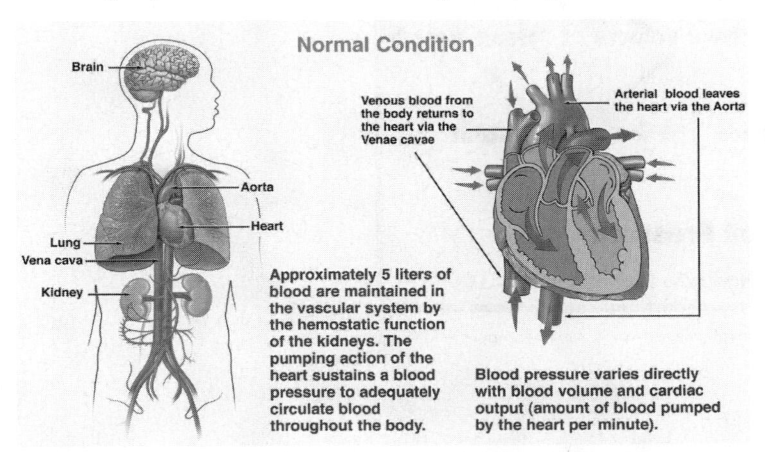

Venous blood from the body returns to the heart via the Venae cavae
Arterial blood leaves the heart via the Aorta
Approximately 5 liters of blood are maintained in the vascular system by the hemostatic function of the kidneys. The pumping action of the heart sustains a blood pressure to adequately circulate blood throughout the body.

These sets of illustrations compare normal blood volume and pressure homeostasis being maintained by normal physiological functions versus the pathophysiology leading to death from hypovolemic shock resulting from massive hemorrhage.
Source: Nucleus Medical Art Inc/Alamy

LO2:

Pathophysiology

Hypovolemic Shock (Macrocirculatory Shock)

- Hypovolemic shock is produced by the loss of circulating or intravascular blood volume (preload), resulting in the loss of blood flow (stroke volume and cardiac output) with consequent inadequate delivery of key nutrients, primarily oxygen.
- Loss of blood volume is not always immediately apparent unless trauma causes visible or massive blood loss.
- The body can compensate for a gradual loss of volume and mask developing hypovolemia without blood pressure changes (see Early, Compensated Hypovolemia image below). Surprisingly, up to 30% of the intravascular volume can be masked before notable drops in blood pressure are apparent.
- Monitoring stroke volume (vigilant observation) for subtle changes in the patient's condition can warn of hypovolemic effects.
- Eventually, untreated hypovolemia leads to circulatory collapse (see Late, Uncompensated Hypovolemia image below).

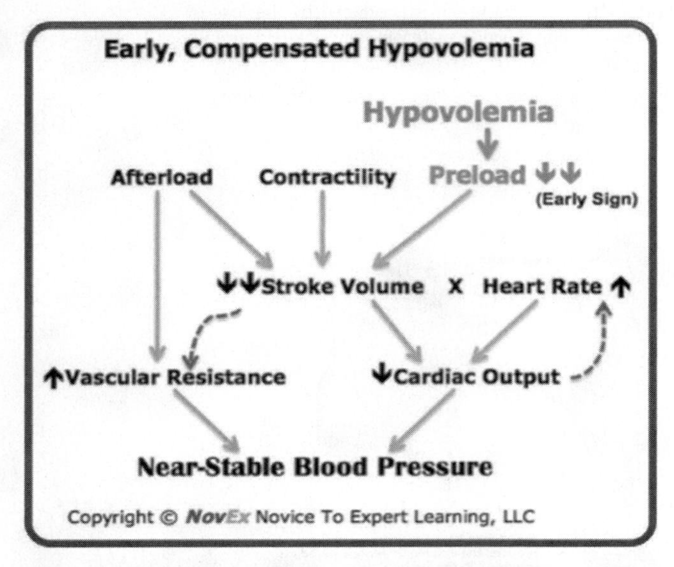

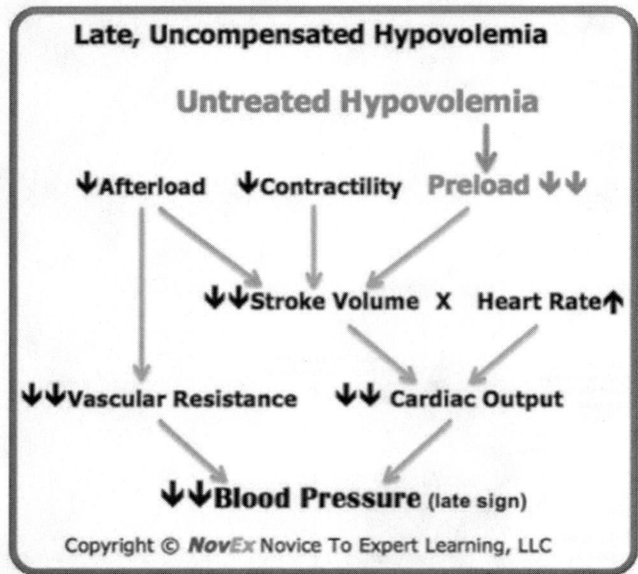

Upper: Early, compensated hypovolemia. Lower: Late, uncompensated hypovolemia.
Source: (*both*) Copyright © 2013, NovEx Novice to Expert Learning, LLC

Concept Check

1. **How much intravascular fluid can be lost before hypovolemic shock occurs?**
   A. At least 50%
   B. 40% to 50%
   C. 25% to 35%
   D. Close to 20%

Answer question

Concept Check

2. **The patient who has lost circulating blood volume has primarily had alteration of which cardiac hemodynamic?**
   A. Preload
   B. Afterload
   C. Systemic vascular resistance
   D. Contractility

Answer question

- Hypovolemic shock presents with "site" control mechanisms, which includes vasoconstriction at the site of the blood loss to slow the loss.
- As the local controls (vasoconstriction) fail, total blood volume further declines. The first macro cardiovascular change is a decrease in stroke volume. Compensatory mechanisms are immediately initiated, including an increase in heart rate and vasoconstriction to maintain cardiac output.
- In this early stage, compensatory mechanisms maintain blood flow and oxygen delivery, as detailed in the Shock States: Overview NovE-lesson.
- The compensatory mechanisms protect blood flow (or shunt blood) to vital organs (e.g., brain, heart), to the detriment of nonvital organs, for a period of time (depending on the amount of blood loss).

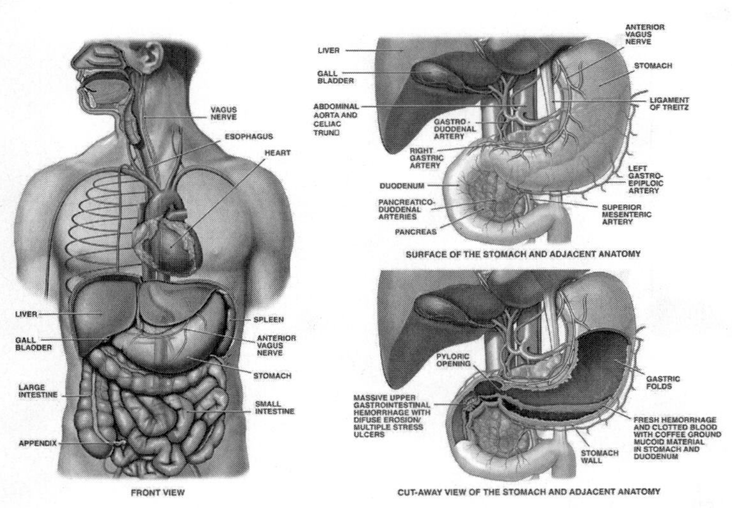

This picture depicts a massive gastric hemorrhage. Erosion of the stomach lining from several ulcers can lead to hemorrhage and hypovolemic shock.
Source: Nucleus Medical Art Inc/Alamy

- Eventually, reduced blood flow to vital organs produces organ dysfunction, as described in all Shock States NovE-lessons.
- If shock is not reversed, cellular dysfunction results, including disruption of essential ion control activities, which can lead to cell death:
  - o Lactate levels rise in shock. Monitoring lactate becomes an important indicator of change in peripheral perfusion and effectiveness of treatment.
  - o $ScvO_2$ and StO_2 levels can also be used to track the severity of shock. $ScvO_2$ and StO_2 levels should return to normal (e.g., more than 70%) as shock is alleviated.
  - o Metabolic acidosis hastens the loss of compensatory vasoconstriction and produces circulatory collapse.

Internal Abdominal Bleeding

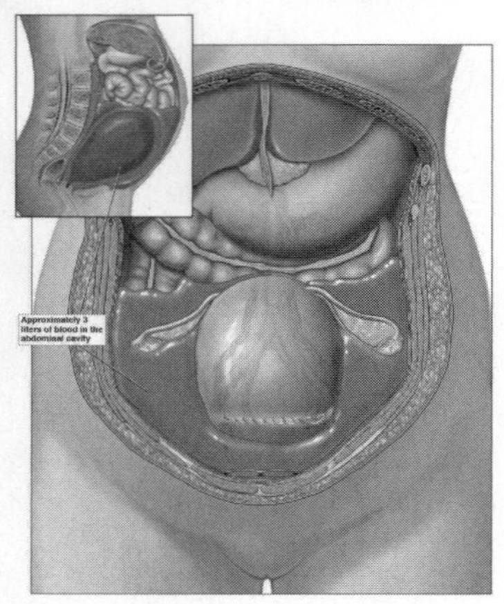

This diagram shows internal abdominal bleeding secondary to injury. Local vasoconstriction can sometimes slow the bleeding, but when severe bleeding is present, hypovolemic shock will ensue.

Concept Check

3. Which organ is one of the best perfused during the compensatory phase of hypovolemic shock?

A. Heart

B. Bowel

C. Skin

D. Stomach

Answer question

Concept Check

4. Which finding indicates that hypovolemic shock is resolving?

A. $S_{CV}O_2$ decreases

B. Lactate level rises

C. StO_2 increases

D. Metabolic acidosis occurs

Answer question

Causes and Risk Factors

- Causes and risk factors of hypovolemic shock include anything that causes loss of blood volume from the vascular system.
- The first type of causes and risk factors include any trauma or medical condition producing significant blood loss or bleeding:
  - Traumas and injuries: These include penetrating or blunt trauma of the chest or abdomen, injury or rupture of any major blood vessel (e.g., aortic aneurysm, carotid artery).
  - Internal bleeding conditions: OB/GYN conditions (e.g., miscarriage, ruptured ectopic, placenta previa, placental abruption, uterine rupture), GI bleeding, retroperitoneal, and peritoneal bleeding (e.g., pelvic fracture, post cardiac cath, trauma) which can be missed.
- A second type of hypovolemia involves fluid rather than actual blood loss:
  - Gastrointestinal (GI) or GI-related fluid loss: diarrhea, vomiting, ascites, peritonitis, pancreatitis, cirrhosis, intestinal obstruction
  - Severe dehydration: excessive perspiration, poor fluid intake
  - Burns (significant insensible loss)

Normal Anatomy

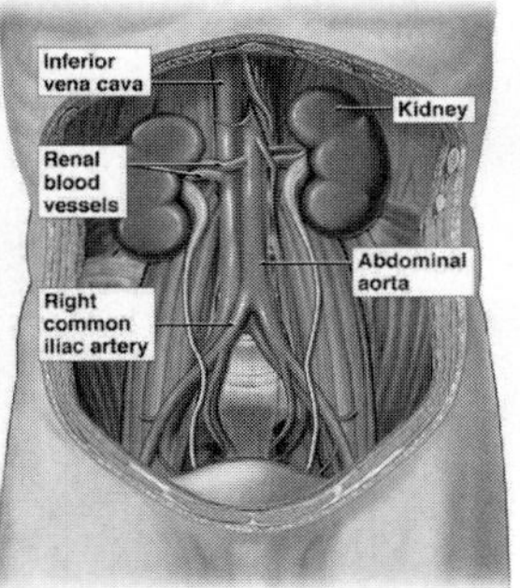

Abdominal Aortic Aneurysm

Abdominal aortic aneurysm

Anterior cut-away view

Eventual Condition

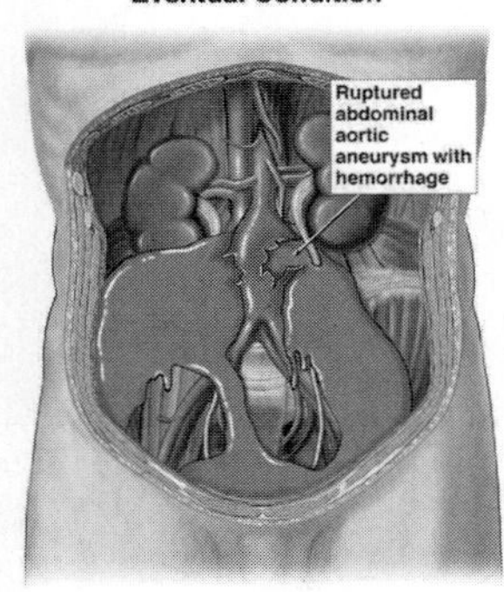

CT Colorizations of Abdomen

Blood
Inferior vena cava
Kidney
Abdominal aorta

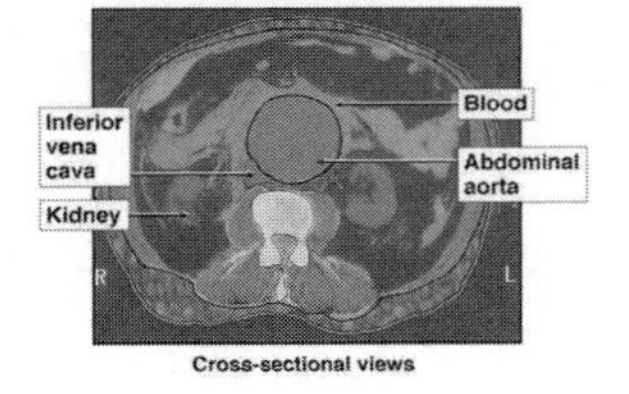

Cross-sectional views

A ruptured abdominal aortic aneurysm is an emergency. This series of pictures shows an aneurysm with subsequent rupture, hemorrhaging, filling the intra-abdominal cavity. Additionally, the actual CT prints of two patients are shown with color highlighting abdominal hemorrhage.
Source: Nucleus Medical Art Inc/Alamy

Concept Check

5. How does pancreatitis result in hypovolemic shock?
   A. The pancreas cannot produce normal clotting factors.
   B. The pancreas becomes so inflamed that it bleeds into the abdominal cavity.
   C. Pancreatitis causes massive urinary diuresis.
   D. Pancreatitis results in fluid shifting to outside the circulatory system.

Answer question

Assessment Findings

Early Stage of Hypovolemic Shock

Due to effective compensatory mechanisms, there are few helpful or clear findings in the early stage of hypovolemic shock:

- Elevated blood lactate levels
- Decreased $ScvO_2$, SvO_2, and StO_2
- Possible tachycardia
- Dropping CVP or preload
- Hypovolemic shock is typically recognized when its late symptoms present (e.g., tachycardia, hypotension, tachypnea, decreased urine output, altered mental status, cool, clammy skin). However, prior to these late symptoms, stroke volume and cardiac output are reduced while vascular resistance and heart rate are increased in the early phase.
- The increased vascular resistance produces vasoconstriction that shunts blood flow away from the periphery (nonvital organs), producing the typical cold, clammy skin.

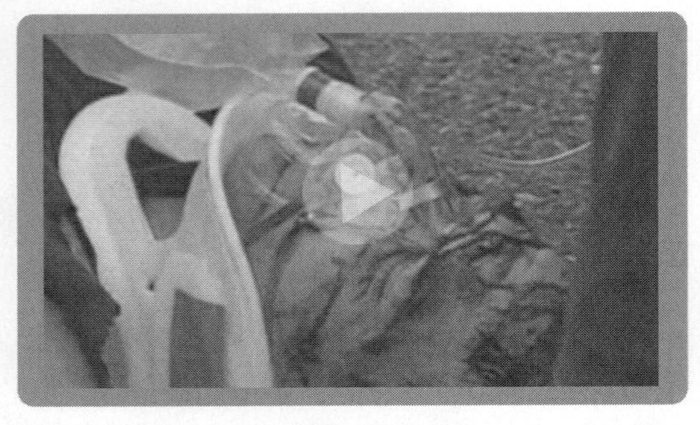

This video gives a brief overview of the signs and symptoms of acute blood volume loss leading up to hypovolemic shock.

Late Stage of Hypovolemic Shock

As the patient's blood volume loss exceeds 30%, the compensatory mechanisms gradually fail. The patient deteriorates into the progressive stage of hypovolemic shock and, without effective treatment, into the irreversible stage. Signs and symptoms are not longer subtle and include:

- Tachycardia with thready pulse
- Hypotension: Systolic BP <90 mmHg or drop >25% of presenting BP
- Marked tachypnea
- Decreased urine output
- Altered mental status
- Cool, clammy skin
- Delayed capillary refill
- Low stroke volume and cardiac output
- High lactate levels
- Low preload or CVP reading (<2–4 mmHg)

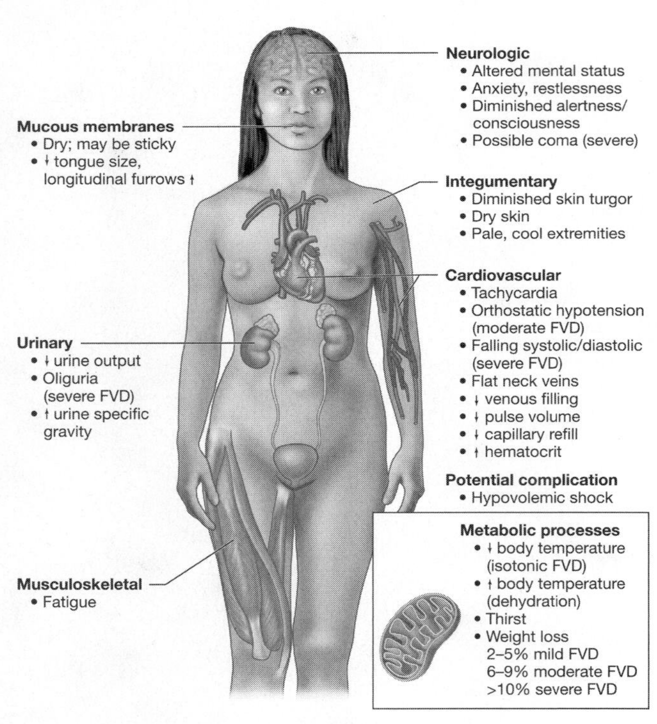

This chart lists the late effects on multiple organ systems secondary to fluid volume deficit (FVD) and hypovolemic shock.

- Unlike cardiogenic shock, hypovolemic shock often produces no other remarkable clinical signs in the early stage. Occult hypoperfusion, defined as hypoperfusion while vital signs are normal, is likely to develop prior to clinical signs of hypovolemic shock.
- Again, unlike cardiogenic shock, pulmonary function may be normal. Venous engorgement is absent because the drop in blood volume reduces preload and, therefore, reduces pulmonary capillary wedge pressure (PCWP) and central venous pressure (CVP). The body's compensatory mechanisms, with their ability to mask symptoms, make hypovolemic shock difficult to detect early.
- Urine may be concentrated and contain low sodium levels as the kidneys try to compensate for the reduced blood flow.
- Hypovolemic shock from severe dehydration can present with dry skin, poor turgor, and dry mucous membranes. However, in acute blood or volume loss, these symptoms are not present.
- Early recognition that blood volume loss can lead to hypovolemia is the first and most important role of the clinician in preventing this major complication. Vigilance around volume replacement is key.

Diagnostics

- Blood lactate: Lactate is often high (>2.5) in hypovolemic shock.
- Blood chemistry panel: Blood urea nitrogen/creatinine (BUN/Cr) ratio may be elevated (>20:1) in hypovolemic shock due to GI hemorrhage or severe dehydration. Dehydration may present with hypernatremia (normal level is 135–140 mEq/L). The most clinically relevant chemistries in most situations of hypovolemic shock are BUN, creatinine, and sodium, although others may hold importance with confounding problems.
- Complete blood count: Even in severe hemorrhage, hemoglobin (Hgb) and hematocrit (Hct) may be normal at first before they begin to drop. Dehydration may present with elevated Hgb and Hct (normal levels are 13–16 g/dL and 38–46 g/dL).
- Central venous pressure: CVP decreases with hypovolemic shock (normal is 2–6 mmHg).

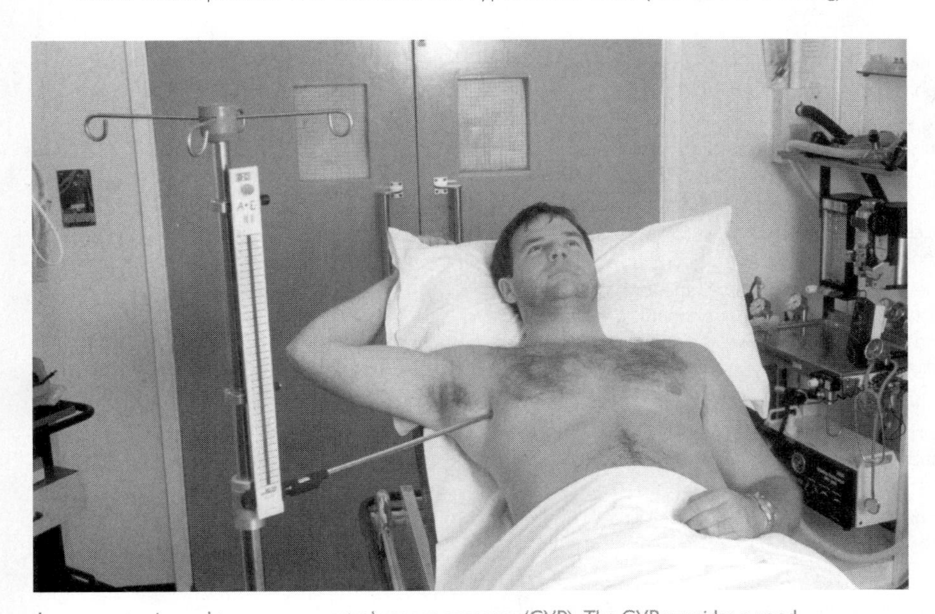

A manometer is used to measure central venous pressure (CVP). The CVP provides a good understanding about the degree of blood loss or volume depletion in hemorrhagic shock.
Source: Medical-on-Line/Alamy

Priority Patient Concerns and Desired Collaborative Care Outcomes

Prior to caring for patients with hypovolemic shock, it is important to prioritize the patient's concerns that must guide the nursing care plan and interventions. Care for the patient is ordered and organized in accordance with the patient's priority and urgent needs. Desired collaborative care outcomes in patients with hypovolemic shock typically include:

1. Patient will have normal stroke volume and cardiac output.
2. Patient will be normovolemic.
3. Patient will have adequate to normal tissue perfusion.
4. Patient will exhibit a calm demeanor and experience a relief of fear and anxiety.

Considering these important care outcomes, prepare a list of the major 3–6 priority patient concerns or nursing diagnoses for patients with hypovolemic shock. Be prepared to participate in a discussion of this list and/or to submit them as an assignment, as determined by your faculty. Resources you may find helpful in this assignment can include this lesson, the references, resources on nursing care plans, and standard nursing diagnoses manuals.

Concept Check

6. Which chemistry value is typically most clinically relevant in patients with hypovolemic shock?

A. Hemoglobin

B. Hematocrit

C. BUN

D. Blood glucose

Answer question

LO3:

Collaborative Interventions

Evidence-Based Practice: Hypovolemic and/or Hemorrhagic Shock

- Goals in managing hypovolemic and/or hemorrhagic shock are: blood or fluid replacement, maintain tissue delivery and oxygenation, and identify and correct the cause or problem (e.g., hemorrhage).
- Evidence-based practice for hypovolemic and/or hemorrhagic shock is fluid replacement (and blood as needed); however, the specific fluid to use or recommendations for blood use should include the following:
  - N — Rapid infusion requires reliable IV access with large-bore lines (e.g., 14 gauge venous catheter), often two, and possibly a central line.
  - M N — Intravenous fluids are good for volume replacement, normally in the form of crystalloids (e.g., normal saline). No evidence exists regarding superiority of one fluid type over another, despite extensive research. Normal saline is as effective as albumin and is considerably less expensive. However, either can be used.
  - M N — Colloids, such as albumin or hetastarch, tend to achieve volume replacement faster.
  - M N — Concurring studies show that blood products (e.g., whole blood, packed red blood cells) benefit patients with fewer complications when given if the hemorrhagic loss is severe and continuing (e.g., a hemoglobin level of <7 g/dL).
  - M N — Since no fluid except blood carries oxygen, fluids such as normal saline and albumin achieve their effect by increasing blood flow (stroke volume [SV] and cardiac output) and tissue perfusion.
- M N — Fluid replacement end points: Fluid should be given until stroke volume has normalized or does not increase more than 10% after the bolus (e.g., 500 mL) or subsequent boluses, are given. A bolus is a large volume of fluid that is rapidly infused. If stroke volume cannot be measured, give fluids until the mean arterial pressure (MAP) is >65 mmHg.
  - M N — Improvement in urine output to >0.5 mL/kg/hr is another end point for volume resuscitation.
  - M N — Lactate is a good measure of improvement in tissue oxygenation, although it is slow to respond, meaning that the lactate level may not show improvement for hours. Measuring lactates often and noting a decreasing "trend" to near normal is a good resuscitation end point (<2.5 mmol).
- M N — Keep in mind, the definitive management of blood or fluid volume loss is to find the cause and correct it.

- o If the person has trauma-induced bleeding, surgery is the likely treatment of choice.
- o If nontrauma (e.g., dehydration), the patient can be managed by giving both IV and oral fluid. Using fluids that are similar to vascular components is best (e.g., normal saline).
- o If medical conditions are causing intravascular volume loss to third spacing, treating the medical condition to control or reduce hypovolemia is needed.

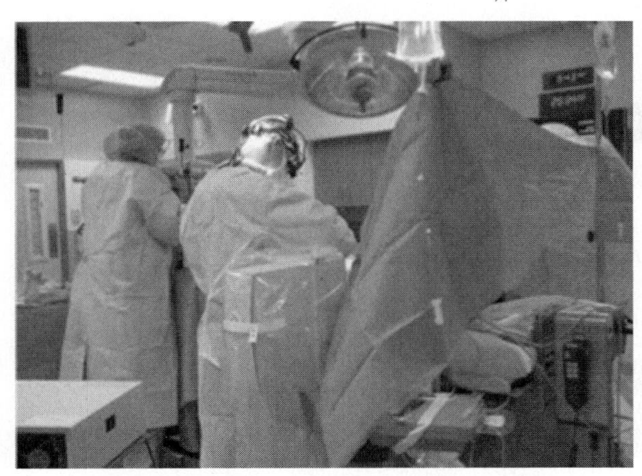

Surgery is often needed following traumatic injury to repair the cause of the volume loss.

Collaborative Symptom Management and Comfort Care

Depending on the patient's responses to volume replacement, the following interventions may need to be concomitantly administered:

- Best practice for the treatment of hemorrhage, moderate or massive, is yet to be determined, but volume replacement is necessary.
- M N Common, early, and often effective practice includes placing the patient in a supine position with his or her feet elevated one foot higher than their body. This maneuver increases blood return to the heart and circulation to the vital organs.
- N Monitor the patient's core temperature during rapid volume replacement to prevent hypothermia. Keep patient warm. Warm infusions if feasible.
- If fluid resuscitation does not correct hypotension and tissue hypoxia, vasopressors can be used with caution. These are *not* primary or early treatments. Norepinephrine (Levophed), dopamine, vasopressin, and phenylephrine are among the drugs used:
  - N o Vasopressors are aimed at improving stroke volume and tissue oxygenation (SvO_2 greater than 70%). If stroke volume and SvO_2 levels are not available, reestablishing **MAP greater than or equal to 65 mmHg** is a common target.
  - M N o **Vasopressors should only be given if adequate fluid (volume) has not restored blood flow and tissue oxygenation.**
  - N o Vasopressors are infused with close, continuous monitoring and caution.
  - N o Vasopressors can cause severe local reactions from their strong vasoconstrictive effects. **Do not infuse peripherally; infuse only in a large central vein.** Stop a vasopressor infusion immediately if it has extravasated or leaked out of the vein.
  - M N o Blood pressure is not always a good indicator of improved perfusion. Use stroke volume and tissue oxygenation end points (SvO_2) to help gauge the impact of vasopressors whenever possible.

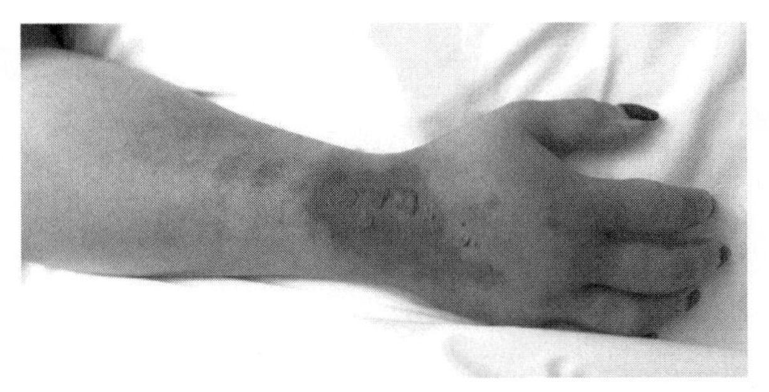

Tissue necrosis can result in peripheral extraversion.
Source: Courtesy of K. Kyriakidis

Concept Check

7. What situation should be present before vasopressor medications are infused?

A. Patient's BUN should be normal.

B. Patient should receive adequate fluid resuscitation.

C. Patient should be normotensive.

D. Patient or family should sign a release.

Answer question

Summary of Interventions

1. Hypovolemic shock is a medical emergency. Do not delay intervention. The Rapid Response Team is needed.
2. Rapid fluid replacement (or blood products with hemorrhage), sometimes massive, is the treatment of choice.

   End points for volume resuscitation include improving stroke volume, tissue oxygenation (e.g., $ScvO_2$, lactate), mean arterial pressure, and urine output. Useful parameters:

   a. The SV does not increase more than 10% after a bolus or subsequent boluses of fluid.

   b. MAP >65 mmHg

   c. Lactate trending to <2.5 mmol, although lactate may not decline for hours after successful resuscitation. A downward trend can be a useful indicator.

   d. $ScvO_2$ (or StO_2) >70%

   e. Urine output >0.5 mL/kg/hr
3. Finding the source of the blood or fluid volume loss and correcting the problem is the only definitive treatment in hypovolemic shock.

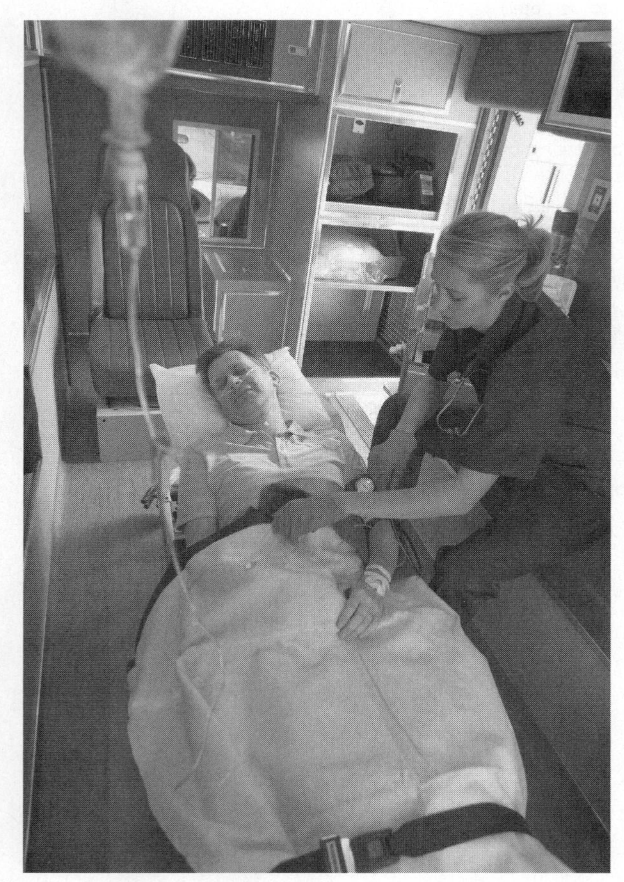

Shock can be mitigated by rapidly treating the cause and can be helped with early first aid. The severity of this emergency depends on the pathologies, the stage of shock, and age. Older adults generally have poorer outcomes.

Source: Monkey Business/Fotolia

LO4:

Evaluation of Desired Collaborative Care Outcomes

Evaluation and reassessment should reveal attainment of previously established patient outcomes. In summary:

- Patient's blood pressure is within normal limits and pulse is full and regular.
- Patient's urine output is balanced with fluid intake and blood pressure is at normal level.
- Patient's skin is warm and dry, mentation is at pre-illness level, and tissue oxygenation is normal.
- Patient expresses feeling less anxious about treatments and state of health.

References

Gonzales, E. A. (2008). Fluid resuscitation in the trauma patient. *J Trauma Nurs, 15*(3), 149–157.

Knight, A. R., Fry, L. E., Clancy, R. L., & Pierce, J. D. (2011). Understanding the effects of oxygen administration in haemorrhagic shock. *Nurs Crit Care, 16*(1), 28–35.

Moore, K. (2011). Managing hemorrhagic shock in trauma: are we still drowning patients in the field? *J Emerg Nurs, 37*(6), 594–596.

Myburgh, J. A., & Mythen, M. G. (2013). Resuscitation fluids. *N Engl J Med, 369*, 1243–1251. DOI: 10.1056/NEJMra1208627.

Pacagnella, R. C., Souza, J. P., Durocher, J., et al. (2013). A systematic review of the relationship between blood loss and clinical signs. *PLoS One, 8*(3), e57594. DOI: 10.1371/journal.pone.0057594

Vincent, J.L., Ince, C., & Bakker, J. (2012). Clinical review: circulatory shock—an update: a tribute to Professor Max Harry Weil. *Critical Care*, 16(6), 239. **ccforum.com/content/16/6/239**

Wang, J., Liang, T., Louis, L., Nicolaou, S., & McLaughlin, P. D. (2013). Hypovolemic shock complex in the trauma setting: a pictorial review. *Can Assoc Radiol J, 64*(2), 156–163.

Patient Education

http://www.nlm.nih.gov/medlineplus/ency/article/000167.htm

http://www.uptodate.com/contents/treatment-of-severe-hypovolemia-or-hypovolemic-shock-in-adults?source=search_result&search=hemorrhagic+shock&selectedTitle=1~143#PATIENT_INFORMATION

Learning Outcomes for Anaphylactic Shock

When you complete this lesson, you will be able to:

1. Recognize the clinical relevance of anaphylactic shock.
2. Consider the pathophysiology, etiology, risk factors, and clinical presentation of anaphylactic shock that determine the priority patient concerns.
3. Determine the most urgent and important nursing interventions and patient education required in caring for a patient with anaphylactic shock.
4. Evaluate attainment of desired collaborative care outcomes for a patient with

LO1:

What Is Anaphylactic Shock?

- Anaphylaxis is a potentially fatal immunologic response by the whole body to an allergen. It is a response to a previously encountered allergen to which the immune system has already developed antibodies.
- Anaphylactic shock is a potentially fatal circulatory manifestation of anaphylaxis.
- Anaphylaxis develops rapidly (onset, minutes to hours) and can quickly progress to anaphylactic shock and death.
- It is unclear which patients with anaphylaxis will progress to shock or recover spontaneously.

Fatal Anaphylaxis with Fulminant Pulmonary Edema

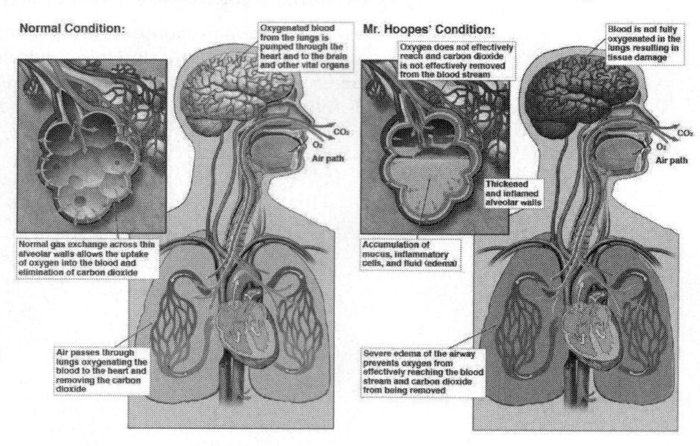

This exhibit depicts fatal anaphylaxis with fulminant pulmonary edema.

Concept Check

1. **Which statement about anaphylaxis is accurate?**
   A. Damage from anaphylactic shock is limited to the respiratory system.
   B. Anaphylaxis is an immunological response.
   C. Criteria predict those who will progress from anaphylaxis to shock.
   D. Anaphylaxis can occur on initial exposure to an allergen.

Answer question

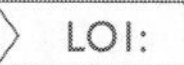

Clinical Relevance

- Anaphylaxis is a medical emergency and can occur in any setting. Nurses need to be able to recognize and initiate treatment for this condition promptly.
- Deaths from anaphylaxis usually occur from development of anaphylactic shock or airway obstruction.
- 80–86% of patients who died from anaphylaxis never received epinephrine prior to arrest. Mortality was very high among patients receiving epinephrine too late.

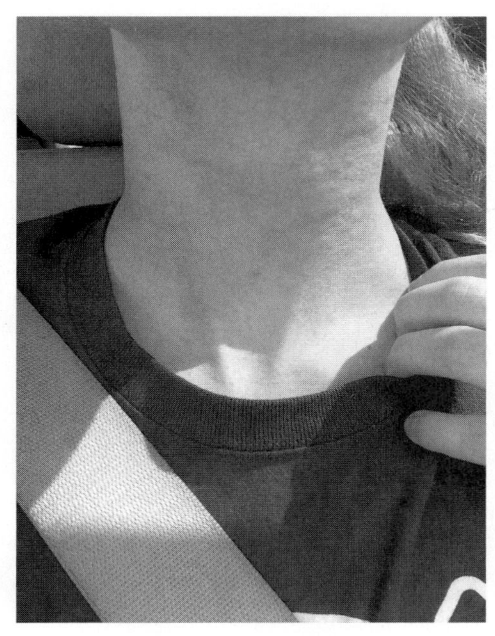

This patient is highly allergic to cats. At a swim meet, her friend, who has a cat, offered the patient a towel to dry off and the patient broke out in hives within a short time. In hindsight, the friend realized that the cat is often on the bed where the towel had been.
Source: Courtesy of K. Kyriakidis

LO2:

Pathophysiology

Anaphylaxis

- Anaphylaxis is a severe and potentially fatal immune response that occurs when the immune system develops sensitivity to a previously exposed allergen.
- Upon initial exposure to the allergen (e.g., a bee sting, peanuts) the immune system forms IgE antibodies to that antigen (allergen).
- After a subsequent exposure to the allergen, the IgE binds to the antigen.
  The IgE-antigen then binds to receptors on mast cells and basophils, triggering the release of numerous cytokines, including histamine. These cytokines produce dangerous effects (e.g., vasodilation, hypotension, bronchospasm).
- Histamine acts by binding to H_1 and H_2 receptors on target cells. Antihistamines can counter the effects of histamine release.

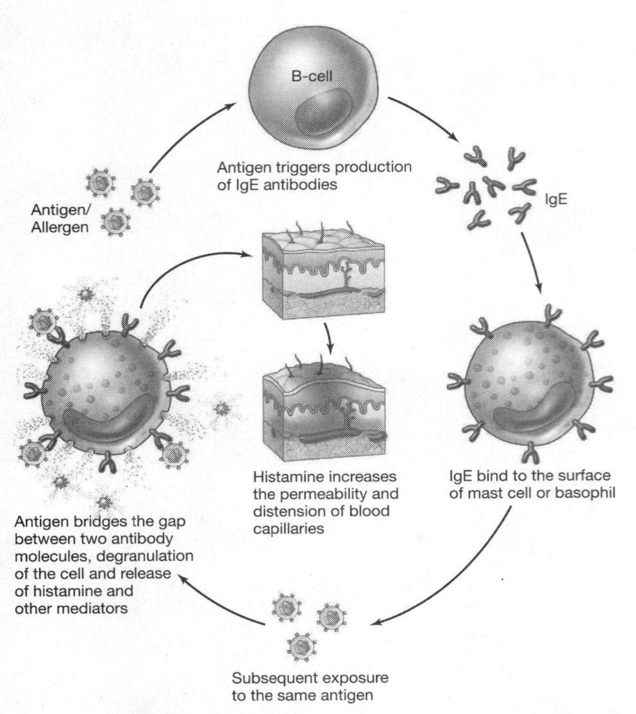
B-cell
Antigen triggers production
of IgE antibodies
IgE
Antigen/
Allergen
IgE bind to the surface
of mast cell or basophil
Histamine increases
the permeability and
distension of blood
capillaries
Antigen bridges the gap
between two antibody
molecules, degranulation
of the cell and release
of histamine and
other mediators
Subsequent exposure
to the same antigen

Allergic reaction cascade leading to a total body anaphylactic response.

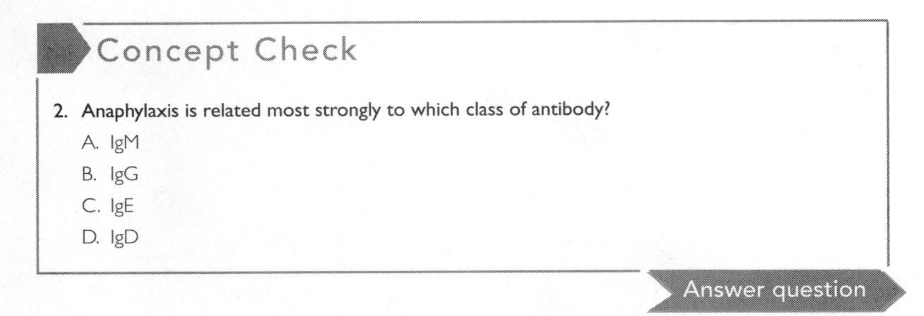
Concept Check
Answer question

2. Anaphylaxis is related most strongly to which class of antibody?
   A. IgM
   B. IgG
   C. IgE
   D. IgD

- With a severe reaction, the following can rapidly occur:
  1. Severe vasodilation, with excessive pooling of blood in the veins and capillaries, leads to sudden and severe hypotension with resultant loss of blood flow. Without blood flow, oxygen is not delivered to the tissues and microcirculatory shock ensues. This explains why:
     a. A supine position with the legs elevated can return the pooled blood back into the central circulation.
     b. A vasoconstricting medication is imperative.
  2. Severe capillary permeability causes massive fluid shifts from the intravascular to extravascular spaces. This shift, which can involve 50% of the vascular volume in ten minutes, creates a significant "loss" of intravascular blood volume, similar to hemorrhage but without actual blood loss from the body.
     a. Reversing the capillary permeability is crucial to reverse the intravascular blood loss.
     b. "Loss" of blood volume requires large and rapid volume replacement.
  3. Tachycardia and severe hypotension follow, due to the shifting of blood volume from the central or core circulation.

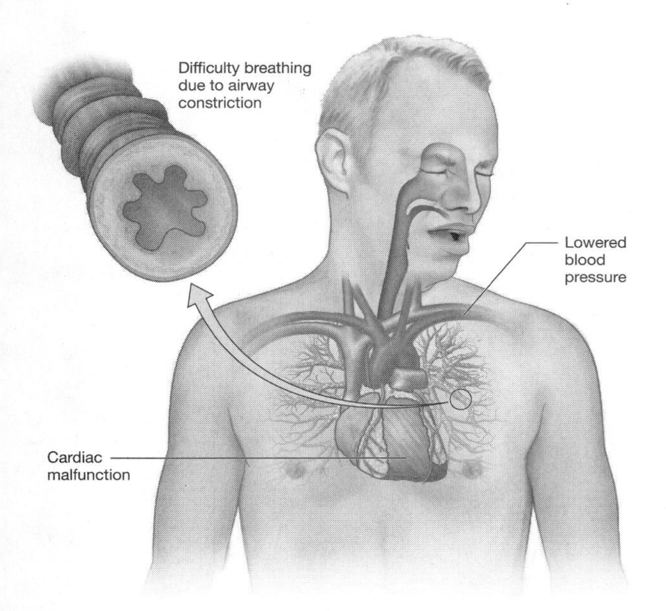

Anaphylactic crisis occurs during immediate serious allergic reactions.

- The circulatory effects that result in arterial vasodilation and increased capillary permeability may result in anaphylactic shock and inadequate perfusion of tissue.
- Cardiac output in this type of shock may be normal or increased.

Risk Factors

- Patients with the following conditions are at increased risk of anaphylaxis:
  - o Asthma
  - o Eczema
  - o Allergic rhinitis

Causes

Anaphylactic shock is an extreme allergic response.

- Almost any foreign substance can cause an allergic response. However, some are more commonly associated with allergic reactions and anaphylaxis and include:
  - o Venoms (e.g., bee stings)
  - o Foods (e.g., peanuts, shellfish)
  - o Medications (e.g., penicillin)

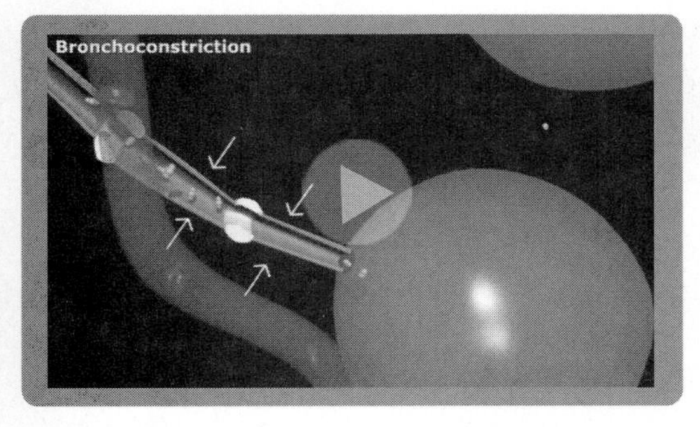

This animation depicts a secondary (anamnestic) immune response to a hymenoptera (stinging insect) venom. These kind of allergic reactions can be rapid and fatal.

Assessment Findings

Findings That Signal Danger

Depending on the severity and rapidity of the patient's allergic reaction, signs and symptoms may develop immediately or over time. Signs that warn of immediate danger and require emergency, lifesaving treatment include:

- Respiratory distress: Stridor (caused by spasm of the larynx), wheezing, bronchospasm, labored breathing, shortness of breath, hypoxemia, cyanosis
- Circulatory problems or collapse: Hypotension from vasodilation and capillary permeability or leak, severe tachycardia, dysrhythmias, chest pain, vascular collapse
- Mucocutaneous: Angioedema is edema that develops rapidly in the subcutaneous tissue and mucosa (swollen lips, uvula, tongue, face).
- Rapid onset and progression of these or even more minor symptoms may prove fatal.

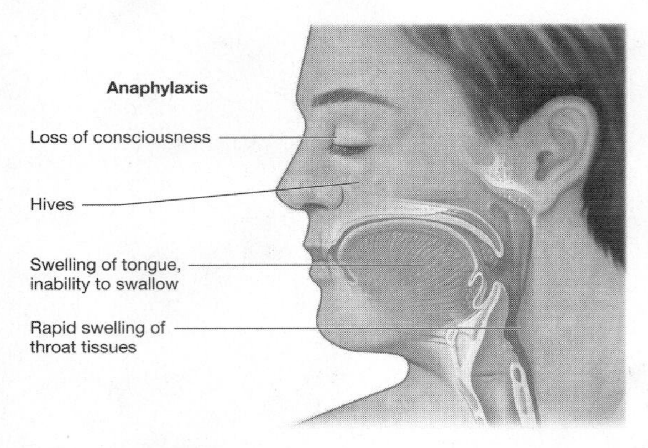

After being exposed to a substance such as bee sting venom, the person's immune system becomes sensitized to it

Additional Findings

More common signs and symptoms include:

- Headache
- Mucocutaneous:
    - o Pruritis (itching)
    - o Urticaria (hives) is a rash with raised pale red bumps
    - o Flushing
- Gastrointestinal: abdominal cramping, nausea, vomiting, diarrhea

Symptoms like hives usually begin within 5–30 minutes from the time the culprit antigen is injected but can occur within seconds. If the antigen is ingested, symptoms usually occur within minutes to 2 hours. In rare cases, symptoms can be delayed in onset for several hours.

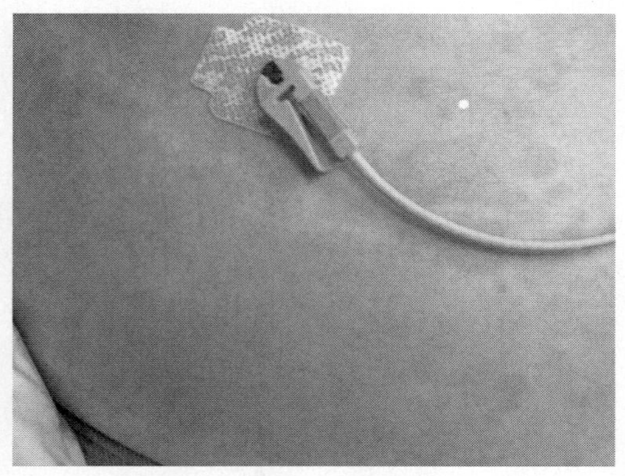

Hives from a systemic allergic reaction are common in anaphylaxis.
Source: Courtesy of K. Kyriakidis

Inconspicuous Finding

Some types of anaphylactic shock may not be immediately visible, but may produce significant dysfunction of an organ system, including disturbances in coagulation that cause bleeding.

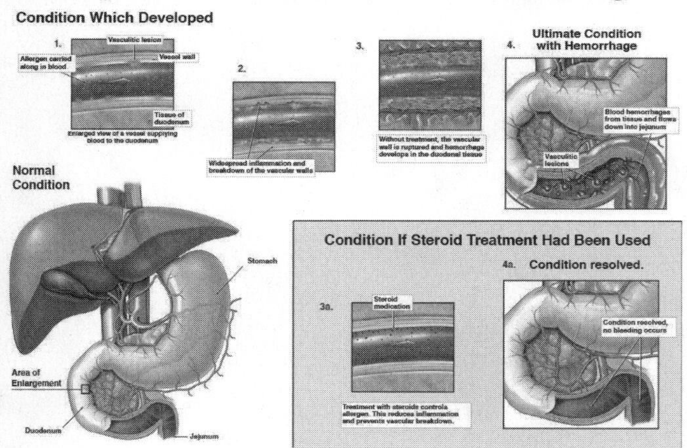

This exhibit depicts the development of allergic vasculitis with massive intestinal hemorrhage.
Source: © 2013 Nucleus Medical Media, All rights reserved

Concept Check

3. What causes the stridor associated with anaphylaxis?
   - A. Collapse of alveoli
   - B. Spasm of the larynx
   - C. Edema of nasal passages
   - D. Decreased perfusion to lung tissue

Answer question

Concept Check

4. The nurse reports that a patient has developed angioedema after receiving an IV antibiotic. What finding is present?
   - A. Shortness of breath
   - B. Swollen lips
   - C. Flushing
   - D. Severe itching

Answer question

Diagnostics

- Anaphylaxis is a diagnosis that is made clinically. It is important to obtain a history of possible exposures to inciting allergens over the prior several hours. The presence of one of the following criteria (World Allergy Organization Guidelines*) makes anaphylaxis highly likely. Recommendations are to treat for anaphylaxis immediately if the patient has any one of the following three:

**J Allergy Clin Immunol, 127(3)*

1. Sudden onset of skin or mucosal symptoms and at least one of the following:
   a. Sudden onset of respiratory symptoms
   b. Sudden onset of decreased BP or end organ dysfunction (e.g., syncope, incontinence)
2. Exposure to likely allergen and at least two of the following four:
   a. Sudden onset respiratory symptoms
   b. Sudden onset of mucosal and skin symptoms
   c. Sudden onset of decreased BP or end organ dysfunction (e.g., syncope, incontinence)
   d. Sudden onset of gastrointestinal symptoms
3. Sudden decreased BP after exposure to an allergen that the patient is known to be sensitive to.

- Decreased BP is defined as a systolic BP (SBP) of <90 or SBP that drops more than 30% mmHg from baseline.
- Additional findings that aid in the diagnosis of anaphylactic shock include:
  - o Elevated lactate levels >2.5 mmol
  - o Confusion, decreased level of consciousness
  - o Decreased urine output

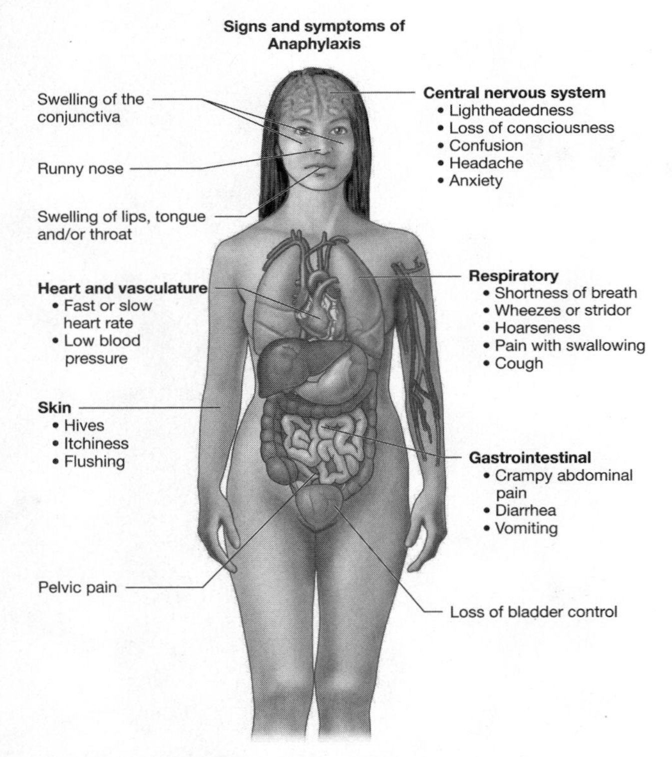

Diagnosis of anaphylaxis is heavily based on the physical findings when examining the patient. If one is clinically uncertain, treatment with epinephrine is recommended, as one dose has not been known to harm a patient.

Priority Patient Concerns and Desired Collaborative Care Outcomes

Prior to caring for patients with anaphylactic shock, it is important to prioritize the patient's concerns that must guide the nursing care plan and interventions. Care for the patient is ordered and organized in accordance with the patient's priority and urgent needs. Desired collaborative care outcomes in patients with anaphylactic shock typically include:

1. Patient will have a clear airway.
2. Patient's cardiac output will return to pre-episode level.
3. Patient will have no findings associated with ineffective tissue perfusion.
4. Patient will breathe easily and will report feeling less anxious and scared.

Considering these important care outcomes, prepare a list of the major 3–6 priority patient concerns or nursing diagnoses for patients with anaphylactic shock. Be prepared to participate in a discussion of this list and/or to submit them as an assignment, as determined by your faculty. Resources you may find helpful in this assignment can include this lesson, the references, resources on nursing care plans, and standard nursing diagnoses manuals.

LO3:

Collaborative Interventions

Evidence-Based Practice

In anaphylaxis or shock, there are typically multiple, simultaneous, emergency interventions. If the patient is unresponsive, the following need to be initiated urgently *and simultaneously*:

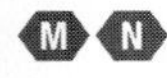

1. As in *every* emergency, follow the CABs: CIRCULATION, AIRWAY, BREATHING, and call for help (Rapid Response Team). Shock and death can rapidly ensue.

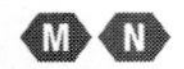

2. Epinephrine is the crucial, first treatment for anaphylaxis and reduces mortality from shock and airway obstruction:
   a. Epinephrine 0.3–0.5 mg IM (thigh), repeat in 5–15 min as needed
   b. Epinephrine IV, if severe
   c. Epinephrine can improve blood flow and pressure due to its ability to reduce inflammation via inflammatory mediators.
   d. Although epinephrine can be given subcutaneously in other conditions, anaphylaxis and shock require faster absorption, particularly when peripheral circulation is compromised.

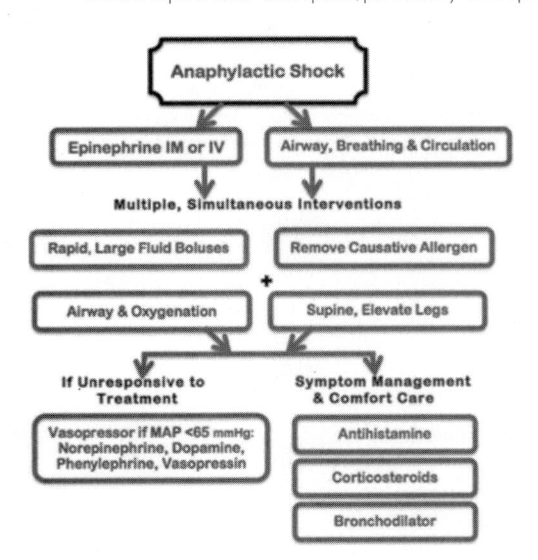

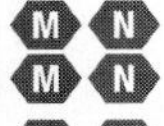

3. Remove the causative agent (e.g., discontinue antibiotic, food allergen, blood product).

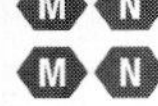

4. Symptom management that is fundamental to protecting the patient's vital functions:

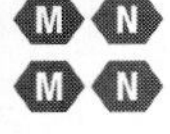

   - Airway management, which may include BiPap or intubation (especially for angioedema) if needed, depends on the patient's level of consciousness.
   - Administer oxygen if O_2 saturation is ≤92%.

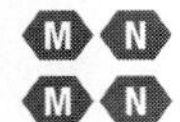

   - Rapid fluid administration to support hemodynamics (e.g., stroke volume, cardiac output BP). Bolus infusions in large amounts may be necessary to treat significant hypotension along with massive shifts of intravascular volume to interstitial spaces.

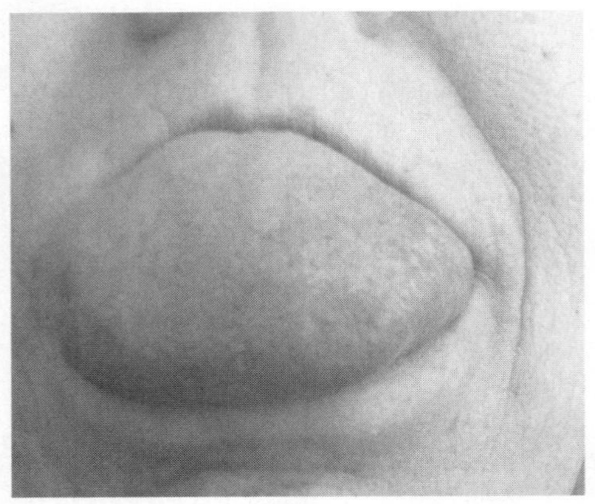

Angioedema can cause rapid and often severe swelling. This patient's tongue occludes his mouth. Immediate airway management is crucial.
Source: Courtesy of K. Kyriakidis

M N **5.** Vasopressors, if fluid alone does not restore hemodynamics:

a. Epinephrine infusion, 2–10 mcg/min

b. Norepinephrine, dopamine, or phenylephrine as needed: add if unresponsive to epinephrine.

c. Vasopressors are used with close, continuous monitoring and caution!

d. Vasopressors should be aimed at improving stroke volume and tissue oxygenation (SvO_2 levels). If stroke volume and SvO_2 levels are not available, mean arterial pressure (MAP) >65 mmHg is a common target.

e. Vasopressors should only be started if fluid infusions do not restore blood flow, BP, and tissue oxygenation.

f. Vasopressors can have intense local reactions from strong vasoconstrictive effects. **Do not infuse peripherally, but only in a large central vein**. Immediately stop a vasopressor infusion if it extravasates or leaks out of the vein and into the surrounding tissues.

g. Blood pressure is not always a good indicator of perfusion status. Use tissue oxygenation end points (SvO_2) to help gauge the impact of vasopressors whenever possible.

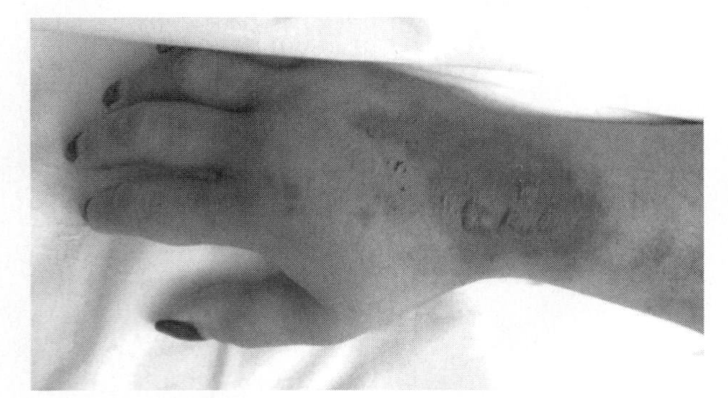

Tissue necrosis can result in peripheral extraversion.
Source: Courtesy of K. Kyriakidis

M N **6.** Placement in a supine position *with legs elevated* improves blood return to the heart in the face of significant pooling of blood in the periphery.

M N **7.** Reliable IV (or IVs) access is essential in the presence of this shock emergency. Use large bore or gauge IVs (14 gauge) for multiple and rapid infusions.

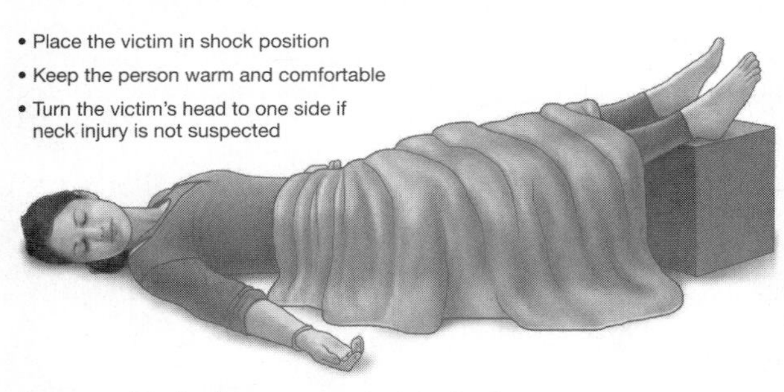

• Place the victim in shock position
• Keep the person warm and comfortable
• Turn the victim's head to one side if neck injury is not suspected

Proper positioning for a person who is in shock.

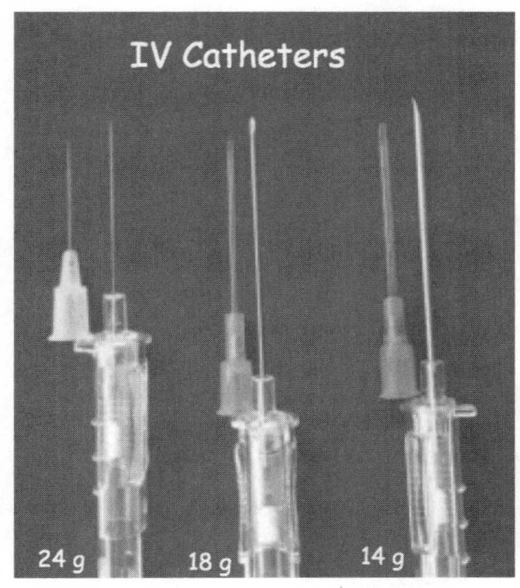

Reliable IV access in shock emergencies include: (1) Peripheral intravenous 14 gauge catheters, seen at the right, and (2) Central venous access device or a catheter, which is placed in a large central vein under sterile conditions in order to give medication, fluids, or blood products.
Source: Copyright © 2013, NovEx Novice to Expert Learning, LLC

Collaborative Interventions (continued)

Collaborative Symptom Management and Comfort Care

Additional treatments are not currently evidence based and have not been shown to reduce mortality, but may help to relieve symptoms and provide comfort:

M N **1.** Antihistamines, both H_1 and H_2 blockers (PO or IV) may be given to relieve histamine initiated symptoms: itching, flushing, hives, rhinorrhea. Antihistamines do not prevent airway obstruction or anaphylactic shock. Diphenhydramine and ranitidine are an appropriate combination. Antihistamines have a much slower onset of action and should not be administered alone as treatment for anaphylaxis. Intravenous administration can be used in urgent situations to avoid oral and IM absorption concerns.

M N **2.** Corticosteroids: Steroids have a longer onset of action and do not relieve symptoms immediately and have no immediate effect on anaphylaxis. However, steroids may help shorten the course of prolonged symptoms. The most commonly used corticosteroid is prednisone (usual dose is 1 mg/kg/day in divided doses).

M N **3.** To treat shortness of breath that has not responded to epinephrine:

   a. Inhaled beta2-adrenergic agonists, such as albuterol, are an option. Beta2 agonists, however, do not prevent shock or laryngeal spasm.

   b. While there is little evidence to support its use, racemic epinephrine via a nebulizer can be used to reduce laryngeal swelling.

M N **4.** Bronchodilator (albuterol): if bronchospasm is unresponsive to epinephrine.

M **5.** Follow-up testing is indicated if allergen is unknown.

Patient Education

Patient education should include prevention and treatment issues, depending on the patient's particular situation:

N • Avoidance of triggering allergens. If allergic to particular food, become a label reader.

N • Educate about signs, symptoms, increased risk of future anaphylactic reactions, and action plan.

M N • Patient should have epinephrine autoinjector available and should be educated about its use:

  o Keep a current pen on hand.

  o Grip injector without touching either end.

  o Remove covers.

  o Press firmly into outer thigh.

  o Hold for 10 seconds.

N

- Educate patient and family about:
  - o Urgency of administering epinephrine as soon as symptoms appear, even if not yet certain
  - o Dangers of delay. Time matters.
  - o Suggest wearing a Medical Alert bracelet.

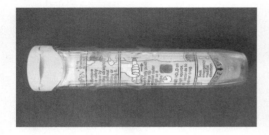

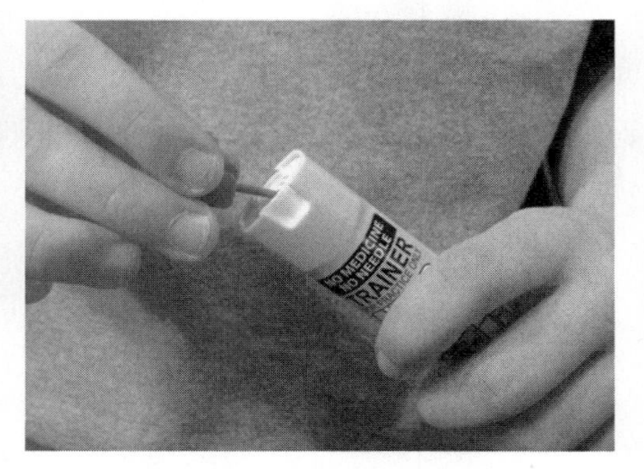

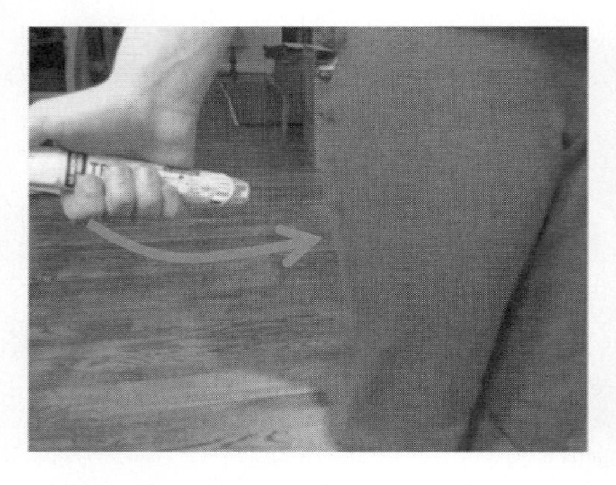

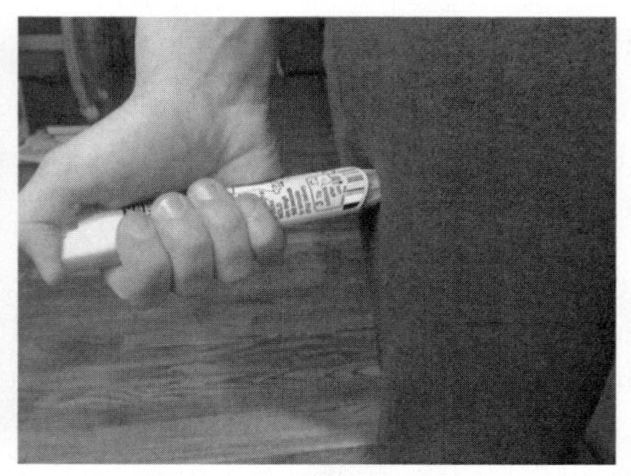

1. Flip open the yellow cap. Remove epinephrine auto-injector from its carrier. 2. Remove blue safety release from epi auto-injector. Needle comes out orange end. Place thumb where blue cap was. 3. Aim epi pen toward mid-outer thigh. Swing and firmly push orange end at 90° angle onto thigh so it clicks. 4. While continuing to press, hold onto outer thigh 10 seconds while drug is delivered. Remove needle. Massage area 10 seconds. Call your HCP.

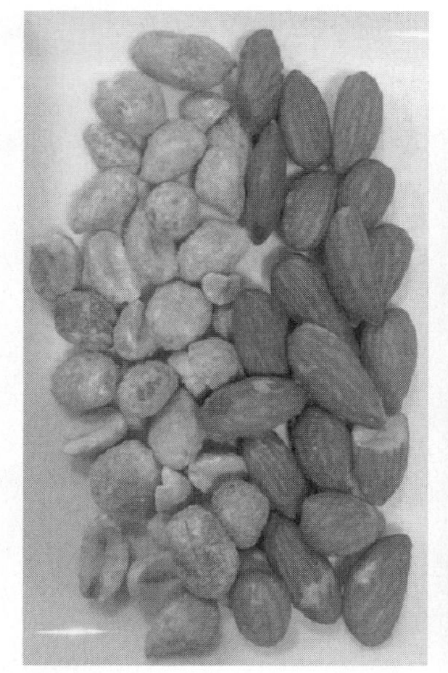

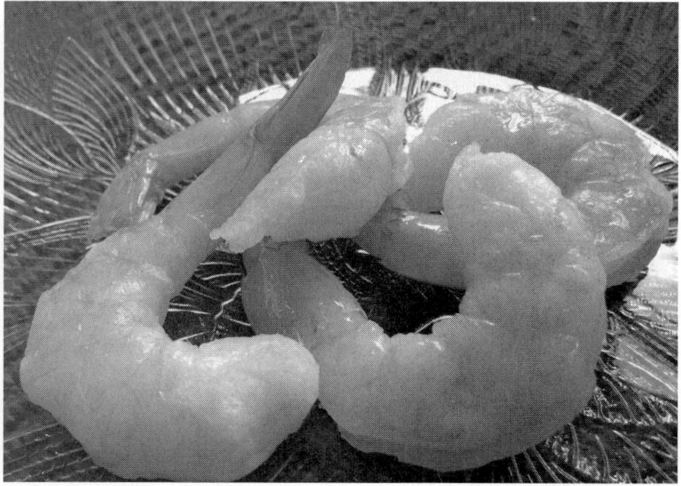

Common allergies include foods (e.g., peanuts, shellfish, and eggs). Nonfood causes include wasp or bee stings, penicillin, sulfa, or any other drug or injection.

Concept Check

5. How should vasopressors be administered?

A. Intravenously into a peripheral catheter

B. Subcutaneously

C. Intravenously into a central catheter

D. Intramuscularly

Answer question

Concept Check

6. Where is the epinephrine autoinjector placed for injection?

A. Against the upper arm

B. Against the abdomen

C. Against the buttock

D. Against the thigh

Answer question

Concept Check

7. Which medication is indicated to treat anaphylaxis-induced shortness of breath refractory to epinephrine?

A. An intravenous H_1 blocker

B. An intravenous H_2 blocker

C. An oral corticosteroid

D. An inhaled $beta_2$-adrenergic blocker

Answer question

Summary of Interventions

- Anaphylaxis is a medical emergency that may progress to anaphylactic shock and death.
- Epinephrine is the first and most important lifesaving treatment in anaphylaxis and may help prevent development of anaphylactic shock or airway obstruction.
- Treatment must first, and simultaneously, address the triggering allergen. Removal of the allergen causing the anaphylactic response is critical.
- Supporting vital signs and functions is a critical step to save the patient's life:
  - o Airway management: Intubation and ventilatory support may be necessary.
  - o Hemodynamic support with fluids can help sustain tissue oxygenation.
  - o Place patient in supine position with legs elevated.
- Other treatments are not evidence based and may not decrease mortality but may help relieve symptoms:
  - o Vasopressors may help if unresponsive to epinephrine and fluids.
  - o Beta agonists (e.g., albuterol) may help with bronchospasm.
  - o Antihistamines, such as diphenhydramine and ranitidine, may help with flushing, itching, and hives.
  - o Steroids take several hours to start working but may shorten the duration of symptoms.

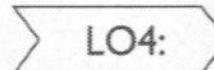

Evaluation of Desired Collaborative Care Outcomes

Evaluation and reassessment should reveal attainment of previously established patient outcomes. In summary:

- Patient respirations are even, easy, and effective.
- Patient's heart rate and blood pressure are normal, and pulses are full and even.
- Patient's skin is warm, dry, and intact; mentation is clear; and urine output is adequate.
- Patient expresses resolution of anxiety regarding air hunger and immediate fear of dying.

References

Hirayama, F. (2013). Current understanding of allergic transfusion reactions: incidence, pathogenesis, laboratory tests, prevention and treatment. *Br J Haematol, 160*(4), 434–44.

Sicherer, S. H., & Leung, D.Y. (2013). Advances in allergic skin disease, anaphylaxis, and hypersensitivity reactions to foods, drugs, and insects in 2012. *J Allergy Clin Immunol, 131*(1), 55–66.

Simons, F. E., & Sheikh, A. (2013). Anaphylaxis: the acute episode and beyond. *BMJ, 346*, f602.

Clinical Practice Guidelines

National Institute for Health and Clinical Excellence (NICE). (2011). Anaphylaxis: Assessment to confirm an anaphylactic episode and the decision to refer after emergency treatment for a suspected anaphylactic episode. London (UK): NICE Clinical Guideline 134, 1–95.

Simons, F. E., Ardusso, L. R., Bilo, M. B., et al. (2012). 2012 update: World Allergy Organization Guidelines for the assessment and management of anaphylaxis. *Curr Opin Allergy Clin Immunol, 12*(4), 389–399. doi: 10.1097/ACI.0b01e328355b7e4.

Patient Education

http://www.nlm.nih.gov/medlineplus/ency/article/000844.htm

www.uptodate.com/contents/epinephrine-auto-injectors-the-basics?source=searchresult&search=patient+information+anaphylaxis&selectedTitle=5~150

STOP

Go to the online course and complete the NovE-Cases assigned by your instructor for this module.

Learning Outcomes for Sepsis

When you complete this lesson, you will be able to:

1. Recognize the clinical relevance of sepsis.
2. Consider the pathophysiology, etiology, risk factors, and clinical presentation of sepsis that determine the priority patient concerns.
3. Determine the most urgent and important nursing interventions and patient education required in caring for a patient with sepsis.
4. Evaluate attainment of desired collaborative care outcomes for a patient with sepsis.

LO1:

What Is Sepsis?

Sepsis is the body's systemic immune response to an infection. The response is initially designed to help contain an invader, whether it be a bacteria, virus, or other pathogen, from harming the person. However, the response of the immune system is extremely powerful and can present a threat to survival as well as saving the patient's life (see photo). A quote from Dr. Lewis Thomas illustrates the power of the immune system in fighting infections:

> "Our arsenals for fighting off bacteria are so powerful, and involve so many different defense mechanisms, that we are more in danger from them than from the invaders.... We live in the midst of explosive devices; we are mined!"
>
> *Germs, New England Journal Of Medicine, 1972*

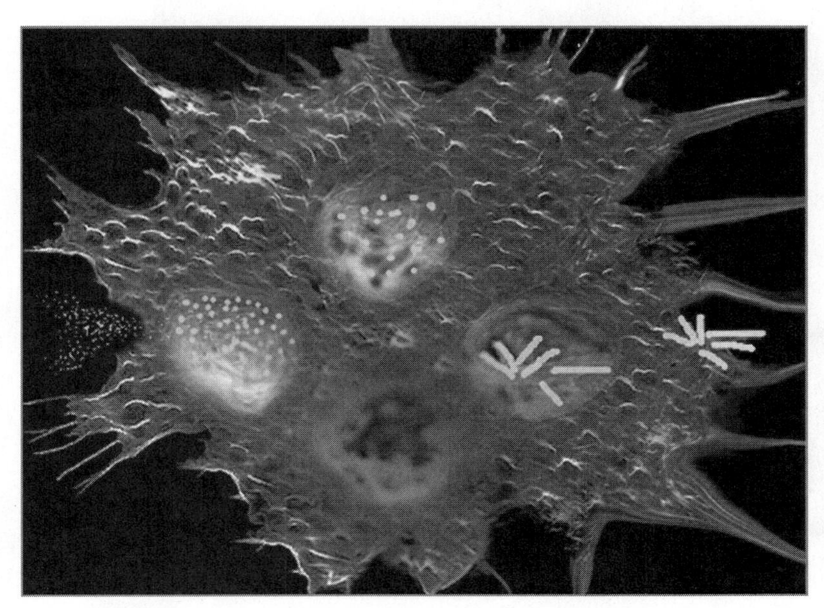

Electron micrograph type photo of a macrophage engulfing foreign organisms (yellow), ingesting them, and releasing the microscopic debris (yellow dust like particles).
Source: Courtesy of George Kyriakidis/Santa Ana, CA

What Is Sepsis? (continued)

As recognized by Dr. Thomas, the greater threat to survival is not the infection to be eradicated in severe sepsis; rather, it is the body's or host response to the infection. Of course, treating and eradicating the pathogens or source of the infection (such as an abscess or pneumonia) is important. However, it is also very important to address treatment of the systemic immune response to the infection.

The most important point in sepsis is to remember that an infection is at the center of sepsis development. Everyone with an infection should routinely be screened for sepsis.

Brown Recluse Bite Resulting in Sepsis

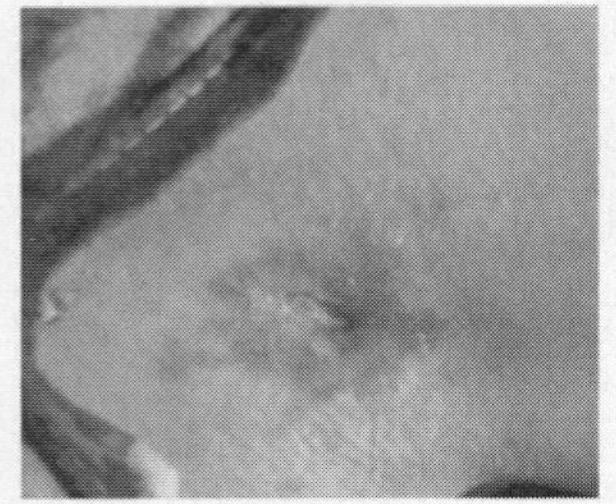

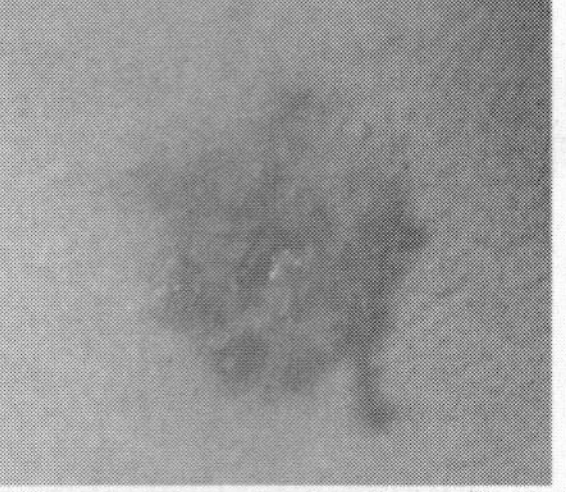

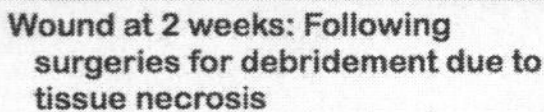

Wound at 2 weeks: Following surgeries for debridement due to tissue necrosis

Wound at 3 weeks: Healing well except for allergic skin reaction to topical antibiotic

A young woman was bitten by a brown recluse spider, which caused extensive tissue damage, necrosis, and sepsis due to infection. After several surgeries and hospitalization for 10 days, the patient recovered from sepsis and her wound eventually healed. Left: Photo taken 2 weeks post-recluse bite, after the surgeries when the deep wound is progressively healing. Right: Wound healing is almost complete at 3 weeks, except for antibiotic-induced inflammation.

Source: Copyright © 2013, NovEx Novice to Expert Learning, LLC

In Aimee's story, a relatively small injury from a home-made zipline became infected following the injury. She developed widespread tissue damage that required multiple surgeries. The damage eventually led to leg, foot, and bilateral hand amputations from necrotizing fasciitis (flesh-eating bacteria) and sepsis. This courageous, positive 24-year-old was determined to beat the odds.

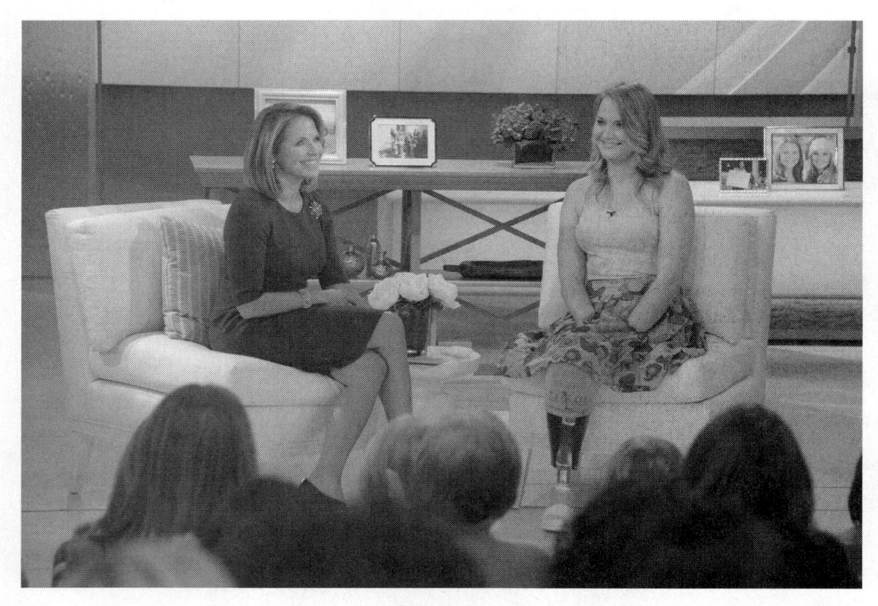

Aimee was interviewed by Katie Couric about her experience and energetic outlook. Her dad reports that the world-class medical care and compassion made survival possible.

Source: AP Photo/Disney-ABC Domestic Television/Ida Mae Astute

LO1:

Clinical Relevance

- The clinician's skill at recognizing sepsis in its early stages can make the difference in patient survival and level of suffering. Effective treatment of sepsis in its early stages improves survival rates and shortens hospitalizations.
- Hospital systems that recognize the importance of rapid identification of sepsis most often establish:
  - Education for nurses to recognize early warning signs of sepsis
  - Rapid response teams that are prepared to act quickly
  - ED and ICU protocols for treating sepsis at the earliest possible time
- Delayed identification, and therefore treatment, can negatively affect any organ. This delayed identification can result in progression of multiple organ dysfunction, often manifested by:
  - Respiratory failure
  - Cardiovascular hypotension
  - End-organ dysfunction (e.g., central nervous system or renal dysfunction) of any organ

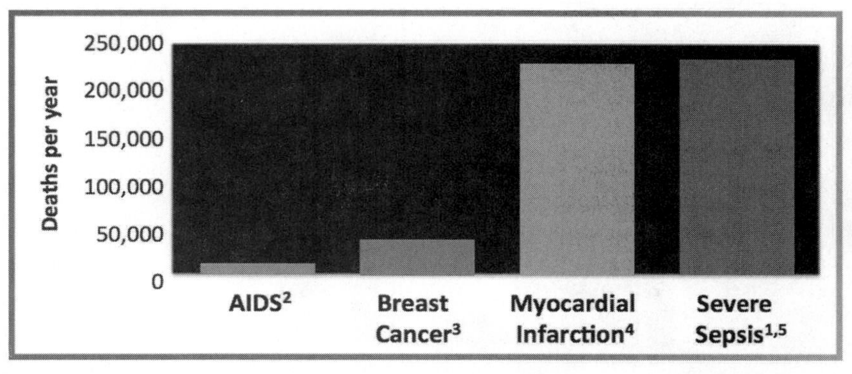

1. Dombrovskiy V. Y., et al. (2007). *Crit Care Med, 35*, 1414–1415
2. Centers for Disease Control and Prevention. (2010).
3. American Cancer Society. (2011).
4. American Heart Association. (2008).
5. National Center for Health Statistics. (2011).

Comparison of deaths from sepsis versus other leading causes.

- Sepsis is the leading cause of death in noncardiac ICUs. About 750,000 patients in the United States have severe sepsis each year, and 30–50% die (see graph).
- One of the challenges with sepsis is that clinicians often fail to identify it. For example, in causes of death, clinicians often attribute death to an infection, such as pneumonia, when sepsis is the actual cause of death.
- Patients aged 85 or older are 30 times more likely to be hospitalized from sepsis than patients under age 65.
- Sepsis diagnosis is too often delayed until near-shock state. This late diagnosis limits success in treatment.
- Due to the high frequency of sepsis, substantial effort by clinicians and hospitals are necessary to limit sepsis' impact.
- More patients die of severe sepsis annually than those from AIDS and breast cancer combined.
- Sepsis is currently the single most expensive condition treated in hospitals, costing more than $20 billion yearly in the United States alone.
- The increasing prevalence of multidrug-resistant organisms is contributing to the growing development of sepsis.

Concept Check

1. **What factor is present in all cases of sepsis?**
   A. Elevated body temperature
   B. Infection
   C. Decreased heart rate
   D. Pain

Answer question

LO2:

Pathophysiology

- Sepsis is not an infection, but rather the presence of an infection that triggers a complex, self-propagating immune system response to an infection.
- Every patient with an infection should be considered at risk for sepsis.
- Not all infections lead to sepsis, but each infection can lead to sepsis, particularly in patients with significant comorbid conditions.

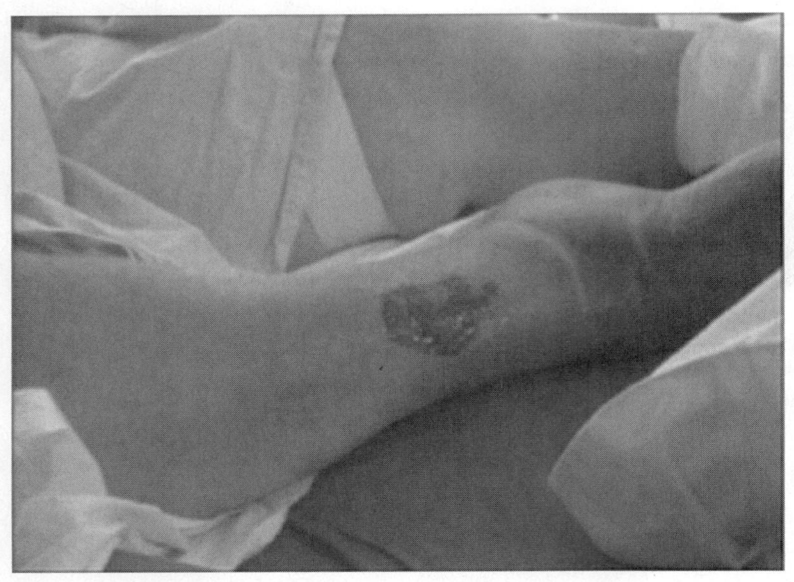

Unexpected infections such as this leg ulcer can lead to sepsis in vulnerable patients.
Source: Copyright © 2013, NovEx Novice to Expert Learning, LLC

A Body's Normal Response to Infection

When an infection invades the body, a normal immune response is initially activated. Macrophages recognize and extend their pseudopods (long thin arms) to grab infectious organisms (see photo on left). They then bind with the pathogens, pull them into the macrophage, and engulf microorganisms so that digestive enzymes destroy the pathogen (see animation on right). This normal process is called phagocytosis.

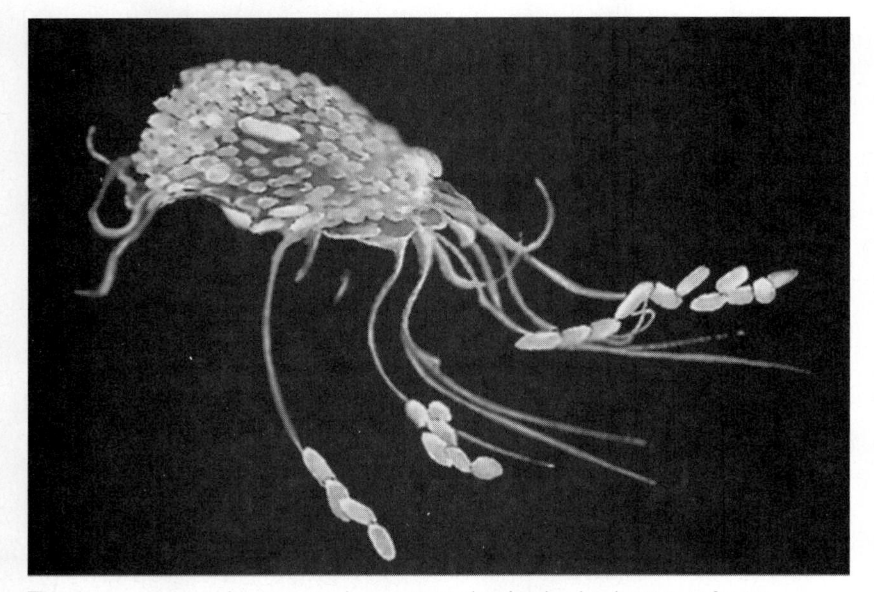

This electron micrograph type image shows a macrophage's role when bacteria or foreign organism is present. A macrophage (green) is extending its many long thin pseudopods (or arms) out to bind with multiple bacteria (beige rods), pull them in, engulf them, and lyse them. Note that some of the organisms are on the surface of the macrophage, ready to become engulfed.
Source: Courtesy of George Kyriakidis/Santa Ana, CA

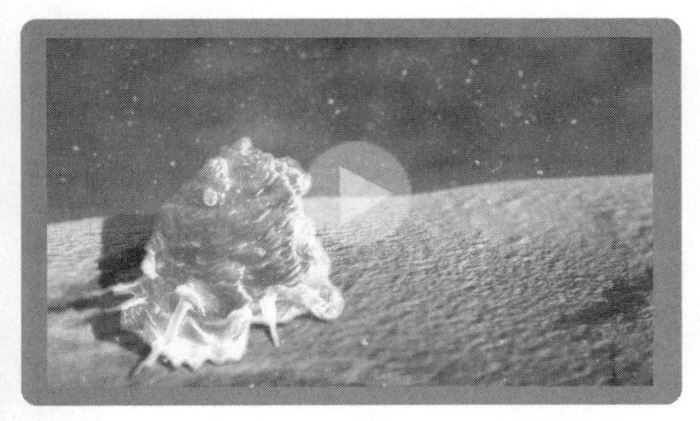

This animation shows a macrophage, a white blood cell, engulfing bacteria (green). Phagocytosis is a major mechanism by which the immune system normally removes pathogens and cell debris from the body.
Source: Polymime Animation Co./Science Photo Library/Science Source

- In addition to phagocytosis, the macrophages secrete pro-inflammatory and anti-inflammatory mediators that regulate and balance the immune response to the infection.
- Pro-inflammatory mediators signal the influx of more macrophages and strengthen the immune response whereas anti-inflammatory mediators suppress the immune response by inhibiting the production of cytokines.
- In a normal immune response, the anti-inflammatory mediators balance the pro-inflammatory ones to regulate the inflammatory response, restore homeostasis, and prevent the damaging evolution of sepsis.

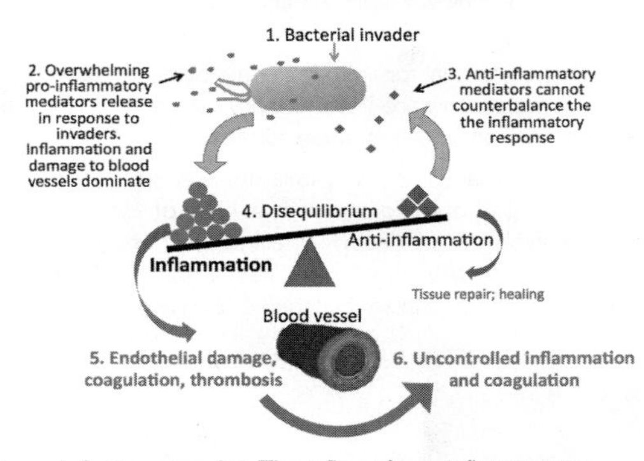
Normal Inflammatory Response: Balanced
1. Bacterial invader
2. Pro-inflammatory mediators are released in response to invaders, causing inflammation and death to the invader
3. Anti-inflammatory mediators are then released to counteract the inflammation
Inflammation
Anti-inflammation
4. Equilibrium
5. Endothelial damage
6. Tissue repair; healing
Inflammatory Response in Sepsis: Imbalanced
1. Bacterial invader
2. Overwhelming pro-inflammatory mediators release in response to invaders. Inflammation and damage to blood vessels dominate
3. Anti-inflammatory mediators cannot counterbalance the the inflammatory response
4. Disequilibrium
Anti-inflammation
Inflammation
Tissue repair; healing
Blood vessel
5. Endothelial damage, coagulation, thrombosis
6. Uncontrolled inflammation and coagulation

Left: This image depicts how the immune system normally responds to an infectious invader. The influx of pro-inflammatory mediators is balanced by the anti-inflammatory mediator response to create an equilibrium in the body. Endothelial damage caused by the pro-inflammatory mediators (e.g., cytokines) is repaired by the anti-inflammatory mediators. Right: This image indicates how sepsis develops following an infection. It demonstrates the pro- and anti-inflammatory imbalances that occur, the continued endothelial wall damage, and the negative cycle of coagulation leading to disseminated intravascular coagulation (DIC) throughout the body.
Source: *(both)* Copyright © 2013, NovEx Novice to Expert Learning, LLC

Pathophysiology (continued)

Early Development of Sepsis

- Many disturbances in homeostasis occur with sepsis. A key problem is the overproduction of pro-inflammatory cytokines.
- Evidence suggests that increased levels of pro-inflammatory cytokines occur that cause sepsis and are responsible for the organ damage sequelae in septic shock.
- Once the imbalance evolves, the patient's condition transitions from a normal and more localized immune response to the invading organism to a generalized or *systemic* inflammatory response syndrome (SIRS). SIRS is a syndrome that then has widespread, damaging effects on organs that were not involved in the initial or local infection.
- Several known problems occur with the pro-inflammatory over-response (imbalance and overproduction) that evolves into SIRS:
  1. Excessive microvascular coagulation, known as disseminated intravascular coagulation (DIC) (see photo)
  2. An impairment to fibrinolysis
  3. Altered endothelial function, including damage and increased permeability

An example of pro-inflammatory response is reduced tissue perfusion.

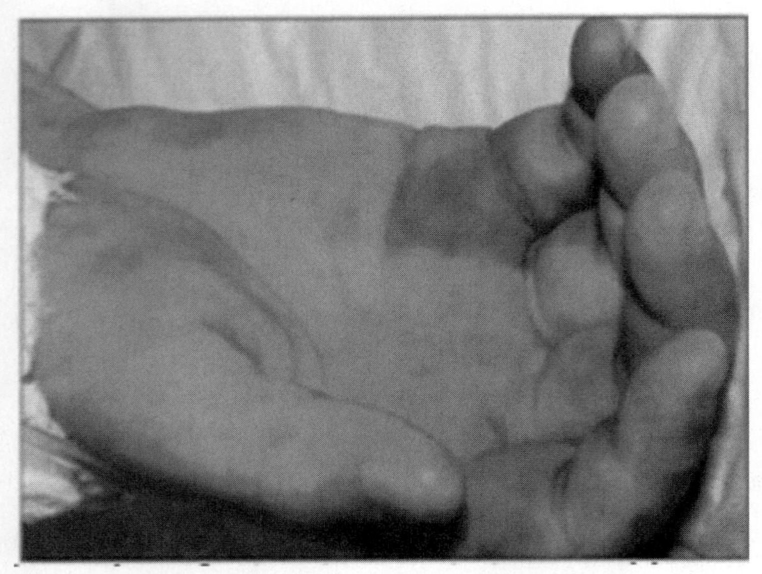

Altered perfusion in sepsis is noted by disseminated intravascular coagulation of the hand. The purplish areas reveal microvascular clotting.
Source: Copyright © 2013, NovEx Novice to Expert Learning, LLC

Conversely, anti-inflammatory response may cause the following:

1. Inhibition of the pro-inflammatory response and mediator production
2. Anergy (decreased oxygen utilization) and cell stunning, where the cells become dysfunctional but may not die
3. Apoptosis (preprogrammed cell death): This is essential for limiting the abnormal immune response as it does not further trigger or stimulate the pro-inflammatory response. It is a major mechanism to eliminate dysfunctional cells once inflammation subsides.
4. Repair of injured tissue: Healing effects that balance the pro-inflammatory response. However, sepsis is extremely complex in its pathophysiology with a host of cytokine release and feedback loops attempting to isolate and destroy the invader. When the local response fails and the systemic response (sepsis) occurs, the pathophysiologic response can become overwhelming and complex as excessive cytokine release becomes uncontrolled (see animation).

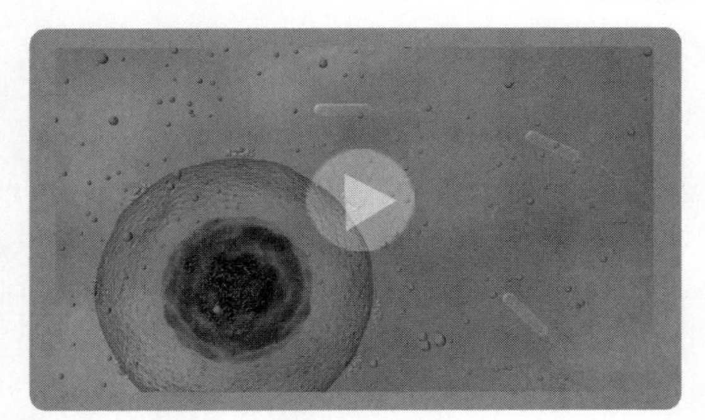

This animation shows the mechanism of the receptor immune response. White blood cells in blood bear toll-like receptors (green) on their surface, which detect a specific molecule (purple) on pathogenic bacterial (yellow) cell walls. When receptors bind to the molecule, the cell releases large amounts of cytokines (red). Cytokines then attract more macrophages. Macrophages are white blood cells that engulf and lyse pathogenic invaders. This process first helps prevent serious infection, but when excessive, begins to damage normal body tissues.
Source: Flix Productions Medical Animation/Science Photo Library/Science Source

- When macrophages release excessive pro-inflammatory cytokines that stimulate a continued immune response, the cytokines not only cause increased phagocytosis of the infecting organisms and the injured tissue debris, they also begin injuring cells in uninvolved multiple organs.
- This process sets up the uncontrolled and devastating cycle of continued injury.
- Sepsis is thus referred to as a malignant intravascular inflammation.
- Additionally, the toxins released from the invading organisms additively damage cells leading to the cycle in this schematic:

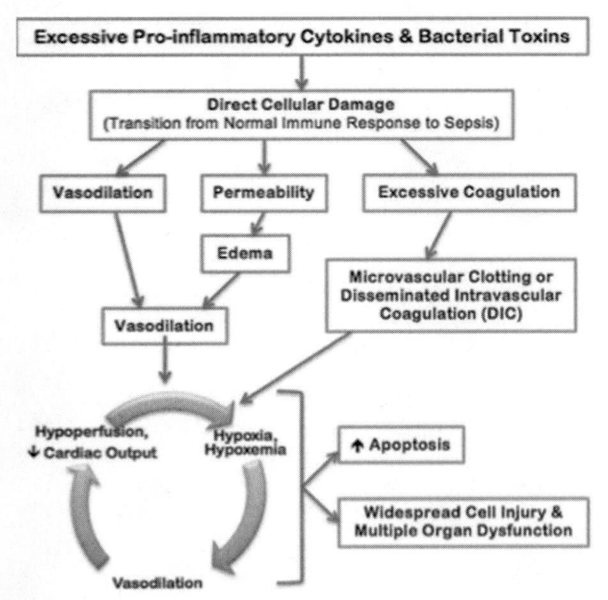

This schematic depicts pathophysiologic process that results in the feedback loop leading to the body's transition or deterioration into severe sepsis and septic shock.

Pathophysiology (continued)

Transition into Severe Sepsis and Septic Shock

If sepsis or the systemic inflammatory response goes untreated, or if the treatment used is unsuccessful, the potentially fatal pathophysiological sequelae intensify far beyond the site of the infection:

- Excessive endothelial damage, causing loss of autoregulation with systemic vasodilation, may not respond to therapy, such as vasopressors, leading to severe circulatory dysfunction and collapse (see illustration).
- Cardiac myocytes are directly damaged, leading to depressed myocardial function and reduced cardiac output.
- Hypotension may be unresponsive to fluid replacement.
- Increased capillary permeability may continue to cause excessive interstitial edema and greatly reduce vascular volume (further hindering cardiac output and blood flow). Edema affects all organs, causing complications such as pulmonary edema with consequent hypoxemia, renal failure, etc.
- Excessive microcirculatory clotting may cause widespread lack of microcirculatory blood flow.
- Reduced oxygen extraction from the blood by the tissues (tissue hypoxia) may cause multi-organ damage.

Progressive Vasodilation to Vascular Collapse: Mechanism of Shock

1. In this normal arteriole, a constant blood volume and flow sustain a constant blood pressure (BP).

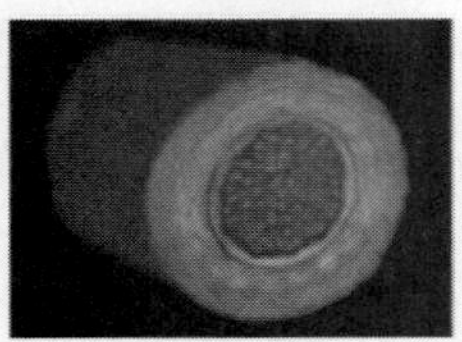

2. Early vasodilation occurs due to toxins that damage vessels. Lumen widens as the wall thins. Without increased volume, BP begins to drop.

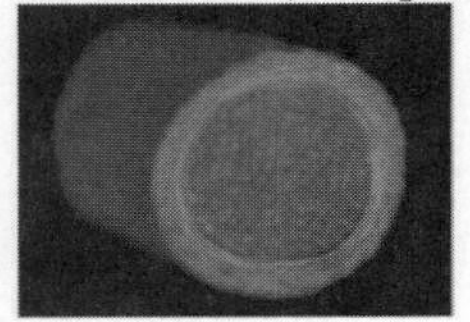

Note the changing vessel (1-4) diameter and muscle thinning as it expands. Blood flow gradually slows, becomes sluggish, and disseminated intravascular coagulation (microcoagulation) results.

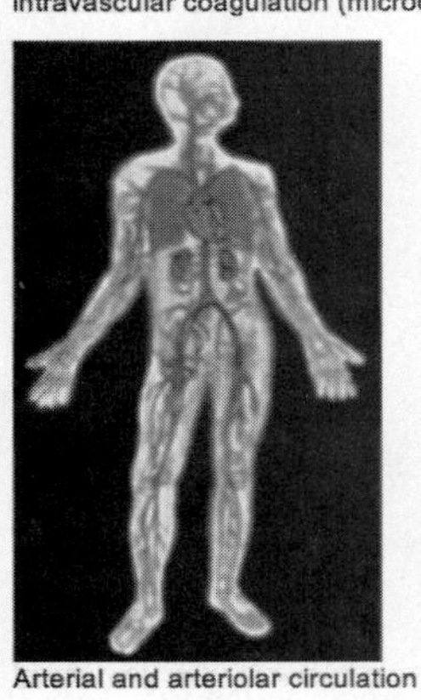

Arterial and arteriolar circulation

3. Worsening sepsis causes extreme vasodilation with a severe drop in BP, perfusion, and oxygenation.

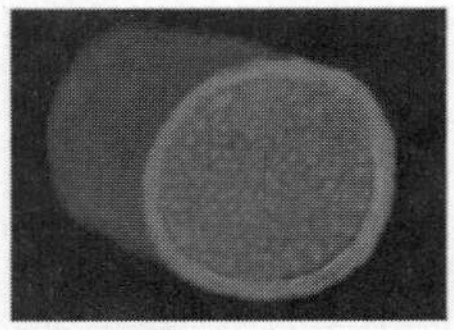

4. As septic shock ensues, vascular collapse and blood clotting result.

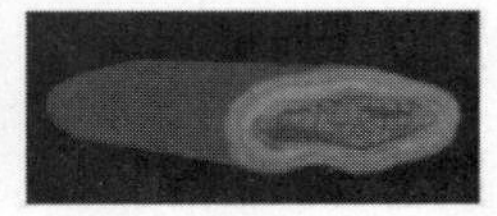

This picture illustrates the process of vasodilation and subsequent shock.

Source: Courtesy of George Kyriakidis/Santa Ana, CA

These sequelae of the systemic inflammatory response, manifested as organ dysfunction, hypotension, and/or poor tissue perfusion, signal the development of or transition into **severe sepsis**. If the hypotension persists after adequate fluid resuscitation, the patient is understood to be in **septic shock**. Clinically this distinction is not necessarily easy to recognize. There is a change in sepsis' clinical presentation.

The early phase of sepsis is characterized by hypodynamic hemodynamics:

1. Low Cardiac Index: normal is 2.5–4.0 $L/min/m^2$
2. Low Stroke Index: normal is 33–47 $mL/m^2/beat$
3. Low $ScvO_2$ levels: normal is greater than 70%

However, if treatment is delayed, sepsis can change to a more resistant, hyperdynamic phase:

1. High Cardiac index
2. High Stroke index
3. High $ScvO_2$ levels
    - The hyperdynamic response is called "warm shock" because a patient's skin can feel warm. Warm shock is often more resistant to treatment.
    - Understanding the pathophysiology of sepsis and septic shock explains why the mortality rate is so high.

Concept Check

2. **Which condition suppresses the immune system?**
    A. Release of pro-inflammatory mediators
    B. Increased production of cytokines
    C. Increased anti-inflammatory mediator
    D. Impairment of fibrinolysis

Answer question

Concept Check

3. Why is sepsis sometimes referred to as malignant intravascular inflammation?

A. It only affects the intravascular tissues.
B. It results in a cycle of continued injury.
C. It occurs primarily in patients with cancer.
D. It results in unregulated apoptosis.

Answer question

Causes and Risk Factors

- An infection is always the trigger that initiates the inflammatory response of sepsis.
- SIRS is a set of symptoms resulting from a severe systemic inflammatory response that may have other causes, such as burns, pancreatitis, autoimmune disorders.
- There are some general factors that may predispose patients to sepsis:
  - o Age (very young and older adults)
  - o Immunosuppresssion
  - o Prior, recent antibiotic use
  - o Chronic diseases
  - o Presence of central lines, urinary catheters, and intubation
  - o Recent severe injury, prolonged ICU care, and ventilator-related pneumonia
  - o Substance abuse and/or malnutrition

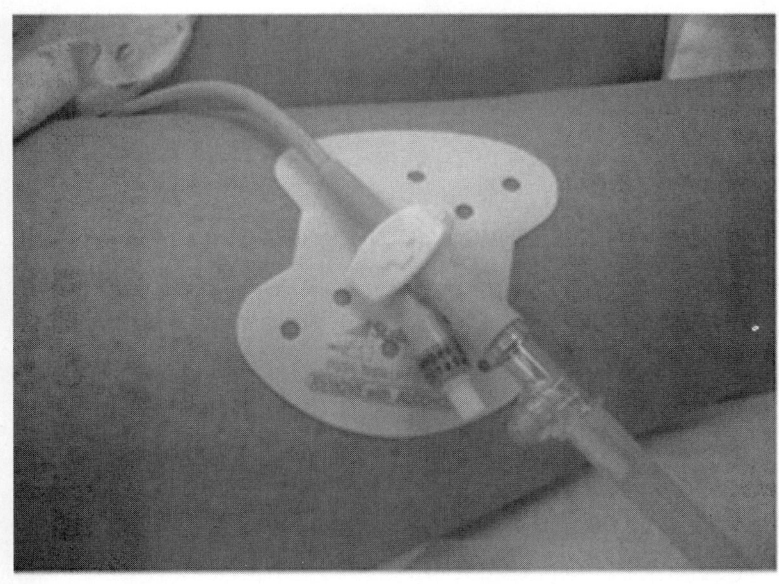

Indwelling catheters are a primary source for culprit pathogen growth and sepsis.
Source: Copyright © 2013, NovEx Novice to Expert Learning, LLC

Concept Check

4. Which patient is at greatest risk for developing sepsis?

A. 34-year-old who is pregnant
B. 2-month-old with pneumonia
C. 50-year-old with dehydration
D. 64-year-old who smokes two packs of cigarettes a day

Answer question

- Certain infections, such as meningococcal meningitis, are more likely to develop into sepsis than other infections such as cellulitis.
- Sudden onset of infection and rapid development of sepsis suggests a worse outcome.

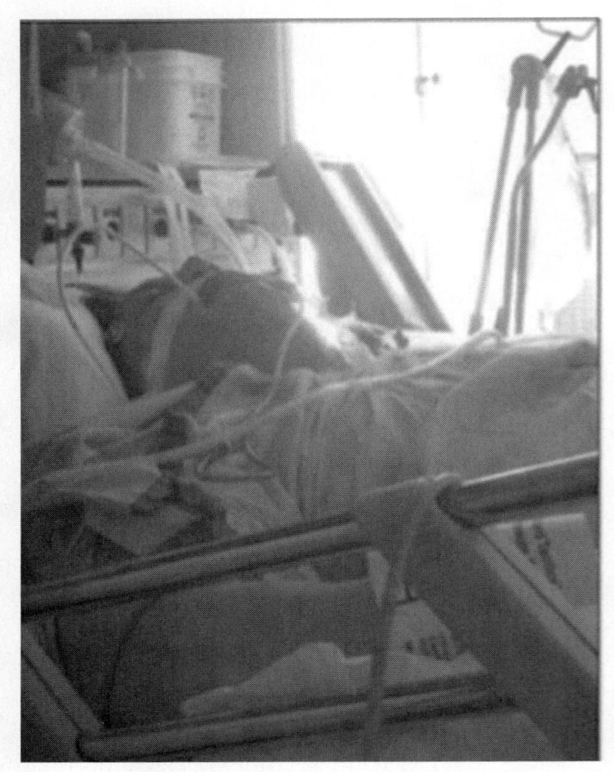

Patients on mechanical ventilation are at higher risk for ventilator-associated pneumonia and sepsis.

Assessment Findings

The Surviving Sepsis Campaign gives clear guidelines that can be followed by all clinicians to identify and diagnose sepsis. Sepsis is identified when the following are present:

1. Patient has, or is suspected of having, an infection.
2. Patient has two or more signs of SIRS. The SIRS criteria are:
    - o Core temperature >100.4°F or <96.8°F (>38°C or <36°C)
    - o Tachycardia (>90 bpm)
    - o Tachypnea (>20 breaths/min)
    - o WBC count >12,000/mm^3 or <4,000/mm^3 or >10% immature neutrophil

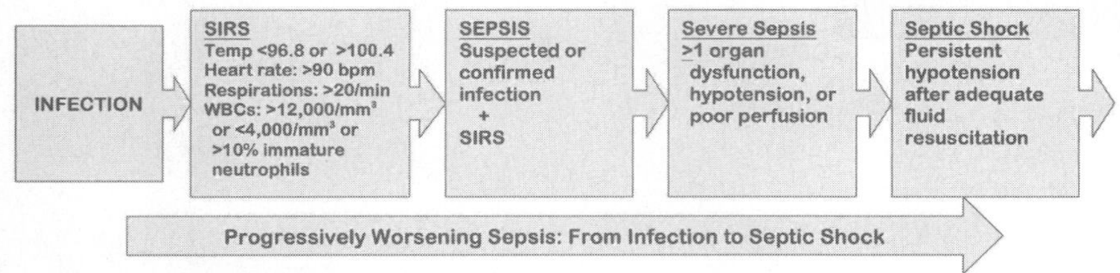

Comparison of stages in sepsis development.

- If signs of SIRS are present, obtain a blood lactate level to assess for tissue hypoxia. Normal lactate levels are 1–2 mmol.
- Severe sepsis is recognized when SIRS symptoms are present, but one or more organs are also showing signs of dysfunction (e.g. hypoxemia in a patient without a pulmonary infection).
- Septic shock occurs when the patient has sepsis, which is accompanied by hypotensive (mean arterial pressure [MAP] <65 mmHg) or the lactate is >4 mmol/L.

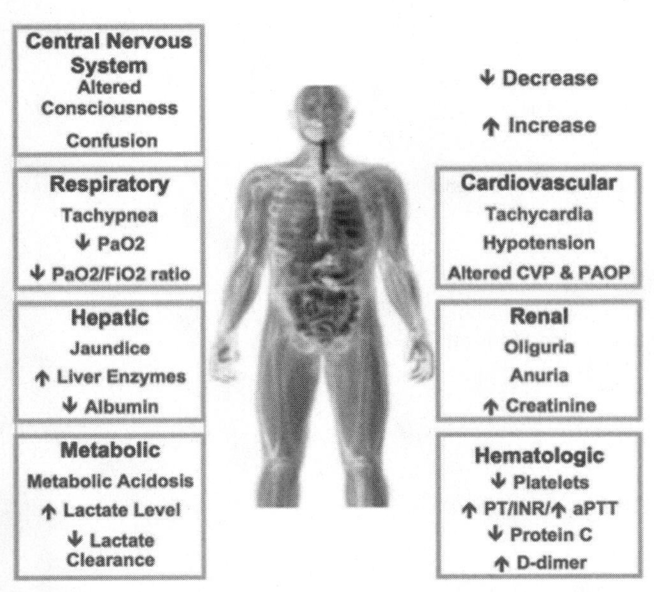

When sepsis evolves, most body systems are affected or potentially damaged, as seen in the diagram.

Source: Copyright © 2013, NovEx Novice to Expert Learning, LLC

Diagnostics

SIRS and Sepsis

- Sepsis is diagnosed using clinical signs (i.e., if the patient has a real or suspected infection) and two or more signs of SIRS.
- The site of a known infection may provide important clues about the infecting organism.
- The source and type of infection may be suggested by risk factors (e.g., the presence of an arterial line predisposes to sepsis with *Staphylococcus aureus*).
- Blood cultures (and sputum when indicated) are the best way to identify the infectious agents.
- Any necessary radiology or ultrasound imaging should be done promptly in order to confirm and sample any source of infection if safe to do so.

Priority Patient Concerns and Desired Collaborative Care Outcomes

Prior to caring for patients with sepsis, it is important to prioritize the patient's concerns that must guide the nursing care plan and interventions. Care for the patient is ordered and organized in accordance with the patient's priority and urgent needs. Desired collaborative care outcomes in patients with sepsis typically include:

1. Patient will not develop or will recover from end-organ damage.
2. Patient will not develop or will sufficiently recover from shock.
3. Patient's skin will remain intact or progressively heal with improved oxygenation.
4. Patient's temperature will return to normal following effective treatment of infection.
5. Patient will be normovolemic or return to normal fluid balance with effective fluid resuscitation.
6. Patient will express less anxiety when conscious or experience quiet, restful periods and constant, caring reassurance when noncommunicative.

Considering these important care outcomes, prepare a list of the major 3–6 priority patient concerns or nursing diagnoses for patients with sepsis. Be prepared to participate in a discussion of this list and/or to submit them as an assignment, as determined by your faculty. Resources you may find helpful in this assignment can include this lesson, the references, resources on nursing care plans, and standard nursing diagnoses manuals.

LO3:

Collaborative Interventions

Due to our limited understanding of sepsis' root causes, there is difficulty in treating sepsis. However, sepsis recognition in order to begin early treatment is a major responsibility of all nurses.

Best Sepsis Treatment Is to Avoid Infections

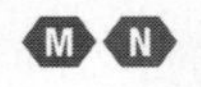

Basics in the prevention of infections should be meticulously followed, including but not limited to:

- Good handwashing
- Isolation of patients with contagious diseases
- Protocols to avoid preventable nosocomial infections (or Never Events) are needed (recommeded by the Surviving Sepsis Campaign and the Institute for Healthcare Improvement) and should minimally include:
    - o Bloodstream infections
    - o Ventilator-associated pneumonia: oral chlorhexidine gluconate (2B)
    - o Surgical site infection
    - o Urinary catheter infections
    - o Pressure ulcers
    - o Deep vein thrombosis
- Removal of lines, catheters, endotracheal tube, and other invasive therapies as soon as they are not necessary

These guidelines should be high priorities in hospital quality initiatives, as they will reduce the incidence of sepsis and better protect patients.

Evidence-Based Practices

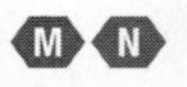

- The best in-depth evidence-based practice guide for treating sepsis is from the Surviving Sepsis Campaign (SSC). The following guidelines are from the Surviving Sepsis Campaign Pocket Guide.
- Visit their web site at www.survivingsepsis.org for more information about sepsis management.
- The SSC has graded the treatments according to the strength of the research. Strength of recommendation and quality of evidence have been assessed using the GRADE criteria presented in brackets after each guideline.
- For added clarity:
    - o 1A, 1B, and 1C: Indicate a strong recommendation or "we recommend"
    - o 2A, 2B, and 2C: Indicate a weak recommendation or "we suggest"

Patient and Family Communication; Honoring Treatment Preferences

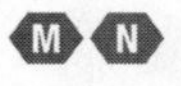

- Before administering treatment to a patient with sepsis, understanding the patient's treatment preferences is necessary. Discuss treatment options, prognosis, and goals with patients and family. (1B)

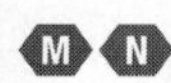

- Honoring patient's wishes for treatment is a core concept for all clinicians. Talking with patients and families prevents ethical dilemmas later during hospitalizations. If patients opt for comfort care versus curative care, treatment plans may be substantially altered. Any treatment can be withheld or stopped if it is in accordance with the patient's wishes. (1B)

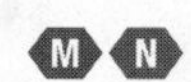

- The patient's wishes should be formally documented as the advanced directives, placed in the patient's chart, and shared with the health care team.

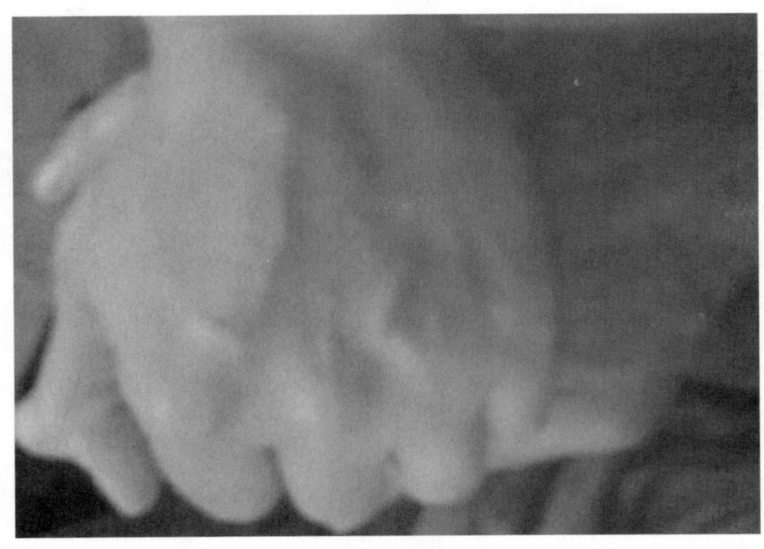

End-of-life decisions are difficult for both families and clinician. Compassion and caring are important ways of supporting families through decisions.
Source: Courtesy of Sarah S. Dresen

Collaborative Interventions (continued)

Brief Overview of the Key Treatments

The following information regarding treatment reviews the detailed guidelines from the SSC. This quick summary of treatment for sepsis is essential for nurses to know:

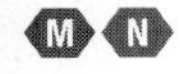

1. To identify the infectious agent causing sepsis, obtaining blood, sputum, or other cultures before starting antibiotics is critical, provided this does not significantly delay starting antibiotics. The SSC also suggest the following regarding blood cultures:
   - Obtain blood cultures ASAP on any patient with sepsis.
   - Obtain two or more blood cultures (BCs).
   - One or more BCs should be percutaneous.
   - One BC from each vascular access device in place >48 hours.
   - Culture other sites as clinically indicated.

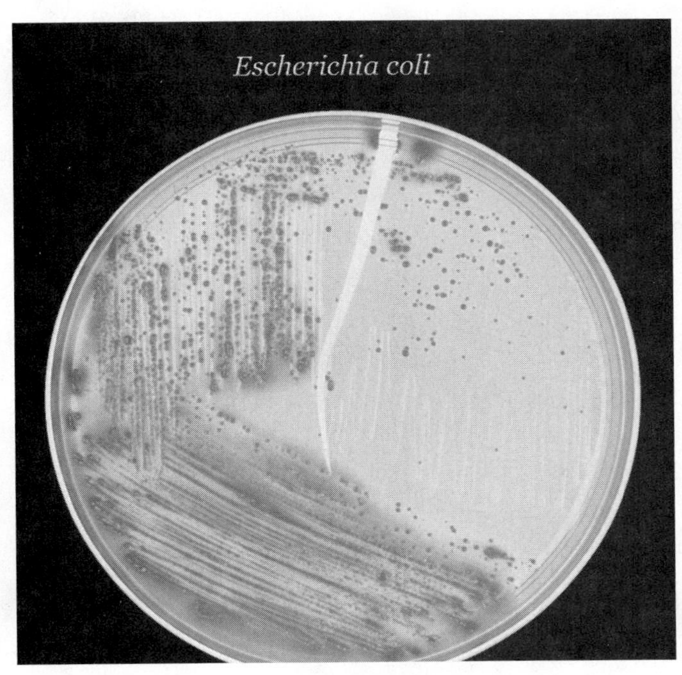

This is a photo of a culture growing *E. coli* bacteria, a common infectious culprit.
Source: CDC

Concept Check

5. Which criterion determines the need for a culture of a vascular access device in a patient with sepsis?

A. Age of the patient

B. Credentials of the person placing the device

C. Length of time the device has been in place

D. Area of the body in which the device is placed

Answer question

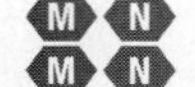

2. Obtain lactate levels on any patient with sepsis.

3. Begin broad spectrum antibiotic therapy immediately.

4. If hemodynamically unstable (e.g., mean arterial pressure <65 mmHg), give 20–30 mL/kg of fluid (e.g., normal saline) until hemodynamics are stabilized.

5. If fluids do not produce hemodynamic stability, administer a vasopressor (e.g., norepinephrine), and as needed, an inotrope.

6. If fluids and vasopressors do not produce hemodynamic stabilization, start steroid therapy.

7. Keep blood glucose levels <180 mg/dL, but >90 mg/dL.

Collaborative Interventions (continued)

Specific Treatment

A detailed description of the Surviving Sepsis Guidelines follows to provide the necessary understanding for clinical reasoning and judgment in the care of the septic patient and those in septic shock. Specific interventions include:

- Initial resuscitation (first 6 hours)
- Antibiotic (antimicrobial) therapy
- Infection source identification and control
- Fluid therapy
- Vasopressors and inotropes
- Low-dose steroids
- Glucose control

Initial Resuscitation (First 6 Hours)

Begin resuscitation immediately in patients with hypotension or elevated serum lactate greater than or equal to 4 mmol/L. Do not delay obtaining the lactate level awaiting ICU admission. (1C)

- Treatment goals within the first 6 hours include (1C):
  - o Central venous pressure: 8–12 mmHG
  - o Mean arterial pressure (MAP): greater than or equal to 65 mmHg
  - o Urine output: greater than or equal to 0.5 mL/kg/hr
  - o Scv02: greater than or equal to 70%

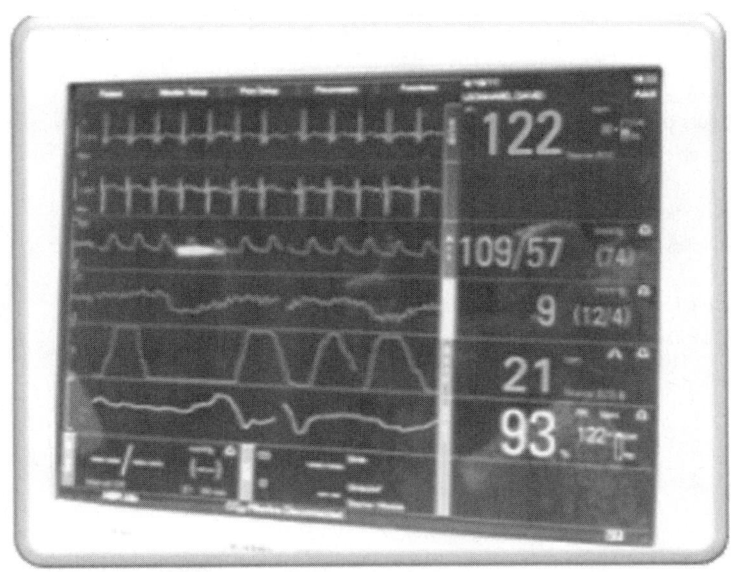

Vital signs require continuous monitoring. Transfer to ICU is common.
Source: Copyright © 2013, NovEx Novice to Expert Learning, LLC

M N Antibiotic (Antimicrobial) Therapy

- Begin intravenous antibiotics as early as possible, and always within the first hour of recognizing severe sepsis (1C) and septic shock. (1B)
- Broad-spectrum: one or more agents active against likely bacterial, fungal, or viral pathogens and with good penetration into presumed source. (1B)
- Reassess antimicrobial regimen daily to optimize efficacy, prevent resistance, avoid toxicity, and minimize costs. (1B)
- Low procalcitonin levels or similar biomarkers can be used to help guide the clinician's judgment about discontinuing empiric antibiotics in those who appeared septic with no subsequent evidence of infection. (2C)
- Combination therapy (when used empirically) for no more than 3–5 days. De-escalation to the single most appropriate therapy when organism susceptibility is known. (2B)
- Duration of (combination and/or single) therapy typically limited to 7–10 days; longer if response is slow, undrainable foci of infection, immunologic deficiencies (including neutropenia), S. aureus bacteremia, or some fungal/viral infections. (2C)
- Antiviral therapy is started immediately in patients with severe sepsis or shock of viral origin. (2C)
- Stop antimicrobial therapy if cause is found to be noninfectious. (UG)

Concept Check

6. What is the maximum length of time a patient with sepsis should be empirically receiving two different antibiotics?

A. 2 days
B. 5 days
C. 7 days
D. 10 days

Answer question

Collaborative Interventions (continued)

M N **Source Identification and Control**

- A specific anatomic site of infection should be established as rapidly as possible and intervention started for source control within the first 12 hours of diagnosis. (1C)
- Formally evaluate patient for a focus of infection amenable to source control measures (e.g., abscess drainage, tissue debridement). (1C)
- Use the most effective intervention with the least physiologic insult possible.
- Implement source control measures as soon as possible following successful initial resuscitation. (1C)
  - o Exception: infected pancreatic necrosis, where surgical intervention is best delayed. (2B)
- Remove intravascular access device promptly if potentially infected. (1C)

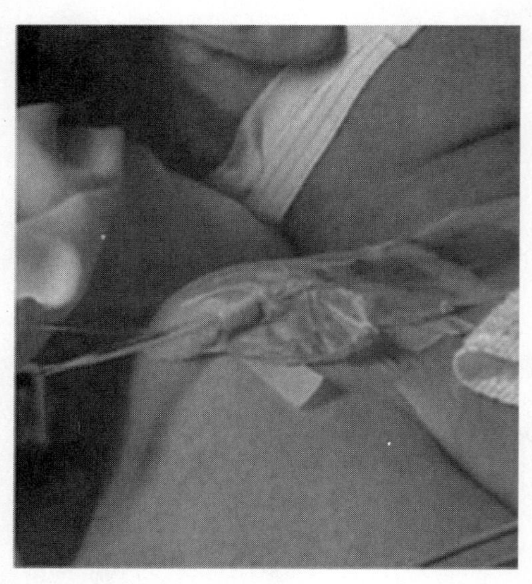

Central lines should be an immediate concern as a probable source.
Source: Copyright © 2013, NovEx Novice to Expert Learning, LLC

M N **Fluid Resuscitation Therapy**

- Fluid-resuscitate using crystalloids in initial resuscitation of severe sepsis (1B) and adding colloids, as needed. (2C)
- Goal is to keep the mean arterial pressure (MAP) >65 mmHg.
- If a central line is present, target a CVP of greater than or equal to 8 mmHg (greater than or equal to 12 mmHg if mechanically ventilated). (1C)
- Give fluid challenges of 1000 mL of crystalloids or 300–500 mL of colloids over 30 minutes with a minimum of 30 mL/kg within the first 4–6 hours. More rapid and larger volumes may be required in sepsis-induced tissue hypoperfusion. (1C)
- Rate of fluid administration should be reduced if cardiac filling pressures increase without concurrent hemodynamic improvement. (1D)
- Hydroxyethyl starches are not recommended for use in fluid resuscitation of severe sepsis or shock. (1B)

M N Vasopressors and Inotropic Therapy

Surviving Sepsis Campaign Updated Guidelines for 2012—Vasopressors:

- If fluids do not raise the MAP, vasopressors can be used to maintain MAP greater than or equal to 65 mmHg. (1C)
- Norepinephrine (NE) was strongly recommended as the first choice of vasopressors (1B). Vasopressin infused at 0.03 units/min can be added concomitant to NE to either raise MAP or lower NE. (2A)
- Use epinephrine as the first alternative agent in septic shock when blood pressure is poorly responsive to norepinephrine or added as a second vasopressor to support MAP. (2B)
- Dopamine centrally administered was also suggested as an alternative vasopressor but primarily in selected patients with low stroke volume and relatively low heart rate *who were not at high risk for dysrhythmias*. (2C)
- Phenylephrine should not be used to treat septic shock except when: (1) NE causes serious dysrhythmias, (2) high cardiac output with persistently low BP, and (3) salvage therapy is needed after inotrope/vasopressor drugs combined with low dose vasopressin therapy fail to maintain MAP >65 mmHg. (1C)
- Do not use low-dose dopamine for renal protection. (1A)
- In patients requiring vasopressors, insert an arterial catheter as soon as practical. (1D)

Surviving Sepsis Campaign Updated Guidelines for 2012—Inotropes:

- A trial of dobutamine is recommended, infused up to 20 mcg/kg/min, alone or concomitant with a vasopressor when:
    1. Myocardial dysfunction occurs with elevated cardiac filling pressures and low stroke volume or cardiac output.
    2. Poor myocardial function causes persistent hypoperfusion after adequate intravascular volume is achieved and MAP is >65 mmHg. (1C)
- Do not recommend attempting to increase cardiac index to supranormal levels. (1B)

M N Low-Dose Steroids

- Avoid hydrocortisone use in septic shock patients if fluid resuscitation and vasopressor therapy restore hemodynamic stability. (2C)
- Consider intravenous hydrocortisone for adult septic shock when hypotension responds poorly to adequate fluid resuscitation and vasopressors. (2C)
- Hydrocortisone dose should be 200 mg/day. (2C)
- Corticosteroids should not be used to treat sepsis in the absence of shock. (1D)

Collaborative Interventions (continued)

Glucose Control

- There is insufficient information from randomized controlled trials to determine the optimal target range of blood glucose in the severely septic patient. The NICE-SUGAR trial is the largest most, compelling study to date on glucose control in ICU patients, given its inclusion of multiple ICUs and hospitals, and a more general patient population.
- M N Based on the results of this trial, we recommend against intravenous insulin therapy titrated to keep blood glucose in the normal range (80–110 mg/dL) in patients with severe sepsis. It is clear that attempts to normalize blood glucose with IV insulin during critical illness results in higher rates of hypoglycemia. Until additional information is available, teams seeking to implement glucose control should:
    - o Consider initiating insulin therapy when two consecutive blood glucose levels exceed 180 mg/dL with a goal blood glucose <180 mg/dL. (1A)
    - o Use IV insulin to control hyperglycemia in patients with severe sepsis following stabilization in the ICU. (1B)
    - o Provide a glucose calorie source and monitor blood glucose values every 1–2 hours (4 hours when stable) in patients receiving intravenous insulin. (1C)

M N *Insulin Dose in Glucose Control (GC)*

- One common dose for insulin is 0.04 units/kg.
- Before glucose and insulin values stabilize, monitor blood glucose values every 1–2 hours; monitor every 4 hours once stable. (1C)
- Point of care measurement of blood glucose levels, via capillary blood samples, may overestimate blood glucose levels.
- Other methods to monitor glucose and initiate insulin exist. The following is an example from one hospital of a standard dosing protocol based on insulin level.

Blood Glucose Level	130-170 mg/dl	171-220 mg/dl	221-279 mg/dl	280-239 mg/dl	330-379 mg/dl	380-430 mg/dl	>430 mg/dl
Dose of Insulin	No IVP infusion @ 1 unit/hr	Give 2 units IVP infusion @ 1 unit/hr	Give 4 units IVP infusion @ 2 unit/hr	Give 6 units IVP infusion @ 2 unit/hr	Give 8 units IVP infusion @ 2 unit/hr	Give 10 units IVP infusion @ 2 unit/hr	Call MD for orders
References: Taylor, BE, Schallom, ME, Sona, CS, et. al., (2006). Efficacy and safety of an insulin protocol in a surgical ICU. J AM Coll Surg, 202(1): 1-9.							

Parameters for insulin in glucose control.

Concept Check

7. Which intervention should be part of the care of a patient in septic shock?
   A. Fluids to keep MAP below 65 mmHg
   B. High-dose steroid therapy
   C. Administration of vasopressor agents
   D. Insulin administration to keep blood glucose under 125 mg/dL

Answer question

M N ***Titration of Insulin***

Example of glucose control guideline:

Blood Glucose (BG)	If blood glucose is decreasing	If blood glucose is increasing
< 60 mg/dl	Discontinue Insulin infusion. Give 25 ml D50% IV push immediately. Check BG in 15 minutes. If BG remains <60 mg/dl, repeat D50% 25 ml. Notify physician.	
60-90 mg/dl	Stop insulin infusion	Continue to hold infusion.

Titration of insulin infusions.

M N ***Verifying Glucose Control Success or Failure***

- Blood glucose should stabilize between 180 and 90 mg/dL.
- Generally, by normalizing blood glucose levels the patient will not show any signs of immediate improvement in their septic condition.

N ***Glucose Control and Hypoglycemia***

- Hypoglycemia is the most serious potential side effect of glucose control.
- Symptoms of hypoglycemia manifest when blood glucose levels fall below 60 mg/dL, including:
  - Changes in behavior
  - Decreased consciousness
  - Coma and death with level below 30 mg/dL
- Avoid hypoglycemia with frequent blood glucose monitoring. Hourly monitoring may be needed when glucose falls dangerously low.

Summary of Interventions

- Sepsis is the leading cause of death in noncardiac ICUs and is one of the leading causes of death in the world. Early recognition and treatment are essential to prevent poor outcomes.
- Evidence-based treatment guidelines are provided by the Surviving Sepsis Campaign (www.survivingsepsis.org). The best way to treat sepsis is to prevent infection. However, if sepsis is present, the evidence-based treatments are:
  - o Measure serum lactate.
  - o Obtain blood cultures prior to antibiotic administration.
  - o Administer broad-spectrum antibiotics.
  - o Treat hypotension and/or elevated lactate with fluids.
  - o Use vasopressors for persistent hypotension.
  - o Administer low-dose steroids if hemodynamic instability persists.
  - o Maintain adequate glycemic control.
- This schematic provides an abbreviated summary of the major nursing and medical interventions for patients who develop sepsis and/or septic shock.
- Advanced directives are important in guiding interventions and should be discussed as early as possible.

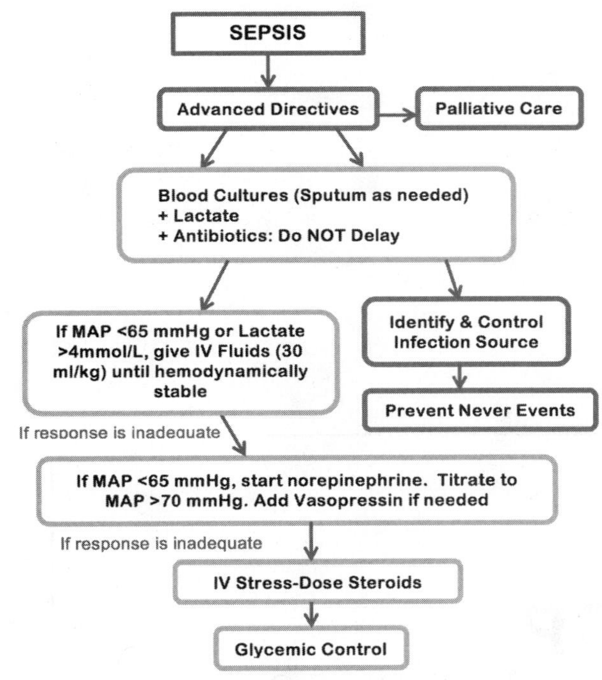

Summary of interventions for sepsis.

LO4:

Evaluation of Desired Collaborative Care Outcomes

Evaluation and reassessment should reveal attainment of previously established patient outcomes. In summary:

- Patient is awake and alert, normotensive, has adequate urine output or renal supportive treatment, and minimal to no other findings associated with untreated end-organ damage upon discharge.
- Patient has avoided or sufficiently recovered from the shock state.
- Patient's skin is warm, dry, and intact or has sufficiently healed to warrant home care upon discharge.
- Patient's temperature is normal.
- Patient's fluid intake is balanced with urine output or with kidney injury treatments.
- Patient calmly discusses illness and treatment plans upon discharge.

References

Ahrens, T., & Tuggle, D. (2004). Surviving severe sepsis: Early recognition and treatment. *Critical Care Nurse, Suppl*, 2–15.

Angus, D. C. & van der Poll, T. (2013). Severe sepsis and septic shock. *N Engl J Med. 369*, 840–851. doi: 10.1056/NEJMra1208623.

Cohen, J., Cristofaro, P., Carlet, J., & Opal, S. (2004). New method of classifying infections in critically ill patients. *Crit Care Med, 32*(7), 1510–1526.

Hoesel, L. M., Gao, H., & Ward, P. A. (2006). New insights into cellular mechanisms during sepsis. *Immunol Res, 34*(2), 133–141.

Hotchkiss, R. S., & Karl, I. E. (2003). The pathophysiology and treatment of sepsis. *N Engl J Med, 348*, 138–150.

Clinical Practice Guidelines

Update: **http://www.survivingsepsis.org/guidelines/Pages/default.aspx**

http://pulmccm.org/main/2012/critical-care-review/surviving-sepsis-guidelines-updated-at-sccm-meeting/

Dellinger, R. P., Levy, M. M., Carlet, J. M., et al. (2008). Surviving sepsis campaign: International guidelines for management of severe sepsis and septic shock. *Crit Care Med, 36*(1), 296–327.

SCCM/ESICM/ACCP/ATS/SIS International Sepsis Definitions Conference. (2003). *Crit Care Med, 31*, 1250–1256.

Vincent, J. L., Habib, A. M., Verdant, C., & Bruhn, A. (2006). Sepsis diagnosis and management: Work in progress. *Minerva Anestesiol, 72*(3), 87–96.

Patient Education

Sepsis Alliance. (2015). Patient education information. **www.sepsisalliance.org/medical_professionals/nurses/patient_ed/**

http://www.mayoclinic.com/health/sepsis/DS01004

http://emedicine.medscape.com/article/168689-overview

STOP

Go to the online course and complete the NovE-Cases assigned by your instructor for this module.

Learning Outcomes for Fluid and Electrolyte Disturbances

When you complete this lesson, you will be able to:

1. Recognize the clinical relevance of fluid and electrolyte disturbances.
2. Consider the pathophysiology, etiology, risk factors, and clinical presentation of fluid and electrolyte disturbances that determine the priority patient concerns.
3. Determine the most urgent and important nursing interventions and patient education required in caring for a patient with fluid and electrolyte disturbances.
4. Evaluate attainment of desired collaborative care outcomes for a patient with fluid and electrolyte disturbances.

LO1:

What Are Body Fluids?

- Fluids in the body are made up primarily of water (approximately 60% water).
- Bodily fluids are distributed where about 67% is in the intracellular space and around 8% is in the intravascular space or bloodstream.
- Homeostasis requires that the amount of water intake equals the water loss (e.g., excretion, sweat).
- When water loss exceeds fluid intake, dehydration or volume depletion occurs.
- When water intake exceeds water loss, overhydration or volume overload occurs.

LO1:

Clinical Relevance: Fluids

- Many complications including patient mortality are linked to fluid and electrolyte abnormalities.
- Dehydration is one of the top diagnoses in hospital admissions among older adults.
- IV fluids can be either crystalloids or colloids.
- Electrolytes are electrically charged elements.
- Fluid and electrolytes are closely associated and work together to achieve homeostasis in the body.

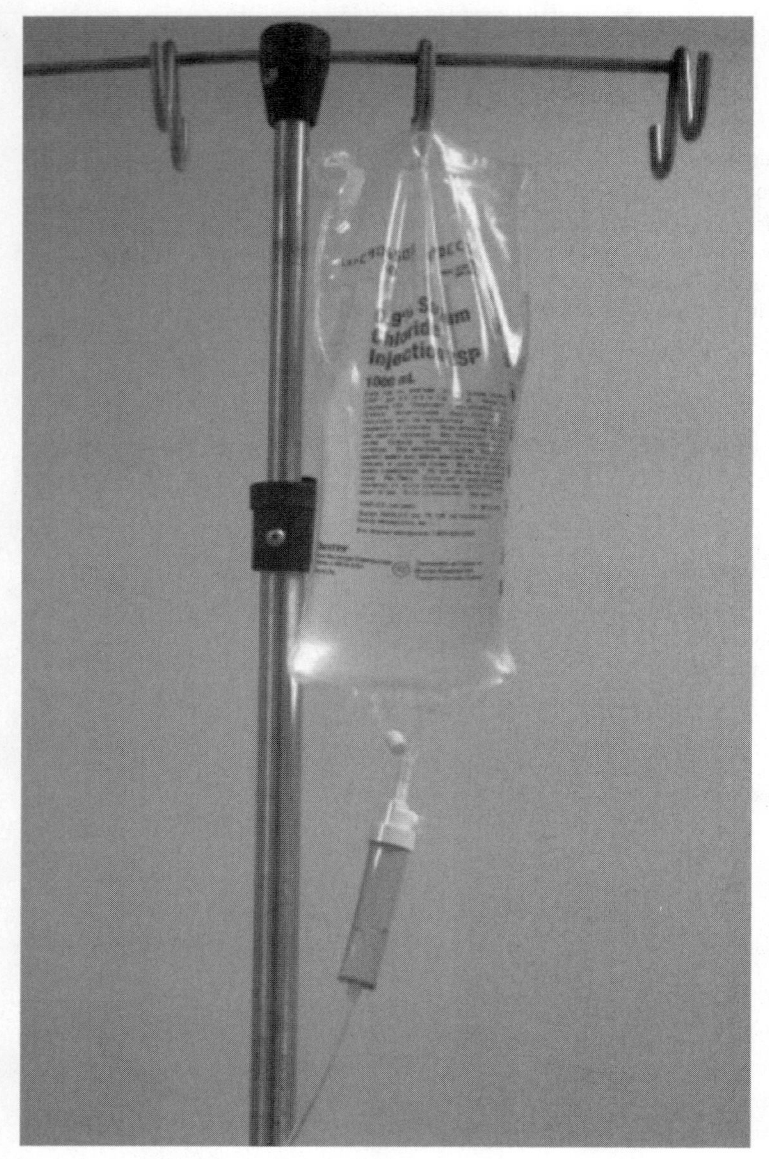

Source: Courtesy of Sarah Dresen/Charlottesville, VA

LO2:

Pathophysiology: Fluids

Homeostasis and Equilibrium

- Equilibrium occurs when both sides of a membrane are in an isotonic state, meaning there is no movement of solutes or water across the membrane (as with blood vessels and cell walls).
- The body's responses always strive to achieve physiological equilibrium. Once achieved, the patient is considered to be in homeostasis. Similarly, the clinical team strives to meet this natural physiologic goal.
- When fluid and electrolyte levels are within normal limits and are maintained, homeostasis and equilibrium have occurred, and the clinical team has achieved this important goal.

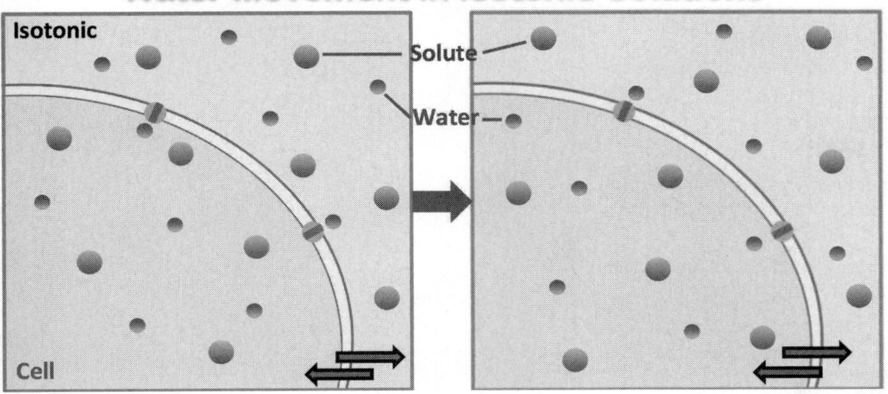

The images from left to right show the movement of water molecules through protein channels in the cell membrane in isotonic solution. Note that the number of water molecules on both sides of the membrane remains essentially unchanged.

Source: Copyright © 2014, NovEx Novice to Expert Learning, LLC

- Several body systems contribute to the regulation of the fluid and electrolyte balance:
  - o Hypothalamus
  - o Pituitary gland
  - o Adrenal cortex
  - o Renal system
  - o Cardiac regulation
  - o Gastrointestinal system
  - o Insensible water loss
- When one of these systems is not working properly, fluid and/or electrolyte imbalances may occur.

Concept Check

1. **What is the most important fact to remember about electrolyte imbalances?**
   A. If left untreated, they can be lethal.
   B. They are uncommon after hospitalization.
   C. They are easy to treat.
   D. They increase cost of hospitalization.

Answer question

Concept Check

2. **Which term describes physiological equilibrium?**
   A. Homeostasis
   B. Isotonic
   C. Insensible
   D. Isoelectric

Answer question

IV Fluid Concentration and Tonicity: Crystalloids

- Crystalloids are IV water solutions with electrolytes or other substances such as glucose added.
  - o Examples: 0.9% sodium chloride (normal saline) and D5W (water with 5% dextrose added)
- Crystalloids are categorized as isotonic, hypotonic, and hypertonic. This is in relation to the normal concentration of solutes in body cells. A normal concentration is equivalent to a concentration of 0.9% sodium chloride.
- Concentration and tonicity are often measured with osmolarity and osmolality. Sodium levels are usually used to estimate the tonicity of plasma.
- Crystalloids are readily available and less expensive to administer compared to colloids.

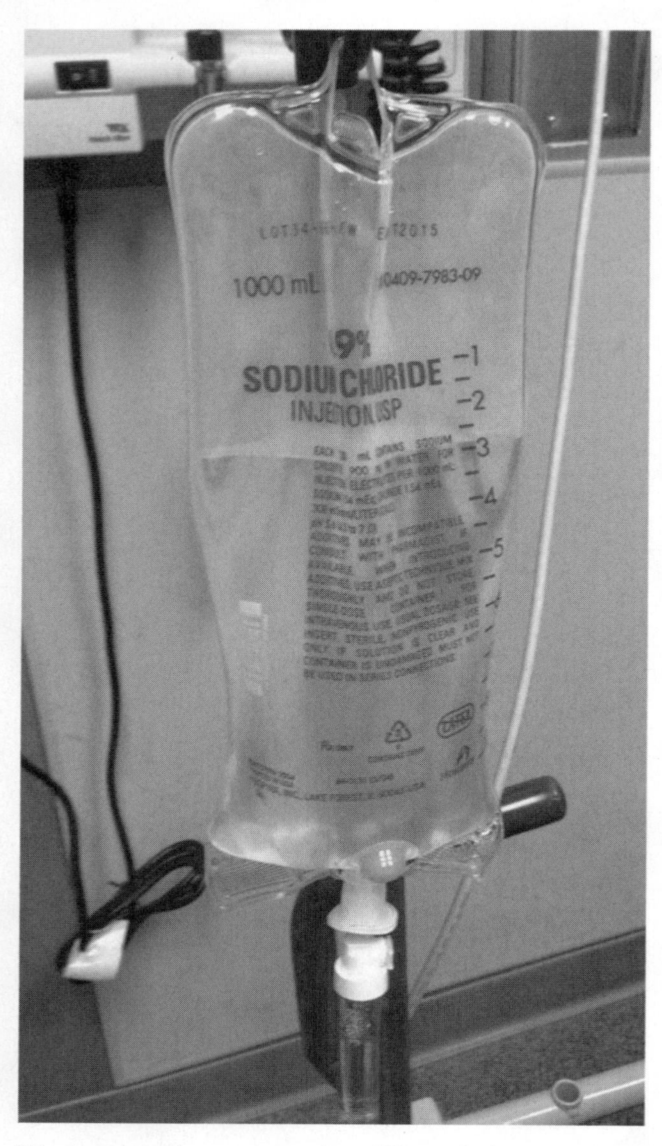

This photo shows the most commonly used IV crystalloid, isotonic saline, or sodium chloride. It is composed of water and dissolved crystals, which are able to diffuse across cellular membranes.
Source: Courtesy of K. Kyriakidis

- Crystalloids have tonicity, which impacts the patient's fluid and electrolyte status.
- Tonicity is the relationship between the amount of water on both sides of a membrane (such as the inside and outside of vascular walls or cell walls). When concentrations on both sides of the membrane are equal or in an equilibrium, an isotonic state is achieved (note that an isotonic state can be achieved even if the solution on both sides is either hypotonic or hypertonic). If the concentration of the fluid is lower on one side of a membrane than the other, it is called hypotonic (middle example below). If the concentration is higher, it is called hypertonic (right example) and can dehydrate and even damage the cell.
- The tonicity of the patient and the tonicity of the IV fluid are important as the clinician strives to achieve homeostasis. Hypotonic, hypertonic, and isotonic fluids are available, depending on the patient's need. The tonicity of IV fluids is described in relationship to the tonicity in a normal cell.

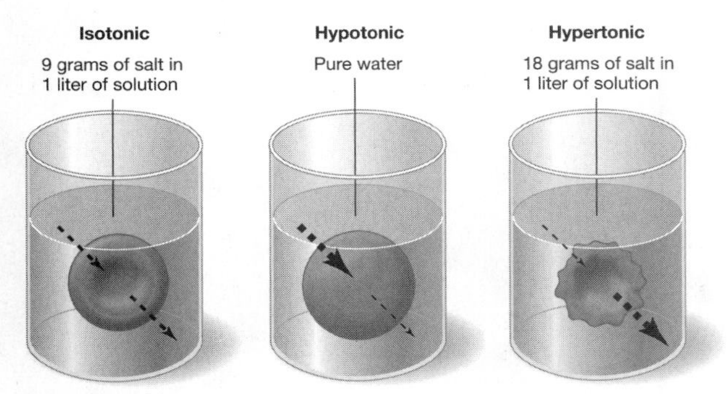

Comparison of tonicity with relative salt concentrations and effects of red blood cells.

Pathophysiology: Fluids (continued)

Hypotonic Conditions

- Hypotonic conditions occur when there is a lower concentration of solutes than is considered normal.
- Patients in fluid overload are often hypotonic because there is too much fluid diluting their solute (e.g., glucose, electrolytes), allowing their cells to expand and often dysfunction.
- Conditions with fluid overload that result in hypotonicity include failure of the liver, heart, and/or renal systems.
- Patients who are dehydrated may also be hypotonic. This occurs if both fluid and electrolytes are lost and replaced with only water. This may occur in patients with diarrhea and/or vomiting who are drinking free water to stay hydrated. Patients on certain types of diuretics can also become hypotonic if the diuretic causes a loss of sodium out of proportion to loss of fluids.
- Hypotonic patients may exhibit symptoms such as headache, confusion, twitching, irritability, hypertension, edema, and bounding pulses due to too much fluid and too few electrolytes.

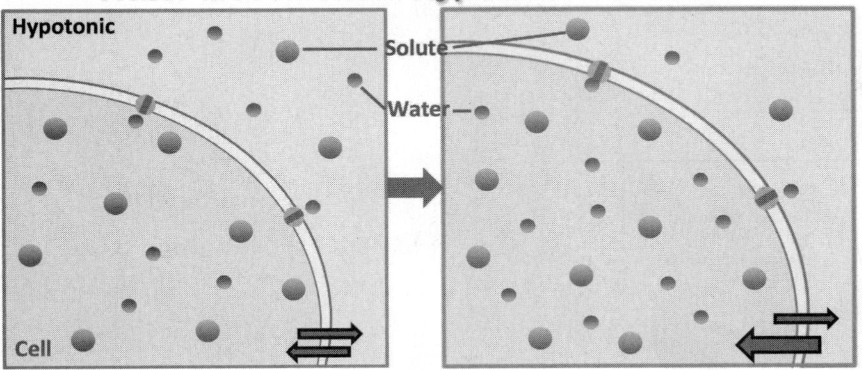

The images from left to right show the movement of water molecules across the cell membrane in hypotonic solution. Note that the number of water molecules inside the cell increases with time, and the cell swells as a result.

Hypertonic Conditions

- Hypertonic conditions occur when there are higher concentrations of solutes in fluid than is considered normal.
- Patients who are hypertonic are deficient in extracellular fluid volumes.
- Conditions leading to hypertonicity include diabetic ketoacidosis (DKA), burns, prolonged vomiting and diarrhea, nasogastric or other GI suctioning, surgical patients, excessive use of diuretics, excessive diaphoresis, and inadequate fluid intake with dehydration.
- Hypertonic patients may exhibit symptoms such as nausea, vomiting, decreased tearing with dry eyes, dry skin, rapid (but clear) respirations, thirst, pale skin, dry mucous membranes, decreased urine output, tachycardia, increased hematocrit, postural hypotension, elevated BUN and creatinine, irritability, and restlessness.

Water Movement in Hypertonic Solutions

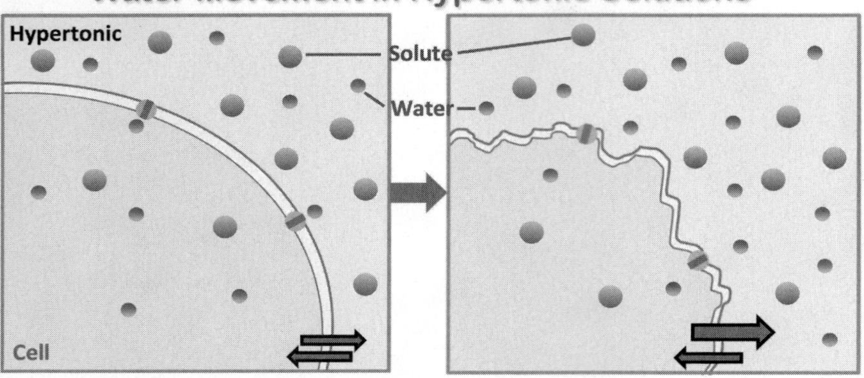

The images from left to right show the movement of water molecules across the cell membrane in hypotonic solution. Note that the number of water molecules inside the cell increases with time, and the cell swells as a result.

Comparison of Hypertonicity and Hypotonicity

These diagrams demonstrate how tonicity looks inside the body. Note the changes (top diagrams) in the amount of fluid compared to the amount of solutes based on tonicity. In the diagrams below, note the potential corresponding effect on vital body cells (e.g., red blood cells).

Comparsion of IV Fluid Concentration & Tonicity

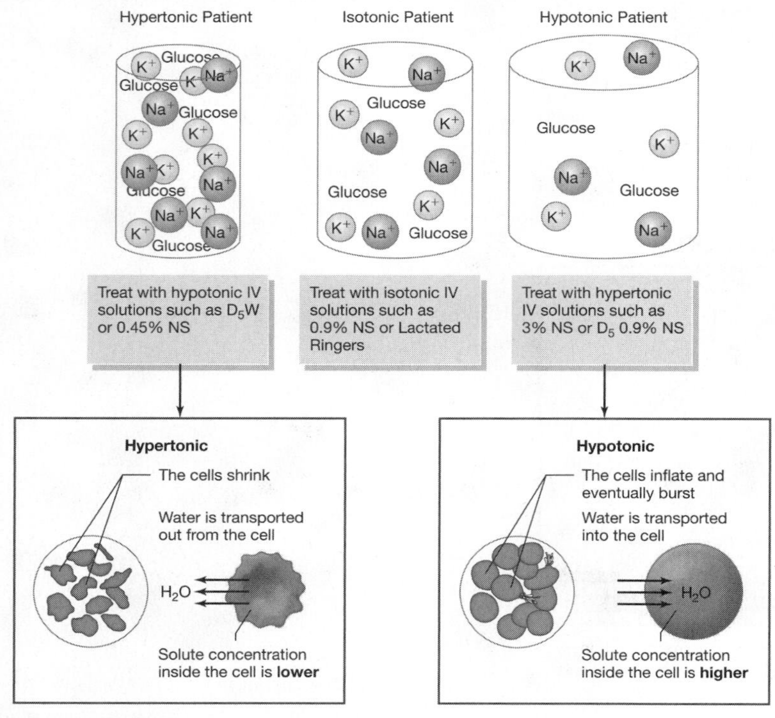

Summary

- This series of photos shows what happens to red (top) and white blood cells (bottom) in different tonicities, from isotonic to hypertonic, and finally to hypotonic (distilled water). The tonicity is labelled and shows the comparative results of exposure to different solutions.
- In isotonic solution (left), the cells display normal shape and size with no change.
- In hypertonic solution (middle), the red and white cells shrink as water is pulled out of the cells. In real life, the cells will re-expand when exposed to isotonic solutions again.
- In hypotonic distilled water (right), both red and white cells expand until they burst. The upper red blood cells burst, disintegrate, and become "ghosts" as they disappear. The white cells undergo a vivid burst or rupture.
- These visual images can assist clinicians to better imagine what is happening in the body when they infuse various IV fluids or have a patient with particular types of fluid and electrolyte imbalances.

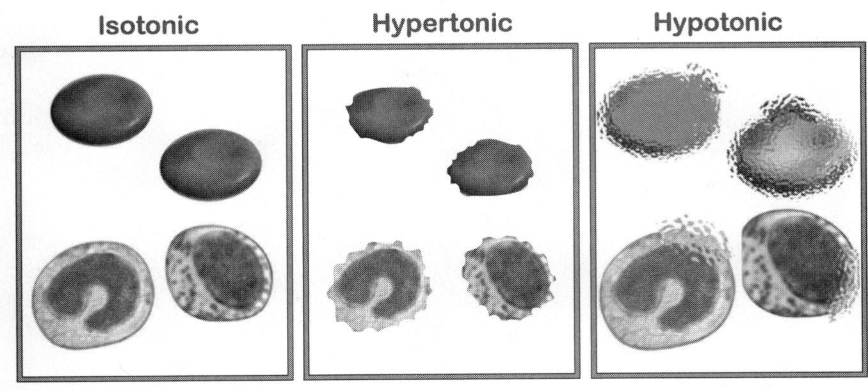

Cellular responses to extracellular solutions.
Source: Courtesy of George Kyriakidis/Santa Ana, CA

Total Body Water: 50–70%

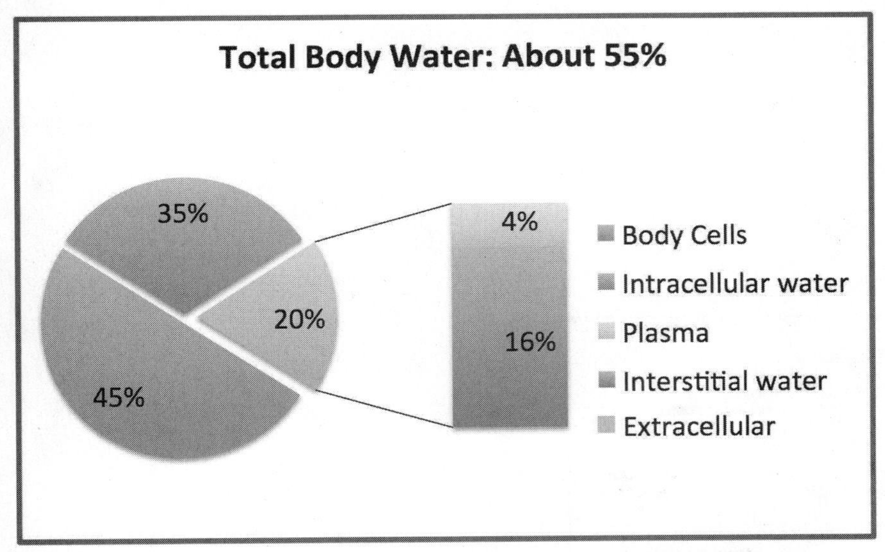

This diagram represents the normal distribution of water in the body with the approximate percentages of total body water located in each compartment. If hypertonic solution is infused into the vascular system, water will be drawn from the intracellular into the extracellular space. If hypotonic solution is infused water will move across the cell membranes into the cells (i.e., from extracellular to intracellular space). An isotonic solution will cause no movement of fluid. So the percentage can fluctuate slightly.
Source: Copyright © 2014, NovEx Novice to Expert Learning, LLC

Clinical Implications

- IV fluids also have tonicity, and it is important for the nurse to understand tonicity in order to give the correct fluid solutions to his or her patient.
- As a general rule, patients should receive the IV tonicity that is the opposite of their body's tonicity. For example, a hypertonic patient usually benefits from a hypotonic IV solution.
- It is important to remember that isotonic IV solutions do not cause osmosis or diffusion and do not change the composition of body fluids.

Pathophysiology: Fluids (continued)

IV Fluid Concentration and Tonicity: Colloids

- Colloids are the other type of IV fluids.
- Colloids are volume expanders because they have large molecules (e.g., albumin, blood, and blood products).
- Colloids are more expensive than crystalloids but require much less volume to produce the same effect.
- Colloids generally increase the osmotic gradient and are useful for pulling fluid from the interstitial spaces (edematous areas) into the intravascular spaces.

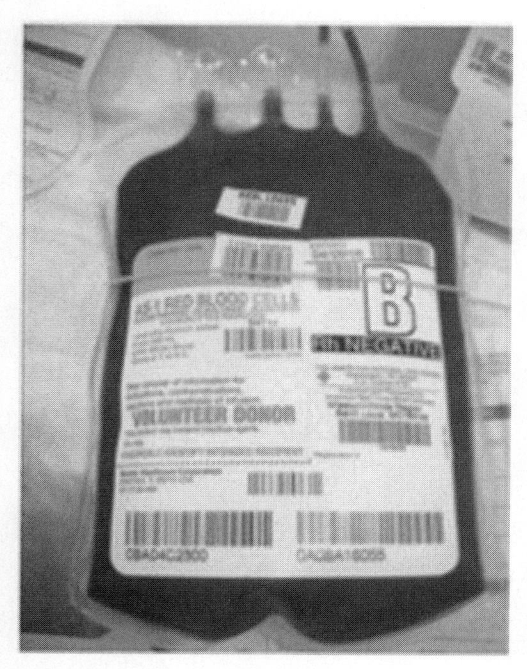

Blood transfusion therapy involves transfusing whole blood or blood components (specific portion or fraction of blood lacking in patient). One unit of whole blood consists of 450 mL of blood collected into 60–70 mL of preservative or anticoagulant. Whole blood stored for more than 6 hours does not provide therapeutic platelet transfusion, nor does it contain therapeutic amounts of labile coagulation factors (factors V & VIII).
Source: Copyright © 2014, NovEx Novice to Expert Learning, LLC

Comparison of Crystalloids and Colloids

	Crystalloids			Colloids
Type	Isotonic	Hypotonic	Hypertonic	
Examples	0.9% Normal Saline Lactated Ringers	0.45% Normal Saline Dextrose 5% In Water* D_5.45% Normal Saline	3.0% Saline D_5.9% Normal Saline D5LR Dextrose 10% TPN	Whole blood Albumin Fresh frozen plasma Dextran 40 Artificial Colloids
Properties	No fluid shifts between spaces	Causes fluid shift into cells	Causes fluid shift from intracellular into intravascular space	Increases intravascular volume expansion without excess fluid volume.
Useful for	Hemorrhage Hypovolemia Shock Hypotension Dehydration	Dehydration Diuretic overuse Renal Dysfunctions DKA Hypernatremia	Head Trauma with ↑ ICP Hyponatremia Edema Acid/base disturbances	Reducing edema Vascular volume expansion Improving tissue perfusion Vasospasm prevention Severe anemia
Caution In	Heart Failure Hypertension Avoid LR in: DKA COPD Hyperthermia Liver Disease Febrile conditions Head Injuries Metformin Use	SIADH Hyponatremia Increased ICP (Head trauma, Stroke, neurosurgery) Heart Failure Increased CVP Pulmonary Edema Edema Burns Liver disease	Pulmonary congestions Increased CVP JVD Hemoconcentration DKA Cardiac or renal dysfunction	Heart Failure Volume Overload Hemoconcentration

*D_5W is isotonic in the bag but quickly becomes hypotonic when administered intravascularly.
Source: Copyright © 2014, NovEx Novice to Expert Learning, LLC

Oral Fluids

- Not all fluid replacement needs to be intravenous.
- Often, oral intake can correct or prevent fluid and electrolyte imbalances.
- Free water and electrolyte beverages are useful and inexpensive ways to ensure people, particularly athletes, stay well hydrated.
- Oral water is an excellent choice to maintain hydration. Six to eight glasses of water per day are recommended.
- Beverages with electrolytes are good choices for athletes and people working in hot climates where electrolytes are lost through sweating.

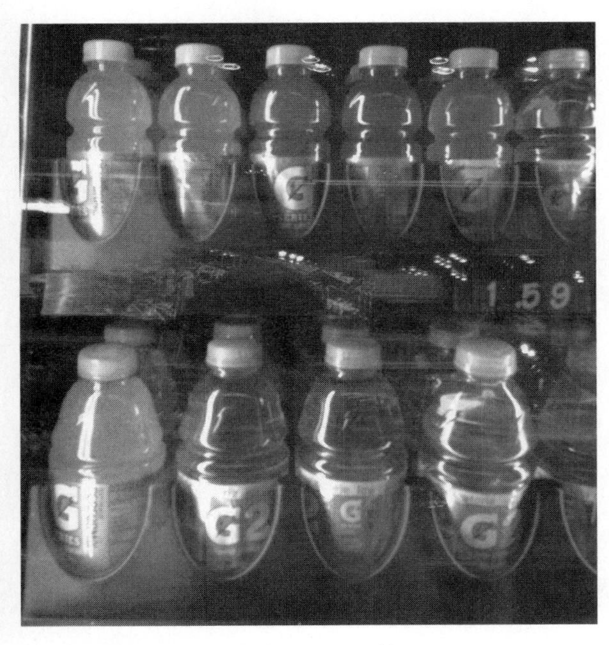

Oral hydration is preferred whenever possible.

Concept Check

3. What is the benefit of using colloids for volume expansion?

A. They are less expensive.
B. They require less volume to give.
C. They pull fluids from intravascular spaces to interstitial spaces.
D. They do not require intravenous access.

Answer question

Concept Check

4. Which fluid is isotonic?

A. D5, 9% NS
B. D5, 45% NS
C. 10% dextrose
D. Lactated Ringers

Answer question

LO2:

Assessment Findings: Fluid Disturbances

Volume Deficit or Dehydration

Major signs and symptoms of hypovolemia or dehydration include:

- Tachycardia
- Hypotension, if moderate to severe dehydration
- Thready or weak pulse
- Dry skin
- Loss of skin turgor
- Tachypnea
- Sunken eyes
- Orthostatic hypotension

Volume Overload or Hypervolemia

Key signs and symptoms of fluid overload include:

- Shortness of breath; orthopnea
- Tachycardia
- Bounding pulses
- Pulmonary edema; crackles on auscultation
- Edema
- Restlessness; anxiety
- Neck vein distension

LO1:

What Are Electrolytes?

- An electrolyte is a substance with an electrical charge that dissociates into ions when placed in water.
- Positively charged electrolytes are called cations and include sodium (Na^+), potassium (K^+), calcium (Ca^{++}) and magnesium (Mg^{++}).
- Negatively charged electrolytes are called anions and include chloride (Cl^-) and phosphate (PO_4^{3-})
- The electrolytes maintain fluid balance between the membranes throughout the body. They play a key role in muscle contraction and nerve impulse transmission.
- The major electrolytes outside the cells, in the extracellular fluid, are Na^+ and Cl^-.
- The major electrolytes inside the cells, in the intracellular spaces, are K^+ and PO_4^{3-}.

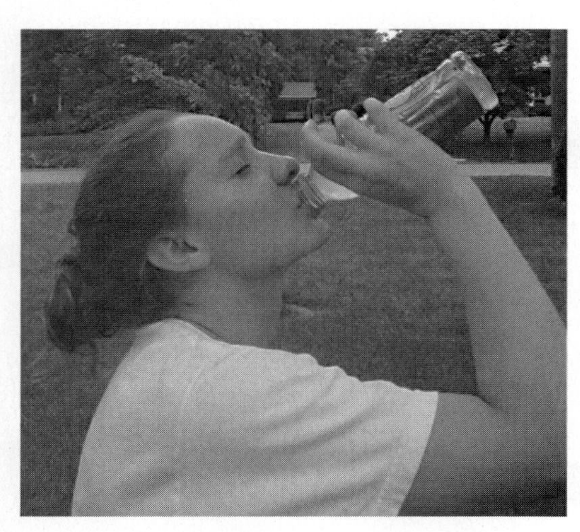

Electrolyte is a "medical/scientific" term for salts, specifically ions. The term *electrolyte* means that this ion is electrically charged and moves to either a negative or positive electrode: Ions that move to the cathode (cations) are positively charged and ions that move to the anode (anions) are negatively charged. For example, your body fluids–blood, plasma, interstitial fluid–are like seawater and have a high concentration of sodium chloride.

Source: Copyright © 2014, NovEx Novice to Expert Learning, LLC

LO1:

Clinical Relevance: Electrolytes

- Electrolyte imbalances are common in most patients who are ill.
- Imbalances can be caused as a direct result of the disease process (e.g., left-sided heart failure, diabetic ketoacidosis, and burns), or as a result of therapeutic interventions (e.g., IV fluid replacement or diuretic use).
- It is important for the nurse to anticipate and to assess for signs and symptoms of electrolyte imbalances and intervene quickly to restore proper balance.

LO2:

Pathophysiology: Electrolytes

- Electrolytes and fluid move between membranes through a variety of mechanisms, including:
  - o Diffusion
  - o Oncotic pressure
  - o Osmosis
  - o Active transport
  - o Facilitated diffusion
  - o Hydrostatic pressure

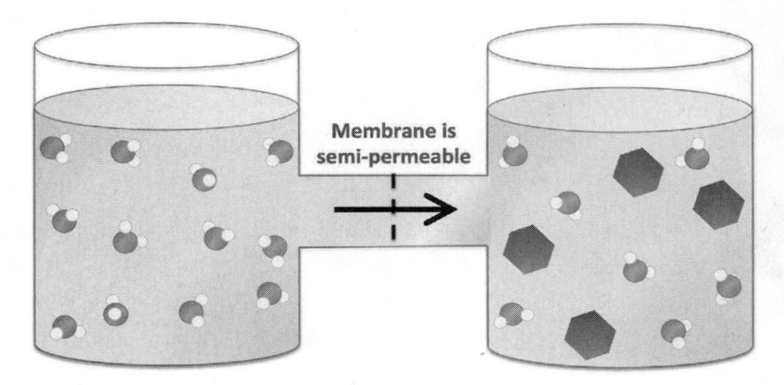

This movement of water (yellow dots) would continue until the water concentration on both sides of the membrane is equal, and will result in a change in volume of the two sides. The side that contains sugar (purple hexagons) will end up with a larger volume.

- Many nursing and pharmacologic interventions use these transportation mechanisms to improve patient health. For example, protein is a colloid that increases oncotic pressure. Increased oncotic pressure pulls fluid from the interstitial into the intravascular spaces and thus assists in reducing edema. Mannitol is an osmotic diuretic that pulls fluid from the intracellular spaces, to reduce brain swelling, back into the blood vessels, where the excess fluid can then be eliminated via the kidneys.

Concept Check

5. **Which electrolytes are primarily within cells?**
   A. Sodium and chloride
   B. Chloride and phosphate
   C. Potassium and sodium
   D. Potassium and phosphate

Answer question

Sodium Imbalances

- Sodium (Na^+) is a major extracellular ion. It helps regulate intravascular volume and pressure, helps maintain the body's fluid balance, is involved in transmission of neural impulses, and facilitates muscle contraction. Numerous body processes (e.g., muscles, nerve cells) require electrical conduction of signals. Movement of sodium and potassium are among the most critical.
- Normal sodium levels are considered to be between 135–145 mEq/L but can vary slightly between different labs.
- Insufficient amounts of sodium are often caused by sodium-free or hypotonic IV fluids. Patients experiencing excessive dehydration, vomiting, diarrhea or hypervolemia may become hyponatremic (<135 mEq/L).
- Excess sodium (hypernatremia) can occur with water loss or with increased sodium retention. Patients with Cushing's syndrome, diabetes insipidus, and hyperaldosteronism are prone to hypernatremic states (>145 mEq/L).

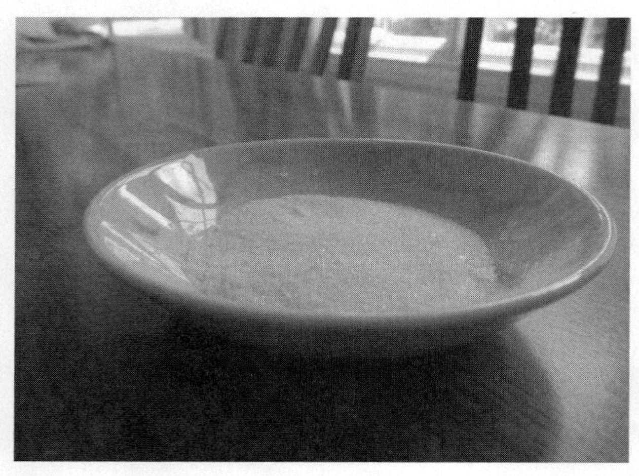

Sodium chloride or salt.
Source: Copyright © 2014, NovEx Novice to Expert Learning, LLC

Pathophysiology: Electrolytes (continued)

Potassium Imbalances

- Potassium (K^+) is the major intracelluar cation and is intricately involved in the communication process between nerves and muscles.
- Normal potassium levels vary slightly between different labs but are generally considered normal between 3.5–5.0 mEq/L.
- Hypokalemia (K^+ <3.5 mEq/L) may be due to chronic diarrhea, vomiting, diuretic use, or renal artery stenosis.
- Hyperkalemia (K^+ >5.0 mEq/L) may be due to kidney failure, crushing injuries, or blood transfusions.

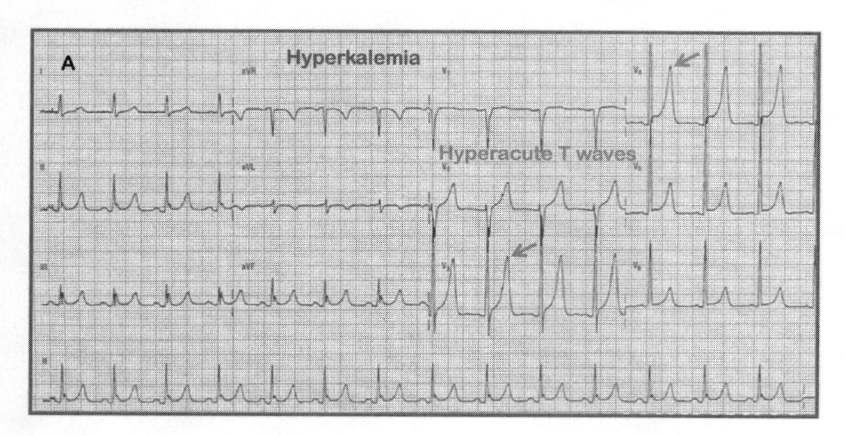

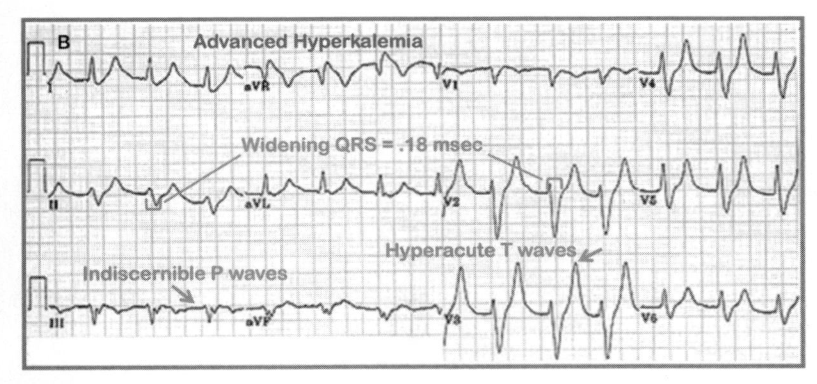

Upper: Because of the large T-waves (arrow), this ECG was interpreted as "hyperacute T-waves" commonly seen in mild–moderate hyperkalemia. However, these T waves are pathognomonic of hyperkalemia because they are peaked, "tented," come to point, and have a very flat ST segment. Note that the QRS remains within normal limits. Lower: This EKG shows progression into advanced hyperkalemia. The hyperacute T-waves persist, but note that the QRS is abnormally and dangerously widened. Sluggish or prolonged electrical depolarization of the heart causes abnormal cardiac contraction and hinders cardiac output. The P waves can no longer be recognized.

Source: *(both)* Courtesy of Chris Janowiecki

Calcium Imbalances

- Calcium (Ca^{++}) is an important electrolyte that is essential in building strong bones and teeth. It is also necessary for normal cardiac function, muscle contraction, nerve transmission and blood clotting.
- Normal calcium levels are considered to be between 8.5–10.2 mg/dL but can vary slightly between different labs.
- Hypocalcemia (<8.5) can be caused by kidney and liver failure, pancreatitis, osteomalacia, and by vitamin D deficiency.
- Hypercalcemia (>10.2) can be caused by prolonged bed rest, excessive calcium intake, HIV/AIDS, and some cancers.

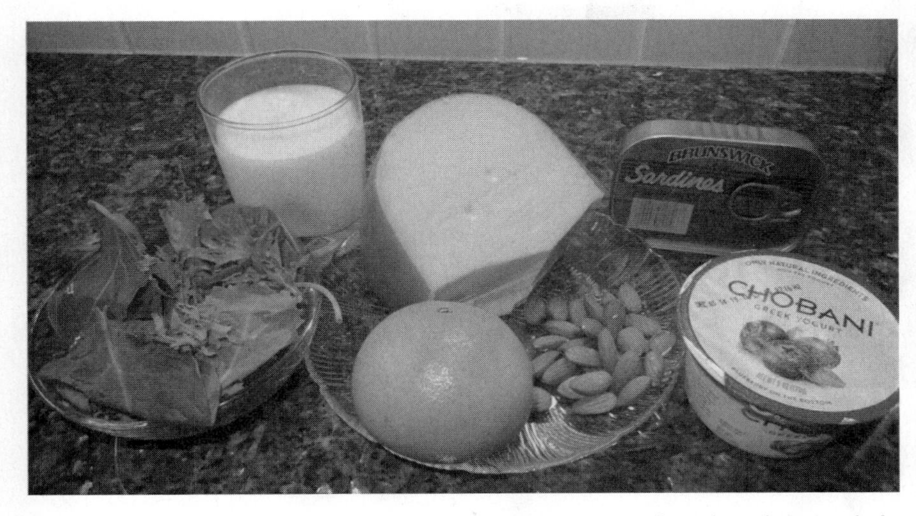

The photo shows many of the top 10 calcium-rich foods: cheese, yogurt, milk, sardines, dark green leafy greens, fortified orange juice, and almonds.

Source: Copyright © 2014, NovEx Novice to Expert Learning, LLC

Eliciting Chvostek's Sign

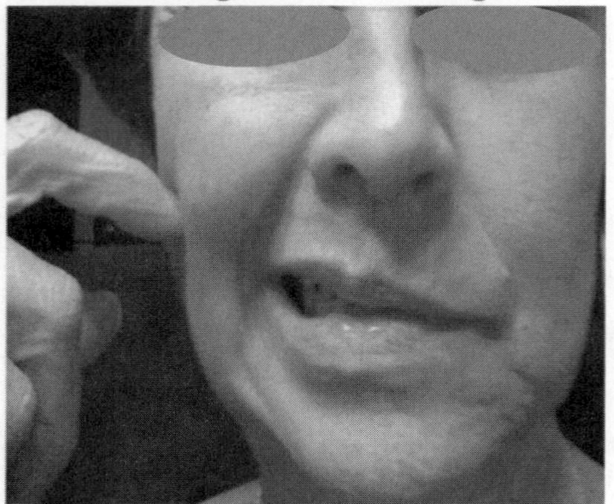

To check for Chvostek's sign, ask the patient to relax her face. Standing in front, tap on the facial nerve either anterior to the earlobe and below the zygomatic arch OR between the corner of the mouth and the zygomatic arch. If positive, note responses can range from twitching of the lip at the corner of the mouth to facial muscle spasms, depending on the severity of hypocalcemia.
Source: Courtesy of K. Kyriakidis

- Evaluation for calcium abnormalities includes two simple tests: Chvostek Sign and Trousseau Sign. These are quick and inexpensive tests that clinicians can readily perform.

Relaxed Hand

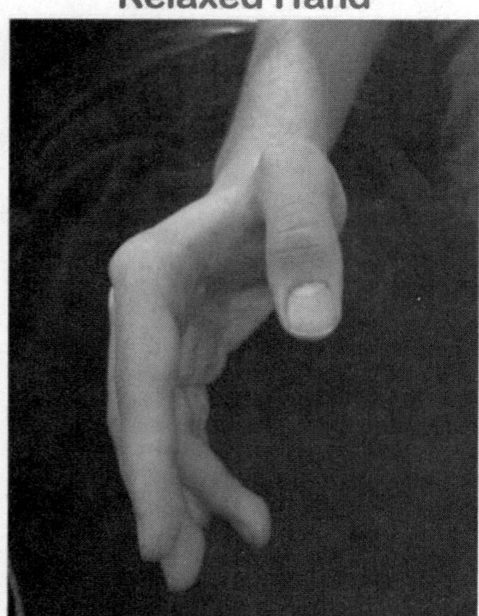

Positive Trousseau's Sign

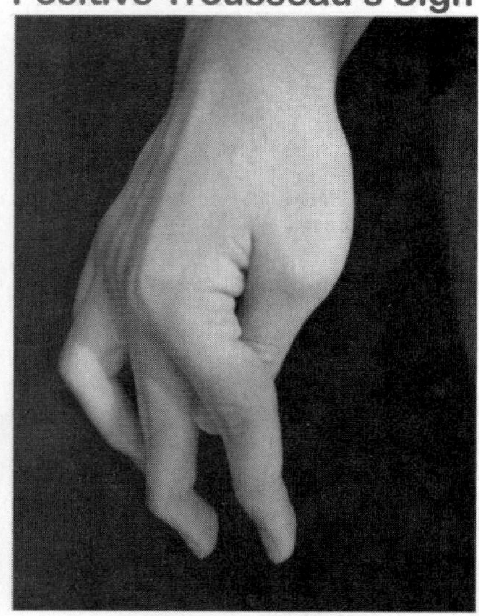

Trousseau's sign is positive when carpal spasm is induced by occluding the brachial artery for 3 minutes with an inflated blood pressure cuff. It is often an indication of hypocalcemia.
Source: Courtesy of K. Kyriakidis

Concept Check

6. A patient's serum potassium is 4.0 mEq/L. What is the condition?

A. Hypokalemia
B. Hyperkalemia
C. Normokalemic
D. Not enough information to determine

Answer question

Pathophysiology: Electrolytes (continued)

Magnesium Imbalances

- Magnesium (Mg^{++}) is an important electrolyte required for the maintenance of normal muscle and nerve functioning. It is also necessary for adequate bone strength, cardiac regulation, blood pressure maintenance, and proper glucose control and is a component of the body's defense system.
- The normal range for magnesium is between 1.7–2.2 mg/dL but can vary between laboratories.
- Hypomagnesemia (<1.7) is often noted in patients with alcoholism, hemodialysis, chronic diarrhea, cirrhosis, pancreatitis and ulcerative colitis.
- Hypermagnesemia (>2.2) may be the result of dehydration, oliguria, chronic kidney failure, DKA, or Addison's disease.

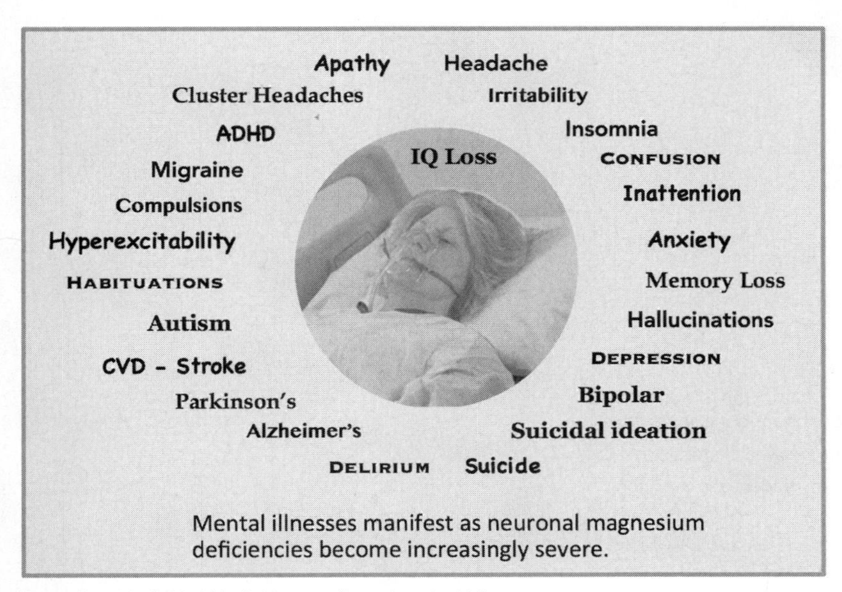

Chloride Imbalances

- Chloride (Cl^-) is the major extracellular fluid cation.
- It is utilized in conjunction with other electrolytes such as potassium, sodium, and carbon dioxide to maintain proper acid–base balance.
- Normal chloride is between 96–106 mEq/L.
- Hypochloremia (<96 mEq/L) can be seen in Addison's disease, burns, dehydration, excessive sweating, prolonged GI suctioning, or in metabolic alkalosis.
- Hyperchloremia (>106 mEq/L) is often seen in metabolic acidosis, renal tubular acidosis, and bromide poisoning.

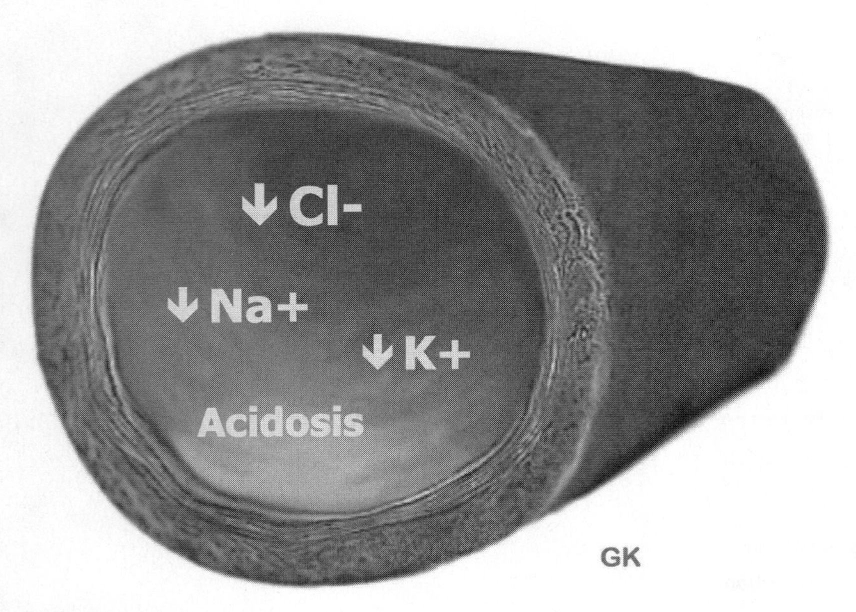

What is Hypochloremia? Hypochloremia is abnormal chlorine ion depletion in the blood. However, a chloride level <98mEq/L is often associated with hypokalemia, hyponatremia and metabolic acidosis.
Source: Courtesy of George Kyriakidis/Santa Ana, CA

Phosphate Imbalances

- Phosphorus exists as the ion phosphate (PO_4^{3-}) in the blood. Phosphate is the major intracellular anion, is a buffering agent, and is utilized in the process that develops bone and teeth.
- Normal phosphate levels are between 2.4–4.1 mg/dL but may vary between laboratories.
- Hypophosphatemia (<2.4 mg/dL) may be caused by alcoholism, inadequate nutrition, hypercalcemia, and insufficient intake of phosphate.
- Hyperphosphatemia (>4.1 mg/dL) may be caused by disease processes such as DKA, liver and kidney disease, and overuse of phosphate-containing laxatives.

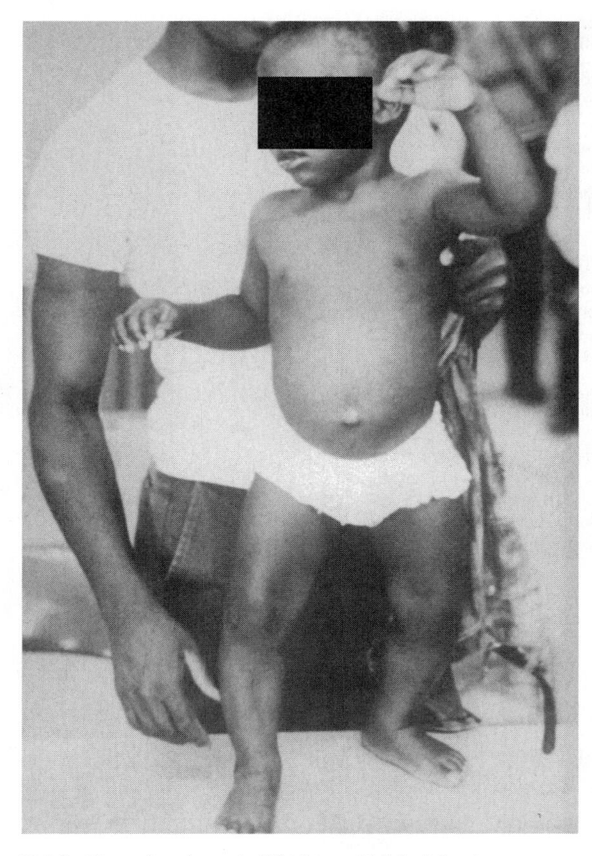

X-linked hypophosphatemia (XLH) is an X-linked dominant disorder characterized by growth retardation, rickets (softening and weakening of the bones), and hypophosphatemia due to kidney defects in phosphate reabsorption and vitamin D metabolism.
Source: Centers for Disease Control and Prevention

LO2:

Assessment Findings: Electrolyte Imbalances

- It is important for the nurse to assess for signs and symptoms of fluid and electrolyte imbalance in his or her patient in order to provide rapid and appropriate interventions.
- Some assessment findings are common with either excessive or deficient levels of the electrolytes and are shown in the following tables.

Electrolyte	Excess	Deficit
Sodium (Na+)	Cardiac: ↓ cardiac output Thirst Dry Mucous membranes Dehydration, ↓ Urine output CNS changes, muscle twitching	Cardiac: tachycardia, BP alterations Neuro changes such as confusion, lethargy, irritability, personality changes, and loss of consciousness Nausea, diarrhea
Potassium (K+)	Cardiac Dysrhythmias & EKG change (can be lethal such as ventricular fibrillation Death can be first sign Muscle weakness Tingling sensations, twitches Fatigue Nausea, diarrhea	Dysrhythmias Orthostatic hypotension Constipation Polyuria, ↓ urine concentration Mental status changes Muscle weakness, spasms Shallow breathing
Calcium (Ca++)	Cardiac: EKG changes, ↑ BP Nausea, vomiting, anorexia Thirst, dehydration Bloating, constipation Confusion, lethargy, coma Muscle & joint pain /aching	Syncope with Hypotension ↓ Cardiac output with CHF Muscle cramps (tetany), numbness + Chvostek's & Trousseau's signs Dysphagia, Diarrhea Neuro changes (irritability, depression, personality changes, fatigue, seizures Dermatologic changes

Source: Copyright © 2014, NovEx Novice to Expert Learning, LLC

Electrolyte	Excess	Deficit
Magnesium (Mg++)	Hypotension EKG changes, cardiac arrest Loss of Deep tendon reflexes Depressed CNS / neuromuscular functioning, drowsy, lethargic Facial paresthesias **Very rare clinically: kidneys eliminate magnesium by reducing reabsorption in the tubules*	Hypertension, dysrhythmias, Sudden death Personality changes, hallucinations Vasospasm Abnormal eye twitch- nystagmus Fatigue Hyperactive deep tendon reflexes + Babinski, Trousseau & Chvostek's signs
Chloride (Cl-)	Hypertension Weakness, altered mental status Intense thirst Kussmaul's breathing Poor sugar control (diabetics)	Hyponatremia Tremors Muscle Twitching, spasticity Diarrhea, dehydration
Phosphate (PO4-3)	Hypocalcaemia signs & symptoms EKG changes, Dysrhythmias Hypotension Calcium deposits in connective tissues (cardiac valves & organs) Twitching, weakness, paresthesias Irritability, psychosis	Hypocalcaemia signs & symptoms Increased Bleeding Weak muscles, shallow respirations Dysphagia Reduced cardiac output Altered mental status: Irritability, confusion, seizures

LO2:

Diagnostics: Fluid and Electrolyte Imbalances

- Obtain a good medical history and physical exam are key to honing in on the problem.
- Perform electrolyte-specific physical tests, such as Chvostek sign and Trousseau sign in calcium disturbances.
- Examine laboratory data to establish the diagnosis:
  - o Complete metabolic panel (includes electrolytes)
  - o Serum and urine osmolality
  - o Arterial blood gases
- Examine EKG.

Priority Patient Concerns and Desired Collaborative Care Outcomes: Fluid and Electrolyte Imbalances

Prior to caring for patients with fluid and electrolyte imbalances, it is important to prioritize the patient's concerns that must guide the nursing care plan and interventions. Care for the patient is ordered and organized in accordance with the patient's priority and urgent needs. Desired collaborative care outcomes in patients with fluid and electrolyte imbalances typically include the following:

1. Patient will return to normal fluid volume status.
2. Patient's excessive or deficient electrolyte levels will be restored to within normal limits.
3. Patient will have intact skin and mucous membranes.
4. Patient will demonstrate knowledge of and the ability to follow a collaborative health maintenance regimen.
5. Patient will remain free of injury.

Considering these important care outcomes, prepare a list of the major 3–6 priority patient concerns or nursing diagnoses for patients with fluid and electrolyte imbalances. Be prepared to participate in a discussion of this list and/or to submit them as an assignment, as determined by your faculty. Resources you may find helpful in this assignment can include this lesson, the references, resources on nursing care plans, and standard nursing diagnoses manuals.

LO3: Collaborative Interventions

Fluid and Electrolytes

- In all cases of fluid and electrolyte abnormalities, the goal is to identify and correct the underlying cause.
- Fluid boluses, maintenance fluids, increasing or decreasing oral intake, or diuretics may be needed for patients with fluid volume abnormalities. These are discussed in detail in specific disease condition NovE-lessons.
- Restrict, or increase, oral or IV electrolytes if necessary to correct electrolyte abnormalities.
- For patients with fluid and/or electrolyte disturbances, care of the patient should include the following:
  - o Immediately discontinue any fluids, medications, or supplements that exacerbate the abnormality.
  - o Monitor cardiac rate and rhythm via bedside EKG, as indicated.
  - o Monitor vital signs, physical exam, and patient's responsiveness to interventions.
  - o Measure and record daily weight, intake, and output to achieve a balance.
  - o Assess for signs and symptoms of over- or undertreatment.
- When fluid and/or electrolyte imbalances are suspected, continued assessments and diagnostic procedures may include:
  - o Electrolytes, blood counts, and urine chemistries
  - o Use caution in patients with comorbid conditions that may confound or alter therapy or rapidity of therapy to avoid complications, including patients with cardiac, renal, hepatic, neuro, or diabetic conditions.
- Provide or encourage frequent mouth care.

Concept Check

7. **Chvostek sign is a test for imbalance of which electrolyte?**
   A. Potassium
   B. Calcium
   C. Chloride
   D. Sodium

Answer question

Fluid Disturbances

Volume Deficit

- Identify and treat the underlying cause.
- Monitor for vital signs and orthostatic hypotension. Implement fall precautions as needed.
- Force fluids: Encourage patients who can tolerate oral intake to drink 1.0–1.5 liters per day. Fluids should include:

  - o Water or primarily water solutions for mild to moderate dehydration situations where electrolyte loss was minimal. Water is the best treatment to avoid worsening vomiting and diarrhea, if present.

  - o Glucose and electrolyte solutions for severe dehydration (e.g., vomiting, diarrhea, strenuous or prolonged exercise, high fever, excessive sweating) to replace water and electrolytes and provide an energy source to meet metabolic needs

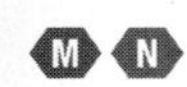

- Intravenous infusion: Provide fluid rehydration intravenously for those who are unable to take orally or are NPO. (See Fluid Therapy table.)

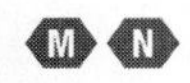

- Do not administer specific fluids to patients who are vulnerable or at high risk for complications. (See the Comparison of Crystalloids and Colloids of IV Fluids table below.)

Comparison of IV Fluids: Nursing Interventions

Type	Crystalloids: Isotonic	Crystalloids: Hypotonic	Crystalloids: Hypertonic	Colloids
Examples	0.9% Normal Saline Lactated Ringers	0.45% Normal Saline Dextrose 5% In Water* D_5.45% Normal Saline *Isotonic, but hypotonic after glucose is metabolized	3.0% Saline D_5.9% Normal Saline D5LR Dextrose 10% TPN	Whole blood Albumin Fresh frozen plasma Dextran 40, 70, or 75 Artificial Colloids
Useful for	Hemorrhage Hypovolemia Shock Hypotension Dehydration	Dehydration Diuretic overuse Renal Dysfunctions DKA Hypernatremia	Head Trauma with ↑ ICP Hyponatremia Edema Acid/base disturbances	Reducing edema Vascular volume expansion Improving tissue perfusion Vasospasm prevention Severe anemia
Nursing Interventions (fluid-specific)	Use caution in patients with hepatic disease who cannot metabolize the lactate. Avoid using if pH >7.50	Monitor sodium levels closely Consider central venous access due to vein irritation and inflammation in peripheral sites Avoid in patients with increased intracranial pressure (stroke, head trauma, infectious disorder, neurosurgery)	Monitor sodium levels closely Consider central venous access due to vein irritation and inflammation in peripheral sites Avoid in cardiac, diabetic, or renal patients	Use caution in patient with cardiac disease Consider cost effective alternatives if colloids are not specifically needed as a volume expander

Volume Overload

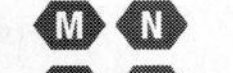

- Identify and treat the underlying cause.

- Restrict fluids and sodium as determined, including those taken in meals and with medications.

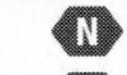

- Family requires education to assist in restricting fluids.
- Collaborate with patient on fluid management. Subtract required fluid volumes (meals, medications) from total allotted fluids; then divide the remainder according to patient preferences. Suggested amounts: 50–55% during the day, 30–35% during the evening, and 10–20% during the night. Collaborate with patient on the type of fluid. Suggest ice chips as a replacement since one cup of ice equals half a cup of water.

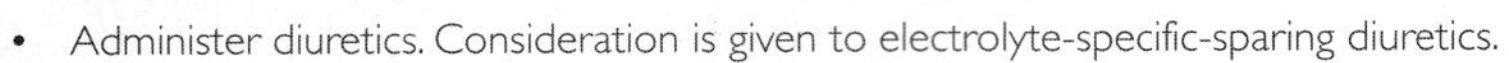

- Administer diuretics. Consideration is given to electrolyte-specific-sparing diuretics.

- Monitor for fluid overload or symptoms of rapid fluid shifts.

Collaborative Interventions (continued)

Sodium Disturbances

Hyponatremia

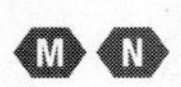

Depending on severity of the hyponatremia, patients may be managed as outpatients or in the ICU. Interventions may vary but include the following:

- Identify and treat the underlying cause.
- If mild to moderate, encourage increased oral intake of salt and foods high in sodium.
- Restrict free water intake which exacerbates hyponatremia.
- If severe and accompanied by hypovolemia, sodium IV infusions are typically needed (e.g., isotonic Ringer's or saline, 0.9%). Caution and continuous monitoring are needed with this therapy to avoid undercorrection of the hyponatremia. Collaborate with the health care provider to calculate the formula for infusion.
- If overt manifestations of low sodium are present, hypertonic saline is indicated. Caution and continuous monitoring are needed with this therapy as complications can be rapid and dire. Collaborate with the health care provider to calculate the formula for infusion.
- Consider diuretics to increase free water excretion.
- Vasopressin receptor antagonists may be considered but are new, expensive, and should be used as monotherapy.

Hypernatremia

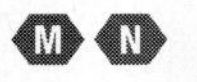

Collaborative interventions for patients with hypernatremia typically include the following:

- Identify and treat the underlying cause.
- If asymptomatic with concurrent hypovolemia, water replacement correction with hypotonic fluids can be used but should not reduce sodium levels to exceed 0.5 mEq/L/hour to avoid cerebral edema.
- If very symptomatic with concurrent hypovolemia, water replacement is increased until symptoms subside. Monitor neurologic responses and sodium levels frequently.
- If symptomatic with concurrent hypervolemia, administer a diuretic to increase sodium and water loss. Restrict fluid intake.
- Consider dialysis or blood ultrafiltration in patients with kidney failure.

Potassium Disturbances

Hypokalemia

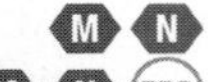

- Identify and treat the underlying cause.

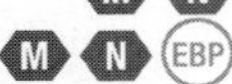

- Provide oral potassium if patient is able to drink and hypokalemia is not severe. Should supplement with dietary intake of potassium-rich foods (Cohn, et al., 2000).

- Offer a flavored beverage when administering oral potassium, for the patient to drink with or after the potassium. Oral potassium has a strong and bitter taste.

- If mild to moderate (K^+ 3.0–3.4 mEq/L) and without continued potassium loss, give 10–20 mEq orally, two to four times daily (Cohn, et al., 2000).

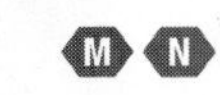

- If severe (K^+ <2.5–3.0 mEq/L) or symptomatic (e.g., dysrhythmias, significant muscle weakness), give oral potassium 40 mEq, three to four times daily or 20 mEq IV every 2–3 hours.

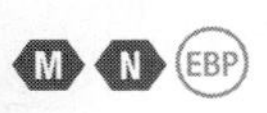

- If symptoms are severe and patient is unable to take orally, infuse potassium 20 mEq IV every 2–3 hours (Cohn, et al., 2000). Use of a central line is preferred due to potential phlebitis.

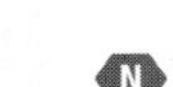

- Safety issues with potassium:
  - o Never administer potassium through IV push, intramuscularly or subcutaneously, which will likely cause tissue necrosis.
  - o Never administer potassium undiluted.
  - o Potassium infusions should not exceed 20 mEq/hr due to risk of life-threatening cardiac dysrhythmias and arrest.
  - o Discontinue infusion immediately if IV infiltration occurs until a new IV site is established.
  - o Avoid giving oral potassium when patients have an empty stomach due to nausea and vomiting.

Potassium Must Be Given with Caution

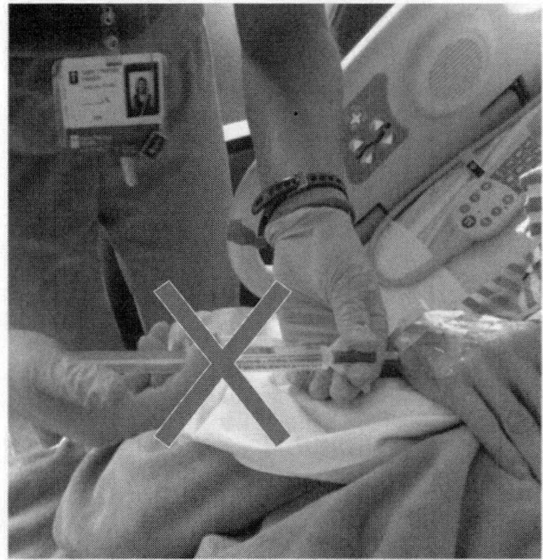

Always use great caution when administering potassium. Never give potassium IV push or undiluted.

Source: Courtesy of Sarah Bateman/Nashville, TN

Hyperkalemia

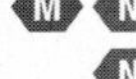

- Identify and treat the underlying cause (e.g., dietary).

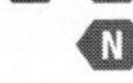

- Monitor patient's heart rhythm with EKG for toxic cardiac dysrhythmias and cardiac arrest. Monitor for neurologic and muscular control abnormalities. Monitor vital signs and patient responsiveness continuously.

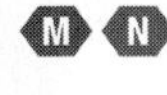

- Treat life-threatening hyperkalemia (e.g., widening QRS) with rapid acting but transient interventions:

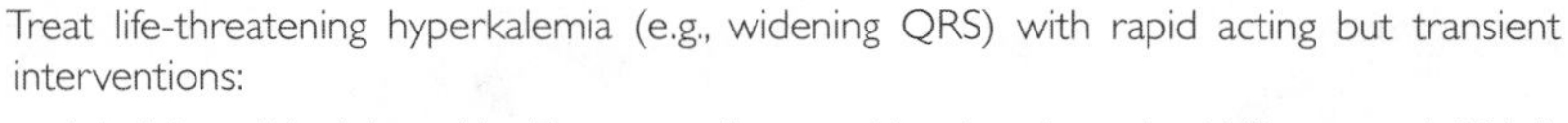

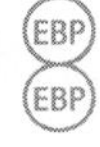

  - o Administer IV calcium chloride as an adjuvant with other therapies (Alfonzo, et al., 2014).
  - o Begin insulin and IV glucose infusion in severe situations to drive extracellular potassium back into the cells (Alfonzo, et al., 2014). Insulin must accompany this infusion in diabetic patients. Give insulin alone if blood glucose is >250 mg/dL.
  - o Consider sodium bicarbonate in combination with other interventions if metabolic acidosis exists.
  - o Consider giving a loop or thiazide diuretic to remove excess potassium.

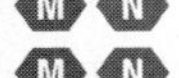

- Deliver Kayexalate orally or rectally if hyperkalemia is not life-threatening.
- Initiate dialysis, particularly hemodialysis, if hyperkalemia is life-threatening and/or other rapid acting interventions are inadequate.

Collaborative Interventions (continued)

Calcium Disturbances

Hypocalemia

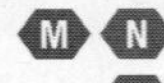

- Identify and treat the underlying cause.
- Safety precautions, which are specific to hypocalcemia, include the following:
  - o Emergency and code cart nearby
  - o Seizure precautions: padded side rails on the bed
  - o Oxygen, airway, and suction equipment at the patient's bed
  - o Endotracheal tray and tubes readily accessible in case of laryngeal spasm from tetany
  - o Never give calcium IV push rapidly, which can cause severe bradycardia or cardiac arrest. Never give by intramuscular or subcutaneous injection, which will damage tissues and lead to necrosis with subsequent sloughing.
  - o Never infuse via a leaking IV site. Prefer infusion via a central line.
  - o Observe the patient for digitalis toxicity and monitor heart rhythm via EKG.
  - o Patients with long-term and/or severe hypocalcemia are at high risk for fractures when moving and lifting them. Use a sheet to lift, lift carefully and gently, and don't pull on patients to move them.

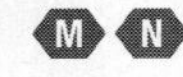

- Management with calcium:
  - o If severely symptomatic (e.g., tetany, seizures, cardiac dysfunction), rapidly begin IV calcium.
  - o If asymptomatic with Ca^{++} <7.6 mg/dL, begin IV calcium therapy.
  - o If asymptomatic and with renal disease, evaluate and first correct probable hyperphosphatemia and low vitamin D abnormalities.
  - o If Ca^{++} >7.5 mg/dL and with mild neurologic symptoms, initiate oral calcium supplements.
  - o If hypomagnesemia present, correct hypomagnesemia first.

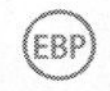

  - o If permanent hypoparathyroidism is present, give calcitriol in addition to calcium supplements (Winer, et al., 2003).

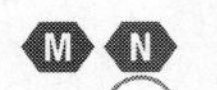

- Management with vitamin D:

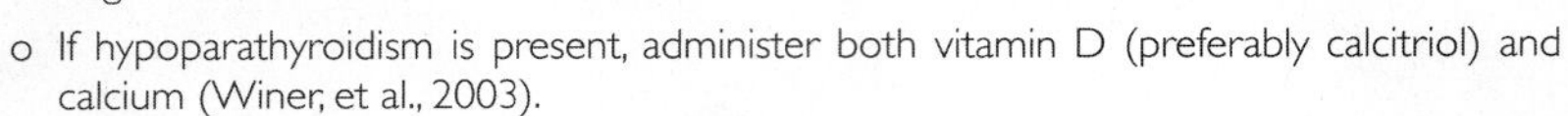

  - o If hypoparathyroidism is present, administer both vitamin D (preferably calcitriol) and calcium (Winer, et al., 2003).
  - o If vitamin D deficiency present, administer vitamin D.

Hypercalcemia

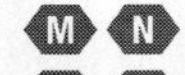

- Identify and treat the underlying cause.

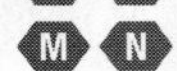

- If asymptomatic or mild symptoms with calcium levels <12 mg/dL:
  - o Observe without necessary medical intervention.
  - o Force fluids if volume depleted.
  - o Instruct the patient and/or alter treatments to avoid aggravating hypercalcemia: avoid calcium-rich foods or supplements, change diuretic to other than thiazide if used, and avoid long periods of bed rest or inactivity.

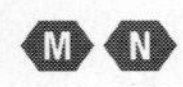

- If moderate to severe (Ca^{++} >14 mg/dL) and symptomatic:
  - o Give orally or infuse IV isotonic saline solutions for rehydration (a common factor in hypercalcemia).

  - o Administer calcitonin along with isotonic saline solution for immediate and short-term care (Berenson, 2002).

  - o Consider administering bisphosphonate, preferably zoledronic acid, for long-term management of hypercalcemia (Rosen, et al., 2003).
- Dialyze only if necessary in severe hypercalcemia.

Magnesium Disturbances

Hypomagnesemia

- Identify and treat the underlying cause.
- If at high risk for hypomagnesemia with concurrent, unexplained low calcium and potassium, administer magnesium empirically.
- If asymptomatic with hypomagnesemia, provide oral replacement with sustained-release properties to avert sudden hypermagnesemia.
- If severe symptoms are present, administer IV magnesium. Monitor heart rhythm continuously via cardiac monitor and check deep tendon reflexes every 1–2 hours.
- Safety issues:
    - o Avoid giving magnesium via intramuscular injection as it can damage tissues and is very painful.
    - o Avoid giving oral magnesium. Diarrhea ensues and further lowers magnesium levels.
    - o Never give IV magnesium undiluted.

Hypermagnesemia

- Identify and treat the underlying cause.
- Discontinue patient's intake of magnesium-containing foods or substances. In most patients, magnesium levels will return to normal.
- Treat concurrent hypocalcemia, which commonly occurs with hypomagnesemia.
- Infuse magnesium-free fluids intravenously.
- Administer loop diuretics which help to excrete magnesium.
- If severe (e.g., cardiac dysfunction), administer calcium to help alleviate the cardiac problems.
- Administer IV isotonic fluids, a loop diuretic, and discontinuing magnesium-containing drugs can be used in combination in patients with renal failure.
- If severe and symptomatic (e.g., severe neurologic or cardiac symptoms), initiate dialysis. While preparing for dialysis, administer IV fluids, IV calcium, and loop diuretic.
- Safety issue: Do not give patients with renal failure magnesium-containing medications.

Collaborative Interventions (continued)

Patient Safety: Fluid and Electrolytes

Safety precautions are important due to neurologic and hemodynamic instability. The nurse must take the following precautions:

- Know the patient's history and current medications as a fluid or electrolyte disturbance can increase or decrease the effectiveness of medications (e.g., digoxin).
- Use caution and monitor carefully when infusing high concentrations or volumes of fluid and electrolytes to prevent physiologic complications, pain, and phlebitis.
- Evaluate orthostatic hypotension prior to patient's getting out of bed.
- Implement fall precautions in those evaluated to be at high risk. Re-evaluate fall risk often if neuro or muscular function worsens.
- Position the bed to lowest position with bed brakes in locked position.
- Instruct about use of call light prior to getting out of bed, as needed, and keep it within the patient's reach.
- Ensure airway device is at the bedside. Locate emergency equipment for patients with severe fluid and electrolyte imbalances.
- Monitor for changes in mental status and neurologic and muscular function.
- Move frequently needed items (e.g., eye glasses, urinal) close to patient to prevent unnecessary reaching and getting up.
- Use a night-light to improve seeing in the dark.
- Use bedrails without increasing the patient's risk (making them crawl around rails) in those who can safely get up without assistance.
- Check on patient frequently.
- Use a gait belt with patients who experience neuromuscular weakness when they are walking.
- Prevent medication or infusion errors by being attentive to the fluid and electrolyte calculations, dosage administering, infusion rates, and patient responses.
- Prevent common never events in these patients with the following:

- o Catheter-associated urinary tract infections
- o Central line-associated bloodstream infections
- o Pressure ulcers
- o Deep vein thrombosis
- o Air embolism
- o Ventilator-associated pneumonia

Patient Education: Fluid and Electrolytes

- N • Educate the patient about the cause and how to avoid future problems.
- N • Instruct, and consult a dietician as needed, about specific foods that are electrolyte-rich or depleting to assist patient in increasing or decreasing intake as instructed.
- N • Educate the patient regarding specific effects that the electrolyte may have on medication effectiveness or other comorbid conditions (e.g., hypertension, diabetes).
- N • Instruct the patient to become a label reader when shopping.
- N • Educate patient and family about how to substitute herbs, wine, spices, lemon or lime juice, and vinegars as good flavor replacements for electrolyte-rich (e.g., salt) seasonings in cooking.
- N • Instruct the patient on taking electrolyte supplements that are to be taken with meals, with large amounts of water, on an empty stomach, or in conjunction with other supplements.
- N • Educate the patient about signs and symptoms of concern and when to call the health care provider.
- N • Educate patient and family about any needed safety precautions that should continue upon discharge.

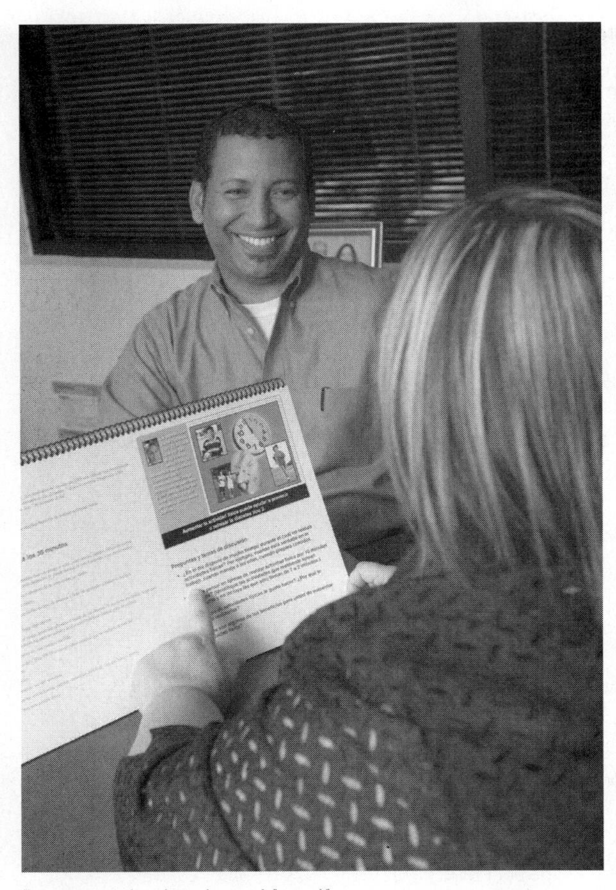

Patients need to be educated for self management to promote wellness at every opportunity.

Source: Amanda Mills/Centers for Disease Control and Prevention

LO3: Summary of Interventions: Fluid and Electrolytes

- The nurse must regularly assess for signs of fluid status and tonicity in each patient.
- In general, patients commonly receive needed fluids that have an IV tonicity opposite of their body's tonicity in order to return the body to an isotonic state.
- Examples of fluid overload signs and symptoms include crackles, edema, increased central venous pressures, and bounding pulses. These patients benefit from hypertonic solutions, which draw excess fluid into their intravascular space for removal by the kidneys. Other collaborative treatments include the use of diuretics or fluid restriction.
- Examples of fluid deficit signs and symptoms include thready pulse, dry skin, loss of skin turgor, tachypnea, and sunken eyes. These patients often benefit from hypotonic solutions that dilute the blood and restore an isotonic state. Fluid boluses, an increase in the IV rate, or free intake of oral fluids can be implemented as well.

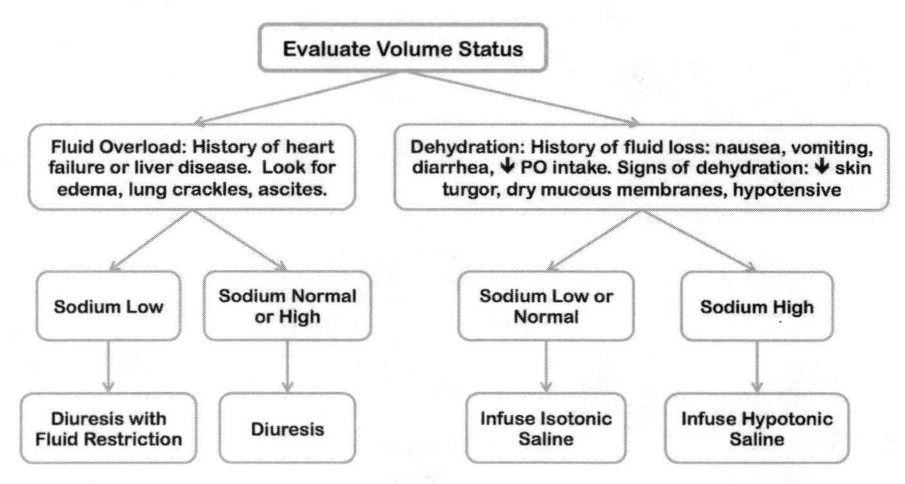

Achieving homeostasis involves balancing fluids and electrolytes. Ideally, the patient is euvolemic (normal volume) with normal concentration of electrolytes. Note that if the patient is stable, fluids and electrolytes can be administered orally.

- Colloids are more expensive than crystalloids for fluid replacement but require much less volume to mobilize fluid from the interstitial into the intravascular spaces.
- The nurse must be aware of signs and symptoms of electrolyte imbalance in the patient and monitor closely for patients at risk of developing electrolyte imbalances.
- Electrolyte abnormalities are best corrected by identifying and correcting the underlying cause. Delay in correcting electrolyte problems can complicate the patient's primary conditions.
- Any patient with an illness, disease process, or injury or who is admitted to the hospital is at risk for developing an electrolyte abnormality.
- It is a nursing responsibility to monitor, assess, and collaboratively intervene in order to maintain or to restore homeostasis to the patient.

LO4: Evaluation of Desired Collaborative Care Outcomes: Fluid and Electrolytes

Evaluation and reassessment should reveal attainment of previously established patient outcomes. In summary:

- Patient's blood pressure is within expected range, skin turgor is appropriate for age, mental status is clear, and fluid intake is balanced with urine output.
- Patient's mental status is clear, no seizure activity has occurred, lab results are within expected range, and cardiac rhythm is regular.
- Patient has intact skin and mucous membranes.
- Patient reports a greater understanding of disease process and demonstrates the ability to balance fluids and electrolytes.
- Patient has no signs of injury and no known falls.

References

Alfonzo, A., Soar, J., MacTier, R., et al. (2014). Clinical practice guidelines: Treatment of acute hyperkalaemia in adults. United Kingdom: UK Renal Association. **www.renal.org/docs/default-source/guidelines-resources/joint-guidelines/treatment-of-acute-hyperkalaemia-in-adults/hyperkalaemia-guideline---march-2014.pdf?sfvrsn=2**

Berenson, J. R. (2002). Treatment of hypercalcemia of malignancy with bisphosphonates. *Seminars in Oncology, 29*(6 Suppl 21), 12–18.

Criss, E. (2007). *A comparison of normal saline and lactated Ringer's IV solution in the treatment of shock (Master's thesis).* **w3.nursing.arizona.edu/Library/Criss_E.pdf**

Daniels, R. (2010). *Nursing fundamentals: Caring and clinical decision-making.* Clifton Park, NY: Delmar Cengage Learning.

Daniels, R., & Nicoll, L. (2012). Fluid, electrolyte and acid-base imbalances. In R. Daniels, & L. Nicoll, *Contemporary medical-surgical nursing* (2nd ed., pp. 240–267). Clifton Park, NY: Delmar Cengage Learning.

Grossman, R., Mukherjee, D., Chaichana, K., et al. (2010). Complications and death among elderly patients undergoing pituitary tumour surgery. *Clinical Endocrinology, 73*, 361–368. doi: 10.1111/j.1365-2265.2010.03813.x

Kee, J. L., Paulanka, B. J., & Polek, C. (2010). *Fluids and electrolytes with clinical applications: A programmed approach* (8th ed.). Clifton Park, NY: Delmar Cengage Learning.

Pantanwala, A. E., Amini, A., & Erstad, B. (2010). Use of hypertonic saline injection in trauma. *American Journal of Health-System Pharmacy, 67*(22), 1920–1928. doi:10.2146/ajhp090523

Philips, C. R., Vinecore, K., Hagg, D. S., et al. (2009). Resuscitation of haemorrhagic shock with normal saline versus lactated Ringer's: Effects on oxygenation, extravascular lung water, and haemodynamics. *Critical Care, 13*(2), R30. doi:10.1186/cc7736

Phillips, L. D. (2005). *Manual of IV therapeutics* (4th ed). Philadelphia, PA: F.A. Davis Company.

Rosen, L. S., Gordon, D., Kaminski, M., et al. (2003). Long-term efficacy and safety of zoledronic acid compared with pamidronate disodium in the treatment of skeletal complications in patients with advanced multiple myeloma or breast carcinoma. *Cancer, 98*(8), 1735–1744. doi:10.1002/cncr.11701

Science and Nature. (2008). *What are diffusion, osmosis and tonicity?* **www.ananyoo.com/article/news-society/science-nature/what-are-diffusion-osmosis-tonicity.html**

Shafiee, M. A., Bohn, D., Hoorn, E. J., & Halperin, M. L. (2003). How to select optimal maintenance intravenous fluid therapy. *QJM: An International Journal of Medicine. 96*(8), 601–610. doi:10.1093/qjmed/hcg101

The Joint Commission. (2015). *National patient safety goals.* **www.jointcommission.org/standards_information/npsgs.aspx**

Thompson, R. C. C. (2005). Physiologic 0.9% saline in the fluid resuscitation of trauma. *Journal of the Royal Army Medical Corps, 151*(3), 146–151.

Tzamaloukas, A. H., Malhotra, D., Rosen, B. H., et al. (2013). Contemporary reviews: Principles of management of severe hyponatremia. *Journal of the American Heart Association.* 2, e005199. doi:10.1161/JAHA.112.005199

Winer, K. K., Ko, C. W., Reynolds, J. C., et al. (2003). Long-term treatment of hypoparathyroidism: a randomized controlled study comparing parathyroid hormone-(1-34) versus calcitriol and calcium. *The Journal of Clinical Endocrinology and Metabolism, 88*(9), 4214–4220.

Clinical Practice Guidelines

(Refer to Guidelines related to the cause of the Fluid and Electrolyte imbalance.)

Cohn, J. N., Kowey, P. R., Whelton, P. K., & Prisant, L. M. (2000). New guidelines for potassium replacement in clinical practice: a contemporary review by the National Council on Potassium in Clinical Practice. *Archives of Internal Medicine, 160*, 2429–2436. **fm.mednet.ucla.edu/IMG/download/NewGuidelinesForPotassiumReplacement.pdf**

Patient Education

Cleveland Clinic Foundation. (2013). *Diseases & conditions: Hyperkalemia.* **my.clevelandclinic.org/disorders/hyperkalemia/hic-hyperkalemia.aspx**

Mayo Clinic Staff. (2011). *Diseases and conditions: Dehydration.* **www.mayoclinic.org/diseases-conditions/dehydration/basics/treatment/con-20030056**

STOP

Go to the online course and complete the NovE-Cases assigned by your instructor for this module.

CARE OF PATIENTS WITH PLATELET AND COAGULATION DISORDERS: DISSEMINATED INTRAVASCULAR COAGULATION AND THROMBOCYTOPENIA

Learning Outcomes for Platelet and Coagulation Disorders

When you complete this lesson, you will be able to:

1. Recognize the clinical relevance of platelet and coagulation disorders.
2. Consider the pathophysiology, etiology, risk factors, and clinical presentation of platelet and coagulation disorders that determine the priority patient concerns.
3. Determine the most urgent and important nursing interventions and patient education required in caring for a patient with platelet and coagulation disorders.
4. Evaluate attainment of desired collaborative care outcomes for a patient with platelet and coagulation disorders.

LO1:

What Are the Disorders of Hemostasis?

- Hemostasis is the response that limits blood loss after blood vessel damage. Properly functioning platelets and coagulation factors present in the blood are responsible for hemostasis.
- Disorders of hemostasis result from:
    - o Thrombocytopenia and platelet dysfunction: acquired or congenital
    - o Disorders of coagulation factors: acquired, congenital, or induced as complication of another condition

LO1:

Clinical Relevance: Hemostasis

- With increasing use of antiplatelet agents, warfarin, and coagulation pathway inhibitors to prevent development of thrombosis, there is a corresponding increase in hemorrhage.
- Other causes for disorders of hemostasis include common clinical conditions such as sepsis and liver disease.

LO2:

Pathophysiology: Platelet and Coagulation Disorders

- Blood contains factors and platelets that promote coagulation. These factors normally circulate in an inactive form.
- Endothelial cells that line blood vessel lumen are in contact with blood. Healthy endothelial cells prevent adhesion of platelets and clotting with a number of anticoagulant factors.
- Damage to the endothelium of blood vessels, however, exposes tissue such as collagen that promotes clot formation. This damage results in a cascade of events that can result in clot formation.
- Disruption in the balance of coagulation and anticoagulation can result in either clot formation or excessive bleeding.

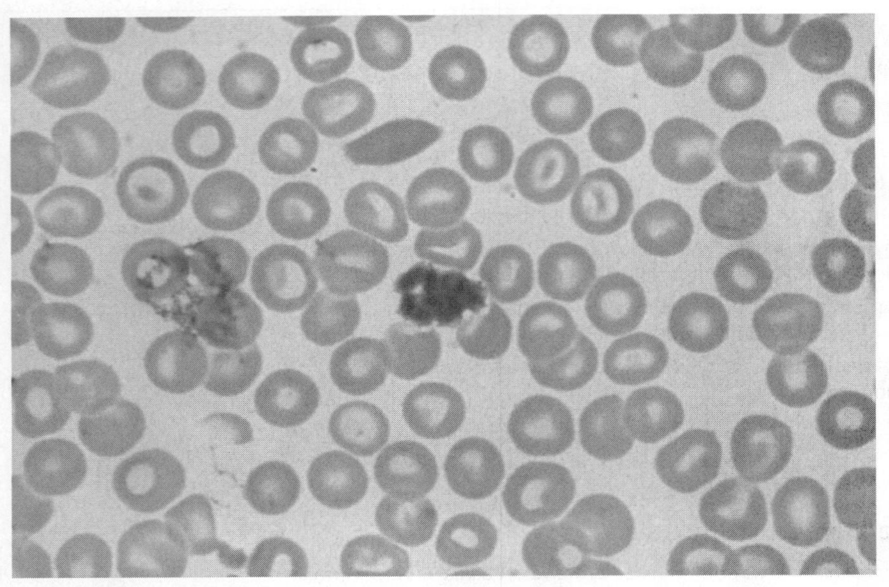

The blood smear shows a clump of platelets that can be mistaken for a foreign body.
Source: CDC/Dr. Mae Melvin

- When damage to the endothelium occurs, it results in vasoconstriction, which can limit blood loss.
- Exposed tissue such as collagen causes platelets to adhere and release substances (degranulation) that promote vasoconstriction. The buildup of platelets with further degranulation causes continued adherence of more platelets and more clotting factors. This process promotes clot formation.
- Damaged tissue also activates the procoagulant factors, ultimately resulting in a clot consisting of a mesh of fibrin and platelets.

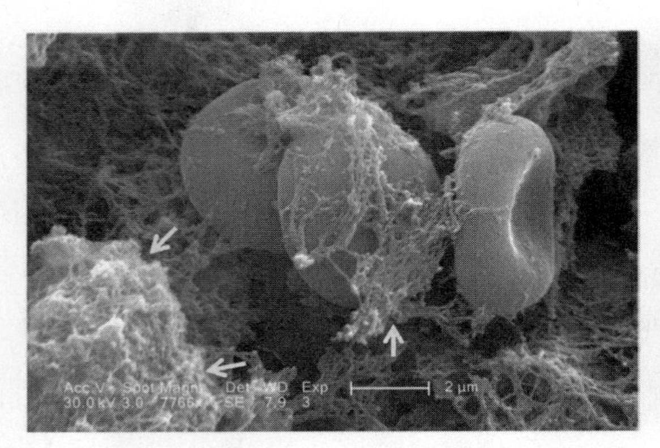

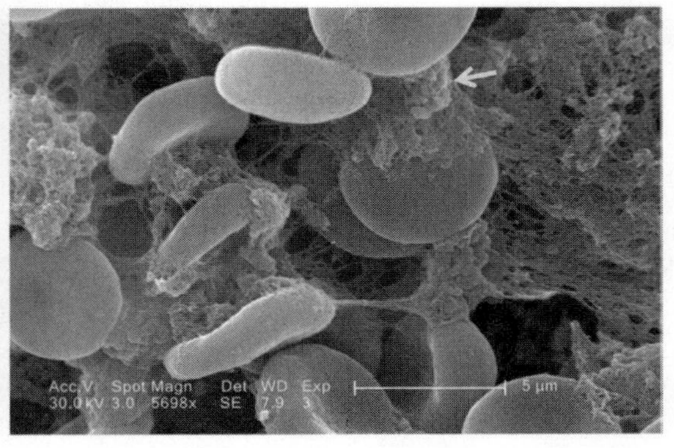

Left: Red blood cells are the three circular cells in the middle. They are trapped in the chunks of debris-appearing fibrin clumps (arrows), which are key components in blood clot formation. They form the mesh-like latticework that strengthens the clot. Right: Over time, the clot grows and strengthens. Platelets are the smaller whitish specks (arrow) caught in the fibrin mesh.
Source: *(both)* CDC/Janice Haney Carr

Coagulation Cascade

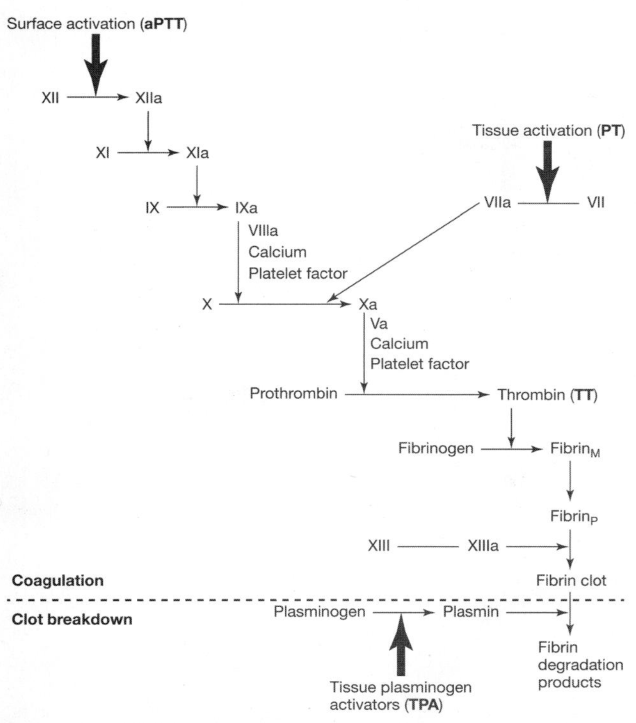

Diagram from NIH illustrating the progression of substances involved in coagulation and clot breakdown.

Pathophysiology: Platelet and Coagulation Disorders (continued)

Hemostasis

Hemostasis is the body's mechanism to stop bleeding after a blood vessel is damaged. Hemostasis requires:

- Vasoconstriction
- Activation of platelets to adhere, degranulate, and release cytoplasmic granules like serotonin, thromboxane A_2, and adenosine diphosphate (ADP).
- ADP attracts more platelets. Thromboxane A_2 causes more platelet aggregation and degranulation. The positive feedback cycle continues and creates a platelet plug.
- Activation of coagulation factors and cascade is initiated. A fibrin mesh results.
- RBCs and platelets are caught in the fibrin mesh to form a blood clot.

Injury & Vasoconstriction

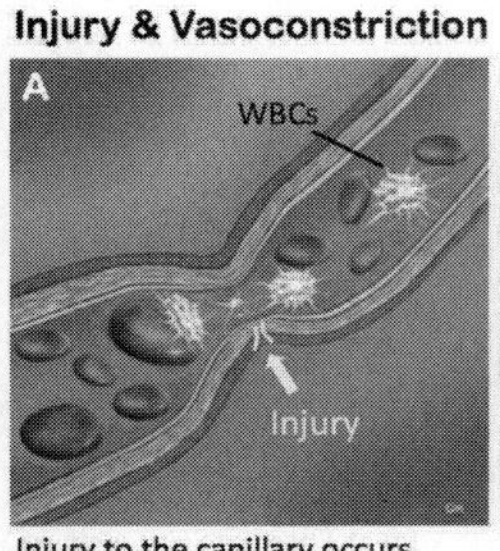

Injury to the capillary occurs. Reflex vasoconstriction is the first mechanism activated to stop the bleeding.

Platelet Adhesion

B
Thromboxane A2
Serotonin
ADP
Granules
Platelets

Collagen is exposed and promote platelet adhesion and aggregation at the injury site. Platelets release granules that attract more platelets and aggregation.

Platelet Plug Forms

C

Positive feedback loop of platelets releasing granules which in turn attract more platelets creates a platelet plug in the vessel.

Coagulation

Clotting cascade activate

Intrinsic and extrinsic clotting factors become activated to initiate the coagulation cascade, turning fibrinogen into fibrin to form a loose mesh.

Blood Clot Formation

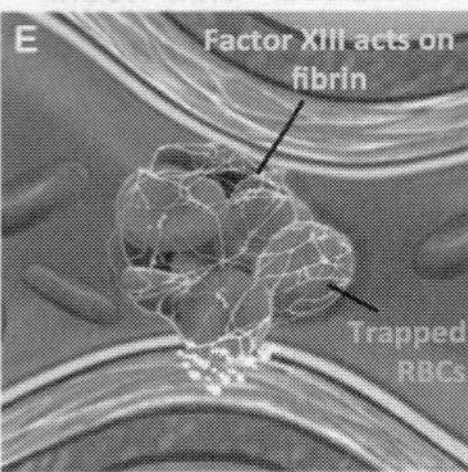

Factor XIII converts fibrin threads (yellow) into a tight mesh of fibers that "glue" the hemostatic plug together. RBCs and platelets continue to get caught to form the blood clot.

Recirculation

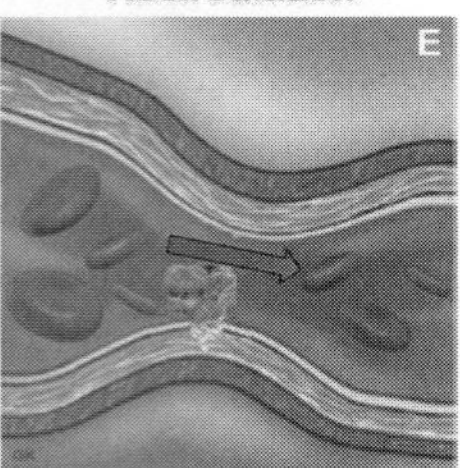

If the clot resolves, circulation may be reestablished if tissue ischemia is not severe.

This series of images describes normal hemostasis or the body's mechanism for the formation of blood clots. A damaged blood vessel initiates the clotting cascade as described in detail.

Source: Courtesy of George Kyriakidis/Santa Ana, CA

Propensity for Bleeding

The following conditions result in a propensity toward excessive bleeding:

- Inhibition or lack of clotting factors:
  - Von Willebrand syndrome is an inherited or rarely acquired deficiency or defect in a key clotting factor; failure to produce the von Willebrand factor can lead to excessive bleeding.
    - It can be experienced for the first time as life-threatening blood loss during a menstrual period or childbirth.
    - It is additionally problematic because it is commonly underdiagnosed in women, on average for 16 years.
    - Heavy bleeding is a common female menstrual symptom, but is commonly dismissed as "normal" by women who have it and don't know.
    - It is the most common bleeding disorder among women.
  - Hemophilia: This is an inherited disorder that is caused by a lack of sufficient amounts of clotting factor VIII (hemophilia A) or clotting factor IX (hemophilia B or Christmas disease). Hemophilia A is most common and about 60% of patients have a severe form.
  - Although primarily inherited, one-third of patients have no family history of hemophilia and experience a spontaneous genetic mutation.
  - Excessive bleeding can result from a major injury to spontaneous bleeding episodes, depending on severity of the defect.
- Platelet dysfunction or low platelets (thrombocytopenia)
- A combination of both
- If coagulation factors are normal, bleeding is uncommon if platelet counts are >50,000.

Concept Check

1. **Hemostasis requires activation of platelets and coagulation factors. What other mechanism is required?**

   A. Vasoconstriction

   B. Thrombocytopenia

   C. Fibrin degradation

   D. Tissue plasminogen activation

Answer question

LO2:

Risk Factors: Platelet and Coagulation Disorders

Risk factors can vary, depending on the type of bleeding disorder that a patient is predisposed to. Risk factors, in general, include:

- Inherited coagulation disorders (e.g., von Willebrand, hemophilia)
- Medications such as heparin or antibiotics
- Sepsis, major injury, or trauma
- Complications with labor and delivery
- Cancer
- Blood transfusion
- Severe liver disease
- Vitamin K deficiency

LO2:

Causes: Platelet and Coagulation Disorders

Coagulation Factor Disorders

- **Liver disease:** The liver synthesizes many of the coagulation factors. Patients with liver disease are often deficient in multiple clotting factors, resulting in a predisposition to bleeding.
- **Von Willebrand disease (vWD):** The lack of this protein, a clotting factor, is essential in the coagulation cascade. Degrees of severity depend on the type of defect in the protein and on the level of its production.
- **Hemophilia:** This lack of clotting factor VIII (hemophilia A) or clotting factor IX (hemophilia B or Christmas disease) causes this clotting disorder.
- **Disseminated intravascular coagulation:** DIC is an unregulated activation of coagulation factors that is widespread and causes clotting as well as depletion of coagulation factors and bleeding.
- **Medications:**
  - o **Thrombin inhibitors:** Dabigatran
  - o **Factor Xa inhibitors:** Rivaroxaban, apixaban
  - o **Warfarin** works by preventing recycling of vitamin K, which is needed for several coagulation factors (factors II, VII, IX, and X).
  - o **Heparin** binds and activates antithrombin III, which inactivates several clotting factors, including thrombin and factor Xa.

Platelet Disorders

- **Low platelets** (thrombocytopenia)
  - o Decreased production due to
    - ■ Chemotherapy
    - ■ Alcohol
    - ■ Infections (e.g., HIV)
    - ■ Radiotherapy
    - ■ Bone marrow problems
  - o Increased platelet destruction by antibodies
    - ■ **Immune or idiopathic thrombocytopenia (ITP)**
    - ■ Heparin-induced antibodies with platelet destruction
- **Platelet dysfunction caused by:**
  - o Uremia from kidney failure
  - o Sepsis
  - o Medications
    - ■ Aspirin
    - ■ Nonsteroidal medications (e.g., ibuprofen)

LO2:

Assessment Findings: Platelet and Coagulation Disorders

Patients with disorders of hemostasis, either coagulation disorder or platelet dysfunction (e.g., thrombocytopenia), may bleed spontaneously or may develop excessive bleeding from relatively small lesions:

- Brain hemorrhage
- Skin: petechiae, ecchymosis
- Bleeding from mucous membranes or gums. Recurrent nosebleeds are common.
- Excessive bruising
- Heavy bleeding
- Gastrointestinal bleeding
- Bleeding into muscle or joints

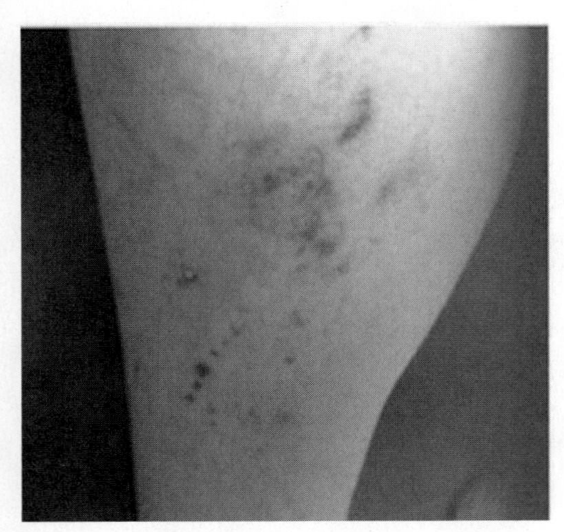

Petechial hemorrhages, seen in this photo, can warn of a coagulation problem.
Source: Courtesy of K. Kyriakidis

Concept Check

2. **Which factor has not been demonstrated to increase risk for platelet disorders?**
   A. Alcohol use
   B. Tobacco use
   C. Infection
   D. Chemotherapy

Answer question

LO2:

Diagnostics: Platelet and Coagulation Disorders

- Prothrombin time (PT) and international normalized ratio (INR): measure activity of factors X, VII, thrombin, and fibrinogen. They can be elevated with liver disease, warfarin therapy, and DIC.
- Activated partial thromboplastin time (PTT): measures activity of fibrinogen, thrombin, and factors V, VIII, IX, X, XI, and XII. It may be elevated with heparin, hemophilia, or DIC.
- Complete blood count (CBC): determines platelet count
- Bleeding time to assess platelet function: This is a crude test to measure how long it takes for bleeding to completely stop after a small incision is made in the forearm or the ear lobe.

Priority Patient Concerns and Desired Collaborative Care Outcomes: Platelet and Coagulation Disorders

Prior to caring for patients with platelet and coagulation disorders, it is important to prioritize the patient's concerns that must guide the nursing care plan and interventions. Care for the patient is ordered and organized in accordance with the patient's priority and urgent needs. Desired collaborative care outcomes in patients with platelet and coagulation disorders typically include:

1. Patient will explain and take precautions to prevent bleeding.
2. Patient will experience decreased pain.

Considering these important care outcomes, prepare a list of the major 3–6 priority patient concerns or nursing diagnoses for patients with platelet and coagulation disorders. Be prepared to participate in a discussion of this list and/or to submit them as an assignment, as determined by your faculty. Resources you may find helpful in this assignment can include this lesson, the references, resources on nursing care plans, and standard nursing diagnoses manuals.

LO3:

Collaborative Interventions: Platelet and Coagulation Disorders

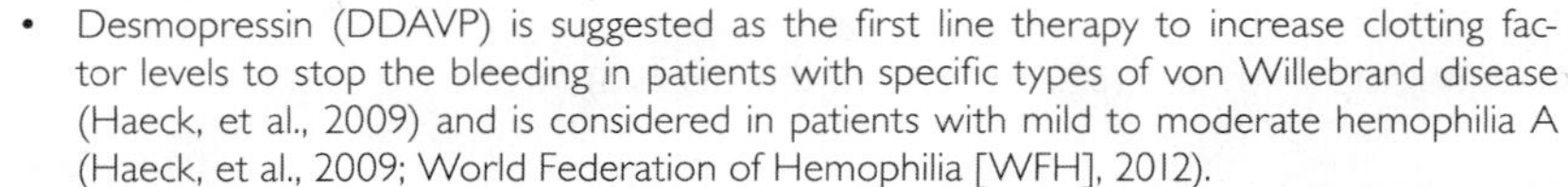

- Desmopressin (DDAVP) is suggested as the first line therapy to increase clotting factor levels to stop the bleeding in patients with specific types of von Willebrand disease (Haeck, et al., 2009) and is considered in patients with mild to moderate hemophilia A (Haeck, et al., 2009; World Federation of Hemophilia [WFH], 2012).
- Replacement therapy in patients not responding to DDAVP include clotting factor VIII (for hemophilia A), clotting factor IX (for hemophilia B), or von Willebrand factor.
- Fresh frozen plasma for coagulation disorders
- Regular infusions, depending on severity include clotting factor VIII (for hemophilia A), clotting factor IX (for hemophilia B), or von Willebrand factor.
- Prophylactic factor replacement infusions are recommended to prevent bleeding and joint destruction. Short-term prophylaxis, which may be combined with intensive physiotherapy, can interrupt bleeding (WFH, 2012).
- Educate the patient and/or family to monitor the environment for safety issues:
  - Select lower impact sports and activities.
  - Choose organized sports activities (e.g., supervised, necessary safety equipment) over "pick up" games; choose low contact sports, especially when injuries worsen during teens.
  - Strengthening, conditioning, and stretching exercises are central in injury prevention.
- Assess for and manage pain related to bleeding into tissues and joints:
  - Analgesics as needed
  - Cyclooxygenase-2 (COX-2) inhibitors may be useful.
- Safety issues include avoiding the use of nonsteroidal anti-inflammatory (NSAIDs) medications.
- Monitor for caregiver role strain and implement interventions for relief.
- Vitamin K (oral or IV) to reverse anticoagulation with warfarin.
- Platelet transfusion for thrombocytopenia and platelet dysfunction

Patient Education

Patient education should include:

- How to deal with minor bleeds, including clean the cut, apply prolonged pressure until bleeding subsides, and cover with bandage or dressing
- When bleeding requires medical attention, including deep cuts, bleeding that appears internal, and bleeding in joints, so that treatment can be administered
- Instruction about bruising easily, having recurrent and prolonged nosebleeds, potential for excessive after procedures (e.g., tooth extraction, childbirth, minor surgery, menstrual bleeding)
- Caution about using aspirin or any medication that aggravates bleeding. Instruct the patient about the safety of using acetaminophen for pain.
- In severe bleeding disorders, routine clotting factor replacements may be used (possibly administered by the patient) as prophylaxis.
- Clotting factors that are not from human blood sources (known as recombinant factors) are safer as they do not place the patient at risk for blood borne diseases (e.g., HIV, hepatitis).
- Home therapy should be considered in those who may need immediate clotting factors. It can reduce pain and hospitalization. Supervision and education are key in the initiation of home therapy (WFH, 2012).
- Collaborative efforts are needed between health care providers and dentists to develop a homeostasis management plan prior to invasive dental extractions or surgery (WFH, 2012).
- Exercise to promote health, fitness, and self-esteem. If exercise is not possible, weight-bearing activities can help preserve bone density (WFH, 2012).
- Genetic counseling for patients with hereditary disorders (e.g., von Willebrand, hemophilia) prior to pregnancy when possible
- Support regarding psychosocial issues because bleeding disorders can impact the patient's work, social, physical, emotional, and financial aspects of life. Support groups may be helpful to many.

LO4:

Evaluation of Desired Collaborative Care Outcomes: Platelet and Coagulation Disorders

Evaluation and reassessment should reveal attainment of previously established patient outcomes. In summary:

- Patient reports adopting lifestyle modifications to reduce risk of bleeding caused by ineffective protection.
- Patient reports preventive measures and prompt recognition of pain onset with prompt treatment have reduced episodes of pain.

Specific Coagulation Disorders

The following coagulation disorders are discussed in more detail:

- Disseminated intravascular coagulation (DIC)
- Platelet disorders

LO1:

What Is Disseminated Intravascular Coagulation (DIC)?

- DIC is a syndrome that involves the unregulated activation of the clotting system that results in thrombosis, particularly in the microvasculature, as well as bleeding complications.
- The activation of the clotting cascade is widespread (disseminated) or systemic.
- DIC often leads to multiple organ dysfunction syndrome (MODS).
- DIC is always a complication of other underlying illnesses (e.g., sepsis) that trigger this abnormal clotting cascade.
- DIC can be acute and rapidly progressive or chronic and insidious.
- Chronic DIC is commonly related to the presence of tumors or aortic aneurysms.

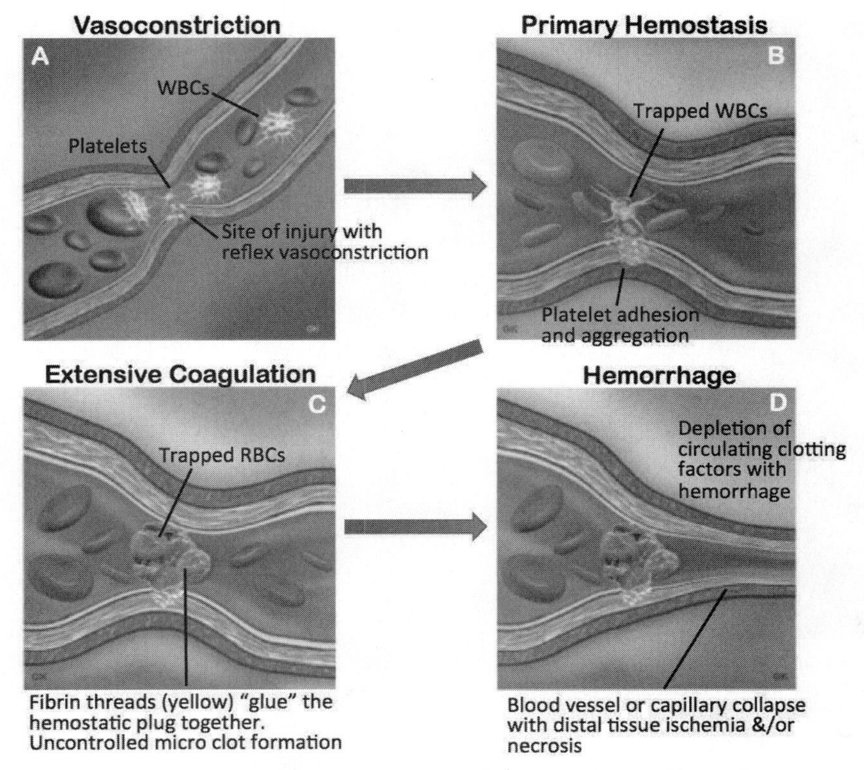

This series depicts the progression from normal blood flow to coagulation and hemorrhage.
Source: Courtesy of George Kyriakidis/Santa Ana, CA

LO1:

Clinical Relevance: DIC

- The incidence of DIC is about 1% in hospitalized patients.
- It is associated with a high mortality rate.
- DIC is always a complication that can result from a large variety of illnesses. The most prominent include cancers, infections, and particularly sepsis.

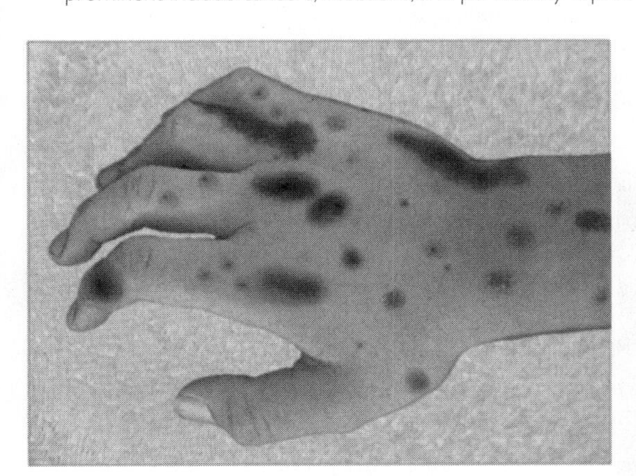

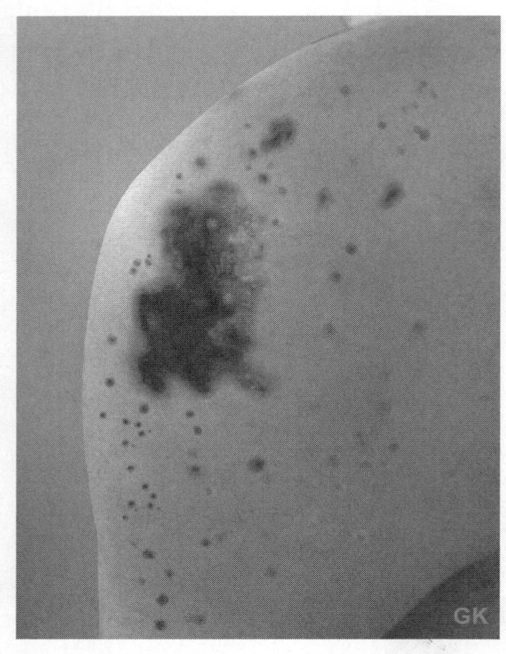

Both photos show purpura that manifests in patients with DIC. The photos of a hand (top) and shoulder (bottom) are of a patient who is afflicted with disseminated intravascular coagulation that is associated with Meningococcal septicemia.
Source: *(both)* Courtesy of George Kyriakidis/Santa Ana, CA

LO2:

Pathophysiology: DIC

- The clotting cascade can be triggered by the release of cytokines from tissue or endotoxins from infections. DIC occurs as a complication of other conditions that trigger the release of cytokines or endotoxins rather than being a specific disease.
- Normally, there is a balance between clotting (or coagulation) and anticoagulation (or fibrinolysis which breaks down blood clots). Clotting tends to be localized to areas of trauma or bleeding. However, in DIC, there is an overwhelming widespread activation of clotting factors that leads to formation of microthrombi.
- Microvascular blood clots occur systemically and are deposited throughout the small blood vessels of tissues and organs. The microcirculatory interference with perfusion causes tissue and organ hypoxia, ischemia, and tissue damage.
- This process can lead to multiple organ dysfunction syndrome (MODS).

DIC with Distal Tissue Necrosis

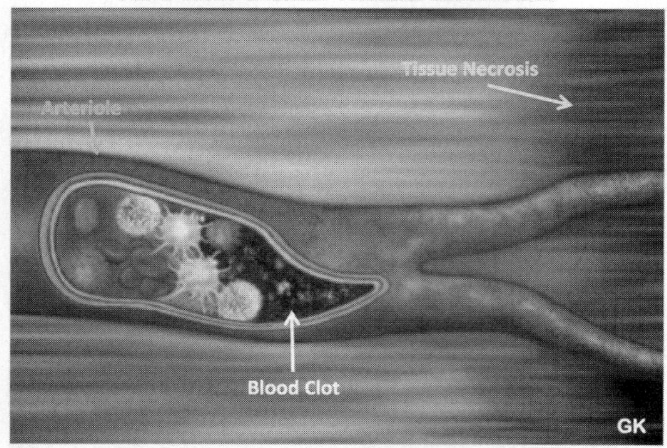

This image depicts DIC with arteriolar blood clotting off the blood flow. The darkening tissue distal to the clot reveals prolonged oxygen deprivation with necrosis.

Source: Courtesy of George Kyriakidis/Santa Ana, CA

- Large amounts of thrombin are produced and fibrin is deposited throughout the blood vessels (see photo).
- Platelet count drops when DIC is unrecognized, untreated, and/or extensive because platelets are consumed in formation of thrombi.
- Red blood cells are damaged by fibrin strands.
- Depletion of clotting factors, which become consumed in the disseminated clotting, can subsequently result in bleeding. Bleeding can be excessive and widespread.
- Patients may bleed from gums, orifices, IV sites, and/or incisions. They may also develop spontaneous hemorrhages in the brain or spinal cord, and bruise easily.

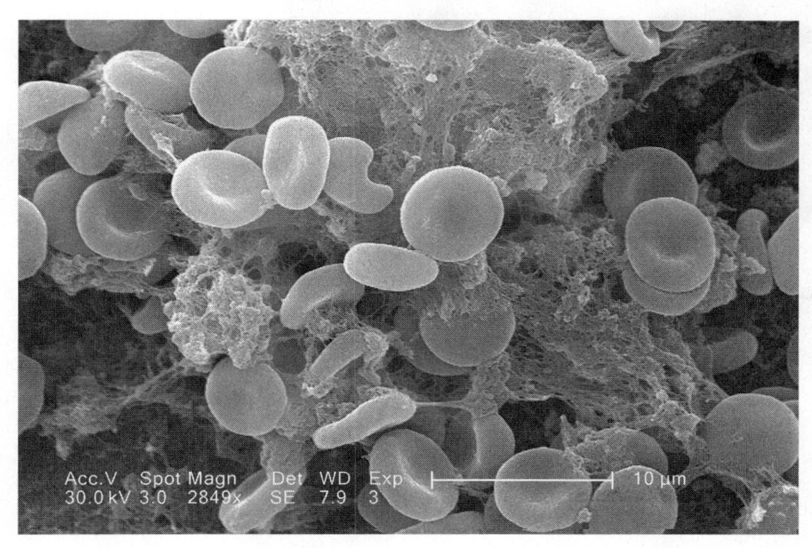

The unregulated activation of the clotting cascade results in large amounts of thrombin production and deposition of fibrin throughout the vasculature. Red blood cells can be destroyed by fibrin strands. When the extensive microcoagulation (photo) binds up large amounts of clotting factors, the patient can bleed profusely from all over the body, internally and externally. Here, large numbers of RBCs are trapped in fibrin, platelets, and other clotting factors.
Source: CDC/Janice Haney Carr

LO2:

Risk Factors and Causes: DIC

- **Sepsis and septic shock (most common)**
- Infections
- Obstetric diseases and complications (e.g., low platelets syndrome [HEELP], abruptio placentae, amniotic fluid emboli, retained placenta)
- Trauma or severe burns
- Severe brain injury
- Toxic reactions (e.g., transfusion reactions, organ transplant rejection)
- Liver disease and/or failure
- Pancreatitis
- Hyperthermia and heatstroke
- Malignancies
- Aortic aneurysms
- Snake bites

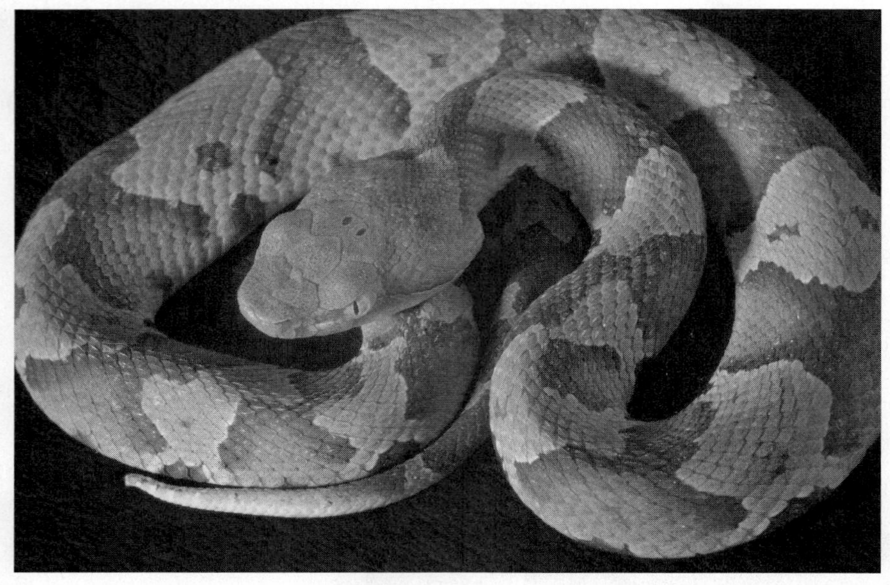

Poisonous snake bites, like one from this Copperhead, commonly disrupt the clotting cascade and cause hemorrhage. The consequences can lead to DIC.
Source: CDC/James Gathany

LO2:

Diagnostics: DIC

Diagnostics include a number of tests because there is no single diagnostic that is capable of diagnosing DIC. Diagnostics can include:

- Patient history and physical exam findings commonly suggest both the presence of DIC as well as the underlying cause.
- **Labs:**
  - CBC: typically low platelet count
  - Smear may show fragments of RBCs (schistocytes) caused by fibrin strands.
  - Clotting studies: PT and PTT are usually elevated.
  - Fibrin degradation products, D-dimer: Elevation of both is highly suggestive of DIC.
  - Chemistry with potential hyperkalemia, hypocalcemia, and hypomagnesium
  - Lactate level may be elevated from sepsis or ischemia caused by DIC.
  - Blood gases may reveal metabolic acidosis due to poor perfusion.
- **Blood cultures**, if sepsis is source
- **Imaging:** x-ray, CT
  - Useful only in detecting underlying causes, complications, or locations of internal bleeding

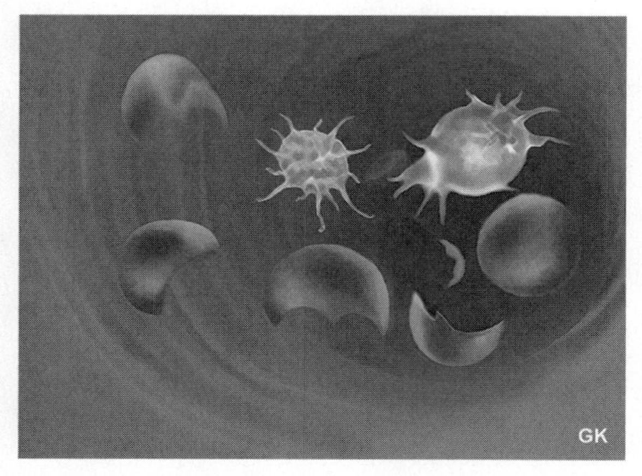

Fragments of red cells (schistocytes or helmet cells) are seen in a blood smear from a patient with hemolytic anemia and associated DIC.
Source: Courtesy of George Kyriakidis/Santa Ana, CA

Concept Check

3. What is the most common cause of DIC?

A. Abruptio placentae

B. Pancreatitis

C. Sepsis

D. Malignancy

Answer question

Priority Patient Concerns and Desired Collaborative Care Outcomes: DIC

Prior to caring for patients with DIC, it is important to prioritize the patient's concerns that must guide the nursing care plan and interventions. Care for the patient is ordered and organized in accordance with the patient's priority and urgent needs. Desired collaborative care outcomes in patients with DIC typically include:

1. Patient will remain normovolemic.
2. Patient will not experience bleeding.
3. Patient will report adequate pain control.
4. Patient will not experience shock.
5. Patient will demonstrate adequate perfusion.

Considering these important care outcomes, prepare a list of the major 3–6 priority patient concerns or nursing diagnoses for patients with DIC. Be prepared to participate in a discussion of this list and/or to submit them as an assignment, as determined by your faculty. Resources you may find helpful in this assignment can include this lesson, the references, resources on nursing care plans, and standard nursing diagnoses manuals.

LO3:

Collaborative Interventions: DIC

Evidence-based practice guideline recommendations are included below and are helpful in most patients except those with solid cancers (Wada, et al., 2013):

- Care and management of the patient varies and is focused on treating the underlying cause (e.g., antibiotics for sepsis) (Wada, et al., 2013).
- The primary goal of care is reduction in morbidity and mortality.

Interventions can include:

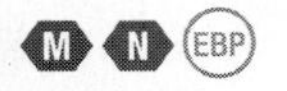

- Blood, fresh frozen plasma, platelets, and clotting factor replacements for those who have evidence of significant hemorrhage

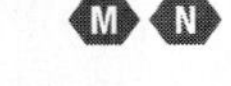

- Correcting laboratory abnormalities such as a high PT or PTT is not an indication for transfusion unless the patient is actively bleeding.

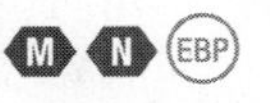

- Heparin for those with thrombosis without hemorrhage. Low molecular weight heparin is preferred.

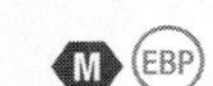

- Antifibrinolytic agents are not generally suggested.

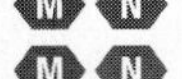

- Antibiotics, if infection is present or suspected

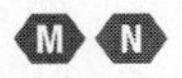

- Surgical intervention, if indicated

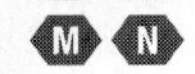

- Serial monitoring of lab tests provides information about dynamic changes, the degree of clotting factor activation and consumption, and the patient's responsiveness to therapies.

Symptom Management and Comfort Care

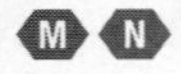

- Hemodynamic stabilization: Patients with DIC are critically ill and quickly become hemodynamically unstable. Symptom management, in addition to routine nursing care, can include:
    - IV fluid infusions and monitoring the patient's responses
    - Vasopressors may be needed if perfusion and cardiac output are not supported by fluids.
    - Oxygen therapy and/or mechanical ventilation may be necessary if oxygenation and/or ventilation become compromised.
    - Warming blankets may be needed for hypothermia.
    - Continuous monitoring for early recognition should include pain, cardiac rhythm, vital signs, mental status, hemodynamics as indicated, intake and output, physical exam changes, signs of bleeding and/or bruising (e.g., abdominal distention, petechiae), peripheral circulation (e.g., capillary refill, warmth, pulses), signs of any organ dysfunction, and discontinue oral feedings if the patient is unable to tolerate.

- Safety and bleeding precautions need to include care that prevents unnecessary bleeding:
    - Avoid IM injections.
    - Avoid unnecessary venopuncture sticks.
    - Minimize or postpone invasive procedures.
    - Avoid strong adhesive tapes that can tear the skin when removed.
    - Avoid the use of a rectal thermometer.
    - Avoid administration of medications that cause a propensity to bleed (e.g., aspirin, ibuprofen, warfarin).
    - Hold direct pressure on bleeding sites for 5–10 minutes to prevent bleeding.
    - Use care when turning or moving the patient. Use a drawsheet to move the patient and avoid skin tears from shearing.
    - Use a soft toothbrush for mouth care. Avoid mouthwash.
    - Moisten lips with lip balm or petroleum jelly.

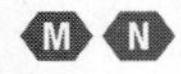

- Prevention of never events as patients with DIC are at high risk for such events (e.g., urinary catheter-associated infections, ventilator associated pneumonia, pressure ulcer)

- Comfort care may include:
    - Schedule the patient's care to provide rest and sleep. Recruit family members to assist in ensuring that the patient is not disturbed during sleep.
    - Minimize noise while supporting meaningful interaction with friends and family as tolerated to manage sensory overload and deprivation.
    - Provide emotional support and reassurance in an honest, open, and comforting manner.
    - Educate the patient and family about the patient's condition, therapies, constant care, and changes in the patient's condition.
    - Ongoing explanations are needed to respond to the myriad of questions.
    - Discuss advanced directives to receive guidance in situations where curative treatments may become futile.

LO4:

Evaluation of Desired Collaborative Care Outcomes: DIC

Evaluation and reassessment should reveal attainment of previously established patient outcomes. In summary:

- Patient's blood pressure is within expected range, mentation is returning to pre-DIC state, skin turgor is as expected, and urine output balances with fluid intake.
- Patient shows no signs of bleeding.
- Patient reports that measures to control pain are adequate.
- Patient is hemodynamically stable.
- Patient's skin is intact, mentation is returning to pre-DIC state, and kidney and gastrointestinal function are as expected.

LO1:

What is Thrombocytopenia?

- Platelets are the smallest and lightest blood cells. The small size tends to push the platelet toward the endothelial layer of the blood vessel.
- Thrombocytopenia is defined as a decreased number of <100,000 circulating platelets. (This definition varies by organization.)
- Normal platelet count is between 130,000 to 400,000.
- The main danger of thrombocytopenia is bleeding. Platelets are a key component of clotting, and any reduction can interfere with control of bleeding.

LO1: Clinical Relevance: Thrombocytopenia

- The key reason to know about thrombocytopenia is the bleeding risk that is present with low platelets.
- Thrombocytopenia is common with chemotherapy, radiation, and certain types of cancers, such as blood cancers.
- Many other conditions cause thrombocytopenia.
- Patients are typically referred to and evaluated by a hematologist.

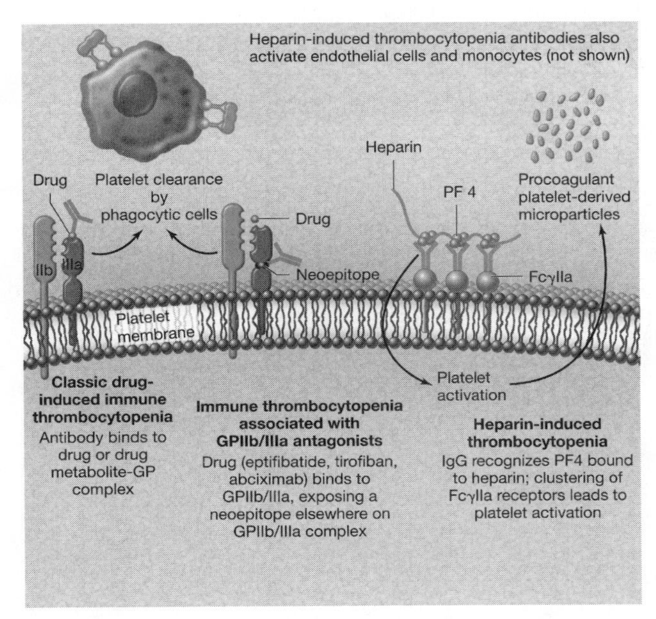

This image illustrates the various mechanisms by which thrombocytopenia can be induced by the use of drugs.

LO2: Causes: Thrombocytopenia

- Thrombocytopenia may be due to either decreased production or increased destruction of platelets.
- Bleeding is uncommon if the platelet count is 50,000 or higher.
- Platelet concentrations of <10,000 are frequently associated with episodes of spontaneous bleeding.
- Hemorrhages can be severe with platelet counts in the range of 5,000 to 10,000.

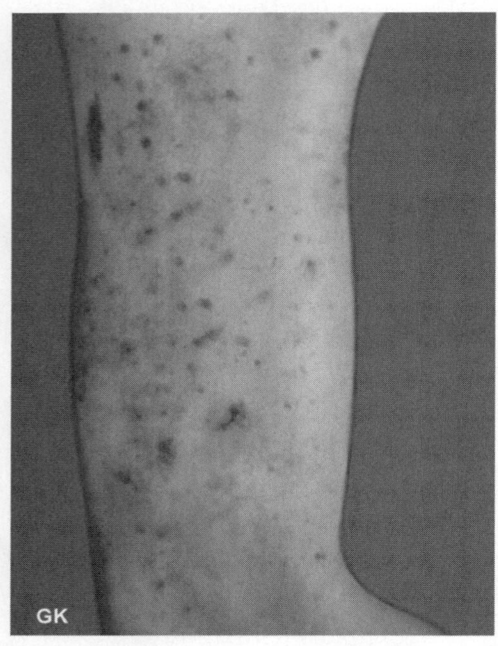

This patient has ITP with purpura and petechiae on his arm.
Source: Courtesy of George Kyriakidis/Santa Ana, CA

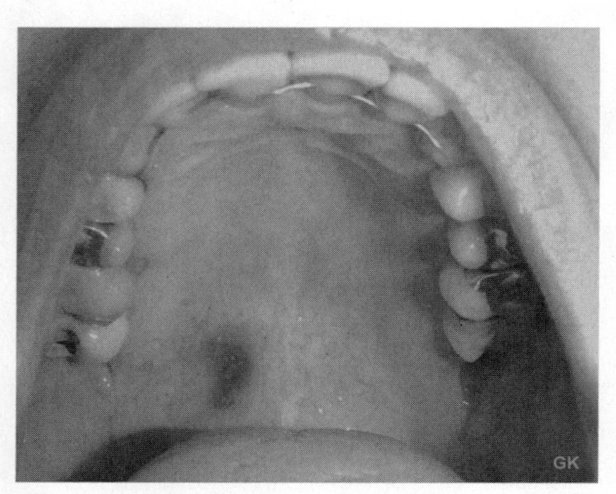

Patient is shown with his mouth open and you are looking at a hematoma of the soft palate. Bleeding within the oral cavity is not unusual in thrombocytopenia.
Source: Courtesy of George Kyriakidis/Santa Ana, CA

Decreased Production

Conditions that cause a decrease in the number of circulating platelets essential for clotting are numerous:

- Inborn causes:
  - Inherited thrombocytopenias (rare)
  - Fanconi anemia
- Acquired causes:
  - Aplastic anemia
  - Bone marrow infiltration (carcinoma, leukemia, myelofibrosis, myelodysplasia, tuberculosis)
  - Ionizing radiation and other causes of myelosuppression
  - Cytotoxic chemotherapy
  - Drugs (trimethoprim-sulfamethoxazole, gold, thiazide diuretics, estrogens, interferons)
  - Deficiency of vitamins and other essential trace elements or nutrients (B_{12}, folate, iron)
  - Viral infections
  - Prolonged heavy alcohol consumption
  - Pregnancy

Increased Consumption or Destruction

The following causes result in the destruction of platelets in the body so that they cannot be used to form clots:

- **Inborn causes**
  - o Nonimmunologic: hemolytic disease of the newborn, prematurity, maternal preeclampsia, infections
  - o Immunologic: alloimmune neonatal thrombocytopenia, maternal idiopathic thrombocytopenia purpura (ITP)
- **Acquired causes**
  - o Nonimmunologic: infections, disseminated intravascular coagulation, thrombotic thrombocytopenic purpura, hemolytic-uremic syndrome, drug-induced overconsumption of platelets
  - o Immunologic: drug-induced, following blood transfusion, chronic and acute ITP
  - o Antibody production in response to heparin: heparin-induced thrombocytopenia (HIT)
  - o Sequestration of platelets by the spleen in patients with a large spleen (e.g., patients with liver cirrhosis)

LO2:

Assessment Findings: Thrombocytopenia

- Symptoms of thrombocytopenia can be any that are related to bleeding:
  - o Nosebleeds
  - o Petechiae
  - o Easy bruising
  - o Spontaneous bleeding

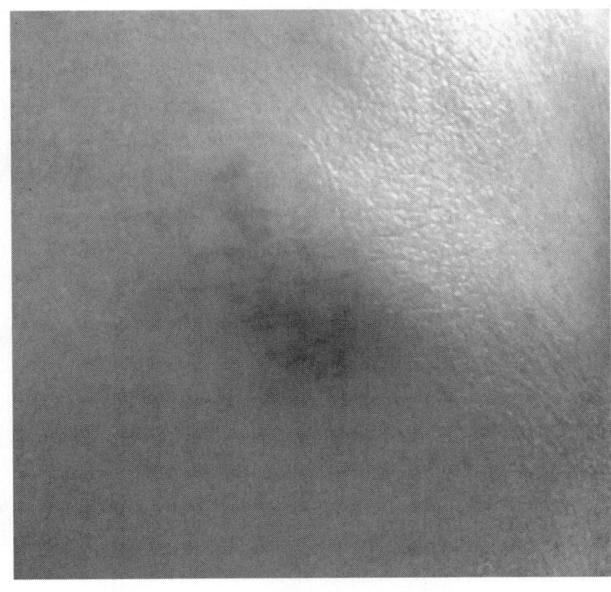

LO2:

Diagnostics: Thrombocytopenia

- CBC showing low platelet count. Anemia and leukopenia may suggest a condition suppressing the bone marrow.
- Blood smear showing small platelets may suggest problems with production. Large platelets are more likely due to increased destruction of platelets. Presence of schistocytes may indicate DIC.

- Hepatitis C virus and HIV tests are recommended in patients newly diagnosed with immune thrombocytopenia (Neunert, et al., 2011).

EBP

- Bone marrow biopsy may be done but is not recommended in patients where the cause of thrombocytopenia is unclear (Neunert, et al., 2011).

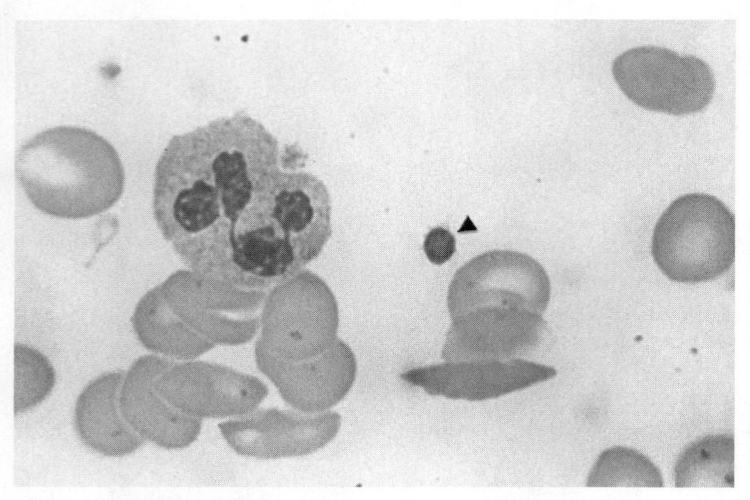

This photo shows an aggregation of platelets (arrow), which are very small elements in the blood. The large, purple-stained cell is a leukocyte and there are numerous red blood cells (pale, pinkish-beige cells). Blood smears like this can assist in diagnostics.
Source: Centers for Disease Control and Prevention/Dr. F. Gilbert

Concept Check

4. Which condition leads to thrombocytopenia due to increased destruction?

A. Faconi anemia

B. Heavy alcohol consumption

C. Blood transfusion

D. Leukemia

Answer question

Priority Patient Concerns and Desired Collaborative Care Outcomes: Thrombocytopenia

Prior to caring for patients with thrombocytopenia, it is important to prioritize the patient's concerns that must guide the nursing care plan and interventions. Care for the patient is ordered and organized in accordance with the patient's priority and urgent needs. Desired collaborative care outcomes in patients with thrombocytopenia typically include:

1. Patient will report adequate pain control.
2. Patient's peripheral tissue perfusion will remain adequate.

Considering these important care outcomes, prepare a list of the major 3–6 priority patient concerns or nursing diagnoses for patients with thrombocytopenia. Be prepared to participate in a discussion of this list and/or to submit them as an assignment, as determined by your faculty. Resources you may find helpful in this assignment can include this lesson, the references, resources on nursing care plans, and standard nursing diagnoses manuals

LO3: Collaborative Interventions: Thrombocytopenia

- Goal: The most important goal in the care of patients with thrombocytopenia is to prevent serious bleeding. Returning platelet counts to normal is not a realistic goal, but interventions include increasing platelets.
- Interventions for thrombocytopenia are commonly directed at:
  - o Increasing the number of platelets, such as platelet transfusion (Damron, et al., 2009)
  - o Administering first line therapy drugs (Haeck, et al., 2009; Neunert, et al., 2011) that can increase the bone marrow production of platelets, prolong life span, or promote better platelet function include:
    - Platelet growth factors, which stimulate the marrow to produce more platelets

    - Corticosteroids that are used for presumed autoimmune causes and considered in most patients with thrombocytopenia

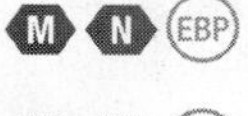

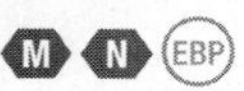

    - Intravenous immune globulin (IVIg) is used in immune thrombocytopenia (ITP), particularly if corticosteroids are contraindicated. IVIg is considered in most patients with thrombocytopenia.

- Safety issues:
  - o Discontinue heparin when heparin-induced thrombocytopenia is suspected as the culprit.
  - o Discontinue aspirin or NSAIDs that aggravate bleeding.
- Monitor patient for blood loss and bleeding continuously to identify complications at the earliest possible time.
- Plasmapheresis is used; however, to date, evidence does not support this therapy.

Transfusion

Indications for transfusion may include:

- Platelet transfusion is recommended for urgent management of severe cases with critical bleeding (Damron, et al., 2009).
  - o Therapeutic platelet transfusion (to stop active bleeding):
    - ■ Patients with active bleeding and platelets <50,000 should be transfused with platelets. Patients with hemorrhage usually respond to a transfusion of 5 units of platelets to stop bleeding. Other factors can affect response, such as conditions that disrupt platelet function (e.g., uremia [kidney failure], sepsis, and drugs).
- Prophylactic transfusion (to prevent bleeding):
  - o Transfuse for platelets <10,000. (Patients with autoimmune destruction of platelets, such as with ITP, may not benefit from platelet transfusion since platelets are rapidly destroyed.)
  - o For invasive surgical procedures with a platelet count <50,000
  - o For neurosurgical procedures with a platelet count <100,000
- Patients with platelet dysfunction may need to be transfused to higher platelet counts.
- Platelet transfusions carry the risk of a transfusion reaction. As with all blood product administration, care includes:
  - o Do not administer medications or other infusions with blood products.
  - o Do not piggyback the administration of blood products and other infusions into blood administration lines.
  - o Utilize a blood filter whenever indicated during infusion of blood products. Follow the specific hospital procedure.
  - o Begin administration of blood products slowly for 15 minutes to evaluate the patient's response.
  - o If an adverse reaction to the blood administration is observed: Immediately stop the infusion, evaluate the patient, call the rapid response team or health care provider urgently.

Follow-Up to Transfusion

- One unit of platelets should increase platelet count by 5,000–10,000 in a patient weighing 70 kg.
- Follow-up platelet count should be checked immediately after transfusion and, again, within 24 hours.
- A possible reason for the platelet count not increasing by the amount expected includes the autoimmune destruction of platelets that were transfused.
- Patients with persistent bleeding, despite transfusion, may have a coagulation factor deficiency and can sometimes respond to the following:
  - o Cryoprecipitate
  - o Clotting factor concentrates
  - o Recombinant factor VIIa (Damron, et al., 2009)

Types of Platelets Available for Transfusion

- Single donor platelets are derived from one donor.
- Random donor platelets are platelets that come from different donors.
- Single donor platelets are preferred so as to decrease the risk of alloimmunization.
- Specially matched platelets may be ordered for those who have many antibodies to platelets.

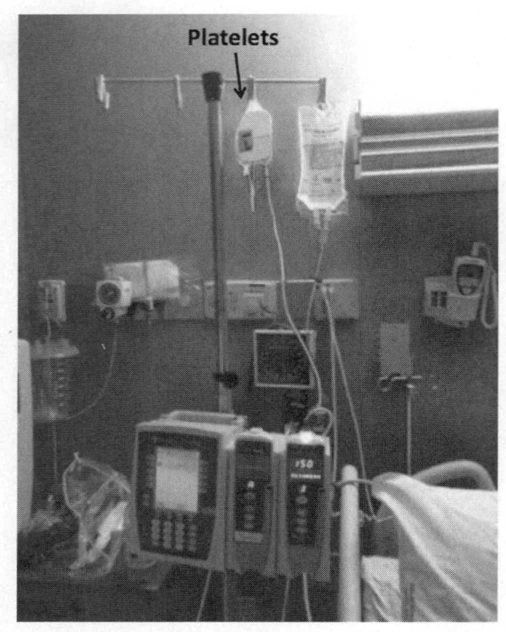

This photo shows platelets ready for transfusion. Note the yellowish milky color, which differs from whole blood or packed red cells.
Source: Courtesy of K. Kyriakidis

Collaborative Interventions: Thrombocytopenia (continued)

Patient Education

Patient education commonly includes precautions that are not evidence-based, primarily because they have not been studied. Some "common sense" interventions that may help prevent bleeding episodes should be taught to patients:

- Educate about a diet high in green leafy vegetables.
- Avoid rectal suppositories.
- Trim and cut nails.
- Caution the patient to avoid falls in the home by using preventive measures, such as to suggest removing throw rugs, clutter, and objects in walking pathways.
- Avoid contact sports, particularly ones that are not supervised or don't have protective equipment.
- Instruct about essential dental care and hygiene. Gum disease and tartar buildup increase the risk of bleeding:
  - Brush with a soft to medium toothbrush twice per day.
  - Gently floss teeth and use interdental cleaning aids.
  - Limit high sugar-containing drinks and foods.
- Use skin lotion to prevent dryness and breaks in skin.
- Shave using an electric razor.
- If bleeding occurs, apply pressure for at least 10–15 minutes.
- Patients with known bleeding condition should wear or carry easily recognizable identification such as an alert bracelet.

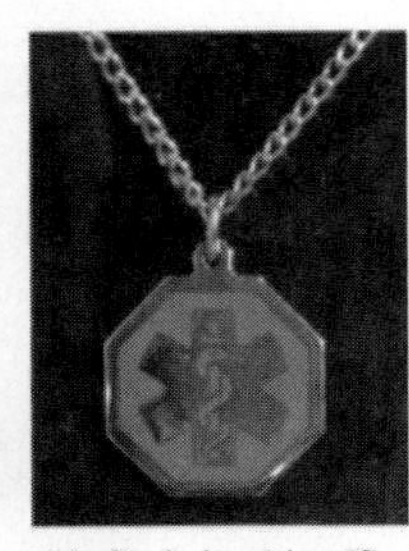
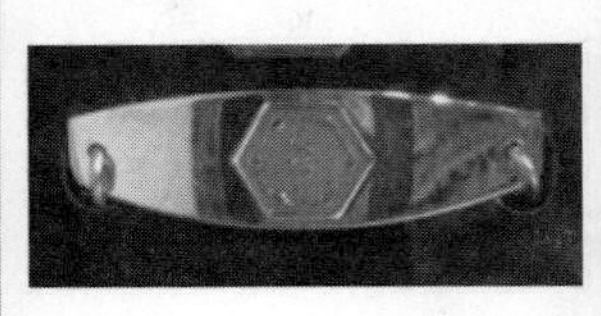
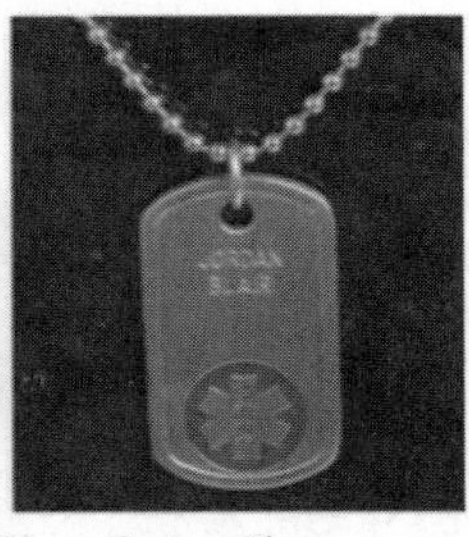

Medical alert identifications (examples above) are convenient to patients, with an array of necklaces or bracelets. Most simple ones are fairly inexpensive and can be found in drug stores. More sophisticated medical alert IDs can also be purchased to include a jump drive with the patient's medical records to expedite care and safety of the patient.

Medical alert identification bracelets.

Source: Copyright © 2014, NovEx Novice to Expert Learning, LLC

Concept Check

5. Which finding indicates that treatment for thrombocytopenia is effective?

A. Bleeding has stopped.

B. Platelet levels are normal.

C. Level of consciousness is improved.

D. Vital signs are stable.

Answer question

Concept Check

6. Random donor platelet administration may result in which complication?

A. Continued bleeding

B. Development of antibodies against subsequent infusions

C. Hemophilia

D. Disseminated intravascular coagulation

Answer question

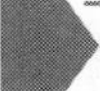

Concept Check

7. What bleeding precautions are recommended for patients with platelet disorders?

A. Use a new razor or new razor blade each time you shave.

B. Use firm-bristled toothbrushes.

C. Apply skin lotion regularly.

D. Use an emery board instead of cutting nails.

Answer question

LO3:

Collaborative Care Summary: Major Hemorrhage with Coagulation Disorders

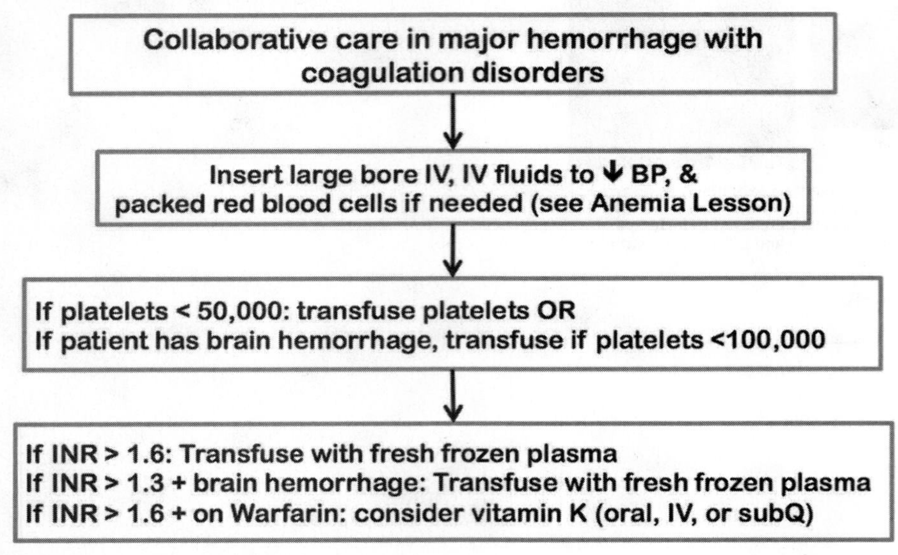

Collaborative care in major hemorrhage with coagulation disorders
Insert large bore IV, IV fluids to ↓ BP, & packed red blood cells if needed (see Anemia Lesson)
If platelets < 50,000: transfuse platelets OR
If patient has brain hemorrhage, transfuse if platelets <100,000
If INR > 1.6: Transfuse with fresh frozen plasma
If INR > 1.3 + brain hemorrhage: Transfuse with fresh frozen plasma
If INR > 1.6 + on Warfarin: consider vitamin K (oral, IV, or subQ)

Source: Copyright © 2014, NovEx Novice to Expert Learning, LLC

LO4:

Evaluation of Desired Collaborative Care Outcomes: Thrombocytopenia

Evaluation and reassessment should reveal attainment of previously established patient outcomes. In summary:

- Patient reports that pain control measures have resulted in adequate relief.
- Patient's skin is warm, dry, and intact with capillary refill in <5 seconds.

LO3:

Summary of Interventions: Platelet and Coagulation Disorders

- In general, patients do not need to be acutely treated unless they have a hemorrhage. However, patients with a platelet count of <10,000 have a high risk of spontaneous hemorrhage and platelet transfusion should be considered.
- Fresh frozen plasma may be used to treat patients with coagulation disorders and profuse bleeding.
- Give vitamin K to reverse anticoagulation with Coumadin.
- Therapeutic transfusion (to stop active bleeding):
  - o Patients with active bleeding and a platelet count of <50,000 should be transfused platelets. Patients with hemorrhage will usually respond to a transfusion of 5 units of platelets to stop bleeding.
  - o Consider factors that disrupt platelet function and can affect response (e.g., sepsis).
- Prophylactic transfusion (to prevent bleeding):
  - o Transfuse for platelets <10,000.
  - o For invasive surgical procedures, transfuse for a platelet count of <50,000.
  - o For neurosurgical procedures, transfuse for a platelet count of <100,000.
- Patients with platelet dysfunction may need to be transfused to higher platelet counts.
- In DIC patients, blood, platelets, and clotting factor replacements are required for those who have evidence of significant hemorrhage.
- Correcting laboratory abnormalities, such as a high PT or PTT, is not an indication for transfusion.
- Regular infusions of factor VIII (for hemophilia A), or IX (for hemophilia B) are needed.

References

Backhouse, R. (2004). Understanding disseminated intravascular coagulation. *Nursing Times, 100*, 36–38. **www.nursingtimes.net/nursing-practice/specialisms/wound-care/understanding-disseminated-intravascular-coagulation/204139.article**

Cooney, M. (2006). Heparin-induced thrombocytopenia: Advances in diagnosis and treatment. *Crit Care Nurse, 26*(6), 30–36. **ccn.aacnjournals.org/content/26/6/30.full**

Dressler, D. (2012). Coagulopathy in the intensive care unit. *Crit Care Nurse, 32*(5), 48–59. **ccn.aacnjournals.org/content/32/5/48.full**

Frazier, T. (2012). Disseminated intravascular coagulation and implications for medical-surgical nurses. *Med-Surg Matters, 21*(3-4), 8–11.

Munro, N. (2009). Hematologic complications of critical illness: anemia, neutropenia, thrombocytopenia, and more. *AACN AdvCrit Care, 20*(2), 145–154. **www.nursingcenter.com/lnc/pdfjournal?AID=859302&an=01256961-200904000-00007&Journal_ID=&Issue_ID=**

Sisson, E. M. (2007). Delayed-onset thrombocytopenia induced by heparin. *Am J Nurs, 107*(10), 29–30. **journals.lww.com/ajnonline/citation/2007/10000/Delayed_Onset_Thrombocytopenia_Induced-By_Heparin.20.aspx**

Wada, H., & Hatada, T. (2008). Pathophysiology and diagnostic criteria for disseminated intravascular coagulation associated with sepsis. *Crit Care Med 36*(1), 348–349

Clinical Practice Guidelines

Damron, B. H., Belansky, H. B., Friend, P. J., et al. (2009). Putting evidence into practice: prevention and management of bleeding in patients with cancer. *Clin J Oncol Nurs, 13*(5), 573–783. **www.guidelinecentral.com/summaries/putting-evidence-into-practice-prevention-and-management-of-bleeding-in-patients-with-cancer/#h2_scope**

Haeck, P. C., Swanson, J. A., Achechter, L. S., et al. (2009). Evidence-based patient safety advisory: blood dyscrasias. *PlastReconstrSurg, 124*(4 Suppl), 82S–95S. **www.guidelinecentral.com/share/summary/52d5681acefd9/#h2_scope**

Neunert, C., Lim, W., et al. (2011). The American Society of Hematology 2011 evidence-based practice guideline for immune thrombocytopenia. *Blood, 117*(16): 4190–4207. **bloodjournal.hematologylibrary.org/content/117/16/4190.full**

Wada, H., Thachil, J., DiNicio, M., et al., & the Scientific and Standardization Committee on DIC of the ISTH. (2013). Guidelines for diagnosis and treatment of disseminated intravascular coagulation from harmonization of the recommendations from three guidelines. *J Thrombosis Haemostasis, 11*, 761–767. **onlinelibrary.wiley.com/doi/10.1111/jth.12155/pdf**

World Federation of Hemophilia. (2012). *Guidelines for the management of hemophilia* (2nd ed). Motreal, Quebec: World Federation of Hemophilia. **www.guideline.gov/content.aspx?id=39323&search=hemophilia**

Patient Education

Centers for Disease Control and Prevention. (2015). *Blood disorders in women*. **www.cdc.gov/ncbddd/bloooddisorders/aboutus.html**

Levi, M. (2013). *Disseminated intravascular coagulation*. **emedicine.medscape.com/article/199627-overview**

National Hemophilia Foundation and Grifols' Patient Services in collaboration with the Centers for Disease Control and Prevention. (2013). *Victory for women with blood disorders*. **www.hemophilia.org/NHFWeb/MainPgs/MainNHF.aspx?menuid=339&contentid=1564&rptname=women**

Learning Outcomes for Anemia

When you complete this lesson, you will be able to:

1. Recognize the clinical relevance of acquired hemolytic and nutritional anemia.
2. Consider the pathophysiology, etiology, risk factors, and clinical presentation of acquired hemolytic and nutritional anemia that determine the priority patient concerns.
3. Determine the most urgent and important nursing interventions and patient education required in caring for a patient with acquired hemolytic and nutritional anemia.
4. Evaluate attainment of desired collaborative care outcomes for a patient with acquired hemolytic or nutritional anemia.

LO1:

What Is Anemia

- Anemia is an inadequate number of fully formed (adult) healthy red blood cells. However, hemoglobin is the most important component of the oxygen delivery system, along with cardiac output. Hemoglobin is the protein that delivers oxygen to the tissues from the lungs and is primarily found in red blood cells (RBCs).
- The primary nursing actions for patients with anemia is to aid the patient with symptom relief, and, if possible, help reverse the cause of the anemia.
- This lesson covers common causes of anemia. The key points focus on symptom relief and reversal of the cause of anemia.

LO1:

Clinical Relevance

- Anemia can result in decreased oxygen delivery to the tissues.
- Without adequate oxygenation, cells cannot function properly or for long periods. Clinically, oxygen delivery is fundamental to life.
- There are approximately 30 million transfusions of blood products yearly in the United States. Someone needs blood every 2 seconds.
- The blood for these transfusions is supplied by 9.5 million donors. Less than 25% of eligible donors give blood.
- The average cost of transfusing one unit of blood is $1,000.
- There were only 58 transfusion-related fatalities in 2011 with 72,000 transfusion-related reactions in 2006.

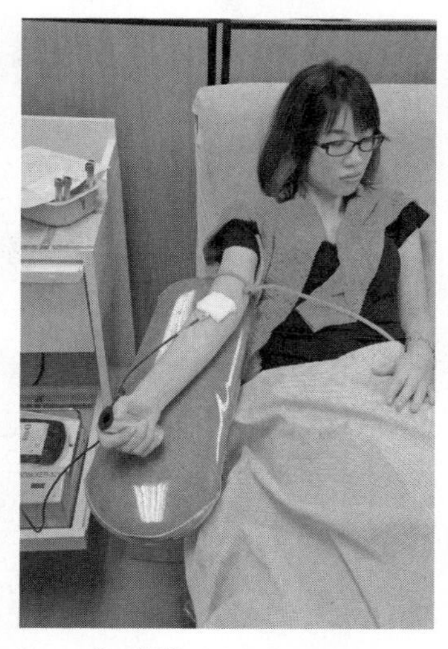

Source: Gow27/Shutterstock

LO2:

Pathophysiology

Erythropoiesis

- Blood is primarily produced in the red marrow of flat bones and the proximal ends of long bones.
- Bone marrow initially produces stem cells that then mature and differentiate into RBCs or erythrocytes, white blood cells (WBCs), and platelets.
- The maturation of stem cells into RBCs is called erythropoiesis.
- The trigger for regulation of erythropoiesis is tissue oxygenation. Thus, when tissue oxygenation drops, the bone marrow is signaled, via endogenous erythropoietin, to produce more RBCs.

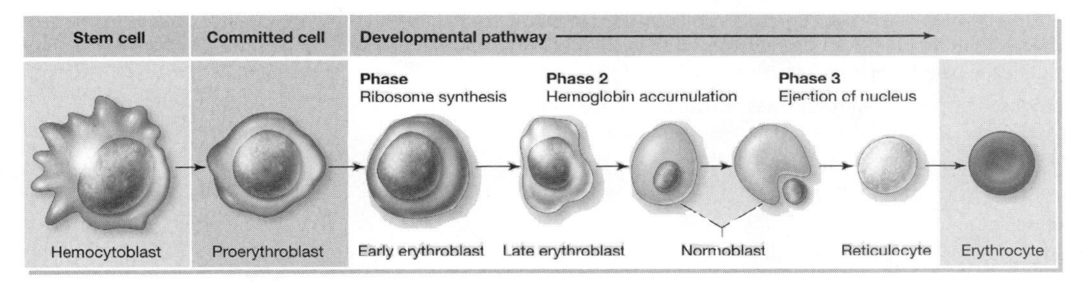

This chart demonstrates the evolutionary path from the beginning stem cell to the end product of a circulating RBC. This process is called Erythropoiesis and takes about 5 days.

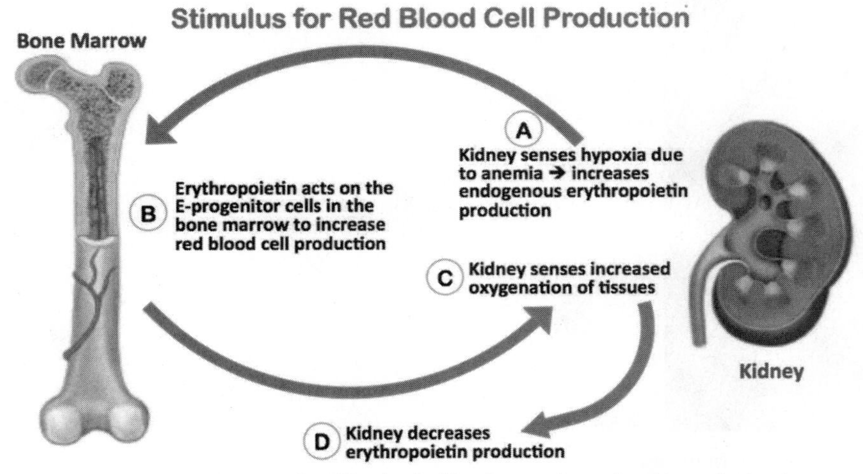

Erythropoiesis is the production of red blood cells. The diagram shows that this mechanism is mediated between the kidneys and bone marrow where numerous chemicals regulate production of red cells. Erythropoietin has a major role in signaling production when hypoxia is detected.

Sources: Courtesy of George Kyriakidis/Santa Ana, CA, & Copyright © 2014, NovEx Novice to Expert Learning, LLC

Anemia

- Hemoglobin is the protein that carries oxygen to tissues and is found primarily in red blood cells. Hemoglobin combines with oxygen to form oxyhemoglobin and carries oxygen from the lungs to the tissues, where it is released.
- Normally, the percent of hemoglobin that is saturated with oxygen, SaO_2, is >95%. However, at higher altitudes the normal percent saturation is lower. For example, in Denver a normal arterial SO_2 (SaO_2) is 93–97%.
- Other types of hemoglobin that cannot carry oxygen can form as a result of medication or toxin exposures. For example, carboxyhemoglobin forms when carbon monoxide attaches to hemoglobin and cannot carry oxygen.
- Hereditary abnormalities of hemoglobin include sickle cell disease (SCD). There are several types of SCD, depending on the genotype inherited. The thalassemias are a type of mutation in SCD. These abnormalities in hemoglobin result from mutations in DNA that are protective against malaria. Sickle cell disease is most common in African Americans and thalassemias are most common in patients of Mediterranean origin.
- Abnormal hemoglobin produced by patients with sickle cell disease results in abnormalities in the shape of red blood cells. The abnormal sickle-shaped cells have shorter life spans and can produce occlusions in the small blood vessels causing ischemia.

Anemia may result from:

- Decreased production of RBCs
- Increased destruction of RBCs
- Blood loss (e.g., gastrointestinal bleeding)

Large Duodenal Ulcer: Temporarily Stopped Bleeding

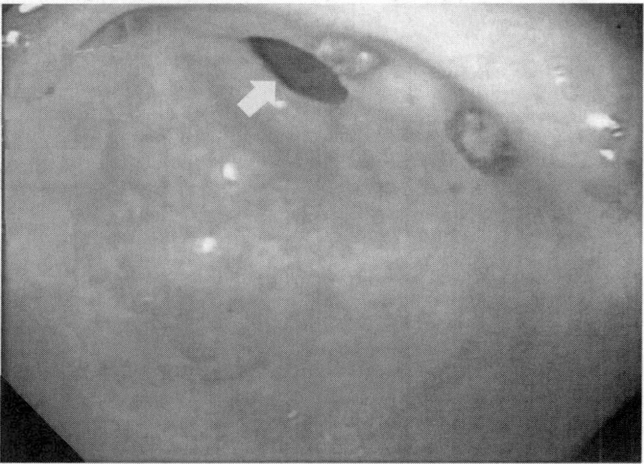

Endoscopy: This patient has a large duodenal ulcer that caused extensive gastrointestinal bleeding. It resulted in anemia secondary to blood loss and necessitated surgical treatment for control of bleeding.
Source: Courtesy of K. Kyriakidis

Pathophysiology (continued)

Sickle Cell Anemia

- Sickle cell anemia is caused by a genetic condition known as sickle cell disease (SCD). Patients with sickle cell disease inherit two genes, one from each parent, that cause the abnormal sickle hemoglobin.
- Some people inherit only one sickle cell gene and are known to have sickle cell trait. Those with the trait typically live normal lives without experiencing the illness described in this NovE-lesson. However, in extreme situations, people with sickle cell trait can develop a crisis.
- SCD refers to all the various genotypes (such as thalassemia) that cause the characteristic clinical syndrome, whereas sickle cell anemia refers to the most commonly seen SCD.
- SCD is much more common in people of African (affecting about 8%), Hispanic, and Mediterranean descent.
- Sickle cell anemia affects 70,000–100,000 people yearly in the United States alone.
- It is caused by the production of an abnormal type of hemoglobin called hemoglobin S (HbS). Red blood cells with HbS have an abnormal shape and are less flexible in moving through the microcirculation, especially when the cells are exposed to low oxygen levels.
- The red blood cells become shaped like crescents or sickles when triggered by particular conditions such as during infection, inflammation, hypoxia, hypothermia, stress, acidosis, high-intensity exercise, or dehydration.
- The sickle-shaped cells deliver less oxygen to the body's tissues.
- The sickle cells can also get trapped more easily in small blood vessels, break into pieces or rupture (hemolysis), obstruct the blood vessels, and interrupt blood flow. Blood flow is often restored but the reperfusion process releases chemicals that result in vascular endothelial damage with further organ damage.
- Occlusion of the small vessels can cause a sickle cell pain crisis, which is a sudden episode of excessive and sometimes prolonged pain. Pain is common in the spine, pelvis, ribs, abdomen, and long bones in the arms and legs. Patients can develop leg ulcers as a result of the occlusions.
- Vascular occlusion results in pain due to tissue ischemia. Each episode of ischemia has consequent tissue damage throughout the various organs. Over time, repeated sickle cell crises can cause significant damage to every body organ and lead to infarction and organ failure. Patients with SCD are at risk for acute kidney failure, pulmonary and systemic hypertension, acute chest pain, liver failure, cerebrovascular disease with neurologic disorders, cholelithiasis, and priapism.
- When the causative factor for sickle cell crisis is treated or resolved, most of the sickle cells can recover their normal shape.
- By adulthood, patients eventually develop fibrosis of the spleen from the repeated episodes of splenic infarction during childhood SCD crises. Without splenic function, patients are less capable of mounting a strong immune response and are, therefore, more susceptible to infections with encapsulated organisms, especially with *streptococcus*.

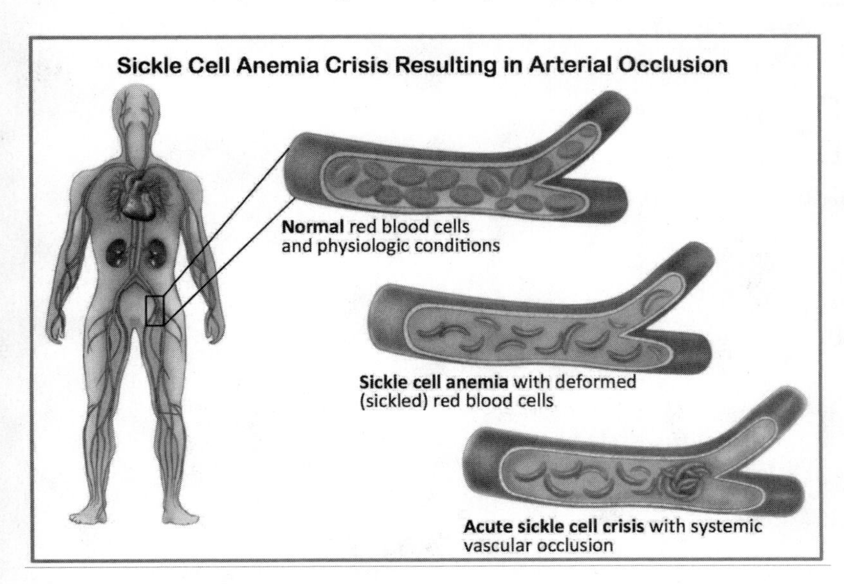

Arterial blockage due to sickle cell disease.
Source: Courtesy of George Kyriakidis/Santa Ana, CA

- Anemia in SCD is additionally exacerbated by sickle cells dying after only 15 days, on average, instead of living for the normal 120 days. The reduced life span results in a hemolytic anemia. The bone marrow simply cannot produce RBCs rapidly enough to replace those that are dying.

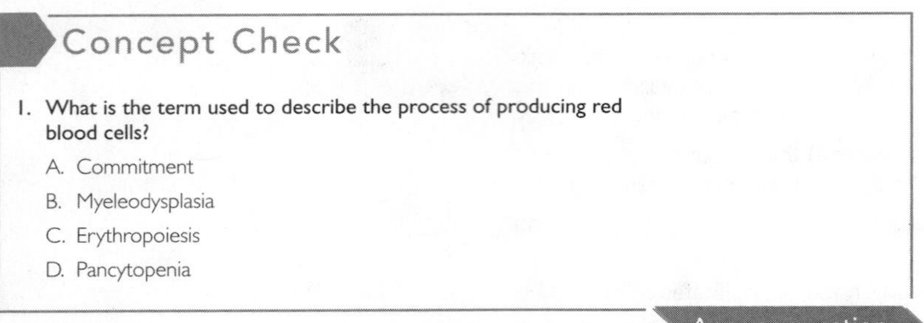

Concept Check

1. **What is the term used to describe the process of producing red blood cells?**
   A. Commitment
   B. Myeleodysplasia
   C. Erythropoiesis
   D. Pancytopenia

Answer question

LO2:

Risk Factors

People of all ages, ethnic backgrounds, and genders may have anemia. However, those who are particularly prone to anemia are:

- Pregnant women with lower folic acid and iron levels
- Women of childbearing age who are menstruating
- Infants and toddlers who do not receive iron-fortified milk or dietary intake of iron
- Adults, particularly older adults, with iron and vitamin deficiencies in their diet
- Patients with chronic or serious illnesses that compromise healthy nutritional intake, digestion, and/or absorption, such as bowel diseases, liver conditions, cancer, diabetes, heart failure, kidney failure, HIV/AIDS, severe dementia, infections, and COPD.
- Patients who had surgery, trauma, or injury with significant blood loss
- Patients with hereditary diseases (e.g., sickle cell, thalassemia)

LO2:

Causes

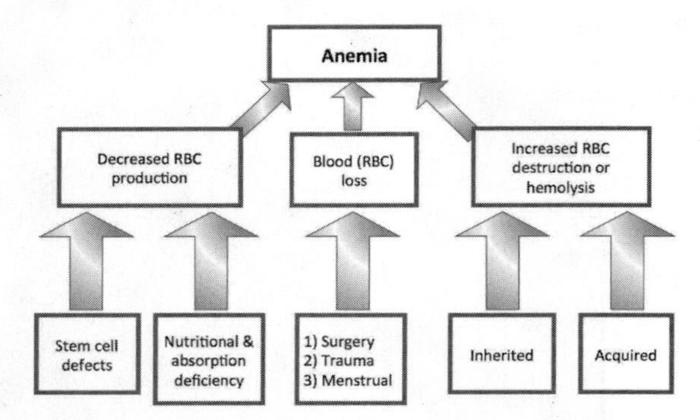

Major causes and their mechanisms of anemia are depicted in this diagram.
Source: Copyright © 2014, NovEx Novice to Expert Learning, LLC

Impaired Production

Several factors can interfere with RBC production, including:

- Chemotherapy
- Primary involvement of bone marrow (aplastic anemia, myelodysplasia, tumor infiltration, infection, toxins, e.g., ETOH)
- Folate deficiency
- Iron deficiency (e.g., infection, pregnancy)
- B_{12} deficiency
  - o Protein malnutrition
  - o Aplastic anemia
  - o Chronic kidney failure (decreased erythropoietin)
  - o Anemia of chronic disease (e.g., malabsorption syndromes)

Concept Check

2. **What is the major cause of sickle cell anemia?**
   A. Poor nutrition in infancy
   B. Alcohol use in the mother while pregnant
   C. Genetic predisposition
   D. Low birth weight

Answer question

Decreased Production in Aplastic Anemia

- Aplastic anemia is a stem cell failure to produce blood cells, that is, a pancytopenia (decreased red blood cells, white blood cells, and platelets). Causes of aplastic anemia include:
  - o Viruses (e.g., hepatitis C, parvovirus, Epstein-Barr)
  - o Various types of drugs, chemicals (e.g., benzene, alkylating agents, insecticides), and radiation
  - o Immune disorders

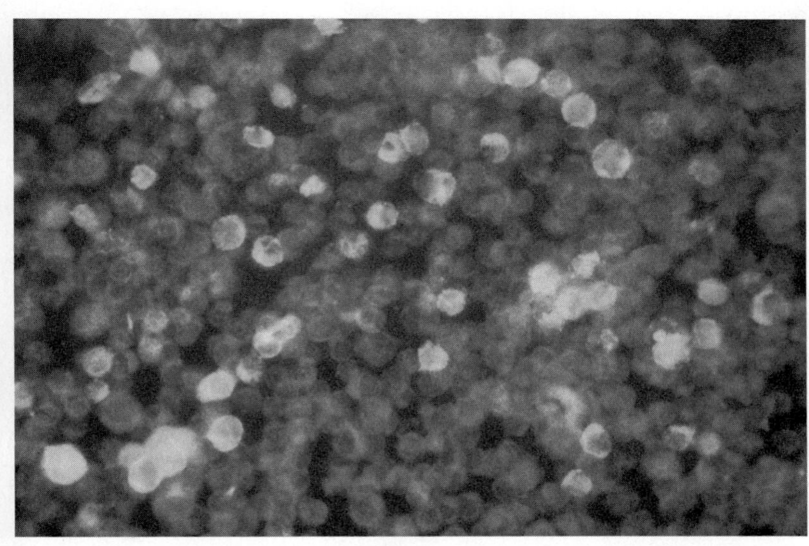

This photomicrograph shows Epstein-Barr virus (EBV) in the blood cells. It is a common human virus that often causes infectious mononucleosis and is known to be a cause of aplastic anemia.
Source: CDC/Dr. Paul M. Feorino

- In infrequent situations, an infection may be the cause of simultaneous anemic episodes. For example, an infection (e.g., parvovirus) may both trigger sickle cell crisis and invade the bone marrow to cause aplastic anemia.

Decreased Production in B_{12} Deficiency

- Lack of B_{12} is commonly associated with disorders of absorption of B_{12} and leads to anemia.
- Etiology of B_{12} deficiency (pernicious anemia) includes:
  - o Gastric bypass
  - o Gastric cancer surgery
  - o Other disruptions of the gastrointestinal track (e.g., Crohn's disease).
  - o Chemotherapy agents such as pemetrexed (Alimta)

Concept Check

3. Aplastic anemia results in decreased numbers of red blood cells. What other blood components are reduced?

A. Serum and white blood cells

B. Lymph and platelets

C. Serum and lymph

D. White blood cells and platelets

Answer question

Causes (continued)

Decreased Production in Folate Deficiency

- Etiology
  - o Folate deficiency is common in conditions such as poor nutrition and alcoholism.
  - o Chemotherapy agents such as methotrexate and pemetrexed (Alimta) can cause folate deficiency.
  - o Women who are pregnant are at greater risk for RBC folate deficiency and resultant anemia. These mothers are at high risk for neural tube defects (serious congenital anomaly) in their infants.

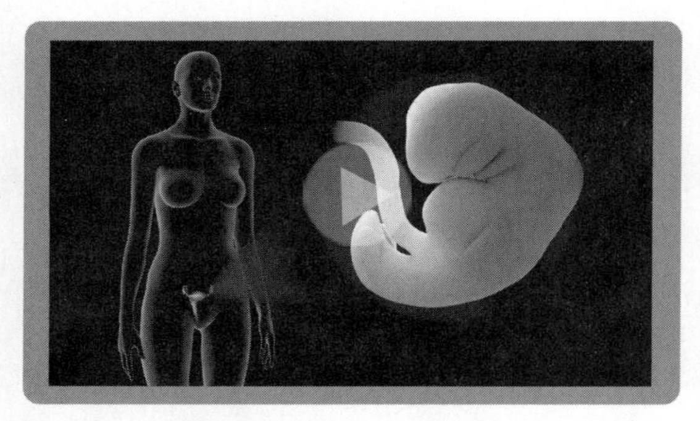

This animation explains the important role that folic acid serves in the production of new cells in the body, including those comprising the vascular system. A deficiency of folic acid can generate severe depression of essential components of the body's cells.

Concept Check

4. Vitamin B_{12} deficiency results in which condition?

A. Thalassemia

B. Ricketts

C. Thrombocytopenia

D. Pernicious anemia

Answer question

Decreased Production Due to Chemotherapy

- Chemotherapy commonly suppresses bone marrow function and often results in decreased production of red blood cells as well as platelets and white blood cells.
- The mechanism for depressed bone marrow function is the toxic effect on stem cells in the marrow as well as the depletion of folate.
- Some chemotherapeutic drugs are toxic to the kidneys and may additionally cause low erythropoietin levels.

Causes (continued)

Decreased Production in Chronic Kidney Disease

- Hypoxemia is the normal trigger to release erythropoietin, which is a hormone produced by the kidneys. Erythropoietin reaches the bone marrow and stimulates increased production of RBCs.
- Chronic hypoxemia can occur in patients who have chronic diseases, such as lung diseases, and can continuously trigger the release of erythropoietin. This subsequent overproduction of RBCs by the bone marrow can result in high levels of hemoglobin and hematocrit.
- Patients with chronic kidney disease usually have low levels of erythropoietin and, therefore, develop anemia.

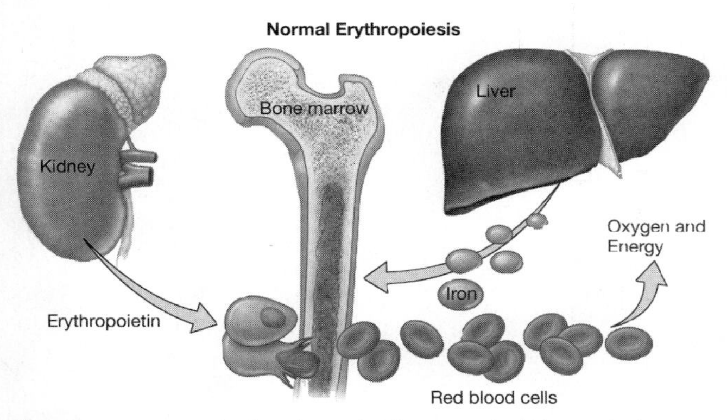

This illustration reveals the relationship between the kidneys, the bone marrow, and the liver acting in conjunction in the normal erythropoiesis process, generating red blood cells. Chronic kidney disease severely limits this process.

Decreased Production in Chronic Disease

- Patients with chronic diseases may have anemia due to decreased RBC production. This may include infections, severe trauma, type 2 diabetes, and inflammatory disorders (e.g., lupus). The mechanism may be due to the circulation of cytokines that are released, which then suppress red blood cell production in the marrow.
- Changes in the hematopoietic system that occur with chronic disease:
  - o Red blood cells have a slightly shortened life span.
  - o Iron is sequestered in macrophages.
  - o There is a decreased availability of iron for red cell production.
- Because attention is focused on the primary disease, symptoms of anemia may not be noticed.
- Women who are pregnant are at greater risk for iron deficiency and resultant decreased RBC production and therefore anemia.

Causes (continued)

Blood Loss

Blood loss is usually obvious and can include conditions such as:

- Surgery
- Acute bleeding
  - o Trauma/injury
  - o Aneurysm
- GI bleeding
  - o Ulcers
  - o Cancer
  - o Inflammatory conditions (e.g., Crohn's disease)
- Anticoagulant therapy side effect
  - o Heparin
  - o Warfarin
  - o NSAIDs
- Disseminated intravascular coagulation (DIC) leads to bleeding due to:
  - o Increase in fibrin split products
  - o Loss of clotting factors, fibrinogen, and platelets

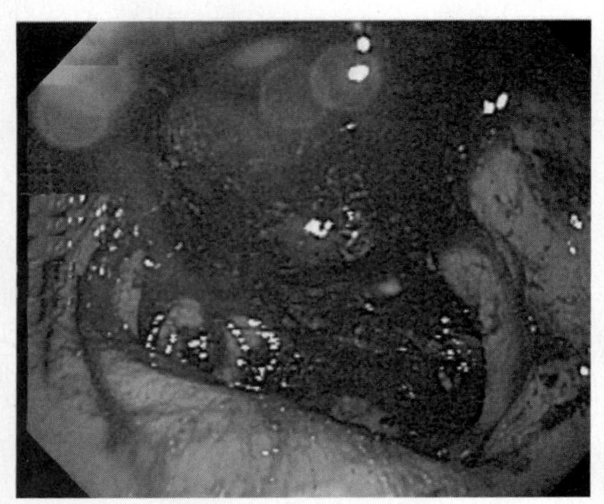

A gastric ulcer with massive GI bleeding is seen here. It is a cause of blood loss anemia.
Source: Courtesy of K. Kyriakidis

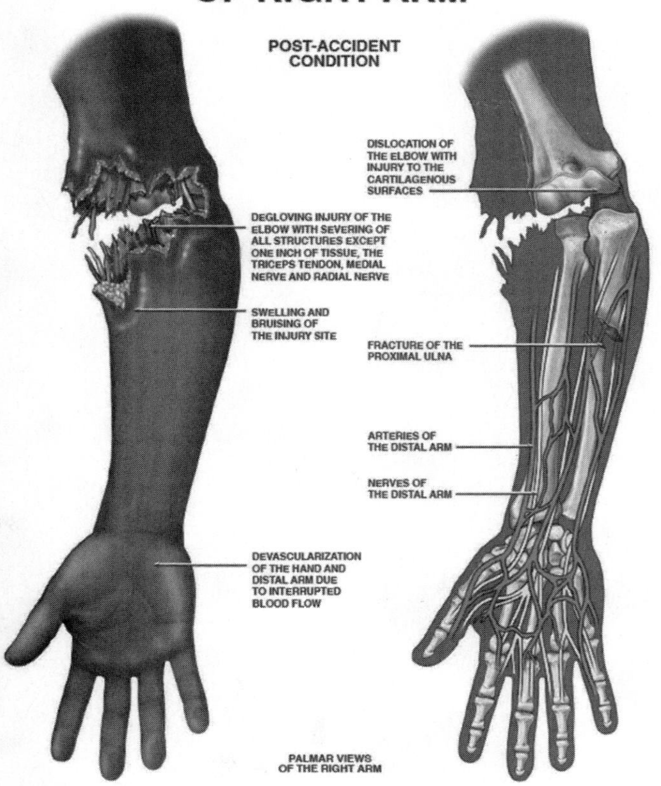

Major trauma can cause large blood losses.
Source: © 2014 Nucleus Medical Media, All rights reserved

Causes (continued)

Hemolysis

- In hemolytic anemia, RBCs are destroyed and removed prior to the end of their natural life span. Because the bone marrow cannot replace RBCs at this accelerated rate of destruction, anemia ensues. Many conditions or factors can cause the hemolysis of RBCs.
- Inherited causes include those that were genetically passed down. A faulty gene causes the production of RBCs with an abnormality in the hemoglobin, cellular metabolism, or cell membrane, resulting in fragile and easily fragmented RBCs. Inherited or intrinsic causes include:
  - o Abnormal hemoglobin production: sickle cell disease
  - o Enzyme deficiency: G6PD deficiency results in abnormally shaped RBCs.
  - o Thrombotic thrombocytopenia purpura (TTP): a coagulation disorder but causes extensive microvascular clotting, which consumes RBCs
- Acquired or extrinsic causes are those that prompt early destruction of RBCs but are not genetically linked:
  - o Drugs, chemicals, and toxins
    - ■ Cephalosporins, NSAIDs, and other drugs can trigger an immune response that targets destruction of RBCs.
    - ■ Lead poisoning
    - ■ IIb/IIIa inhibitors
  - o Autoantibodies are produced in immune hemolytic anemia where the immune system mistakes its own RBCs as a foreign substance and attacks them. Examples are systemic lupus erythematosus or rheumatoid arthritis.
  - o Infections (e.g., mycoplasma, malaria)
  - o Transfusion reactions

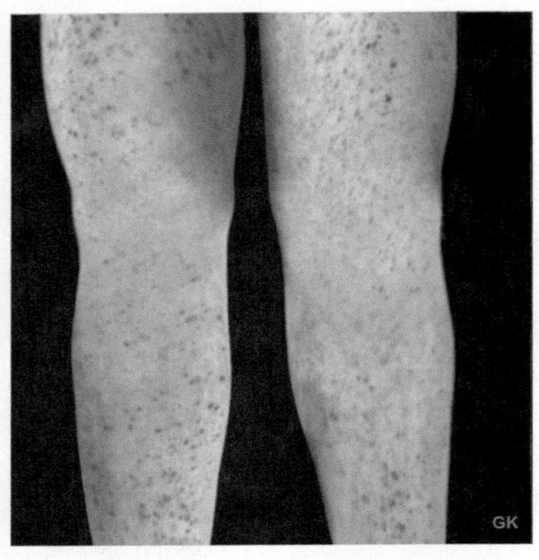

The picture is of the thighs and knees of a person who is afflicted with idiopathic thrombocytopenic purpura resulting in a myriad of subcutaneous hemorrhages afflicting the entire body.
Source: Courtesy of George Kyriakidis/Santa Ana, CA

- o Physical damage (e.g., damage by prosthetic cardiac valves, burns)
- o Disseminated intravascular coagulation, as in sepsis
- o Cancer, particularly in blood cancers

LO2:

Assessment Findings

- Signs and symptoms of anemia arise from the loss of oxygen delivery to the tissues. Findings that are common include:
  - o Fatigue
  - o Pale skin and conjunctival pallor
  - o Tachypnea
  - o Tachycardia
- The cardiac output increases in an attempt to offset the loss of hemoglobin, producing the classic sign of sinus tachycardia with anemia.
- Patients may feel shortness of breath or have dyspnea, particularly if the cardiac output cannot increase to offset the loss of hemoglobin.
- Loss of intravascular volume, because it occurs with acute bleeding, can also result in hypotension.

Sickle Cell Anemia

- Clinical manifestations differ somewhat from those caused by other anemias. Depending on the severity of illness, the signs and symptoms can vary from mild to severe but can include:
  - o Typical anemia signs and symptoms
  - o Dizziness
  - o Headaches
  - o Dark-colored urine
  - o Edema in extremities
  - o Cold extremities
  - o Jaundice
  - o Sudden and prolonged pain in the bones, joints, lungs, and abdomen
  - o Stunted growth in children
  - o Organ damage such as stroke and pulmonary hypertension

LO2:

Diagnostics

Hemoglobin (Hgb) is typically measured along with hematocrit (Hct). These two measurements are central in identifying the presence and extent of anemia:

- The hematocrit is volume percent of RBCs, a measure of the space in blood that is occupied by the red blood cells.
- The normal Hct values are:
  - o 41.0–53.0% in men younger than 65 years old
  - o 37.0–51.0% in men older than 65 years old
  - o 36.0–46.0% in women younger than 65 years old
  - o 35.0–46.0% in women older than 65 years old
  - o "Normal" is based on averages for Caucasians
- The normal hemoglobin value is about one-third of the hematocrit. Normal values are:
  - o 14–18 gm/dL in men younger than 65 years old
  - o 12.6–17.4 gm/dL in men older than 65 years old
  - o 12–16 gm/dL in women younger than 65 years old
  - o 11.7–16.1 gm/dL in women older than 65 years old
- Smokers and people living at high altitudes have a higher than normal baseline hemoglobin.

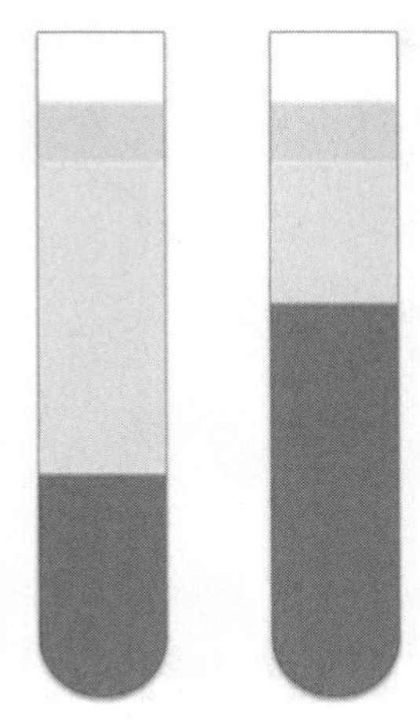

This image compares a normal hematocrit with one that is abnormally high to provide a better understanding of the meaning of a hematocrit level.

Diagnostics (continued)

Defining Grades of Anemia

	NCI	WHO
Grades	**Hgb level (gm/dL)**	**Hgb level (gm/dL)**
0	Normal	> 11
1	10 - normal	9.5 – 10.9
2	8.0 – 10.0	8.0 – 9.4
3	6.5 – 7.9	6.5 – 7.9
4	< 6.5	< 6.5

*14–18 g/dL for men and 12–16 g/dL for women
WHO = World Health Organization
NCI = National Cancer Institute

Laboratory Values

The following values are used in the evaluation of anemia:

- Mean corpuscular volume (MCV)
  - o MCV refers to the size of the blood cell.
  - o Normal: 80–100 μm^3
  - o Large is macrocytic.
  - o Small is microcytic.
- Mean corpuscular hemoglobin (MCH)
  - o The average weight of hemoglobin per red cell
  - o Normal: 27–32 pg (picograms)
- Mean corpuscular hemoglobin concentration (MCHC)
  - o Normal: 32–36%
  - o Refers to the color of the cell

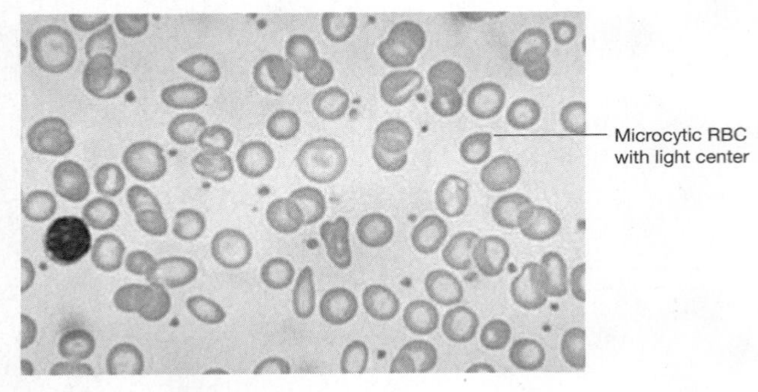

Peripheral blood smear demonstrating microcytic erythrocytes of iron deficiency anemia.

Concept Check

5. A patient's hemoglobin level is 6.6 gm/dL. Which grade of anemia is present?

A. Grade 0

B. Grade 1

C. Grade 3

D. Grade 4

Answer question

Diagnostics (continued)

Blood Volume and Anemia

- Blood volume status affects hemoglobin and hematocrit (H&H) measurements and the interpretation:
  - o Increases in blood volume can dilute normal RBC quantities and make them appear to be abnormally low (e.g., fluid overload or a patient receiving crystalloids [e.g., normal saline] in large amounts).
  - o Dehydration can cause hemoconcentration and make the H&H appear high.
  - o Low blood volume can also mask anemia by making the H&H appear to be normal.
  - o In early pregnancy, the blood volume expands and can create a dilutional effect in relation to the RBCs. So, the woman may appear to be anemic at a time when she is actually producing more RBCs than normal.
- The only way to assess if anemia (or any problem) is affecting tissue oxygenation is to obtain a lactate (normally 1–2 mmol/L) or a venous oxyhemoglobin (normally 75–85%). These are, in fact, the only two measures that reveal what is happening at the tissue level. Without sufficient oxygen for aerobic metabolism, cells must revert to anaerobic metabolism, which produces lactate as a by-product.

Lactate: Potential Sign of Tissue Oxygen Deprivation in Anemia

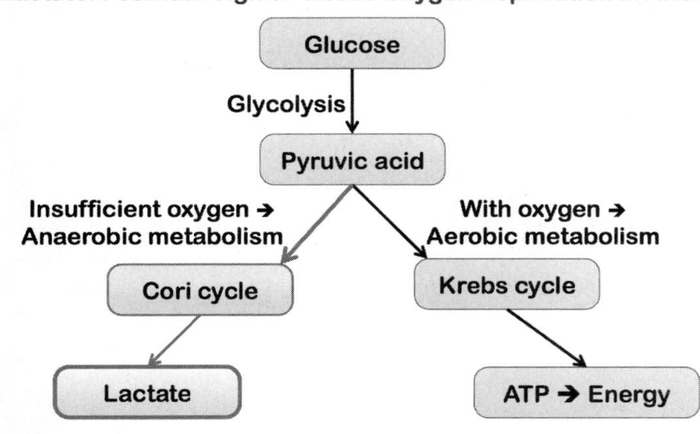

Severe anemia results in failure to deliver adequate oxygen to tissues. Without oxygen, cellular metabolism reverts to anaerobic processes that produce lactate. The higher the lactate levels, the poorer is the tissue oxygenation.
Source: Copyright © 2014, NovEx Novice to Expert Learning, LLC

Type and Crossmatch

- Blood must be typed and crossmatched before a patient receives blood from a donor.
- Each person has one of four types of blood: A, B, AB, or O. Each person's blood type has either Rh-positive or Rh-negative factor.
- The blood types are therefore:

A Rh+ or A+	B Rh+ or B+	AB Rh+ or AB+	0 Rh+ or O+
A Rh− or A−	B Rh− or B−	AB Rh− or AB−	0 Rh− or O−

- If blood is incompatible (meaning the wrong type is infused into the patient), a severe blood reaction occurs where the patient's blood attacks the donor blood. Blood incompatibility causes a rapid or acute intravascular hemolytic reaction. This reaction massively destroys the RBCs and the patient is likely to die.
- The first step in assessing whether blood from a donor is safe to transfuse into a patient is by typing. Typing determines antigens that are present on the surface of a person's RBCs. Blood typing determines ABO compatibility or matching. Blood from the donor (type A, B, AB, or O) should match the blood type from the recipient or it should be compatible.
- The last step is crossmatching. Crossmatching tests for additional antigens and antibodies to make sure that the recipient has no antibodies against any of the donor's antigens that could react. This is one more comprehensive step to ensuring blood compatibility.
- Blood that **matches** means that the donor and recipient are both the same blood type and Rh factor.
- Blood that is **compatible** means that the patient can receive the donor's blood, which may be a different type, without a blood reaction occurring.
- Everyone can safely receive type O blood. Donors with type O blood are known as "universal donors" for that reason. People with type AB blood can receive any type of blood, making them "universal recipients."
- People with Rh-positive blood can receive both Rh-positive and Rh-negative blood. However, people who are Rh-negative must receive only Rh-negative blood. Therefore, Rh-negative blood can be received in an emergency when there is no time to confirm the Rh factor.
- Given that type O and Rh-negative blood can be universally received, in an emergency when there is no time to type and crossmatch, blood type O Rh negative may be safely administered.

Diagnostics (continued)

Lab Values Interpretation

Decreased Production

Lab values are interpreted to evaluate for decreased RBC production:

- **Reticulocytes** are immature RBCs that circulate for approximately one day before losing residual RNA and becoming a mature RBC. The normal value is 0.5–2.5% of all RBCs. When there is decreased production, the reticulocyte count is low.
- **Fe (Iron)**, which is required for Hgb production has a normal value of 30–160 μg/dL.
- **Ferritin** is a protein in which iron is stored. Serum levels reflect iron stores.
  - o 30–300 ng/mL is normal for men.
  - o 10–200 ng/mL is normal for women.
- **B_{12}** is a vitamin that is required for normal RBC production. The normal value is 160–925 pg/mL.
- **Folate**, in conjunction with B_{12}, is required for normal RBC production. The normal value is 3.1–17.5 ng/mL.
- **Transferrin** transports iron in the blood to where it is needed. Normal value is 230–390 mg/dL.
- **Total iron binding capacity (TIBC)** is a direct, quantitative measurement of transferrin.
- **Erythropoietin** may be low in kidney disease.
- **Bone marrow biopsy** can evaluate the health of stem cells.
  - o Biopsy can be useful in detecting bone marrow problems such as cancer and infection.
  - o It can also assess iron stores.

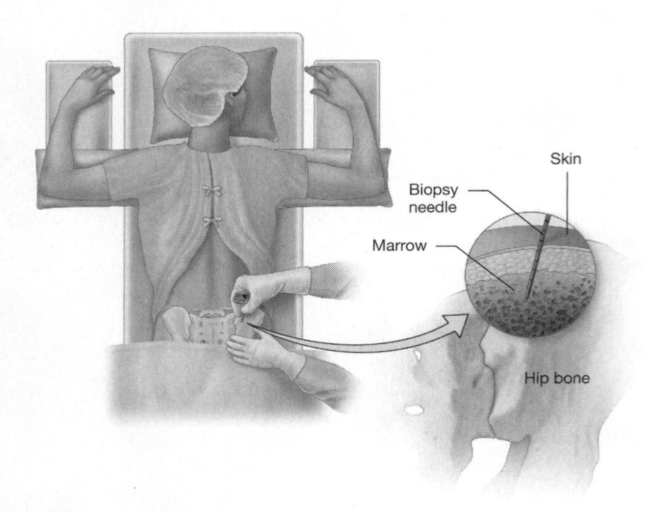

These two images illustrate the essential elements of a bone marrow aspiration. The marrow is usually taken from the large bone in the hip. On the right is shown the detail of needle insertion into the bone.

Concept Check

6. Initial typing of patient blood will place it into one of how many categories or types?
   A. 2
   B. 4
   C. 6
   D. 8

Answer question

Increased Destruction (Hemolysis)

Lab values are interpreted to evaluate for hemolysis:

- **Haptoglobin**
  - o Glycoproteins are produced by the liver and are hemoglobin-binding proteins. When RBCs are broken apart or destroyed, haptoglobin attaches to the released hemoglobin.
  - o Therefore, in hemolysis, freely floating haptoglobin levels are decreased since they are bound to the released hemoglobin.
- **Coombs Test**
  - o The direct Coombs test measures antibodies on the RBCs.
  - o The indirect Coombs measures antibodies in the blood system. These antibodies fight normal healthy RBCs and kill them.
  - o In uncrossed, unmatched blood (as in an emergency), the presence of this antibody could cause a transfusion reaction.
- **LDH** is elevated when cells are broken down or hemolyzed.
- **Bilirubin** is released from hemolyzed blood cells.

Priority Patient Concerns and Desired Collaborative Care Outcomes

Prior to caring for patients with anemia, it is important to prioritize the patient's concerns that must guide the nursing care plan and interventions. Care for the patient is ordered and organized in accordance with the patient's priority and urgent needs. Desired collaborative care outcomes in patients with anemia typically include:

1. Patient will have sufficient energy to perform activities of daily living.
2. Patient's arterial blood gas measurements or oxygen saturation levels will return to desired range.
3. Patient will have stools with a frequency and consistency that provide physical comfort.
4. Patient will be free of signs and symptoms of infection.
5. Patient will have intact oral mucous membranes and maintain hygienic practices that help prevent oral problems.
6. Patient will report adequate pain control, with or without complementary alternative therapies.
7. Patient will have no findings associated with inadequate tissue perfusion.
8. Patient will select and consume a nutritionally adequate diet.

Considering these important care outcomes, prepare a list of the major 3–6 priority patient concerns or nursing diagnoses for patients with anemia. Be prepared to participate in a discussion of this list and/or to submit them as an assignment, as determined by your faculty. Resources you may find helpful in this assignment can include this lesson, the references, resources on nursing care plans, and standard nursing diagnoses manuals.

LO3:

Collaborative Interventions

RBC Production

Patients with impaired RBC production primarily require supportive care, symptom management, and patient education:

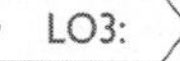

- Treat the underlying causes.
- Prevent or treat folate deficiency:

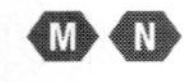

  - o Administer folate supplement.
  - o Educate patient to eat foods with large amounts of folic acid such as green leafy vegetables, nuts, beans, peas, eggs, seafood, and meats.

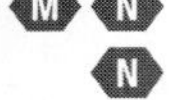

  - o Educate women of childbearing age that folate deficiency and anemia can result in serious neurologic birth defects (Kapur, et al., 2002).
- Prevent or treat B_{12} deficiency:

M N o Administer monthly intramuscular B_{12} or instruct the patient about high oral doses of daily B_{12}. The route of administration depends on the need and urgency.

N o Educate the patient to consume larger amounts from natural sources such as fish, meat, eggs, poultry, dairy (e.g., milk, yogurt, cheese) or foods fortified in B_{12}.

M N o Educate the patient about paresthesias (altered sensations like tingling, burning, prickling) and neuropathies (loss of sensation) that can accompany B_{12} deficiency, primarily affect the spinal cord, and cause sensorimotor problems.

N o Instruct the patient about the risk and avoidance of injuries sustained because of the patient's diminished sensations to heat and pain.

M N • Evaluate the patient for gastric carcinoma frequently by observing for abdominal pain after a small meal, dark stools, difficulty swallowing, loss of appetite, excessive belching, weight loss, and hematemesis.

N • Monitor labs that require frequent checks by using bedside or point of care devices, which require a fraction of the amount of blood to produce hematologic or blood chemistry information.

N EBP • Minimize or prevent unnecessary blood loss to prevent anemia and reduce the need for blood transfusions (Liumbruno, et al., 2011) due to procedures. Examples include:

- o Collaborate with the lab techs to minimize phlebotomy-related blood loss for tests. Aim for reduction in specimen volumes or minimum volumes for specimens.
- o Collaborate with medical team to order all needed labs in clusters to minimize blood loss.
- o Limit iatrogenic blood loss when withdrawing and/or discarding blood with IVs or arterial lines.
- o Closely monitor patients at high risk for bleeding to identify early warning signs if bleeding or rebleeding occurs.

• Prevent or treat iron deficiency:

M N o Administer iron supplement with oral or intravenous iron, depending on urgency and the patient's condition.

M N o Intravenous iron is more effective and is administered to those who cannot take it orally (e.g., GI bleeding, GI inflammatory disease, on dialysis).

M N o Parenteral (IM or IV) iron solutions include several types, like iron dextran, sodium ferric gluconate, and iron sucrose. The type of parenteral iron determines the administration concerns and patient education, but anaphylaxis is possible.

N o Educate the patient to increase oral intake of iron from food sources or oral iron supplements taken between meals for increased absorption.

N o Educate the patient to consume larger amounts of red meat (e.g., liver, lean sirloin), fish, dark green leafy vegetables, pumpkin seeds, dark chocolate, dried apricots, lentils, and beans.

• Care for the patient needing erythropoietin (EPO):

M N o Administer erythropoietin as prescribed. Patients with low EPO levels (e.g., patients with kidney disease) can be treated with erythropoietin or darbepoetin.

N o Monitor patient response (e.g., physical exam, labs) to these drugs as they may vary. A minority of patients show little or no response.

N o Monitor for physical findings, vital signs, for possible adverse effects such as hypertension, edema, fever, nausea, vomiting, sudden headache, and dizziness.

N o Monitor and take precautions to prevent complications:

- ■ Venous thromboembolism: Consider sequential compression device if patient is hospitalized and not ambulatory. Mobilize patient early and frequently, particularly if at home. Ensure patient is educated to stay well hydrated.
- ■ Serious or life-threatening complications such as acute coronary syndrome, pulmonary embolism, stroke, peripheral arterial occlusion, hypertension, and heart failure
- ■ Allergic reaction to the EPO

M N o Monitor EPO levels. Many studies have shown that in patients without underlying disease or active bleeding, EPO can raise the hemoglobin by 1 g/dL in as little as 1 week.

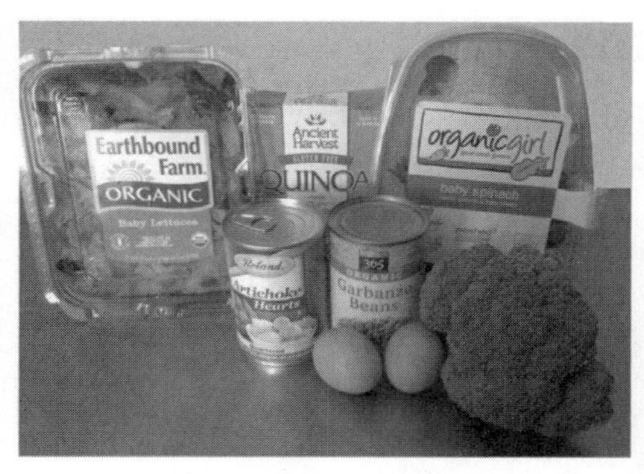

Encourage patients to consume foods high in iron. Meats, particularly red meats, are well known as being rich in iron. However, dark green vegetables, some grains, and eggs are excellent sources.

Source: Copyright © 2014, NovEx Novice to Expert Learning, LLC

Collaborative Interventions (continued)

Chemotherapy-Induced Anemia

Care of the patient involves the same prevention, patient education, and treatment measures as for anemia caused by chronic diseases (as mentioned earlier):

- Treat the cause (e.g., vitamin-related)
- Iron supplements
- Erythropoietin (EPO)
- The types of blood transfusions may differ for blood-related cancers due to multiple transfusions and risks of graft-versus-host disease (GVHD) and excess antibodies. Care and safety of the patient can include:
    - GVHD is rare but most often fatal if a transfusion reaction occurs as there is no effective treatment.
    - Team collaboration is paramount to ensure prevention of GVHD when transfusions are ordered and administered.
    - Infuse irradiated blood products so that lymphocytes and lymphocyte-containing components have been inactivated prior to transfusion, thereby preventing GVHD.
    - Instruct patients to also advocate for themselves by asking their health care providers if transfusions have been irradiated prior to infusion.
    - Monitor for cytomegalovirus (CMV) exposure and avoid giving CMV-positive products to CMV-negative patients.

Blood Loss Anemia

Depending on the cause, amount, patient's symptoms, and illness regarding the blood loss, interventions, supportive and safety care, and symptom management are considered:

- If the patient is postop, or has a history of bleeding (e.g., GI bleeding), monitor the hemoglobin, hematocrit, and RBCs frequently.
- Collaborate with the health care provider to consider reversing coagulation abnormalities in patients with bleeding.
- Consider discontinuing anticoagulant medications in patients with bleeding.

Abdominal Aortic Aneurysm, Rupture, and Hemorrhage

Normal Anatomy

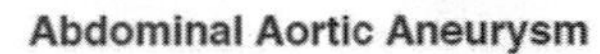

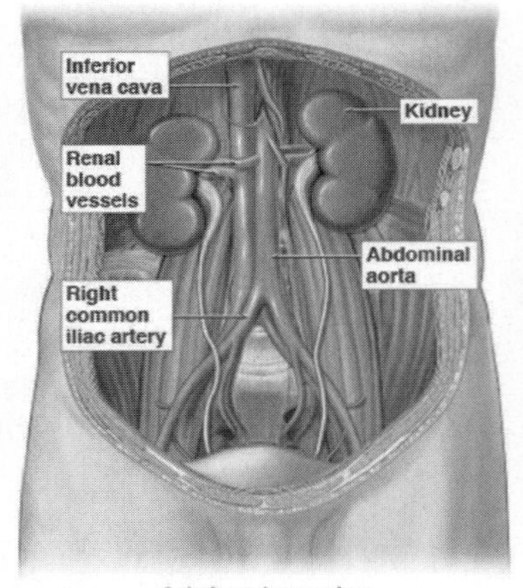

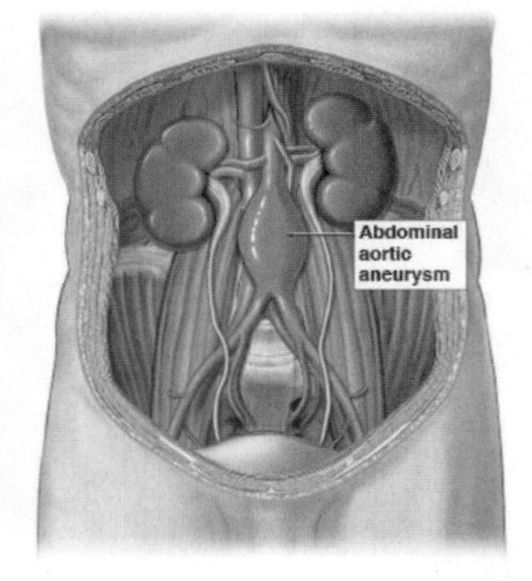

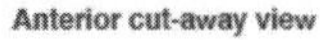

Eventual Condition

CT Colorizations of Abdomen

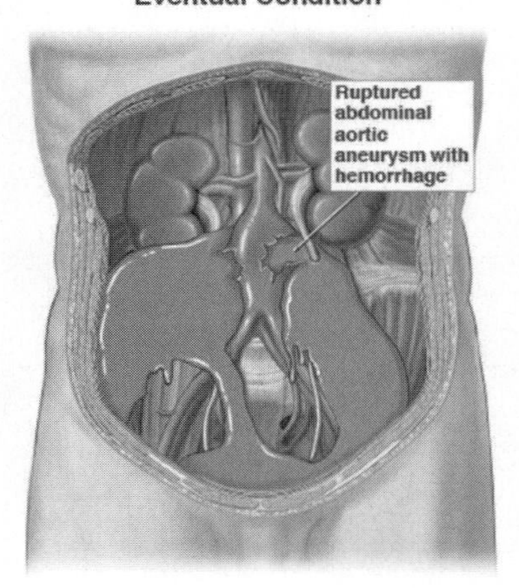

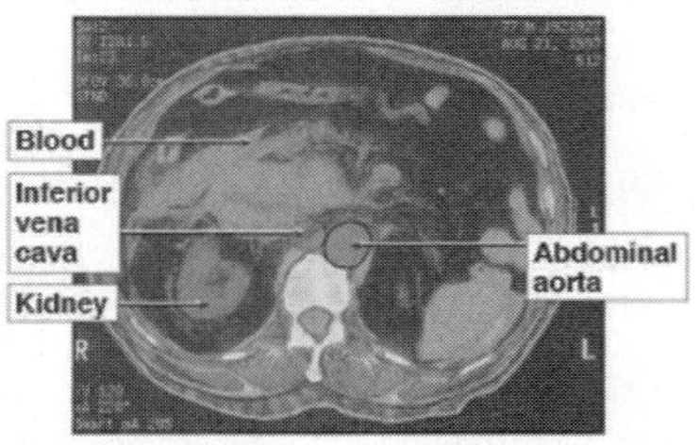

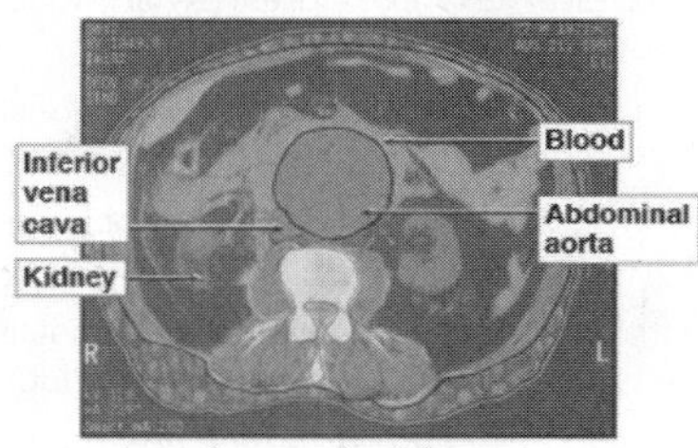

Cross-sectional views

This series of illustrations depicts the progression of an abdominal aortic aneurysm as it ruptures and causes extensive intra-abdominal bleeding with a resulting serious threat to the patient's continuing survival.

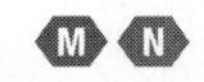

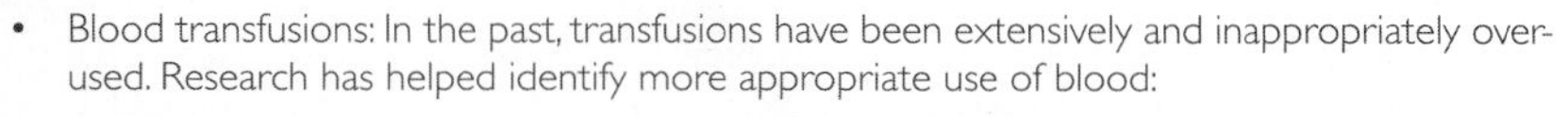

- Blood transfusions: In the past, transfusions have been extensively and inappropriately overused. Research has helped identify more appropriate use of blood:

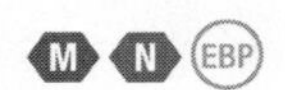

  - Blood transfusions are strongly recommended for patients with hemoglobin levels <7–8 gm/dL and who have active bleeding (American Society of Hematology, 2012; Carson, et al. and AABB, 2012).
  - However, because the guidelines were recently updated and have become even more conservative, it is not uncommon for transfusions to be ordered outside this guideline based on old habits of practice.
  - Transfusions have a host of issues, ranging from increased infections to blood reactions; so caution should be used and blood should never be given unnecessarily.

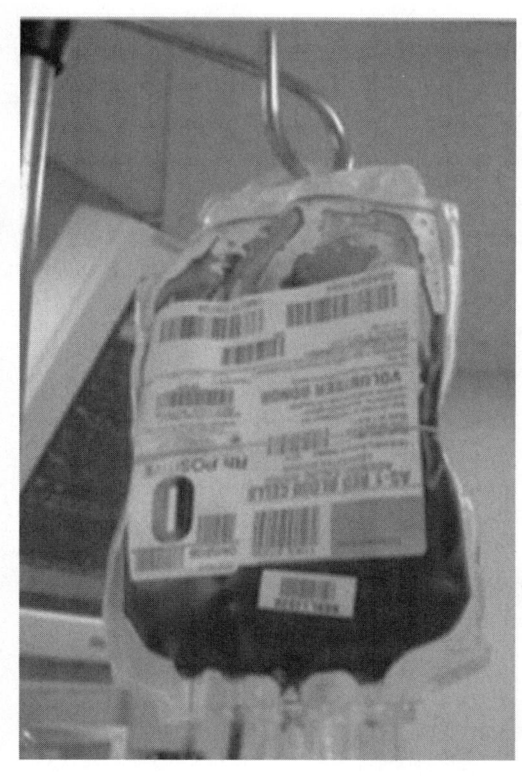

Blood transfusion.

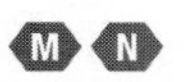

- Iron supplements:
  - o While these will not work quickly, they may be effective over time.
  - o IV or oral iron supplements can be used.
  - o IV iron supplements have better outcomes.
- Erythropoietin can be used to stimulate RBC production. However, it can take several weeks to achieve optimal impact.

Collaborative Interventions (continued)

Transfusions

In recent years, the high cost and limited supply of donor blood has added to the need to determine the efficacy of blood or blood product transfusions. Multiple medical specialty associations and societies are reevaluating or have reevaluated the appropriate use of blood and blood products, and there is a transition from liberal to restrictive practices.

Liberal Versus Restrictive Transfusion

Studies	Liberal Transfusion	Restrictive Transfusion	Summary: Landmark Studies
Upper GI bleeding[1]	Hemoglobin of trigger of 9 g/dl target of 9-11 g/dl	Hemoglobin trigger 7g/dl with target of 7-9 g/dl	Mortality was lower in the restrictive group vs the liberal group 5% vs 9 %. Further bleeding was also lower in the restrictive group 10 vs 16%. The restrictive group had a decreased length of stay and fewer complications (e.g. pulmonary edema).
After Hip surgery[2]	Hemoglobin trigger of 10g/dl	Hemoglobin trigger 8g/dl	No significant difference in death or inability to walk at 60 day follow-up.
In the ICU[3]	Target of 10-12g/dl	Target of 7-11g/dl	Restrictive strategy resulted in decreased mortality at 30 days, rates of cardiac complications, and rates of organ dysfunction.

1. Villanueva, C., Colomo, A., Bosch, A., et al. (2013). Transfusion strategies for acute upper gastrointestinal bleeding. *N Engl J Med, 368*(1), 11–21.
2. Carson, J. L., Terrin, M. L., Noveck, H., et al. (2011). Liberal or restrictive transfusion in high-risk patients after hip surgery. *N Engl J Med, 365*, 2453–2462
3. (1999). A multicenter, randomized, controlled clinical trial of transfusion requirements in critical care. *N Engl J Med, 340*, 409–417.

The American Society of Hematology (ASH) (2012) and/or AABB (2012) made recommendations for clinical practice:

M N EBP
- Strongly recommended transfusion for massive hemorrhage

M N EBP
- Strongly recommended transfusion for acute bleeding and hemoglobin ≤7 gm/dL

M N EBP
- If the patient is not responding to the treatment of the underlying condition and the patient remains symptomatic (dyspnea, tachycardia, fatigue), consider RBC transfusion.

M N
- May be considered in patients who have not responded to EPO, iron, or B_{12}.

N
- Safe administration of blood products requires:
  - o Ensuring ABO compatibility
  - o In an emergency, infusion of unmatched blood should be O negative.
  - o Begin infusion slowly for the initial 15 minutes.
  - o Complete transfusion of a single unit of blood within 4 hours.

N
- Care and safety of the patient when transfusing blood or blood products involves:
  - o Obtaining a set of vital signs and physical exam prior to, at 15 minutes after start of infusion, and hourly during and after the transfusion(s)
  - o Beginning transfusion slowly; the rate may be increased after 15 minutes if patient is tolerating it well
  - o Using precautions in patients with heart disease, heart failure, or other conditions where fluid overload is a concern
  - o Collaborating with the health care provider if patient is at risk for a mild reaction to have PRN orders for diphenhydramine or acetaminophen, if needed
  - o Instructing the patient to immediately report and observe for any signs and symptoms warning of a blood reaction, acute hemolysis, anaphylaxis, volume overload, or sepsis:
    - ■ Severe: hives, flushing, hypotension, chest pain, fever and chills, dyspnea, shock, wheezing, tachycardia, tightness in throat restricting ventilation, rigors, vomiting, and sudden bleeding.
    - ■ Moderate: itching, localized redness, low grade fever, restlessness, low back pain, nausea, or diarrhea
    - ■ Stop the infusion at any sign of an adverse response, call the rapid response team and the health care provider, switch the IV infusion to normal saline, prepare for emergency interventions, recheck to verify correct blood unit for that patient, notify the blood bank, and monitor the patient continuously or transfer to ICU if indicated. Administer diphenhydramine if reaction is mild.

Transfusion-Related Reactions

Reaction	Cause	Signs and Symptoms	Treatment (stop infusion)
Hemolytic reaction	Transfusion of an incompatible blood type resulting in hemolysis.	Fever, flank pain, hemoglobinuria. Severe cases with kidney failure, DIC. May occur from initiation of transfusion and up to first 24 hours.	Stop transfusion immediately. O2 for sat<93% IVF (avoid glucose) Call rapid response
Febrile, nonhemolytic reactions	Cytokines that are released in stored blood	Fever chills up to four hours after infusion.	Stop transfusion. Antipyretics
Allergic reactions	Antibodies in the person receiving the blood transfusion against an allergan in the donor blood.	Pruritis, hives	Stop transfusion for severe reaction. Antihistamine PO, IV
Anaphylactic reactions	Antibodies in the person receiving the blood transfusion against an allergan in the donor blood.	Rapid onset within minutes. Hives, wheeze, dyspnea, hypotension	O2 for SpO_2 <93% Epinephrine 0.3 ml 1:1000 solution IM IV fluids Call rapid response
Transfusion Related Acute Lung Injury	Activation of neutrophils in the recipient.	Shortness of breath, tachypnea, bilateral infiltrates on chest X-ray, hypoxia. No evidence of circulatory overload. Within six hours of blood transfusion.	Stop Transfusion. O2, supportive care
Transfusion Associated Circulatory Overload (TACO)	Excess volume transfused	Shortness of breath, tachypnea, crackles at bases, elevated jugular venous pulsations, bilateral infiltrates on chest X-ray, hypoxia, elevated BNP	Slow or stop transfusion or IVF, Use of diuretic, O2, raise head of bed

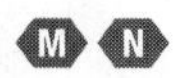

- Removal of WBCs (leukoreduction) from packed red blood cells (PRBC) transfusions should result in decreased incidence of adverse reactions to transfusions.

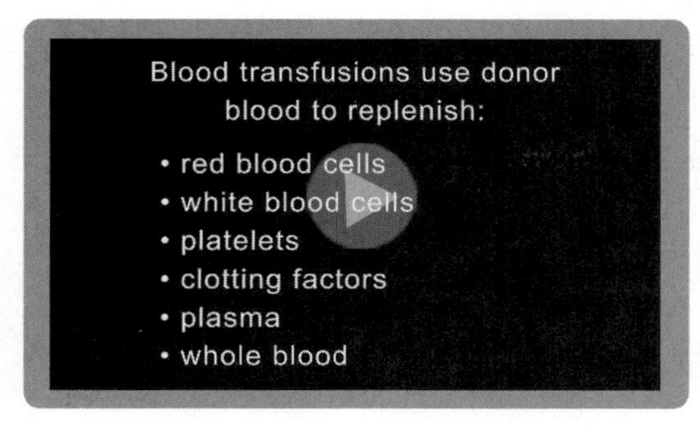

Blood transfusions use donor blood to replenish:
• red blood cells
• white blood cells
• platelets
• clotting factors
• plasma
• whole blood

This animation adequately describes and portrays the process of blood transfusion. Blood components are addressed, safeguards are enumerated, and the precautions and monitoring of the patient are described with the goal of protecting the patient.
Source: © 2014 Nucleus Medical Media, All rights reserved

Collaborative Interventions (continued)

Hemolytic Anemia

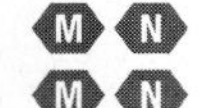

- Treat the underlying disease or cause if one is known.
- Avoid any blood transfusion, if at all possible, due to the potential for a hemolytic reaction resulting in anemia and other serious consequences.

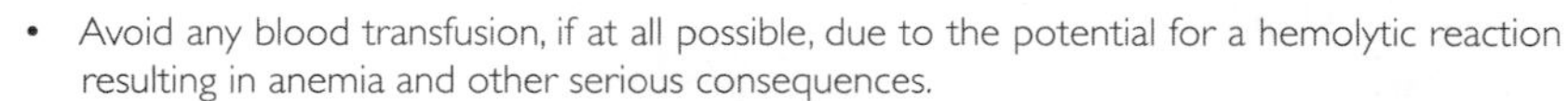

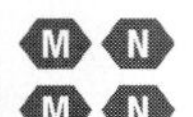

- Intravenous immunoglobulin (IVIG) may be indicated, particularly, in oncologic conditions.
- Steroids may be needed to reduce inflammation.

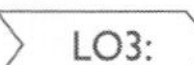

LO3:

Sickle Cell Disease

Although hematopoietic stem cell transplantation is showing potential curative results in very limited numbers of patients, most patients will not experience the possibility of cure at this time. Without cure, care of patients with SCD focuses on symptom management, prevention, and patient education:

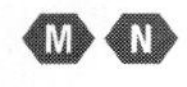

- Pain medications and complementary alternative therapies:
  - o Treat a sickle cell crisis as a medical emergency.
  - o For patients in the ED and in the hospital, pain should be treated with intravenous opioids.
  - o Reassess pain and administer additional doses as needed.
  - o Assess patients on opioids for the need for:
    - ■ Antiemetics if nausea and/or vomiting arise
    - ■ Stool softeners or laxatives for constipation
  - o Complementary and alternative therapies may be incorporated to provide a holistic and safer approach to care and comfort. Meeting patient's emotional and physical needs can improve the overall state of well-being. Comfort may be enhanced to reduce stress, mitigate anxiety, and alter the experience of discomfort. Some therapies include:
    - ■ Warm room
    - ■ Distraction (e.g., conversation, music, or activity)
    - ■ Relaxation (e.g., massage, Reiki)
    - ■ Positioning
    - ■ Aromatherapy
    - ■ Warm soaks on a painful area

- Hydration for patients that are hypovolemic:
  - o Hydration of at least 200 mL/hour oral or IV intake during a sickle cell crisis
- Oxygen for patients that are hypoxic with an SpO_2 of <93%
- Antibiotics for infections
- Prevention, safety, and early detection strategies:
  - o Wash hands frequently and thoroughly.
  - o Prophylactic antibiotics, when indicated
  - o Use strict aseptic technique if invasive procedures are required.
  - o Monitor patients' SpO_2, intake and output, vital signs, peripheral circulation, chest pain, and escalating oxygen requirements after treatment.
  - o Avoid constrictive clothing.
  - o Avoid extremities in dependent position to reduce venous stasis.
  - o Instruct patient not to use the bed's knee gatch.
  - o Avoid cold environmental temperatures.
  - o Monitor blood counts.

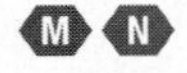

- Folic acid supplement should be given to all SCD patients. Educate the patient as above regarding folic acid deficiency.

- Hydroxyurea should be considered for all symptomatic SCD patients to minimize severe clinical episodes (National Heart, Lung, & Blood Institute [NHLBI], 2002).

- Patient education and safety should include:
  - o Avoid high altitudes due to less available oxygen.
  - o Avoid extreme temperatures unless dressed appropriately.

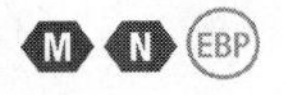

  - o Get pneumonia and influenza vaccinations annually (NHLBI, 2002). Receive meningitis and hepatitis B vaccines as the health care provider advises.
  - o Teach for early detection and prevention of complications from recurrent sickle cell episodes (e.g., pulmonary hypertension, kidney failure, neurologic deficits).
  - o Use over-the-counter medication for pain when mild.
  - o When a sickle cell episode is mild, treat with hydration, rest, and heating pad.
  - o Stay well hydrated at all times to prevent episodes.
  - o Instruct patient how to begin self-treatment at home.
  - o Routinely follow-up with the health care provider.
  - o Encourage a healthy lifestyle: healthy diet, weight management, stop smoking, moderate alcohol use, manage comorbid conditions, exercise, reduce stress.
  - o Avoid decongestants.
  - o Discuss effective ways that the patient may cope if anxious, stressed, depressed, or fearful (e.g., support group). Counseling or social services may be helpful as many patients are undereducated (from missing school during repeated illnesses), underemployed due to frequently missed work, isolated, or seek self-destructive means of coping with the SCD or its consequences.
  - o Involve a social worker as needed to work with school or employer about ways of supporting the patient. Additionally, vocational counseling may be helpful.
  - o Seek medical attention if fever exceeds 101°F; hands, feet, or stomach swell; severe fatigue develops; or penile erection persists.
  - o Discuss the importance of genetic counseling.

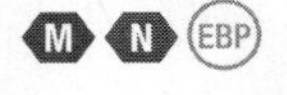

- Transfusions should be considered to improve oxygenation according to guidelines (e.g., preoperative, stroke, multiorgan failure, acute chest syndrome) (NHLBI, 2002).

- Hematopoietic stem cell transplant may be considered in some patients.

Collaborative Interventions (continued)

Patient Education: All Anemias

Instructions for patients and safety that are condition-specific were included above. But many issues that patients should understand are common across the various types of anemia and include:

- Instruct the patient to stay well hydrated during episodes of hemolysis to avoid tubular obstruction in the kidneys by RBC debris.
- Educate the patient about the importance of taking prescribed medications and supplements and how to deal with problems:
  - o If discomfort arises due to medications, do not stop taking them but call your health care provider about making some adjustments.
  - o Collaborate with the health care provider about possibly reducing the dose temporarily and gradually increasing it to full dose so that the body may acclimate.
  - o Collaborate with the health care provider about dividing the dosage and taking half at another time of day.
  - o Take medicines with food to reduce side effects.
  - o Collaborate with a pharmacist about changing the brand or type of medication (e.g., iron comes in various types) to try to reduce adverse effects.
- Educate the patients with B_{12} deficiency to consume larger amounts from natural sources such as fish, meat, eggs, poultry, dairy (e.g., milk, yogurt, cheese), or foods fortified in B_{12}.
- Educate the patients with iron deficiency to consume larger amounts of red meat (e.g., liver, lean sirloin), fish, dark green leafy vegetables, pumpkin seeds, dark chocolate, dried apricots, lentils, raisins, and beans.
- Encourage patients with iron deficiency to make modifications with meals to improve iron absorption:
  - o Consume vitamin C-rich foods to improve iron absorption. These include foods such as oranges (or juice), strawberries, all citrus, broccoli, kiwi, and parsley.
  - o Avoid drinking caffeine at meals as it interferes with iron absorption.
  - o Avoid consuming calcium with foods high in iron as it reduces iron absorption.
  - o Avoid dieting unless the diet is high in iron.
- Instruct patient about potential constipation, stomach irritation, indigestion and bloating if taking iron supplements: Stay well hydrated (8–10 glasses of water daily), increase fruits and vegetables, and exercise.
- Encourage a healthy lifestyle: disease, recognition of early warning signs, when to call the health care provider, follow-up care, healthy diet, weight management, medications, smoking cessation, moderate alcohol use, manage comorbid conditions, exercise, and reduce stress.
- Educate the patient about the need to balance rest with activity to avoid setbacks in recovery from overactivity.
- Discuss and assist patient to identify healthy ways that may help them emotionally cope with the challenges of a chronic illness.
- Educate patients who are at a higher risk of bleeding for fall precautions.
- Prepare the patient to monitor for any of the following signs of a blood reaction that may be delayed and occur within days post-transfusion:
  - o Chest or back pain, shortness of breath, fever, chills, tachycardia, rash, dizziness, dark urine, nausea, fainting, diarrhea, jaundice, sudden bleeding within 1–2 weeks, blood in stool, unexpected vagina bleeding, or sudden onset of headache may all be signs of a blood reaction, hemolysis, or infection. The patient should know to call the health care provider or seek medical care.
  - o Fever, rash, and diarrhea should trigger concern by anyone who has received a stem cell transplant, warning of a graft-versus-host condition.
- Instruct patients who do not want to receive blood products to make their preferences and concerns known and documented. This is particularly important prior to surgery. Inform patients that autologous transfusions are possible by banking and then receiving their own blood.
- Educate those at higher risk for anemia about the potential for anemia and preventive alteration that can be made in the diet:
  - o Patient with a low but still normal RBC count, hemoglobin or hematocrit
  - o Young women who are considering pregnancy
  - o Women (or the parents of a teen) who may have very heavy menstrual periods
  - o Women who are pregnant. Pregnancy increases the demand for iron by about 33–50%.
- Consult a nutritionist if needed or desired. This is particularly important for vegetarians or vegans if their diet is deficient in essential RBC building factors (e.g., iron, vitamins).
- Inform all patients about the benefits of advanced directives and encourage discussion with loved ones.

Summary: Anemia

Types of Anemia	Causes	Diagnostics	Treatment
B12	Decreased absorption due to Crohn's disease, gastric bypass surgery.	Macrocytic (high MCV mean corpuscular volume) Low reticulocyte count	Monthly B12 injections, or daily high dose B12
folate	Poor nutrition, alcoholism, some types of chemotherapy e.g. methotrexate	Macrocytic Low reticulocyte count	Folate PO or IV
Iron deficiency	Chronic bleeding e.g. colon cancer, or heavy menstrual bleeding; poor iron absorption, (e.g. celiac disaese, crohn's disease); decreased iron in diet	Microcytic (low MCV) Low iron, low ferritin, High iron binding capacity Low iron stores on bone marrow biopsy Stool ± occult blood Low reticulocyte count	Intravenous or oral iron supplementation. Intravenous iron may useful in patients that have decreased absorption
Chronic disease	Chronic illness: e.g. infection, diabetes, cancer, inflammatory disorders e.g. lupus	Normocytic or microcytic Iron (Fe) low or normal Ferritin high TIBC low or normal Low reticulocyte count	Treat underlying problems e.g. diabetes, infection. Treat iron deficiency if present. May use SQ erythropoeitin or darbopoeitin
Chronic Kidney disease	Chronic Kidney disease	Elevated BUN and creatinine Normocytic Low reticulocyte count Low erythropoeitin levels	Erythropoietin or darbopoeitin SQ or IV. Evaluate iron stores
Aplastic anemia	Viral infections Autoimmune toxins	Macrocytic Pancytopenia- low platelets, WBCs and RBCs Bone marrow shows decreased cellularity.	Erythropoietin. Blood transfusions if symptomatic

Types of Anemia	Causes	Diagnostics	Treatment
Chemotherapy induced Anemia	Chemotherapy	Evaluate kidney function BUN/Cr Fe, Ferritin Reticulocyte count low	Erythropoietic stimulating agents for Hgb <10g/dl and goal 10-12 g/dl. Supplemental iron. Consider transfusion for symptomatic anemia not responding to erythropoietin agents. Folate for chemotherapies that deplete folate.
Bleeding, acute	Trauma Menstrual bleeding Gastrointestinal bleeding	Normocytic anemia. If bleeding is acute hemoglobin levels may be normal initially	IV fluids to maintain blood pressure. Transfuse for massive bleeding or Hg < 7
Bleeding, chronic	Menstrual bleeding Colon cancer, gastritis, gastric cancer, bleeding polyp	Microcytic (low MCV) Low iron, low ferritin High iron binding capacity Low iron stores on bone marrow biopsy Stool ± for occult blood Low reticulocyte count	Evaluate and treat cause of bleeding. Oral iron supplementation. Intravenous iron may be useful in patients that have decreased absorption.
Hemolytic	Enzyme deficiency e.g., G6PD, cancer, Hemolytic idiopathic thrombocytopenia purpura, Drugs e.g., heparin, IIb/IIIa inhibitors Autoantibodies Infections: e.g. mycoplasma, malaria Disseminated Intravascular coagulation. Transfusion reactions	Haptaglobin low Positive Coombs test Elevated LDH Elevated Total Bilirubin Elevated Indirect Bilirubin	Depends on the cause. Steroids, withdrawal of medications that are causing problem, treatment of infection.

Summary: Anemia (continued)

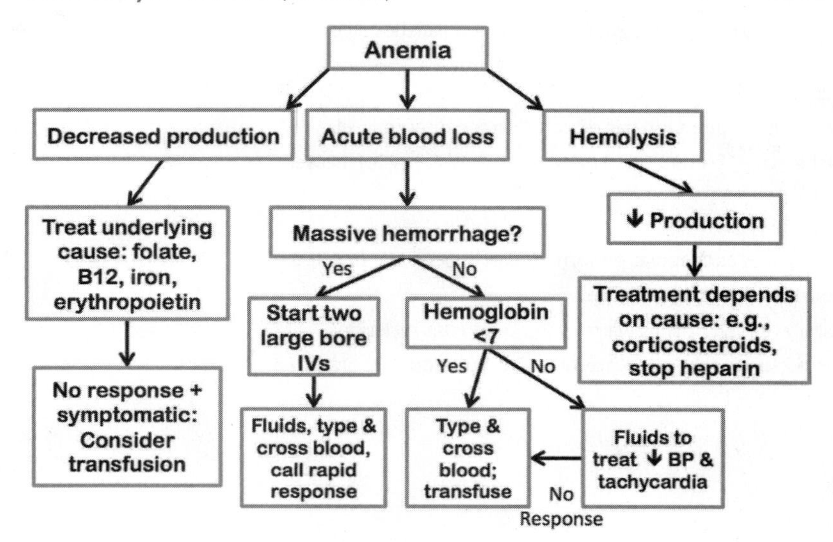

Source: Copyright © 2014, NovEx Novice to Expert Learning, LLC

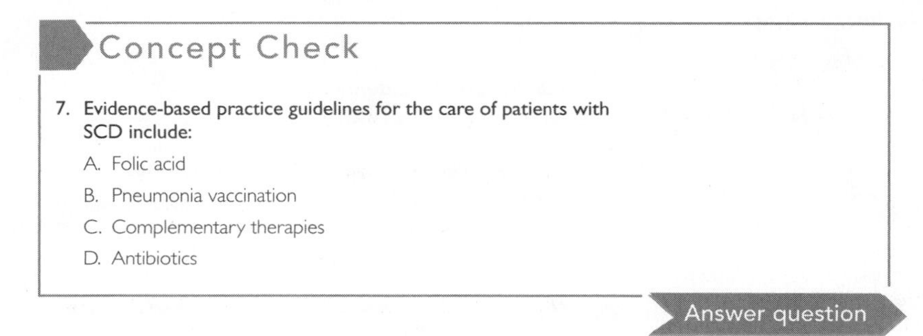

Concept Check
7. Evidence-based practice guidelines for the care of patients with SCD include:
A. Folic acid
B. Pneumonia vaccination
C. Complementary therapies
D. Antibiotics
Answer question

LO3:

Summary of Interventions

- For anemia due to impaired production of RBCs, treat the underlying deficiencies or causes (e.g., B_{12}, folate, or iron).
- Anemia due to chronic kidney disease is commonly treated with erythropoietin.

Indications for transfusion:

- Massive hemorrhage
- Acute bleeding and hemoglobin <7 gm/dL
- If patients are not responding to treatment of underlying conditions and the patient remains symptomatic (dyspnea, tachycardia, fatigue), consider RBC transfusion. Examples include patients that have not responded to erythropoietin, iron, or B_{12}.

LO4:

Evaluation of Desired Collaborative Care Outcomes

Evaluation and reassessment should reveal attainment of previously established patient outcomes. In summary:

- Patient reports adequate endurance for daily activities.
- Patient's arterial blood gas and/or oxygen saturation has returned to the desired level.
- Patient reports being comfortable with current frequency and consistency of bowel movements.
- Patient is infection free.
- Patient has intact oral mucous membranes and reports performing oral hygiene as instructed.
- Patient reports that measures to control pain are effective.
- Patient has uncompromised capillary refill and skin is warm with no necrosis or lesions.
- Patient demonstrates consuming a nutritionally adequate diet, and nutritional laboratory values are trending toward expected range.

References

Adegbola, M., Barnes, D., Opollo, J., et al. (2012).Voices of adults living with sickle cell disease pain. *J Natl Black Nurses Assoc, 23*(2), 16–23. **www.ncbi.nlm.nih.gov/pmc/articles/PMC3804106/**

Annibale, B., Lahner, E., & Fave, G. D. (2011). Diagnosis and management of pernicious anemia. *Curr Gastroenterol Rep, 13*(6), 518–24.

Brown, M. (2012). Managing the acutely ill adult with sickle cell disease. *Brit J Nurs, 21*(2), 90–96.

Carson, J. L., Terrin, M. L., Noveck, H., et al. (2011). Liberal or restrictive transfusion in high-risk patients after hip surgery. *N Engl J Med, 365*(26), 2453–2462. doi: 10.1056/NEJMoa1012452.

Kapur, B., Soldin, O. P., & Koren, G. (2002). Potential prevention of neural tube defects by assessment of women of childbearing age through monitoring of folate. *The Drug Monit, 24*(5), 628–630.

Liebman, H. A. (2008). Heparin-induced thrombocytopenia: diagnosis and management. *Vascular, 16*(Suppl 1), S71–S76.

Michel, M. (2011). Classification and therapeutic approaches in autoimmune hemolytic anemia: an update. *Expert Rev Hematol, 4*(6), 607–618.

National Institute for Health and Clinical Excellence (NICE). (2012). *Sickle cell acute painful episode: management of an acute painful sickle cell episode in hospital.* London, UK: National Institute for Health and Clinical Excellence (NICE clinical guideline #143).

Rees, D., Williams, T., & Gladwin, M. (2010). Sickle-cell disease. *Lancet, 376*, 2018–2031. doi: 10.1016/S0140-6736(10)61029-X

Simmons, S. (2010). Anemia. *Nursing, 40*(6), 34. doi: 10.1097/01.NURSE.0000376295.75723.4d

Tolich, D., Blackmur, S., & Stahorsky, K. (2013). Blood management: best-practice transfusion strategies. *Nursing, 43*(1), 40–48. doi: 10.1097/01.NURSE.0000423955.22755.b1

United States Department of Health and Human Services. *The 2007 National Blood Collection and Utilization Survey Report.* **www.aabb.org/research/hemovigilance/bloodsurvey/Documents/07nbcusrpt.pdf#search=The%202007%20National%20Blood%20Collection%20and%20Utilization%20Survey%20Report**

Villanueva, C., Colomo, A., Bosch, A., et al. (2013). Transfusion strategies for acute upper gastrointestinal bleeding. *N Engl J Med, 368*(1), 11–21. doi: 10.1056/NEJMoa1211801

Clinical Practice Guidelines

American Medical Directors Association. (2011). *Anemia in the long-term care setting.* Columbia, MD: America Medical Directors Association. **http://www.guideline.gov/content.aspx?id=10830**

Carson, J., Brossman, B., Kleinman, S., et al., and the Clinical Transfusion Medicine Committee of the AABB. (2012). Red blood cell transfusion: a clinical practice guideline from the AABB. *Ann Intern Med, 157*(1), 49–58. doi: 10.7326/0003-4819-157-1-201206190-00429

Glassberg J. (2011). Evidence-based management of sickle cell disease in the emergency department. *Emerg Med Pract, 13*(8): 1–20.

National Heart, Lung, and Blood Institute. (2002). *Management of sickle cell disease.* **www.nhlbi.nih.gov/health/prof/blood/sickle/sc_mngt.pdf**

Weinstein, R. (2012). 2012 Clinical practice guide on red blood cell transfusion. *Ann Intern Med, 157*, 49–58. **www.hematology.org/Practice/Guidelines/2934.aspx**

Patient Education

American Society of Hematology. (2013). *Anemias.* **www.hematology.org/Patients/Blood-Disorders/Anemia/5225.aspx**

Harvard Sickle Cell Program. **Sickle.bwh.harvard.edu/outpatient.html**

Mayo Clinic Staff. (2014). *Iron deficiency anemia.* **www.mayoclinic.org/diseases-conditions/iron-deficiency-anemia/basics/definition/con-20019327**

Womenshealth.gov, U.S. Department of Health and Human Services. (2012). *Anemia.* **www.womenshealth.gov/publications/our-publications/fact-sheet/anemia.html#g**

Learning Outcomes for Blood Cancers

When you complete this lesson, you will be able to:

1. Recognize the clinical relevance of blood cancers.
2. Consider the pathophysiology, etiology, risk factors, and clinical presentation of blood cancers that determine the priority patient concerns.
3. Determine the most urgent and important nursing interventions and patient education required in caring for a patient with blood cancer.
4. Evaluate attainment of desired collaborative care outcomes for a patient with blood cancer.

LO1:

What Are Blood Cancers?

- Blood cancers, including leukemia, lymphoma, and myeloma, are diseases that can affect the bone marrow, the blood cells, the lymph nodes, and other parts of the lymphatic system.
- A review of the types of blood cancers will illustrate their similarities and differences in symptoms and treatment.

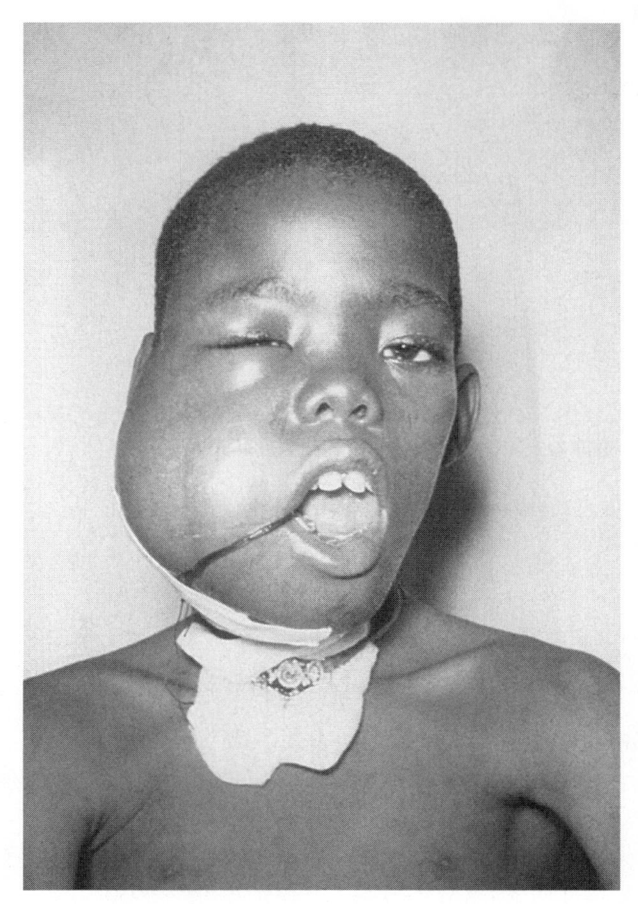

Blood cancer can manifest with solid tumor formation. This photo shows a patient with Burkitt's lymphoma, which is a type of non-Hodgkin's lymphoma. Like leukemia, it is a malignant and very aggressive cancer. Abnormal B cells predominantly make up the tumor mass.

Source: Centers for Disease Control and Prevention/Robert S. Craig

LO1: Clinical Relevance

- Blood cancers, as a group, occur in more than 130,000 patients per year.
- Patients with blood cancers can present in nononcology settings with rapid progression before diagnosis.
- Blood cancers can be very aggressive and often have many complications, including septic shock, that lead to the patient being admitted to an intensive care unit.
- These patients often live well, despite their disease; so they are seen in the community for care or admitted to hospitals for other health reasons.

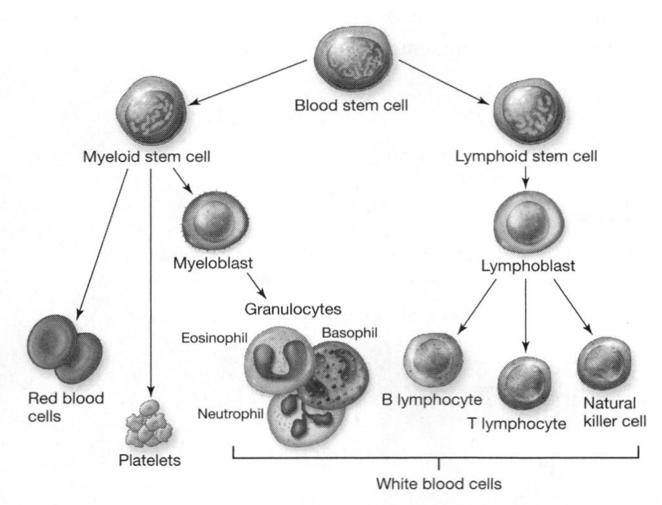

This drawing illustrates the formation of the different types of red and white blood cells. Originating as a parent stem cell that gives rise to myeloid and lymphoid stem cells, the final products are the many and varied cells that occupy the vascular systems of humans throughout the world.

LO2: Pathophysiology

Blood cancers are all related to one another in that they all result from DNA mutations of blood-forming stem cells.

- The abnormal stem cell produces clones, generating rapid growth in the numbers of abnormal cells.
- The cancer cells grow without the usual controls that are in place for normal blood cells. Production of normal blood cells is decreased as normal cells in the bone marrow are replaced.
- These abnormal cells proliferate in the blood, lymphatic system, and bone marrow.
- The abnormal cells often produce cytokines that can cause systemic symptoms such as fevers.
- The most clinically important types of blood cancers include:
    - o Leukemia
    - o Lymphoma
    - o Myeloma

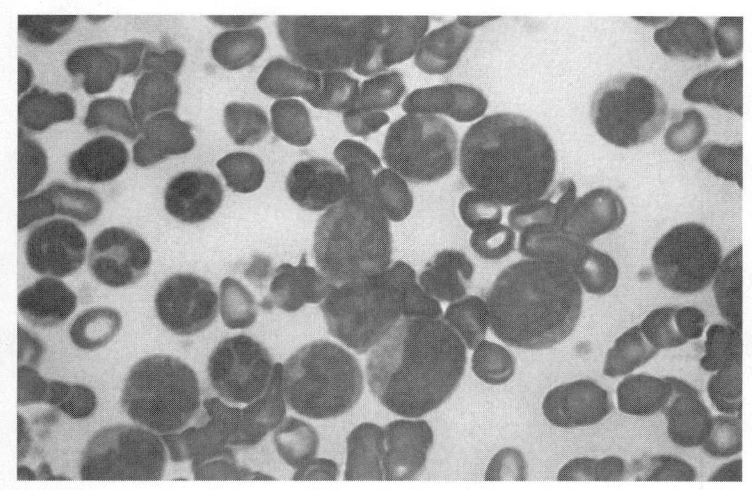

This histology smear shows the marked and unregulated growth of white blood cells (WBCs) or specifically myeloblasts in chronic myelogenous leukemia. Note the number of large purple-stained WBCs in the photo reveals a "blast crisis." Also note the characteristic disproportionate nucleus versus cytoplasm areas in the WBCs ... much less cytoplasm seen in cancer cells.
Source: Centers for Disease Control and Prevention/Stacy Howard

Concept Check

1. **Blood cancer cells are not shown to proliferate in which tissue?**
   A. Blood
   B. Lymphatic
   C. Bone marrow
   D. Muscle

Answer question

Pathophysiology (continued)

Leukemia

- Leukemia is a cancer of the blood/bone marrow. The word "leukemia" comes from the Greek *leukos* (or "white") and *aima* (meaning "blood"). In leukemia, the patient has abnormal production of blood cells, generally immature leukocytes (blasts).
- Blast cells can become markedly elevated in leukemia. Blasts are not typically found in the peripheral blood. So, in leukemia, you may see blasts circulating in the blood. The white blood cell (WBC) count of a patient with leukemia may be markedly elevated or severely decreased.
- In leukemia, blast cells grow and divide chaotically.
- The abnormal blood cells do not die easily and, therefore, accumulate, occupying more and more space. As increasing space is occupied by these faulty blood cells, there is less space for the normal cells.
- Certain leukemias (acute leukemias) can develop quickly and proceed with a rapid decline in the patient's health.
- Chronic leukemia is much more subtle and not as quick to cause symptoms.

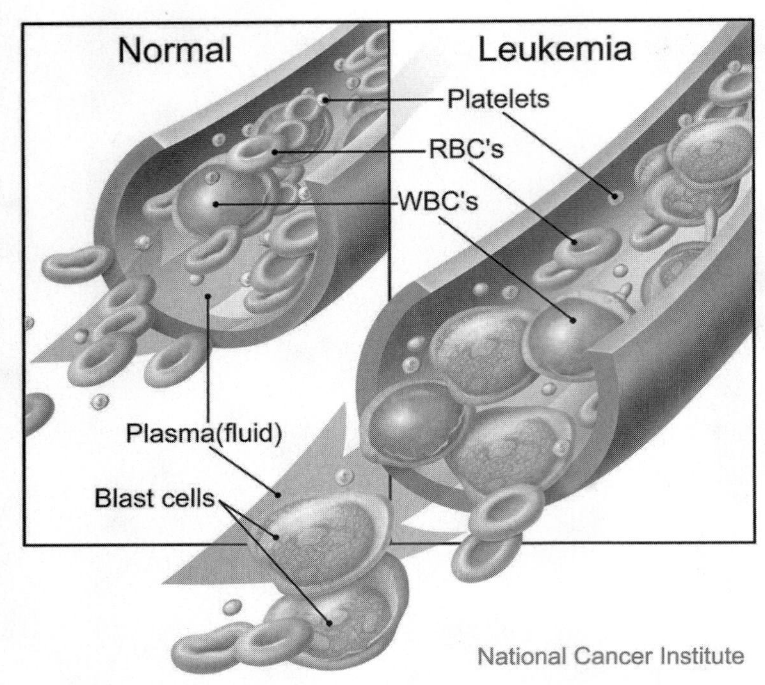

The drawings compare the blood composition of normal versus leukemia. Note the uncontrolled increase in blast cells in leukemia.
Source: Alan Hoofring/National Cancer Institute, www.cancer.gov

Types of Leukemia

- Leukemia presents as one of four distinct types, with subtypes within each major type depending on the cells they are derived from or on whether onset is acute and rapid.
  - Acute myeloid leukemia (AML) is derived from myeloid cells (WBCs that are not lymphocytes).
    - In the United States, there are 12,950 cases per year with 9,050 deaths.
    - Rapid onset with high risk of death can occur if not treated quickly.
  - Chronic myeloid leukemia (CML) arises from bone marrow overproduction of granulocytes, a type of WBCs that are not healthy.
    - In the United States, there are 5,150 cases per year with 270 deaths.
    - Slow disease progression
  - Acute lymphocytic leukemia (ALL) is derived from the lymphocyte line of cells.
    - In the United States, there are 5,730 cases per year with 1,420 deaths.
    - Much more prevalent and curable in children
  - Chronic lymphocytic leukemia (CLL) arises from the bone marrow overproducing lymphocytes (a type of WBC).
    - In the United States, there are 14,570 cases per year with 4,380 deaths.
    - Most common leukemia with the slowest clinical course, often not requiring any treatment

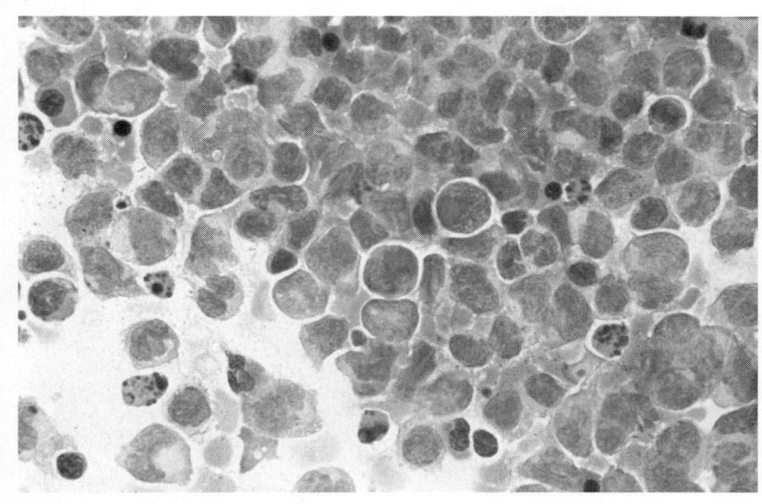

This histology blood smear shows acute myelocytic leukemia (AML). Note the abundance of WBCs or leukocytes (purple-stained, large cells).
Source: Dr. Lance Liotta Laboratory/National Cancer Institute, www.cancer.gov

Concept Check

2. Which cells, not typically found in blood, are present in the blood of a patient with leukemia?
   A. A cells
   B. Erythrocytes
   C. Blast cells
   D. Lymphocytes

Answer question

Pathophysiology (continued)

Lymphoma

- Lymphoma is a general term for blood cancers that originate in the lymphatic system.
- Malignant lymphocytes accumulate in the following body parts with lymphatic tissue:
  - o Lymph nodes
  - o Liver
  - o Spleen
  - o Bone marrow

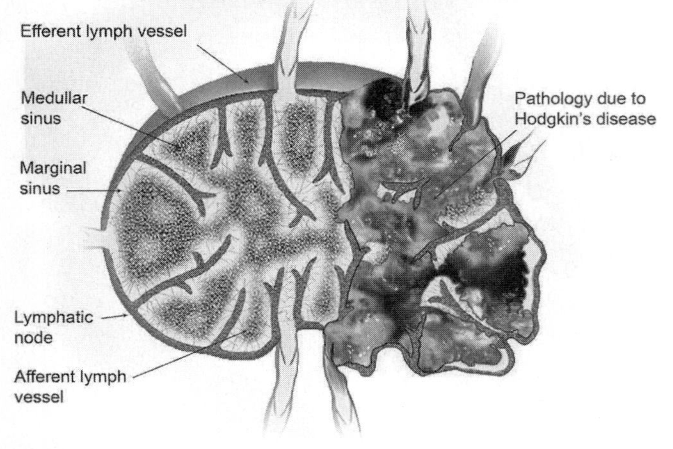

Depicted above is the normal anatomy of a lymph node on the left and an abnormal one on the right as it is afflicted with Hodgkin Disease.
Source: © 2014 Nucleus Medical Media. All rights reserved

- Lymphoma is the leading blood cancer in the United States with more cases annually than any other type of blood cancer.
- There are two distinct types of lymphoma:
  - o Hodgkin's disease
    - In the United States, there are 8,830 cases per year with 1,300 deaths.
    - Has a specific cell type called the Reed-Sternberg Cell
    - Usually affects people 20–40 years of age
  - o Non-Hodgkin's lymphoma
    - In the United States, there are 66,360 cases per year with 19,320 deaths.
    - Over 40 different types of non-Hodgkin's lymphoma have been identified.

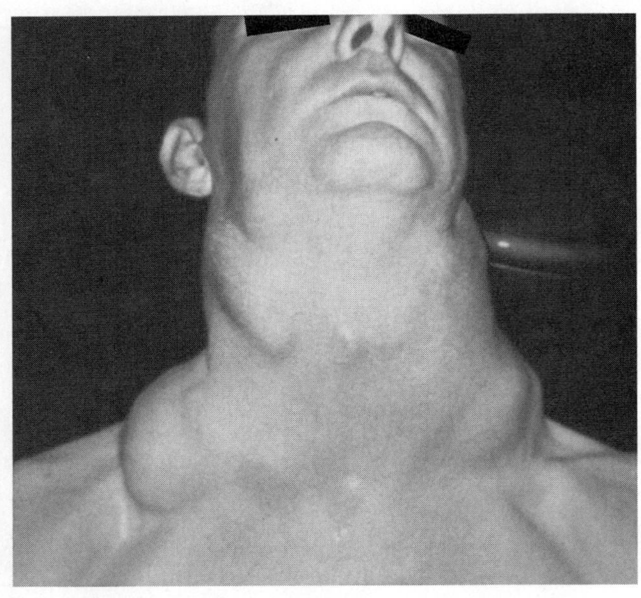

This young man experienced painless enlargement of his cervical lymph nodes and was found to have Hodgkin's lymphoma.
Source: Centers for Disease Control and Prevention/Robert E. Sumpter

Myeloma

- Myeloma is a cancer of the plasma cells (the end of B lymphocyte differentiation).
  - o Plasma cells make immune globulins in the blood.
  - o Immune globulins are antibodies and are made of proteins.
- In myeloma, the plasma cells become malignant, resulting in overproduction of one clone of immunoglobulins (antibodies).
  - o The patient will then overproduce one of the following:
    1. IGG
    2. IGM
    3. IGA
    4. Light chains (Lamda or Kappa)

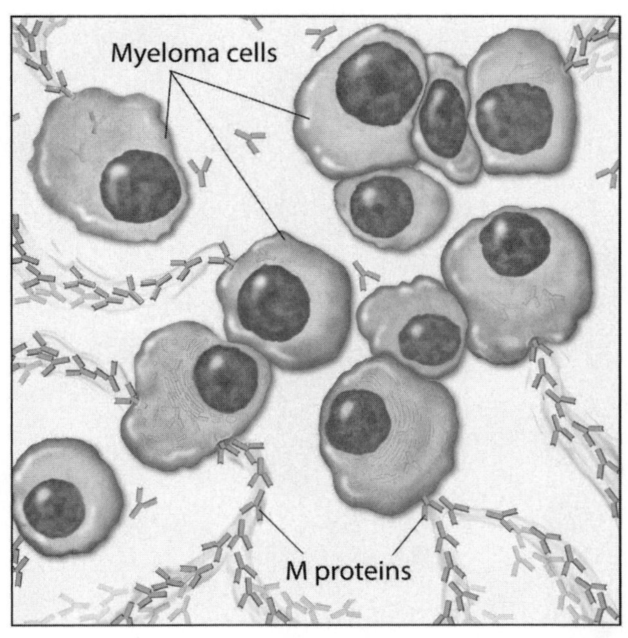

The above drawing depicts myeloma cells making an overabundance of M proteins. M proteins are antibodies made by myeloma cells, abnormal plasma cells.
Source: Lydia Kibiuk/National Cancer Institute

Concept Check

3. **Which type of blood cancer is most common in the United States?**
   A. Leukemia
   B. Hodgkin's lymphoma
   C. Non-Hodgkin's lymphoma
   D. Myeloma

Answer question

LO2:

Risk Factors

- Radiation
- Chemotherapy
- Weak immune system
- Older age
- Particular infections (e.g., HIV, Epstein-Barr virus, *H. pylori*, human T-cell leukemia/lymphoma virus type 1, hepatitis C)
- Race, dependent on type of blood cancer
- Heredity
- Smoking
- Chemicals such as benzene, herbicides, pesticides
- Geographic location
- Body weight
- Dietary intake

LO2: Causes

- Radiation
- Genetics
- Viruses: human T-lymphotropic virus and HIV
- Chemicals such as benzene

Radiation Exposure Pathways

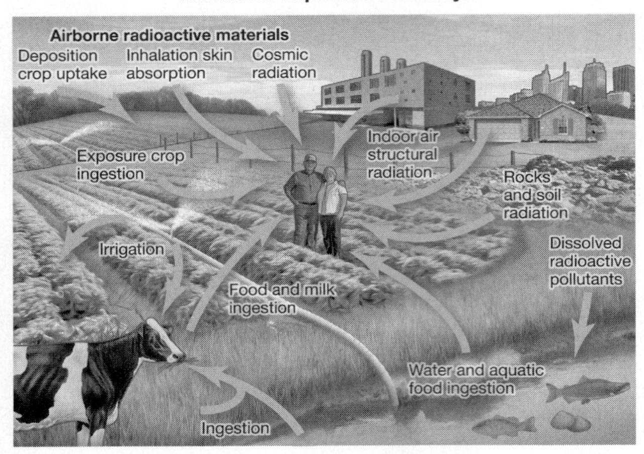

Total body radiation has many environmental sources of which we are not usually aware. However, over the period of a lifetime, there is a cumulative dose to a person that becomes a risk factor for developing cancer, especially of the blood-forming elements of our system that can result in leukemia, myeloma, and lymphoma.

LO2: Assessment Findings

- The different blood cancers often produce similar symptoms due to the overproduction of WBCs that is common in all. The WBCs crowd out all other blood cells and not only the red cells. Signs and symptoms, therefore, reflect the consequences of the abnormally high WBC affects, which lead to anemia, thrombocytopenia, and neutropenia.
    - o Anemia impairs oxygen delivery to tissues and causes fatigue.
    - o Thrombocytopenia causes easy bruising or bleeding.
    - o Neutropenia predisposes to infection.
- Lymphomas often have symptoms called "B symptoms" that result from cytokines that B cells produce:
    - o Fever
    - o Night sweats
    - o Weight loss
- In myeloma, patients often present with bone pain, renal dysfunction, and electrolyte abnormalities, namely high calcium levels in the blood.

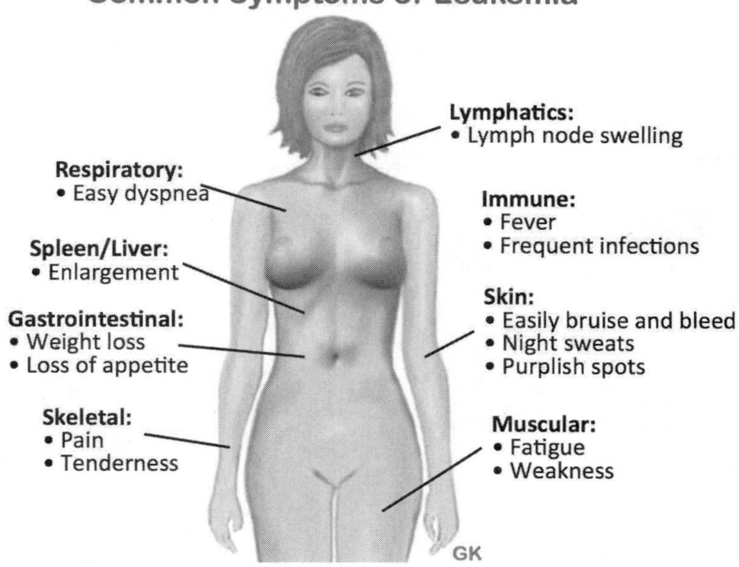

Common symptoms of leukemia.
Source: Courtesy of George Kyriakidis/Santa Ana, CA

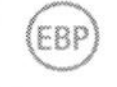

Diagnostics

- (EBP) For leukemia, a diagnosis is made by doing a test on the bone marrow sample (Alberta Provincial Hematology Tumour Team [APHTT], 2009).
  - o The procedure consists of a biopsy of the bone marrow with aspiration of the blood within.
  - o The blood and marrow are sent off for special testing to identify genetic abnormalities.
- For lymphoma, diagnosis may include:
  - o Special scanning, particularly CT and PET scans, which assist in staging and restaging the lymphoma
  - o (EBP) A full lymph node dissection and evaluation (APHTT, 2012)
  - o (EBP) Immunohistochemical and fluorescence in situ hybridization (FISH) test to confirm a specific diagnosis (e.g., Hodgkin lymphoma, diffuse large B-cell lymphoma) (APHTT, 2012)
  - o A bone marrow biopsy
- For multiple myeloma, diagnosis is made by blood testing, looking for the overproduced antibody immune globulin.
  - o A bone marrow biopsy is also done at initial diagnosis.

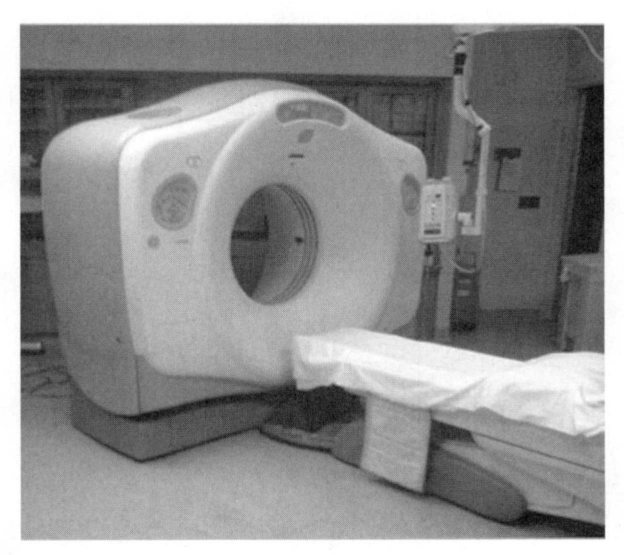

CT scan.
Source: Courtesy of K. Kyriakidis

Concept Check

4. Which finding is common in patients with lymphoma?

A. Night sweats
B. Bone pain
C. Kidney dysfunction
D. High serum calcium

Answer question

Prognosis

- Prognosis of the blood cancers is dependent on how many chromosomal abnormalities are found on the bone marrow and lymph node biopsy.
    - o The more chromosomal abnormalities are found, the worse the prognosis tends to be.
    - o There are some genetic alterations (AML with 11q23 genetic abnormalities) that have very well-established and poor prognoses.

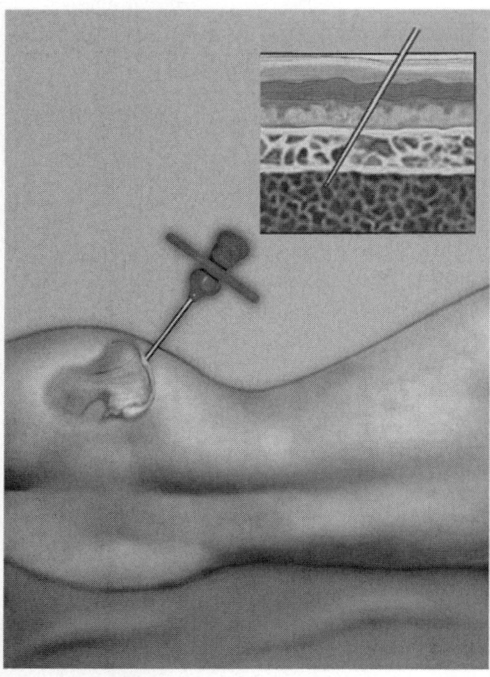

A bone marrow biopsy is usually performed on the back of the hip bone in adults. A long needle is inserted into the bone to remove bone marrow.
Source: Copyright © 2014, NovEx Novice to Expert Learning, LLC

Priority Patient Concerns and Desired Collaborative Care Outcomes

Prior to caring for patients with blood cancers, it is important to prioritize the patient's concerns that must guide the nursing care plan and interventions. Care for the patient is ordered and organized in accordance with the patient's priority and urgent needs. Desired collaborative care outcomes in patients with blood cancers typically include:

1. Patient will remain free of infection and will not experience bleeding episodes.
2. Patient's fluid volume will remain in balance.
3. Patient will have sufficient energy to maintain daily activities as desired.
4. Patient will verbalize fears and demonstrate healthy coping behaviors.

Considering these important care outcomes, prepare a list of the major 3–6 priority patient concerns or nursing diagnoses for patients with blood cancers. Be prepared to participate in a discussion of this list and/or to submit them as an assignment, as determined by your faculty. Resources you may find helpful in this assignment can include this lesson, the references, resources on nursing care plans, and standard nursing diagnoses manuals.

LO3:

Collaborative Interventions

Collaborative interventions, particularly the nursing monitoring and interventions that are common in most cancers, are detailed in the Oncology Care of the Cancer Patient NovE-lessons. This section includes collaborative interventions that are more specific to the care of patients with blood cancers and also includes recommendations from the clinical practice guidelines (APHTT, 2009, 2012; Imrie, et al., 2009; Oscier, et al., 2010):

- Blood cancers are "liquid," meaning they are fluid throughout the body. For this reason:

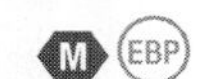
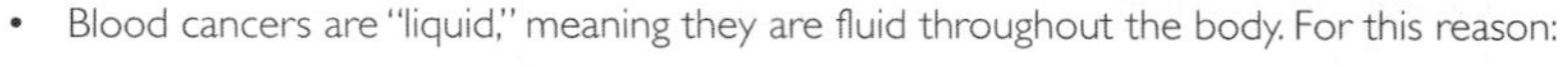

  - Surgery is not a typical treatment modality for blood cancers.

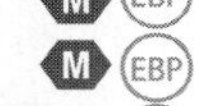

  - Radiation is not a typical treatment modality for most blood cancers.
  - Exceptions may include very early stage Hodgkin lymphoma and solitary lesions in myeloma.
- Chemotherapy is the main treatment modality because it is a systemic treatment.
  - Chemotherapy is very aggressively used. It has side effects that include bone marrow suppression, hair loss, mouth sores, and nausea. (See the Overview of the Care of Cancer Patients NovE-lessons for care of the patients with these complications.)
  - Rituximab is recommended in combination with fludarabine and cyclophosphamide to treat patients with relapsed or refractory chronic lymphocytic leukemia in most conditions (National Institute for Health and Clinical Excellence [NICE], 2010).
- Stem cell transplantation is a very common treatment modality used in patients with blood cancers for:
  - Relapse
  - High risk diseases that have a high risk for recurrence. Stem cell transplantation attempts to prevent the disease from coming back.

For greater detail, refer to clinical practice guidelines in the specialty care of these patients (Oliansky, et al., 2012). (See the Care of Cancer Patients and Treatment Toxicities NovE-lessons.).

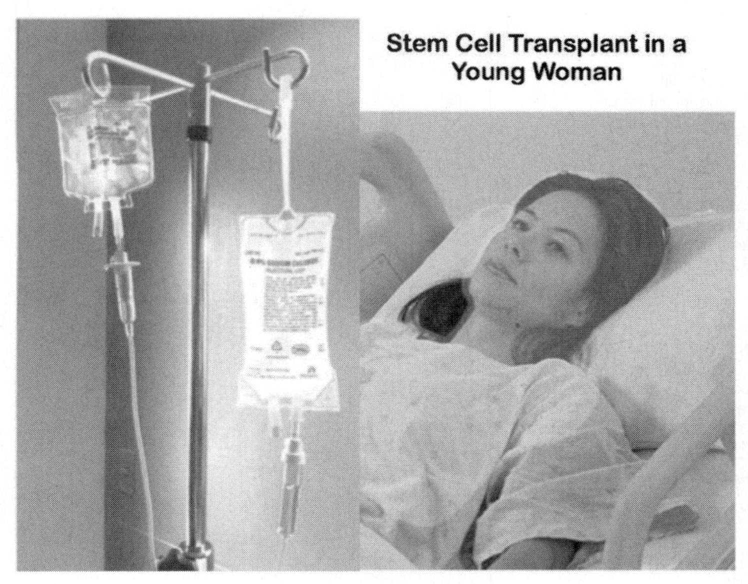

Following recurrence of her blood cancer, this young patient received a stem cell transplant.

Collaborative Interventions (continued)

Hematopoietic Stem Cell Transplantation (HSCT)

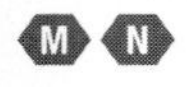

HSCT, also known as bone marrow transplant, is an increasingly common procedure. It includes the transplantation of donor stem cells from bone marrow harvest, peripheral blood, or umbilical cord blood. HSCT involves a multistage process with differing patient care needs at each stage:

Hematopoietic Stem Cell Transplantation Process	
Process Stages	**Collaborative Interventions**
Stem cell harvest or collection	
• Bone marrow may be harvested from the patient's or donor's iliac crest by aspirating marrow multiple times.	Routine postoperative care of the donor is needed with emphasis on: • IV fluid replacements • Recovery from anesthesia • Airway protection and management • Management of postoperative pain • Wound care • Monitoring vital signs • Monitoring for bleeding
• Peripheral stem cells may be collected by pheresis, which entails filtering the stem cells from the donor's whole blood.	Care of the donor during the 2–4 hour pheresis includes: • Anticoagulation with potential hypocalcemia • Prevention of vascular catheter clotting • Management of hypovolemia and hypotension
• High concentrations of stem cells may also be obtained from the umbilical cord before detachment from the placenta.	(Phlebotomy procedure and blood is sent to a Cord Blood Registry for processing.)
Conditioning or Preparative Regimen: 2–7 days prior to transplantation	
• Before receiving the donor stem cells, the patient receives doses of chemotherapy to suppress the bone marrow and immune system, to eradicate cancer cells (myeloablation), and prevent the patient's rejection of the stem cells. This is the conditioning or preparative phase. • Total body irradiation (TBI) may also be used in the regimen. • Newer approaches, such as nonmyeloablative stem cell transplantation, are being studied to reduce the intensity of the conditioning regimen and decrease the morbidity and mortality.	Care of the patient centers on: • Prevention, early recognition, and management of the treatment-induced toxicities, particularly infections and sepsis. • Toxicities from this intensive regimen cause all the side effects of both treatments, particularly o Nausea and vomiting; loss of appetite o Capillary leakage (e.g., edema, orthopnea) o Bleeding from thrombocytopenia o Diarrhea and abdominal pain o Fatigue from anemia and toxic drugs o Mucositis o Severe neutropenia with vulnerability to bacterial, viral, and fungal infections. o (See the Oncology Care of the Cancer Patient with Treatment Toxicities NovE-lesson for details.) • Administration of hematopoietic growth factor to improve recovery time, boosts RBC production, reduces infections, and lowers severity and duration of mucositis. Additional care includes managing the side effects, such as injection site pain, flu-like effects, bone pain, muscle aching, hypertension, headaches, and fever. • Management of polypharmaceutical administration • Emotional support of the patient during this period of toxicities, severe illness, and isolation
Transplantation or Stem Cell Infusion: 30 minutes; considered Day 0	
• Transplantation involves thawing the stem cells or frozen marrow and infusing them in a simple infusion via a central venous catheter.	Care of the patient during stem cell transfusion involves: • Early recognition, prevention, and management of fever and hypertension with pretreatment acetaminophen, hydrocortisone, and diphenhydramine • Early recognition and management of hypertension with diuretics and antihypertensive medications • Recognition of hemorrhagic cystitis (red urine), cardiomyopathy with heart failure, INFECTION, and acute kidney injury
Engraftment: 8–12 days post-HSCT	
• Stem and bone marrow cells discover and inhabit the patient's marrow-forming sites in the bone where they struggle to survive, grow, and produce blood cells (e.g., RBCs, platelets, WBCs). This process is known as engraftment.	Similar care of the patient continues due to: • High risk for infections • Continued complications of treatment-induced toxicities • High risk for bleeding • Administration of hematopoietic growth factor • Potential need for parenteral nutrition • Fluid and electrolyte imbalances • Management of polypharmaceutical administration • Emotional support of the patient during this prolonged period of toxicities, severe illness, isolation, body image changes, threat of death, dependence, and family role changes. • Consult chaplain, social worker, psychologist, family members, friends, and support groups in collaboration with the patient and preferences.

Collaborative Interventions (continued)

Symptom Management and Comfort Care

Interventions for blood cancers, as well as for most cancers, cause multisystem toxicities (e.g., anorexia, diarrhea, mucositis, nausea) in patients. Symptom management and comfort care due to these toxicities require extensive nursing care, which is detailed in the Oncology Care of the Cancer Patient NovE-lessons. Care that is more specific to patients with blood cancers includes:

- Aggressive support to prevent or treat myelosuppression

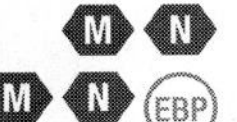

- Prevention, assessment for risk of, early recognition, and treatment of infections (early initiation of antimicrobials at first sign of infection) is strongly recommended. This should be ongoing but is particularly important prior to initiation of treatment (Oscier, et al., 2012).

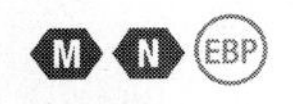

- Screen all patients for Hepatitis B and C prior to immunosuppressive therapy (Oscier, et al., 2012).
- Monitoring for less typical signs of infection. Pus may not be a reliable sign of infection in patients with blood cancers. The production of pus requires neutrophils and these patients commonly have few neutrophils, making the identification of infection more challenging.
- Prevention, early recognition, and treatment of bleeding. The highest risk of bleeding occurs during procedures when the platelet count drops below 50,000. Danger of spontaneous bleeding occurs when the platelet count falls below 10,000.

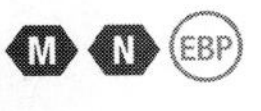

- A central venous catheter should be considered in patients undergoing chemotherapy (APHTT, 2009).
- Treatment of fatigue by encouraging activity balanced with energy conservation
  - o Encourage patient to guide plans on activity and rest.
  - o Encourage adequate nutritional intake.
  - o Collaborate with patient and family to ensure protected rest and sleep periods.
  - o Collaborate with patient to allow appropriate numbers of visitors.
  - o Incorporate diversions that enhance rest (e.g., music, massage).
  - o Teach patient and family how to compassionately guide visitors to limit number and duration of visits.

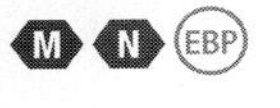

- Antifungal prophylaxis should be considered for patients receiving chemotherapy (APHTT, 2009).
- Provide ample opportunities for and support the patient to share any fear, concern, or anxiety about their illness or potential consequences of the illness.
- Educate the patient about tests, procedures, limitations, and medications needed to provide good care.
- Offer and explain the various types of alternative therapies (e.g., massage, music, guided imagery, acupuncture) that may complement or substitute for pharmacologic interventions for pain and discomfort.
- Transfusion of packed red blood cells, if needed for symptomatic anemia (APHTT, 2009)

Concept Check

5. What is the most common treatment modality for leukemia?

A. Surgery
B. Chemotherapy
C. Brachytherapy
D. External beam radiation

Answer question

Concept Check

6. When is stem cell transplantation most often used in blood cancers?

A. Upon relapse
B. If myelosuppression occurs
C. As initial therapy
D. If chemotherapy adverse effects are not tolerated

Answer question

Collaborative Interventions (continued)

Complications

- Oncologic emergencies are complications that should be recognized as soon as possible and treated immediately:
  - o Tumor lysis syndrome occurs when aggressive cancers, such as acute leukemias and lymphomas, are rapidly growing, are treated, and treatment results in the lysis of large numbers of cancer cells. Lysis of the cancer cells releases their intracellular contents into the bloodstream. High levels of potassium, phosphorus, and uric acid, the most common manifestations of tumor lysis syndrome, signal this complication. The goal of treatment for tumor lysis is to reduce the circulating uric acid and abnormal electrolytes. Uric acid can be managed by administering rasburicase or allopurinol. For electrolyte management, see the NovE-lesson on Fluid and Electrolytes.
  - o Sepsis can evolve very rapidly and can be deadly within hours due to the abnormally low neutrophil count. Monitor for and intervene immediately with early signs of sepsis in a neutropenic patient; signs include a slight drop in blood pressure, rise in heart rate, and a very low grade fever of 100.5°F (38°C).
- Monitor for and educate the patient to observe for long-term issues with blood cancers:
  - o Recurrence can occur in any of these diseases.
  - o Myeloma is not considered curable.
  - o There are several support programs available to these patients:
    - ▪ Leukemia/Lymphoma Society offers patient education, support groups, and financial support.
    - ▪ Lymphoma Network offers patient education, support groups, and financial support.
    - ▪ Myeloma Foundation offers patient education and support groups.

Patient Education

Education for patients with cancers is extensive and detailed in the Oncology Care of the Cancer Patient NovE-lessons. Additionally, education that is specific to patients with blood cancers and follows the APHTT clinical guidelines (2012) should include the following tasks:

- Educate regarding neutropenic precautions (see the Care of Cancer Patient with Treatment Toxicities NovE-lesson for details).
- Educate the patient to discuss antimicrobial prophylaxis with their health care provider when in an immunosuppressed state.
- Encourage the patient to keep immunizations current (Oscier, et al., 2012):
  - o Recommend pneumonia and flu vaccines at the time of diagnosis and annually.
  - o Avoid exposure to live vaccines.
  - o Avoid vaccinations 2 weeks prior, during, or within 6 months after chemotherapy.
- Stress the importance of routine follow-up care and treatment.
- Educate the patient about advanced directives.
- Consult pastoral care according to patient preferences.
- Educate the patient and family about how to politely and caringly limit visitors to minimize fatigue and risk of infection.
- Educate the patient regarding increased risk for complications, depending on the type and location of treatment: dental caries, infertility, relapse, hypothyroidism, secondary neoplasms.

Summary of Interventions

- Chemotherapy is the primary treatment for blood cancers, with radiation being occasionally and selectively used.
- Stem cell transplantation is a common treatment, depending on the type of blood cancer.
- Patients often develop anemia, thrombocytopenia, and neutropenia from blood cancers or from the treatment of blood cancers.
  - o Anemia may be severe enough to require transfusion.
  - o Thrombocytopenia can necessitate platelet transfusion if bleeding occurs and should be considered for a platelet count that is <10,000.
  - o Neutropenia leads to the development of infections. These infections or possible infections should be treated quickly and aggressively with antibiotics to prevent the development of sepsis.
- Symptom management and patient education should include prevention and early recognition.

Concept Check

7. Tumor lysis syndrome is highly associated with which finding?

A. Increased uric acid

B. Decreased potassium

C. Increased hematocrit

D. Decreased blood glucose

Answer question

LO4:

Evaluation of Desired Collaborative Care Outcomes

Evaluation and reassessment should reveal attainment of previously established patient outcomes. In summary:

- Patient has no signs of infection or bleeding.
- Patient's skin is warm and dry, blood pressure is within desired range, skin turgor is normal for the particular patient, and fluid intake is balanced with fluid output.
- Patient performs expected daily activities without excessive fatigue.
- Patient discusses fears related to diagnosis and demonstrates healthy coping.

References

Breed, C. (2003). Diagnosis, treatment, and nursing care of chronic leukemia. *SeminOncol Nursing, 19*(2), 109–117.

Devine, H., & DeMeyer, E. (2003). Hematopoietic cell transplantation in the treatment of leukemia. *SeminOncol Nursing, 19*(2), 118–132. **www.seminarsoncologynursing.com/article/S0749-2081(03)00008-1/fulltext**

Fairman, B. (2007). Clinical updates and nursing considerations for patient with multiple myeloma. *Clin J Oncol Nurs, 11*(6), 831–840. doi: 10.1188/07.CJON.831–840.

King, J. (2008). What is tumor lysis syndrome? *Nursing, 38*(5), 18.

Long, J., & Versea, L. (2006). Treatment approaches and nursing considerations for non-Hodgkin's lymphoma. *SeminOncol Nursing, 22*(2), 97–106. **www.seminarsoncologynursing.com/article/S0749-2081(06)00044-1/fulltext**

Saria, M. G., & Gosselin-Acomb, T. K. (2007). Hematopoietic stem cell transplantation: implications for critical care nurses. *Clin J Onco lNurs, 11*(1), 53–63. **www.researchgate.net/publication/6388044_Hematopoietic_stem_cell_transplantation_implications_for_critical_care_nurses**

Viele, C. (2003). Diagnosis, treatment, and nursing care of acute leukemia. *SeminOncol Nursing, 19*(2), 98–108 **www.seminarsoncologynursing.com/article/S0749-2081(03)00006-8/fulltext**

Clinical Practice Guidelines

Alberta Provincial Hematology Tumour Team. (2009). *Acute myeloid leukemia (Clinical practice guideline, no. LYHE-006).* Edmonton, Alberta: Alberta Health Services, Cancer Care.

Alberta Provincial Hematology Tumour Team. (2012). *Lymphoma (Clinical practice guideline, no. LYHE-002).* Edmonton, Alberta: Alberta Health Services, Cancer Care.

Imrie, K., Rumble, R. B., Crump, M., Advisory Panel on Bone Marrow and Stem Cell Transplantation, Hematology Disease Site Group. (2009). *Stem cell transplantation in adults: recommendations.* Toronto, Ontario: Cancer Care Ontario Program in Evidence-based Care.

National Institute for Health and Clinical Excellence (NICE). (2010). *Rituximab for the treatment of relapsed or refractory chronic lymphocytic leukaemia (no. 193).* London, UK: National Institute for Health and Clinical Excellence (NICE).

Oliansky, D. M., Larson, R. A., Weisdorf, D., et al. (2012). The role of cytotoxic therapy with hematopoietic stem cell transplantation in the treatment of adult acute lymphoblastic leukemia: update of the 2006 evidence-based review. *Biol Blood Marrow Transplant, 18*(1), 18–36.e6.

Oscier, D., Dearden, C., Erem, E., et al. (2012). *Guidelines on the diagnosis, investigation and management of chronic lymphocytic leukaemia.* London, England: British Society of Haematology.

Patient Education

Dana-Farber Cancer Institute. (2015). *Health library.* **www.dana-farber.org/Health-Library/**

International Myeloma Foundation. (2014). *About myeloma.* **myeloma.org/IndexPage.action?tabId=1&indexPageId=107&parentTabId=1&categoryId=0**

Mangan, P. (2006). Teach your patient about multiple myeloma. *Nursing, 36*(4), 64hn1–64hn4.

Memorial Sloan Kettering Cancer Center. (2015). *Cancer & treatment.* **www.mskcc.org/cancer-care/cancer-treatment**

National Cancer Institute at the National Institutes of Health. (2015). *Blood-forming stem cell transplants.* **www.cancer.gov/cancertopics/treatment/types/stem-cell-transplant/stem-cell-fact-sheet**

STOP

Go to the online course and complete the NovE-Cases assigned by your instructor for this module.

Learning Outcomes for Cancer

When you complete this lesson, you will be able to:

1. Recognize the clinical relevance of cancer.
2. Consider the pathophysiology, etiology, risk factors, and clinical presentation of cancer that determine the priority patient concerns.
3. Determine the most urgent and important nursing interventions and patient education required in caring for a patient with cancer.
4. Evaluate attainment of desired collaborative care outcomes for a patient with cancer.

LO1:

What Is Cancer?

- Cancer results from the loss of regulation of normal tissue growth and from cell division.
- Tissues grow when cells replicate themselves and then divide, a process known as mitosis.
- A normal cell may contain a proto-oncogene, which when activated by a cancer-causing agent, transforms the normal cell into a cancer cell as shown in the illustration.

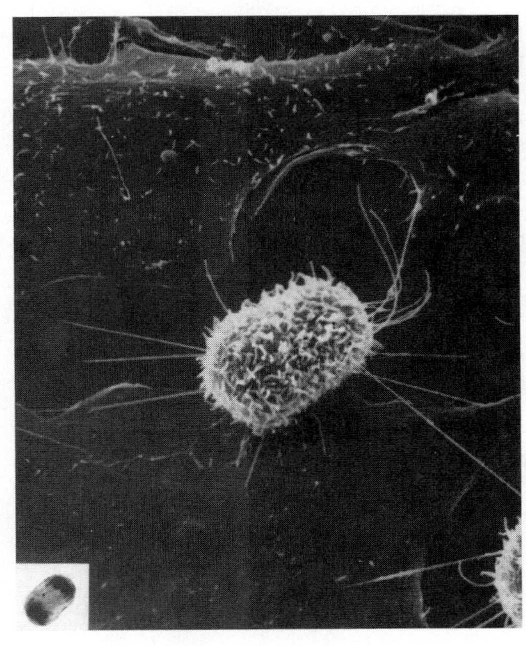

This electron micrograph shows mitosis in the anaphase stage, prior to cell cleavage. This early stage of cell division is when the chromosomes migrate to opposite poles.

Source: Courtesy of George Kyriakidis/Santa Ana, CA

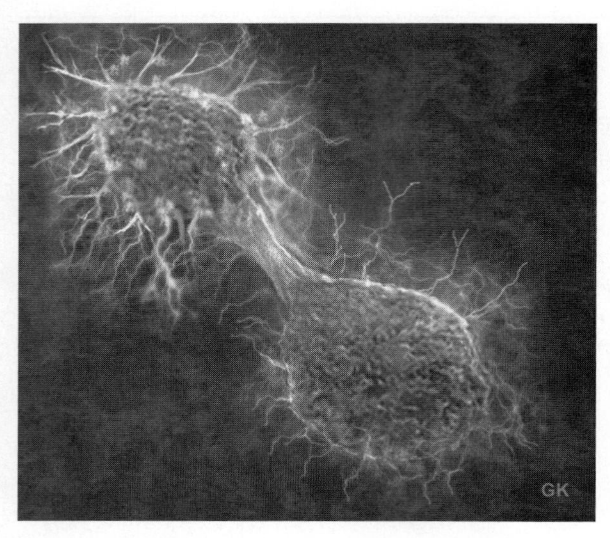

Electron micrograph of dividing cancer cells in the final stage of mitosis. Note its elongated shape.
Source: National Cancer Institute, www.cancer.gov

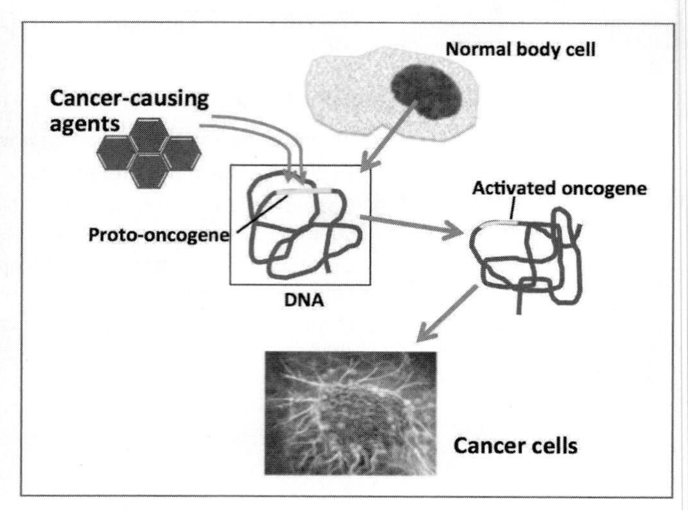

A cancer-causing agent initiates the transformation of a normal cell into an abnormal cancer cell.
Source: Copyright © 2014, NovEx Novice to Expert Learning, LLC

LO1:

Clinical Relevance

- Based on statistics from 2013, 41% of men and women born today will be diagnosed with a cancer at some point during their life.
- Currently, there are approximately 13,028,000 people in the United States with some form of cancer. About 66% of patients with cancer survive at least 5 years.
- One out of every five deaths is related to cancer.
- Chronic pain is one of the most common symptoms of cancer and is present in up to 50% of patients undergoing treatment for cancer and up to 90% in those with advanced disease.
- However, pain is undertreated in many patients.
- Nurses have a major role in providing comfort care for these patients and in educating them regarding management of pain.

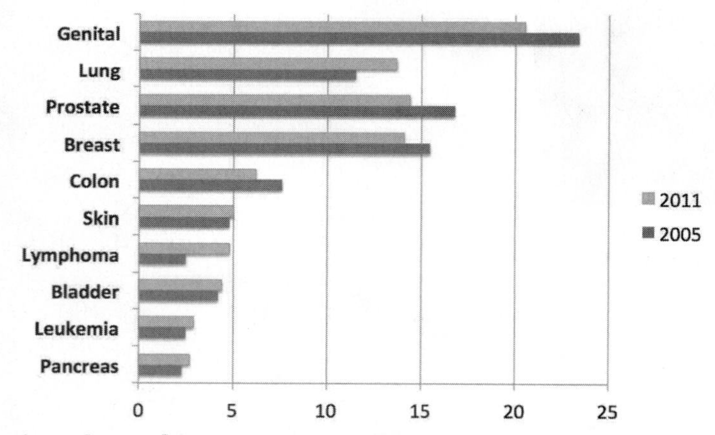

Source: Copyright © 2014, NovEx Novice to Expert Learning, LLC

LO2:

Pathophysiology

Loss of Regulation

- Cancer results when there is a loss of regulation of normal tissue growth and cell division. Normal cell growth and division is controlled by genes that promote growth (called proto-oncogenes) and genes that suppress cell division (called tumor-suppressor genes).
- Proto-oncogenes can be altered by mutations in such a way that cell division is promoted. These altered genes are called oncogenes.
- Mutations in tumor-suppression genes that turn these genes off can also result in unregulated cell division.
- Damage to DNA is normally repaired by DNA repair genes. When DNA repair genes are damaged, it can be detrimental to the cell and increases the possibility of mutations of the proto-oncogenes and tumor-suppressor genes.
- Cancer, the uncontrollable division of cells, can be the result of a single mutation or more commonly the result of several mutations of proto-oncogenes and tumor-suppressor genes.
- There are approximately 400 gene mutations that have been identified as being related to cancer.
- The patient's immune system also plays a role in suppressing cancer since cancer cells may be recognized as abnormal or foreign and destroyed by the immune system.

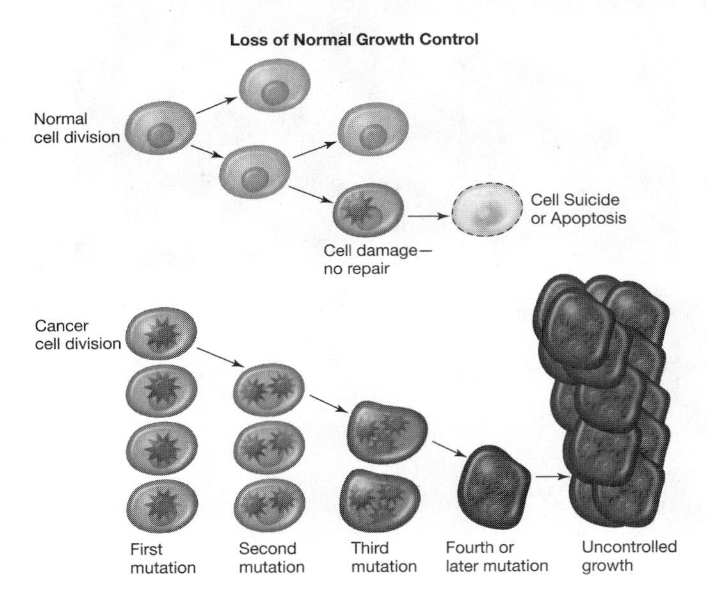

Pathophysiology (continued)

Undifferentiation

- Cancer cells can often be recognized under the microscope because they develop large nuclei with a large amount of DNA and they also divide so frequently.
- Also, cancer cells often start to lose the characteristics of the tissue from which it originated.
- In an undifferentiated tumor, the cells eventually lose all those characteristics, and it may be impossible to tell from which tissue it was derived.
- Several grading systems have been developed based on these factors.

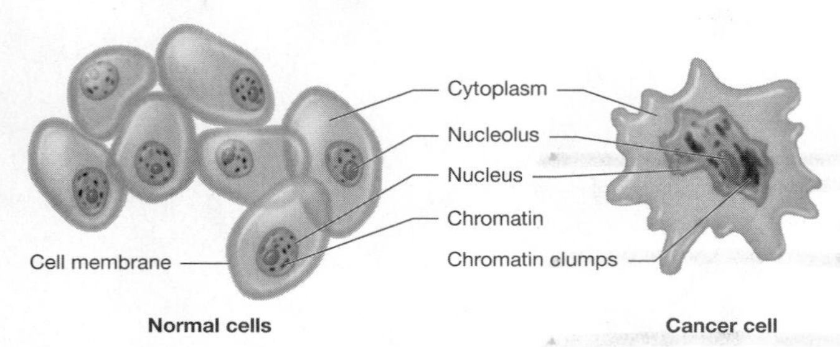

A cluster of normal cells is seen (left). Normal cells have a relatively large amount cytoplasm, a clear nuclear stain, a small nucleolus with fine chromatin granules in the nucleus, and smooth borders on the nucleus. In contrast, the cancer cell (right) has a large nucleus with relatively less cytoplasm, a darker staining nucleus, larger chromatin clumps with a larger nucleolus, and irregular borders on the nucleus.

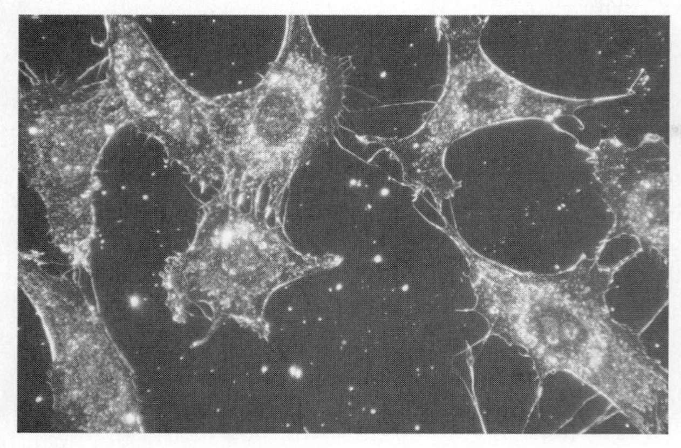

Normal cells.
Source: Dr. Cecil Fox/National Cancer Institute, www.cancer.gov

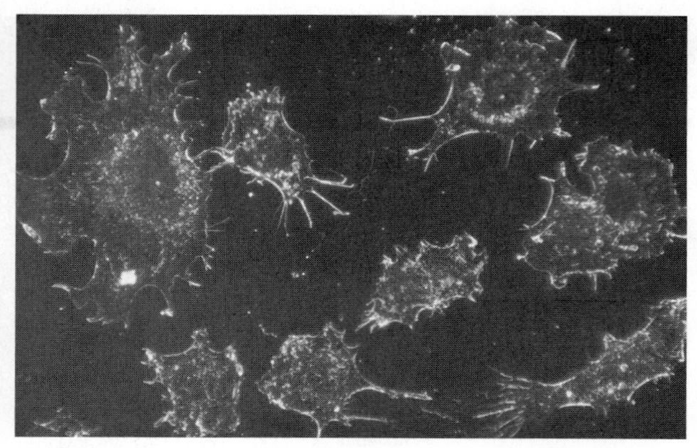

Cancer cells.
Source: Dr. Cecil Fox/National Cancer Institute, www.cancer.gov

The American Joint Committee on Cancer recommends the following guidelines for grading tumors:

Grade	
GX	Grade cannot be assessed (Undetermined grade)
G1	Well-differentiated (Low grade)
G2	Moderately differentiated (Intermediate grade)
G3	Poorly differentiated (High grade)
G4	Undifferentiated (High grade)

Pathophysiology (continued)

Tumors

- Uncontrolled growth of cells usually results in the formation of a solid dense mass called a tumor, which invades local tissue.
- Cytokines are released by cancer cells that trigger blood vessel growth and vascularization of the tumor.
- However, the tumor may outgrow its blood supply and develop areas of necrosis.
- These characteristics of tumor growth usually result in formation of masses that are dense, invading surrounding tissue and resulting in unclear borders and areas of necrosis.
- Some cancers, such as blood cancers (leukemia), may not be associated with the formation of tumors.

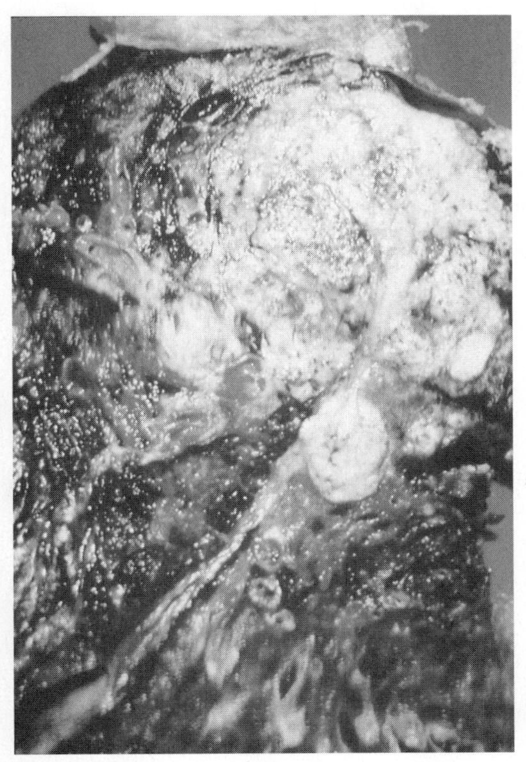

The lung tumor (yellow, upper right) shows the huge overgrowth of cells that invaded the tissue.
Source: National Cancer Institute, www.cancer.gov

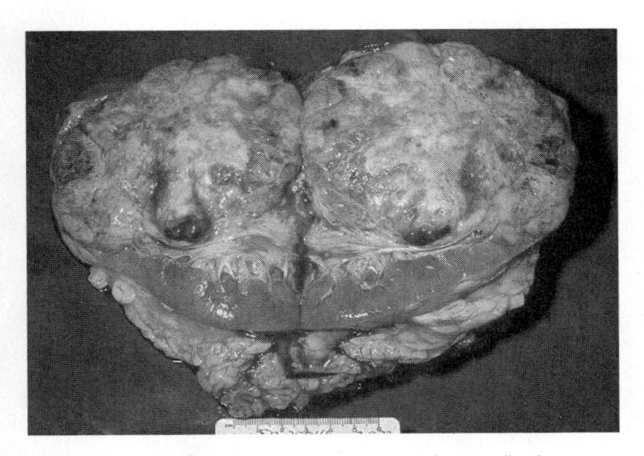

When the enlarged kidney was dissected (opened), the yellow and gray tumor from the renal cell carcinoma had replaced most of the kidney tissue. Normal kidney tissue is burgundy red in color.
Source: CDC/Dr. Edwin P. Ewing, Jr.

Concept Check

1. The GX-G4 tumor grading system is based upon which characteristic?
   A. Tumor size
   B. Tumor location
   C. Cell differentiation
   D. Cell color

Answer question

Pathophysiology (continued)

Metastatic Disease

- Malignant cells may invade local tissue or metastasize (invade) to other parts of the body.
- Metastasis can take place when malignant cells detach from the tumor and enter either the lymphatic or the venous system.
- After systemic tumors (tumors excluding the lung, brain, or heart) develop their own blood supply, malignant cells can detach into the systemic venous system and travel through the right ventricle to the lungs.
- The first capillary bed that the malignant cell encounters is in the lungs. The lungs are therefore a common area of metastasis of systemic cancers.

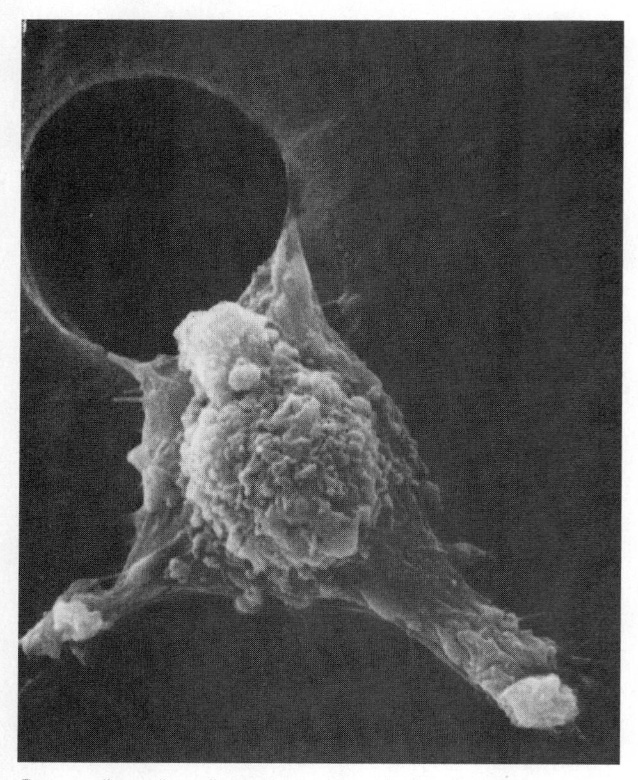

Cancer cells can "grow" arm-like pseudopodia that allow them to migrate and therefore metastasize.

Source: Susan Arnold/Dr. Raouf Guirgus/Dr. Liotta's Laboratory/National Cancer Institute

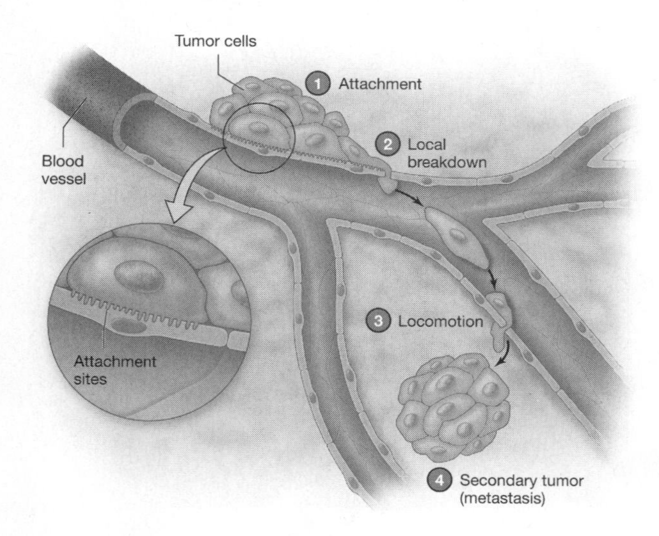

This image presents the stages of metastasis.

This image presents the stages of metastasis.

- Malignancies of the gastrointestinal system (e.g., colon cancer) can also enter the portal venous system and travel to the liver. The liver is, therefore, a common area of metastasis originating from the gastrointestinal tract.
- Lung cancer malignant cells may enter the pulmonary veins and can travel to the brain.
- Metastasis can also occur through the lymphatic system through which malignant cells may eventually enter the venous circulation.

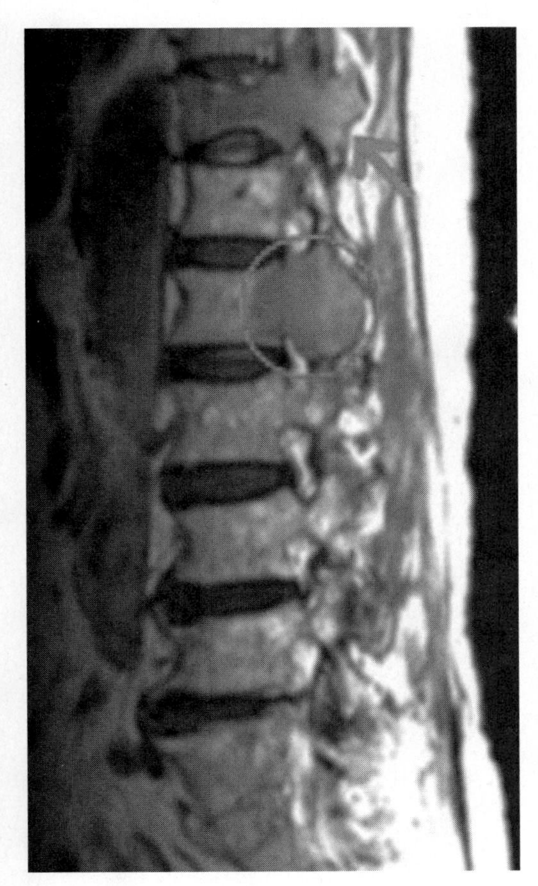

This CT scan of the spine reveals metastatic cancer invading the spine at T12 (arrow) and L2 (circle). The extensive metastatic lesion at T12 is replacing the bone marrow.
Source: Courtesy of K. Kyriakidis

Concept Check

2. What organ is a common first site of metastasis?

A. Brain

B. Spine

C. Kidney

D. Lung

Answer question

Pathophysiology (continued)

Pain

Pain is a very common problem in patients with cancer. Cancer pain can be divided into two categories:

1. Nociceptive pain caused by tissue damage.
2. Neuropathic pain caused by impairment of the nervous system. Neuropathic pain tends to be described more vaguely as a burning, itching, crawling sensation, or a loss of sensation. An example of neuropathic pain is phantom pain that is experienced in a limb after amputation, as if the limb were present.

Cancer pain has multiple causes:

- Tumors secrete cytokines that cause local and systemic inflammation and pain. Tumors also cause acidosis locally, which triggers local pain fibers.
- Malignant cells can infiltrate sensory nerves, causing damage to the nerve tissue.
- Tumors can also mechanically press on sensory nerve fibers.
- Tumors may cause obstructions resulting in the stretching of viscera (e.g., colon cancer) causing colon obstruction.
- Metastatic spread of cancer to bone is one of the most common causes of cancer pain. Pain can be caused by infiltration of nerves in the bone or by fractures or microfractures that can develop. Bone metastasis also triggers spasm of the adjacent muscles.
- Pain can also result from treatment. Chemotherapy and radiation therapy can cause nerve damage, resulting in pain.

Thrombophilia

- Patients with cancer are in a hypercoagulable state (i.e., they develop blood clots easily).
- Tumor cells can activate the blood clotting cascade.
- Systemic inflammation caused by cytokine release results in platelets and vascular endothelial cells becoming more thrombogenic.
- Other factors that contribute to clot formation in cancer patients include:
  - o Vascular invasion by the tumor
  - o Immobility of the patient
  - o Placement of central venous catheters
- Patients may develop deep venous thrombosis (DVT), pulmonary emboli, and/or arterial occlusions.

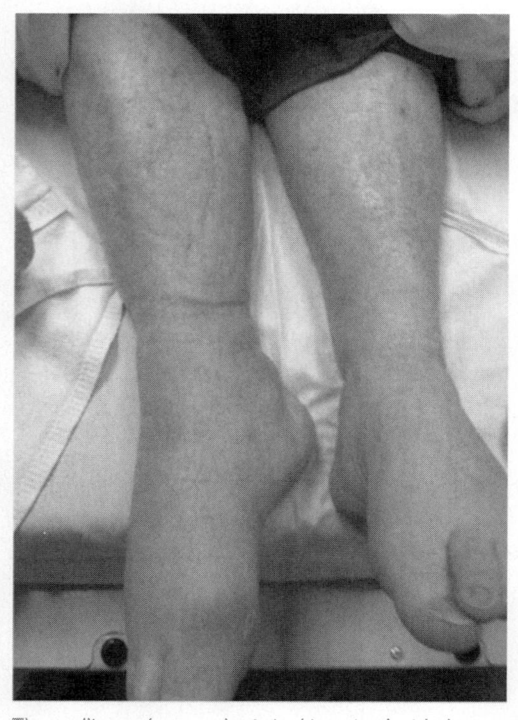

The swelling, redness, and pain in this patient's right leg signals the development of a DVT.
Source: Courtesy of K. Kyriakidis

Pathophysiology (continued)

Cachexia

- Tumor cells release cytokines and cause the release of hormones that are catabolic (resulting in the breakdown of muscle).
- Some cancer patients may also have an increased metabolism (energy expenditure). The reasons for this are unclear but may be, in part, due to the increased energy demand of rapidly dividing and growing cancer cells.

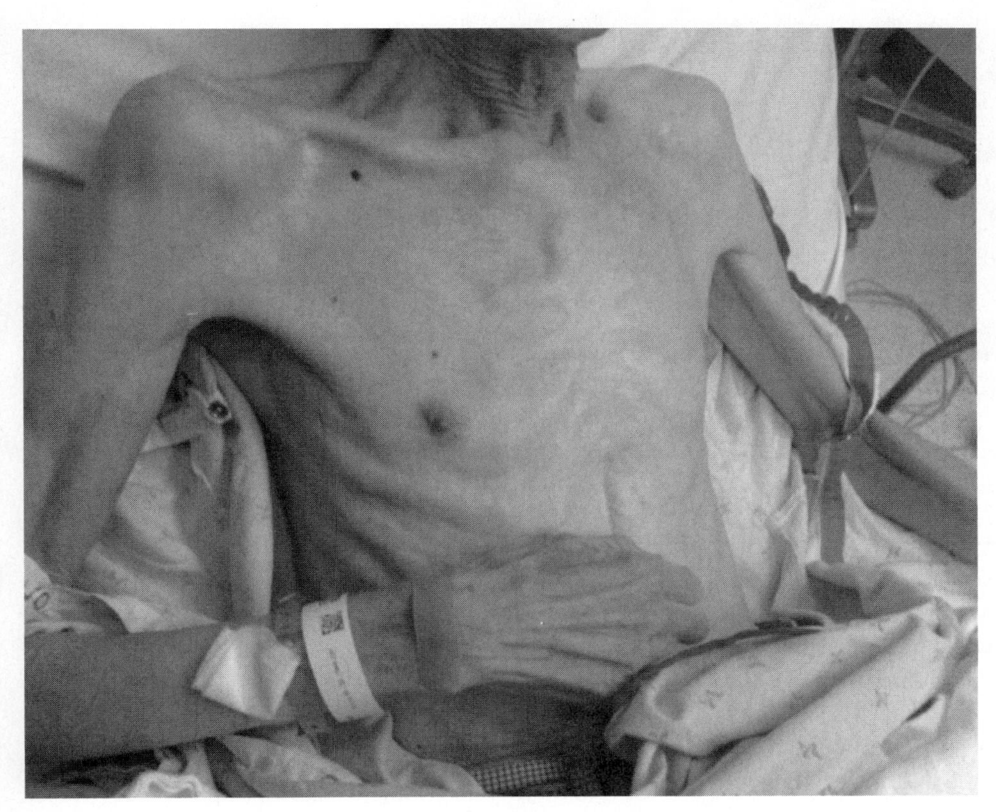

With the increased metabolism and gastrointestinal problems experienced by cancer patients, nutrition therapy is an important discussion. These patients need to understand how to minimize cachexia, the loss of lean body mass, and the nutritional impact of cancer and its treatments. Cachexia significantly increases the risk of complications and death from cancer.
Source: Courtesy of K. Kyriakidis

Paraneoplastic Syndromes

- Paraneoplastic syndromes refer to disorders that are caused by neoplastic cells that are not directly related to the mass effect or invasion of the tumor itself.
- Almost every type of neoplastic cell is able to produce hormones and cytokines, or can cause an immune response that can have many effects.
- Effects include electrolyte abnormalities, skin manifestations, and neurologic manifestations. A common example is small cell carcinoma of the lung causing a syndrome of inappropriate antidiuretic hormone (SIADH), a condition that results in low serum sodium.
- Another example is paraneoplastic cerebellar degeneration. The tumor triggers an autoimmune response that is targeted against the cerebellum and causes gait imbalance and problems with coordination.

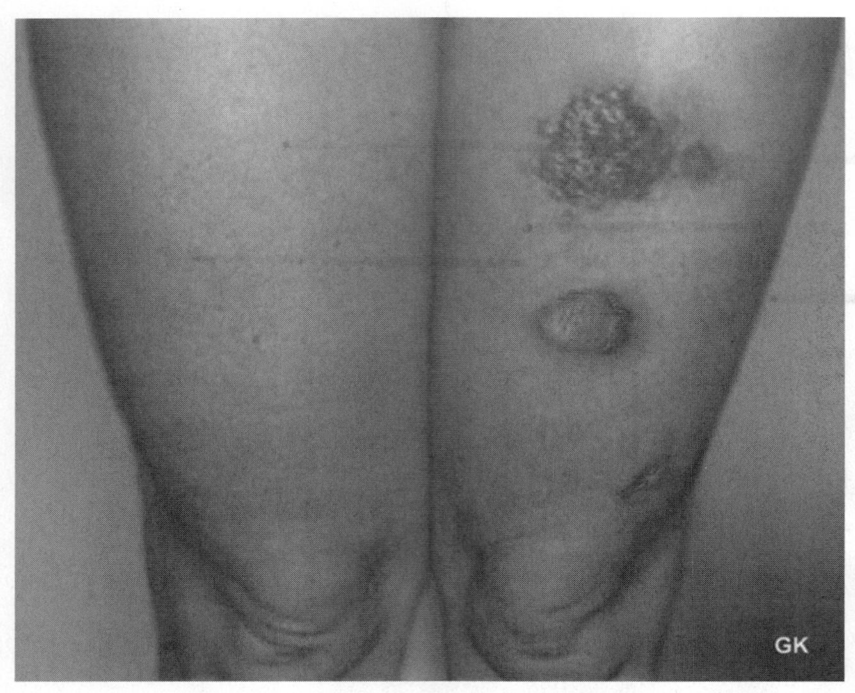

Sweet syndrome is often the first manifestation of acute myelogenous leukemia. The pathogenesis of Sweet syndrome, though unclear, may be a hypersensitivity response to tumor antigens.

Source: Courtesy of George Kyriakidis/Santa Ana, CA

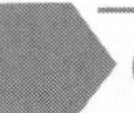

Concept Check

3. **A patient with lung cancer has developed SIADH. This is an example of which complication?**

   A. Metastasis

   B. Thrombophilia

   C. Cachexia

   D. Paraneoplastic syndrome

Answer question

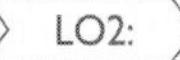

LO2:

Risk Factors and Causes

Modifiable

- One third of cancer deaths are linked to tobacco and one third are linked to diet, obesity, and sedentary lifestyle.
- Obesity is linked to breast cancer, colon cancer, endometrial cancer, and pancreatic cancer.
- Smoking causes mouth and throat cancer, renal cancer, lung cancer, pancreatic cancer, and bladder cancer.
- Sedentary lifestyle is linked to breast cancer.
- Diet: Consumption of red meat and saturated fat has been linked with breast, colon, and prostate cancer. Diets high in fruits and vegetables may lower risk.
- Alcohol is a risk factor for esophageal, colon, pharyngeal, laryngeal, liver, and breast cancer.
- Sun exposure: Exposure to ultraviolet light is linked to skin cancers.
- HPV virus infection acquired through sexual intercourse is the cause of all cervical cancers.

Nonmodifiable

- Genetic predisposition and family history
- Age
- Gender
- Race/ethnicity
- Prior cancer treatment: Chemotherapy and radiation therapy that damages DNA increases the risk of future cancer development.
- Immunosuppressed patients
- Radiation exposure: To some extent, a patient's radiation exposure can be decreased by decreasing the number of unnecessary radiologic tests.
- A complete list of all known and probable carcinogens can be found at the American Cancer Society website: http://www.cancer.org/cancer/cancercauses/othercarcinogens/generalinformationaboutcarcinogens/known-and-probable-human-carcinogens.

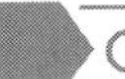

Assessment Findings

Generalized Manifestations

Some signs and symptoms are common to many cancers:

- Constitutional symptoms are weight loss, cachexia/muscle wasting, unexplained fatigue, and fever in some cancers (especially lymphoma) from the systemic inflammation.
- Nausea may be caused by brain tumor or tumors directly affecting the gastrointestinal system.
- DVT may present with leg edema and pain.
- Pain

Localized Manifestations

Other assessment findings are related to the location of cancer. Examples include the following:

- Brain malignancies may produce changes in behavior, stroke symptoms, or ataxia.
- Lung cancers may cause large pleural effusions or obstruction of a bronchus causing shortness of breath.
- Malignancies causing obstruction of the common bile duct may cause jaundice and abdominal pain.
- Renal malignancies may produce hematuria and flank pain.
- Colon cancers can produce symptoms of obstruction with nausea, vomiting, and abdominal pain.

Concept Check

4. A patient who drinks alcohol is at increased risk for which cancer?
   A. Breast
   B. Renal
   C. Lung
   D. Bladder

Answer question

Manifestations of Cancer Emergencies

Patients may present with the following conditions that are emergencies.

- **Tumor lysis syndrome** is a potentially fatal complication that results when extensive numbers of cancer or tumor cells are rapidly killed by anticancer treatments and release an overwhelming amount of intracellular and metabolic by-products. The numerous by-products or the magnitude of particular by-products creates life-threatening or lethal metabolic disturbances.
- **Superior vena cava syndrome** results from tumor compressing the superior vena cava. Venous flow is impeded from the head and upper extremities, resulting in headache, edema of the face, neck and upper extremities, cough, engorgement of the neck, and chest veins.

Emergency Due to Increased Intracranial Pressure from Metastatic Lesions

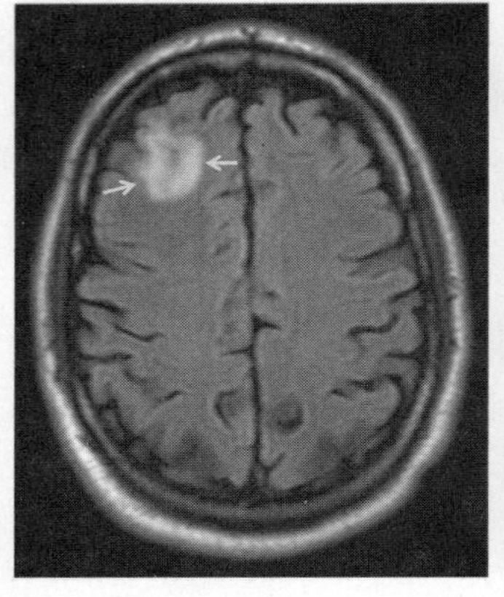

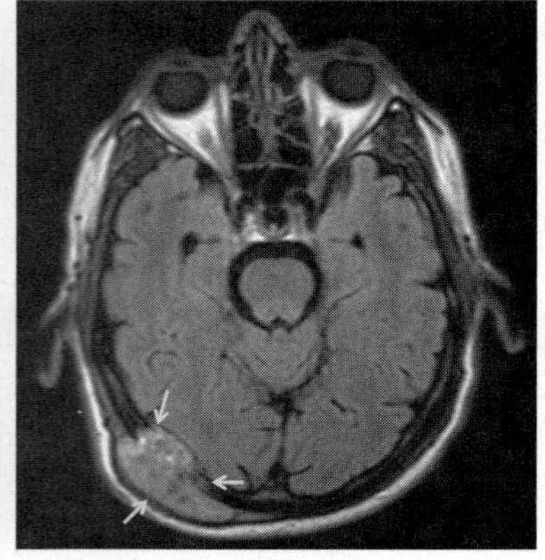

This patient with lung cancer presented with symptoms of increased intracranial pressure. On CT scan, multiple metastatic brain tumors were discovered. The patient's deteriorating condition warranted immediate intervention.
Source: Courtesy of K. Kyriakidis

- **Spinal cord compression** is due to metastasis or primary tumor invading the spine and compressing the cord. Symptoms include leg weakness, paresthesias, and urinary and fecal incontinence or retention. Leg weakness may progress to paralysis if left untreated.
- **Increased intracranial pressure** due to brain metastasis can present with headache, decreased consciousness, confusion, and unequal pupils.

These conditions require vigilance to:

- o Identify those at high risk for specific complications.
- o Be attentive to recognize early warning signals (e.g., metabolic and/or renal imbalances) of the complication.
- o Collaborate with the team to initiate appropriate treatment.

LO2:

Diagnostics

- **Laboratory testing:**
  - o CBC: Patients with most types of cancer may have a slightly elevated white count. In contrast, patients with blood cancers may have a very elevated white count.
  - o Elevation in transaminases (SGOT/SGPT, AST/ALT) indicates liver damage and may indicate a primary liver cancer or metastasis to the liver.
- **Cancer markers:** These are substances found in serum, urine, or stool. They are produced by cancer cells. Levels of these markers are often used to monitor response to treatment. A drop is usually associated with improvement. They can sometimes be used for screening (e.g., PSA), but are often not specific (other conditions may cause an increase in these markers) enough to make a diagnosis. Examples include:
  - o Alpha-fetoprotein: liver cancer and germ cell tumor
  - o CA-125: ovarian cancer
  - o Carcinoembryonic antigen (CEA): colon and breast cancer
  - o Prostate-specific antigen (PSA): prostate cancer
  - o Thyroglobulin: thyroid cancer
- **Urinalysis:** RBCs may be present with renal cancer.
- **Gene testing:** Genetic mutations for some types of cancer have been identified. Presence of these genes in an individual increases the risk of cancer. For breast cancer, two genes, BRCA1 and BRCA2, can be detected by blood testing. Not everyone with these abnormal genes will develop cancer. Testing is also expensive and is not recommended for the general population. It may be useful for patients with a strong family history of breast cancer (i.e., multiple relatives with breast cancer). Patients should be counseled before and after the test is performed. For a variety of reasons, not everyone will want to know their risk for cancer.

Imaging in Cancers

- Chest x-rays may be helpful in assessing the presence of a primary malignancy or metastatic disease to the lungs. X-rays, however, are not very sensitive.
- CT scans and MRI are more sensitive and can also be used for staging.
- Positron emission tomography (PET scan) produces a 3-D image of the body showing areas of cancer with increased metabolic activity. This is because cancer cells are dividing faster, resulting in a higher metabolic rate. PET scans are accomplished by using a nuclear tracer, an analogue of glucose, injected into the veins. The tracer is then taken up by active tissue. Unlike CT scans that show only structure, a PET scan may help determine if an area has cancer. It may also show lesions too small to appear on a CT scan.

Common Locations of Metastatic Cancers

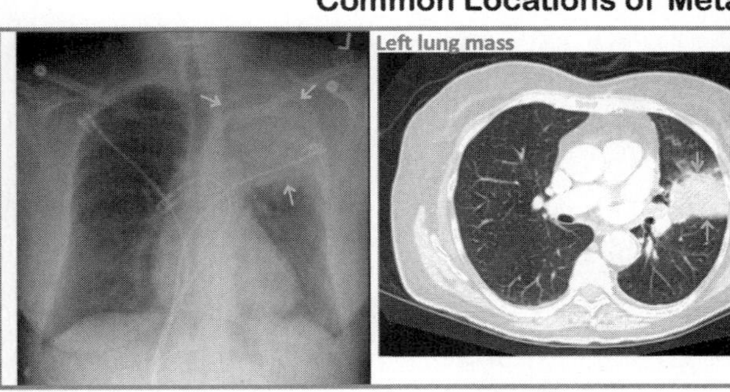

This patient had breast cancer as the primary malignancy. Unfortunately, following complaints of pulmonary symptoms, xray (left) revealed left upper lung mass that was suspicious for metastasis. CT scan (middle) confirmed the metastatic tumor.

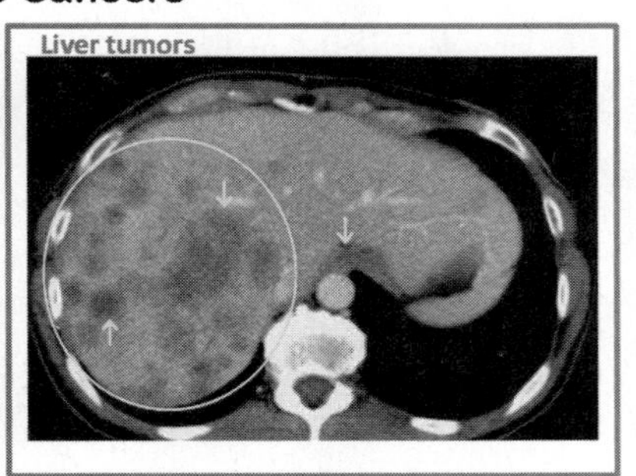

Numerous metastatic lesions (tumors) were found in this 59 year old male's liver at the time he was diagnosed with colon cancer.

Source: Courtesy of K. Kyriakidis

Endoscopy

Some areas of the body are amenable to visualization by endoscopy. These include:

- Lung: bronchoscopy
- Stomach and duodenum: endoscopic gastroduodenoscopy (EGD)
- Colon: colonoscopy
- Bladder: cystoscopy

Visualized suspicious areas can also be biopsied.

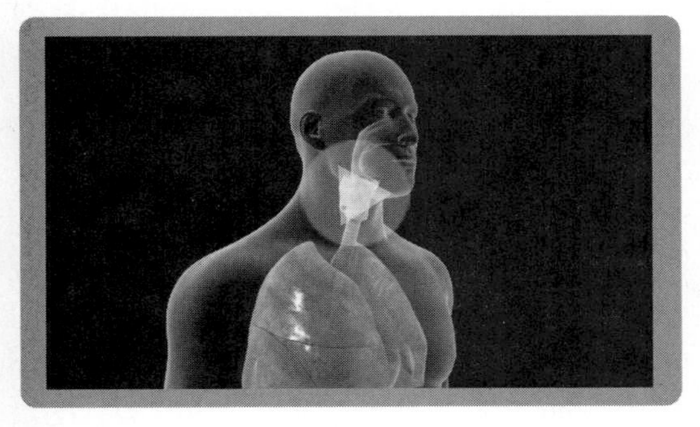

This animation demonstrates a bronchoscopy, which is a procedure in which a physician inserts a scope into the bronchus to evaluate suspected problems.
Source: © 2014 Nucleus Medical Media, All rights reserved

Diagnostics (continued)

Obtaining Tissue

- Obtaining abnormal cells either by endoscopy, fine needle aspiration of tissue, aspiration of fluid (pleural or ascites), or by surgery is essential for making a diagnosis and developing a treatment plan.
- The decision on how to obtain this tissue is usually based on what is possible, which will be the safest method for the patient, and which will yield the most accurate results.

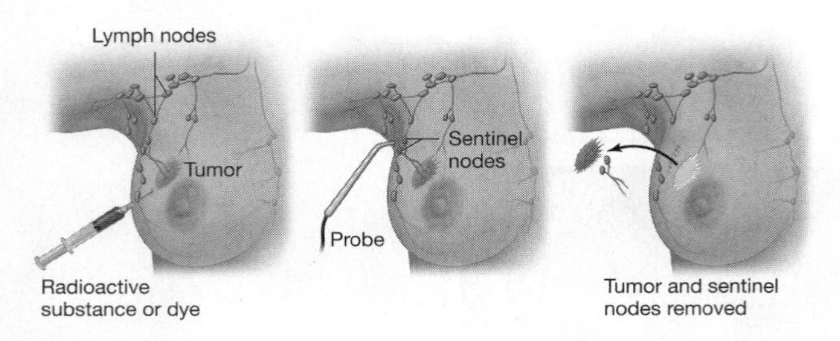

Concept Check

5. **Patients with a strong family history of which type of cancer may want to consider genetic testing?**

   A. Renal

   B. Lung

   C. Colon

   D. Breast

Answer question

Staging System

- The extent of tumor invasion is determined through physical examination, imaging, and pathology reports. This knowledge can help determine the prognosis for a patient and guide in the development of a treatment plan.
- When needed, the stage of the cancer can help identify if and which clinical trial may be helpful to a patient.
- Different staging systems have been developed and used, but the TNM system is common.
- It is based on these factors:

  (T) What is the extent (size, severity, and how extensive) of the tumor?

  (N) Has it spread to nearby lymph nodes?

  (M) Is there metastasis?

Primary Tumor (T)

- TX: Primary tumor cannot be evaluated.
- T0: No evidence of primary tumor
- T1, T2, T3, T4: Size and/or extent of the primary tumor

Regional Lymph Nodes (N)

- NX: Regional lymph nodes cannot be evaluated.
- N0: No regional lymph node involvement
- N1, N2, N3: Number of lymph nodes and extent of spread

Distant Metastasis (M)

- MX: Distant metastasis cannot be evaluated.
- M0: No distant metastasis found
- M1: Distant metastasis is present.

Staging System I–IV

Another common staging system that is used designates stages from I–IV:

- Stage 0: Carcinoma in situ; this means it is an early stage of cancer and the tumor cells have not invaded the surrounding tissue.
- Stage I, Stage II, and Stage III: Higher numbers indicate more advanced disease and is defined differently with each type of cancer. These stages are determined by the size of the tumor and whether or not it has invaded adjacent organs or lymph nodes.
- Stage IV: Metastatic disease

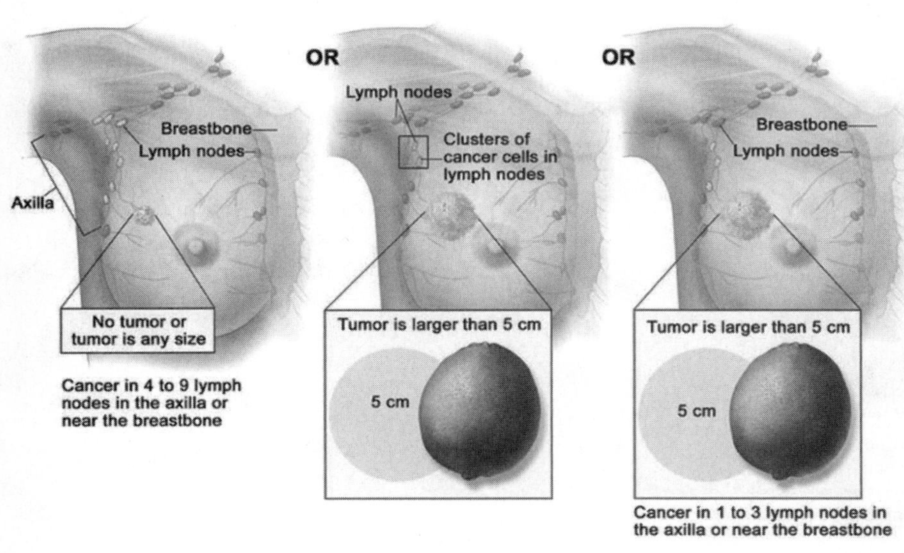

Criteria that qualifies cancer as Stage III breast cancer.
Source: National Cancer Institute, www.cancer.gov.

Priority Patient Concerns and Desired Collaborative Care Outcomes

Prior to caring for patients with cancer, it is important to prioritize the patient's concerns that must guide the nursing care plan and interventions. Care for the patient is ordered and organized in accordance with the patient's priority and urgent needs. Desired collaborative care outcomes in patients with cancer typically include:

1. Patient will be free of pain or report that pain is at a tolerable level with treatment.
2. Patient's skin will be free of breakdown or be progressively healing.
3. Patient's oral mucous membranes will return to pre-illness state.
4. Patient will remain free of infection.
5. Patient will maintain body mass index in normal range.
6. Patient will report medications are effective in decreasing nausea.
7. Patient will report having sufficient energy to engage in desired daily activities.
8. Patient will discuss fears and engage in coping behaviors to help manage fear.
9. Patient will describe actual change in body function, demonstrate acceptance of appearance, and maintain close social interaction and personal relationships.
10. Patient will identify actions that are within his or her control, verbalizing any feelings of powerlessness.

Considering these important care outcomes, prepare a list of the major 3–6 priority patient concerns or nursing diagnoses for patients with cancer. Be prepared to participate in a discussion of this list and/or to submit them as an assignment, as determined by your faculty. Resources you may find helpful in this assignment can include this lesson, the references, resources on nursing care plans, and standard nursing diagnoses manuals.

LO3:

Collaborative Interventions

Interventions that are commonly needed in patients who have cancer include:

- Chemotherapy
- Radiation therapy
- Surgery
- Pain control
- DVT prophylaxis
- Cancer emergencies
- Communication
- End-of-life discussions/hospice
- Screening
- Prevention

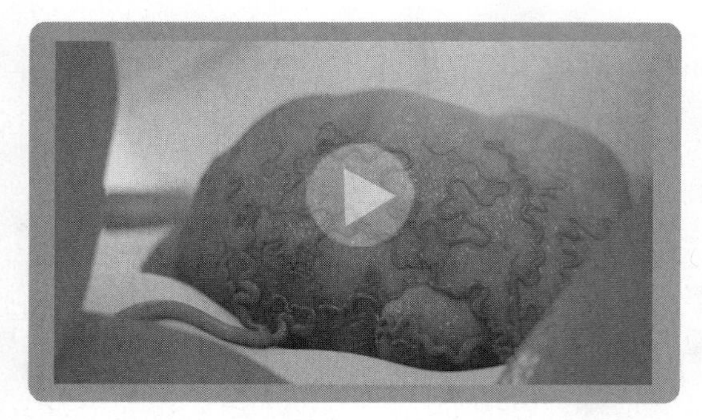

This animation on chemotherapy explains normal cell division and the pathophysiology of cancer development, growth, and metastasis. Chemotherapy and its effects on the body and cancer cells are reviewed. Numerous treatments related to symptom management and care are explained.

Collaborative Interventions (continued)

Chemotherapy

- The purpose of chemotherapy is to improve the patient's condition by disproportionately destroying cancer cells relative to healthy cells.
- M N Complete specialized education must be provided to patients prior to administering chemotherapeutic medications. Many chemotherapy treatments have very toxic effects. One type of chemotherapeutic agent, nitrogen mustard, was first developed to be used in chemical warfare.
- The way chemotherapy works is by targeting the toxic effects on the characteristics of cancer cells that make them more susceptible to destruction than normal cells. One susceptible characteristic of cancer cells is that they divide rapidly; so chemotherapy targets rapidly dividing cells. As a result, bone marrow, which is also very active in producing new blood cells, is critically affected by chemotherapy. New blood cells are rapidly dividing.
- M N Administer chemotherapy with strict adherence to the specific organization's standards and clinical practice guidelines.
- M N Observe for anemia, thrombocytopenia and neutropenia. Close observation is needed to identify the early, but common side effects. For the same reason, hair loss is also a common side effect.
- M N Observe for adverse effects in multiple organs. All tissue is also affected to some extent, and patients can develop damage to heart, lungs, and kidneys.
- M N Use a central venous access device to deliver chemotherapy drugs. Extravasation of chemotherapeutic drugs can cause serious damage to tissues. If extravasation is noted or suspected, the infusion should be stopped and an experienced clinician should gently try to aspirate as much of the drug as possible.
- Chemotherapy drugs can be divided into categories based on how they work and how they are derived.
- Several chemotherapy drugs are often used in combination and administered at intervals.

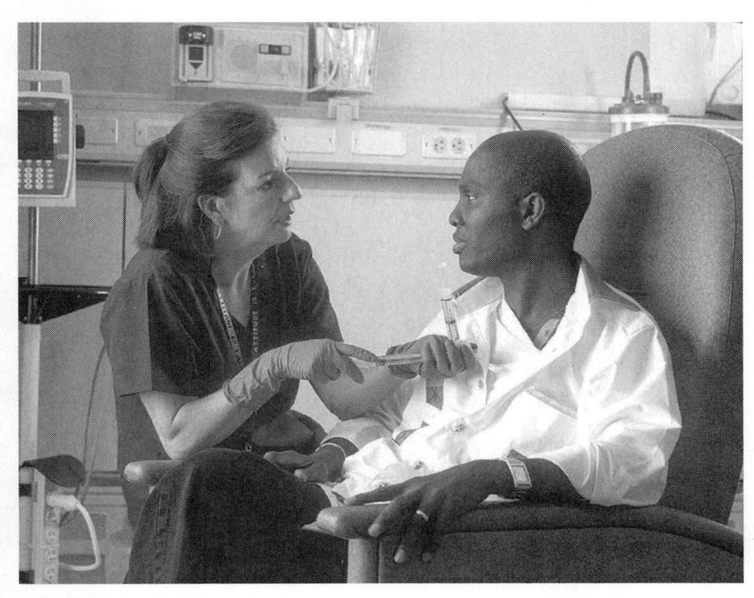

Patient receiving chemotherapy.
Source: National Cancer Institute

Categories of Chemotherapy Drugs

- **Alkylating agents** are the oldest class of cancer drugs. They damage the DNA by binding to it to prevent division and, thus, cause cell death. Damage to DNA can lead to secondary cancers, commonly, acute leukemia. These agents are used in leukemia, lymphoma, Hodgkin lymphoma, multiple myeloma, sarcoma, breast, lung, and ovarian cancer. Examples include nitrogen mustard and cyclophosphamide.
- **Antimetabolites** work by inhibiting normal metabolic pathways in cells. For example, methotrexate works by inhibiting a pathway that is necessary for DNA production. These drugs are used in head and neck cancers, breast cancer, colon cancer, esophageal cancer, hepatoma, pancreatic, and colon cancer. Other examples include 5-Fluorouracil, 6-mercaptopurine, hydroxyurea, and cytarabine.
- The **platinum drugs** work by cross-linking DNA within a strand or between two strands, interfering with the function of DNA. Some will cause renal toxicity. These drugs are used in lung, testicular cancer, and colon cancer, and examples are cisplatin and carboplatin.
- **Antitumor antibiotics and anthracyclines** are peptides derived from naturally occurring fungi that act as cancer antibiotics. They work by producing oxygen radicals that damage DNA and the repair mechanism. Some can damage the heart and lung. Examples include doxorubacin and bleomycin. Their uses include treatment of Hodgkin's lymphoma and testicular cancer.
- **Topoisomerase inhibitors** are drugs that inhibit topoisomerase, which is needed for DNA repair. An example is etoposide.
- **Taxanes** are naturally derived from plants and interfere with cell division. They are used in the treatment of lung cancer, breast cancer, leukemia, myeloma, and lymphoma. Paclitaxel is an example.
- **Corticosteroids** are naturally occurring hormones that are used to treat leukemia, lymphoma, and multiple myeloma. Examples include methylprednisolone and dexamethasone.

Collaborative Interventions (continued)

Side Effects of Chemotherapy

Common side effects listed below are discussed in more detail in the Care of Cancer Patients with Treatment Toxicities NovE-lesson:

- Anemia
- Thrombocytopenia
- Neutropenia
- Infection
- GI side effects:
  - o Nausea and vomiting
  - o Mucositis
  - o Stomatitis
  - o Esophagitis
- Hair loss

Candida Esophagitis

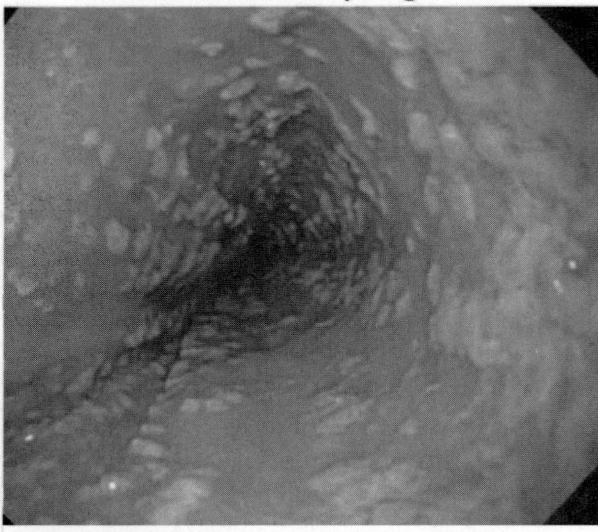

Esophagitis and stomatitis are painful and uncomfortable side effects of chemotherapy. Inflammation of the mucosa commonly allows fungal infections, like *Candida*, to invade. This photo shows candida esophagitis (extensive whitish patches) in this cancer patient.

Source: Courtesy of K. Kyriakidis

Some of the chemotherapy medicines that tend to cause hair loss:

- Adriamycin
- Cactinomycin
- Cyclophosphamide
- Doxorubicin
- Docetaxel
- Etoposide
- Irinotecan
- Ifosfamide
- Paclitaxel
- Vinorelbine
- Topotecan

Patient Education: Chemotherapy

Patients with cancer require extensive educational preparation, as some patients have years of treatments to improve survival. Clinicians who specialize in oncology are more extensively prepared to care for these patients. Patient education typically includes:

N
- Educate the patient to report any burning or pain in the mediastinum, pleural, chest, or neck areas that may warn of extravasation during chemotherapy infusions.

M N
- Educate regarding the disease, recognition of symptoms, prevention of recurrence or complications, medications, when to seek medical attention, follow-up care, exercise and activity balanced with rest, smoking and substance cessation, weight management, and flu and pneumonia vaccines when approved by the physician.

N
- Instruct the patient and family about infection prevention measures, particularly those who may have a communicable illness.

N
- Instruct the patient on the various situations when it is appropriate to call their health care provider regarding evidence of toxicity or other urgent matters related to the chemotherapy.

M N
- Consult a social worker who may need to be involved and available with, in some instances, regular visits and consultation. A social worker is particularly helpful when chemotherapy impacts work and financial obligations.

N
- Ensure that the patient has a copy, or procure a copy, of general advanced directives and suggest consideration of and discussion with appropriate family members, significant others or close friends if desired, and religious counselor.

N
- Discuss the patient's and family's preference about visits from pastoral services or from their own minister regarding spiritual well-being, faith, hope, and spiritual questions or distress.

N
- Suggest following a bland diet, frequent small meals, and avoiding spicy and hard-to-digest foods.

N
- Instruct to avoid consumption of alcohol and mouth rinses containing alcohol.

N
- Prepare the patient about balancing activity with periods of rest. Teach the patient to cluster activities to allow for longer and uninterrupted rest periods.

N
- Suggest options or obtain dietician recommendations for optimal nutritional intake and stress the importance maintaining adequate nutrition is spite of lack of desire for food and diminished appetite.

N
- Consider referrals for coping strategies related to depression, body image, family relationships, or any other stressful situations that may be encountered.

M N
- Collaborate with the health care provider to refer the patient for genetic counseling when a cancer may have a genetic link.

N
- Refer the patient to a local cancer support group.

N
- Provide local contacts for Meal Train, Meals-on-Wheels, or a similar organization that could provide home-delivered meals when needed.

N
- Provide information regarding reliable websites, blogs, or other Internet addresses where patients might find more information relating to their specific diagnosis. Blogs such as Caring Bridge can help with communication overload and allows the patient and family to communicate when convenient without constant, inconvenient interruptions.

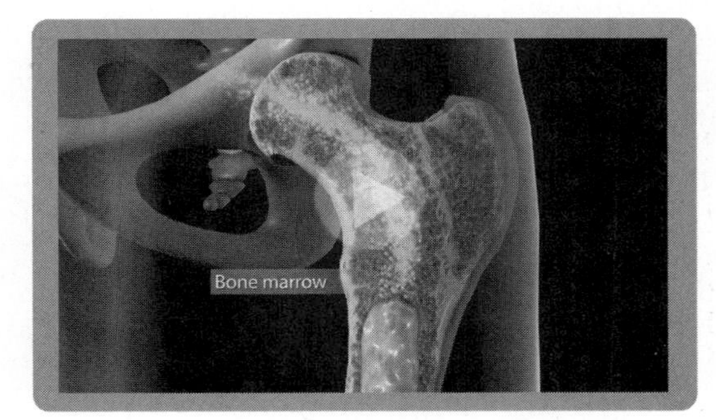

This animation provides an in-depth explanation of how chemotherapy affects the cancer cells and the normal cells of the body. Not only are cancer cells destroyed but cells that are essential for the normal functioning of the body can be severely damaged, producing adverse effects that must be addressed so that the patient can survive.

Collaborative Interventions (continued)

Additional Systemic Medications

M N • Administer **targeted therapies** when ordered and educate the patient about the medication, actions, and side effects. Targeted therapies are drugs that work more specifically against cancer cells. Examples include imatinib, gefitinib, and sunitinib.

M N • Administer or teach the patient how to take **hormone therapy**. Exogenous hormones affect the production or function of sex hormones. These are used to treat prostate and breast cancer. Examples include tamoxifen, anastrozole, flutamide, and leuprolide.

M N • Administer **immune therapies** as prescribed and educate the patient about the medication, actions, and side effects. Immune therapy uses the immune system to respond to cancer cells. This can be achieved by stimulating the immune system or by introducing an antibody to proteins expressed on the surface of abnormal cells. An example is trastuzumab (Herceptin). This is an antibody that attaches to HER receptors on a type of breast cancer cell.

• Future research will concentrate on finding more specific treatments for cancers that will have fewer side effects. One example is the use of nanotechnology. Nanotechnology is revolutionizing the fight against cancer. It provides a unique ability to detect cancer cells in an early stage, diagnose the cancer, and treat it more precisely with technology that is smaller than a single human cell.

Collaborative Interventions (continued)

Radiation Therapy

M N • Prepare patient for radiation therapy. Radiation kills cells by damaging their DNA. Rapidly dividing cells such as cancer cells are more susceptible but healthy cells are also affected. To minimize damage to healthy cells, radiation may be delivered as beams that are focused on the tumor or on small beads that are implanted in the malignant tissue. The radiation in the beads travels only a short distance and is called brachytherapy.

M N • Instruct the patient about combination therapy and how it is scheduled. Radiation therapy may be used alone or in conjunction with chemotherapy and/or surgery.

M N • Inform the patient about the purpose of using radiation in the specific case. Radiation is commonly used as a palliative therapy to treat pain produced by bone metastases. Assist the patient to understand what might be expected as a result of the radiation.

M N • Inform the patient about an invading cancer that is creating complications and how radiation may reduce the risk. Radiation is often used to treat cancer emergencies such as spinal cord compression, SVC syndrome, and increased intracranial pressure in an attempt to shrink the tumor(s) that is causing the problem.

Collaborative Symptom Management and Comfort Care: Radiation

- N Monitor for skin breakdown or radiation burns.
- N Provide wound care as needed for radiation burns.
- N Provide comfort care for stomatitis (sores in the mouth) and mucositis (irritation or ulceration anywhere in the lining of the digestive tract) if damaged from radiation. Patients commonly have painful swallowing.
- N Protect from infectious exposure due to immunosuppression.
- N Support the patient, provide comfort, and discuss any concerns regarding emotional or psychological distress. Carefully listening to the patient can help identify the patient's primary stressors or concerns.
- M N Manage symptoms and provide comfort care for side effects: chills, fever, nausea, vomiting, diarrhea, urinary or bladder changes.
- N Administer antidiarrheal, as needed.

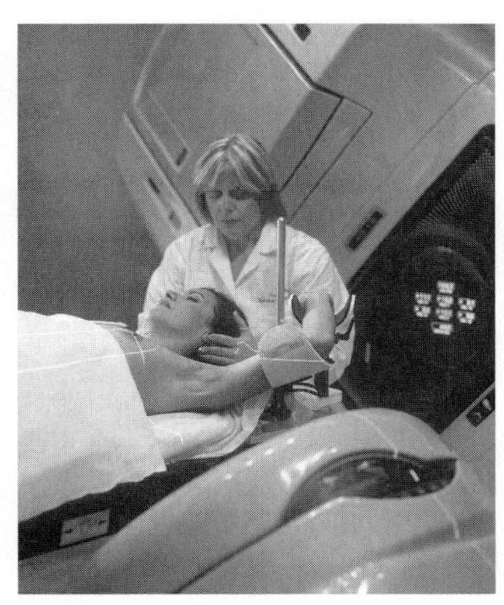

Preparing for radiation.
Source: National Cancer Institute

Complications of Radiation

- N Observe for and treat radiation dermatitis, which is a skin reaction in the area being treated. Its appearance may be similar to a sunburn (e.g., red, itchy, edematous, and peel) or it may be worse and ulcerate, bleed, blister, and be painful.
- N Identify brain function changes that can result as a complication. Brain changes can include disturbances or deficits in memory, mobility, calculations, continence, thinking and reasoning, and possibly, personality. Changes can persist for months to years. Collaborate with the health care provider to consult speech, occupational, or physical therapists as indicated.
- M N Identify mucositis as early as possible and begin treatment. Mucositis is inflammation and damage to the GI mucosal lining in patients receiving x-ray therapy to the head, ears, eyes, neck, throat, and/or upper GI tract areas.
- M N Manage diarrhea, nausea, and vomiting in patients with radiation therapy to the abdominal area.
- M N Prepare the patient for potential infertility if the lower abdomen is involved in or near targeted treatment areas. Educate patients prior to radiation so that they are fully aware and can potentially "bank" sperm or eggs for the future. Patients should be informed, if interested, of additional options (e.g., donors, adoption) so that they understand that infertility does not necessarily mean never having children.
- M N Inform the patient about potential secondary cancers that can be caused by the radiation therapy. These may arise years later, necessitating routine check-ups for early detection.

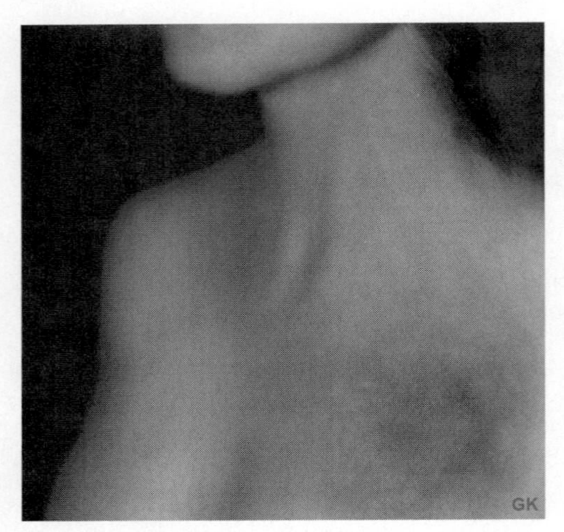

Radiation dermatitis is a skin reaction that commonly occurs as a side effect of radiation therapy.
Source: Courtesy of George Kyriakidis/Santa Ana, CA

Patient Education: Radiation

- Educate the patient about radiation therapy:
  - o Radiation therapy is the use of high dose x-rays to kill cancer cells.
  - o Internal radiation comes from a source that is put inside the body.
  - o Radiation is usually received in the hospital, but the patient can return home after the treatment.
  - o Radiation is not painful. The treatment lasts for 1–5 minutes, and the machine sends x-rays into and around the tumor.
- Explain that the health care provider will advise what to wear while receiving treatment, usually avoiding bandages, jewelry, and other items on the skin where treatment occurs.
- Instruct that skin and organs being treated may suffer some damage. The skin may blister or turn red.
- Educate regarding side effects and the potential impact on quality of life and social life because of avoiding close contacts during treatments.
- Educate regarding hygiene, skin, and wound care, cleaning only with water, and precautions to be taken in the radiation site.
- Educate not to use lotions, harsh soaps, perfumes, and powder on the skin but creams may be used. Instruct the patient to wear long sleeves, a hat, and use sunblock to protect skin. Instruct the patient not to scratch.

Products to Use

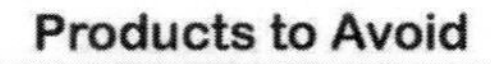

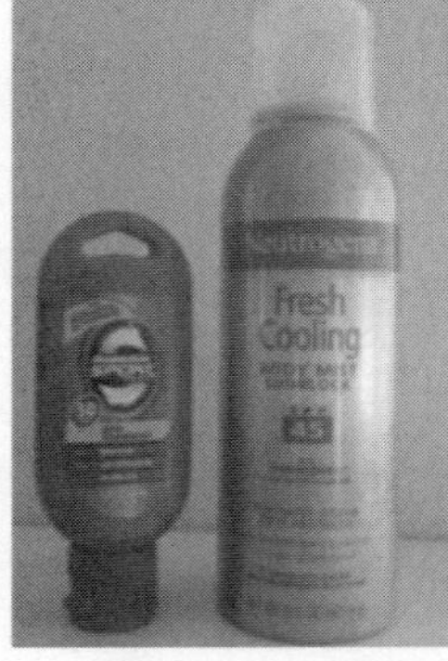

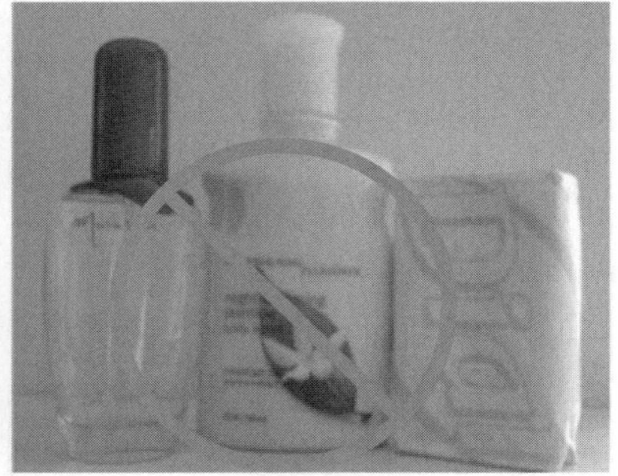

Source: Copyright © 2014, NovEx Novice to Expert Learning, LLC

- Prepare the patient that feeling weak and tired with no energy is common and may worsen during treatment.
- Teach the proper method of disposal of bodily wastes that are affected by internal radioactive contamination but are not affected by external radiation.
- Direct the patient to nutritionists for consultation regarding meal planning, with small frequent meals.
- Encourage the patient to verbalize fears and concerns.
- Make the patient aware of general advanced directives and encourage the patient to discuss their feelings with family members.

Collaborative Interventions (continued)

Management of Chemotherapy and Radiation Side Effects

Managing the toxic effects of both chemotherapy and radiation has important implications for nurses. As important, patients and their caregivers should be educated about these management strategies because toxic effects continue even after discharge of the patient:

M N
- **Nausea/vomiting:**
  - o Teach the patient to eat/drink when not nauseated.
  - o (EBP) Administer antiemetics or combinations of antiemetics (e.g., ondansetron, Zofran, dexamethasone are recommended on a scheduled basis). Guidelines provide the type of antiemetic combination that may be the most effective, based on the type of chemotherapy used (Roila, et al., 2010).
  - o Encourage diversional activities as appropriate.

N
- **Anorexia:**
  - o Advise the patient to eat small frequent meals of high-protein, high-calorie foods.
  - o Don't nag—gently encourage.
  - o Serve food in a pleasant environment.

M N
- **Diarrhea:**
  - o Give antidiarrheal agents.
  - o Encourage the patient to eat a low-fiber, low-residue diet.
  - o Insist on maintaining a fluid intake of at least 3 liters per day.

M N
- **Stomastitis, mucositis, and/or esophagitis:**
  - o Assess oral mucosa daily.
  - o Encourage intake of nutritional supplements.
  - o Create awareness that eating may be painful, requiring analgesia.
  - o Assist with diet selection of soft, bland, moist foods.
  - o Advise use of frequent oral rinses to keep the mouth moist.
  - o Discourage the use of oral irritants (tobacco, alcohol).
  - o Advise application of topical anesthetics.

M N
- **Constipation:**
  - o Give stool softeners.
  - o Advise intake of high-fiber foods.
  - o Recommend increased fluid intake.

M N
- **Hepatotoxicity:**
  - o Monitor liver function tests.

M N
- **Anemia:**
  - o Monitor hemoglobin and hematocrit levels.
  - o Administer iron supplements, erythropoietin.
  - o Encourage foods that promote RBC production.

N
- **Fatigue:**
  - o Encourage rest when fatigued.
  - o Encourage that usual lifestyle be maintained as much as possible.
  - o Pace activities.
  - o Encourage moderate exercises as tolerated.
  - o Assess for reversible causes (e.g., electrolyte imbalance).

M N
- **Thrombocytopenia:**
  - o Monitor platelets.
  - o Observe for signs of bleeding.

M N
- **Leukopenia** (especially neutropenia):
  - o Vigilant monitoring and early recognition are critical due to the significant morbidity and mortality rates from neutropenia.
  - o Monitor WBC, especially neutrophils.
  - o Report temperature elevations and any other manifestations of infection.
  - o Recommend avoiding large crowds and people with infections.
  - o Administer filgrastrim and Neupogen.

M N
- **Hyperuricemia:**
  - o Monitor uric acid levels.
  - o Administer allopurinol/Zyloprim prophylactically.
  - o Encourage increased fluid intake.

N
- **Alopecia:**
  - o Suggest ways to cope (by using a scarf, hat, hair piece, wig).
  - o Suggest that long hair be cut before therapy.
  - o Suggest avoidance of excessive shampooing, brushing, combing of hair.
  - o Discuss impact of hair loss on self-image.

M N
- **Reproductive dysfunction:**
  - o Discuss possibility with patients before treatment.
  - o Offer opportunity for sperm and ova banking.

M N
- **Nephrotoxicity:**
  - o Monitor BUN and serum creatinine.
  - o Avoid drugs that will potentiate effects.
  - o Alkalinize the urine with sodium bicarbonate.
  - o Administer allopurinol for Tumor Lysis Syndrome prevention.

M N
- **Increased intracranial pressure:**
  - o Monitor the neuro status.
  - o Control intracranial pressure with corticosteroids.

M N
- **Peripheral neuropathy:**
  - o Monitor for neuropathic symptoms (e.g., temperature sensitivity, pain, numbness, burning).
  - o Administer antiseizure drugs (gabapentin and Neurontin).

N
- **Cognitive changes:**
  - o Teach patients to use a detailed daily planner.
  - o Suggest that the patient gets enough sleep and rest.
  - o Suggest exercises for the brain.
  - o Encourage the patient to focus on one thing at a time (no multitasking).

N
- **Pneumonitis:**
  - o Monitor for respiratory symptoms of dry hacking cough, fever, and exertional dyspnea.

N
- **Pericarditis and myocarditis:**
  - o Monitor for clinical symptoms such as dyspnea and chest pain.

M N
- **Cardiotoxicity:**
  - o Monitor heart with ECG and EF.
  - o Modify drug therapy according to symptoms or deteriorating cardiac function studies.

Collaborative Interventions (continued)

Surgery

M

Surgery performed in the treatment of cancer can serve several purposes:

- Diagnosis. Surgery is one way by which a tissue can be obtained for diagnosis.
- Removal of tumor. If cancer is localized in one area, the surgery may be curative.
- Decreasing the size of the tumor. The remaining cancer cells can sometimes be treated with radiation or chemotherapy.
- Palliative surgery. The purpose is to help relieve the patient's symptoms rather than cure. Examples include surgery for urinary or colon obstruction or to treat a fractured bone due to bone metastasis.
- Reconstructive surgery. The purpose is to restore appearance or function after treatment. A common example is breast reconstruction after breast cancer and mastectomy.

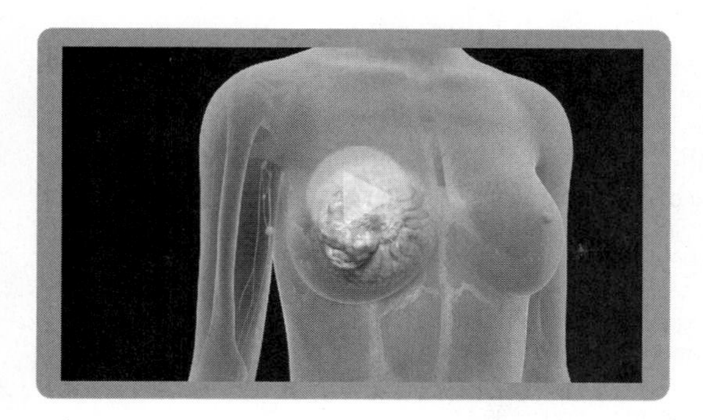

This animation reviews several breast cancer surgeries: lumpectomy, simple mastectomy, modified radical mastectomy, and radical mastectomy surgery.
Source: © 2014 Nucleus Medical Media, All rights reserved

Postoperative Care

- Assist the patient to adapt to functional changes and activities of daily living. Cancer surgery involves the loss of a specific body part and/or its function. Sometimes, whole organs are removed. Any organ loss reduces function.
- Provide emotional support as the patient adapts to bodily changes. Some surgery results in major scarring or disfigurement. Patients may be anxious about the chances of surviving the cancer and also may be grieving about the loss of body image or a change in lifestyle.
- Postoperative care is similar to that of any surgery with additional priority care needs of psychosocial support and assisting the patient to achieve or maintain maximum function:
  - o Assess patient's ability to cope with cancer treatment, changes in body image, and role.
  - o Coordinate with the health care team to provide support for the patient and family. Encourage the patient to look at, touch, and participate in dressing changes for the surgical site.
  - o Specific exercises after surgery can minimize functional loss, for example, arm exercises after mastectomy. Patient needs encouragement as exercises can be painful and need to progress in intensity. Physical and occupational therapists and family members should be engaged.

Concept Check

6. A patient will have surgery to remove lung cancer even though there is no hope for a cure. What type of procedure is this?

A. Reconstructive
B. Diagnostic
C. Palliative
D. Exploratory

Answer question

Collaborative Interventions (continued)

Collaborative Symptom Management and Comfort Care: Pain

- Quality of life in cancer patients can be adversely affected by many factors:
  - o Physical impairments
  - o Depression
  - o A multitude of symptoms, the most prominent being pain
- Pain management is one of the most important components of caring for cancer patients. Pain relief is possible for almost all patients with the use of medications. However, the following barriers prevent this from happening.
  - o Patient, caregiver, or health care provider concerns regarding addiction and side effects of opioids
  - o Patient noncompliance with analgesic pain management
  - o A focus on cancer treatment rather than treatment of cancer symptoms
- Education of patients and health care providers can help overcome some of these barriers.

Management of Cancer Pain Guidelines

Evidence-based recommendations to provide an overview of pain management are based on clinical practice guidelines from the Agency for Health Care Policy and Research (Jacox, et al., 1994) and the European Society of Medical Oncology (Ripamonti, et al., 2012):

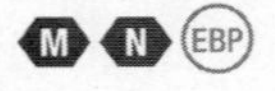

1. **Assessment** of quality, severity, onset of pain. Determining the cause of pain is crucial in initiating the right kind of therapy. For example, a patient presents with right hip pain due to bone metastasis to the hip with a fracture. This patient is more likely to benefit from surgery rather than an increase in analgesics. The quality of pain may guide the health care provider to choose the right medication for pain. Numbness and burning may suggest a neuropathic pain, which will not respond well to typical analgesics. Worsening pain may indicate progression of the cancer. Patients should be reassessed routinely after adjustments or initiation of analgesics for response. Pain not adequately responding to treatment may require an increased dose. Assessment must include all components of suffering. Validated visual, verbal, and numeric analogue or rating scales can be helpful in accurately assessing pain.

2. **Medications**

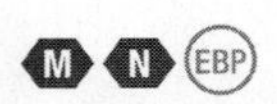

   Analgesic use should progress in accordance with the World Health Organization's (WHO) analgesic ladder, which is as follows:

   - NSAIDs (e.g., ibuprofen, naproxen) and paracetamol are strongly recommended for mild pain (should not be used in patients with high risk for bleeding). NSAIDs can only be used up to a ceiling dose beyond which toxicities prohibit further increases.
   - NSAIDs and paracetamol are also strongly recommended for use in treating all pain intensities and in combination with opioids.
   - Opioids are strongly recommended for moderate to severe pain. Opioids do not have a maximum dose. Doses may be titrated up according to need. Dosing may be limited, however, by sedation or suppression of breathing. Opioids may be given around the clock with doses for breakthrough pain. The preferred method is oral but they may be administered IV, transdermally, or rectal.
   - Adjuvant treatments may include corticosteroids, antidepressant, and anticonvulsive medications. For example, antidepressant (e.g., amitryptiline and duloxetine) and antiseizure medications (e.g., carbamazepine, gabapentin) can be useful for neuropathic pain.
   - For specific cancers, there are additional cancer type-specific pain interventions (e.g., use of denosumab or bisphosphonates in treatment of metastatic bone tumors).

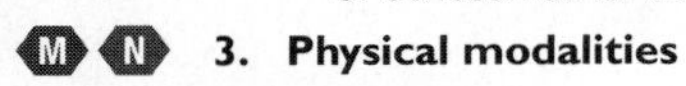

3. **Physical modalities**
   - Heat, cold, exercise, temporary immobilization, electrical stimulation, and vibration can help relieve pain caused by muscle spasm or muscle tension.

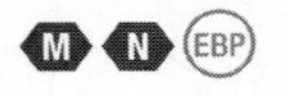

4. **Psychosocial interventions**
   - Educating patients and caregivers about management of pain and side effects of treatment can be helpful.
   - Assessing psychological distress as a component of cancer pain is strongly associated with the adequacy of pain control.
   - Encouraging patients to actively participate in their pain management can be helpful.

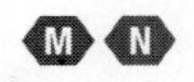

5. **Alternative or complementary therapies**
   - Offer and explain the various types of alternative therapies (e.g., massage, music, guided imagery, hypnosis, biofeedback, acupuncture) that may complement or substitute for pharmacologic interventions for pain and discomfort.

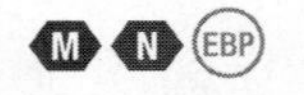

6. **Invasive interventions** for situations when noninvasive interventions do not work:
   - Surgery can be used for palliative reasons for obstruction or bleeding.
   - Neuroablation (ablating nerves) and implantation of electrical stimulator can help relieve pain.
   - Radiation can help with tumor-associated pain by shrinking tumors. It is especially helpful for bone pain. Evaluation for radiation is strongly recommended in patients with bone metastasis. Radiation therapy is used for palliative reasons in about one third of patients with cancer.
   - Nerve blocks usually involve the destruction of nerves to relieve pain in areas that a tumor has invaded. This is achieved by using chemical, heat or radio frequency delivered by a catheter to specific areas along the nerve pathway. Neurolytic or destructive interventions are used for intractable pain.

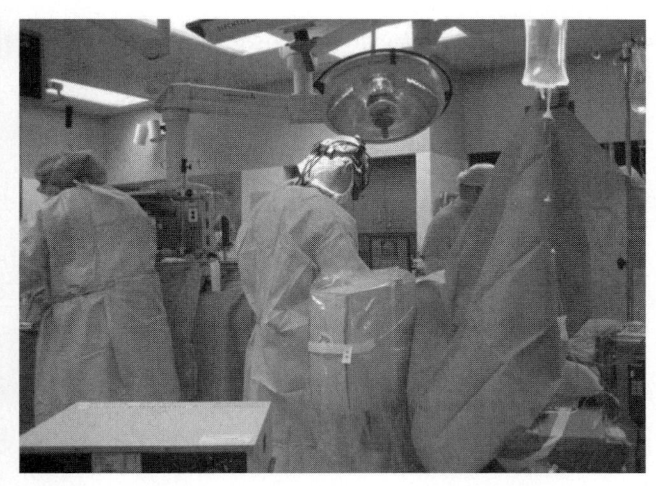

Surgery may be needed for tumor removal or relief of pain.

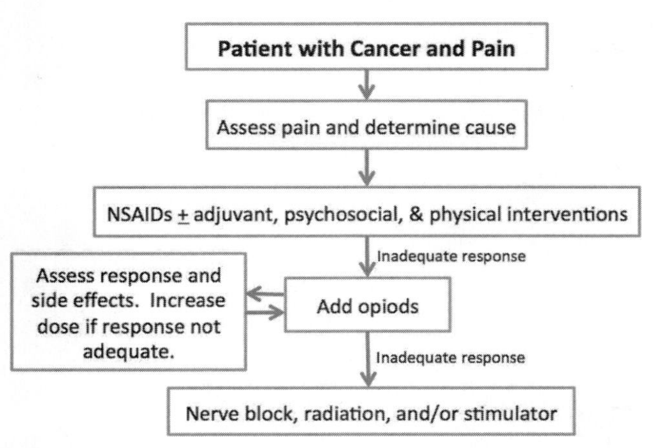

Collaborative Interventions (continued)

Common Side Effects of Opioids

M N
- Administer laxatives for any patient on opioids, as needed, to prevent or manage opioid-induced constipation, which is a problem in almost all patients taking opioids.

M N
- Provide antiemetics on a fairly regular basis to reduce or eliminate nausea and vomiting.

N
- Anticipate that mild sedation commonly fails to be effective after several days.

M N
- Collaborate to temporarily discontinue the opioid or effectively reverse it with the opioid-antagonist Narcan if more severe sedation and/or respiratory depression ensue. Alternative pain management may be necessary.

M N
- Gradually increase the dose of opioids over time to control pain when and if tolerance to opioids develops.

N
- Be attentive to early warning signs and symptoms of withdrawal if opioids are abruptly discontinued or the dose is rapidly decreased. Symptoms include anxiety, muscle aches, insomnia, diaphoresis, abdominal cramping, diarrhea, nausea, and vomiting.

M N
- Avoid undertreatment of pain in cancer patients. Although concerns about addiction are common and influence the administration of opioids, addiction to opioids in cancer patients is rare.
- To assist health care providers, the World Health Organization (WHO) developed an algorithm to guide the management of acute pain in cancer patients. To date, clinicians who care for cancer patients have relied on the WHO algorithm for guidance in non-opioid and opioid treatment.

M N
  - o The approach depends on the intensity of pain a patient reports and is then matched with appropriate medication.

M N
  - o As with any algorithm, the health care provider must use good clinical judgment and account for the various acute and chronic aspects of the patient's pain and responses.

Recommended WHO Analgesic Ladder with Suggested Adaptation

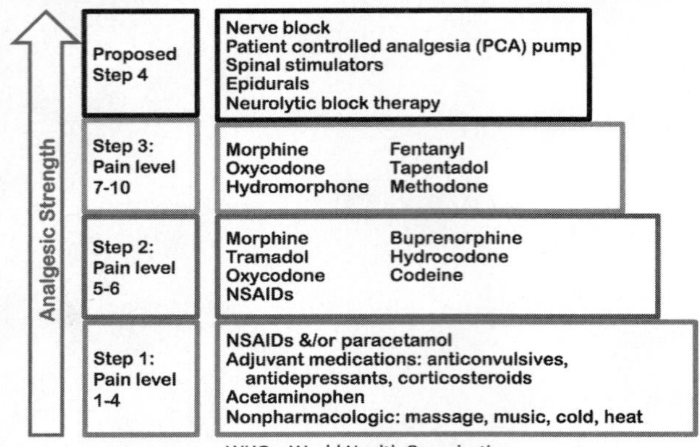

WHO = World Health Organization

Source: Copyright © 2014, NovEx Novice to Expert Learning, LLC

Venous Thromboembolism Prophylaxis

Prevention of venous thromboembolism is especially important for cancer patients. The European Society of Medical Oncology (Mandala, et al., 2011) recommendations for clinical practice include:

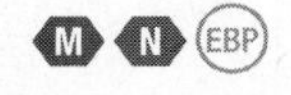

- Treat patients with cancer with either low molecular weight heparin (LMWH) or unfractionated heparin (UFH) if:
  - o Having major pelvic or abdominal surgery. Treat during and after hospitalization.
  - o Immobilized in bed due to medical complications
  - o Receiving chemotherapy with combinations of adjuvant medications for myeloma
- Avoid extensive, routine prophylaxis in cancer patients who:
  - o Receive hormone and/or chemotherapy.
  - o Have central venous catheters to prevent venous thromboembolism (VTE).
- Recommend prevention using postoperative prophylaxis is imperative.
- Use sequential compression device in conjunction with thromboprophylaxis.
- Avoid using compression stockings and sequential compression devices as monotherapy. Evidence does not support the effectiveness of mechanical without pharmacologic thromboprophylaxis (e.g., LMWH).
- Consider inferior vena cava filter in patients with cancer to prevent recurrent pulmonary emboli despite adequate anticoagulation or when anticoagulants are contraindicated.
- Consider continuing anticoagulant treatment at home in patients who have already developed thrombosis—either Coumadin or low molecular weight heparin subcutaneously.
- Advocate for additional interventions (e.g., early mobilization, hydration), which are not specific to patients with cancer but are important in all patients at risk for VTE

DVT and Pulmonary Embolism - Greenfield Filter Placement

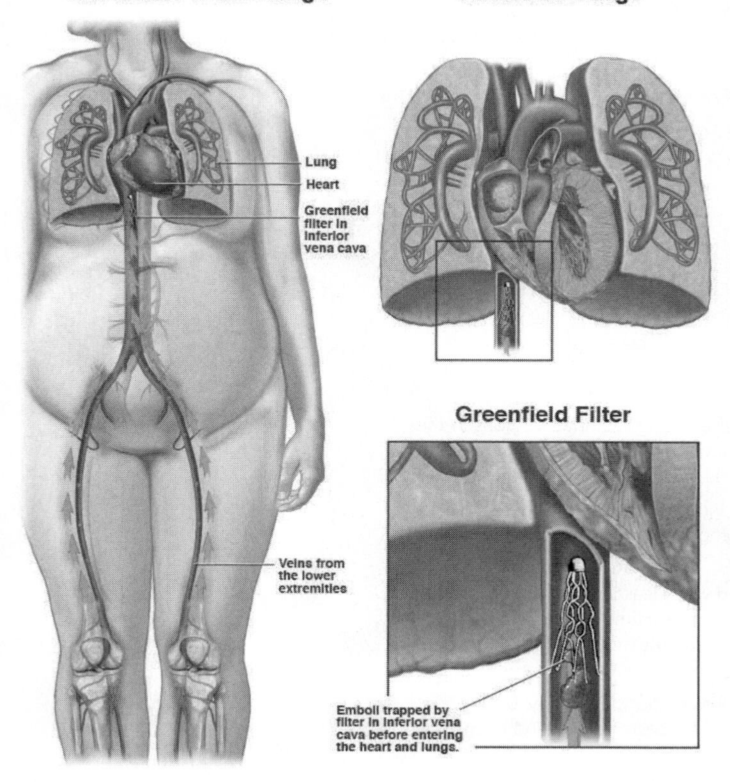

This image depicts how a deep vein thrombosis (DVT) forms and can then embolize to the lungs (pulmonary embolism). A Greenfield filter is often inserted into the inferior vena cava to prevent blood clots from reaching the heart and lungs.

Collaborative Interventions (continued)

Cancer Emergencies

Cancer emergencies can be unexpected and/or can occur rapidly. For this reason, clinicians caring for patients with cancer must be mindful of the patient's advanced directives or preferences regarding the kind of extent of interventions. Adhering and advocating to the patient's preferences guide the team's clinical judgments. In non-DNR or noncomfort care only situation, immediate interventions for patients experiencing major cancer emergencies until the team arrives and a plan of care is determined include:

- **Tumor lysis syndrome:**
  - o Initiate continuous cardiac monitoring and be alert for cardiac dysrhythmias.
  - o Anticipate the need for hemodialysis due to acute renal failure.
  - o Prepare for insertion of central venous catheter and/or dialysis catheter.
  - o Anticipate and prepare for treatment of heart failure, hyperkalemia, and hypocalcemia.
- **Superior vena cava syndrome:**
  - o Raise the head of the bed or have the patient sit to keep the upper body higher than the lower body.
  - o Support the patient to reduce anxiety to improve breathing until more definitive intervention is determined.
  - o Anticipate and prepare for (1) watchful waiting in patients with very mild symptoms; (2) medications to be administered if the patient has mild to moderate symptoms; and (3) possible surgical (e.g., thrombectomy, stent placement, vascular bypass) intervention if the vessel is blocked.

N • **Spinal cord compression:**

- o Thoroughly evaluate the pain, neurological symptoms (e.g., weakness, mobility changes, paresis, paresthesias, incontinence, urinary retention.
- o Immobilize the spine until the evaluation is completed.
- o Medicate for pain as soon as the complication has been evaluated.
- o Carefully monitor vital signs, bladder and bowel function as indicators of the degree of compression injury.
- o Prevent pressure ulcer development due to immobilization.
- o Implement safety precautions, such as fall precautions if not immobilized, to prevent injury.
- o Depending on the location and degree of dysfunction, such as palliative care in most situations, but anticipate the need for medications and/or surgical intervention.

N • **Increased intracranial pressure:**

- o Anticipate the need to administer glucocorticoids.
- o If severe, anticipate and prepare for potential intubation if respiratory depression is observed. Hyperventilation and/or mannitol may be needed.

M N These conditions require early intervention to prevent long-term or fatal consequences.

Communication and Patient Education

Multiple evidence-based clinical practice guidelines emphasize that crucial interventions in the care of patients with cancer are good and frequent communication and education. Clinicians are challenged to learn to be honest while being compassionate, supportive, and encouraging so that the patient maintains realistic hope.

- M N Educate the patient about the illness, which is a key component in caring for patients with cancer.
- M N First and foremost, recognize that patients are distressed when learning about their diagnosis. It is a very stressful time for a patient and the family. It is extremely difficult for patients to understand the consequences of their disease and treatment when educated just after learning of the prospect that they may die.
- N Empathize that patients often have multiple other considerations that may be financial, spiritual, family, or relational in nature. Consider the need for pastoral care and counseling sessions with a social worker or counselor.
- M N Be sensitive to the patient's cultural norms and practices. Ask if unfamiliar, as cultural barriers are common. Cancer is a stigma in many cultures, and family members often request that the patient not find out about their diagnosis. It can be understood as a death sentence and suicide has resulted, though rarely, when clinicians ignore the family's adamancy not to tell. Despite the American norms around the patient's rights, cultural considerations must be in the best interest of the patient.
- M N Provide adequate time for the patient to assimilate the information that they are hearing. Overwhelming the patient causes more stress.
- N Encourage the patient to identify and have the appropriate support of those who may help the patient make the best decisions. This may include spouse, friends, other family members, and spiritual advisors.
- N Provide ample opportunities for and support the patient to share any fear, concern, or anxiety about their illness or potential consequences of the illness, particularly related to small children. Prepare ahead of time for potentially emotional interactions. Seek a mentor who may help with what to expect and how to respond. Listening and being fully present for the patient and/or family are critical skills.
- N Help the patient learn to best cope with their illness and its consequences requires that the clinician explore and listen to how the patient effectively copes with other stressors in life. Avoid "telling" the patient how to cope, but rather encourage the patient to grasp what he/she finds most helpful or point out those strategies that they identify as helpful.
- N Ensure that a professional translator is accessible if there is a language barrier. It is important to keep in mind that, in some cultures, the family may not convey information (e.g., difficult, emotional-evoking, prognostic) to the patient if they are used as translators.
- M N Respect the family's wishes if they are resistant to sharing the diagnosis with the patient. It is important to acknowledge that it is difficult information for the patient to hear. Explore the cultural differences, explain the patient's essential role in planning care, but respect and observe the family's wishes. Collaborate with the health care provider and the ethics committee when necessary.
- M N Discuss end-of-life issues, including whether the patient wants resuscitative interventions and life-prolonging measures, such as feeding tubes.
- M N Educate the patient and family about advanced directives and encourage them to reach an understanding about the patient's preferences.

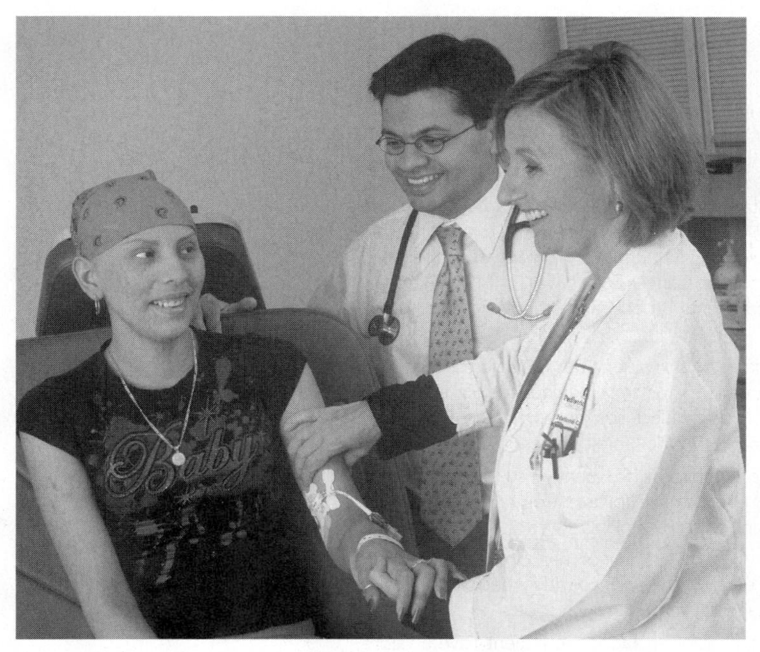

Communication and support of patients, particularly those with cancer who are receiving chemotherapy, is central in the care of the patient.
Source: Rhoda Bae/National Cancer Institute, www.cancer.gov

Collaborative Interventions (continued)

Hospice and Palliative Care

- Palliative care provides comfort care and management of symptoms at any point in a life-threatening illness. It is typically provided by a team to meet the patient's multiple and complex physiologic, emotional, social, and spiritual needs. Hospice always provides palliative care but differs by caring primarily for patients who are no longer receiving curative interventions. Most hospice patients are within 6 months of the end of life.
- The palliative care team may be very helpful to patients who require ongoing care while receiving treatments.
- M N Provide comfort care to patients who decide that their main goal is not to prolong life after they have weighed the benefits versus toxicities of treatment.
- M N Discuss and provide symptom management and comfort care to patients who may not be offered treatment by their health care provider because their underlying health is too poor and is likely to deteriorate with treatments such as surgery and chemotherapy.
- M N Collaboratively explore hospice as an option for patients whose survival is expected to be less than six months. A major goal of hospice is to keep the patient comfortable and as symptom free as possible.
- M N Consider hospice early. Hospice is underutilized, and many patients do not enroll until the last several days or weeks of their lives. One barrier to the use of hospice is the fear that when enrolled, patients die faster. Research has shown the opposite to be true. Patients enrolled in hospice tend to live longer than those who are not.
- N Educate patients that hospice focuses on the control of symptoms, including pain, nausea, and shortness of breath.
- N Educate patients that a benefit of hospice is to allow patients who prefer to be at home in familiar surroundings to remain at home. Hospice offers the resources to make this possible and to educate the caregivers. There are usually nurses who make home visits and work with a team that includes health care providers, pharmacists, and pastoral care.
- N Inform patients who cannot be cared for at home to be cared for in a hospital or skilled nursing facility in conjunction with hospice or can be admitted to inpatient hospice units.

Collaborative Interventions (continued)

Prevention

Incidence of cancer can be significantly decreased if patients engage in modifying key risk factors or participate in early screening.

Modifiable Risk Factors

Many of the modifiable risk factors are also important for the general well-being of a patient and should demand wider public education. In general, of the risk factors, no one factor is applicable to or relevant for all cancers, but each does have strong implications for many of the cancers. The National Cancer Institute (2014) and the American Cancer Society (ACS) (2014) strongly advocates for prevention and recommends that patients be educated about evidence-based preventive practices:

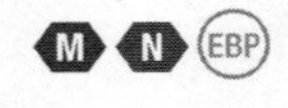

- Stop smoking and using tobacco, which are strongly associated with multiple cancers, such as lung, oropharyngeal, esophageal, renal, pancreatic, gastric, renal, bladder, cervical and blood cancers. Research shows that lung cancers closely reflect smoking practices. Smoking is understood to cause 30% of all deaths from cancer in the United States.

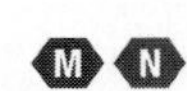

  - o Simply telling patients to stop smoking or using tobacco is frequently insufficient to change behavior. Although some patients comply, many smoke for a reason and may need to adopt new ways of coping or self-comforting to stop smoking.

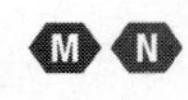

  - o Encourage patients to explore potential ways of relaxing or reducing stress without replacing one risk factor for another (e.g., eating). The ACS provides multiple strategies that can help smokers overcome cravings and get through rough spots.

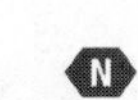

  - o Explore the patient's thoughts about quitting smoking. Does the patient have a desire to quit? Has the patient ever tried to stop in the past? What caused resuming smoking? What made or makes it hard to stop? Understanding the addiction, social, and coping issues related to smoking is helpful.

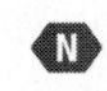

  - o If patients desire to stop smoking, collaborate with them to imagine what it will involve. Research shows that imagining, preparing, and forecasting is very helpful in moving into a change.

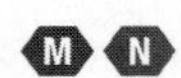

  - o Suggest a starting point such as cutting back if the patient is interested but unable to stop smoking altogether. Explore the patient's openness to nicotine patches or gum.
  - o Refer a willing patient to a smoking cessation program nearby, preferably with a brochure that provides contact information and program description.

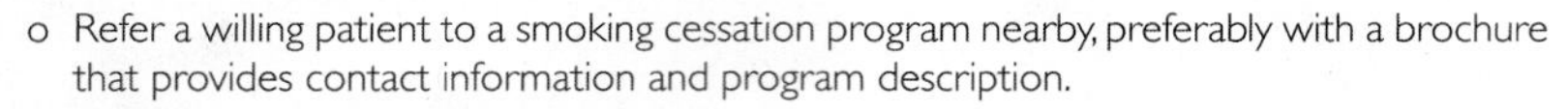

  - o Be warm, compassionate, and understanding rather than judgmental, harsh, or adamant.

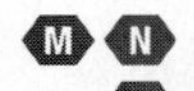

  - o Request and provide follow-up on their progress in cutting back on tobacco use or in making a decision about what to do.

  - o Empathize and acknowledge that it can feel impossible to stop smoking. Provide affirmation, encouragement, and positive examples of success.

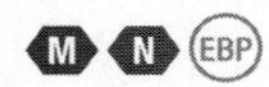

- Increased physical activity and exercise can likely lower the risk of certain cancers (e.g., breast, colorectal, endometrial).

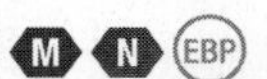

- Achieving a healthy weight, particularly reducing obesity
- Improved diet: a healthy diet that is high in fruits and nonstarchy vegetables, low in red meat, and low in fat

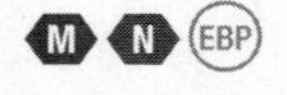

- Limiting alcohol: The strongest evidence available reflects the increased risk of cancers (e.g., oral, esophageal, colorectal, and breast) in those who drink alcohol.

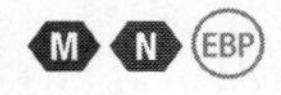

- Prevent or treat infections that place the patient at high risk for cancers. Safer sex practices and HPV vaccine, for example, can specifically help avoid hepatomas and prevent penis, vaginal, oropharyngeal, cervical, and anal cancers. Preventing hepatitis B and C greatly lowers the risk of liver cancers.

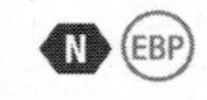

- Avoid excess radiation from sun exposure and use sunblock lotions and clothing for protection (e.g., hats, long-sleeve shirts).

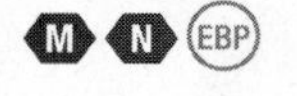

- Avoid living in areas where environmental pollutants are known (e.g., air, smoke, arsenic in water, pesticides, radon, asbestos) as these are well-established associations to cancers.

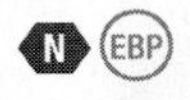

- Use of vitamins or dietary supplements is not supported by the evidence in reducing cancer risks at this time.

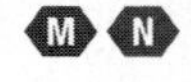

- Participate in cancer screening tests.

Collaborative Interventions (continued)

Screening for Cancers

Prevention and early detection of cancer are superior interventions over treatment after cancer is detected. Screening tests for early detection include the following:

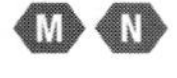

- Complete a physical examination with special attention devoted to achieving a healthy weight, abnormal lymph nodes, masses, and any other indications of cancer.

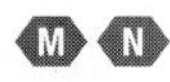

- Monitor laboratory tests for blood and urine, noting any abnormalities that may indicate cancer.

- Initiate imaging procedures such as a virtual colonoscopy (an MRI of the colon), when indicated.

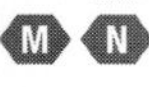

- Collaborate with the health care provider to refer patients with genetically associated cancer for genetic tests to determine abnormal genes in patients at high risk for certain types of cancer (e.g., breast).

- Initiate invasive screening tests when necessary, but these may have risks associated with them. Even tests that appear benign, such as MRI, CT, and PSA, may lead to further testing and procedures that are invasive in a patient that may, otherwise, be healthy.

Clinical Practice Guidelines for Screening

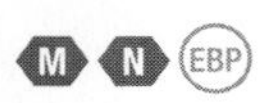

The American Cancer Society (2013) recommends the following screening tests for early detection of specific cancers:

- Breast cancer
  - o Yearly mammograms are recommended starting at age 40 and continuing for as long as a woman is in good health.
  - o Clinical breast exam (CBE) about every 3 years for women in their 20s and 30s and every year for women 40 years and older.
  - o Women should know how their breasts normally look and feel and report any breast change promptly to their health care provider. Breast self-exam (BSE) is encouraged for women, starting in their 20s.
  - o Some very high-risk women should be screened with MRI in addition to mammograms.
- Colorectal cancer and polyps: Beginning at age 50, both men and women should follow one of these testing schedules:
  - o Flexible sigmoidoscopy every 5 years or
  - o Colonoscopy every 10 years or
  - o Double-contrast barium enema every 5 years or
  - o CT colonography (virtual colonoscopy) every 5 years
- Endometrial (uterine) cancer
  - o At the time of menopause, all women should be told about the risks and symptoms of endometrial cancer.
  - o Women should report any unexpected bleeding or spotting to their doctors.

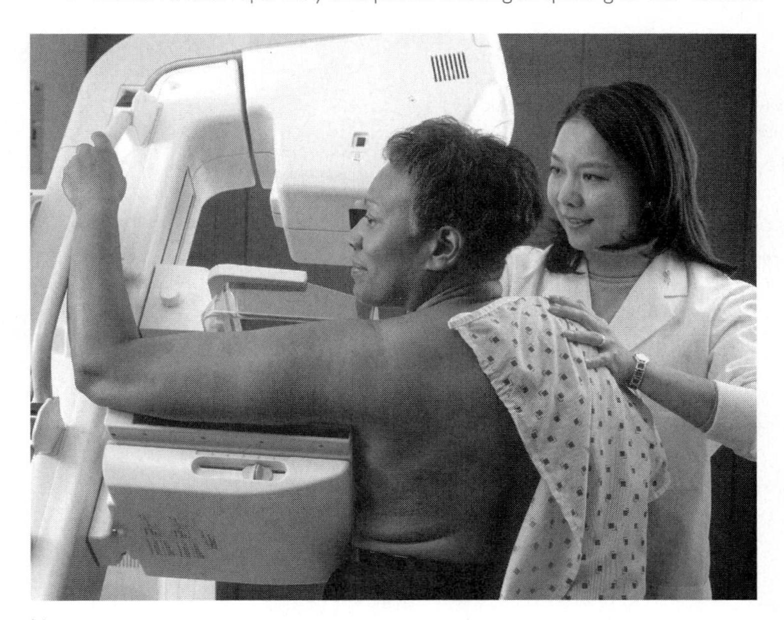

Mammogram.
Source: Rhoda Baer/National Cancer Institute

- Cervical cancer
  - o Cervical cancer screening (testing) should begin at age 21. Women under age 21 should *not* be tested.
  - o Women between ages 21 and 29 should have a Pap test done every 3 years.
  - o The preferred approach for women between 30–65 years is to be evaluated every 5 years with both Pap and HPV tests. If Pap test only, test every 3 years.
  - o Women over age 65 who have had regular cervical cancer testing with normal results should *not* be tested for cervical cancer. Once testing is stopped, it should not be started again. Women with a history of a serious cervical precancer should continue to be tested for at least 20 years after that diagnosis, even if testing continues past age 65.
  - o **A woman who has had her uterus removed (and also her cervix)** for reasons not related to cervical cancer and who has no history of cervical cancer or serious pre-cancer should not be tested.
  - o **A woman who has been vaccinated against HPV** should still follow the screening recommendations for her age group.
  - o Some women—because of their history—may need to have a different screening schedule for cervical cancer.
- Prostate cancer
  - o Starting at age 50, men should talk to a doctor about the pros and cons of testing so they can decide if testing is the right choice for them.
  - o If they are African American or have a father or brother who had prostate cancer before age 65, men should have this talk with a doctor starting at age 45. If men decide to be tested, they should have the PSA blood test with or without a rectal exam. How often they are tested will depend on their PSA level.

Concept Check

7. Typically, screening for colorectal cancer should begin at what age?
   A. 40
   B. 45
   C. 50
   D. 60

Answer question

Summary of Interventions

- Patients diagnosed with cancer are treated with chemotherapy, radiation, and surgery.
- Pain is the most prominent symptom of cancer and is treated with various modalities including psychosocial and physical interventions with medications.
  1. First line treatment is, commonly, NSAIDs followed by opioids if NSAIDs fail. NSAIDs may be used adjuvantly with opioids.
  2. Adjuvant medications may be used to treat the neuropathic component of pain.
  3. Surgical interventions may be used for patients not responding to medications.
- Hospice and palliative care may be very helpful for patients who primarily want to be comfortable or who are not candidates for chemotherapy and surgery.

LO4:

Evaluation of Desired Collaborative Care Outcomes

Evaluation and reassessment should reveal attainment of previously established patient outcomes. In summary:

- Patient reports that pain is tolerable and does not interfere with rest or desired activities.
- Patient's skin is free of lesions or that lesions are progressively healing.
- Patient's oral mucous membranes are intact and not inflamed or are being effectively treated and are progressively healing.
- Patient is infection free and is actively participating in practices that reduce the risk.
- Patient's body mass index is within normal range or is steadily improving toward normal.
- Patient reports decrease in nausea and can eat.
- Patient reports engaging in daily activities without excessive fatigue and balances rest with activity.
- Patient reports being less fearful.
- Patient accurately describes body changes, reports changes have not prevented socialization, and/or is comfortable with level of current social interactions.
- Patient reports acclimating to treatments and their side effects, and having better control of the effects of toxicity.

References

American Cancer Society. (2013). *Chemotherapy principles: an in-depth discussion of the techniques and its role in cancer treatment.* **www.cancer.org/treatment/treatmentsandsideeffects/treatmenttypes/chemotherapy/chemotherapyprinciplesanin-depthdiscussionofthetechniquesanditsroleintreatment/**

American Joint Committee on Cancer. (2002). *AJCC Cancer Staging Manual.* 6th ed. New York, NY: Springer.

Christakis, N. A., & Escarce, J. J. (1996). Survival of medicare patients after enrollment in hospice programs. *N Engl J Med, 335*, 172–178. doi: 10.1056/NEJM199607183350306

Connor, S. R., Pyenson, B., et al. (2007). Comparing hospice and nonhospice patient survival among patients who die within a three-year window. *J Pain SympManag, 33*(3), 238–246.

Lewis, M. A., Hendrickson, A. W., & Moynihan, T. J. (2011). Oncologic emergencies: pathophysiology, presentation, diagnosis, and treatment. *CA Cancer J Clin, 61*, 287–314. **Onlinelibrary.wiley.com/doi/10.3322/caac.20124/pdf**

Miaskowski, C., Dodd, M. J., et al. (2001). Lack of adherence with the analgesic regimen: asignificant barrier to effective cancer pain management. *J Clin Oncol, 19*(23), 4275–4279.

Myers, J. S. (2013). Cancer- and chemotherapy-related cognitive changes: the patient experience. *Semin Oncol Nursing, 29*(4), 300–307. **www.seminarsoncologynursing.com/article/S0749-2081(13)00058-2/fulltext**

National Cancer Institute at the NIH. (2013). *Cancer staging.* **http://www.cancer.gov/cancertopics/factsheet/detection/staging**

National Cancer Institute at the NIH, Surveillance, Epidemiology, and End Results Program. (2013). *SEER stat fact sheets: all cancer sites.* **seer.cancer.gov/statfacts/html/all.html**

Roila, F., Herrstedt, J., Aapro, M., et al. on behalf of ESMO/MASCC Guidelines Working Group. (2010). Guideline update for MASCC and ESMO in the prevention of chemotherapy- and radiotherapy-induced nausea and vomiting: results of the Perugia consensus conference. *Annals Oncolog, 21* (Suppl 5), v232–v243.

Stein, C. J., & Colditz, G. A. (2004). Modifiable risk factors for cancer. *Br J Cancer, 90*(2), 299–303.

World Cancer Research Fund. (2007). *Food, nutrition, physical activity, and the prevention of cancer. A global perspective.* Washington, DC: American Institute of Cancer Research.

Clinical Practice Guidelines

American Cancer Society. (2013). *Stay healthy.* **www.cancer.org/healthy/index**

American Cancer Society. (2014). *ACS guidelines on nutrition and physical activity for cancer prevention.* **www.cancer.org/healthy/eathealthygetactive/acsguidelinesonnutritionphysicalactivityforcancerprevention/nupa-guidelines-toc**

American Cancer Society (2014). *American Cancer Society guidelines for the early detection of cancer.* **www.cancer.org/healthy/findcancerearly/cancerscreeningguidelines/american-cancer-society-guidelines-for-the-early-detection-of-cancer**

Jacox, A., Carr, D. B., & Payne, R. (1994). New clinical practice guidelines for the management of pain in patients with cancer. *N Engl J Med, 330*, 651–655. doi: 10.1056/NEJM199403033300926

Mandala, M., Falanga, A., & Roila, F. (2011). Management of venous thromboembolism (VTE) in cancer patients: ESMO clinical practice guidelines. *Annals Oncolog, 22*(Suppl 6), vi85–vi92.

National Cancer Institute at the NIH. (2014). *Cancer prevention overview: description of the evidence.* **http://www.cancer.gov/cancertopics/pdq/prevention/overview/HealthProfessional/page2#Section_132**

Ripamonti, C. I., Santini, D., Maranzano, E., et al. on behalf of the ESMO Guidelines Working Group. (2012). Management of cancer pain: ESMO clinical practice guidelines. *Annals Oncology, 23*(Suppl 7), vii139–vii154. doi: 10.1093/annonc/mds233

Patient Education and Support (support groups, advanced directives, end-of-life, home care, hospice)

National Cancer Institute. *NCI facts by topic.* **www.cancer.gov/cancertopics/factsheet**

Stanford Health Care Cancer Institute. (2015). *Managing chemotherapy side effects.* **stanfordhealthcare.org/medical-treatments/c/chemotherapy/side-effects.html**

Learning Outcomes for Cancer Toxicities

When you complete this lesson, you will be able to:

1. Recognize the clinical relevance of cancer treatment toxicities.
2. Consider the pathophysiology, etiology, risk factors, and clinical presentation of cancer treatment toxicities that determine the priority patient concerns.
3. Determine the most urgent and important nursing interventions and patient education required in caring for a patient with cancer treatment toxicities.
4. Evaluate attainment of desired collaborative care outcomes for a patient with cancer treatment toxicity.

LO1:

What Are Treatment Toxicities?

- The most common and frequent treatments for cancers that kill malignant cells unfortunately also harm normal cells, and therefore damage organs.
- Treatment toxicities are the toxic side effects that result when effective and therapeutic dosages of anticancer treatments are delivered.
- Anticancer effects can vary between patients, even if given the same dosage. Further, anticancer drugs attack and injury normal cells while they attack cancer cells. Therefore, it is difficult to gauge the anticancer dosage in each patient that can eradicate the cancer without producing lethal side effects that irreparably damage body organs.
- Treatment combinations frequently create additive toxicities since many treatments target the same cellular characteristics for eradication. Combinations can therefore compound the severity and extent of the toxic effects.
- The threshold for treatment toxicities should be determined based on the goals of treatment:
    - If cure is an attainable goal, a higher level of toxicity may be reasonable and endured.
    - If cure is not possible and treatment is palliative, the level of toxicity suffered must be weighed against the benefits to try to prolong life or improve the quality of life.

LO1:

Clinical Relevance: Toxicities

- Toxicities and/or side effects that patients experience from cancer treatments can be worse than the symptoms of cancer.
- Every organ system can be affected.
- Survival can require multiple rounds of treatments, without a patient attaining full recovery from one round before requiring another.
- It is important to be aware that many symptoms may be the result of the cancer or may be the result of the treatment of the cancer. Sometimes, treatment regimens can be adjusted to minimize side effects that are so severe that patients either cannot tolerate or cannot continue the treatment.

LO2:

Pathophysiology: Toxicities

- The majority of side effects related to cancer treatments are due to the toxic effects of radiation and chemotherapy on healthy cells.
- These effects are most profound in rapidly dividing cells such as finger and toenails, hair, the lining of the gastrointestinal (GI) track, and bone marrow. However, all organs may be affected.
- Some chemotherapy treatments are more toxic to particular organs (e.g., anthracyclines may cause heart damage).
- Radiation is more likely to affect only the organs that are most exposed to the radiation.
- Fatigue is a common side effect of both chemotherapy and radiation.

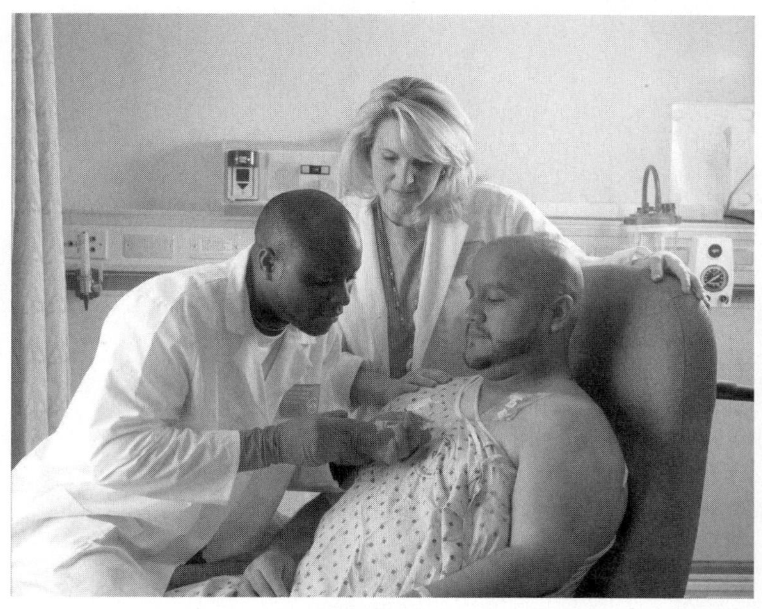

This photo shows a Hispanic patient receiving chemotherapy through his central venous catheter. Toxic effects on the blood vessel walls are reduced when these toxic drugs are infused into a major vessel.
Source: Rhoda Baer/National Cancer Institute

Concept Check

1. **Treatment toxicities most profoundly affect which tissues?**
   A. Muscle
   B. Bone
   C. Lining of GI tract
   D. Retinal

Answer question

LO2:

Risk Factors: Toxicities

There are factors that place patients at a higher risk for developing treatment-induced toxicities. These can include:

- Older age
- Chronic comorbidities
- Prolonged or repeated radiation or chemotherapy
- Gastrointestinal or hepatic disease
- Renal disease
- Prior chemotherapy-related toxicities
- Neutropenia

LO2:

Causes: Toxicities

- Chemotherapy
- Radiation therapy
- Medications used to treat symptoms of cancer (e.g., narcotics used to treat pain)

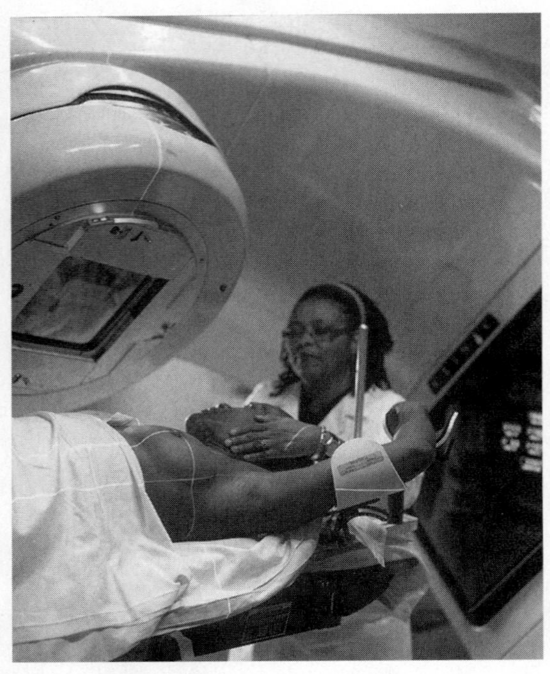

Toxicities are very common in patients who undergo not only radiation therapy, as the patient in this photo, but also chemotherapy.
Source: Rhoda Baer/National Cancer Institute

Priority Patient Concerns and Desired Collaborative Care Outcomes: Toxicities

Prior to caring for patients with cancer treatment-related toxicities, it is important to prioritize the patient's concerns that must guide the nursing care plan and interventions. Care for the patient is ordered and organized in accordance with the patient's priority and urgent needs. Desired collaborative care outcomes in patients with cancer treatment-related toxicities typically include:

1. Patient will report soft, formed stools according to usual daily schedule.
2. Patient will consume balanced diet to maintain desired nutritional level.
3. Patient's oral mucous membranes will be intact.
4. Patient's white blood cell count and red blood cell count will be within the desired range.
5. Patient will participate in decision making regarding treatment regimen.

Considering these important care outcomes, prepare a list of the major 3–6 priority patient concerns or nursing diagnoses for patients with cancer treatment-related toxicities. Be prepared to participate in a discussion of this list and/or to submit them as an assignment, as determined by your faculty. Resources you may find helpful in this assignment can include this lesson, the references, resources on nursing care plans, and standard nursing diagnoses manuals.

Overview: Diagnostics, Assessment Findings, and Collaborative Interventions

System Affected	Diagnostics	Assessment Findings	Collaborative Interventions
General	CBC to evaluate for anemia	Fatigue	Taking short naps, light exercise, support Home Health: assist in ADLs
Respiratory	Chest x-ray to rule out pneumonia or heart failure Pulse ox to evaluate oxygen status	Shortness of breath, cough	Supplemental oxygen for hypoxia or to improve oxygenation to keep SpO_2 >92%
Cardiovascular	Echocardiogram may show depressed ejection fraction, BNP may be elevated	Shortness of breath, orthopnea, edema	Diuretics and sodium restriction
Renal	Elevated BUN and creatinine, hyperkalemia	Edema due to fluid retention	Diuretics and sodium restriction
Gastrointestinal	Elevated BUN, creatinine due to volume depletion; electrolyte abnormalities such as hypokalemia from diarrhea	Anorexia, nausea, vomiting, mucosal ulcerations, muscle cramping, mental status changes, taste changes, painful mouth, mucositis, diarrhea, constipation	Antiemetics, corticosteroids, smaller meals, encourage fluid consumption, antidiarrheals for diarrhea, ice chips or magic mouthwash for mucositis, assess for acidosis / alkalosis, fluid and electrolyte imbalances Nutritional consult: dietary support
Neurologic	CT or MRI of to r/o metastatic disease to the brain	Confusion/delirium, paresthesias, numbness in extremities, difficulty walking, using hands.	Support, use of assistive devices for walking.
Hematologic	Anemia, Neutropenia, Thrombocytopenia	Fever due to infection, petechiae, and bruising from thrombocytopenia	Antibiotics for infections, transfusions
Skin/ hair		Hair loss/ dry skin	Wigs, support

LO1:

Overview: Toxicities

- The following topics are discussed in greater detail in this lesson:
  - o Gastrointestinal (GI) toxicities
  - o Neutropenia
- Additional side effects and toxicities that are discussed in separate lessons:
  - o Anemia (see the Care of Patients with Anemia NovE-lesson)
  - o Thrombocytopenia (see the Care of Patients with Platelet and Coagulation Disorders NovE-lesson)

Concept Check

2. A patient who is receiving chest radiation for pulmonary cancer is most likely to have toxicities associated with which organ?
   A. Brain
   B. Lungs
   C. Liver
   D. Heart

Answer question

Gastrointestinal Toxicities Unique to Cancer and Its Treatment

The most frequent and debilitating gastrointestinal toxicities that patients experience as a result of cancer treatments include:

- Anorexia
- Mucous membrane inflammations and infections
- Xerostomia (dry mouth)
- Nausea and vomiting
- Constipation
- Diarrhea

To best anticipate, recognize, and manage treatment-induced toxicities, it is helpful for patients to keep a diary of the onset of toxicities and their responses to treatment. This information can assist clinicians, patients and caregivers with information about how to better prepare, prevent, and/or mitigate the discomfort and adverse effects of treatments for cancers.

GI Toxicities: Anorexia

Anorexia is the involuntary loss of appetite that complicates the suffering and recovery of those with cancer.

- It may be related to the cancer.
- It may be related to chemotherapy or radiation, which can cause nausea and changes in taste.
- Anorexia is a universal complication in metastatic cancers.
- It accelerates the development of cachexia, which is the progressive wasting of body muscle, fat, and weight. Cachexia is estimated to be the cause of death in 20–40% of patients with cancers.
- Complications of anorexia include:
  - o Loss of >10% of weight, which contributes to a worse prognosis
  - o Muscle wasting, resulting in generalized weakness, which can affect ambulation
  - o Compromised immune function
  - o Poor wound healing
  - o Depression

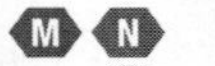

- Drugs may be needed to treat anorexia by stimulating the appetite.
  - EBP o Dexamethasone, prednisolone, or methylprednisolone may be used for a short term (Adams, et al., 2012) to stimulate appetite and improve quality of life, but this will cause loss of muscle mass in the long term.
  - EBP o Progestins: Megestrol acetate (Adams, et al., 2012) may stimulate appetite and increase body fat to increase weight, but does not improve lean body mass.
  - o Dronabinol: A cannabinoid (component of marijuana) may improve appetite in some patients but is not recommended in patients with refractory cachexia.

Poor Wound Healing

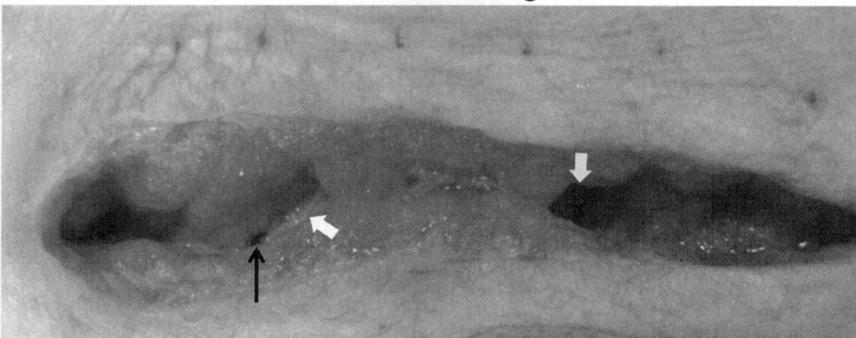

This photo reveals poor abdominal wound healing in a postoperative cancer patient. Fluid seeping from the wound resulted in removal of the staples. Although the wound is not infected, anemia and malnutrition interfered with normal healing. Whitish fibrin (white arrow) can be seen deep in the wound but healthy granulating tissue (glistening reddish, dark pink) is covering most of the slowing healing tissues. The opening to one of three wound tunnels (yellow arrow) is visible. A black peritoneal suture (black arrow) is seen deep inside the wound.

Source: Courtesy of K. Kyriakidis

- The Oncology Nursing Society recommendations (Adams, et al., 2012) are as follows:
  - o Consult a dietician for individualized nutritional counseling to optimize the patient's daily intake.
  - o Additional medications may be used on an individual basis (e.g., ghrelin, erythropoietin).
  - o Medications that are less likely to improve appetite are hydralazine and melatonin.
- Malnutrition screening may be completed to identify those at high risk for anorexia.
- Stabilizing the patient's weight is an appropriate goal for patients with anorexia and/or cachexia.
- Plan with the patient on improving protein and caloric intake as an initial nutritional intervention. The patient's preferences must be taken into account.
- Educate patients who experience early satiety to (Rock, et al., 2012):
  - o Eat smaller and more frequent meals and restrict liquids during meals.
  - o Drink nutritionally dense supplements under the direction of the health care provider to avoid replacing meals with supplements.
- Set caloric goals at around 120 kJ/kg/day (Bauer, et al., 2006).
- Set protein intake goals at about 1.4 g/kg/day and assist in identifying high protein foods (Bauer, et al., 2006).
- Review and re-educate the patient regularly about their nutrition because regular intervention shows improved nutritional outcomes (Bauer, et al., 2006).

Gastrointestinal Toxicities Unique to Cancer and Its Treatment (continued)

GI Toxicities: Mouth and Mucous Membrane Changes

- Chemotherapy or radiation to the oral cavity and chest can affect the fast growing cells lining the GI tract.
- This causes mucositis, which is an inflammation of the mucosal lining of the mouth, esophagus, or intestine (stomatitis, esophagitis, enteritis).
- Stomatitis is common and is inflammation involving the oral tissues.
- Mucositis commonly occurs within 7–10 days after chemotherapy and leads to the following problems:
  - o Pain and sores, sometimes severe
  - o Infections, especially thrush and herpes simplex
  - o Dry mouth (xerostomia)
- Chemotherapy, its intensity, duration and route of administration affect the risk for mucositis. Combination therapy (e.g., radiation), malnutrition, and xerostomia (dry mouth) further increase the risk.
- The mucosal effects last as long as the treatment continues, but improves when treatment is complete.

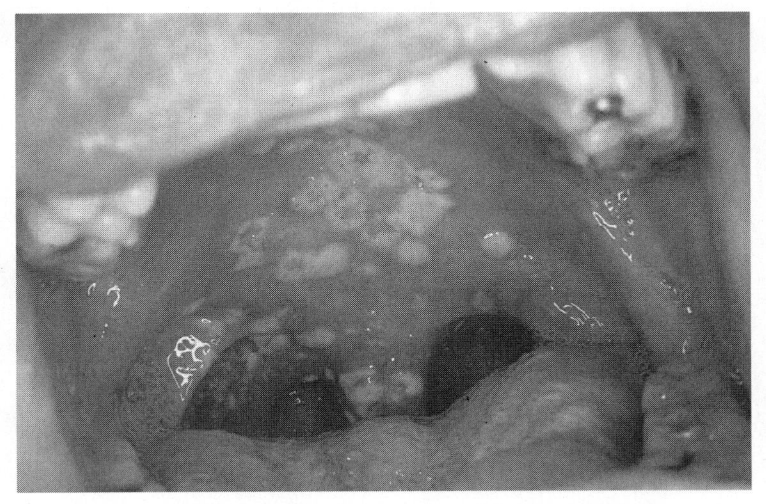

The image shows stomatitis in the open mouth of an adult. It appears as inflammation, irritation, pain, and/or ulcers in the mucous lining.

Source: Centers for Disease Control and Prevention/Sol Silverman, Jr., DDS

GI Toxicities: Xerostomia

- Xerostomia is an abnormal or excessive dryness of the mouth and characterized by a decrease in saliva.
- Disease-related xerostomia results from direct tumor invasion of salivary glands.
- Treatment-related xerostomia results from radiation to the neck or total body irradiation.
- The higher the dose of radiation (quantified as Gy [gray]), the greater the risk of xerostomia or the occurrence of dry mouth.
- More than 40 Gy may result in permanent, progressive inflammation and degeneration of the acinar ductal cells, which are then replaced with fibrinous connective tissue.
- Other drugs like diuretics, anticholinergics, opioids, decongestants, antidepressants, and antihistamines can add to the risk of dry mouth.
- Other conditions that can contribute to dry mouth are diabetes, infection, candida, OCD, and anxiety.

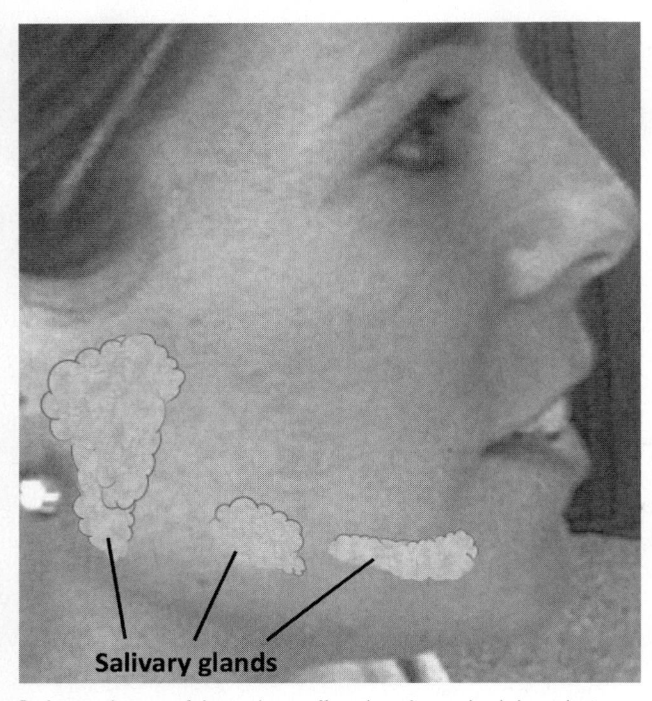

Radiation therapy of the neck can affect the salivary glands by reducing their ability to function.
Source: Courtesy of R. Murphy

Gastrointestinal Toxicities Unique to Cancer and Its Treatment (continued)

Collaborative Interventions and Prevention: Mucositis

- Prevention of mucositis (Harris, et al., 2008; MASCC/ISOO, 2014):
  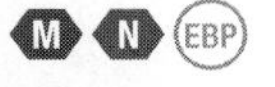
  - o Good oral hygiene with a soft bristle toothbrush is recommended. Avoid rotary electric toothbrushes that can tear the mucosa. Good hygiene includes thoroughly cleaning and storing the toothbrush where it can dry.
  - o Oral cryotherapy is recommended by placing ice in the mouth to constrict the mucous membranes and prevent the damage or by eating ice chips for 30 minutes prior to chemotherapy.
  - o Special growth factor drugs (e.g., palifermin) are recommended to induce cell growth in the mouth as a means to enhance healing or prevent mouth sores.
  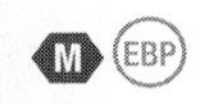
  - o Low-level laser therapy is recommended to help prevent mucositis in high-dose chemotherapy.
  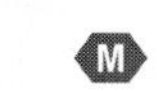
  - o Other medications such as allopurinol, anti-inflammatory rinses, immunoglobulin, honey, oral aloe vera have not been suggested as helpful.
  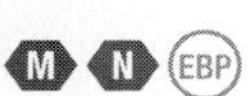
  - o Substances that are *not* suggested in preventing mucositis include: chlorhexidine with alcohol base, misoprostol mouthwash, systemic pentoxifyline, granulocyte macrophage-colony stimulating factor mouthwash, and systemic pilocarpine.

  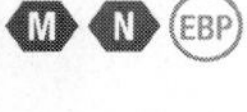
  - o Strong evidence leading to recommendations *against* use include: antimicrobial lozenges, antimicrobial paste, antimicrobial mouthwash, sucralfate mouthwash, systemic sucralfate, and IV glutamine due to lack of effectiveness.
  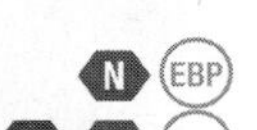
  - o Educate the patient on ways they may help prevent mucositis:
    - ■ Benzydamine mouthwash is recommended to prevent mucositis in patients with cancers of the head or neck who receive radiation therapy.
    - ■ Avoid irritants like hot, acidic, spicy, sour, and hard foods and beverages. Avoid sugar-rich foods.
    - ■ Use a mild, unflavored, or nonirritating toothpaste.
    - ■ Rinse with saline mixed with peroxide mouthwash.
    - ■ Use waxed floss that slides easily between teeth. Avoid sore or bleeding areas.
    - ■ Limit or avoid alcohol.
    - ■ Avoid wearing dentures when mucositis is present. Avoid denture adhesives and loose-fitting dentures.
    - ■ Keep lips moist using lanolin products.

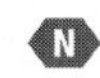

- Prevent infection in the mouth or attempt to minimize the risk of infection from the inflammation of the oral mucosa (overlaps prevention of mucositis). In addition, educate the patient about the following:
  - o Dental exam and pretreatment with the goal of repairing any damage in the gums/teeth prior to treatment
  - o Oral care protocol and education teaches the patient to rinse the mouth after meals and at bedtime with salt water or salt and baking soda water.

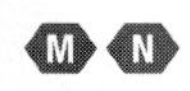

- Treatment, once problems arise (infection in the mouth or pain), consists of:
  - o Treating the specific type of infection (e.g., bacterial, viral, fungal). It is common to get thrush or herpes simplex virus in the mouth.
  - o Apply topical agents for pain.
  - o Continue all preventive measures detailed earlier.

  - o Provide pain medication: analgesics may be needed. If required, patient-controlled analgesia using morphine is recommended (Harris, et al., 2008; MASCC/ISOO, 2014).

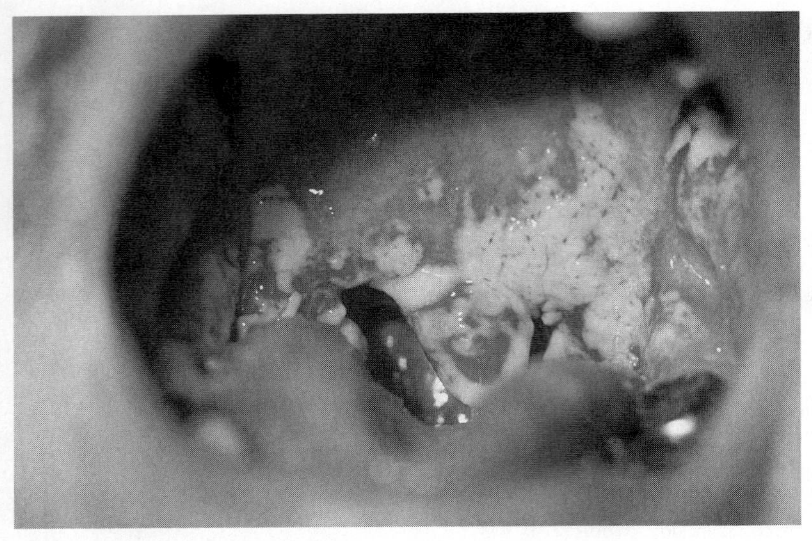

This photo shows a patient with oral thrush on the roof of his mouth and throat.
Source: Centers for Disease Control and Prevention

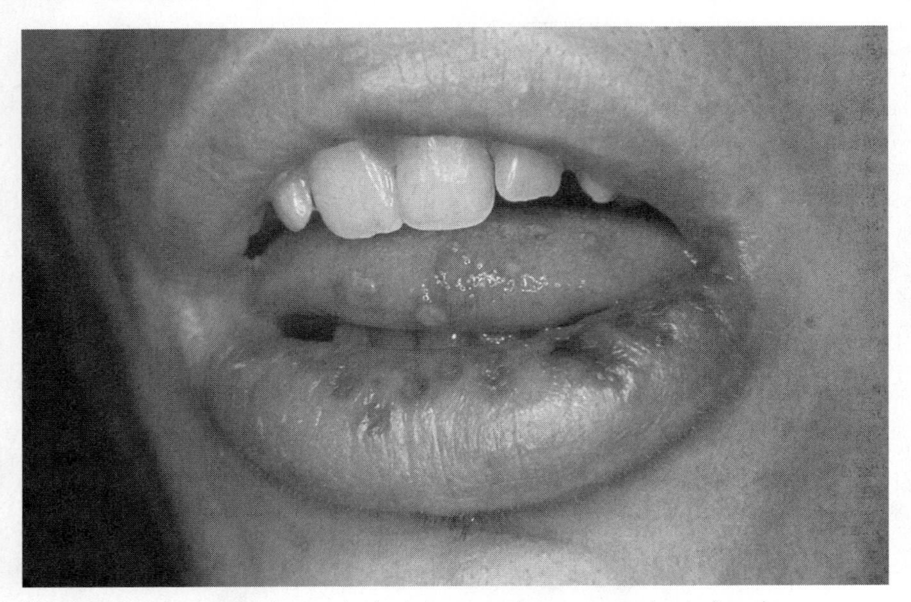

This photo reveals numerous herpes simplex lesions or canker sores covering the lip and tongue.
Source: CDC/Robert E. Sumpter

Concept Check

3. **How is cryotherapy to prevent stomatitis achieved?**
   A. Holding ice in the mouth
   B. Swishing aloe vera juice in the mouth
   C. Systemic pilocarpine
   D. Honey-containing lozenges

Answer question

Gastrointestinal Toxicities Unique to Cancer and Its Treatment (continued)

GI Toxicities: Nausea and Vomiting

- Nausea is a feeling of discomfort in the stomach associated with an urge to vomit.
- Vomiting is the forceful expulsion of the contents of the stomach out through the mouth, resulting in emesis.
- Nausea and vomiting are major reasons patients fear chemotherapy.

Pathophysiology: Nausea and Vomiting

- The vomiting center and chemoreceptor trigger zone (CTZ) are two sites in the brainstem responsible for the nausea and vomiting that produce emesis.
- As an overview, chemotherapy causes a release of serotonin from the gastrointestinal tract, which binds with the 5-HT_3 receptors seen in the image to stimulate the CTZ.
- The CTZ then stimulates the vomiting center so that emesis ensues.
- Therapy is targeted at jamming the neurotransmitted signal anywhere along this pathway to mitigate emesis.

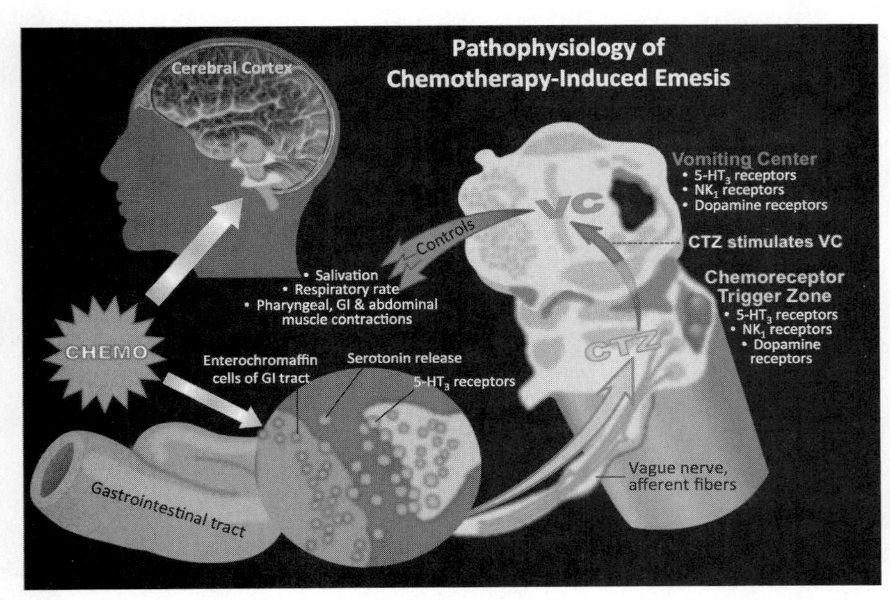

Causes: Nausea and Vomiting

Causes of nausea and vomiting in cancer patients:

- Drugs (chemotherapy and others)
- Radiation (especially in the abdomen and brain)
- Cancer, obstructing the gastrointestinal tract
- Constipation, a frequent problem in patients with cancer
- Contributing factors such as inactivity and medications (e.g., narcotics and anticholinergic medications)
- Brain tumors, by causing increased intracranial pressure

Collaborative Interventions: Nausea and Vomiting

The goal in preventing and controlling nausea and vomiting is to block the signal sent to the brain that causes nausea.

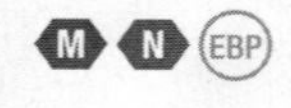

- Prophylaxis: The frequency of nausea and vomiting due to treatment-related toxicity or the effects of a cancer are expected. Prevention and management improve the care of patients and recommendations include (Naeim, et al., 2008):
    - o Evaluate the emetic potential (e.g., high, moderate) of the chemotherapeutic medications. For a list of the drugs, see Cancer.net, 2014.
    - o Use a medication or drug combination to prevent acute emesis.

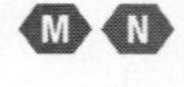

- Pharmacologic agents: Administer prescribed antiemetics, which are medications that may mitigate or control nausea and vomiting. These may include:

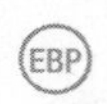

    - o NK1 antagonist (aprepitant): Use aprepitant in combination with other drugs for patients at moderate and high risk for emesis (Naeim, et al., 2008).
    - o 5-HT_3 (serotonin antagonists)
        - ■ Ondansetron
        - ■ Granisetron
        - ■ Dolesetron
        - ■ Palonosetron

    - o Dexamethasone: Start with dexamethasone to prevent emesis in patients at low risk for emesis (Naeim, et al., 2008).
    - o Dopamine antagonist
        - ■ Prochlorperazine
        - ■ Metoclopromide
    - o Cannabioids
        - ■ Dronabinol
        - ■ Nabilone
    - o Scopolamine: acts in the central nervous system (CNS) by blocking cholinergic transmission from the vestibular nuclei to higher centers in the CNS and from the reticular formation to the vomiting center
    - o Others
        - ■ Lorazepam

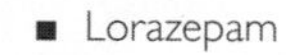

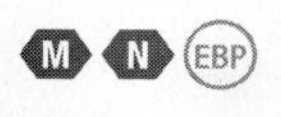

- Evaluate the patient's response at each patient visit and potential need for a different medication to manage emesis because patients do not all respond the same to each drug. A combination of medications may be needed.

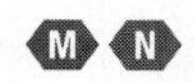

- **Nonpharmacologic interventions**: When drug therapy is not fully effective, there may need to be additional or adjuvant treatment to help reduce nausea. Or, nonpharmacologic therapies may be used to prevent or minimize the use of medications if the patient prefers or responds well. The addition of nonpharmacologic interventions helps many patients and is recommended by the Oncology Nursing Society (2011). They include those in which:
    - o Effectiveness is likely:
        - ■ Music therapy
        - ■ Progressive muscle relaxation for anticipatory nausea
        - ■ Guided visual imagery

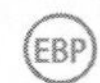

        - ■ Electroacupuncture: Manual acupuncture is not recommended for reducing nausea or vomiting. However, sufficient evidence supports the use of electroacupuncture when performed by a competent acupuncturist. Despite the evidence, this method has not been incorporated into most clinical guidelines at this point.
    - o Effectiveness not established but may be useful in some:
        - ■ Massage
        - ■ Reiki
        - ■ Distraction
        - ■ Exercise
        - ■ Acustimulation with a wristband or watch-like device
        - ■ Chinese traditional or herbal medicines
        - ■ Ginger
        - ■ Yoga
        - ■ Hypnosis
        - ■ Aromatherapy

Concept Check

4. Which substance is commonly suggested as an oral rinse for patients to prevent mucositis?
   A. Alcohol-based mouthwashes
   B. Baking powder
   C. Molasses
   D. Salt

Answer question

Gastrointestinal Toxicities Unique to Cancer and Its Treatment (continued)

GI Toxicities: Constipation

Constipation is a nagging problem that makes a patient who is already feeling bad feel even worse.

- Constipation can be disease-related:
  - o GI tumors
  - o Abdominal tumors
- Constipation can be treatment-related:
  - o Certain chemotherapy will cause constipation (e.g., vinca alkaloids)
  - o Opioids
- Constipation can be situational due to:
  - o Immobility
  - o G-tubes or other alteration in GI function
  - o Dehydration

Pathophysiology: Constipation

- Several pathophysiologic mechanisms may be responsible for constipation:
  - o Reduction in peristalsis is not uncommon when patients are immobile or take numerous types of medications (e.g., narcotics) in cancer.
  - o Decreased sensory awareness of rectal filling reduces the patient's attempts to defecate.
  - o Changes in motor control of the anal sphincter and rectal capacity can lead to constipation.

Collaborative Interventions: Constipation

The following interventions may help with treating constipation:

- N Encourage increased dietary fiber.
- N Encourage and educate the patient to increase fluid intake.
- N Advise the patient to participate in regular exercise and activity as much as capable.
- N Provide the proper environment for toileting:
  - o Sufficient privacy
  - o Unhurried and uninterrupted time periods
  - o Comfortable place: A bedpan is not always comfortable.
- N Provide and demonstrate how to perform abdominal massage to stimulate peristalsis, which may be helpful to some patients.

Massage to Stimulate Peristalsis

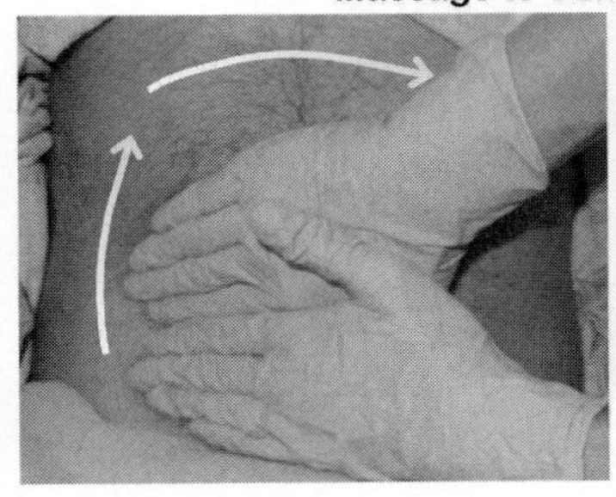

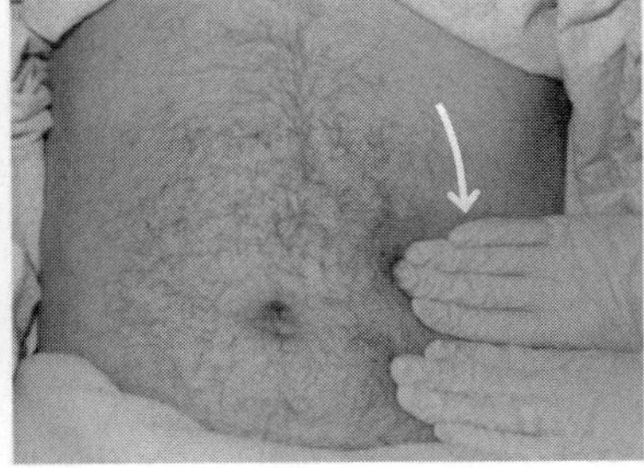

Massaging the abdomen is a technique shown in this series of photos that can help stimulate peristalsis. It is considered by many to be beneficial while others question its effectiveness.

Source: Copyright © 2014, NovEx Novice to Expert Learning, LLC

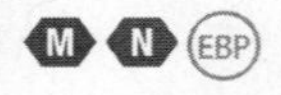

- Suggest trying osmotic laxatives if results are needed (e.g., GoLYTELY, glycolax, MiraLax, polyethylene glycol) (Woolery, et al., 2008).
- Minimize the use of laxatives whenever possible.
- If other interventions fail, educate the patient about pharmacologic management of constipation, which can be addressed progressively, from stool softeners through peristalsis-stimulating laxatives:
  - o Lubricants (e.g., mineral oil, stool softener)
  - o Bulk laxatives (e.g., psyllium, kelp, agar, Metamucil, FiberCon, Benefiber)
  - o Saline laxatives (e.g., magnesium, citrate, milk of magnesia)
  - o Stimulant laxatives (e.g., cascara, senna, castor oil, bisacodyl, Senokot, Ex-Lax, Dulcolax)
  - o Detergent laxatives (e.g., soapsuds enema)
  - o Suppositories

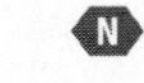

- Ensure adequate fluid intake with laxatives because some (e.g., bulking agents) can lead to intestinal obstruction by forming a viscous mass within the bowel.
- For opioid-induced constipation (Woolery, et al., 2008):
  - o Administer methylnaltrexone to relieve constipation.
  - o Rotate opioids to switch between different medications (e.g., morphine, fentanyl, sustained-release oral medications, transdermal medications, methadone).
  - o Suggest naloxone.
  - o Opioid receptor antagonists are not recommended (e.g., nalmefene, naltrexone).

Gastrointestinal Toxicities Unique to Cancer and Its Treatment (continued)

GI Toxicities: Diarrhea

To best understand and plan for patients with diarrhea, a good and thorough assessment is needed. The assessment should entail:

- Number of stools in a 24-hour period
- Characteristics of stools
- Dietary history
- Medications
- Signs of dehydration
- Stool culture
- Vital signs
- Physical examination

Diarrhea can be a side effect from multiple cancer treatments. Evaluate the treatments that the patient is on to determine what is needed in order to provide good care.

Acute Causes: Diarrhea

Key causes of diarrhea in patients with cancer are as follows:

- Graft versus host disease, an immune-mediated diarrhea that occurs after stem cell transplant
- Radiation
- Chemotherapy
- Infectious process, like C. difficile

Chronic Causes: Diarrhea

- Bowel surgery
- Pancreatic insufficiency

Symptom Management: Diarrhea

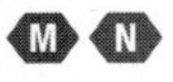

- Fluid and electrolyte replacement, either oral or intravenous, may be necessary to correct imbalances.
- Fiber content of diet may need to be increased, and can be particularly helpful with chronic diarrhea.
- The patient should be instructed to avoid foods that can exacerbate diarrhea.
- A dietician may be consulted to help educate the patient on food choices.
- Probiotics containing lactobacillus are suggested and may help many patients in preventing diarrhea (MASCC/ISOO, 2014).
- Antimotility agents can be very useful.
- Octreotide, twice daily, is recommended to treat diarrhea due to chemotherapy (MASCC/ISOO, 2014).
- Perianal and perineal skin care is extremely important to avoid skin breakdown and to improve patient comfort. Provide good skin care and educate the patient on how to care for perineal skin area.

Concept Check

5. What is the primary treatment modality for nausea and vomiting associated with cancer treatment?
   A. Medication administration
   B. NPO status
   C. Abdominal massage
   D. Visual imaging

Answer question

LO1:

What Is Neutropenia?

- Neutrophils are the centerpiece of the body's ability to protect itself from invaders. These are present in the bloodstream and normally make up 50–70% of all white blood cells.
  - A normal white blood cell count is between 5,000–10,000.
  - A normal absolute neutrophil count is between 2,500–7,000, depending on the white blood cell count.
- Neutropenia is a decreased number of circulating neutrophils.

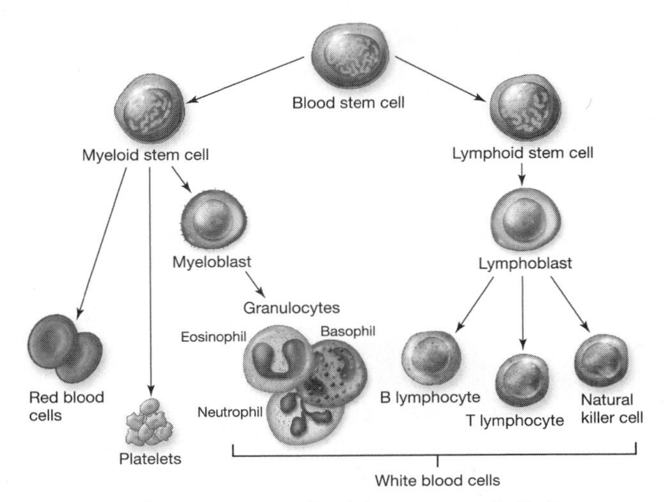

This diagram illustrates a stem cell and the vast array of cells that can derive from this single source.

LO1:

Clinical Relevance: Neutropenia

- The main reason neutropenia is important is that it will increase the risk of the patient developing a dangerous infection. Infections may progress to sepsis rapidly because of delayed immune response.
- Neutropenia is important, particularly in oncology, for several reasons such as:
  - o It can be a manifestation of blood cancers.
  - o It can be a side effect of chemotherapy and radiation to the bone marrow.
  - o It is a very common side effect of cancer treatments, especially due to aggressive chemotherapy regimens.

LO2:

Pathophysiology: Neutropenia

- Apart from the skin and mucous membrane, neutrophils are the first line of response to invading organisms.
- Invading bacteria, viruses, or fungi cause an inflammatory response, which attracts neutrophils. Neutrophils then phagocytose the invading organisms and release cytokines to attract more inflammatory cells.
- With diminished numbers of neutrophils, the body's response is markedly impaired.

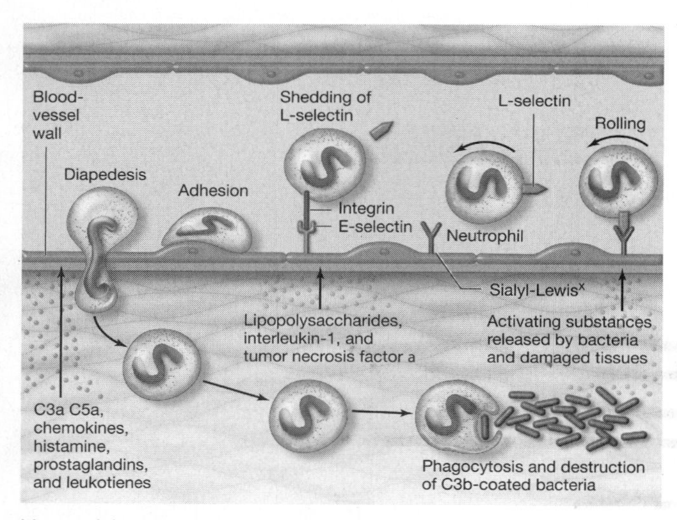

Neutrophils are one of the first components of the immune system to identify and attack any tissue that is foreign to the individual.

LO2:

Causes: Neutropenia

- Alteration of bone marrow function can make the WBCs decrease in number and function.
- Blood cancers, chemotherapy, and radiation therapy are common reasons for the development of neutropenia.
- Nononcologic causes
  - o Benign idiopathic "cyclic neutropenia"
  - o Inherited or acquired diseases
  - o Congenital neutropenia
  - o Autoimmune neutropenia
  - o Chronic disease and infection
- Certain drugs can cause reduction in white blood cells.

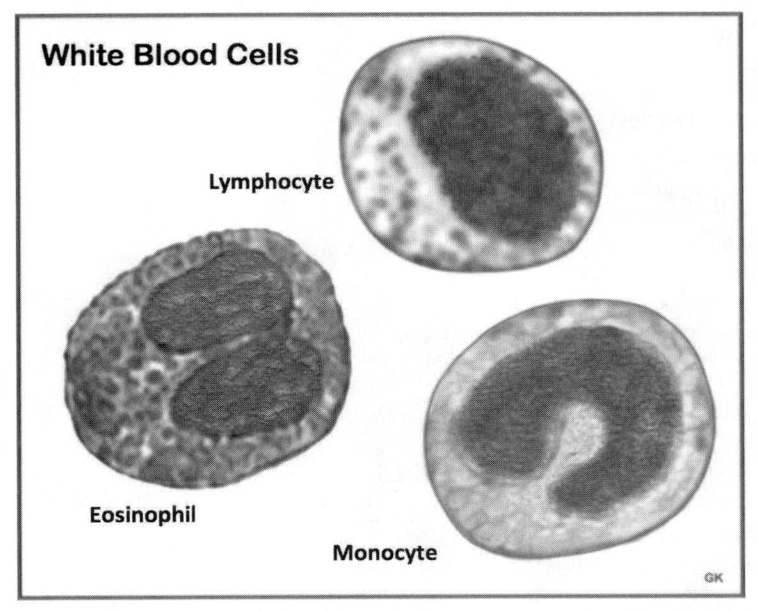

Three of the most common types of white blood cells are depicted above: monocyte, lymphocyte, and eosinophil.
Source: Courtesy of George Kyriakidis/Santa Ana, CA

LO2:

Assessment Findings: Neutropenia

- Neutropenia is often silent with no obvious symptoms.
- Patients may not show signs of a normal inflammatory response.
- Normal cues for infection may be absent. For example, patients with a urinary tract infection may not have leukocytes in their urine. Patients will also not form pus. Fever may be delayed and temperature may be low rather than high.
- Early identification of infection is essential, including assuming infection without obvious signs. Some signs to watch for include:
  - o Very low grade fever of 38°C (100.3°F) or higher
  - o A decreasing trend in blood pressure
  - o An increasing trend in heart rate
  - o An increasing trend in respiratory rate

LO2:

Diagnostics: Calculating the Absolute Neutrophil Count (ANC)

- Neutrophils may be reported as its subspecies:
  - o Segmented neutrophils (segs): the mature, most capable neutrophils
  - o Banded neutrophils (bands): slightly less mature than a seg
  - o Polymorphoneucleated cells, or PMNs (polys)
- Determining the ANC:
  - o Calculate using this formula: (% segs + % bands [or polys]) × total white blood count = ANC
  - o ANC is often calculated by an automated CBC/differential.
    For example, if the neutrophil percentage is 70% and the total WBC is 5,000, then the ANC is 3,500.
  - o Typically, the laboratory calculates both the ANC as well as the subspecies and reports it.

LO3:

Collaborative Interventions: Neutropenia

The key to managing patients with neutropenia is to protect them from potential sources of infection. Recommendations for clinical practice include (Centers for Disease Control and Prevention [CDC], 2014; Oncology Nursing Society [ONS], 2011):

M N EBP
- Washing hands prior to any contact is the single best way to prevent infection.

M N EBP
- A private room is sufficient for patients with neutropenia. Research evidence does NOT support the use of barrier or reverse isolation as a method to protect the patient.

M N EBP
- Wearing gloves, gowns, and masks while in the patient's room does not reduce the risk of infection but only serves to isolate the patient.

N
- Body hygiene and excellent wound care are important because infections in neutropenic patients often come from their own normal flora (gut, oral mucosa, skin breaks, central catheters, previous exposure to pulmonary infections that now flare when the neutrophils are low).

M N EBP
- Antibiotic prophylaxis (specifically quinolone) is recommended in neutropenic patients and has reduced the risk for infection, bacteremia, and infection-related death.

M N EBP
- Antifungal prophylaxis is recommended and has reduced the rate of infection, infection-associated deaths, and the need for treatment of fungal infections.

M N EBP
- Antiviral prophylaxis is recommended and effective in preventing herpes infections.

M N EBP
- Growth factors (also known as colony stimulating factors) help stimulate the growth of neutrophils and are recommended to reduce the risk of neutropenia, neutropenic fever, infections, treatments needed for infections, infection-related death, and hospitalizations:
  - o Filgastrim (neupogen)
  - o Pegfilgastrim (neulasta)
  - o Sargramostim (leukine)

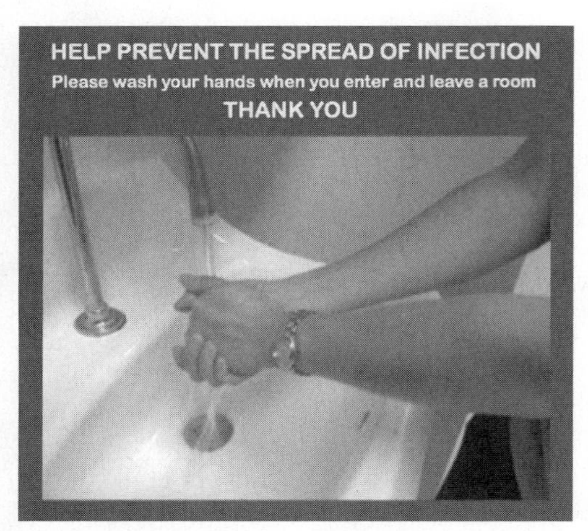

Neutropenic Fever (or Presumed Infection)

At the first sign of infection (typically fever ≥38°C [100.3°F] or abnormal trends in vital signs), the following should be done:

M N
- Perform a clinical assessment of the patient.

M N
- Obtain blood cultures 2 times.

M N
- Obtain urine cultures.

M N
- Obtain a chest x-ray if not done recently.

M N
- Start broad-spectrum antibiotics that cover the most virulent and lethal infections in the neutropenic patient:
  - o Cefepime/ceftazadime
  - o Piperacillin/tazobactim
  - o Imipenem cilastatin/meropenem
  - o Antibiotics should be based on institution sensitivities.

M N EBP
- Oral antibacterial medications can be safely administered instead of IV in most stable patients (de Naurois, et al., 2010).

M N EBP
- Consider early discharge of low-risk patients once they are stable for 24 hours and have improved symptoms (de Naurois, et al., 2010).

M N
- Addition of vancomycin for gram-positive infection prevention is not recommended unless microbiologic and/or clinical findings suggest the need.

Follow-Up Care

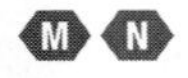

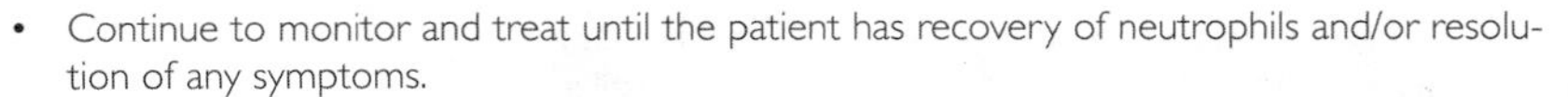

- Continue to monitor and treat until the patient has recovery of neutrophils and/or resolution of any symptoms.

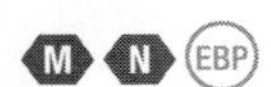

- If fever persists and/or there is hemodynamic worsening (de Naurois, 2010):
  - o Consider changing antibiotics (often blood culture's are negative because of low bacterial yield).
  - o Consider adding antifungal treatment.
  - o Consider adding treatment for other opportunistic infections.

Collaborative Interventions: Neutropenia (continued)

Preventing Infection

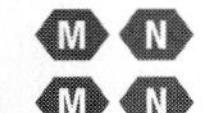

- Preventing infection is **the** essential intervention when caring for the neutropenic patient.
- Understanding the patient's susceptibility and providing safeguards may best be guided by considering the patient's relative risk, as noted in the following table:

Risk of Infection Based on Absolute Neutrophil Count (ANC)

Absolute Neutrophil Count (ANC)	Neutropenia	Risk of Infection
ANC greater than 1500	Normal	No increased risk of infection
ANC 1000-1500	Mild	Slight increase in risk of infection
ANC 500-1000	Moderate	Moderate increase in risk of infection
ANC 100- 500	Severe	High risk of infection
ANC below 100	Extreme	Extremely high risk of infection

Source: Copyright © 2014, NovEx Novice to Expert Learning, LLC

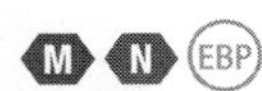

- Key evidence-based nursing actions to help protect the patient include (CDC, 2014; ONS, 2011):
  - o Wash hands prior to encounters.
  - o Have the patient and family wash hands and body to prevent infection.
  - o Have the patient avoid known sources of infection.
    - Do not eat raw eggs or meat if food is brought to the patient. Educate the patient for discharge to cook meats and eggs while neutropenic.
    - People who are ill: Friends and family with a communicable disease should avoid contact with the patient.
    - Wash all fruits and vegetables prior to eating.

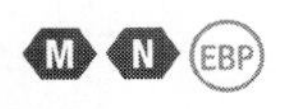

- Patients, families, and health care providers should be vaccinated against common communicable infections such as the flu (CDC, 2014).

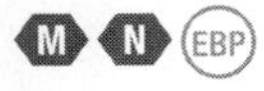

- Current research does NOT support the 20-year practice of a neutropenic diet (CDC, 2014; ONS, 2011). For instance, fresh fruits and vegetables are not considered to be a danger for neutropenic patients. The former neutropenic diet was based on theoretical suppositions (or guesses) that exposure to organisms would increase infection rates in neutropenic patients. In contrast, randomized trials have now disproved the need of the former severe restriction; yet, 78% of hospitals continue to use the neutropenic diet.
- Educate the patient and family about preventing infections (see Prevention of Infections under Patient Education).
- Plants and flowers (fresh or dried) should not be in a neutropenic patient's hospital room.

Safe Care to Prevent Infections

The CDC (2011) published evidence-based guidelines and recommendations for the safe care of patients with cancer. The recommendations are intended to help prevent infection as well as protect clinicians:

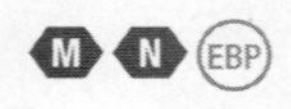

- Develop, provide, and maintain infection prevention policies and procedures, appropriate supplies (e.g., protective equipment), education and competency checks of clinicians on infection prevention, regular education and competency checks on patient and clinician safety, and reporting on disease and outbreaks.

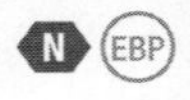

- Adhere to standard infection prevention precautions, which include:
    - Good hand hygiene, even with glove use, before touching the patient, upon exiting the room, after contact with blood or bodily fluids, before performing aseptic procedures, and after removing gloves. Soap and water must be used when hands are soiled or after caring for patients with diarrhea, particularly with *C. diff* or norovirus.
    - Appropriate availability, use, disposal, and changing of personal protective equipment, such as masks, gloves, and gowns
    - Safe injections should include aseptic technique, proper administration, safe disposal, and protection of clinicians.
    - Maintain policies and procedures that adhere to standards of good practice for routine cleaning and disinfection of the environment.
    - Proper training, cleaning, disinfection, handling, and sterilization of all reusable medical equipment between patient uses
    - Provide signs to instruct and educate personnel on good respiratory hygiene. Provide signs with instructions, tissues, disposal receptacles, antibacterial solutions for hand hygiene, masks as needed, and provide separate waiting areas.

Concept Check

6. **What is the best way to protect a patient who is neutropenic from cancer treatments?**
    A. Wash your hands.
    B. Place patient in a private room.
    C. Restrict visitors.
    D. Prophylactic antibiotic administration

Answer question

Concept Check

7. **Which substance(s) should not be present in the food of a patient with neutropenia?**
    A. Fresh peaches
    B. Raw carrots
    C. Raw egg in salad dressing
    D. Raw broccoli

Answer question

Collaborative Interventions: Neutropenia (continued)

Patient Education

Prevention of Infection

Many patients with cancer have neutropenia or are immunocompromised. Special attention is needed to prevent infection:

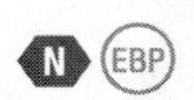

- Instruct patient and those caring for the patient about proper hand washing, oral intake, food preparation, handling pets, with toileting, and after interacting with others (CDC, 2014; ONS, 2011).

- Take precautions to prevent exposure to communicable illnesses (CDC, 2014):
  - o Avoid crowds.
  - o Avoid contact with anyone who is sick.
  - o Do not share food, drinks, or utensils with others.
  - o Never share toothbrushes.
  - o Prepare patient and family on how to handle the number of visitors and screen those who may have any communicable illness.
- Educate the patient and family about food safety precautions. Despite 70% of organizations that continue to teach about use of a neutropenic diet, research does not support the restriction (CDC, 2014):
  - o Cook all meats, seafood, fish, and eggs.
  - o Thoroughly wash fruits and vegetables but there is no restriction on what to consume.
  - o Consume only pasteurized dairy products and juices.
  - o Wash hands and utensils after handling raw foods or anything not clean.
  - o Dispose of foods that are not within the expiration date.
  - o Prevent raw meat juices from contaminating other foods, surfaces, or utensils used for cooking.
- Use mild soap (e.g., Jergens mild, Dove, baby soaps) and shower or bathe daily.
- Instruct about protecting personal and hygienic items from being shared with others.
- Avoid handling pet excrement and reptiles (CDC, 2014).
- Use gloves if gardening (CDC, 2014).
- Check for fever twice each day.
- Report any signs of infection to the health care provider:
  - o New or changing cough
  - o Sore throat
  - o Fever >100.3°F (38°C) for over 1 hour or fever anytime >101°F (38.3°C)
  - o Pus
  - o Chills with sweating
  - o Mouth sores
  - o Shortness of breath
  - o Chest pain
  - o Mental changes or decreased level of consciousness
  - o Stiff neck
  - o Pain, urgency, frequency or burning on urination
  - o Inflammation of a wound
  - o Unexpected vomiting and diarrhea
- Clinical manifestations of opportunistic infections (e.g., pneumocystis, herpes infections) should be taught.

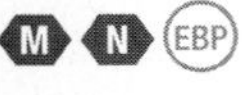

- Antifungal prophylaxis should be considered for patients receiving chemotherapy (APHTT, 2009).

- Avoid environments with poor sanitation.

- Educate the patient to discuss antimicrobial prophylaxis with their health care provider when in an immunosuppressed state (de Naurois, et al., 2010).

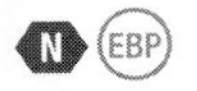

- Encourage the patient to keep immunizations current (CDC, 2014; ONS, 2011):
  - o Recommend pneumonia and flu vaccines at the time of diagnosis and annually.
  - o Avoid exposure to live vaccines.
  - o Avoid vaccinations 2 weeks prior, during, or within 6 months after chemotherapy.
  - o Consider the high dose flu vaccine for older adults because it contains the inactivated vaccine and provides better protection for those with weaker immune defenses.
- Educate on appropriate dressing technique for central venous access line.

- Instruct patients post-stem cell transplant that despite normalized WBC and neutrophil counts, the immune system recovers only beyond 6 months or more, placing them at continued high risk for infection.

Safety and Comfort

N • Educate patient about bleeding precautions in those who have thrombocytopenia (see Care of Patients with Platelet and Coagulation Disorders NovE-lesson).

N • Avoid contact with environmental toxins or chemicals whenever possible.

N • Instruct about preparation of the environment to prevent injury or falls (e.g., remove objects obstructing paths and loose throw rugs).

M N • Encourage patients to prepare and document their advanced directives.

N • Inform patient and family about local support groups to better cope with illness, treatments, and caregiver burdens.

N • Encourage patient and family to open up opportunities for and support all involved to share any fear, concern, or anxiety about their illness or potential consequences of the illness.

N • Encourage patient and family members to openly discuss the role changes that necessarily occur during major illnesses and intense treatments. Prepare them for lifestyle changes, the loneliness of protective isolation, impact on work, and alterations in independence.

N • Consult pastoral care, social worker, counselor, and dietician as indicated.

Summary of Interventions: Treatment Toxicities

- Nausea/vomiting may be treated with antiemetics.
- Treat dehydration caused by diarrhea, or decreased oral intake, with oral or intravenous fluids.
- Constipation may be treated with laxatives, stool softeners, and increased fluid intake.
- Mucositis may be treated with topical pain medications such as magic mouthwash.* Associated infections should be treated.
- Start broad-spectrum antibiotics that cover the most virulent and lethal infection in the neutropenic patient (gram negative species).

Magic mouthwash contains a combination of ingredients that may include: an antibiotic, tetracycline or erythromycin; sucralfate, a coating agent; nystatin, an antifungal; lidocaine, a local anesthetic; Maalox, a coating agent; glucocorticoids to reduce inflammation; diphenhydramine, an antihistamine. There are some commercial products on the market. The physician can specify the ingredients and amounts. A popular combination contains lidocaine, diphenhydramine, and Maalox.

LO4:

Evaluation of Desired Collaborative Care Outcomes: Treatment Toxicities

Evaluation and reassessment should reveal attainment of previously established patient outcomes. In summary:

- Patient reports that stools are soft and easy to pass and occur on previously established schedule.
- Patient weight has remained within 10% of baseline level.
- Patient's oral mucous membranes are intact and without infection.
- Patient's white blood cell and red blood cell counts are at levels considered normal for gender and age.
- Patient is an active participant in decisions regarding treatment regimen and follows regimen identified.

References

American Society of Clinical Oncology (ASCO). (2014). *Cancer.net: preventing vomiting caused by cancer treatment.*

Avila, J. G. (2004). Pharmacologic treatment of constipation in cancer patients. *Cancer Control, 11*(3, Suppl 1), 10–18.

Jubelirer, S. (2011). The benefit of the neutropenic diet: Fact or fiction? *The Oncologist, 16*(5): 704–707. **www.ncbi.nlm.nih.gov/pmc/articles/PMC3228185/**

Kornblau, S., Benson, A. B., Catalano, R, et al. (2000). Management of cancer treatment-related diarrhea: Issues and therapeutic strategies. *J Pain Symptom Manage, 19*(2), 118–129. **www.jpsmjournal.com/article/S0885-3924(99)00149-9/fulltext**

Rock, C. L., Doyle, C., Demark-Wahnefried, W., et al. (2012). Nutrition and physical activity guidelines for cancer survivors. *CA Cancer J Clin, 62*(4), 242–274. **www.guideline.gov/content.aspx?id=37279&search=nutrition+and+physical+activity+cancer**

Clinical Practice Guidelines

Adams, L. A., Shepard, N., Caruso, R. A., et al. (2012). Putting evidence into practice: evidence-based interventions to prevent and manage anorexia. *Clin J Oncol Nurs, 13*(1), 95–102. **www.guideline.gov/content.aspx?id=15691&search=adams+shepard+caruso**

Bauer, J. D., Ash, S., Davidson, W. L., et al. (2005). *Evidence based practice guidelines for the nutritional management of cancer cachexia.* **eprints.qut.edu.au/6766/1/6766.pdf**

Centers for Disease Control and Prevention. (2014). *Cancer Prevention and Control.* **www.cdc.gov/cancer/index.htm**; **www.cdc.gov/cancer/preventinfections/providers.htm**

deNaurois, J., Novitzky-Basso, I., Gill, M.J., et al. and ESMO Guidelines Working Group. (2010). Management of febrile neutropenia: ESMO Clinical Practice Guidelines. *Ann Oncol, 21* (suppl 5): v252–256. doi: 10.1093/annonc/mdq196

Harris, D. J., Eilers, J., Harriman. A., et al. (2008). Putting evidence into practice: evidence-based interventions for the management of oral mucositis. *Clin J Oncol Nurs, 12*(1), 141–152. **www.guideline.gov/content.aspx?id=15700&search=harris+eilers+harriman**

Multinational Association of Supportive Care in Cancer (MASCC) and International Society of Oral Oncology (ISOO). (2014). *MASCC/ISOO evidence-based clinical practice guidelines for mucositis secondary to cancer therapy.* **www.mascc.org/assets/Guidelines-Tools/mascc%20isoo%20mucositis%20guidelines%20summary%207nov2014.pdf**

Naeim, A., Dy, S. M., Lorenz, K. A., et al. (2008). Evidence-based recommendations for cancer nausea and vomiting. *J Clin Oncol, 26*(23), 3903–3910. **jco.ascopubs.org/content/26/23/3903.full#T1**

National Comprehensive Cancer Network (NCCN). (2009). *NCCN guidelines.* **www.nccn.org/professionals/physician_gls/f_guidelines.asp#supportive**

Oncology Nursing Society. (2011). *ONS putting evidence into practice systematic review/meta-analysis table 4-13.* **www.ons.org/practice-resources/pep/prevention-infection/prevention-infection-general**

Woolery, M., Bisanz, A., Lyons, H. F., et al. (2008). Putting evidence into practice: evidence-based interventions for the prevention and management of constipation in patients with cancer. *Clin J Oncol Nurs, 12*(2), 317–337. **www.guideline.gov/content.aspx?id=15694**

Patient Education

Centers for Disease Control and Prevention. (2014). *3 steps toward preventing infections during cancer treatment.* **www.preventcancerinfections.org/health-tip-sheets**

National Neutropenia Network. (2014). *Awareness, education, research and support.* **www.neutropenianet.org**

U.S. Department of Agriculture. (2011). *Food safety for people with cancer.* **www.fda.gov/Food/FoodborneIllnessContaminants/PeopleAtRisk/ucm312565.htm**

STOP

Go to the online course and complete the NovE-Cases assigned by your instructor for this module.

OVERVIEW OF THE CARE OF PATIENTS WITH UPPER AND LOWER GASTROINTESTINAL (GI) BLEEDING

Learning Outcomes for GI Bleeding

When you complete this lesson, you will be able to:

1. Recognize the clinical relevance of gastrointestinal bleeding.
2. Consider the pathophysiology, etiology, risk factors, and clinical presentation of gastrointestinal bleeding that determine the priority patient concerns.
3. Determine the most urgent and important nursing interventions and patient education required in caring for a patient with gastrointestinal bleeding.
4. Evaluate attainment of desired collaborative care outcomes for a patient with gastrointestinal bleeding.

LO1:

What Is GI Bleeding?

- Gastrointestinal (GI) bleeding is defined as loss of blood from the GI tract.
- It is commonly divided into upper GI (from the mouth to the first part of the duodenum) and lower GI bleeding (from the lower duodenum to the rectum).
- Depending on the cause and location, GI bleeding may be rapid and cause extensive blood loss or can be slow and gradually cause anemia.
- Conditions causing GI bleeding can include ulcerations, perforations, infections, malformations, neoplasms, and ruptured blood vessels.

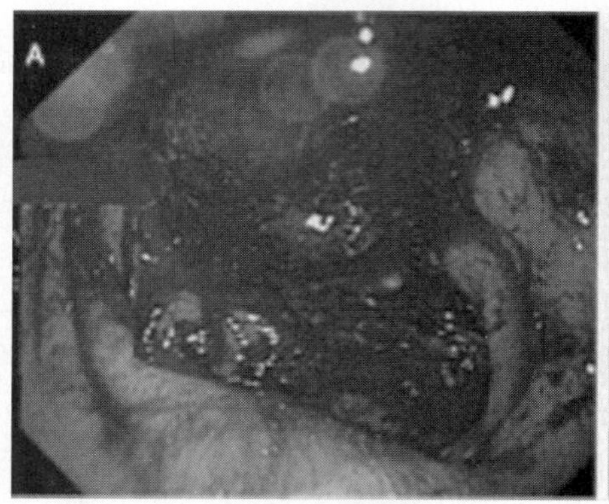

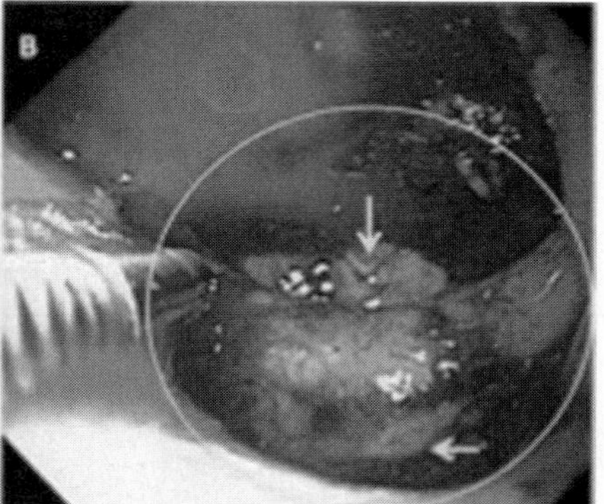

This patient was admitted to the hospital with an upper GI bleed. On urgent endoscopy, a very large and deep ulcer was diagnosed. Photo A: This photo shows a view looking down into the ulcer that was found to be profusely bleeding and required treatment. Photo B: Looking down into the ulcer, the tip of the lavage instrument (to wash the blood away) is seen and the large deep ulcer is now visible (yellow circle). Treatment with epinephrine resulted in hemostasis. The arrows point at the deepest areas of the ulcer.

Source: Courtesy of K. Kyriakidis

LO1: Clinical Relevance

- GI bleeding is a common problem in adult medicine.
- The condition spans the spectrum from chronic problems to acute, life-threatening emergencies.
- This lesson is presented as an overview for numerous conditions that first present as patients with GI bleeding. When a patient first presents, the diagnosis simply is not known in most situations. Thus, this overview precedes the many NovE-lessons that detail various GI conditions with GI bleeding because the clinician must provide good care while working to identify the cause of the bleeding. This lesson is intended as an overview of all patients with GI bleeding to assist in the clinician's general understanding about what may be occurring. It also lays the foundation for how to care for patients with GI bleeding until a definitive diagnosis is made and condition-specific interventions can be initiated.
- This overview is intended to assist in the development of good clinical thinking and reasoning, the way a real nurse must learn to think and reason, from presentation to diagnosis. At the point of diagnosis, the condition-specific NovE-lessons (e.g., Care of Patients with Peptic Ulcer Disease) are the most helpful.
- Learning an approach to problem solve an unknown illness, such as GI bleeding, the way that excellent nurses problem solve in real life can better prepare a learner to become a practice-ready nurse with good clinical thinking and reasoning skills.

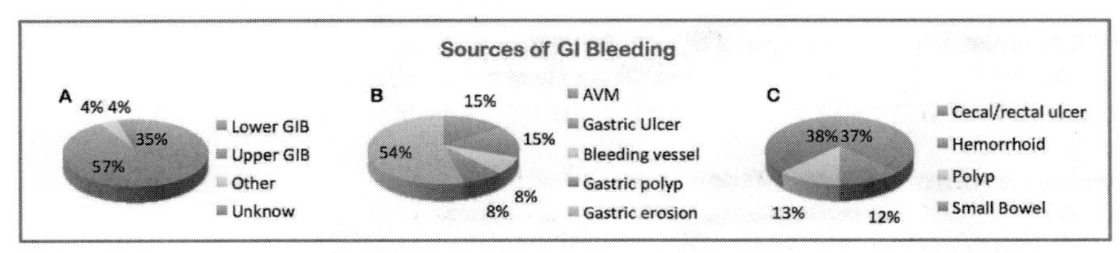

The charts show the sources of GI bleeding. (A) Overall distribution of causes. (B) Causes of upper GI bleeding (UGIB) and (C) lower GI bleeding (LGIB). AVM = arteriovenous malformation.
Source: Copyright © 2014, NovEx Novice to Expert Learning, LLC

LO2: Pathophysiology: Sequela After GI Bleeding

GI bleeding can be caused by a diverse array of conditions of the GI tract, which are discussed in detail in many of the GI NovE-lessons. The primary finding in all patients with GI bleeding is the abnormal loss of blood into the lumen.

- Acute blood loss reduces intravascular volume and results in a decreased stroke volume and cardiac output. Depending on the severity and rapidity of blood loss, the decreased cardiac output can cause a drop in arterial blood pressure.
- If blood loss is slow, the patient's hydration may replace the fluid loss, but can dilute the blood and result in anemia.
- The effects of acute blood loss activate compensatory mechanisms and the consequent hypovolemia is counterbalanced by activation of the sympathetic nervous system (SNS). The SNS causes arterial vasoconstriction and tachycardia in an attempt to increase cardiac output to maintain perfusion and normotension.
- A prototypical example of acute blood loss is gastric ulceration, in which an ulcer forms in the stomach, erosion extends into local blood vessels, and blood leaks into the lumen of the stomach.

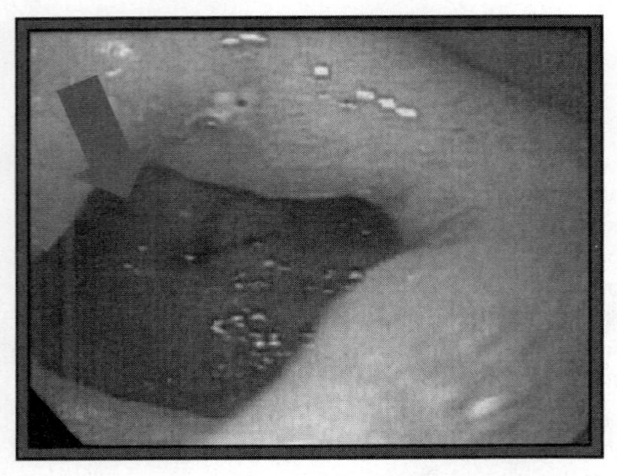

Endoscopy shows a deep acute gastric ulcer with a "punched out" ulcer appearance near the gastroesophogeal junction. Notice how the edges protrude outward. A blood clot is seen in the deep middle area of the ulcer.
Source: Courtesy of K. Kyriakidis

- Tachycardia may not be seen in patients until they experience >15% blood loss. When blood loss exceeds 15%, some patients begin to experience a drop of blood pressure and an increase in pulse of >20 beats/minute. So, tachycardia and hypotension are not early warning signs.
- However, with >30% blood loss, patients may experience hypovolemic shock with associated decreased venous return to the heart. Stroke volume and cardiac output can drop by 50%. These patients become hypotensive even when lying supine (see the Care of Patients with Hypovolemic Shock NovE-lesson).
- In contrast, patients with chronic slower bleeding usually have normal intravascular volumes but may be anemic. These patients often have an increased cardiac output and increased pulse rate to compensate for the decreased oxygen carrying capacity. These patients are usually not hypotensive.

Concept Check

1. **The majority of GI bleeding occurs from a source in which position?**
   A. Above the duodenum
   B. Below the duodenum
   C. At the duodenum
   D. Equally spread across the GI tract

Answer question

LO2:

Risk Factors

Upper GI Bleeding

- Helicobacter pylori colonization
- Nonsteroidal anti-inflammatory drugs (NSAIDs)
- Alcohol misuse and/or cirrhosis
- GE reflux disease
- Anticoagulant drugs
- Factors that increase susceptibility to ulcers (not causes) and bleeding from *H. pylori*: chronic stress and smoking

Lower GI Bleeding

- History of diverticulosis
- Age
- Anticoagulant drugs
- History of inflammatory bowel disease

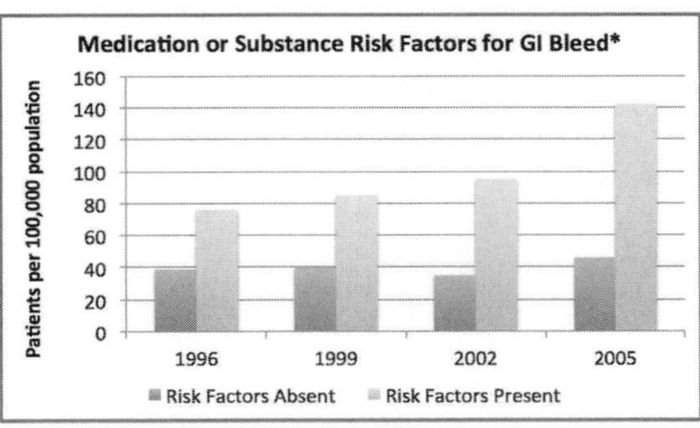

* Anticoagulants, NSAIDs, alcohol misuse

During 1996–2005, there was an increase in the overall incidence of UGIB. *This increase was almost exclusively linked to patients with one or more medication or substance risk factors for UGIB (anticoagulant drugs, such as low-dose aspirin, NSAIDs or alcohol abuse).*

LO2:

Common Causes

Upper GI Bleeding

- Gastric or duodenal ulcers
- Erosive esophagitis
- Mallory–Weiss tear, which is a tear or laceration in the gastroesophageal region
- Esophageal varices

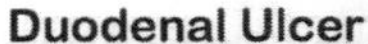

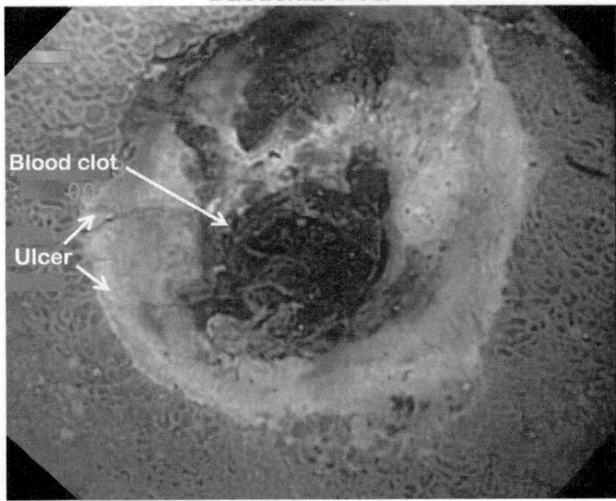

This endoscopic photo shows the most common site for peptic ulcer is the duodenal bulb, the junction where the stomach and duodenum join. It may be referred to as duodenal ulcer as it anatomically lies in the duodenum. During upper GI endoscopy, this large duodenal ulcer was found. Note the large overlying blood clot (brown) that could not be dislodged for treatment.

Source: Courtesy of K. Kyriakidis

Lower GI Bleeding

- Diverticulosis
- Colon polyps and cancer
- Angiodysplasia (a small vascular malformation)
- Ischemic colitis
- Infectious or inflammatory colitis (e.g., Crohn's disease)
- Hemorrhoids

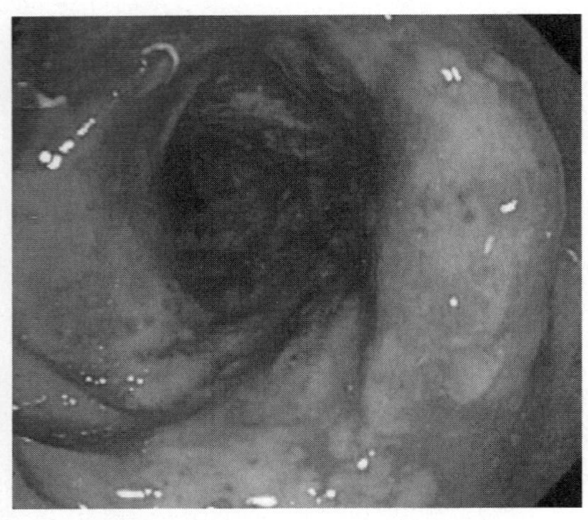

This photo is taken in the sigmoid colon. The yellowish appearance was infectious in origin, the inflamed colon is deep pinkish red, and this resulted in GI bleeding.
Source: Courtesy of K. Kyriakidis

Concept Check

2. Which findings are early signs of GI bleeding?

A. Tachycardia
B. Hypotension
C. Tachypnea
D. Early GI bleed often has no symptoms.

Answer question

LO2:

Assessment Findings

Upper GI Bleeding

- Hematemesis
- Melena: dark black, tarry appearing stool that is foul smelling. Iron in blood becomes oxidized and altered by gastric acid and intestinal bacteria, which turn it black. Exposure to gastric acid indicate upper GI bleed as the origin. It is distinguished from hematochezia, which is more typically red or maroon and indicates a lower GI bleed.
- Anemia
- Abdominal pain
- Altered stroke volume (SV): Hypovolemia from bleeding causes reduced SV or cardiac output. Low SV compromises peripheral perfusion, which is reflected in low $ScvO_2$. Compromised perfusion is also reflected by increasing lactate levels.
- Altered mental status: Mental status changes (e.g., disoriented, agitated, confused, drowsiness) can occur when there is inadequate cerebral perfusion due to hypovolemia or hypoperfusion from the bleeding. Changes in mental status signal a problem and should be taken seriously, as it is not an early sign but it signals progression of shock.
- Tachycardia
- Hypotension: This reflects hypovolemia beyond which the body can compensate, therefore, it is a late sign when compensatory mechanisms start to fail and shock is looming.
- Orthostatic symptoms: dizziness or syncope with standing

Lower GI Bleeding

- Hematochezia, which ranges in color from bright to dark red, is blood passed from rectum, typically associated with abdominal pain. This differs from the black, tarry, foul-smelling stool seen in melena. Hematochezia presents abruptly and can vary from stool that is formed and blood-streaked to stool that is bloody, liquid, and diarrhea-appearing. Hematochezia indicates a lower GI bleed because the blood has less exposure time to the GI acids and is therefore brighter red.
- Anemia
- Abdominal pain
- Decreased stroke volume
- Altered mental status
- Tachycardia
- Hypotension: a late sign
- Orthostatic symptoms: dizziness or syncope with standing

Hematemesis

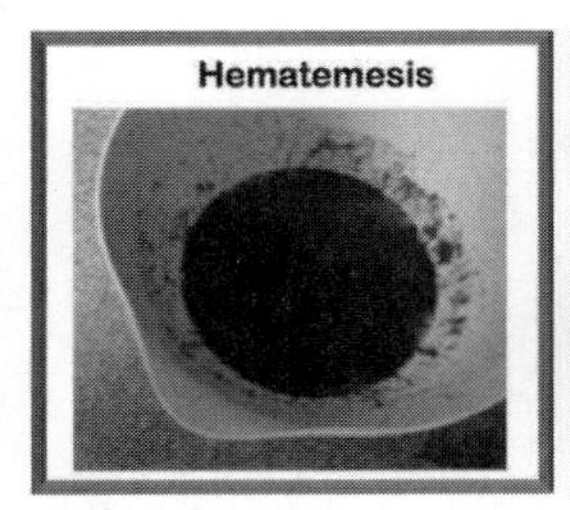

Hematochezia or Bloody Stool

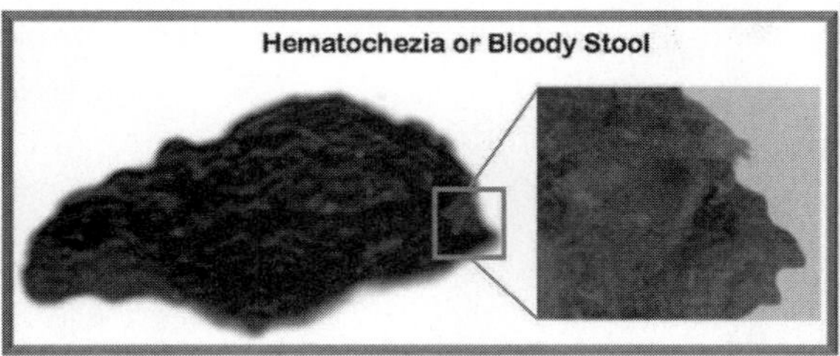

Hematemesis is emesis that contains old dark blood that has a coffee ground appearance. At first glance, the vomitus appears to be a solid color. Upon close inspection, the blood separates out and a clearer fluid is noted. Right: Hematochezia ranges from formed, blood-streaked stools to liquid, bloody stools that may be bright red, dark mahogany, or maroon in color. This sign usually develops abruptly and is heralded by abdominal pain. It is distinguished from melena, which is stool with blood that has been altered by reaction with stomach acids and bacteria and appears jet black or "tarry" (black, sticky, and foul smelling). It is also different from bright-red blood per rectum. Hematochezia is commonly associated with lower (distal) gastrointestinal bleeding, but can be seen in brisk upper gastrointestinal bleeding. Generally, the closer the bleeding site is to the anus, the blood will be a brighter red. Thus, bleeding from the anus, rectum, and the sigmoid colon tend to be bright red.

Concept Check

3. **Which factor is causative of gastrointestinal bleeding?**

   A. Smoking

   B. Stress

   C. Alcohol abuse

   D. Obesity

Answer question

LO2:

Diagnostics

Upper GI Bleeding

- Laboratory: CBC and platelet count. These may vary from normal to low, depending on the duration and rapidity of blood loss.
- Coagulation studies: PT/INR. Findings can vary depending on the source and duration of the bleeding but can indicate the presence of coagulopathy or thrombocytopenia.
- Esophagogastroduodenoscopy (EGD)
- Check vomitus and gastric aspirate for blood
- Checking stool for occult blood (also known as guaiac or hemoccult test)

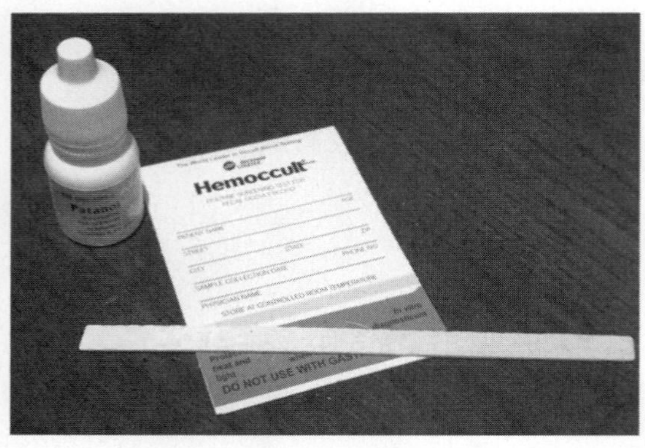

A noninvasive test to detect the presence of small or imperceptible amounts of blood in the stool is a fecal occult blood test. Detection of blood in the stool that is not noticeable is commonly the earliest, and in many patients, the sole warning sign of colorectal disease, including colon cancer.
Source: Courtesy of K. Kyriakidis

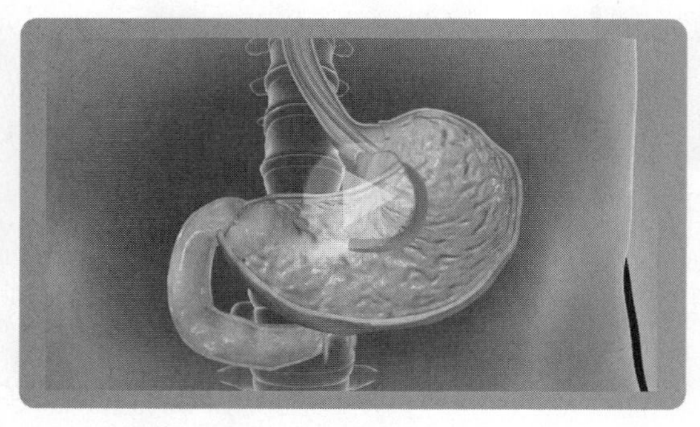

This animation shows an upper GI endoscopy procedure to diagnose the presence of helicobacter pylori causing a gastric ulcer. It also includes the treatment of a bleeding ulcer using endoscopic tools.
Source: © 2014 Nucleus Medical Media, All rights reserved

Lower GI Bleeding

- Laboratory: CBC, platelet count, and coagulation studies
- Checking stool for occult blood
- Colonoscopy
- Nuclear medicine tagged RBC scan: This is helpful only if the patient is actively bleeding. The patient's RBCs are tagged with a radioisotope. The patient is then scanned to locate the leakage from the tagged RBCs.
- Angiography

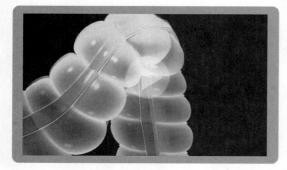

This animation shows endoscope use in the large bowel during a colonoscopy. A biopsy is sometimes performed to distinguish between benign and cancerous tissue. If polyps are found, a polypectomy is generally preformed.
Source: © 2014 Nucleus Medical Media, All rights reserved

Priority Patient Concerns and Desired Collaborative Care Outcomes

Prior to caring for patients with GI bleeding, it is important to prioritize the patient's concerns that must guide the nursing care plan and interventions. Care for the patient is ordered and organized in accordance with the patient's priority and urgent needs. Desired collaborative care outcomes in patients with GI bleeding typically include:

1. Patient will have findings that are associated with normal circulating blood volume.
2. Patient will not experience significant rebleed from GI disorder.
3. Patient will state ways to prevent bleeding episode.
4. Patient will have sufficient or show improving levels of energy to sustain activities of daily living.
5. Patient will avoid falls and demonstrate safety strategies (such as dangling at bedside before rising slowly from seated position).

Considering these important care outcomes, prepare a list of the major 3–6 priority patient concerns or nursing diagnoses for patients with GI bleeding. Be prepared to participate in a discussion of this list and/or to submit them as an assignment, as determined by your faculty. Resources you may find helpful in this assignment can include this lesson, the references, resources on nursing care plans, and standard nursing diagnoses manuals.

Concept Check

4. Which test is performed to identify occult blood in the stool?

A. Guaiac

B. INR

C. Angiography

D. Grote

Answer question

LO3:

Collaborative Interventions

When patients present with GI bleeding, particularly if significant, it can take time and testing to locate the site or cause of the bleeding. However, care of the patient is required until definitive therapy is possible. Although specific and detailed interventions are provided for different GI conditions in separate NovE-lessons, that information is helpful only **AFTER** one understands which specific condition the patient has. This lesson targets how one may generally care for a patient with GI bleeding until a cause is identified and is therefore predictably more vague or nonspecific:

Upper GI Bleeding

- Immediately evaluate the patient to identify the source and cause of the bleeding, the patient's hemodynamic stability, and the need for immediate resuscitation (Barkun, et al., 2010; Laine & Jensen, 2012). Patients who should elicit the greatest concern include those who are older than 60 years of age, show evidence of hemodynamic compromise (e.g., tachycardia, hypotension), have evidence of gross (obvious) bleeding, are on anticoagulants, and/or have significant comorbid conditions.
- Make the patient nothing per os (NPO) until problem is identified.
- Continuously monitor the patient's clinical status, cardiac rhythm, vital signs, intake and output, airway, and oxygen saturation. Provide oxygen per nasal cannula if needed.
- Initiate fluid resuscitation as indicated. Urgent and aggressive resuscitation is necessary if signs of shock are noted. Fluid management is guided by volume of blood lost, hematocrit and hemoglobin, hemodynamic stability and perfusion, and tissue oxygenation. Colloid or crystalloid solutions are effective, although colloids are far more expensive (Palmer, et al., 2008).
- Administer acid suppression drugs (proton pump inhibitors) if and as prescribed (Barkun, et al., 2010; Palmer, et al., 2008).
- Transfuse the prescribed blood products (Barkun, et al., 2010):
    - o Carefully follow the many safety precautions for transfusions according to hospital protocol (e.g., double check the patient's identity and the correct blood product, infuse with normal saline).
    - o Monitor patient closely and be attentive to any signs of allergic reaction.
    - o Document expected vital signs and exam findings.
    - o Mentally rehearse what to do in case of a transfusion reaction and locate all needed emergency equipment (e.g., stop the transfusion, switch to saline, care for patient).
    - o Instruct the patient to call immediately if they have any signs of an allergic reaction (e.g., dyspnea, dizziness, palpitations, rash or hives, chills, fever, itching).
    - o Carefully monitor patients with cardiac disease to prevent fluid overload or heart failure.

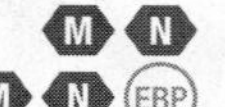

- Administer pain medications as prescribed and as indicated.
- Withhold anticoagulants, NSAIDs, and aspirin (ASA). Consider reversing anticoagulants (Barkun, et al., 2010; Palmer, et al., 2008).
- Collaborate about the need for an NG tube (Barkun, et al., 2010). If placed, ensure correct tube placement and secure the NG position. Maintain it on low, intermittent suction. May check for presence of blood with hemoccult or guaiac test. Document NG output.
- Contact GI specialist for consultation as requested for the diagnosis and treatment of GI bleeding source.
- Administer prescribed octreotide or somatostatin for patients with bleeding varices (Barkun, et al., 2010; Palmer, et al., 2008).
- Avoid gastric lavage via NG tube, a traditionally common intervention, with or without iced saline. Evidence reveals it does not improve clinical outcomes and is not recommended (Barkun, et al., 2010; Laine & Jensen, 2012).
- Prepare patient for possible endoscopic interventions, including cauterization and stapling (use of clip or staple to occlude a bleeding blood vessel), if needed to stop the bleeding (Barkun, et al., 2010). Administer an antibiotic and/or a proton-pump inhibitor (PPI) prior to procedure as prescribed (Laine & Jensen, 2012).
- If endoscopic intervention fails, prepare patient for percutaneous embolization if determined as the next step to stop the bleeding (Barkun, et al., 2010; Palmer, et al., 2008).
- If endoscopic and/or embolization intervention fails, prepare patient for surgical intervention (rare, such as a perforated ulcer) (Barkun, et al., 2010; Palmer, et al., 2008).
- Consider transferring patients who are actively bleeding to the ICU.

Collaborative Interventions (continued)

Lower GI Bleeding

- Immediately evaluate the patient to identify the source and cause of the bleeding, the patient's hemodynamic stability, and the need for immediate resuscitation (Barkun, et al., 2010; Laine & Jensen, 2012).
- Make the patient NPO until problem is identified.
- Continuously monitor the patient's clinical status, cardiac rhythm, vital signs, intake and output, airway, and oxygen saturation. Provide oxygen per nasal cannula if needed.
- Initiate fluid resuscitation as indicated. Urgent and aggressive resuscitation is necessary if signs of shock are noted. Fluid management is guided by volume of blood lost, hematocrit and hemoglobin, hemodynamic stability and perfusion, and tissue oxygenation. Colloid or crystalloid solutions are effective, although colloids are far more expensive (Palmer, et al., 2008).
- Collaborate with team about transfusion in patients in need (Palmer, et al., 2008).

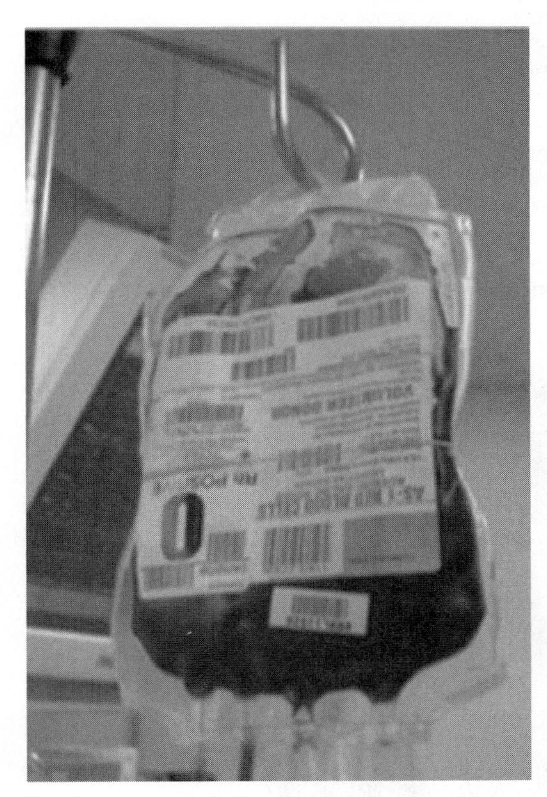

Transfusion with whole blood is relatively uncommon in recent times. The preference is to transfuse the specific components needed. One must always focus on the primary goal: to identify the cause if unknown and stop the bleeding.

- Withhold anticoagulants, NSAIDs, and aspirin (ASA). Consider reversing anticoagulants (Barkun, et al., 2010; Palmer, et al., 2008).
- Administer pain medications as prescribed and as indicated.
- Prepare and educate patient for colonoscopic interventions if needed (insertion of a scope to identify and treat cause of bleeding) (Palmer, et al., 2008).
- Prepare and educate patient for angiography, if needed, to locate the bleeding and for embolization to nonsurgically stop the bleeding with minimally invasive microcatheterization (Barkun, et al., 2010; Palmer, et al., 2008).
- If nonsurgical procedures fail, prepare the patient for surgical intervention to stop the bleeding (Barkun, et al., 2010; Palmer, et al., 2008).
- Consider transferring patients who are actively bleeding to the ICU.

Symptom Management and Comfort Care

The care of patients with specific GI conditions is addressed in separate NovE-lessons. However, general care of most patients who have a GI bleed can include:

N
- Provide emotional support to the patient as most people are frightened by seeing themselves bleeding. Collaborate with patient to identify their best source(s) of support, which may include involvement from pastoral services, family or friends. Support should be guided by the patient's preferences.

M N EBP
- Resume feedings within 24 hours post-endoscopy in patients at low risk for rebleed (Barkun, et al., 2010).

M N EBP
- Suspect and test for *H. pylori* and treat if confirmed (Barkun, et al., 2010; Laine & Jensen, 2012). If positive for *H. pylori*, see the Care of Patients with Gastric Ulcer Disorders NovE-lesson for detailed treatment and care.

N
- Depending on the extent of the bleeding and procedure done, frequently or continuously monitor the patient's vital signs and physical exam for cues of rebleeding or deterioration (e.g., emesis and stool for traces of blood, hemodynamic changes, labs, altered mental status). Pain from esophageal spasm, esophageal reflux, and heartburn are possible. Although rare, be alert for signs of perforation with abdominal distension as it can be life threatening (see the Care of Patients with Abdominal Pain NovE-lesson).

N EBP
- Call the Rapid Response Team: If GI bleeding recurs or worsens or if the patient's condition deteriorates, be prepared to intervene. The Rapid Response Team should be called whenever the severity or the demands of the patient's condition require assistance (Palmer, et al., 2008). (See the Care of Patients in Hypovolemic Shock NovE-lesson for details.)

N EBP
- Provide ongoing and critical hemodynamic and airway monitoring and support: Sudden and large bleed in the stomach can lead to significant blood loss and hypovolemia. Repeated rapid fluid administration and advanced airway support may be needed (Palmer, et al., 2008).

Active GI Bleeding in Stomach

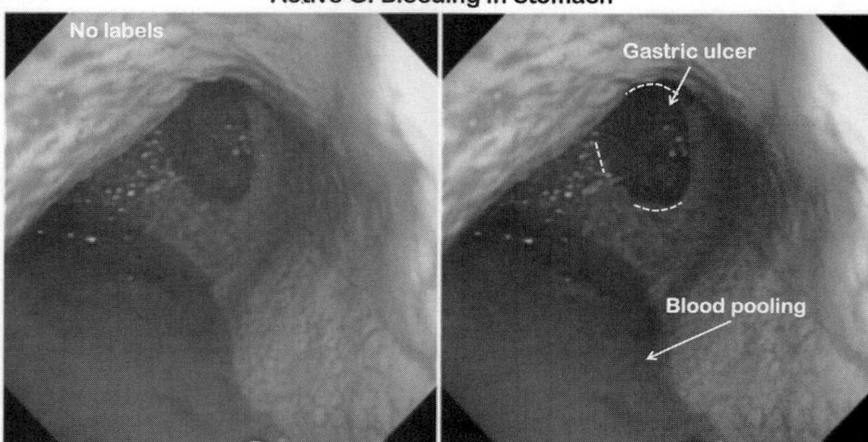

Courtesy of K. Kyriakidis

M N EBP
- Initially, chronic bleeding may not be life threatening but may require fluids and/or blood transfusion (Palmer, et al., 2008).

M N EBP
- Collaborate with the health care provider to avoid administering NSAIDs and aspirin if the patient is on NSAIDs or aspirin and the bleeding was related to the medication. Confer with the health care provider if the patient has known acute coronary syndrome, which warrants continued use of aspirin (Laine & Jensen, 2012).

N
- Educate the patient about safety precaution as needed if blood loss is significant enough to impact tissue perfusion. Significant anemia and/or hypovolemia may result in orthostatic hypotension, dizziness, or being unsteady while standing or walking. All of these consequences place the patient at risk for falls.

M N EBP
- Prepare patients who are at high risk (e.g., active bleeding) that observation and care is preferably 3 days if bleeding does not recur (Laine & Jensen, 2012).

Concept Check

5. Which medication is withheld when gastrointestinal bleeding occurs?
   A. Vitamin K
   B. Acetaminophen
   C. Opioids
   D. Aspirin

Answer question

Collaborative Interventions (continued)

Evidence-Based Interventions: When to Transfuse

The new restrictive transfusion guidelines are strongly recommended when making clinical judgments about who and when to transfuse. The evidence revealed significantly improved mortality when the guidelines are followed (Villanueva, et al., 2013).

Stable Patients

Patients are considered stable when they show no signs of abnormal hemodynamic or physiological function, except for a mild tachycardia (heart rate <120 beats/min):

M N EBP
- Communicate and collaborate to consider transfusion with packed red blood cells (PRBC) when hemoglobin is <7 mg/dL or when the hemoglobin is <8 mg/dL in a patient with symptoms (Laine & Jensen, 2012; Liumbruno, et al., 2011; Rezale, 2014).

M N
- Anticipate that each unit of transfused PRBC usually raises the hemoglobin level by 1 mg/dL or the hematocrit by 3 mg/dL.

M N EBP **Unstable Patients**

Patients are considered unstable if they have symptoms of hypoxia. Hypoxic symptoms are thought of as physiological transfusion triggers and may include altered stroke volume (early sign) reflected in decreased perfusion or measured using hand-held ultrasound device, mental status changes reflecting altered cerebral perfusion, tachycardia >120 beats/min, ischemic changes on EKG, lactic acidosis or elevated lactate, or hypotension (later sign) (Barkun, et al., 2010; Liumbruno, et al., 2011).

N
- Insert two large bore IVs: Large bore IVs are required in unstable patients when bleeding is severe in order to effectively and rapidly replace blood if needed.

M N EBP
- Initiate IV fluid boluses if the patient's symptoms warrant treatment (Villanueva, et al., 2013). Those not responding to IV boluses need transfusion of PRBC.

N EBP
- May temporarily place these patients in a supine position with legs elevated 20 degrees until fluids have been infused. Avoid a Trendelenburg position because evidence shows no benefit, but it has caused harmful effects in particular patient groups (Makic, et al., 2011). (A safety precaution when elevating the legs: continuously evaluate the patient's breathing for potential respiratory and cardiovascular compromise.)

N
- Use extreme care in patients who have symptoms of shock, require temporary leg elevation position, but are also vomiting. These patients are at high risk for aspiration. A high priority is to protect the airway. If supine or legs elevated positions are required due to severe hypotension, make certain to keep the patient's head turned to the side to prevent aspiration. Make certain to have suction equipment ready for immediate use. Consider intubation to protect the airway if hematemesis persists.

M N EBP
- Prepare for transfusions, which are indicated in patients with uncontrolled, persistent bleeding or hemorrhaging (Palmer, et al., 2008).

M N EBP
- Rapidly recognize and intervene if the patient has >30% blood loss (>1500 mL) because hypovolemic shock may develop (see the Care of Patients with Hypovolemic Shock NovE-lesson). These patients require urgent transfusion, and they may emergently need uncrossmatched blood if perfusion is severely compromised (Palmer, et al., 2008).

M N
- When massive transfusion is needed from uncontrolled hemorrhage, uncrossmatched group O Rh (D) negative red cells is ordered. Due to potential coagulation abnormalities (e.g., thrombocytopenia, dilutional coagulopathies) and complications (e.g., disseminated intravascular coagulation [DIC]), clinicians should vigilantly monitor vital signs, blood gases, electrolytes, physical exam, and type and cross match as soon as possible.

M N
- In patients with acute bleeding, anticipate and gauge clinical thinking to keep in mind that hemoglobin and hematocrit (H&H) are not always reliable in evaluating the need for transfusion. H&H can temporarily appear to be normal, even after massive blood loss. It may take some time for H&H to drop after blood loss (e.g., until after the plasma volume is restored).

- As importantly, anticipate and adjust thinking to account for the dilutional effect that administration of large volumes of IV fluids can have on the H&H.
- Use blood warming device whenever possible on blood, packed cells, and fresh frozen plasma. Platelets may be room temperature upon arrival.
- Carefully document intake and output balances to "stay ahead" of the patient's blood volume needs.
- Be alert for early warning of likely complications such as:
  - o Fever, chills, and/or urticarial, which signal a hemolytic transfusion reaction, anaphylaxis, or bacterial contamination
  - o Hypothermia from infusion of many cold units of blood. Consider warming blood prior to infusion when possible.
  - o Electrolyte imbalances, particularly hypocalcemia, hyperkalemia, and hypokalemia
  - o DIC due to abnormal coagulation reactions (e.g., microvasular bleeding), which should trigger concern and collaboration with the health care provider
  - o Acid-base imbalances
- Provide ongoing emotional support and include the family as support if they are coping well. Pastoral services may be helpful, depending on the patient's preferences.
- Provide ongoing information to the patient about what is happening and inform the patient about what is being done to help. Determine whether or not more or less information helps the patient cope better. Inform the patient that lots of communication among the team is important so the environment may be noisy at times.

Collaborative Interventions (continued)

Clinical Judgment When Determining Who Is Stable or Unstable

- Despite typical definitions of stable and unstable, the clinician who is caring for the patient serves as the eyes and ears for the team to help determine which patients are stable without transfusion and which are unstable. The following clinical parameters should be taken into account when the team is evaluating and identifying who to transfuse with a hemoglobin >7 mg/dL (Liumbruno, et al., 2011):
  - o Patient's age: Older adult patients may not tolerate the same hemoglobin as well as a younger patient.
  - o Rapidity of blood loss: Patients who lose blood quickly may not adapt to the loss as well as patients who lose blood slowly and can compensate.
  - o Volume of blood loss: The body can only compensate for about 30% blood loss before compensatory mechanisms begin to fail and transfusion is needed.
  - o Symptomatic anemia: Despite other factors and the hemoglobin level, a patient's inability to tolerate their anemia from blood loss should guide clinical judgment about the patient's need for transfusion. Symptoms include the physiological transfusion triggers, as these indicate hypoxia with failing compensatory mechanisms. Additional symptoms that signal hypoxia and the need to transfuse include:
    - ■ Dyspnea
    - ■ New ST elevation or depression on 12-lead EKG
    - ■ New onset of dysrhythmia
    - ■ New cardiac ischemic changes
    - ■ Orthostatic hypotension
    - ■ $ScvO_2$ <60%
    - ■ SvO_2 <50%
    - ■ Lactate >2 mmol/L with acidosis.
  - o Comorbid conditions: The presence of significant comorbid conditions, such as cardiac or lung conditions prevents a patient from tolerating a lower hemoglobin, so transfusion may need to occur earlier. Earlier transfusion should be considered, particularly in patients with ischemic heart disease, heart failure, and cerebrovascular disease.
  - o Medications that may alter the patient's ability to compensate for blood loss (e.g., some cardiac meds that interfere with compensatory mechanisms, chemotherapy, anticoagulants).
- Abnormal findings of these parameters should compel the nurse to collaborate with the health care provider for more immediate consideration of the need for transfusion.
- Transfusions have a host of issues, ranging from increased infections to blood reactions, so caution should be used. Always weigh the potential benefits against the potential risks and then make a judgment about what is best for the patient at the time (Barkun, et al., 2010).
- Collaborate with the health care provider routinely to discuss how the patient is tolerating the level of anemia, particularly lower levels, to determine who and when to transfuse.

Blood loss	Pathophysiological Response	Advocate Need to Transfuse
<15%	No notable symptoms	No need unless physiological transfusion triggers* are present
15-30%	Tachycardia	No need unless physiological transfusion triggers* or significant comorbid conditions are present
30-40%	Hypoxia: dyspnea, ↓ cardiac output, ↓ mental status, ischemia, ↑ lactate, ↓ BP, ST changes, dysrhythmias, ↓ $ScvO_2$, ↓ SvO_2, possible shock	Collaborate with team about probable need for transfusion
>40%	Shock, possibly severe	Urgent transfusion needed and can be life-saving

* Physiological transfusion triggers signaling hypoxia: tachycardia, decreased stroke volume altered mental status, ischemic ST changes on EKG, dyspnea, new onset of dysrhythmia, $ScvO_2$ less than 60%, SvO_2 less than 50%, lactate over 2 mmol/L with acidosis or elevated lactate, and/or hypotension

Despite the best guidelines, nurses must make good clinical judgments about the responses of individual patients who may not fit a guideline. This table can help guide good clinical evaluation and judgment.

Collaborative Interventions (continued)

Safety and Prevention to Reduce Blood Transfusions

Patients with GI bleeding often require frequent monitoring of labs and commonly have comorbid conditions. Care of these patients can sometimes inadvertently exacerbate blood loss. Precautions are needed to prevent anemia, reduce unnecessary blood loss, and minimize the need for blood transfusions, which expose the patient to higher risk:

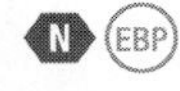
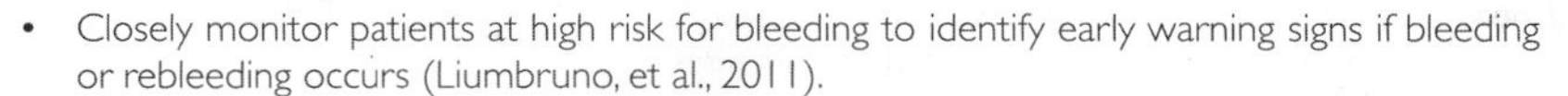

- Closely monitor patients at high risk for bleeding to identify early warning signs if bleeding or rebleeding occurs (Liumbruno, et al., 2011).

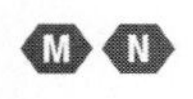

- Monitor labs that require frequent checks by using bedside or point of care devices, which require a fraction of the amount of blood to produce hematologic or blood chemistry information.

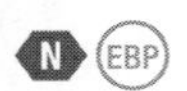

- Minimize or prevent unnecessary blood loss to prevent anemia and reduce the need for blood transfusions (Liumbruno, et al., 2011) due to procedures. Examples include:
  - o Collaborate with the lab techs to minimize phlebotomy-related blood loss for tests. Aim for reduction in specimen volumes or minimum volumes for specimens.
  - o Collaborate with the medical team to order all needed labs in clusters to minimize blood loss.

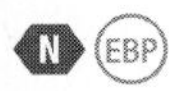

- Limit iatrogenic blood loss when withdrawing and/or discarding blood with IVs, arterial lines, or other samples (Liumbruno, et al., 2011).

- Collaborate with the team to consider prophylaxis for GI bleeding (e.g., antacids, H_2 receptor antagonists, or PPI) in high-risk patients, such as those on mechanical ventilation (Liumbruno, et al., 2011).

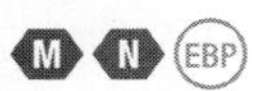

- Use intra-op or postoperative blood salvage (collecting the patient's own blood for reinfusion to avoid use of allogeneic sources) when possible (Liumbruno, et al., 2011). Follow institutional policy on the type of blood collection device used and procedures before and for autotransfusion (transfusion with one's own blood).

Liberal Versus Restrictive Blood Transfusion in Acute GI Bleeding

Study: Upper Gastrointestinal bleeding [1]	Liberal Transfusion	Restrictive Transfusion
Hemoglobin level triggering transfusion	Hemoglobin of trigger of 9 g/dl target of 9-11 g/dl	Hemoglobin trigger 7g/dl with target of 7-9 g/dl
Mortality	Higher: 9%	Lower: 5%
Further Bleeding	Higher: 16%	Lower: 10%
Length of Stay		Decreased
Complications	Greater (e.g. pulmonary edema): 48%	Fewer: 40%
Conclusion: The restrictive strategy (transfused given at a lower hemoglobin level), when compared to liberal or more traditional hemoglobin triggers, improved patient outcomes in patients with acute GI bleeding.		

[1] Villanueva, et al. (2013). Transfusion strategies for acute upper GI bleeding. *NEJM, 368*(1), 11-21.

Summary of landmark study comparing liberal versus restrictive transfusion strategies in patients with upper GI (UGI) bleeding.

Collaborative Interventions (continued)

Anticoagulation

- **Discontinue anticoagulants:**
  - o Stop or withhold all anticoagulant medication that can exacerbate the bleeding (e.g., NSAIDs, aspirin, heparin, Coumadin) (Palmer, et al., 2008).
  - o Interruption in anticoagulation places the patient at risk for thrombotic complications that this med was preventing. Collaborate with the health care provider if patient has a comorbid condition in which the anticoagulant is strongly needed (e.g., coronary artery disease). Resuming anticoagulation within a week post-bleed is recommended (Barkun, et al., 2010).
- Consider reversing the effects of heparin in situations of massive bleeding. Even though heparin's anticoagulant effect lasts only 3 hours, reversal may be warranted. Protamine is administered to reverse heparin but should be given very slowly and cautiously due to the potential anaphylactic reaction by some patients. Mortality from protamine-related anaphylaxis is about 30%.
- **Consider reversing the effects of warfarin if the patient is hemorrhaging or bleeding severely or recurrently:**
  - o Administer vitamin K, which is the first line therapy to accomplish reversal. It may take 12–24 hours to start lowering INR.
  - o Simultaneously infuse fresh frozen plasma (FFP) or prothrombin complex concentrates (PCC), which can have immediate effects. Infuse with care and constant monitoring as FFP is known to cause fluid overload and can cause acute lung injury (ALI). PCC achieves a more rapid and complete INR recovery than FFP and with far less volume. PCC, therefore, minimizes the risk of fluid overload and ALI.

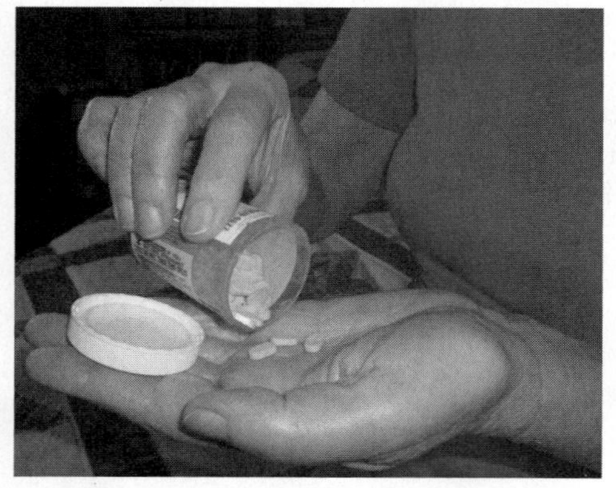

A recent study reveals that patients on warfarin (anticoagulation) who experienced a GI bleed had significantly lower risk of thrombotic complications and mortality if they either continued or resumed taking warfarin within 1 week post-bleed. Recurrent GI bleed was not increased. Researchers suggest that benefits of restarting warfarin within 1 week outweigh potential risks.
Source: Courtesy of George Kyriakidis/Santa Ana, CA

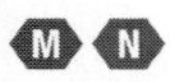

- Because aspirin irreversibly blocks platelet function for the life of the platelet, reversal is not possible. Transfuse normal platelets to achieve normal coagulation.

Collaborative Interventions (continued)

Patient Education

Educating patients with a GI bleed is important because, for most, it is a scary situation. Detailed education depends on the specific condition or cause; however, early education can include general explanations about:

- Upper or lower GI bleeding

- Diagnostics to identify and interventions to manage the bleeding

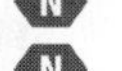

- Specific procedures (and what the patient may experience) that are ordered to identify and treat the bleeding or that may protect the patient (e.g., NPO, NG tube)

- More specific information that will be provided when a definitive diagnosis is confirmed

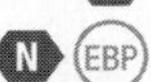

- Ways to prevent bleeding, especially when known risk factors exist such as peptic ulcer or colitis (NICE, 2012). Nursing management of GI bleeding is focused on prevention.

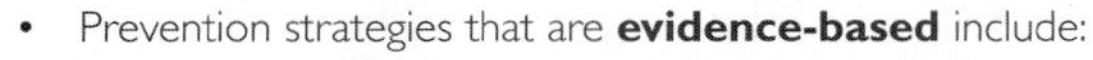

- Prevention strategies that are **evidence-based** include:

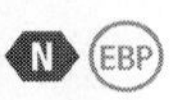

  - o Teaching about the importance of adhering to prescribed medical regimens, such as acid reducers or proton pump inhibitors (NICE, 2012)

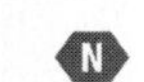

  - o Instruction on proper diet and nutrition choices has recently changed:
    - ■ More than 3 cups of coffee daily may increase susceptibility to *H. pylori* infection.
    - ■ Moderating intake of acidic and spicy foods did not prove harmful in studies.
    - ■ Limit or, preferably, avoid alcohol.

  - o Fruits, vegetables, and olive oil are particularly protective against both ulcer formation and/or *H. pylori* infection leading to ulcer.

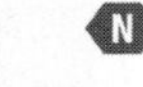

  - o Avoid large meals; however, a bland diet and small frequent meals make no difference in ulcer formation or bleeding

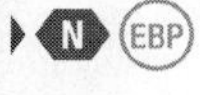

  - o Educate regarding over-the-counter therapies to avoid, such as NSAIDs (e.g., ibuprofen, ketoprofen, naproxen) and aspirin-containing drugs (NICE, 2012).

  - o Preferentially use alternative pain reliever, such as acetaminophen.
  - o Use antacids if helpful.

  - o Teach about the compounding effects of tobacco. Offer support in resources for smoking cessation.

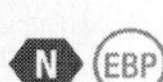

  - o Teach about how to identify early warning signs and symptoms of anemia such as fatigue, palpitations, and shortness of breath (NICE, 2012).

Concept Check

6. Which dietary instruction should be provided to patients with GI bleed?

A. Avoid spicy foods.

B. Drink milk between meals.

C. Eat several small meals throughout the day.

D. Drink no more than three cups of coffee each day.

Answer question

Nursing and Medical Interventions: Priorities

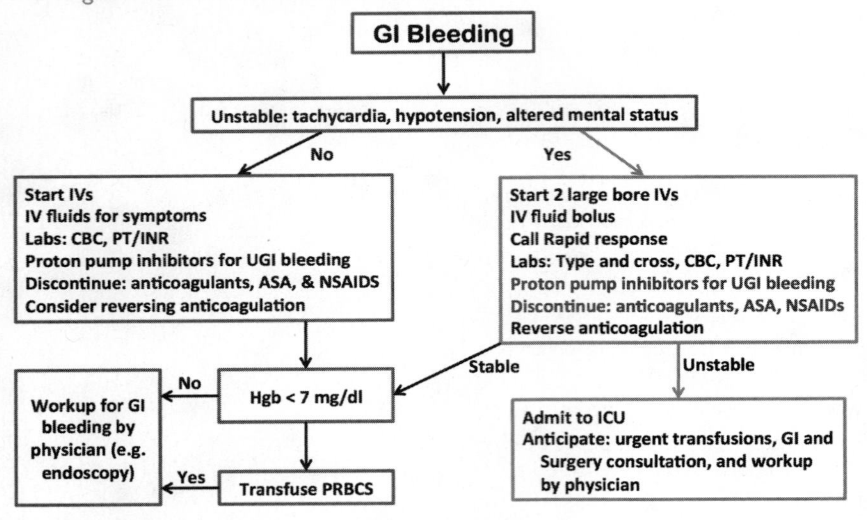

Source: Copyright © 2014, NovEx Novice to Expert Learning, LLC

Summary of Interventions

- Assess patient's hemodynamic stability as a priority.
- Identify the source or cause of the bleeding.
- Give the patient nothing by mouth until evaluation completed.
- Continuously monitor the patient's clinical status.
- Rapid volume and/or blood product resuscitation is indicated for the unstable patient.
- Administer acid suppression therapy for upper GI bleeding sources and for GI bleeding where source is not immediately known.
- Patients at risk for further bleeding or unstable patients should have two large bore IVs in place, be typed and crossmatched for blood transfusion, have aggressive volume repletion, be considered for transfusion with PRBC.
- Administer pain medication to provide relief.
- Discontinue anticoagulation temporarily.
- Contact GI physician for consultation as requested for the diagnosis and treatment of GI bleeding source.
- Prepare the patient for endoscopy, arterial embolization, and/or surgery as needed.

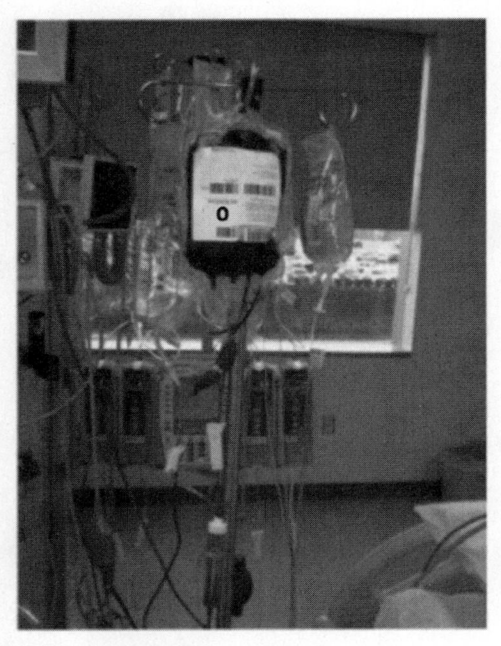

Rapid fluid and blood product resuscitation can be life-saving in patients who are hemorrhaging.
Source: Copyright © 2014, NovEx Novice to Expert Learning, LLC

Concept Check

7. Vitamin K lowers INR within ________ of administration.

A. 5 minutes

B. 20–30 minutes

C. 10 hours

D. 12–24 hours

Answer question

LO4:

Evaluation of Desired Collaborative Care Outcomes

Evaluation and reassessment should reveal attainment of previously established patient outcomes. In summary:

- Patient's skin is warm and dry with their normal elastic turgor, blood pressure is within desired range, urine output is >30 mL per hour, and mentation is normal for the patient.
- Patient shows no discernible bleeding.
- Patient can discuss lifestyle changes (e.g., limited alcohol intake) that are being adopted to prevent bleeding episodes.
- Patient reports having sufficient or improving levels of energy to sustain desired daily activities.
- Patient demonstrates precautions and safety strategies necessary to avoid falls.

References

Bjorkman, D. J. (2013). Cirrhosis increases mortality risk in peptic ulcer bleeding. *Gastroenterology*. **www.jwatch.org/na32645/2013/11/01/cirrhosis-increases-mortality-risk-peptic-ulcer-bleeding**

Dworzynski, K., Pollit, V., Kelsey, A., et al., and the Guideline Development Group. (2012). Management of acute upper gastrointestinal bleeding: Summary of NICE guidance. *Brit Med J, 344*, e3412. **www.bmj.com/content/344/bmj.e3412?view=long&pmid=22695897**

Hwang, J. H., Fisher D. A., Ben-Menachem, T., et al. (2012). The role of endoscopy in the management of acute non-variceal upper GI bleeding. *Gastrointest Endosc, 75*(6), 1132–1138. **www.guideline.gov/content.aspx?id=37851&search=peptic+ulcer**

Krumberger, J. M. (2005). How to manage an acute upper GI bleed. *Modern Medicine*. **www.modernmedicine.com/modern-medicine/news/how-manage-acute-upper-gi-bleed.**

Clinical Practice Guidelines

Barkun, A., Bardou, M., Kuipers, E., et al. (2010). International consensus recommendations on the management of patients with nonvariceal upper gastrointestinal bleeding. *Ann Intern Med, 152*(2), 101–113. **annals.org/article.aspx?articleid=745521**

Laine, L., & Jensen, D. M. (2012). Management of patients with ulcer bleeding. *Am J Gastroenterol, 107*, 345–360. doi: 10.1038/ajg.2011.480

Liumbruno, G. M., Bennardello, F., Lattanzio, A., et al. (2011). Recommendations for the transfusion management of patients in the peri-operative period. III. The post-operative period. *Blood Transfus, 9*(3), 320–335. **www.ncbi.nlm.nih.gov/pmc/articles/PMC3021395/**

Makic, M. B., VonRueden, K. T., Rauen, C., et al. (2011). Evidence-based practice habits: Putting more sacred cows out to pasture. *Crit Care Nurs, 31*(2), 38–62. **www.aacn.org/wd/cetests/media/c1123.pdf**

NICE. (2012). *Acute upper gastrointestinal bleeding: Management. NICE Clinical Guideline 141*. **www.nice.org.uk/nicemedia/live/13762/59549/59549.pdf**

Palmer, K., Balfour, R., et al., and the Guideline Development Group. (2008). Management of acute upper and lower gastrointestinal bleeding: A national clinical guideline. *Scottish Intercollegiate Guidelines Network*, 105. Edinburgh, UK: Scottish Intercollegiate Guidelines Network. **www.sign.ac.uk/pdf/sign105.pdf**

Rezale, S., (2014). Upper gastrointestinal bleeding: evidence-based treatment. *ALiEM*, March 12. **academiclifeinem.com/upper-gastrointestinal-bleeding-treatment/**

Villanueva, C., Colomo, A., Bosch, A., et al. (2013). Transfusion strategies for acute upper gastrointestinal bleeding. *NEJM, 368*(1), 11–21. **www.ncbi.nlm.nih.gov/pubmed/23281973.**

Patient Education

Dugdale, D. C., & MedlinePlus of the U.S. National Library of Medicine. (2011). *Gastrointestinal bleeding*. **www/nlm.nih.gov/medlineplus/ency/article/003133.htm**

National Heart, Lung, and Blood Institute. (2012). *Blood transfusion*. **www.nhlbi.nih.gov/health/health-topics/topics/bt/**

www.uptodate.com/contents/peptic-ulcer-disease-genetic-environmental-and-psychological-risk-factors-and-pathogenesis?source=preview&anchor=Patient_Information&Selectedtitle=13~150#Patient_Information

Learning Outcomes for Abdominal Pain

When you complete this lesson, you will be able to:

1. Recognize the clinical relevance of abdominal pain.
2. Consider the pathophysiology, etiology, risk factors, and clinical presentation of abdominal pain that determine the priority patient concerns.
3. Determine the most urgent and important nursing interventions and patient education required in caring for a patient with abdominal pain.
4. Evaluate attainment of desired collaborative care outcomes for a patient with abdominal pain.

LO1:

What Is Abdominal Pain?

- Abdominal pain is a symptom caused by a myriad of conditions.
- Some conditions are life threatening and require urgent intervention while others may resolve without significant treatment.
- Some of the many conditions that are commonly presented as abdominal pain include:
  - Pancreatitis
  - Esophageal varices
  - Hepatitis
  - Gastric ulcer disease
  - Cirrhosis
  - Ulcerative colitis
  - Constipation
  - Crohn's disease
  - Colon cancer
  - Mallory–Weiss esophageal tear
  - Diverticulitis
  - Gastroesophageal reflux disease
  - Irritable bowel syndrome
  - Gallbladder diseases
  - Peritonitis
  - Appendicitis

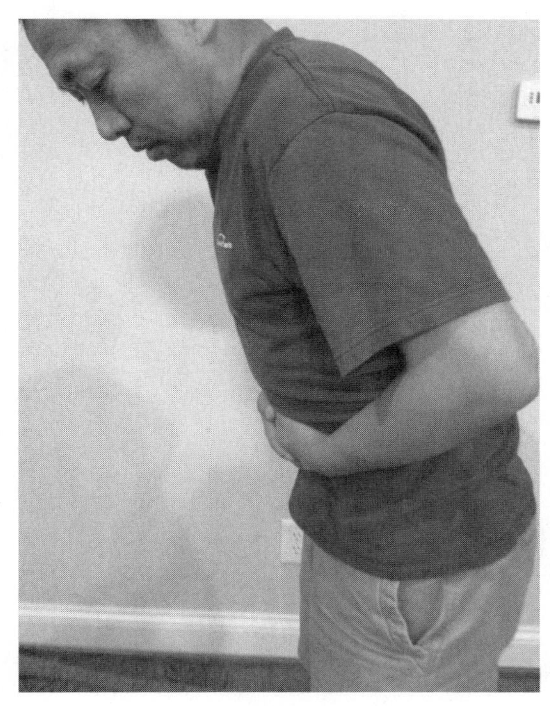

Concern about abdominal pain depends on its location, quality (sharp or dull), duration, severity, constancy, and associated symptoms (e.g., nausea, vomiting, fever). Each characteristic assists in better identifying the potential cause. It is important to notice, ask, and note if the patient recently had a bowel movement, ate a meal, or is doubled over due to pain.

LO1:

Clinical Relevance

- Abdominal pain is a common symptom encountered in adult medicine.
- The symptom can indicate a range of conditions from a severe life-threatening condition to a benign self-limited one.
- A clinician's challenge is to reliably and accurately recognize what the nature or source of the problem is when most patients present with pain of unknown origin. Where do they start?
- This NovE-lesson (and the lesson on GI Bleeding) introduces an overview of abdominal pain that is consistent with the way a real nurse has to think, reason, make judgments, and evaluate a patient, starting with pain of unknown cause. It clinically presents the problem the way a nurse is confronted by it when he or she meets the patient.
- Approaching abdominal pain the way excellent nurses problem solve it in real life can better prepare a learner to become a practice-ready nurse with good clinical thinking.
- Once the condition causing the pain is identified, the condition and its treatment are easily understood. However, until the cause is known, patients require supportive care. This NovE-lesson, therefore, provides an overview of the general care that most patients with abdominal pain need while waiting for diagnosis. When the specific condition is recognized, the numerous NovE-lessons present detailed information about and interventions for the different conditions, which can cause abdominal pain.

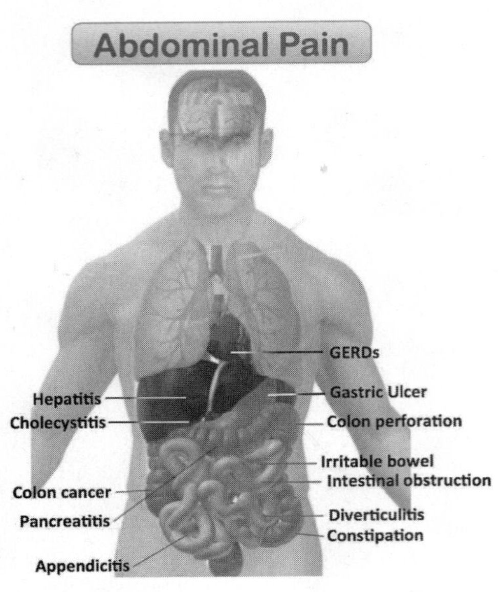

Source: Copyright © 2014, NovEx Novice to Expert Learning, LLC

LO2:

Pathophysiology

- The abdominal viscera are innervated by nerve fibers with nociceptors that transmit pain sensation to the brain but are more primitive and nonspecific than other parts of the body.
- The nociceptors can sense pain from distension of abdominal organs, ischemia, or other types of tissue damage.
- The pain sensations are often diffused and not readily localized. Therefore, regions of pain are often experienced.
- At times, organ damage outside the abdomen may present with referred pain to the abdominal area. The pathophysiology of referred pain sensations is poorly understood.

LO2:

Risk Factors

- Risk factors for abdominal pain are specific to the etiology of the cause. An example being NSAID exposure is a risk factor for peptic ulcer disease, which may cause upper abdominal pain.
- Lifestyle behaviors can increase the risk of epigastric pain. For instance, excessive alcohol use can lead to gastric discomfort. Other factors include smoking, excessive or continual stress, unhealthy or spicy diet, and use of medications that cause GI irritation (anti-inflammatories).

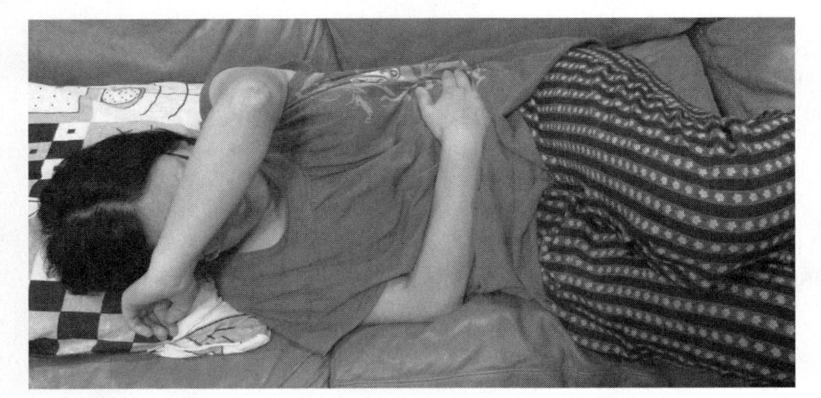

Many lifestyle behaviors can be modified to reduce the risk and incidence of abdominal pain and discomfort.
Source: Copyright © 2014, NovEx Novice to Expert Learning, LLC

LO2:

Common Causes

Upper Abdominal Pain

- Gastric or duodenal ulcers
- Esophagitis
- Abdominal aortic aneurysm
- Gallbladder stones
- Liver diseases
- Pancreatic diseases
- Bowel obstruction or inflammation

Lower Abdominal Pain

- Diverticulitis
- Bowel obstruction
- Bowel ischemia
- Appendicitis
- Renal disease
- Kidney stones

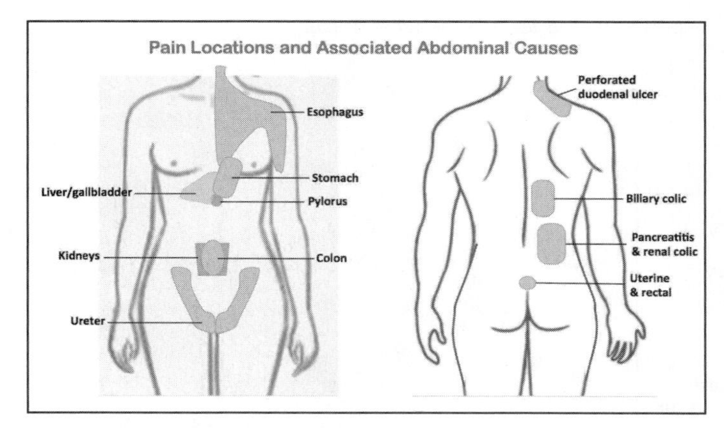

The diagrams show the body surface location of pain associated with abdominal causes.
Source: Copyright © 2014, NovEx Novice to Expert Learning, LLC

Non-Abdominal Causes of Abdominal Pain		
Systemic	**Infectious**	**Thoracic**
Uremia	Rocky mountain spotted fever	Pneumonia
Diabetic ketoacidosis	Strep pharyngitis	Pulmonary embolism
Alcoholic ketoacidosis	Mononucleosis	Myocardial infarction
Lupus erythematosus		Unstable angina
Porphyria		Abdominal aortic aneurysm
Vasculitis	**Toxic**	Herniated thoracic disc
Hyperthyroidism	Heavy metal toxicity	
Sickle cell disease	Scorpion bite	**Abdominal Wall**
Glaucoma	Black widow spider bite	Muscle spasm
	Methanol poisoning	Herpes zoster
Genitourinary		Muscle hematoma
Renal colic		
Testicular torsion		

Important extra-abdominal cause of abdominal pain.
Source: Copyright © 2014, NovEx Novice to Expert Learning, LLC

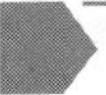

Concept Check

1. What is a common characteristic of abdominal pain?

   A. It is discrete.

   B. It is well-localized.

   C. It is vague.

   D. It is sharp.

Answer question

LO2:

Assessment Findings

- Among the numerous and often similar assessment findings, three key symptoms or symptom clusters should stand out as urgent in terms of the patient's safety. These warn of life-threatening conditions until proven otherwise:
  1. Pulsatile abdominal mass, which should trigger concern about a dissecting or ruptured abdominal aortic aneurysm
  2. Symptom cluster of hemodynamic instability with fever, tachycardia, and/or hypotension
  3. Peritoneal signs describe severe abdominal pain with associated inflammation of the lining of the abdominal cavity:
     - o Rebound tenderness is the severe pain elicited when the examiner removes his hand abruptly after applying pressure during palpation of the abdomen.
     - o Guarding is the tensing of the abdominal muscles that occurs during abdominal palpation
     - o Rigidity is spasm and marked tension noted in abdominal wall muscles during exam and has been referred to as "washboard abdomen."
- Patients with gastrointestinal (GI) conditions typically present with either abdominal pain or bleeding, or both.
- There are numerous GI conditions that cause pain. A nurse's specific understanding and communication about the patient's pain can help mobilize the team in the most helpful direction at the earliest time.

Causes of Abdominal Pain

More common in Patients >50:	**Left Lower Quadrant:**
Cholecystitis	Diverticulitis
Bowel obstruction	Irritable Bowel
Pancreatitis	
Diverticular disease	**Lower Quadrants:**
Cancer	Salpingitis
Hernia	Ectopic pregnancy
	Inguinal hernia
More common in Patients <50:	Nephrolithiasis
Appendicitis	
	Epigastric:
Right Upper Quadrant:	Peptic Ulcer Disease
Hepatitis	Gastroesophageal reflux
Cholecystitis	Gastritis
Cholangitis	Pancreatitis
Pancreatitis	Aortic Aneurysm
Pneumonia	
	Diffuse:
Left Upper Quadrant:	Gastroenteritis
Spleen	Bowel ischemia
Gastritis or ulcer	Bowel obstruction
Pancreatitis	Peritonitis
	Irritable Bowel
Right Lower Quadrant:	Inflammatory Bowel
Appendicitis	

Causes of abdominal pain.

Concept Check

2. A nurse should be concerned about which of the following conditions when a patient reacts with rebound tenderness:

A. Chron's disease

B. Colon cancer

C. Peritonitis

D. Cirrhosis

Answer question

LO2:

Diagnostics

When patients with abdominal pain present, it is important to hone in on the region of the problem to avoid unnecessary testing and discomfort to the patient. A good history and physical examination can help guide and prioritize the diagnostic testing. Location and radiation of the pain, pain acuity, duration, and symptom clusters guide diagnostics. Diagnostic testing in patients with abdominal pain can include any combination of the following tests after the history and physical examination:

- History and physical examination: Physical findings can provide immediate clues to urgent conditions. Abdominal rigidity should trigger great and urgent concern. Among the most common causes of involuntary abdominal rigidity are:
    - o Peritonitis
    - o Appendicitis
    - o Cholecystitis
    - o Dissecting abdominal aortic aneurysm: misdiagnosed in 30% of patient and is life threatening
    - o Mesenteric artery occlusion or ischemia
    - o Toxin released from insect bite: A spider bite (see photo) can provide a clue about the cause.

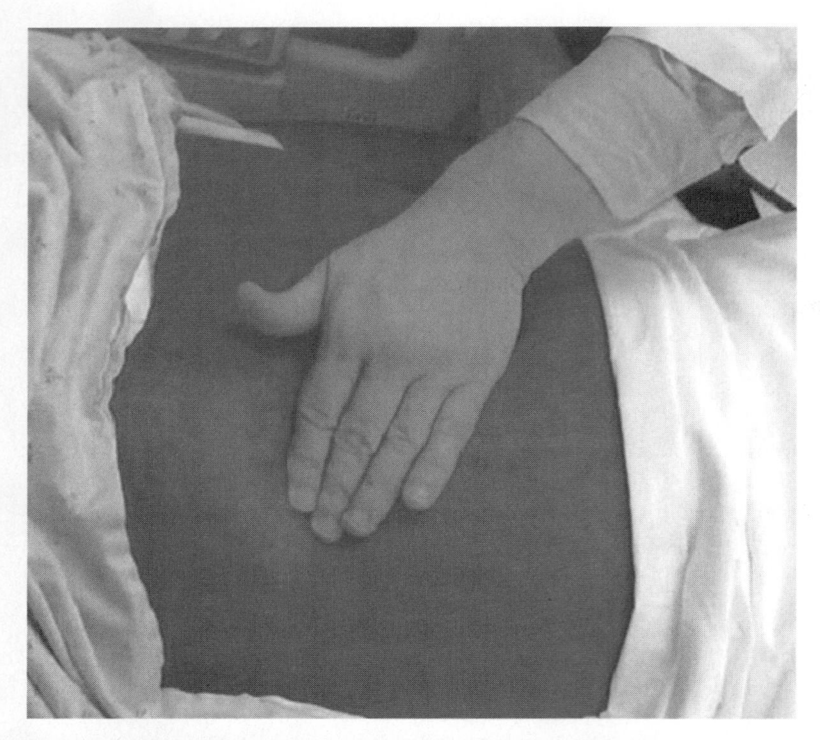

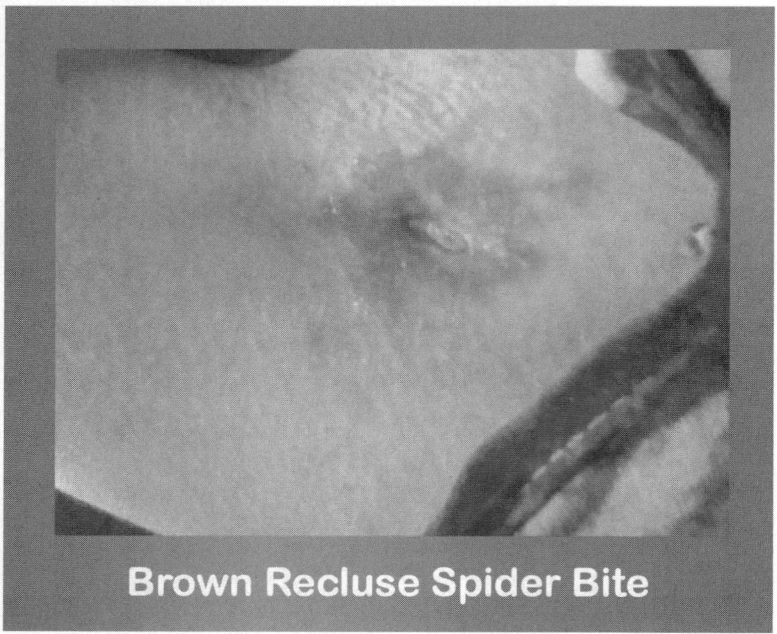

What is abdominal rigidity? It refers to abdominal inflexibility that presents as abnormal muscle tone. There are two types of abdominal rigidity: voluntary or involuntary. Voluntary is reflected in the patient's anxiety and fear when the abdomen is examined by the clinician. Involuntary rigidity arises with peritoneal irritation, which can be life threatening. It may also accompany toxic effects of insect bites or respiratory, GI, and vascular disorders. Involuntary rigidity often presents with abdominal pain, tenderness, rebound tenderness, guarding (peritoneal signs) and nausea, fever, and vomiting.

Source: Copyright © 2014, NovEx Novice to Expert Learning, LLC

- With upper abdominal pain, cardiac-related causes must always be ruled out as a priority in care because referred pain can be present. Possible myocardial infarction requires urgent evaluation.
- Labs that include CBC, liver function tests, amylase, lipase, and coagulation tests. These tests provide indicators about liver, pancreas, gallbladder, inflammatory, and infective processes that may be abnormal.
- Urine analysis and pregnancy (if possible) tests
- Abdominal and chest x-rays: can be helpful in detecting calcifications (gallstones), structural abnormalities (bowel obstruction), abnormal air (perforations) and fluid (ascites)
- CT scan:
  - o Enables 3-D visualization of bone and soft tissue
  - o Enhances detection of fractures, tumors, infection, blood clots, cancer, nodules, masses, internal injuries, and internal bleeding
  - o Because MRI is most useful in detecting injuries of tendons, ligaments, spinal cord, brain, small subtle lesions, and is a more expensive test, it is not as helpful or as commonly used.
  - o CT scan is often preferable over MRI as CT takes 5–10 minutes to complete whereas an MRI can take 45 minutes. In an emergency situation, a CT scan is commonly preferable.
  - o In patients with fever of 100.4°F (38°C) or higher and who have flank pain and/or only one kidney, urgent imaging is recommended (Bader, et al., 2010). Nurses are often best situated to recognize the symptoms early and mobilize the team to respond.
- Ultrasound: May be useful when select conditions are suspected, including gallbladder disease, hepatic abscess, appendicitis, some malignancies, diverticulitis or small bowel inflammation. False negatives are a drawback, as ultrasound is blind to many areas, particularly if there is gas or free air (never a good sign) in the abdomen.
- Endoscopy: allows visualization of structural abnormalities, inflammation, infection, and bleeding as well as exact location
- Surgical exploration

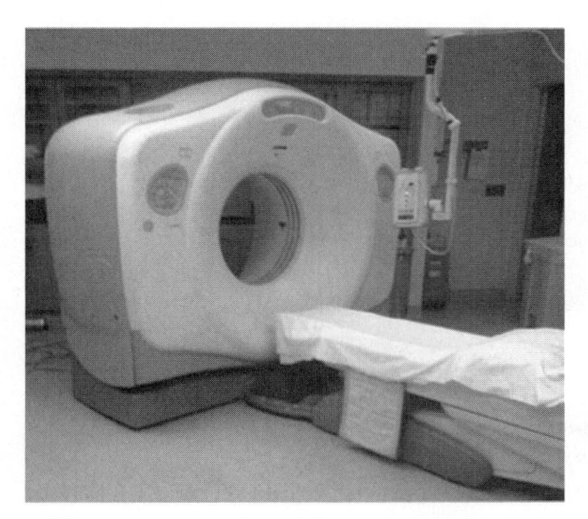

A CT scan is a commonly used diagnostic technology in patients with abdominal pain. It frequently assists in locating and/or verifying the source of the patient's illness.
Source: Courtesy of K. Kyriakidis

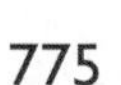

Priority Patient Concerns and Desired Collaborative Care Outcomes

Prior to caring for patients with abdominal pain, it is important to prioritize the patient's concerns that must guide the nursing care plan and interventions. Care for the patient is ordered and organized in accordance with the patient's priority and urgent needs. Desired collaborative care outcomes in patients with abdominal pain typically include:

1. Patient will report tolerable level of discomfort.
2. Patient will have normal bowel movements and remain free of emesis.
3. Patient will consume sufficient calories to meet metabolic requirements.
4. Patient will report reduction in fear and anxiety.
5. Patient will demonstrate understanding of pending diagnostic procedures.

Considering these important care outcomes, prepare a list of the major 3–6 priority patient concerns or nursing diagnoses for patients with abdominal pain. Be prepared to participate in a discussion of this list and/or to submit them as an assignment, as determined by your faculty. Resources you may find helpful in this assignment can include this lesson, the references, resources on nursing care plans, and standard nursing diagnoses manuals.

Concept Check

3. A patient tenses abdominal muscles while being assessed. Which term describes this finding?

A. Voluntary rigidity

B. Rebound tenderness

C. Washboard abdomen

D. Pruning

Answer question

LO3:

Collaborative Interventions

General care of a patient with abdominal pain is needed while the patient is undergoing work-up to determine the problem. Evidence-based practices are detailed in the condition-specific NovE-lesson (e.g., Care of Patients with Pancreatitis). Many patients with abdominal pain, but not all, may receive the following interventions, depending on the severity, duration, location, and associated symptoms:

M N
- Allow nothing by mouth (NPO) status if the patient has nausea, vomiting, may go for emergency surgery, or is severely ill.

M N
- Initiate IV placement and IV fluids to maintain good hydration while NPO or if nausea and vomiting has been persistent.

N
- May call the Rapid Response Team (RRT) if the patient has early or later signs of instability, such as fever, tachycardia, hypotension, and abnormal tissue oxygenation. Call RRT immediately if patient has signs of peritonitis or severe illness, such as severe pain, rebound tenderness, guarding, involuntary abdominal rigidity, melena, or hemodynamic instability.

M N EBP
- Initiate pain control: Many patients require analgesics, possibly IV opioids, as needed. Judicious administration of pain medication is needed to make the patient comfortable without hindering the ability to obtain important history and physical exam information. Evidence supports analgesia appears to be safe, appropriate, and in the patient's best interest (McHale & LoVecchio, 2001; Thomas & Silen, 2003).

M N
- Consider inserting an NG tube if nausea and vomiting are persistent, particularly with refractory vomiting (e.g., bowel obstruction) (see photo).

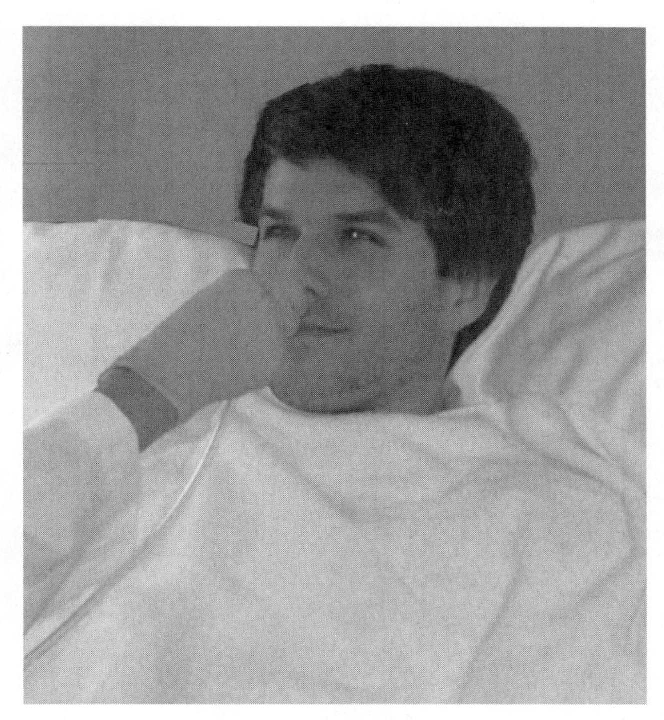

An NG tube is inserted to help alleviate nausea, vomiting, and some abdominal discomfort, particularly distention.
Source: Courtesy of K. Kyriakidis

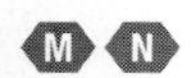

- Consider surgical evaluation: The most dangerous and rapidly deteriorating GI conditions require urgent surgery and are, therefore, considered, detected as early as possible, and ruled out first:
  - o Peritonitis
  - o Dissecting abdominal aortic aneurysm
  - o Bowel obstruction

If these conditions are ruled out, additional diagnostic tests and ongoing assessment findings are obtained. If physical exam and diagnostic tests indicate that surgical exploration is required, conditions that may be uncovered by exploratory laparotomy include:

- Acute appendicitis
- Acute or chronic pancreatitis
- Abscess
- Endometriosis
- Salpingitis
- Adhesions
- Cancer
- Diverticulitis
- Intestinal perforation
- Ectopic pregnancy
- Hodgkin's lymphoma

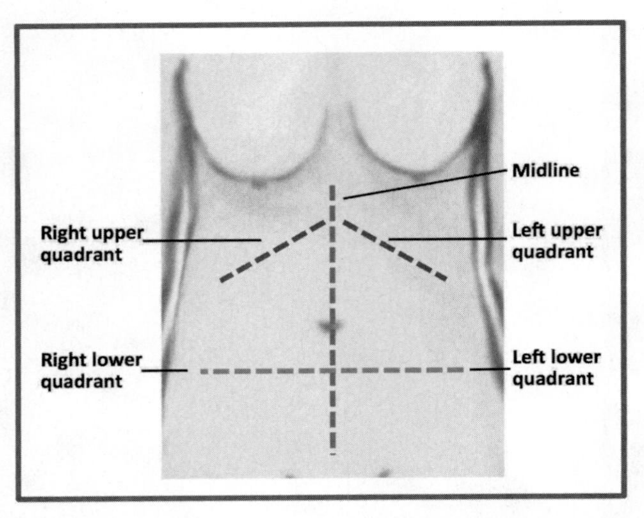

This diagram points out common surgical incision sites for abdominal pain in the different quadrants.
Source: Courtesy of George Kyriakidis/Santa Ana, CA

Concept Check

4. A patient presents to the ED with nausea and vomiting. Which diet order is correct?
   A. NPO
   B. Ice chips
   C. Clear liquids
   D. Soft

Answer question

Collaborative Interventions (continued)

Symptom Management and Comfort Care

Management of symptoms and discomfort are condition and patient-specific, but some general interventions may help most patients:

N
- Manage the patient's pain using medication-specific and dose-appropriate drugs. Collaborative care of patients with abdominal discomfort requires considerable thought due to such varied and vague etiologies. For example, administering ibuprofen might be an excellent intervention for patients experiencing menstrual cramps but may be risky due to increased risk of bleeding in patients with a suspected gastric ulcer. Frequent evaluation of the patient's discomfort enables a good understanding about what medication and how much is needed without hindering the patient's ability to communicate. Traditionally, there was caution about treating pain for fear of masking important symptoms. However, patients with rebound tenderness, for instance, continue to have it despite pain management.

M N
- Obtain a detailed history, which can significantly contribute to honing in on the cause of the discomfort. Once a medical diagnosis is made (or ruled out), nursing interventions can be more specific to the cause.

N
- Avoid repeated exams that cause pain, whenever possible: Once the medical diagnosis is made, it can guide ongoing physical exam to avoid repeated palpation of painful areas unless repeated exam provides valuable insights. For example, palpating the lower right abdominal quadrant in a patient with known appendicitis does not yield additional information and creates unnecessary discomfort for the patient.

- May offer nonpharmaceutical interventions (e.g., music therapy; massage of unaffected areas; distraction techniques such as reading or television; and dark, quiet, restful environments) can yield excellent results in reducing discomfort and pain, providing an adjuvant benefit to pain medications, or helping the patient cope better with the discomfort while awaiting definitive intervention.
- Provide emotional support to patients who have ongoing pain. Compassionate and engaged listening allows the patient and family time to express their feelings, especially if the pain persists without an identifiable cause. Unknown sources of pain can cause frustration for the patient. Listening also provides the opportunity to learn how the patient best copes with pain and distress and may disclose ways of caring for the patient that were otherwise unknown.
- Reassurance and teaching regarding pending diagnostic or interventional procedures can assist in reducing the patient's fear, questions, and anxiety.

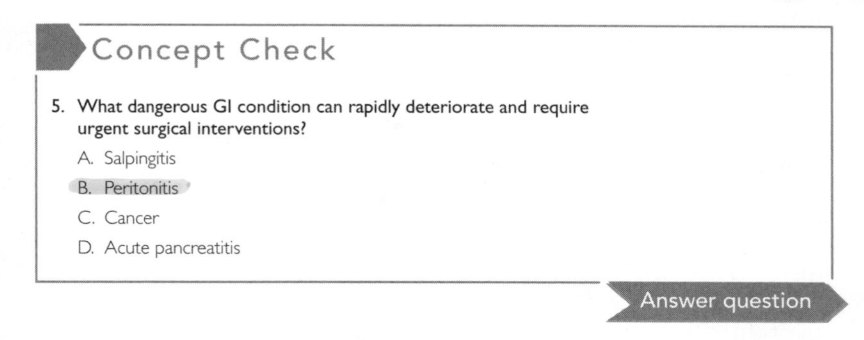

Concept Check
5. What dangerous GI condition can rapidly deteriorate and require urgent surgical interventions?
A. Salpingitis
B. Peritonitis
C. Cancer
D. Acute pancreatitis
Answer question

Collaborative Interventions Summary

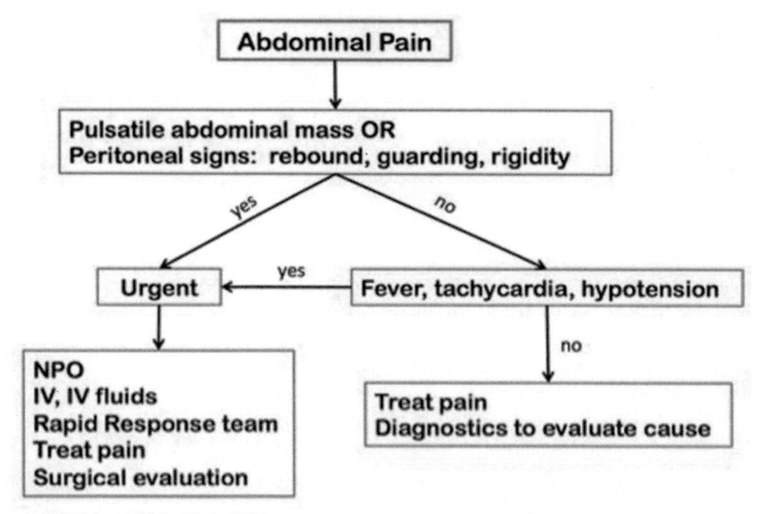

Source: Copyright © 2014, NovEx Novice to Expert Learning, LLC

Summary of Interventions

Depending on the cause of the patient's abdominal pain, some, if not all, of the following interventions may be helpful while awaiting definitive diagnosis:

- A good history and abdominal examination is important to determine urgency of the patient's condition, particularly if obstruction or peritoneal signs are present.
- Should the patient's condition deteriorate, call the Rapid Response Team for assistance.
- Depending on the cause, restricted oral intake, NG tube, and/or IV fluids may be needed.
- Pain management is essential.
- Urgent surgical evaluation is indicated for peritoneal signs and/or unstable vital signs.
- Surgical exploration is commonly needed for treatment.

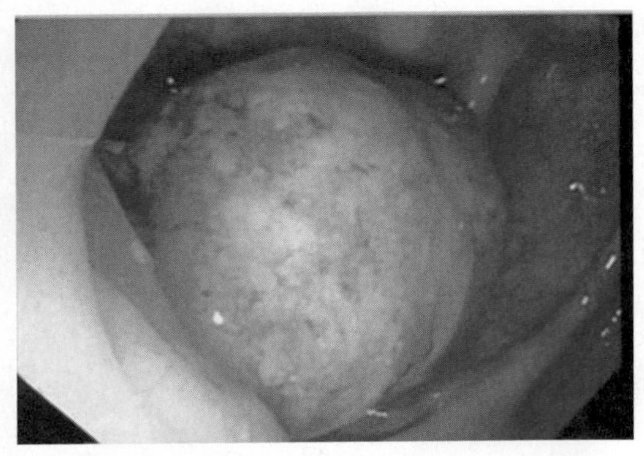

Colonoscopy revealed a large, ulcerated mass in the cecum in a patient with abdominal pain. Evaluation for surgical intervention was required.
Source: Courtesy of K. Kyriakidis

LO4:

Evaluation of Desired Collaborative Care Outcomes

Evaluation and reassessment should reveal attainment of previously established patient outcomes. In summary:

- Patient reports discomfort has decreased to a tolerable level that allows for patient participation in desired activities.
- Patient has soft, formed stools according to pre-illness pattern and is not having emesis.
- Patient's weight has returned to pre-illness or desired range.
- Patient reports feeling confident and calm regarding personal health.
- Patient accurately describes treatment regimen and modalities.

Concept Check

6. **Which finding is a peritoneal sign?**
   A. Nausea
   B. Guarding
   C. Tenderness to palpation
   D. Vomiting

Answer question

Concept Check

7. **A diagnosis of appendicitis has been made. How often should the nurse palpate the abdomen while awaiting surgery?**
   A. Every 15 minutes
   B. Every 30 minutes
   C. Every hour
   D. Never

Answer question

References

Bader, M. K., & Littlejohns, L. R. (2010). *AANN core curriculum for neuroscience nursing* (5th ed). Glenview, IL: American Association of Neuroscience Nurses.

Cartwright, S. L., & Knudson, M. P. (2008). Evaluation of acute abdominal pain in adults. *Am Fam Physician, 77*(7), 971–978. **www.med.upenn.edu/gastro/documents/AmFamPhysacuteabdominalpain.pdf**

Holcomb, S. S. (2008). Acute abdomen: What a pain! *Nursing, 38*(9), 34–40. doi: 10.1097/01.NURSE.0000334644.51961.47

Saccomano, S. J., & Ferrara, L. R. (2013). Evaluation of acute abdominal pain. *Nurs Practioner Amer J Primary Health Care, 38*(11), 46–53. **www.nursingcenter.com/lnc/journalarticleprint?tid=812422**

Clinical Practice Guidelines

McHale, P. M., & LoVecchio, F. (2001). Narcotic analgesia in the acute abdomen—a review of prospective trials. *European J Emergency Med, 8*(2), 131–136.

Thomas, S. H., & Silen, W. (2003). Effect on diagnostic efficiency of analgesia for undifferentiated abdominal pain. *Brit J Surgery, 90*(1), 5–9. **onlinelibrary.wiley.com/doi/10.1002/bjs.4009/full**

Patient Education

MedlinePlus, U.S. National Library of Medicine. (2011). *Abdominal pain.* **www.nlm.nih.gov/medlineplus/ency/article/003120.htm**

RelayHealth. (2011). *Abdominal pain.* **www.patienteducationconnect.com/files/AbdominalPain_Dx.pdf**

University of Maryland Medical Center. (2011). *Abdominal pain.* **www.umm.edu/ency/articles/abdominal-pain**

Learning Outcomes for Esophageal Disorders

When you complete this lesson, you will be able to:

1. Recognize the clinical relevance of esophageal disorders.
2. Consider the pathophysiology, etiology, risk factors, and clinical presentation of esophageal disorders that determine the priority patient concerns.
3. Determine the most urgent and important nursing interventions and patient education required in caring for a patient with esophageal disorder.
4. Evaluate attainment of desired collaborative care outcomes for a patient with esophageal disorder.

LO1:

What Are Esophageal Disorders?

Esophageal disorders discussed in this section include:

- Gastroesophageal reflux disease (GERD):
  - o Esophagitis
  - o Esophageal strictures
  - o Barrett's esophagus
- Esophageal food bolus obstruction
- Mallory–Weiss tear
- Esophageal varices and bleeds

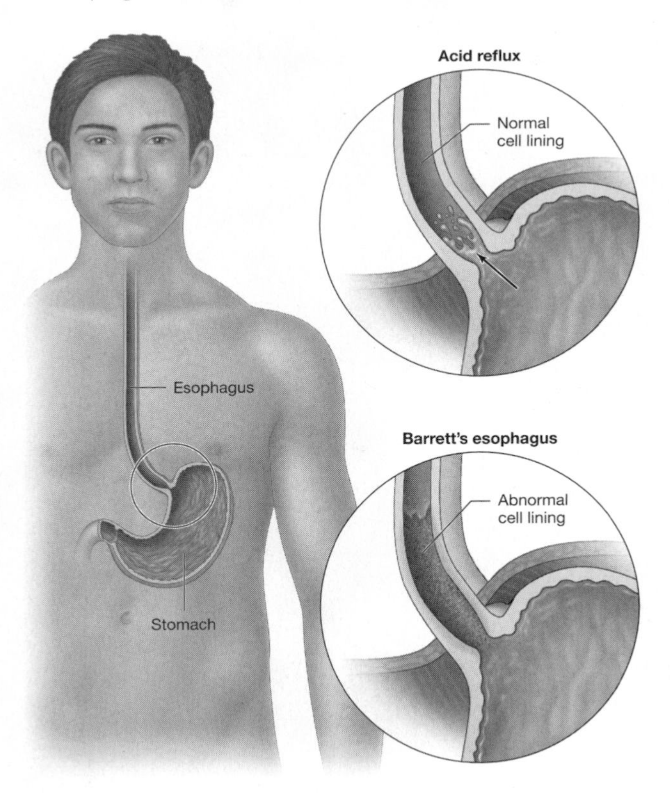

This illustration shows disorders of the esophagus.

LO1:

Clinical Relevance

- Esophageal disorders are common problems in adult medicine.
- It is estimated that 10–20% of adults in the western world suffer from GERD.
- Barrett's esophagus is an increasingly diagnosed condition that places patients at higher risk for esophageal cancer. The incidence of esophageal cancer is rapidly rising in the United States, outpacing breast cancer.
- Over half of adults aged 50 and older have hiatal hernias.
- Esophageal variceal bleeding is a medical emergency with high mortality.

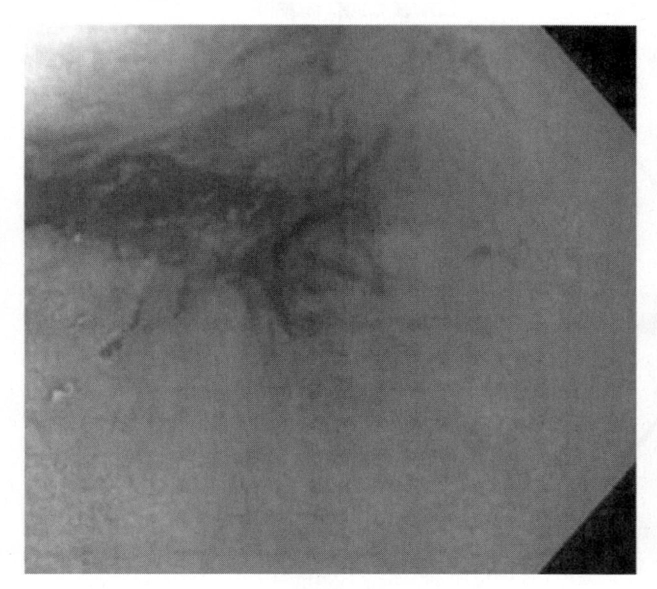

Esophagitis is seen as the area with inflammation commonly seen in GERD.

Sources: Courtesy of K. Kyriakidis & George Kyriakidis/Santa Ana, CA

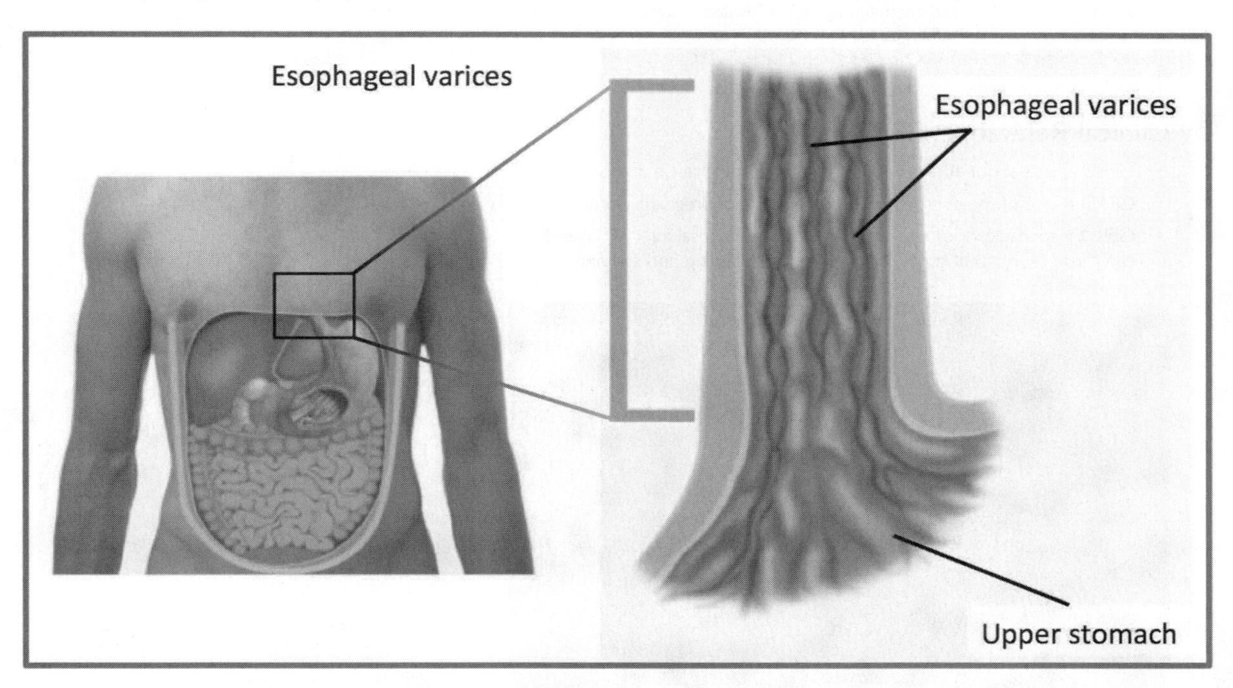

Esophageal varices are fragile, swollen veins at the base of the muscular tube (esophagus) that serve as the conduit between the mouth and the stomach.

Source: Copyright © 2014, NovEx Novice to Expert Learning, LLC

LO1:

What Is GERD?

- GERD results when gastric contents move backwards into the esophagus, causing irritation of the esophagus.

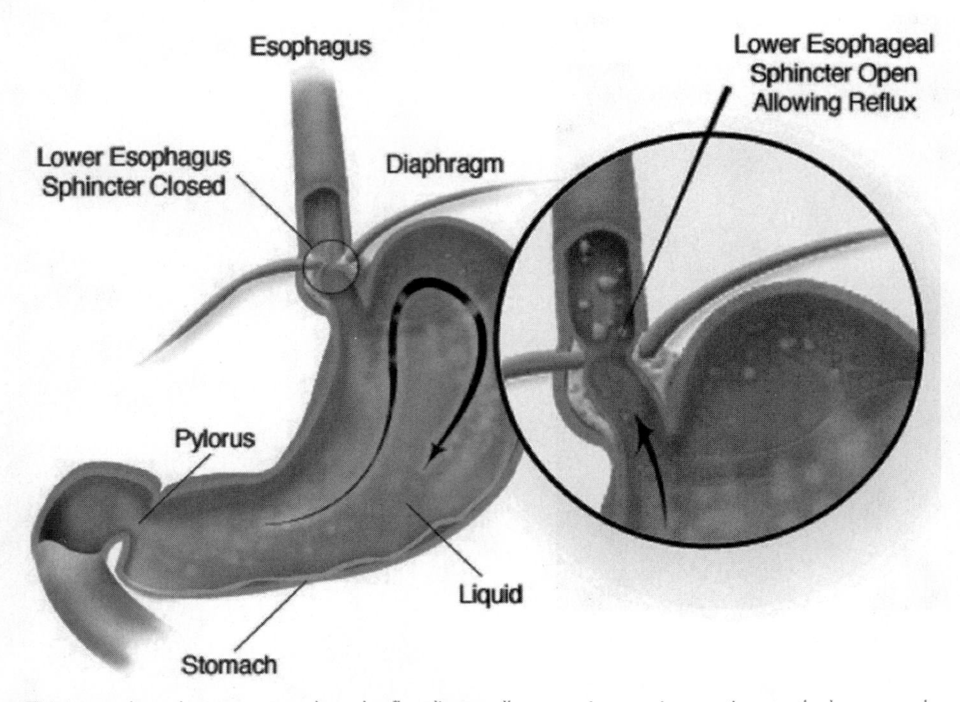

This image shows how gastroesophageal reflux disease allows erosive gastric secretions to the lower esophagus and causes inflammation of esophageal mucosa.
Source: Copyright © 2014, NovEx Novice to Expert Learning, LLC

LO1:

Clinical Relevance: GERD

- GERD affects about 40% of adults and is the leading cause of esophageal stricture (70–80%).
- GERD is one of the most common complaints of pregnant women.
- GERD, if sporadic, does not necessarily cause mucosal injury. If consistent and untreated, it can cause esophageal irritation (esophagitis), bleeding, and scarring.

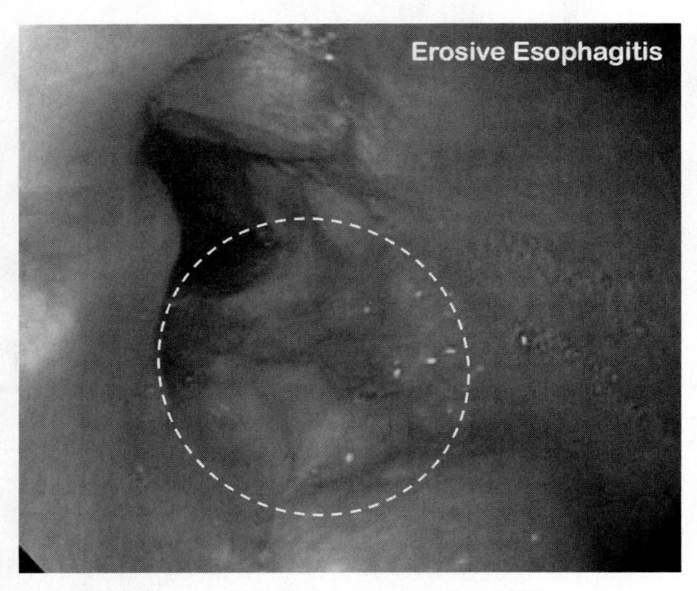

Esophagitis (esophageal inflammation) that can result from GERD.
Source: Courtesy of K. Kyriakidis

Concept Check

1. Which statement regarding the incidence of hiatal hernia is accurate?

A. It is an uncommon condition except among the very old.

B. Less than 5% of those in the United States will have a hiatal hernia.

C. Over half of people over 50 have hiatal hernias.

D. The condition is much more common in infants and toddlers.

Answer question

LO2:

Pathophysiology: GERD

GERD—The role of the LES

- The lower esophageal sphincter (LES) joins the esophagus to the stomach and is responsible for keeping stomach contents from reentering the esophagus.
- The sphincter opens to allow food to pass into the stomach, then closes to keep stomach contents in place.

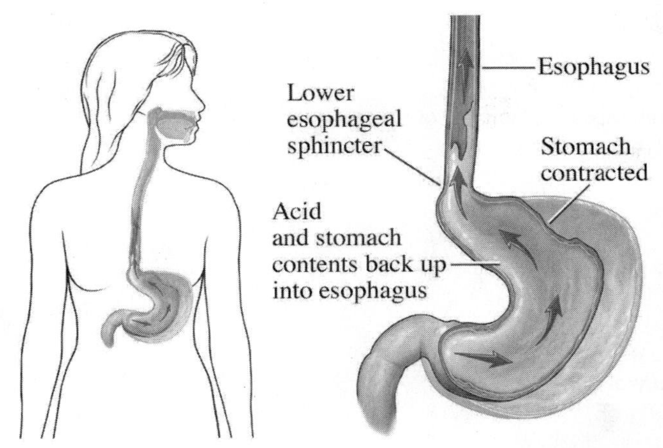

GERD heartburn. This medical illustration pictures a body outline with the stomach and esophagus with the mechanism of gastroesophageal reflux. With the stomach contracted, the stomach contents are shown pushing past the weakened lower esophageal sphincter into the esophagus. Labels identify the esophagus, lower esophageal sphincter, acid and stomach contents backing up into esophagus, and the stomach contracted.

Several factors can contribute to stomach contents entering the esophagus:

- **Dysfunction of the esophageal sphincter.** When the LES relaxation becomes more frequent or when the LES is weak and does not close tightly, backflow of stomach contents can occur, resulting in GERD.
- **Delayed emptying of stomach contents.** Delayed gastric emptying can contribute to distention and reflux. Influences related to delayed gastric emptying include:
  - o Critical illness
  - o Diabetes (diabetic gastroparesis)
  - o Diet high in fat
  - o Gastric outlet obstruction
  - o Head injury
  - o Medications (e.g., narcotics, anesthetics, and neuromuscular blocking agents)
- **Hiatal Hernia.** Occurs when part of the top of the stomach protrudes up through the opening in the diaphragm (esophageal hiatus). Hiatal hernias may be fixed or may slide up and down through the esophageal hiatus. Some people are asymptomatic. The exact cause is unknown but may result from a weakening of supportive structures or from a congenital origin.

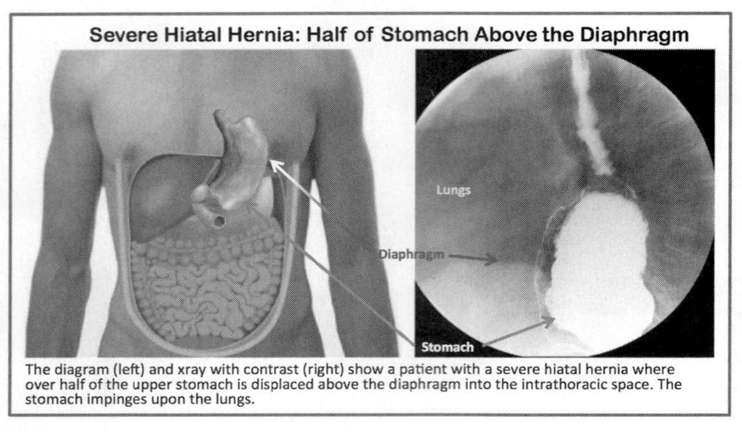

Severe Hiatal Hernia: Half of Stomach Above the Diaphragm
Lungs
Diaphragm
Stomach
The diagram (left) and xray with contrast (right) show a patient with a severe hiatal hernia where over half of the upper stomach is displaced above the diaphragm into the intrathoracic space. The stomach impinges upon the lungs.

Sources: Copyright © 2014, NovEx Novice to Expert Learning, LLC & Courtesy of Erick Kyriakidis

LO2:

Pathophysiology: GERD and Barrett's Esophagus

Stomach contents that contain gastric acid and bile can be irritating to the esophagus and can cause inflammation, bleeding, ulceration, and scarring. Resulting conditions include:

- **Esophagitis.** Inflammation that occurs from GERD is termed esophagitis. If it is severe enough, it can cause bleeding.
- **Esophageal stricture** can occur from repeated inflammation and formation of scar tissue.
- **Barrett's esophagus** results from prolonged and untreated GERD. GERD accounts for the majority of people with Barrett's, but Barrett's can occur without GERD being present.

When GERD is present, it is thought that the repeated exposure of the esophageal mucosa to stomach acid causes the damage that leads to Barrett's.

- As a result, the esophageal lining is replaced by tissue similar to the lining of the intestines (dysplasia, or intestinal metaplasia).
- An increased risk of esophageal cancer exists when dysplasia is present.

Barrett's Esophagus

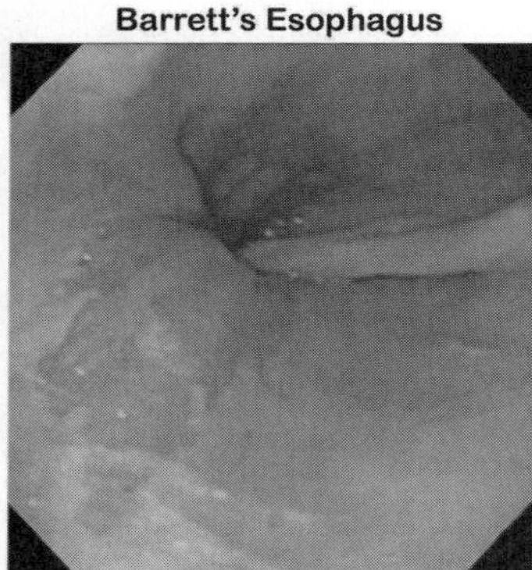

Esophageal Cancer

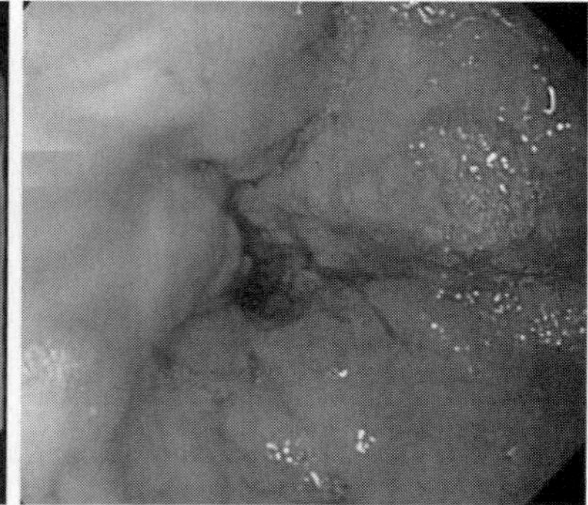

Endoscopic pictures show Barrett's esophagus on the left and esophageal cancer (poorly differentiated adenocarcinoma) on the right. Barrett's esophagus can develop into esophageal cancer as the dysplastic cells proliferate.
Source: Courtesy of K. Kyriakidis

LO2:

Cause and Risk Factors: GERD

The cause of GERD is acid reflux of gastric contents into the esophagus. The risk factors for reflux include:

- Alcohol use
- Obesity
- Food choices (e.g., spicy foods, coffee, chocolate, peppermint)
- Specific diseases (e.g., diabetes, asthma, scleroderma)
- Hiatal hernia
- Pregnancy
- Smoking
- Stress and fatigue
- Medications—particular types of drugs such as:
  - o Anticholinergics
  - o Narcotics
  - o NSAIDs
  - o Beta blockers
  - o Bronchodilators, such as theophylline
  - o Calcium channel blockers
  - o Tricyclic antidepressants
  - o Sedatives

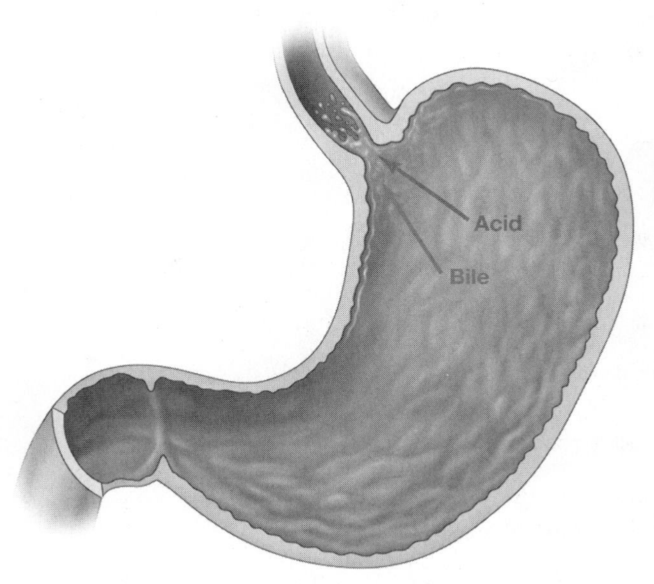

GERD can be aggravated by other factors in addition to a malfunctioning valve. Some factors include obesity, slow stomach emptying, weak muscular contractions in the esophagus, exercise, pregnancy, smoking, certain hormones, many foods, and some medications.

Concept Check

2. How are GERD and Barrett's esophagus related?

A. Barrett's esophagus only exists in those with a history of GERD.

B. Exposure to stomach acid due to GERD can result in Barrett's esophagus.

C. Esophageal dysplasia is another name for both GERD and Barrett's esophagus.

D. Barrett's esophagus increases the patient's risk for GERD.

Answer question

LO2:

Assessment Findings: GERD

Symptoms include:

- Heartburn (burning pain in chest and/or throat) at night, sour taste, dysphagia, hiccups, nausea, regurgitation of stomach contents into the mouth, feeling that food is stuck in the lower esophagus (may occur with inflammation or stricture), difficulty or pain when swallowing, flatulence, and atypical chest pain
- Aspiration of gastric contents can cause pneumonia, hoarse voice, chronic cough, wheezing, sore throat, bad breath, asthma or asthma exacerbation, and pneumonia.

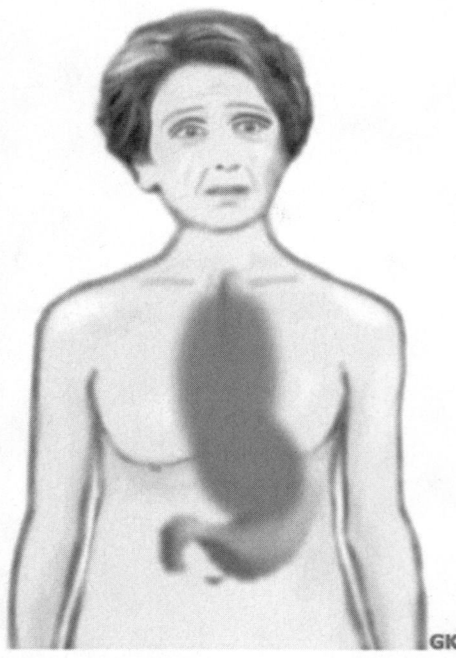

This image depicts the regions in the chest and esophagus where patients experience burning sensations due to heartburn or reflux.
Source: Courtesy of George Kyriakidis/Santa Ana, CA

- Symptoms can worsen with bending, stooping, or lying down.
- Antacids commonly relieve the symptoms temporarily.
- Symptoms of severe pain, protracted nausea and vomiting, blood in vomitus, and/or fever, require immediate attention.
- Since cardiac ischemia and infarction can mimic symptoms associated with upper gastrointestinal disorders, ruling out a cardiac origin is essential in any patient with risk factors or a history of cardiac disease.

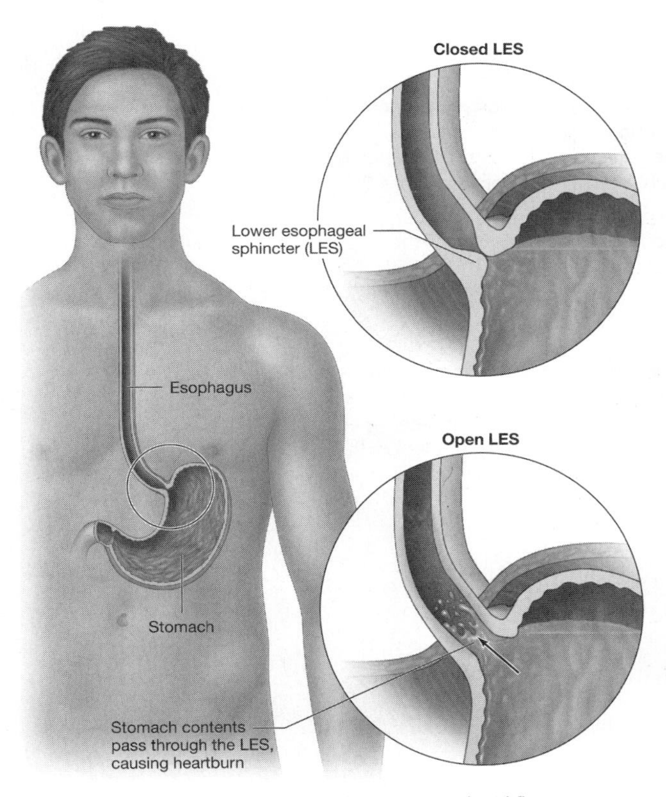

This set of images depicts how stomach contents and acid flow backwards, up the esophagus, to cause esophageal burning. Due to the reflux of harmful and irritating gastric contents, heartburn is a common and gradually worsening symptom.

LO2:

Diagnostics: GERD

Cardiac origin of symptoms of epigastric pain and heartburn should be ruled out first with an EKG and troponin test for patients with risk factors or a history of cardiac disease.

Labs/Testing:

- CBC
- CMP
- PT/PTT
- Stool guaiac (simple test for the presence of blood) or hemocult
- Lactate if signs of SIRS are present
- Esophageal pH monitoring
- Esophageal manometry

Imaging:

- Barium swallow/upper GI

Endoscopy:

- Esophagogastroduodenoscopy (EGD). (Please see the Upper GI Bleed animation in the Diagnostic section of the GI Bleeding NovE-lesson.)

Priority Patient Concerns and Desired Collaborative Care Outcomes: GERD, Hiatal Hernia, and Esophagitis

Prior to caring for patients with GERD, hiatal hernia, or esophagitis, it is important to prioritize the patient's concerns that must guide the nursing care plan and interventions. Care for the patient is ordered and organized in accordance with the patient's priority and urgent needs. Desired collaborative care outcomes in patients with GERD, hiatal hernia, or esophagitis typically include:

1. Patient will discuss lifestyle alterations to prevent esophageal disorder exacerbations.
2. Patient will report decrease or absence in painful symptoms.
3. Patient will not aspirate gastric contents.
4. Patient will have no findings associated with aspiration.

Considering these important care outcomes, prepare a list of the major 3–6 priority patient concerns or nursing diagnoses for patients with GERD, hiatal hernia, or esophagitis. Be prepared to participate in a discussion of this list and/or to submit them as an assignment, as determined by your faculty. Resources you may find helpful in this assignment can include this lesson, the references, resources on nursing care plans, and standard nursing diagnoses manuals.

LO3:

Collaborative Interventions: GERD, Hiatal Hernia, and Esophagitis

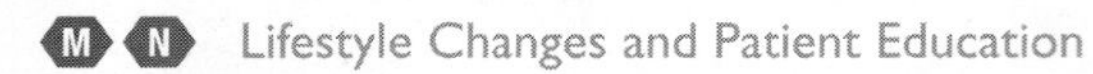

Lifestyle Changes and Patient Education

All EBP listings under the above heading are referenced: (Kahrilas, et al., 2008; Katz, et al., 2013; Moraes-filho, et al., 2010)

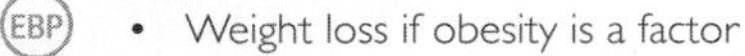

- Weight loss if obesity is a factor

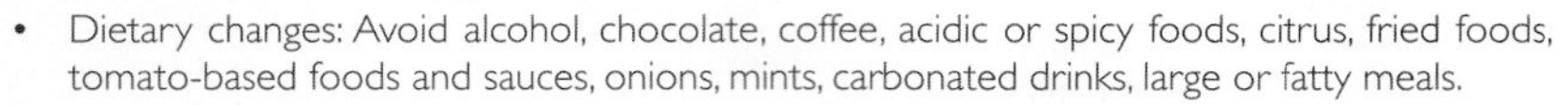
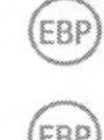

- Dietary changes: Avoid alcohol, chocolate, coffee, acidic or spicy foods, citrus, fried foods, tomato-based foods and sauces, onions, mints, carbonated drinks, large or fatty meals.
- Avoid NSAIDs and aspirin.

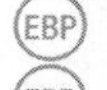

- Wait 2–3 hours after eating before lying down.
- Eat smaller meals. Avoid large meals.
- Stop smoking and avoid tobacco products.

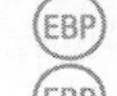

- Elevate head of bed if heartburn or regurgitation occur when reclined.
- Avoid or reduce stress and fatigue, which trigger reflux.

Medications

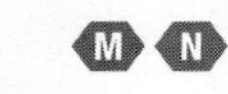

- **Administer antacids:** Neutralize gastric acid for heartburn (e.g., Maalox) as needed. Have limited duration of effectiveness.

- **Administer proton pump inhibitors (PPI):** Block the hydrogen pump that produces acid (e.g., omeprazole, pantoprazole, esomeprazole) (Moraes-filho, et al., 2010).

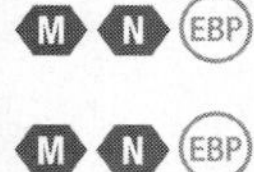

  - o Recommend empiric PPIs for medical treatment because PPIs have proven to be more effective than H_2 blockers (Kahrilas, et al., 2008).

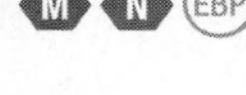

  - o Recommend PPI long-term use in patients with esophagitis if effective. Recommend tapering the dose to the lowest clinically effective dose possible once controlled (Kahrilas, et al., 2008).

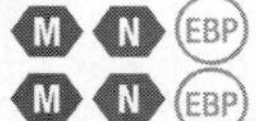

  - o PPIs are strongly recommended over antireflux surgery (Kahrilas, et al., 2008).

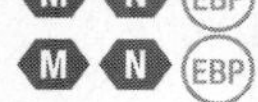

  - o Recommend antireflux surgery when patients cannot tolerate PPIs (Kahrilas, et al., 2008).
  - o Recommend an empirical trial on PPIs in patients with cardiac-like epigastric pain after cardiac origin has been ruled out (Kahrilas, et al., 2008).

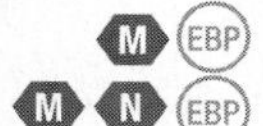

  - o Optimize PPI therapy in patients who are not initially responsive (Katz, et al., 2013).

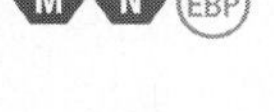

  - o Use caution when administering PPIs to vulnerable patients as PPIs increase the risk of *C. diff* infection (Katz, et al., 2013).
- **Administer histamine (H_2) antagonists:**

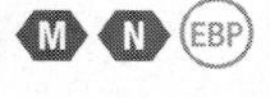

  - o May be administered as first-line agents (e.g., famotidine, ranitidine, cimetidine) that block acid production for mild to moderate symptoms; typically safe (Moraes-filho, et al., 2010).

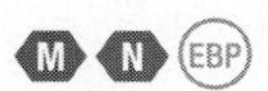

  - o May be administered long term in patient with heartburn and who get relief but do not have erosive disease (Katz, et al., 2013).

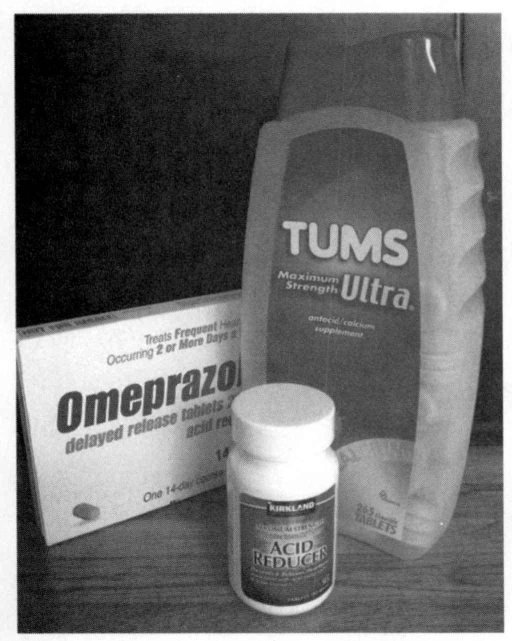

Antacids are commonly used by patients prior to seeking medication care. When antacids are unhelpful, histamine antagonists and PPIs are then trialed.
Source: Copyright © 2014, NovEx Novice to Expert Learning, LLC

Collaborative Interventions: GERD, Hiatal Hernia, and Esophagitis (continued)

Surgical Management

Surgical management is indicated in a number of situations to alleviate pain and symptoms:

- **GERD:**
  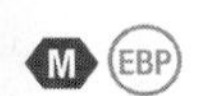
  - Strongly recommend surgical intervention as an option in patients with long-term GERD (Katz, et al., 2013).
  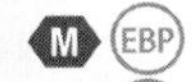
  - Not recommended in patients who are responsive to PPI therapy (Katz, et al., 2013)
  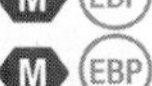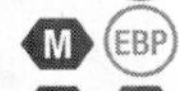
  - Surgical effectiveness is associated with the experience of the surgeon (Katz, et al., 2013).

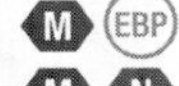

- **Hiata l hernia:** Several different techniques may be used for surgical repair, depending on the situation. Consider these options and educate the patient about which is selected, the postoperative expectation, and potential complications, including:
  - Nissen fundoplication: open surgery that wraps the upper part of the stomach around the lower end of the esophagus
  - Toupet: partial fundoplication performed by laparoscopy that partially wraps the upper portion of the stomach around the esophagus to create a valve. The valve reduces or prevents reflux of gastric contents up into the esophagus. It provides fewer risks than the Nissen surgery.
  - Stretta procedure: Radio frequency energy is applied to the lower esophageal sphincter (LES), causing it to contract and tighten.
- **Routine postoperative care** with special attention to:

  - Individualize pain management; although pain is typically mild.
  - Early mobilization with light activity
  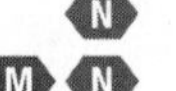
  - Instruct patient that swallowing may be difficult for up to 1–2 months.
  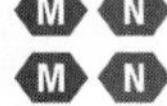
  - Consuming a soft, pureed, or mashed food diet for the first week and advancing slowly (e.g., to pasta or fish and later to poultry)

  - Monitor for and collaborate with the health care provider regarding nausea, vomiting, abdominal swelling, unusual or persistent pain, bleeding, signs of infection, signs of systemic inflammatory response syndrome (preceding sepsis), unexpected wound drainage or inflammation, or signs of cardiac or respiratory distress.

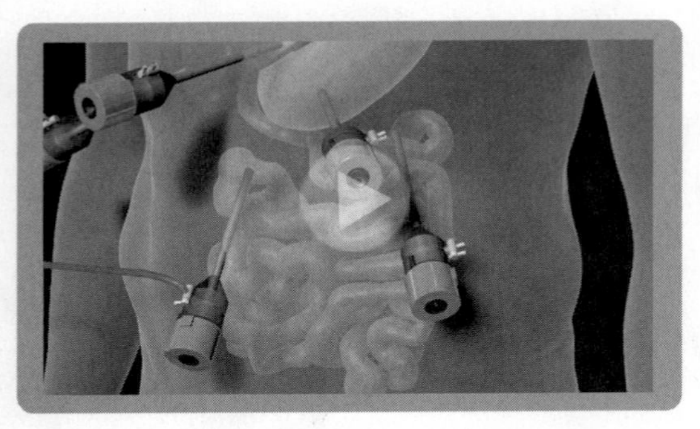

This animation shows a surgical procedure in which the upper portion of the stomach is wrapped around the lower esophagus to strengthen the cardiac sphincter of the stomach. This helps prevent GERD. Hiatal hernia repair is also depicted. This involves pulling a portion of the stomach that has protruded from the diaphragm back into place.

Concept Check

3. Which symptom associated with GERD indicates immediate medical attention is necessary?

A. Pain worsens with stooping.

B. There is blood in the vomitus.

C. Hiccups have developed.

D. The voice suddenly becomes hoarse.

Answer question

Patient Education

Patient education is a key nursing role in the treatment of esophageal disorders. Interventions should include:

N
- Assess for risk and contributing factors. Educate or advise the patient to:
  N EBP
  - Achieve a healthy weight if obese. If contributing to GERD, weight reduction strategies should be encouraged and taught, and/or patient should be referred locally to helpful programs (Kahrilas, et al., 2008).
  N
  - Stop smoking and instruct patients who smoke about the contributory effects on esophageal disorders. Provide direction about smoking cessation programs and the benefits.

N
- Consistently adhere to the prescribed medication regimen to improve compliance and reduction in symptoms.

N
- Prepare patient for diagnostic testing by discussing and describing with the patient prior to the procedure to improve compliance and reduce anxiety relating to unknown medical procedures.

N
- Assist patients to understand the interventions. Improved patient understanding tends to lead to their improved compliance and better outcomes, making this an important nursing intervention.

LO1: What Is Esophageal Food Bolus Obstruction?

- Esophageal food bolus obstruction occurs when food becomes lodged in the esophagus.
- Esophageal obstruction is sometimes referred to as "steakhouse syndrome."

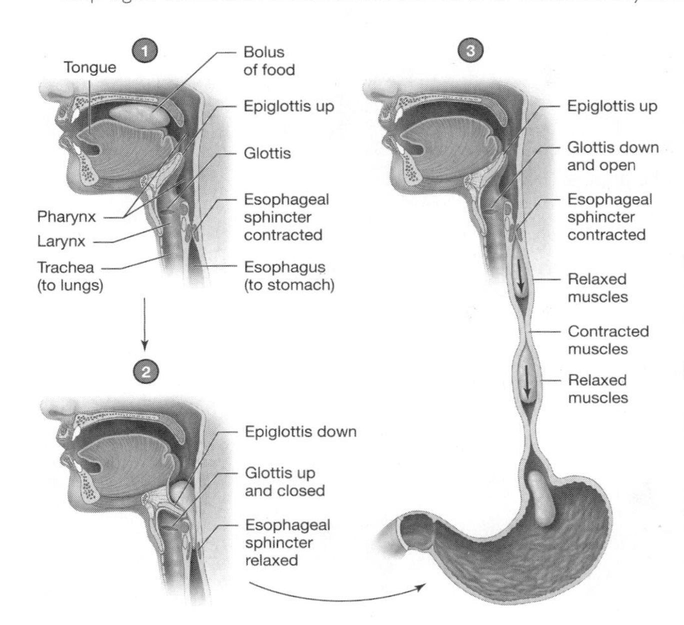

From mouth to stomach: the swallowing reflex and esophageal peristalsis.

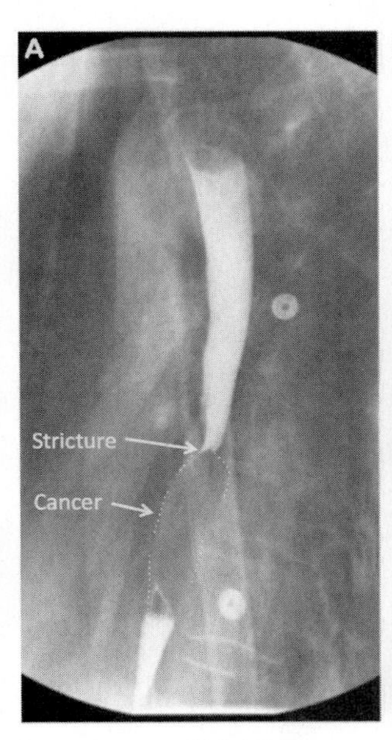

Esophageal Stricture with Obstruction

The xray (A) shows severe esophageal narrowing, or stricture, caused by suspected cancer. Endoscopy (B) reveals that esophageal cancer has severely narrowed the esophagus, causing obstruction.

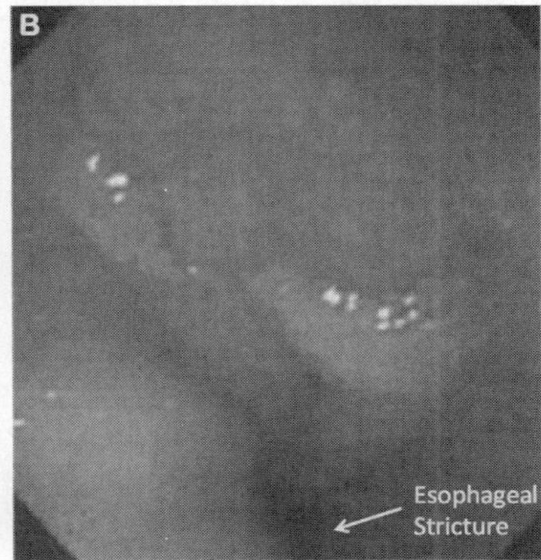

Source: Courtesy of K. Kyriakidis

LO2: Risk Factors and Causes: Esophageal Food Bolus Obstruction

- Not chewing food completely may occur in patients with:
  - o Excessive alcohol intake
  - o Ill-fitting dentures
- Conditions that affect the movement of food through the esophagus
  - o Schatzki's ring is a ring of mucosal or muscular tissue that forms in the lower part of the esophagus.
  - o Esophageal stricture is a narrowing of the esophagus caused by scar tissue.
  - o Eosinophilic esophagitis is a chronic allergic inflammation of the esophagus.
  - o Foods that commonly cause obstruction are meat products.
  - o Esophageal cancer

LO2:

Assessment Findings: Esophageal Food Bolus Obstruction

Rule out airway obstruction—patient should be able to speak and have normal O_2 saturation with absence of stridor or cyanosis.
Assessment findings include:

- History of eating just prior to event
- Foreign body sensation in esophagus
- Epigastric discomfort—can be severe, often at night
- Painful swallowing
- Inability to swallow anything, even saliva; drooling may be present
- Repeated regurgitation of saliva, or any other oral intake

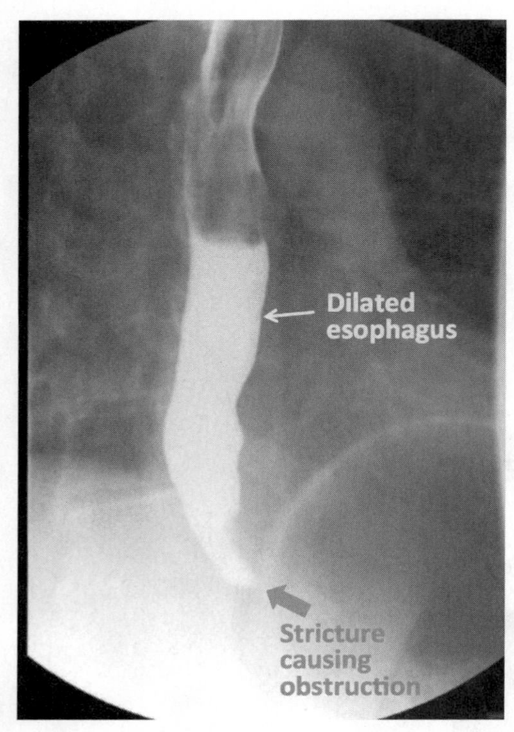

This x-ray highlights why symptoms of esophageal obstruction are manifest in this patient with a stricture due to achalasia, an esophageal motility disorder. Notice the upper esophageal passage is very dilated but then narrows so severely that food can no longer pass into the stomach.
Source: Courtesy of K. Kyriakidis

Priority Patient Concerns and Desired Collaborative Care Outcomes: Esophageal Obstruction or Risk for Esophageal Obstruction

Prior to caring for patients with esophageal obstruction, it is important to prioritize the patient's concerns that must guide the nursing care plan and interventions. Care for the patient is ordered and organized in accordance with the patient's priority and urgent needs. Desired collaborative care outcomes in patients with esophageal obstruction typically include:

1. Patient will report that episodes of pain related to esophageal obstruction have been eliminated.
2. Patient will not aspirate gastric contents.
3. Patient will consume appropriate foods to meet caloric demands.
4. Patient will describe ways to prevent and demonstrate practices that prevent recurrent esophageal obstructions.

Considering these important care outcomes, prepare a list of the major 3–6 priority patient concerns or nursing diagnoses for patients with esophageal obstruction. Be prepared to participate in a discussion of this list and/or to submit them as an assignment, as determined by your faculty. Resources you may find helpful in this assignment can include this lesson, the references, resources on nursing care plans, and standard nursing diagnoses manuals.

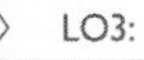

Collaborative Interventions: Esophageal Food Bolus Obstruction and Esophageal Strictures

Food bolus obstructions can resolve spontaneously as evidenced by patient feeling relief and being able to keep fluids down, although some discomfort may still be present. If the obstruction is not resolved, interventions may be needed:

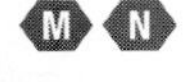

- Assess, protect, and manage the airway as indicated. Anticipate and be prepared for possible endotracheal intubation.
- Thoroughly interview the patient or family, quickly and if possible, to identify the object. Identification and expedient removal of the object is imperative due to potential for injury, necrosis, erosion, perforation, complete obstruction, overdose (e.g., drug packet rupture), toxic poisoning, and death.
- Prevent aspiration of or perforation, particularly if patient is unable to manage secretions.
- Administer prescribed medication: IV glucagon is given slowly to reduce LES sphincter pressure for obstruction. If unsuccessful, a GI consult is necessary.
- Educate and prepare the patient for endoscopic procedure: Upper GI endoscopy is used to relieve esophageal obstruction, diagnose and treat esophageal strictures, and to identify other structural lesions (ACP Paper, 2014).

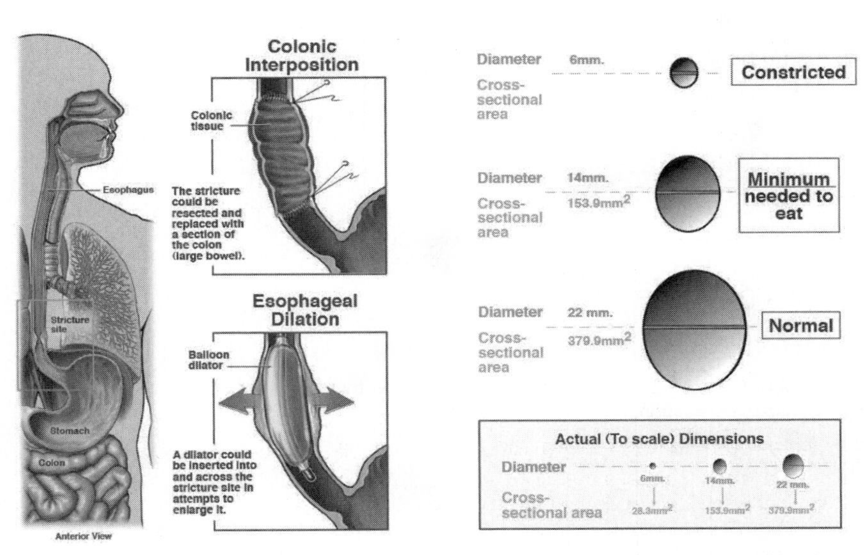

This illustration shows examples of surgical procedures that are designed to relieve esophageal strictures.

Source: © 2014 Nucleus Medical Media. All rights reserved

Endoscopic view of Esophageal Stricture Before and After Stenting

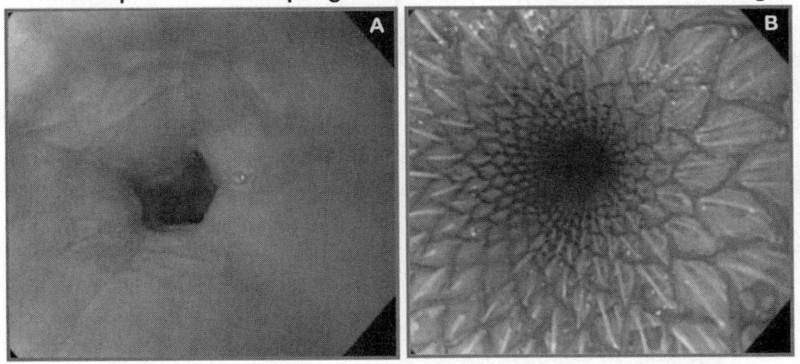

Esophageal stricture (A) caused from scarring due to recurrent esophagitis. The patient experienced significant discomfort with eating. An esophageal stent (B) was placed to alleviate the obstruction.

Source: Courtesy of K. Kyriakidis

- o Situations requiring emergency intervention include esophageal obstruction, ingested disk batteries in the esophagus, sharp objects in esophagus.
- o Situations requiring urgent endoscopy include objects in esophagus that are not sharp, impaction without complete obstruction, sharp objects in the stomach, objects longer than 6 cm, and magnets within endoscopic reach.

M EBP
- Remove food impactions by en bloc removal, piecemeal removal, or by gently pushing (American Society for Gastrointestinal Endoscopy, 2011).

Nursing Interventions and Patient Education: Esophageal Obstruction

Prevention of esophageal obstructions is the priority nursing intervention for patients at risk.

N
- Teach the patient prevention strategies, which may include:
  - o Adequate mastication (chewing) of food
  - o Minimal alcohol intake
  - o Diet restriction to soft or thick liquids for patients with known strictures
  - o Well-fitting comfortable dentures
  - o Prevention from putting foreign objects in the mouth (especially common in children)

N
- Monitor for symptoms of esophageal obstruction and notify the health care provider if suspected and unable to dislodge spontaneously.

Concept Check

4. Which substance is most commonly associated with development of esophageal obstruction?

A. Cigarette smoke

B. Meat

C. Sugar

D. Caffeine

Answer question

LO1:

What Is Mallory–Weiss Tear?

- Mallory–Weiss tear is described as upper GI bleeding caused by longitudinal tears in the esophageal mucosa at the gastroesophageal connection.
- The tears can be precipitated by forceful vomiting, retching, hiccuping, chronic coughing, convulsions, blunt trauma, or CPR.
- Hiatal hernia is a predisposing factor along with excessive alcohol and aspirin use.

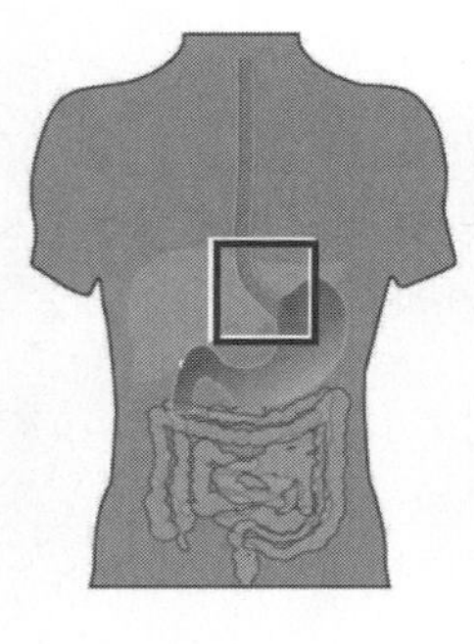
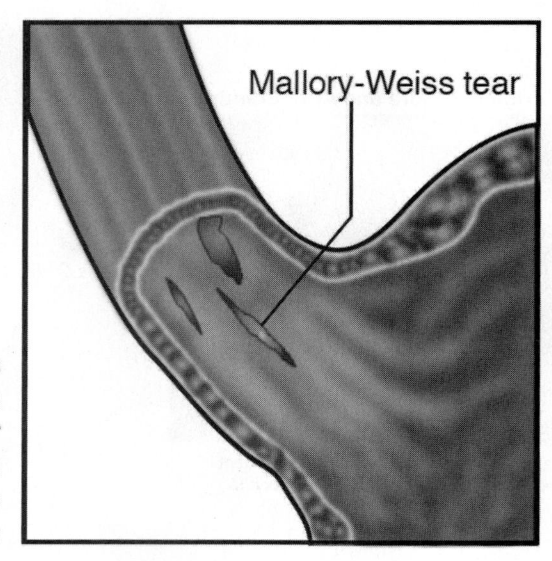
Mallory-Weiss tear
A Mallory-Weiss tear is a tear in the mucosal layer at the junction of the esophagus and stomach

This is the second most common cause of stomach bleeding. The tear occurs at the gastroesophageal junction (where the esophagus meets the stomach) and is a result of excessive pressure or force on the stomach.

Source: Copyright © 2014, NovEx Novice to Expert Learning, LLC

LO2:

Assessment Findings: Mallory–Weiss Tear

- Hematemesis occurs in the majority of patients (85%).
- There is often a history of excessive alcohol or aspirin use.
- Abdominal pain
- Forceful vomiting
- Symptoms are related to degree of blood loss and can include:
  - o Hypotension
  - o Tachycardia
  - o Fatigue
  - o Melena (black blood in stool)

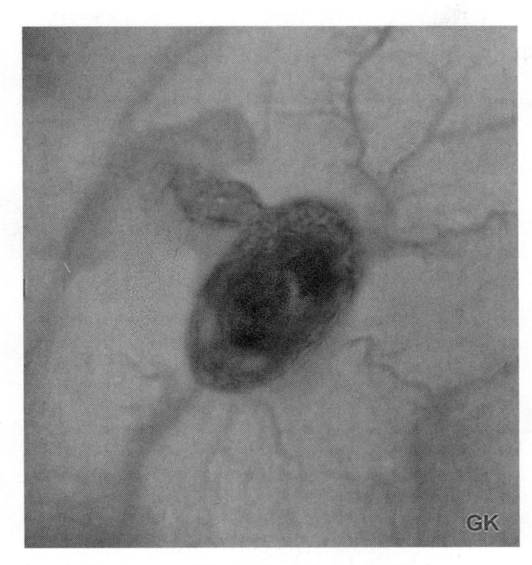

Longitudinal mucosal lacerations that occur in the distal esophagus and proximal portion of the stomach are characteristic of Mallory–Weiss syndrome. These tears are commonly associated with forceful retching. Significant lacerations frequently disrupt submucosal arteries and lead to bleeding.
Source: Courtesy of George Kyriakidis/Santa Ana, CA

LO2:

Diagnostics: Mallory–Weiss Tear

Labs:

- CBC
- CMP
- PT/PTT
- Type and cross match if blood loss is significant
- Cardiac enzymes to assess myocardial ischemia from blood loss and/or as a cause of symptoms

EKG:

- To assess for potential myocardial ischemia

Endoscopic procedures:

- Upper endoscopy to identify active bleeding or tear(s)
- About 80% of patients will demonstrate a single 2–3 cm tear just below the gastro-esophageal connection.

Priority Patient Concerns and Desired Collaborative Care Outcomes: Mallory–Weiss Tear

Prior to caring for patients with Mallory–Weiss tear, it is important to prioritize the patient's concerns that must guide the nursing care plan and interventions. Care for the patient is ordered and organized in accordance with the patient's priority and urgent needs. Desired collaborative care outcomes in patients with Mallory–Weiss tear typically include:

1. Patient's bleeding will stop.
2. Patient will maintain tissue perfusion within desired range.
3. Patient will not aspirate.
4. Patient will recover and maintain an acceptable fluid balance.
5. Patient will report feeling calmer and more confident about personal health.

Considering these important care outcomes, prepare a list of the major 3–6 priority patient concerns or nursing diagnoses for patients with Mallory–Weiss tear. Be prepared to participate in a discussion of this list and/or to submit them as an assignment, as determined by your faculty. Resources you may find helpful in this assignment can include this lesson, the references, resources on nursing care plans, and standard nursing diagnoses manuals.

Concept Check

5. Risk factors for a Mallory–Weiss tear include which condition?
   A. Obesity
   B. Surviving CPR
   C. Hypertension
   D. Drinking alcohol

Answer question

LO3:

Collaborative Interventions: Mallory–Weiss Tear

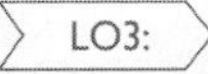
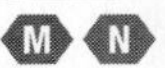

Medications and fluids:

- Maintain hemodynamic stability. Evaluate the need for blood replacement.
- Maintain NPO status for active bleeding.
- Administer antiemetics (e.g., ondansetron, metoclopramide) for persistent nausea and vomiting.
- Provide acid suppression with proton pump inhibitors (i.e., omeprazole, esomeprazole).

M N **Endoscopic procedures:**

- Five to thirty-five percent of patients may require endoscopic intervention.
- Prepare patient for interventions that may include a combination of: contact thermal treatment (through an endoscope), epinephrine injection, sclerosant injection, argon plasma coagulation, band ligation, and hemoclipping.

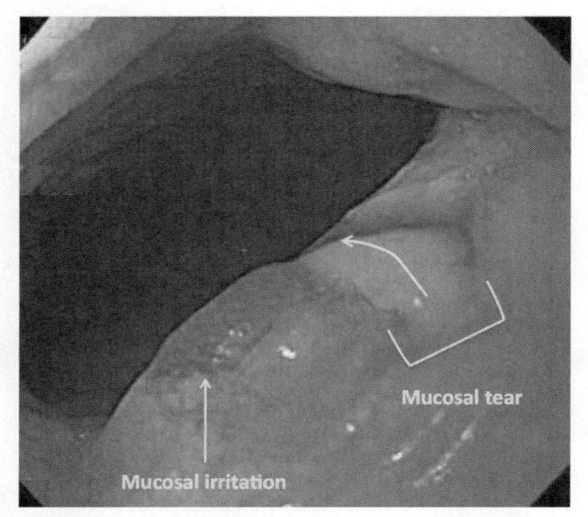

This endoscopic view is looking down the esophagus (dark center) toward the stomach. A wide tear is noted, next to an area of mucosal irritation of the esophagus. A tear this large helps to understand how patients can lose blood quickly and require resuscitation.
Source: Courtesy of K. Kyriakidis

M **Angiotherapy (e.g., arterial embolization) and surgery:**

- Reserved for situations when endoscopic measures have failed

Nursing Interventions and Patient Education

M N
- Manage rapid fluid resuscitation, which may be warranted in patients whose tear continues to bleed despite other interventions.

N
- Prevent aspiration when patient is actively bleeding and may be vomiting.

N
- Monitor vital signs, hemodynamic status, fluid and electrolyte balance, mental status, oxygenation, and perfusion until patient is hemodynamically stable and bleeding is stopped.

N
- Provide frequent, comforting emotional support while answering patient's questions with honesty.
- Once bleeding is controlled:

N
  - Monitor the patient closely for any changes. Early detection and prevention of excessive bleeding is critical in patients with Mallory–Weiss tears.

N
  - Assess vital signs frequently as increased heart rate and decreased blood pressure may be indicators of bleeding and subsequent shock (inadequate tissue perfusion).

M N
  - Assess signs and symptoms of anemia such as fatigue, lethargy, and shortness of breath and follow lab values.

N
  - Instruct patients with known tears about complying with ordered medical interventions, such as medications and diagnostic testing.

LOI:

What Are Esophageal Varices?

- Esophageal varices are varicose veins in the esophagus and are caused by increased portal hypertension.
- Bleeding is the major concern.
- Bleeding from esophageal varices accounts for about 10% of upper GI bleeds.

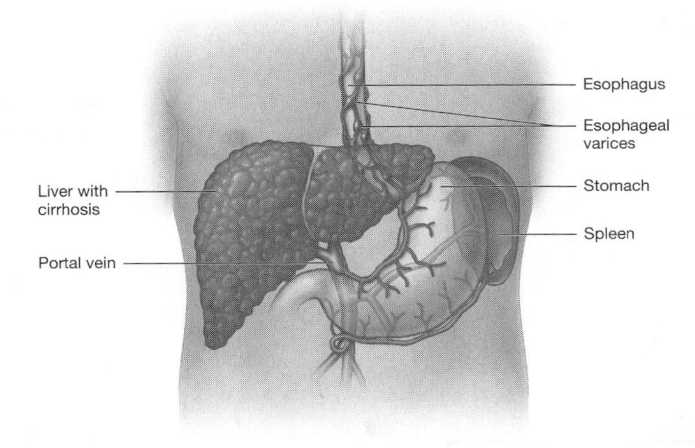

Cirrhosis can cause the blood vessels around the esophagus to swell. This is called "esophageal varices." In severe cases, these blood vessels can burst and cause internal bleeding.

LOI:

Clinical Relevance: Esophageal Varices

- Bleeding esophageal varices is a medical emergency and requires immediate intervention and resuscitation.
- Having an episode of esophageal bleeding greatly increases the patient's risk of having another episode.
- Bleeding from esophageal varices can create a life-threatening condition.

LO2:

Pathophysiology: Esophageal Varices

- The portal vein carries blood to the liver from the esophagus, small bowel, colon, and spleen.
- With development blood flow impedance to the liver, in conditions such as liver cirrhosis, pressure in the portal vein and lower esophagus results in distension of esophageal veins.
- Extreme dilation and swelling of the veins is the condition known are varices.
- These esophageal varices are susceptible to rupturing and bleeding.
- Bleeding tends to be compounded by the coagulopathy that patients with liver cirrhosis develop. (See Care of Patients with Hepatic Diseases NovE-lesson for details.)

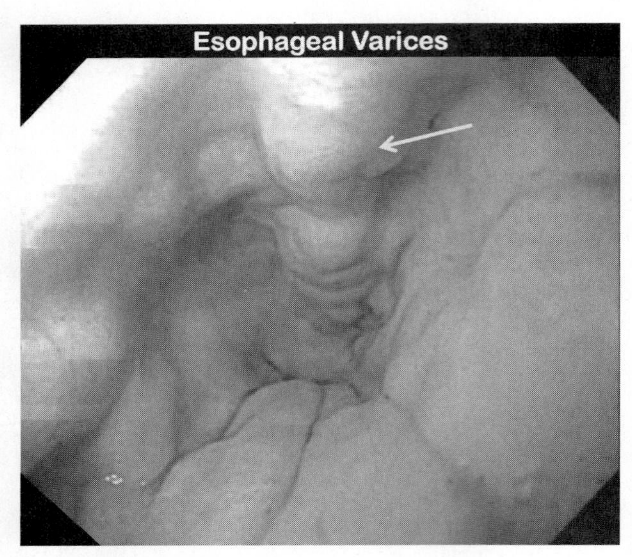

An endoscopic exam in this patient revealed swollen esophageal varicose veins (varices) as the source of the bleeding. The varices will progress to become blue swollen veins without intervention and/or lifestyle modifications. Esophageal varices signal advancing liver disease. Rupture and hemorrhage can cause massive blood loss. The arrow points out one of many varices.

Source: Courtesy of K. Kyriakidis

LO2:

Risk Factors: Esophageal Varices

- Risk factors are related to developing liver cirrhosis.
  - o Viral (hepatitis B and C)
  - o Alcoholic cirrhosis
  - o IV drug abuse
  - o Alcohol abuse
- Alcohol and hepatitis are the leading causes of esophageal varices in the United States.

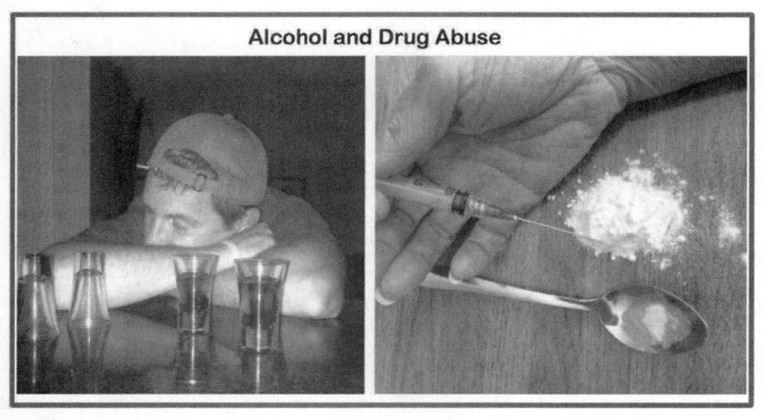

Alcohol and drug abuse lead to liver damage or infections like hepatitis C, which cause liver damage. In all situations, portal hypertension places the patient at high risk for esophageal varices.

Sources: *(left)* Copyright © 2014, NovEx Novice to Expert Learning, LLC; *(right)* Courtesy of R. Murphy

LO2:

Assessment Findings: Esophageal Varices

- Symptoms are usually related to bleeding. Bleeding tends to be profuse, sudden, and commonly results in shock.
- Other symptoms are usually related to liver disease.
- Symptoms of cirrhosis and liver disease causing portal hypertension are:
  - o Fatigue
  - o Loss of appetite
  - o Nausea/vomiting
  - o Weight loss
  - o Jaundice
  - o Edema
  - o Abdominal swelling (ascites)
  - o Pruritus
  - o Bruising easily
  - o Mental status changes
- Past medical history is often suggestive of liver disease (e.g., excessive alcohol intake, IV drug abuse, previous history of hepatitis, known varices).

Normal Condition Versus Stage Four Cirrhosis of the Liver

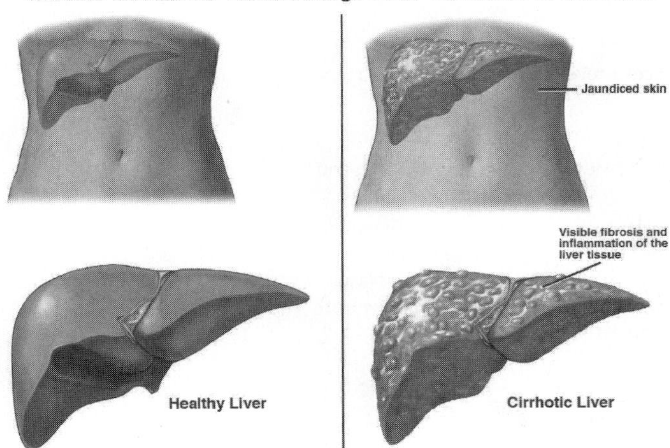

These images display a comparison of the normal anatomy of the liver to a liver with late-stage cirrhosis. It depicts some features of the physical exam and the liver itself.

LO2:

Diagnostics: Esophageal Varices

Labs:

- CBC
- CMP
- PT/PTT
- Hepatitis panel
- Arterial blood gas
- Type and cross for blood replacement

Physical examination:

- Stool guaiac or hemocult
- Presence of jaundice

Imaging:

- Ultrasound of upper abdomen to evaluate for liver cirrhosis or ascites.

Endoscopy:

- Used to diagnose and treat variceal bleeding

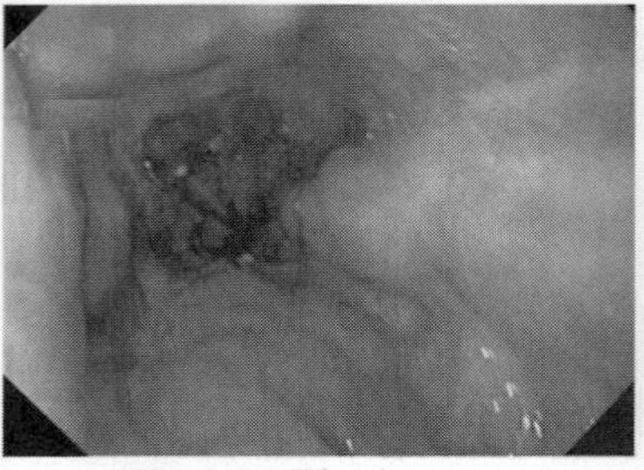

Endoscopy is an excellent tool for identifying and diagnosing esophageal varices and bleeding.
Source: Courtesy of K. Kyriakidis

Priority Patient Care and Desired Collaborative Care Outcomes: Esophageal Varices

Prior to caring for patients with esophageal varices, it is important to prioritize the patient's concerns that must guide the nursing care plan and interventions. Care for the patient is ordered and organized in accordance with the patient's priority and urgent needs. Desired collaborative care outcomes in patients with esophageal varices typically include:

1. Patient will not experience or will satisfactorily recover from a shock state.
2. Patient will explain probable cause of esophageal varices, prevention strategies, and plan for emergency management.
3. Patient will experience a reduction in fear related to the serious illness.
4. Patient will demonstrate modifications being made in lifestyle to improve overall health and prevent complications.

Considering these important care outcomes, prepare a list of the major 3–6 priority patient concerns or nursing diagnoses for patients with esophageal varices. Be prepared to participate in a discussion of this list and/or to submit them as an assignment, as determined by your faculty. Resources you may find helpful in this assignment can include this lesson, the references, resources on nursing care plans, and standard nursing diagnoses manuals.

LO3:

Collaborative Interventions: Esophageal Varices

EBP recommendations are included throughout this section (Jalan & Hayes, 2000).

Medications/fluids:

- Administer a beta blocker, if not contraindicated, which can decrease risk of initial bleeding.
- Manage octreotide infusion, which can reduce portal pressures and slow variceal bleeding.
- Use a long acting nitrite if the beta blocker is contraindicated.
- For active bleeding, use large bore IV access.
- Type and cross match. Try to restore blood volume with blood transfusions and fluids.
- Correct clotting factor deficiencies with fresh frozen plasma or vitamin K1.
- Call the **Rapid Response Team** if a significant amount of blood loss occurs with variceal bleeding. Call the Rapid Response Team for sudden increase in bleeding, decreased level of consciousness, and/or hemodynamic instability. Note: Variceal bleeding may not be controlled, even after large amounts of blood products. Some patients will die despite the best possible care.

Endoscopic intervention:

- Prepare patient for sclerotherapy (varices are injected with a sclerosing agent) or variceal ligation.

Surgical intervention:

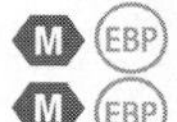

- Portosystemic shunt to decrease portal hypertension
- Liver transplantation

Therapeutic radiologic procedures:

- Educate the patient for TIPS (transjugular intrahepatic portosystemic shunt) to decrease portal hypertension.

Banding of a Bleeding Esophageal Varix

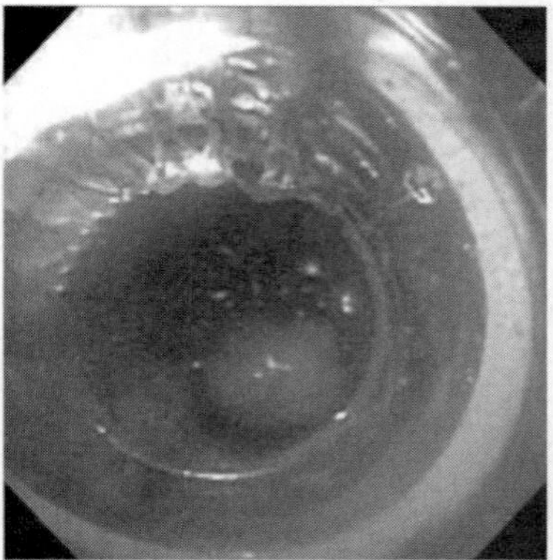
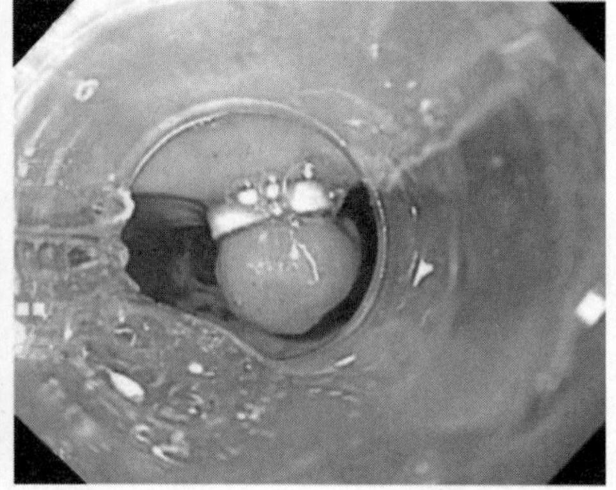

Left: A bleeding varix is isolated for intervention. Right: A band is successfully tightened around the bleeder. Water (lower left) cleanses the area.

Source: Courtesy of K. Kyriakidis

Patient Education

- Because the presence of esophageal varices puts the patient at risk for esophageal bleeding, the nurse must educate the patient and family on prevention strategies to avoid rupture of the varices (such as reduction in blood pressure, avoiding stress, and complying with prescribed medical regimen).
- Educate the patient and family about when to call 911 quickly in the event of an esophageal bleed. A quick response is imperative in order to maintain and restore fluid status and prevent shock.
- Educate patients with known varices to avoid alcohol, enter alcohol cessation programs, seek assistance to help stop IV drug usage, and comply with hepatitis treatment. These patient-dependent interventions are needed to prevent further liver deterioration, reduce portal hypertension, and alleviate esophageal congestion.
- Educate patients and their families about the importance of complying with prescribed medical regimens in order to reduce the risk of a bleed and improve symptoms.
- Initiate discussion about advanced directives with patient and family early. Advanced directives are intended for everyone, not only those with terminal or life-threatening illnesses.

Key Complication: Esophageal Varices

Hypovolemic/Hemorrhagic Shock

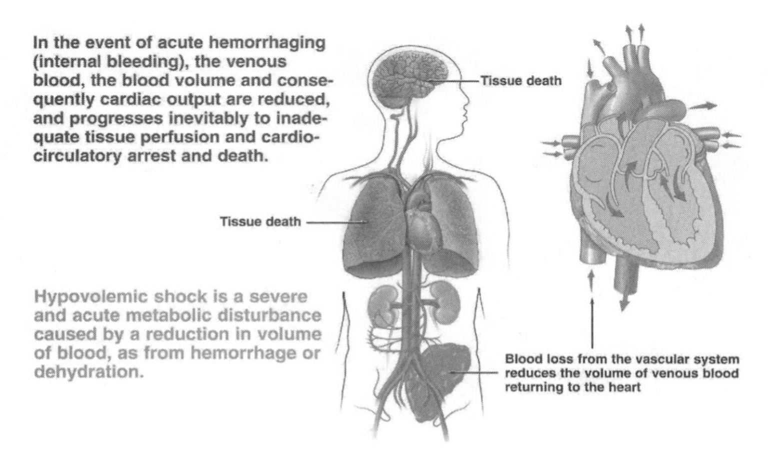

In the event of acute hemorrhaging (internal bleeding), the venous blood, the blood volume and consequently cardiac output are reduced, and progresses inevitably to inadequate tissue perfusion and cardiocirculatory arrest and death.
Tissue death
Tissue death
Hypovolemic shock is a severe and acute metabolic disturbance caused by a reduction in volume of blood, as from hemorrhage or dehydration.
Blood loss from the vascular system reduces the volume of venous blood returning to the heart

This image depicts the sequence of events when hypovolemic (low blood volume) shock occurs. Death is a potential outcome.

Source: Nucleus Medical Art Inc./Alamy

Concept Check

6. Which lifestyle change is most likely to reduce the risk of esophageal varices rupture?

A. Patient has increased intake of green, leafy vegetables.

B. Patient has enrolled in a stress management course.

C. Patient has started a smoking cessation program.

D. Patient has started taking a statin drug regularly.

Answer question

Concept Check

7. Sclerotherapy is most commonly used for which condition?

A. Esophagitis

B. Barrett's esophagus

C. Esophageal obstruction

D. Esophageal varices

Answer question

Summary of Interventions

- GERD is usually treated with acid lowering agents, such as antihistamines or proton pump inhibitors.
- Mallory–Weiss tears are treated with proton pump inhibitors. Patients who are bleeding need to be stabilized. They may require IV fluids and/or transfusion.
- Esophageal food bolus obstruction may be treated with IV glucagon and/or endoscopic removal of the bolus.
- Acute esophageal variceal bleeding is a life-threatening situation that can result in hemorrhagic shock. Treatment consists of stabilizing the patient with blood transfusions, IV hydration and, possibly, correction of coagulopathy with fresh frozen plasma. Endoscopic intervention to stop the bleeding is commonly required. Patient education to prevent further liver damage is central to the care of the patient.

LO4: Evaluation of Desired Collaborative Care Outcomes

Evaluation and reassessment should reveal attainment of previously established patient outcomes. In summary:

GERD

- Patient describes techniques and lifestyle modifications necessary to prevent GERD.
- Patient reports being pain free.
- Patient has not experienced aspiration
- Patient's lungs are clear to auscultation, voice is normal, and no sore throat or cough is present.

Esophageal Obstruction

- Patient reports painful episodes of esophageal obstruction have stopped occurring.
- Patient's lungs are clear to auscultation, voice is normal, and no sore throat or cough is present.
- Patient's weight is within or improving toward the desired range.
- Patient accurately describes techniques for preventing recurrent esophageal obstruction.

Mallory–Weiss Tears

- Patient's bleeding stopped with no recurrence.
- Patient's oxygen saturation remains within desired range.
- Patient's lungs are clear, voice is normal, and no sore throat or coughing is present.
- Patient's blood pressure and heart rate are stable, mentation is clear, and urine output balances fluid intake.
- Patient reports feeling calmer and more confident about personal health.

Esophageal Varices

- Patient's mentation is clear and blood pressure and urine output are within desired range.
- Patient accurately discusses the probable cause of esophageal varices, prevention strategies, and verbalizes a plan for emergency management.
- Patient reports feeling less fearful regarding potential complications from the serious illness.
- Patient is demonstrating lifestyle modification to improve overall health and prevent complications.

References

Carlson, D, & Pfadt, E. (2011). Mallory-Weiss syndrome. *Nursing, 41*(10), 72.

Garcia-Tsao, G., Sanyal, A. J., Grace, N. D., & Carey, W. (2007). Prevention and management of gastroesophageal varices and variceal hemorrhage in cirrhosis. *Am J Gastroenterol, 102*, 2086–2192. doi: 10.1111/j.1572-0241.2007.01481.x

Kortas, D. Y., Haas, L., Simpson, W., et al. (2001). Mallory-Weiss tear: Predisposing factors and predictors of a complicated course. *Am J Gastroenterol, 96*, 2863–2865. doi: 10.1111/j.1572-0241.2001.04239.x

Rayhorn, N. (2004). Gastroesophageal reflux disease (GERD). *Nursing 2014, 34*(7), 54–55.

Smith, M. M. (2010). Emergency: Variceal hemorrhage from esophageal varices associated with alcoholic liver disease. *Amer J Nursing, 110*(2), 32–39. doi: 10.1097/01.NAJ.0000368049.57482.00

Clinical Practice Guidelines

American College of Physicians. (2014). *American College of Physicians: Upper endoscopy is overused in patients with heartburn.* **www.acponline.org/pressroom/upper_endoscopy_overused.htm**

American Society for Gastrointestinal Endoscopy. (2011). Guideline: Management of ingested foreign bodies and food impactions. *Gastrointestinal Endoscopy, 73*(6), 1085–1091. **www.asge.org/uploadedFiles/Publications_and_Products/Practice_Guidelines/Management%20of%20ingested%20foreign%20bodies%20and%20food%20impactions.pdf**

Jalan, R, & Hayes, P. (2000). UK guidelines on the management of variceal haemorrhage in cirrhotic patients. *Gut, 46*, iii1–iii15. doi: 10.1136/gut.46.suppl_3.iii1 **http://gut.bmj.com/content/46/suppl_3/iii1.full**

Kahrilas, P. J., Shaheen, M. J., & Vaezi, M. F. (2008). American Gastroenterological Association Institute technical review on the management of gastroesophageal reflux disease. *Gastroenterology, 135*(4), 1392–1413.e5. **www.gastrojournal.org/article/S0016-5085(08)01605-3/fulltext#sec4.1**

Katz, P. O., Gerson, L. B., & Vela, M. F. (2013). Diagnosis and management of gastroesophageal reflux disease. *Am J Gastroenterol, 108*, 308–328. **gi.org/guideline/diagnosis-and-managemen-of-gastroesophageal-reflux-disease/**

Moraes-filho, J., Navarro-Rodriguez, T., Barbuti, R., et al. (2010). Guidelines for the diagnosis and management of gastroesophageal reflux disease: An evidence-based consensus. *Arq. Gastroenterol, 47*(1). **www.ncbi.nlm.nih.gov/pubmed/20520983**

Patient Education

Carale, J. (2013). *Portal hypertension.* **emedicine.medscape.com/article/182098-overview**

Patti, M. G. (2014). *Gastroesophageal reflux disease.* **emedicine.medscape.com/article/176595-overview**

Runyon, B. A. (2014). *Patient information: Esophageal varices.* **www.uptodate.com/contents/esophageal-varices-beyond-the-basics?source=search_result&search=esophageal+varices+beyondthe+basics&selectedTitle=7~150**

Song, L. (2013). *Mallory-Weiss tear overview of Mallory-Weiss syndrome.* **emedicine.medscape.com/article/187134-overview**

Learning Outcomes for Peptic Ulcer Disease

When you complete this lesson, you will be able to:

1. Recognize the clinical relevance of peptic ulcer disease.
2. Consider the pathophysiology, etiology, risk factors, and clinical presentation of peptic ulcer disease that determines the priority patient concerns.
3. Determine the most urgent and important nursing interventions and patient education required in caring for a patient with peptic ulcer disease.
4. Evaluate attainment of desired collaborative care outcomes for a patient with peptic ulcer disease.

LO1:

What Is Peptic Ulcer Disease?

- Peptic ulcer disease (PUD) is an ulceration of the esophagus, stomach, duodenum or upper portion of the small intestines.
- Ulceration is the breakdown of the normal lining and may cause pain and/or bleeding.
- Gastric ulcers are those occurring within the stomach.
- Duodenal ulcers are those occurring within the upper region of the small intestines.
- Traditionally, PUD was primarily understood as an abnormality of pepsin and gastric acid oversecretion.
- Although hypersecretion remains a relevant factor in causing PUD, the identification of *Helicobacter pylori* as a primary cause of PUD greatly informed our understanding, diagnosis, treatment, and prevention effort in patients with PUD.

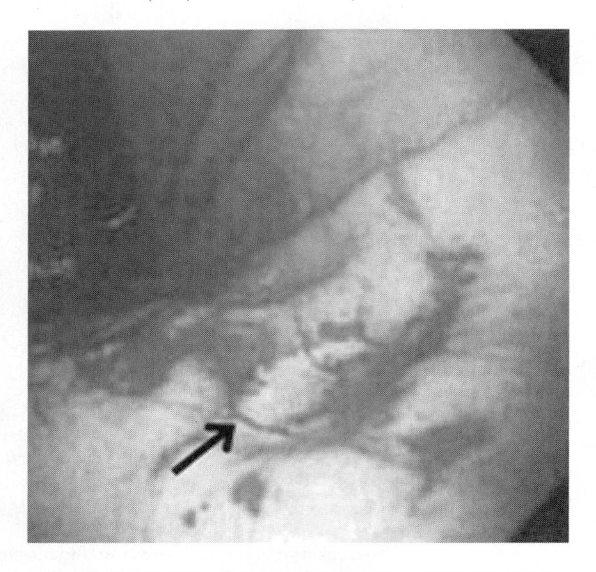

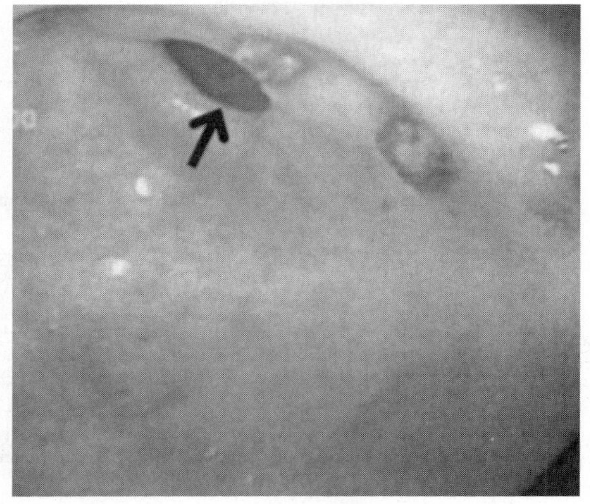

Both images are from upper GI endoscopies. Upper: The gastric ulcer is 1–1.5 cm deep, has been bleeding, and lies in the upper portion of the stomach. Lower: Note the large ulcer covered by a clot.
Source: *(both)* Courtesy of K. Kyriakidis

LO1:

Clinical Relevance

- Peptic ulcer disease is a common disorder encountered in patient care.
- The prevalence of peptic ulcer disease is thought to be about 4 million active cases in the United States.
- Peptic ulcer disease, if left untreated may cause pain, bleeding, strictures, and perforation.

LO2:

Pathophysiology

- Some cells lining the stomach secrete gastric acid and pepsin (a protease). This gastric fluid can be harmful to living cells. However, other cells produce mucous-containing bicarbonate, which protects the stomach and duodenum from damage. Bicarbonate neutralizes gastric acid. In addition, any disruption of the epithelial cell lining is normally rapidly filled by adjacent cells.
- This balance keeps the lining of the stomach and duodenum intact.
- The lining can however be disrupted by several factors. These factors include nonsteroidal anti-inflammatory drugs (NSAIDs), alcohol, smoking, and/or *Helicobacter pylori* (*H. pylori*) infection that can damage the epithelial lining, allowing gastric fluid to cause damage, producing erosion, and eventually ulceration.

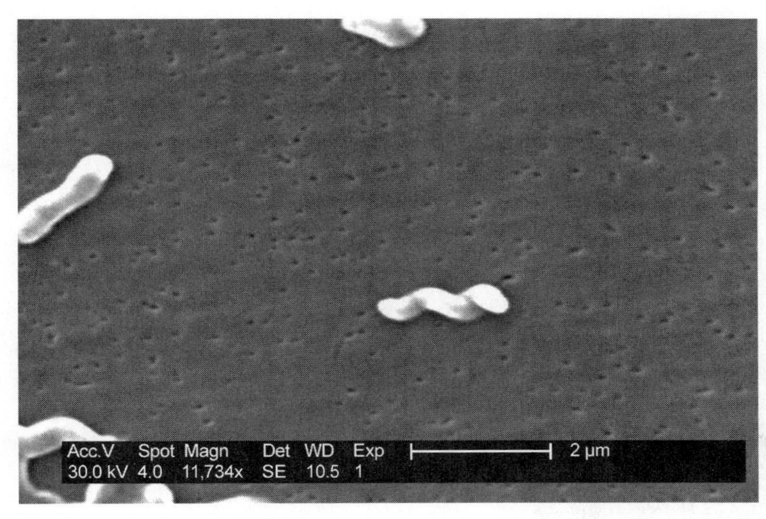

H. pylori are slender, often spiral-looking gram-negative rods that are motile and invade the gastric lining to cause inflammation and infection.
Source: CDC/Dr. Patricia Fields/Dr. Collette Fitzgerald/Photo: Janice Carr

- The mechanisms of injury typically differ between gastric and duodenal ulcers. NSAID use has arisen as a major cause or factor in gastric ulcers, while *H. pylori* is the primarily causative factor in duodenal ulcers.
- When an *H. pylori* infection is present and NSAID use is added, there can be a synergistic or additive effect to increase the risk or inflammation leading to PUD.
- Ulcerations can cause pain, bleeding, and scar formation. An ulceration can involve small blood vessels but can also erode into larger arteries, causing profuse bleeding. Perforation occurs when an ulceration penetrates the wall.
- Other factors that affect this balance include inadequate nutrition and hypoperfusion (e.g., sepsis). Patients who are in the ICU are, therefore, susceptible to "stress ulcers."

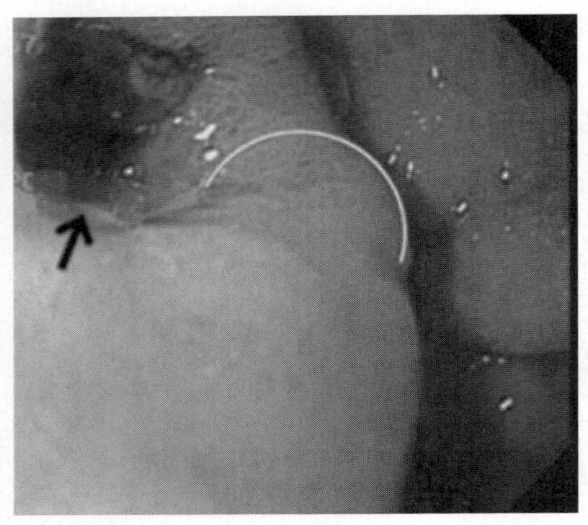

This photo is an endoscopic view of a large, deep gastric ulcer (arrow) in the prepyloric area. It is covered by a dark blood clot. The edges of the ulcer are edematous (yellow arch) and raised.
Source: Courtesy of K. Kyriakidis

Complications

- Pain
- Bleeding may be mild to severe.
- Perforation
- Obstruction of the opening from the stomach to the duodenum (pylorus) can occur from inflammation surrounding a nearby ulcer or development of a stricture from scarring.

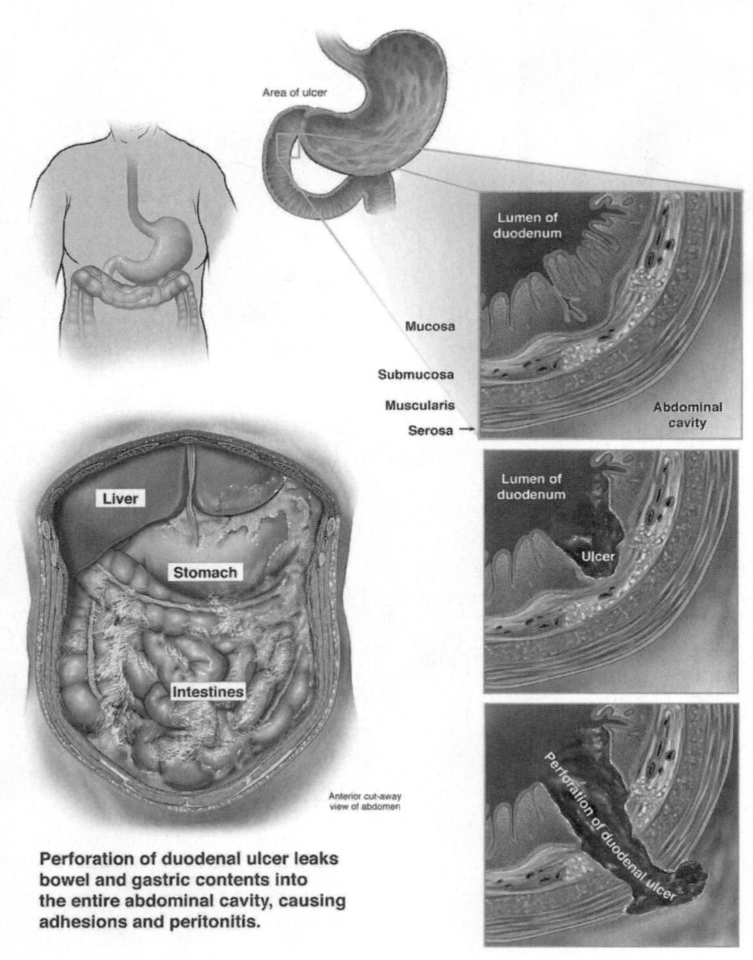

This series of images depicts a perforated duodenal (small intestine) ulcer. The ulcer allows bile to leak into the peritoneal cavity, resulting in extensive peritonitis (peritoneal infection). Mortality from this complication is high.
Source: Nucleus Medical Art Inc./Alamy

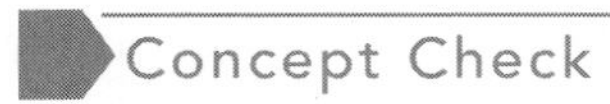

Concept Check

1. If left untreated, PUD may cause which condition?
   A. Perforation
   B. Ulcerative colitis
   C. Venous thrombosis
   D. Irritable bowel syndrome

Answer question

LO2:

Risk Factors and Causes

Peptic Ulcer Diseases: gastric and duodenal ulcers

- Gastric and duodenal ulcers are most commonly (about 90%) caused by bacterial infection known as *H. pylori* and/or NSAID use.
- This bacterium produces substances that weaken the lining of the stomach or duodenum, making it more susceptible to acid erosion. Not everyone who has the infective organism develops PUD.
- Examples of NSAIDs include: aspirin, ibuprofen, naproxen, indomethacin, piroxicam, and celecoxib.
- Other causes of gastric and duodenal ulcers:
  - o Medications, such as potassium supplements, bisphosphonates
  - o Alcohol abuse
  - o Cigarette smoking
  - o Cancer

Acute Gastric Ulcer

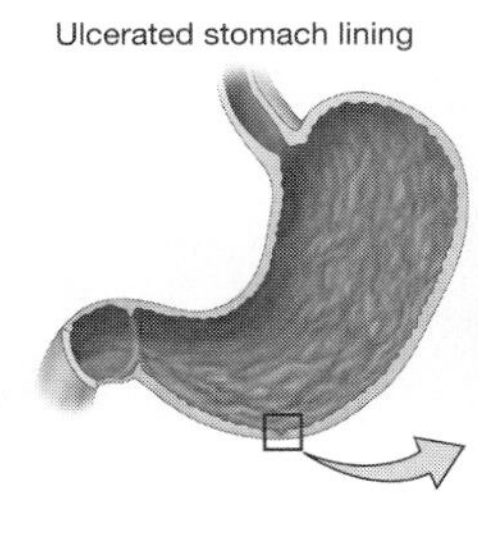

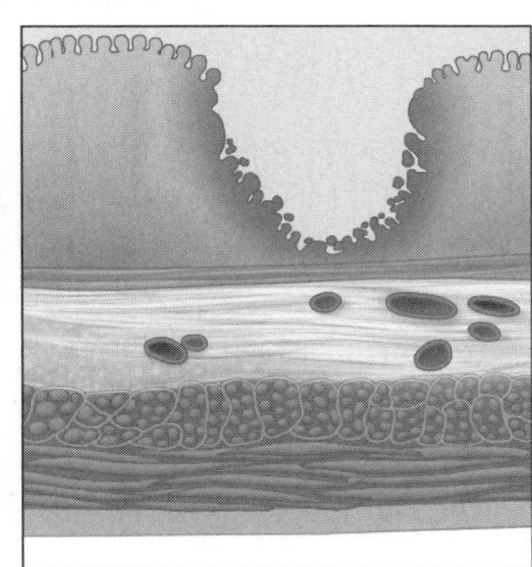

This image shows an acute gastric (peptic) ulcer.

LO2:

Assessment Findings

Symptoms of heart disease can be very similar to PUD. **Cardiac origin of symptoms of epigastric pain and heartburn should be ruled out first** with an EKG and troponin for patients with risk factors or history of cardiac disease.

PUD signs and symptoms include:

- Pain: burning (heartburn), gnawing, and/or epigastric pain
- Belching
- Nausea and vomiting
- Anorexia
- Weight loss
- Fatigue
- Hematemesis (vomiting blood)
- Melena (blood in stool)
- Hypovolemia

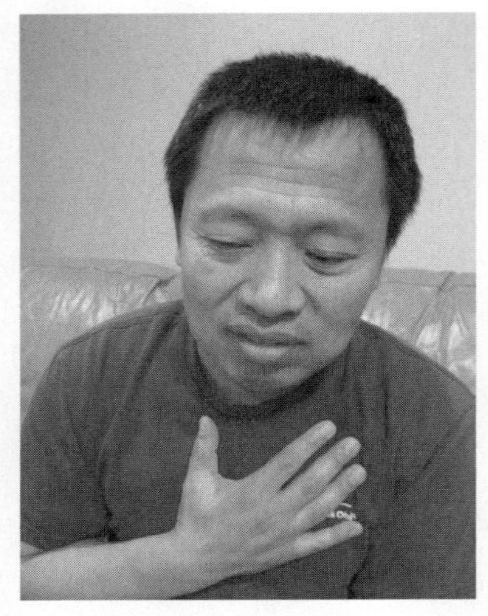

Cardiac symptoms can mimic gastric ulcer discomfort. If overlooked, the patient may suffer serious consequences, including death. Thus, cardiac concerns warrant urgent and first priority.

Concept Check

2. Gastric ulcers may be caused by which lifestyle choice?

A. Caffeine consumption

B. Drinking alcoholic beverages

C. Eating spicy foods

D. High fat diet

Answer question

LO2:

Diagnostics

Labs:

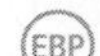

H. pylori tests. American Society of Gastrointestinal Endoscopy (ASGE) recommends that all patients with PUD be tested for *H. pylori* due to its frequency (ASGE, 2010).

- CBC to evaluate for anemia
- Complete metabolic panel (CMP)
- PT and PTT
- Type (blood) and cross match if active bleeding present or suspected
- Checking stool for occult blood

Imaging:

- Upper GI series

Endoscopy:

- Esophagogastroduodenoscopy (EGD) usually requires that the patient is NPO. Endoscopy is strongly recommended for patients who are unresponsive to treatment and for those with bleeding peptic ulcers (ASGE, 2010; Laine & Jensen, 2012). Endoscopy is very helpful in diagnosing, predicting, and treating bleeding peptic ulcers.

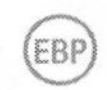

- Endoscopic intervention (e.g., cauterization) is strongly recommended in patients during EGD who are actively spurting blood, visibly oozing, or have a nonbleeding but visible vessel (Laine & Jensen, 2012).

- EGD is recommended in patients with suspected gastric outlet obstruction (ASGE, 2010)

- EGD is not recommended as a method of evaluating uncomplicated or benign-appearing dyspepsia or duodenal ulcers. Similarly, biopsy is not recommended in duodenal ulcers since malignancy is highly unlikely (ASGE, 2010; North of England Dyspepsia Guideline Development Group or NEDGDG, 2004).

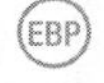

- EGD is not recommended in patients with suspected perforation (ASGE, 2010).

*Please reference the animation in the Diagnostics section of the Overview of GI Bleeding NovE-lesson.

H. Pylori Testing

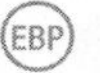

Testing for *H. pylori* can be by (Koletzko, et al., 2011):

- Blood test: blood serum to detect *H. pylori* antibody

- Gastric biopsy specimen should be obtained during EGD to determine the presence of *H. pylori* organisms.
- Breath test is a reliable test to identify the presence of *H. pylori*: The patient is asked to drink a small amount of fluid containing C14-labeled urea. If *H. pylori* is present, it breaks the urea into CO_2 and ammonia. The labeled CO_2 is then measured when the patient breathes out.
- Stool (feces) is tested for *H. pylori* antigens.

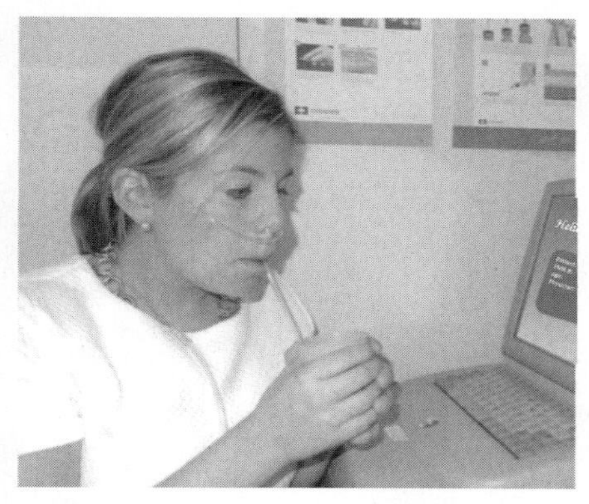

The breath test is noninvasive and can be an easy test to perform to identify the presence of *H. pylori*.
Source: Courtesy of R. Murphy

Priority Patient Concerns and Desired Collaborative Care Outcomes

Prior to caring for patients with PUD, it is important to prioritize the patient's concerns that must guide the nursing care plan and interventions. Care for the patient is ordered and organized in accordance with the patient's priority and urgent needs. Desired collaborative care outcomes in patients with PUD typically include:

1. Patient will state ways to prevent, avoid, and treat gastrointestinal ulcer.
2. Patient will experience reduction in pain.
3. Patient will be able to perform activities of daily living without excessive fatigue.
4. Patient will be able to consume sufficient calories to meet body requirements.
5. Patient will not experience GI bleed.

Considering these important care outcomes, prepare a list of the major 3–6 priority patient concerns or nursing diagnoses for patients with PUD. Be prepared to participate in a discussion of this list and/or to submit them as an assignment, as determined by your faculty. Resources you may find helpful in this assignment can include this lesson, the references, resources on nursing care plans, and standard nursing diagnoses manuals.

Concept Check

3. Duodenal ulcer is associated with which infection?

A. *Staphylococcus aureus*
B. *H. pylori*
C. *Candida albicans*
D. *H. influenzae*

Answer question

Concept Check

4. *H. pylori* can be demonstrated by which technique?
   - A. Scrapings from oral mucosa
   - B. Stool sample
   - C. Urine sample
   - D. Hair sample

Answer question

Concept Check

5. The pain associated with peptic ulcer may mimic which other condition?
   - A. Angina
   - B. Spinal injury
   - C. Appendicitis
   - D. Pneumothorax

Answer question

LO3:

Collaborative Interventions and Patient Education

Collaborative interventions are also important teaching points to discuss with the patient and family regarding prevention and treatment of PUD:

- M N Rule out cardiac-related disease, which can be a life-threatening cause of gastric-like discomfort.
- M N Identify and remove the cause if possible. Examples of potential causes include nitrates (e.g., nitroglycerin, Isordil, Nitrostat), bisphosphonates (e.g., Fosamax, Reclast, Boniva, Actonel), calcium antagonists, theophylloines (e.g., Theo-Dur, Slo-Bid), steroids, and NSAIDs.
- M N EBP Consider managing patients on an outpatient basis if they are at low-risk for bleeding, are hemodynamically stable, and can be helped by a responsible adult (Hwang, et al., 2012). Patients need to be educated about medications, early warning signs for seeking follow-up care, regular diet, and lifestyle changes (Laine & Jensen, 2012).
- M N EBP Assess patients who require hospitalization for hemodynamic stability. Patients who are actively bleeding need immediate fluid resuscitation and ICU admission may be indicated (Laine & Jensen, 2012).
- M N EBP Consider patients with stigmata of recent hemorrhage (e.g., actively spurting ulcer, non-bleeding but visible vessel, ulcer with active oozing, ulcer with adherent clot) to be at higher risk of further bleeding (Laine & Jensen, 2012).

Medications

To care for patients with PUD who have an infection:

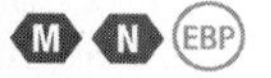

- Initiate antibiotics if positive for *H. pylori* (e.g., amoxicillin, tetracycline, metronidazole, and clarithromycin). Usually a combination of antibiotics is used together with a proton pump inhibitor (PPI) (Laine & Jensen, 2012).

To decrease gastric acid production:

- Prepare patients who are to have endoscopy that they should not take the H_2 blockers or PPIs within 2 weeks prior to the procedure (NEDGDG, 2004).
- H_2 blockers: first line agent for mild to moderate symptoms (e.g., famotidine, ranitidine, cimetidine)
- Initiate or continue proton pump inhibitors (PPIs) in patients with PUD, with suspected PUD, and after successful hemostasis (Hwang, et al., 2012; Laine & Jensen, 2012):
  - o Examples include omeprazole, pantoprazole, and esomeprazole.

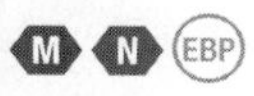

  - o Patients with an actively bleeding ulcer, a nonbleeding but visible vessel, or an adherent clot on the ulcer should receive a PPI bolus with subsequent IV infusion (Laine & Jensen, 2012).

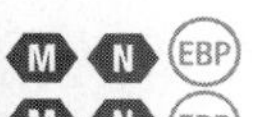

  - o Patients with lower risks should receive oral PPIs (Laine & Jensen, 2012).
  - o Patients with or with suspected PUD who are bleeding should be given PPIs while waiting for EGD (Hwang, et al., 2012).
  - o Advise patient to seek medical attention if any of the following occur prior to routine follow-up visit: difficulty in swallowing, GI bleeding noticed in vomitus or stool, unintended weight loss, or abdominal swelling (Laine & Jensen, 2012).

Symptom Management and Comfort Care

For hospitalized patients with PUD, pain, nausea, and vomiting can create considerable discomfort. If needed, be prepared or collaborate with the health-care provider to manage discomfort:

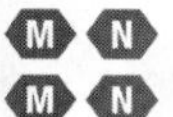

- Administer pain medications, including opioids.
- Provide antiemetics, such as ondansetron, prochlorperazine, or metoclopramide.
- Continuous monitoring for early recognition of rebleeding or complications should include vital signs, SpO_2, hematemesis, melena, and any signs of hemodynamic compromise.

For Patients Who Are Bleeding

- Urgently assess hemodynamic status and begin resuscitative interventions (Laine & Jensen, 2012).

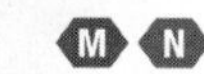

- Depending on hemoglobin, initiate fluid replacement with normal saline.

- Administer blood transfusion for acute bleeding if hemoglobin falls to or below 7 gm/dL (Carson, et al., 2012). Consider blood transfusion at a higher hemoglobin if indicated (e.g., coronary artery disease, hypovolemia).

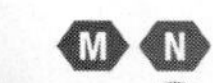

- Replace clotting factors using fresh frozen plasma, if needed.

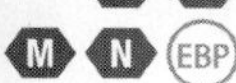

- Do not perform nasogastric lavage with or without iced saline. It is not recommended as a way to stop gastric bleeding (Laine & Jensen, 2012).

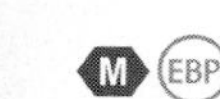

- Repeat EGD is recommended prior to further intervention in patients who rebleed after initial endoscopic hemostasis (ASGE, 2010; Hwang, et al., 2012; Laine & Jensen, 2012).

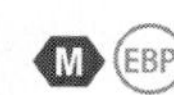

- Epinephrine injection to stop peptic ulcer bleeding should accompany another endoscopic procedure, such as clips or cautery. Epinephrine should not be used as the sole intervention (Hwang, et al., 2012; Laine & Jensen, 2012).

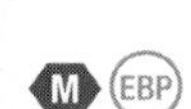

- Evidence strongly supports use of thermal therapy with bipolar electrocoagulation with injection of sclerosant. This intervention has reduced recurrent bleeding, decreased the need for surgery, and lowered mortality (Laine & Jensen, 2012).

Surgical Intervention

- Consider laparoscopic surgery if the patient's bleeding is recurrent or if hemostasis is not successful. Surgeries include vagotomy, antrectomy, and pyloroplasty (rarely used since the advent of effective medical therapies).

Lifestyle Changes

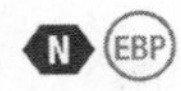

Educate the patient and caregiver about the important role lifestyle has on health and wellness. Care of patients with PUD should include (NEDGDG, 2004):

- Encourage smoking cessation: Smoking causes delayed healing and can cause recurrence of PUD.
- Avoid use of aspirin and NSAID medication with history of ulcer disease.
- Educate the patient about transitioning into healthier eating habits. Eating more often or increasing dairy intake is not recommended.
- Collaborate with patient about maintaining a healthy weight.
- Explore stress reducing strategies with patients when stress may be either a causative or complicating factor.
- Avoid caffeinated beverages, chocolate, and spicy foods. Eliminate midnight snacks.
- Decrease alcohol consumption.

Prevention of PUD

- Educate patient about self-care with over-the-counter antacids and alginates (e.g., Gaviscon, Bisodol) to relieve early symptoms, if no prescription medications are required. Collaborate with the health care provider and/or pharmacists to ensure there is no drug interactions in those taking prescribed medications for comorbid conditions. Be particularly vigilant with older adults who are commonly on multiple medications.

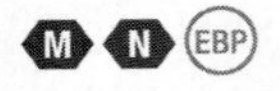

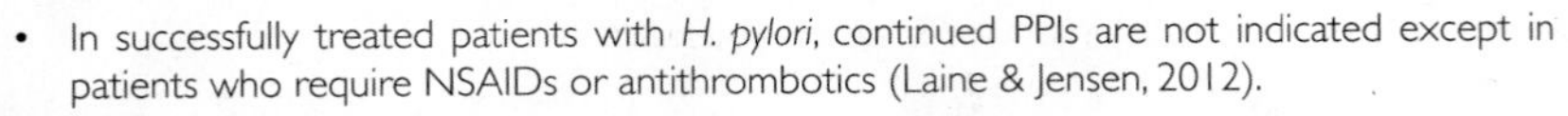

- In successfully treated patients with *H. pylori*, continued PPIs are not indicated except in patients who require NSAIDs or antithrombotics (Laine & Jensen, 2012).

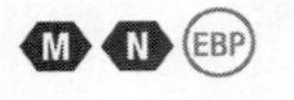

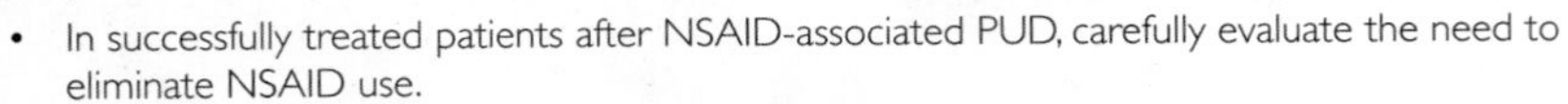

- In successfully treated patients after NSAID-associated PUD, carefully evaluate the need to eliminate NSAID use.

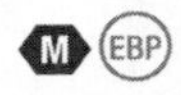

  - o If the patient is at high risk for further PUD events and it is not possible to eliminate NSAIDs, a COX-2 selective NSAID is recommended in conjunction with a PPI (Laine & Jensen, 2012; Lanza, et al., 2009).

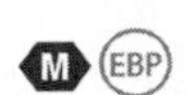

  - o If the patient is at moderate risk, evidence supports using a COX-2 inhibitor alone or with a PPI plus a nonselective NSAID (Lanza, et al., 2009).

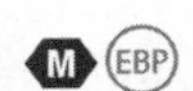

  - o If the patient is at low risk, a nonselective NSAID may be used (Lanza, et al., 2009).

  - o For patients at all risk levels, consider testing for and treating *H. pylori* if starting on any long-term NSAID treatment (Lanza, et al., 2009).

Summary of Interventions

- Since cardiac ischemia and infarction can mimic symptoms associated with upper gastrointestinal disorders, ruling out a cardiac etiology is essential in any patient with risk factors or a history of cardiac disease.
- Identify, remove, and/or treat the cause.
- Medical therapy (antacids, H_2 blockers, PPIs, diet, and lifestyle changes) is the primary treatment for patients at low risk of bleeding.
- Antibiotics are used for the treatment of patients with *H. pylori*.
- Patients with pain or nausea and vomiting may require pain relievers, such as opioids and antiemetics.
- Nasogastric lavage is not recommended to stop bleeding.
- Fluid resuscitation is needed for hemodynamically unstable patients.
- Blood or blood product infusions are administered if hemoglobin falls to or below 7 mg/dL.
- Surgical intervention is rarely used and is usually reserved for perforated ulcers or for ulcer disease that is refractory to medical treatments.
- Educate the patient about preventing recurrent: smoking cessation, NSAID use, healthy diet and weight, stress reduction, avoiding caffeine, and limiting alcohol intake.

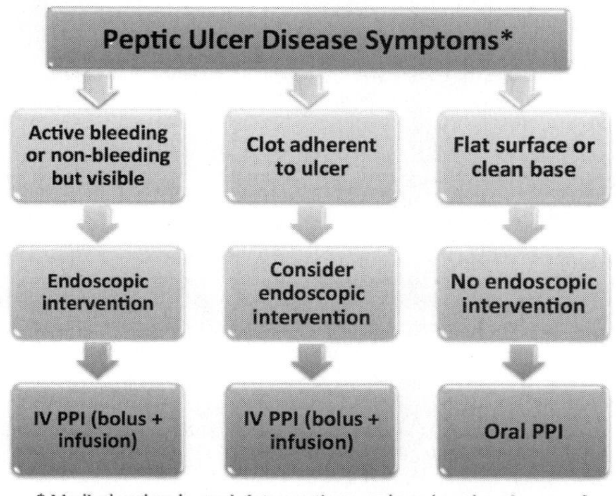

Source: Copyright © 2014, NovEx Novice to Expert Learning, LLC

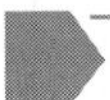

LO4: Evaluation of Desired Collaborative Care Outcomes

Evaluation and reassessment should reveal attainment of previously established patient outcomes. In summary:

- Patient accurately discusses methods for prevention of new ulcers and for treatment of existing ulcers.
- Patient reports pain has been eliminated or is controlled at an acceptable level.
- Patient reports being able to perform desired daily activities without fatigue.
- Patient's weight is at the desired level.
- Patient has not experienced GI bleed.

Concept Check

6. Which factor has been shown to delay healing of gastric ulcers?
   A. Eating spicy foods
   B. Dividing food intake into three large meals per day
   C. High fat diet
   D. Smoking

Answer question

Concept Check

7. Which medication should be avoided by those with peptic ulcers?
   A. Maalox
   B. Famotidine
   C. Tetracycline
   D. Aspirin

Answer question

References

Barba, K., Fitzgerald, P., & Wood, S. (2007). Hospital nursing: Managing peptic ulcer disease. *Nursing 2014, 37*(7), 56hn1–56hn4.

Brock, J., Sauala, A., Ahnen, D., et al. (2001). Process of care and outcomes for elderly patients hospitalized with peptic ulcer disease: Results from a quality improvement project. *JAMA, 286*(16), 1985–1993. doi: 10.1001/jama.286.16.1985

Moayyedi, P., Talley, N. J., Fennerty, M. B., et al. (2006). Can the clinical history distinguish between organic and functional dyspepsia? *JAMA, 299*(13), 1566–1576. doi: 10.1001/jama.299.13.1566

O'Malley, P. (2003). Gastric ulcers and GERD the new "plagues" of the 21st century update for the clinical nurse specialist. *Clin Nurs Specialist: J Adv Nurs Pract, 17*(6), 286–289.

Yuan, Y., Padol, I. R., & Hunt, R. H. (2006). Peptic ulcer disease today. *Nat Clin Pract Gastroenterol Hepatol, 3*(2), 80–89. **www.medscape.com/viewarticle/522900**

Clinical Practice Guidelines

ASGE Standards of Practice Committee, Banerjee, S., Cash, B. D., et al. (2010). The role of endoscopy in the management of patients with peptic ulcer disease. *Gastrointest Endosc, 71*(4), 663–668. **www.guideline.gov/content.aspx?id=37862**

Carson, J., Brossman, B., Kleinman, S., et al., & the Clinical Transfusion Medicine Committee of the AABB. (2012). Red blood cell transfusion: A clinical practice guideline from the AABB. *Ann Intern Med, 157*(1), 49–58. doi: 10.7326/0003-4819-157-1-201206190-00429

Hwang, J. H., Fisher D. A., Ben-Menachem, T., et al. (2012). The role of endoscopy in the management of acute non-variceal upper GI bleeding. *Gastrointest Endosc, 75*(6), 1132–1138. **www.guideline.gov/content.aspx?id=37851&search=peptic+ulcer**

Koletzko, S., Jones, N. L., Goodman, K. J., et al. and Working Groups of ESPGHAN and NASPGHAN. (2011). Evidence-based guidelines from ESPGHAN and NASPGHAN for Helicobacter pylori infection in children. *J Pediatr Gastroenterol Nutr, 53*(2), 230–243. doi: 10.1097/MPG.0b013e3182227e90

Laine, L., & Jensen, D. M. (2012). Management of patients with ulcer bleeding. *Am J Gastroenterol, 107*(3), 345–360. doi: 10.1038/ajg.2011.480

Lanza, F. L., Chan, F. K., Quigley, E. M., & Practice Parameters Committee of the American College of Gastroenterology. (2009). Guidelines for prevention of NSAID-related ulcer complications. *Am J Gastroenterol, 104*(3):728–738. doi: 10.1038/ajg.2009.115

North of England Dyspepsia Guideline Development Group (NEDGDG). (2004). *Dyspepsia: Managing dyspepsia in adults in primary care.* Newcastle upon Tyne, NE2 2AA: Centre for Health Services Research. **www.nice.org.uk/nicemedia/pdf/CG017fullguideline.pdf**

Palmer, K., Balfour, R., et al., Guideline Development Group. (2008). Management of acute upper and lower gastrointestinal bleeding: a national clinical guideline. *Scottish Intercollegiate Guidelines Network,* 105. Edinburgh, UK: Scottish Intercollegiate Guidelines Network. **www.sign.ac.uk/pdf/sign105.pdf**

Patient Education

Anand, B., Katz, J., Aziz, F., et al. (2012). *Peptic ulcer disease treatment and management.* **emedicine.medscape.com/article/181753-treatment**

Crowe, S. E. (2013). *Patient information: Peptic ulcer disease.* **www.uptodate.com/contents/peptic-ulcer-disease-beyond-the-basics**

Longstreth, G. (2013). *Peptic ulcer.* **www.nlm.nih.gov/medlineplus/ency/article/000206.htm**

Patti, M. G. (2014). *Gastroesophageal reflux disease.* **emedicine.medscape.com/article/176595-overview**

STOP

Go to the online course and complete the NovE-Cases assigned by your instructor for this module.

Learning Outcomes for GI Infections

When you complete this lesson, you will be able to:

1. Recognize the clinical relevance of infectious gastrointestinal disorders.
2. Consider the pathophysiology, etiology, risk factors, and clinical presentation of infectious gastrointestinal disorders that determine the priority patient concerns.
3. Determine the most urgent and important nursing interventions and patient education required in caring for a patient with an infectious gastrointestinal disorder.
4. Evaluate attainment of desired collaborative care outcomes for a patient with an infectious gastrointestinal disorder.

LO1:

Gastrointestinal Disorders: Lower GI Tract

Gastrointestinal bowel disorders consist of:

- **Infectious Disorders**
- Inflammatory Disorders
- Functional Disorders
- Structural Disorders

This NovE-lesson focuses on infectious disorders.

LO1:

What Are Infectious Gastrointestinal Disorders?

- Infectious gastrointestinal (GI) disorders are problems that can arise from exacerbation of inflammatory bowel diseases (e.g., Crohn's disease or ulcerative colitis) or from structural bowel diseases (e.g., diverticulitis), which can progress to infection, abscess formation, or perforations in the bowel.
- Rectal fissures and fistulas can also lead to abscess formation in the perianal area.
- Key GI disorders include:
  - o Peritonitis
  - o Diverticulitis
  - o Appendicitis

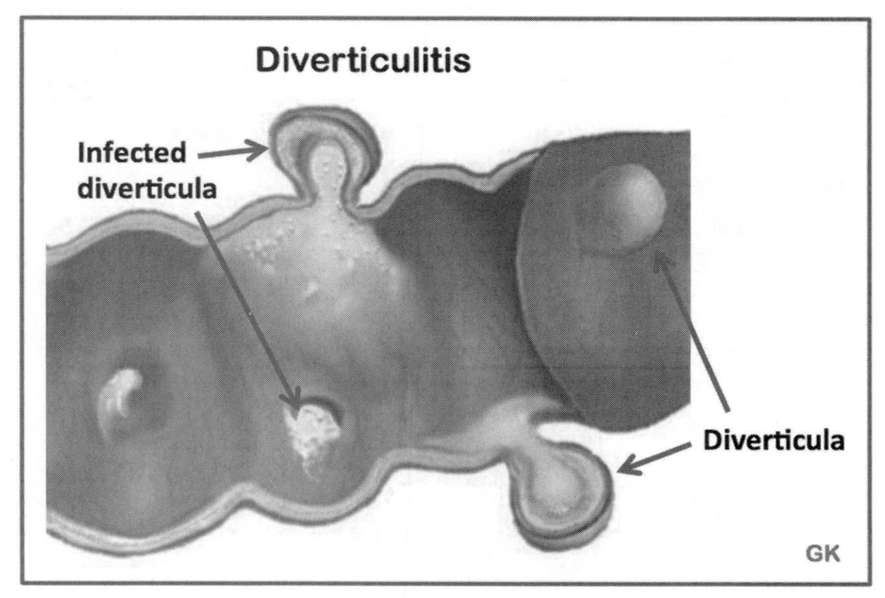

This exhibit shows the presence of diverticulitis, an infectious disorder, affecting the colon (yellow area). The surface of the colon is typically hyperemic because of inflammation as a result of diverticulitis. The erosion of the mucosa by the stool in the diverticula can produce inflammation and hemorrhage.

Source: Courtesy of George Kyriakidis/Santa Ana, CA

LO1:

What Is Peritonitis?

- Peritonitis is inflammation of the inner lining that surrounds the abdominal organs and is typically the result of an infection.
- Of the two peritoneal layers (parietal and visceral), the visceral peritoneum that surrounds the abdominal organs in the intraperitoneal cavity is often affected by peritonitis.

Fatal Colon Perforation

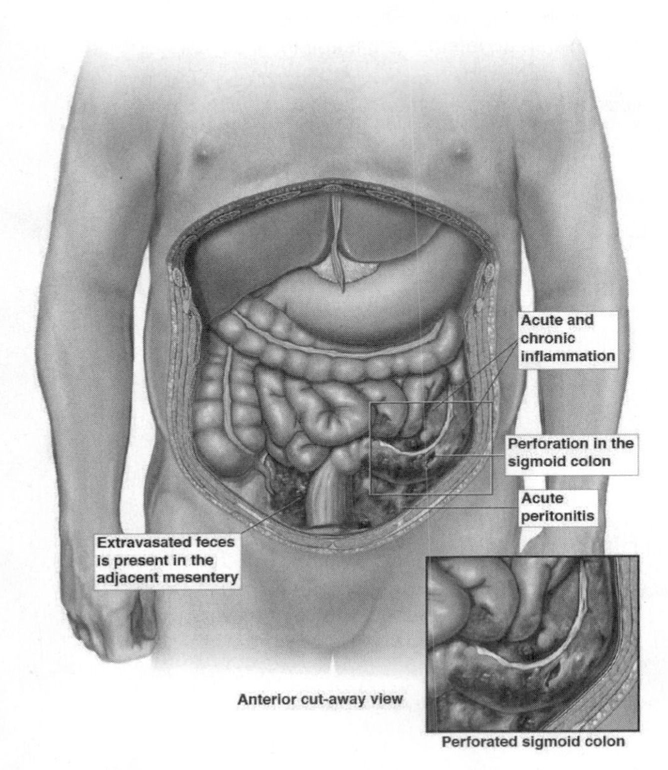

The image shows a perforation in the sigmoid colon where feces has extravasated, creating inflammation and peritonitis. The perforation that is significant enough to be fatal.

Source: © 2014 Nucleus Medical Media, All rights reserved

LO1:

Clinical Relevance: Peritonitis

- Peritonitis is a sign of an abdominal infectious process, or a perforation of the gastrointestinal tract with leakage of bacteria-filled contents into the peritoneal space.
- Peritonitis signals a potentially life-threatening condition and prompt treatment is required.
- Intra-abdominal infections account for 3.5 million cases per year with approximately 60% mortality in patients whose infections are well established and result in organ failure.

RUPTURED APPENDIX WITH PERITONITIS

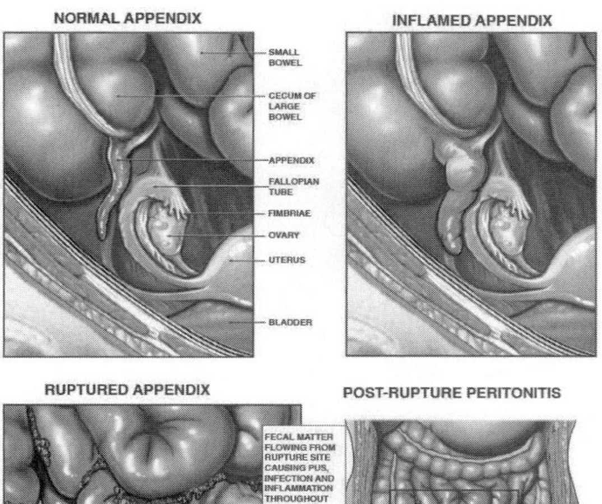

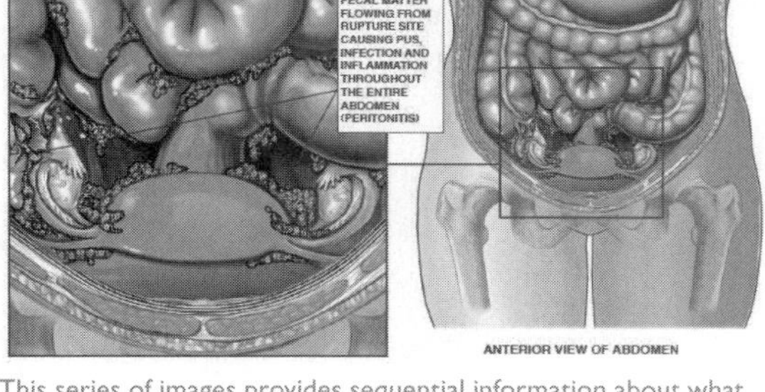

This series of images provides sequential information about what happens if an inflamed appendix ruptures and peritonitis develops. The subsequent peritonitis can be fatal.

Source: © 2014 Nucleus Medical Media, All rights reserved

LO2:

Pathophysiology: Peritonitis

- Typically, infectious material comes into contact with the normally sterile environment of the peritoneum.
- Following exposure, an inflammatory response is initiated with the influx of white blood cells (neutrophils).
- If the inflammatory response continues, it may spread throughout the peritoneum. Sepsis syndrome may then progress, causing hypotension, organ dysfunction, and death.

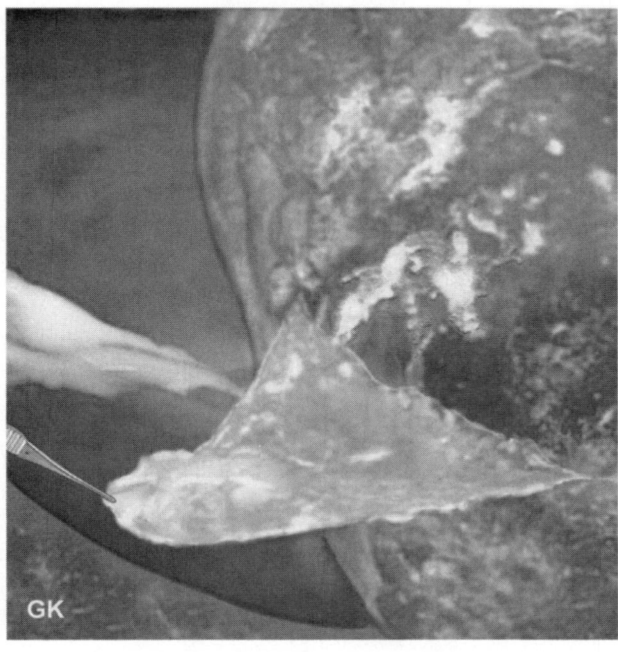

Perforation of the GI tract can result in a peritonitis as seen here in this intra-abdominal view. A thick, yellow purulent exudate covers the peritoneal surfaces. Unless treated early, the patient is at high risk for death.

Source: Courtesy of George Kyriakidis/Santa Ana, CA

LO2: Causes and Types: Peritonitis

- **Primary** or spontaneous bacterial peritonitis: rare; most often associated with chronic liver disease and ascites
- **Secondary:** most common; over 90% are associated with colon perforation, as in appendicitis or diverticulitis rupture, or colon abscess formation. It is also associated with inflammatory bowel disease, especially Crohn's disease. Other causes of secondary peritonitis include:
  - o Perforations of stomach or gallbladder
  - o Pelvic inflammatory disease
  - o Introduction of pathogens during surgery or postoperatively
  - o Pathogens from penetrating trauma to the abdomen
- **Tertiary:** Peritonitis can describe a recurrent or persistent infection.

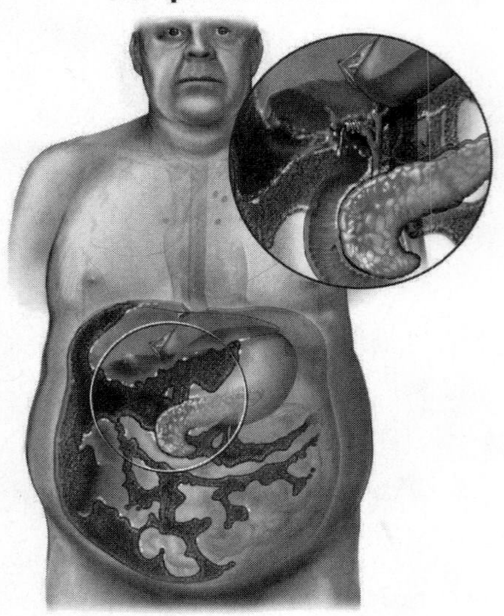

This image depicts a situation of jaundice and peritonitis. A detailed enlargement of the biliary region further reveals a continued bile leak with onset of acute pancreatitis, representing how peritonitis can spread and affect multiple organs.

Concept Check

1. Which peritoneal layer is most often affected by peritonitis?
   A. Parietal
   B. Mucosal
   C. Submucosal
   D. Visceral

Answer question

LO2:

Assessment Findings: Peritonitis

- **Pain:** very tender; pain is worse with *any* movement, sneezing, coughing, or palpation. May have knees bent in fetal position to alleviate pain.
- Abdominal muscle tensing known as "guarding," which is an instinctive protective response to pain. Guarding is elicited when pain is caused by pressing on the abdomen during an exam.
- Abdomen can be rigid.
- Abdominal distention
- Rebound tenderness may be present: Pain is worse with release of pressure on abdomen during palpation.
- Fever
- Chills
- Fatigue
- Decreased stool and gas production
- Nausea and vomiting
- Anorexia
- Leukocytosis
- Sepsis: lactic acidosis

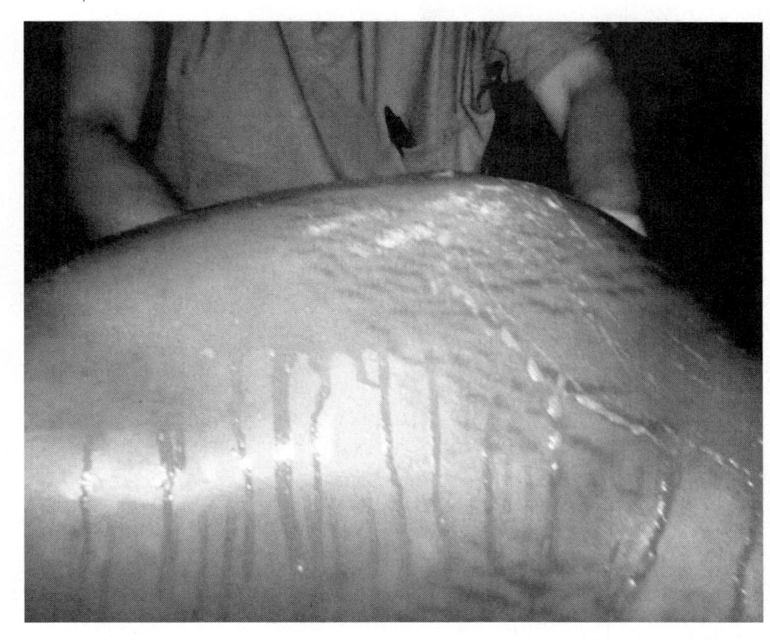

This female patient (ready for surgery) presented with disseminated peritonitis throughout her abdominal and pelvic cavity. She was originally diagnosed with pelvic inflammatory disease and developed an abscess, which initiated the peritoneal inflammatory over-response. Note the severe abdominal distention. A poor outcome is expected with this presentation.
Source: CDC/Dr. James Curran

LO2:

Diagnostics: Peritonitis

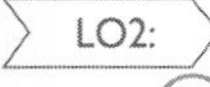

Physical Exam (Solomkin, et al., 2010):

- Signs of peritoneal irritation: can be localized or generalized:
  - o Abdominal wall tenderness
  - o Rebound tenderness
  - o Involuntary contraction of the abdominal wall (involuntary guarding)
- Absence of bowel sounds

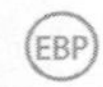 **Labs** (Solomkin, et al., 2010):

- CBC: leukocytosis
- CMP: Baseline chemistries are essential.
- **Obtain lactate:** sepsis severity indicator/tissue hypoxia
- Blood cultures: for specific pathogen identification and guide to correct antibiotic therapy
- Sedimentation rate: nonspecific measure of inflammation
- C-reactive protein: Levels rise when there is inflammation.

Imaging:

- X-ray: may show intestinal distention due to ileus or free air in abdomen (usually evidence of a perforation)
- 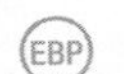 CT scan: more specific for inflammatory processes or perforations (Solomkin, et al., 2010)

CT Scans Suggestive of Bowel Perforation, Peritonitis, & Necrosis

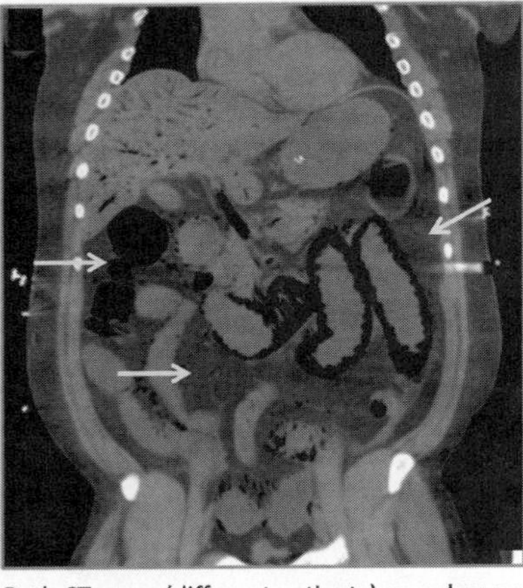

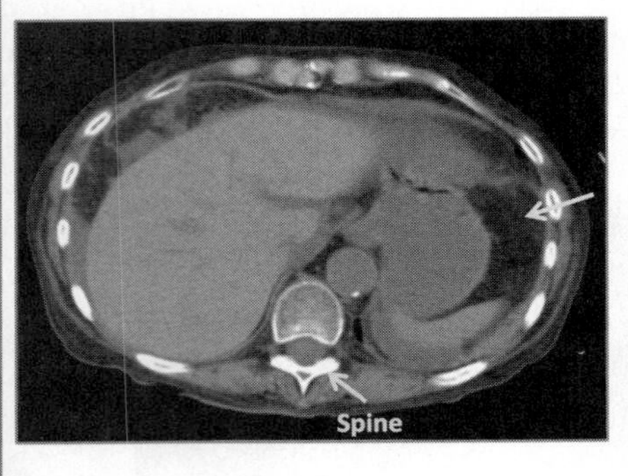

Both CT scans (different patients) reveal pneumatosis (gas bubbles around, not just inside, the intestines) which can be a sign of perforation. The patient on the left shows severe pneumatosis throughout the small bowel. Further, both patients' free intraperitoneal air (black space is air where yellow arrows point) is consistent with perforation and necrosis. Clinically, the severe abdominal distension and pain point to peritonitis.

Source: Courtesy of K. Kyriakidis

Priority Patient Concerns and Desired Collaborative Care Outcomes: All Infectious GI Disorders

Prior to caring for patients with GI infections, it is important to prioritize the patient's concerns that must guide the nursing care plan and interventions. Care for the patient is ordered and organized in accordance with the patient's priority and urgent needs. Desired collaborative care outcomes in patients with GI infections typically include:

1. Patient and family will practice or demonstrate ways to prevent spread of organisms to others.
2. Patient's assessment findings will indicate a balance in body fluids.
3. Patient will not have findings associated with electrolyte imbalance.
4. Patient will state pain has diminished or disappeared.
5. Patient will state understanding of disease process and recommended therapeutic interventions.

Considering these important care outcomes, prepare a list of the major 3–6 priority patient concerns or nursing diagnoses for patients with GI infections. Be prepared to participate in a discussion of this list and/or to submit them as an assignment, as determined by your faculty. Resources you may find helpful in this assignment can include this lesson, the references, resources on nursing care plans, and standard nursing diagnoses manuals.

LO3: Collaborative Interventions: Peritonitis

Urgent treatment is required, as this is a life-threatening situation. Delays in treatment can lead to death. Multiple simultaneous interventions can include:

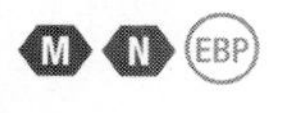

- **Sepsis screening** should be done for any infectious disorder with signs of systemic inflammatory response syndrome (SIRS) and infection: physical exam, history, lab studies (listed in diagnostics) (Solomkin, et al., 2010).

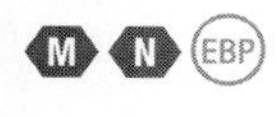

- **Microbiological cultures:** Take prior to antibiotics if possible, but do not delay antimicrobial treatment; cultures guide antibiotic selection. Cultures are especially important in high-risk patients with prior antimicrobial exposure who have greater potential for harboring resistant or multiresistant organisms (Solomkin, et al., 2010).

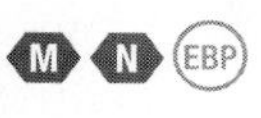

- **Fluid resuscitation** immediately for hemodynamic stability, particularly if hypotension and/or septic shock are present (Solomkin, et al., 2010).
- **Oxygen** to maintain SpO_2 >92%
- **Medications** that may be needed can include:

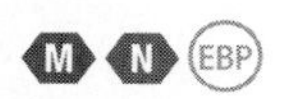

  - **Antibiotics:** Urgent need to begin antimicrobial treatment. Administer empiric, broad-spectrum, systemic antibiotic therapy as soon as an intra-abdominal infection is suspected. Cultures are needed to later guide specific treatment due to organism and organism-resistant variations. Additional antimicrobials may be necessary before initiation of procedures (Solomkin, et al., 2010).

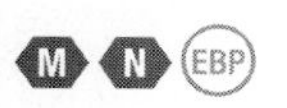

  - Collaborate with clinical pharmacists on the selection of most appropriate antimicrobials, which must take into account how the infection was acquired, the severity, the anatomic location of the infection, dosages, and the type of pathogen (Solomkin, et al., 2010).
  - **Pain medication** (i.e., morphine, fentanyl, hydromorphone)
  - **Antiemetics** (e.g., ondansetron, metoclopramide, prochlorperazine)

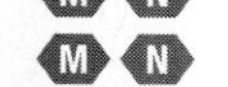

- **Nasogastric tube** insertion: bowel decompression if obstruction is present

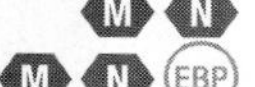
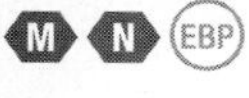

- Because peritonitis is most effectively treated with medications or surgery, administering ordered antibiotics quickly or preparing the patient for surgery is a priority nursing intervention (Solomkin, et al., 2010).
- The nurse must also be vigilant to communicate lab results to the health care providers.

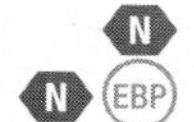

- Vigilant monitoring and collaboration are imperative to track the patient's responsiveness to therapy within the expected time period. Treatment failure needs to be identified as early as possible to initiate alterative interventions (Solomkin, et al., 2010).

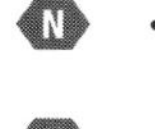

- Fluids, antipyretics, and antiemetics are also helpful for patient comfort and symptom management. These are commonly administered based on standing orders.
- Patients and families may also require information, reassurance, and a better understanding of peritonitis and the recommended treatment plan.
- Discussion with patient and family about advanced directives can assist health care providers in caring for patients in accordance with their wishes.

Surgical Intervention

Surgery is the *cornerstone* of treatment if the cause is a perforation of the GI tract or if there is abscess formation.

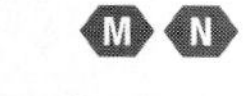

- Patients with peritonitis should be evaluated immediately by a surgeon. Collaborate at the earliest possible indication.

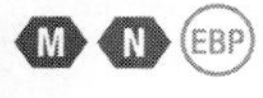

- Emergency surgery is indicated for diffuse peritonitis (Feingold, et al., 2014; Solomkin, et al., 2010). Early recognition allows immediate preoperative preparation of patient and family.

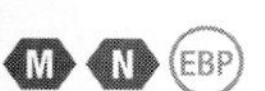

- Postoperative care of the patient depends, in part, on the extent of the surgery. The peritoneum is usually irrigated, infected foci drained, and the perforation or infection is located and repaired. This may be known as "source control." Diversion of the GI tract may be needed to control peritoneal contamination (Solomkin, et al., 2010).
- Early identification of the source and timely intervention are essential for best outcomes.

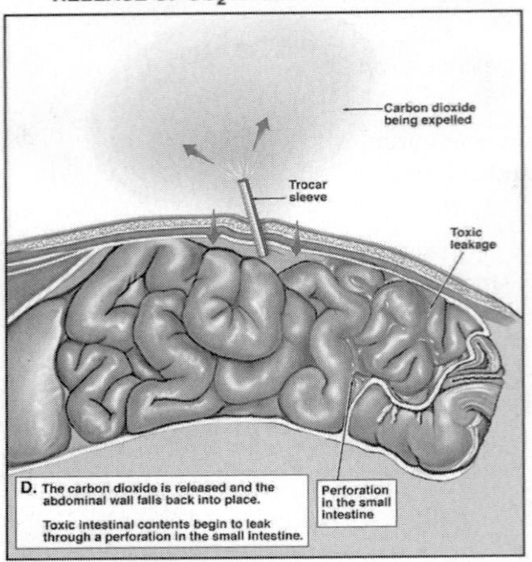

Laparoscopic surgery requires skillful surgeons. Perforation is possible. This image shows a perforation of the small intestine (iatrogenic perforated bowel injury) with widespread peritonitis and purulence.
Source: Nucleus Medical Art Inc./Alamy

Concept Check

2. Which finding would raise suspicion that a patient's peritonitis is related to intestinal perforation?
   A. Free air in the abdomen
   B. Rebound tenderness
   C. Guarding
   D. Increased sedimentation rate

Answer question

LO1:

What Is Diverticulitis?

- Diverticula are pouch-like protrusions that form along the intestinal wall, typically the colon or large intestines.
- The formation of the pouches, if they do not become inflamed, is diverticulosis.
- Diverticulitis can occur in patients with diverticulosis if these pouch-like protrusions become inflamed or infected.
- Although there is no clarity about why, diverticulitis is more common in developed nations where there is less fiber in the diet.

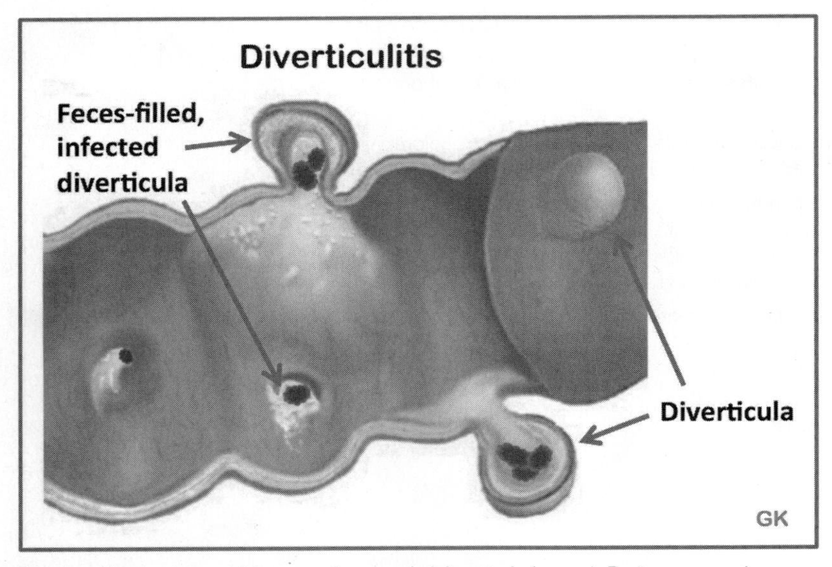

The sigmoid colon has multiple protruding rounded diverticula (arrows). During surgery, the diverticula are often bluish-gray. Note how fecal matter is pushed inside to set up infection and inflammation.
Source: Courtesy of George Kyriakidis/Santa Ana, CA

LO2: Pathophysiology: Diverticulitis

- Fecal material can get caught in and may cause an impaction of the diverticula. Trapped feces causes the inflammation.
- Distension can result from mucous produced that cannot exit the diverticula, resulting in increased pressure within the diverticula.
- In addition, bacterial overgrowth may occur and contribute to distension as well as cause more inflammation and infection. This may eventually lead to abscess formation, perforation, or fistulas.
- Inflammation typically causes systemic symptoms such as fever, as well as local symptoms of pain.

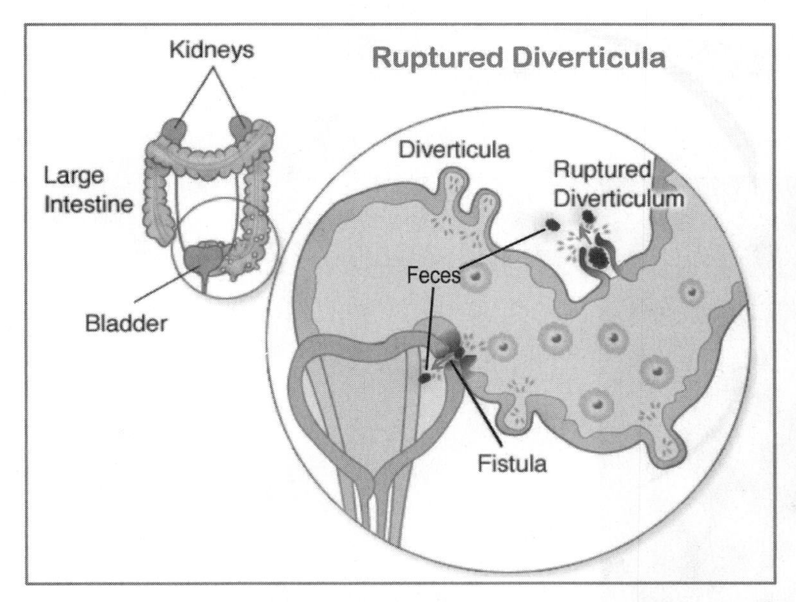

These diverticula became inflamed and ruptured outward, seen as the dark, ruptured, irregular tract extending into the peritoneal space (upper) and into the bladder via a fistula (lower).

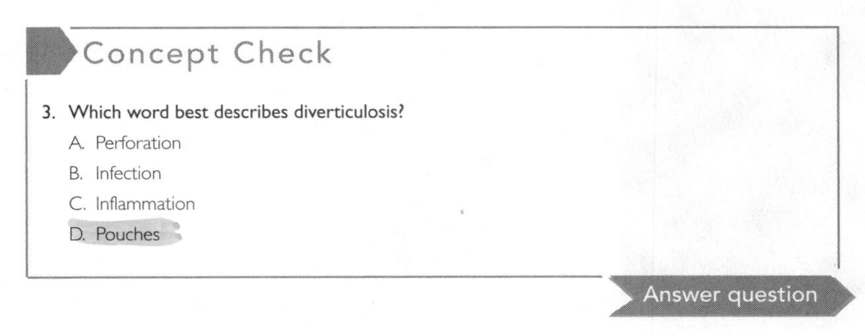

Concept Check

3. Which word best describes diverticulosis?
   - A. Perforation
   - B. Infection
   - C. Inflammation
   - D. Pouches

Answer question

LO2: Risk Factors and Causes: Diverticulitis

- **Risk factors:**
  - o Age: Wall of the bowel becomes weaker and less elastic with aging.
  - o Low-fiber diet: High fiber content in the diet keeps stools softer with more bulk, which moves easily.
  - o Lack of exercise: Diverticula are more common in people with a sedentary lifestyle.
  - o Obesity: Presence of diverticula and incidence of bleeding is greater in the obese.
  - o Smoking: Cigarette use contributes to a higher incidence of diverticulosis.
  - o Constipation
- **Hypothesized causes:**
  - o Weak areas of the colon protrude under pressure and become infected.
  - o Diverticula trap feces and become infected.

LO2:

Assessment Findings: Diverticulitis

- Presentation varies with the area of involvement and can be misdiagnosed as appendicitis, ulcer disease, pancreatitis, or cholecystitis.
- Left lower quadrant pain is the most common complaint.
- Other complaints include:
  - o Cramping abdominal pain
  - o Nausea and vomiting
  - o Constipation and diarrhea
  - o Flatulence
  - o Bloating
  - o Anorexia
  - o Peritonitis: A sign of intestinal perforation includes rebound tenderness (or increased pain with release of pressure on the abdomen).
  - o Palpable mass may be present.

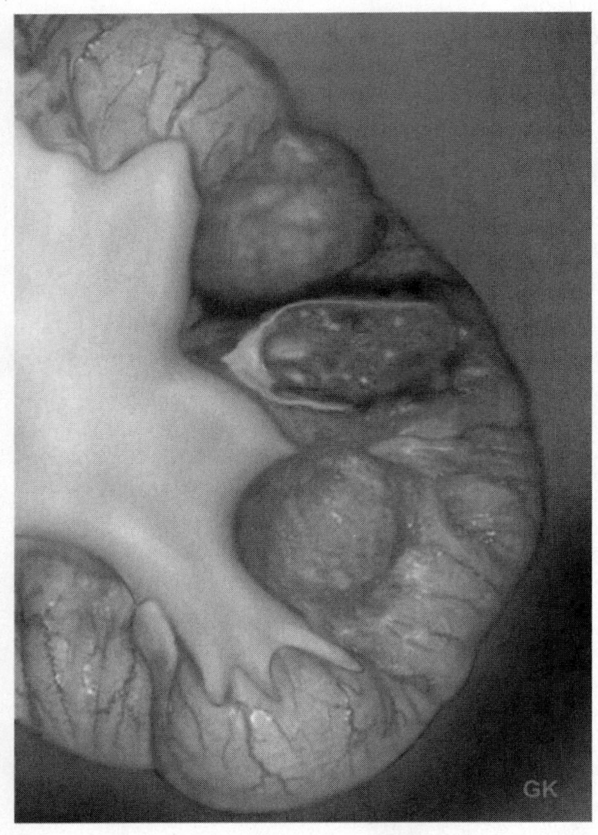

This image depicts a close up of severe diverticulitis with rupture. The pain of diverticulitis is then compounded by the pain of peritonitis as fecal contents seep into the peritoneal cavity and cause dangerous infection.

Source: Courtesy of George Kyriakidis/Santa Ana, CA

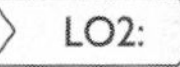
LO2:

Diagnostics: Diverticulitis

Problem-specific history and physical exam

Labs:

- CBC: leukocytosis, although 20–40% of patients have a normal WBC level
- Urinalysis
- Pregnancy test to rule out ectopic pregnancy for women of childbearing age
- Blood cultures
- Lactate: sepsis indicator of tissue hypoperfusion
- Chemistry: tests for electrolyte imbalance and liver function

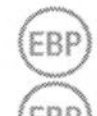

Imaging:

- X-rays to determine bowel obstruction, ileus, or perforation
- CsT scan: most accurate for diagnosis (Feingold, et al., 2014)

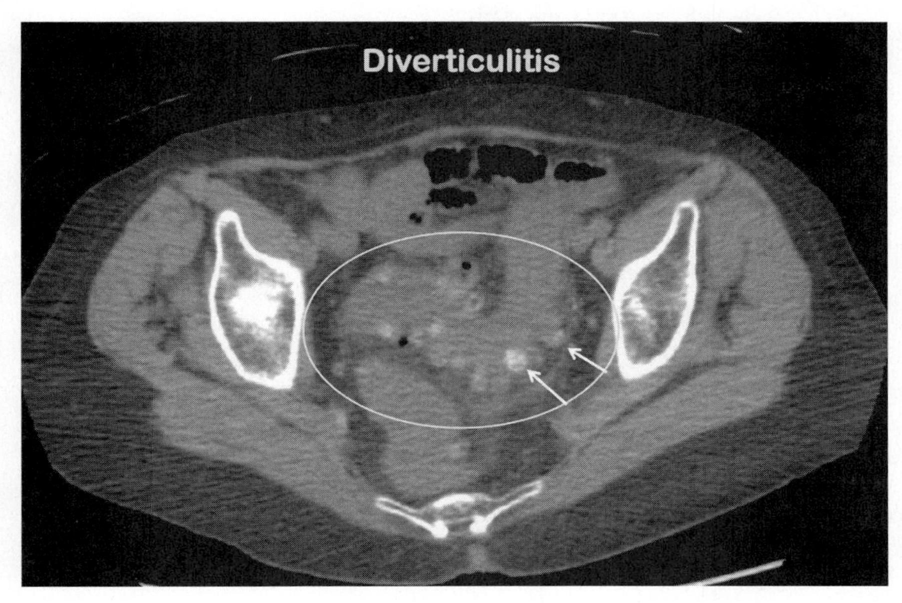

Abdominal CT scan reveals findings consistent with moderate sigmoid diverticula (cloudy, white, round spots within the yellow circle) without abscess formation.
Source: Courtesy of K. Kyriakidis

Endoscopy:

- Not recommended during acute inflammatory episode. Useful after diverticulitis has abated to evaluate the degree of diverticulosis and/or to rule out malignancy.

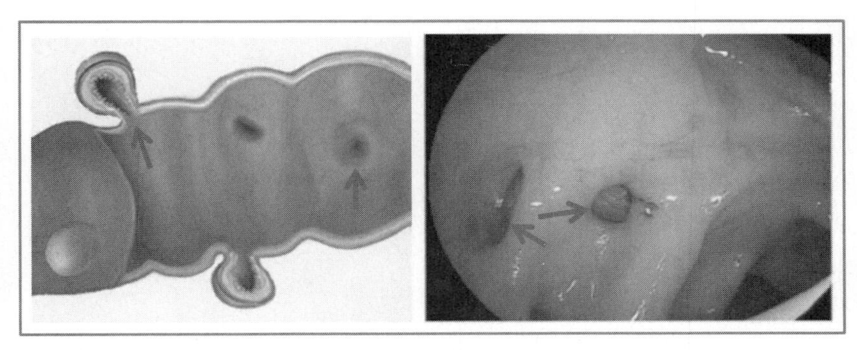

This set of images shows what diverticula look like via endoscopy. Left: Diverticula shown protruding from colon with narrow opening into the colon. Right: During endoscopy, diverticular openings (arrow) are noted. It is clear from this photo to understand how feces gets trapped and initiates inflammation.
Sources: Courtesy of K. Kyriakidis & George Kyriakidis/Santa Ana, CA

LO3:

Collaborative Interventions: Diverticulitis

Medical Interventions

M N EBP 70–100% of patients with uncomplicated diverticulitis can be successfully treated with conservative or medical management (Feingold, et al., 2014).

- M N EBP **IV fluids:** Maintain good hydration with IV fluids if patient is NPO (Feingold, et al., 2014).
- **Medications**
  - o M N EBP Antibiotics: Anticipate and administer ordered antibiotics to reduce or minimize symptoms of worsening diverticulitis to include broad spectrum with anaerobic coverage (i.e., clavulanic acid, moxifloxacin, amoxicillin). For signs of peritonitis or severe diverticulitis: Beta-lactamase inhibiting antibiotics (i.e., piperacillin or tazobactam) (Feingold, et al., 2014).
  - o M N EBP Multiple drug regimens for inpatients may include metronidazole and a third generation cephalosporin or fluoroquinolone such as ceftriaxone, cefotaxime, levofloxacin (Feingold, et al., 2014).
  - o M N Pain management: For severe pain, parenteral narcotics may be needed.
- **Diet**
  - o M N EBP Clear liquid diet for uncomplicated diverticulitis (Feingold, et al., 2014)
  - o M N NPO for signs of bowel perforation or peritonitis
  - o N High-fiber diet in the long term can help prevent recurrence of diverticulitis (e.g., fruits, grains, vegetables).
- N EBP Educate the patient to prevent future episodes and for symptom management (Feingold, et al., 2014).
  - o Diet modifications
  - o Exercise
  - o Avoid enemas and laxatives, which can exacerbate the pain.
  - o Pain management, which may include a heating pad to relieve mild abdominal cramping, over-the-counter pain relievers (e.g., acetaminophen), relaxation techniques
- M N EBP **Image-guided percutaneous drainage:** This is the recommended intervention in a stable patient with a large diverticular abscess (Feingold, et al., 2014).

Surgical Intervention

M N EBP Surgery may be required due to diffuse peritonitis, bowel obstruction, abscess formation, fistula, uncontrolled sepsis (Feingold, et al., 2014).

Concept Check

4. **Can a person with diverticulitis present with a normal white blood cell count (WBC)?**
   - A. No, the inflammation will increase WBC.
   - B. Only if antibiotic therapy has been started.
   - C. Yes, and this occurs in 20–40% of cases.
   - D. Only if the patient's immune system is compromised.

Answer question

LO1:

What Is Appendicitis?

- The appendix consists of a finger-like pouch that extends from the cecum in the lower right quadrant of the abdomen.
- The exact function or purpose of the appendix is unknown.
- Appendicitis occurs when the appendix becomes inflamed.

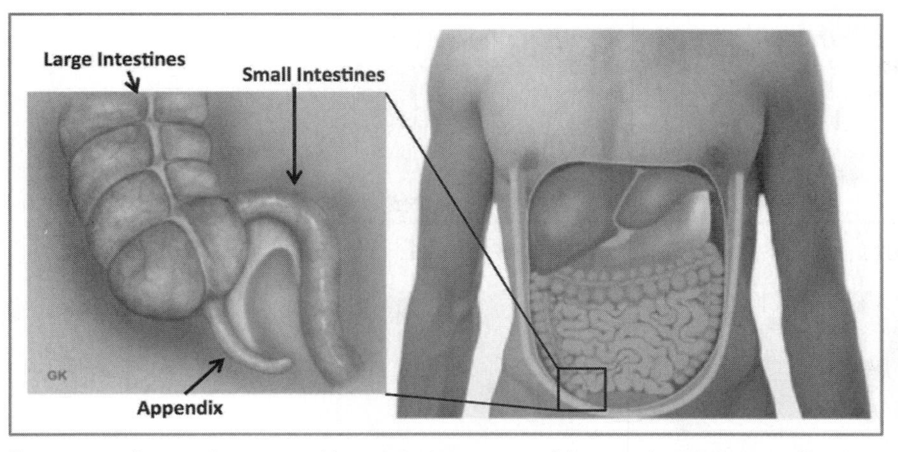

These images illustrate the anatomical location and appearance of the appendix, which is just off and below the large intestines, at the cecum.
Sources: Courtesy of George Kyriakidis/Santa Ana, CA, & Copyright © 2014, NovEx Novice to Expert Learning, LLC

LO1:

Clinical Relevance: Appendicitis

- Appendicitis is a medical emergency and requires immediate surgery.
- Appendicitis is the leading cause of emergency abdominal surgeries.
- Appendicitis occurs more commonly in individuals ages 10–30.

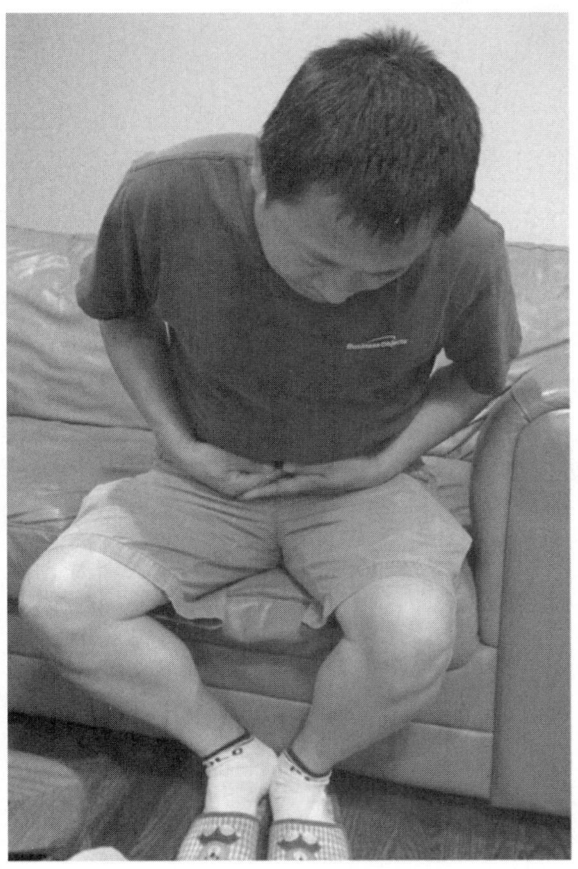

Abdominal pain.
Source: Copyright © 2014, NovEx Novice to Expert Learning, LLC

LO2:

Pathophysiology: Appendicitis

- Obstruction of the appendiceal lumen can occur. It is caused by a variety of sources (e.g., mucus that does not drain, feces, parasitic infections, or other growths).
- Obstruction initiates inflammation, which is accompanied by mucus and pressure increasing in the appendix. The subsequent thrombosis and occlusion of the small blood vessels causes ischemia that progresses into necrosis, typically within 24 hours.

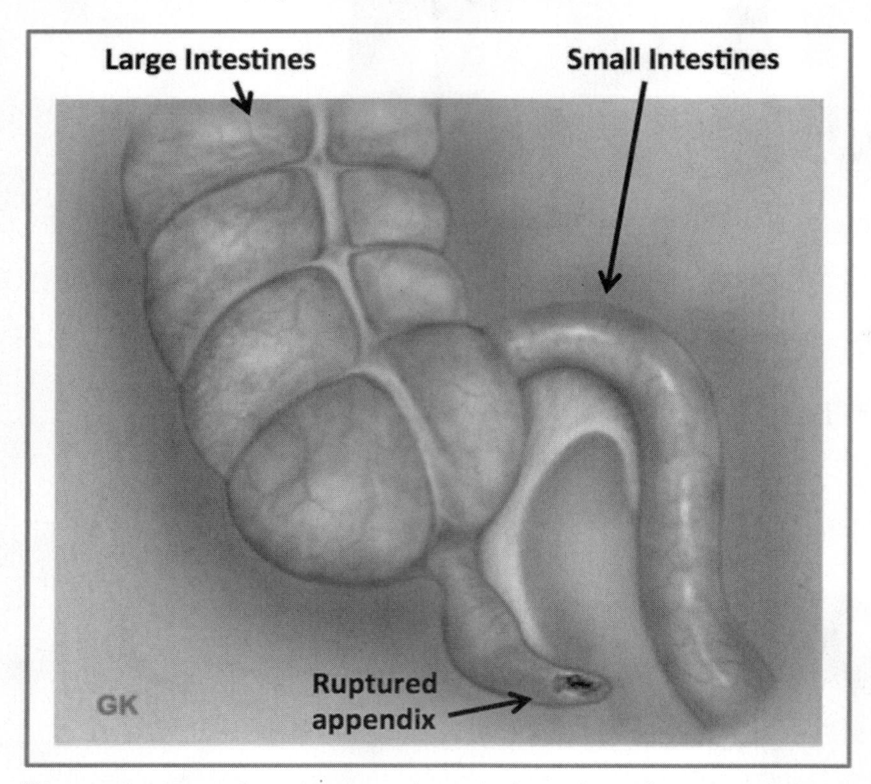

This image depicts appendicitis with a ruptured appendix. As seen here, inflammation and infection can lead to perforation and rupture.
Source: Courtesy of George Kyriakidis/Santa Ana, CA

Complications: Perforation or Rupture

- Once ischemia and necrosis develop, the appendix is prone to infection, abscess formation, perforation, and/or rupture, causing peritonitis.
- Up to 20% of patients experience perforation within 24 hours of onset.
- Patient is at high risk for perforation if fever exceeds 103°F, WBC >15,000, and fluid collection is seen on imaging.

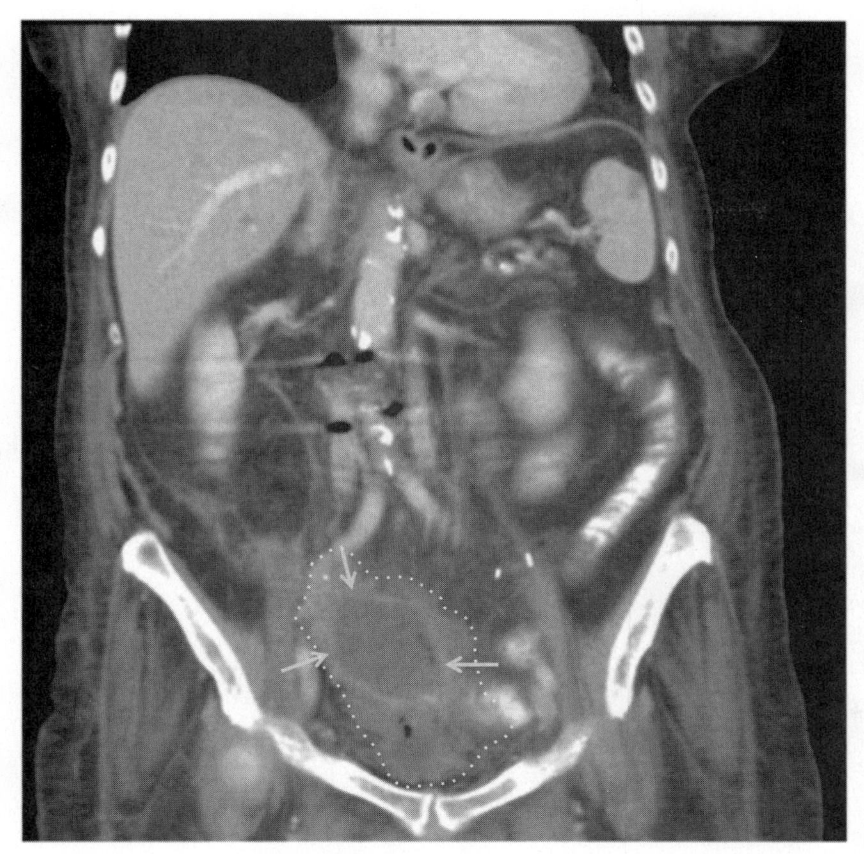

This CT scan shows an acute appendicitis and the consequences of rupture. A severely inflamed and enlarged appendix (arrows) is shown with probably fluid collection. Rupture is seen by the enlarged area that has also created an abscess (yellow, dotted line). Peritonitis is likely.
Source: Courtesy of K. Kyriakidis

LO2:

Risk Factors and Causes: Appendicitis

Risk Factors

- Age 11–20: Children and young adults at these ages are at higher risk. The reason for a higher incidence is not known.
- Infection: GI infection in the recent past increases likelihood of appendicitis.
- Appendiceal trauma: Recent injury to the appendix for whatever reason somewhat increases risk.
- Family history of appendicitis: Parents or siblings who have had appendicitis increase the risk for an individual.
- Male gender: Boys and young men have a higher incidence than young girls or adult females.

Causes

- Obstruction of the appendix opening
- Inflammation or infection of the appendix

LO2:

Assessment Findings: Appendicitis

Classic signs and symptoms are:

- Sudden onset of periumbilical abdominal pain that eventually localizes in the right lower quadrant. McBurney's point is the most common location.
- Anorexia
- Nausea and/or vomiting within a short time after the pain onset

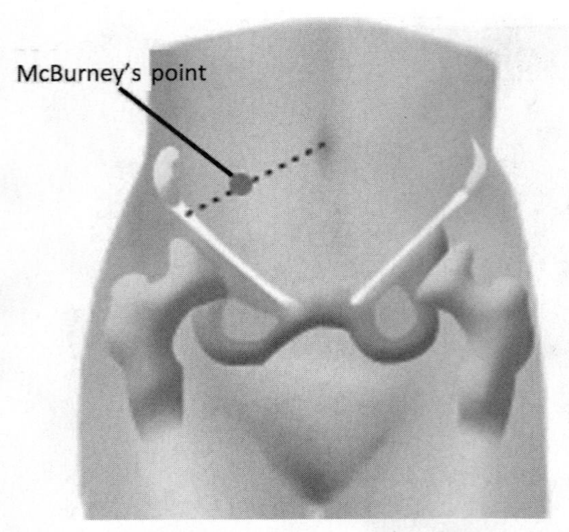

McBurney's point (red dot) is located one third of the distance up from the right anterior superior iliac spine to the umbilicus.
Source: Copyright © 2014, NovEx Novice to Expert Learning, LLC

After initial onset, additional symptoms often occur:

- Fever: 99–102°F
- Pain worsens in a short period of time (12–24 hours).
- Pain worse with movement, coughing, or sneezing
- Abdominal swelling
- Constipation or diarrhea with gas
- Inability to pass gas
- Painful urination
- The patient may experience a *temporary* relief of pain with the rupture of the appendix.

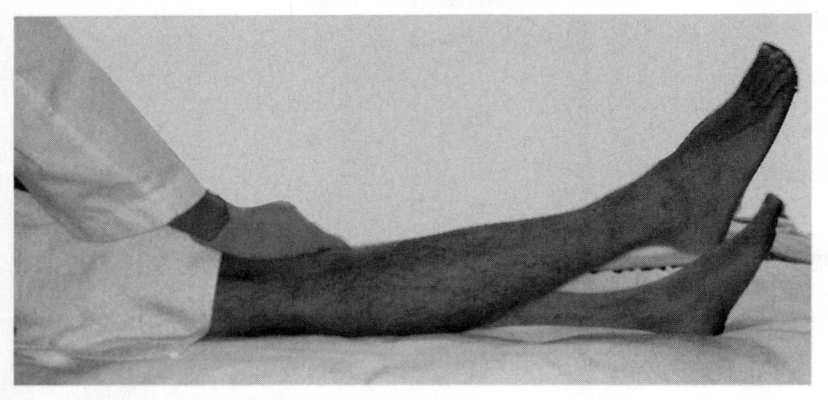

Test for Psoas sign: Perform this test when lower abdominal pain is present and you suspect appendicitis. With the patient in the supine position, place your left hand just above the level of the client's left knee. Ask the client to raise the leg to meet your hand. Flexion of the hip causes contraction of the psoas muscle. Normally, there is no abdominal pain associated with this maneuver. Pain during this maneuver is indicative of irritation of the psoas muscle associated with the peritoneal inflammation or appendicitis.
Source: Courtesy of K. Kyriakidis

LO2:

Diagnostics: Appendicitis

Labs:

- CBC: Leukocytosis with WBC >10,000 is expected. Appendicitis is not expected if WBC is normal. WBCs typically exceed 13,500 if appendix is gangrenous and exceed 15,800 if perforated.
- Complete metabolic panel (CMP)
- Urinalysis
- Lactate: sepsis indicator of tissue hypoperfusion

Imaging:

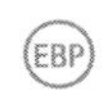

- CT scan can show appendiceal thickening, inflammation, and abscess formation. CT scan should include abdominal and pelvic areas (Howell, et al., 2010).

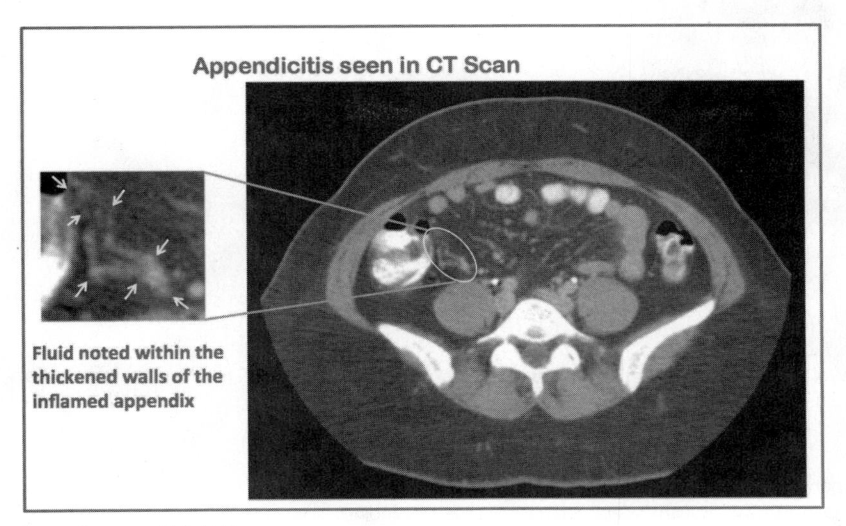

Appendicitis seen in CT Scan
Fluid noted within the thickened walls of the inflamed appendix

Source: Courtesy of K. Kyriakidis

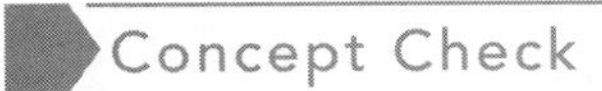

Concept Check

5. The pain of appendicitis often first appears in which area?
   A. Periumbilical
   B. Right shoulder
   C. Mid epigastric
   D. Right costal margin

Answer question

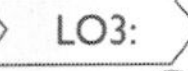

LO3:

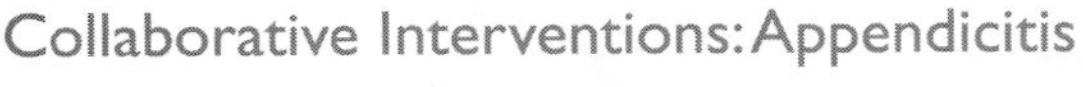

Collaborative Interventions: Appendicitis

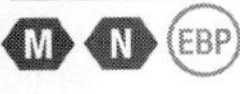

Goals in care of patients with acute appendicitis include early diagnosis and prompt surgical intervention (Solomkin, et al. 2010).

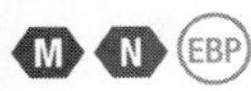

- **Surgical intervention:** Surgery, by laparoscopic or open laparotomy, for appendectomy is the primary and only definitive treatment for appendicitis (Solomkin, et al. 2010). Almost always performed on an emergency basis. Early recognition assists in preventing rupture of the appendix and consequent peritonitis.

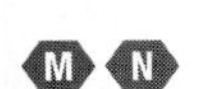

- **Dietary**
  - o Preoperative: NPO
  - o Postoperative: clear liquids and advance as tolerated
- **Medications/fluids:**

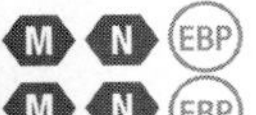
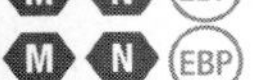
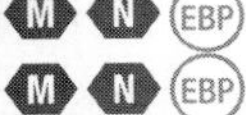
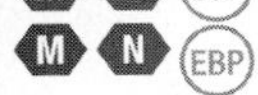

  - o Antibiotics IV: Start preoperatively (Solomkin, et al. 2010).
  - o IV fluids for hydration and meds (Solomkin, et al. 2010)
  - o Pain medications IV (Solomkin, et al. 2010)
  - o Antiemetics IV (Solomkin, et al. 2010)

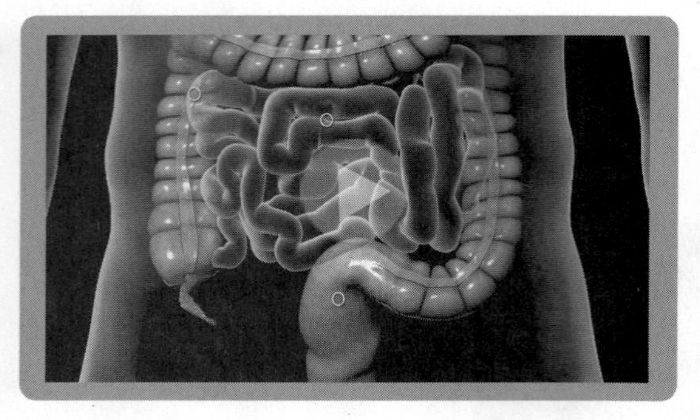

This animation provides an overview of a laparoscopic appendectomy. Pre- and postoperative care of the patient are detailed.

- N After diagnosis of appendicitis, avoid palpating the right lower quadrant or performing the psoas test, which will not yield additional information and will cause undue pain in the patient. However, ice packs to the area may help alleviate inflammation and promote comfort.
- N Monitor vital signs, including temperature, at least every 4 hours. Despite the benefits of laparoscopic (less invasive) over laparotomy approach for appendectomy, research findings point at the continued vigilance required for early recognition of complications.

Beneficial outcomes of laparoscopy	Worse outcomes of laparoscopy
Wound infection: lower	Intra-abdominal abscess: higher
Postoperative pain: lower	Operative time: longer
Duration of hospital stay: shorter	Operative costs: higher
Return of bowel function: faster	In-hospital costs: higher
Obese and/or older patients	

Chart comparing beneficial versus worse outcomes of laparoscopy.

- N Educate the patient regarding surgical procedure. Provide information and reassurance to the patient and family.

Concept Check

6. What is the primary treatment for appendicitis?
   A. Insertion of a nasogastric tube
   B. Antibiotic therapy
   C. Surgery
   D. Anti-inflammatory medications

Answer question

LO1:

What Is Viral Gastroenteritis?

- Acute gastroenteritis (AGE) is inflammation that affects the stomach and small and large intestines and is most commonly caused by a virus. It is characterized by development of nausea, vomiting, diarrhea, and abdominal pain.
- Rotaviruses, adenoviruses (types 40 and 41), noroviruses, astroviruses, and sapoviruses can all cause gastroenteritis.
- AGE is commonly called "stomach flu" but is not caused by the influenza viruses.
- Intestinal bacterial infection is mainly caused by *Salmonella*, *Shigella*, *Staphylococcus*, *Campylobacter jejuni*, *Clostridium*, *Escherichia coli*, *Yersinia*, and *Vibrio cholera*, among others.
- This lesson focuses on the most common types of gastroenteritis, those caused by viruses.

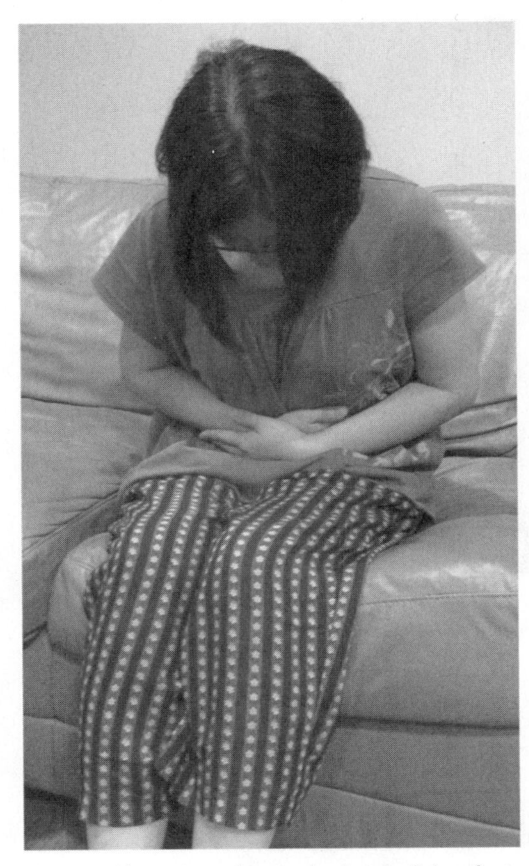

Viruses and bacteria can damage the digestive lining of both stomach and the intestine. In additional to viruses and bacteria, gastroenteritis can be caused by excessive ingestion of particular medications (e.g., antibiotics, nonsteroidal anti-inflammatory drugs) and food-borne elements.
Source: Copyright © 2014, NovEx Novice to Expert Learning, LLC

LO1:

Clinical Relevance: Gastroenteritis

- Nearly 179 million people in the United States are infected yearly with AGE.
- Outbreaks are significant public health problems because they spread rapidly from person to person.
- Norovirus is the leading cause of gastroenteritis in the United States in adults.
  - o It affects about 23 million people per year.
  - o There are multiple strains of noroviruses.
  - o Outbreaks especially complicate illness in those who are hospitalized, chronically ill, in long-term facilities, immunosuppressed, and/or vulnerable.

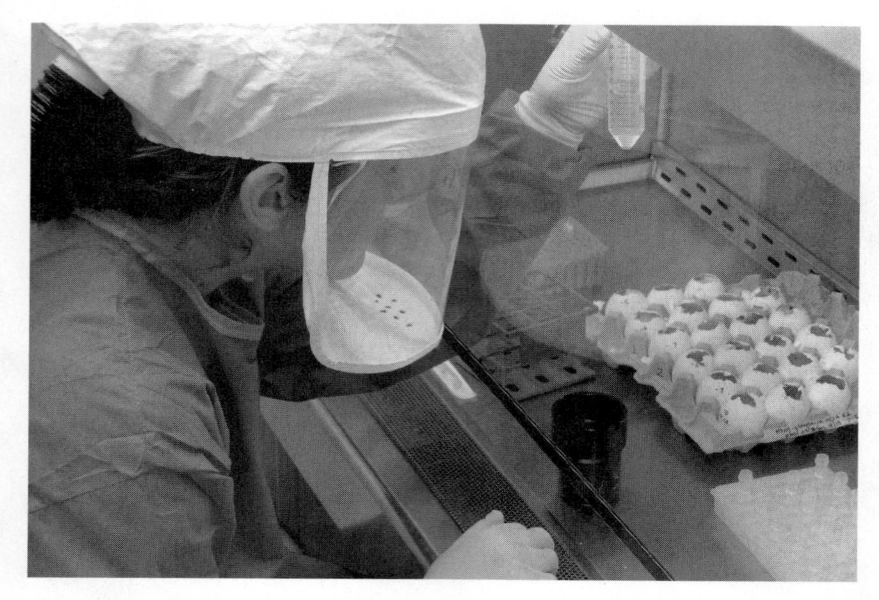

Like many viruses, noroviruses can mutate. Those patients who harbor the mutated virus are then reservoirs for infecting others. Research continues in order to discover the ever-changing organisms.
Source: CDC/Douglas E. Jordan

LO2:

Pathophysiology: Norovirus

- The norovirus is a virulent gastrointestinal infection that is highly contagious.
- Incubation time is 24–48 hours after exposure, and the infection lasts about 2–3 days in otherwise healthy individuals.
- Individuals are contagious as long as they have symptoms for up to 2 weeks afterward.
- Individuals who are immunocompromised can continue to shed the virus (be contagious) for months.
- Transmission of the norovirus occurs by various means—that is, fecal–oral, person-to-person, fecal contamination of food or water, contaminated object or surface to person, and by aerosolized vomit.
- Immunity from the norovirus is only temporary, and reinfection can occur.

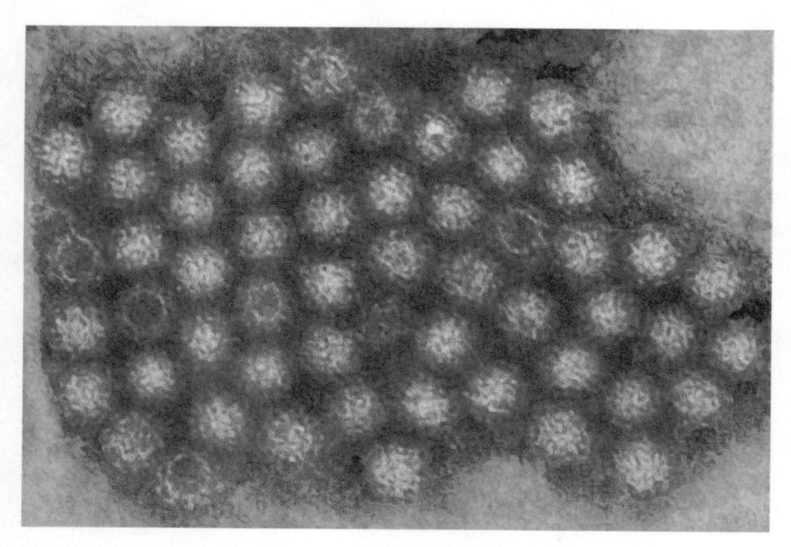

Noroviruses belong to the genus Norovirus. They are a group of related, single-stranded RNA viruses that cause acute gastroenteritis in humans. Norovirus was recently approved as the official genus name for the group of viruses provisionally described as "Norwalk-like viruses" (NLV).
Source: CDC/Charles D. Humphrey

- The norovirus does not multiply in food as bacteria do and is destroyed by thorough cooking at 212°F.
- It takes as little as 10 viral particles to cause an infection.
- The norovirus can remain alive for days on surfaces; however, disinfection with appropriate solutions eradicates the virus.
- **Hand sanitizers are not effective against the norovirus** (Centers for Disease Control and Prevention [CDC], 2013).
- The norovirus can withstand freezing as well as acidic conditions and will survive in saltwater for up to 6 days.
- The U.S. Food and Drug Administration (FDA) reported that there is evidence of "person to person" transmission of the norovirus; however, the "norwalk (same virus) gastroenteritis" is commonly transmitted through fecal–oral contamination of water and foods. Contaminated water from wells, lakes, water storage tanks (cruise ships), municipal supplies and pools are likely sources of the norovirus.

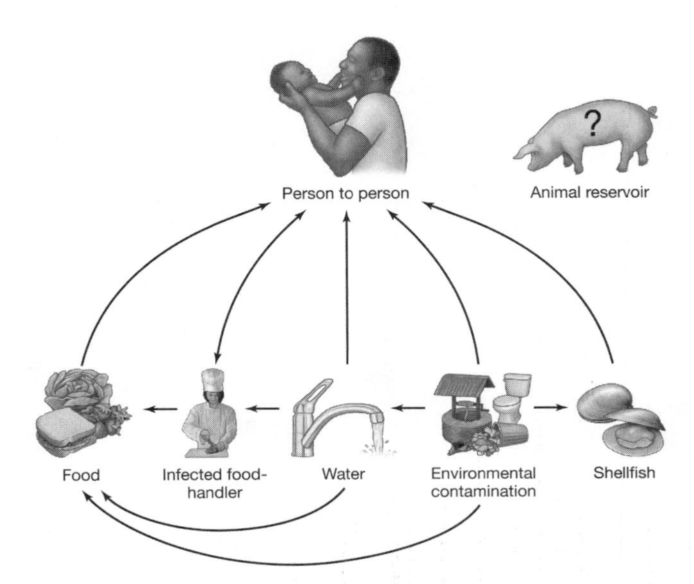

This diagram suggests some of the various ways that humans become infected by the norovirus and develop acute gastroenteritis.

LO2:

Assessment Findings: Gastroenteritis

Common symptoms of AGE include:

- Diarrhea: varies in character and frequency depending on infecting agent, usually watery
- Vomiting
- Cramping low abdominal or periumbilical pain
- Dehydration: dry mucous membranes, poor skin turgor, decreased urination; hypotension and tachycardia if severe
- Hypokalemia
- Fever occurs in up to half of infected individuals.
- Muscle aches
- Headache
- Most symptoms for norovirus last 2–3 days, longer with other infecting agents, in otherwise healthy individuals. The noroviruses do not typically produce blood or pus in the stool like a bacterial infection such as *Shigella* or *Campylobacter* can.

Concept Check

7. For how long can an otherwise healthy person be contagious after contracting a norovirus?
   A. Until fever is resolved
   B. For the length of time the patient has diarrhea
   C. For up to 2 weeks after symptoms clear
   D. For several months after having the disease

Answer question

LO2:

Diagnostics: Gastroenteritis

Labs:

- CBC: Look for leukocytosis.
- CMP: electrolyte imbalance
- Urinalysis
- Stool for ova and parasites
- Fecal leukocytes strong indicator of inflammatory diarrhea
- Lactate: sepsis indicator for tissue hypoperfusion

Imaging:

- Abdominal x-rays and CT scan indicated if bowel obstruction, perforation, or toxic megacolon is suspected.

Endoscopy:

- Sigmoidoscopy for inflammatory bowel disease, if suspected

LO3:

Collaborative Interventions: Gastroenteritis

Care of patients with gastroenteritis focuses on symptom management, comfort care, and prevention of spread to others:

- M N EBP Fluids: IV isotonic or oral hydration, if tolerated, are focal in treatment (CDC, 2011; Cincinnati Children's Hospital, 2011).
- M N EBP Electrolyte replacement, guided by lab results if needed, are the second focus of treatment (CDC, 2011; Cincinnati Children's Hospital, 2011).
- M N EBP Antimicrobials: Management with antimicrobial agents depends on identifying or ruling out a specific infecting agent (Cincinnati Children's Hospital, 2011).
- M N Antipyretics may be used for fever, aching, and mild to moderate pain relief (e.g., acetaminophen)
- M N Pain medications (e.g., ketorolac, hydrocodone, morphine)
- M N Antidiarrheals: loperamide, diphenoxylate with atropine
- M N Antiemetics: metoclopramide, ondansetron
- N EBP Disinfect surfaces and objects with bleach solutions or other approved disinfectants as specified by each facility (CDC, 2011).
- M N EBP Implement strict contact isolation precautions, which are imperative to prevent the spread of infectious organisms (CDC, 2011).
- M N EBP Isolation precautions include (CDC, 2011):
  - Private room
  - Gown and gloves for all person entering the room
  - M N EBP Stringent hand washing with soap and water with any encounter (Cincinnati Children's Hospital, 2011).
- N EBP Ensure the clinicians and families adhere to strict hand hygiene with soap and water. **Hand sanitizers are NOT effective alone** against the norovirus or *Clostridium difficile* (*C. diff*) (CDC, 2011).

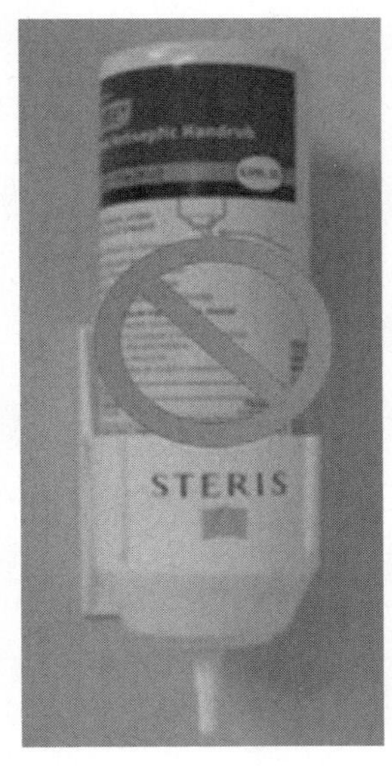

Do not rely on hand sanitizers for *C. diff* and norovirus precautions. Always use soap and water.

Safety, Prevention, and Education

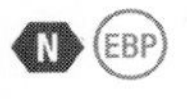

- The highest priority intervention in caring for patients with gastroenteritis and for the community is to prevent the spread of the virus. Strict adherence to soap and water for good hand hygiene and isolation of sick persons are imperative (CDC, 2011; Cincinnati Children's Hospital, 2011).

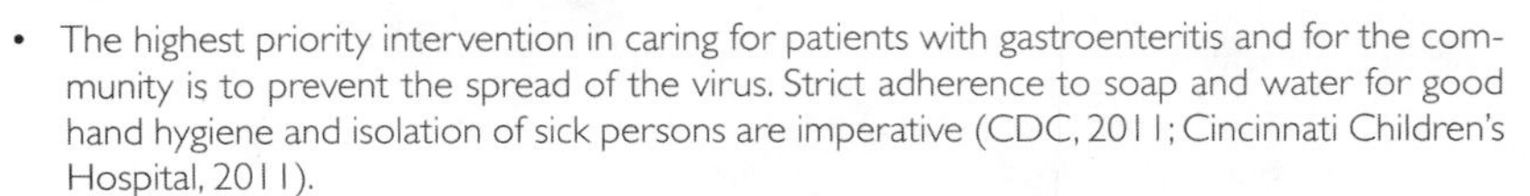

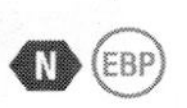

- Education for the patient and family about ways to prevent the spread of the virus is also important (see Patient Education section) (CDC, 2011; Cincinnati Children's Hospital, 2011).

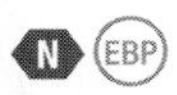

- Careful assessment of fluid and electrolyte status is important as diarrhea and vomiting can cause significant imbalances. Dry mucous membranes, sunken eyes, poor skin turgor, and decreased urine output may indicate dehydration or hypovolemia. Lethargy, irritability, confusion, weakness, and muscle twitching may indicate hyponatremia, which is often caused by gastroenteritis (Cincinnati Children's Hospital, 2011).

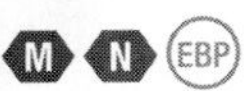

- Health care providers who have been sick should not return to work for a minimum of 48 hours after symptoms are absent (CDC, 2011).

Concept Check

8. Which intervention is most likely to help prevent the spread of the norovirus?

A. Liberal use of alcohol-based hand sanitizers

B. Private room for infected patients

C. Use of gowns and masks by all caregivers

D. Hand washing with soap and water

Answer question

Collaborative Interventions: Gastroenteritis (continued)

Patient Education

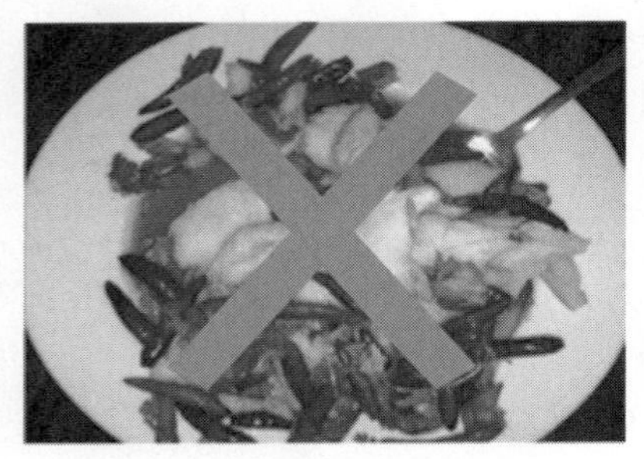

Source: Copyright © 2014, NovEx Novice to Expert Learning, LLC

- Withhold food and liquids for several hours to allow gastric upset to subside.

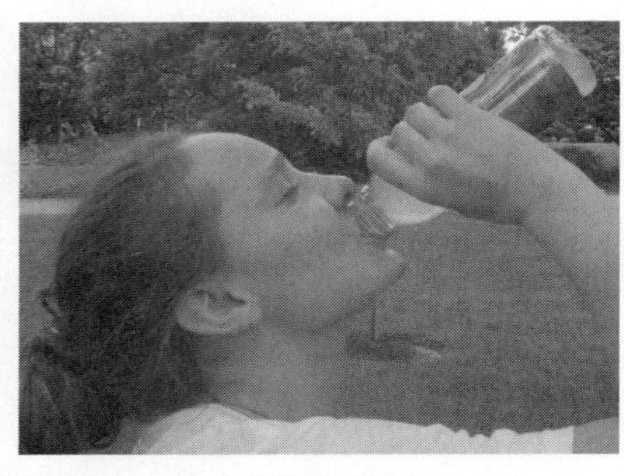

Source: Copyright © 2014, NovEx Novice to Expert Learning, LLC

- To avoid dehydration, replace fluids with dilute electrolyte drinks (e.g., Pedialyte, Ceralyte), rehydration salt solutions (e.g., rehydration salt packets mixed in water), or water. Colas, juices, chicken broth, and sports drinks should be avoided in severe vomiting and diarrhea. Rehydration solutions are easy to make using 2 tablespoons of sugar and one-half teaspoon of salt mixed into a quart or liter of water.

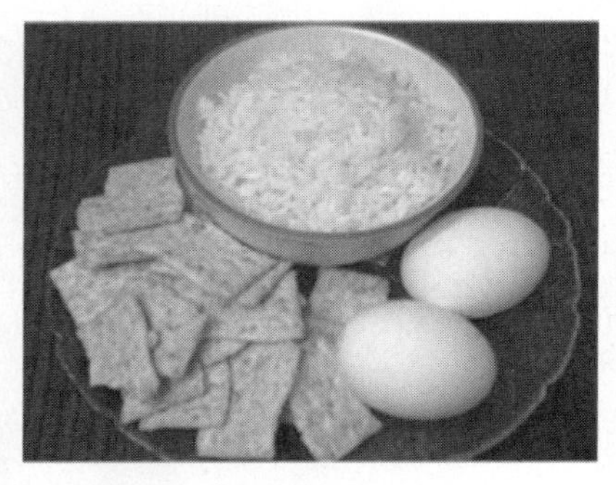

Source: Copyright © 2014, NovEx Novice to Expert Learning, LLC

- Twenty-four hours after onset, slowly eat bland, simple foods (e.g., rice, toast, crackers, gelatin, dry rice cereal, or bananas).

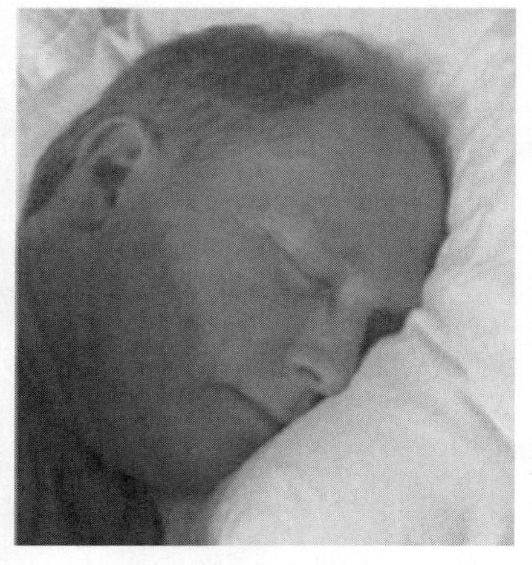

Source: Copyright © 2014, NovEx Novice to Expert Learning, LLC

- Getting plenty of rest will help alleviate fatigue and weakness.

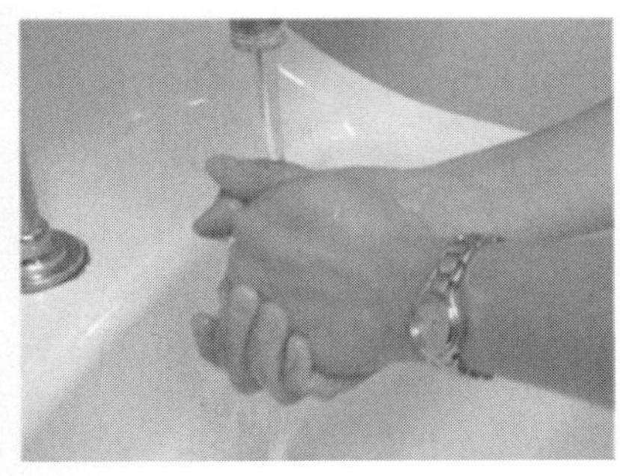

Source: Copyright © 2014. NovEx Novice to Expert Learning, LLC

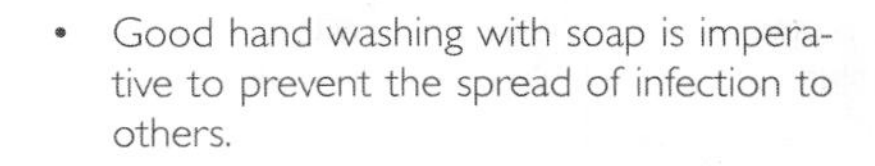

- Good hand washing with soap is imperative to prevent the spread of infection to others.

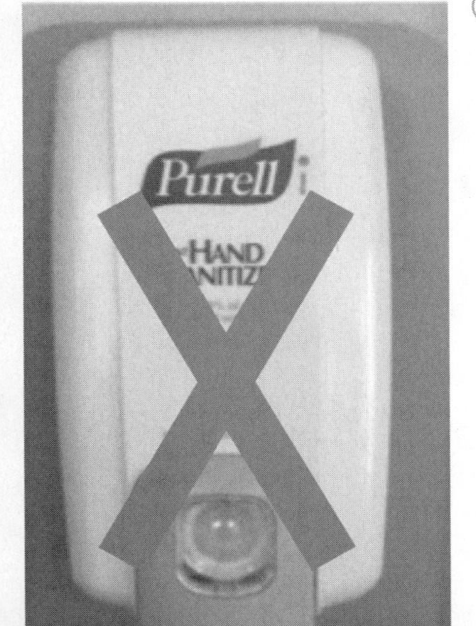

Source: Copyright © 2014, NovEx Novice to Expert Learning, LLC

EBP

- Hand sanitizers are not effective alone against the norovirus or *C. diff.* Use soap and water (CDC, 2011).

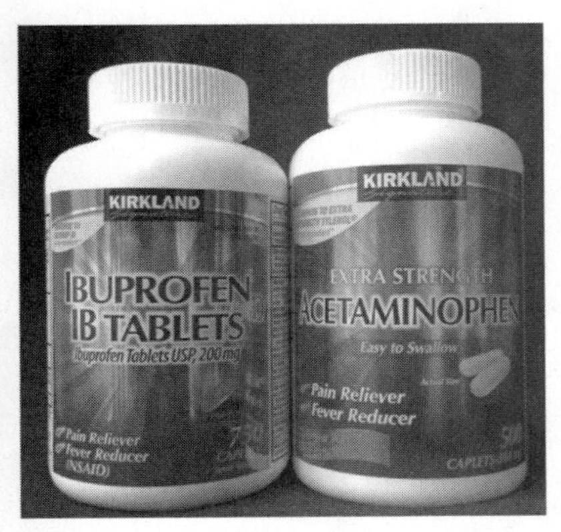

Source: Copyright © 2014, NovEx Novice to Expert Learning, LLC

- Antipyretics may be needed to control fever and reduce aching and discomfort.

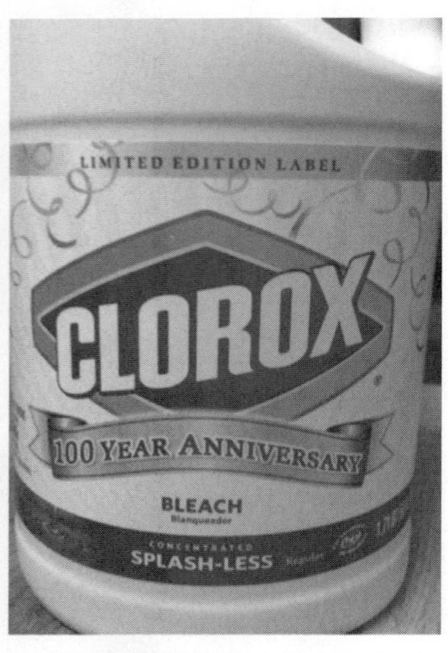

Source: Copyright © 2014, NovEx Novice to Expert Learning, LLC

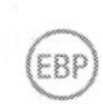

- Disinfect surfaces and objects with bleach solutions to kill virulent strains of viruses or organisms (CDC, 2011).

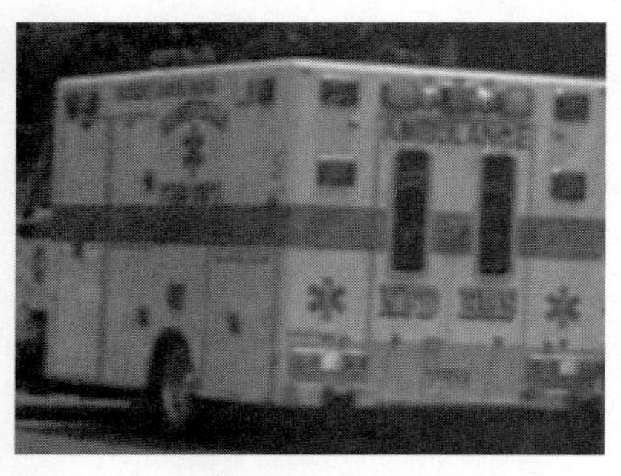

Source: Copyright © 2014, NovEx Novice to Expert Learning, LLC

- If severe or persistent diarrhea, dehydration, and vomiting occur, seek medical attention. Bloody diarrhea should trigger concern. Antiemetics and/or antidiarrheals may be needed. Also, instruct family to seek medical attention if three or four of these symptoms are seen in combination: very drowsy, eyes are very sunken, tongue is dry, tears are absent, and skin is cold or sweaty.

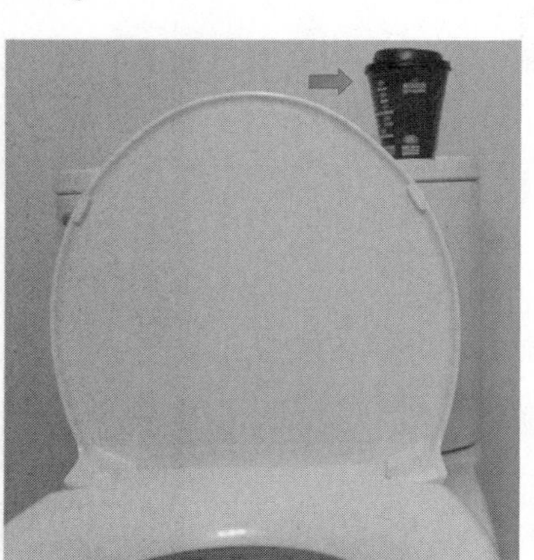

Source: Copyright © 2014, NovEx Novice to Expert Learning, LLC

- Make sure foods are cooked and from sources not contaminated by sewage, such as food in the bathroom.

Concept Check

9. Which finding would indicate possible hyponatremia as a complication of gastroenteritis?

A. Poor skin turgor

B. Fever

C. Stomach cramping

D. Muscle twitching

Answer question

LO1:

What Is Infectious Colitis?

- Infectious colitis is a bacterial infection of the colon causing severe diarrhea and fever.
- Infections of the colon are commonly caused by bacteria and protozoa. Viruses more typically invade the small intestines.
- Depending on the type of infection and the severity, complications may develop quickly.

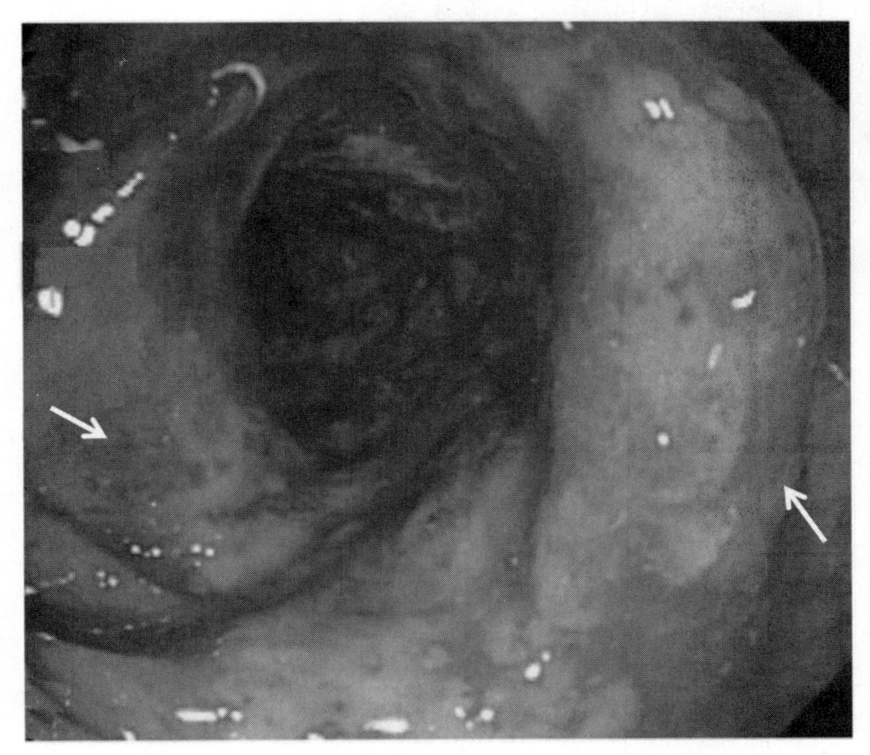

This photo shows diffuse inflammation (white arrows) throughout the entire colon of a 37-year-old male. He has experienced chronic ulcerative colitis. Seeing the condition of the patient's GI tract helps one understand why the patient experiences abdominal cramping, diarrhea, and even bleeding.
Source: Courtesy of K. Kyriakidis

LO2:

Pathophysiology: Infectious Colitis

- Pathogens that infect the colon cause inflammation.
- Inflammation leads to damage, denuding of the mucosa, and ulceration of the colon wall, with subsequent bleeding, increased mucous production, and diarrhea.
- Release of cytokines by inflammatory cells as well as toxins by the pathogens cause systemic symptoms, such as fever and sepsis.

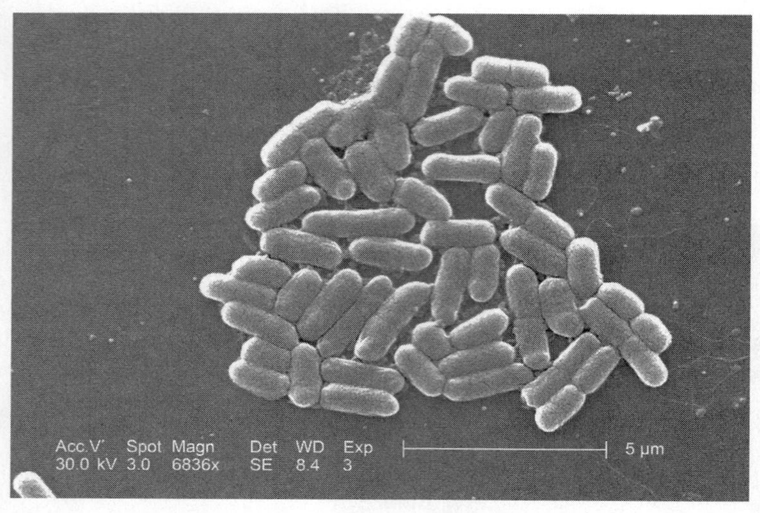

There are hundreds of strains of harmless *E. coli*, some of which reside as normal GI flora. The one in this photo, however, causes severe colitis with bloody diarrhea in humans by producing a powerful toxin. Upon close inspection, the flagella (thin, whip-like tail) can be seen on the *E. coli* bacteria.
Source: CDC/Janice Haney Carr

Concept Check

10. Which organisms are likely to cause infectious colitis?

A. Protozoa
B. Viruses
C. Prions
D. Parasites

Answer question

LO2:

Risk Factors and Causes: Infectious Colitis

Risk Factors

- Currently on antibiotics, which suppress normal bacterial flora and enable overgrowth of infectious organisms
- Hospital stay or residence in long-term care facility
- Age, over 65
- Immunocompromised patient
- Intestinal surgery
- Chemotherapy
- Colon inflammation or infection

Causes

Most of the following causes are transmitted through the fecal–oral route by eating contaminated food:

- Enterohemorrhagic *E. coli* is food borne and commonly associated with undercooked meat and contaminated vegetables.
- *Shigella* is transmitted from human to human only.
- *Salmonella* can be human- or nonhuman-to-human transmission and is caused by consuming contaminated raw or undercooked food, especially poultry. It has also been linked to reptiles.
- *Campylobacter* is commonly caused by consuming contaminated food or water and/or raw meat.
- Protozoans, such as *Entamoeba histolytica*, can also cause infections.
- *Clostridium difficile* is a well-known cause (discussed in the following text).

LO2: Assessment Findings: Infectious Colitis

- Patients present with:
  - o Fever
  - o Abdominal cramping
  - o Diarrhea
  - o Blood in stool
  - o Mucous and/or pus in stool
- Patients can present with sepsis.
- Patients should be screened for severe sepsis (see sepsis guidelines).

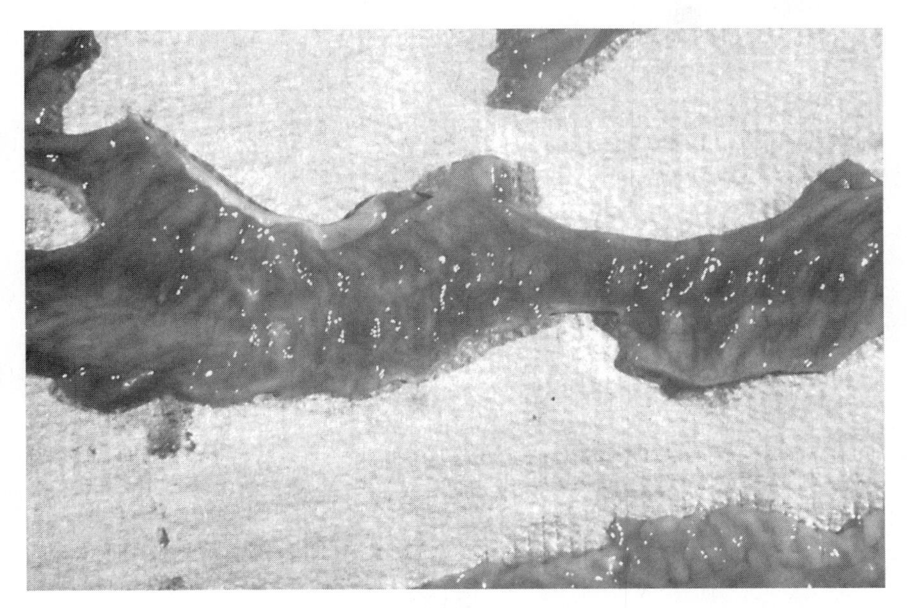

This photo demonstrates the effects of infectious colitis from *Shigella* (bacteria) on the colon. This specimen is from a Rhesus monkey, but the effects are the same in humans. Note the diffuse inflammation, infection, and bloody mucous that appears as bloody diarrhea. The photo can assist in anticipating what signs and symptoms would manifest from this condition.
Source: Centers for Disease Control and Prevention

LO2: Diagnostics: Infectious Colitis

- Stool testing for WBCs, which are elevated
- Stool culture for pathogenic organisms
- Electrolytes may show evidence of volume depletion with increased blood urea nitrogen-to-creatinine (BUN/Cr) ratio.
- CBC to evaluate for anemia and leukocytosis

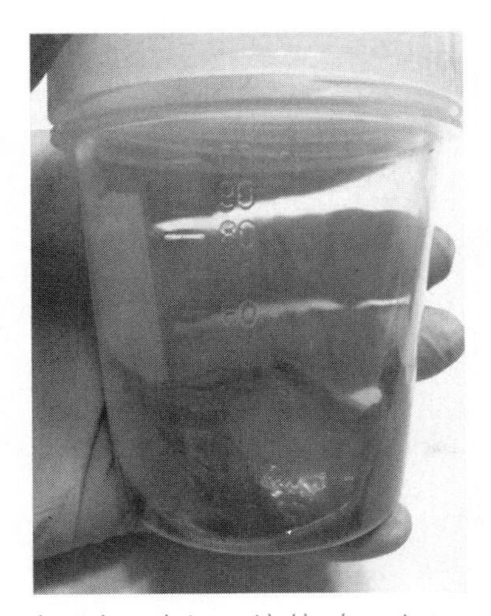

A stool sample is provided by the patient for testing.
Source: Copyright © 2014, NovEx Novice to Expert Learning, LLC

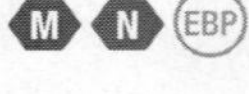

Collaborative Interventions: Infectious Colitis

- Care and treatment are primarily supportive with fluid and electrolyte replacement (Guerrant, et al., 2001).
- Rehydration: To avoid dehydration, replace fluids with dilute electrolye drinks (e.g., Pedialyte, Ceralyte), rehydration salt solutions (e.g., rehydration salt packets mixed in water), or water. Sodas, juices, chicken broth, and sports drinks should be avoided in severe vomiting and diarrhea (Guerrant, et al., 2001). Rehydration solutions are easy to make using 2 tablespoons of sugar and one-half teaspoon of salt mixed into a quart or liter of water. IV isotonic rehydration may be needed in hospitalized patients who are unable to keep oral fluids down.
- Fecal testing: Cultures to identify specific organisms are needed to guide treatment if diarrhea is persistent, blood is noted in stool, or antibiotics or chemotherapy have recently been taken. Test for parasites (e.g., *Giardia*, *Cryptosporidium*) if diarrhea persists for more than 7 days.
- Patients can be treated with antimicrobials (e.g., azithromycin). The antimicrobials are tailored after stool culture results are obtained (e.g., quinolone for shigellosis; macrolide for resistant *Campylobacter*) (Guerrant, et al., 2001).
- Collaborate with and consult an infectious disease specialist in instances of drug resistant organisms. Multidrug-resistant organisms (MDROs) are increasing and challenging the ability to adequately treat infections.
- Antibiotics should be avoided with enterohemorrhagic *E. coli* (EHEC) because the increased release of toxins from dying *E. coli* may place the patient at higher risk for life-threatening hemolytic uremic syndrome. EHEC is typically self-limiting, runs its course, and resolves (Guerrant, et al., 2001).
- Antidiarrheal agents should not be used, especially without antimicrobial treatment, because they can allow overgrowth of bacteria (Guerrant, et al., 2001).
- Collaborate to ensure infectious diseases, particularly outbreaks, are swiftly reported to public health agencies for surveillance, detection, prevention, source control, and public education (Guerrant, et al., 2001).

Concept Check

11. Which type of infectious colitis is only transmitted person to person?

A. *Shigella*

B. *Salmonella*

C. *E. coli*

D. *Campylobacter*

Answer question

Concept Check

12. Which treatment strategy is incorrect for a patient with enterohemorrhagic *E. coli*?

A. IV fluids

B. Antibiotic therapy

C. Fecal sampling

D. Avoidance of antidiarrheals

Answer question

LO1:

What Is *Clostridium Difficile* Colitis?

- *Clostridium difficile* (*C. diff*) is a gram-positive, anaerobic, spore-forming bacillus and is a major cause of antibiotic-associated diarrhea and colitis.
- Any patient who has been on antibiotics in the past 2 months or develops diarrhea within 72 hours of hospital admission should be suspect for *C. diff* infection.
- Hospitalized patients are most commonly infected with *C. diff*. It can affect up to 3 million patients per year and is more prevalent in older adults.

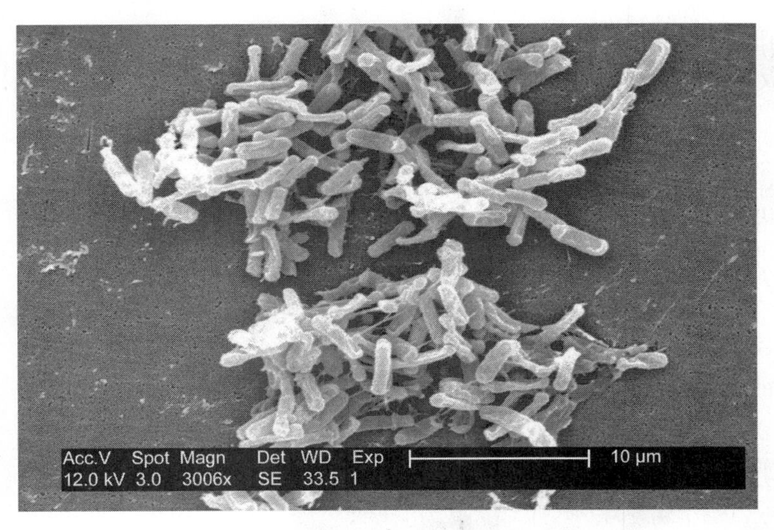

This electron micrograph captures the gram-positive *C. diff* bacteria from a fecal culture.
Source: CDC/Lois S. Wiggs

LO2:

Pathophysiology: *C. Difficile* Colitis

- Normal intestinal bacteria keep *C. diff* in check.
- Antibiotics upset the normal intestinal bacteria composition, allowing colonization of *C. diff*, which multiplies and releases toxins.
- Most patients develop diarrhea soon after taking antibiotics, although as many as 40% may not have symptoms for as long as 10 weeks following antibiotic therapy.
- Pathogenic strains of *C. diff* produce both an enterotoxin and a cytotoxin.
- Hospitalized patients and patients in long-term care facilities are prime targets for this infection.

Perioperative View of C. diff | **Colonoscopy: Severe C. diff**

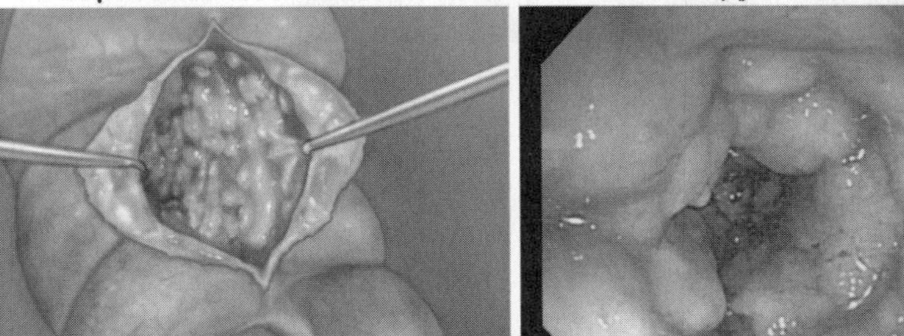

Left: This image depicts the inflamed and edematous mucosa with multiple discrete, nodular, and polypoid lesions covered with yellowish exudates. Right: A colonoscopy revealed severe *C. diff* infection throughout the colon. A cytotoxic assay of a stool specimen for *C. difficile* toxin B was positive.
Sources: Courtesy of George Kyriakidis/Santa Ana, CA, & K. Kyriakidis

Concept Check

13. Which person is at greatest risk for development of *C. difficile* colitis?
    A. College student living in a dorm
    B. Older adult who had a screening colonoscopy
    C. Middle adult who has diabetes type 2
    D. Preschool child taking medications for asthma

Answer question

LO2:

Risk Factors and Causes: *C. Difficile* Colitis

- Although the majority of patients develop *C. diff* while in health care facilities, it is now spread in the general population, primarily from person-to-person contact with contaminated hands.
- Hands, toilets, sinks, stethoscopes, blood pressure cuffs, items set on the floor (purse, backpacks), bedside tables, bedrails, remote controls, telephones, house slippers, and socks also worn into the bed are some of the sources of contamination.
- Those at highest risk:
    - o Older adults, especially in long-term care
    - o Recent antibiotic use
    - o Recent or current hospitalization, especially for GI diseases or conditions
    - o Immunosuppressed patients or those with serious medical conditions
    - o Abdominal surgery or GI procedure

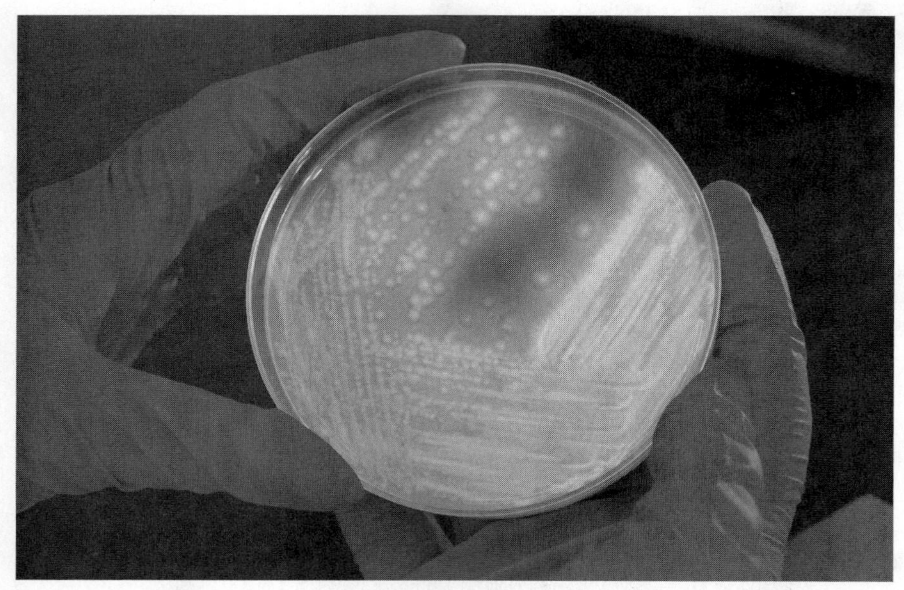

This photo shows a culture of *C. diff* taken from sources obtained in an infected patient's room. Clinicians must stay cognizant that their gloved hand, after examining or caring for a patient infected with *C. diff*, can contaminate objects that others touch and can spread. *C. diff* organisms are potentially deadly bacteria and are responsible for at least 300,000 infections a year in U.S. hospitals. Gloves are protective only when used properly and disposed of after every use and before handling anything that may cross contaminate.

Source: Centers for Disease Control and Prevention

LO2:

Assessment Findings: *C. Difficile* Colitis

- Cramp-like abdominal pain; low abdominal tenderness
- Diarrhea: watery
- Loss of appetite
- Malaise and lethargy
- Fever
- Dehydration with electrolyte imbalances: dry mucous membranes, poor skin turgor, and thirst
- Relapse is common and occurs in about 27% of cases in 3 days to 3 weeks after treatment.
- *C. diff* is more prominent in older people.
- Mortality rates in patients who are acutely ill can range between 10–30%.

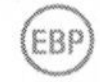

- The use of proton pump inhibitors (PPIs) can increase susceptibility to *C. diff* (Surawicz, et al., 2013).

Proton-Pump Inhibitors

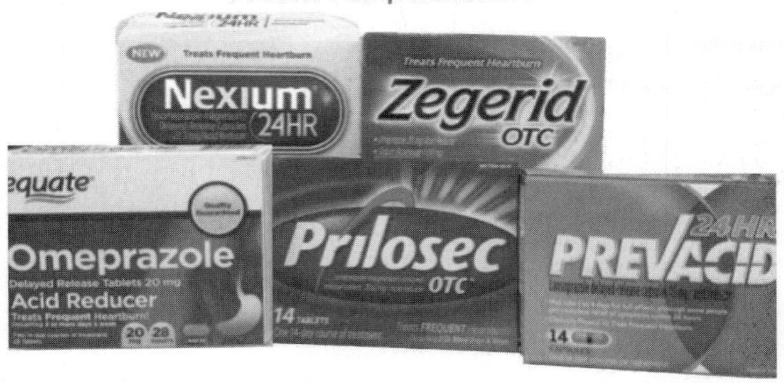

A meta-analysis from Harvard Health Publication involved over 300,000 patients and revealed a statistical correlation between the development of *C. diff* and the use of PPIs. Patients taking PPIs for upper GI conditions have a 65% higher risk of *C. diff*, particularly those who are taking antibiotics, living in long-term care institutions, and hospitalized.

Source: Copyright © 2014, NovEx Novice to Expert Learning, LLC

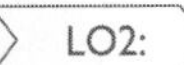

Diagnostics: *C. Difficile* Colitis

Labs:

- CBC: Leukocytosis is often prominent and can be very high.
- CMP: electrolyte imbalance
- Albumin: hypoalbuminemia

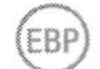

- Stool culture: sensitivity in 90–100% (Cohen, et al., 2010; Surawicz, et al., 2013)
- Fecal leukocytes may be present in about 50% of cases.
- Hemoccult positive without grossly bloody stools

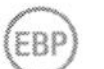

- Stool is positive for *C. diff* toxin (Cohen, et al., 2010; Surawicz, et al., 2013).

Endoscopy:

- Raised yellow-white plaques (2–10 mm) with erythematous mucosa (pseudomembranous plaques), most evident with severe infection (see photos)

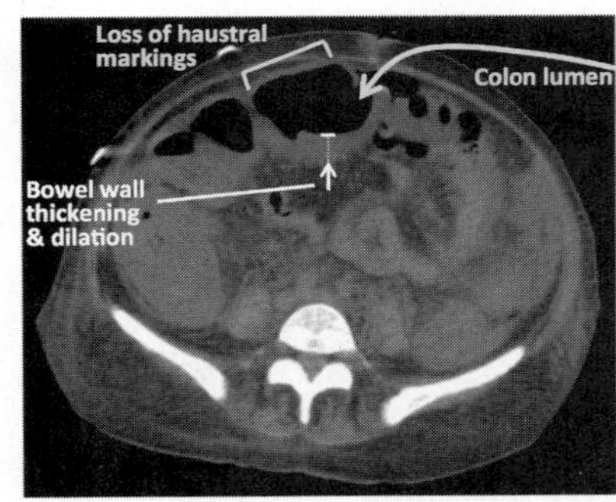

In patients with C. difficile, CT scan reveals several important clues: 1) the abnormal extent and degree of bowel distention (black space inside the bowel lumen, 2) the bowel wall thickening, and 3) the loss of haustral markings (folds in the lumen) leaving a smooth wall appearance.

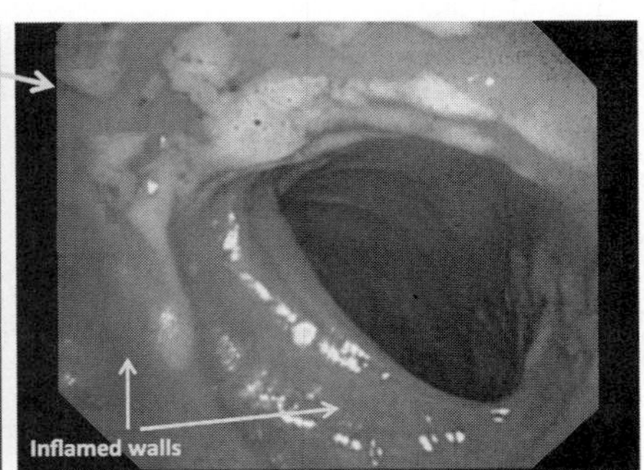

On endoscopy of the colon, characteristic yellowish white lesions are visible and can become extensive in severe disease. Note the inflamed mucosal walls of the intestines typically seen in patients with C. difficile. Endoscopy is cautiously used due to the friable nature of the intestinal walls.

Source: Courtesy of K. Kyriakidis

LO3: Collaborative Interventions: *C. Difficile* Colitis

***C. diff* is identified as a major nosocomial infecting agent.** Interventions include:

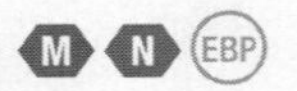

- **Strict contact isolation precautions** are imperative to prevent the spread (Surawicz, et al., 2013).
- Isolation precautions include private room, gown and gloves for everyone entering the room, and stringent hand hygiene with any encounter with anything in the room. Maintain contact precautions until diarrhea ceases (Surawicz, et al., 2013).
- For suspected or known *C. diff* infections, strict hand hygiene with soap and water as opposed to gel hand sanitizer is required (Cohen, et al., 2010; Surawicz, et al., 2013).
- Hand sanitizers do not destroy *C. diff* spores (Cohen, et al., 2010; Surawicz, et al., 2013).

Medications and fluids are initially recommended (Cohen, et al., 2010; Surawicz, et al., 2013):

- Antibiotics: oral or IV metronidazole, oral vancomycin, fidaxomicin, cholestyramine (Surawicz, et al., 2013). There is a significant cost difference that may be considered when the exact antimicrobial is not an issue (e.g., metronidazole = $0.73/dose versus fidaxomicin = $140/dose).

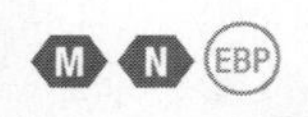

- Metronidazole is the antimicrobial of choice in mild to moderate *C. diff* infection (Cohen, et al., 2010; Surawicz, et al., 2013).

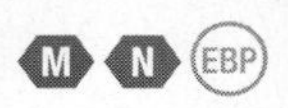

- Repeat fecal testing to evaluate antimicrobial effectiveness is not recommended (Cohen, et al., 2010; Surawicz, et al., 2013).

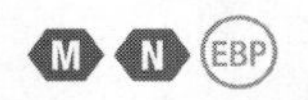

- **Fecal transplant** is proving to be much more effective (approximately 90% cure) than antibiotic treatment for recurrent *C. difficile* colitis. Donor feces is infused using a variety of methods: nasoduodenal infusion, colonoscopy, endoscopy, sigmoidoscopy, or enema. The FDA classified fecal matter as an investigational new drug in 2013. It is a low-cost, low-risk intervention (van Nood, et al., 2013).

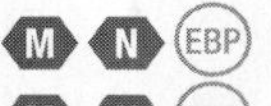

- IV fluids for hydration (Surawicz, et al., 2013)
- Electrolyte replacement (Surawicz, et al., 2013)
- **Antidiarrheal** agents should be avoided to prevent masking symptoms and reduce the risk of toxic megacolon (Cohen, et al., 2010; Surawicz, et al., 2013).

Surgical intervention:

Toxic megacolon or perforated colon can occur in a small percentage of patients (about 3%).

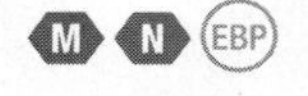

- Colectomy should be considered in patients who are complicated and/or severely ill (Cohen, et al., 2010; Surawicz, et al., 2013). These minimally include patients with:
    - Hypotension, tachycardia, and are unstable
    - Vasopressor support for hypotension
    - Physical examination findings indicating systemic inflammatory response syndrome, sepsis, or multiorgan dysfunction
    - Decreased level of consciousness
    - Abnormally high lactate level and/or white blood cell count
    - Failure to satisfactorily respond to medical management

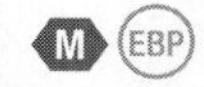

- Evaluate the patient for sepsis prior to surgery using lactate levels and peripheral white blood counts. Abnormally high results is associated with higher surgical morbidity and mortality (Cohen, et al., 2010).

Clostridium Difficile Colitis and Toxic Megacolon

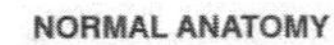

PRE-OPERATIVE CONDITION

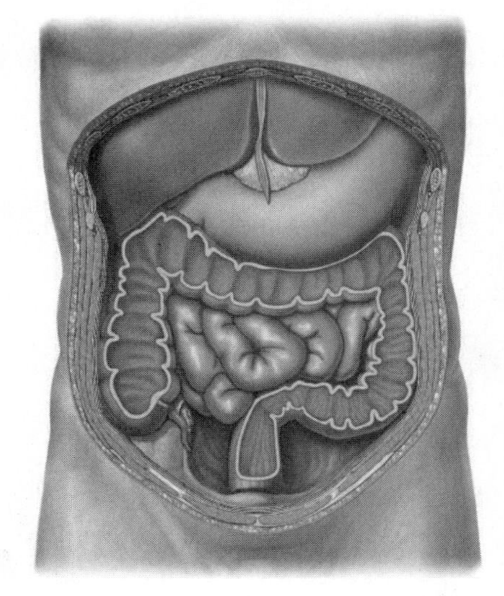

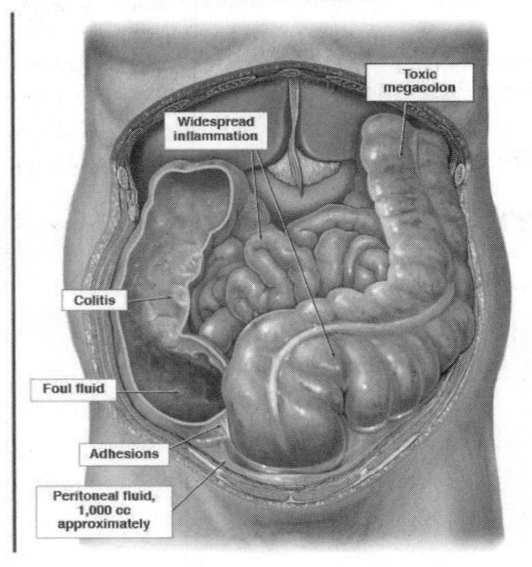

Comparison of these two images points out the difference between a normal colon versus a toxic megacolon condition as a result of *C. diff.*

Safety and prevention practices are essential in infection control. Strong recommendations in caring for patients includes:

- Similar to gastroenteritis, prevention of the spread of the disease is paramount (Surawicz, et al., 2013).
- Excellent and strict hand hygiene and prevention precautions are important to follow and implement (Cohen, et al., 2010; Surawicz, et al., 2013).
- Careful assessment of the patient's fluid and electrolyte status is an important nursing assessment. Early and rapid intervention is a high nursing priority (Cohen, et al., 2010; Surawicz, et al., 2013).
- Early and rapid administration of ordered antibiotics may help reduce the duration of the illness and prevent worsening of symptoms (Surawicz, et al., 2013).
- Clean with chlorine-containing or sporicidal products (Cohen, et al., 2010; Surawicz, et al., 2013).
- Prevention: Team should minimize the use of antimicrobials (duration, frequency, number) in other conditions to reduce the risk of developing *C. diff.* This is commonly known as "antibiotic or antimicrobial stewardship" (Cohen, et al., 2010; Surawicz, et al., 2013).
- Clinical leadership: Collaborate with team to evaluate the earliest possible, safe time to discontinue antimicrobials that impact a patient's risk for *C. diff* (Surawicz, et al., 2013).

Concept Check

14. Which type of isolation is necessary when caring for a patient with *C. difficile* colitis?

   A. Wound
   B. Droplet
   C. Contact
   D. Reverse

Answer question

Summary of Interventions: All Infectious GI Disorders

- Sepsis screening should be done for any infectious disorder when there are signs of systemic inflammatory response syndrome (SIRS), infection, or sepsis.
- Patients with symptoms of peritonitis or appendicitis need to be quickly evaluated by a surgeon. Patients should receive antibiotics, be NPO, given IV fluids, and medicated for pain.
- Patients with diverticulitis should receive antibiotics, be NPO, given IV fluid, and pain medication.
- Patients with viral gastroenteritis primarily require supportive care: IV fluids, electrolyte replacement, and antiemetics.
- Patients with infectious colitis should be treated with rehydration, fecal testing, and antibiotics (except with enterohemorrhagic *E. coli*) and IV fluids.
- Patients with *C. diff* should be treated with IV fluids and oral or IV metronidazole or oral vancomycin.
- Strict hand hygiene is the critical preventative intervention.

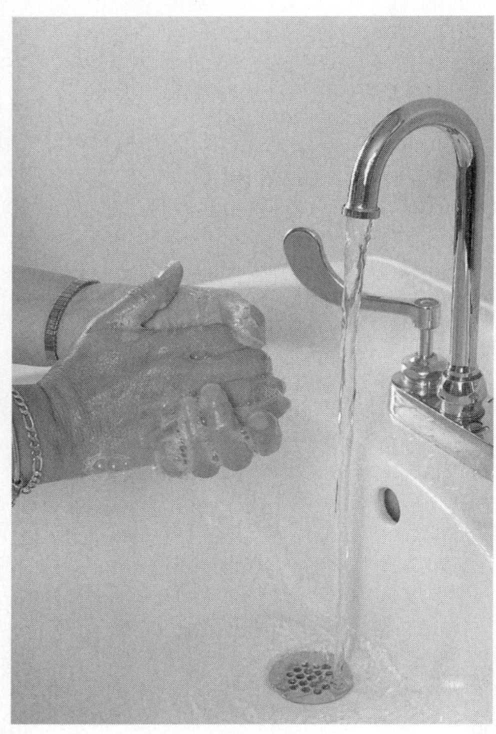

Source: Centers for Disease Control and Prevention/Amanda Mills

LO4: Evaluation of Desired Collaborative Care Outcomes: All Infectious GI Disorders

Evaluation and reassessment should reveal attainment of previously established patient outcomes. In summary:

- Patient and family accurately describe and routinely demonstrate practices that prevent spread of organisms to others.
- Patient's mentation is clear or at the patient's preadmission "normal," blood pressure is within desired range, skin turgor is elastic, and fluid intake is balanced with fluid losses.
- Patient has no neuromuscular, cardiovascular, or other findings associated with electrolyte imbalance.
- Patient reports that pain is reduced to a tolerable level.
- Patient accurately explains disease process and the recommended therapeutic interventions.

References

Amerine, E. (2007). Preventing and managing acute diverticulitis. *Nursing 2007, 37*(9), 56hn1–56hn6.

Beckett, G., & Bright, J. (2013). Prevention and control of viral gastroenteritis. *Nursing & Residential Care, 15*(6), 426–430.

Higgins, R. (2009). Abdominal assessment and diagnosis of appendicitis. *Emergency Nurse, 16*(9), 22–24.

Holzheimer, R. G. (2001). *Surgical treatment: Evidence-based and problem-oriented: Management of secondary peritonitis.* **www.ncbi.nlm.nih.gov/books/NBK6950/**

Horinek, E., & Fish, D. (2009). Spontaneous bacterial peritonitis. *AACN Advanc Crit Care, 20*(2), 121–125. **www.aacn.org/wd/cetests/media/acc2021.pdf**

Jabbar, U., Leischner, J., Kasper, D., et al. (2010). Effectiveness of alcohol-based hand rubs for removal of *Clostridium difficile* spores from hands. *Infect Control Hosp Epidemiol, 31*(6), 565–570.

Nitzan, O., Elias, M., Chazan, B., et al. (2013). *Clostridium difficile* and inflammatory bowel disease: Role in pathogenesis and implications in treatment. *World J Gastroenterol, 19*(43), 7577–7585.

Ordoñez, C., & Puyana, J. (2006). Management of peritonitis in the critically ill patient. *Surgical Clinics Of North America, 86*(6), 1323–1349.

Pfadt, E., & Carlson D. (2009). Acute appendicitis. *Nursing 2009, 39*(12), 72.

Schweon, S. J. (2012). Recognizing and preventing norovirus infection. *Nursing 2012, 42*(6), 68–69.

Seaward-Hersh, A. (2004). Case study: Ensuring best practice in the treatment of peritonitis and exit site infection. *Nephrology Nursing Journal, 31*(5), 585–586.

van Nood, E., Vrieze, A., Nieuwdorp, M., et al. (2013). Duodenal infusion of donor feces for recurrent Clostridium difficile. *N Engl J Med, 368*(5), 407–415. **www.nejm.org/doi/full/10.1056/NEJMoa1205037**

Watkins J. Recognizing the signs of acute appendicitis. *British Journal of School Nursing* 2010; 5(10):488–491.

Clinical Practice Guidelines

Centers for Disease Control and Prevention Healthcare Infection Control Practices Advisory Committee. (2011). *Guideline for the prevention and control of norovirus gastroenteritis outbreaks in healthcare settings, 2011.* **www.cdc.gov/norovirus/index.html** and **www.cdc.gov/norovirus/hcp/diagnosis-treatment.html#treatment**

Cincinnati Children's Hospital Medical Center. (2011). *Evidence-based care guideline for prevention and management of acute gastroenteritis.* **www.cincinnatichildrens.org/workarea/linkit.aspx?linkidentifier=id&itemid=93672&libid=93365** or **www.guideline.gov/content.aspx?id=34025&search=gastroenteritis**

Cohen, S. H., Gerding, D. N., Johnson, S., et al. (2010). Clinical practice guidelines for *Clostridium difficile* infection in adults: 2010 update by the Society of Healthcare Epidemiology of America (SHEA) and the Infectious Disease Society of America (IDSA). *Infection Control Hosp Epidemiol, 31*(5), 431–455. **www.cdc.gov/HAI/pdfs/cdiff/Cohen-IDSA-SHEA-CDI-guidelines-2010.pdf**

Guerrant, R., Van Gilder, T., Steiner, T., et al. on behalf of the Infectious Diseases Society of America. (2001). Practice guidelines for the management of infectious diarrhea. *Clinical Infectious Diseases,* 32(3), 331–351. **www.uphs.upenn.edu/bugdrug/antibiotic_manual/idsadiarrhea.pdf**

Howell, J. M., Eddy, O. L., Lukens, T. W., et al. & American College of Emergency Physicians (2010). Clinical policy: Critical issues in the evaluation and management of emergency department patients with suspected appendicitis. *Ann Emerg Med, 55*(1), 71–116. **www.guideline.gov/content.aspx?id=15598&search=appendicitis**

Feingold, D., Steele, S.R., Lee, S., et al. (2014). Practice parameters for sigmoid diverticulitis. *The American Society of Colon and Rectal Surgeons, 57*(3), 284–294. **www.fascrs.org/sites/default/files/downloads/publication/practice_parameters_for_the_treatment_of_sigmoid.2.pdf.**

Solomkin, J., Mazuski, J., Bradley, J., et al. (2010). Diagnosis and management of complicated intra-abdominal infection in adults and children: Guidelines by the Surgical Infection Society and the Infectious Diseases Society of America. *Clinical Infectious Diseases, 50*(2), 133–164. **www.idsociety.org/uploadedFiles/IDSA/Guidelines-Patient_Care/PDF_Library/Intra-abdominal%20Infectin.pdf**

Surawicz, C., Brandt, L., Binion, D., et al. (2013). Guidelines for diagnosis, treatment, and prevention of clostridium difficile infections. *Am J Gastroenterol, 108*:478-498. **gi.org/guideline/diagnosis-and-management-of-c-difficile-associated-diarrhea-and-colitis/**

Patient Education

Centers for Disease Control and Prevention. (2012). *Clostridium difficile infection.* **www.cdc.gov/hai/organisms/cdiff/Cdiff-patient.html**

Centers for Disease Control and Prevention, Division of Viral Diseases. (2011). *Viral gastroenteritis.* **www.cdc.gov/ncidod/dvrd/revb/gastro/faq.htm**

Centers for Disease Control and Prevention Healthcare Infection Control Practices Advisory Committee. (2013). *Norovirus.* **www.cdc.gov/norovirus/about/overview.html**

Daller, J. A. (2013). *Appendectomy.* **www.nlm.nih.gov/medlineplus/ency/article/002921.htm**

Shahedi, K. (2014). *Diverticulitis.* **emedicine.medscape.com/article/173388-overview**

Learning Outcomes for GI Inflammatory Disorders

When you complete this lesson, you will be able to:

1. Recognize the clinical relevance of gastrointestinal inflammatory disorders.
2. Consider the pathophysiology, etiology, risk factors, and clinical presentation of gastrointestinal inflammatory disorders that determine the priority patient concerns.
3. Determine the most urgent and important nursing interventions and patient education required in caring for a patient with a gastrointestinal inflammatory disease.
4. Evaluate attainment of desired collaborative care outcomes for a patient with a gastrointestinal inflammatory disease.

LO1:

Gastrointestinal Disorders: Lower GI Tract

Gastrointestinal bowel disorders consist of:

- Infectious Disorders
- **Inflammatory Disorders**
- Functional Disorders
- Structural Disorders

This NovE-lesson focuses on inflammatory disorders.

LO1:

What Are GI Inflammatory Disorders?

- **GI inflammatory disorders** are conditions that cause chronic inflammation of the bowel with episodes of acute exacerbations that can lead to abscess formation and perforation. This can result in gastrointestinal infection.
- Frequently referred to as inflammatory bowel disease (IBD)
- Examples of inflammatory diseases of the bowel are:
  - Crohn's disease
  - Ulcerative colitis
  - Ischemic colitis
  - Radiation colitis

Endoscopic Image of Crohn's Disease

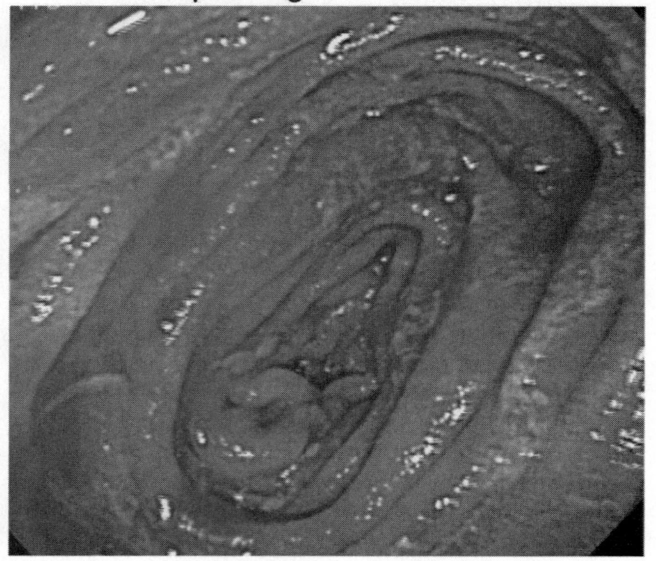

Crohn's disease is pictured above in the small intestines. Note the hyperemic mucosal surface with the multiple areas of ulceration. The pain associated with Crohn's disease is understandable.

Source: Courtesy of K. Kyriakidis

LO1:

Clinical Relevance

- There are approximately 1.4 million patients with inflammatory bowel disease in the United States.
- Health care costs related to inflammatory bowel disease total more than $1.7 billion annually.
- Inflammatory bowel disease is not curable and requires lifelong care.
- Nearly 75% of patients with Crohn's disease and 25% of patients with ulcerative colitis require surgery for their condition at some point.

LO2:

Pathophysiology

- **Crohn's disease** is a chronic inflammatory process, which can extend through the entire thickness of the wall of the bowel. It may involve any portion of the gastrointestinal tract.
- **Ulcerative colitis (UC)** is another inflammatory disorder that commonly involves the rectum and colon in an uninterrupted pattern involving part or the entire colon.
- **Ischemic colitis** results from limited blood flow that causes inadequate oxygenation of GI tissues.
- **Radiation colitis** is the inflammation and injury to the lower GI tract caused by radiation therapy.

Ulcerative Colitis Covered with Mucopurulent Exudate

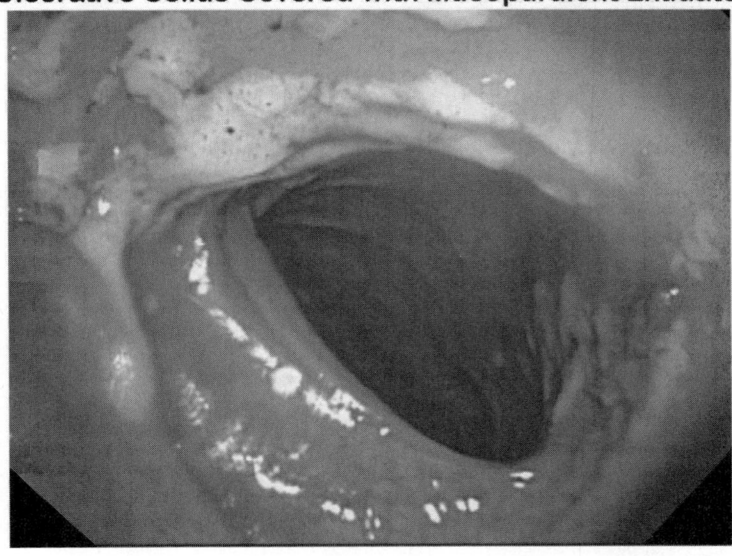

The photo presents severe ulcerative colitis where numerous pseudopolyps (masses of scar tissue that have the appearance of a polyp) are seen and cover the ulcerations. The pseudopolyps are also referred to as mucopurulent exudate. The intestinal mucosa is eroded, and hyperemic (engorged with blood).

Source: Courtesy of K. Kyriakidis

Concept Check

1. Which treatment may result in inflammatory GI diseases?

   A. Radiation treatments for cancer

   B. NPO status

   C. Respiratory treatment with albuterol

   D. Bedrest

Answer question

Pathophysiology (continued)

Crohn's Disease

- While the exact cause is unknown, genetic defects together with environmental factors likely result in an imbalance of the immune system.
- Crohn's disease is thought to produce a defect in the GI mucosal barrier against pathogens, causing too many bacterial antigens to cross the mucosal barrier.
- Bacterial antigens that penetrate the mucosal barrier are presented to T cells, which produce proinflammatory cytokines (e.g., TNF-alpha). The overabundance of antigens results in uncontrolled mucosal inflammation of the gut. (*Proinflammatory* means promoting inflammation.)
- More inflammatory cells are "called to" or attracted into the bowel wall, causing further disruption of the mucosal barrier and greater inflammation.

Endoscopic Images of Crohn's Disease in the Ileum

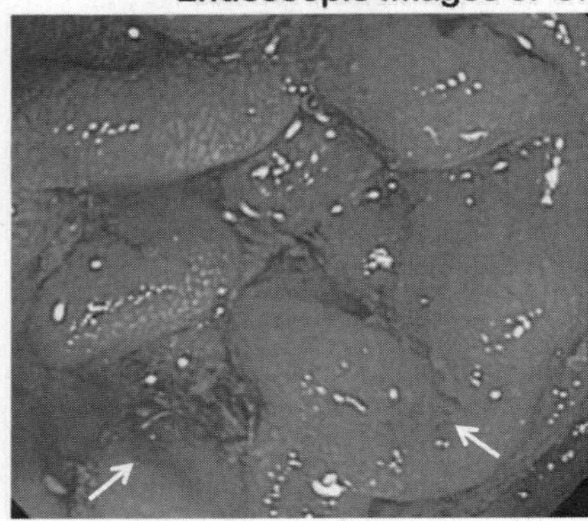

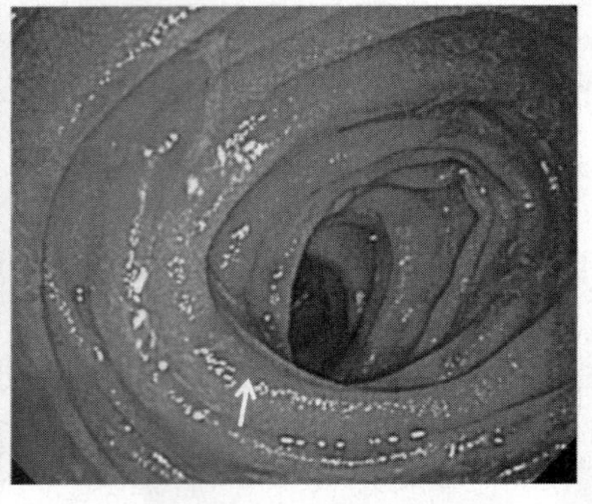

This endoscopic photo shows the inflamed, edematous intestinal walls with ulcerations (arrows). The yellowish orange appearing strands of "creeping fat" are hyperplasia of the adipose tissue.
Source: Courtesy of K. Kyriakidis

- This uncontrolled inflammatory process frequently leads to edema of the bowel mucosa and subsequent spasms, microperforations, fibrosis, obstructive symptoms, abscess, and fistula formation.
- The inflamed bowel with its many circumferential ulcers and fissures create a cobblestone street appearance known as cobblestoning. Cobblestoning is not pathognomonic for Crohn's disease, but it is common.
- As in every systemic inflammatory response, this can also cause inflammation in distant organs (e.g., arthritis, conjunctivitis).
- The segment of the GI tract affected by Crohn's disease is approximately:
  - o 30% in the small bowel
  - o 30% in the colon
  - o 40% in both the small bowel and the colon
- Inflammation results in malabsorption of water, electrolytes, fat (steatorrhea) and nutrients.
- Intestinal obstruction can result from strictures, abscesses, and perianal fistulae.

CT Scan of Crohn's Disease

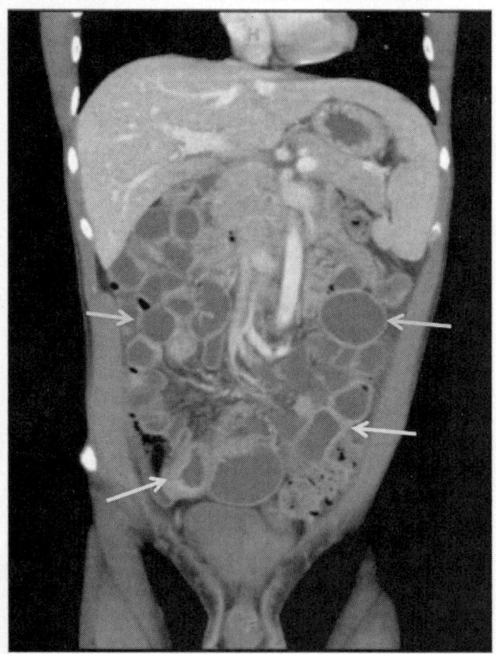

CT scan reveals this patient has Crohn's disease. Note the small intestines appear as numerous circles. The lower intestines show thickening of the intestinal walls (yellow arrows) seen in Crohn's as compared to the thin walls of the normal intestinal areas (blue arrows).

Source: Courtesy of K. Kyriakidis

Pathophysiology (continued)

Ulcerative Colitis

- Ulcerative colitis is also thought to be due to an abnormal immune response, similar to Crohn's disease.
- However, the resulting inflammation involves primarily the mucosa (the entire wall is involved in Crohn's disease).
- Obstruction, abscess formation, and fistula formation is much less common than in Crohn's disease.
- Ulcerative colitis commonly involves the entire colon and most of the rectum, but not the small bowel.
- Contributing factors include genetics, immune reactions, altered intestinal flora, NSAID use, and vitamin A and E deficiencies.

Ulcerative Colitis

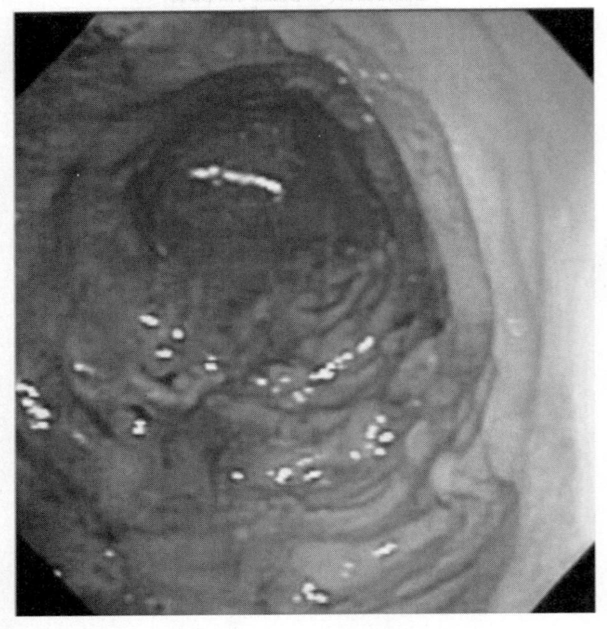

This image shows how ulcerative colitis can be widespread, throughout the transverse, descending, and sigmoid regions of the colon. This ulceration pattern is typical of ulcerative colitis. Notice here that the exudate covering the ulcerations on the mucosal wall is extensive.

Source: Courtesy of K. Kyriakidis

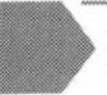

Concept Check

2. **Crohn's disease is most likely to occur in which part of the gastrointestinal tract?**
   A. Esophagus
   B. Small bowel
   C. Large bowel
   D. Small bowel and large bowel together

Answer question

LO2:

Risk Factors

Crohn's Disease

- Smoking: This leads to other health problems and increases the risk for surgery. It is the most controllable risk factor.
- Family history: Approximately 20% of those affected have a close relative who also has the disease.
- Ethnicity: Caucasians have a higher risk. Ashkenazi Jews have an even higher risk.
- Age: Most cases are diagnosed prior to age 30 but can occur at any age.
- Geography: A slightly higher risk exists for residents of northern climates and people living in cities and industrial areas.

Ulcerative Colitis

- Smoking: This does not seem to be a factor.
- Family history: Diagnosis of the disease in a close relative (e.g., parent, sibling, child) increases the risk.
- Age: Onset usually occurs before age 30, but onset is not uncommon at age 50 to 60.
- Ethnicity: Higher incidence in Caucasians and still higher in Ashkenazi Jews
- It has been suggested, but not confirmed, that the use of isotretinoin (e.g., Amnesteem, Sotret, Claravis, Accutane) for the treatment of acne increases risk.

LO2:

Causes: Crohn's Disease and Ulcerative Colitis

- Not yet understood; stress and diet are no longer considered to be causes.
- Hypothesis: A microorganism triggers an immune response.
- Hypothesis: Heredity plays a role due to the strong familial incidence.

LO2:

Assessment Findings

Inflammatory bowel diseases share many similar characteristics and assessment findings; however, there are clinical differences. For instance, patients with Crohn's disease more commonly present with abdominal pain whereas patients with ulcerative colitis more commonly present with GI bleeding.

Crohn's Disease

- Cramping abdominal pain in the right lower quadrant and periumbilical area that may feel better after defecating
- Diarrhea is intermittent; may have mucous, pus, and/or blood in stool.
- Abdominal distension, severe abdominal pain, and intractable nausea and vomiting occur in patients with obstruction.
- Low grade fever
- Weight loss
- Malaise
- Anorexia
- Severe abdominal pain, rebound tenderness (increased pain with release of pressure rather than with pressure), and fever in patients with peritonitis due to perforation
- Vaginal discharge as a result of fistula formation

Ulcerative Colitis

- Gastrointestinal bleeding in many patients presenting as bloody diarrhea
- Colicky, cramping abdominal pain in right lower quadrant and periumbilical area that may feel better after defecating
- Urgency and/or tenesmus (constant urge to defecate) despite an empty colon
- Low grade fever
- Diarrhea is intermittent; may have mucous, pus, and/or blood in stool.
- Weight loss is less common but present in more severe cases.
- Perforation and obstruction are much less common than in patients with Crohn's disease.

Extraintestinal Assessment Findings

Crohn's Disease

- Erythema nodosum is a painful inflammatory disorder of the subcutaneous fat. It often signals the presence of a systemic disease. It presents as red, tender nodules under the skin.
- Eye involvement (i.e., conjunctivitis)
- Pericarditis or myocarditis
- Gallstones
- Renal stone formation

Ulcerative Colitis

- Uveitis or painful inflammation of the uvea (middle layer) of the eye wall is associated with ulcerative colitis.
- Sclerosing cholangitis with fibrosis and inflammation of the bile ducts

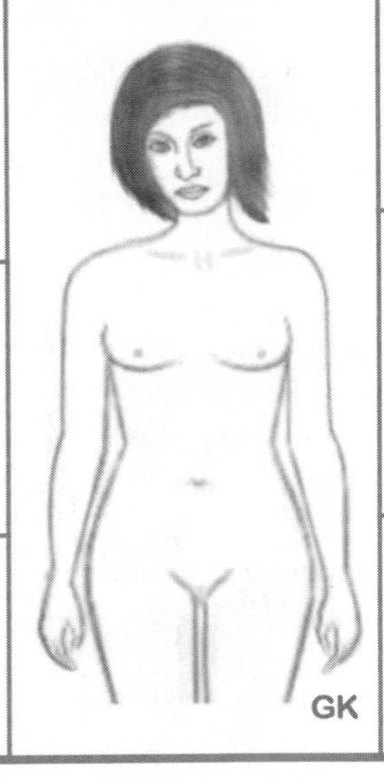

This illustration indicates the numerous systemic effects of inflammatory bowel disease.
Source: Courtesy of George Kyriakidis/Santa Ana, CA

Concept Check

3. Which situation is a risk factor for developing Crohn's disease?
   A. Smoking
   B. Aging past 50 years
   C. Stressful living conditions
   D. Poor diet

Answer question

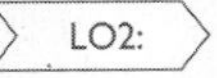
LO2:

Diagnostics

Labs:

- CBC
- Complete metabolic panel (CMP)
- Sed rate and C-reactive protein to detect inflammatory process
- Lactate: sepsis indicator of tissue hypoperfusion

Imaging:

- Upper and lower GI with barium
- CT scan to evaluate for abscess formation and extent of involvement of the colon

Endoscopy:

- Colonoscopy (see the animation in the Diagnostics: Polyps section in the GI Structural Disorders NovE-lesson)

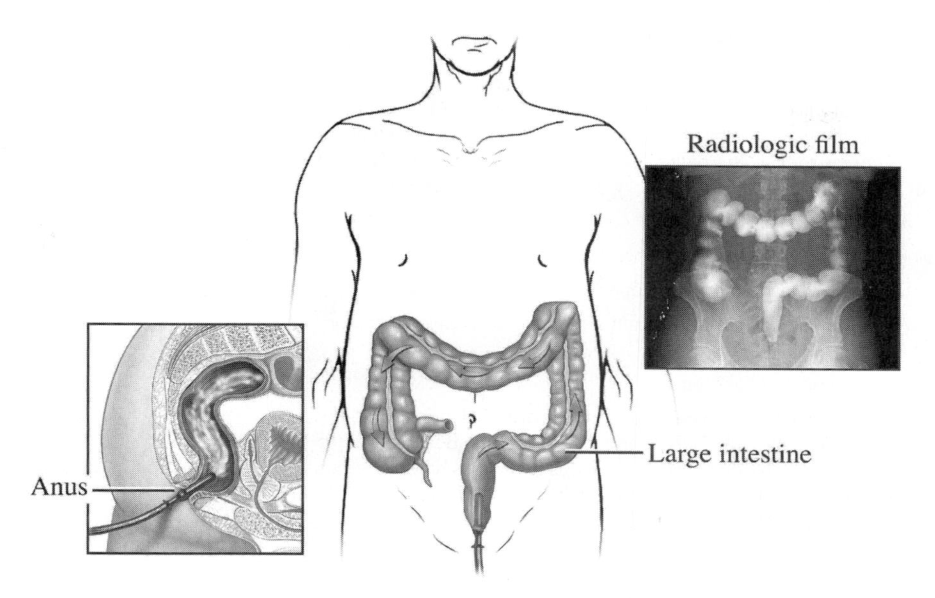

To perform a barium enema, an endoscope is inserted into the rectum and the barium is instilled into the colon and pushed up and around to fill the entire colon. A radiograph is then taken and the result is the film that you see on the right.
Source: Nucleus Medical Art Inc./Alamy

Diagnostics: Differentiating Crohn's Disease and Ulcerative Colitis

	Ulcerative Colitis	**Crohn's Disease**
Location	Limited to colon	Whole GI tract
	Continuous inflammation from rectum	Noncontinuous lesions
Imaging	Continuous inflammation from rectum	Noncontinuous lesions
	Limited to colon	Whole GI tract
	Mucosal involvement only	Obstruction, abscess, fistula, fibrosis, toxic megacolon
Pathologic findings	Mucous membranes only	Full thickness involvement
	Granulomas absent	Granulomas common
Physical Exam		
Weight loss/malnutrition	Unusual	Expected
Bleeding	Expected	Sometimes
Fistula formation	No	Expected
Perianal involvement	Rare	Expected
Intestinal obstruction	Unusual	Common
Risk for Cancer	Slight to none	Higher risk

Source: Copyright © 2014, NovEx Novice to Expert Learning, LLC

Concept Check

4. The patient with Crohn's disease should be monitored for the development of what associated disorder?
   A. Arthritis
   B. Venous ulcers on the legs
   C. Liver cancer
   D. Pericarditis

Answer question

Priority Patient Concerns and Desired Collaborative Care Outcomes

Prior to caring for patients with GI inflammatory disorders, it is important to prioritize the patient's concerns that must guide the nursing care plan and interventions. Care for the patient is ordered and organized in accordance with the patient's priority and urgent needs. Desired collaborative care outcomes in patients with GI inflammatory disorders typically include:

1. Patient will experience reduction in pain.
2. Patient will report feeling more comfortable in social situations.
3. Patient will state or demonstrate increased ability to cope.
4. Patient will state ways to improve, prevent, and ameliorate symptoms from GI inflammatory processes.
5. Patient will maintain or return to normal fluid status.

Considering these important care outcomes, prepare a list of the major 3–6 priority patient concerns or nursing diagnoses for patients with GI inflammatory disorders. Be prepared to participate in a discussion of this list and/or to submit them as an assignment, as determined by your faculty. Resources you may find helpful in this assignment can include this lesson, the references, resources on nursing care plans, and standard nursing diagnoses manuals.

LO3:

Collaborative Interventions

Goals of Care: The main goals of treatment for GI inflammatory disease are the reduction of inflammation and symptom management. [Note that radiation colitis is a toxic effect of treating cancer. See detailed care of the patient under Diarrhea in the Care of Cancer Patients with Treatment Toxicities NovE-lesson]

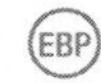

- Treatment and combinations of treatment vary, depending on the location and extent of the disease (Carter, et al., 2004).

Acute GI Inflammatory Bowel Exacerbation

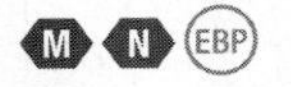

- When a patient presents with an acute exacerbation, the priority is to evaluate the patient for any urgent or life-threatening complication (Carter, et al., 2004).

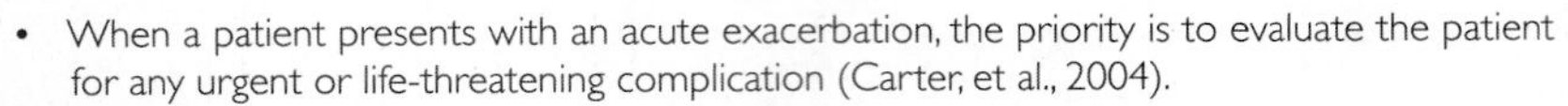

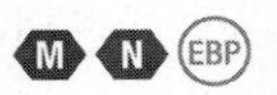

- Patients with fever >38.5°C (101.3°F), hypotension, and tachycardia should be evaluated immediately for sepsis (see the Care of Patients with Sepsis NovE-lesson). Perforation leading to peritonitis and/or sepsis is an emergent situation. Call the Rapid Response Team and/or the health care provider (Carter, et al., 2004).

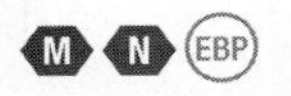

- Infection resulting from abscess formation or perforation must be treated with antibiotics (e.g., fluoroquinolone, metronidazole). Patients with perforation and/or abscess formation commonly require surgery and/or abscess drainage (Carter, et al., 2004).

- Anticipate and prepare for immediate surgery, start IV fluids, restrict oral intake, and collaborate with team if the patient has findings suggesting abscess, fistula, hemorrhage, toxic megacolon, or obstruction.

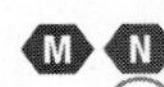

- If the patient is without urgent complications:

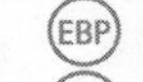

  - o Initiate IV fluids for rehydration (Carter, et al., 2005).

  - o Replace electrolytes to correct imbalances (Carter, et al., 2005).

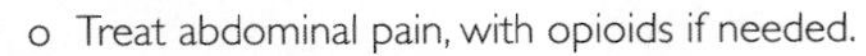

  - o Treat abdominal pain, with opioids if needed.
  - o Permit no oral intake (NPO) if nauseated and vomiting.
- If the patient does not respond to initial care, administer ordered:

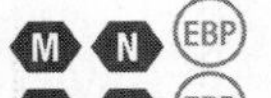

  - o Corticosteroids (oral or IV) (Travis, et al., 2007)

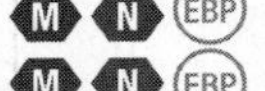

  - o Antibiotics (Travis, et al., 2007)

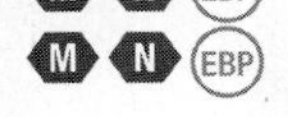

  - o Both corticosteroids and antibiotics (Travis, et al., 2007)
- Surgery may be required if the patient still does not respond to conservative medical treatments.

Necrotizing Fasciitis and Enterocutaneous Fistula with Intra-Abdominal Sepsis

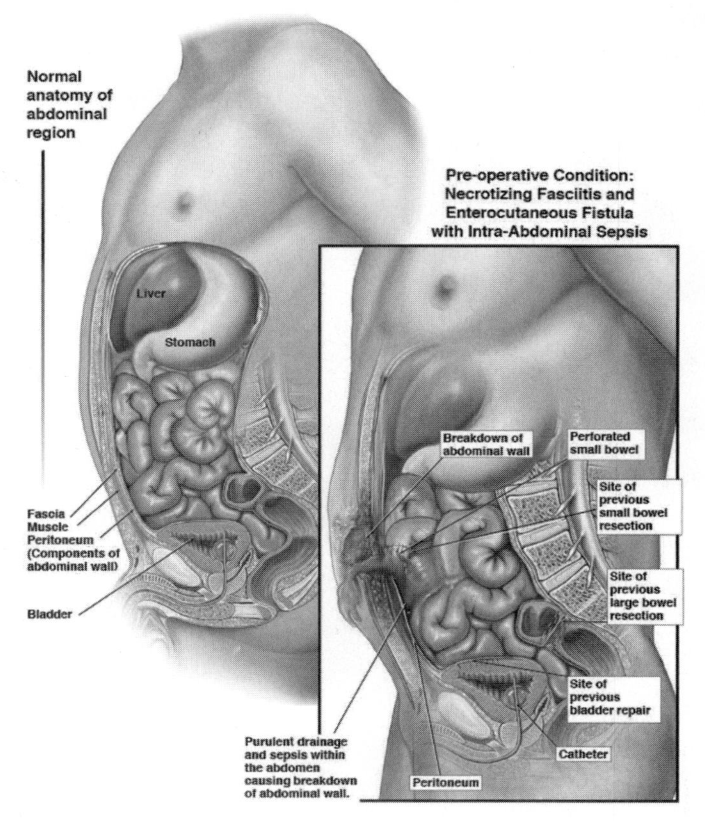

This image depicts a bowel perforation, leakage of contaminated wastes into the peritoneum, and development of severe sepsis with necrotizing effects. Early intervention is essential.

Collaborative Interventions (continued)

Symptom Management After Mild Exacerbations

- Once the patient has achieved remission for the acute episode, the goal is to stabilize the patient on maintenance therapy.
- One of the primary symptoms of patients with GI inflammatory disease is pain, which may be chronic with acute exacerbations. Symptoms with **mild exacerbations**, particularly pain, may be treated with:
  - Antispasmodics may be helpful (e.g., hyoscyamine, dicyclomine) for mild colitis without symptoms of systemic toxicity.
  - Antidiarrheals may be helpful for mild intermittent diarrhea without symptoms of systemic toxicity:
    - Loperamide (Imodium)
    - Diphenoxylate and atropine (Lomotil)
    - Cholestyramine

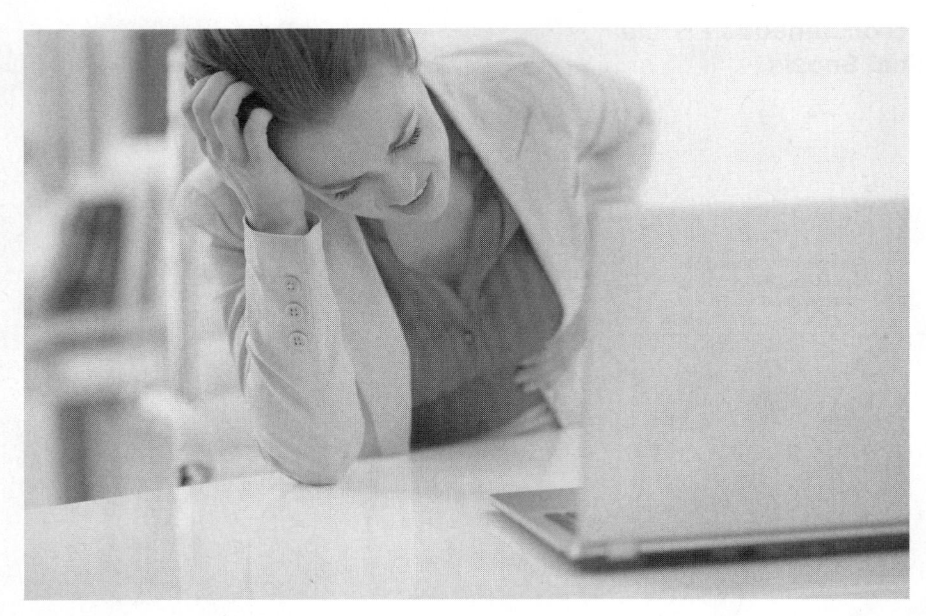

This young female presents the typical picture of a person suffering with the pain of inflammatory bowel disease: a cramping, bloated feeling of intense discomfort.
Source: Alliance/Fotolia

Concept Check

5. A patient with acute exacerbation of an inflammatory bowel disorder is most likely to require which intervention?
   A. Intravenous fluids
   B. Surgery
   C. NPO status
   D. Blood transfusion

Answer question

Symptom Management After Moderate–Severe Exacerbation

When a patient with moderate-to-severe GI inflammatory disease achieves remission, maintenance therapy is more complex. Interventions (and combinations) to manage symptoms can include:

- Administer anti-inflammatory meds and educate the patient about these meds:
  - o 5-aminosalicylic acid (5-ASA) derivatives act on epithelial cells of the intestines to modulate proinflammatory cytokines in order to treat mild–moderate disease and maintain remission (e.g., mesalamine, sulfasalazine) (Talley, et al., 2011).
  - o Corticosteroids (IV or oral) to treat mild-to-moderate disease (e.g., prednisone, methylprednisolone, budesonide, hydrocortisone) (Talley, et al., 2011)

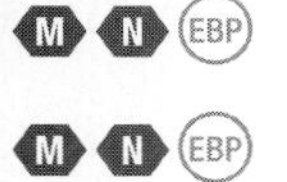

  - o Corticosteroid enemas are sometimes used to treat ulcerative colitis when the rectum is mostly involved (Travis, et al., 2007).
- Immunosuppressant agents may be considered: azathioprine (Imuran), 6-mercaptopurine (Purinethol), methotrexate (Rheumatrex), tacrolimus (Prograf) (Talley, et al., 2011).
- Biologic therapy:

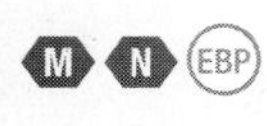

  - o Treatments can more specifically target the pathway that causes Crohn's disease. For example, infliximab is an antibody to tumor necrosis factor alpha (cytokine) (Talley, et al., 2011).
  - o Other biologic agents include:
    - Adalimumab
    - Certolizumab
    - Natalizumab

    (Talley, et al., 2011)

If the patient is not responsive to the combinations of medications, additional care and treatments are aimed at managing symptoms and infections that may develop:

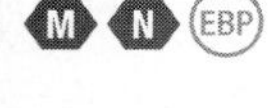

- Antibiotics are used to treat abscess and fistula formation (e.g., metronidazole, ciprofloxacin) and may be tried in patients who cannot tolerate or do not improve on 5-ASA (Talley, et al., 2011).

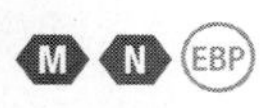

- Opiates may be used for patients with severe acute pain or for chronic pain that does not improve after other treatment (Carter, et al., 2004).

- Tricyclic antidepressants (e.g., *amitriptyline*, imipramine) can help decrease the need for opiate pain medication.

Small Bowel Perforations with Resulting Abdominal and Pelvic Abscesses

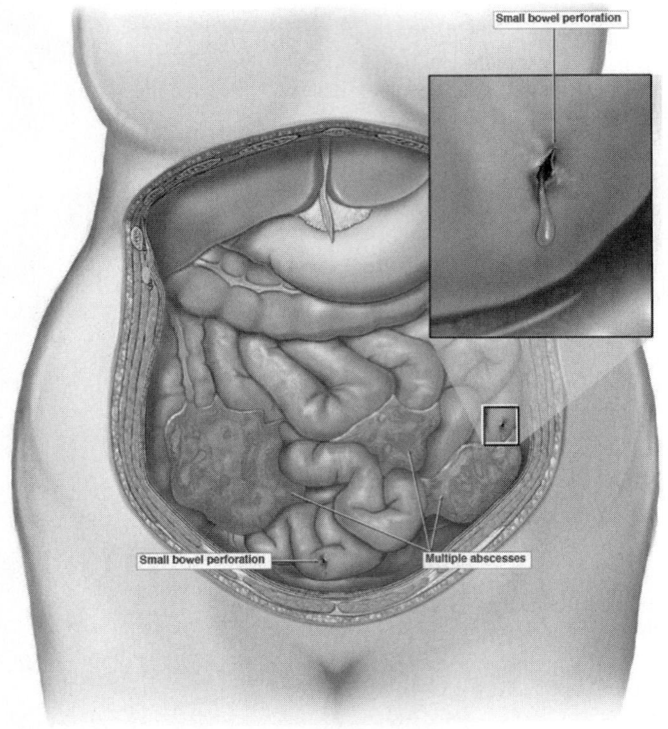

Bowel perforation caused by Crohn's disease can lead to intra-abdominal abscesses that require immediate antibiotics and aggressive surgical debridement.

Collaborative Interventions (continued)

Surgery in GI Inflammatory Disease

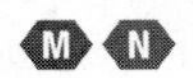

- The goal of surgical intervention is to preserve function and length of the bowel. Collaboration of the team is needed to orchestrate and prepare patients for intervention. Surgery, sometimes emergent, is indicated for (Travis, et al., 2007):

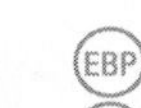

  - o Bowel perforation (Travis, et al., 2007)
  - o Intra-abdominal abscesses (Travis, et al., 2007)

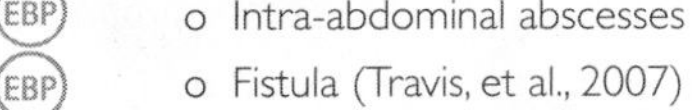

  - o Fistula (Travis, et al., 2007)
  - o Bowel obstruction (intractable nausea, vomiting, abdominal distention) (Talley, et al., 2011)
  - o Severe hemorrhage (Travis, et al., 2007)

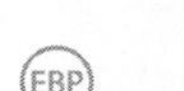

  - o Toxic megacolon (sudden, severe dilation of the colon with associated severe pain, distension, shock) (Travis, et al., 2007)

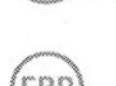

  - o Cancer (Travis, et al., 2007)
  - o Curative intervention for ulcerative colitis (Travis, et al., 2007)

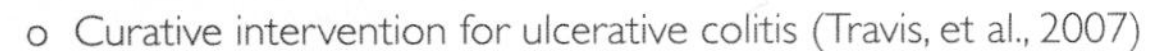

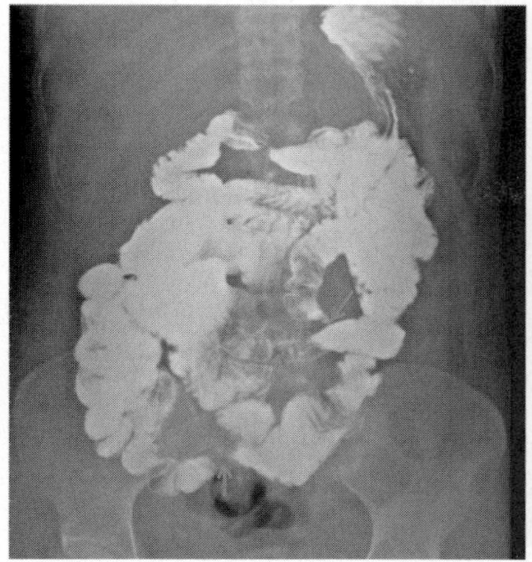

The arrows point to several of the multiple strictures caused by Crohn's disease. The xray shows strictures that caused fecal blockage, small bowel distension, pain, and necessary surgery.

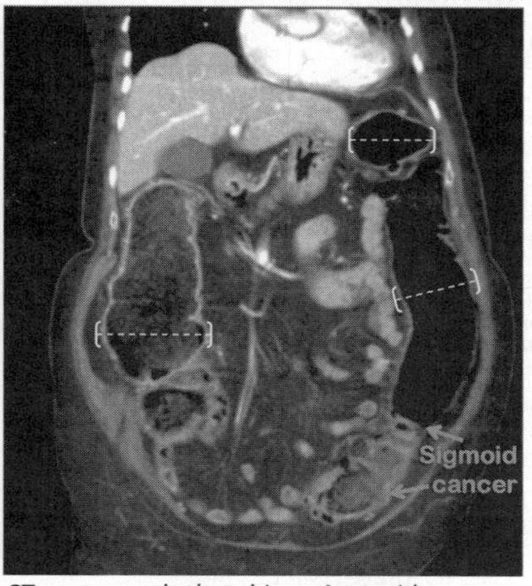

CT scan reveals that this patient with ulcerative colitis also has a sigmoid cancer in the lower large colon causing an obstruction. Note the remarkable large bowel distension (yellow) with accumulation of feces, fluid and air. This condition warrants surgical intervention for relief.

Source: Courtesy of K. Kyriakidis

Patient Education and Prevention

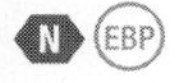

Patient education and prevention are aimed at helping the patient to sustain remission (Travis, et al., 2007).

Diet

- **Diet** does not cause GI inflammatory disease but can exacerbate symptoms.
- **Dietary recommendations** include:
  - o Staying hydrated, especially when diarrhea is present
  - o Avoiding certain foods:
    - ■ High-fiber foods (bran, beans, nuts, seeds, and popcorn)
    - ■ Fatty, greasy, or fried foods and sauces (butter, margarine, and heavy cream)
  - o Being alert and tracking particular foods that exacerbate symptoms
  - o Limiting dairy products if lactose intolerance develops
  - o Consulting a nutritionist (Carter, et al., 2004)

Educate and Support Patient

- About disease, treatment, medications, coping, body image changes, fear, when to seek help, and healthy diet

Supplements

- Iron supplements for anemia due to bleeding
- Calcium and vitamin D for patients who must decrease dairy intake
- Vitamin B_{12} supplement is sometimes necessary in patients with Crohn's disease involving the ileum, where B_{12} is normally absorbed.

Stress and Coping

- Stressful incidents or major changes in life, such as relationship problems, moving, a new job, or the loss of a job, can contribute to digestive problems.
- Assist with strategies to help patient manage stress and learn to cope with significant changes in lifestyle.
- Collaborate for referral if patient can benefit from more in-depth psychological support or additional strategies for coping with altered body function and image.

Prevention

- Due to increased risk:
  - o Vaccinations for flu and pneumonia (strongly encouraged)
  - o Smoking cessation (Carter, et al., 2004)
  - o Routine colorectal screening
  - o Routine cervical cancer screening
  - o Osteoporosis screening

Collaborative Interventions Summary: Maintenance Therapy, Patient Education, and Prevention

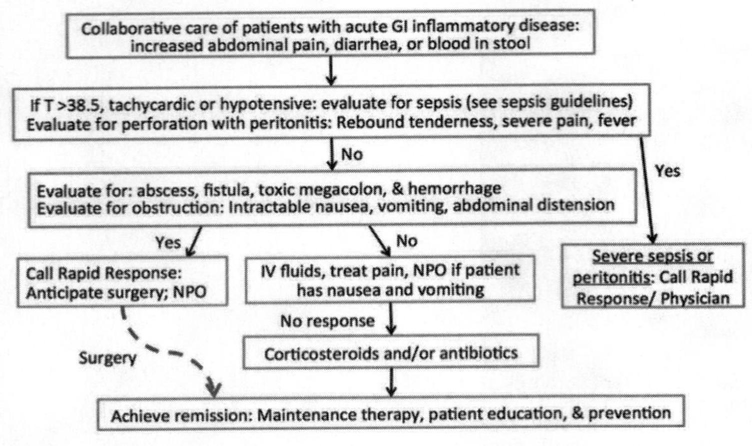

Summary: Acute GI Inflammatory Exacerbation

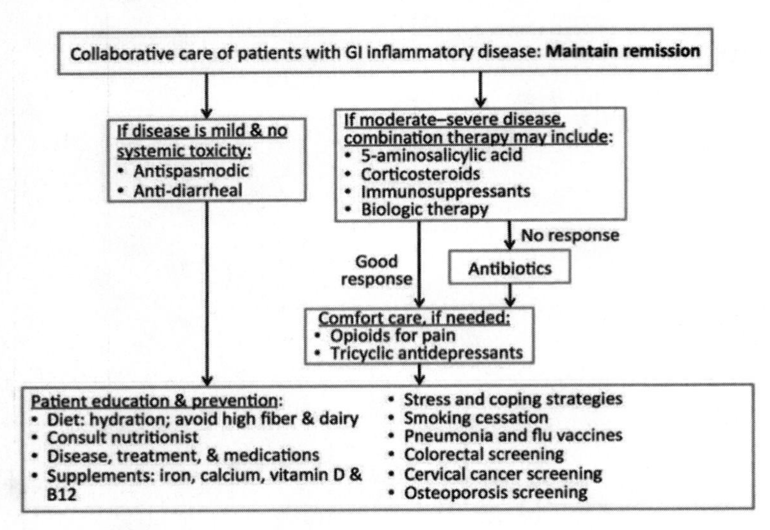

Summary of Interventions

For Exacerbations

- IV fluids, electrolyte replacement, pain treatment, and NPO if nauseated and vomiting
- Evaluate for sepsis in patients with fever >38.5°C (101.3°F), tachycardia, and hypotension (see the Care of Patients with Sepsis NovE-lesson, guidelines).
- Anticipate and rapidly prepare the patient for surgery for bowel perforation, hemorrhage, obstruction, abscess, and malignancy.

Maintenance Management

- Mild disease: antidiarrheals and antispasmodics
- Moderate-to-severe: Treatment of inflammation with anti-inflammatory meds:
  - o 5-aminosalicylic acid (5-ASA) derivative
  - o Corticosteroids
  - o Immunosuppressant agents
  - o Biologic therapy
- Treatment of pain with:
  - o Opiates
  - o Tricyclic antidepressants
- Antibiotics for patients with:
  - o Infection, abscess formation, or sepsis
  - o No response to treatment
- Dietary recommendations
  - o Consult nutritionist.
- Patient education and prevention

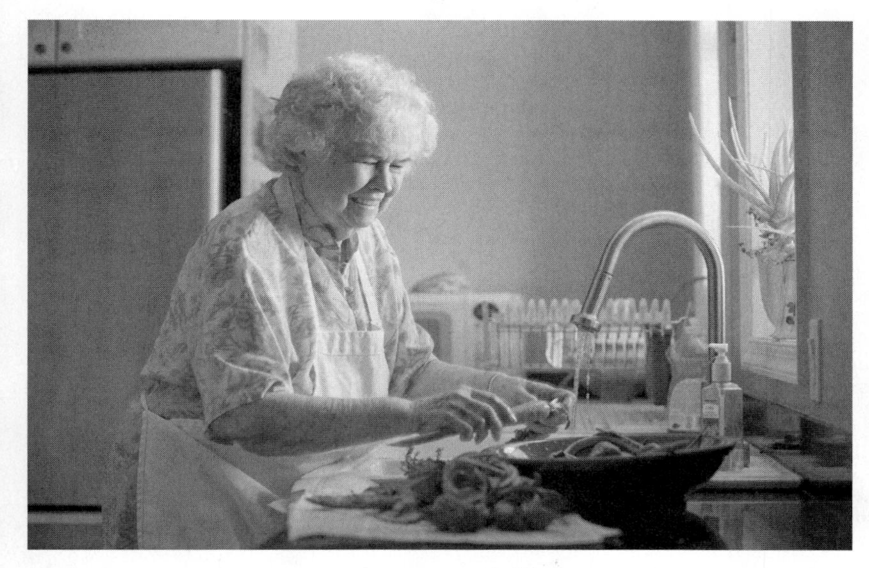

Specific dietary instructions are essential in patients with GI inflammatory diseases. A nutritionist or dietician can help provide disease-specific instructions on what foods to avoid. Because patients vary in what foods affect them, keeping track of what foods exacerbate the disease is important.
Source: CDC/Cade Martin/Dawn Arlotta

Concept Check

6. Which dietary supplement is needed by patients with inflammatory bowel disease?

A. Vitamin A
B. Potassium
C. Magnesium
D. Iron

Answer question

Concept Check

7. Which of the following interventions can cure Crohn's disease?

A. Reduction of stress and improved coping skills
B. Surgery
C. Biologic therapy combined with immunosuppressants
D. None of the above

Answer question

LO4:

Evaluation of Desired Collaborative Care Outcomes

Evaluation and reassessment should reveal attainment of previously established patient outcomes. In summary:

- Patient reports that adherence to treatment plan has resulted in decreased number and severity of painful episodes.
- Patient reports feeling confident and enjoying participation in social events.
- Patient describes strategies being used that are improving the ability to cope with body changes.
- Patient accurately discusses and demonstrates methods to improve, prevent, and ameliorate symptoms from GI inflammatory processes.
- Patient is alert, with elastic skin turgor, blood pressure within desired range, and fluid intake that is equal to fluid losses.

References

Amplo, K., & Nelson, D. (2009). Care of the patient with irritable bowel disease. *AORN J, 90*(6), 909–918.

Anastasi, J. K., Capili, B., & Chang, M. (2013). Managing irritable bowel syndrome. *Amer J Nurs, 113*(7), 42–54.

Chadda, S. (2013). Nurse perspectives in ulcerative colitis: An approach to individualised care. *Gastrointestinal Nursing, 11*(5), 24–29.

Collins, P., & Rhodes, J. (2006). Ulcerative colitis: Diagnosis and management. *British Med J, 333*(7563), 340–343. **www.ncbi.nlm.nih.gov/pmc/articles/PMC1539087/**

Darlin, A. (2008). Caring for the patient with Crohn's disease: Practical do's and don'ts to improve patients' quality of life. *Gastroenterology Nursing, 31*(5), S2–S4.

Day, M. (2014). Fight back against inflammatory bowel disease. *Nursing 2014, 38*(11), 34–40. **www.nursingcenter.com/lnc/CEArticle?an=00152193-200811000-00034&Journal_ID=54016&Issue_ID=825443**

Fraser, A. (2008). New treatment options for patients with ulcerative colitis. *Gastrointestinal Nursing, 6*(1), 27–31.

Holmes, S. (2014). *Caring for the patient with Crohn's disease.* **nursing.advanceweb.com/Article/Caring-for-the-Patient-with-Crohns-Disease-3.aspx**

Mayer, E. A. (2008). Clinical practice: Irritable bowel syndrome. *N Engl J Med, 358*(16), 1692–1699.

O'Connor, M., Bager, P., Duncan, J., et al. (2013). Consensus/Guidelines: N-ECCO consensus statements on the European nursing roles in caring for patients with Crohn's disease or ulcerative colitis. *J Crohns Colitis, 7*(9), 744–764. **download.journals.elsevierhealth.com/pdfs/journals/1873-9946/PIIS1873994613002080.pdf**

Registered Nurses Association of Ontario (RNAO). (2005). *Prevention of constipation in the older adult population.* **rnao.ca/sites/rnao-ca/files/storage/related/611_BPG_Prevent_Constipation_Summary_rev05.pdf** [no real EBP for constipation].

Toner, F., & Claros, E. (2012). Preventing, assessing and managing constipation in older adults. *Nursing 2012, 42*(12), 32–40.

Clinical Practice Guidelines

Carter, M., Lobo, A., Travis, S., et al. (2004). Guidelines for the management of inflammatory bowel disease in adults. *Gut, 53*(suppl 5), v1–v16. **gut.bmj.com/content/53/suppl_5/v1.full#ref-93**

Kornbluth, A., Sachar, D., and the Practice Parameters Committee of the American College of Gastroenterology. (2010). Ulcerative colitis in adults. *Amer J Gastroenterol, 105*, 500. **gi.org/guideline/ulcerative-colitis-in-adults/**

Lichtenstein, G. R., Hanauer, S. B., Sandborn, W. J., and the Practice Parameters Committee of the American College of Gastroenterology. (2008). Management of Crohn's disease in adults. *Amer J Gastroenterol.* **gi.org/guideline/management-of-crohn%E2%80%99s-disease-in-adults/**

Talley, N., Abreu, M., Achkar, J., et al. (2011). An evidence-based systematic review on medical therapies for inflammatory bowel disease. *Am J Gastroenterol, 106*, S2–S25. **s3-patients.gi.org/files/2011/10/AJG-IBD-supplement-0411.pdf**

Travis, S., Stange, E., Lemann, M., et al. (2007). European evidence-based consensus on the management of ulcerative colitis: Current management. *Journal of Crohn's and Colitis, 2*, 24–62. **ugcg.me/files/GIT/Consensus_UC.pdf**

Patient Education

Mayo Clinic Staff. (2011). *Crohn's disease.* **www.mayoclinic.com/health/crohns-disease/DS00104/DSECTION=risk-factors**

Mayo Clinic Staff. (2011). *Ulcerative colitis.* **www.mayoclinic.com/health/ulcerative-colitis/DS00598/DSECTION=risk-factors**

Rendi, M. (2013) *Crohn disease.* **emedicine.medscape.com/article/1986158-overview#a1**

Learning Outcomes for Structural and Obstructive GI Disorders

When you complete this lesson, you will be able to:

1. Recognize the clinical relevance of structural and obstructive gastrointestinal disorders.
2. Consider the pathophysiology, etiology, risk factors, and clinical presentation of structural and obstructive gastrointestinal disorders that determine the priority patient concerns.
3. Determine the most urgent and important nursing interventions and patient education required in caring for a patient with a structural or obstructive gastrointestinal disorder.
4. Evaluate attainment of desired collaborative care outcomes for a patient with a structural or obstructive gastrointestinal disorder.

LO1:

Gastrointestinal Disorders: Lower GI Tract

Gastrointestinal bowel disorders consist of:

- Infectious Disorders
- Inflammatory Disorders
- Functional Disorders
- **Structural Disorders**

This NovE-lesson focuses on structural disorders.

LO1:

What Are Structural Gastrointestinal Disorders?

- **Structural disorders** are problems that include an abnormal appearance of the bowel with impaired functioning.
- Colon polyps, rectal prolapse, hernias, adhesions, hemorrhoids, rectal fissures and fistulas, tumors, and diverticulosis are the most common causes of structural disorders of the intestinal tract.

Examples of GI Structural Disorders

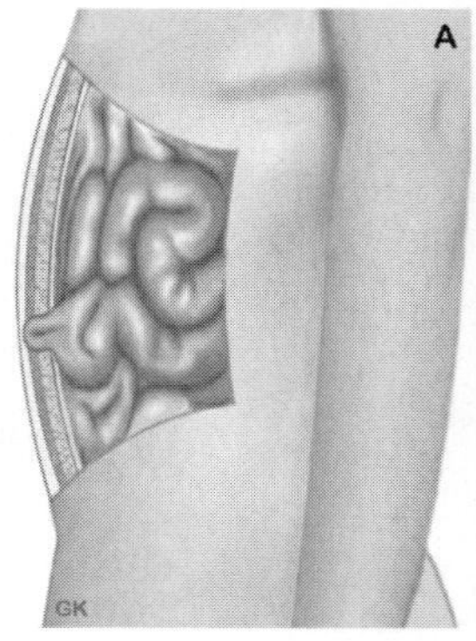

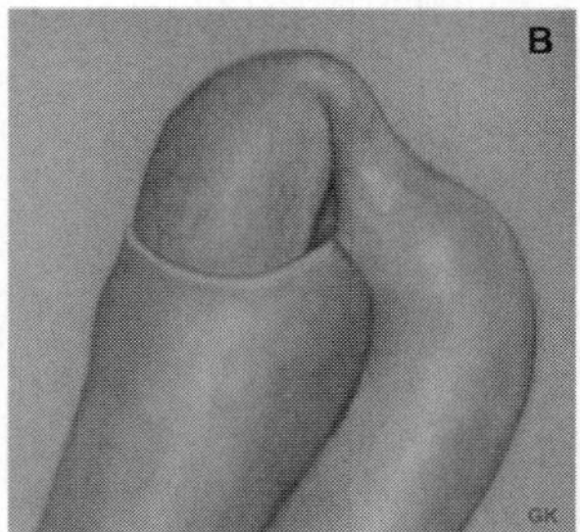

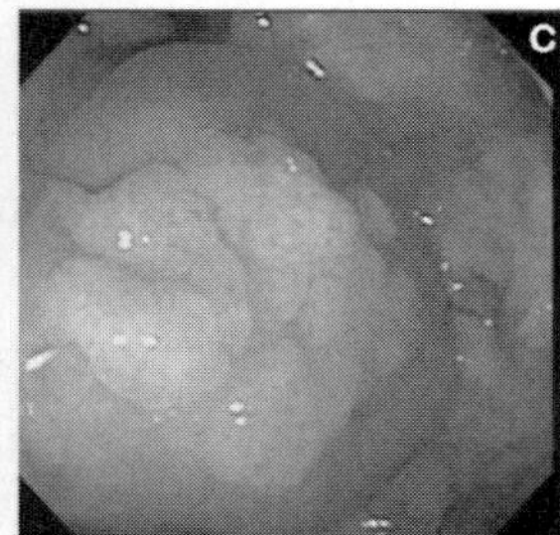

These images illustrate a few of the many abnormal structural disorders that may occur in the gastrointestinal system: A) umbilical hernia where a loop of intestines protrudes through the abdominal wall, B) intussusception where a section of bowel is invaginated into another, and C) tubular adenoma type polyp in the colon.

Sources: Courtesy of George Kyriakidis/Santa Ana, CA, & K. Kyriakidis

LO1:

What Is Intestinal Obstruction?

- Colonic obstruction can be a result of tumor growth, an anatomical anomaly such as volvulus, an incarcerated hernia, adhesions, stricture, inflammatory bowel disease, or obstipation.
- Colonic obstruction is more common in older adults.
- Determining the cause of the obstruction and distinguishing obstruction from ileus is imperative in determining the management.

Small Bowel Obstructions Caused By Adhesions

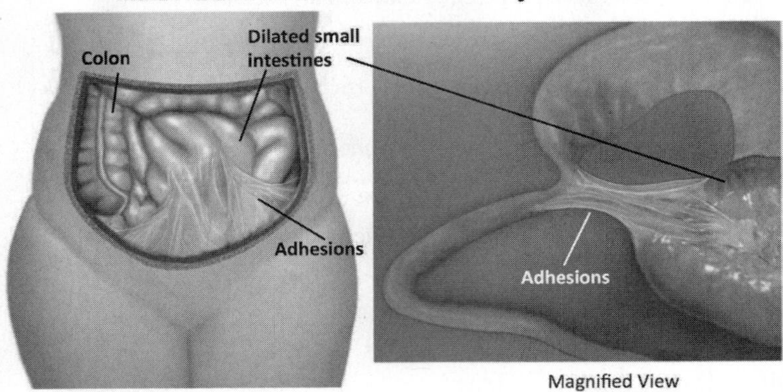

Left: This woman has an adhesive band that has caused a small bowel obstruction with dilated small bowel above the adhesion obstruction. Right: A magnified view shows how adhesions can cause small bowel obstruction.
Source: Courtesy of George Kyriakidis/Santa Ana, CA

LO1:

Clinical Relevance: Intestinal Obstruction

Small Bowel Obstruction

- Small bowel obstruction (SBO) accounts for 20% of all acute surgical admissions, with approximately a 40% rate of strangulation, which is a surgical emergency.
- Morbidity and mortality are related to timely diagnosis and treatment.
- Treatment in <36 hours results in a mortality of 8%, >36 hours increases mortality up to 25%. If left untreated, the mortality rate reaches 100%.

Large Bowel Obstruction

- Morbidity and mortality in patients with large bowel obstruction (LBO) are closely related to the patient's overall health, comorbid conditions, and surgical procedure. Almost 60% of LBOs are related to malignancies.
- Early treatment generally results in a good outcome.
- There is generally 20% mortality in patients with LBO. Mortality rises to 40% in patients with perforation or ischemia of the colon.

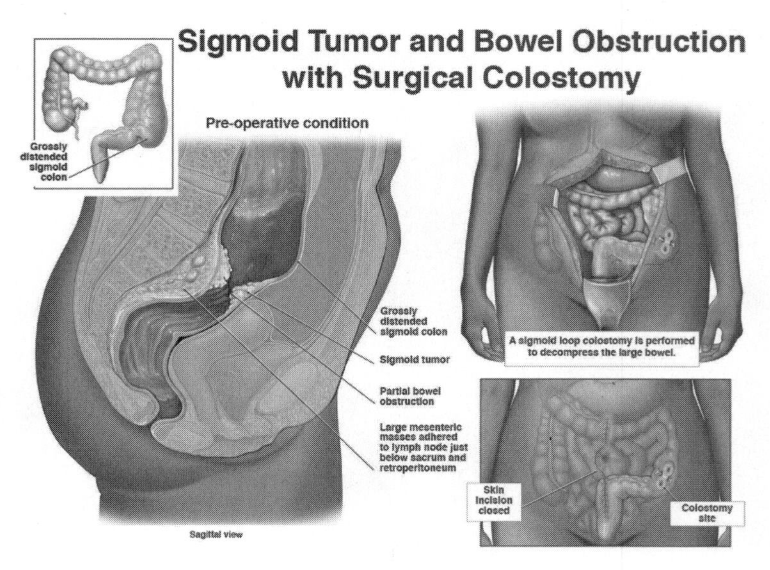

A tumor in the sigmoid colon, plus a large mass in the mesentery, supposedly metastatic lymph nodes, produces an obstruction that is treated with a colostomy devised from a loop of the sigmoid that is proximal to the tumor.

LO2:

Pathophysiology: Intestinal Obstruction

- **Obstruction:** Gas and fluid accumulate, and the intestine becomes dilated proximal to the obstruction. Bacterial overgrowth can then take place proximal to the obstruction (even in the small bowel, which is normally sterile) that can lead to the production of gas and further distension. If dilation becomes severe, the intestine can perforate. The segment of bowel beyond the obstruction collapses. There is an increase in the peristaltic movement of the intestine proximal to the obstruction. The increased intraluminal pressure in the intestine causes a collapse of the veins and edema of the intestinal wall, which can exacerbate obstruction.
- **Simple obstruction:** The blood flow to the intestine is not compromised.
- **Strangulated obstruction:** Arterial blood flow is compromised. Arterial blood flow is commonly compromised because of compression of the arterial supply. This occurs, for example, in a volvulus or hernia. This results in ischemia and necrosis of the bowel tissue within several hours. Release of cytokines quickly follows ischemia and necrosis. The cytokines can cause a systemic inflammatory response syndrome (SIRS) with hypotension and hypoperfusion. Eventually, the affected area may perforate or become gangrenous (see details about peritonitis in the Care of Patients with Infectious GI Disorders NovE-lesson). Perforation can cause leakage of intestinal contents and peritonitis as well as infection. A strangulated obstruction is a medical emergency requiring rapid surgical intervention.
- Intestinal obstruction can be either partial or complete.

LO2:

Risk Factors and Causes: Intestinal Obstruction

Small Bowel (Intestine)

- Most often caused by postoperative adhesions: 60% from colorectal surgeries, appendectomy, hernia repair, and GYN surgery
- Malignancy (20%)
- Hernias (10%)
- Crohn's disease

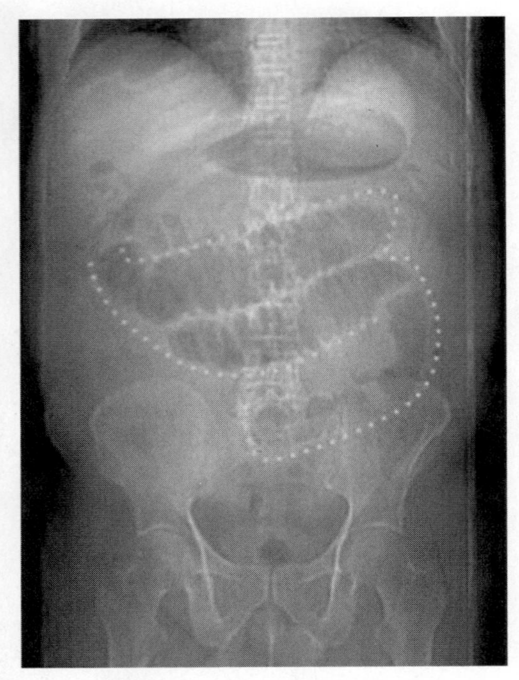

This radiograph of the abdomen shows the markedly dilated loops of the jejunum (dark structures within dotted lines), characteristic of small bowel obstruction. The remainder of the intestine is collapsed beyond the site of obstruction. The small bowel is so distended that an untrained eye may mistake it for the large bowel.
Source: Courtesy of K. Kyriakidis

Large Bowel (Colon or Intestine)

- Malignancy (60%)
- Obstipation
- Volvulus
- Intussusception
- Incarcerated hernia
- Adhesions

Strangulated intestinal obstruction is most commonly caused by:

- Adhesions
- Strangulated hernia
- Volvulus or the intestine becomes twisted and occluded
- Intussusception, which is a condition where a segment of the intestine becomes invaginated or pulled into itself

Mechanical Causes of Intestinal Obstruction

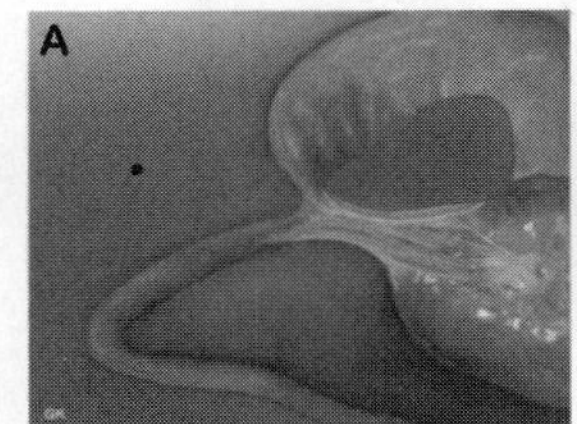

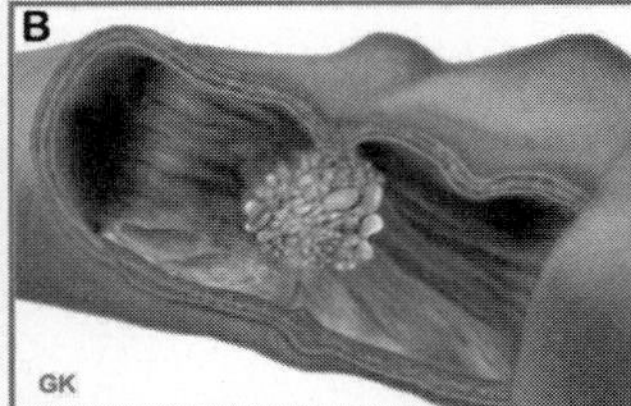

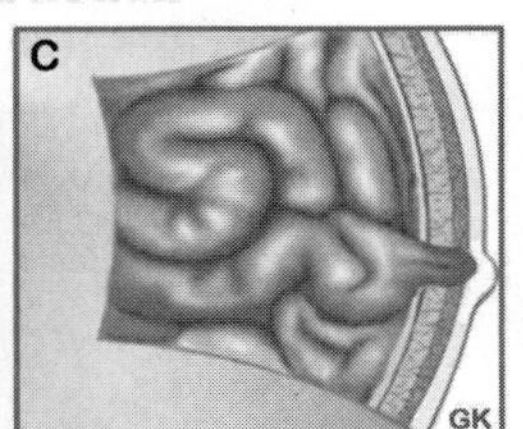

Causes of mechanical intestinal obstruction can include: A) adhesions, B) cancers or tumors, and C) strangulated hernias.

Source: Courtesy of George Kyriakidis/Santa Ana, CA

Concept Check

1. Which distinguishing pathophysiologic sequela occurs that indicates an intestinal obstruction is simple rather than strangulated?
   A. There is only one section of the bowel involved.
   B. Bowel sounds above the obstruction are hyperactive.
   C. The patient is still able to pass mucous per rectum.
   D. The arterial flow to the bowel is not compromised.

Answer question

LO2:

Assessment Findings: Intestinal Obstruction

Small Bowel Obstruction (SBO)

- Abdominal pain: crampy and colicky, progressive, can last for days
- Abdominal distention with distal obstruction
- Nausea
- Diarrhea: early sign
- Vomiting: more prominent with proximal obstruction and can be feculent from bacterial overgrowth
- High-pitched bowel sounds
- Constipation: late sign
- Fever: late sign
- Tachycardia: late sign
- Abdominal scars from previous surgery or radiation, which can cause adhesions where bands of thick, fibrous scarring form and mechanically block the intestine
- Peritoneal signs (usually due to perforation): involuntary guarding, abdominal rigidity, rebound tenderness

Large Bowel Obstruction (LBO)

- Abdominal distention and pain
- Fever
- Tachycardia
- Inability to move bowels or pass gas with complete obstruction
- No stool in rectal vault with complete blockage
- Diarrhea with partial obstruction
- Nausea
- Anorexia
- Vomiting is a late sign.
- Borborygmus: loud abdominal growling noises
- Peritoneal signs (usually due to perforation): involuntary guarding, abdominal rigidity, rebound tenderness (pain when pressure on abdomen is released)

Concept Check

2. What is the best description of a volvulus?
   A. A section of bowel has telescoped into itself.
   B. The bowel has twisted.
   C. The bowel is stuck to itself.
   D. A bowel section has died.

Answer question

LO2: 

Diagnostics: Intestinal Obstruction

Labs:

- CBC: leukocytosis; Anemia may be present.
- Complete metabolic panel: electrolyte imbalance from vomiting
- PT and PTT
- Urinalysis
- Lactic acid: sepsis indicator for tissue hypoxia
- ABG if abnormal anion gap is present.
- Type and cross match

Imaging:

- Abdominal x-ray: Look for air and fluid levels or colon dilation.
- CT scan: Rule out other intra-abdominal processes or detect abscess formation, inflammatory process, and extraluminal pathology (e.g., tumor).
- CT scan of both pelvis and abdomen in all patients with SBO should be performed because informational benefits surpass x-rays (Maung, et al., 2012).
- Ultrasound: less costly for SBO than CT scan; high accuracy for SBO

Colonoscopy Confirms Suspicious Air, Fluid, & Density Seen on CT Scan

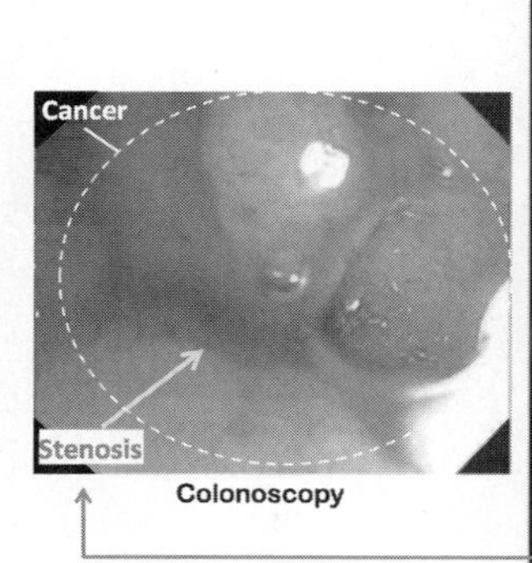

Colonoscopy

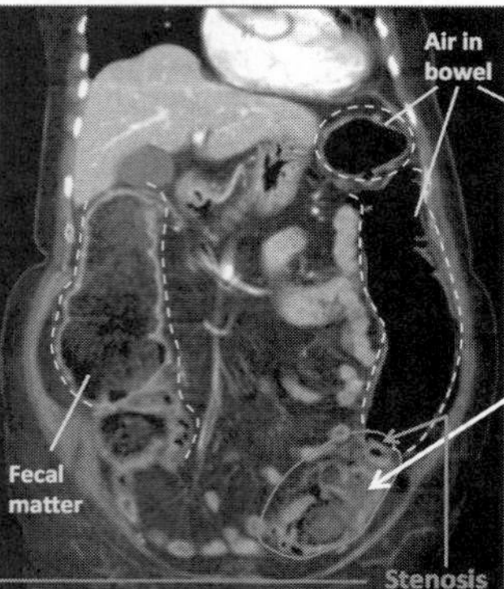

CT Scan

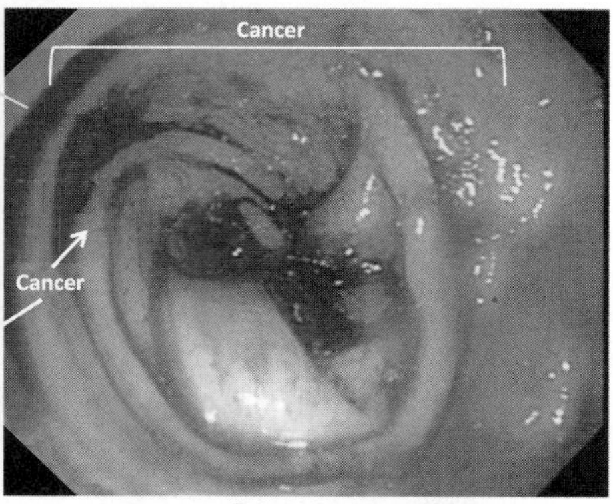

Colonoscopy

Middle: CT scan suggests mass (cancer in red circle) obstructing the sigmoid colon. The distended colon (yellow outlines) is filled with air, fluid, and fecal matter that cannot be eliminated. *Right*: In the same patient, colonoscopy confirms a large cancerous mass (white arrows and bracket) invading the colon and creating obstruction. *Left:* This close-up photo from colonoscopy clearly shows the colon lumen is stenosed and obstructing passage of all bowel contents. With complete stenosis, air and fecal matter are propelled backwards toward the stomach.

Source: Courtesy of K. Kyriakidis

Concept Check

3. Which assessment finding is an early sign of small bowel obstruction?

A. Fever

B. Tachycardia

C. Constipation

D. Diarrhea

Answer question

Priority Patient Concerns and Desired Collaborative Care Outcomes: Intestinal Obstruction

Prior to caring for patients with intestinal obstruction, it is important to prioritize the patient's concerns that must guide the nursing care plan and interventions. Care for the patient is ordered and organized in accordance with the patient's priority and urgent needs. Desired collaborative care outcomes in patients with intestinal obstruction typically include:

1. Patient will demonstrate no findings associated with impairment of arterial blood flow to the gastrointestinal tissues.
2. Patient will report that pain has resolved or abated to a tolerable level.
3. Patient will have no findings associated with fluid imbalance or associated electrolyte or acid–base imbalance.
4. Patient's weight will remain at or return to desired level.
5. Patient will remain free of infection.

Considering these important care outcomes, prepare a list of the major 3–6 priority patient concerns or nursing diagnoses for patients with intestinal obstruction. Be prepared to participate in a discussion of this list and/or to submit them as an assignment, as determined by your faculty. Resources you may find helpful in this assignment can include this lesson, the references, resources on nursing care plans, and standard nursing diagnoses manuals.

LO3:

Collaborative Interventions: Intestinal Obstruction

Upon Admission

Before and while the patient is being evaluated, care should include:

- M N EBP The patient should be NPO (Di Saverio, 2013).
- M N EBP NG tube placement (Di Saverio, 2013)
- M N EBP Aggressive IV fluid resuscitation: normal saline or lactated Ringer's with potassium if renal function is adequate (Di Saverio, 2013)
- M N Immediately evaluate for strangulation, perforation, and peritonitis. These emergencies require surgical evaluation.
- N Monitor vital signs for shock.
- M N Supplemental oxygen for SpO_2 (oxygen sats) that is <93%
- M N Pain medications (e.g., morphine, hydromorphone)
- M N Antiemetics
- M N Enema and fecal disimpaction for LBO if obstipation is the suspected cause of a severe fecal impaction

M N ***Caution: Oral laxatives are contraindicated for SBO and LBO.*** Laxative use with obstruction can result in complications, such as intussusception.

Intestinal Obstructions That Can Require Surgical Intervention

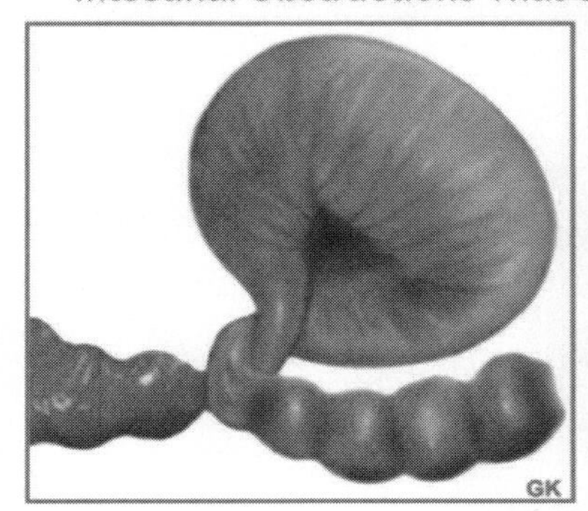

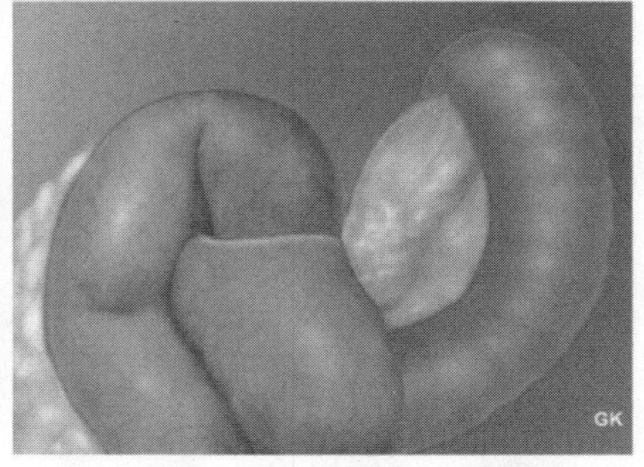

These two images depict volvulus or intestinal twisting (left) and intussusception, which occurs when one section of intestine is invaginated into another (right). These types of mechanical obstructions can require surgical intervention to correct. Visually seeing the obstructions, which additionally causes constipation, can improve understanding about why laxatives for constipation can potentially be harmful or lead to bowel rupture in these patients.

Source: Courtesy of George Kyriakidis/Santa Ana, CA

Subsequent Interventions

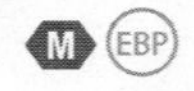

- Surgical correction may be needed, depending on the cause (Di Saverio, 2013). Examples include:
  - o Bowel resection, if a segment of the bowel is ischemic or necrosed
  - o Colostomy, if portions of the bowel require temporary bypass while healing or portions of the bowel require removal that prevent normal fecal evacuation
- Endoscopy for reduction of volvulus or intussusception is sometimes an option.
- Dilation of colon with stenting for partial obstruction or for large bowel obstruction in patients with malignancies that are terminal.
- Care of patients who do not require surgery (patients with no peritonitis, strangulation, perforation, persistent vomiting, negative CT scans) but are being followed and observed include (Di Saverio, et al., 2013):
  - o NPO
  - o Medication for pain
  - o Hydration to replace lost fluids and electrolytes; total parenteral nutrition (TPN) is an option.
  - o Gastric decompression: NG tube insertion; Placement should always be confirmed by chest x-ray.
  - o Nasogastric tube helps decompress the intestine and helps with discomfort, distension, nausea, and vomiting.

Surgical Intervention

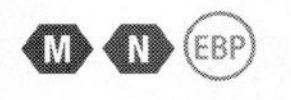

- Patients requiring urgent surgery include those with:
  - o Peritoneal signs (abdominal guarding, tenderness, or continuous pain), which suggest perforation (Maung, et al., 2012)
  - o Fever (Maung, et al., 2012)
  - o Hypotension and tachycardia not resolving with fluid replacement (Maung, et al., 2012)
  - o Leukocytosis (Maung, et al., 2012)
  - o Incarcerated or strangulated hernia
  - o Deteriorating status (e.g., metabolic acidosis) (Maung, et al., 2012)
- Patients with LBO typically require surgical intervention if obstruction is mechanical. Mechanical obstructions are less likely to resolve without surgery.
- About 25% of patients with SBO require surgery (most may spontaneously resolve). Many patients with SBO respond to nonoperative interventions.
- Patients with peritoneal signs, hypotension, fever, and unresponsive to IV hydration should be treated with IV antibiotics that cover aerobic and anaerobic gram negative organisms (i.e., clindamycin, metronidazole, aztreonam, cefotetan, cefoxitin).
- Laparoscopic surgery is preferable over open laparotomy whenever possible due to shorter recovery, lower risk of complications, shortened hospitalization, and lower costs.

Obstruction due to Colon Cancer That Requires Surgical Intervention

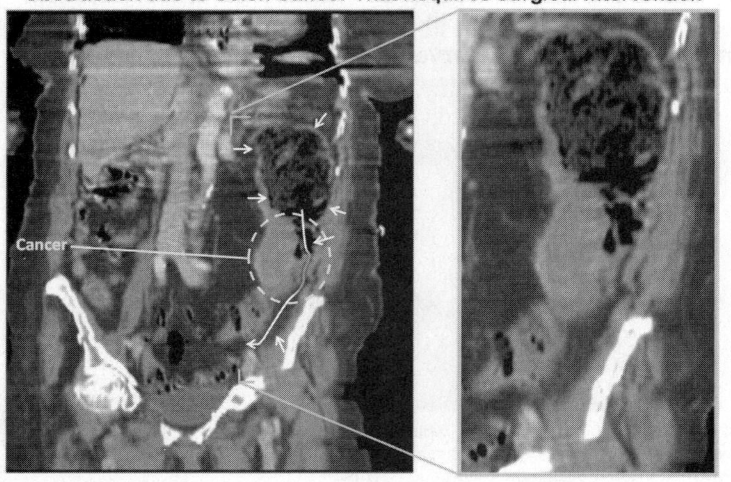

Left: **A CT scan, with accompanying enlarged area, shows a large cancer (yellow outline) that has grown around and into the descending colon. The white arrows point at the distended colon. The long white arrow shows the lumen of the bowel, with reddish segment highlighting and passing through the obstructed area.** ***Right*****: This enlarged area allows closer examination of the cancer, abnormally distended colon, and obstruction (red arrow). Surgical intervention is required.**

Source: Courtesy of K. Kyriakidis

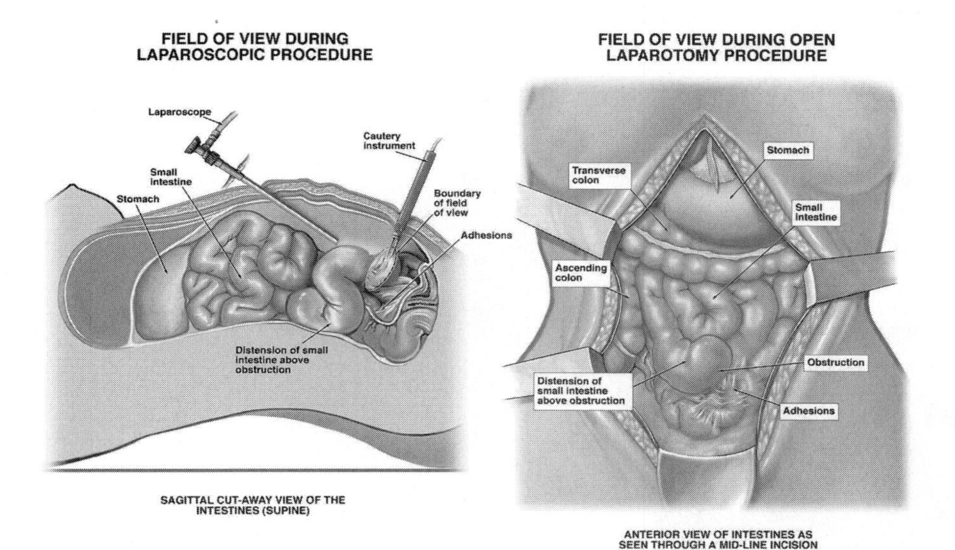

Left: The image depicts how the less invasive laparoscopic surgery is performed. Right: An open laparotomy is demonstrated. There are obvious advantages and disadvantages to both procedures. A better view is seen on the right, but a much smaller wound and potentially less risk for complications are afforded by laparoscopy.
Source: Nucleus Medical Art Inc./Alamy

Collaborative Interventions: Summary for Intestinal Obstruction

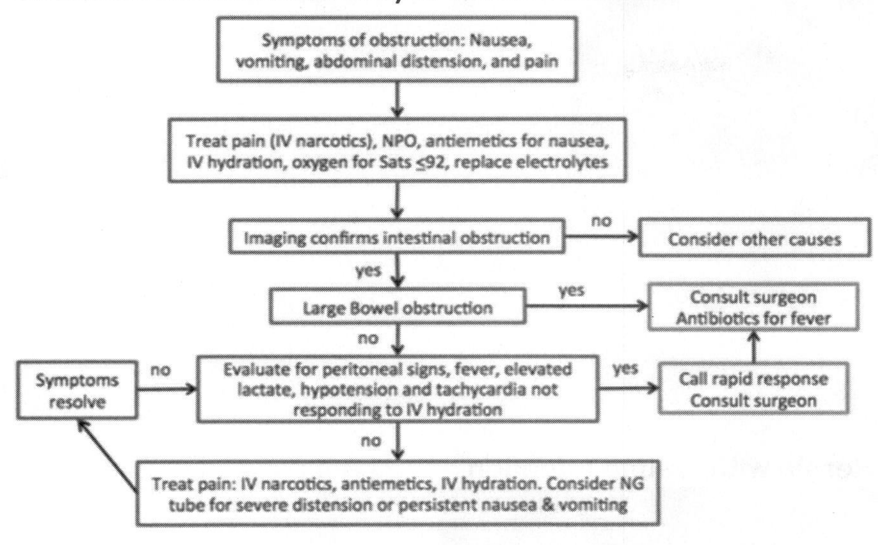

Source: Copyright © 2014, NovEx Novice to Expert Learning, LLC.

LO4:

Evaluation of Desired Collaborative Care Outcomes: Intestinal Obstruction

Evaluation and reassessment should reveal attainment of previously established patient outcomes. In summary:

- Patient's obstruction is resolved and there is no indication of continued gastrointestinal tissue damage.
- Patient reports minimal to no pain.
- Patient has clear mentation, elastic skin turgor, and fluid intake that is balanced with output.
- Patient's weight has returned to pre-illness or desired level.
- Patient is free of infection or is responding well to intervention.

LO1:

What Are Hernias?

A hernia is a structural disorder that is defined as a projection of viscera from its appropriate location.

Location of Hernias

- Epigastric
- Umbilical
- Inguinal
- Femoral

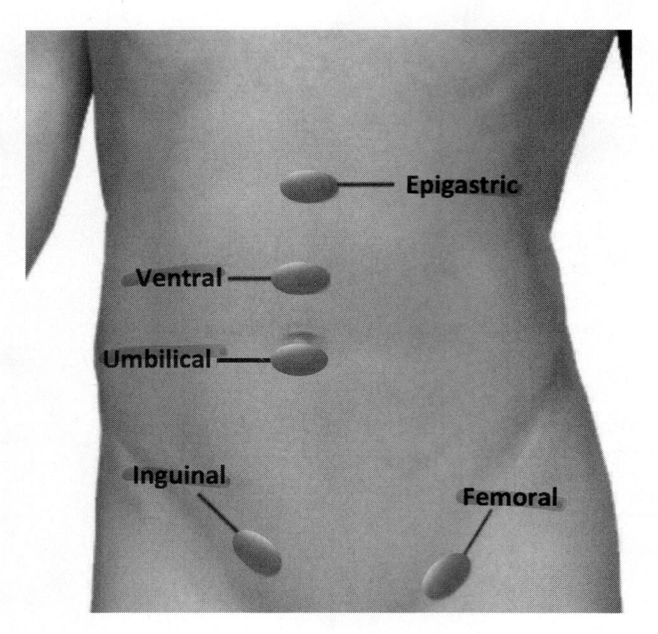

Locations (ventral or incisional) of abdominal wall and inguinal hernias are shown.

Source: Copyright © 2014, NovEx Novice to Expert Learning, LLC

Types of Hernias

- Reducible
- Incarcerated
- Strangulated

Repaired Inguinal Hernia with Wound Infection

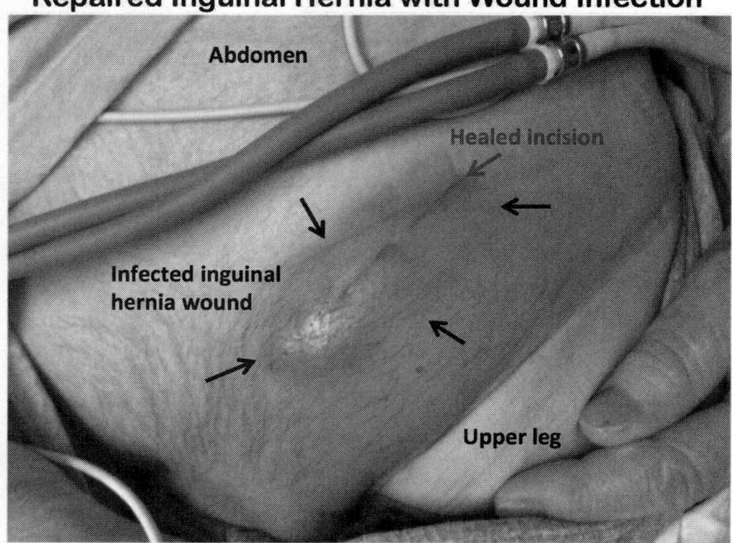

An inguinal hernia that has been repaired is seen in this patient. The incision itself healed well; however, the surrounding tissues involving the hernia repair are infected. The black arrows point to the raised, edematous, and red infected areas.

Source: Courtesy of K. Kyriakidis

LO2:

Pathophysiology: Types of Hernias

- **Reducible:** Hernia can be manually or spontaneously returned to its cavity.
- **Incarcerated:** Hernia is no longer reducible but the vascular supply of the bowel is intact and bowel obstruction is typically seen.
- **Strangulated:** Vascular supply is compromised as a result of the incarceration.

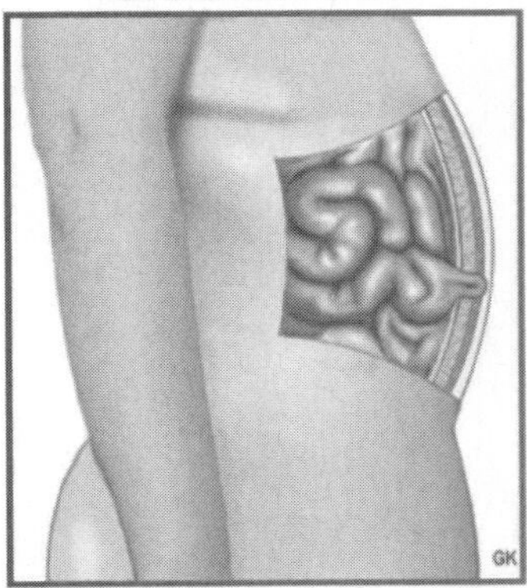

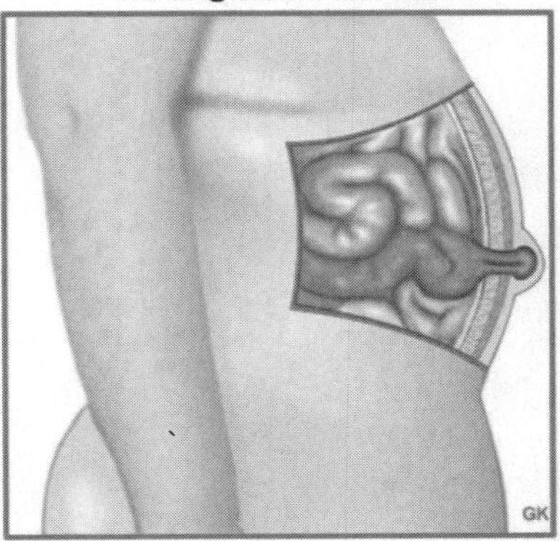

This illustration depicts two different types of hernias. The patient on the left shows a reducible hernia where the vascular supply remains intact and manual manipulation of the bowel is possible. However, on the right, a larger segment of bowel is protruding as an umbilical hernia. Note that strangulated bowel is seen where ischemia and subsequent necrosis are occurring.
Source: Courtesy of George Kyriakidis/Santa Ana, CA

LO2:

Risk Factors and Causes: Hernias

- **Contributing factors** include situations that increase intra-abdominal wall pressure:
  - o Heavy lifting
  - o Obesity
  - o Coughing
  - o Straining to urinate or defecate
  - o COPD
  - o Peritoneal dialysis
  - o Ascites

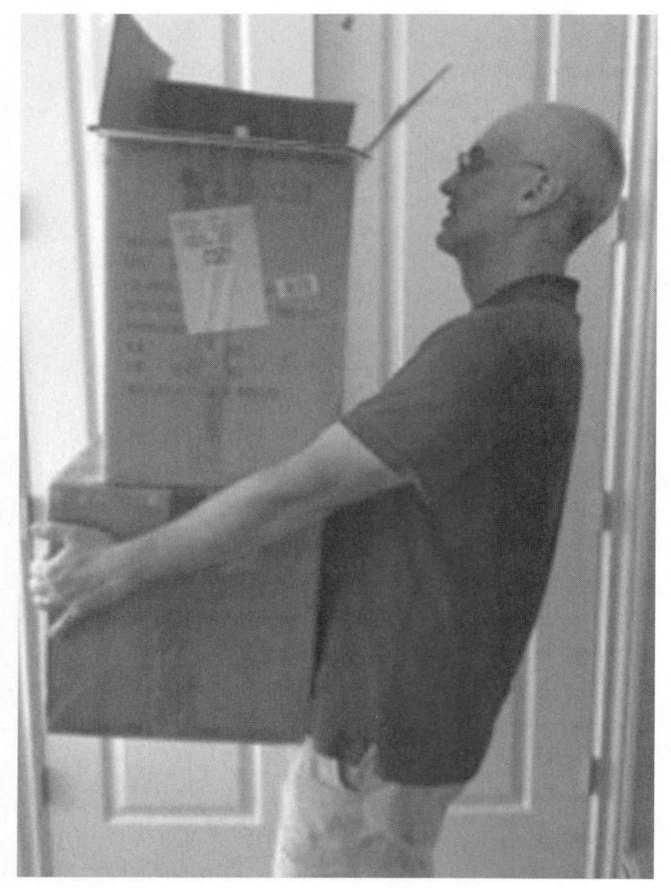

Abdominal pressure created by lifting heavy objects is a common cause of hernias.
Source: Copyright © 2014, NovEx Novice to Expert Learning, LLC

LO2:

Assessment Findings: Hernias

Benign Hernia

- Swelling or a bulge at the site of the hernia
- Slight ache but generally painless
- Enlarges with increased intra-abdominal pressure or position
- Easily reducible

CT Scan Confirms Physical Assessment Findings

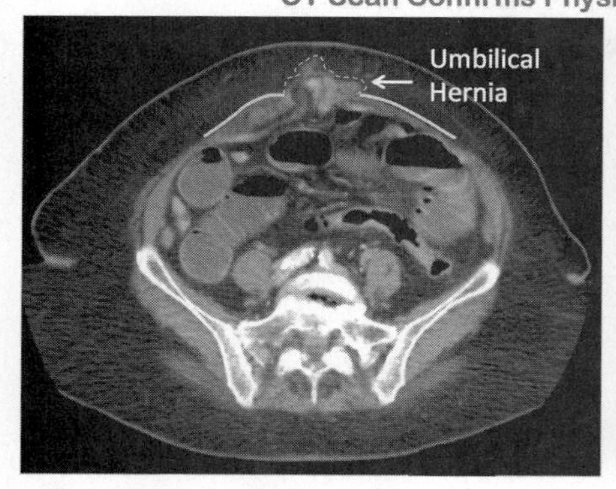

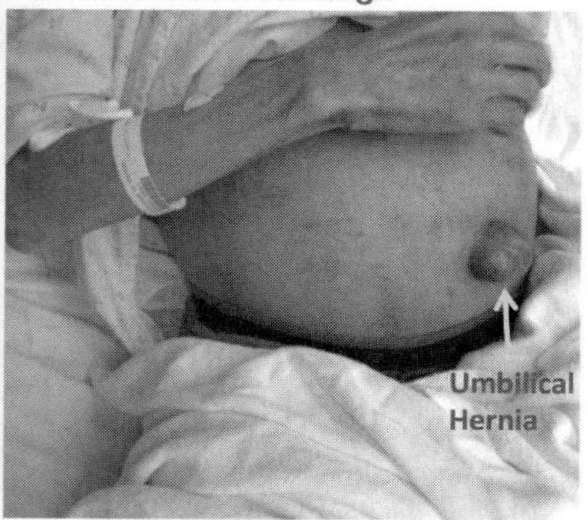

A CT scan is performed (left) to better evaluate the status of the bowel and vascular supply. Right: A large umbilical hernia is found on physical exam.
Source: Courtesy of K. Kyriakidis

Incarcerated Hernia

- Pain and increased size of previous hernia
- Cannot be reduced manually or spontaneously through the abdominal wall defect.
- Bowel obstruction is common.

Strangulated Hernia

- Abdominal pain
- Symptoms similar to incarcerated hernia
- Symptoms of sepsis (e.g., elevated lactate, tachycardia, worsening hypotension, elevated WBCs) due to bowel ischemia

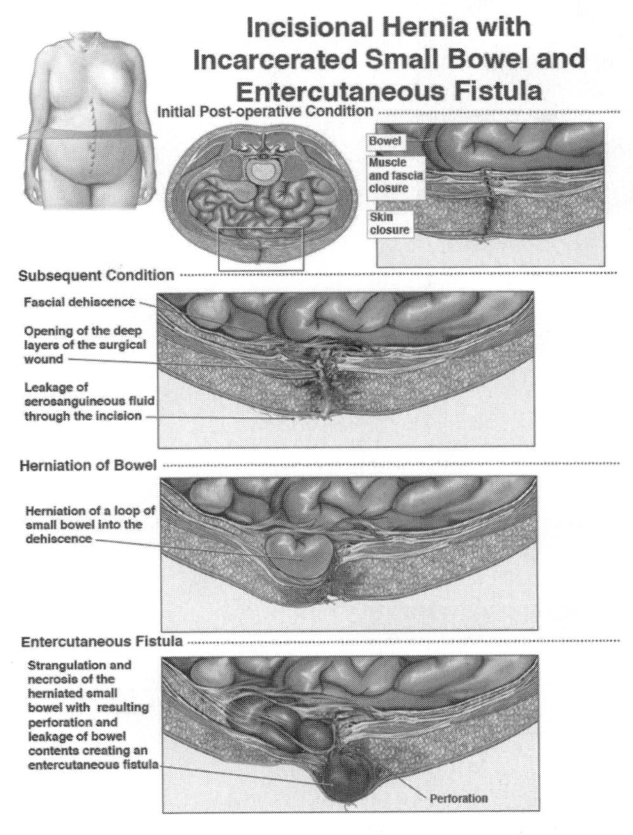

This series of images denotes a progression of a hernia from the surgical closure of an operative incision. There is a gradual breakdown of tissue layers that finally allows a small portion of the intestine to herniate so that it is covered only by skin. The extruded portion of the intestine becomes trapped, incarcerated, and finally strangulated, giving rise to a surgical emergency and life-threatening situation.

LO2:

Diagnostics: Hernias

Labs:

Labs for suspicion of incarceration or strangulation:

- CBC
- Complete metabolic panel (CMP)
- Lactate: sepsis indicator
- Urinalysis

Imaging:

- Ultrasound
- Abdominal x-rays to determine bowel obstruction
- CT scan

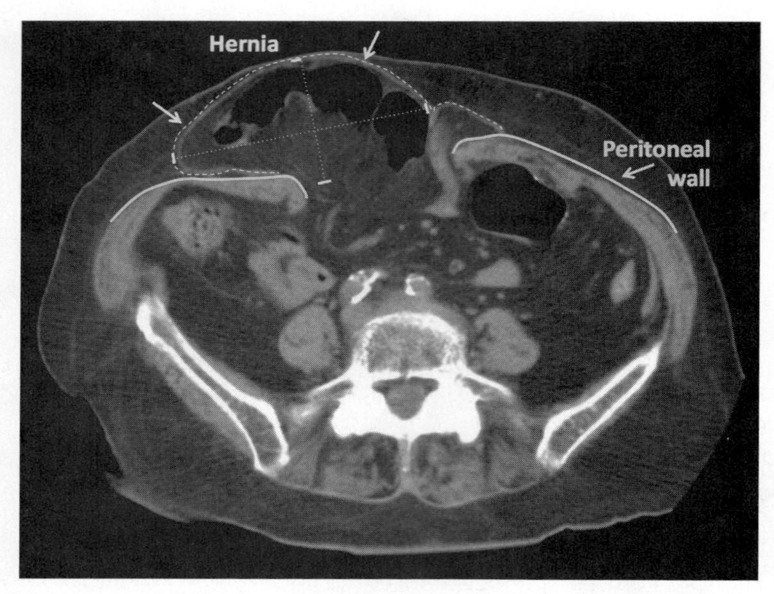

CT scan shows a large ventral hernia (yellow arrows) of the small bowel. Note how large the protruding intestinal loop is beyond the peritoneal wall.
Source: Courtesy of K. Kyriakidis

Concept Check

4. **A patient has a bulge in his inguinal area that increases with increased intra-abdominal pressure. This is most likely which type of hernia?**
   - A. Benign
   - B. Incarcerated
   - C. Strangulated
   - D. Malignant

Answer question

Priority Patient Concerns and Desired Collaborative Care Outcomes: Hernias

Prior to caring for patients with hernias, it is important to prioritize the patient's concerns that must guide the nursing care plan and interventions. Care for the patient is ordered and organized in accordance with the patient's priority and urgent needs. Desired collaborative care outcomes in patients with hernias typically include:

1. Patient will have minimal to no pain.
2. Patient will accurately discuss medical management of the disorder.
3. Patient will accurately discuss expected surgical management of the disorder.
4. Patient will demonstrate control of ability to urinate.

Considering these important care outcomes, prepare a list of the major 3–6 priority patient concerns or nursing diagnoses for patients with hernias. Be prepared to participate in a discussion of this list and/or to submit them as an assignment, as determined by your faculty. Resources you may find helpful in this assignment can include this lesson, the references, resources on nursing care plans, and standard nursing diagnoses manuals.

LO3:

Collaborative Interventions: Hernias

Medical Management (when appropriate)

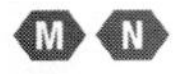

- **Medications**
  - o Administer pain medications as needed.
  - o Start antibiotics (e.g., cefoxitin) if ischemic bowel is suspected secondary to strangulation.
- **Assist in manual maneuvers.** Manual reduction may be attempted by physician (can also be done with sedation)
- **Assist with truss.** Used only when deemed necessary and appropriate, a truss is like an athletic support and is the only nonsurgical alternative. Its use is not encouraged as it can lead to complications such as prolonged pressure on the spermatic cord, hernia sac damage, or impingement on hernia contents. If necessary to hold hernia contents in the abdomen, instruct the proper use of a truss and check for skin irritation at the site where truss makes contact with the skin.

Surgical Intervention

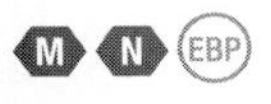

- **Nonurgent** outpatient surgery may be scheduled in patients for benign hernias. Some patients may choose to not undergo surgery because they are asymptomatic or because of their underlying health and/or comorbid conditions (Simons, et al., 2009).

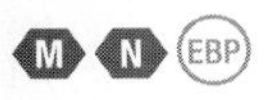

- **Prepare patient for immediate** surgical intervention if required for incarcerated or strangulated hernia presentation (Simons, et al., 2009).

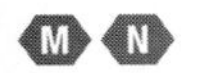

- Begin sepsis management if signs of SIRS or sepsis are present. Call the Rapid Response Team to assist.

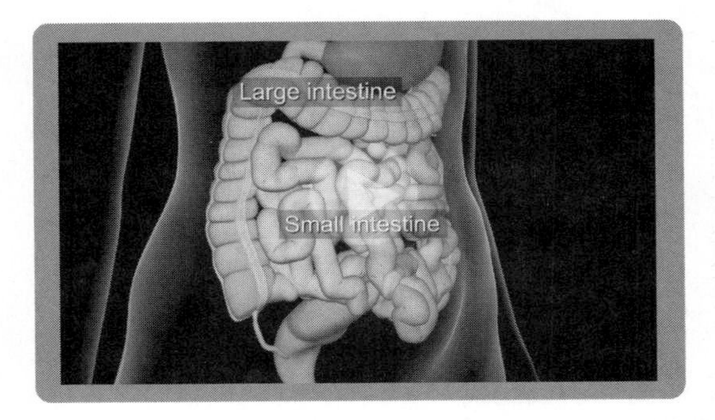

This animation describes the laparoscopic repair of a ventral hernia.
Source: © 2014 Nucleus Medical Media. All rights reserved

- Provide postoperative patient education:
  - o Instruct patient about proper postoperative care, including scrotal support and ice bag to relieve swelling and pain.
  - o Educate to avoid coughing as much as possible.
  - o If coughing or sneezing is necessary, instruct the patient to splint the incision and keep the mouth open.
  - o Instruct patient to frequently deep breathe.
  - o Assist with early mobilization (ambulate, turn in bed, sit in a chair).
  - o Educate the patient about no heavy lifting for 6–8 weeks.

LO4:

Evaluation of Desired Collaborative Care Outcomes: Hernias

Evaluation and reassessment should reveal attainment of previously established patient outcomes. In summary:

- Patient reports that pain has resolved.
- Patient accurately demonstrates medical management of the disorder such as use of a truss.
- Patient accurately discusses postoperative self-management.
- Patient is able to void and has no postvoiding residual urine.

LO1: What Are Colon Polyps?

- **Colon polyps** are slow growing intestinal mucosa overgrowths.
  - o Hyperplastic polyps account for 90% of colon polyps.
  - o They are usually benign. However, hyperplastic polyps can have some malignant potential, particularly in the setting of hyperplastic polyposis syndrome (syndrome characterized by multiple polyps, ranging from 6 up to 100).
- **Adenomatous polyps** harbor the potential to become malignant.
  - o This potential increases with increasing polyp size. Not all adenomatous polyps develop into cancer, but almost all colon cancers are thought to arise from adenomatous polyps. Familial adenomatous polyposis (hereditary) is the most common form of adenomatous polyposis syndrome.

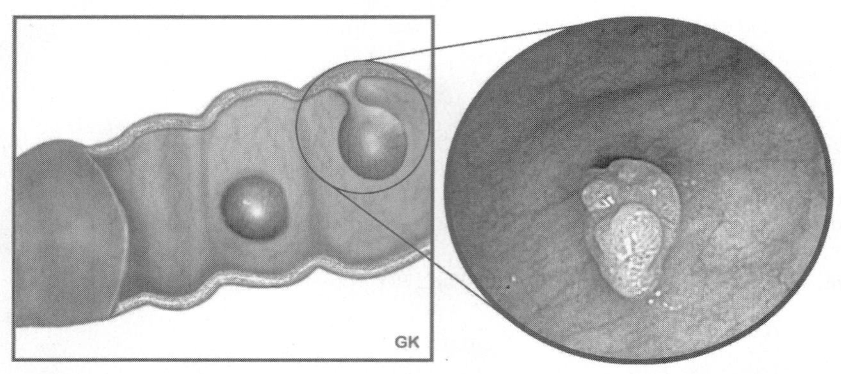

Left: This image depicts two common types of polyps that can be found on the colon wall: sessile and peduncular. Right: This photo reveals a peduncular polyp in the distal sigmoid colon, which was resected and retrieved during a colonoscopy. As seen, polyps may be found in varying shapes.
Sources: Courtesy of George Kyriakidis/Santa Ana, CA, & K. Kyriakidis

- **Malignant polyps** are cancer.
- **Shapes of Polyps:**
  - o Pedunculated polyps have peduncles or stalks of overgrown tissue that connects the polyps to the intestinal surface. It has a mushroom-like appearance. These polyps are often precursors to cancer.
  - o Sessile polyps also grow on the surface of the intestinal mucosa and have a mushroom-like appearance but have no peduncle. They may become cancerous.
  - o Flat polyps develop on the mucosal surface but are flat.

LO2: Assessment Findings: Colon Polyps

- Colon polyps are most often asymptomatic and incidentally found on a screening colonoscopy.
- Polyps may cause bleeding, which is more likely to be visible in the stool, only when they are close to the rectum.
- Some types of polyps may cause diarrhea (large villous adenomas close to the rectum).

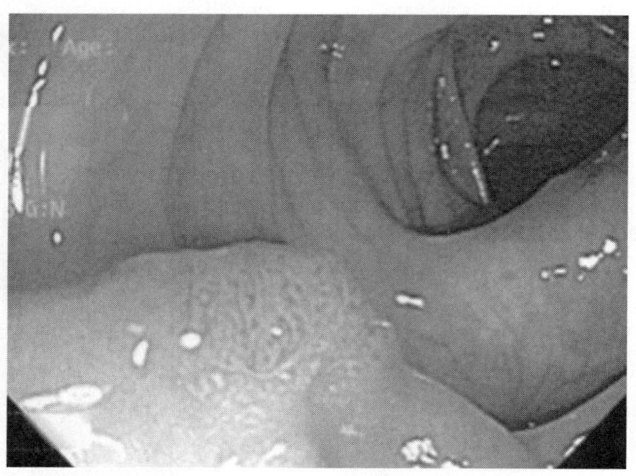

This illustration depicts a sessile type of colon polyp. Unlike the peduncular polyps, which are commonly found in the sigmoid colon, this sessile polyp is found nearer the rectum.
Source: Courtesy of K. Kyriakidis

LO2:

Diagnostics: Colon Polyps

Labs:

- CBC if bleeding is present
- CMP
- Stool guaiac to evaluate for occult blood

Imaging:

- Virtual colonoscopy by CT or MRI
- Flexible sigmoidoscopy
- Colonoscopy
- Capsule endoscopy

Colonoscopy Reveals Colon Polyps

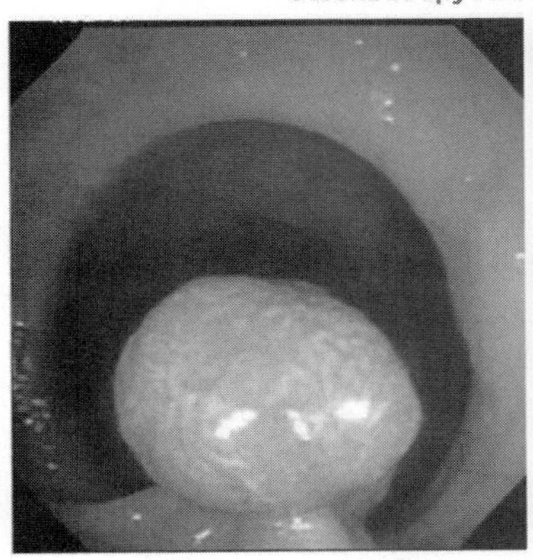

Peduncular Polyp

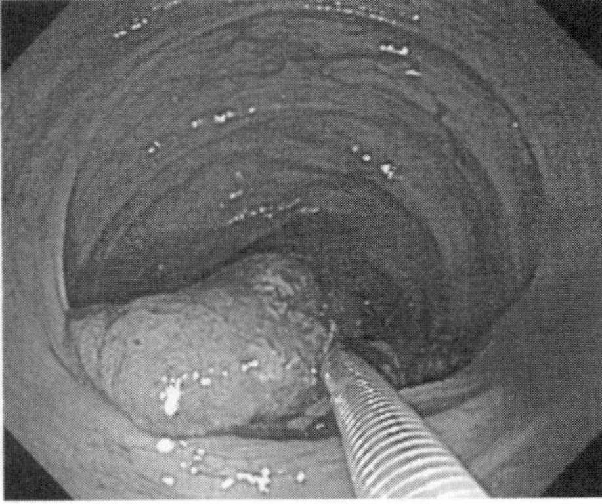

Villous Adenoma

Colonoscopy offers an excellent method to visualize and sometimes remove polyps. The animation in the GI Bleeding lesson shows the procedure. Left: This endoscopic photo shows a close-up view of a penduncular polyp in the colon. Right: A villous adenoma (which are neoplastic) was diagnosed in this patient.

Source: Courtesy of K. Kyriakidis

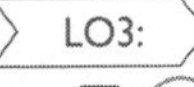

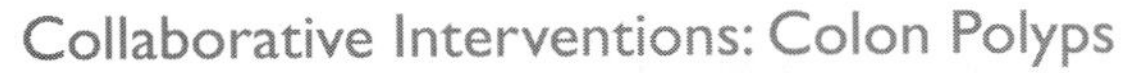

Collaborative Interventions: Colon Polyps

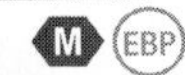

- **Endoscopy:** Endoscopic polypectomy and biopsy to detect pathology (Bond, 2000)

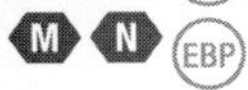

- **Surgical intervention:** Colon resection for familial adenomatous polyposis or partial resection for large polyps not amenable to polypectomy (Galiatsatos, Foulkes, 2006)

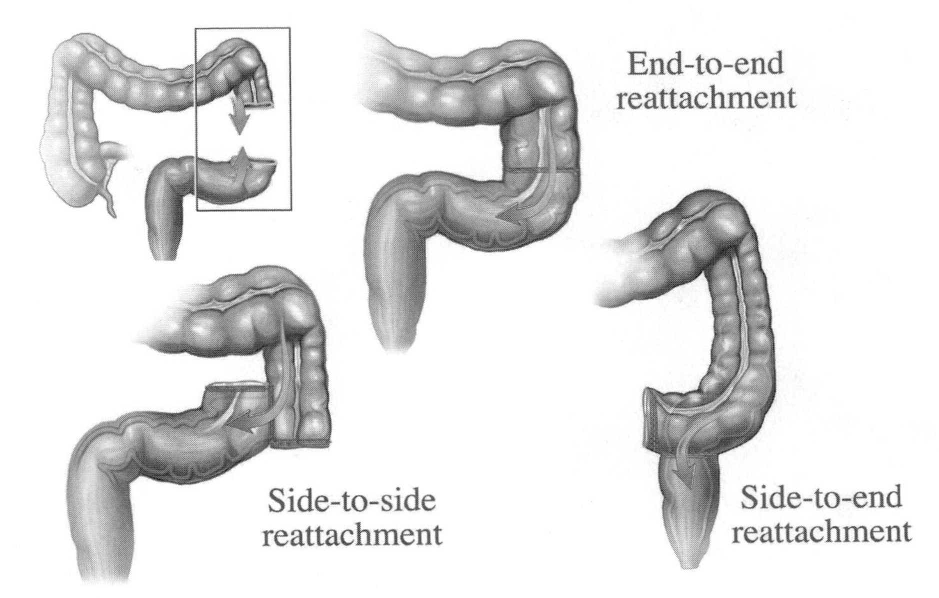

This collection of drawings details three different techniques that might be used to rejoin the two ends after a segment of the colon has been removed.

Source: Nucleus Medical Art Inc./Alamy

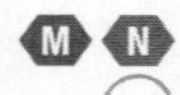

- **Patient education** for surveillance (Lieberman, et al., 2012):

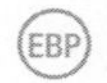

  - Ten-year follow-up for reexamination in patients with:
    - No adenomas
    - No small benign hyperplastic polyps (<10 mm)
    - EBP First-degree relative >59 years old with colorectal cancer or high-risk adenoma (Lieberman, et al., 2012)
  - Five- to 10-year follow-up in patients with 1–2 adenomas of <10 mm
  - EBP First-degree relative <60 years old with colorectal cancer or high-risk adenoma (Lieberman, et al., 2012)
  - Three-year follow-up in patients with:
    - Three to 10 adenomas
    - Any tubular adenomas ≥10 mm
    - Any adenomas with villous features
    - Any adenomas with high-grade dysplasia
    - Sessile serrated polyp ≥10 mm
    - Sessile serrated polyp with dysplasia
  - Less than 3 years follow-up in patients with >10 adenomas
  - One-year follow-up in patients with serrated polyposis syndrome

Concept Check

5. **Which endoscopic procedure examines only the rectum and descending colon?**

A. Esophagogastroduodenoscopy

B. Sigmoidoscopy

C. Colonoscopy

D. Protoscopy

Answer question

LO1:

What Are Hemorrhoids?

Hemorrhoids are the protrusions caused by the enlargement and displacement of veins in the lower portion of the rectum and anus.

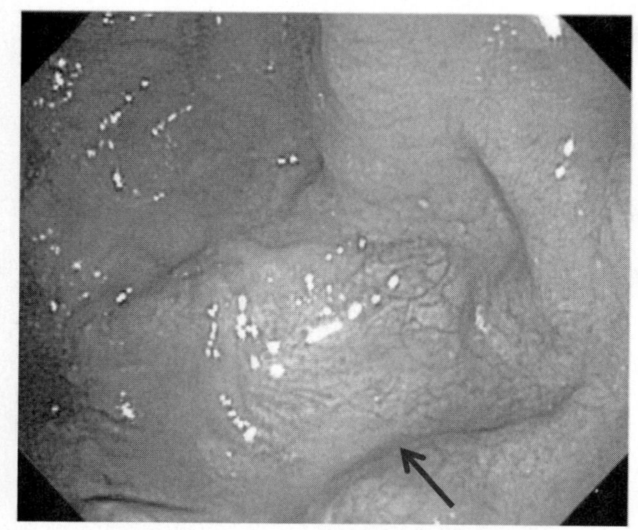

Internal, non-thrombosed hemorrhoid

This photo reveals a very large internal hemorrhoid inside the anal region. It is not bleeding but is uncomfortable.

Source: Courtesy of K. Kyriakidis

LO1:

Clinical Relevance: Hemorrhoids

- In the United States, 10.4 million people currently complain of having hemorrhoids.
- Hemorrhoids can cause bleeding and anal discomfort.

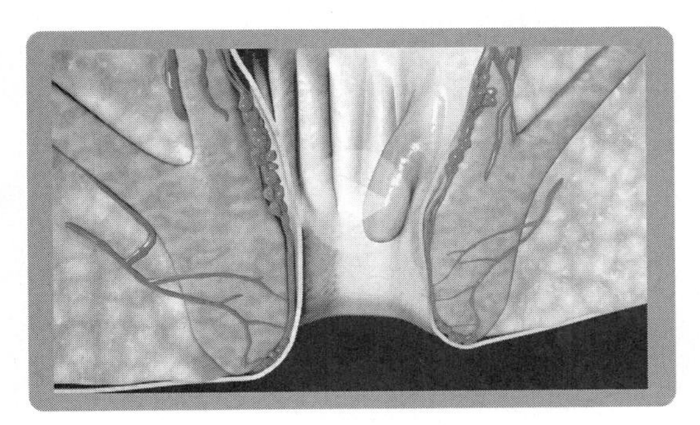

Hemorrhoids are shown in this animation with an explanation of types. A visual presentation of where and how they form is provided.

Source: © 2014 Nucleus Medical Media, All rights reserved

LO2:

Pathophysiology: Hemorrhoids

- Anal cushions are submucosal structures that consist of blood vessels, smooth muscle, and elastic connective tissue. Prior to defecation, the anal sphincter relaxes, and the anal canal opens. The anal cushions fill with blood and expand, acting as a cushion. When the anal sphincter contracts and closes, the anal cushions are again compressed.
- In hemorrhoids, there is a weakening of the smooth muscle and fibrous tissue of the anal cushions. This is accompanied by dilation of the veins in the tissue that are displaced into the anal canal and distally.
- The vascular walls become inflamed and may become thrombosed, meaning that blood clots form. Blood vessels may become ulcerated and bleed.

Classification of Hemorrhoids

Grade I: Internal

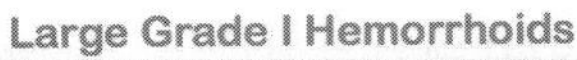

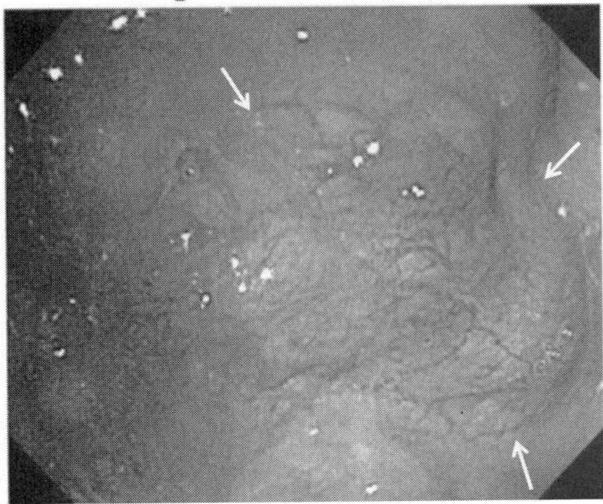

Source: Courtesy of K. Kyriakidis

Grade II: Exits rectum with defecation then retracts on its own

Grade II Hemorrhoids

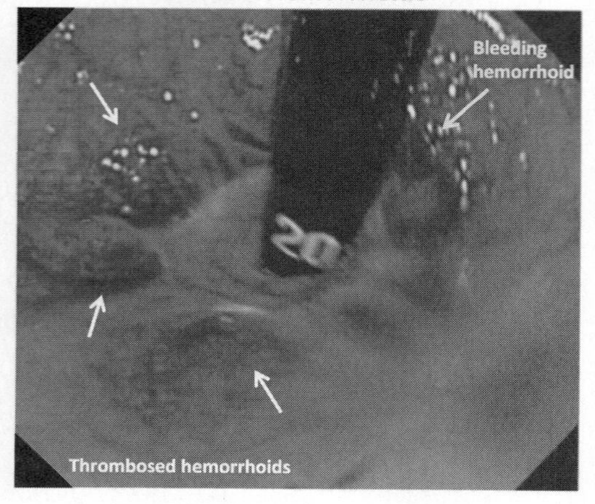

Source: Courtesy of K. Kyriakidis

Grade III: Exits rectum with defecation, stays out, but can be pushed in

Grade IV: External that do not retract and cannot be pushed in

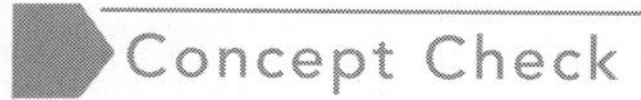

6. Which tissues are involved in the development of hemorrhoids?

A. Perianal muscles

B. Intestinal mucosa

C. Rugae of the large intestine

D. Anal cushions

Answer question

LO2:

Risk Factors and Causes: Hemorrhoids

Conditions that increase the pressure in the pelvic area are thought to contribute to hemorrhoid formation:

- Low-fiber diet
- Straining and constipation
- Inflammatory bowel disease
- Pregnancy
- Anorectal varices
- Obesity
- Chronic diarrhea
- Rectal surgery
- Episiotomy
- Anal intercourse

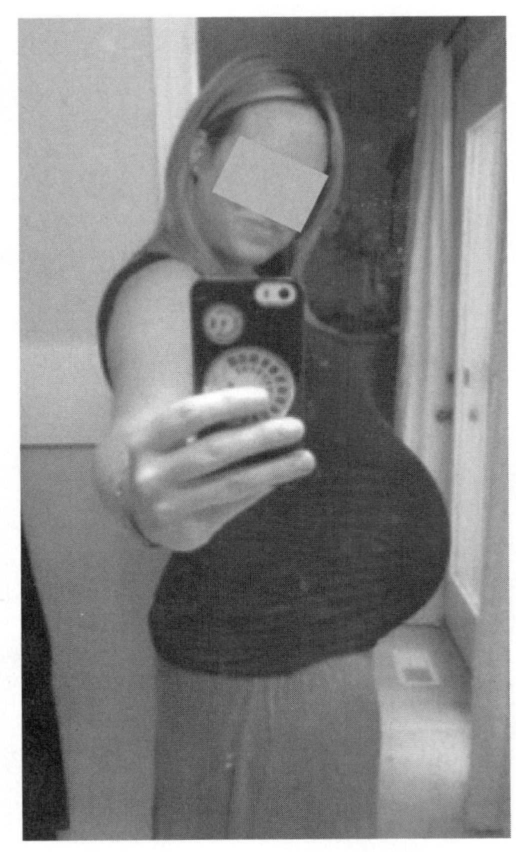

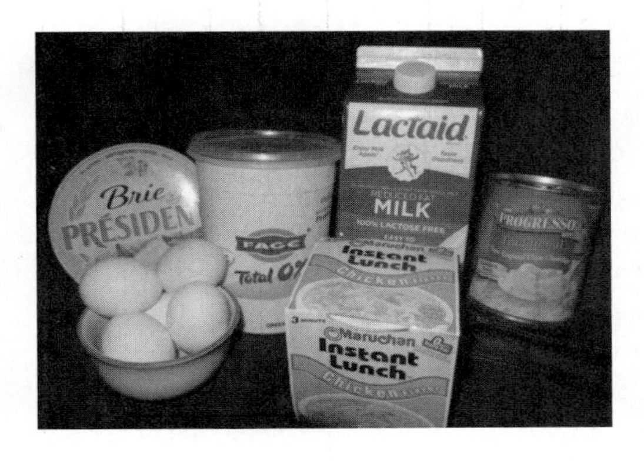

Well-known causes of hemorrhoids are shown in these photos. Left: The continuous pressure on the rectal area during pregnancy commonly causes hemorrhoids. Right: Low fiber diets are associated with hemorrhoids.

Sources: (*left*) Courtesy of R. Murphy; (*right*) Copyright © 2014, NovEx Novice to Expert Learning, LLC

LO2:

Assessment Findings: Hemorrhoids

- Rectal bleeding
- Rectal pain: Severe pain can occur if hemorrhoid is thrombosed.
- Rectal itching
- Prolapse
- Visible hemorrhoids on exam of Grade 3 and 4 hemorrhoids

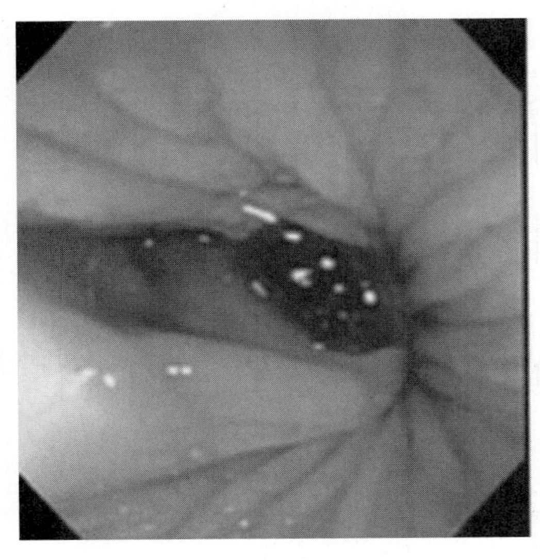

This image of the anal region during colonoscopy demonstrates an external hemorrhoid with a blood clot on its surface.

Source: Courtesy of K. Kyriakidis

Priority Patient Concerns and Desired Collaborative Care Outcomes: Hemorrhoids

Prior to caring for patients with hemorrhoids, it is important to prioritize the patient's concerns that must guide the nursing care plan and interventions. Care for the patient is ordered and organized in accordance with the patient's priority and urgent needs. Desired collaborative care outcomes in patients with hemorrhoids typically include:

1. Patient will collaborate on and express an understanding of the management plan.
2. Patient will have minimal to no pain.

Considering these important care outcomes, prepare a list of the major 3–6 priority patient concerns or nursing diagnoses for patients with hemorrhoids. Be prepared to participate in a discussion of this list and/or to submit them as an assignment, as determined by your faculty. Resources you may find helpful in this assignment can include this lesson, the references, resources on nursing care plans, and standard nursing diagnoses manuals.

LO3:

Collaborative Interventions: Hemorrhoids

Management varies according to symptomatology despite the classification. However, general conservative treatment involves:

Grade I and II:

- Focuses on dietary changes:
  - N EBP o Increase dietary fiber (Lohsiriwat, 2012).
  - N EBP o Avoid spicy and fatty foods (Lohsiriwat, 2012).
- Medications:
  - M N o Consider stool softeners (e.g., docusate).
  - M N o Avoid NSAIDs.
  - M N EBP o Consider flavonoids, which have been shown to decrease risk of bleeding, pain, and symptoms (Lohsiriwat, 2012).
  - M N EBP o Consider calcium dobesilate, which has been shown to decrease bleeding and inflammation, particularly when used in conjunction with fiber supplements (Lohsiriwat, 2012).
  - M N EBP o Topical steroid products in cream, foam, or suppository form (e.g., Anusol-HC) (Lohsiriwat, 2012)
- M EBP Nonsurgical treatments can include (Lohsiriwat, 2012):
  - o Sclerotherapy involves the injection of chemicals (such as vegetable oil, hypertonic salt solution) into the submucosal tissue at the base of the hemorrhoid.
  - o Radiofrequency ablation attempts to reduce the vascular mass within the hemorrhoid.
  - o Rubber band ligation results in hemorrhoidal necrosis, scarring, and fixation of the underlying tissue to the rectal wall.

Grade III and IV:

- N EBP Increase dietary fiber (Lohsiriwat, 2012).
- N EBP Use fiber supplements (e.g., Metamucil, Citrucel) (Alonso-Coello, Castillejo, 2003; Lohsiriwat, 2012).
- N EBP Reduce spicy and fatty foods in the diet (Lohsiriwat, 2012).
- M N EBP May require surgical intervention for hemorrhoid removal through plication, ligation, laser, stapling, or hemorrhoidectomy (Alonso-Coello, Castillejo, 2003; Lohsiriwat, 2012)

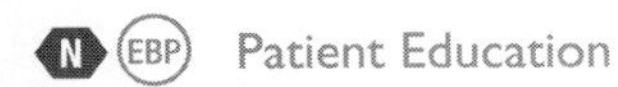

Patient Education

Recommendations to reduce, control, or prevent hemorrhoids include (Lohsiriwat, 2012):

- Add more bulk to the diet with fiber. Explain that it can reduce or even eliminate straining during defecation over a 6–8 week time period. It has been shown to reduce bleeding by 50%.
- Reduce straining during toileting.
- Educate about lifestyle changes that can be helpful:
  - o Increase fluid intake, particularly water.
  - o Reduce fat consumption.
  - o Exercise.
  - o Improve anal hygiene.
  - o Abstain from reading on the toilet.
  - o Avoid medications whenever possible that cause diarrhea or constipation. Talk with the health care provider if prescribed medications cause problems.
- Avoid prolonged standing or sitting.
- Use over-the-counter drugs and products appropriately.
- Contact the health care provider if pain and bleeding are persistent or excessive.
- Sit in warm, sitz bath to alleviate pain and swelling.

LO4:

Evaluation of Desired Collaborative Care Outcomes: Hemorrhoids

Evaluation and reassessment should reveal attainment of previously established patient outcomes. In summary:

- Patient accurately discusses ways of managing hemorrhoids conservatively.
- Patient has minimal to no pain postoperatively.

LO1:

What Is Diverticulosis?

- A colonic structural disorder that occurs from small mucosal herniations in the wall of the colon creating pouch-like and outward protrusions, called diverticula.
- **Diverticulosis** is the term used for noninflamed diverticula, while inflamed diverticula are known as **diverticulitis**.
- The presence of diverticula appears to have some association with a low-fiber diet, constipation, and obesity.
- Incidence is 5% before age 40 and >65% by age 85 in the United States.

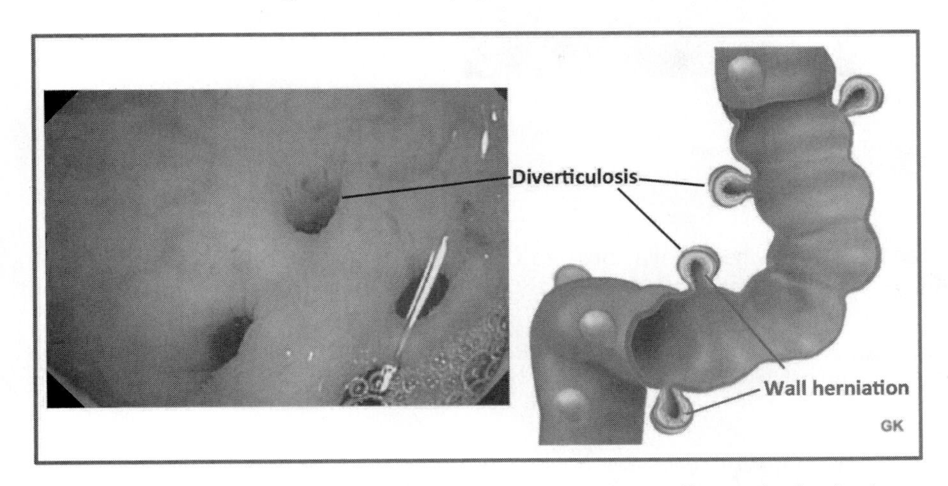

This illustration depicts the small mucosal herniation of the large intestines (diverticulosis) and a photo of the diverticula.

Sources: Courtesy of K. Kyriakidis & George Kyriakidis/Santa Ana, CA

LO2: Diagnostics: Diverticulosis

Imaging:

- X-ray is a primary imaging diagnostic used in patients with diverticulosis. A barium enema can highlight the presence of colonic diverticula.

Endoscopy:

- Colonoscopy provides direct visualization used for confirmation of diverticulosis.

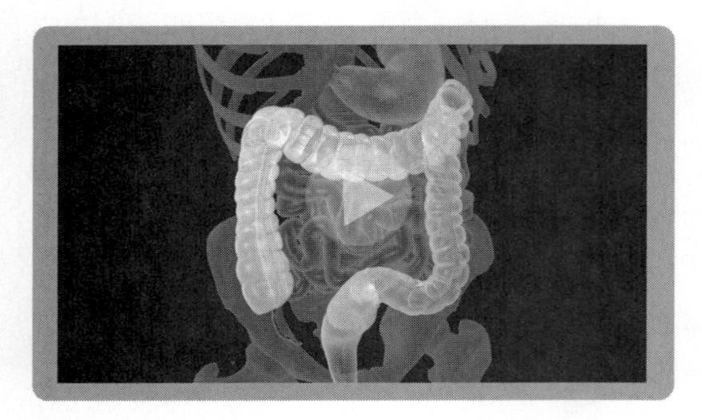

This animation provides an overview of the gastrointestinal anatomy. It details the administration of a barium enema that provides multiple views of the colon, making it possible to take x-rays of any segment desired. The animation also shows the types and reasons for x-rays as barium flows through and illuminates the colon.

- During an endoscopy, a series of photos can be made to visualize the presence and extent of diverticula throughout the entire colon.

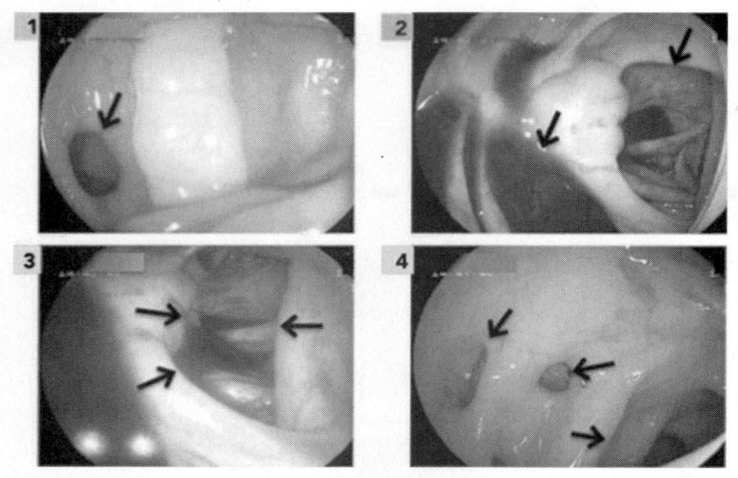

This series of photos verified the extensive small and large-mouthed diverticula (arrows) and blood found throughout the entire colon. The terminal ileum appeared normal. Locations: 1. Ascending colon. 2. Cecum. 3. Cecum. 4. Sigmoid colon.

Source: Courtesy of K. Kyriakidis

Priority Patient Concerns and Desired Collaborative Care Outcomes: Diverticulosis

Prior to caring for patients with diverticulosis, it is important to prioritize the patient's concerns that must guide the nursing care plan and interventions. Care for the patient is ordered and organized in accordance with the patient's priority and urgent needs. Desired collaborative care outcomes in patients with diverticulosis typically include:

1. Patient will accurately discuss treatment plans.
2. Patient will monitor stool for signs of bleeding and notify the health care provider of blood in stool.

Considering these important care outcomes, prepare a list of the major 3–6 priority patient concerns or nursing diagnoses for patients with diverticulosis. Be prepared to participate in a discussion of this list and/or to submit them as an assignment, as determined by your faculty. Resources you may find helpful in this assignment can include this lesson, the references, resources on nursing care plans, and standard nursing diagnoses manuals.

LO3: Collaborative Interventions: Diverticulosis

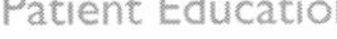

Patient Education

Dietary management is the most common recommendation for diverticulosis and includes:

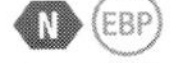

- Increase dietary fiber (Stollman, Raskin, 1999).
- Maintain adequate hydration.

- Exercise on a regular basis.
- Manage weight within desired and healthy range.
- Avoid increased intra-abdominal pressure (tight clothing, bending, lifting, and straining during defecation).

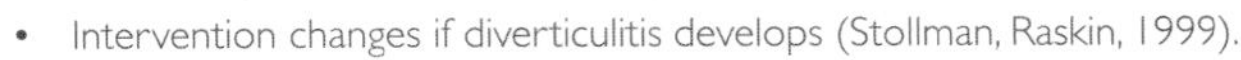

- Intervention changes if diverticulitis develops (Stollman, Raskin, 1999).

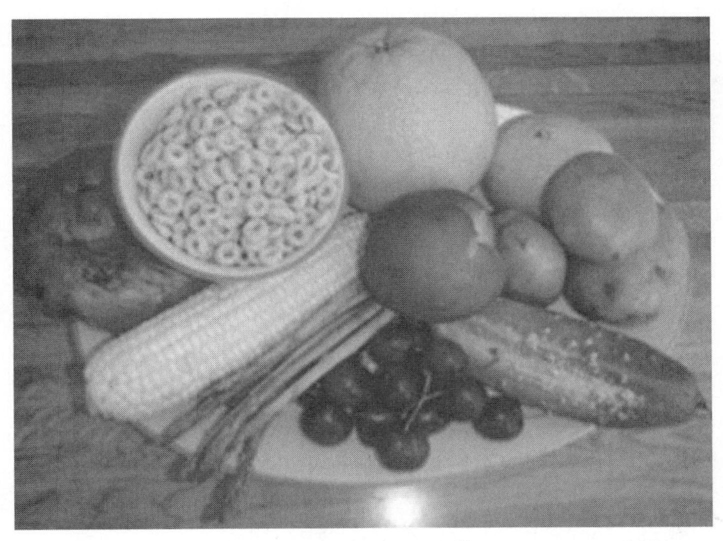

Fiber refers to carbohydrates that cannot be digested. The two types are soluble and insoluble. Soluble fiber partially dissolves in water while insoluble fiber does not. Current recommendations suggest consuming at least 20 grams of dietary fiber daily (not from supplements). Teenagers and males may require 30–35 grams daily. Most American only consume 15 grams of dietary fiber.

- **Diverticular Bleeding**
  - o This is usually managed by volume resuscitation (IV fluids and transfusion) and observation.
  - o Severe bleeding or persistent bleeding often requires surgical intervention to stop the hemorrhage.
  - o After the site of bleeding is localized by colonoscopy, a nuclear red cell tagged study or angiography may be conducted.
- **Diverticulitis**
  - o Diverticulitis is an inflammation or infection that affects the diverticula.
  - o Treatment for diverticulitis is discussed in the GI Infections NovE-lesson.

Bleeding Diverticula Leading to Lower GI Bleeding

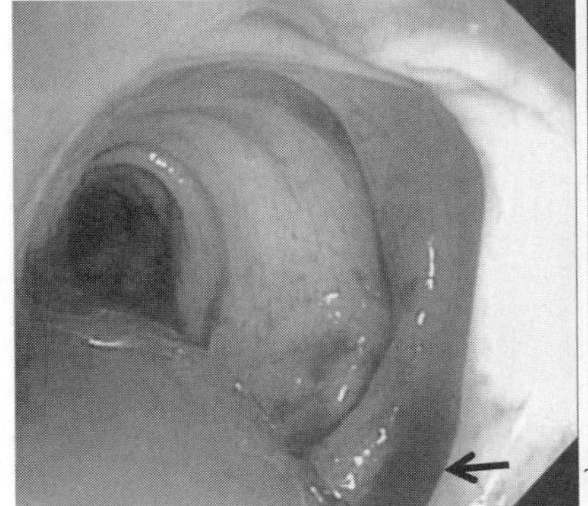

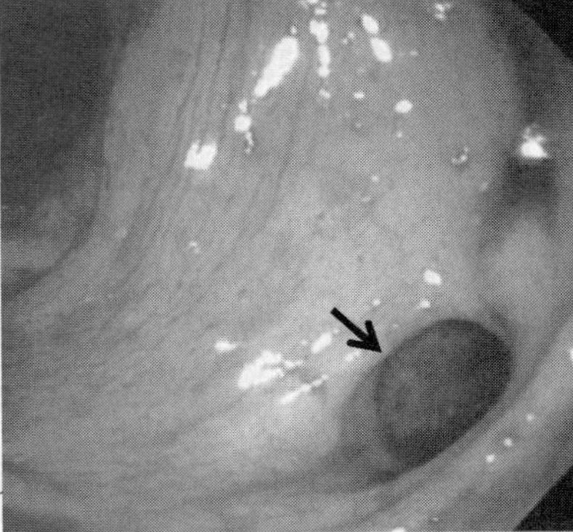

Extensive diverticulitis is seen above with the formation of diverticula (intestinal bulges) on both sides of the intestine. Note the flow of blood in the lower left photo from bleeding diverticula.

Source: Courtesy of K. Kyriakidis

LO4:

Evaluation of Desired Collaborative Care Outcomes: Diverticulosis

Evaluation and reassessment should reveal attainment of previously established patient outcomes. In summary:

- Patient accurately describes the prescribed treatment regimen and is adhering to same.
- Patient discusses importance of monitoring stool for signs of bleeding and notifying the health care provider of blood in stool.

Concept Check

7. **A patient with infection of out-pouching in the intestinal wall has what disorder?**
   A. Strangulated hernia
   B. Diverticulitis
   C. Internal hemorrhoids
   D. Adenomatous polyps

Answer question

Summary of Interventions: Structural Disorders

- Patients with intestinal obstruction are usually treated with NPO, IV narcotics, hydration to replace lost fluids, and electrolytes.
- Some patients may require a nasogastric tube.
- Patients may require surgery urgently and intravenous antibiotics if they have:
  - o Peritoneal signs (sign of perforation), fever, hypotension, and tachycardia not resolving with fluid replacement
  - o Incarcerated or strangulated hernia
  - o No improvement with treatment may also require surgery.
- **Hemorrhoids** are treated by increasing fiber in the diet and stool softeners. Topical corticosteroids can help with inflammation and itching. More severe hemorrhoids can be surgically treated with band ligation, laser, sclerotherapy, stapling, or surgical removal.
- **Colon polyps** are usually treated with polypectomy via colonoscopy.
- Colon resection for familial adenomatous polyposis or partial resection for large polyps not amenable to polypectomy may be required.
- **Diverticular bleeding** is usually managed by volume resuscitation (IV fluids and transfusion) and observation. Severe bleeding or persistent bleeding often require surgery. After site of bleeding is localized by colonoscopy, nuclear red cell tagged study or angiography may be needed.

References

Gaye, K. (2008). How to perform a digital removal of faeces. *Continence Essentials, 1*, 126–130. **www.continence-uk.co.uk/essentials_2008/Continence_Essentials_2008_Digital_Removal_of_Faces.pdf**

Harold, B. (2011). Urgent treatment of patients with intestinal obstruction. *Emergency Nurse, 18*(11), 28–31.

Madoff, R. D., & Fleshman, J. W. (2004). American Gastroenterological Association technical review on the diagnosis and management of hemorrhoids. Clinical Practice Committee, American Gastroenterological Association. *Gastroenterology, 126*(5), 1463–1473. **www.gastrojournal.org/article/S0016-5085%2804%2900355-5/fulltext**

Massey, R. L. (2012). Return of bowel sounds indicating an end of postoperative ileus: Is it time to cease this long standing nursing tradition? *MEDSURG Nursing, 21*(3), 146–150.

Clinical Practice Guidelines

Alonso-Coello, P., & Castillejo, M. M. (2003). Office evaluation and treatment of hemorrhoids. *J Fam Pract, 52*(5), 366–374. **www.ecardiologynews.com/fileadmin/jfp_archive/pdf/5205/5205JFP_AppliedEvidence.pdf**

Bond, J. H. (2000). Polyp guideline: diagnosis, treatment, and surveillance for patients with colorectal polyps. *Amer J Gastroenterol, 95*(11), 3053–3063. **67.192.160.122/physicians/guidelines/NonfamilialColorectalPolyps.pdf**

Di Saverio, S., Cocolini, F., Galati, M., et al. (2013). Bologna guidelines for diagnosis and management of adhesive small bowel obstruction (ASBO): 2013 update of the evidence-based guidelines from the world society of emergency surgery ASBO working group. *World J Emergency Surg, 8*, 42. doi:10.1186/1749-7922-8-42. **www.wjes.org/content/pdf/1749-7922-8-42.pdf**

Galiatsatos, P., & Foulkes, W. (2006). Familial adenomatous polyposis. *Amer J of Gastroenterology, 101*, 385–398. **www.fapinfo.com/Galiatsatos%202006%20-%20Review%20FAP.pdf**

Lieberman, D. A., Rex, D. K., Winawer, S. J., et al. (2012). Guidelines for colonoscopy surveillance after screening and polypectomy: A consensus update by the US Multi-Society Task Force on colorectal cancer. *Gastroenterology, 143*, 844–857. **www.med.upenn.edu/gastro/documents/JCarticle10-1-12.pdf**

Lohsiriwat, V. (2012). Hemorrhoids: From basic pathophysiology to clinical management. *World J Gastroenterol, 18*(17), 2009–2017. **www.ncbi.nlm.nih.gov/pmc/articles/PCM3342598/**

Maung, A., Johnson, D., Piper, G., et al. (2012). Eastern Association for the Surgery of Trauma. Evaluation and management of small-bowel obstruction: An Eastern Association for the Surgery of Trauma practice management guideline. *J Trauma Acute Care Surg, 73*(Suppl 4), S362–S369. **www.east.org/education/practice-management-guidelines/small-bowel-obstruction%2c-evaluation-and-management-of**

Simons, M., Aufenacker, T., Bay-Nielsen, M., et al. (2009). European Hernia Society guidelines on the treatment of inguinal hernia in adult patients. *Hernia, 13*, 343–403. doi: 10.1007/s10029-009-0529-7. **link.springer.com/article/10.1007/s10029-009-0529-7#page-53**

Stollman, N., & Raskin, J. (1999). Diagnosis and Management of diverticular disease of the colon in adults. *Amer Jour of Gastroenterology, 94*(11). **s3.gi.org/physicians/guidelines/DiverticularDiseaseoftheColon.pdf**

Patient Education

Enders, G. H. (2014). *Colonic Polyps.* **emedicine.medscape.com/article/172674-overview**

Nicks, B. A. (2014). *Hernias.* **emedicine.medscape.com/article/775630-overview**

Noble, B. A. (2014). *Small bowel obstruction.* **emedicine.medscape.com/article/774140-overview**

Thornton, S. C. (2012). *Hemorrhoids.* **emedicine.medscape.com/article/775407-overview**

STOP

Go to the online course and complete the NovE-Cases assigned by your instructor for this module.

Learning Outcomes for Hepatic Disorders

When you complete this lesson, you will be able to:

1. Recognize the clinical relevance of hepatic disorders.
2. Consider the pathophysiology, etiology, risk factors, and clinical presentation of hepatic disorders that determine the priority patient concerns.
3. Determine the most urgent and important nursing interventions and patient education required in caring for a patient with hepatic disorder.
4. Evaluate attainment of desired collaborative care outcomes for a patient with hepatic disorder.

LO1:

What Are the Primary Hepatic Disorders?

- Hepatitis is an inflammation of the liver due to viruses, toxins, drugs, or autoimmune process. It can be chronic or acute.
- Cirrhosis is scarring of the liver that causes diminished function. It is usually the result of chronic liver disease.
- Liver cancer:
  - o Hepatocellular carcinoma is a malignant cancer that is often fatal.
  - o Cholangiosarcomas are tumors of the connective tissues of the bile ducts.
  - o Metastatic disease from other locations in GI tract

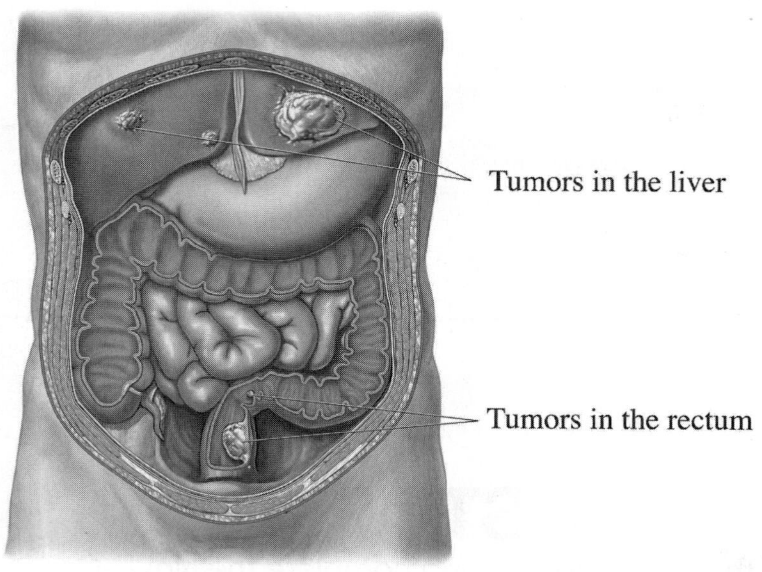

This picture shows rectal (colon) cancer with metastatic tumors in the liver.
Source: Nucleus Medical Art Inc./Alamy

LO1:

Clinical Relevance: Hepatic Disorders

The liver is a vital organ, the largest gland in the body, and is responsible for a multitude of functions such as detoxification, protein synthesis, and production of biochemicals needed for digestion.

- Many medications administered are metabolized by the liver and may require dosage adjustment or may be contraindicated with hepatic insufficiency or failure.
- Chronic liver disease and cirrhosis cause 35,000 deaths in the United States every year and are the ninth leading cause of death.
- Hepatitis C is now the nation's leading cause of both chronic hepatitis and cirrhosis, ahead of alcoholic liver disease, which is second.
- Acetaminophen, a commonly used medication, is the leading cause of acute liver failure in the United States.
- In many cases of liver failure, liver transplant may be the only definitive treatment.
- Patients with cirrhosis can develop esophageal varices and die from massive hemorrhage.
- Cirrhosis is the most common reason for liver transplantation.

LO1:

Liver Anatomy and Function

- The liver is located in the right upper abdomen and protected by the lower ribcage.
- The liver is divided into two large sections—the right and left lobes, with segments in each lobe.
- The gallbladder is situated beneath the liver and assists in the digestive process by storing bile, which is manufactured in the liver and is instrumental in the metabolism of fat.

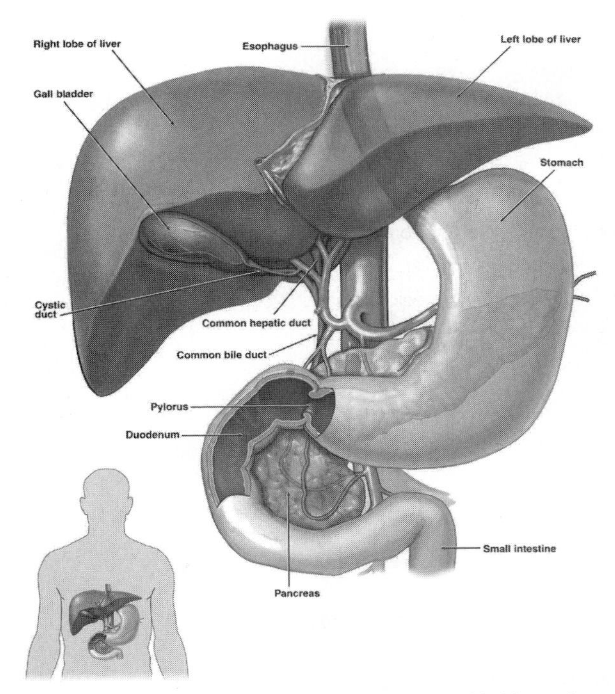

This illustration displays the anatomy of the liver, gallbladder, and biliary system. Surrounding structures for digestion and important vasculature are labeled.

Source: Nucleus Medical Art Inc./Alamy

- The primary function of the liver is to filter blood arriving from the digestive tract, carrying the products of digestion, before the blood is circulated to the rest of the body.
- The liver metabolizes carbohydrates, fats, and proteins, along with hormones, vitamins, and minerals.
- It has a key role in detoxifying or inactivating many substances before elimination through the bile and urine.
- The liver contains about 13% of the body's blood supply at any given moment.

Vital Functions of the Liver

Most vital (of 500) liver functions include:

- Provides immunity against infection
- Regulates blood clotting
- Produces proteins and cholesterol
- Metabolizes drugs, chemicals, & alcohol
- Filters wastes and excretes through bile
- Converts excess glucose to starch for storage
- Excretes bile for fat digestion

Source: Copyright © 2014. NovEx Novice to Expert Learning, LLC

Concept Check

1. **What is the leading cause of acute liver failure in the United States?**
   A. Cirrhosis
   B. Acetaminophen
   C. Cancer
   D. Hepatitis C

Answer question

LO2:

Pathophysiology: Hepatic Disorders

- Seventy-five percent of liver cells are hepatocytes with multiple important functions:
  - o Synthesizing proteins such as albumin and those required for clotting of blood
  - o Metabolizing toxic substances (especially those produced by the gut) and medications
  - o Storing carbohydrates (gluconeogenesis)
  - o Production of cholesterol
  - o Production and secretion of bile
- Damage to hepatocytes can be caused by toxins, viruses, or autoimmune processes.
  - o Regardless of the cause, damage to hepatocytes results in the release of cytokines plus the attraction and activation of inflammatory cells.
  - o Inflammation of the liver is termed **hepatitis**.
  - o Hepatocytes that are damaged by viruses or toxins have the ability to regenerate, and most patients with acute hepatitis will completely recover.
  - o However, if the damage is rapid and extensive, with insufficient time for regeneration, the patient may suffer a sudden loss of liver function.
  - o This extensive inflammation of the liver is termed **fulminant hepatitis**.
  - o The loss of function is termed liver failure and can be fatal.
  - o Hepatitis can also be chronic and long term; viruses or toxins can cause damage and inflammation that persists for years.
  - o This chronic inflammation usually results in replacement of liver cells by scar tissue, and hepatocytes become unable to regenerate.
  - o Diffuse scarring of the liver is termed **cirrhosis**.
  - o Over time, these patients lose function of the liver and evolve into chronic liver failure.
- Loss of liver function causes:
  - o Toxin accumulation, resulting in a condition termed **hepatic encephalopathy**
  - o Decreased lactate clearance, resulting in **metabolic acidosis**
  - o Loss of production of proteins, resulting in **coagulopathy** (inability to clot)
  - o Release of bile into the systemic circulation, resulting in **jaundice** due to blockage of the intrahepatic bile ductuli, thus producing jaundice, dark urine, itching, and light-colored stools
  - o Loss of production of albumin, resulting in a decreased ability to retain fluids in the vascular system, causing edema
- In end-stage liver disease, severe vasodilatation affects the splanchnic (gut) circulation and triggers intense renal vasoconstriction in an attempt to increase renal perfusion. However, intense renal artery vasoconstriction can cause renal failure (secondary to liver failure) and is termed **hepatorenal syndrome**.

Cirrhosis

With liver cirrhosis, there is disruption of blood flow through the liver. The disruption results in increased pressure in the portal system (**portal hypertension**) as well as shunting of blood from the portal system to the systemic circulation. Effects include:

- Development of dilated blood vessels in the portal system, termed **varices**, which are commonly seen in the esophagus or stomach. These blood vessels are susceptible to rupturing and bleeding.
- Bypassing of blood flow from the GI tract to the liver results in decreased toxin clearance.
- Development of fluid retention manifested by ascites and lower extremity edema

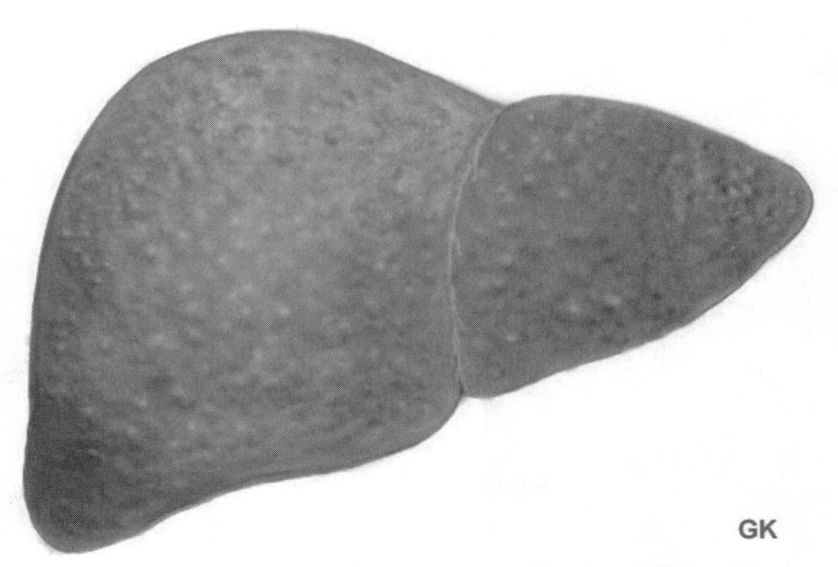

This image shows the coarse, tuberous liver cirrhosis, resembling that of a 30-year-old male patient. His liver was removed. A liver transplant was performed and he has been living for more than 10 years without any negative side effects.
Source: Courtesy of George Kyriakidis/Santa Ana, CA

Concept Check

2. **Patients in liver failure are at risk for which condition?**
   A. Deep vein thrombosis
   B. Respiratory acidosis
   C. Hemorrhage
   D. Increased albumin level

Answer question

Pathophysiology: Hepatic Disorders (continued)

Hepatic Infections

- Patients with liver cirrhosis are at risk for infections due to a suppressed immune system.
- This is exacerbated by the presence of ascites, which is a medium for bacterial growth.
- Bacteria from the gut that pass into the peritoneal space may cause an infection called **spontaneous bacterial peritonitis**.
- Inflammation produces pain and can cause sepsis and shock.

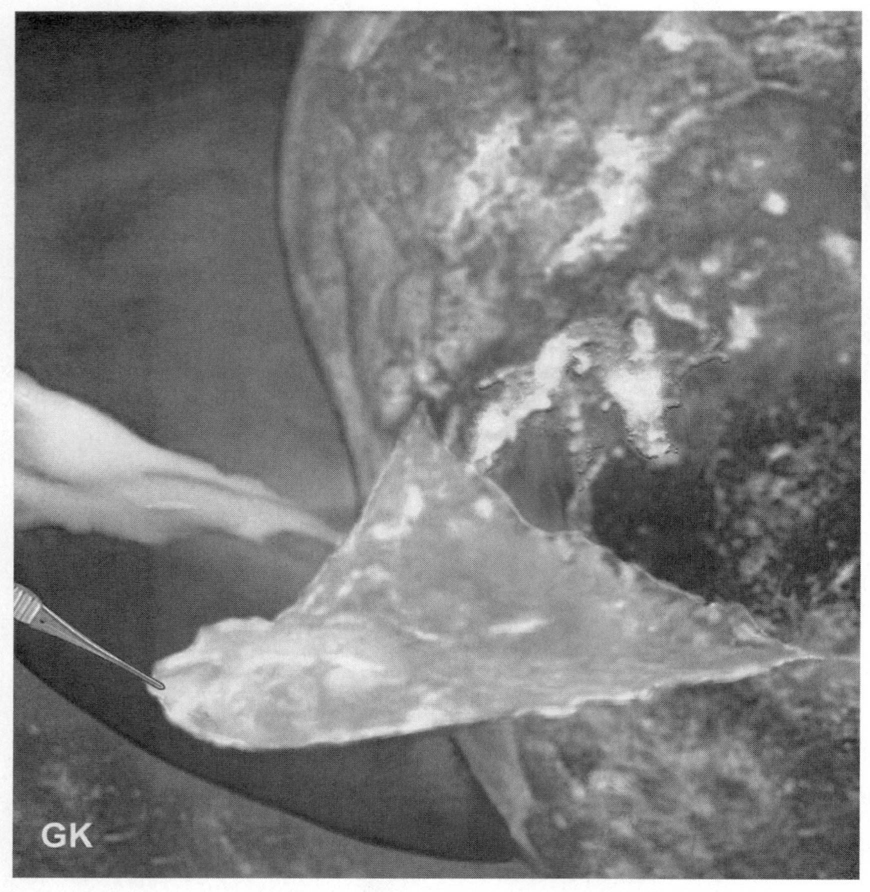

Acute bacterial peritonitis is depicted above. A surgical instrument is holding a flap of the peritoneum open for viewing. The yellowish areas demonstrate purulent accumulations. In contrast, spontaneous bacterial peritonitis usually occurs in patients with ascites and is not purulent.
Source: Courtesy of George Kyriakidis/Santa Ana, CA

Hepatic Viral Infections

Hepatitis viruses infect and damage liver cells:

- Viruses replicate inside infected hepatocytes and then infect other cells.
- Viruses can cause acute hepatitis as well as cirrhosis when the body is unable to clear the infection and the infection becomes chronic.
- Enteral forms of the hepatitis virus A and E are transmitted by the fecal–oral route.
- Parenteral forms B, C, and D are transmitted by blood exposure (e.g., IV drug abuse with shared needles) or sexual contact.
- Chronic infections occur when the immune system is unable to clear the viral infection.
- Chronic infections are caused by B, C, and D.
- Chronic infection of hepatocytes with the hepatitis B or C viruses also causes damage to the DNA of hepatic cells, increasing the probability of the development of hepatic cancer.

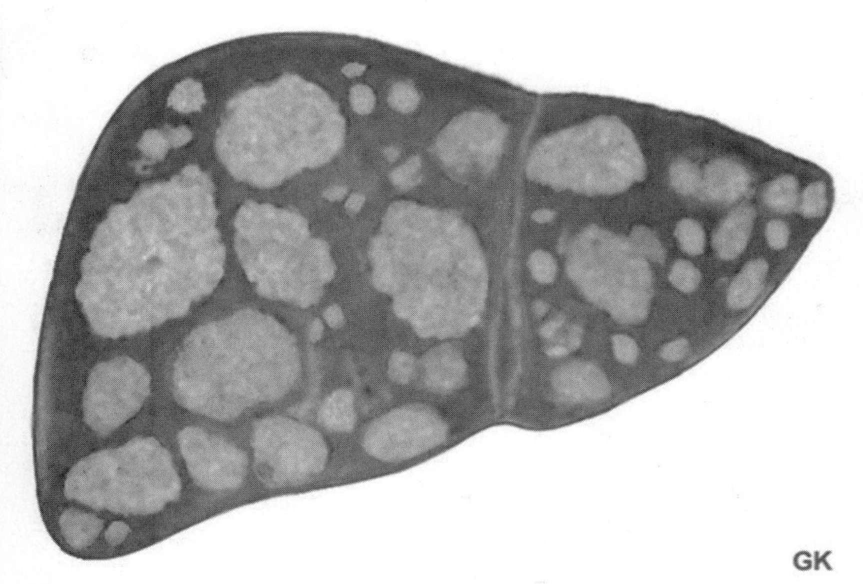

This photo shows the liver infected by hepatitis B, which is spread through infected blood or bodily fluids. Note the liver inflammation, scarring, and fatty accumulation.
Source: Courtesy of George Kyriakidis/Santa Ana, CA

Pathophysiological Consequences of Liver Failure

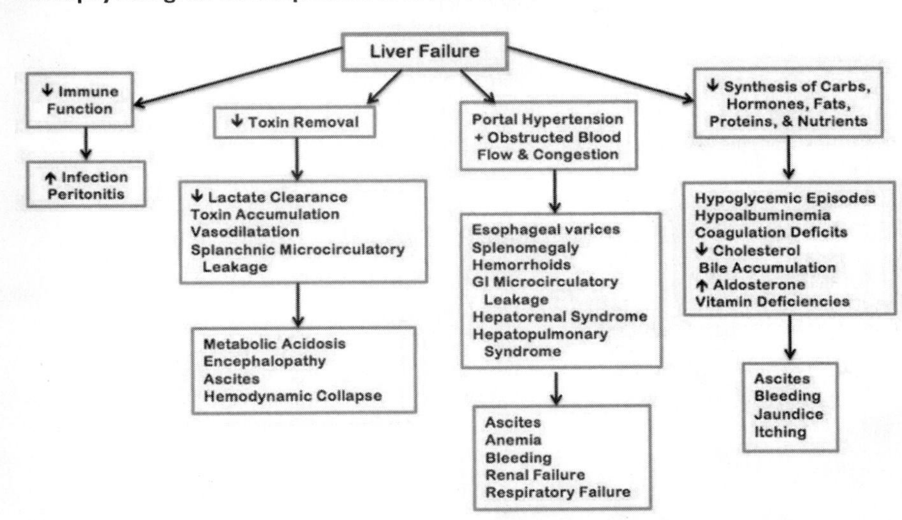

Source: Copyright © 2014, NovEx Novice to Expert Learning, LLC

LO2:

Causes: Hepatic Disorders

Liver disorders may result from:

- A virus, such as hepatitis
- Exposure to toxic substances
  - o Alcohol or other toxins (poisons)
  - o Drugs, such as acetaminophen
- Metabolic disorders
- Surgery
- Vascular causes
  - o Portal vein thrombosis
  - o Hepatic vein thrombosis (Budd–Chiari syndrome)
  - o Veno-occlusive disease
  - o Ischemic hepatitis (may occur with hypoperfusion in a patient with shock)
- Autoimmune or hereditary factors
- Cancer

Acute Liver Failure

- Acetaminophen (Tylenol) overdose
- Viruses, including hepatitis A, B, and C (especially in children)
- Reactions to certain prescription and herbal medications
- Ingestion of poisonous wild mushrooms (*Amanita phalloides,* or Death Cap, responsible for majority of deaths worldwide)

Chronic Liver Failure and Cirrhosis

- Alcohol abuse
- Chronic hepatitis B, C, or D (chronic inflammation from these viruses can cause progressive liver damage and scarring)
- Autoimmune hepatitis (destruction of liver cells by the immune system)
- Steatohepatitis (fatty liver causing chronic inflammation) is caused by alcohol ingestion, diabetes, and obesity.
- Liver damage from drugs, toxins, or infections
- Chronic biliary cirrhosis (bile duct obstruction, bile stasis, hepatic fibrosis)

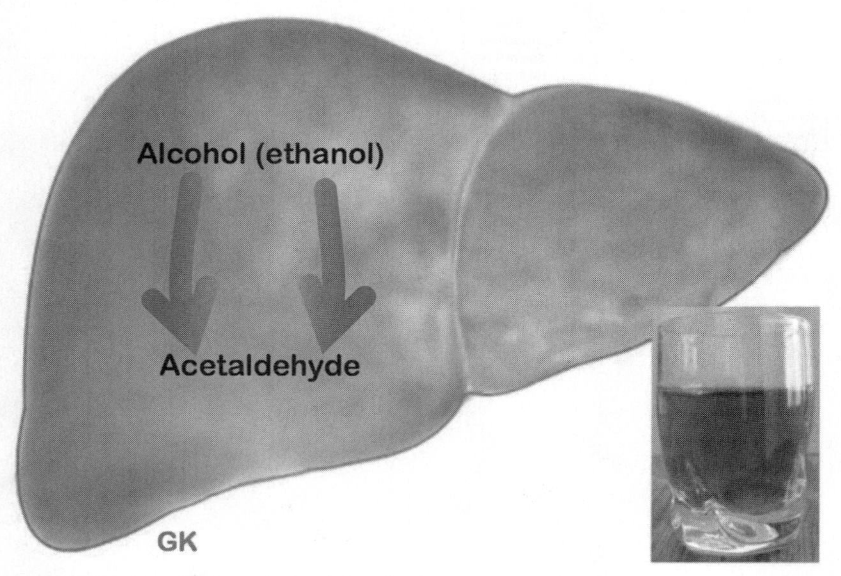

How damage occurs: When alcohol (ethanol) is broken down by the liver, it produces fat and a chemical called acetaldehyde, which is toxic to the liver but is processed into water and carbon dioxide.

Source: Courtesy of George Kyriakidis/Santa Ana, CA

LO2:

Assessment Findings: Hepatic Disorders

Acute Viral Hepatitis

- Onset of symptoms in acute hepatitis are usually sudden, appear in predictable phases, and range from mild to very severe.
- Incubation or preclinical phase (10–50 days) involves viral replication and spread, typically without symptoms. Transmission of the virus is greatest during this phase, before patients are aware that they are contagious.
- Pre-icteric or prodromal phase is when nonspecific symptoms appear and include:
  - o Loss of appetite, sometimes profound
  - o Nausea and vomiting
  - o General malaise
  - o Fever
  - o Smokers may have an aversion to cigarettes
  - o Pain in the upper right abdomen
  - o Itching (urticarial) due to hyperbilirubinemia
  - o Joint pains (arthralgias)
  - o Skin rash
- Icteric phase evolves after 3–10 days of initial symptoms appearing and presents with:
  - o Dark urine due to bilirubin
  - o Jaundice develops and worsens:
    - ■ Jaundice usually appears within days of onset at which point most other symptoms start to improve.
    - ■ Jaundice typically peaks at 1–2 weeks but may last up to a month.
  - o Hepatic enlargement and tenderness
  - o Splenomegaly in some patients
- Recovery, convalescent, or post-icteric phase may last 2–4 weeks as the jaundice resolves. It resolves slowly and relapse is possible.
- Hepatitis due to toxins has similar symptoms (except for joint pains).

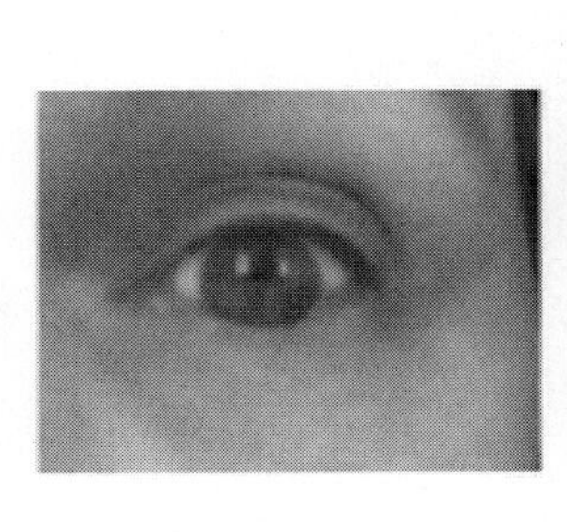
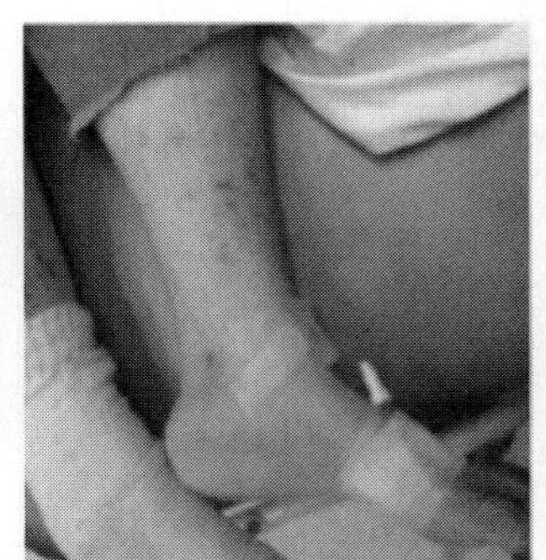
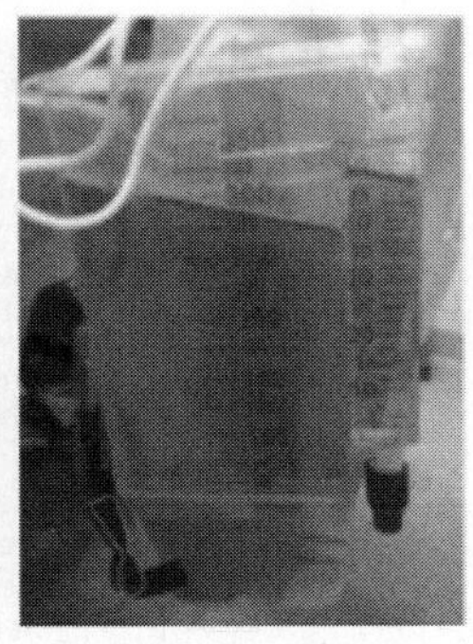

This patient exhibits classic signs of hepatitis, a few shown in photos here: a) scleral jaundice (yellowish discoloration), b) excoriation due to skin rash covering his legs and abdomen, and c) dark urine discolored by bilirubin.

Sources: Courtesy of K. Kyriakidis & George Kyriakidis/Santa Ana, CA

Concept Check

3. Which finding signals the beginning of the icteric stage of hepatitis?
   A. Fever
   B. Dark-colored urine
   C. Skin rash
   D. Loss of appetite

Answer question

Multisystem Effects: Hepatitis Versus Liver Cirrhosis

Multisystem Effects of Hepatitis

Hepatitis and Its Possible Manifestations

Neurologic
Memory loss
Hallucinations
Stroke
Paranoia

Musculoskeletal
Swollen legs & muscles
Numbness
Tingling

Skin
Jaundice

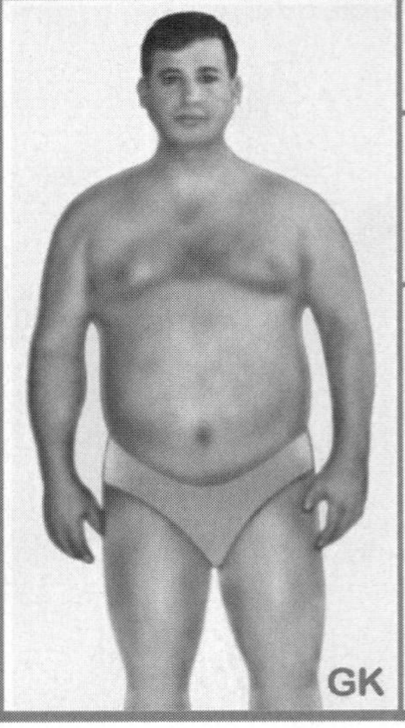

Eyes
Jaundiced

Hepatic
Enlarged liver
Splenomegaly

Gastrointestinal
Esophagus
Inflammation
Bleeding

Stomach
Inflammation
Bleeding

Source: Courtesy of George Kyriakidis/Santa Ana, CA

Multisystem Effects of Cirrohsis

Neurologic
Sensory alterations
Paresthesias
Asterixis (liver flap)
Portal systemic encephalopathy with progressive agitation to lethargy to stupor to coma

Hepatic
Atrophic, nodular
Splenomegaly
Possible liver cancer

Respiratory
Dyspnea

Hematologic
Thrombocytopenia
Anemia
Reduced clotting factors

Endocrine
Male gynecomastia
Possible diabetes mellitus

Immune
Susceptibility to infection
Leukocytopenia

Reproductive
Atrophy of testicles (men)
Oligomenorrhea (women)

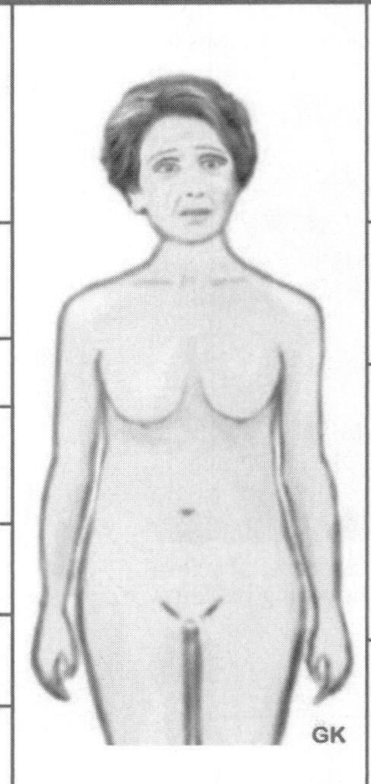

Skin
Jaundice
Spider angioma
Pruritis
Palmar erythema
Reduced body hair
Ecchymosis
Caput medusae

Cardiovascular
Portal hypertension
Dysrhythmias
Pulmonary hypertension
Bounding pulses

Gastrointestinal
Esophageal varices
Abdominal pain
Nausea
Anorexia
Ascites
GI bleeding
Peptic ulcer
Clay-colored stools
Hemorrhoids

Metabolic
Malnutrition
Muscle wasting
Fluid & electrolyte disturbances

Source: Courtesy of George Kyriakidis/Santa Ana, CA

Liver Cirrhosis

- Personality changes
- Ascites, sometimes severe
- Caput medusa or visible dilation of the superficial abdominal veins
- Jaundice
- Hyperventilation
- Palmar erythema
- Spider nevi: spider web-like bruising
- Lower extremity edema and weight gain
- Asterixis or "liver flaps": flapping tremor of the hand
- Increased abdominal girth due to ascites
- Shortness of breath due to ascites pushing up on the diaphragm and limiting full lung expansion
- Striae (stretch-like marks)

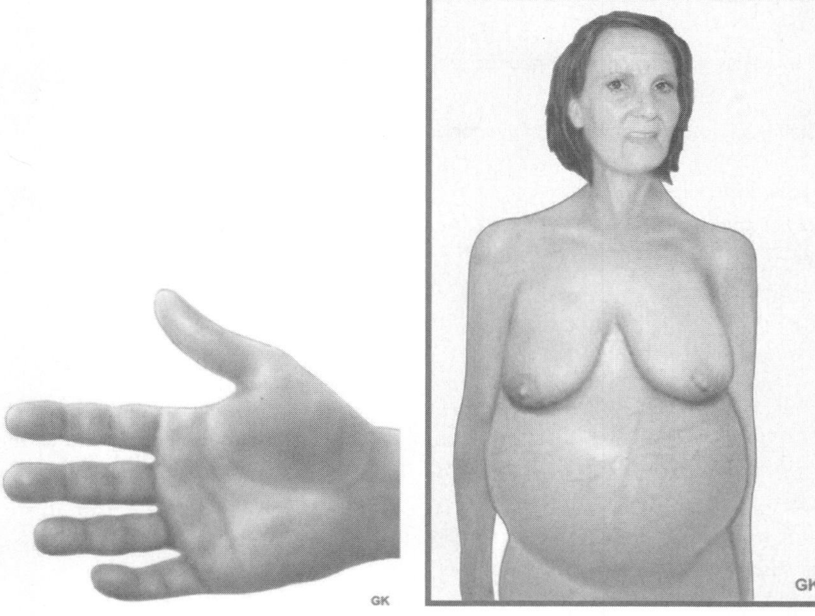

Left: Palmer erythema. Right: The abdomen of a person with cirrhosis showing massive ascites and caput medusae.
Source: *(both)* Courtesy of George Kyriakidis/Santa Ana, CA

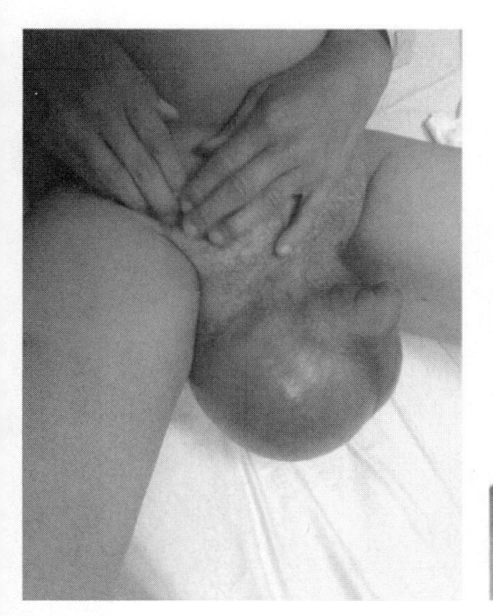

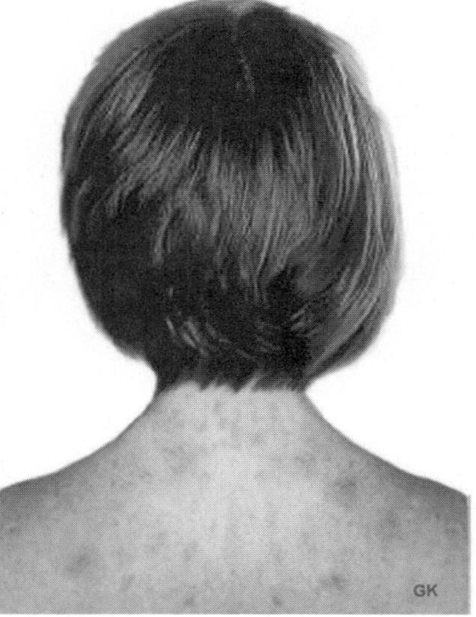

Left: Scrotal enlargement due to ascites. Right: Spider nevi are seen on the neck and back of a patient with liver cirrhosis.
Sources: *(left)* Courtesy of K. Kyriakidis; *(right)* Courtesy of George Kyriakidis/Santa Ana, CA

LO2:

Diagnostics: Hepatic Disorders

Labs:

- Serum liver function tests (LFTs) are commonly elevated:
  - o ALT (alanine transaminase) is most definitive for assessing **liver** tissue damage.
  - o AST (aspartate transaminase) is nonspecific and found in many tissues.
  - o GGT (gamma-glutamyl transferase)
- Alkaline phosphatase to detect cholestasis or metastatic cancer
- Serum bilirubin is commonly elevated:
  - o Direct (conjugated)
  - o Indirect (unconjugated)
  - o Total
- Serum proteins and albumin: decreased due to decreased hepatic synthesis
- Clotting factors: prothrombin time/INR prolonged due to decreased synthesis of prothrombin
- Acetaminophen levels for suspected overdose:
  - o Four hours after a single ingestion
  - o Toxic ingestion is 150 mg/kg or 7–10 grams for an average-sized adult in a 24-hour period.
- Serum lactate due to impairment of clearance
- Ammonia can increase in patients with encephalopathy because the conversion of ammonia to urea is altered.
- Hepatitis serology markers and antibody testing to evaluate for viral hepatitis
- Serum creatinine elevation in severe liver disease (*hepatorenal syndrome)*
- Alpha-fetoprotein (AFP) is elevated in liver cancer.
- TSH: may see mild elevation in liver enzymes with hypothyroidism
- Lipid levels may be decreased.

Imaging:

- Abdominal x-ray may reveal hepatomegaly, ascites, or spleen enlargement.
- Ultrasound is used to detect cancer, evidence of cirrhosis, and ascites.
- CT scan may detect cancer, ascites, or cirrhosis and may also show evidence of portal or hepatic vein thrombosis.

Endoscopy:

- Esophagogastroduodenoscopy (EGD) can detect esophageal varices secondary to liver dysfunction. Review the animation in the Diagnostics section of the Care of Patients with GI Bleeding NovE-lesson.

CT Scan of Liver Cirrhosis

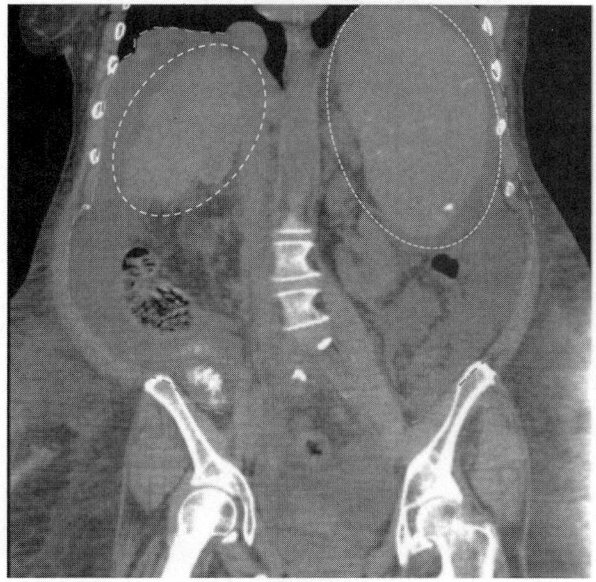

This CT scan of the abdomen reveals liver cirrhosis by the atrophied, abnormally shaped, nodular-appearing liver (yellow outline). The spleen is grossly enlarged (blue outline) and the red outline denotes how ascites fills the abdominal cavity.

Gastric Varices from Cirrhosis

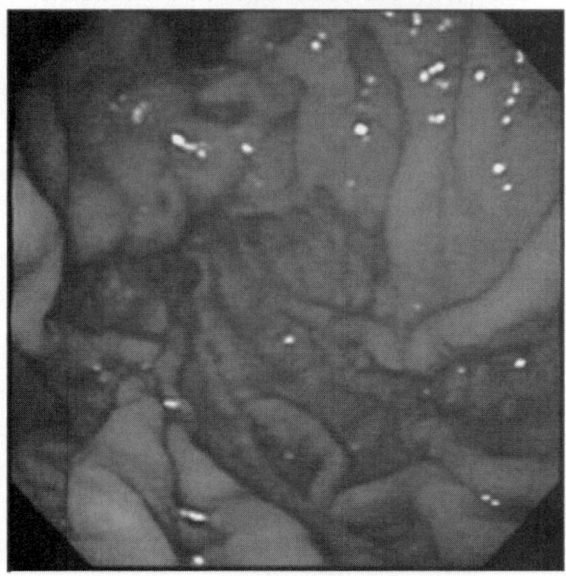

Gastric varices are noted during endoscopy. Varices are the distended and numerous veins bulging from the gastric mucosa.

Source: *(both)* Courtesy of K. Kyriakidis

Paracentesis

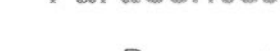

- Paracentesis is a procedure to aspirate fluid from the peritoneal space.

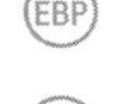

- Fluid analysis can help determine if there is an infection (spontaneous bacterial peritonitis) and cause of ascites (Runyon, 2012).
- Paracentesis is also used to remove excess fluid and may be repeated (Runyon, 2012).

Indications for abdominal paracentesis:

- o Ascites (new-onset or malignant) for diagnostic or therapeutic means (relieve cardio-respiratory compromise secondary to tense ascites)
- o Suspected infection

Contraindications:

- o Coagulopathy when there is evidence of disseminated intravascular coagulation (DIC) or thrombocytopenia
- o Acute abdomen requires immediate surgery.

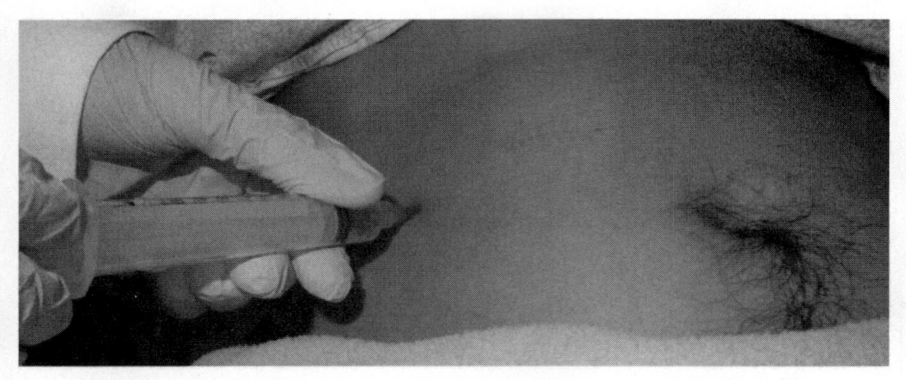

Ascites can prompt the need for paracentesis. Paracentesis is performed using needle aspiration to draw off fluid accumulation. Typical ascites aspirate is yellowish peritoneal fluid. Paracentesis may result in temporary relief. Note here that the abdomen is no longer bulging after several syringes of fluid were discarded.
Source: Courtesy of K. Kyriakidis

Diagnostics: Hepatic Disorders (continued)

Biopsy

Liver biopsy can identify infection, if present, tissue damage, or cancer cells.

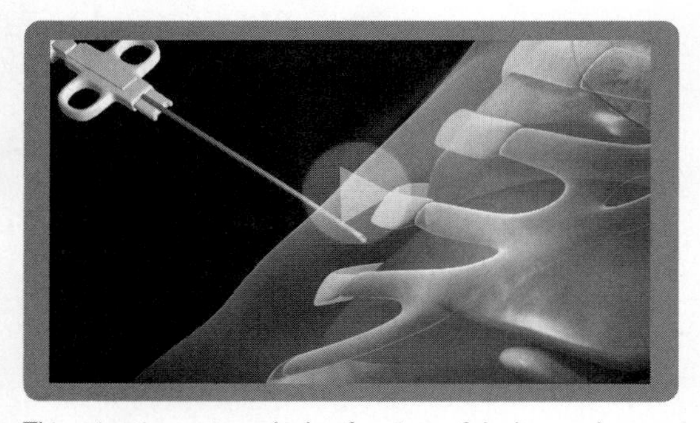

This animation reviews the key functions of the liver and describes how a liver biopsy is performed. It depicts the removal of a small sample of liver tissue (or biopsy). The purpose of the liver biopsy is usually performed to diagnose suspected abnormal conditions that may be caused by hepatitis, cancers, or infections.
Source: © 2014 Nucleus Medical Media, All rights reserved

Concept Check

4. Which test is considered the most definitive for liver tissue damage?

A. AST

B. GGT

C. Total bilirubin

D. ALT

Answer question

Priority Patient Concerns and Desired Collaborative Care Outcomes: Hepatic Disorders

Prior to caring for patients with hepatic disorders, it is important to prioritize the patient's concerns that must guide the nursing care plan and interventions. Care for the patient is ordered and organized in accordance with the patient's priority and urgent needs. Desired collaborative care outcomes in patients with hepatic disorders typically include:

1. Patient will be able to perform daily activities without fatigue.
2. Patient will increase understanding of disease process and treatment.
3. Patient will maintain normal fluid volume status with minimal fluid volume shifts.
4. Patient will maintain adequate intake to meet metabolic demands.
5. Patient will not experience bleeding from esophageal varices.
6. Patient will remain alert and oriented.
7. Patient will remain free of additional infections.
8. Patient's skin and mucous membranes will remain intact.

Considering these important care outcomes, prepare a list of the major 3–6 priority patient concerns or nursing diagnoses for patients with hepatic disorders. Be prepared to participate in a discussion of this list and/or to submit them as an assignment, as determined by your faculty. Resources you may find helpful in this assignment can include this lesson, the references, resources on nursing care plans, and standard nursing diagnoses manuals.

Concept Check

5. **Which technique is typically used to obtain a liver biopsy?**
   A. Insertion of a needle into the liver
   B. An open surgical procedure requiring general anesthesia
   C. Insertion of an endoscopic tube with tissue sampling capability
   D. A laparoscopic surgical procedure requiring conscious sedation

Answer question

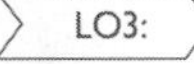

LO3:

Collaborative Interventions: Hepatic Disorders

Acute Hepatitis

Care of patients with acute hepatitis is most commonly guided by patient-specific presentation and test data. Care may include:

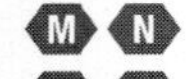

- Management is usually supportive with fluids and antiemetics for patients with nausea.
- Discharging patients with acute viral hepatitis to be followed at home whenever possible.

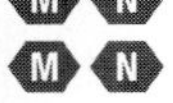

- Typically admit patients with severe (acute fulminant hepatitis) or patients at risk of worsening (e.g., patients with acetaminophen overdose or mushroom poisoning) to the hospital. These patients may develop liver failure and should be monitored for early warning signs (e.g., coagulopathy, encephalopathy).

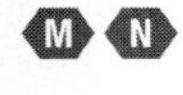

- Some of the patients with poisoning may require liver transplant. Monitor for signs of progressive liver failure (e.g., hemodynamic instability, liver function decline, renal failure) that is unresponsive to treatment.

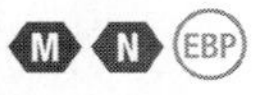

- Collaborate to refer patients with alcoholic hepatitis to counseling on abstaining from alcohol (O'Shea, et al., 2010).
- Instruct all patients to avoid hepatotoxins (e.g., acetaminophen, alcohol).

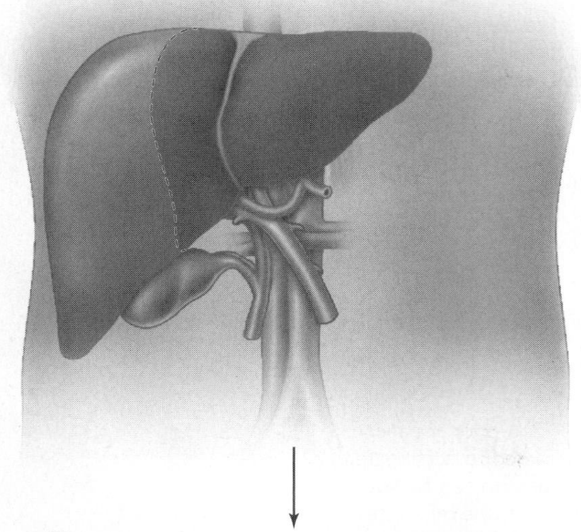
1 A portion of the donor liver is removed.

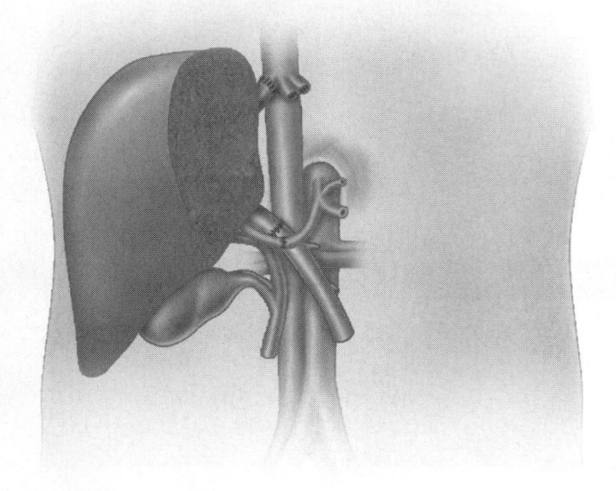
2 The donor liver is transplanted to the recipient.

Living donor transplants shed light on the amazing nature of the liver is as an organ. Transplantation of the liver from a living donor entails transplanting a portion of the donor's liver into the recipient. The liver is then able to regenerate new liver tissue in both the living donor and the recipient until it reaches a normal size. The new liver tissue can take up normal liver functions.

Chronic Viral Hepatitis

- Chronic viral hepatitis (B and C) can be treated with medications that stimulate the immune system to clear the viral infection.
- The goal of treatment is to diminish inflammation and prevent progression to cirrhosis or liver cancer.
- M N Treatment may include:
  - o Interferon therapy
  - o Ribavirin
- M N Patients should be instructed to avoid hepatotoxins (e.g., alcohol, acetaminophen, select chemotherapy medications).

Liver Cirrhosis

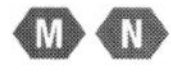

- Management of liver cirrhosis consists of managing the individual problems that arise from liver failure:
  - o Encephalopathy
  - o Esophageal bleeding from varices (see details in the Care of Patients with Esophageal Disorders NovE-lesson)
  - o Ascites
  - o Spontaneous bacterial peritonitis (see details in the Care of Patients with GI Infections NovE-lesson)
- Depending on the patient's severity of illness and recovery, patients may need to be educated about the potential need for transplantation.
- Educate patients to avoid hepatotoxins, such as alcohol.
- Encourage vaccination against viral hepatitis, which may help prevent further deterioration.

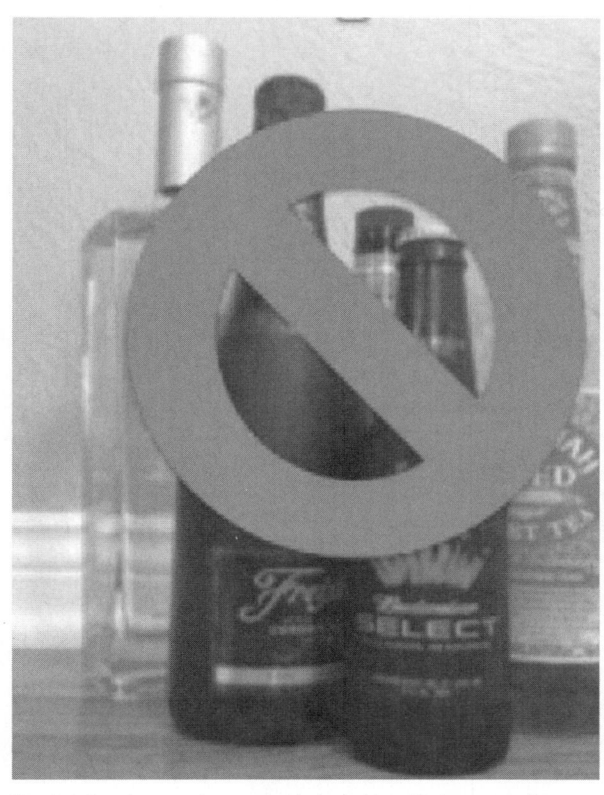

Simply informing a patient to avoid alcohol is unlikely to transform harmful habits. Counseling and additional resources are likely needed for lasting lifestyle changes. Family involvement is often essential.

Collaborative Interventions: Hepatic Disorders (continued)

Encephalopathy

- Encephalopathy can occur in patients who have hepatic disorders and:
  - o Are not compliant with treatment
  - o Experience GI bleeding
  - o Have worsening hepatic function

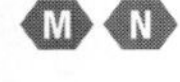

  - o High protein restrictions are not supported by evidence. Patients on high-protein diets showed significant improvement, particularly because so many patients with liver failure are malnourished.

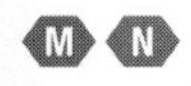

- Treatment and prevention of encephalopathy consists of removal of nitrogenous waste (e.g., ammonia) from the large intestine.

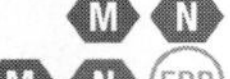

- Lactulose, which results in bowel movements, is the primary therapy (see schematic).

- Antibiotics that remain in the intestinal lumen, such as neomycin and rifaximin, are also used to treat this condition (Bass, et al., 2010).

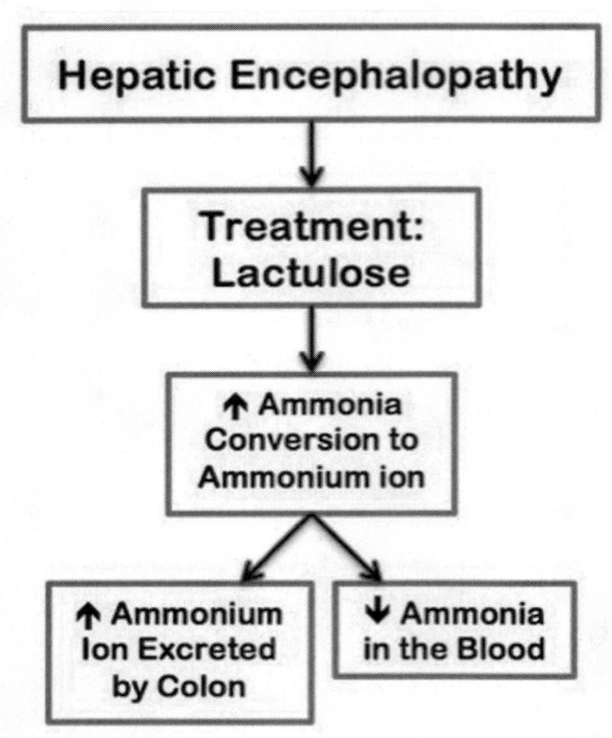

Source: Copyright © 2014, NovEx Novice to Expert Learning, LLC

Ascites

Massive ascites is uncomfortable and can interfere with breathing by pressing up on the diaphragm.

- Treat by removing ascitic fluid by paracentesis and repeat as necessary (Runyon, 2012).
- Removal of large amounts of ascitic fluid causes a shift of fluid from the intravascular space into the abdominal cavity and creates hemodynamic instability. Caution is important.
- With severe splanchnic vasodilation, blood flow to the kidneys can diminish and compromise kidney function. Monitor for hepatorenal syndrome.
- Patients with ascites are at risk for developing hypotension as fluid shifts. Close monitoring is needed.
- Milder ascites that does not cause a lot of discomfort may be treated with diuretics (e.g., furosemide, spironolactone) and sodium restriction (Runyon, 2012).
- Spontaneous bacterial peritonitis is diagnosed by paracentesis and treated with intravenous antibiotics (Runyon, 2012).

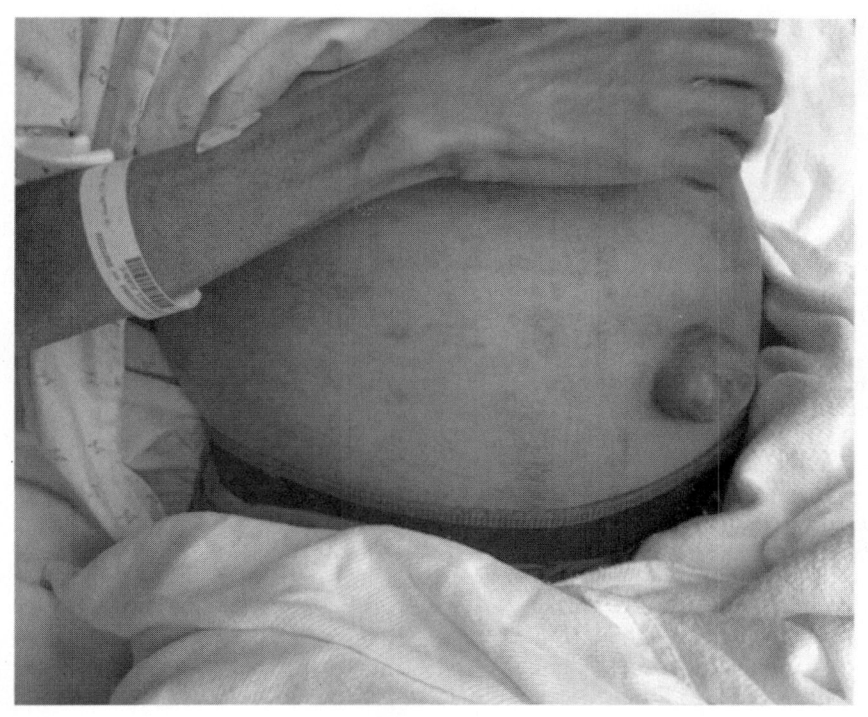

This patient has fluid accumulation in his abdomen due to cirrhosis. Note that an umbilical hernia is exacerbated by the abnormally high intra-abdominal pressure. The pressure compromises lung expansion and interferes with respirations.
Source: Courtesy of K. Kyriakidis

Concept Check

6. **Patients with chronic hepatitis should avoid which of the following to prevent exacerbation or progression of liver failure?**
   A. Furosemide (Lasix)
   B. Ribavirin
   C. Alcohol
   D. Cigarette smoking

Answer question

Collaborative Interventions: Hepatic Disorders (continued)

Bleeding

Patients with liver cirrhosis are predisposed to massive hemorrhage because they have a combination of coagulopathy and varices (see details in the Care of Patients with Esophageal Disorders NovE-lesson). Treatment for bleeding includes:

- Vitamin K, fresh frozen plasma (FFP), and/or packed red blood cells to replace losses (Garcia-Tsao, et al., 2007).

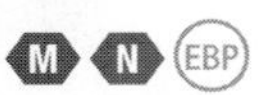

- Octreotide for variceal bleeding as well as endoscopic banding or ligation of the varices (see video) are used to halt the hemorrhage (Garcia-Tsao, et al., 2007).

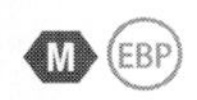

- Endoscopy with injection sclerotherapy endoscopically may stop the variceal bleeding. This employs injection of a substance that causes clotting and scarring of the varices. A combination of methods may be used (Garcia-Tsao, et al., 2007).
- Methods to decrease pressure in varices and decrease chance for bleeding include shunts from the portal system to the systemic veins:

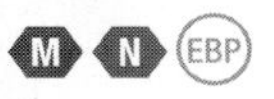

  - o Beta blockers (e.g., propranolol) can lower portal pressure. These are usually started prophylactically or after a variceal bleed when the patient is stable and ready for discharge (Garcia-Tsao, et al., 2007).

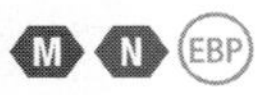

  - o Transjugular intrahepatic portosystemic shunt (TIPS) and surgical bypass shunting procedure lower portal pressures and can be used for patients with recurrent hemorrhage despite other treatments. These procedures can worsen encephalopathy since blood flow through the liver is bypassed (Garcia-Tsao, et al., 2007). Closely monitor for early clinical cues or worsening encephalopathy.

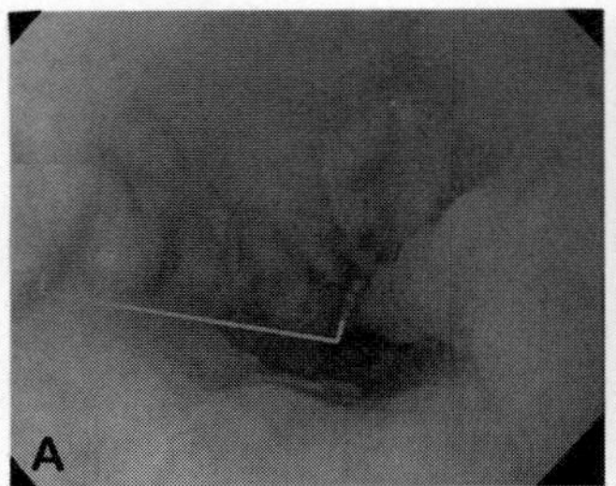

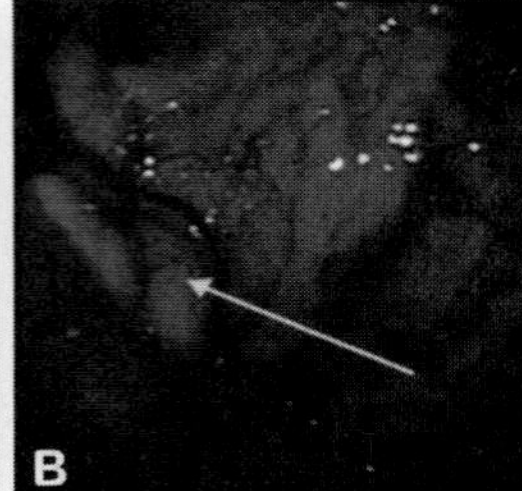

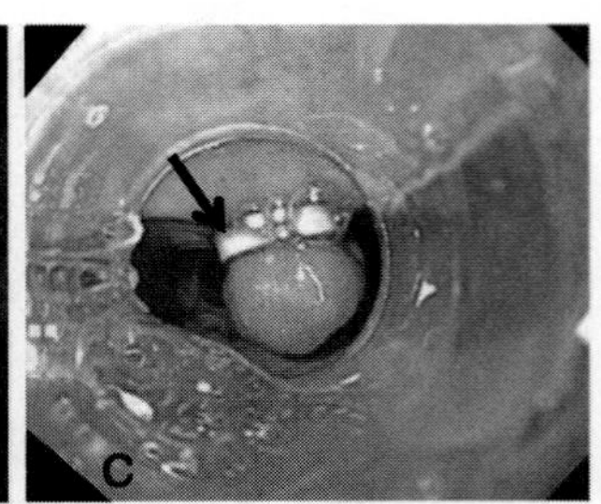

This series of endoscopic photos depicts the complication and treatment of esophageal varices that is common in patients with cirrhosis. (A) Esophageal varices in the red bracket appear like varicose veins in the leg. It is a distended, engorged, and contorted vessel. (B) This photo reveals the esophageal varix (arrow) that is bleeding and can cause significant blood loss, left untreated. (C) The black arrow points at the banding ligator that clamps off the bleeding vein to establish hemostasis.

Source: Courtesy of K. Kyriakidis

N
- For patients on a medical or surgical floor, call the **Rapid Response Team** if any signs of uncontrolled bleeding or deterioration are detected to evaluate the need for a more intensive level of care in the ICU.

N
- Collaborate with the health care provider about the need for ICU care if patient has:
  - o Moderate–large blood loss
  - o Signs of sepsis or organ failure
  - o PaO_2 ≤94%
  - o Sustained tachycardia
  - o Hypotension
  - o Altered mental status

Collaborative Interventions: Hepatic Disorders (continued)

Supportive Care

N
- Prevent complications:
  - o Surveillance for infection
  - o Maintenance of nutrition
  - o Prompt recognition of early signs and symptoms of gastrointestinal bleeding
  - o Prevent never events (e.g., DVT, hospital acquired infections, central line and urinary catheter-related infections, pressure ulcers).

M N
- Manage multisystem involvement.

N
- Prepare family for needed ongoing care.

N
- Maintain safe environment.

M N
- Collaborate with the health care team regarding liver transplant if applicable.

Patient Education

Nursing care for patients with hepatic disorders can be complicated. Patient education is imperative to prevent the disease occurrence, prevent spread of disease, and/or to delay onset of complications.

Hepatitis

N
- Educate patients, families, groups, and community on ways to prevent hepatitis. Hepatitis A and E are especially prevalent in developing countries and close proximity situations (e.g., dormitories, crowded living).

N EBP
- Community health nurses need to educate the public on the importance of good hand washing and hygiene, proper food preparation and appropriate disposal of waste (Siegel, et al., 2007).

N EBP
- Nurses are also instrumental in educating people on the importance of safe sexual practices. Condom use should be emphasized when the nurse is educating people about hepatitis (CDC, 2008).

M N EBP
- Educate about cessation of IV drug use. In situations of IV drug use, educate the patient on the risks of spreading or obtaining the hepatitis virus (B and C) through needle sharing (CDC, 1998).

Prevention of Acute or Chronic Hepatitis

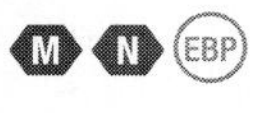

All persons who are potentially infected or colonized and pose a risk to others cannot be readily identified. Thus, excellent care minimally requires implementation of **evidence-based universal precautions** detailed by the CDC (Siegel, et al., 2007) in all patients at all times. Similarly, there are disease-specific precautions in some forms of hepatitis that may not be applicable to other forms. However, we recommend adhering to precautions in all patients since those who are infected or colonized and pose a risk are not always clearly known. Adhere to the following standards and educate patients and their families to:

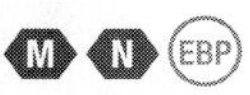

- Strictly adhere to all hand hygiene standards before and after caring for every patient or coming in contact with patient environments (Siegel, et al., 2007).
- Hepatitis vaccine or an immunoglobulin shot is given to prevent hepatitis A and B. Vaccination is the most effective preventive measure to infection and its sequelae, including cirrhosis, cancer, liver failure, and death (Mast, et al., 2006).

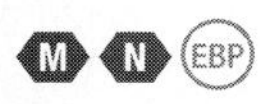

- Vaccinate adults for hepatitis B is especially recommended in persons who are at risk from (Mast, et al., 2006):
  - o Sexual exposure (e.g., STD treatment, sexually active persons not in a monogamous relationship)
  - o Mucosal or percutaneous exposure to blood (e.g., IV drug use, close contact with hepatitis B-positive person, tattoos, body piercing, persons with end-stage renal disease)
  - o Exposure during international travel to areas with moderate-to-high levels of endemic HBV infections
  - o Exposure to patients with chronic liver disease
  - o HIV positive persons

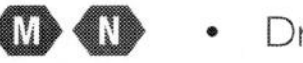

- Drink alcohol in moderation. Avoid alcohol when taking acetaminophen (Tylenol).
- Do not exceed 4 grams of acetaminophen daily or 2 grams with alcohol intake.

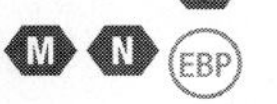

- Do not handle any blood or blood products without universal precautions (Siegel, et al., 2007).

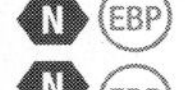

- Do not share personal toiletry items, such as toothbrushes and razors (CDC, 2008).

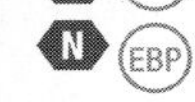

- If getting a tattoo or body piercing, make sure that the equipment is properly sanitized (CDC, 1998).

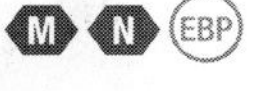

- Adhere to safe sex practices: Use protection (condoms) when having sex if infected, if not monogamous, or if one's partner is unknown and/or not monogamous (CDC, 1998).

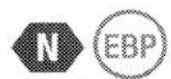

- If using illegal IV drugs, do not share or reuse needles or syringes.

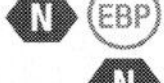

- Do not eat wild mushrooms. Even experts often cannot tell the difference between poisonous and nonpoisonous species. Urgent liver transplant is commonly the only effective intervention.

Cirrhosis

Because cirrhosis is most often preventable, clinicians should focus on preventative education for those at risk.

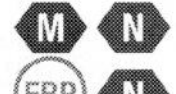

- Stress the importance of alcohol cessation in people prone to excessive alcohol consumption.

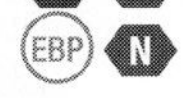

- Fatty liver can also lead to cirrhosis. Educate at-risk patients (e.g., diabetics, obese, alcohol misuse) on the damage excessive fat can cause to the liver (Powell, et al., 1990).

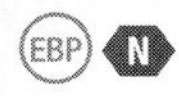

- Weight reduction programs should be stressed for patients with a fatty liver. Early evidence suggests improvement (Promrat, et al., 2010).

- When cirrhosis has progressed beyond restoration, educate the patient on ways to treat symptoms of the disease such as abdominal ascites, frequent rest periods, adequate fluids, lower limb edema, and cessation of alcohol.

Collaborative Interventions: Hepatic Disorders (continued)

Advanced Directives

Liver cirrhosis is a terminal disease without transplantation.

- There is a very high mortality rate associated with many of the complications including:
  - o Esophageal varices bleeding
  - o Spontaneous bacterial peritonitis
- Many patients die even with the best possible care.
- Variceal bleeding in a patient may not be controlled, even with large amounts of blood products (e.g., FFP, RBCs, and platelets).

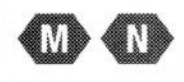

- Discussions regarding advanced directives should be initiated early. Advanced directives are intended for everyone, not only those with terminal or life-threatening illnesses.

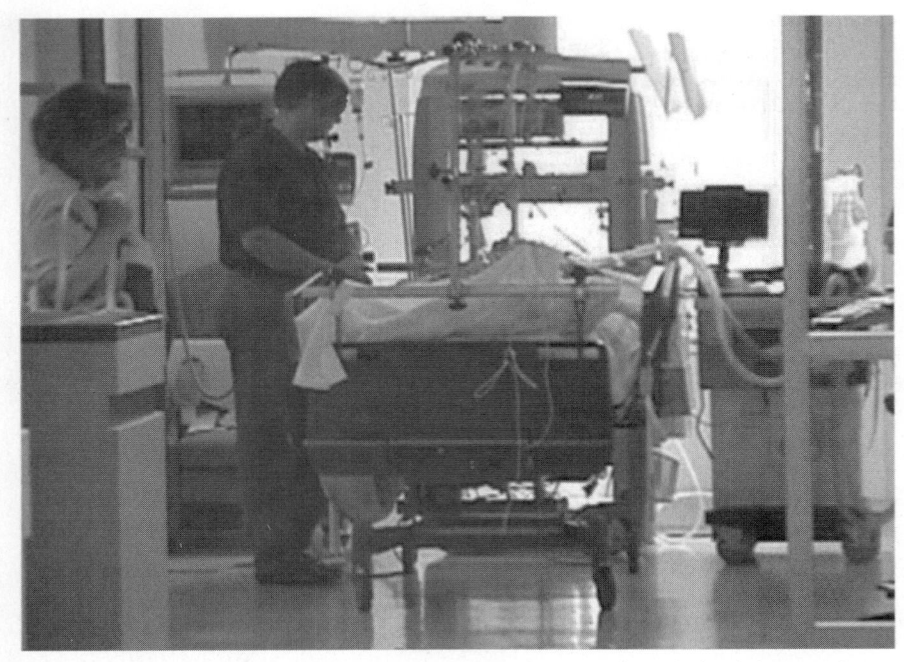

This terminally ill patient has advanced directives, alleviating his parents from the harsh decisions that need to be made on his behalf as aggressive care is futile. An advance directive serves as a written guide or instructions which specify a person's preferences about the type of medical care desired in the event that communication is not possible. An advance directive is a critical guide for healthcare providers to ensure that the patient's wishes are respected and implemented. A living will is a way of making these directives a legal document. Advanced directives should be shared with physicians and family to make one's wishes known.

Hepatic Impairment

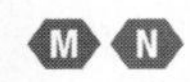

- Avoid alcohol, acetaminophen, and/or toxins. Ask your HCP about other medications.

- Medication metabolized by the liver may need to be altered:
  - o Diuretics
  - o Stress ulcer medication or H2 receptor antagonist
  - o Lactulose to promote excretion of ammonia in stool
  - o Neomycin and rifaximin remove intestinal bacteria that produce ammonia.
- Diet: Low sodium diets are important for patients with ascites. Avoidance of high-protein diets are no longer recommended for patients with liver failure.
- Provide education regarding:
  - o Rehabilitation
  - o Chronic illness
  - o Support groups
  - o Alcohol addiction treatment
  - o Preventing recurrence

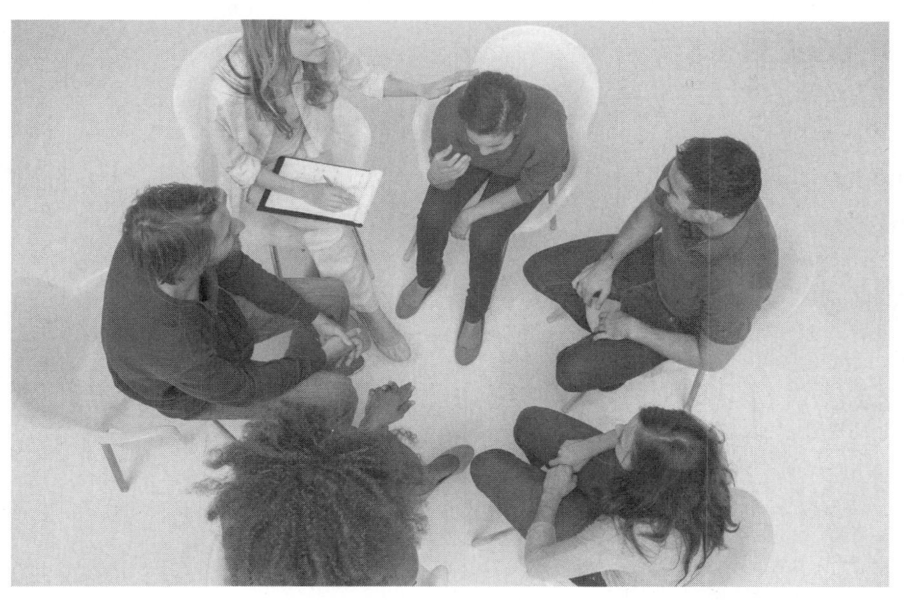

Successful treatment for substance abuse is relatively poor without support. Rehabilitation and support groups improve success of recovery.
Source: WavebreakmediaMicro/Fotolia

LO1:

Clinical Relevance: Acetaminophen Toxicity and Acute Hepatic Failure

- Acetaminophen (APAP) is the most commonly used medication for pain relief and fever control in the world.
- APAP is one of the most common medications used for intentional and unintentional overdoses.
- APAP toxicity is the single most common cause of acute hepatic failure requiring a liver transplant.
- APA at near normal levels can cause hepatotoxicity when used with alcohol.
- Any patient presenting with an intentional or unknown overdose, should have an APAP level done, no matter what medication the patient claims to have taken.
- Toxicity occurs at 150 mg/kg or higher or about 7–10 grams in an adult in a 24-hour period.
    - o This equals 14–20 500 mg APAP tablets or capsules.
- APAP is an ingredient in more than 100 over-the-counter products.
- Use the **Rumack-Matthew nomogram** (see Interventions section) for any acute ingestion within a 24-hour period.

LO2:

Pathophysiology: Acetaminophen Hepatotoxicity

- The toxic metabolite of APAP is N-acetyl-p-benzoquinone imine (NAPQI).
- High levels of NAPQI quickly deplete the glutathione stores in the liver that detoxify this metabolite.
- At toxic levels, this metabolite leads to an inflammatory response, followed by hepatocellular damage, cellular death, and centrilobular hepatic necrosis.
- Since the Rumack-Matthew nomogram is for calculating acute ingestions only, chronic acetaminophen poisoning hepatotoxicity is determined by the AST, ALT, and serum acetaminophen levels.

Tylenol Injury to Liver

Normal Anatomy

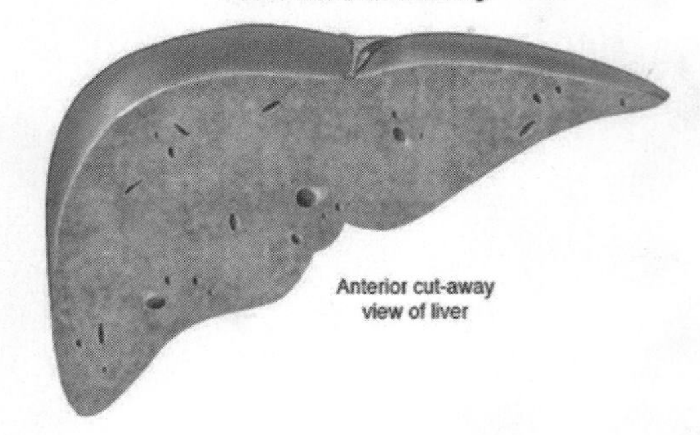

Cirrhosis

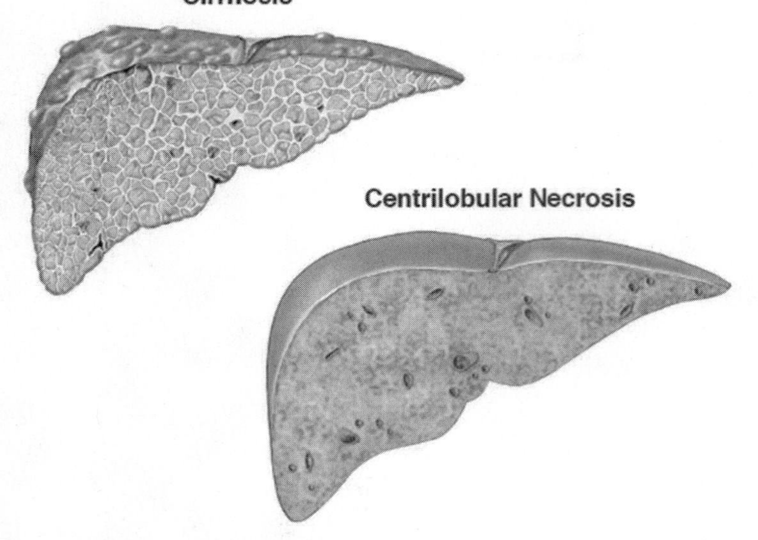

This drawing illustrates the effects of Tylenol on the liver. The first image is shown to compare a normal liver to ones with disease. The second image depicts cirrhosis of the liver while the lower image depicts centrilobular necrosis due to acetaminophen toxicity.

Stages of Acetaminophen Toxicity

Stage	Findings	Day
Stage 1	• Abdominal pain, diaphoresis, nausea & vomiting, pallor, generalized discomfort • Liver function tests can be normal	Day 0-1
Stage 2	• Injury to liver develops • Upper right quadrant pain evolves • Liver function test abnormalities (AST, ALT, INR, bilirubin)	Day 1-3
Stage 3	• Liver toxicity peaks • Hepatic failure is rapid and severe • Glucose, phosphate and lactate abnormalities evolve • Encephalopathy and hypoglycemia manifest • Coma and even death may occur	Day 3-5
Stage 4	• If the patient survives, recovery progresses	Day 5-8

LO2:

Risk Factors: Acetaminophen Toxicity

- Patients at risk for taking too much APAP are those with:
  - o Depression and suicidal ideations
  - o Chronic pain who are prescribed APAP in combination with a narcotic and take more than is prescribed.

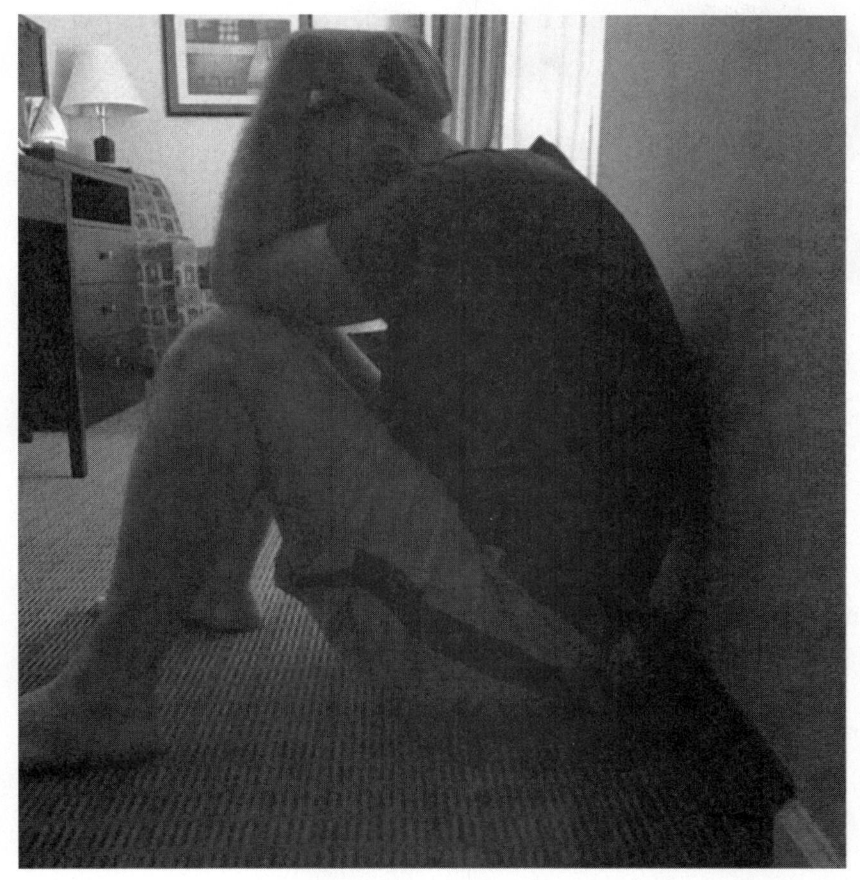

Suicidal ideation is having thoughts of suicide. It can range from momentary to deliberate planning. The majority of people who have suicidal ideation do not attempt to harm themselves, but the clinician should not take it lightly. Depression commonly accompanies suicidal ideation. It is linked to mental disturbances, stressful life or family situation, and other forms of significant stress.

LO3:

Collaborative Interventions: Acetaminophen Hepatotoxicity

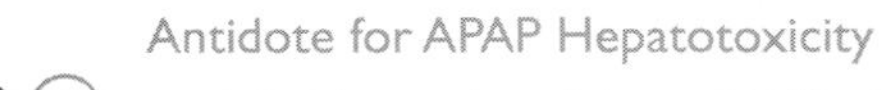

Antidote for APAP Hepatotoxicity

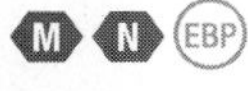
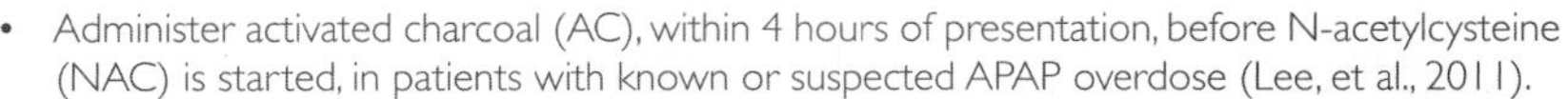

- Administer activated charcoal (AC), within 4 hours of presentation, before N-acetylcysteine (NAC) is started, in patients with known or suspected APAP overdose (Lee, et al., 2011).

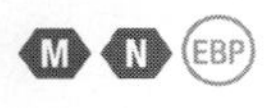

- Initiate NAC, the recommended antidote for APAP hepatotoxicity or for impending liver injury, immediately. It is a glutathione precursor that can be given orally, through a nasogastric tube, or intravenously (Lee, et al., 2011). NAC decreases acetaminophen toxicity by increasing hepatic glutathione stores.

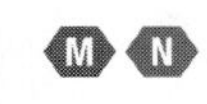

- Do not delay administration of NAC in order to give AC. Early administration of NAC takes precedence over gastric decontamination with AC in overdose situations. However, AC renders NAC less bioavailable so NAC is given IV in situations where AC administration, or multiple dosages of AC, is needed.

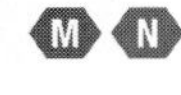

- Further hepatic toxicity is prevented by NAC through deactivating the toxic APAP metabolite, NAPQI, before it causes further damage to liver cells. NAC will not reverse already damaged liver cells.

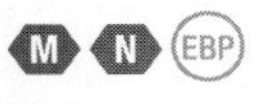

- Consider AC for out-of-hospital patients if it is <2 hours after ingestion of a toxic dose of APAP (Dart, et al., 2006).

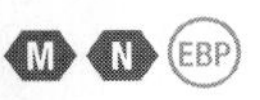

- It is strongly recommended that cimetidine not be administered as an antidote (Dart, et al., 2006).

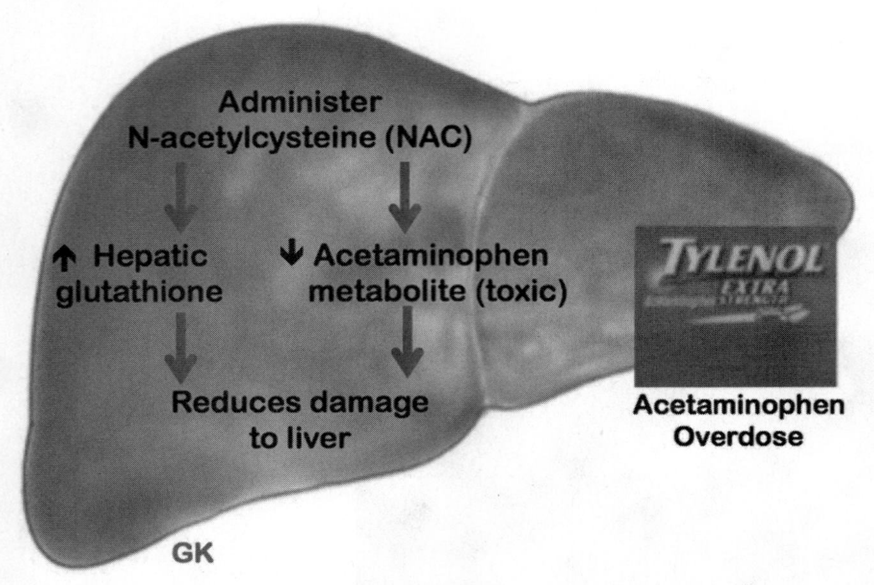

Exceeding the recommended dose of acetaminophen, a key ingredient in over-the-counter medications such as Tylenol® and Tempra®, may result in acute liver failure. The mechanism of action for the antidote is depicted to reduce liver damage and failure.

Source: Courtesy of George Kyriakidis/Santa Ana, CA

Collaborative Interventions: Acetaminophen Hepatotoxicity (continued)

APAP Toxicity

M N
- Administer NAC for APAP overdose to decrease hepatic damage.

M N
- NAC is maximally hepatoprotective when given within 8 hours of ingestion. The Rumack-Matthew nomogram provides guidance for clinical intervention.

M N
- If significant ingestion is suspected, NAC should be given regardless of time of ingestion and should be started before an APAP level is back.

M N
- IV NAC, not oral, has been shown to decrease mortality rates even when given late in the process, with fulminant hepatic failure from acetaminophen overdose, when serum levels are not detectable.

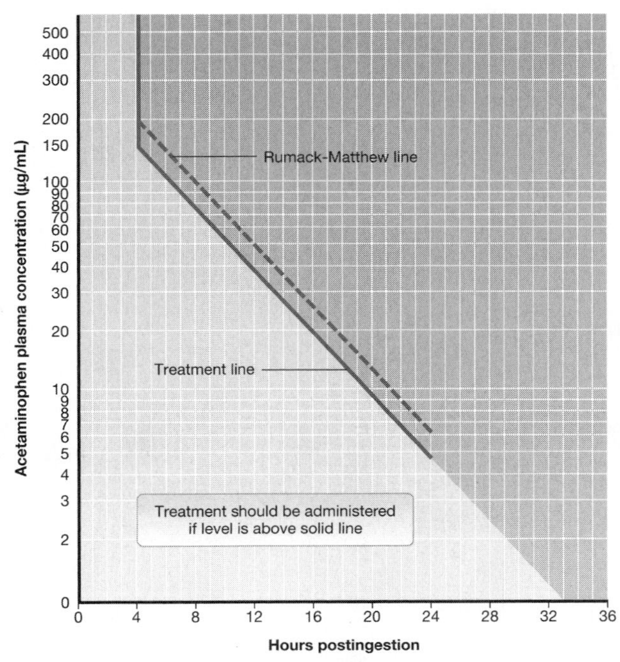

Rumack-Matthew nomogram: acetaminophen plasma concentration versus time after acetaminophen ingestion (adapted from Rumack, B.H, and Matthew, H. (1975). Acetaminophen poisoning and toxicity. *Pediatrics, 55*, 871–876, with permission). The nomogram has been developed to estimate the probability of whether a plasma acetaminophen concentration in relation to the interval post ingestion will result in hepatotoxicity and, therefore, whether N-acetylcysteine therapy should be administered.

M N

- NAC IV doses:
  - o If giving AC or the patient has persistent vomiting despite antiemetics, administer intravenously.
  - o IV loading dose: 150 mg/kg in 200 mL of D5W given over 15 minutes
  - o Maintenance dose: 50 mg/kg in 500 mL of D5W given over 4 hours
  - o Then 100 mg/kg in 1000 mL D5W infused over 16 hours

M N

- Oral or NG tube doses:
  - o Oral loading dose: 140 mg/kg
  - o Maintenance doses: 17 doses of 70 mg/kg every 4 hours

N

- Oral NAC is foul-tasting and may be given in juice or soda.

N

- Collaborate with the health care provider if vomiting limits oral administration.

Patient Education

N

A key nursing intervention is to educate the patient on ways to prevent or restore effective liver functioning. Some of the following educational teachings are useful in health restoration with patients who have hepatic disorders.

- Importance of rest
- Weight management: Notify the health care provider if weight gain exceeds 2 lbs or if noticeable, unintended weight loss occurs because it is likely to be fluid.
- Diet teaching: low sodium and low protein
- Restrict fluid intake if the patient becomes hyponatremic.
- Alcohol, smoking, and substance cessation
- Refer for rehab.

Concept Check

7. Which medication is administered for treatment of APAP overdose?
   A. NAC
   B. Lactulose
   C. Neomycin
   D. Rifaximin

Answer question

Summary of Interventions: Hepatic Disorders

- Management is usually supportive with fluids plus antiemetics for patients with nausea.
- Management of liver cirrhosis consists of managing the individual problems that arise from liver failure. Treat:
  - o Encephalopathy with lactulose
  - o Esophageal variceal bleeding with:
    - ■ Transfusions of fresh frozen plasma and packed red blood cells
    - ■ Endoscopy with banding, ligation, or sclerotherapy of varices
    - ■ Beta blockers to prevent further bleeding
  - o Ascites with paracentesis or diuretics depending on the severity
  - o Spontaneous bacterial peritonitis with IV antibiotics
- NAC for APAP toxicity
- Liver transplant for patients with advanced liver cirrhosis and some patients with acute fulminant hepatitis
- Patient education:
  - o Hepatotoxic substances
  - o Substance cessation
  - o Diet restrictions
  - o Hygienic practices
  - o Prevention of acute or chronic hepatic conditions
  - o Safe sex
  - o Rehab and/or support groups

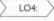

Evaluation of Desired Collaborative Care Outcomes: Hepatic Disorders

Evaluation and reassessment should reveal attainment of previously established patient outcomes. In summary:

- Patient reports being able to complete desired activities of daily living without excessive fatigue.
- Patient accurately discusses ways to prevent complications or worsening of disease process, including need for ETOH abstinence.
- Patient is alert, blood pressure is within desired range, skin turgor is elastic, urine output is balanced with fluid intake, and there is little or no ascites.
- Patient's weight remains within desired range.
- Patient has not experienced bleeding from esophageal varices and reports taking measures to prevent future episodes of bleeding.
- Patient is awake, alert, conversant, and aware of surroundings.
- Patient is free of additional infections.
- Patient's skin and mucous membranes are intact.

References

Bass, N. M., Mullen, K. D., Arun Sanyal, A., et al. (2010). Rifaximin treatment in hepatic encephalopathy. *N Engl J Med, 362*, 1071–1081. doi: 10.1056/NEJMoa0907893

Casey, L., & Lee, W. (2013). Hepatitis C virus therapy update 2013. *Curr Opin Gastroenterol, 29*(3), 243–249.

Centers for Disease Control and Prevention (CDC). (2014). *Viral Hepatitis—Resource Center for Health Professionals.* **www.cdc.gov/hepatitis/**

Dentinger, C. (2009). Emerging infections. Hepatitis A: An update. *Amer J Nurs, 109*(8), 29–33.

Green, J., Heard, K., Reynolds, K., et al. (2013). Oral and intravenous acetylcysteine for treatment of acetaminophen toxicity. *Western J Emerg Med, 14*(3), 218–226.

Hoofnagle, J .H., & DiBisceglie, A. M. (1997). The treatment of chronic viral hepatitis. *New Engl J Med, 336*, 347–356.

O'Malley, P. (2013). Tattoos and piercings: Reasons, risks, and reporting: Update for the clinical nurse specialist. *Clin Nurs Special: J Advanced Nurs Prac, 27*(1), 14–16.

O'Malley, G. F., & O'Malley, R. (2013). *Acetaminophen poisoning.* **www.merckmanuals.com//professional/injuries_poisoning/poisoning/acetaminophen_poisoning.html**

O'Neal, H., Olds, J., & Webster, N. (2006). Managing patients with acute liver failure: Developing a tool for practitioners. *Nurs Crit Care, 11*(2), 63–68.

Poole, S. (2009). Update on the treatment and management of patients with hepatitis. *J Infusion Nurs, 32*(5), 269–275.

Powell, E. E., Cooksley, W. G. E., Hanson, R., et al. (1990). The natural history of nonalcoholic steatohepatitis: A follow-up study of forty-two patients for up to 21 years. *Hepatology, 11*(1): 74–80. doi: 10.1002/hep.1840110114

Promrat, K., Kleiner, D. E., Niemeier, H. M., et al. (2010). Randomized controlled trial testing the effects of weight loss on nonalcoholic steatohepatitis. *Hepatology, 51*(1): 121–129. doi: 10.1002/hep.23276

Rustgi, V., Carriero, D., Bachtold, M., & Zeldin G. (2010). Update on chronic hepatitis B. *J Nurs Practitioners, 6*(8), 631–639.

Tujios, S. & Lee, W. (2013). Update in the management of chronic hepatitis B. *Curr Opin Gastroenterol, 29*(3), 250–256.

Werner, K. T., & Perez, S. T. (2012). Role of nurse practitioners in the management of cirrhotic patients. *J Nurs Practitioners, 8*(10), 816–821.

Clinical Practice Guidelines

Centers for Disease Control and Prevention (CDC). (1998). Recommendations for prevention and control of hepatitis C virus (HCV) infection and HCV-related chronic disease. *MMWR, 47*(RR19), 1–54.

Centers for Disease Control and Prevention (CDC). (2008). Recommendations for partner services programs for HIV infection, syphilis, gonorrhea, and chlamydial infection. *MMWR, 57*(RR09), 1–63. **www.cdc.gov/mmwr/preview/mmwrhtml/rr5709a1.htm**

Dart, R. C, Erdman, A. R., Olson, K. R., et al., & American Association of Poison Control Centers. (2006). Acetaminophen poisoning: An evidence-based consensus guideline for out-of-hospital management. *Clin Toxicology, 44*(1), 1–18. **Informahealthcare.com/doi/pdf/10.1080/15563650500394571**

Garcia-Tsao, G., Sanyal, A. J., Grace, N. D., Carey, W., & the Practice Guideline Committee of the American Association for the Study of Liver Diseases and the Practice Parameters Committee of the American College of Gastroenterology. (2007). AASLD practice guidelines: Prevention and management of gastroesophageal varices and variceal hemorrhage in cirrhosis. *Hepatology, 46*(3), 922–938. **www.aasld.org/sites/default/files/guideline_documents/GastroVaricesand2009Hemorrhage.pdf**

Lee, W. M., Larson, A. M., & Stravitz, T. (2011). *AASLD position paper: the management of acute liver failure: Update 2011.* Baltimore, MD: American Association for the Study of Liver Diseases. **www.guideline.gov/content.aspx?id=36894&search=evidence+based+practice+acetaminophen+overdose+and+acetaminophen+overdose**

Mast, E. E., Weinbaum, C. M., Fiore, A. E., et al. (2006). A comprehensive immunization strategy to eliminate transmission of hepatitis B virus infection in the United States: Recommendations of the Advisory Committee on Immunization Practices (ACIP) Part II: Immunization of adults. *MMWR, 55*(RR16), 1–25.

O'Shea, R. S., Dasarathy, S., McCullough, A. J., & the Practice Guideline Committee of the American Association for the Study of Liver Diseases and the Practice Parameters Committee of the American College of Gastroenterology. (2010). AASLD practice guidelines: Alcoholic liver disease. *Hepatology, 51*(1), 307–328. **www.aasld.org/sites/default/files/guideline_documents/AlcoholicLiverDisease1-2010.pdf**

Runyon, B. A. (2012). AASLD practice guidelines: Management of adult patients with ascites due to cirrhosis: Update 2012. *Hepatology, 49*(6), 2087–2107. **www.aasld.org/sites/default/files/guideline_documents/adultascitesenhanced.pdf**

Siegel, J. D., Rhinehart, E., Jachson, M., Chiarello, L., & the Healthcare Infection Control Practices Advisory Committee. (2007). *2007 Guideline for isolation precautions: Preventing transmission of infectious agents in healthcare settings.* **www.cdc.gov/ncidod/dhqp/pdf/isolation2007.pdf**

www.aasld.org/practiceguidelines/pages/default.aspx

www.hepatitis.va.gov/provider/guidelines/index.asp

s3.gi.org/physicians/guidelines/HepaticEncephalopathy.pdf

gi.org/guideline/diagnosis-management-and-treatment-of-hepatitis-c-an-update/

gi.org/guideline/prevention-and-management-of-gastroesophageal-varices-and-variceal-hemorrhage-in-cirrhosis/

Patient Education

Buggs, A. M. (2014). *Viral hepatitis.* **emedicine.medscape.com/article/775507-overview**

Centers for Disease Control and Prevention (CDC). (2014). *Viral hepatitis—resource center: Patient education.* **CDC.gov/hepatitis/Resources/PatientEdMaterials.htm**

Farrell, S. E. (2014). *Acetaminophen toxicity.* **emedicine.medscape.com/article/820200-overview**

Mayo Clinic. (2014). *Cirrhosis.* **www.mayoclinic.org/diseases-conditions/cirrhosis/basics/definition/con-20031617**

Sood, G. K. (2014). *Acute liver failure.* **emedicine.medscape.com/article/177354-overview**

Wolf, D. C. (2014). *Cirrhosis.* **emedicine.medscape.com/article/185856-overview**

Learning Outcomes for Pancreatitis

When you complete this lesson, you will be able to:

1. Recognize the clinical relevance of pancreatitis.
2. Consider the pathophysiology, etiology, risk factors, and clinical presentation of pancreatitis that determine the priority patient concerns.
3. Determine the most urgent and important nursing interventions and patient education required in caring for a patient with pancreatitis.
4. Evaluate attainment of desired collaborative care outcomes for a patient with pancreatitis.

LO1:

What Is Pancreatitis?

- Acute pancreatitis is a severe inflammation of and sudden swelling in the pancreas.
- Chronic pancreatitis refers to chronic inflammation that fails to heal or improve. It also includes recurrent inflammation of the pancreas that results in fibrosis and permanent damage of the pancreas.
- Damage can result from trapped digestive secretions, which can:
  - o Digest pancreatic tissues
  - o Erode blood vessel and cause hemorrhage
  - o Cause necrosis

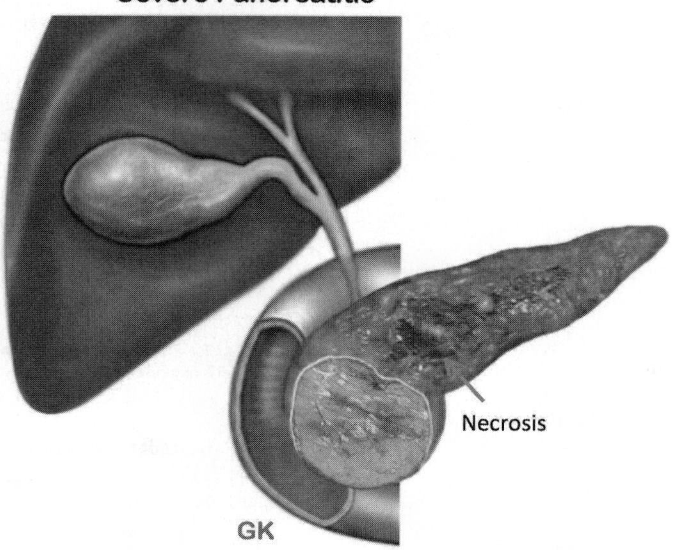

This illustration depicts severe pancreatitis with areas of hemorrhage and necrosis.
Source: Courtesy of George Kyriakidis/Santa Ana, CA

LO1:

Clinical Relevance

- Annually, about 210,000 people in the United States are admitted to the hospital with acute pancreatitis.
- An acute pancreatitis attack can range from a mild, short-term event to a severe event leading to a systemic inflammatory response syndrome (SIRS), multisystem organ dysfunction (MODS), and death.
- Chronic pancreatitis is common in patients between 30–40 years old.
- Overall mortality is 10–15%.

Severe Pancreatitis

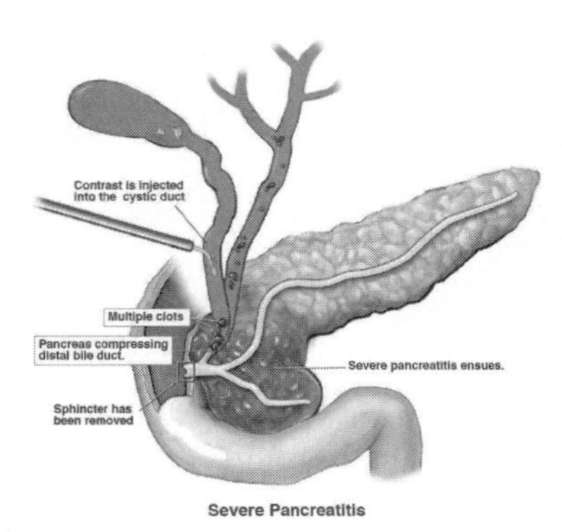

This exhibit demonstrates severe pancreatitis as a result of bile duct compression and clot blockage.

LO2:

Pathophysiology

Digestive enzymes are produced and stored by pancreatic acinar cells. These enzymes are normally activated in the gastrointestinal tract. When these enzymes are activated within the pancreas, autodigestion of the pancreatic tissue can occur. Pancreatic enzymes, released and activated in the pancreatic tissue, cause damage to the vascular endothelium and other cells of the pancreas. This causes impairment to the microcirculation, leading to ischemia and inflammation of the pancreas. Bleeding, hemorrhage, and/or necrosis (necrotizing pancreatitis) may occur. One or all of these problems can lead to shock and/or death.

- Inflammation results in cytokine release that can also produce SIRS.
- Systemic capillaries become leaky, and fluid moves from the intravascular space to the extravascular space, causing ascites, acute lung injury, and generalized edema. This movement of fluid is often referred to as third spacing.
- More severe cases of pancreatitis can result in multiorgan dysfunction (e.g., acute lung injury, renal failure, and hepatic failure), any one of which can be life threatening. Multiorgan failure carries a high mortality rate.

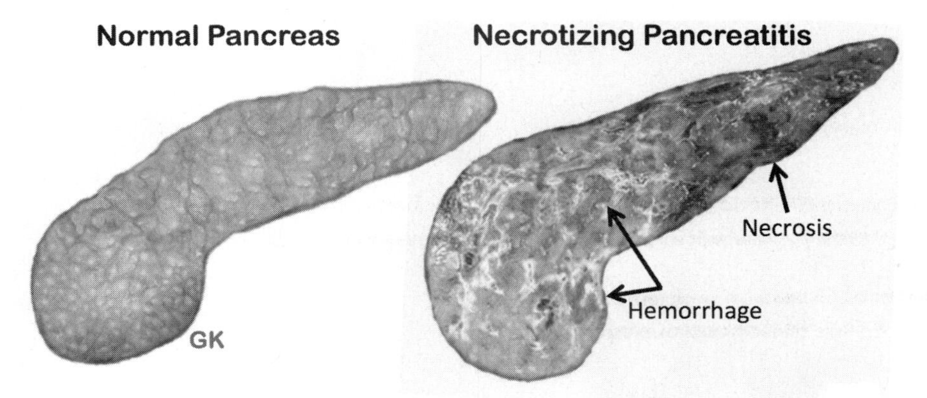

This comparison of a normal pancreas shows the numerous pathologic changes that occur in severe pancreatitis. Inflammation and bleeding lead to hemorrhage, dysfunction, and then necrosis. The inflammatory process leads to generalized edema of the diseased organ.

Source: Courtesy of George Kyriakidis/Santa Ana, CA

- It is unclear what first triggers this process of acinar cell injury, but the mechanism may be related to the cause.
- Gallstone pancreatitis results from a gallstone lodging at the sphincter of Oddi and blockage of the pancreatic duct blocking pancreatic outflow.
- Alcohol causes intracellular accumulation of digestive enzymes and premature activation and release of these enzymes, initiating autodigestion of the pancreas.
- Alcohol can also cause the accumulation of protein in the pancreatic secretions, leading to the formation of protein plugs in the duct, blocking pancreatic outflow.

Passing off a Gallstone with Trauma and Swelling Leading to Pancreatitis

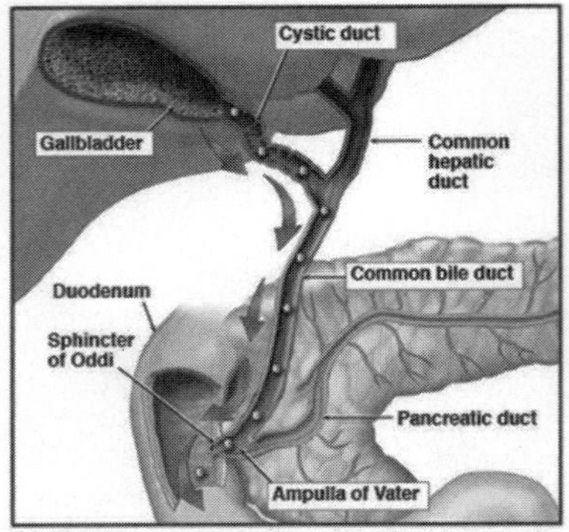

Gallstones can move out of the gallbladder, into the cystic duct, down the common bile duct, through the ampulla of Vater and out the sphincter of Oddi.

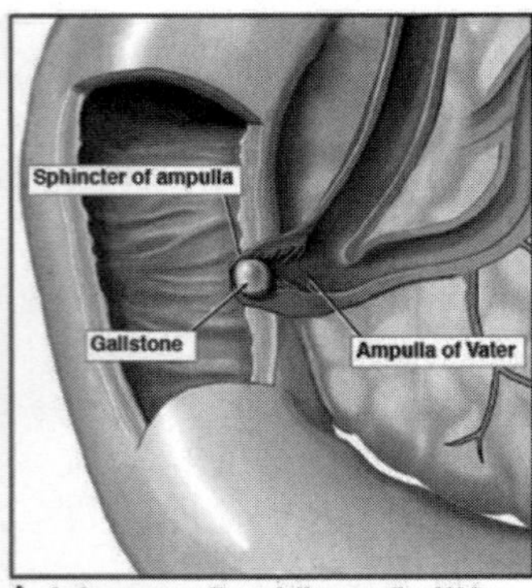

A. A stone passes through the ampulla of Vater and out the sphincter of Oddi which causes trauma and inflammation.

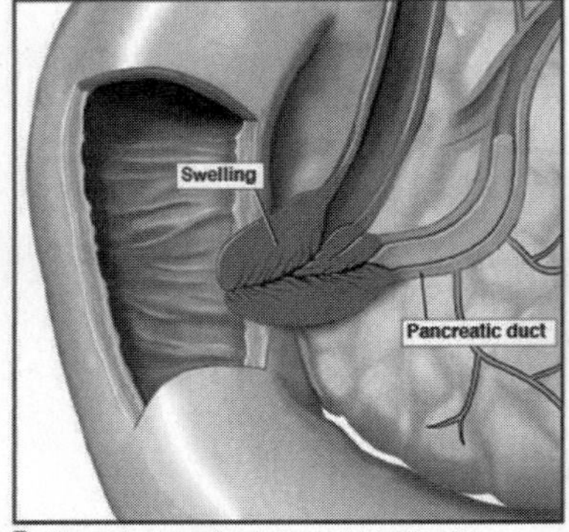

B. The sphincter and ampulla swell, blocking the pancreatic duct.

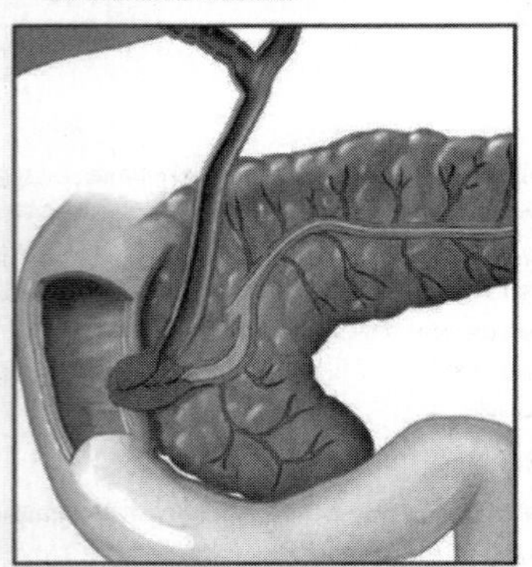

C. Pancreatic fluid backs up. This leads to widespread pancreatitis.

This illustration shows the passing of a gallstone with trauma and swelling leading to pancreatitis.

Pathophysiology (continued)

Chronic Pancreatitis

- Chronic pancreatitis occurs after recurrent bouts of acute pancreatitis or chronic inflammation.
- There is permanent damage to the pancreas with fibrosis and impairment of both exocrine and endocrine function.
- Hyperglycemia (diabetes) is caused by loss of insulin-producing capacity.
- Weight loss and malabsorption are caused by loss of exocrine function.

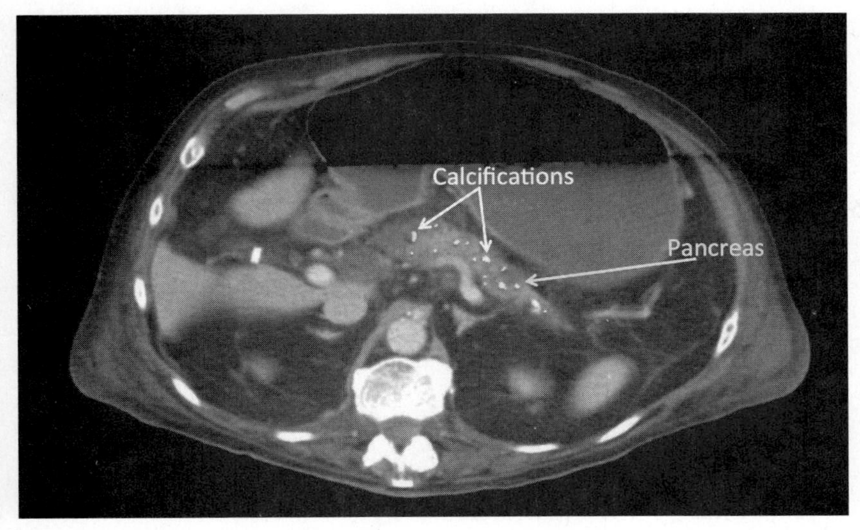

This axial CT scan shows multiple calcifications (solid, white specks) in the pancreas in a patient who has chronic pancreatitis.
Source: Courtesy of K. Kyriakidis

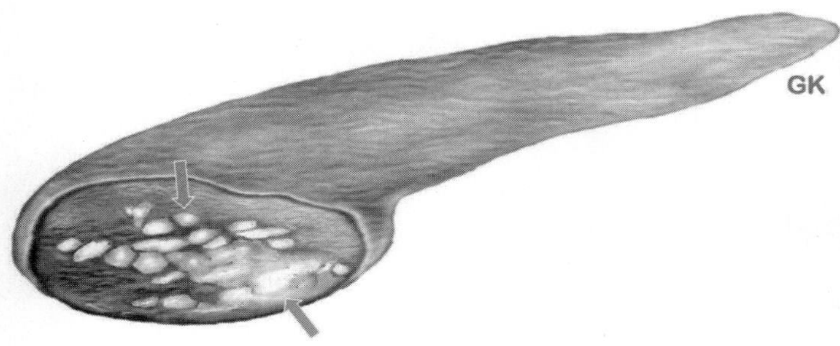

This chronic pancreatitis specimen is shrunken, fibrotic, and the arrows point to calcified secretions.
Source: Courtesy of George Kyriakidis/Santa Ana, CA

Concept Check

1. What information regarding pancreatitis is accurate?

A. It is easy to treat once diagnosed.
B. It almost always results in patient death.
C. Many patients are living with chronic pancreatitis.
D. The most common diagnosis occurs during routine examinations.

Answer question

Concept Check

2. Gallstone pancreatitis results from gallstone blockage of which structure?

A. Duodenum
B. Cardiac sphincter
C. Common hepatic duct
D. Sphincter of Oddi

Answer question

LO2:

Causes and Risk Factors

Most common:

- Gallstones
- Idiopathic or unknown cause
- Alcohol misuse

Other causes:

- Trauma to abdomen and pancreas
- Trypsin activation while still in the pancreas (digest pancreatic cells)
- Hypertriglyceridemia
- Family history
- Autoimmune diseases
- Congenital abnormalities of pancreatic ducts or biliary ducts
- Hypercalcemia
- Malignancy
- Certain drugs (e.g., antiretroviral cocktails to treat HIV/AIDS, estrogens, diuretics, steroids, antihypertensives, opiates)
- Endoscopic retrograde cholangiopancreatography (ERCP)

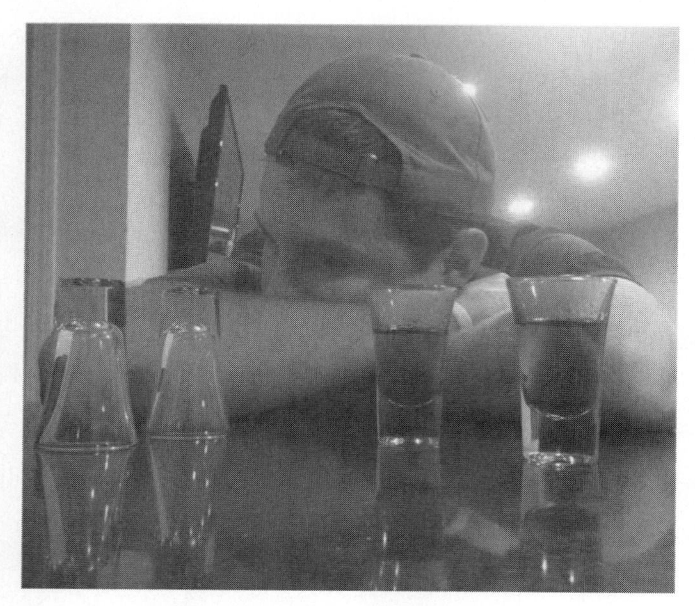

Alcoholism is a leading cause of and risk factor for pancreatitis.
Source: Courtesy of R. Murphy

Concept Check

3. Which common disorder may be caused by chronic pancreatitis?
   A. Diabetes mellitus
   B. Gastric ulcer
   C. Pulmonary embolism
   D. Appendicitis

Answer question

LO2:

Assessment Findings

- Sudden onset of dull steady pain in the upper abdomen that radiates to the back
- Pain progresses to severe, constant, and lasting for several days. Exacerbated by food and alcohol intake.
- Pain may improve with supine position or curling up.
- Abdominal distension, tenderness, and guarding
- Fever in 76% and tachycardia in 65% of patients
- Nausea and vomiting, anorexia, diarrhea
- Jaundice is present in 28% of patients.
- 10% of patients exhibit hemodynamic instability.

Poor prognostic indicators 48 hours after admission:

- Hematocrit decreased by >10%
- Arterial oxygen pressure <60 mmHg
- Serum urea increased by >5 mg/dL over baseline
- Serum calcium <8 mg/dL
- Base deficit >4 mEq/L
- Fluid sequestration estimated to >6 liters

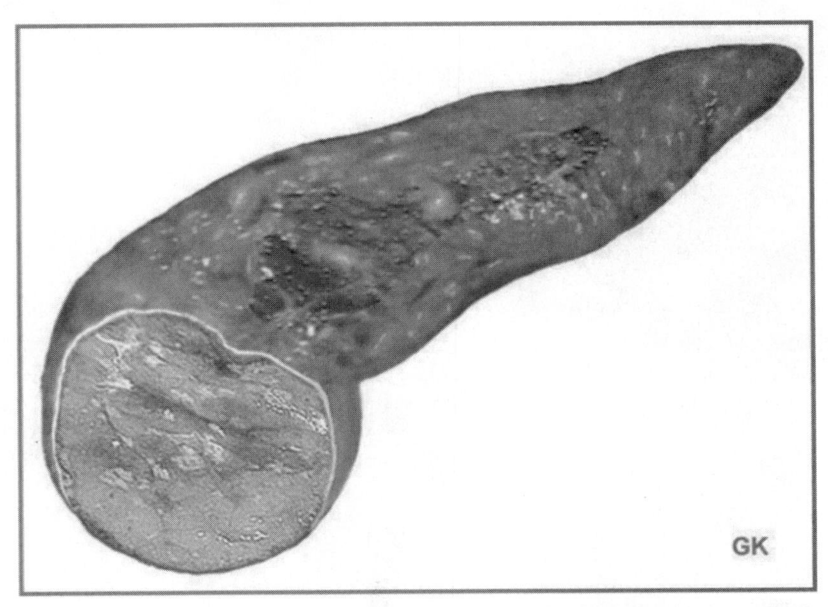

Acute pancreatitis is seen with dark, blackish hemorrhagic and necrotic areas. It is common for a pus-filled pseudocyst to form, which is liquified necrotic pancreatic tissue.
Source: Courtesy of George Kyriakidis/Santa Ana, CA

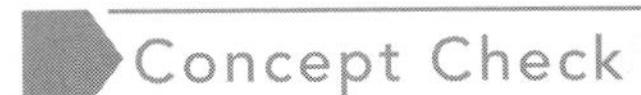

Concept Check

4. **Which procedure may result in the development of pancreatitis?**
   A. ERCP
   B. Abdominal ultrasound
   C. MRI
   D. CT scan of the abdomen

Answer question

Chronic Pancreatitis

- Chronic epigastric pain
- Diabetes
- Diarrhea

Additional symptoms of chronic pancreatitis:

- Jaundice
- Nausea and vomiting
- Fatigue and weakness
- Fatty stools
- Digestive discomfort and problems

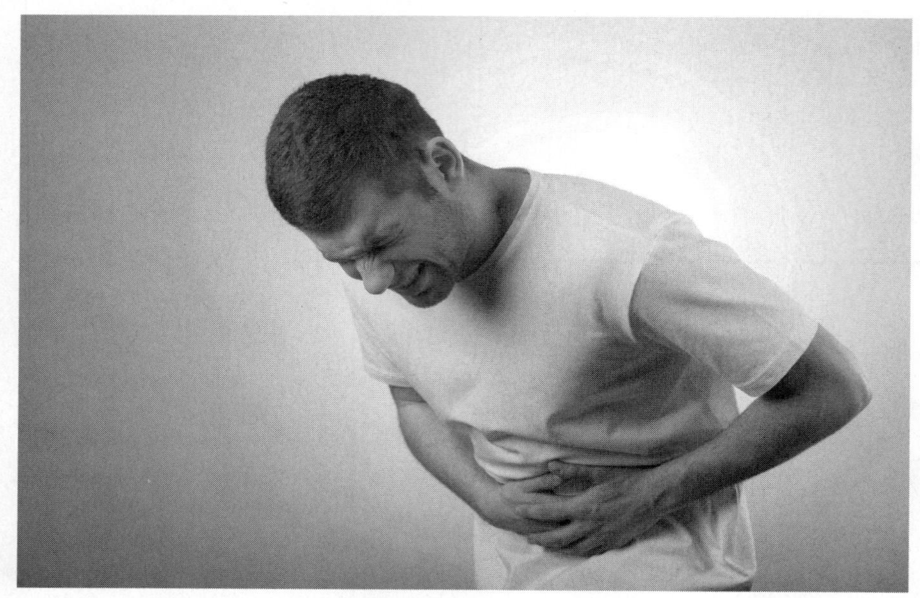

Alcohol consumption is the primary cause of chronic pancreatitis, contributing 70% of the total cases. A prolonged period (i.e., 10 years or more) of alcoholism increases the risk of chronic pancreatitis.
Source: Photographee.eu/Fotolia

LO2:

Diagnostics

Labs:

- Amylase and lipase are usually elevated in acute pancreatitis with lipase being the most sensitive and specific marker.
- These are usually normal in chronic pancreatitis.
- CBC: Leukocytosis is commonly present in pancreatitis.
- Patients may also develop bleeding, resulting in anemia.
- Comprehensive metabolic panel (CMP), including liver function tests
- Lactate is a key sepsis marker for tissue hypoperfusion.
- C-reactive protein is normally done 24–48 hours after onset to determine severity of pancreatitis and potential organ dysfunction.

Imaging:

- Abdominal ultrasound to assess for gallstones and/or pancreatic inflammation
- Computerized tomography (CT) scan with contrast to visualize pancreatitis, pseudocyst formation, and/or necrosis
- Endoscopic ultrasound (EUS), using an ultrasound attached to an endoscope to visualize the pancreas and bile ducts
- Magnetic resonance cholangiopancreatography (MRCP), a noninvasive test with intravenous contrast to visualize the pancreas, gallbladder, and ducts

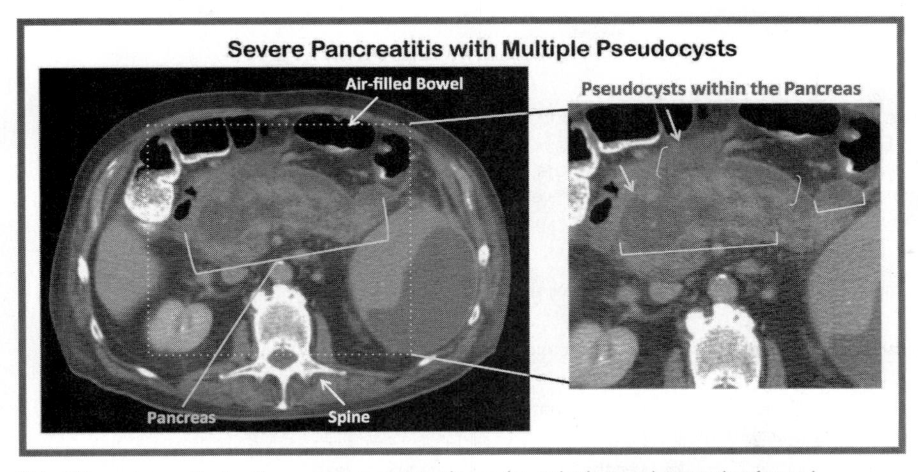

This CT scan in a patient with severe pancreatitis shows the multiple pseudocysts that formed around the pancreas (cutout). Pseudocysts are the pancreatic fluids that leak and collect around the pancreas.
Source: Courtesy of K. Kyriakidis

Definition of Severity of Acute Pancreatitis

Determination of the severity of illness can help guide the type, extent, and aggressiveness of intervention. The Atlanta revised criteria (Tenner, et al., 2013) are often used:

- Mild acute pancreatitis:
    - Lack of organ failure
    - Lack of complications
- Moderate acute pancreatitis
    - Transient organ dysfunction and/or
    - Complications
- Severe acute pancreatitis
    - Organ failure that persists over 48 hours

Concept Check

5. Which laboratory test is most specific for acute pancreatitis?

A. Amylase
B. Lipase
C. Lactate
D. C-reactive protein

Answer question

Priority Patient Concerns and Desired Collaborative Care Outcomes

Prior to caring for patients with pancreatitis, it is important to prioritize the patient's concerns that must guide the nursing care plan and interventions. Care for the patient is ordered and organized in accordance with the patient's priority and urgent needs. Desired collaborative care outcomes in patients with pancreatitis typically include:

1. Patient will experience reduction in or elimination of pain.
2. Patient will demonstrate assessment findings of normal fluid volume.
3. Patient will report nausea has abated.
4. Patient will report diarrhea has abated.
5. Patient will demonstrate understanding of lifestyle changes necessary to maintain health.

Considering these important care outcomes, prepare a list of the major 3–6 priority patient concerns or nursing diagnoses for patients with pancreatitis. Be prepared to participate in a discussion of this list and/or to submit them as an assignment, as determined by your faculty. Resources you may find helpful in this assignment can include this lesson, the references, resources on nursing care plans, and standard nursing diagnoses manuals.

LO3:

Collaborative Interventions

Pancreatitis

Care of patients with pancreatitis focuses on supportive interventions. If pancreatitis is mild (organ dysfunction is absent), three interventions may be all that is necessary: withhold oral intake, IV rehydration, and analgesia for pain control. However, if the patient has moderate to severe pancreatitis, intervention focus on supportive care to prevent hypoxia, provide fluid resuscitation, and control pain:

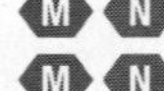

- Remove causative agent (e.g., alcohol, toxic medication).
- Give oxygen for hypoxemia (SpO_2 <93%). Monitor oxygen saturation closely when administering narcotics.

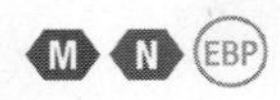

- Aggressively administer IV hydration, particularly with hemoconcentration (Tenner, et al., 2013):
  - o This is critical in patients with severe or necrotizing pancreatitis because intravascular fluid moves to the extravascular space (third spacing).
  - o Fluid requirements are approximately 20 mL/kg over the first hour followed by at least 250 mL/hr. This rate may not be tolerated by patients with heart failure.
  - o Lactated Ringer's infusion is associated with lower systemic inflammation as compared to normal saline solutions.
  - o Early aggressive fluid resuscitation is associated with lower sepsis, length of stay, and mortality rates.
  - o Aggressive but uncontrolled fluid administration is related to twice the mortality rate.

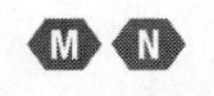

- If patients do not respond to fluid or shock state persists, administer vasopressors (e.g., norepinephrine)

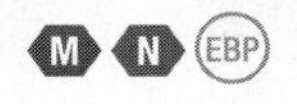

- Continuously or frequently monitor vital signs, SpO_2, pain, impact of pain medication on vital signs, fluid balance, arterial blood gases, and lactate levels, as these patients are often very ill. Collaborate with team that transfer to ICU may be warranted if danger signs persist (Banks, et al., 2006):
  - o Sustained hypoxemia
  - o Hypotension unresponsive to aggressive fluid resuscitation
  - o Renal insufficiency that fails to respond to fluid; oliguria (urine output <50 cc/hr)
  - o Respiratory distress requiring intubation with mechanical ventilation
  - o Metabolic disorders
  - o Obesity with BMI >30
  - o Signs of encephalopathy

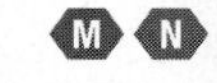

- Monitor for coagulopathy or low albumin levels. Infuse fresh frozen plasma and/or albumin as needed.

- Make all patients with pancreatitis NPO initially. The goal is to decrease pancreatic enzyme release to minimize pain and inflammation. In severe pancreatitis, early enteral nutrition (within 72 hours) with a nasojejunal tube is recommended (Tenner, et al., 2013).

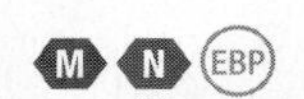

- Provide pain control, usually with IV narcotics (e.g., morphine) (Banks, et al., 2006).

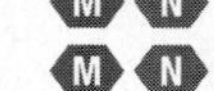

- Monitor and manage electrolyte imbalances (e.g., hypocalcemia).
- Closely monitor for early warning signs of respiratory distress, shock, heart failure, or other organ dysfunction.

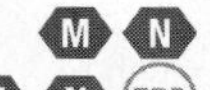

- Initiate DVT prophylaxis.

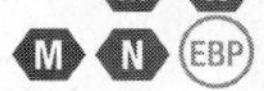

- Administer antibiotics, only if infection or substantial necrosis is present, >30% on CT scan (Tenner, et al., 2013).
- Provide nutritional support, depending on the severity of pancreatitis:

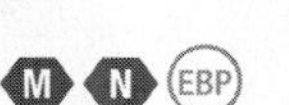

  - o In mild pancreatitis, oral diet can usually be initiated after the pain resolves (Tenner, et al., 2013.

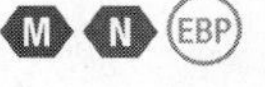

  - o In severe pancreatitis, early enteral nutrition (within 72 hours) with a nasojejunal tube is recommended (Tenner, et al., 2013).

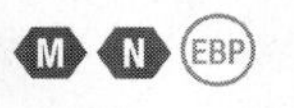

- Employ parenteral nutrition is only indicated if unable to achieve nasojejunal access (Tenner, et al., 2013).

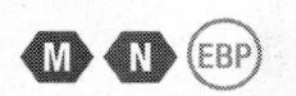

- Prioritize enteral nutrition, which is superior to parenteral nutrition:
  - o Decreased infectious complications
  - o Maintains gut barrier integrity, decreasing bacteria in GI tract from migrating into bloodstream (Tenner, et al., 2013)

Collaborative Interventions (continued)

- Carefully observe hospitalized patients with pancreatitis as they may deteriorate and progress to severe sepsis, shock, or organ failure.
- Watch for warning signs:
  - o Mental status change
  - o Dyspnea and tachypnea
  - o Hypotension unresponsive to fluids
  - o Lactate level >4
  - o Low PaO_2 <95%
- Call the Rapid Response Team if any early warning signs emerge. It is essential to evaluate the patient's needs for a higher level of care and monitoring in the ICU.
- Collaborate to consider an endocrinologist consult, as indicated.
- Consider surgical intervention, particularly for urgent situations, which include:
  - o Blockage of the pancreatic duct (Tenner, et al., 2013)
  - o Removal of a portion of the pancreas for serious conditions, such as infected necrotizing pancreatitis (Tenner, et al., 2013)
  - o Transplantation of islet cells

Large bile leak, massive ascites and pancreatitis

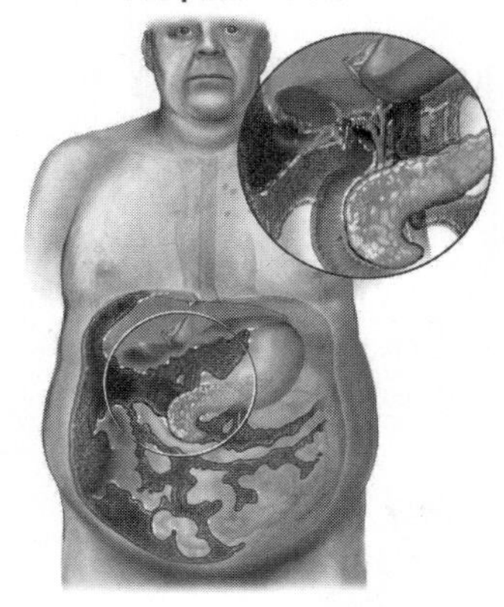

This exhibit depicts a man with jaundice and peritonitis. A detailed enlargement of the biliary region further reveals a continued bile leak with onset of acute pancreatitis.
Source: © 2014 Nucleus Medical Media, All rights reserved

Complications of Pancreatitis

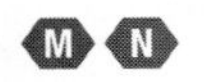

Observe for and immediately alert medical team if serious and/or life-threatening complications develop in pancreatitis:

- Necrotizing pancreatitis is severe acute pancreatitis in which pancreatic tissue is no longer viable and dies. The necrotic tissue can be sterile or infected. Surgery is recommended if signs of sepsis appear or if infection is present.
- Pseudocyst is a collection of pancreatic fluids, particularly pancreatic enzymes, and tissue debris. Pseudocysts may require percutaneous or endoscopic drainage to prevent or treat infection, bleeding, and/or rupture.
- Abscess is a collection of pus that accumulates from tissue necrosis and debris, infection, and liquefaction of tissue. Percutaneous or surgical drainage may be necessary.
- Compartment syndrome is a rare but urgent complication in severe pancreatitis is abdominal compartment syndrome. It may manifest at the time when other organs reveal signs of failure. Pancreatic inflammation can cause retroperitoneal edema to the point that ascites and paralytic ileus result. Mortality is high. Additional supportive care includes decompression with nasogastric tube, fluid restriction, diuretics to lower the abdominal pressures. Decompression is essential, whether noninvasively, percutaneously, or surgically. Continued compression on the bowel, leading to ischemia, is associated with an almost 100% mortality rate.

Collaborative Interventions (continued)

Gallstone Pancreatitis

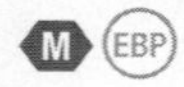

- Endoscopic retrograde cholangiopancreatography (ERCP) within 24 hours to remove stones to lessen the severity of gallstone pancreatitis (Tenner, et al., 2013). ERCP is not recommended unless patient has cholangitis (infection of common bile duct).
- Patients should be instructed and informed consent obtained regarding complications of ERCP, which can include pancreatitis, bleeding, intestinal perforation, and cholangitis.

What is ERCP?

Examination of the Common Bile Duct and Pancreatic Duct

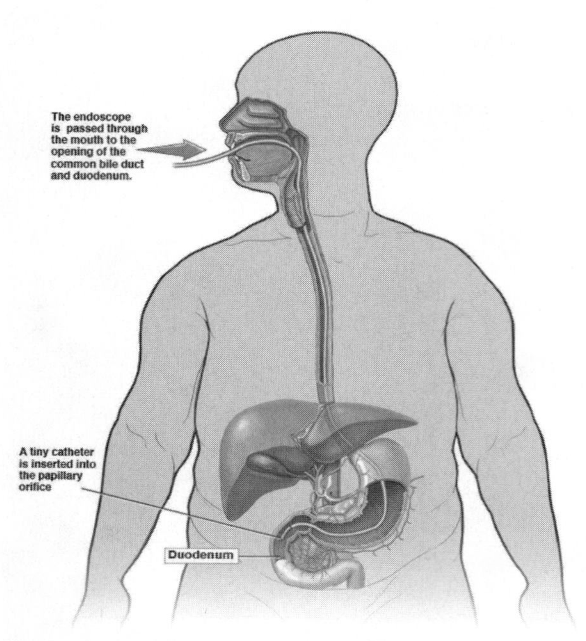

This illustration depicts the examination of the bile duct and the pancreatic duct utilizing an ERCP.
Source: © 2014 Nucleus Medical Media, All rights reserved

Endoscopic Retrograde Cholangiopancreatography

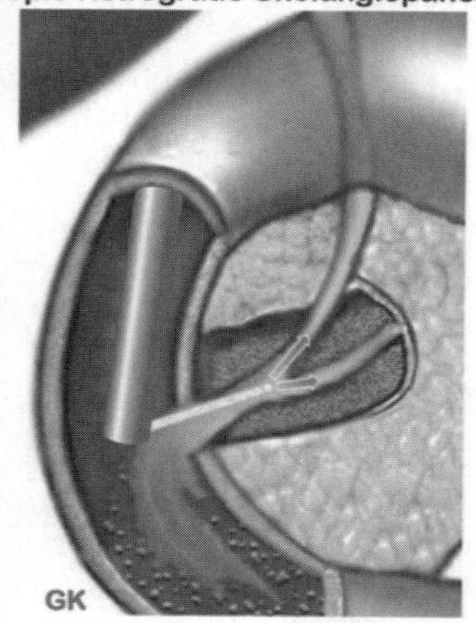

This illustration shows an ERCP. A duodenoscope is seen in the duodenum, with a catheter protruding through the end of the duodenoscope into the pancreatic duct. Dye is injected into the pancreatic duct from the end of the catheter.
Source: Courtesy of George Kyriakidis/Santa Ana, CA

- Closely monitor the patient for any signs of these complications.
- Cholecystectomy should be performed after recovery from pancreatitis and prior to discharge, when possible (Tenner, et al., 2013).
- Patient should be instructed that cholecystectomy is done to decrease the risk of recurrent episodes of pancreatitis and to prevent further hospitalizations.

Gallbladder Removal Surgery - Open and Laparoscopic Cholecystectomy

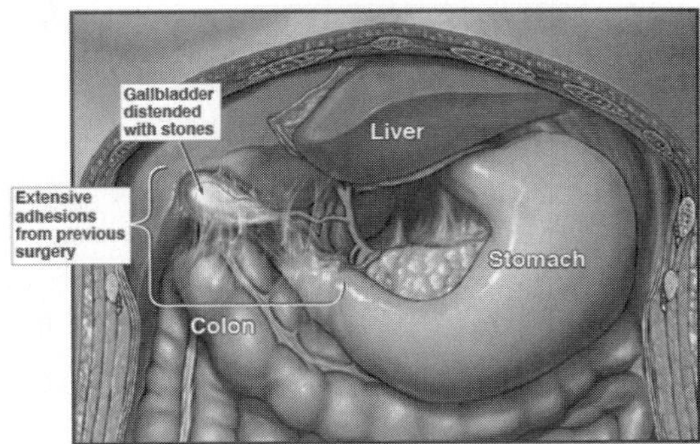

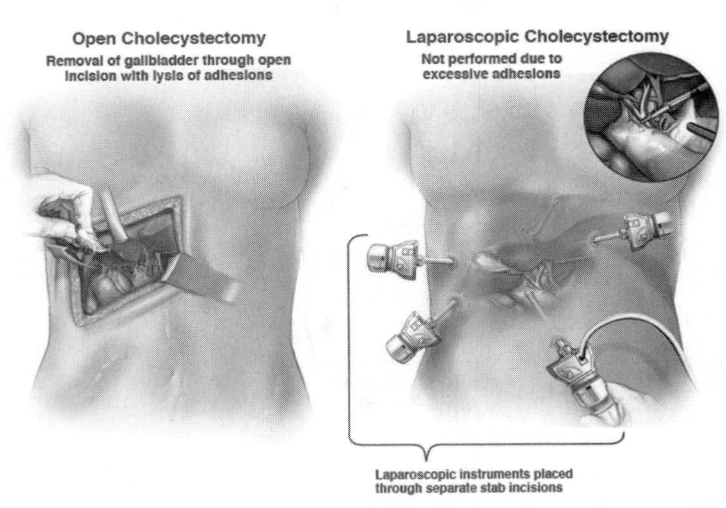

This series depicts two gallbladder removal surgeries: an open cholecystectomy where the surgeon exposes the gallbladder through an incision in the abdominal wall; and a laparoscopic cholecystectomy, where the surgeon uses a laparoscope and surgical instruments to conduct a minimally invasive removal of the gallbladder.

Collaborative Interventions (continued)

Pancreatic Cancer

Pancreatic cancer is hard to detect during its early stages so care of patients with pancreatic cancer is often aggressive. Like the care of all patients with cancer (see the NovE-lesson on Overview of the Care of Patients with Cancer), interventions may involve:

- Radiation therapy
- Chemotherapy
- Surgery
- Combination radiation and chemotherapy
- Targeted drug therapy
- Support, comfort care, symptom management, and patient education as in all patients with cancers

Patient Education

Patients and families should be educated about how to best care for the patient during and after this condition:

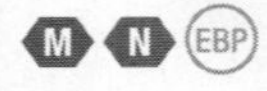

- Avoid alcohol in patients with alcoholic pancreatitis, patients with recurrent pancreatitis, and with acute pancreatitis (Tenner, et al., 2013). In most patients with nonalcoholic pancreatitis, drinking alcohol in moderation after recovery from the illness is not restricted. For those who are at risk for recurrence, avoid alcohol intake altogether.
- Avoid fatty foods; eat small low-fat meals and drink plenty of fluids.
- Smoking cessation
- Nonsteroidal anti-inflammatory drugs (e.g., ibuprofen) often control pain in mild pancreatitis; however, opioids are commonly needed in less mild cases. Patients with acute pancreatitis who require stronger pain control are commonly hospitalized.
- Pain control in patients with chronic pancreatitis almost always requires analgesics. Low fat diet, alcohol restriction, smoking cessation are essential supportive lifestyle modifications.
- Acupuncture has not shown effectiveness in treating or preventing pancreatitis.
- Reduction in caffeine may be helpful to some patients.
- Pancreatic enzyme supplements can help relieve pain with pancreatitis while reducing the production of enzymes by the pancreas.

Summary of Interventions

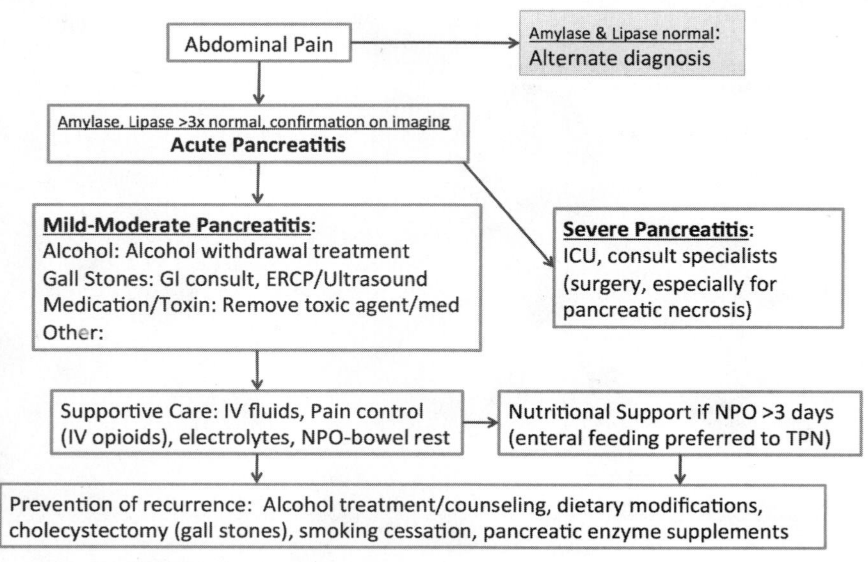

Source: Copyright © 2014, NovEx Novice to Expert Learning, LLC

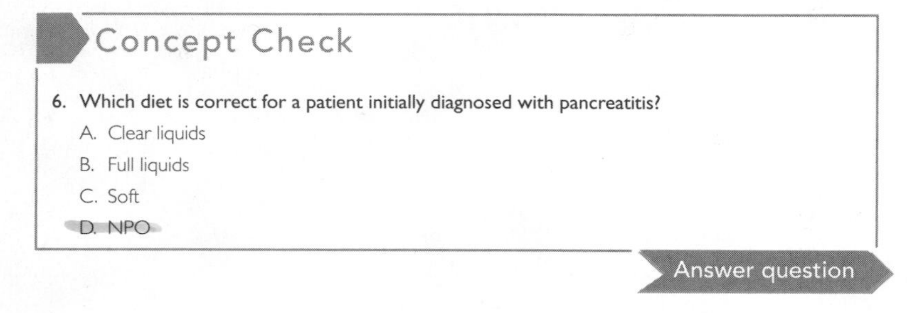

Concept Check

6. Which diet is correct for a patient initially diagnosed with pancreatitis?
   A. Clear liquids
   B. Full liquids
   C. Soft
   D. NPO

Answer question

Summary of Interventions

- Treatment of pancreatitis is primarily supportive. This includes:
  1. Fluid replacement
  2. Initial gastrointestinal rest
  3. Pain management
- Cholecystectomy and ERCP should be considered for gallstone pancreatitis.
- If patients on a medical floor develop signs of deterioration and progression to sepsis, shock, or organ failure, immediate intervention (e.g., Rapid Response Team) is required.
- Avoidance of alcohol for patients with alcoholic pancreatitis
- Smoking cessation

LO4:

Evaluation of Desired Collaborative Care Outcomes

Evaluation and reassessment should reveal attainment of previously established patient outcomes. In summary:

- Patient reports that pain associated with pancreatitis is gone or that pain has reduced to a manageable level.
- Patient's mentation is clear, lungs are clear to auscultation, blood pressure is within expected range, skin turgor is elastic, and urine output is on a desired level.
- Patient reports absence of nausea.
- Patient reports passing soft, formed stools according to pre-illness schedule.
- Patient will accurately discusses appropriate food choices, cessation of alcohol consumption, and plans to adhere to suggested treatment regimen.

Concept Check

7. Which diet is correct for a patient being discharged following treatment for acute pancreatitis?

A. Low residue

B. NPO

C. Low fat

D. Low protein

Answer question

References

Despins, L. (2005). Acute pancreatitis: Diagnosis and treatment of a potentially fatal condition. *Amer J Nursing, 105*(11), 54–57.

Hidalgo, M. (2010). Pancreatic cancer. *N Engl J Med, 362*, 1605–1617. doi: 10.1056/NEJMra0901557

Parker, M. (2004). Acute pancreatitis. *Emergency Nurse, 11*(10), 28–35.

Turner, B. (2003). Acute pancreatitis: Symptoms, diagnosis and management. *Nursing Times, 99*(46), 30–32. **www.nursingtimes.net/Journals/2012/11/23/d/a/c/031118Acute-pancreatitis-symptoms-diagnosis-and-management.pdf**

Whitcomb, D. C. (2006). Clinical practice: Acute pancreatitis. *N Engl J Med, 354*, 2142–2150. doi: 10.1056/NEJMcp054958.

Clinical Practice Guidelines

Banks, P. A., Freeman, M. L., & the Practice Parameters Committee of the American College of Gastroenterology. (2006). Practice guidelines in acute pancreatitis. *Amer J Gastroenterol, 101*, 2379–2400. **gi.org/physicians/guidelines/AcutePancreatitis.pdf**

Tenner, S., Baille, J., DeWitt, J., et al. (2013). American College of Gastroenterology Guideline: Management of acute pancreatitis. *Amer J Gastroenterol, 108*, 1400–1415. **gi.org/guideline/acute-pancreatitis/**

Patient Education

www.emedicinehealth.com/pancreatitis/page2_em.htm

www.uptodate.com/contents/patient-information-pancreatitis-the-basics?source=search_result&search=pancreatitis&selectedTitle=1~150

www.webmd.com/digestive-disorders/digestive-diseases-pancreatitis

Learning Outcomes for Gallbladder Disease

When you complete this lesson, you will be able to:

1. Recognize the clinical relevance of gallbladder disease.
2. Consider the pathophysiology, etiology, risk factors, and clinical presentation of gallbladder disease that determine the priority patient concerns.
3. Determine the most urgent and important nursing interventions and patient education required in caring for a patient with gallbladder disease.
4. Evaluate attainment of desired collaborative care outcomes for a patient with gallbladder disease.

LO1:

What Are Gallbladder Diseases?

Gallbladder diseases are conditions that affect the gallbladder and connecting structures. This lesson focuses on:

- Cholelithiasis: gallstones within the gallbladder, which may remain unnoticed or go on to cause inflammation
- Cholecystitis: inflammation of the wall of the gallbladder
- Choledocholithiasis: Gallstones that exit the gallbladder and become lodged in the common bile duct. It commonly causes and presents along with pancreatitis
- Cholangitis: Infection within the biliary tree that is usually caused by obstruction of the common bile duct. The common bile duct allows bile, which is produced by the liver, to go from the liver into the gallbladder and intestines. When blocked, bacterial infection, which can be life threatening, can develop.

Anatomical Relationships: Gallbladder with Other Organs

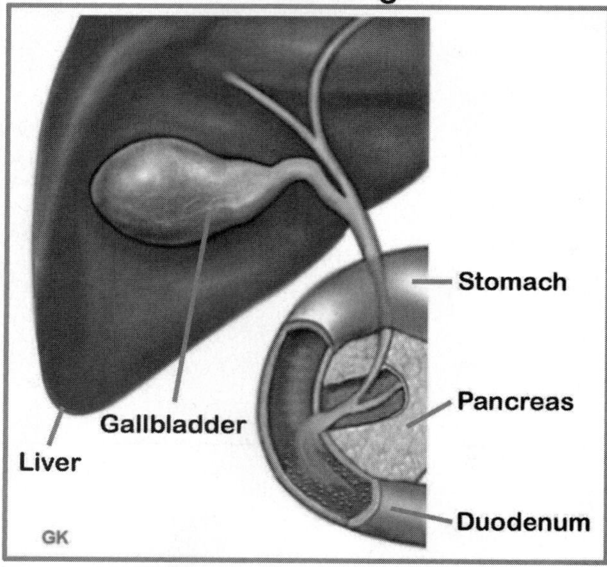

This diagram shows the anatomical structures involved in gallbladder diseases.

Source: Courtesy of George Kyriakidis/Santa Ana, CA

LO1:

Clinical Relevance

- Approximately 5,000–8,000 deaths are caused by complications from acute cholecystitis.
- Thirty percent of Native Americans develop gallstones by age 30, and 80% have gallstones by age 60.
- More than 20,000,000 patients in the United States have gallstones and >750,000 cholecystectomies are performed yearly.
- Early detection and treatment of cholecystitis can reduce morbidity and mortality.

Concept Check

1. **A patient has cholangitis. What condition exists?**
   A. Gallstones within the gallbladder
   B. Inflammation of the gallbladder
   C. Gallstones in the common bile duct
   D. Infection within the biliary tree

Answer question

LO2:

Pathophysiology

- The gallbladder is a small organ that sits just below the liver and concentrates bile secreted by the liver. The gallbladder secretes the concentrated bile into the stomach to aid in the digestion of fats.
- Gallbladder disease is most commonly due to the formation of gallstones. The presence of gallstones within the gallbladder is called **cholelithiasis**.
- Gallstones are stones formed within the gallbladder from the contents of bile.
- Stones may remain in the gallbladder long term and go unnoticed.
- Stones may grow in size and cause inflammation and pain of the gallbladder wall, which is called **cholecystitis**. When inflammation causes pain that is moderate to severe and persists, it is called acute cholecystitis. However, chronic or long term forms of cholecystitis also occur.
- Stones may block the gallbladder outlet, causing inflammation of the gallbladder, which is called **acute cholecystitis**.
- **Choledocholithiasis** occurs if a stone passes beyond the gallbladder and blocks the common bile duct. This can result in acute cholecystitis.

Anatomy of the Gallbladder and the Ducts

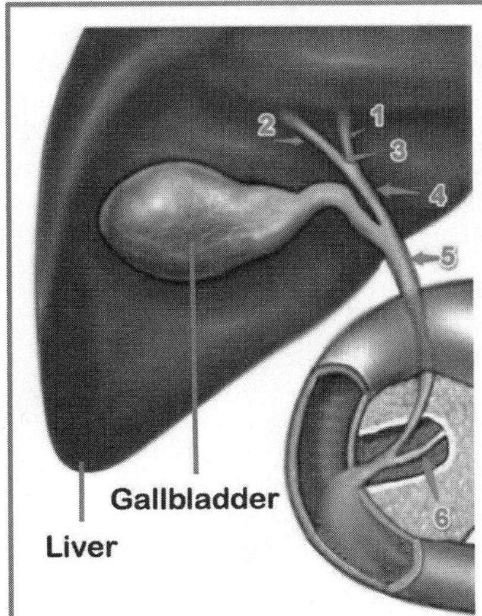

This illustration demonstrates the relationship of the gallbladder to the cystic duct, common bile duct, and cystic artery.
Source: Courtesy of George Kyriakidis/Santa Ana, CA

- Complications of the blockage, which allows bacterial growth and infection, include acute **cholangitis** and acute pancreatitis. Both conditions warrant emergency admission and care due to the high risk of sepsis and life-threatening situation.

Cholelithiasis

- Only about 1–3% of people with gallstones develop symptoms.
- Most gallstones are made from cholesterol found in bile. Bile cholesterol is independent of blood levels of cholesterol.
- Other stones are formed from too much bilirubin in the bile. These tend to occur in patients with hemolysis since bilirubin is a breakdown product of hemoglobin.

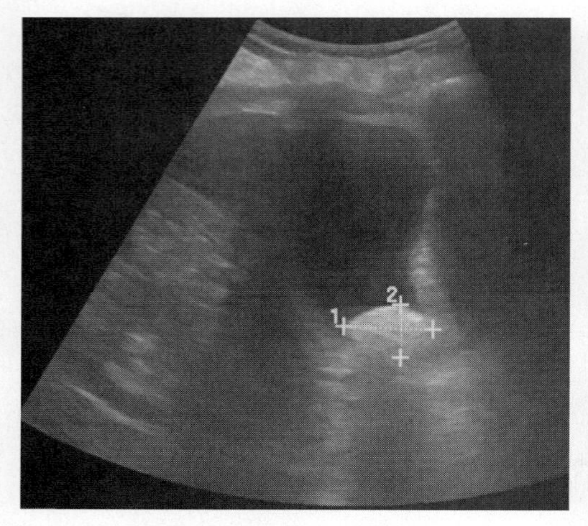

A large gallstone is seen on ultrasound.
Source: Courtesy of K. Kyriakidis

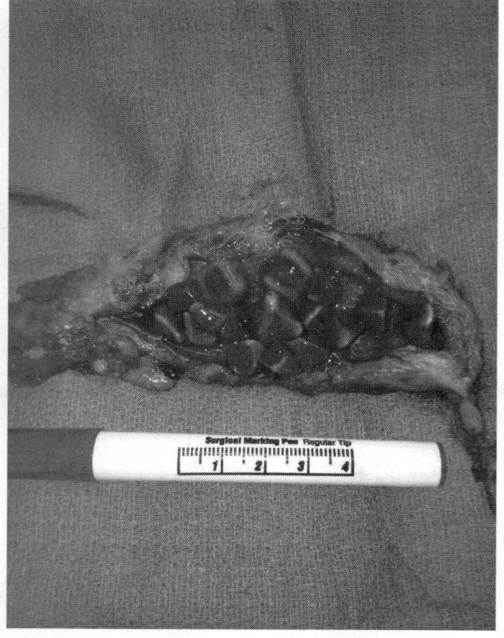

This shows an example of gallstones in a patient following cholecystectomy.
Source: Courtesy of R. Murphy

Concept Check

2. **What is the function of the gallbladder?**
   A. Filters bile to remove cholesterol
   B. Stores bile for future use
   C. Metabolizes bile to deactivate toxins
   D. Produces bile used in fat digestion

Answer question

Pathophysiology (continued)

Cholecystitis

- Acute cholecystitis is inflammation of the gallbladder wall that occurs abruptly. This is usually caused by gallstones that block the outlet (neck or cystic duct) of the gallbladder, causing the gallbladder to become distended.
- If obstruction persists, inflammation ensues and results in the release of cytokines and attraction of inflammatory cells. Capillaries in the gallbladder leak fluid and the gallbladder walls become edematous and thickened.
- Release of cytokines and occasionally infection of the bile within the gallbladder can cause fever.
- Cholecystitis may progress to necrosis and perforation of the gallbladder (see below)

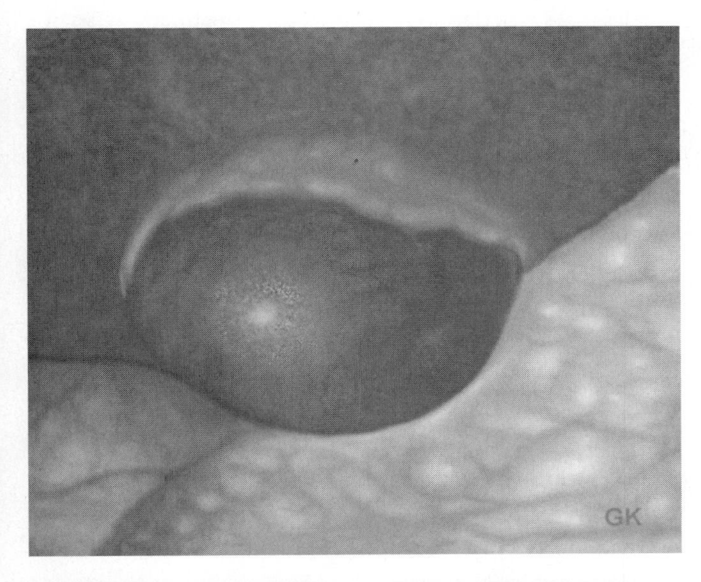

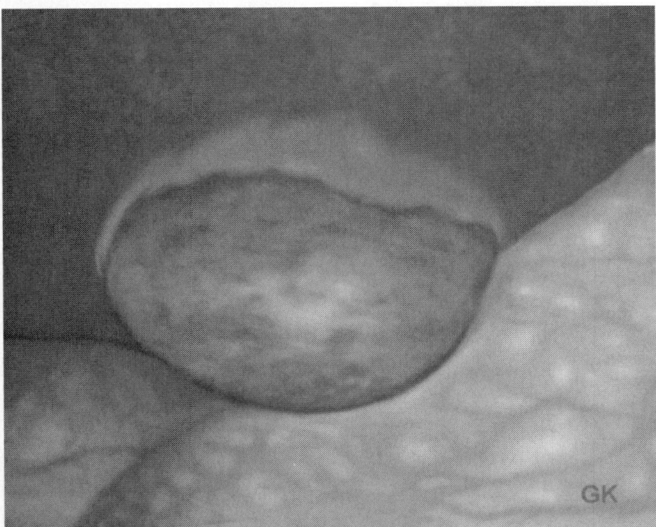

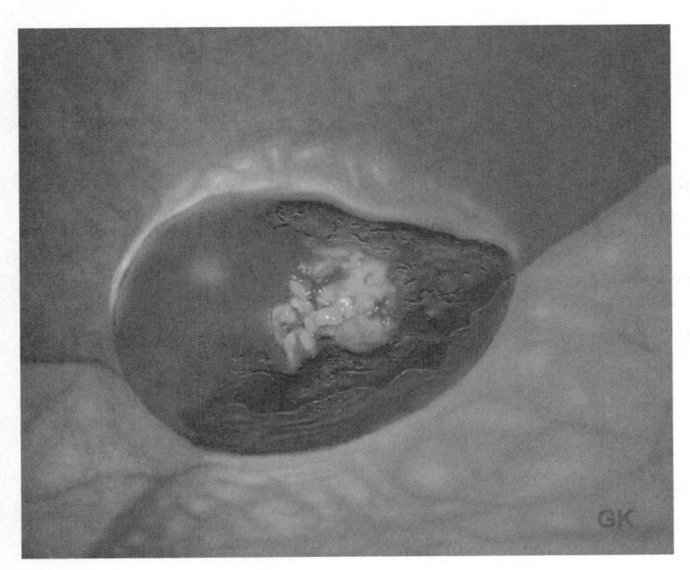

The photos show the early, necrotic and perforated stages of acute cholecystitis. The first (upper) shows a grayish appearance of an edematous gallbladder with swollen walls and is itself edematous. It no longer has the "robin egg blue" appearance of a normal gallbladder. As infection worsens or persists, the walls of the gallbladder develop the red speckles (middle) that signal necrosis. If not removed, it becomes gangrenous (lower) with a dark blackish green appearance and can perforate, as seen in the lower portion of the photo.
Source: (*all*) Courtesy of George Kyriakidis/Santa Ana, CA

- If the gallbladder is perforated, leakage of bile contents into the peritoneum can cause irritation of the peritoneum.
- If the obstruction resolves through movement of the stone, symptoms may subside.
- Repeated episodes of acute cholecystitis can result in chronic inflammation of the gallbladder (chronic cholecystitis).
- Cholecystitis can occur without the presence of gallstones. The mechanism for this is not clear but may have to do with concentration and stagnation of the bile (sludge). The risk for infection of the bile due to sludge is higher in patients with chronic or acute illness, such as sepsis.
- Chronic cholelithiasis or long-term gallstones can eventually lead to obstruction of the bile duct and infection (cholangitis). The chronic presence of bacterial colonies in the gallbladder can also cause a sequence of chronic inflammation, which consequently results in metaplasia, then dysplasia, and can cause neoplasia (malignant cells). Gallbladder cancer is, therefore, commonly accompanied by chronic gallstones.

Ruptured Gallbladder with Abscess

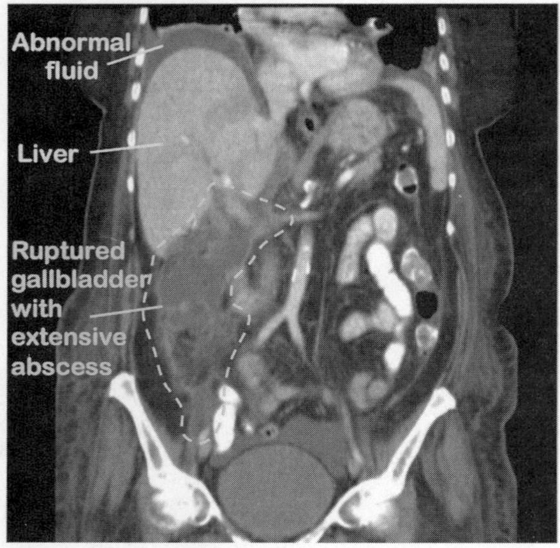

This CT scan reveals a ruptured gallbladder with an abscess leaking into the right abdomen. Fluid is also noted above the liver and is suspicious for abscess.

Source: Courtesy of K. Kyriakidis

Pathophysiology (continued)

Choledocholithiasis

- Stones that pass from the gallbladder into the common bile duct can become obstructive.
- Obstruction commonly occurs at the ampulla of Vater, where the common bile duct empties into the duodenum.
- Obstruction can cause increased pressure within the biliary tree and the pancreatic ducts, resulting in dilatation of the ducts.
- There is an elevation of serum transaminases and bilirubin. Because bile cannot enter the digestive tract and produce the dark color in stools, the stool often turns light in color. Bile excreted into the urine will turn urine a dark color.
- Complications include:
  - Biliary obstruction can result in pancreatitis by preventing pancreatic enzymes from leaving the pancreas and spilling into the small intestines. The enzymes irritate pancreatic cells and cause the inflammation of the pancreas.
  - Cholangitis occurs when a bacterial infection arises from biliary obstruction or blockage in the biliary tree. The static bile grows bacterial colonies.

Obstruction of the Gallbladder by a Stone

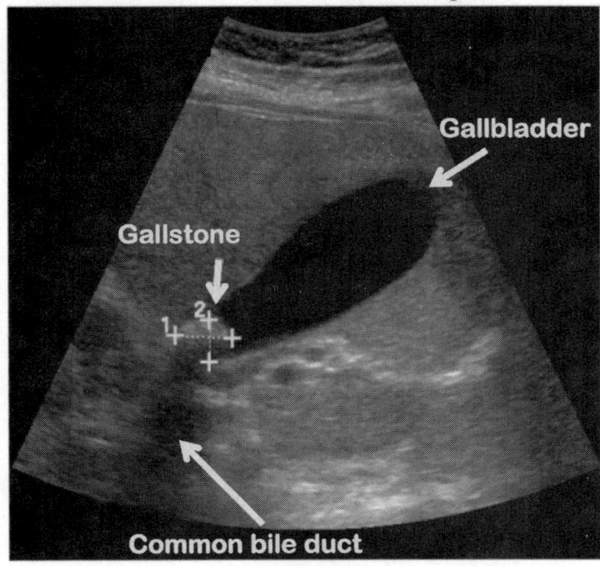

This ultrasound of the gallbladder (solid black oval) shows a gallstone obstructing bile flow into the duct.

Source: Courtesy of K. Kyriakidis

Concept Check

3. **Which condition is thought to predispose the patient to cholecystitis even if gallstones do not exist?**
   A. Hypertension
   B. IV drug abuse
   C. Sepsis
   D. Renal calculi

Answer question

Choledocholithiasis/Cholangitis

- Choledocholithiasis occurs when a gallstone become lodged in and blocks the biliary tree or common bile duct.
- Stagnation of bile in the biliary tree subsequently creates susceptibility to infection from bacteria that may pass up through the ampulla of Vater. The infection can result in a serious condition known as cholangitis.
- Cholangitis is usually associated with fever with hypotension and altered mental status and can progress to sepsis. Thus, hypotension and altered mental state should alert clinicians to potential sepsis.
- Patients with other causes of obstruction (e.g., tumors, strictures) of the common bile duct (CBD) are also at risk for cholangitis.

LO2:

Causes and Risk Factors: Gallstones

Although no specific cause can be cited, risk factors for gallstones (calculi formation) include:

- Female gender
- Native American or Hispanic ethnicity
- Age over 40
- Family history
- Obesity or rapid weight loss
- Drugs (e.g., estrogen therapy in women, clofibrate, fibrate hypolipidemic drugs, somatostatin)
- Lack of exercise
- Pregnancy

Risk factors for acalculous gallbladder disorders include:

- Debilitation
- Major surgery
- Severe trauma
- Sepsis
- Prolonged fasting
- Long-term total parenteral nutrition

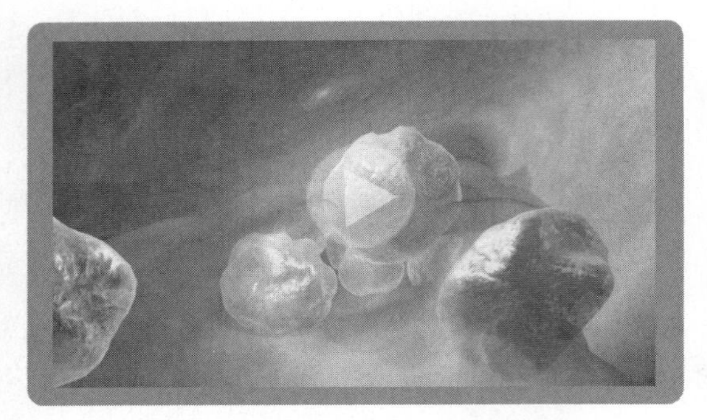

This unnarrated animation demonstrates gallstone formation within the gallbladder, blocking the cystic duct, and causing cholecystitis or inflammation of the gallbladder.

Concept Check

4. Choledocholithiasis is most often caused by obstruction of which structure?
   A. Ampulla of Vater
   B. Duodenum
   C. Pancreatic duct
   D. Hepatic duct

Answer question

LO2:

Assessment Findings

Cholelithiasis

The majority of patients with cholelithiasis are asymptomatic. Key symptoms include:

- **Pain:** may start in the epigastric area and then localize to the right upper quadrant (RUQ)
  - o Onset of pain tends to be abrupt, severe, and constant.
  - o It can last from half an hour to several hours after meals.
  - o Pain may radiate through to the back or to the right shoulder.
  - o The pain can mimic cardiac pain.
- **Nausea and vomiting**

Cholecystitis

Pain is similar to cholelithiasis but lasts over 6 hours.

- There is tenderness in the right upper quadrant (Murphy's sign).
- Pain may be referred to as biliary colic.
- Pain may be less severe (e.g., belching or indigestion).
- It may cause nausea and vomiting.
- Patients with infection of bile within the gallbladder may have fever.
- Tachycardia is usually noted.
- Perforation may result in rebound tenderness and/or sepsis with hypotension and altered mental status.
- Pain suggesting pancreatic involvement is mid-abdomen with radiation into the back. This is a feared and potentially lethal complication.

Chronic and Acute Cholecystitis with Resulting Fatal Sepsis

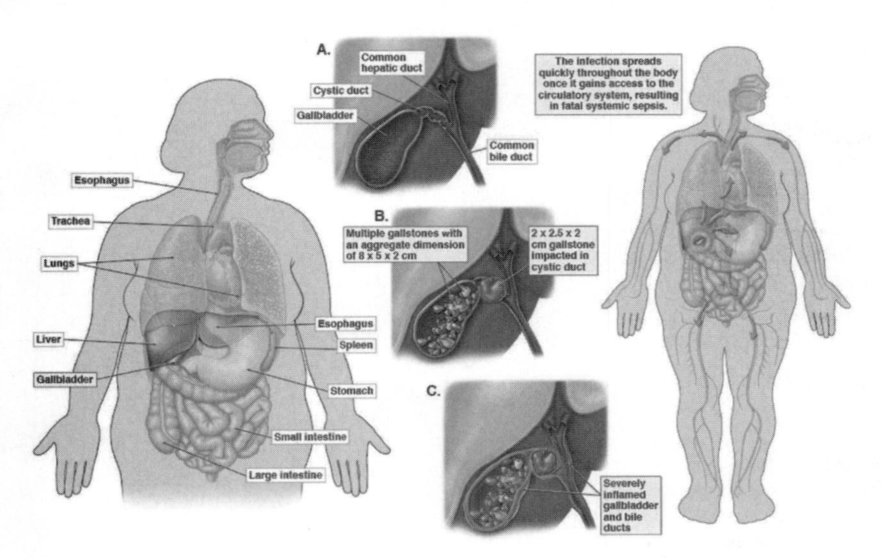

This exhibit depicts chronic and acute cholecystitis with resulting fatal sepsis. The first image is an anterior view of the upper body of a woman, with organs shown transparently beneath the skin. The next three images are cross-sections of the gallbladder and associated ducts, and show the progression of the cholecystitis. The final image shows the infection spreading through the body, resulting in fatal sepsis.

Source:

Choledocholithiasis and Cholangitis

Choledocholithiasis

- Some patients may be asymptomatic if the gallstones in the common bile duct are nonobstructing.
- Pain is located in right upper quadrant (RUQ) with sudden onset, constant, and severe.
- Nausea and vomiting are frequently seen.
- The stool may turn light grayish from absence of bile.
- Urine may turn dark due to increased bile.
- Jaundice is particularly noted in the sclera.

Choledocholithiasis with **cholangitis** (infection of bile in biliary tree):

- Patients additionally have fever and jaundice.
- If sepsis develops, patients may become hypotensive with altered mental status. This is an emergent situation.

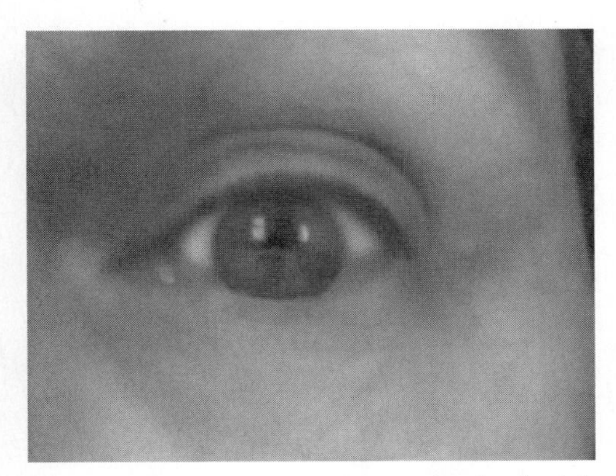

The sclera (white) of the eye and the surrounding facial skin is yellowish or jaundiced.

Source: Courtesy of George Kyriakidis/Santa Ana, CA

LO2:

Diagnostics

Prompt diagnosis is essential to prevent higher morbidity and mortality. While important, lab data are not reliable in identifying patients with cholecystitis.

Labs:

- CBC: Leukocytosis may be present (especially with infection).
- Electrolytes
- Amylase and lipase are elevated if pancreatitis is present. Amylase may also be slightly elevated in cholecystitis.
- Liver transaminases (ALT, AST), alkaline phosphatase, and T bilirubin are usually elevated in the blood in symptomatic choledocholithiasis and cholangitis.
- Urinalysis: Bilirubin may be elevated with symptomatic choledocholithiasis.
- Lactate: Sepsis is indicated if lactate is >4 mmol/L and signals an emergent situation.
- Urine pregnancy test should be performed on all females of childbearing age.

Imaging:

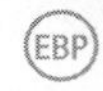

- **Ultrasound imaging** is the primary preferred test in diagnosing acute cholecystitis and cholangitis (Solomkin, et al., 2010). It is performed as soon as possible (90–95% sensitivity). Stones may be visualized in the gallbladder or common bile duct. Gallbladder wall may be thickened and edematous in acute cholecystitis. Common bile duct and biliary tree may be dilated in choledocholithiasis and acute cholangitis.
- **HIDA** (hepatobiliary iminodiacetic acid) **scan** is a procedure that uses a nuclear tracer to track the production and movement of bile through the biliary tree, gallbladder, and small intestine. In patients with acute cholecystitis, bile does not move into the gallbladder since the gallbladder is obstructed.
- **ERCP** (endoscopic retrograde cholangiopancreatography) is an endoscope that has a camera at the tip to transmit pictures as it is passed through the stomach into the duodenum. Contrast can be injected through the ampulla of Vater so that the CBD, biliary tree, pancreatic ducts, narrowings, and blockages can be visualized on fluoroscopy (type of real time x-ray). With ERCP, stones can be retrieved, excess bile drained, and a stent placed in the CBD to keep the lumen patent.
- **CT imaging** with or without IV contrast can identify complications of acute choleycystitis (e.g., perforation or gangrene).
- **MRI:** No contrast used, which limits radiation exposure for pregnant women. It is used when ultrasound is not clear.

Endoscopic Retrograde Cholangiopancreatography

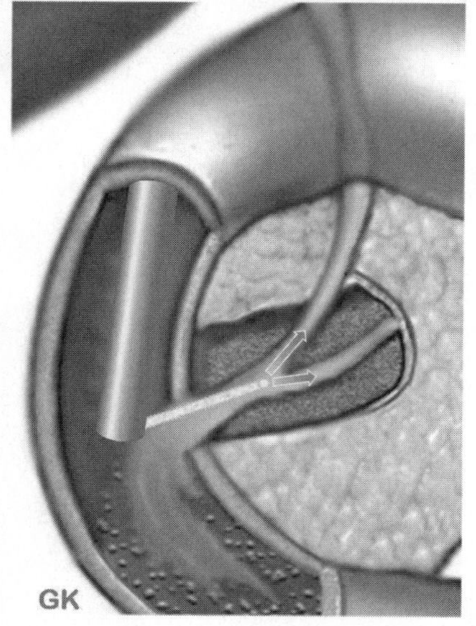

This diagram depicts an ERCP with a catheter (thin, beige tube) extending out of a duodenoscope into the pancreatic duct. Dye can be injected to visualize the duct more clearly.

Source: Courtesy of George Kyriakidis/Santa Ana, CA

Biliary Obstruction by Pancreatic Cancer

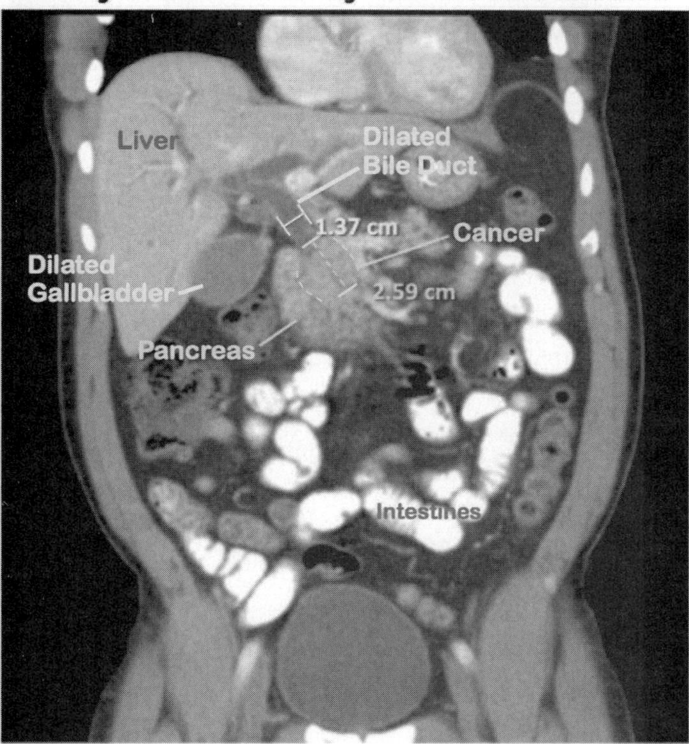

Pancreatic cancer (light blue) is obstructing the biliary duct, causing severe dilation of the bile duct and gallbladder.
Source: Courtesy of K. Kyriakidis

Concept Check

5. Which testing is most useful in determining the presence of cholecystitis?
   A. Serum SGOT level
   B. Serum amylase level
   C. Ultrasonography
   D. Flat plate and upright abdominal x-rays

Answer question

Priority Patient Concerns and Desired Collaborative Care Outcomes

Prior to caring for patients with gallbladder disease, it is important to prioritize the patient's concerns that must guide the nursing care plan and interventions. Care for the patient is ordered and organized in accordance with the patient's priority and urgent needs. Desired collaborative care outcomes in patients with gallbladder disease typically include:

1. Patient will report pain is controlled at a desirable level.
2. Patient will have no illness-related weight loss.
3. Patient will remain infection-free.
4. Patient will report feeling less anxiety.

Considering these important care outcomes, prepare a list of the major 3–6 priority patient concerns or nursing diagnoses for patients with gallbladder disease. Be prepared to participate in a discussion of this list and/or to submit them as an assignment, as determined by your faculty. Resources you may find helpful in this assignment can include this lesson, the references, resources on nursing care plans, and standard nursing diagnoses manuals.

LO3:

Collaborative Interventions

Evidenced-based practice in gallbladder diseases is extensive, particularly regarding antibiotic use and surgical intervention. Key medical practices must be included to understand the collaborative interventions and are based on clinical practice guidelines from the Association of Upper Gastrointestinal Surgeons (AUGIS) (2013), Infectious Diseases Society of America (Solomkin, et al., 2010), the Society for Surgery of the Alimentary Tract (2006), World Gastroenterology Organization (WGO) (2007), Bongala, et al. (2004), and Duncan & Riall (2012). Recommendations to guide patient care are integrated into the following conditions. The seriousness of patient conditions are ordered from mild (cholelithiasis) to serious (choledocholithiasis with cholangitis).

Cholelithiasis

Asymptomatic patients with cholelithiasis are those who have gallstones and are unaware of any problem. Some patients experience mild cholecystitis that does not prompt them to seek emergency or urgent care. Care of asymptomic patients typically includes:

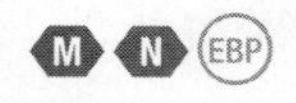

- Watchful waiting (also called expectant management) is recommended in patients whose gallstones are discovered unexpectedly, are asymptomatic, or present with a self-limiting pain episode with short duration. If there are no symptoms or very mild, waiting to see if the gallstones pass on their own and the problem resolves without intervention may be trialed (AUGIS), 2013).

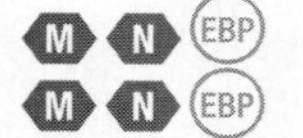

- Asymptomatic patients do not require admission (AUGIS, 2013).

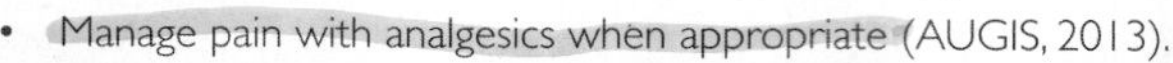

- Manage pain with analgesics when appropriate (AUGIS, 2013).

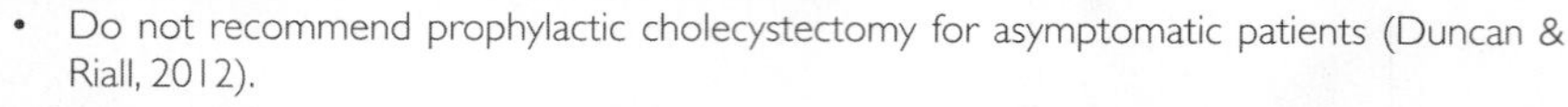

- Do not recommend prophylactic cholecystectomy for asymptomatic patients (Duncan & Riall, 2012).

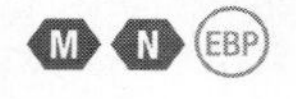

- Refer for emergency hospitalization if pain becomes unmanageable and/or recurs without relief (AUGIS, 2013).

Collaborative Interventions (continued)

Cholecystitis

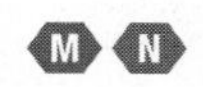

- When the pain of gallbladder disease mimics acute coronary syndrome, one must first rule out cardiac origins.
  - o Obtain a thorough history and perform physical examination.
  - o Obtain a 12-lead EKG to assess for myocardial ischemia or injury.
  - o Evaluate cardiac enzymes.
- The goals of patient care management are to avoid complications and diminish morbidity. Care of patients with gallbladder disease depends on the severity of the disease, the stability of the patient, the presence of complications (e.g., gangrene, sepsis, or perforation) and involves:

Acute Cholecystitis

- **Rapid Response Team:** Call for any significant deterioration in the patient's status (e.g., hypotension, tachycardia, mental status change), which can indicate perforation or sepsis and call for urgent intervention. Early recognition and intervention are critical.
- **Fluid resuscitation:**

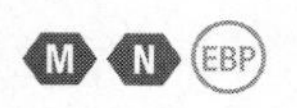

  - o Immediately begin IV fluids using large bore IVs if septic shock is suspected, particularly if hypotension is present (Solomkin, et al., 2010).

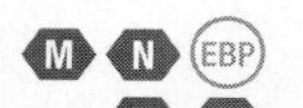

  - o Rapidly resuscitate with IV fluids to attain hemodynamic stability (Solomkin, et al., 2010).
- **NPO:** Make patient NPO or, if uncomplicated cholecystitis, may have liquids. IV(s) required while the patient is NPO or may require fluid resuscitation.

- **Medications:**
  - o Administer analgesics IV for pain (e.g., morphine, hydromorphone, fentanyl).
  - o Administer antibiotics IV which focus on gram-negative and anaerobic pathogens (Solomkin, et al., 2010):
    - ■ In patients with acute and complicated acute cholecystitis with fever or leukocytosis or cholangitis: Examples are ampicillin/sulbactam or piperacillin/tazobactam (Bongala, et al., 2004; Society of American Gastrointestinal and Endoscopic Surgeons [SAGES, 2010]; Solomkin, et al., 2010).
    - ■ If an intra-abdominal infection is highly suspected or diagnosed or if the patient is septic (Solomkin, et al., 2010; SAGES, 2010).
    - ■ During biliary drainage and/or stone removal and prior to procedures (Solomkin, et al., 2010)
    - ■ Preoperatively for prophylaxis in a single dose within 1 hour of skin incision if used prior to laparoscopy (SAGES, 2010)
    - ■ Prophylactically in high-risk patients (e.g., age over 60 years, jaundice, cholangitis, diabetes) who are having laparoscopic surgery (Solomkin, et al., 2010; SAGES, 2010)
    - ■ Prophylactically for patients having surgery who have chronic cholecystitis, such as cefazolin, or cefuroxime (Bongala, et al., 2004)
    - ■ In complicated or life-threatening cases. Recommendations are imipenem/cilastatin or meropenem (Solomkin, et al., 2010).
    - ■ Alternative combinations include metronidazole plus a third-generation antibiotic (cephalosporin, ciprofloxacin, or aztreonam)
  - o Administer antiemetics IV for nausea and vomiting (e.g., ondansetron, promethazine), as needed.
  - o Although used, gallstone dissolution medications and procedures (e.g., ursodiol, lithotripsy) are not recommended. Patients who are not surgical candidates may receive these, but there is no evidence of benefit (AUGIS, 2013).
  - o Do not recommend the use of proton pump inhibitors (PPIs) or hyoscine for gallbladder disease or symptom management (AUGIS, 2013).
- Obtain cultures from infected site in high-risk patients, particularly if the patient had recent antibiotic exposure, due to the higher risk of resistant pathogens. Cultures from lowrisk patients with community-acquired infections are optional (Solomkin, et al., 2010).
- **Surgical intervention:**
  - o Require surgical consultation to determine if removal of the gallbladder (cholecystectomy) is required to relieve pain, remove gallstones, and remove infection (Duncan & Riall, 2012). Collaborate to ensure patient's accurate information is shared and the patient's wishes guide decisions.
  - o Consider placement of a drain if the stone cannot be removed (Duncan & Riall, 2012; Solomkin, et al., 2010).
  - o Avoid routinely placing intraperitoneal drains post-cholecystectomy (Bongala, et al., 2004). If present, collaborate with the health care provider to remove as soon as possible.
  - o Recommend avoiding prophylactic cholecystectomy in asymptomatic patients (Duncan & Riall, 2012).
- Endoscopic Retrograde Cholangiopancreatography (ERCP): Educate and prepare the patient about ERCP as the preferred procedure for diagnosis and stone removal, if possible (Duncan & Riall, 2012).
- The standard of care for removal of the gallbladder (acute or chronic) is laparoscopic procedure in elective, uncomplicated cases (Bongala, et al., 2004; Duncan & Riall, 2012; SAGES, 2010).
  - o Although drains are not recommended after elective, uncomplicated laparoscopic surgery due to higher risk of complications (Bongala, et al., 2004; SAGES, 2010), advocate for drain removal at the earliest possible time if a drain is used and there is little to no drainage.
  - o May discharge patient without complications to home on the day of surgery if pain, nausea, and vomiting are controlled (SAGES, 2010).
  - o Carefully evaluate patients over 50 years of age who are at increased risk for hospital admission rather than discharge to home (SAGES, 2010).
  - o May delay surgical intervention in acute cholecystitis up to 24 hours if patient is hemodynamically stable, has no sign of organ failure, is receiving appropriate antibiotics, and is vigilantly monitored (Solomkin, et al., 2010).

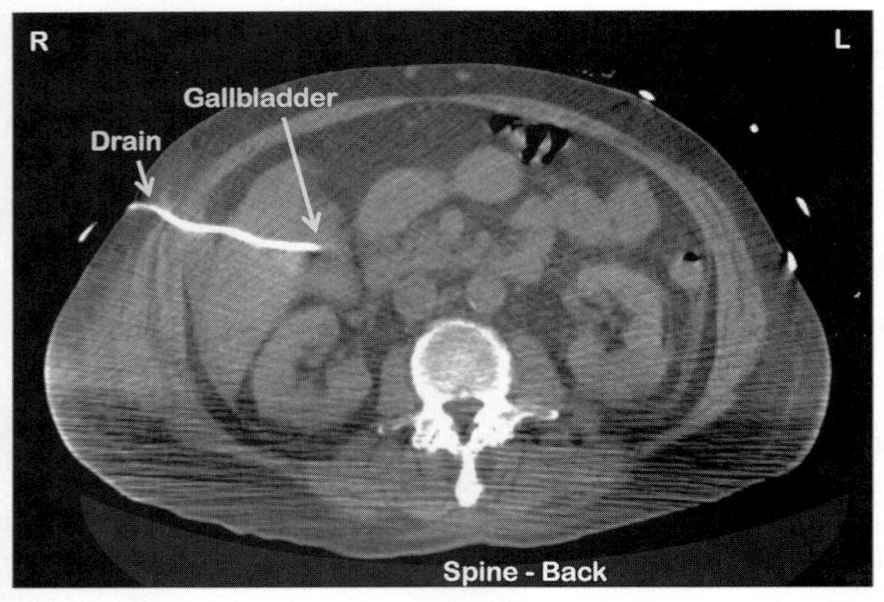

A cholecystostomy drain is being guided for insertion and placement into the gallbladder using CT scan. The patient was in sepsis and had cholecystitis, kidney disease, and pneumonia.
Source: Courtesy of K. Kyriakidis

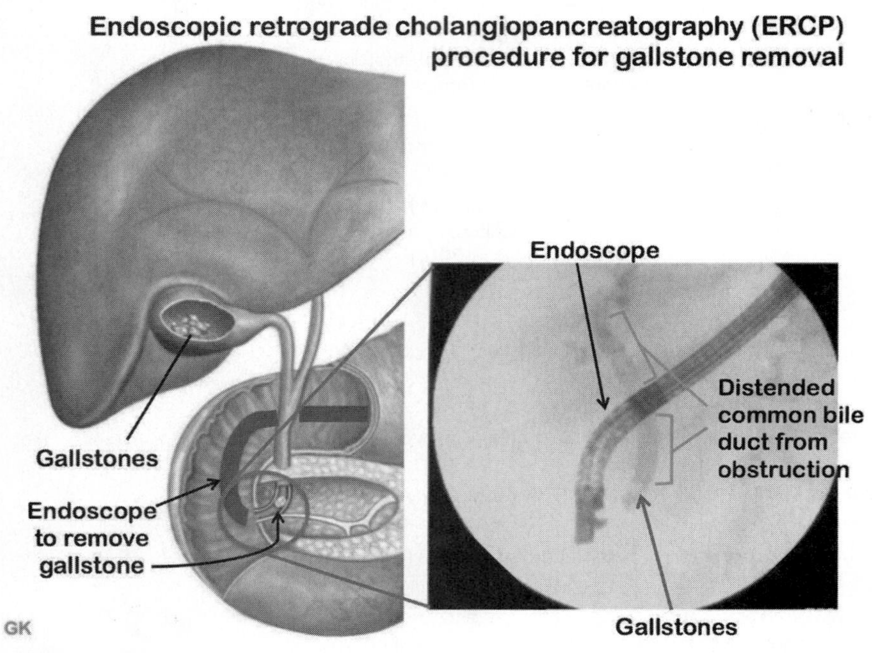

This image features an endoscopic retrograde cholangiopancreatography, or ERCP, procedure for removal of a gallstone that is blocking the common bile duct. Success prevents surgery.
Sources: Courtesy of K. Kyriakidis & George Kyriakidis/Santa Ana, CA

Collaborative Interventions (continued)

Postoperative Care: Symptom Management, Comfort Care, Safety, and Prevention of Complications

Postoperative care of patients with gallbladder disease can vary based on the type and methods of intervention, but should include:

M N
- Maintain fluid and electrolyte balance.

M N
- Control pain, nausea, and vomiting.

M N
- Mobilize the patient as early as possible and encourage self-care activities.

M N
- Resume oral fluids and food after laparoscopy. Graduate to liquids and then bland, soft food if after open abdominal surgery.

N • Provide aseptic wound care of incision and/or drainage (if present) sites, and good skin care around wound and drainage site.

N • Monitor and measure drainage (blood tinged is normal within first day) from T-tube or other drainage device.

N • Provide routine postoperative care, to include:
  - o Turn, cough, deep breathe every 2 hours.
  - o Incentive spirometry or similar inspiratory device
  - o Splint incision to reduce discomfort.
  - o Monitor vital signs, physical exam, intake and output balance.
  - o Monitor labs and correct imbalances as warranted.
  - o Observe for and report early warning of site infection (fever, unusual abdominal pain, or jaundice).

M N • If patient has an NG tube, set on low intermittent suction and monitor drainage.

M N • Use sequential compression device for DVT prophylaxis until the patient is active.

N • Place in semi-Fowler's position for comfort.

• Following **laparoscopic surgery**, postop care for uncomplicated cholecystectomy patients includes:
  - M N o Discharge to home on the same day as surgery or next day for most low-risk patients.
  - N o Educate the patient about the shoulder pain commonly experienced post-laparoscopy. Pain is commonly caused by the carbon dioxide used to expand the abdominal space and improve visualization for surgery. Carbon dioxide becomes trapped against the diaphragm and causes pain that can radiate. Apply heat and analgesics for relief.

N • Assist in returning to normal bowel and bladder function.

N • Observe for systemic infection and blood loss, including hypotension, fever, tachycardia, and abdominal distention.

M N EBP • Consider, or collaborate with team to consider, discontinuing antibiotics if fever is absent for 24 hours, oral intake is tolerated, and WBCs are normal with three or fewer band forms (Bongala, et al., 2004).

M N • Prevent all hospital-acquired conditions or never events, particularly in high-risk patients where they have less resilience. These include infections from surgical sites or urinary and vascular catheters, retained foreign object, ventilator-associated pneumonia, DVTs, pressure ulcers, blood incompatibility, falls, glycemic events, and air embolism.

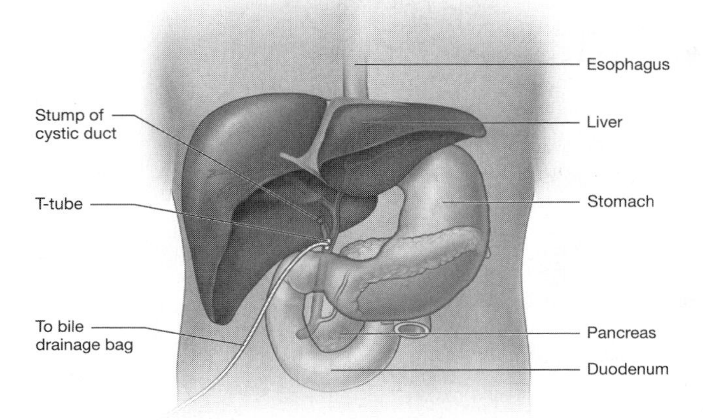

A T-tube, named for its shape, is placed in the common bile duct to drain excess bile postoperatively.

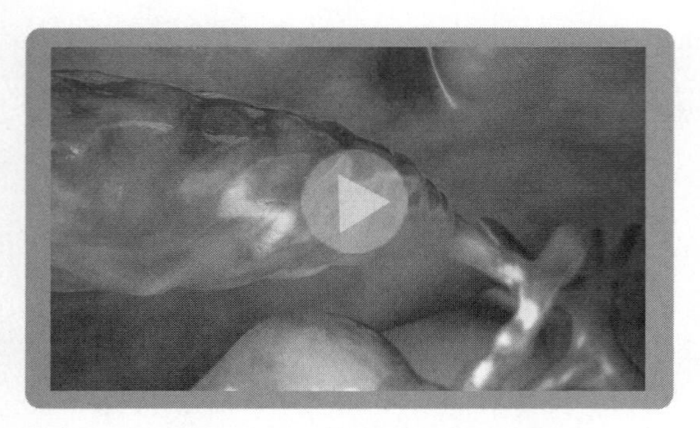

This animation shows gallbladder removal surgery. It shows the normal anatomy of the liver and gallbladder. Over time, gallstones form within the gallbladder, block the cystic duct, and cause the gallbladder to become enlarged and inflamed. As a result, the gallbladder is dissected from the liver and removed from the body.
Source:

Collaborative Interventions (continued)

Patient Education

- If the patient is sent home with watchful wait strategy, education can include:
  - N o Increase activity and exercise to reduce the risk of gallstones.
  - N o Weight management if overweight
  - N o Shift diet to increase fruits and vegetables, reduce sugars and carbohydrates, and evaluate whether or not it improves symptoms.
  - N EBP o Adopt a low-fat diet and avoid fatty meals if these provoke symptoms (AUGIS, 2013). Reducing the release of cholecystokinin, which stimulates gallbladder contraction, may reduce the cholecystitis. Evaluate the benefit based on symptom control.
  - N o Prevent fat-soluble vitamin deficiency due to steatorrhea and malabsorption in patients *who do not have surgery*. Monitor for vitamin A, D, E, and K deficiencies and treat with supplements when indicated.
- If the patient is postoperative:
  - M N o Resume normal diet with no dietary restrictions: Low-fat diet may still be taught but science has *not* concurred that it causes discomfort for most patients, especially after surgery. Many surgeons no longer include this. Collaborate and advocate for a normal diet whenever possible. Fat-soluble vitamin supplements need to be considered if low-fat diet is prescribed.
  - N o Instruct about wound and incision care. Immediately report any signs of bleeding or infection (e.g., severe pain, jaundice, high fever, chills, or odor from drainage).
  - N o Instruct patient about medications, follow-up care, and when to call the health care provider.
  - N o Continue to take full prescription of antibiotics as prescribed.
  - N o Continue pain management: Continue to use opioids as prescribed and as needed. Taper pain medication use and/or transition to nonopioids when tolerated well to prevent opioid-induced constipation.
  - M N o Increase fiber in diet and drink plenty of liquids to prevent constipation if on narcotics.
  - N o Encourage a healthy weight.
  - M N o Avoid tub baths until stitches or staples are removed. May shower on second day after surgery.
  - N o Discuss early mobilization.
- For prevention of gallbladder disease or its recurrence, educational focus is on modifiable risk factors:
  - M N o Avoid medications that are known to increase the risk of cholecystitis in patient who are prone to development of gallstones, such as estrogens, octreotide, and ceftriaxone.
  - N o Avoid rapid weight loss that increases the risk of gallstone formation.
  - N o Avoid parenteral forms for nutrition, which has an association with sludge and consequent stone formation, if enteral nutrition is possible.
  - N o Educate patient to take prescribed medications that can prevent stone formation, such as ursodiol.

Collaborative Interventions (continued)

Cholangitis

(EBP) Patients with acute cholangitis are at high risk for developing sepsis and deterioration with multisystem organ failure. They need to be watched carefully and intervention should be immediate (Duncan & Riall, 2012; Solomkin, et al., 2010). The most urgent and important interventions are:

(N) 1. Monitor carefully for and report the earliest signs of systemic inflammatory response syndrome (SIRS) and sepsis, including hypothermia, fever, tachycardia, tachypnea, leukocytosis, particularly if an infection is present. (See the Care of Patients with Sepsis NovE-lesson for details.)

(M) (N) (EBP) 2. Administer prescribed antibiotics empirically to cover colonic bacterial organisms. Consider the local prevalence of drug-resistant organisms. Adjust antibiotics when blood cultures are available to target the specific organisms identified (Solomkin, et al., 2010).

(M) (N) (EBP) 3. Recommend biliary drainage of infected bile to remove infection and provide decompression. If antibiotics alone are trialed, monitor and report indications for urgent decompression, including persistent or worsening abdominal pain, hypotension after fluid resuscitation, fever exceeding 102°F, or a decreasing level of consciousness (Solomkin, et al., 2010).

(M) (N) (EBP) 4. Remove the gallstone obstruction. If removal is delayed to stabilize the patient, closely monitor and initiate a team response if the patient's condition deteriorates. Recognition of early warning signals and mobilizing the team can be life saving (Duncan & Riall, 2012; Solomkin, et al., 2010).

Care of patients with acute cholangitis additionally includes:

- (M) (N) Make patient NPO during the acute stage.
- (M) (N) Administer IV fluids to correct poor hydration or to resuscitate.
- (M) (N) Monitor and correct electrolyte imbalances.
- (M) (N) Provide pain control and relief from nausea and vomiting.
- (M) (EBP) Removal of stones and bile drainage are required as definitive treatment and may be used to replace surgery (Duncan & Riall, 2012):
  - o Removal of a gallstone obstruction with drainage of bile is common via ERCP. ERCP is considered the gold standard of treatment. Obstruction can cause a persistent source of infection. An endoscope is advanced through the stomach into the duodenum. A stone can then be retrieved in the common bile duct (CBD) and/or a stent placed in the CBD. This procedure provides decompression with relief.
  - (N) o Care of the patient after ERCP involves:
    - ■ Coach the patient about the immediate discomfort due to bloating from air introduced during the procedure.
    - ■ Treat sore throat if too uncomfortable.
    - ■ Offer clear liquids.
    - ■ Observe for and report complications such as abdominal pain suggesting pancreatitis, deterioration suggesting possible perforation or infection.
  - (M) (N) o Percutaneous drainage is important in removing the source of infection and thereby reducing mortality. It is achieved by advancing a catheter through the skin into the biliary tract to drain the bile. Care and education of the patient involves:
    - ■ Examine, empty, and measure bile drainage.
    - ■ Observe for tube patency.
    - ■ Provide meticulous skin care and change dressing whenever soiled to remove irritating bile from skin.
    - ■ Educate the patient about probable loose bowel movements for a few weeks.
    - ■ Notify the health care provider with the following findings: worsening pain, fever, chills, abdominal swelling, nausea, vomiting, incisional redness or failure to heal, foul smell or drainage, or tube becomes dislodged.
  - (M) (EBP) o May perform biliary drainage and stone removal (Duncan & Riall, 2012):
    - ■ Electively if the patient has mild cholangitis (responsive to antibiotics and fluid resuscitation)
    - ■ Within the first 48 hours in patients with moderate cholangitis (no organ dysfunction but unresponsive to fluid resuscitation and antibiotic therapy)
    - ■ Urgently for patients with severe cholangitis (accompanying organ dysfunction)

M N
- Perform blood and bile cultures as early as possible to identify infecting organism, direct or redirect antibiotic therapy, and prevent sepsis development.

M N
- Surgery should be considered after the acute episode is controlled. Emergency surgeries carry much higher mortality and morbidity rates.
    - o Consider cholecystectomy to prevent recurrence.

M N
- Prevent fat-soluble vitamin deficiency due to steatorrhea and malabsorption in patients *who do not have surgery*. Monitor for vitamin A, D, E, and K deficiencies and treat with supplements when indicated.

M N
    - o Manage pruritus, particularly if disabling, with medication such as cholestyramine, colestipol, rifampin, antihistamines, or ursodiol.

M N
    - o Identify patients at high risk for osteoporosis. Prevent osteoporosis in patients with chronic conditions using calcium with vitamin D, ursodiol, calcitonin or bisphosphonate.

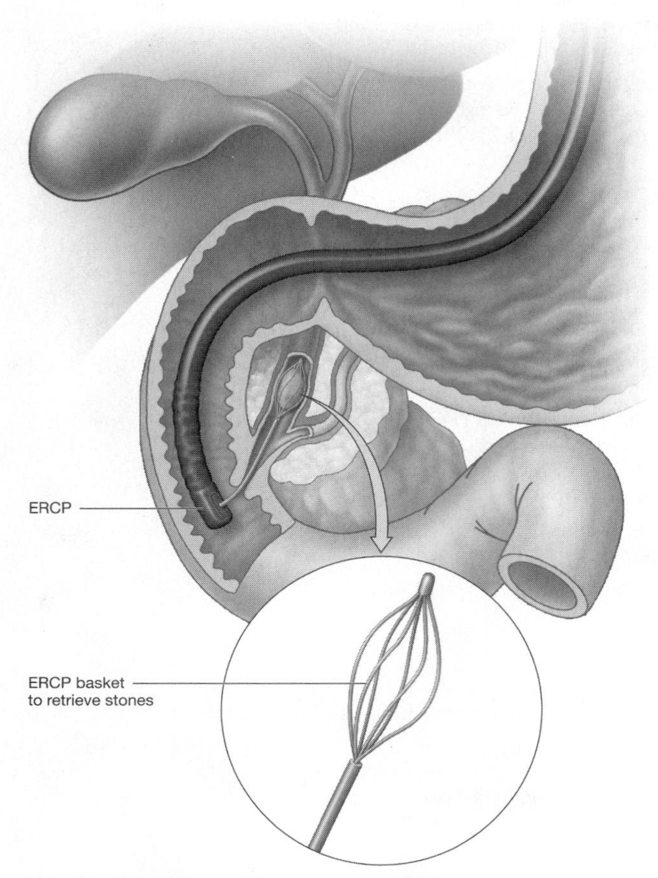

The drawings illustrate ERCP used to retrieve gallstones from the duct using very small extraction baskets.

Collaborative Interventions (continued)

Comparsion: Care of Patients with Gallstone Disease

	Cholelithiasis	Cholecystitis	Choledocholithiasis	Cholangitis
Imaging	Gallstones within gallbladder	Inflammation of gallbladder wall, distended gallbladder, gallstones in gallbladder	Gallstone in common bile duct	Within common bile duct (may have a different source of obstruction)
Signs and Symptoms	Asymptomatic or RUQ pain radiating to right shoulder, nausea.	RUQ pain > 6 hours +/- fever, Nausea, vomiting, Tenderness over RUQ. Patients with perforation or necrosis may have rebound tenderness, hypotension, altered mental status.	RUQ pain, White stool, dark urine. elevation of liver enzymes AST, ALT, Alk phos.	RUQ pain, jaundice, fever, elevation of liver enzymes AST, ALT, Alk phos, WBC's If septic: hypotension and altered mental status
Interventions	Pain control, antiemetics. Consider elective cholecystectomy in symptomatic patients.	IV fluids, NPO, pain control, antiemetics. Antibiotics for fever or leukocytosis. Surgery for cholecystectomy.	NPO, pain control, antiemetics, IV fluids, removal of stone by ERCP. Some stones will spontaneously pass.	IV fluids, NPO, pain control, antiemetics, removal of stone by ERCP.

Concept Check

6. What is the preferred diet for a patient with acute cholangitis?
   A. NPO
   B. Clear liquids
   C. Low-fat, full liquids
   D. Diet as tolerated

Answer question

Concept Check

7. Which finding in a patient discharged after same-day laparoscopic cholecystectomy is most serious?
   A. Shoulder pain
   B. Diarrhea
   C. Tachycardia
   D. Headache

Answer question

Collaborative Interventions (continued)

Summary: Care of Patients with Gallstone Disease

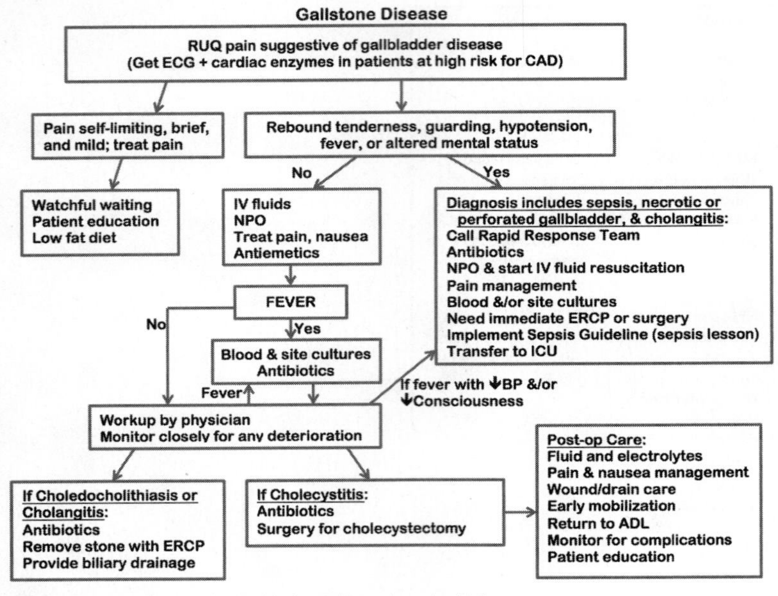

Summary of Interventions

- Management consists of analgesics, antiemetics, and hydration (e.g., limited or no oral intake during the acute phase).
- Antibiotics are prescribed for patients with fever, leukocytosis, or are at higher risk.
- Gallstone removal and biliary drainage are necessary in patients with moderate to severe disease.
- Careful monitoring of the patient is required to detect worsening or deterioration of the patient, particularly sepsis.
- On a medical/surgical unit, the Rapid Response Team should be alerted to assist with patients who show signs of hemodynamic instability, distress or altered mental status.

LO4:

Evaluation of Desired Collaborative Care Outcomes

Evaluation and reassessment should reveal attainment of previously established patient outcomes. In summary:

- The patient reports that pain has disappeared or diminished to a tolerable level.
- The patient's weight remains at or near pre-illness level.
- The patient manifests no findings associated with infection.
- The patient reports confidence in the treatment plan and own ability to manage the treatment regimen as prescribed.

References

Baric, P. S., & Eachempati, S. R. (2010). Acute acalculous cholecystitis. *Gastroenterol Clin North Am, 39*(2), 343–357.

Johnson, A. G., Fired, M., Tytgat, G., et al., & World Gastroenterology Organisation. (2007). *WGO practice guideline: Asymptomatic gallstone disease.* **www.worldgastroenterology.org/assets/downloads/en/pdf/guidelines/10_gallstone_en.pdf**

Kessenich, C. R. (2011). Cholecystitis and HIDA scan. *Nurse Practitioner, 36*(9), 11–12.

Lee, Y. M., Kaplan, M. M., & the Practice Guideline Committee of the ACG. (2002). Management of primary sclerosing cholangitis. *Am J Gastroenterol, 97*, 528–534. **gi.org/guideline/management-of-primary-sclerosing-cholangitis/**

Nursing2014. (2014). Recognizing and responding to gallbladder woes. *Nursing 2014, 37*, 12–15. **journals.lww.com/nursing/pages/articleviewer.aspx?year=2007&issue=04001&article=00002&type=Fulltext3**

Strasberg, S. M. (2008). Clinical practice: Acute calculous cholecystitis. *N Engl J Med, 358*(26), 2804–2811.

Tamhankar, A., Mazari, F., Olubaniyi, J., et al. (2010). Postoperative symptoms, after-care, and return to routine activity after laparoscopic cholecystectomy. *JSLS: J of the Society of Laparoendoscopic Surgeons, 14*(4), 484–489. **www.ncbi.nlm.nih.gov/pmc/articles/PMC3083036/**

Thomas, B. (2009). Cholecystectomy: Take a look at two options. *Nursing 2009, 39*(2), 36–39.

Yusoff, I. F., Barkun, J. S., & Barkun, A. N. (2003). Diagnosis and management of cholecystitis and cholangitis. *Gastroenterol Clin N Am, 32*, 1145–1168. **www.med.upenn.edu/gastro/documents/GastroClinNAcholecystitisandcholangitis.pdf**

Clinical Practice Guidelines

Association of Upper Gastrointestinal Surgeons (AUGIS). (2013). *Commissioning guide: Gallstone disease.* **www.rcseng.ac.uk/healthcare-bodies/docs/published-guides/gallstones**

Bongala, D. S., Santos, R. M., Panaligan, M. M., et al. (2004). *Evidence-based clinical practice guidelines on the diagnosis and treatment of cholecystitis.* **pcs.edgewebmedia.com/wp-content/uploads/files/ebcpg_chole.pdf**

Duncan, C., & Riall, T. (2012). Evidence-based current surgical practice: Calculous gallbladder disease. *J Gastrointestinal Surgery*, (11), 2011–2025. **www.ncbi.nlm.nih.gov/pubmed/22986769**

Society of American Gastrointestinal and Endoscopic Surgeons (SAGES). (2010). *SAGES guidelines for the clinical application of laparoscopic biliary tract surgery.* Los Angeles, CA: Society of American Gastrointestinal and Endoscopic Surgeons (SAGES).

Solomkin, J. S., Mazuski, J. E., Bradley, J. S., et al. (2010). Diagnosis and management of complicated intra-abdominal infection in adults and children: Guidelines by the Surgical Infection Society and the Infectious Diseases Society of America. *Clin Infect Dis, 50*(2), 133–164. **cid.oxfordjournals.org/content/50/2/133.full.pdf+html**

Patient Education

American College of Surgeons. (2009). *Cholescystectomy.* **www.facs.org/public_info/operation/cholesys.pdf**

Bloom, A. (2013). *Cholecystitis.* **emedicine.medscape.com/article/171886-overview**

Elsevier's Clinical Key. (2012). *Cholelithiasis and choledocholithiasis.* **www.clinicalkey.com/topics/surgery/cholelithiasis-and-choledocholithiasis.html#Z1922026511111**

Mayo Clinic Staff. (2011). *Primary sclerosing cholangitis.* **www.mayoclinic.org/diseases-conditions/primary-sclerosing-cholangitis/basics/definition/con-20029446**

Simmons, S. (2010). Gallstones. *Nursing 2010, 40*(11), 37. doi: 10.1097/01.NURSE.0000389020.72770.37

Learning Outcomes for Functional GI Disorders

When you complete this lesson, you will be able to:

1. Recognize the clinical relevance of functional disorders of the gastrointestinal tract.
2. Consider the pathophysiology, etiology, risk factors, and clinical presentation of functional disorders of the gastrointestinal tract that determine the priority patient concerns.
3. Determine the most urgent and important nursing interventions and patient education required in caring for a patient with a functional disorder of the gastrointestinal tract.
4. Evaluate attainment of desired collaborative care outcomes for a patient with a functional disorder of the gastrointestinal tract.

LO1:

Gastrointestinal Disorders: Lower GI Tract

Gastrointestinal bowel disorders consist of:

- Infectious Disorders
- Inflammatory Disorders
- **Functional Disorders**
- Structural Disorders

This NovE-lesson focuses on functional disorders.

LO1:

What Are Functional Disorders of the Gastrointestinal Tract?

- **Functional disorders** of the gastrointestinal (GI) tract consist of problems that cause impaired bowel function while the bowel tissue maintains a normal appearance.
- Constipation and irritable bowel syndrome (IBS) are the most common causes of a functional disorder of the colon and rectum.

This NovE-lesson focuses on these two disorders.

Anatomy of the Large Intestine

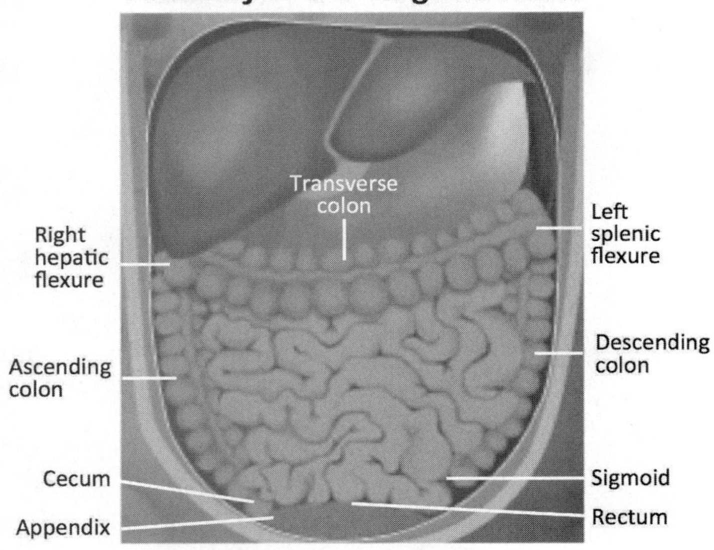

This drawing details the anatomical areas of the large intestine (colon), from the appendix to the rectum. Various functional disorders tend to occur in particular intestinal areas.

Source: Copyright © 2014, NovEx Novice to Expert Learning, LLC

LO1:

What Is Constipation?

- Constipation is generally defined as having fewer than three bowel movements per week or as difficulty having a bowel movement.
- Constipation is a symptom rather than a disease.
- Constipation can result from colon or anorectal dysfunction.
- Prolonged constipation or inability to pass stool can lead to an impaction (fecal obstruction).

Fecal Impaction

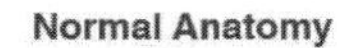

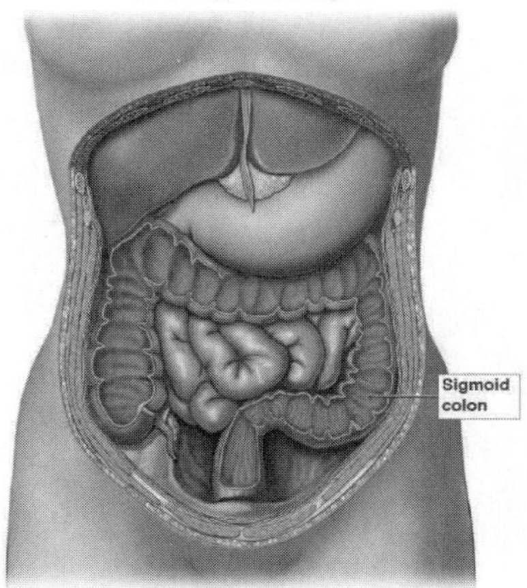

Initial Fecal Impaction

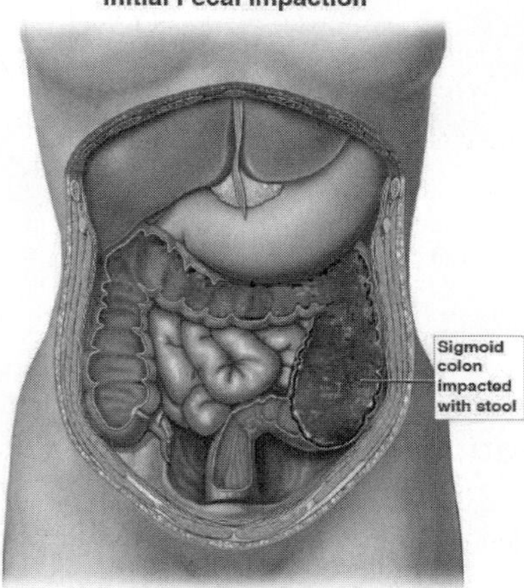

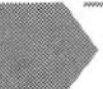

Concept Check

1. **What is the appearance of the bowel on colonoscopy when functional bowel disorder exists?**

   A. Cobblestone-like

   B. General irritation and redness

   C. Skip lesions present

   D. Normal

Answer question

LO1:

Clinical Relevance: Constipation

- Constipation is the most common gastrointestinal complaint.
- Prevalence of this complaint in the population is estimated at 12–19%.
- Incidence of constipation increases with aging.
- Constipation may progress to obstipation and bowel obstruction if not treated.

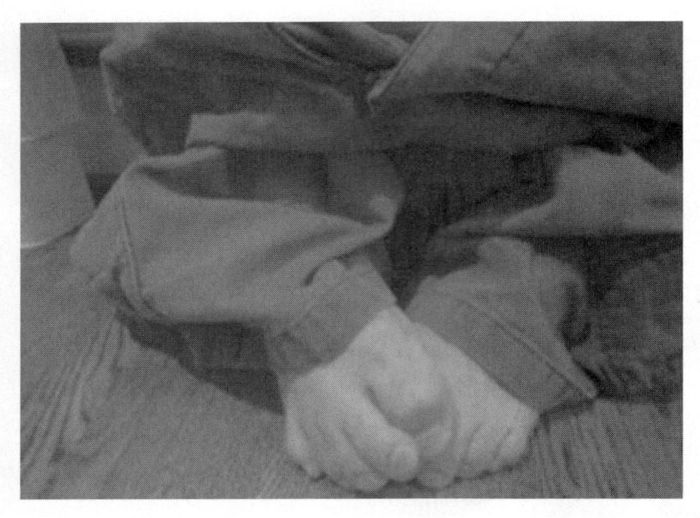

Chronic constipation (known as obstipation) often causes dilation with accumulation of feces in the bowel. Constipation can leave one feeling miserable so natural and regular remedies can prevent longer term problems.

LO2:

Pathophysiology: Constipation

- Movement of stool through the colon is dependent on movement of the colon walls. Movement of the colon walls occurs in the form of peristalsis as well as a mixing or churning movement (haustral contractions).
- Mass movement only occurs several times a day, after meals. Distension of the stomach induces the gastrocolic reflex, and the reflex causes a segment of the colon to contract with a simultaneous relaxation of the distal colon. This coordinated action results in mass movement of stool into the rectum and induces the sensation or urge to defecate.
- If this sensation is ignored for a period of time, the urge to defecate usually goes away until a later time when there is movement of more stool into the rectum.
- The time it takes for stool to move through the colon is called transit time. This is affected by diet, hydration, and activity. Diet that is low in fiber decreases the bulk of stool. Dehydration changes the consistency of stool, making it harder.
- Diminished activity can also decrease the motility of the colon. In addition, a large number of medications (e.g., narcotics) can decrease the motility of the colon.
- Inability to relax the pelvic sphincter and pelvic floor muscles in order to defecate can also cause constipation.
- Patients who have sensory loss (e.g., spinal cord injury patients) may also develop constipation.
- Accumulation of stool in the sigmoid and rectum may eventually cause obstipation with an inability to pass stool or flatus.

Constipation Progression

- **Constipation** diagnosis is based on symptoms and is generally classified as having fewer than three bowel movements a week. Although the patient may have difficulty evacuating feces, constipation does not mean that the patient has a permanent loss of function.
- **Fecal impaction** is characterized by a large amount of hard, dry stool in the rectal vault or sigmoid colon that the patient is unable to pass or eliminate.
- **Obstipation** causes severe constipation with resulting inability to pass stool or flatus. When chronic and persistent, it can lead to intestinal obstruction. It has been referred to as obstinate constipation.
- **Obstruction** represents the most severe stage of this condition, when complete obstruction develops, causing vomiting (along with other lower GI symptoms).

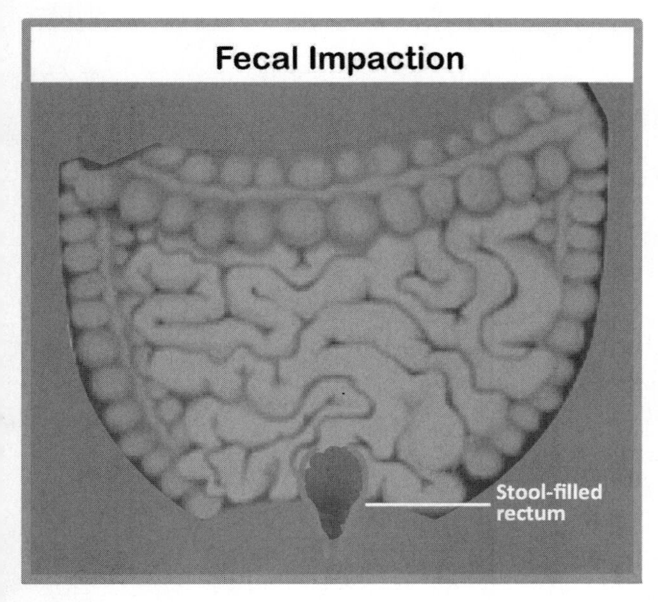

A fecal impaction occurs when the bulk is too large to pass without anal injury and severe pain. Bloody discharge or watery stool leakage without formed stool can occur and mislead one to miss an impaction. However, continued pain, cramping and bloating in the rectal area should trigger concern.

Concept Check

2. Which condition can cause constipation?
   A. Drinking too much fluid
   B. Eating too much fatty food
   C. Not getting enough exercise
   D. Not getting enough sleep

Answer question

Pathophysiology: Constipation (continued)

Complications of Constipation

- Complications can lead to more serious problems and include:
  - Anal fissures
  - Fecal impaction
  - Bowel obstruction
  - Fecal incontinence
  - Megacolon
  - Volvulus
  - Rectal prolapse
  - Urinary retention
  - Syncope, from Valsalva maneuver when bearing down

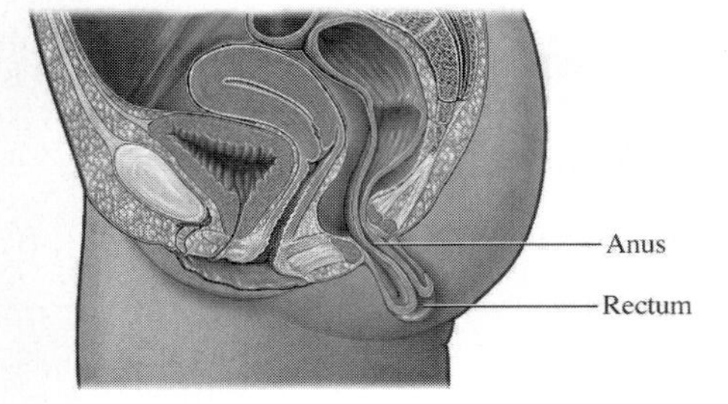

This illustration shows a rectal prolapse.

LO2:

Risk Factors: Constipation

Modifiable Risk Factors

- Low fiber diet: Fiber tends to absorb water and adds bulk to stool, resulting in a softer, larger volume of stool. This allows easy passage of stool.
- Low liquid intake or dehydration, primarily drinking liquids that have diuretic effects (e.g., coffee)
- Physical inactivity
  - o Medications (e.g., opioids, calcium channel blockers) can decrease the motility of the bowel.

Nonmodifiable Risk Factors

- Age
- Gender: Women have a higher incidence of constipation than men.
- Genetics
- Ethnicity
- Family history
- Colonic dysmotility
- Colonic structural disease (e.g., large polyps, tumors)

LO2:

Causes: Constipation

Primary Constipation

- Normal transit constipation: most common type with normal rate of stool movement through the colon with perceived difficulty in defecation
- Slow-transit constipation: infrequent bowel movements with diminished urgency to defecate
- Poor bowel habits: ignoring the urge
- Pelvic floor dysfunction: motility dysfunction of pelvic floor structures or anal sphincter
- Irritable bowel syndrome may present with constipation and abdominal pain (discussed later in this lesson).

Secondary Constipation

- Low fiber diet and inactivity
- Structural problems (e.g., hemorrhoids, anal fissures, colonic strictures)
- Metabolic abnormalities (e.g., pregnancy, hypercalcemia, diabetes, hypokalemia, hypothyroidism)
- Connective tissue disease (e.g., scleroderma, amyloidosis)
- Medications:
  - o Opioids
  - o Antidepressants
  - o Antipsychotics
  - o Antacids
  - o Iron supplements
  - o Calcium channel blockers
  - o H2 blockers
  - o Proton pump inhibitors

LO2:

Assessment Findings: Constipation

- **Constipation** diagnosis is based on symptoms and is generally classified as having fewer than three bowel movements a week.
- A research standard for constipation was developed in 1988 (Rome criteria) and has undergone modifications since (Rome III):
  - o Fewer than three bowel movements/week
  - o Straining
  - o Lumpy and/or hard stools
  - o Sensation of anorectal obstruction
  - o Sensation of incomplete defecation
  - o Manual maneuvering required to defecate

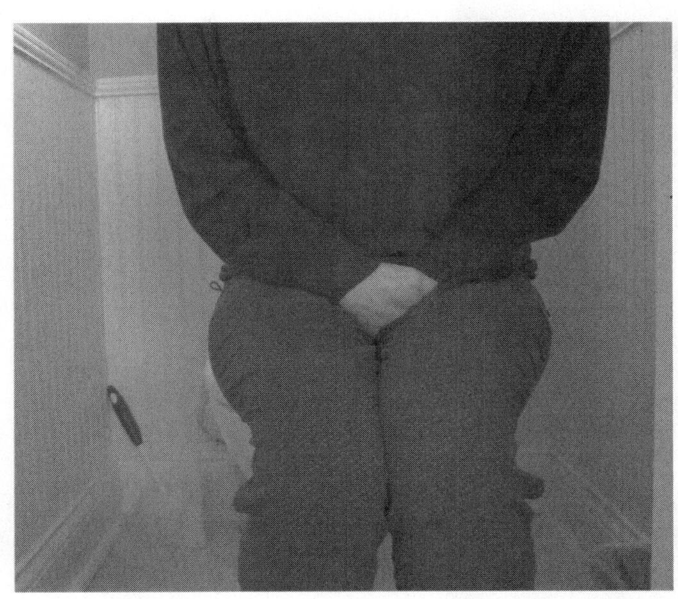

As people age, become less active, have dietary changes, and are not as well hydrated, constipation can be a growing challenge.
Source: Courtesy of K. Kyriakidis

LO2:

Diagnostics: Constipation

Labs:

- Lab tests can be performed to rule out metabolic causes (e.g., complete metabolic panel [CMP], calcium level, thyroid tests, CBC to determine if anemia is present, fecal occult blood test).

Imaging:

- X-rays, barium studies, and endoscopy may be performed to rule out structural causes, inflammatory disease, or tumors. These tests are often reserved for symptoms that do not respond to conservative therapy. They may also show evidence of obstruction.
- CT scan to evaluate for underlying cause such as malignancy

Constipation With Extensive Large Bowel Impaction

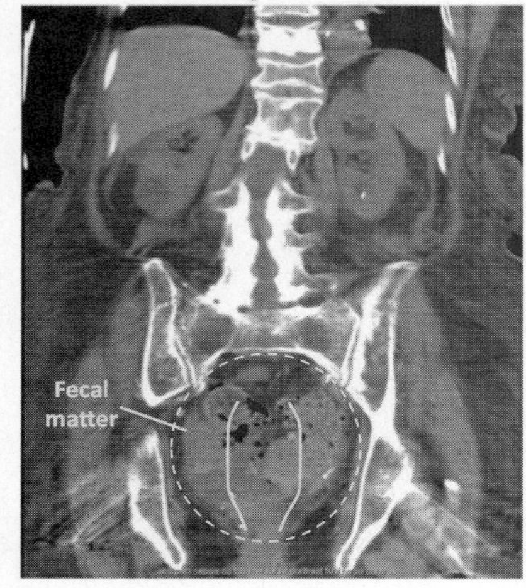

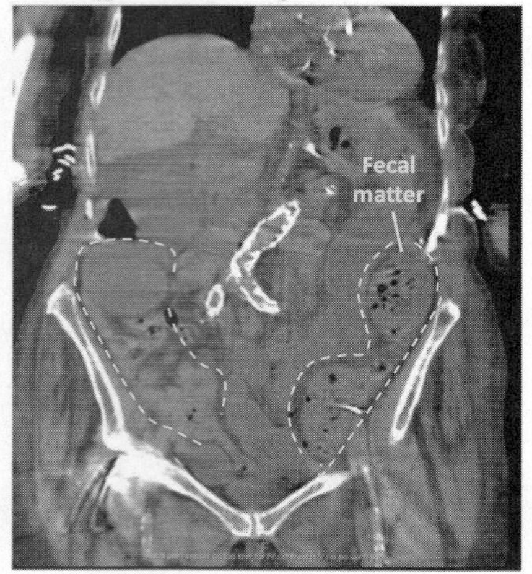

This abdominal CT scan reveals a large amount of fecal material in the rectum (left, in yellow). This shows a megarectum, revealing that this is not a new problem. The blue color outlines the shape of a normal rectum. Right: The second CT scan is the same patient in a closer view to see the colon. Note the extensive fecal material that is backed up throughout the colon, from cecum to rectum. The patient is experiencing an extensive fecal impaction.

Source: Courtesy of K. Kyriakidis

Endoscopy:

- Colonoscopy or endoscopy is helpful to evaluate for underlying cause if symptoms of constipation are new.
- Evaluation with laboratory, imaging, and/or endoscopy is usually reserved for patients who have continued symptoms despite conservative therapy, or whose history and physical indicates probability of secondary cause.

Colonoscopy Confirms the Cause of Constipation Seen on CT Scan

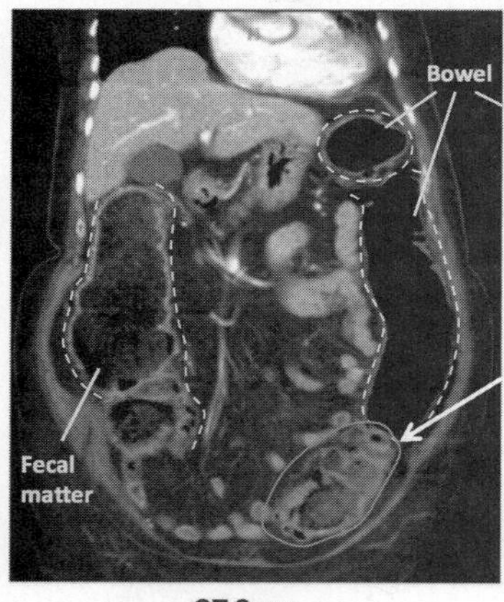

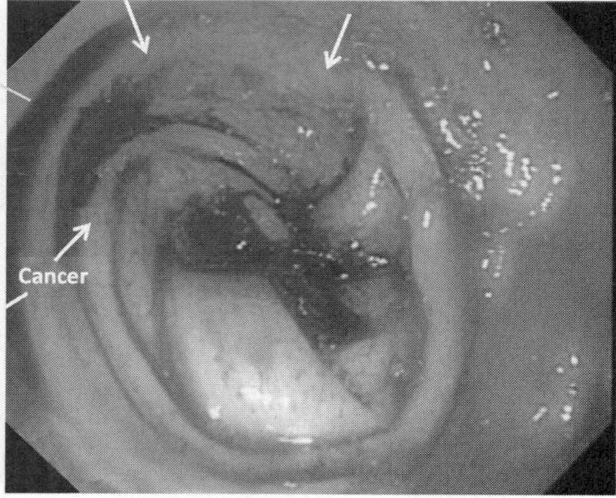

CT Scan **Colonoscopy**

Left: Constipation is seen on CT scan and has caused severe distension in the entire colon (yellow outline). The sigmoid colon mass is suspected to be cancer (red circle). Right: A malignant mass is found on colonoscopy that has invaded the colon and occluded it. Fecal matter cannot move forward, causing constipation.

Source: Courtesy of K. Kyriakidis

Concept Check

3. According to the Rome criteria, when does constipation exist?
   A. When the patient says it does
   B. When the patient reports that stools are hard to pass
   C. When the patient has fewer than three stools each week
   D. When the patient does not have a stool every day

Answer question

Priority Patient Concerns and Desired Collaborative Care Outcomes: Constipation

Prior to caring for patients with constipation, it is important to prioritize the patient's concerns that must guide the nursing care plan and interventions. Care for the patient is ordered and organized in accordance with the patient's priority and urgent needs. Desired collaborative care outcomes in patients with constipation typically include:

1. Patient will have a soft-formed bowel movement every 1–3 days without straining.
2. Patient will not experience abdominal discomfort.
3. Patient will increase dietary fiber, fluids, and daily exercise.
4. Patient will state ways to avoid constipation and prevent fecal impaction.
5. Patient will not experience infection.

Considering these important care outcomes, prepare a list of the major 3–6 priority patient concerns or nursing diagnoses for patients with constipation. Be prepared to participate in a discussion of this list and/or to submit them as an assignment, as determined by your faculty. Resources you may find helpful in this assignment can include this lesson, the references, resources on nursing care plans, and standard nursing diagnoses manuals.

LO3:

Collaborative Interventions: Constipation

Treatment is based on the cause.

- Currently, there is little evidence to show efficacy in interventions as there has been little research on these areas. These recommendations are based on the best expert opinion available in guidelines from respected organizations.
- N **Dietary management:** For uncomplicated primary constipation, dietary management is the cornerstone of treatment: A high fiber diet with adequate hydration is recommended unless the patient does not have adequate fluid intake. Fiber promotes soft stool that may be passed more easily and regularly while water prevents the fiber from becoming dry and hard.
- N EBP **Activity:** Exercise is recommended for those who have a sedentary lifestyle and can tolerate activity (Leung, et al., 2011).
- **Laxatives:**
  - M N EBP Osmotic laxatives work by retaining water in the intestinal tract. Start first with these simple and less expensive agents (e.g., magnesium hydroxide, polyethylene glycol, lactulose, sorbitol, magnesium, and phosphate salts) (Leung, et al., 2011).
  - M N EBP Bulk laxatives or fiber supplements are prescribed if increasing natural fiber in the diet does not work. Laxatives may not always be effective and can cause fecal impaction. They also should not be used with other laxatives (Leung, et al., 2011).
  - M N EBP Stool lubricating agents (e.g., mineral oil) (Leung, et al., 2011)
  - M N EBP Stool softeners (e.g., bisacodyl) (Leung, et al., 2011)
  - N EBP Stimulant laxatives work by stimulating movement in the colon. Stimulants (e.g., senna and bisacodyl) should be used only after the other simple laxatives have failed (Leung, et al., 2011). Note that some laxatives (e.g., bisacodyl) can have two purposes.
  - M N Enemas can assist in bowel evacuations.
  - M N Manual disimpaction may be necessary in some cases.

Patient Education

- The nurse should assess for causes of constipation. Some of the following questions may be useful in determining contributing factors of constipation:
  - o Can you describe your eating and drinking habits? (Dehydration and a low fiber diet can contribute to constipation.)
  - o What medications are you taking? (A side effect of many medications is constipation.)
  - o Tell me about your exercise habits. (Sedentary lifestyles contribute to constipation.)
  - o Have you had any recent abdominal surgeries, trauma, or problems? (Abdominal disorders can lead to bowel obstruction and/or constipation, pain, or fever.)
- The nurse is instrumental in teaching patients and their families about ways to prevent or avoid constipation through diet, exercise, and adequate hydration.
- Collaborating with other members of the health care team may be necessary if contributing factors are related to prescribed medications or procedures.
- Education is also necessary to teach the patient signs and symptoms to watch for and when to notify the health care providers. Symptoms include worsening abdominal distention, no bowel movement in over three days, pain, or fever.

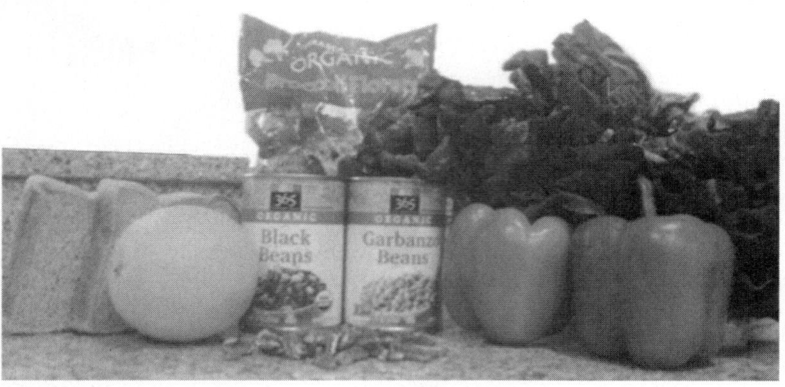

Source: Copyright © 2014, NovEx Novice to Expert Learning, LLC

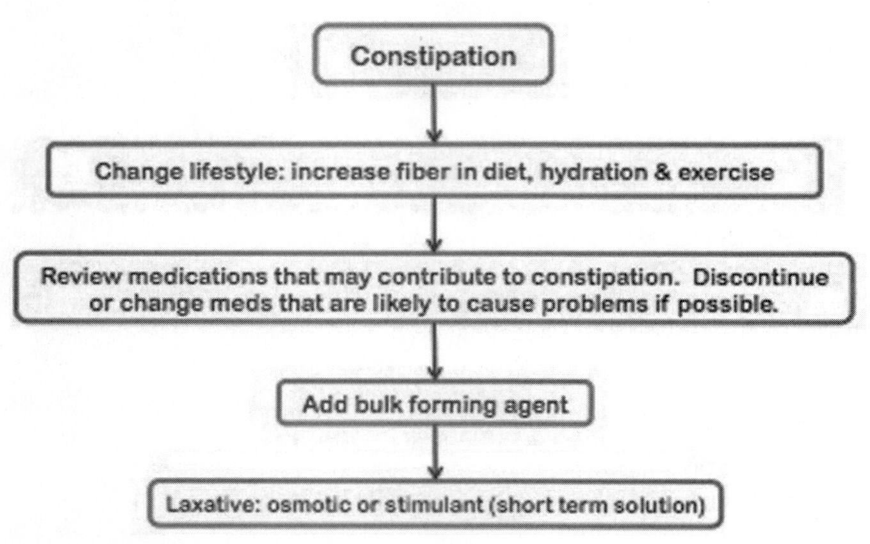

Source: Copyright © 2014, NovEx Novice to Expert Learning, LLC

Concept Check

4. What is the best description of how osmotic laxatives work?

a. Cause water to be retained in the bowel

b. Stimulate movement in the colon

c. Lubricate the stool mass

d. Soften the stool

Answer question

Collaborative Interventions: Constipation (continued)

Prevention

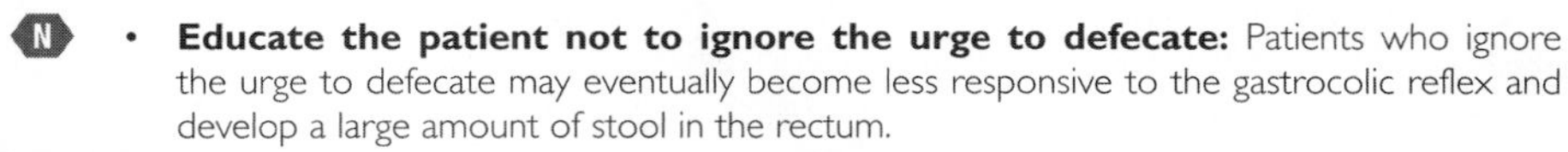

- **Educate the patient not to ignore the urge to defecate:** Patients who ignore the urge to defecate may eventually become less responsive to the gastrocolic reflex and develop a large amount of stool in the rectum.

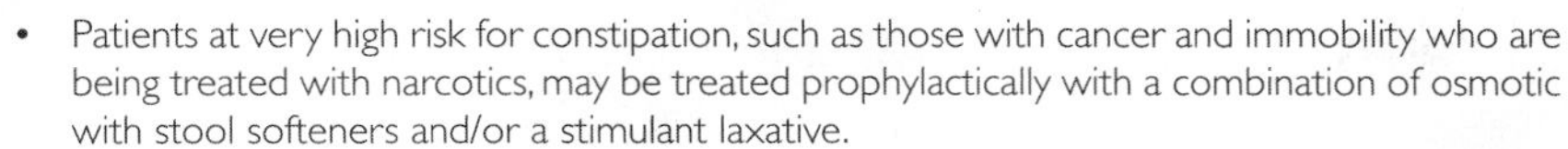

- Patients at very high risk for constipation, such as those with cancer and immobility who are being treated with narcotics, may be treated prophylactically with a combination of osmotic with stool softeners and/or a stimulant laxative.

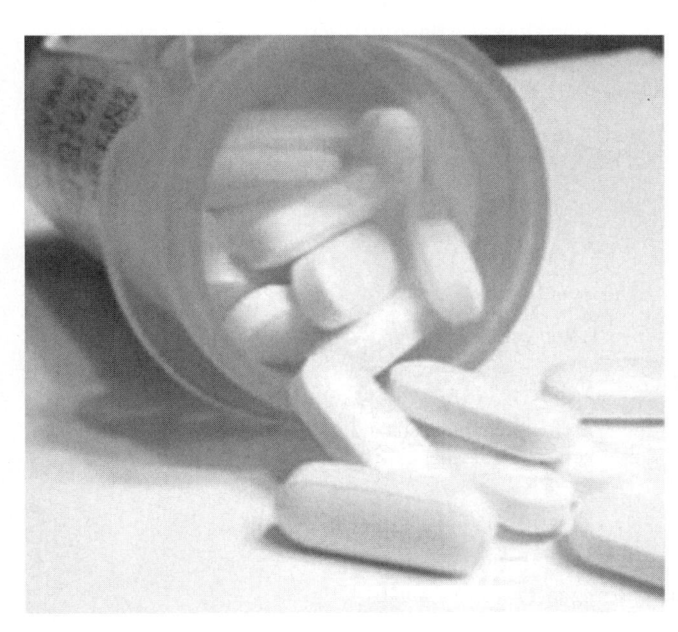

Painkillers, especially opioids or narcotics, can lead to constipation. Many narcotic receptors are in the intestines, so a narcotic can stop peristaltic action in the bowel. In general, a gentle laxative or stool softener should be considered for everyone on a narcotic. Some studies have even suggested that patients who chronically use pain relievers as mild as aspirin or ibuprofen are at a higher risk of constipation.
Source: Copyright © 2014, NovEx Novice to Expert Learning, LLC

Complications

- **Fecal impaction:** Patients with fecal impaction usually require manual disimpaction. Stool in the rectal vault is broken down into smaller pieces for easier passage. If an impaction is present in the sigmoid colon, the patient may require a sigmoidoscopy to help break up the stool. Disimpaction is indicated when diagnostic tests show fecal blockage or when hardened stool is palpated in the rectal vault.
- **Obstipation:** After management of acute episodes of constipation, patients should be treated for chronic constipation.

Pelvic Floor Dysfunction

- Patients with constipation due to pelvic floor dysfunction commonly do not respond as well to lifestyle changes and laxatives.
- These patients often respond to retraining of their pelvic floor muscles with biofeedback.

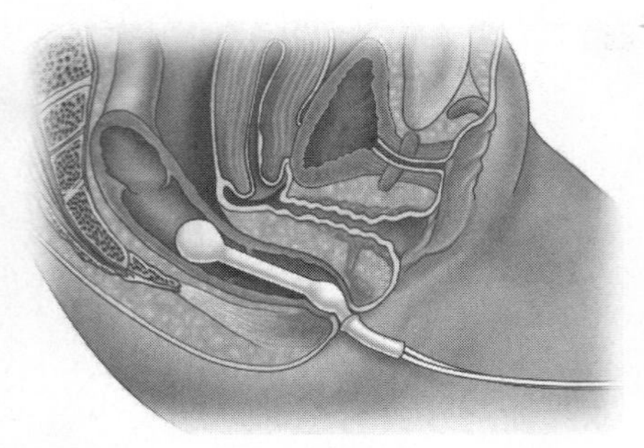

Biofeedback is a treatment that can be used for constipation due to pelvic floor dysfunction. It varies but often involves a few weeks of intensive outpatient training. It educates patients to improve their coordination of their pelvic floor and abdominal muscles in order to accomplish successful defecation.

Summary of Interventions: Constipation

- If initial history does not indicate a secondary cause, treatment is stepwise:
  1. Embrace lifestyle modification by increasing dietary fiber and hydration. Do not ignore the urge to defecate.
  2. Review medications that may cause constipation. Some may be discontinued, and others may be switched to alternatives that are less likely to cause constipation.
  3. Start with bulk laxatives.
  4. Follow with other laxatives, either osmotic or stimulants.
- Fecal impaction usually requires manual disimpaction.
- Patients with pelvic floor dysfunction may improve with retraining these muscles with biofeedback.
- Some patients with very high risk for constipation (e.g., patients being treated with narcotics and patients who are immobile) may be treated prophylactically with a combination of osmotic laxatives, stool softeners, or a stimulant laxative.

LO4:

Evaluation of Desired Collaborative Care Outcomes: Constipation

Evaluation and reassessment should reveal attainment of previously established patient outcomes. In summary:

- Patient reports having soft-formed stools every 1–3 days.
- Patient reports that abdominal discomfort has stopped.
- Patient describes a daily diet that includes additional fluids and fiber-rich foods and reports maintaining a daily exercise routine.
- Patient describes ways to avoid constipation and prevent fecal impaction.
- Patient has remained infection-free.

LO1:

What Is Irritable Bowel Syndrome?

- Irritable bowel syndrome (IBS) is described as a chronic syndrome of abdominal pain with altered bowel function (either frequent and recurrent loose bowel movements or constipation) and pain, with no discernible pathological findings.
- IBS can be debilitating and cause severe impairment in one's quality of life.
- There are subtypes of IBS. Diarrhea predominates in one type. Constipation predominates in another. Diarrhea and constipation may be mixed in the third type.
- The condition can vary throughout life. It may be episodic or continual.

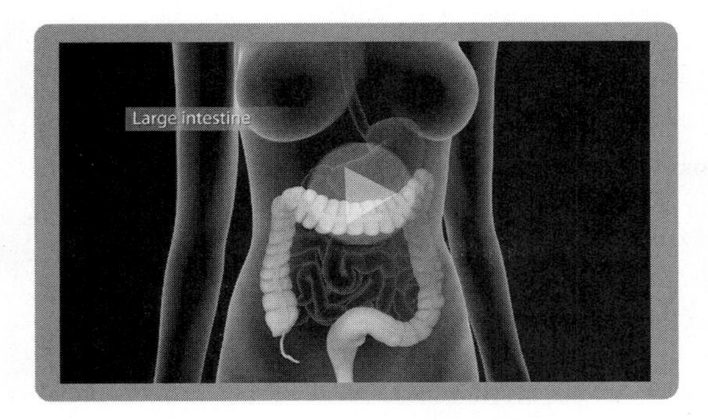

This animation provides an overview of irritable bowel syndrome. It reviews the pathophysiology, symptoms, and exacerbating factors that may aggravate IBS. The most common therapies are described.

LO1:

Clinical Relevance: IBS

- Incidence: IBS is the most common GI disorder.
- Women are 2 times more likely to develop IBS than men.
- The prevalence rate in the United States is 10–20% of the population.
- Fifty percent of patients report symptoms before the age of 35.
- Approximately 20–50% of gastrointestinal referrals are correlated to IBS symptoms.
- IBS does not affect mortality rates, risk of inflammatory bowel disease, or cancer.

LO2:

Pathophysiology: IBS

- IBS is also referred to as spastic colon or nervous colon.
- IBS does not seem to be associated with any structural, inflammatory, or infectious etiology involving the mucosal lining of the bowel. On endoscopy, the mucosal lining appears normal. Hence, a cause remains unidentified.
- Theories point to sensory or motor function impairment in the gastrointestinal system. Components that are theorized, but not conclusive, in the development of IBS include:
    - o Variations in GI motility, particularly with meals. Contractions may be too strong and cause rapid passage.
    - o In other situations, passage is too slow, causing hard, dry stools and constipation.
    - o Both rapid and slow variations in motility cause pain and discomfort.
    - o Increased sensitivity to visceral pain and bloating in the colon.
    - o Psychological component such as anxiety, panic and post-traumatic stress disorders, depression, eating disorders, and/or history of physical or sexual abuse.
- Initial IBS symptoms commonly present in the young adult.

LO2:

Risk Factors: IBS

- Family history: Having a first-degree relative such as a sibling or parent who had the condition places one at higher risk for IBS.
- Gender: female
- Analgesic use

LO2: Causes: IBS

- Exact causes are unknown.
- Common foods that produce symptoms can include caffeine, lactose in dairy products, fatty and/or spicy foods, carbonated drinks, alcohol, gastric stimulants, chocolate, various fruits and vegetables, and sorbitol in sweeteners.
- Individual responses vary but may also be elicited by strong emotions and medications:
  - o Emotions can include stress, mental illness, and anxiety.
  - o Medications can potentially trigger IBS: prolonged antibiotic use, sorbital-containing medications (e.g., cough syrup), antidepressants.
  - o Neurotransmitters, female reproductive hormones, and GI hormones may play a role but are not clearly understood. Menstruating women have more frequent IBS symptoms during their periods.
- Hyper and/or hypo GI motility can lead to IBS

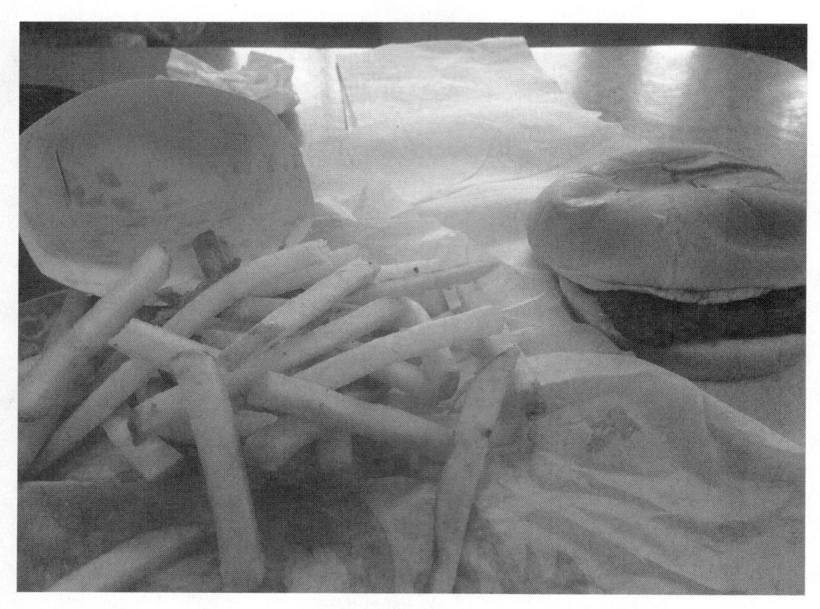

With IBS, patients must learn to avoid irritating foods, which make the bowel work harder to digest (acidic, fried, and processed). These foods become obvious, causing stomach discomfort with diarrhea or constipation, gas, cramping with pain, and bloating. Reducing or minimizing fat (the strongest GI stimulant) intake, meats, dairy, fried and processed food, nut butters, alcohol, smoking, coffee, and carbonated drinks is also recommended.

LO2: Assessment Findings: IBS

- Diarrhea or constipation: The pattern of IBS can vary between diarrhea, constipation, or a mixture of both, and commonly changes over time.
- Abdominal pain or cramping is diffuse in nature and is commonly precipitated by meals and relieved by defecation.
- Bloating and gas
- Clear or white mucous rectal discharge
- Dyspepsia, nausea, vomiting, urinary frequency, and sexual dysfunction have been reported.
- Physical findings are essentially negative except for reported symptomatology.

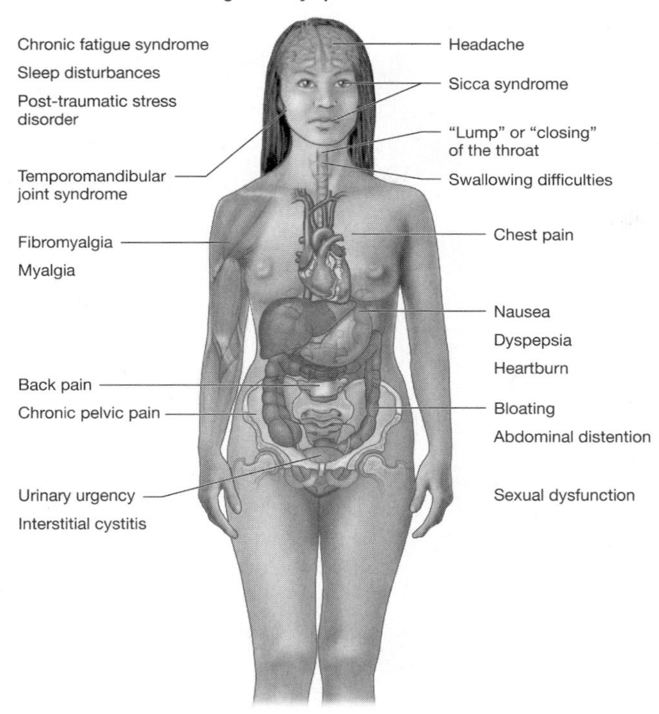

Generally, the signs and symptoms of IBS may wax and wane but begin in one's youth.

LO2:

Diagnostics: IBS

Laboratory testing and imaging is usually normal.
Diagnostics are needed to rule out other causes and abnormalities.

Labs:

- CBC to screen for anemia or infection
- CMP (metabolic panel) to screen for electrolyte imbalance or metabolic disorders
- Stool samples to rule out ova, parasites, Giardia, *Clostridium difficile* (*C. diff*), others
- Enteric pathogens
- Leucocytes
- Thyroid function tests
- Serum calcium to screen for hyperparathyroidism
- C-reactive protein and sedimentation rate as an indication of inflammation

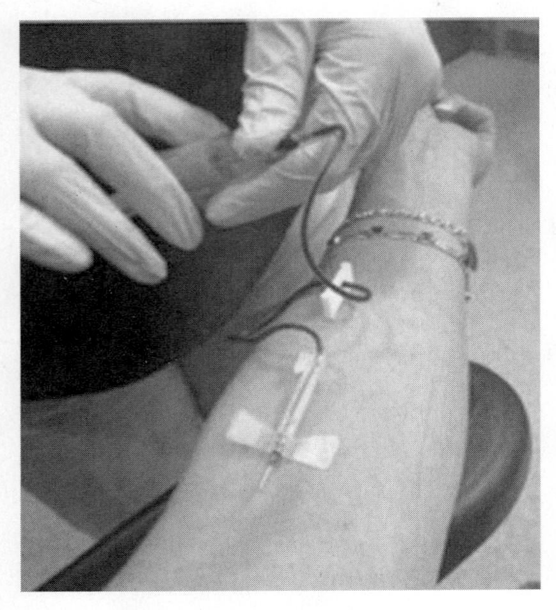

This photo illustrates one method for drawing blood for diagnostics.
Source: Copyright © 2014, NovEx Novice to Expert Learning, LLC

Imaging:

- Upper GI and/or lower GI barium studies to rule out other gastrointestinal diseases (see the animation in the Diverticulosis section of the Care of Patients with GI Structural Disorders NovE-lesson).
- CT scan to detect tumors, abscesses, obstruction, and pancreatic disease.

Endoscopy:

- Colonoscopy
- Esophagogastroduodenoscopy to evaluate for inflammatory bowel disease.
- In IBS, the diagnostic studies are typically normal.

Colonoscopy: Patient with Irritable Bowel

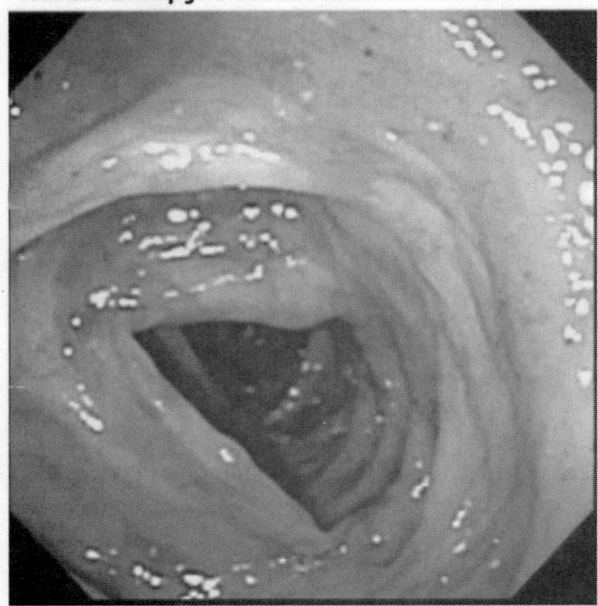

As is common in patients with IBS, this patient's ascending colon appears normal during colonoscopy of the large colon. There is no inflammation.
Source: Courtesy of K. Kyriakidis

Concept Check

5. What is true about the pain associated with irritable bowel syndrome?

A. It is often relieved by defecation.

B. It occurs most often when the patient is hungry.

C. It is sharp and discrete.

D. It is rarely accompanied by nausea.

Answer question

Priority Patient Concerns and Desired Collaborative Care Outcomes: IBS

Prior to caring for patients with IBS, it is important to prioritize the patient's concerns that must guide the nursing care plan and interventions. Care for the patient is ordered and organized in accordance with the patient's priority and urgent needs. Desired collaborative care outcomes in patients with IBS typically include:

1. Patient will experience soft, formed stools once or twice daily (pertains to both **constipation** and **diarrhea** nursing diagnoses).
2. Patient will verbalize effective treatment strategies for managing IBS.
3. Patient will experience reduction or no abdominal discomfort.
4. Patient will verbalize strategies to manage IBS symptoms in public settings.
5. Patient will verbalize feelings of self-acceptance and improvement in self-esteem.

Considering these important care outcomes, prepare a list of the major 3–6 priority patient concerns or nursing diagnoses for patients with IBS. Be prepared to participate in a discussion of this list and/or to submit them as an assignment, as determined by your faculty. Resources you may find helpful in this assignment can include this lesson, the references, resources on nursing care plans, and standard nursing diagnoses manuals.

LO3:

Collaborative Interventions: IBS

Psychological Support and Therapy

In some illnesses, support and/or therapy are often attempted if other interventions fail or fall short. However, these are paramount in IBS patients as these interventions have shown the most effectiveness.

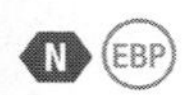

- Explore the patient's concerns, stressors, and anxieties. Naming the concerns can help the patient begin to manage them better (World Gastroenterology Organisation [WGO], 2009).

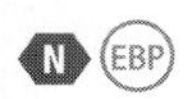

- Acknowledge the significance and impact of the IBS symptoms on the patient with the goal of reducing distress (WGO, 2009).

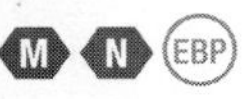

- Psychological support if anxiety, stress, or depression are precipitating factors (Brandt, et al., 2009). Collaborate with the patient to determine if longer term support is needed and assist patient to obtain a referral.

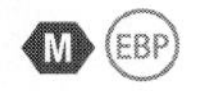

- Counseling, cognitive therapy, psychotherapy and hypnotherapy are often helpful, particularly if abuse or depression are components of the illness (Brandt, et al., 2009). Relaxation therapy has not shown effectiveness.

Patient Education

Educating patients with IBS about triggers is a key intervention in caring for and helping them learn to prevent episodes of pain, particularly in patients who can identify the triggers. Evidence does not show that all patients benefit from diet and lifestyle changes (WGO, 2009). Education needs to be tailored to the individual, but may include teaching about:

- Dietary modifications:

  - o Fiber or bulk supplements if tolerated by the patient to help manage constipation and diarrhea, such as wheat bran, linseeds, nuts, cereals, grains, vegetables, and seeds (McKenzie, et al., 2012); however, evidence does not strongly support the effectiveness.
  - o Avoid caffeine.
  - o Limited lactose, fructose, gas-promoting foods, foods to which patient is allergic
  - o Avoid foods that patient knows will trigger IBS symptoms.
  - o Supplemental calcium

- Regular exercise and activity

Medications

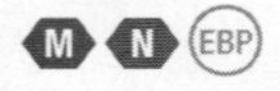

- Complementary therapies: Studies on peppermint oil and probiotics show some efficacy. Evidence supporting acupuncture and specific herbs are inconclusive (American College of Gastroenterology, 2009; McKenzie, et al., 2012).

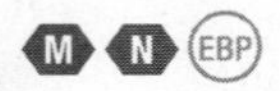

- Antidiarrheals can help reduce diarrheal stools, the urgency often experienced, and stool soiling: Imodium (loperamide), diphenoxylate, atropine (Brandt, et al., 2009). However, evidence does not strongly support the effectiveness.

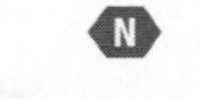

- Bulk laxatives with fiber are used for constipation: Metamucil, methylcellulose, psyllium. Fiber may help some IBS patients.

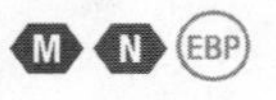

- Tricyclic antidepressants if the patient experiences frequent or severe pain: amitriptyline, chloride-channel activator, that is, lubiprostone (Brandt, et al., 2009).

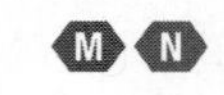

- Antispasmodics/anticholinergics to reduce abdominal pain (e.g., hyoscyamine, dicyclomine, atropine, belladonna). Evidence regarding effectiveness is weak.

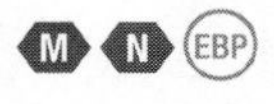

- $5HT_4$ (serotonin) receptor agonists or selective serotonin reuptake inhibitor (SSRI) to relieve IBS symptoms: In patients with severe problems, a gastroenterologist may administer $5HT_4$ receptor agonists (Brandt, et al., 2009).

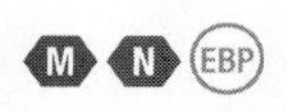

- Analgesics may be required for a few patients with severe pain. Paracetamol is preferred. Opiates place IBS patients at high risk for dependence and should be avoided. NSAIDs are not a drug of choice due to the GI adverse effects (WGO, 2009).

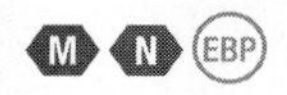

- Antibiotics (e.g., rifaximin), a short course, may have some effectiveness (Brandt, et al., 2009).

Summary of Interventions: IBS

Irritable bowel syndrome is usually managed by treating symptoms:

- Provide psychological support for stressors that trigger IBS flare-ups.
- Providing fiber in the diet may help symptoms of both diarrhea and constipation.
- Modify lifestyle to improve exercise and avoid foods that knowingly precipitate symptoms.
- Peppermint oil and quality probiotics with some to moderate effectiveness.
- Prescription medications can help:
  - o Pain: antispasmodics, tricyclic antidepressants, or SSRI
  - o Constipation: dietary modifications
  - o Diarrhea: bulking agents or antidiarrheals with symptoms of diarrhea.

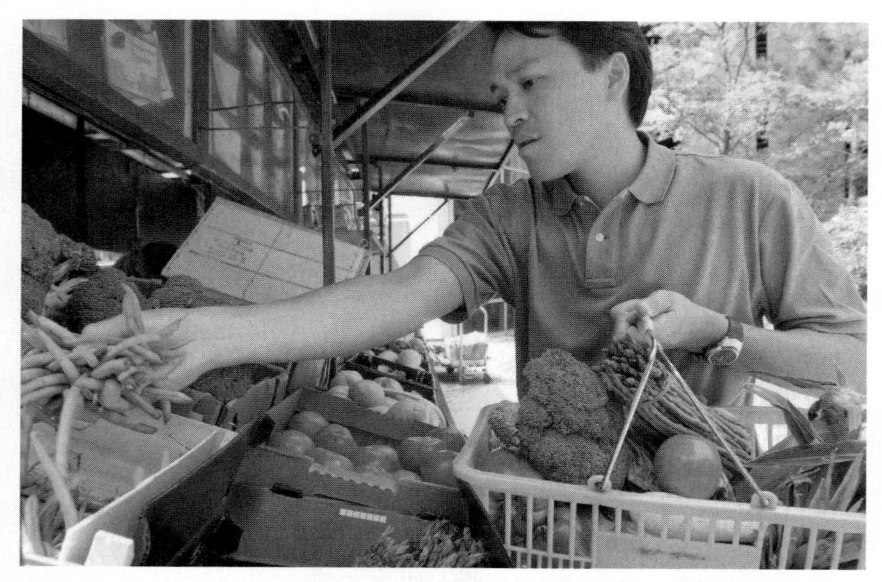

High fiber foods are often effective in a diet for IBS patients. Beans, vegetables, fruits, and whole grain foods should top the list. Fruits that are more acidic may adversely affect the patient unless eaten in small amounts. For patients who are increasing their fiber intake, gradually adding higher fiber foods to the diet can help become acclimated over time.
Source: CDC/Amanda Mills

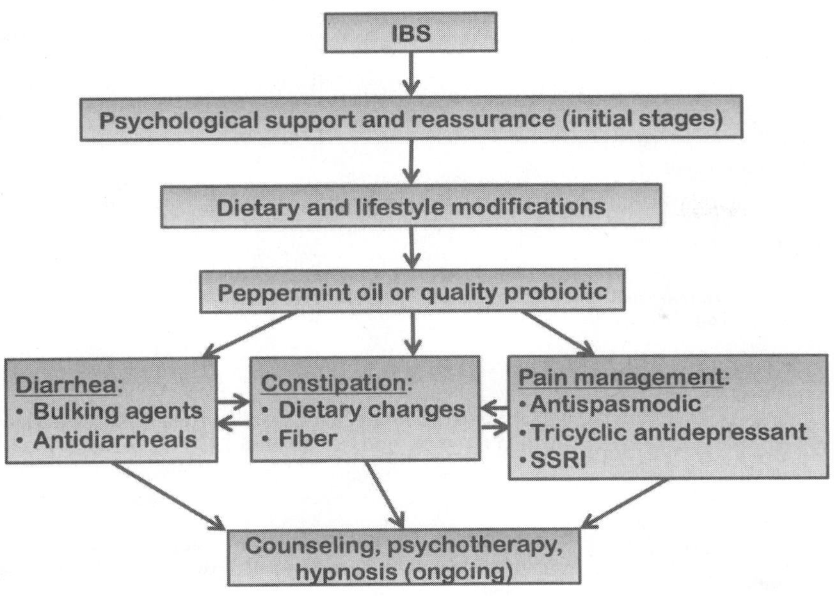

Algorithm of interventions for patients with IBS.

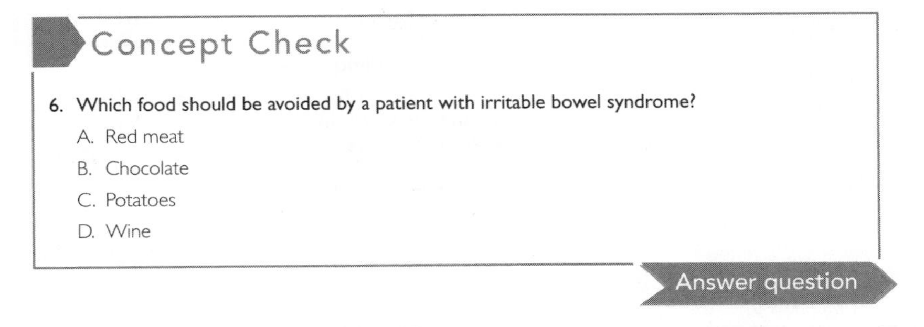

Concept Check

6. **Which food should be avoided by a patient with irritable bowel syndrome?**
   A. Red meat
   B. Chocolate
   C. Potatoes
   D. Wine

Answer question

LO4:

Evaluation of Desired Collaborative Care Outcomes: IBS

Evaluation and reassessment should reveal attainment of previously established patient outcomes. In summary:

- Patient reports having at least one and no more than two soft, formed stools daily.
- Patient discusses methods to decrease IBS symptoms and periods of IBS exacerbations.
- Patient reports less frequent episodes of abdominal discomfort that are of less intensity than before treatments began.
- Patient reports that personal plan to manage IBS in social settings has been successful.
- Patient expresses feeling more self-confident.

Concept Check

7. **What should be included in education for a patient who has irritable bowel syndrome?**
   A. Increasing sleep to no less than 8 hours each day
   B. How to identify foods that exacerbate symptoms
   C. Use of NSAIDs to control discomfort
   D. Need to reduce calcium in the diet

Answer question

References

American Gastroenterological Association. (2002). American Gastroenterological Association Medical position statement: Irritable bowel syndrome. *Gastroenterology, 123*(6), 2105–2107. **www.med.upenn.edu/gastro/documents/AGApositionstatementirritablebowelsyndrome.pdf**

Bassotti, G., Chistolini, F., Sietchiping-Nzepa, F., et al. (2004). Biofeedback for pelvic floor dysfunction in constipation. *Brit Med J. 328*(7436), 393–396. **www.ncbi.nlm.nih.gov/pmc/articles/PMC341393/**

Boivin, M. (2001). Socioeconomic impact of irritable bowel syndrome in Canada. *Can. J. Gastroenterol, 15*(Suppl B), 8B–11B. **www.mayoclinic.org/diseases-conditions/irritable-bowel-syndrome/basics/definition/con-20024578**

Collins, B., & Burch, J. (2009). Constipation, treatment and biofeedback therapy. *British Jour of Community Nursing, 4,* 1, 28, 30, 32–35.

Locke, G. R., Pemberton, J. H., & Phillips, S. F. (2000). American Gastroenterological Association Medical Position Statement: Guidelines on constipation. *Gastroenterology, 119*(6), 1761–1766. **www.med.upenn.edu/gastro/documents/AGApositionstatementconstipation.pdf**

McCallum, I. J. D., Ong, S., & Mercer-Jones, M. (2009). Chronic constipation in adults. *Brit Med J, 338,* b831. **http://dx.doi.org/10.1136/bmj.b831**

Wald, A. (2007). Chronic constipation, advances in management. *Neurogastroenterology and Motility, 19,* 1, 4–10.

Wald, A., Kamm, M. A., Muller-Lissner, S. A., et al. (2006). The BI Omnibus Study: An international survey of community prevalence of constipation and laxative use in adults. *Digestive Disorders Week,* Abstract T1255.

Clinical Practice Guidelines

Brandt, L., Chey, W., Foxx-Orenstein, A. E., et al. (2009). An evidence-based systemic review on the management of irritable bowel syndrome: American College of Gastroenterology task force on IBS. *Amer J of Gastroenterology, 104*(Suppl 1), 1–40. **s3.gi.org/wp-content/uploads/2011/07/institute-IBS_Supplement_AmJGastro.pdf**

Leung, L., Riutta, T., et al. (2011). Chronic constipation: An evidenced-based review. *J Am Board Fam Med, 24,* 436–451. doi:10.3122/jabfm.2011.04.100272. **www.jabfm.org/citmgr?gca=jabfp;24/4/436**

McKenzie, Y. A., Alder, A., Anderson, W., et al., on behalf of the Gastroenterology Specialist Group of the British Dietetic Association. (2012). British Dietetic Association evidence-based guidelines for the dietary management of irritable bowel syndrome in adults. *J Hum Nutr Diet. 25*(3), 260–274. **onlinelibrary.wiley.com/doi/10.1111/j.1365-277X.2012.01242.x/abstract**

World Gastroenterology Organisation (WGO). (2009). *World Gastroenterology Organisation Global guideline: Irritable bowel syndrome: A global perspective.* Munich, Germany: World Gastroenterology Organisation. **www.worldgastroenterology.org/assets/downloads/en/pdf/guidelines/20_irritable_bowel_syndrome.pdf**

Patient Education

Drossman, D. A. (2013). *American Gastroenterological Association Patient Center: Understanding constipation.* **www.gastro.org/patient-center/digestive-conditions/constipation**

Mayo Clinic. (2011). *Irritable bowel syndrome.* **www.mayoclinic.org/diseases-conditions/irritable-bowel-syndrome/basics/definition/con-20024578**

STOP

Go to the online course and complete the NovE-Cases assigned by your instructor for this module.

Learning Outcomes for UTI

When you complete this lesson, you will be able to:

1. Recognize the clinical relevance of urinary tract infection and catheter-associated urinary tract infection.
2. Consider the pathophysiology, etiology, risk factors, and clinical presentation of urinary tract infection and catheter-associated urinary tract infection that determine the priority patient concerns.
3. Determine the most urgent and important nursing interventions and patient education required in caring for a patient with urinary tract infection or catheter-associated urinary tract infection.
4. Evaluate attainment of desired collaborative care outcomes for a patient with urinary tract infection or catheter-associated urinary tract infection.

LO1:

What Is a Urinary Tract Infection?

- A urinary tract infection (UTI) is an infection of the kidney, ureter, bladder, urethra, and/or prostate.
- The Centers for Disease Control and Prevention defines a UTI as a bacteriuria or positive urine culture of "$\geq 10^5$ colony forming units (cfu)/mL" with two or fewer infecting pathogens.
- A catheter-associated urinary tract infection (CAUTI) is a UTI that occurs with an indwelling urinary catheter (IUC) in place. Organisms use the catheter as an entry mechanism into the urinary system.

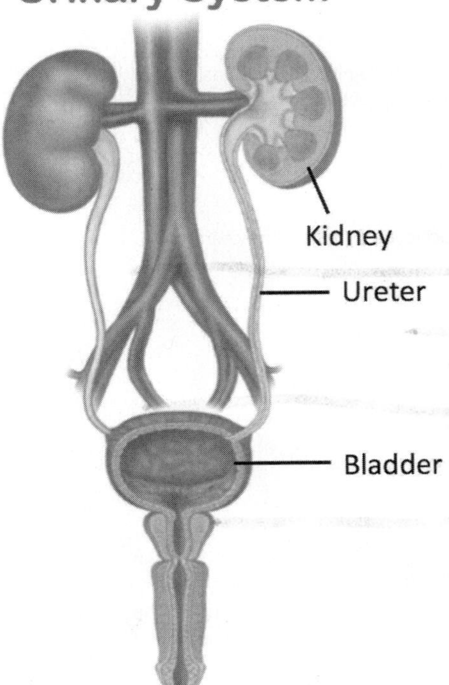

The urinary system tract and its vasculature (with the kidneys) are shown.

LO1:

Clinical Relevance

- A UTI is a frequent problem in the nonhospitalized patient and can often be prevented with simple measures.
- A UTI is also the most common nosocomial (health care acquired) infection, accounting for 20% of hospital-acquired bacteremias.
- Of hospital-acquired UTIs, 75% are associated with indwelling catheters.
- UTIs account for significant hospital complications and costs.
- Most of these nosocomial UTIs are associated with an IUC and are called CAUTI.
- A CAUTI is considered one of the nonreimbursable complications by the Centers for Medicare and Medicaid Services.
- Incidence can be decreased by using urinary catheters only when necessary.

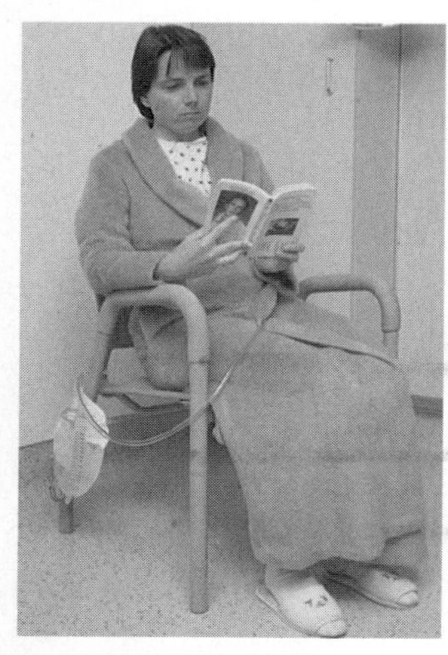

This image represents an indwelling urinary catheter in a bladder, a cause of many UTIs.

- Prevention of UTIs and CAUTIs is among the top 2014 and 2012 Hospital National Patient Safety goals that are proposed by the Joint Commission to improve patient safety.

LO2:

Pathophysiology

- Normally, the urinary tract and urine are sterile. This is achieved by several mechanisms:
  - o Sphincters in the urinary tract allow unidirectional flow of urine toward the urethral opening.
  - o Acidic pH of urine prevents or inhibits bacterial growth.
  - o Immune system responds to fight foreign invaders.
- Due to the close proximity of the rectum, fecal bacteria can colonize the perineum, migrate to the urethra, and then into the bladder.
- In women, the urethra is shorter and the opening is closer to the anus, making women much more susceptible to infections.
- Colonization occurs through the adhesion of bacteria to the lining of the bladder.
- Toxins released by the bacteria cause an inflammatory response. This response results in cytokine release and the attraction of white blood cells (WBCs) into the area, which phagocytize the bacteria. If the immune system is overwhelmed, bacteria eventually enter the bladder to cause an overgrowth of colonies.
- Epithelial cell death then occurs.
- Infection is differentiated from colonization by the presence of damage and inflammation.
- Upper urinary tract infections occur when bacteria ascend the ureters to infect the kidneys. This upper UTI is called pyelonephritis.
- Infections of the lower urinary tract are:
  - o Urethra—urethritis
  - o Prostate—prostatitis
  - o Bladder—cystitis

- Recurrent and/or severe kidney infections can cause damage and scarring with permanent loss of kidney function.
- Bacteria can also infect the urinary tract hematogenously (through the blood), but this is much less common.

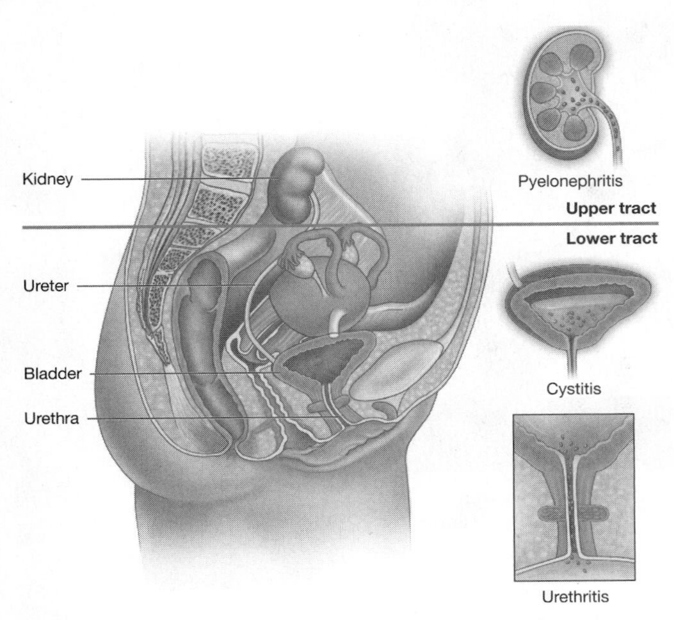

The upper and lower types of UTIs are shown above, as related to the organs affected.

Complicated UTI

- Complicated UTIs are UTIs that occur in the setting of a structural or functional abnormality of the urinary tract.
- Many of these abnormalities are due to mechanical obstruction or neurologic abnormalities that lead to improper emptying of the bladder:
  - o Mechanical obstruction can be due to either congenital abnormalities that interfere with urine flow or acquired mechanical obstructions, such as kidney stones or benign prostatic hypertrophy.
  - o UTIs due to immunosuppression (e.g., patients on chemotherapy or who have diabetes) are also considered complicated.
- Patients with indwelling catheters are at very high risk for infection.
  - o Bacteria are introduced into the urinary tract with the catheters.
  - o Bacteria also grow in colonies on the surface of catheters in a slimy environment that they produce, called a biofilm (see photo).

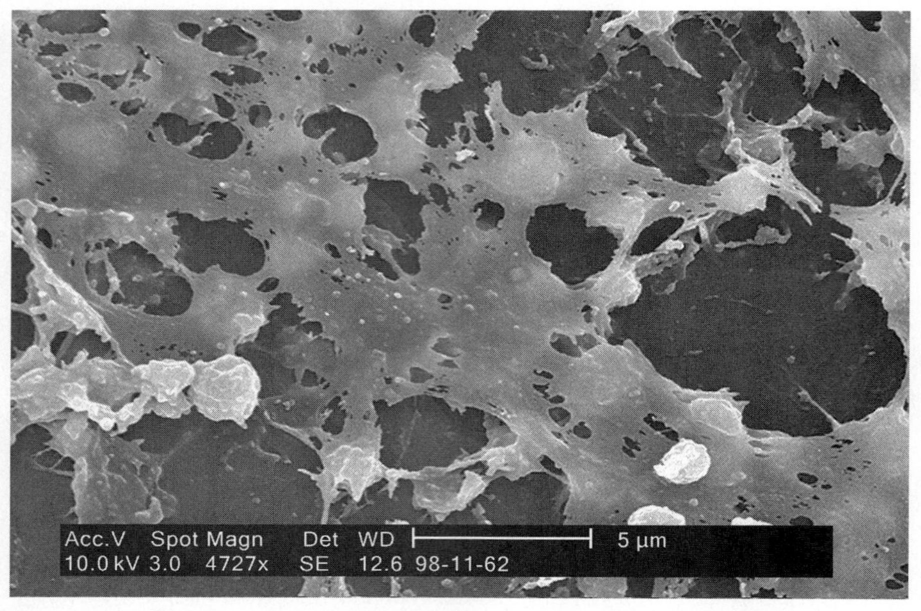

Staphylococcus aureus (whitish, round organisms) are shown on the surface of an IUC. An electron scanning microscope reveals the sticky-looking substance (a biofilm) that the bacteria are woven into and protect them from antibiotic attacks.
Sources: CDC/Rodney M. Donlan, Ph.D., & Janice Carr

- o Bacteria secrete substances that promote growth and protect them from eradication with antibiotics.
- o Biofilms can form on almost any foreign substance (e.g., central line catheters, prosthetic devices, joint prostheses).

Concept Check

1. **A patient hospitalized with pyelonephritis has an infection of which tissues?**
   A. Kidney
   B. Prostate
   C. Bladder
   D. Urethra

Answer question

LO2:

Risk Factors and Causes

UTI

- Kidney stones
- Bacteremia
- Sexual intercourse, frequent or with new partner
- Enlarged prostate
- Wiping from back to front after toileting
- Spermicide use increases susceptibility.
- Incomplete emptying of the bladder
- Enlarged prostates in men over 50 years of age

CAUTI

- Contamination of IUC
- Prolonged use of IUC
- Break in sterile technique during insertion of IUC
- Opening the closed drainage system of IUC
- Reflux of urine from the drainage system of IUC back into the patient

Concept Check

2. Which UTI would be considered complicated?

A. The patient is under 10 years of age.

B. The patient has a stricture in the urethra.

C. The patient is over 70 years of age.

D. The patient just recovered from a respiratory infection.

Answer question

Causative Organisms

Simple UTI

- *E. coli*
- *Staphylococcus saprophyticus*
- *Klebsiella*
- *Enterococcus*
- *Proteus mirabilis*

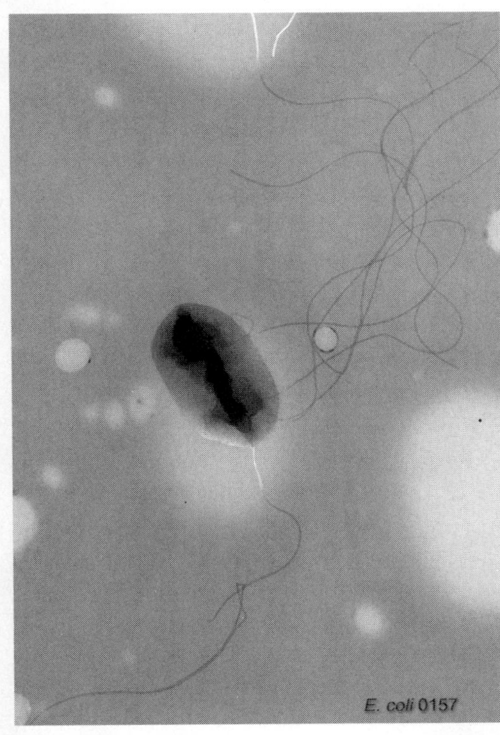

The main causal agent in UTIs is *Escherichia coli*. Although urine contains a variety of fluids, salts, and waste products, bacteria are not normally present. Look up close to see the distinguishing flagella (red tail) on the *E. coli* bacteria.
Source: CDC/Peggy S. Hayes & Elizabeth H. White, M.S.

Complicated

- *Pseudomonas*
- *Enterobacter*
- *Serratia*
- Candida (fungal)
- *Citrobacter*

(in addition to the organisms for uncomplicated UTIs)

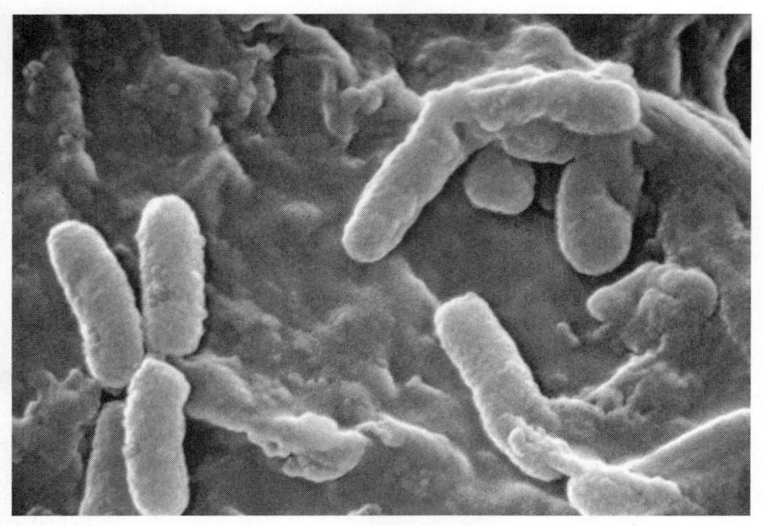

Pseudomonas aeruginosa survives even harsh environments as it is a tough bacterial strain. It is a fairly common in sicker or less healthy patients and is a known opportunistic microorganism. Sick patients can develop a serious urinary infection.
Source: CDC/Janice Haney Carr

Additional Risk Factors

- A key nursing responsibility is identification of high-risk patients on admission.
- Patients with the following risk factors require a higher level of vigilance in monitoring for and prevention of a UTI:
  - Older and immobilized patients
  - Patients who are immunocompromised
  - Patients with diabetes
  - Patients who are catheterized, particularly women
  - Men with enlarged prostate and over 50 years of age
  - Patients with urinary incontinence
- The risk of acquiring a CAUTI depends on:
  - Duration of IUC use
  - The quality of the catheter care
  - Host susceptibility

LO2:

Assessment Findings

UTI

- **Systemic signs** (more common with pyelonephritis and acute bacterial prostatitis) include:
  - Fever >38°C (100.4°F)
  - Nausea or vomiting
  - Altered mental status (a common presenting sign in older adults and patients who are debilitated)
  - Hypotension
  - Systemic inflammatory response (tachycardia, tachypnea, fever, elevated white blood cell count)
- **Cystitis-specific** symptoms include:
  - Dysuria or pain on urination: usually a burning sensation
  - Urinary frequency: abnormal frequent urinating, usually small amounts at a time
  - Urinary urgency: an intense and immediate desire to urinate
  - Pain or tenderness in suprapubic area
  - Bloody, foul smelling, cloudy urine

- **Pyelonephritis:** Patients with pyelonephritis commonly have cystitis. Additional signs and symptoms include:
  - o Costovertebral tenderness (tenderness to percussion over the affected kidney)
- Patients with an IUC do not have symptoms of urgency, dysuria, and frequency.

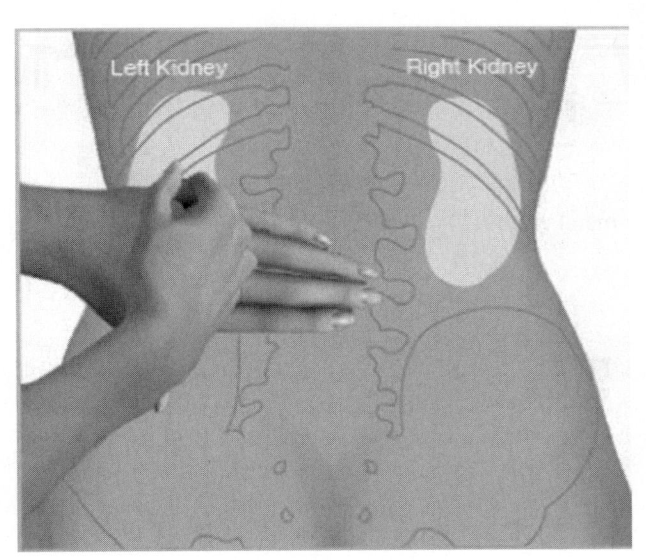

Tenderness to percussion over the flank area is a sign of infection of that kidney.
Source: Copyright © 2014, NovEx Novice to Expert Learning, LLC

Prostatitis

Acute bacterial prostatitis:

- Chills, fever
- Hematuria
- Dysuria
- Urinary frequency
- Pain in the perineal area, lower back, or testicles
- Pain with bowel movement
- Enlarged tender prostate on digital examination
- It is uncommon for men to develop cystitis.

Chronic bacterial prostatitis:

- Signs tend to be more subtle.
- Possible low-grade fever
- Frequency (more often than the patient's normal)
- Dysuria
- Perineal discomfort

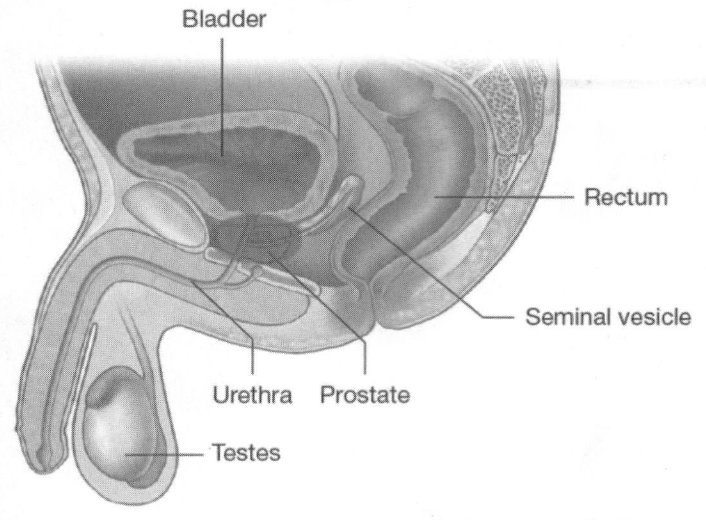

Prostatitis, or inflammation of the prostate gland, mostly affects young and middle-aged men.

LO2:

Diagnostics

Urinalysis

- The presence of signs and symptoms typical of a UTI should lead the clinician to suspect a UTI.
- Urine analysis shows presence of WBCs, a condition called pyuria, indicating an inflammatory process. Analysis may also show RBCs. More than 10 WBCs may indicate an infection.

- Dipstick testing for UTI is not appropriate in catheterized patients (Davey, et al., 2012).
- Urine culture data show the organism(s) that are present. Normally, urine is sterile so the presence of bacteria is considered abnormal.
- Bacteria produce an enzyme that converts nitrates to nitrites. Presence of nitrites in urine is indicative of a bacterial infection.
- WBCs produce leukocyte esterase (LE). The urine LE test detects their presence.
- Caution: The presence of many squamous cells that originate from the skin often indicate that the urine was not collected properly and is contaminated.

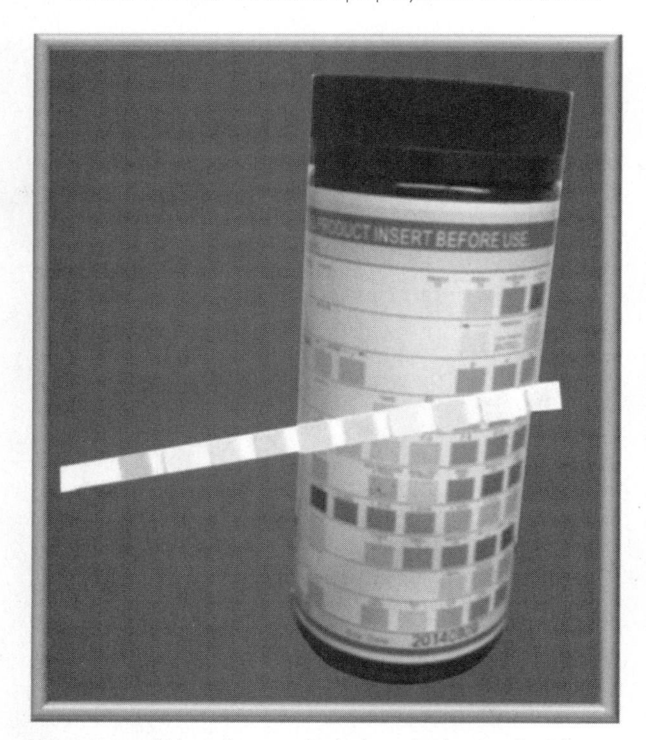

Urine nitrite, which can be recognized using a simple urine dipstick, can help determine the presence of a bacterial infection.

Urine Specimen

- Routine urinalysis and urine cultures from IUCs are unnecessary:
  - o Cloudy or malodorous urine is not necessarily an indication for culture.
  - o Obtain urine for culture based on clinical signs of infection such as fever, chills, and dysuria.
- The quality of the urine specimen is very important when assessing for a UTI.
- The specimen of choice is the first morning void using a midstream, clean catch technique (in a noncatheterized patient).
- Urine collected from a newly inserted catheter is reliable as long as the catheter was inserted aseptically.
- If a CAUTI is suspected and the patient requires a continued indwelling catheter, it is best to remove the old catheter, insert an entirely new IUC system, and obtain a urine specimen from the new catheter. This eliminates the possibility of biofilm (buildup of bacteria on the IUC), which can contaminate the specimen.
- To ensure accuracy of a urine culture taken from the catheter, the urine specimen should be collected aseptically from the sampling port close to the distal end of the urinary catheter. Cleanse the port with a disinfectant and use a sterile syringe/device to obtain the small amount of urine to be tested.
- When larger amounts of urine are needed for nonculture testing, the specimen should be collected by draining it from the collection bag.

Concept Check

3. **What is pyuria?**
   A. A reddish discoloration of the urine
   B. Decreased urine flow
   C. Presence of WBCs in the urine
   D. An increased pH of the urine

Answer question

Diagnostics (continued)

UTI

Asymptomatic Bacteriuria

- Patient is asymptomatic but bacteria counts from collected urine are:
  - o Greater than 100,000 cfu*/mL in a midstream, clean catch specimen **or**
  - o Greater than 100 cfu/mL from a catheterized specimen

*cfu = colony forming unit, a measure of viable bacteria or fungal numbers

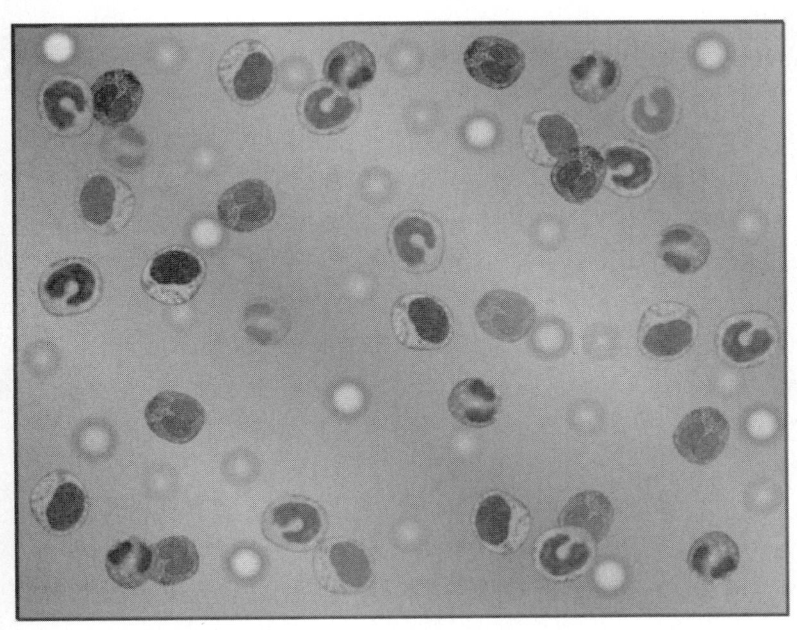

In this microscopic view, numerous white blood cells are seen in the urine sample.
Source: Copyright © 2014, NovEx Novice to Expert Learning, LLC

- Patients with asymptomatic bacteriuria can be divided into two groups:
  - o Those with infection
  - o Those without infection (colonization)
- Those with infection have pyuria with >10 colonies of bacteria/mL of urine.

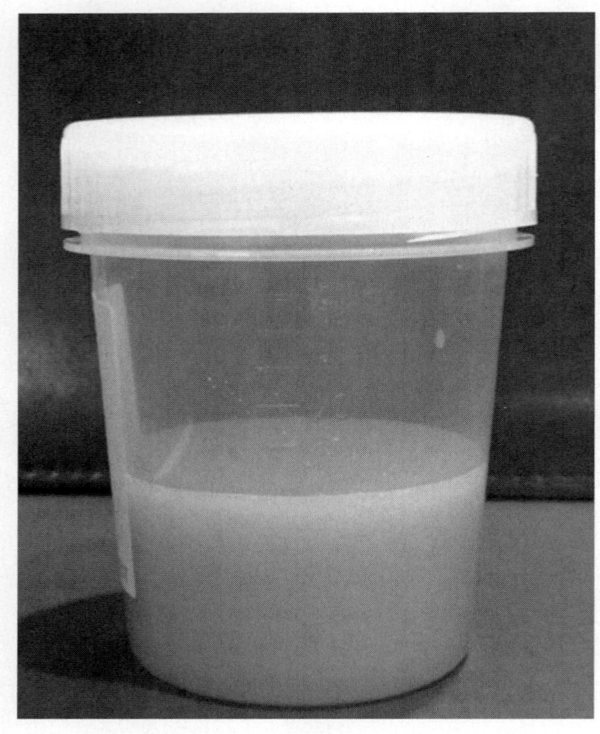

This urine sample is from a patient with pyuria. The cloudy appearance suggests the presence of pus.
Source: Courtesy of K. Kyriakidis

- However, there is no benefit in treating any patient with asymptomatic bacteriuria (except pregnant women).
- Inappropriate use of antibiotics can create antibiotic-resistant bacterial species.
- Nearly 100% of patients with a chronic indwelling urinary catheter have bacteriuria.

Symptomatic Bacteriuria

Defined as patients with both bacteriuria and symptoms.

- Complete blood count (CBC) shows neutrophilic leukocytosis (elevated neutrophils, e.g., >10,000 absolute neutrophils or neutrophils >70% of total WBC). A higher WBC count is more common with pyelonephritis than with cystitis.
- Blood cultures are frequently positive in pyelonephritis with the same organism found in both blood and urine cultures.
- Ultrasound may disclose renal stones, abscess, or hydronephrosis (could indicate an obstruction somewhere).
- CT scan of the abdomen and pelvis or a CT urogram (noncontrast, followed by IV contrast, then delayed images) is used to evaluate for renal obstruction or kidney stones.

Uropathogens	% in Uncomplicated Cases (approximate)
Escherichia Coli (50% are ampicillin resistant)	75-90%
Other gram negative: Proteus, Klebsiella, Citrobacter, Enterobacter, Pseudomonas	5-6%
Coag-negative Staphylococci	7-8%
Other gram positive: Enterococci, Streptococci, Staphylococcus aureus	2-3%

Priority Patient Concerns and Desired Collaborative Care Outcomes

Prior to caring for patients with UTIs, it is important to prioritize the patient's concerns that must guide the nursing care plan and interventions. Care for the patient is ordered and organized in accordance with the patient's priority and urgent needs. Desired collaborative care outcomes in patients with UTIs typically include:

1. Patient will report relief of UTI symptoms and return of baseline urinary elimination patterns.
2. Patient will report pain is absent or reduced to a tolerable level.
3. Patient will be able to perform ADLs without experiencing incontinence.
4. Patient will return to baseline level of social activities.
5. Patient will accurately discuss treatment plan and will use prevention strategies.

Considering these important care outcomes, prepare a list of the major 3–6 priority patient concerns or nursing diagnoses for patients with UTIs. Be prepared to participate in a discussion of this list and/or to submit them as an assignment, as determined by your faculty. Resources you may find helpful in this assignment can include this lesson, the references, resources on nursing care plans, and standard nursing diagnoses manuals.

LO3:

Collaborative Interventions

Cystitis

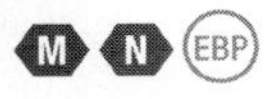

- Do not treat incidental asymptomatic bacteriuria in women (except in the pregnant patient) with an antibiotic (Davey, et al., 2012). This is a strong evidence-based practice (EBP) recommendation.

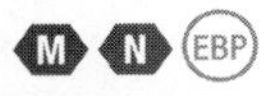

- Administer antibiotics, which are usually necessary to treat the symptomatic infection. It is important to use the urine culture's susceptibility profile to guide antibiotic selection for use (Davey, et al., 2012).

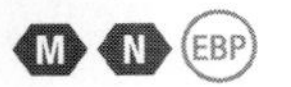

- Administer commonly prescribed antibiotics for cystitis, which include (Davey, et al., 2012):
    - o Trimethoprim-sulfamethoxazole or TMP-SMX (Bactrim, Septra)
    - o Nitrofurantoin, except that caution is needed in older adult patients due to increased risk of toxicity
    - o Ciprofloxacin
    - o Amoxicillin (less effective)

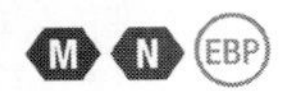

- In pregnant women, due to high risks, perform a urine culture 7 days post-completion of antibiotic treatment to ensure cure (Davey, et al., 2012).

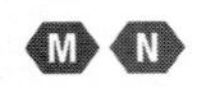

- Administer antispasmodics, such as oxybutynin (Ditropan), to treat bladder spasms caused by inflammation and irritation from the infection.

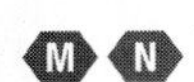

- Administer phenazopyridine (Pyridium) as a painkiller to sooth the lining of the urinary tract. It treats symptoms such as pain, burning, urgency, and frequency caused by the irritation.

- Use nonprescription pain medications such as acetaminophen and ibuprofen, which can be helpful (Davey, et al., 2012).

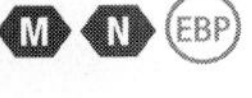

- Strongly encourage drinking plenty of fluids to help ensure normal flushing of bacteria from urinary tract.

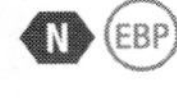

- Carefully monitor for early warning signs of urosepsis (e.g., tachycardia, tachypnea, leukopenia or leukocytosis, fever, hypothermia in older adults) and mobilize the team to respond and manage before severe sepsis develops (Grabe, et al., 2011). See the Care of Patients with Sepsis NovE-lesson for details.

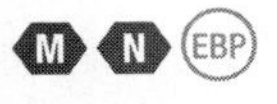

- Recommend daily antibiotic prophylaxis for patients with two or more UTIs within 6 months or for patients with three or more UTIs within 12 months (Epp, et al., 2010).

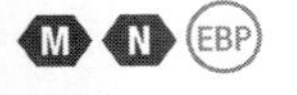

- Consider postcoital antibiotic prophylaxis in patients with recurrent UTIs that are associated with sexual intercourse. This minimizes the risk, cost, and adverse effects of continuous treatment (Epp, et al., 2010).

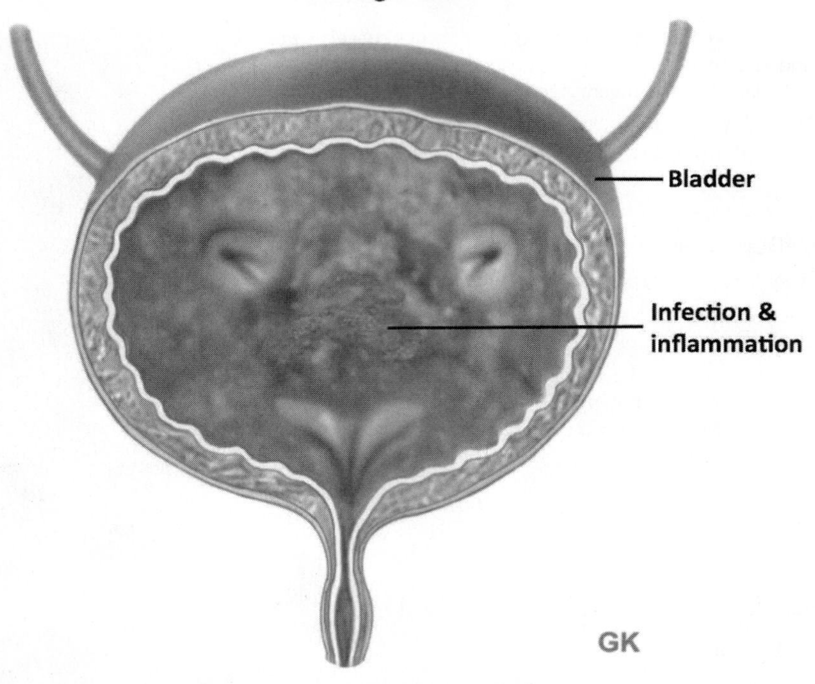

Acute cystitis is noted in this image with inflammation of the bladder, typically caused by a bladder infection. Treatment can help prevent the spread of infection to the kidneys.
Source: Courtesy of George Kyriakidis/Santa Ana, CA

Patient Education for Cystitis Prevention

- Proper care of the perineal area can prevent cystitis, including care such as:
  - o Urinate before and after sexual intercourse.
  - o Wipe the perineum from front to back.
  - o Adequate hydration
  - o Urinate frequently.

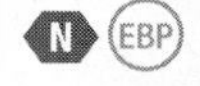

- In patients with recurrent UTI, preventive measures may include (Epp, et al., 2010):
  - o Using an alternative type of contraception if spermicides are associated with recurrent UTI
  - o Consumption of cranberry products, which are effective in reducing recurrent UTIs, particularly in college-age patients

  - o Discussing the potential benefits of vaginal estrogen if postmenopausal
  - o Consider acupuncture as an alternative if antibiotic prophylaxis is ineffective.

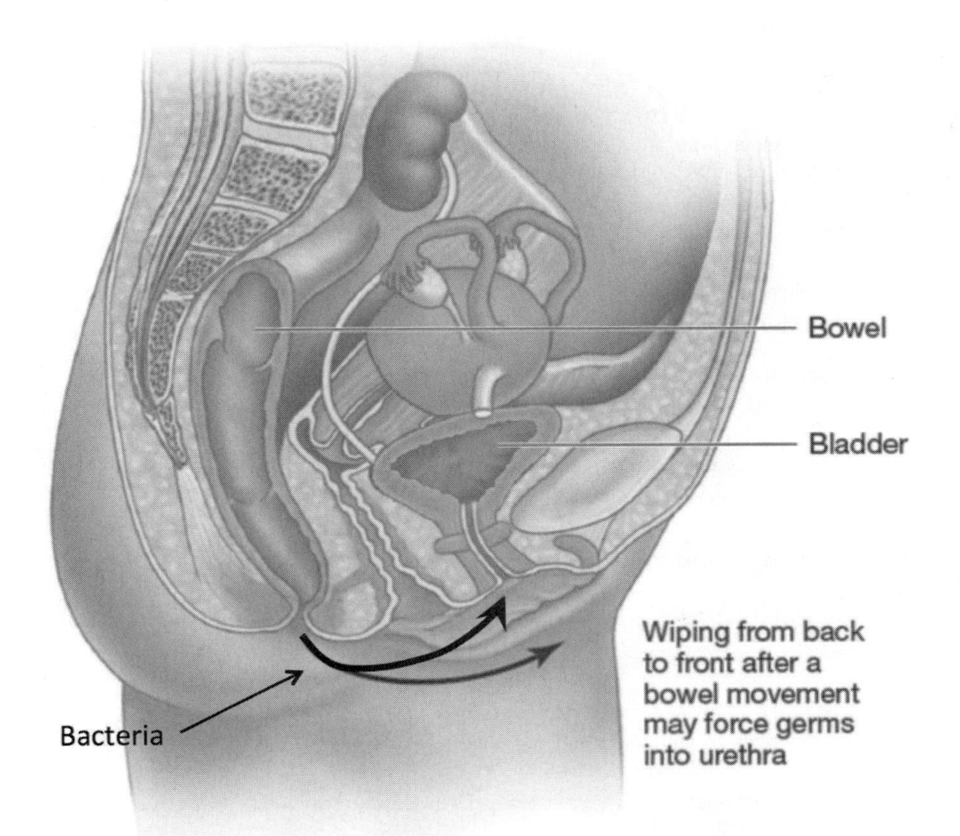
Bowel
Bladder
Wiping from back to front after a bowel movement may force germs into urethra
Bacteria

Good hygiene of the perineal area can mitigate the introduction of bacteria into the urethra, particularly since the rectum is so close in proximity to the urethra. This image emphasizes the importance of wiping from front to back to avoid spreading *E. coli* bacteria from the rectum.

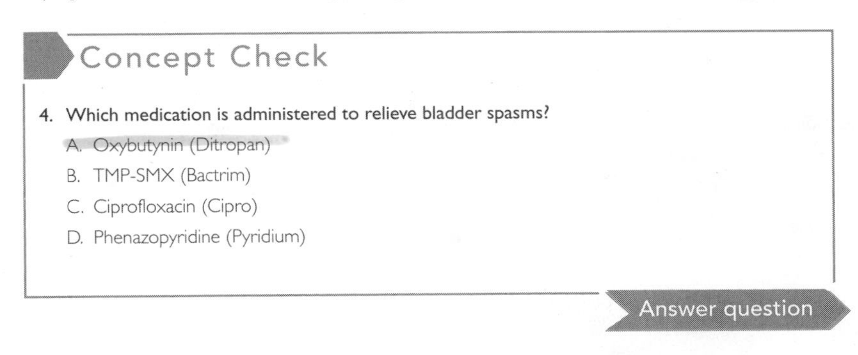

Concept Check

4. Which medication is administered to relieve bladder spasms?
   A. Oxybutynin (Ditropan)
   B. TMP-SMX (Bactrim)
   C. Ciprofloxacin (Cipro)
   D. Phenazopyridine (Pyridium)

Answer question

Concept Check

5. In which patient would asymptomatic bacteriuria be treated?
   A. A child
   B. A pregnant woman
   C. Any woman
   D. A patient who is obese

Answer question

Collaborative Interventions (continued)

Pyelonephritis

- Treat much the same as for other types of UTIs (Davey, et al., 2012).
- Can treat uncomplicated cases of pyelonephritis as an outpatient with oral fluoroquinolones, sulfonamides with trimethoprim, or nitrofurantoin (Davey, et al., 2012).
- Consider hospitalization in complicated cases and treat with IV antibiotics, which should be started immediately after cultures are obtained (Davey, et al., 2012).
- Administer quinolone or ampicillin with gentamicin or tobramycin to provide broad-spectrum coverage. These combinations should be used initially, until cultures and sensitivities are available to guide treatment, as resistant organisms are increasingly common (Davey, et al., 2012).
- When cultures and sensitivities are known, switch, if necessary, to antibiotics that are specific and sensitive to the cultured organisms (Davey, et al., 2012).
- Intervene to relieve obstruction(s) noted on imaging studies.
- Initiate IV antibiotics until signs and symptoms resolve, after 2–5 days, and/or after any obstructive process is relieved, then it is appropriate to switch to oral antibiotics for the remaining 10–14 days.
- Encourage fluids, at least 2 liters per day, including cranberry juice (Epp, et al., 2010).
- Adequate rest is essential.
- Encourage the patient to understand their therapy, which is essential to the patient's compliance and reduces the rate of reoccurrence.

Prostatitis

- Administer trimethoprim-sulfamethoxazole or fluoroquinolone for 4 weeks as the treatment of choice and, usually, the first prescribed (Davey, et al., 2012).
- Consider utilizing other antibiotics if the initial antibiotics are not successful. In severe cases, IV antibiotics may need to be used (Davey, et al., 2012).
- Symptom management and comfort care can include:
  - Administer alpha-adrenergic antagonists to help relax the bladder neck and potentially provide some relief from painful urination.
  - Reduce pain with NSAIDs.
  - Massage prostate with a gloved, lubricated finger, which may give some symptom relief but is not expected to shorten the duration of the infection.
  - Encourage ejaculation to help drain the prostate.
  - Suggest warm baths to help reduce discomfort.
  - Encourage fluid intake.
  - Provide antipyretics for fever relief.

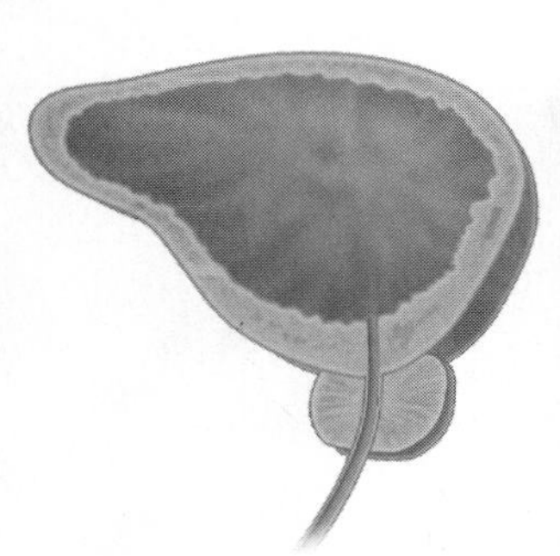

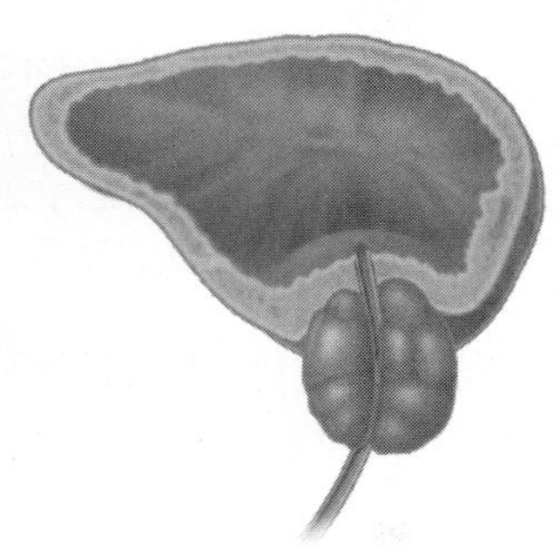

An enlarged prostate from inflammation or infection shows how difficulty emptying the bladder occurs.

UTI Prevention

CDC Recommendations for IUC Use

The recommendations of the Centers for Disease Control and Prevention (CDC) for the use of indwelling urinary catheters, when necessary, include patients who need:

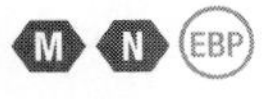

- Surgery and who (Gould, et al., 2010):
  - o Are having genitourinary tract surgery
  - o Are having a prolonged surgical procedure, but remove IUC in PACU
  - o Require hemodynamic or intraoperative urine output monitoring
  - o Receive or are anticipated to receive diuretics or large fluid volumes during the surgical procedure

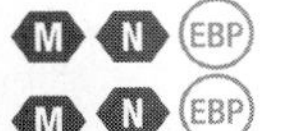

- Monitoring of urine output in critically ill patients (Gould, et al., 2010)
- Management for urinary retention or obstruction (Gould, et al., 2010)
- Protection of a pressure ulcer from urine or fecal incontinence (Gould, et al., 2010)

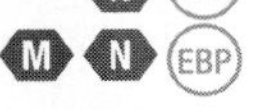

- Prolonged immobilization such as with unstable spinal fractures or multiple traumatic injuries (Gould, et al., 2010)

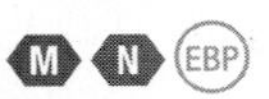

- In special cases, such as to instill medications into the bladder to treat cancer or when the patient requests a catheter for comfort at end of life (Gould, et al., 2010)

Alternatives to IUC

A few alternatives to IUC may be used. Better options than IUCs, when appropriate, include:

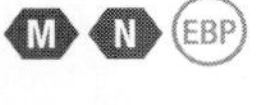

- External catheters (condom caths) in cooperative males who do not have urinary retention or obstruction (Hooten, et al., 2010; Tenke, et al., 2008)
- Intermittent catheterization (also known as straight cath) in certain patients (Hooten, et al., 2010; Tenke, et al., 2008)
- Suprapubic catheterization (Hooten, et al., 2010)
- Also recommended (Saints, et al., 2008; Wald, et al., 2013) is the use of:
  - o Timed or scheduled voiding
  - o Bedside commode or urinal
  - o Incontinence pads or disposable adult briefs

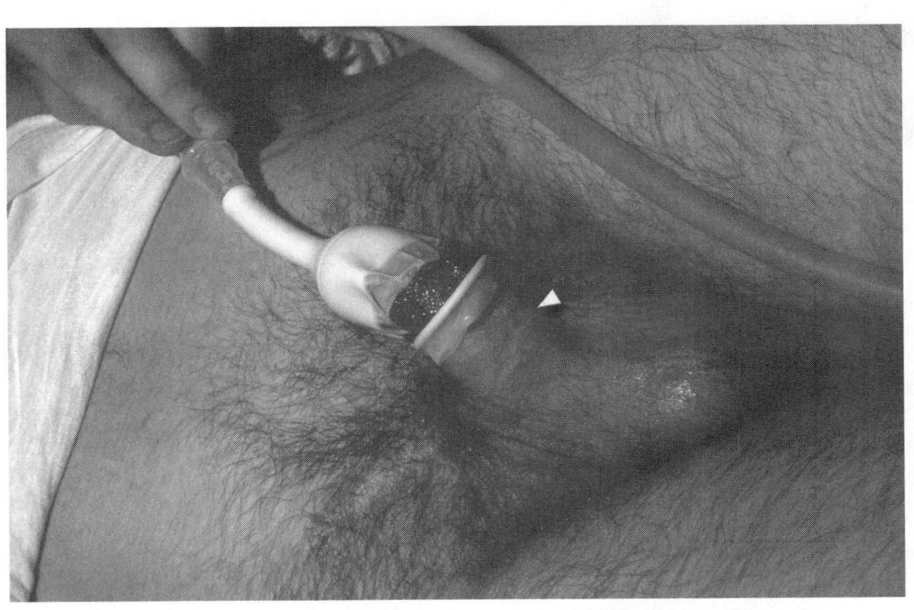

An external or condom catheter shown here is not invasive and provides a better alternative than an indwelling catheter.
Source: CDC/Dr. Thomas M. Hooton

Intermittent Catheterization

Intermittent catheterization involves the temporary insertion of a urinary catheter to drain the bladder with prompt removal. Intermittent catheterization:

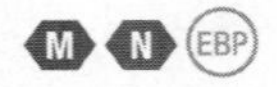

- Is recommended for patients with spinal cord injury, bladder emptying dysfunction, neurogenic bladder, and children with myelomeningocele (Gould, et al., 2010)

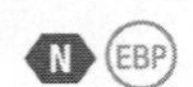

- Should be performed by properly trained persons using sterile technique. The following should also be considered (Hooten, et al., 2010):
    - o In the nonacute setting, clean technique is acceptable (as well as practical).
    - o Perform catheterization at regular intervals, which helps prevent overdistention of the bladder.
    - o Use a bladder scanner to assess when an intermittent catheterization needs to occur.

Bladder Ultra Scan

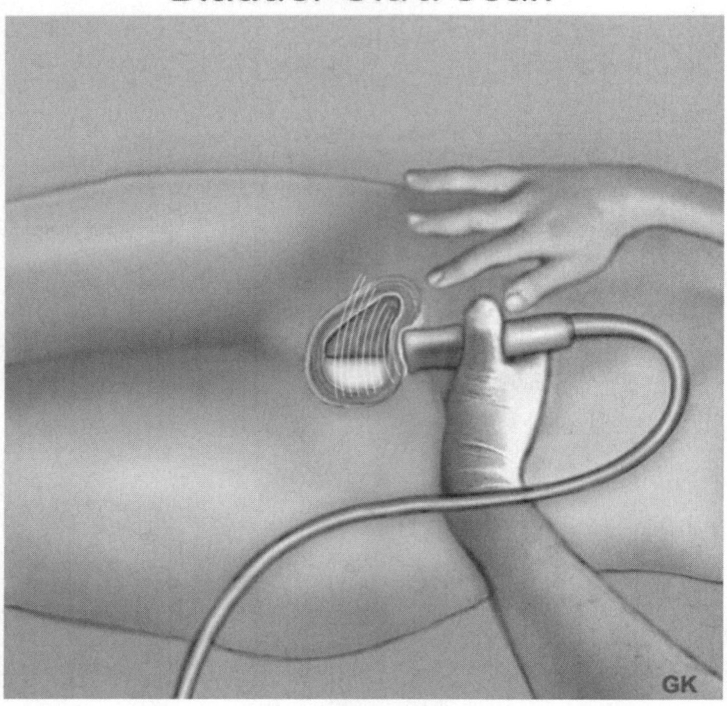

This image depicts how one may scan the bladder to determine residuals and to determine whether or not catheterization is necessary.
Source: Courtesy of George Kyriakidis/Santa Ana, CA

Bladder Scan Use

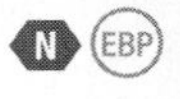

Bedside ultrasound bladder scanning can help the health care provider determine when and if catheterization is indicated (Hooten, et al., 2010). This assessment can help minimize unnecessary use of catheterization:

- Perform a bladder scan if the patient has not or cannot void after 4–6 hours, particularly after removing an IUC.

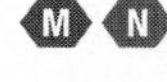

- Use intermittent catheterization to drain the bladder if there is over 500 mL. Intermittent catheterization is recommended over inserting an IUC.

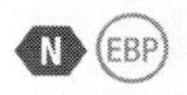

- Ensure the device is properly cleaned between patients to prevent the spread of infections (Gould, et al., 2010).

- Use a condom sheath over the scanner to avoid cross contamination.

Concept Check

6. In which instance are clean techniques used for urinary catheterization?
    - A. At all times
    - B. If the patient self-catheterizes at home
    - C. In the physician's office
    - D. If the patient is a child

Answer question

Collaborative Interventions (continued)

CAUTI Prevention

Overview

- **Keys to prevention:** Once a catheter is inserted, a UTI is considered a CAUTI and prevention becomes paramount. CAUTI is an unnecessary complication, often preventable, and is now a nonreimbursable event in many patients. The keys to preventing CAUTIs are:
  - M N EBP o Limiting the use of IUC is the single most important way of preventing a CAUTI. The single most inappropriate use of an IUC is for urinary incontinence, particularly in non-perioperative patients (Hooten, et al., 2010).
  - M N EBP o If at all possible, remove any IUC at the earliest possible time (Hooten, et al., 2010). Many organizations have implemented or are considering an automatic stop order to remind clinicians to remove unnecessary IUCs.
  - M N EBP o Avoid inappropriate use of antibiotics, which promotes the development of resistant bacterial strains (Davey, et al., 2012).
  - M N EBP o Do not use antibiotics as prophylaxis in preventing UTIs in patients with IUC (Davey, et al., 2012).
  - M N EBP o Do not use antibiotics to treat patients with IUC who have asymptomatic bacteriuria (Davey, et al., 2012).
- M N **Prevention:** Carefully consider the patient's risk for developing a UTI, which is dependent upon the following key factors, before use:
  - o Patient susceptibility
  - o Proper management of the IUC
  - o Duration of catheter usage

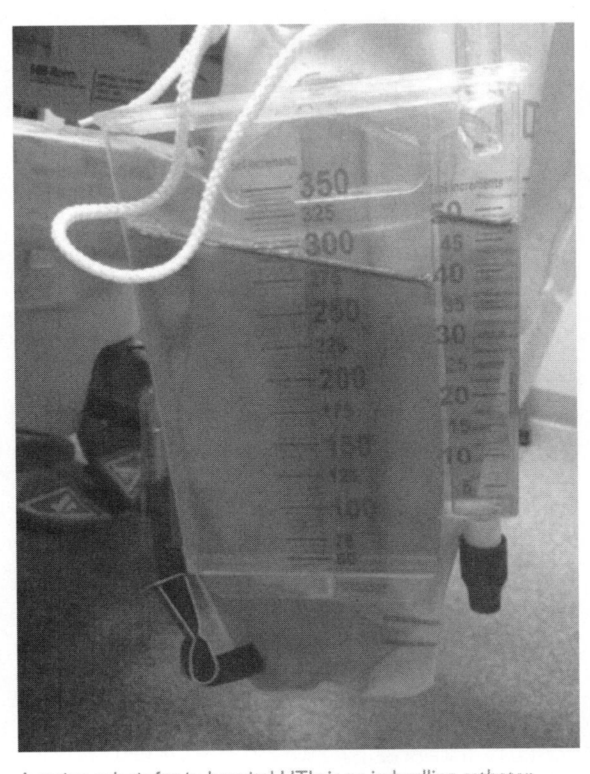

A major culprit for in-hospital UTIs is an indwelling catheter.
Source: Courtesy of K. Kyriakidis

- **Key nursing prevention strategies** can reduce CAUTIs up to 69%:
  - o Catheter avoidance should include use of bedside commode, intermittent catheterization, bladder scanners, condom catheters, toileting schedules (Wald, et al., 2012).
  - o Product selection and routine care that best meets patient's needs, such as smallest possible size catheter, asepsis, soap and water meatus cleansing, securing catheter to leg, closed systems, drainage bag below bladder level, and empty urine bags prior to transport (Wald, et al., 2012).
  - o Removal as soon as possible by frequent evaluation about continued need, stop reminders, and reminders (Wald, et al., 2012).
  - o Surveillance and ongoing education to create constant improvement, reeducation, systems evaluation, outcome measures, and reporting (Wald, et al., 2012).

IUC Precautions

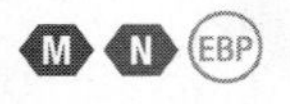

- Perform urinary catheterization only when it is absolutely necessary or the risk is outweighed by the benefits to the patient (Hooten, et al., 2010).
- If an IUC is used, consider an antimicrobial catheter in high-risk patients. A silver alloy or antimicrobial catheter has evidence to support the use for the short term (<14 days) (Hooten, et al., 2010).
- When an IUC is used, remove the catheter as soon as possible, preferably within 24 hours, if manageable (Hooten, et al., 2010).
- Only properly trained persons should insert IUCs (Hooten, et al., 2010).
- Frequently reevaluate the patient's need in prolonged use of IUC in the postoperative patient, as the IUC has been associated with:
  - o Increased occurrence of UTI (Gould, et al., 2010)
  - o Decreased postop activity (causing a possible increase in DVT formation and other inactivity complications)
  - o Increased length of stay
- Many hospitals have developed nurse-initiated protocols for IUC removal (Hooten, et al., 2010).

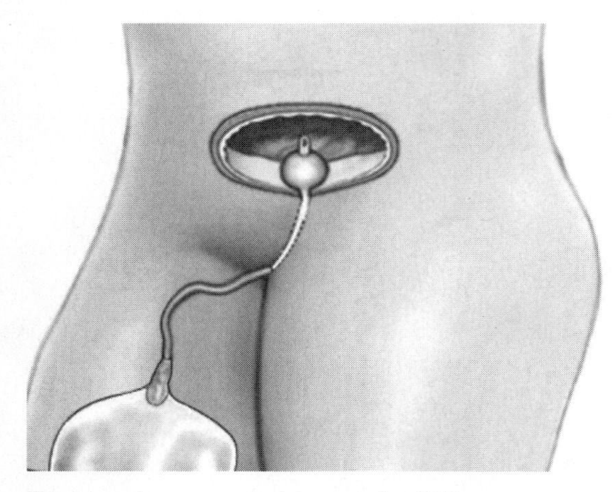

This image shows correct placement of an IUC.
Source: Courtesy of George Kyriakidis/Santa Ana, CA

Hand Hygiene

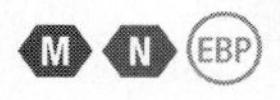

- Hand washing is the key to preventing infections such as a UTI and CAUTI. Use water, soap, and hand friction, particularly if the hands are soiled or contaminated with fluids or particulate matter (Gould, et al., 2010).
- Antiseptic foam or gel can be used in most patients if the hands do not have fluids or other visible contamination on them (CDC, 2013).
- **CAUTION:** Foams and gels *cannot be used* without good hand washing after patients with *Clostridium difficile* or norovirus, as they do not kill these organisms (CDC, 2013).
- Hand washing immediately after contamination is imperative. Avoid touching even inanimate objects or recording patient data before hand washing. Norovirus, for example, can survive for 6 days on objects and transfers to anyone touching them. Prevention of cross contamination is paramount with all infective organisms (Tenke, et al., 2008).

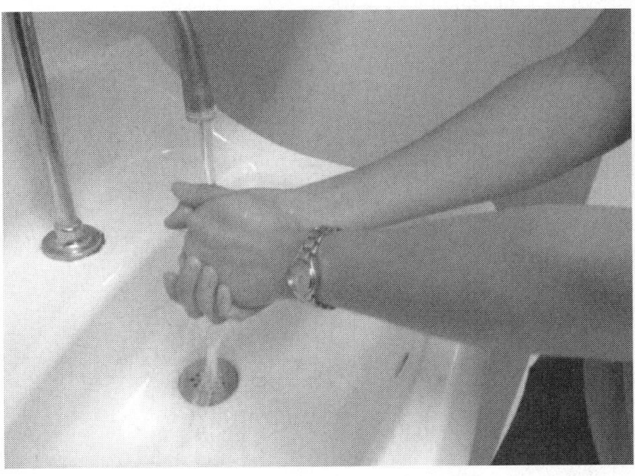

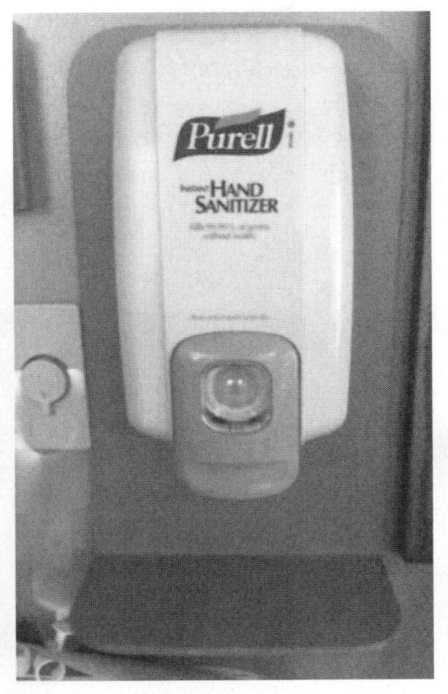

Left: Hand washing is essential in preventing the easy spread of organisms and contaminants, as when touching another person. Microbes are also transmitted to someone if they touch a contaminated object or surface. Food and animals can also transfer germs, particularly salmonella and *E. coli*. Right: One type of foam automatic wall dispenser is shown for hand sanitizer.
Source: *(left)* Courtesy of Sarah Dresen; *(right)* Copyright © 2014, NovEx Novice to Expert Learning, LLC

Insertion and Maintenance

When indwelling catheters are used, **insertion and maintenance** care are of utmost importance:

- Provide meticulous attention to sterile technique is essential (Tenke, et al., 2008).
- Perform hand hygiene immediately before and after catheter insertion (Tenke, et al., 2008).
- Allow catheters to only be inserted by properly trained persons who are aware of aseptic technique (Tenke, et al., 2008).
- Use soap and water for routine meatus care. Avoid daily use of povidone-iodine, green soap, antibiotic ointments or creams, and silver sulfadiazine (Hooten, et al., 2010).
- Decrease trauma to the urethra and bladder neck by:
    - o Securing the catheter to the leg after insertion, to prevent movement and tugging of the catheter (Gould, et al., 2010; Wald, et al., 2013). This was identified as a 2012 Hospital National Patient Safety Goal.
    - o Using the smallest size catheter possible (Tenke, et al., 2008; Wald, et al., 2013).

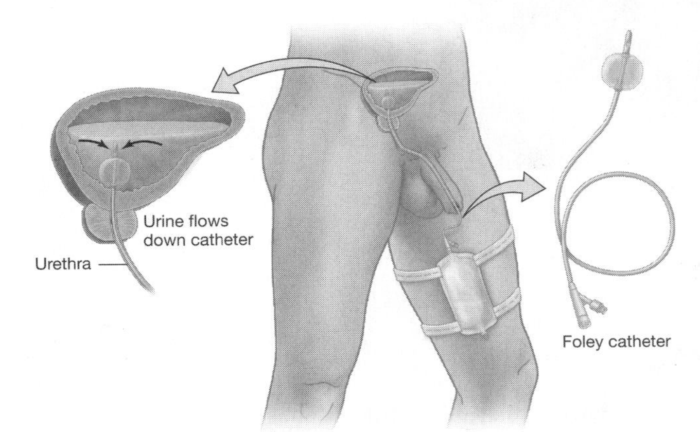

An indwelling urinary catheter and drainage system is depicted showing an IUC in place with the catheter's balloon inflated. Urine can also be drained from the bladder using a straight catheter or "in and out cath" in which the catheter is inserted, the bladder is drained, and the catheter is immediately removed.

Collaborative Interventions (continued)

Closed Catheter-Drainage System

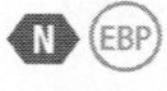
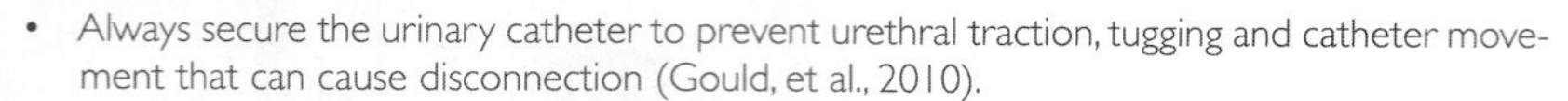

- Always secure the urinary catheter to prevent urethral traction, tugging and catheter movement that can cause disconnection (Gould, et al., 2010).

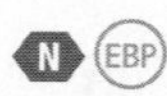

- Never disconnect the catheter and drainage tube unless required for catheter irrigation (Gould, et al., 2010).

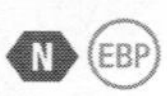

- Avoid irrigation unless done for suspected obstruction. It must be done using sterile technique (Hooten, et al., 2010).

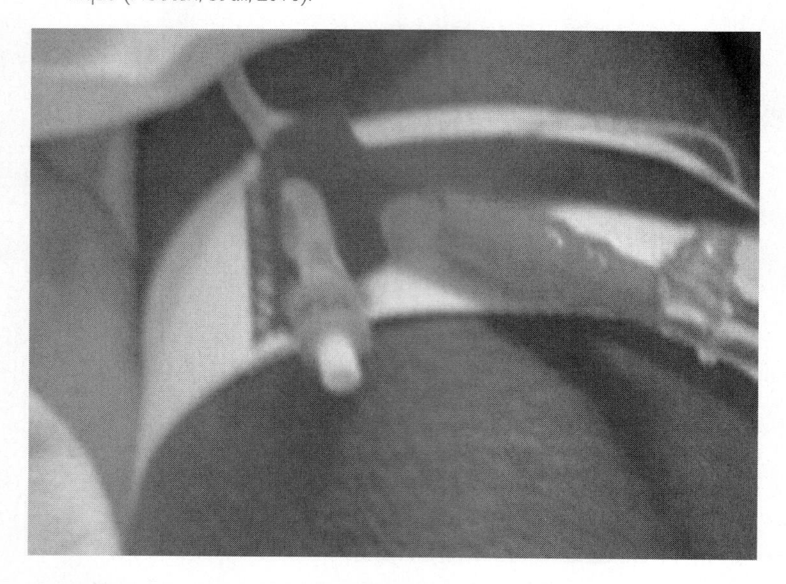

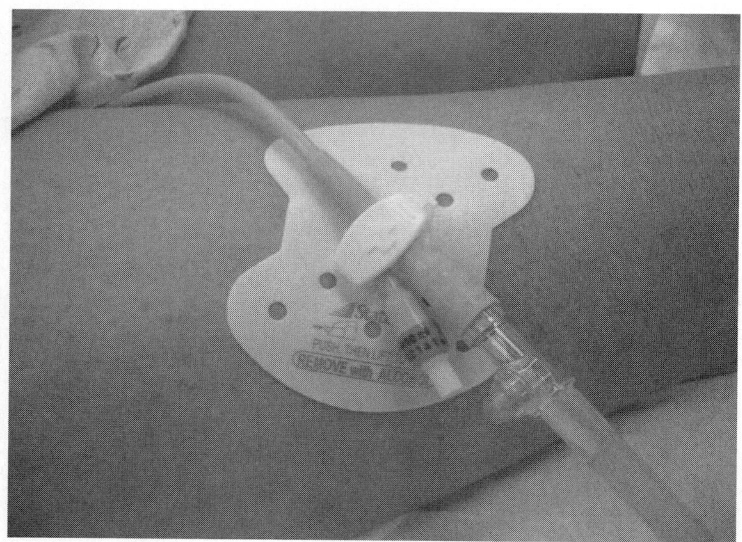

These photos show two examples of securing catheters to prevent traction and movement.

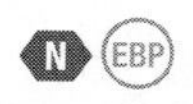
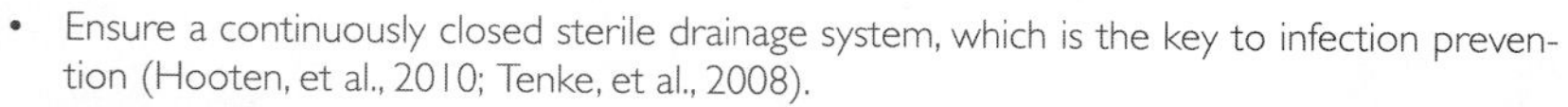

- Ensure a continuously closed sterile drainage system, which is the key to infection prevention (Hooten, et al., 2010; Tenke, et al., 2008).

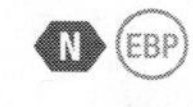
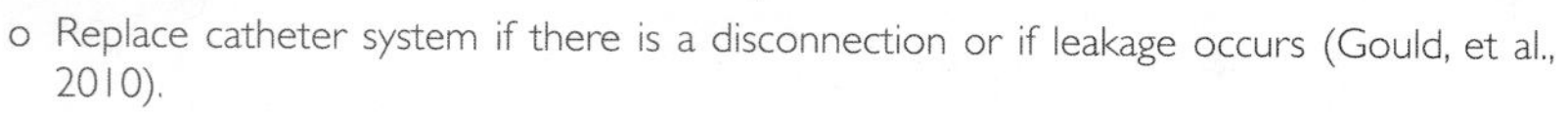

  - o Replace catheter system if there is a disconnection or if leakage occurs (Gould, et al., 2010).

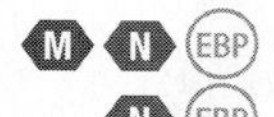

  - o Do not open the system to accommodate clothing when dressing (Hooten, et al., 2010).
  - o Obtain specimens using sterile technique and a distal sampling port when available (Hooten, et al., 2010).

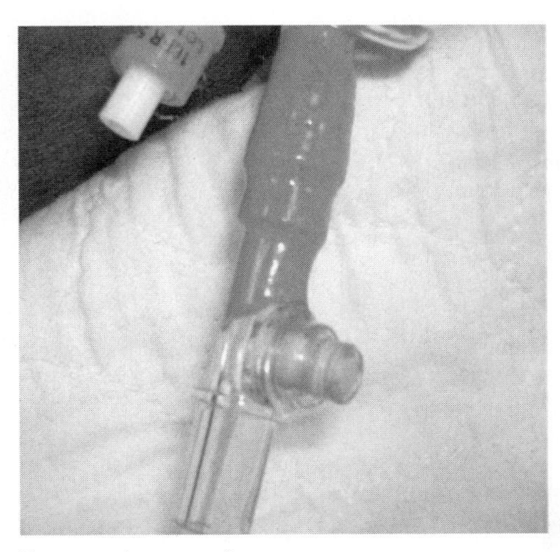

Urinary catheter sampling port.
Source: Copyright © 2014, NovEx Novice to Expert Learning, LLC

Drainage System Care

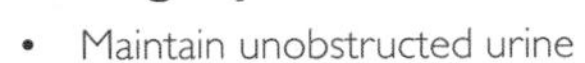

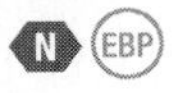

- Maintain unobstructed urine flow and adhere to the following infection prevention care by (Gould, et al., 2010):

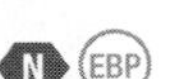

  - o Preventing tubing from kinking (Gould, et al., 2010)

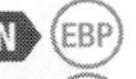
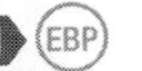
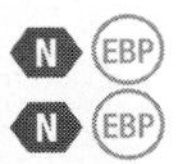

  - o Keeping drainage bag, including the tubing, below the patient's bladder but not on the floor (Gould, et al., 2010). This requires vigilance when lowering the bed.

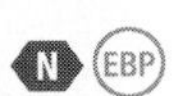

  - o Similarly, ensuring that the urine bag is not placed on the bed during transport and keeping it lower than the patient (Gould, et al., 2010)

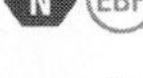
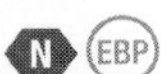

  - o Preventing the backflow of urine back into the bladder (Gould, et al., 2010)

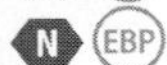

  - o Educating the family about these precautions (Hooten, et al., 2010) because they are frequently involved in assisting the patient get up or walk

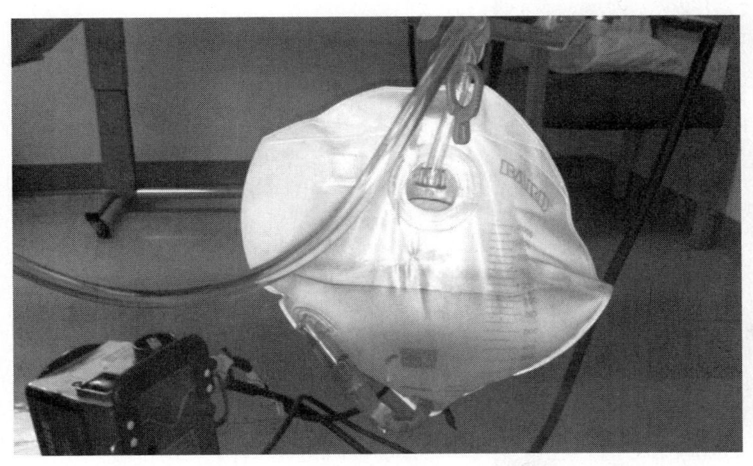

This photo demonstrates a urine collection bag with drainage tubing below the patient level to maintain good urine flow from the bladder.
Source: Copyright © 2014, NovEx Novice to Expert Learning, LLC

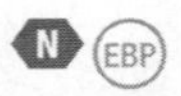

- Use standard precautions (gloves always and gowns when indicated) when handling the urine drainage (Gould, et al., 2010).
- Empty the urine collection bag regularly and note the character of the urine (Gould, et al., 2010).
- Use a single patient use container to empty urine from the bag. Do not share containers between patients (Gould, et al., 2010). For patients with bacteria in their urine, the urine bag is a potential large reservoir of organisms.
- Prevent the drainage spigot on the drainage bag from touching the nonsterile container or floor (Gould, et al., 2010). Ensure that assistive personnel follow these safety and infection control precautions.
- Empty the urine collection bag before transporting the patient to another department or location. Handling the bag during patient movement can easily result in inadvertently raising it above the patient level allowing urine backflow (Wald, et al., 2013).
- Empty urinary contents into approved drainage systems in the dirty utility room.

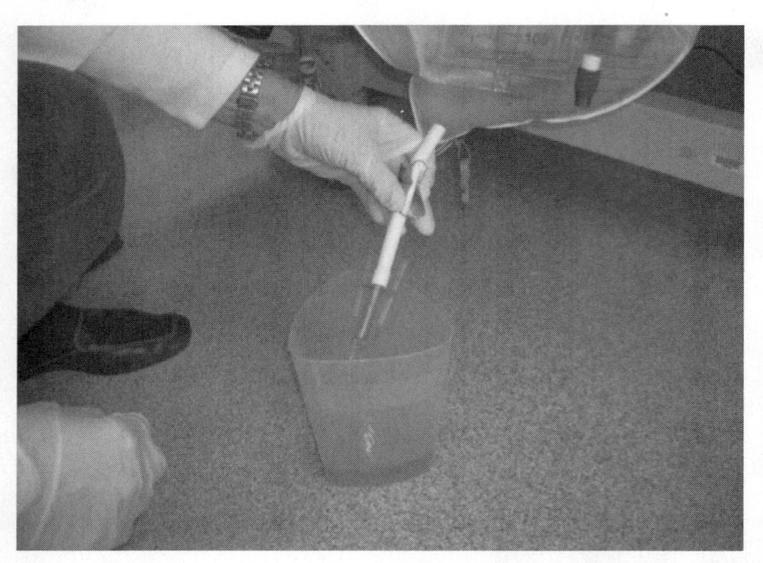

This photo depicts proper handling of the urine drainage system while emptying it.

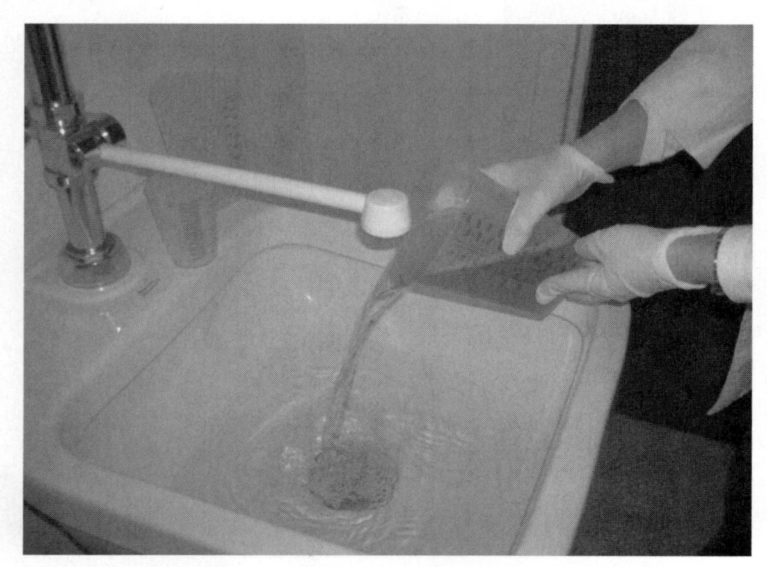

Appropriate disposal of waste in a designated area is essential for infection prevention.

Concept Check

7. **How often should the indwelling urinary catheter of a patient in long-term care be irrigated?**

   A. Every 24 hours

   B. Never

   C. Only if an obstruction occurs

   D. Weekly

Answer question

Collaborative Interventions (continued)

Prevention of CAUTI

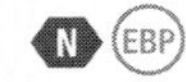

- Do not change an IUC or drainage system at short routine intervals (<4–6 weeks, but this can be hospital-specific) unless (Hooten, et al., 2010):
  - o An infection or obstruction occurs.
  - o The system is not kept intact.
  - o You need to change the collection bag to a urometer (urine measurement device). It is better to change the entire system (replace the IUC with a new catheter and the needed urometer).

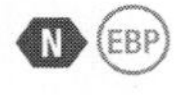

- Use soap and water or perineal cleanser to cleanse the urethral meatus and periurethral area before IUC insertion (e.g., before using Betadine) and, at least, while catheter is in place (Hooten, et al., 2010; Wald, et al., 2013).

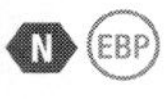

- Avoid use of disinfectants or antibacterial ointments around the meatus to reduce the development of resistant organisms (Hooten, et al., 2010).

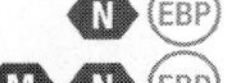

- Use aseptic technique to manipulate and maintain IUC (Hooten, et al., 2010).

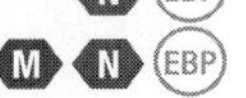

- Do not routinely use systemic antibiotics to prevent CAUTI, but consider in high-risk situations (Davey, et al., 2012).

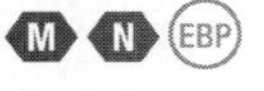

- Assess the need for continued catheter use on a daily basis. Remove IUC as soon as it is no longer essential (Gould, et al., 2010; Tenke, et al., 2008; Wald, et al., 2013).
  - o The longer an IUC is in place, the higher the risk for CAUTI becomes.

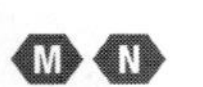

- When long-term catheterization is required, catheter changes every 4–6 weeks may reduce CAUTI incidence.

Patient Education

Educating patients can assist in decreasing the incidence and recurrence of UTIs:

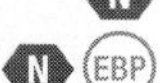

- Encourage fluids, particularly no sugar-filled drinks.

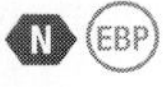

- Increase acidity in diet with unsweetened cranberry juice and cranberry products for UTI prevention (Davey, et al., 2012; Hooten, et al., 2010). Instruct patients that although citrus and citrus drinks may taste acidic, they do not create acidity in the urine.

- Take full course of antibiotics, if prescribed, to avoid the development of resistant organisms. Never take antibiotics unless prescribed by a health care provider, particularly when purchasing medications outside the United States.

- Educate about good hygienic practices, particularly wiping after toileting from front to back and urinating before and after intercourse.

- Empty the bladder regularly, about every 3–4 hours while awake. Drink extra fluids as needed to urinate frequently.

- Women should avoid baths (as distinguished from showers), hot tubs, bubble baths, and vaginal douches, powders, and sprays that can either disrupt the natural, protective vaginal flora or introduce organisms.

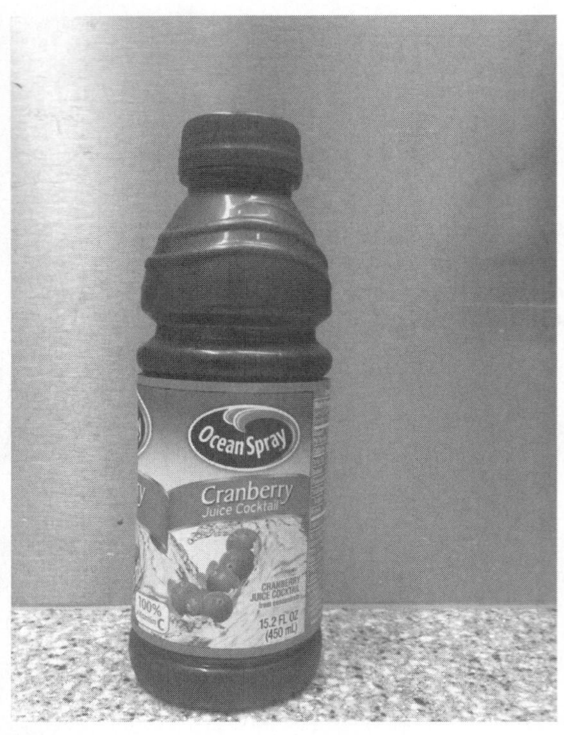

Cranberry juice is preferred to increase urine acidity.
Source: Copyright © 2014, NovEx Novice to Expert Learning, LLC

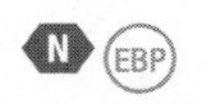

- If intermittent catheterization is needed in nonacute care settings, clean rather than sterile technique is accepted (Hooten, et al., 2010).

- Follow-up care is important. Recurrent symptoms must be further evaluated.

Summary of Interventions

- The most important preventative measure for UTI and CAUTI is avoidance of indwelling urinary catheter use.
- Symptomatic bacteriuria is treated with antibiotics. Asymptomatic bacteriuria should not be treated.
- Evidence-based guidelines state that the use of indwelling urinary catheters and drainage systems:
  - o Should be avoided as much as possible
  - o Should be performed by skilled professionals
  - o Should be limited to specific situations
  - o Should be for the least amount of time possible
  - o Should be cared for using specific procedures
  - o Should include monitoring for early signs of infection
  - o Should maintain a closed catheter-drainage system
  - o Should ensure adherence to known precautions
- Patients depend on the nurse to keep them safe by preventing a UTI.
- Recognition and response to triggers help prevent UTIs.

LO4:

Evaluation of Desired Collaborative Care Outcomes

Evaluation and reassessment should reveal attainment of previously established patient outcomes. In summary:

- Patient reports that feelings of urgency and frequent need to urinate have resolved.
- Patient reports that pain is absent or reduced to a tolerable level.
- Patient reports no episodes of incontinence.
- Patient reports engaging in social activities as before illness.
- Patient accurately discusses treatment plan and reports using suggested prevention strategies.

References

Centers for Disease Control and Prevention (CDC). (2013). *Show me the science—When to use hand sanitizer: Handwashing—clean hands save lives.* **www.cdc.gov/handwashing/show-me-the-science-hand-sanitizer.html**

Grabe, M., Bjerklund-Johansen, T. E., Botto, H., et al. (2011). *Guidelines on urological infections* (pp. 33–39). Arnhem, The Netherlands: European Association of Urology (EAU).

Lo, E., Lindsay, N., Classen, D., et al. (2008). Strategies to prevent catheter-associated urinary tract infections in acute care hospitals. *Infect Control Hosp Epidemiol, 29*(S1), S41–S50. HICPAC/Centers for Disease Control and Prevention. **www.jstor.org/stable/10.1086/591066**

Saint, S., Kowalski, C. P., Kaufman, S. R., et al. (2008). Preventing hospital-acquired urinary tract infection in the United States: A national study. *Clin Infect Dis, 46*(2), 243–250. **cid.oxfordjournals.org/content/46/2/243.long**

Willson, M., Wilde, M., Webb, M. L., et al. (2009). Nursing interventions to reduce the risk of catheter-associated urinary tract infection: Part 2: Staff education, monitoring, and care techniques. *J Wound Ostomy Continence Nurs, 36*(2), 137–154. **www.nursingcenter.com/lnc/static?pageid=930204**

Clinical Practice Guidelines

Davey, P., Byrne, D., Craig, N., et al., and Guideline Development Group. (2012). *Scottish Intercollegiate Guidelines Network (SIGN) 88: Management of suspected bacterial urinary tract infections in adults: A national clinical guideline.* **www.sign.ac.uk/pdf/sign88.pdf**

Epp, A., Larochelle, A., Lovatsis, D., et al. (2010). Recurrent urinary tract infection. *J Obstet Gynaecol Can, 32*(11), 1082–1090. **www.guideline.gov/content.aspx?id=24364&search=urinary+tract+infection**

Gould, C., Umscheid, C., Agarwal, R., et al., and the Healthcare Infection Control Practices Advisory Committee. (2010). Guideline for prevention of catheter-associated urinary tract infections 2009. *Infect Control Hosp Epidemiol, 31*(4), 319–326. **www.cdc.gov/hicpac/pdf/cauti/cautiguideline2009final.pdf**

Hooten, T., Bradley, S., Cardenas, D., et al. (2010). Diagnosis, prevention, and treatment of catheter-associated urinary tract infection in adults. *Clin Infect Dis, 50*(5), 625–663. **cid.oxfordjournals.org/content/50/5/625.long#sec-10**

Tenke, P., Kovacs, B., Johansen, T., et al. (2008). European and Asian guidelines on management and prevention of catheter-associated urinary tract infections. *Internat J Antimicrob Agents, 31* (Suppl 1), S68–S78. **www.ijaaonline.com/article/S0924-8579(07)00418-9/pdf**

Wald, H. L., Fink, R. M., Makic, M. B, et al. (2012). Catheter-associated urinary tract infection prevention. In M. Boltz, E. Capezuti, T. Fulmer, et al. (Eds). *Evidence-based geriatric nursing protocols for best practice (4th ed)*, pp. 388–408. New York, NY: Springer Publishing. **www.guideline.gov/content.aspx?id=43936&search=urinary+tract+infections**

Patient Education

Hooten, T. M. (2014). *Patient information: Urinary tract infections in adolescents and adults.* **www.uptodate.com/contents/urinary-tract-infections-in-adolescents-and-adults-beyond-the-basics**

Mayo Clinic Staff. (2012). *Urinary tract infection (UTI).* **www.mayoclinic.com/health/urinary-tract-infection/DS00286**

Learning Outcomes for Ureteral Calculi or Renal Stones

When you complete this lesson, you will be able to:

1. Recognize the clinical relevance of ureteral calculi.
2. Consider the pathophysiology, etiology, risk factors, and clinical presentation of ureteral calculi that determine the priority patient concerns.
3. Determine the most urgent and important nursing interventions and patient education required in caring for a patient with ureteral calculi.
4. Evaluate attainment of desired collaborative care outcomes for a patient with ureteral calculi.

LO1:

What Are Urinary Tract Calculi?

- Urinary tract calculi are also known as kidney stones or nephrolithiasis. Kidney stones are solid aggregates of minerals that form from minerals in the urinary tract.
- Substances that usually form stones are calcium, oxalate, uric acid, and cystine.
- Stones can form if these substances are at high levels in the urine or if they become concentrated because of low urinary output.
- Stones start as small crystals of these substances. They gradually enlarge as they move through the urinary excretion system and can become excruciatingly painful.

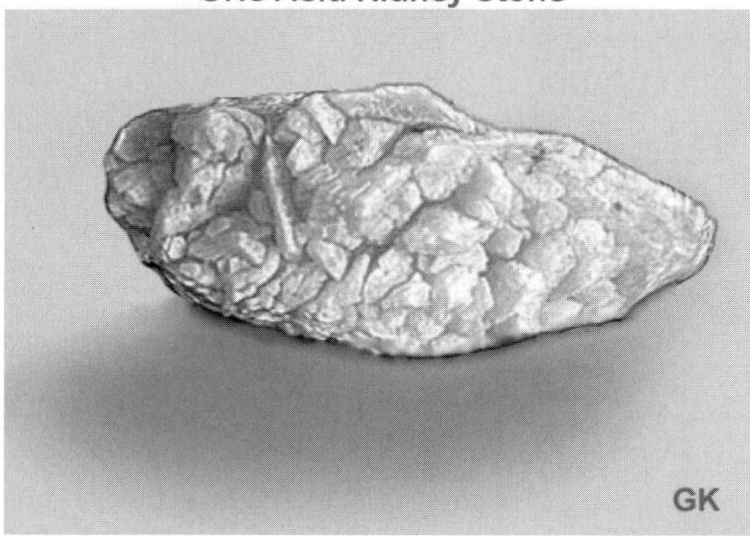

The urinary stones or crystals formed from uric acid. The stones are actually small; however, the jagged edges make them very painful as they scrape against the mucosal membranes.

Source: Courtesy of George Kyriakidis/Santa Ana, CA

LO1:

Clinical Relevance

- Passage of a kidney stone is one of the most painful conditions that humans experience.
- It is common: Lifetime incidence is 10% in men and 6% in women.
- Nephrolithiasis is a common disease that is estimated to produce medical costs of $2.1 billion per year in the United States.
- Pain from renal/ureteral calculi affects approximately 1.2 million people each year and accounts for approximately 1% of all hospital admissions.

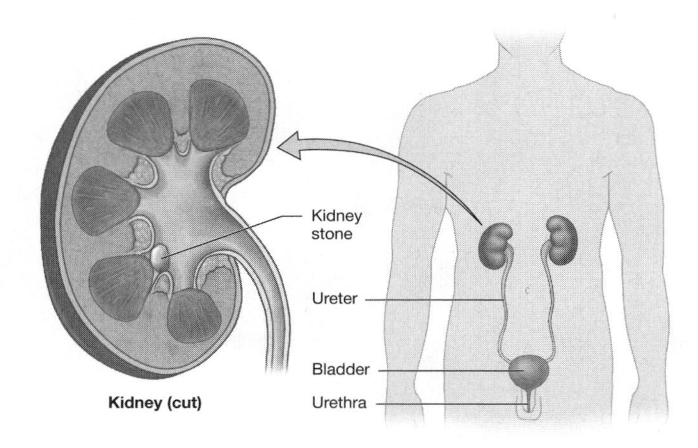

Left: This image of the kidney shows a stone that must dislodge from the kidney into the ureter. Right: This image shows the path that the stone must follow, from the kidney through the urethra, before it can be passed.

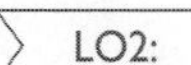

Pathophysiology

- Kidney stones form when dissolved minerals and other substances precipitate to form small crystals.
- These crystals usually first form in the medullary portion of the collecting duct, where the urine is most concentrated.
- As more of the solute precipitates onto the crystals, they grow into larger stones.
- The kidney stones typically pass along the urinary tract down the ureter, and into the bladder before being excreted.
- As the stones pass through the ureters, they cause damage, resulting in bleeding and pain.
- If the stones are too large, they may cause an obstruction to urinary flow with subsequent dilation in the urinary tract prior to the obstruction.
- Pain is produced by dilation and spasm of the ureters.
- Dilation of the renal pelvis due to obstruction may also cause pain by stretching the capsule of the kidney.
- Obstruction can result in acute kidney injury as well as infection since stasis of urine promotes bacterial growth.

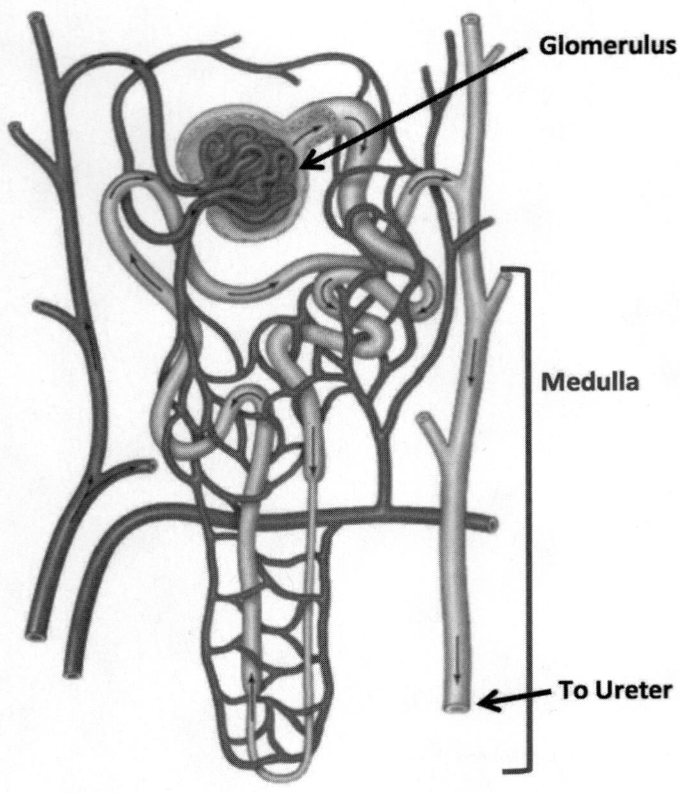

This drawing illustrates the path along which crystals precipitate, grow, and must pass or become lodged within the glomerular-tubular system.

Concept Check

1. In which situation does kidney stone treatment require hospitalization?

A. When the patient is in pain

B. When the patient has fever

C. If the patient cannot tolerate oral fluids

D. If the patient requests hospitalization

Answer question

Pathophysiology (continued)

Types of Kidney Stones

- The following are types of stones, categorized by composition:
  - o Calcium oxalate
  - o Calcium phosphate

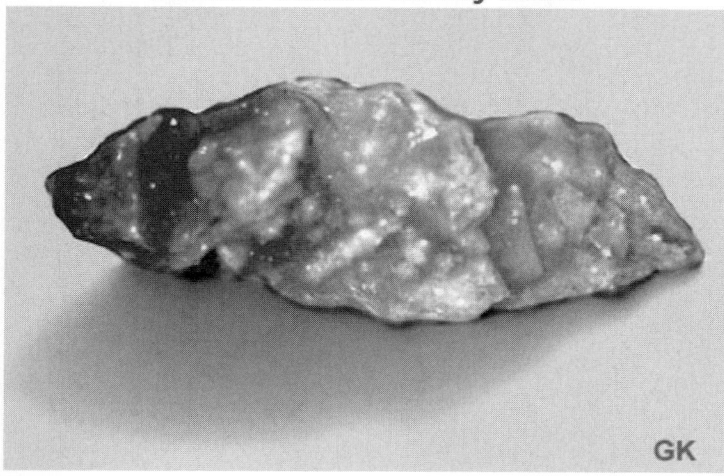

Source: Courtesy of George Kyriakidis/Santa Ana, CA

- o Uric acid
- o Cystine
- o Struvite
- o Indinavir (stones that consist of antiviral medications in patients with HIV)

A number of factors in urine promote stone formation as well as inhibit stone formation.

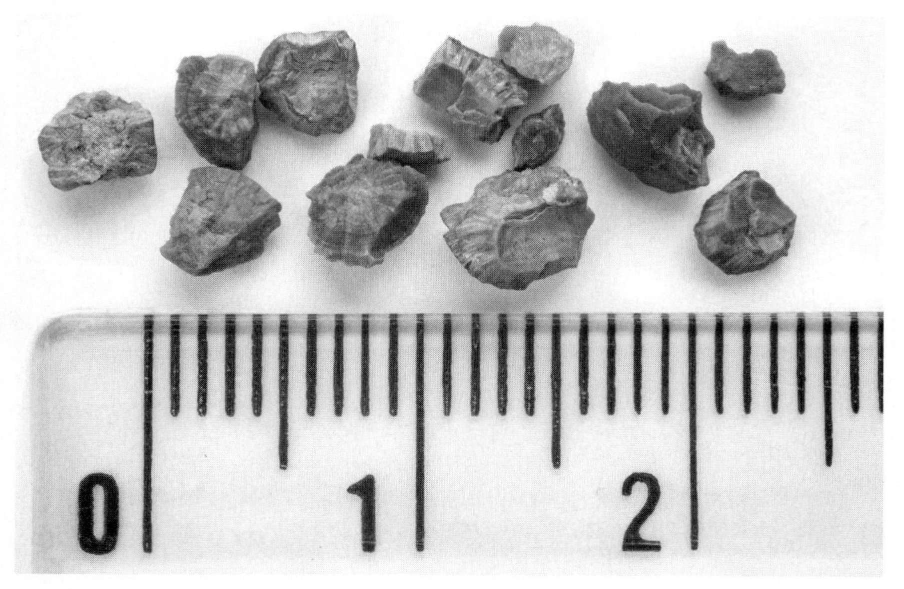

Large bladder stones surgically removed.
Source: airborne77/Fotolia

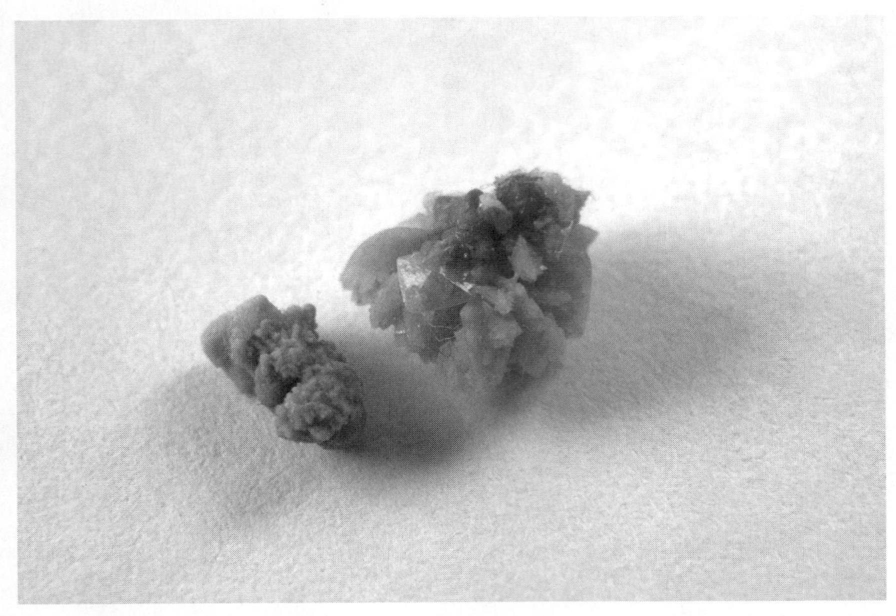

Upon close inspection, the hard calcium oxalate "stones" are actually made up of thousands of tiny crystals with sharp edges that bond together.
Source: remik44992/Fotolia

Pathophysiology (continued)

Promoters of Stone Formation

- Low urine volume, high concentration
- Increased calcium, uric acid, oxalate, or cystine excretion into the urine
- pH determines how soluble minerals are in urine.
  - o Low pH: Calcium oxalate and uric acid are less soluble.
  - o High pH: Calcium pyrophosphate is less soluble.

Inhibitors of Stone Formation

- Citrate in urine
- Magnesium in urine
- Organic inhibitors (e.g., osteopontin, glycosaminoglycans) in urine. When these substances adsorb to the stone's or crystal's surface, growth is inhibited.

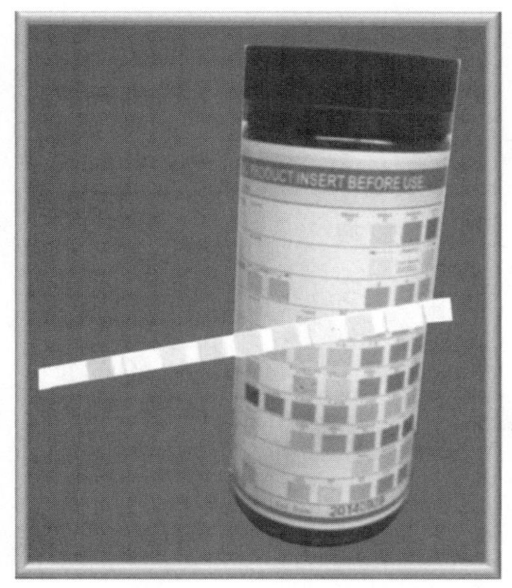

Dipsticks can be used to test the pH levels quickly and easily. The immediate results can help determine if the pH needs attention. As a guide, if urinary pH fluctuates between 6.0 and 6.5 in the morning and between 6.5 and 7.0 in the evening, the patient's body is functioning within a healthy range. The best time to test your pH is about 1 hour before a meal and 2 hours after a meal.

LO2:

Risk Factors

- Dehydration
- Gout
- Prior history of stones
- Being male
- Being an adult—most common after age 40
- Family history
- Obesity
- Diabetes

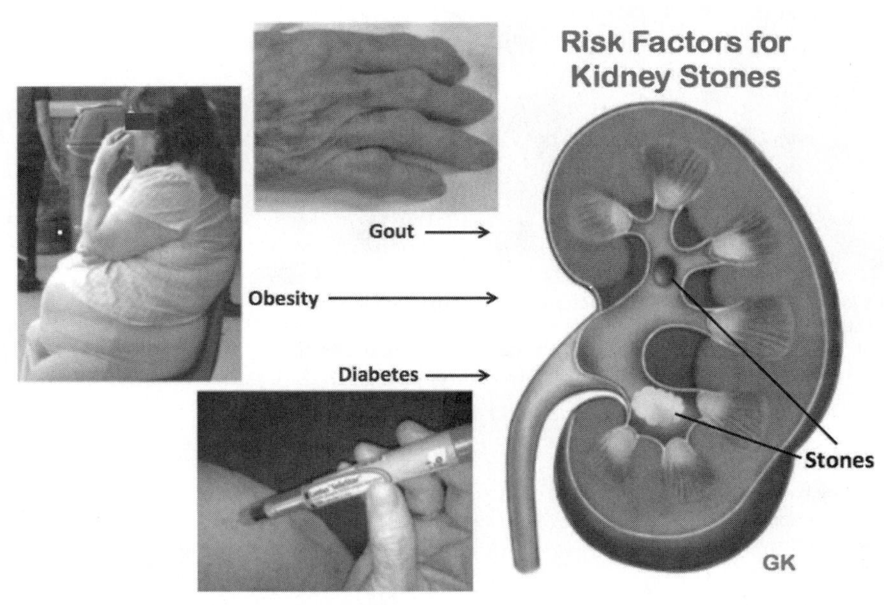

In 2012, the *European Urology Journal* published a study showing a twofold increase in the prevalence of kidney stones in the United States in the past 18 years. Researchers pointed to gout, obesity, and diabetes as key contributors to the surprising increase.

- Bowel surgeries, including bariatric, gastric bypass, and short bowel syndrome
- Hypertension
- Certain diseases and medications

Concept Check

2. Kidney stones are most likely to develop in which age group?

A. Under 16 years
B. 20–30 years
C. 30–40 years
D. Over 40 years

Answer question

LO2:

Causes

- Hypercalciuria (80% of patients)
  - o Hyperparathyroidism
  - o Vitamin D excess
  - o Idiopathic or genetic
  - o Diet high in sodium or protein
- Hyperuricosuria
  - o Gout
- Hyperoxaluria
  - o Dietary intake (e.g., low calcium intake)
  - o Genetic disorders (produced by liver)
  - o Patients with inflammatory bowel disease or post-gastric bypass absorb more oxalate and, therefore, need to excrete more.
- Cystinuria is a genetic disorder in which certain amino acids are not reabsorbed. Cystine is an amino acid that is relatively insoluble and precipitates in the tubules.
- Indinavir is a medication used to treat patients with HIV. It can precipitate in the renal tubules causing stones (see photo).

Gout in the Feet and Hands

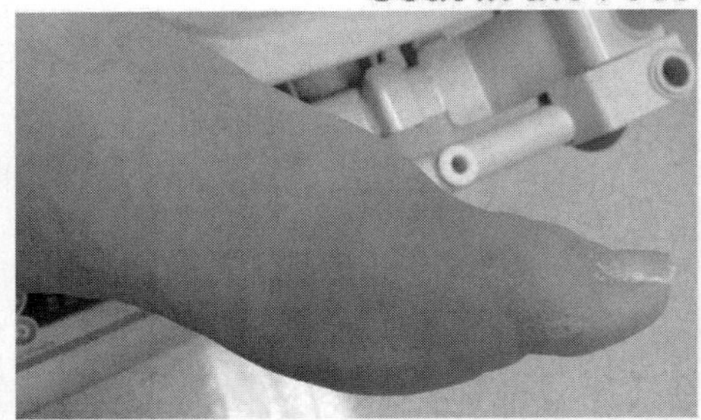

Gout is noted in this patient's joint, one of the most common areas of presentation. The joint is inflamed, swollen, and painful.

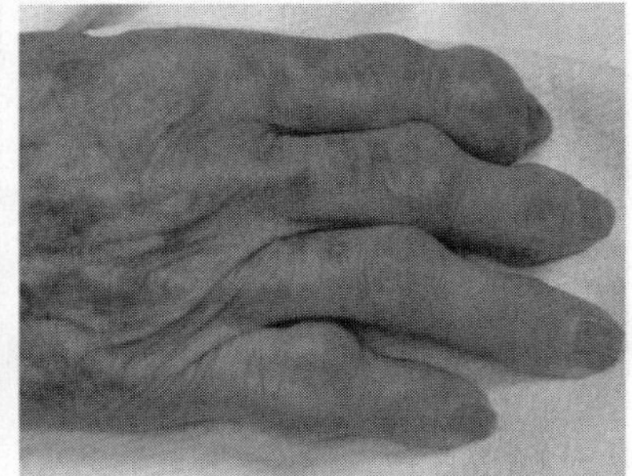

Tophaceous gout is observed in this patient's knuckles. The nodular masses that deform the joints are deposits of uric acid crystals (or tophi).

Source: Courtesy of K. Kyriakidis

- Hypocitraturia
- Urinary tract infections caused by bacteria that can split urea (e.g., Proteus, Klebsiella) into ammonia and carbon dioxide. Ammonia can then precipitate with magnesium and phosphate to form struvite stones.
- Factors that cause metabolic acidosis:
  - o Diarrhea (bicarbonate is lost with stool)
  - o High protein diet, which produces protons (acid)

Concept Check

3. Calcium oxalate kidney stones are more likely to form if the urine is of what pH?

A. Alkaline

B. Acidic

C. Either condition can increase risk for calcium oxalate stone formation.

D. pH level is not a factor in the development of calcium oxalate stones.

Answer question

LO2:

Assessment Findings

- Urinary tract calculi may be asymptomatic if they are not causing obstruction or if they are small enough to easily pass through the ureters.
- Sudden severe pain is felt as the stone travels down the ureter to the bladder.
- Pain may begin in the flank area (back, below the ribs). Pain may also be in the lower abdomen, groin, and above the pelvic arches. Location of the pain may change as the stone moves down the ureter. It is often described by patients as the worst pain they ever experienced, "worse than childbirth." Pain comes and goes in waves (colic).

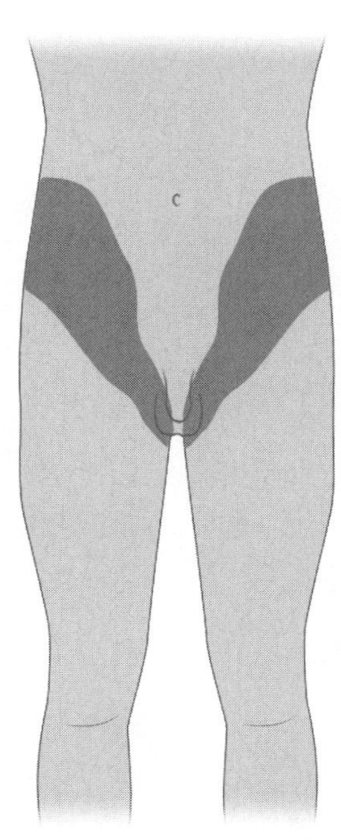

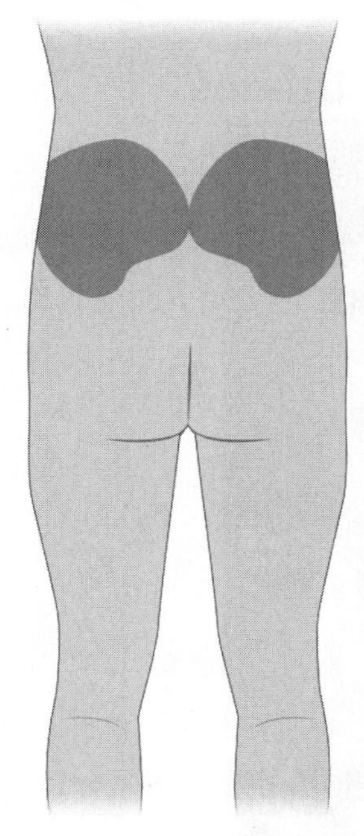

Location of nephrolithiasis-related pain. Pain in the areas on the back and lower abdominal shown above can be caused by kidney stones. Kidney stone pain is usually distinguishable from spinal back pain, which presents as shooting or stabbing pain, radiating down the legs, and with limited range of back motion.

- Pain is unpredictable because it may last weeks while waiting for the stone to pass.
- Hematuria causes the urine to be pinkish red.
- Nausea and/or vomiting may occur due to the intense pain.
- The patient may be diaphoretic and incapacitated.
- Fever may be present if there is an infection.

LO2:

Diagnostics

- Labs/Testing:
  - o CBC: Elevated WBC count may indicate an infection, although a mildly elevated count is not unusual in patients passing stones.
  - o Electrolytes: A low bicarbonate indicates a metabolic acidosis, which can contribute to stone formation.
  - o Serum calcium: Elevated calcium may be present in hyperparathyroidism.
- Urinalysis:
  - o Urine pH can contribute to formation of stone (high or low depending on the stone).
  - o WBCs and bacteria may indicate the presence of infection.
  - o RBCs are usually present with ureteral stones.
  - o Analysis for calcium, oxalate, and uric acid may help to determine the cause.
- Blood and urine cultures should be sent if a patient is febrile or has >10 WBCs in urine.
- Straining urine: Straining urine allows for collection and analysis of stones when passed. The type of stone can guide prevention of recurrence of stones.
- Imaging:
  - o X-ray of abdomen: Calculi containing calcium are radiopaque.
  - o Ultrasound may help visualize obstruction and larger stones.
  - o **CT scan without contrast** (test of choice): may show kidney stones or obstruction. CT scans are typically done without contrast since contrast may hide the radiopaque stones.

Renal Damage From Kidney Stones

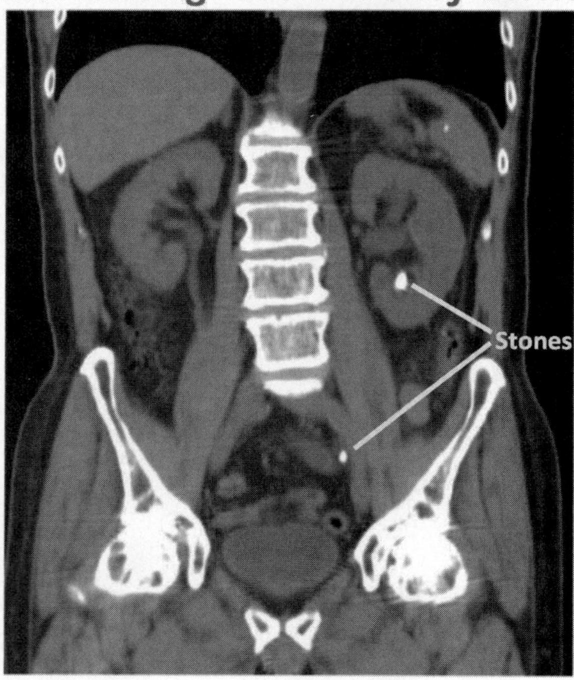

The CT scan reveals multiple calcifications (white spots). The larger stone is in the patient's left kidney. However, the smaller stone caused ureteral obstruction, prevented urine flow, and resulted in hydronephrosis. The kidney enlargement, caused by the hydronephrosis, is notable on CT scan.
Source: Courtesy of K. Kyriakidis

Priority Patient Concerns and Desired Collaborative Care Outcomes

Prior to caring for patients with renal stones, it is important to prioritize the patient's concerns that must guide the nursing care plan and interventions. Care for the patient is ordered and organized in accordance with the patient's priority and urgent needs. Desired collaborative care outcomes in patients with renal stones typically include:

1. Patient will experience effective pain control or relief.
2. Patient will have the free flow of urine without pain or hematuria.
3. Patient will maintain fluid balance.
4. Patient will incorporate lifestyle and dietary changes to prevent stone formation in the future.

Considering these important care outcomes, prepare a list of the major 3–6 priority patient concerns or nursing diagnoses for patients with renal stones. Be prepared to participate in a discussion of this list and/or to submit them as an assignment, as determined by your faculty. Resources you may find helpful in this assignment can include this lesson, the references, resources on nursing care plans, and standard nursing diagnoses manuals.

Concept Check

4. **Why is contrast dye not used during a CT scan for renal stones?**
   A. It increases risk for sepsis.
   B. It increases patient's pain.
   C. Risk for renal failure is increased.
   D. Dye may hide radiopaque stones.

Answer question

LO3:

Collaborative Interventions

As an overview, there are two overall components to care when a patient presents with a kidney stone:

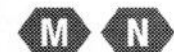

1. Interventions for the patient's acute problem:
   - o Treatment of an obstruction and/or infection

Conservative versus Surgery Management

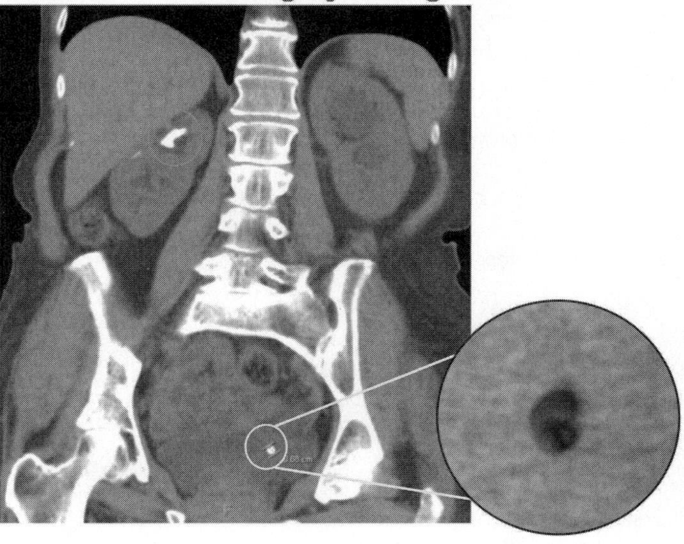

The CT scan shows a large right staghorn calculus in the kidney that is too large to pass (red circle). However, the smaller stone migrated to and blocked the ureter (yellow circle). It was treated conservatively and eventually passed (see enlarged stone).
Source: Courtesy of K. Kyriakidis

- Symptom management

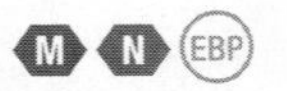

2. Prevention of recurrence, since a patient who has had a kidney stone is at risk for and likely to develop another (Tiselius, et al., 2008).

Care in most patients focuses on:

- Conservative management—pain control and hydration—is the best practice until the kidney stone passes. Determinants of treatment for kidney stones include size, location, obstruction of urine flow out of the kidney, and evidence of infection (Tiselius, et al., 2008).
- If spontaneous stone passage takes weeks, periodic x-rays may be used to track the stone. Urology may be consulted for further intervention or the need for surgical removal (Preminger, et al., 2007).

Pain Management

The key collaborative interventions (particularly nursing measures) in patients with renal calculi focus on pain management and prevention (Tiselius, et al., 2008).

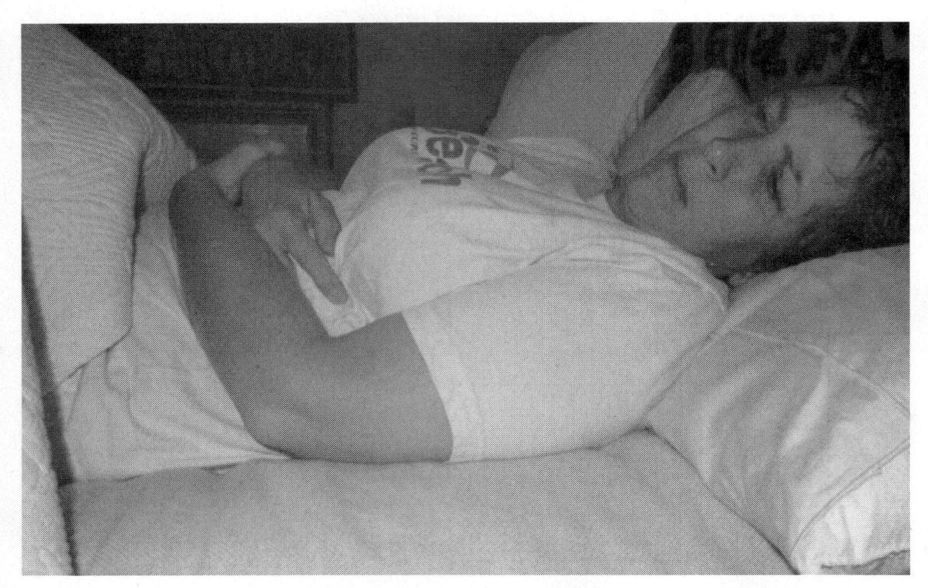

The variable and colicky or intermittent pain of kidney stones may require multiple adjustments in pain management as the stone(s) migrates.
Source: Courtesy of K. Kyriakidis

- If the patient can take oral fluids and medications, care is preferably managed at home.
- Initially treat pain with nonsteroidal anti-inflammatory drugs (NSAIDs). However, the pain can be so severe with renal calculi that narcotics are often required for pain control (Tiselius, et al., 2008).
- Combine opioids (oral or IV) with NSAIDs if needed as the optimal method to achieve pain relief (Tiselius, et al., 2008).
- Wait and observe the patient whenever the situation allows. A stone may take days or possibly weeks to pass.
- Instruct the patient to stop NSAIDs three days prior to lithotripsy (if used) to help minimize any bleeding risk.

Symptom Management

- Encourage oral hydration (or intravenous if the patient has persistent vomiting) with a focus on drinking about 1.5 L of water per day (or one's normal maintenance amount). Forcing fluids has not shown improvements in stone passage or in reducing pain medication requirements as compared to minimal hydration (Tiselius, et al., 2008).
- Administer antiemetics for nausea and vomiting (e.g., ondansetron).
- Instruct the patient to strain urine for kidney stones, which usually pass without medical intervention. Urine is strained in order to catch, analyze, and identify the type of stone passed (Tiselius, et al., 2008).
- Collaborate to consult urology if symptoms exacerbate or complications arise.

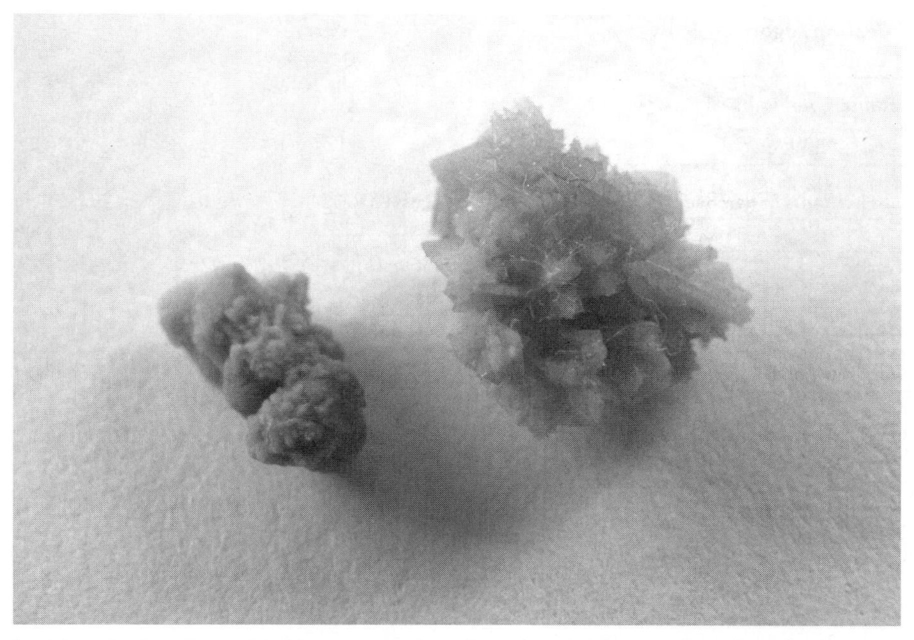

Straining urine in patients with kidneys stones often allows the culprit stone to be collected and identified. The sharp edges help explain the severe pain patients experience.
Source: Remik44992/Shutterstock

Concept Check

5. What is the initial treatment for the pain of kidney stones?

A. Positioning
B. Increasing fluids
C. NSAIDs
D. Opioids

Answer question

Collaborative Interventions (continued)

Obstruction and Infection

- If the patient is febrile or the urinalysis has more than 10 leukocytes (WBCs) that indicate a urinary tract infection (UTI), then the following care is needed:
  - M N EBP o Urine cultures should be obtained and antibiotics should be started (Surviving Sepsis Campaign, 2013).
  - M N EBP o Evaluate the patient immediately for sepsis or severe sepsis (see Surviving Sepsis guidelines in the Care of Patients with Sepsis NovE-lesson). Hypotension, tachycardia, elevated respiratory rate, and/or altered mental status serve as important warning signs for sepsis or severe sepsis (Preminger, et al., 2007).
  - N EBP o Call the Rapid Response Team if the patient has two or more warning signs of sepsis.
- M N An obstruction may be seen on imaging. Spontaneous resolution of the obstruction may occur for stones smaller than 5 mm. However, for stones that are larger than 5 mm, an invasive intervention is usually required. Immediate intervention is also required for patients with infection because of the increased risk of sepsis.
- The algorithm that follows is intended to provide a guide to anticipate and prepare for the care a patient with kidney stone needs.

Renal Obstruction and Infection Algorithm

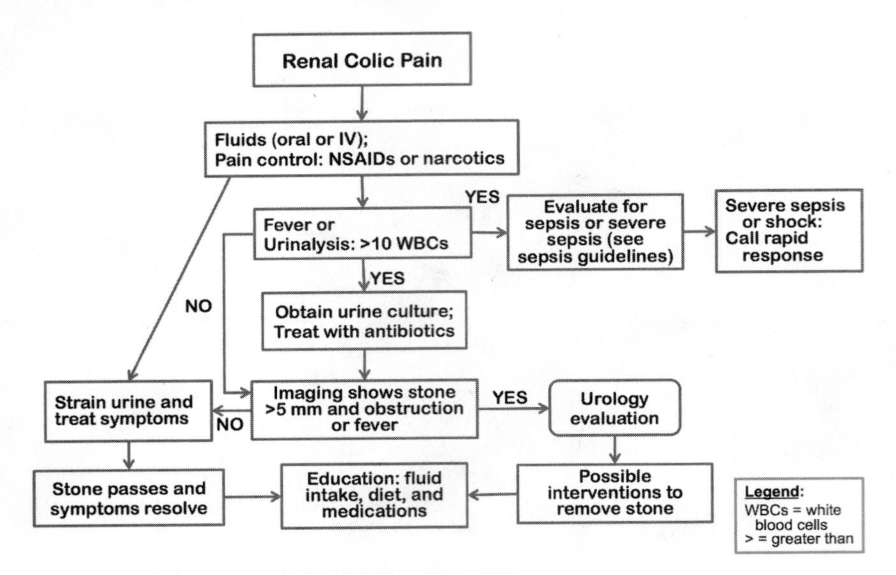

Invasive Interventions

Key invasive procedures include:

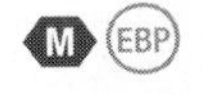

- Extracorporeal shock wave lithotripsy (ESWL) uses shock waves to break up the renal stone into smaller pieces so they can pass more freely through the urinary system (Preminger, et al., 2007).

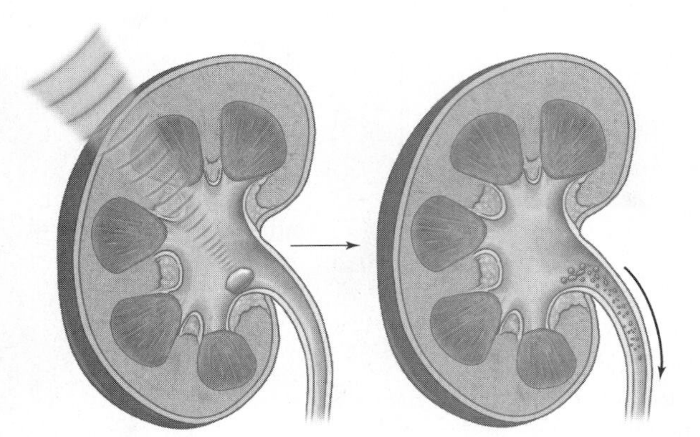

Shock waves are used in the lithotripsy procedure. Note the stone fragments that result and can more easily be passed.

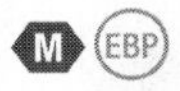

- Ureteroscopy involves the insertion of a small flexible tube into the urinary tract. The stone is then either extracted with instruments, like a small basket, or broken up with a laser into smaller pieces (Preminger, et al., 2007).

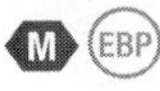

- Ureteral stents may be placed after the ESWL or ureteroscopy to help facilitate passage of the small pieces of stones and healing of the ureter from the inflammation (Preminger, et al., 2007).

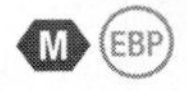

- Urethral stents might also be placed if the patient is septic from the stone. Stents can assist in draining the infected urine. The patient can eventually have the stones removed, after the infection has resolved (Preminger, et al., 2007).

Prevention

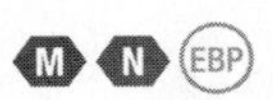

- Educate the patient regarding specific lifestyle and dietary changes as needed; determining the type of stone and urine characteristics of a patient can help guide treatment to prevent further stone formation (Tiselius, et al., 2008).
- In the following tables, note how the characteristics guide the preventative measures.

Type	Frequency	Characteristics	Prevention
Calcium Oxalate	70%	Low urine volume Hypercalciuria due to genetic causes, excess vitamin D or hyperparathyroidism Hyperoxaluria due to increased consumption of foods containing oxalates or GI disorders such as inflammatory bowel disease Hypocitriuria due to metabolic acidosis (e.g. diarrhea, renal tubular acidosis), or idiopathic causes Uricosuria (uric acid may act as a nucleus for crystallization of calcium oxalate) Low urine pH	Increase fluid intake Drug treatment: Thiazide diuretics Treat underlying cause (e.g., hyperparathyroidism) Diet for hyperoxaluria: Increase fuid intake. Do not decrease dietary calcium. Low salt diet. Avoid foods high in oxalate Potassium citrate Allopurinol Low protein diet <8 oz meat/day
Calcium phosphate	8%	Low urine volume Renal tubular acidosis causing high urine pH (since calcium phosphate is very insoluble at high pH), hypocitrauria, and hypercalciuria	Increase fluid intake Potassium citrate
Uric Acid	11%	Low urine volume Hyperuricosuria Low urine pH (since uric acid is very insoluble at low pH) due to renal tubular acidosis. Diarrhea, high protein diet.	Increase fluid intake Allopurinol Low protein diet Potassium citrate
Struvite	10%	Infection by bacteria that split urea (e.g. proteus sp)	Treat infection Removal of stones
Cystine	1%	Cystinuria (genetic)	Increase fluid intake Low protein diet, low salt diet
Other	<1%		

Source: Copyright © 2014, NovEx Novice to Expert Learning, LLC

Concept Check

6. **A 55-year-old male is admitted to the hospital with a kidney stone. He is experiencing nausea, tachycardia, declining mental status, severe flank pain, fever of 101.2°F, and 12 WBCs in his urine. What is your priority intervention?**

   A. Insert an indwelling urinary catheter.

   B. Initiate rapid response team to evaluate for sepsis.

   C. Administer an antiemetic.

   D. Increase oral hydration.

Answer question

Collaborative Interventions (continued)

Fluid Management Education

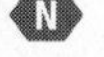

Tips are listed below to reduce the risk of kidney stone formation and include the International Kidney Stone Institute's (2014) tips to increase fluid intake to 1.5–2.0 L daily.

- A 2 L per day goal equals 10 or more glasses of water each day.
- Get a charcoal filter for your pitcher if tap water tastes bad. Water that tastes good is easier to drink.
- Define transitional times during your day and drink 8 oz. of water at those times. Examples include upon waking for the day, at breakfast, when you brush your teeth, when you return from work, after using the bathroom, and before and after exercise.
- Place a water bottle (insulated if you prefer cold) where you work. Sip from a straw, which some people believe encourages them to drink more.
- Good work habits include getting up each hour to stretch. Make going to get water part of your "minute break" routine hourly. Add citrus fruit or pineapple bits for a refreshing flavor. Freeze the fruit and add to water to cool it.
- Challenge family or coworkers to see who can reach water drinking goals daily.
- When you crave a snack, drink a glass of water prior to or with the snack.
- Use a 2-L bottle of water to pour from or fill your water bottle from to track your intake. You should finish the 2 L by the evening.
- Drink a full glass before each meal.
- Take an insulated and/or refillable water bottle with you wherever you go—exercising, outings, shopping, yard work, running errands, or doing chores.
- Select a special container with a comfortable feel to it.
- Fluid intake should be spread out as evenly as possible during the day.
- Drink enough in the evening to get up at least once during the night to urinate.
- Select water-containing foods over drier ones.

Dietary Management

M N EBP **Dietary education is important as a low oxalate diet is key for 70% of patients with kidney stones** (Tiselius, et al., 2008).

- M N Restriction on calcium intake used to be a common practice in patients with a history of calcium oxalate stones.
- M N EBP However, recent evidence has suggested that increasing the intake of calcium may actually reduce the risk of calcium oxalate stone formation. This is likely because calcium binds to oxalate in the gut and prevents absorption of oxalate (Tiselius, et al., 2008).
- N EBP Educate patients to be aware that those who had normal calcium intakes and lower intakes of protein (below 8 oz. per day) and salt had a significantly reduced rate of calcium oxalate stone recurrence (Tiselius, et al., 2008).
- M N EBP Avoid foods high in oxalate (see photo) (Tiselius, et al., 2008).

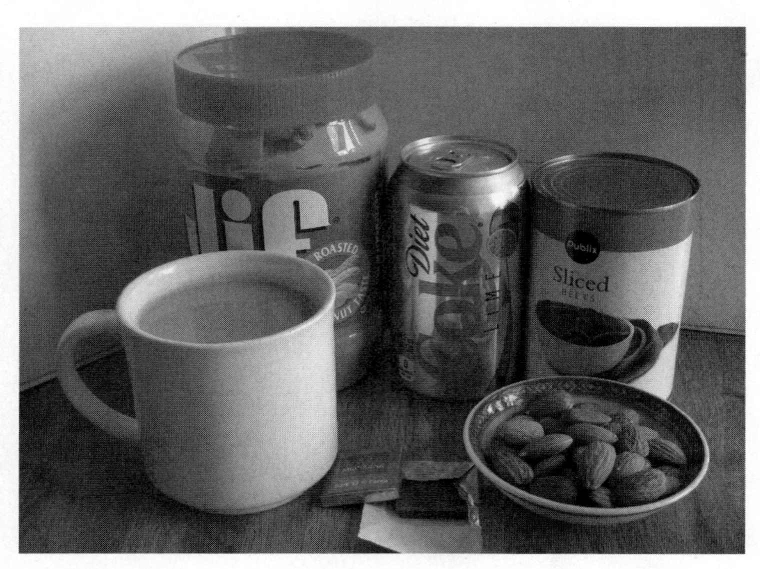

This picture shows oxalate-rich foods to avoid, particularly peanuts, chocolate, almonds, hot chocolate, beets, and colas.

Source: Copyright © 2014, NovEx Novice to Expert Learning, LLC

- M N EBP Simple dietary recommendations may be one of the best ways to reduce the risk of calcium oxalate stones (Tiselius, et al., 2008).
- M N Herbal medications on the market claim to reduce the incidence of kidney stones, but to date there is no evidence to support their use (Chauhan, 2013).

Patient Education

- N **Post-procedure education** may include:
  - o Educate for post-procedure follow-up for renal calculi removal or lithotripsy.
  - o Educate about home care, such as collecting stones by straining the urine.
  - o Educate about postop pain control, antibiotics, and monitoring of urine amount and color (first few voids will be bright red, but then begin to normalize).
  - o Educate regarding the signs and symptoms of the most serious complications of invasive procedures: hemorrhage and infection (of site or of urine).
- Preventive education may include:
  - N EBP o Patient education is essential to help avoid repeat occurrences of renal calculi, including (Tiselius, et al., 2008):
    - ■ Drink plenty of fluid.
    - ■ Reduce animal protein intake.
    - ■ Limit caffeine and alcohol, which are dehydrating.
  - N EBP o Educate about diet to lower risk of calculi formation (uric, purine, oxalate) (Tiselius, et al., 2008).
  - N EBP o Emphasize avoiding acidic foods (Tiselius, et al., 2008).
  - N o Avoid overheating and dehydration (e.g., hard labor, summer weather).
  - N o Improve self-care, particularly diabetes, weight management, hypertension, and significant comorbid conditions.
  - N o Refer patients to helpful websites to review key concepts to guide their understanding and healthier lifestyle management to prevent stones.

Summary of Interventions

- Treatment of symptoms:
  - o NSAIDS and/or narcotics for pain
  - o Hydration—PO or IV
  - o Strain the urine
  - o Antiemetics for nausea and vomiting, as needed
- Patients with fever and/or >10 WBCs in the urine should:
  - o Have urine cultures done.
  - o Start on antibiotics.
  - o Be evaluated for sepsis or severe sepsis.
- If stone is >5 mm or the patient has fever or urinary tract infection, the patient likely needs an intervention to remove the stone or obstruction.
- Interventions include cystoscopy with retrieval of stone or shock wave lithotripsy.
- Prevention of recurrence includes education about increasing fluid intake, diet, and medications. The specific treatment depends on the type of stone and abnormalities detected in urine testing.

Concept Check

7. Which finding is normal immediately following lithotripsy?

A. Sharp increase in abdominal pain intensity
B. Bright red urine
C. Hiccoughs
D. Left shoulder pain

Answer question

LO4:

Evaluation of Desired Collaborative Care Outcomes

Evaluation and reassessment should reveal attainment of previously established patient outcomes. In summary:

- Patient reports that pain is absent or greatly diminished.
- Patient reports no difficulty in starting or maintaining urine stream.
- Patient has clear mentation, elastic skin turgor, and a balance between fluid intake and urine output.
- Patient reports drinking more fluids, limiting alcohol and caffeine, and avoiding foods implicated in specific stone development.

References

Chauhan, V. (2013). Demystifying kidney disease for the average Joe!, *Post Comments.* **www.kidneydoctorbradenton.org/2013/06/can-certain-herbal-medications-treat.html**

International Kidney Stone Institute. (2014). *Tips for increasing your fluid intake.* **www.iksi.org/patients/education/tips-increasing-fluid-intake/**

Massini, L., Han, H., Seifter, J., & Dwyer, J.T. (2014). Diet and kidney stones: Myths and realities. *Nutrition Today, 49*(1), 32–38.

Pearle, M. S., Calhoun, E. A., Curhan, G. C., & Urologic Diseases in America Project. (2005). Urologic Diseases in America Project: Urolithiasis. *J Urol, 173*(3), 848–857.

Teichman, J. M. H. (2004). Acute renal colic from ureteral calculus. *N Engl J Med, 350*(7), 684–693.

Clinical Practice Guidelines

Preminger, G. M., Tiselius, H. G., Assimos, D. G., et al., & American Urological Association Education and Research and European Association of Urology. (2007). 2007 guideline for the management of ureteral calculi. *J Urol, 178*(6), 2418–2434. **www.jurology.com/article/S0022-5347(07)02609-2/fulltext**

Tiselius, H., Alken, P., Buck, C., et al. (2008). *Guidelines on urolithiasis.* Arnhem, The Netherlands: European Association of Urology. **www.guideline.gov/content.aspx?id=45324**

Patient Education

International Kidney Stone Institute. (2014). *Tips for increasing your fluid intake.* **www.iksi.org/patients/education/tips-increasing-fluid-intake/**

Mayo Clinic Staff. (2012). *Diseases & conditions: Kidney stones.* **www.mayoclinic.org/diseases-conditions/kidney-stones/basics/definition/con-20024829**

XPlain Patient Education MedlinePlus Interactive Health Tutorial. (2014). *Kidney stones.* **www.nlm.nih.gov/medlineplus/kidneystones.html**

Learning Outcomes for Urinary Incontinence

When you complete this lesson, you will be able to:

1. Recognize the clinical relevance of urinary incontinence.
2. Consider the pathophysiology, etiology, risk factors, and clinical presentation of urinary incontinence that determine the priority patient concerns.
3. Determine the most urgent and important nursing interventions and patient education required in caring for a patient with urinary incontinence.
4. Evaluate the attainment of desired collaborative care outcomes for a patient with urinary incontinence.

LO1:

What Is Urinary Incontinence?

- Urinary incontinence (UI) is characterized by the involuntary loss of urine.
- Several types of urinary incontinence exist:
    - o Stress urinary incontinence (SUI)
    - o Urgency urinary incontinence (UUI)
    - o Overflow incontinence
    - o Functional incontinence

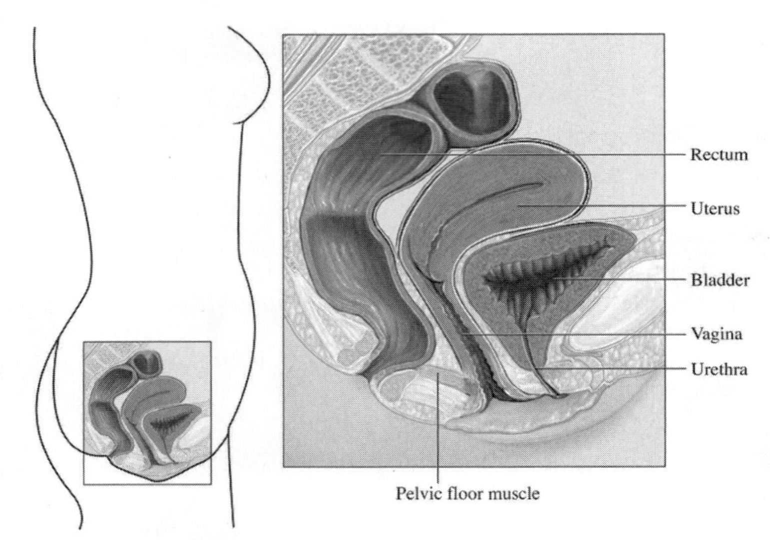

This diagram of the female pelvic anatomy offers a visual image of the organs involved in incontinence of women.

Source: © 2014 Nucleus Medical Media, All rights reserved

LO1:

Clinical Relevance

- Prevalence increases with aging, but is not a normal change. It occurs in:
  - o Twenty-five to thirty percent of older adult women and 10–15% of older adult men living in the community
  - o Fifty percent of older adults living in nursing homes, costing over $3 billion per year
- Often associated with:
  - o Altered mental ability, such as dementia
  - o Stool incontinence
  - o Immobility: unable to walk and move without assistance
- UI and the accompanying odors play a major role in social withdrawal and can lead to activity limitations and depression.
- Patients with UI are at risk for medical complications (e.g., skin breakdown or ulcers, urinary tract infections).
- Without management, patients may have to leave home and move into assisted living institutions.
- UI is the second most common cause for long-term care placement.
- However, the vast majority of UI that patients experience can be improved or alleviated with proper evaluation, intervention, and education.
- Nursing can play a major role in helping patients with UI better adapt and manage their UI problems.

LO2:

Pathophysiology

- Normal micturition occurs through the coordinated relaxation of the smooth muscle of the bladder wall and relaxation of the urethral sphincter muscle by the central nervous system.
- Voiding is under parasympathetic control and retention of urine under sympathetic control.
- A number of factors can affect this normal process:
  - o Obstruction of urine flow through the urethra (e.g., due to enlarged prostate, kidney stone)
  - o Weakening of the pelvic floor
  - o Medications that can affect the urethral sphincter tone and bladder wall function
  - o Under- or overactivity of the bladder wall muscle

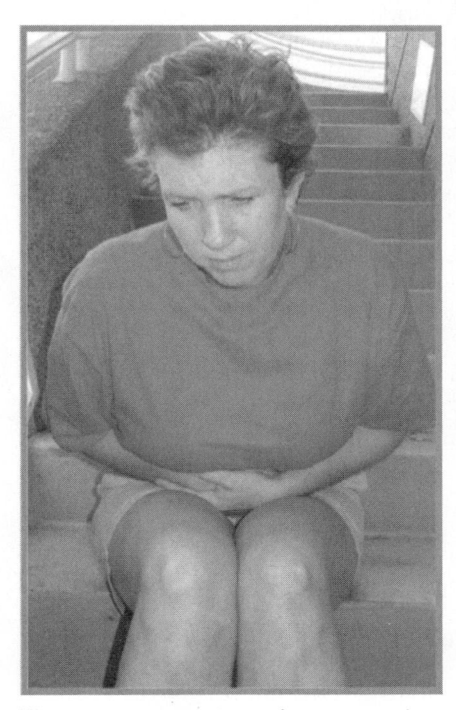

UI occurs in women twice as often as men and affects millions of women. Child bearing, giving birth, and the female anatomy contribute to much of the difference between men and women. Incontinence commonly causes distress due to the unexpected and uncontrollable condition.

Source: Courtesy of K. Kyriakidis

Concept Check

1. **How is aging associated with incontinence?**
   A. It is a part of normal aging.
   B. Aging is a risk factor for developing incontinence.
   C. There is no association.
   D. Incontinence indicates underlying pathology in the older adult.

Answer question

Types of Urinary Incontinence

The type of urinary incontinence dictates the intervention strategies. The major types of UI are:

- Stress urinary incontinence (SUI): involuntary loss of urine that is not caused by bladder contractions. It is usually associated with an activity such as lifting, exercise, sneezing, laughing, or coughing.
- Urgency urinary incontinence (UUI): loss of urine from an involuntary rise in intravesical (bladder) pressure when the bladder contracts
- Overflow urinary incontinence (OUI): loss of urine when the bladder fails to empty. A high post-void residual urine volume leads to overflow.
- Functional urinary incontinence (FUI): urine loss related to cognitive or physical limitations, but not due to urinary tract problems
- Mixed urinary incontinence (MUI): Patients (mostly women) may have more than one type of incontinence.

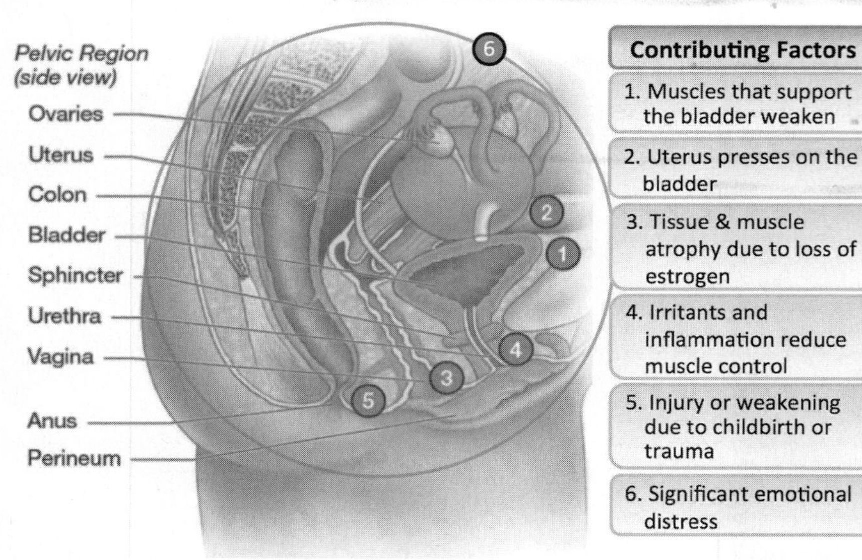

Anatomy of Incontinence
Pelvic Region (side view)
Ovaries
Uterus
Colon
Bladder
Sphincter
Urethra
Vagina
Anus
Perineum
Contributing Factors
1. Muscles that support the bladder weaken
2. Uterus presses on the bladder
3. Tissue & muscle atrophy due to loss of estrogen
4. Irritants and inflammation reduce muscle control
5. Injury or weakening due to childbirth or trauma
6. Significant emotional distress

For women, normal urine control relies on the strength and tone of the pelvic organs and structures (muscles, ligaments). Alterations in the strength, tone, or anatomy of one organ or supporting structure affect others. Changes in the bladder, urinary or digestive systems, aging, and even posture can adversely change the bladder's ability to function properly over time.

Source: Copyright © 2014, NovEx Novice to Expert Learning, LLC

Types and Causes of Stress Incontinence

- Stress incontinence is the most common type of UI and usually occurs in women under the age of 75.
- However, about 20% of women over 40 years old have some degree of SUI.
- It occurs with a sudden increase in abdominal pressure (or normal stress) that exerts pressure on the bladder (e.g., from a sneeze, cough, laugh, or jump).
- Normal stress causes SUI only when the muscles in the pelvic floor become weakened. Pregnancy, vaginal delivery, obesity, diabetes, and smoking are major contributors.
- Hypermotility that occurs in the bladder (both neck and urethra) causes 85% of cases and is related to changing hormones, increasing age, surgery of the pelvis, and childbirth trauma.
- Problems of the intrinsic sphincter cause 15% of cases and are due to surgery for incontinence, traumatic injury, pelvic radiation or surgery, or neurogenic causes.

Stress incontinence
Weakness of the pelvic floor muscles
Coughing, laughing, running etc, causes rise in intra-abdominal pressure
Pelvic floor "sags" and does not support bladder
Bladder neck prolapses through pelvic floor
Pelvic floor fails to contract
Urethra does not tighten
Small amount of urine is passed

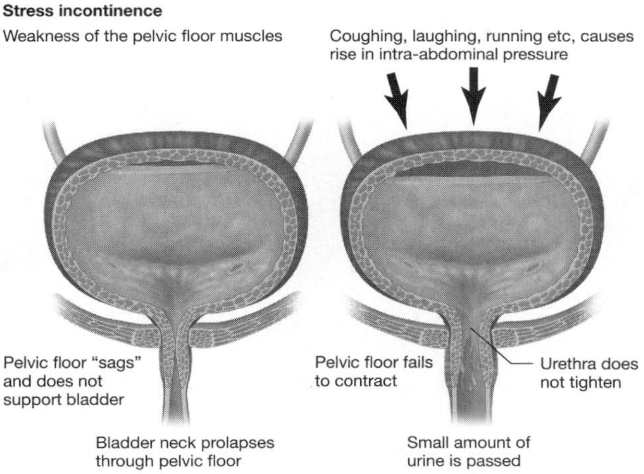

The pathophysiologic changes in the pelvis (left) demonstrate why a patient is vulnerable to stress incontinence. On the right, the process of stress incontinence is shown.

Pathophysiology (continued)

Types and Causes of Urge Incontinence

- Urge or urgency incontinence is a sudden need to void that cannot be suppressed.
- Urge incontinence is also called irritable, overactive, or spastic bladder.
- The most common cause of urge incontinence is aging, particularly past 75 years of age.
- It is usually idiopathic.
- Causes include:
  - Infection
  - Stroke or tumor
  - Dementia
  - Atrophic vaginitis or urethritis
  - Stones
  - Parkinson's disease
- Aggravating factors include:
  - The sound of running water
  - Hand hygiene
  - Being out in the cold

Types and Causes of Overflow Incontinence

- The primary cause of overflow urinary incontinence (OUI) is bladder overdistension.
- Bladder overdistension can be caused by bladder outlet obstruction due to:
  - o Stricture
  - o Benign prostatic hypertrophy
  - o Cystocele (herniation of the bladder through the vaginal wall)
  - o Fecal impaction (stool in rectum pressing on the urethra)
- A noncontractile bladder (also known as hypoactive detrusor or atonic bladder) can result in overflow incontinence secondary to:
  - o Diabetes
  - o Multiple sclerosis
  - o Spinal injury

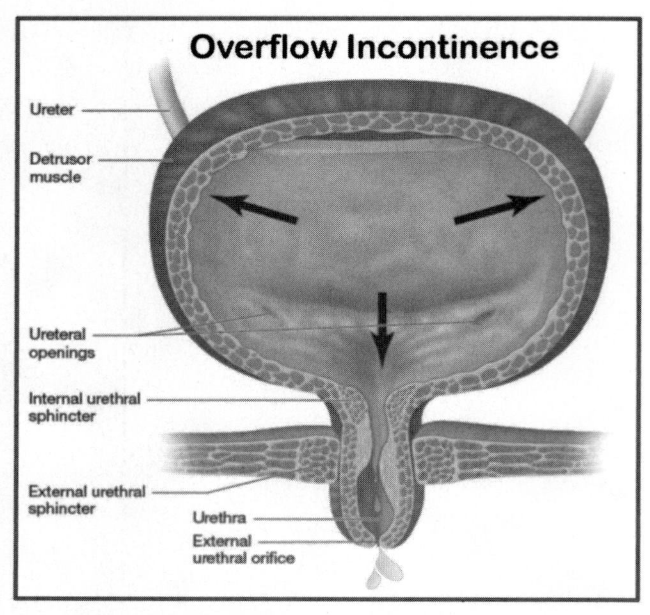

This illustration depicts overflow incontinence. Note the urethral blockage (black deposits) that prevents the bladder from properly emptying. This pathology leads to bladder overdistension (arrows) and leakage (yellow droplets).

Types and Causes of Functional Incontinence

- Functional urinary incontinence (FUI) does not involve the lower urinary tract.
- It is usually the result of physical, psychological, or cognitive impairment:
  - o Inability to walk to a bathroom in time to urinate
  - o Being bedridden
  - o Depression
  - o Alzheimer's disease

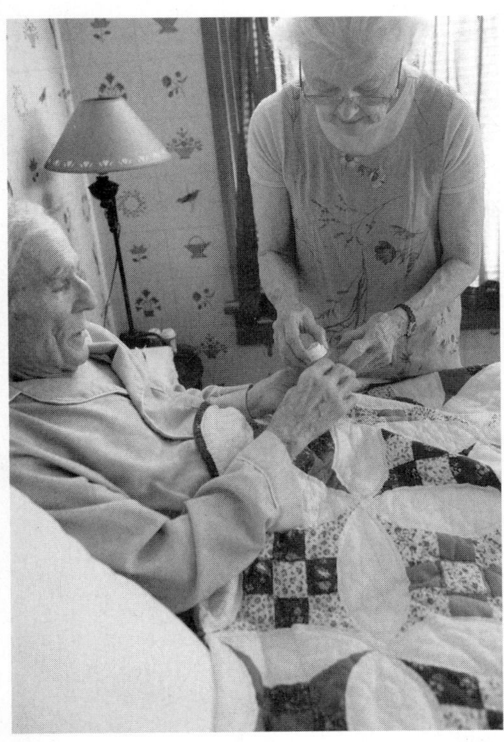

Functional incontinence is a common problem for older bedridden patients. The problem is exacerbated when the primary caregiver is older and may have a great deal of trouble helping the patient to the bathroom.
Source: Purestock/Alamy

Potentially Reversible Causes

- UI has a number of potentially reversible causes.
- The mnemonic **Diapers** can be used to identify reversible causes:

D Drugs
I Infection, especially urinary
A Atrophic vaginitis or urethritis
P Psychological disorders (delirium, depression, dementia)
E Endocrine disorders (hypercalcemia, hyperglycemia)
R Restricted mobility
S Stool impaction

Medications that may cause incontinence can include:

Effect	Causative Drugs
Increased frequency and urge to urinate	Diuretics, caffeine
Interference with bladder function; urinary retention	Anticholinergics, antipsychotics, antihistamines, and antidepressants
Decreased awareness of need to urinate	Sedatives, hypnotics, muscle relaxants, narcotics, alpha- and beta-agonists, and calcium channel blockers
Increased production but decreased awareness of need to urinate	Alcohol
Loss of bladder control	ACE inhibitors

Source: Copyright © 2014, NovEx Novice to Expert Learning, LLC

Concept Check

2. Which type of incontinence is most associated with a high post-void residual urine volume?

   A. Overflow

   B. Urgency

   C. Stress

   D. Functional

Answer question

Concept Check

3. Which drug class may result in incontinence by reducing the patient's awareness of the need to urinate?

   A. ACE inhibitors

   B. Caffeine

   C. Anticholinergics

   D. Calcium channel blockers

Answer question

LO2:

Assessment Findings

- Occasional minor leaks of urine
- Urinary dribbling
- Uncontrolled wetting of one's clothes

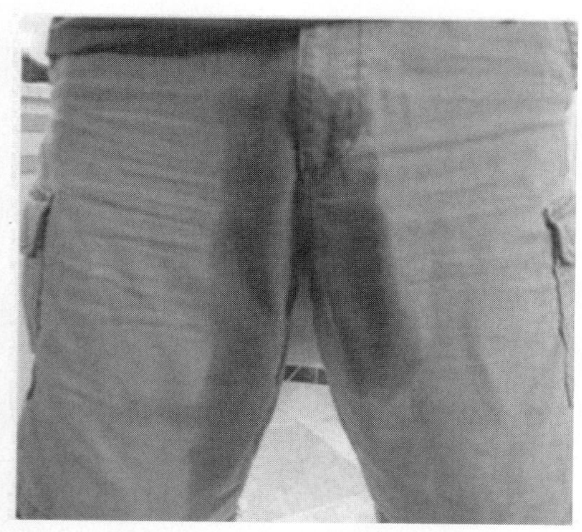

Uncontrolled leakage and wetting are symptoms of UI and commonly create social limitations for those who suffer from it.

Source: Copyright © 2014, NovEx Novice to Expert Learning, LLC

LO2:

Diagnostics

- When diagnosing UI, a few lines of questioning are helpful:
  - o Thorough voiding history is imperative. This may diagnose the problem without further evaluation.
  - o Evaluation of symptoms, including urgency, frequency, dysuria, stress leakage (e.g., with coughing, lifting), along with factors associated with leakage episodes can often point to the diagnosis.
  - o Medical and surgical history, including current medications, the number of pregnancies (for a woman), and caffeine intake are important.
  - o If patient uses urinary pads for protection, note how many per day are used.
  - o On physical examination, look for neurological, abdominal, mobility, dexterity, cognitive function, pelvic or rectal issues that might affect urination.
  - o Laboratory tests focus on trying to find a reason for UI, such as a urinary tract infection or urinary retention from diabetes.
- Post-void residual (PVR) is a measure of the amount of urine left in the bladder after voiding. This measurement is important in helping to determine whether the problem is a failure to store urine or a failure to empty urine from the bladder.
- More advanced studies can also be performed. These are normally not nursing procedures, but the nurse may help get the patient ready for these tests:
  - o Urodynamics: includes the measurement of the force of urine flow. This test can identify an intrinsic sphincter dysfunction.
  - o Radiology studies may include:
    - ■ A voiding cystourethrogram (VCUG), which can be helpful in patients with stress incontinence.
    - ■ For patients with a history of hematuria, persistent infections, or a possible tumor, an intravenous urogram could be obtained.
  - o Cystoscopy includes insertion of a cystoscope through the urethra to examine the bladder. This can be done for patients with hematuria, a possible tumor, persistent infections, or a previous urologic surgical history.

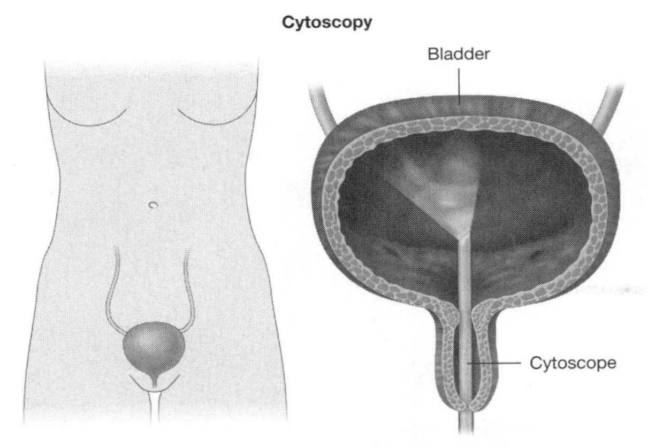

In this image, a cystoscope is shown in the bladder, after insertion into the urethra.

Interpretation of Post-Void Residual (PVR)

- PVR is a useful test to evaluate the incomplete emptying of the bladder.
- PVR is usually measured after a patient voids.
- PVR is obtained by using an ultrasound to scan the residual amount or with a straight catheterization by measuring the residual urine in the bladder.
- Interpretation of a PVR measurement (see table).

If PVR	Needed Intervention or Action
< 50 ml	None, adequate bladder emptying
> 150 ml	Avoid bladder relaxants
> 200 ml	Refer for urology consultation
> 400 ml	Expect urinary incontinence

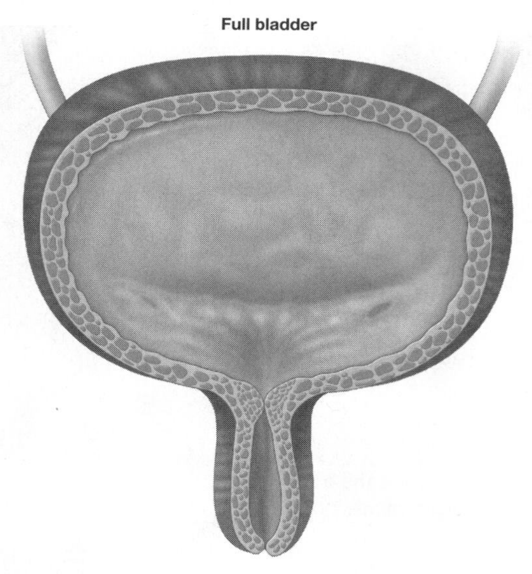

This image of a full bladder illustrates the inability to completely empty, which can cause considerable patient discomfort. If the PVR is high (e.g., >200 mL) immediate relief can be obtained by a straight urinary catheterization (assuming no obstruction is present).

Concept Check

4. Which option describes cystoscopy?
   A. It is done by inserting an endoscope through the urethra into the bladder.
   B. It requires a small incision in the abdomen above the bladder.
   C. It is done by placing a small camera in the ureter.
   D. It requires placement of an indwelling urinary catheter prior to the procedure.

Answer question

Priority Patient Concerns and Desired Collaborative Care Outcomes

Prior to caring for patients with urinary incontinence, it is important to prioritize the patient's concerns that must guide the nursing care plan and interventions. Care for the patient is ordered and organized in accordance with the patient's priority and urgent needs. Desired collaborative care outcomes in patients with urinary incontinence typically include:

1. Patient will participate in activities to improve potential to be continent of urine.
2. Patient will explain and use methods to be safe and independent in toileting.
3. Patient or caregiver will maintain or restore perineal skin to clean, dry, and intact state.
4. Patient or caregiver will demonstrate strategies used to avoid urinary tract infections.
5. Patient will begin to accept or be able to talk about changes in body image.
6. Patient will return or begin to return to previously enjoyed social activities.

Considering these important care outcomes, prepare a list of the major 3–6 priority patient concerns or nursing diagnoses for patients with urinary incontinence. Be prepared to participate in a discussion of this list and/or to submit them as an assignment, as determined by your faculty. Resources you may find helpful in this assignment can include this lesson, the references, resources on nursing care plans, and standard nursing diagnoses manuals.

LO3:

Collaborative Interventions

In SUI, UUI, and MUI, evidence supports nonsurgical interventions such as behavioral therapy, lifestyle changes, supportive devices, and/or medications as first-line therapies to help alleviate or manage urinary incontinence.

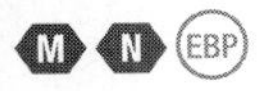

- Pelvic floor muscle training (PFMT) is strongly recommended (American College of Obstetricians and Gynecologists [ACOG], 2015; Abrams, et al., 2010; Thuroff, et al., 2010).
  - o Should be first-line therapy as it improves continence in all groups
  - o Intensive and supervised if possible
  - o Training involves exercises to tighten or squeeze and then release the muscles used to stop urine flow.
  - o Kegel (a name for PFMT) or Aeos exercises: used to strengthen pelvic floor muscles, especially effective during the first year after childbirth
  - o In SUI and mixed UI, PFMT is as effective alone as it is when used with other nonpharmacological interventions.

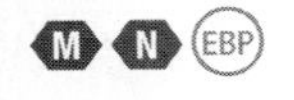

- Bladder training with scheduled or prompted voiding regimen is strongly recommended (Abrams, et al., 2010; ACOG, 2015; Thuroff, et al., 2010).
  - o Involves developing the ability to hold urine for progressively longer periods of time by adhering to a scheduled regimen
  - o A common goal is a 3- to 4-hour duration before emptying the bladder.
  - o The training involves "urge suppression" (or holding one's urine when the urge occurs) to delay bladder emptying.
- Behavioral therapies and lifestyle changes can help:

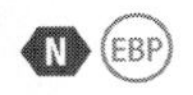

  - o Go to the bathroom on a schedule, such as every 2 hours (ACOG, 2015; Thuroff, et al., 2010).

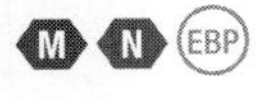

  - o Limit the consumption of caffeine, alcohol, or a lot of fluids before activities (ACOG, 2015; Abrams, et al., 2010; Thuroff, et al., 2010).

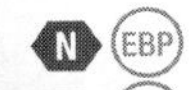

  - o Avoid lifting heavy objects.

  - o Weight reduction if body mass index is >27 (ACOG, 2015; Abrams, et al., 2010; Thuroff, et al., 2010).

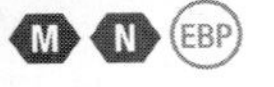

  - o Smoking cessation (Thuroff, et al., 2010)
- Medications: In some situations, medications may be used to improve UI.

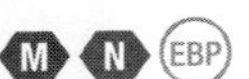

  - o Consider medications to relax the bladder or tighten the sphincter muscles (depending on the cause). High discontinuation rates (58-71% in women, particularly) of medications may provide limited benefits (Abrams, et al., 2010; ACOG, 2015; Thuroff, et al., 2010).

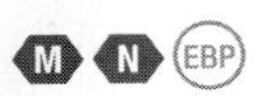

  - o Follow up on medication effectiveness: Up to 50% of women discontinue these medications due to adverse effects such as dry mouth or constipation (Thuroff, et al., 2010).

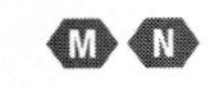

  - o Be alert to medications that predispose patients to incontinence: anticholinergics, beta blockers, antihistamines, antipsychotics, diuretics, alpha blockers, and estrogens.

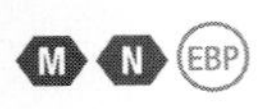

  - o In men with incontinence, if there is no notable PVR, strongly consider antimuscarinic medications for overactive bladder (Thuroff, et al., 2010). Educate the patient about medications.

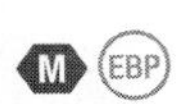

  - o Medications that do not provide significant benefit include oxybutynin and tolterodine (ACOG, 2015).

DRUG CLASS	MECHANISM OF ACTION	EXAMPLES OF DRUG
Muscarinic Receptor Antagonists & Anticholinergics	Reduce overactive bladder contractions	Oxybutynin (Ditropan), tolterodine (Detrol), trospium (Sanctura), darifenacin (Enablex), solifenacin (Vesicare), dicyclomine (Bentyl)
Alpha-Adrenergic Antagonists	Reduce urethral sphincter resistance to urinary outflow	Doxazosin (Cardura), terazosin (Hytrin), tamsulosin (Flomax)
5Alpha-Reductase Inhibitors	Androgen suppression that results in epithelial atrophy and a decrease in total prostate size	Finasteride (Proscar) Durasteride (Avodart)
Alpha-Adrenergic Agonists	Increase urethral resistance	Phenylpropanolamine, pseudephedrine
Tricyclic Antidepressants	Reduce overactive bladder contractions	Imipramine (Tofranil) Amitriptyline (Elavil)
Calcium Channel Blockers	Reduce smooth muscle contraction strength	Nifedipine (Adalat), diltiazem (Cardizem), verapamil (Calan, Isoptin)
Hormone Replacement Therapy	Local application reduces urethral irritation and increases host defenses against UTI	Estrogen cream (Premarin, Estrace), estrogen vaginal ring (Estring), estrogen vaginal tablets (Vagifem)

This table lists medications that may be used and can improve UI.

- Other nonsurgical therapies include:
  - N o Absorbent products that adhere to underwear
  - M N o Alarm notification devices to alert the health care provider of UI episodes in bedridden patients.

Collaborative Interventions (continued)

Interventions for Stress Urinary Incontinence (SUI)

- M N EBP Pelvic floor muscle training (ACOG, 2015; Abrams, et al., 2010; Thuroff, et al., 2010)
- M N EBP Lifestyle modifications (detailed in Patient Education section) (Abrams, et al., 2010; Thuroff, et al., 2010)
- N EBP Anti-incontinence and containment devices (Thuroff, et al., 2010)
- N Skin care (detailed in Patient Education section)
- M N Psychological considerations (detailed in Patient Education section)
- Medications may be needed and include:
  - M N EBP o Consider estrogen therapy to increase sensitivity in the proximal urethra and bladder neck (Estrace vaginal cream three times per week). Not recommended in SUI (Abrams, et al., 2010; Thuroff, et al., 2010). Instruct the patient about its use.
  - o Consider alpha-adrenergic stimulation like ephedrine, midodrine, methoxamine, imipramine, or phenylpropanolamine to increase bladder outlet resistance (Thuroff, et al., 2010).
- M EBP Consider collagen injections: intraurethral and into the bladder neck. Bulking agents work to increase pressure on the walls of the urethra, allowing for better control of urine flow. Studies do not show benefits over PFMT (Abrams, et al., 2010; Thuroff, et al., 2010).

Concept Check

5. **Which medication is commonly prescribed to reduce overactive bladder contractions?**

   A. Tamsulosin (Flomax)

   B. Nifedipine (Adalat)

   C. Estrogen cream (Estrace)

   D. Oxybutynin (Ditropan)

Answer question

Interventions for Urge Urinary Incontinence (UUI)

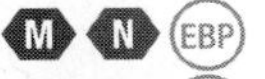

- PFMT are better than medications (ACOG, 2015; Abrams, et al., 2010; Thuroff, et al., 2010).
- Bladder training or scheduled voiding regimen (ACOG, 2015; Abrams, et al., 2010; Thuroff, et al., 2010)
- Caffeine avoidance (ACOG, 2015; Abrams, et al., 2010; Thuroff, et al., 2010)
- Anti-incontinence or containment devices (Thuroff, et al., 2010)
- Skin care
- Psychological considerations
- Medications (e.g., anticholinergics) that relax the bladder muscles and suppress contractions are recommended (Thuroff, et al., 2010).

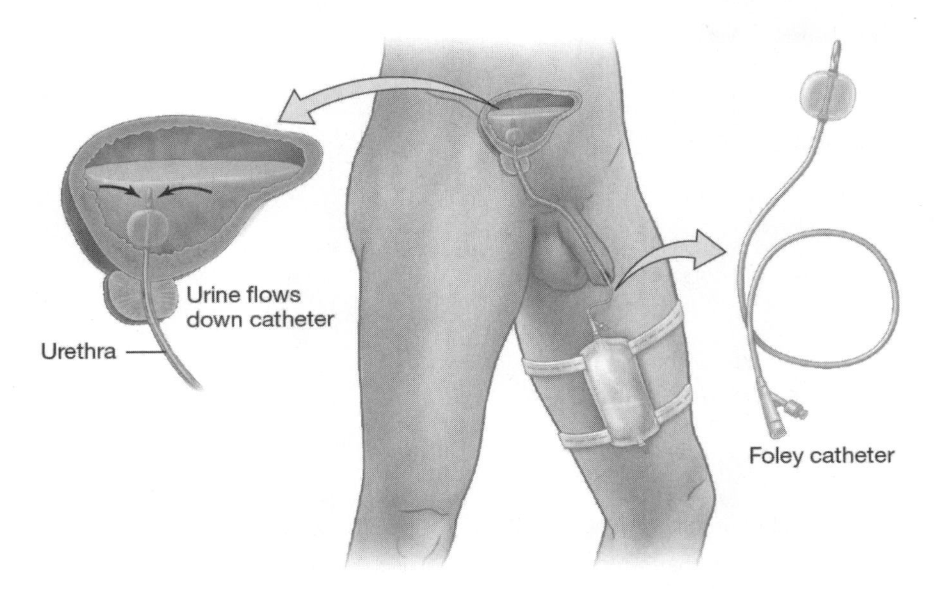

A urinary catheter is shown after placement in a patient. Although it is an effective means of managing UI, it is a major cause of infection and must be used with caution.

Interventions for Overflow Incontinence and Functional Incontinence

Overflow Incontinence

- Overflow incontinence can be temporarily addressed by intermittent self urinary catheterization. Indwelling urinary catheters are not recommended since they can lead to infections.
- Alpha-adrenergic antagonists may be used in male patients with benign prostatic hypertrophy. These drugs work by relaxing smooth muscle in the prostate and the bladder neck, thus improving urine flow (Thuroff, et al., 2010).
- Antimuscarinic medications can have significant benefits and may include fesoterodine, propiverine, trospium, and darifenacin (Abrams, et al., 2010; ACOG, 2015; Thuroff, et al., 2010).
- Skin care
- Psychological considerations

Functional Incontinence

In addition to the general interventions for patients experiencing urinary incontinence:

- Treat the underlying cause if possible.
- Provide prompted or scheduled toileting, individualized for the patient (Abrams, et al., 2010 ACOG, 2015; Thuroff, et al., 2010).

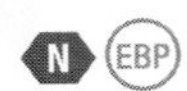

- Modify and declutter the environment and path to the bathroom for easy, rapid, and safe mobility for independent toileting (Abrams, et al., 2010; Thuroff, et al., 2010).

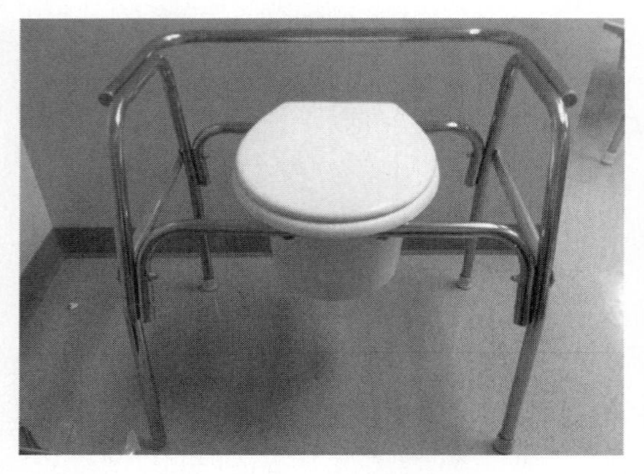

A bedside commode can provide a simple and more desirable alternative for patients with mobility challenges. Minimizing incontinence has social benefits and reduces the risk of skin breakdown and infection caused by repeated exposure to urine and feces.

Source: Copyright © 2014, NovEx Novice to Expert Learning, LLC

- A bedside commode may improve the rapidity and effectiveness of some older or debilitated (e.g., severe arthritis) patients to prevent incontinence.

Collaborative Interventions (continued)

Surgical Interventions

Stress Incontinence

Surgery has shown an 80% "cure" rate, but that success rate falls off to 50% beyond 10 years.

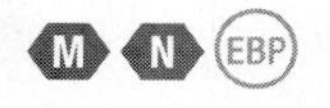
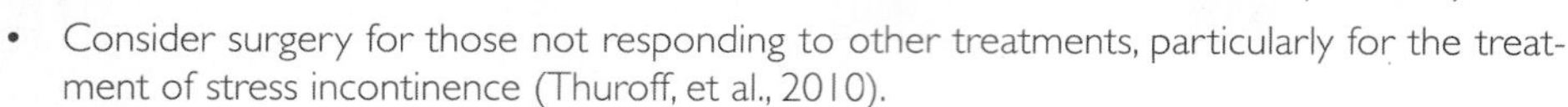

- Consider surgery for those not responding to other treatments, particularly for the treatment of stress incontinence (Thuroff, et al., 2010).

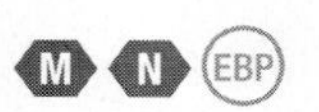

- The most common surgeries that can help return the bladder and urethra to a more normal position and exert pressure on the urethra to assist with urine retention are:
  - o Abdominal bladder suspension
  - o Sling procedure (Thuroff, et al., 2010)

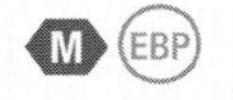

- Artificial urinary sphincter is another type of surgical procedure. It involves the placement of an artificial sphincter to replace a damaged sphincter (Thuroff, et al., 2010).

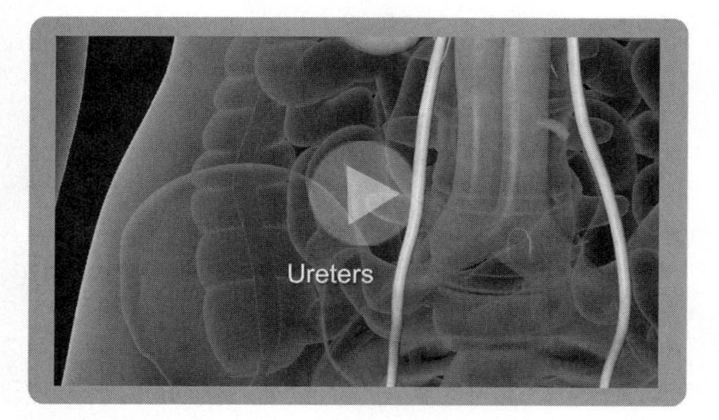

This animation provides a brief overview of the urinary system, stress UI or SUI, and several surgical interventions. The Burch or abdominal bladder suspension is depicted. Additionally, a laparoscopic method of bladder suspension and the sling procedures are shown.

Source: © 2014 Nucleus Medical Media, All rights reserved

Urge Incontinence

If medical management of UUI fails or is inadequate, bladder augmentation may be considered. This surgery:

- Enlarges the bladder
- Involves a cystoplasty to make the bladder larger with a segment of the small bowel
- Is typically a successful cure for UUI
- Can be disappointing for up to 30% of patients who may have to self-catheterize to empty their bladders

Overflow Incontinence

When the cause for overflow incontinence is bladder overdistension from an outlet obstruction, surgery can be helpful. Bladder outlet obstruction may be due to an enlarged prostate or other organ impinging upon, pressing on, or prolapsed onto the bladder. Surgery may include:

- Resection of the prostate
- Repair of an urethral stricture
- Repair of an organ prolapse, such as the uterus

Artificial Urethral Sphincter Placement

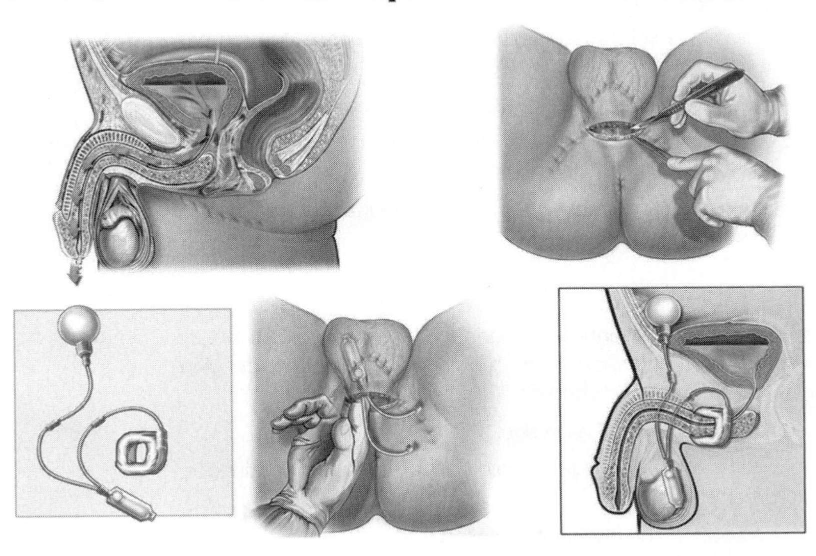

This series of images reviews the preoperative condition and shows how an artificial urethral sphincter is placed to repair a damaged urethral sphincter. Damage is a complication after prostatectomy.

Concept Check

6. What is true regarding surgeries to treat incontinence?

A. It is the major modality to ensure permanent resolution of the problem.

B. The initial success rate is about 80%.

C. The results are usually poor initially, but improve with time and healing.

D. It is no longer used as a treatment for incontinence.

Answer question

Postoperative Care

- Care for most postoperative patients for 1–3 days during hospitalization after an open bladder suspension procedure.
- Care for and prepare patients who have the laparoscopic procedure to go home early, often the same day as the surgery.
- Strongly encourage patients and their care providers to start early ambulation and activity.
- In addition to routine postoperative nursing care (e.g., recovery from anesthesia, vital signs, intake and output, frequent assessments, antibiotics, monitoring for postoperative complications, such as hemorrhage), care includes:
  - o Patients are often instructed to avoid lifting anything heavier than 15 pounds for 3 months.
  - o Monitor for urinary infection and retention, infection, urine leakage noted from the vaginal area (vesicocutaneous fistula), bladder instability, prolonged suprapubic pain, bladder spasms, and peritonitis.
  - o Administer prescribed pain medications for surgical pain and bladder spasms, as needed.
  - o Carefully monitor wounds and dressings near the rectal area. These are challenging to keep clean and intact (Registered Nurses Association of Ontario [RNAO], 2014).
  - o Collaborate to remove a suprapubic or indwelling urinary catheter at the earliest possible time, if present.
  - o Instruct the patient about intermittent self-catheterization should urinary retention become a problem.
  - o Ensure that vaginal packing is removed if placed during surgery.
  - o Ensure DVT prophylaxis is considered with the health care provider in patients with a history of DVT.
  - o Instruct the patient to avoid sexual intercourse for 6–8 weeks or until the health care provider evaluates healing and recovery.

Managing UI Complications: Dermatitis and Altered Skin Integrity

- Pressure wound prevention measures are essential since urinary incontinence can quickly cause wounds to develop. Avoid friction and shear when mobilizing patient. Consider skin sealants or moisture barrier products to protect the skin.
- Cleanse skin to remove caustic ammonia if urine is on skin.
- Maintaining a clean and dry environment is essential to avoid dermatitis from incontinence, particularly when there is skin breakdown.
- Change incontinence products as soon as they are wet or soiled.
- Use mild, dilute soap and water immediately for incontinence episodes. Gently pat area dry.
- Avoid non-soap cleansers that can cause drying or irritation (e.g., scented products, alcohol). Excessive dryness predisposes to infection through skin cracks or fissures. Bacteria counts double every 20 minutes.
- Absorbent and incontinence pads have been associated with a higher rate of urinary tract infections.
- Ensure healthy and sufficient dietary intake of protein and calories.

Complication	Causes	Interventions
Skin breakdown	Prolonged exposure to moisture, ammonia (urine), feces	Protect from pressure, shear and friction damage. Avoid rubbing area which can injure macerated skin. Keep skin ammonia-free to lower pH irritation and bacterial growth.
Bacterial infection	Dry skin exposed to urine and feces	Exposure to bacteria-ridden body wastes must be limited, especially with dry skin. Antibacterial medication to treat infection.
Fungal infection	Warm, damp environment	Clean, dry, environment with anti-fungal agent for healing.
Dermatitis (diaper rash)	Over-exposure to moisture, ammonia, feces	Keep skin clean & dry. Can use protective skin sealant or barrier.

Source: Copyright © 2014, NovEx Novice to Expert Learning, LLC

Collaborative Interventions (continued)

Patient and Care Provider Education

- Pelvic floor muscle training or rehabilitation (Abrams, et al., 2010; ACOG, 2015; Thuroff, et al., 2010):
  - o Should be first-line therapy
  - o Kegel or Aeos exercises to strengthen pelvic floor muscles, especially effective during the first year after childbirth
  - o Consider adding biofeedback if PFMT alone is not effective.

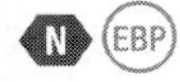

- Lifestyle modifications to improve and prevent UI include:
  - o Smoking cessation is strongly recommended (Thuroff, et al., 2010).
  - o Weight reduction in obese and morbidly obese individuals is strongly recommended (Abrams, et al., 2010; Thuroff, et al., 2010).
  - o Avoid heavy lifting and jumping.
  - o Reduce constipation episodes. Collaborate on constipation management and bowel regimen. Preventing constipation, when present, is key in preventing urinary incontinence (RNAO, 2005).
  - o Reduce bladder irritants such as caffeine, spicy, and acidic foods (Abrams, et al., 2010; Thuroff, et al., 2010).
  - o Reduce fluid intake when excessive (urge incontinence), but maintain a minimum of 6–8 glasses (8 oz) of fluid daily (Thuroff, et al., 2010).
  - o Reduce alcohol intake (Thuroff, et al., 2010).
  - o Environment improvements for safety for patients with impaired mobility
  - o Wear clothing that is comfortable and easy to manage for toileting.
  - o Instruct to bend forward or cross legs when coughing, laughing hard, or in activities that cause leakage (Thuroff, et al., 2010).

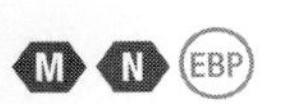

- Bladder training (with scheduled voiding regimens) (Abrams, et al., 2010; ACOG, 2015; Thuroff, et al., 2010):
  - o Good first-line intervention in patients with UUI and may be as effective as antimuscarinic medications
  - o Toileting and reminders for toileting on a regular schedule
  - o Scheduled toileting with adjustments of voiding intervals to retrain bladder.

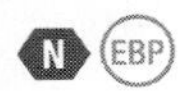

  - o Strongly recommend collaboration with patient to develop an individualized voiding schedule. A 3-day voiding record can provide important information to determine reasonable voiding intervals (RNAO, 2005).

- Supportive nonpharmacologic therapies:
  - o Biofeedback: used to assist the patient to identify, isolate, contract, and relax the pelvic muscles
    - ■ Benefits unknown
  - o Electrical stimulation: low voltage electricity to pelvic muscles to contract and strengthen them (Abrams, et al., 2010; Thuroff, et al., 2010)

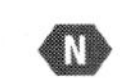

- Skin care is essential, but particularly in the most vulnerable patients:
  - o Keep perineum clean and dry.
  - o Avoid moisture-trapping undergarments and clothing.

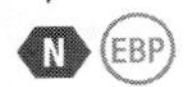

  - o Use moisture-retentive dressings as these can improve the wound environment and healing (RNAO, 2014).
  - o Skin breakdown and pressure ulcer prevention strategies in immobile patients are imperative (e.g., skin barrier ointments).
  - o Alarm notification devices can alert the care provider when a disabled patient needs to be cleaned and changed. When the sensor detects wetness, it alarms to elicit immediate care.

M N
- Anti-incontinence and containment devices:
  - o Intravaginal support devices (pessaries and bladder neck support prostheses)
  - o External collection devices (e.g., condom catheters) (Abrams, et al., 2010) EBP
  - o Absorbent products (e.g., disposable pads and undergarments)
  - o Alarm notification devices to alert care provider of UI episode in bedridden patients

N
- Adhere to medications if prescribed.

M N
- Psychosocial considerations:
  - o Social isolation: need for restroom facilities, caregiver
  - o Body image: stress incontinence while laughing, coughing, sneezing, jogging
    - ■ Affects lifestyle habits
  - o Sexuality: Has this been discussed with partner? What are feelings? Has intimacy been affected?

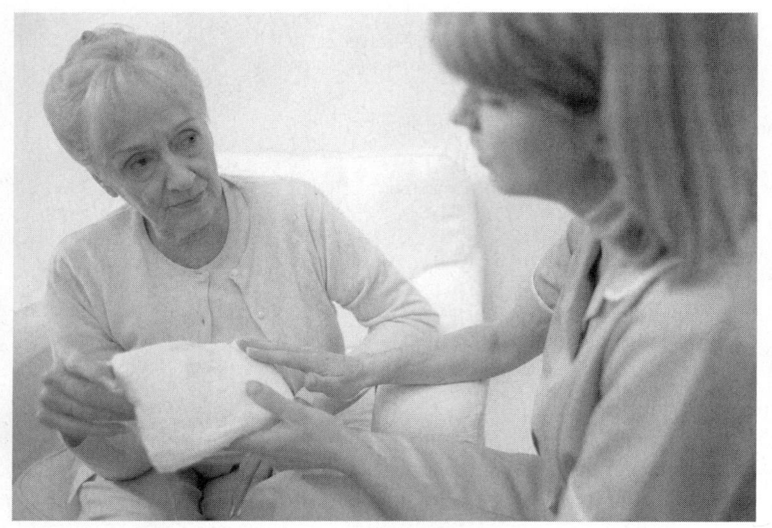

Absorbent pads can allow patients with UI to continue their social interactions. Educate patients to change pads whenever they are wet to protect their skin and to mitigate revealing odors.

Source: Science Photo Library/Alamy

Concept Check

7. Treatment of incontinence includes which strategy?

A. Weight loss

B. Decreased intake of water-rich foods

C. Reduced oral fluid intake

D. Smoking cessation

Answer question

Summary: Comparison of Skin Care—Urinary Incontinence

	Stress	Urgency	Overflow	Functional
Pathophysiology	Incompetent urethral sphincter	Sudden involunatry contraction of bladder causing a sudden need to void. Cause may be idiopathic or due to a bladder infection.	Overdistension of bladder due to bladder outlet obstruction (e.g. enlarged prostate) or to flaccid bladder wall.	Inability to go to the bathroom in time or lack of interest to go to the bathroom.
Symptoms	Incontinence occurs with sneezing, coughing, lifting.	Loss of urine is usually preceded by a sudden intense urge to urinate.	Loss of urine at varying times, dribbling, straining to void, sensation of inability to empty bladder may be present.	Physical immobility such as prior stroke, fracture, depressed mood, confusion (e.g. dementia)
PVR	Normal	Normal	High > 200cc	Normal
Treatment	Kegel exercises, estrogen cream, medications to increase sphincter tone, electrical stimulation, collagen injections, surgery (e.g. bladder suspension)	Treat UTI if present. medications to relax bladder (e.g. oxybutinin).	Intermittent catheterization. Alpha blockers (e.g. flomax) in patients with benign prostatic hypertrophy.	Voiding at regular intervals

Summary of Interventions

- In most cases, nonsurgical treatments can help alleviate urinary incontinence.
- PFMT is a first-line intervention, intensive and supervised if possible.
  - Performing exercises, called Kegel or Aeos exercises, to strengthen the pelvic floor muscle
- Lifestyle modifications should include:
  - Limiting the consumption of caffeine or an excess of fluids before activities
  - Reducing alcohol consumption
  - Smoking cessation
  - Weight reduction if body mass index exceeds 27
- Bladder training
- Behavioral therapies include:
  - Scheduled voiding to go to the bathroom on a schedule, such as every 2 hours
  - Managing constipation
  - Avoiding the lifting of heavy objects
- Other nonsurgical therapies include:
  - Medications to relax the bladder or to tighten the sphincter muscles
  - Absorbent products that adhere to underwear
  - A pessary (a device inserted into the vagina) to support the neck of the bladder and improve urinary control
- Surgery is usually reserved for the treatment of stress incontinence. The most common surgeries for stress incontinence are:
  - Abdominal bladder suspension
  - Sling procedure
- Patient education for improvement and prevention

LO4: Evaluation of Desired Collaborative Care Outcomes

Evaluation and reassessment should reveal attainment of previously established patient outcomes. In summary:

- Patient reports fewer episodes of incontinence.
- Patient reports successful self-toileting.
- Patient's perineal skin is clean, dry, and intact.
- Patient has not developed urinary tract infection.
- Patient reports feeling better about self, has started accepting body changes that cannot be altered, or is talking about feelings experienced due to the changes.
- Patient reports participation in social activities to desired level.

References

Agency for Healthcare Research & Quality. (2012). *Non-surgical treatments for urinary incontinence in adult women: Diagnosis and comparative effectiveness.* **www.effectivehealthcare.ahrq.gov/ehc/products/169/1031/ui_clin_fin_to_post.pdf**

Dowling-Castronovo, A., & Bradway, C. (2008). Urinary incontinence in older adults admitted to acute care. In: Capezuti, E., Zwicker, D., Mezey, M., Fulmer, T., editors, *Evidence-based geriatric nursing protocols for best practice. 3rd ed.* New York, NY: Springer Publishing Company, pp. 309–36.

Fowler, S. B. (2011). Pelvic floor muscle training versus no treatment, or inactive control treatments, for urinary incontinence in women. *Clin Nurse Spec, 25*(5), 226–227. doi: 10.1097/NUR.0b013e31822b41ce

Keyock, K. L., & Newman, D. K. (2011). Understanding stress urinary incontinence. *Nurs Practitioner Amer J Primary Health Care, 36* (10), 24–36. **www.nursingcenter.com/lnc/pdf?AID=1237385&an=00006205-201110000-00007&Journal_ID=54012&Issue_ID=1237343**

Thayer, C., et al., Urinary Incontinence Guideline Development Team. (2013). Urinary incontinence in women guideline. *Group Health Cooperative, 2013.* **provider.ghc.org/all-sites/guidelines/incontinence.pdf**

Clinical Practice Guidelines

Abrams, P., Andersson, K., Birder, L., et al. (2010). Fourth International Consultation on Incontinence recommendations of the International Scientific Committee: Evaluation and treatment of urinary incontinence, pelvic organ prolapse, and fecal incontinence. *Neurourol Urodyn, 29*(1), 213–240. **onlinelibrary.wiley.com/doi/10.1002/nau.20870/pdf**

American College of Obstetricians and Gynecologists (ACOG). (2005; reaffirmed in 2009 & 2015). *Urinary incontinence in women.* Washington (DC): American College of Obstetricians and Gynecologists (ACOG); (ACOG practice bulletin; no. 63). **http://www.aafp.org/afp/2005/0701/p175.html**

Bettez, M., Tu, L. M., Carlson, K., et al. (2012). 2012 update: Guidelines for adult urinary incontinence collaborative consensus document for the Canadian Urological Association. *Can Urol Assoc J, 6*(5), 354–363. **www.ncbi.nlm.nih.gov/pmc/articles/PMC3478335/**

National Collaborating Centre for Women's and Children's Health (UK). (2006). *Urinary incontinence: The management of urinary incontinence in women. NICE clinical guidelines No. 40.* London, UK: RCOG Press.

Registered Nurses Association of Ontario (RNAO). (2014). *Nursing best practice guideline: Assessment and management of stage I to IV pressure ulcers.* **rnao.ca/sites/rnao-ca/files/Pressure_Ulcers_I_to_IV_Summary.pdf**

Registered Nurses Association of Ontario (RNAO). (2005). *Nursing best practice guideline: Promoting continence using prompted voiding.* **rnao.ca/sites/rnao-ca/files/Promoting_Continence_Using_Prompted_Voiding.pdf**

Thuroff, J., Abrams, P., Andersson, K., et al. (2010). EAU guidelines on urinary incontinence. *J European Urology, 59,* 387–400. **uroweb.org/wp-content/uploads/EurUrolarticle_31012011.pdf**

Patient Education

American College of Obstetricians and Gynecologists (ACOG). (2005). *Urinary incontinence.* Atlanta, GA: American College of Obstetricians and Gynecologists. **www.acog.org/~/media/For%20Patients/faq081.pdf?dmc=1&ts=20140517T1225322363**

Markesich, D., Roundtree, A., Workman, T., et al. and the Agency for Healthcare Research and Quality. (2012). *Nonsurgical treatments for urinary incontinence: A review of the research for women.* **www.effectivehealthcare.ahrq.gov/ehc/products/169/1030/ui_cons_fin_to_post.pdf**

UCSF Medical Center. (2014). *Bladder Training.* **www.ucsfhealth.org/education/bladder_training/**

STOP

Go to the online course and complete the NovE-Cases assigned by your instructor for this module.

Learning Outcomes for Acute Kidney Injury

When you complete this lesson, you will be able to:

1. Recognize the clinical relevance of acute kidney injury.
2. Consider the pathophysiology, etiology, risk factors, and clinical presentation of acute kidney injury that determine the priority patient concerns.
3. Determine the most urgent and important nursing interventions and patient education required in caring for a patient with acute kidney injury.
4. Evaluate attainment of desired collaborative care outcomes for a patient with acute kidney injury.

LO1:

What Is Acute Kidney Injury?

- Acute kidney injury (AKI), also known as acute renal failure, is a sudden (acute) decrease in kidney function, which results in a decrease in glomerular filtration rate.
- AKI typically has a rapid onset and progression of renal dysfunction.
- AKI typically causes fluid and electrolyte imbalance, particularly resulting from the retention of electrolytes that are normally excreted.
- Due to the rapid deterioration in AKI, patients may require emergent treatment for a number of complications.

LO1:

Clinical Relevance

- AKI is one of the most common medical conditions encountered in the hospital.
- The incidence of community-acquired AKI is approximately 1 case per 10,000 people per year, but only 1% of patients are diagnosed on hospital admission.
- AKI comprises 8% of hospital patients and 50% of ICU patients.
- The incidence of hospital-acquired AKI is high. There are several contributing factors: high use in hospitals of nephrotoxic agents (meds, contrast dyes), increasing risks for AKI in our aging population, and increasing complexity and severity of illness with comorbid conditions.
- Some types of AKI (e.g., prerenal or postrenal) can be managed quickly and effectively if the cause is diagnosed appropriately and timely.
- AKI due to intrarenal dysfunction carries a mortality rate that may be as high as 50%.
- The cost of AKI is high because many patients with kidney failure require intensive care management.
- Use of renal replacement therapy (e.g., dialysis) is both difficult for the patient and very costly.
- With dialysis use, mortality in AKI is most commonly caused by complications. The leading problems include: sepsis, heart failure, and respiratory failure. Age does not seem to impact mortality rates in AKI.
- Nurses must be skillful and vigilant in identifying patients at risk for AKI in order to reduce mortality and morbidity from this condition.

LO2:

Pathophysiology

Three major types of AKI exist:

- **Prerenal** is caused by decreased perfusion of the kidney from dehydration or heart failure. It is often reversible.
- **Intrarenal** is usually due to an insult to the kidney, such as severe hypotension. However, kidney disease or toxic substances, such as radiographic dye and nephrotoxic drugs, can also cause AKI.
- **Postrenal** is usually due to an obstruction past the kidneys (e.g., in the ureters).

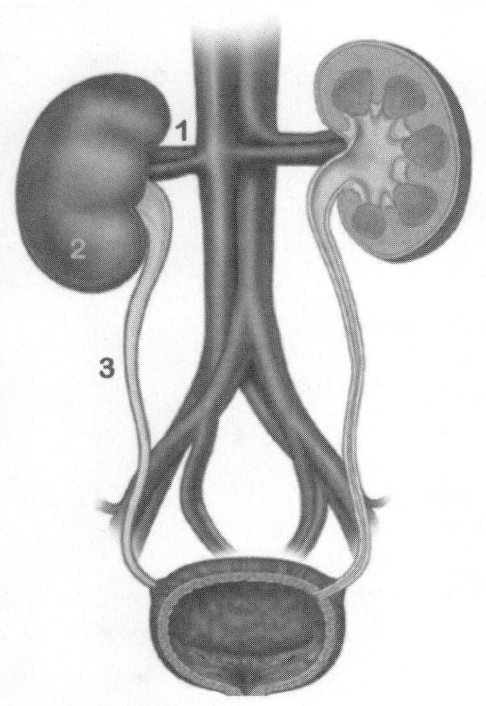

This illustration of the urinary system is labeled to point out the general location where the three types of acute kidney injury occur: 1 = prerenal, 2 = intrarenal, and 3 = postrenal.

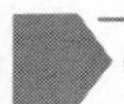

Concept Check

1. Which common treatments used in hospitals are potentially nephrotoxic?

A. Intravenous fluids

B. X-rays

C. Respiratory therapy

D. Medications

Answer question

Prerenal AKI

- Prerenal acute kidney injury is caused by inadequate renal perfusion, usually from a decrease in cardiac output or loss of blood flow. This is commonly the result of either heart failure or volume depletion due to dehydration or bleeding.
- The hypoperfusion causes ischemia, which compromises glomerular filtration and allows the accumulation of nitrogenous wastes. Short-term hypoperfusion commonly results in prerenal acute tubular necrosis (ATN), which is completely reversible. The kidney recovers. However, if hypoperfusion and ischemia are prolonged, intrarenal ATN may ensue.
- Occlusion of the renal artery can also cause decreased perfusion.
- Decreased perfusion results in enhanced sodium and water reabsorption in the renal tubules. Urine output drops.
- In prerenal AKI, the kidneys retain their ability to function. Glomerular filtration rate (GFR) quickly recovers with improvement of perfusion (e.g., with hydration).

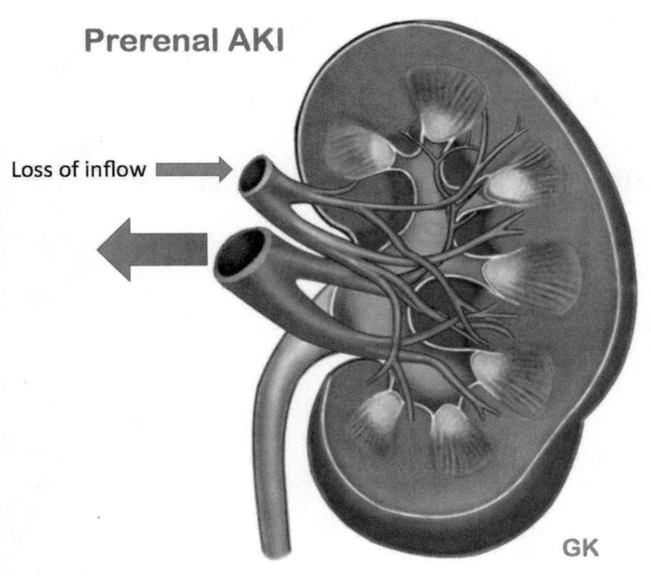

This diagram illustrates the anatomy of the kidney. The red arrow points to the renal artery receiving the inflow of blood with waste products that require filtration and removal. Prerenal AKI with reduced blood flow results in failure to remove waste products.
Source: Courtesy of George Kyriakdis/Santa Ana, CA

Pathophysiology (continued)

Intrarenal AKI

- AKI results from an acute parenchymal injury causing tubular cell damage. The renal parenchymal area is the functional portions of the kidney that filter blood and form urine.
- This is often precipitated by an inflammatory process (e.g., kidney infection), hypoperfusion, or nephrotoxic injury.
- Causes include:
  - o Acute tubular necrosis (ATN)
  - o Acute glomerulonephritis
  - o Acute interstitial nephritis

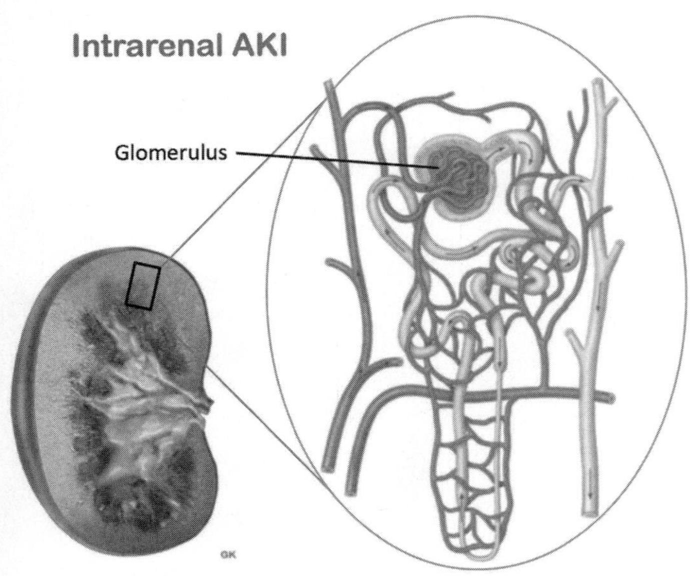

Damage to the glomerulus or any of the many types of renal tubules results in intrarenal kidney injury.

Source: Courtesy of George Kyriakdis/Santa Ana, CA

Intrarenal ATN

ATN is the most common type of intrarenal AKI acquired in hospitals.

- The initial injury to the kidney is commonly due to an acute condition such as severe hypotension, sepsis, myoglobin from necrotic cells, and trauma, or damage from a nephrotoxic medication.
- Hypotension and nephrotoxins are the major causes of the necrosis and sloughing of cells lining the kidney tubules.
- Glomerular filtration rate drops and the ability to reabsorb sodium decreases.
- Some patients develop oliguria (decreased urine output) because the tubules become blocked by necrotic epithelial cells.
- Other patients do not develop oliguria because the ability to concentrate urine and reabsorb water also diminishes.
- Recovery, if it occurs, may take several weeks.

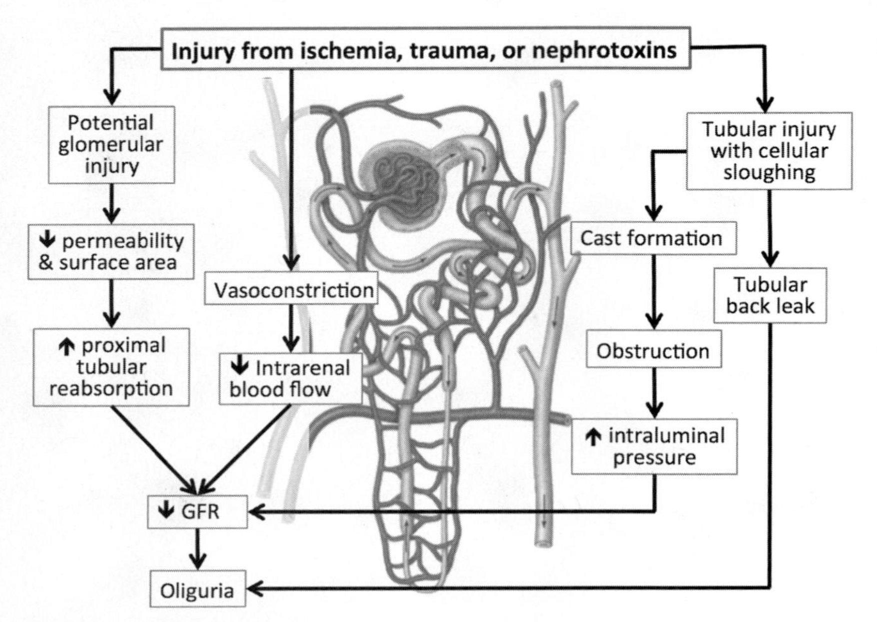

In ATN, injury may damage the glomeruli, capillaries, or tubules. Injury can result from hypotension, sepsis, or hemorrhage, as examples. All consequences of injury typically lead to decreased glomerular filtration and oliguria.

Source: Copyright © 2014, NovEx Novice to Expert Learning, LLC

- Glomerulonephritis is a type of intrarenal ATN that:
  - o Is caused by autoimmune damage to the nephrons
  - o Results in leakage of RBCs and protein into the urine due to the autoimmune damage
  - o See the images below that depict pathophysiology of glomerulonephritis after an infection.
- Interstitial nephritis is also a type of intrarenal ATN that:
  - o Is caused by an inflammatory response involving the tissues in the renal tubules
  - o Commonly results from an allergic reaction to drugs (e.g., sulfa)

Pathophysiology: Acute Post-Infectious Glomerulonephritis

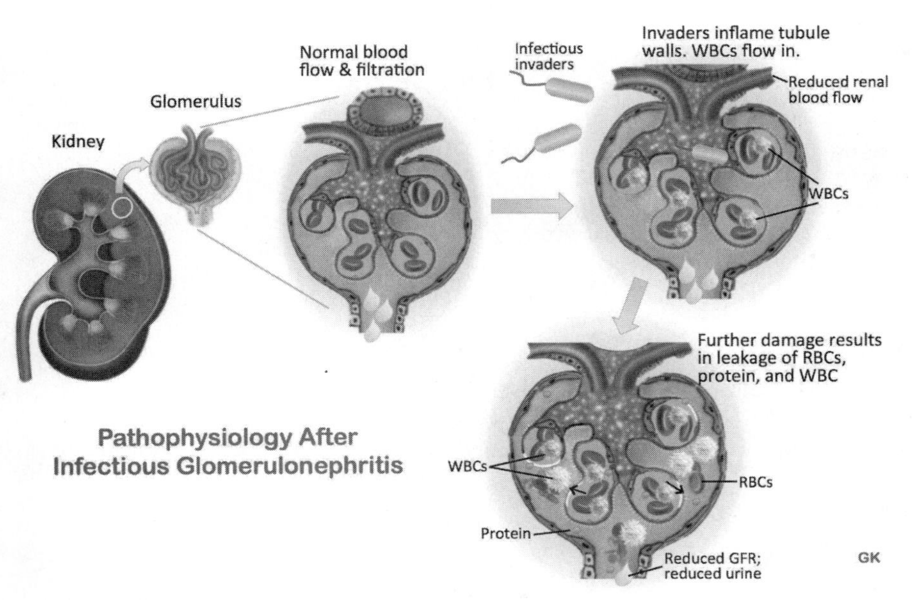

The multiple images on this slide demonstrate the pathophysiology of acute glomerulonephritis and how an infection damages the anatomical structure of the kidneys.
Source: Courtesy of George Kyriakdis/Santa Ana, CA

Pathophysiology (continued)

Postrenal AKI

- Obstruction of urine flow results in increased water and pressure inside the kidney (hydronephrosis) and in the urinary tract proximal to the obstruction.
- Obstruction of the urethra causes obstruction of both kidneys.
- Pressure increases in the tubules causing dysfunction of the nephrons and GFR drops.
- Necrosis of nephron cells may occur.
- After obstruction resolves, the patient may develop a large diuresis because the affected tubules have trouble reabsorbing sodium and water.

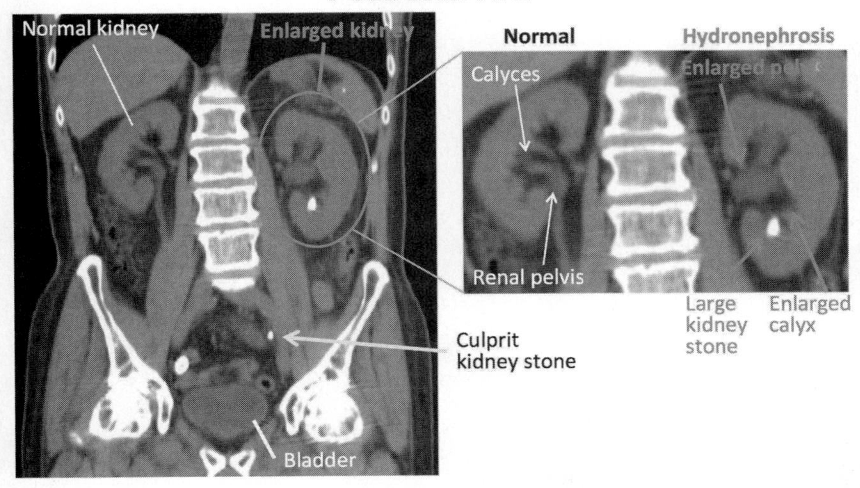

CT scan shows hydronephrosis (red circle) with dilated calyx and renal pelvis of the kidney. The dilated ureter cannot be seen in this view. Note the large kidney stone in the kidney. However, the smaller culprit stone (yellow arrow) is the cause of ureteral blockage, hydronephrosis, and postrenal AKI.
Source: Courtesy of K. Kyriakidis

Concept Check

2. What is the most common type of intrarenal AKI?

A. Acute tubular necrosis

B. Renal stones

C. Acute glomerulonephritis

D. Hypovolemia

Answer question

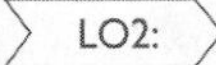

Risk Factors

- Renal failure is less likely to develop in healthy individuals, even when causes described previously are present.
- Underlying kidney disease and the presence of comorbid conditions predispose patients to the development of acute kidney injury.
- Risk factors for the development of AKI include:
  - o Diabetes mellitus
  - o Increasing age
  - o Chronic kidney disease
  - o Heart failure
  - o Hypertension
  - o Illness (e.g., hypovolemia, sepsis, cardiac surgery, liver failure) requiring intensive care (up to 50% of patients in the ICU develop AKI)

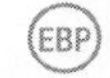

- These risk factors place patients having post-percutaneous coronary intervention at greater risk for contrast-induced nephropathy (Tepel, Aspelin, & Lameire, 2006).

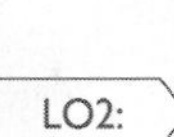

Causes

Prerenal AKI

Prerenal AKI results from decreased perfusion of the kidneys. The most common conditions to cause this are hypovolemia and heart failure.

- Hypovolemia can be due to many factors:
  - o Dehydration from diarrhea, vomiting, diuretics, or decreased oral intake of fluids
  - o Hemorrhage
  - o Systemic vasodilation and hypotension from sepsis
- Heart failure can be caused by a variety of conditions that include:
  - o Myocardial infarction/ischemia
  - o Cardiac tamponade
  - o Hypothyroidism
  - o Chronic heart failure
- Occlusion of the renal arteries can also result in decreased perfusion of the kidneys and can be caused by:
  - o Vasoconstriction of the renal arteries from sepsis
  - o Aortic dissection involving the renal artery
  - o Atherosclerosis of the renal arteries
  - o Thrombosis of the renal arteries
  - o A mass pressing on the renal arteries, such as a malignancy

Intrarenal AKI

- Ischemic injury:
  - o Most commonly results from severe or prolonged hypotension
  - o Causes acute tubular necrosis (ATN) when decreased perfusion of the kidneys is severe
- Nephrotoxins
  - o Nephrotoxic drugs (e.g., aminoglycosides, NSAIDs)
  - o Contrast dye: Contrast dye is used in many procedures in the hospital, including coronary angiography and CT scans. AKI due to contrast dye is called contrast-induced nephropathy.
  - o Myoglobinuria occurs in rhabdomyolysis (breakdown of muscle with release of myoglobin). Myoglobin blocks the tubules, causing AKI.
- Acute glomerulonephritis is an autoimmune response to the glomeruli (see the Care of Patients with Glomerulonephritis NovE-lesson).
- Acute interstitial nephritis is usually caused by an allergic reaction to medications. Bactrim is a common cause.

Postrenal AKI

Causes of urinary obstruction (see illustrations below):

- Within the ureters:
  - o Renal stones
  - o Malignancy
  - o Peritoneal or retroperitoneal tumor or obstruction pressing on the ureters
  - o Retroperitoneal fibrosis
  - o Ureteropelvic junction obstruction
  - o Postsurgical or traumatic obstructions
- Bladder outlet:
  - o Benign prostatic hyperplasia
  - o Strictures
  - o Renal stones
  - o Tumors
  - o Bladder neck contractures

Renal Cancer: Cause of Intrarenal & Postrenal AKI

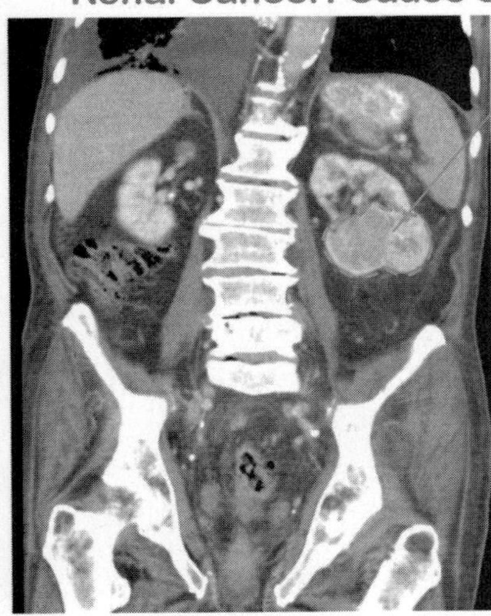

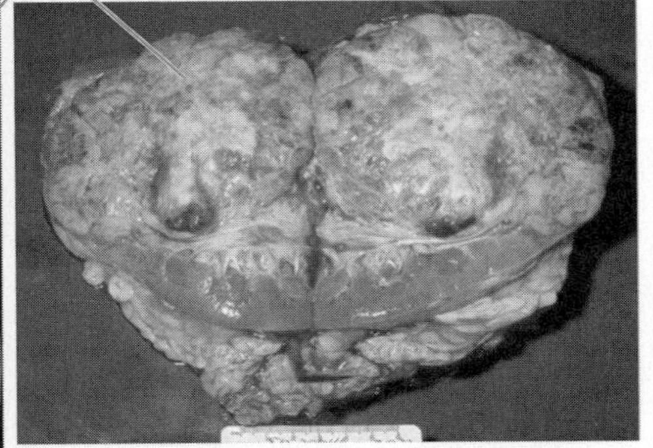

The CT scan (left) reveals a large invasive renal cancer causing intrarenal AKI. On autopsy, a renal cancer shows extensive renal destruction.

Sources: Courtesy of K. Kyriakidis & Dr. Edwin P. Ewing, Jr./Centers for Disease Control and Prevention

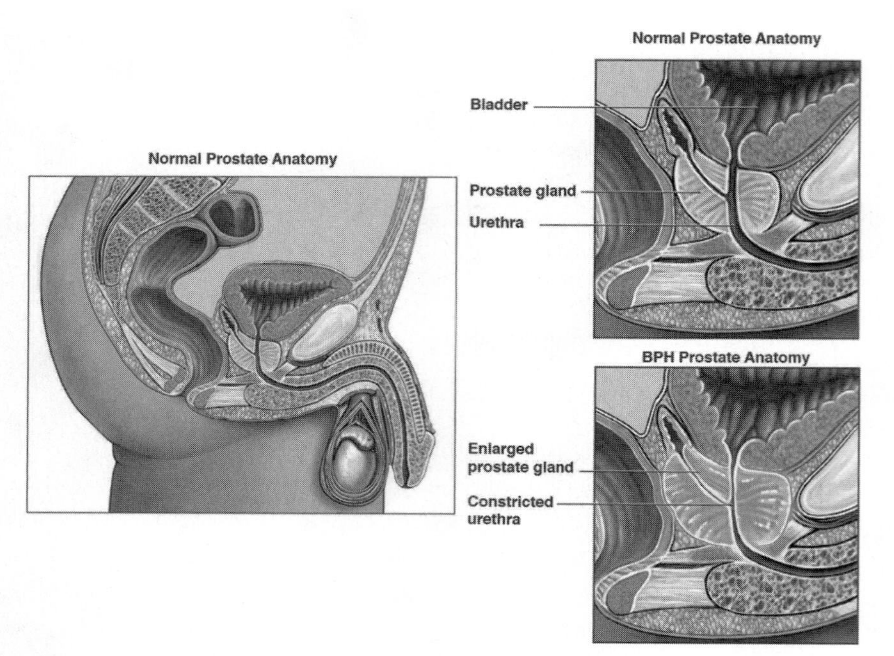

This example illustrates how pressure on the ureter (postrenal) can obstruct urine flow to cause postrenal AKI.

Concept Check

3. Contrast dyes may cause which type of renal failure?
   A. Prerenal
   B. Intrarenal
   C. Postrenal
   D. Extrarenal

Answer question

LO2:

Assessment Findings

Symptoms for acute renal failure include:

- Anorexia
- Fluid retention (e.g., peripheral edema, pulmonary edema)
- Confusion
- Other assessment findings may also be present, depending upon the etiology of AKI.

Prerenal

- Volume depletion
  - o Sepsis: fever, hypotension, tachycardia, decreased urine output
  - o Hypovolemia or bleeding: thirst, dizziness, overt weight loss, dry mucous membranes, decreased skin turgor, tachycardia, hypotension
- Heart failure: shortness of breath, dyspnea, leg swelling, tachycardia

Intrarenal

The patient may have only a few symptoms since intrarenal failure is abrupt in onset. Symptoms are primarily due to renal failure itself. These include:

- Possible weight gain
- Changes in mentation, including level of consciousness
- Pain, particularly in the flank region
- Urine output: may be normal or low volume; oliguria (e.g., <0.5 mL/kg/hr)
- Dangerously high potassium levels due to the inability to clear potassium

Urine Samples

When the urine output is low, the urine should be concentrated if the kidneys are functioning properly.

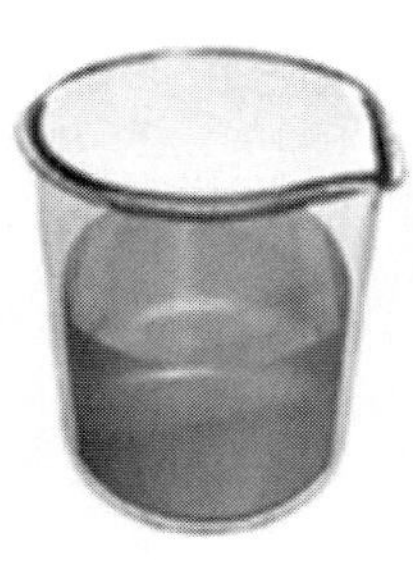

Dilute urine in face of low urine output is a warning of kidney injury.

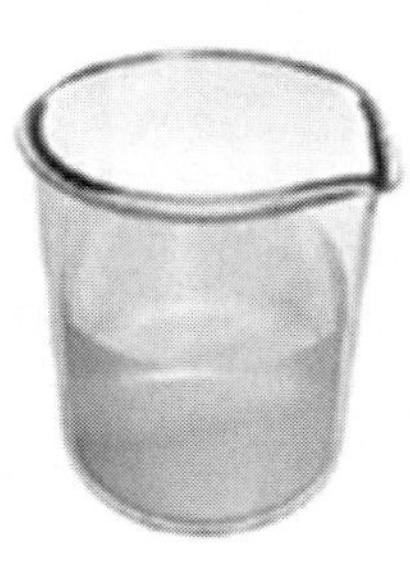

The kidneys lose their ability to reabsorb water and concentrate urine in intrarenal AKI.

Postrenal

- Difficulty or inability to urinate; dribbling
- Suprapubic discomfort from enlarged bladder
- Suprapubic tenderness or mass
- Anuria (no urine output)

LO2:

Diagnostics

Glomerular Filtration Rate (GFR)/Creatinine Clearance

- GFR is an indicator of kidney function that measures the amount of fluid filtered by the kidneys. Normal rate is ≥90 mL/hr.
- In AKI, there is a sudden decrease in GFR.
- Creatinine clearance is used to approximate the GFR.
- Measuring creatinine clearance requires a 24-hour urine collection, which is not always convenient in a hospital setting.
- However, there are a number of ways to estimate GFR based on serum creatinine, age, sex, and weight.
- Creatinine clearance can be estimated with the formula:

$$\text{Creatinine clearance} = \frac{(140 - \text{age}) \times \text{weight (kg)} \times (0.85 \text{ if female})}{72 \times \text{serum creatinine (in mg/dL)}}$$

- Calculations are accurate only if creatinine is stable. If creatinine is increasing, these calculations underestimate the drop in GFR.

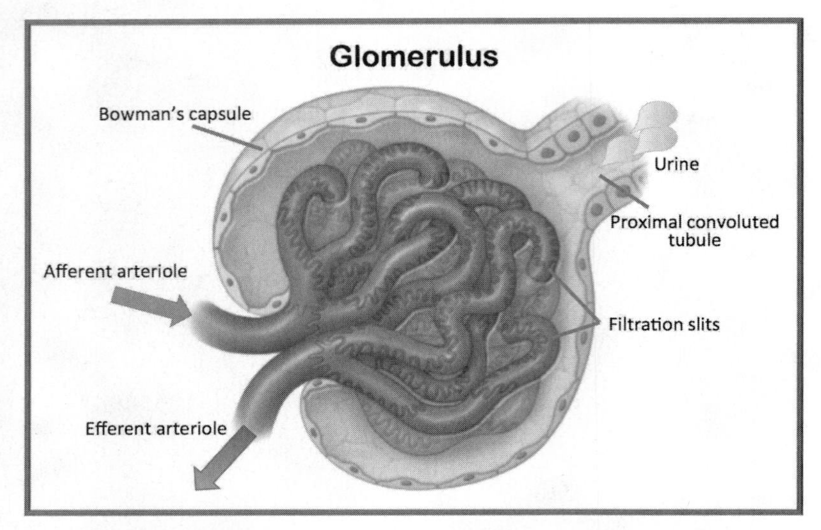

Each glomerulus is a cluster of blood capillaries surrounded by a Bowman's capsule. Blood enters the glomerulus and pressure forces fluid out of the blood through the filtration slits, creating a cell-free fluid that enters the renal tubule. Waste products, like creatinine, are then excreted.

Creatinine

- Serum creatinine measurement is an estimation of glomerular filtration rate and is the most commonly used measure of renal function. Creatinine is a by-product of muscle cells and is normally released in the course of muscle function.
- Creatinine is released from the muscle cells at a relatively constant rate and is filtered through the glomerulus and is not reabsorbed. Therefore, muscle mass is a determinant of creatinine production.
- The higher the muscle mass, the higher the creatinine. The level is, therefore, a function of how fast it is produced (related to muscle mass) and how fast it is filtered (related to GFR and kidney function).

↑Muscle → ↑ Serum Creatinine → ↑ Urine Creatinine

- A patient's age, gender, and weight influence muscle mass and should always be factors in interpreting the serum creatinine, even though these are often overlooked in clinical practice.
- A creatinine level at the upper limits of normal can be as high as 1.9 mg/dL in a large muscular patient. A creatinine of 1, on the other hand, could be abnormally high in a patient with low muscle mass (e.g., an older adult woman).
- Men generally have a higher muscle mass per kilogram of body weight and thus a higher serum creatinine level than women.
- Serum creatinine is used to estimate changes in kidney function and GFR.
- If creatinine of 1 mg/dL is baseline for a given patient with normal GFR, then:
  - o A creatinine of 2 mg/dL = 50% reduction in GFR.
  - o A creatinine of 4 mg/dL = 70–85% reduction in GFR.
  - o A creatinine of 8 mg/dL = 90–95% reduction in GFR.
- After the age of 40, the GFR decreases by 1% per year. However, serum creatinine level generally remains stable because muscle mass usually decreases with age.

Blood Urea Nitrogen (BUN)

- The correlation between BUN concentration and GFR is poor.
- In prerenal failure, the serum BUN-to-creatinine ratio (normally 10:1–20:1) rises and can have ratios that typically exceed 15:1.

Concept Check

4. What is the most important determining factor in what is a normal creatinine level?
   A. Age
   B. Muscle mass
   C. Ethnicity
   D. Weight

Answer question

Fractional Excretion of Sodium

- While most nurses do not calculate this value, some clinicians believe it is a helpful tool for assessing renal injury.
- The fractional excretion of sodium (FE_{Na}) is calculated using:

$$FeNa = 100 \times \frac{sodium_{urinary} \times creatinine_{plasma}}{sodium_{plasma} \times creatinine_{urinary}}$$

- Interpretation of FE_{Na} results:
  - o FE_{Na} of less than 1% indicates prerenal acute renal failure (AKI) may be suspected.
  - o FE_{Na} that exceeds 1% leads to concern about ATN.
- Pathophysiologic interpretation:
  - o A low FE_{Na} suggests the kidney is retaining sodium and that the cause is likely prerenal (e.g., hypovolemia, heart failure, sepsis).
  - o A high FE_{Na} points to sodium wasting that is expected with conditions that cause direct renal damage, such as acute tubular necrosis.
  - o Caution is needed when interpreting FE_{Na} when diuretics are used. Diuretics alter renal reabsorption of sodium and can, therefore, skew the results.

Diagnostics (continued)

RIFLE System in AKI

- RIFLE is an in-depth classification of AKI that is useful because the traditional markers are often late indicators of severe AKI.
- The development of the RIFLE classification system has become the basis for defining acute renal failure or AKI.
- Changes from the patient's baseline, in GFR, serum creatinine level, or urine output are the basis for the RIFLE classification and are as follows:

		Serum Creatinine	Decrease in GFR	Urine Output
R	Risk	Increase x 1.5	25%	<0.5 mL/kg/hr x 6 hrs
I	Injury	Increase x 2.0	50%	<0.5 mL/kg/hr x 12 hrs
F	Failure	Increase x 3.0	75%	
		≥4 mg/dL + acute increase >0.5 mg/dL		<0.3 mL/kg/hr x 24 hrs or anuria x 12 hrs
L	Loss	Persistent AKI; Complete loss of kidney function >4 weeks		
E	End-Stage	Loss of kidney function >3 months		

RIFLE classification of AKI.
Source: Copyright © 2014, NovEx Novice to Expert Learning, LLC

Prerenal AKI

- Patients with all types of prerenal AKI usually have a low volume of urine (e.g., <0.5 mL/kg/hr).
- However, since the kidneys still function, the urine can be concentrated (the kidneys try to conserve fluid elimination based on decreased renal perfusion).
- The result is:
  - o Concentrated urine is reflected by an increased urine specific gravity (>1.025; normal is 1.010–1.025)
  - o Urine sodium is decreased (<20 mEq/L; normal is 40–220 mEq/L) as the kidneys try to retain sodium to increase extravascular volume
  - o BUN-to-creatinine ratio increased (>15:1; normal is 10:1)
  - o FE_{Na} <1%

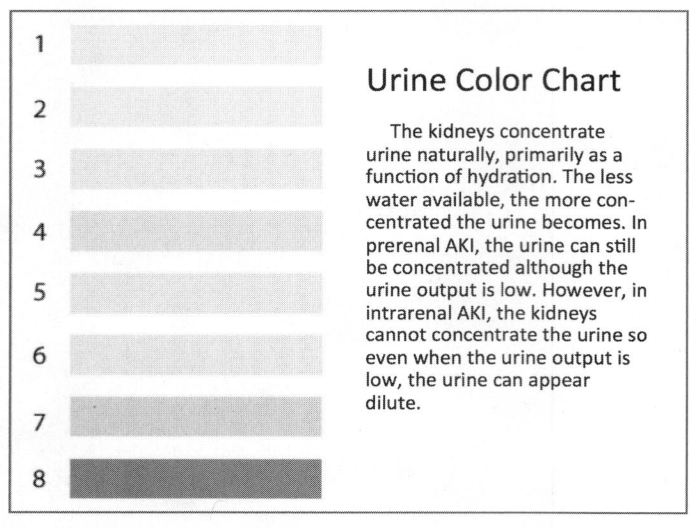

1
2
3
4
5
6
7
8
Urine Color Chart
The kidneys concentrate urine naturally, primarily as a function of hydration. The less water available, the more concentrated the urine becomes. In prerenal AKI, the urine can still be concentrated although the urine output is low. However, in intrarenal AKI, the kidneys cannot concentrate the urine so even when the urine output is low, the urine can appear dilute.

Intrarenal AKI

In AKI of intrarenal origin, the kidneys are damaged. The result is a failure to concentrate the urine. The findings include:

- A dilute urine and decreased urine specific gravity (<1.010; normal is 1.010–1.025)
- BUN-to-creatinine ratio remains normal, although both are elevated (normal ratio is 10:1)
- Urine sodium is normal or high (>40 mEq/L)
- FE_{Na} >1%

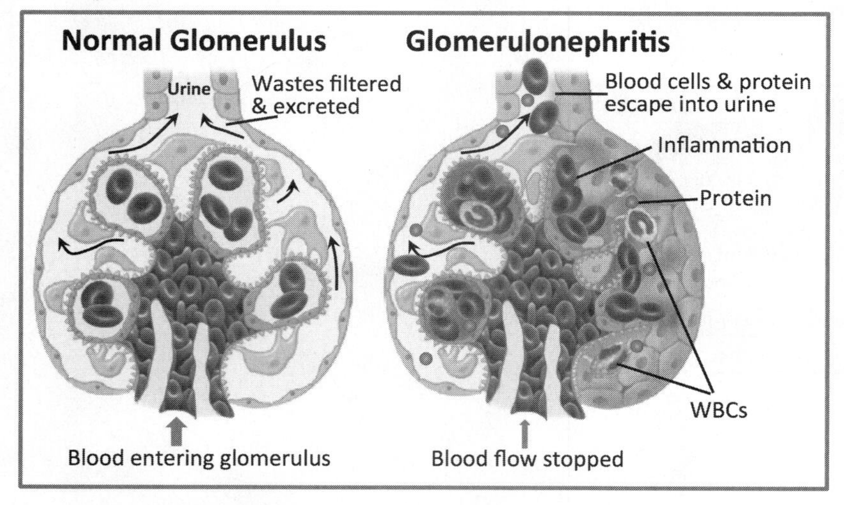

This image compares a normal glomerulus and glomerulonephritis. The right image depicts a severely inflamed glomerulus that no longer allows blood flow or filtration. Red blood cells, white blood cells, and proteins escape through the damaged renal tubules, resulting in many abnormal urine lab findings.

Postrenal AKI

- Bladder ultrasound may show a distended bladder.
- Intermittent catheterization (may be referred to as an "in and out" cath) may show a large post-void residual (the amount of urine left in the bladder after voiding).
- Renal ultrasound may show a dilated upper renal collecting system characteristic of hydronephrosis.
- Cystoscopies or retrograde urethrogram could reveal urethral obstruction.

Priority Patient Concerns and Desired Collaborative Care Outcomes

Prior to caring for patients with acute kidney injury (AKI), it is important to prioritize the patient's concerns that must guide the nursing care plan and interventions. Care for the patient is ordered and organized in accordance with the patient's priority and urgent needs. Desired collaborative care outcomes in patients with AKI typically include:

1. The patient will achieve and maintain normal fluid and electrolyte balance.
2. The patient will remain free of signs and symptoms of infection.
3. The patient will ingest an adequate amount of calories to meet metabolic needs within the guidelines of dietary restrictions.
4. The patient will express feelings related to fatigue and convey plans for fatigue management.
5. The patient will discuss anxiety as related to disease process, prognosis, and therapeutic interventions.
6. The patient will begin to discuss lifestyle changes in terms of their benefit.
7. The patient will verbalize ways to avoid AKI in the future and will comply with follow-up care.

Considering these important care outcomes, prepare a list of the major 3–6 priority patient concerns or nursing diagnoses for patients with AKI. Be prepared to participate in a discussion of this list and/or to submit them as an assignment, as determined by your faculty. Resources you may find helpful in this assignment can include this lesson, the references, resources on nursing care plans, and standard nursing diagnoses manuals.

LO3:

Collaborative Interventions

Care of patients with AKI can be complex and a number of interventions may necessarily occur simultaneously or are overlapping:

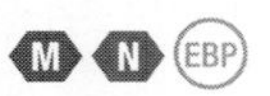
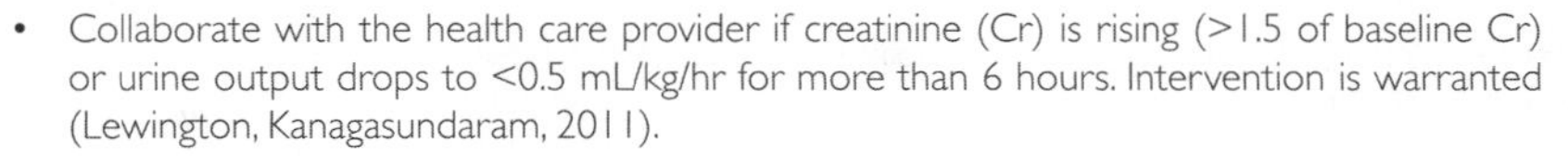

- Collaborate with the health care provider if creatinine (Cr) is rising (>1.5 of baseline Cr) or urine output drops to <0.5 mL/kg/hr for more than 6 hours. Intervention is warranted (Lewington, Kanagasundaram, 2011).

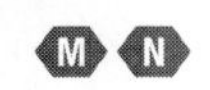

- Evaluate for postrenal AKI causes and treat if present:
  - o Exclude postrenal AKI by obtaining a post-void residual (PVR) in patients who present with abdominal bloating, suprapubic discomfort, or trouble urinating.
  - o If PVR is >400 mL, postrenal AKI cause of renal failure is likely. Insert a Foley catheter to relieve the obstruction and continue to monitor urine output and electrolytes.
- Evaluate for prerenal AKI causes of hypoperfusion and treat if present:

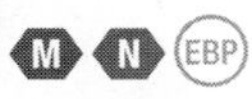

  - o Assess for hypovolemia as the prerenal cause (e.g., dehydration, diarrhea, bleeding, burns, injury) (Fliser, et al., 2012).

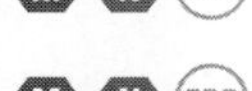

    - ■ Examine the patient for hemorrhage or severe dehydration (Fliser, et al., 2012).

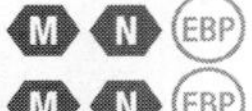

    - ■ If the patient is volume depleted, hydrate with continuous IV fluids or fluid boluses (Fliser, et al., 2012).

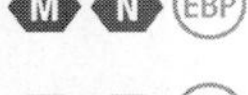
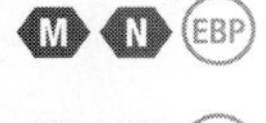

    - ■ Infuse isotonic crystalloids instead of colloids (e.g., albumin) as the initial and primarily volume expander (Kellum, et al., 2012).

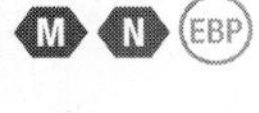

    - ■ Optimize patient's hemodynamics (e.g., blood pressure) with IV fluids and vasopressors if necessary. Vasopressors are appropriate in volume-resuscitated patients (Fliser, et al., 2012; Kellum, et al., 2012; Lewington & Kanagasundaram, 2011).

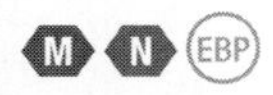

    - ■ Avoid IV diuretics to increase urine output to prevent or treat AKI, as diuretics can be very harmful (Kellum, et al., 2012). Diuretics are indicated to treat an underlying condition (e.g., heart failure) that is causing AKI.
    - ■ If fluid depleted, patients with prerenal AKI fully recover after hydration.

M N EBP o Assess for heart failure (e.g., shortness of breath, dyspnea, lung crackles, and leg edema). If present:

M N EBP ■ Treat with diuretics if patient is in heart failure (Kellum, et al., 2012) (see the Care of Patients with Heart Failure NovE-lesson for details).

M N EBP ■ May consider inotropes (e.g., dobutamine) in severe heart failure (Lewington & Kanagasundaram, 2011).

M N EBP o Assess for and treat other underlying cause (e.g., sepsis, conditions that cause fluid shifts with subsequent hypoperfusion) (Lewington & Kanagasundaram, 2011).

M N • Monitor urine output and creatinine as indicators of improvement because both should improve quickly when the cause is treated in patients with prerenal and postrenal AKI:

o Urine output (UO) usually improves within hours.

o Creatinine usually improves within 12–24 hours.

M N • If UO and creatinine do not improve, consider intrarenal AKI as a cause.

• Most intrarenal AKI causes are due to previous injury and primarily require supportive care until kidney function starts to improve:

M N EBP o Assess the patient for any recent episodes of hypotension or exposure to nephrotoxic drugs (Kellum, et al., 2012).

M N EBP o Stop nephrotoxic drugs (e.g., ACE inhibitors) and maintain hydration. If the patient is in heart failure and has pulmonary edema, diuretics may be needed (Kellum, et al., 2012; Lewington & Kanagasundaram, 2011).

M N EBP o Treat hyperkalemia in symptomatic patients (Alfonzo, et al., 2012).

N EBP o Observe for signs that should trigger concern about the need for dialysis: severe confusion, severe hyperkalemia, hyperkalemia resistant to treatment with medication, and severe metabolic acidosis (Pannu, et al., 2008).

M N o Anticipate that renal recovery, if it occurs, can sometimes take weeks.

M N EBP • Avoid diuretics to prevent or treat AKI. Patients with AKI who are oliguric have worse outcomes, including mortality and renal recovery, than nonoliguric patients. Nonoliguric patients have >0.5 mL/kg/hr of urine output (Kellum, et al., 2012). Poor outcomes in oliguric patients has led some clinicians to mistakenly attempt to administer diuretics to convert oliguric to nonoliguric renal failure.

M N EBP • Research indicates that diuretics are useful only in management of fluid-overloaded patients (Kellum, et al., 2012).

M • Consider dialysis, which can be more effective in oliguric renal failure when diuretics do not work.

M N EBP • Avoid using low-dose dopamine, fenoldopam, or atrial natriuretic peptide to prevent or treat AKI (Fliser, et al., 2012; Kellum, et al., 2012).

M N EBP • Avoid glycemic events, particularly hyperglycemia (Kellum, et al., 2012).

M N EBP • Consult nutritionist to support the patient with needed dietary modifications: Achieve intake of 20–30 kcal/kg/day (Kellum, et al., 2012).

M N EBP • Avoid limiting protein intake, particularly in patients who are at risk for protein-energy malnutrition (Kellum, et al., 2012). Collaboration with the nutritionist can assist the patient to avoid the unappetizing, traditional low-protein diet and assist the patient to eat healthier protein-controlled diet without causing AKI progression. However, a high-protein diet should be avoided.

M N EBP • Modify drug dosages, in collaboration with pharmacist as needed, to correct for altered renal function (Lewington & Kanagasundaram, 2011).

Summary of Interventions: Acute Kidney Injury

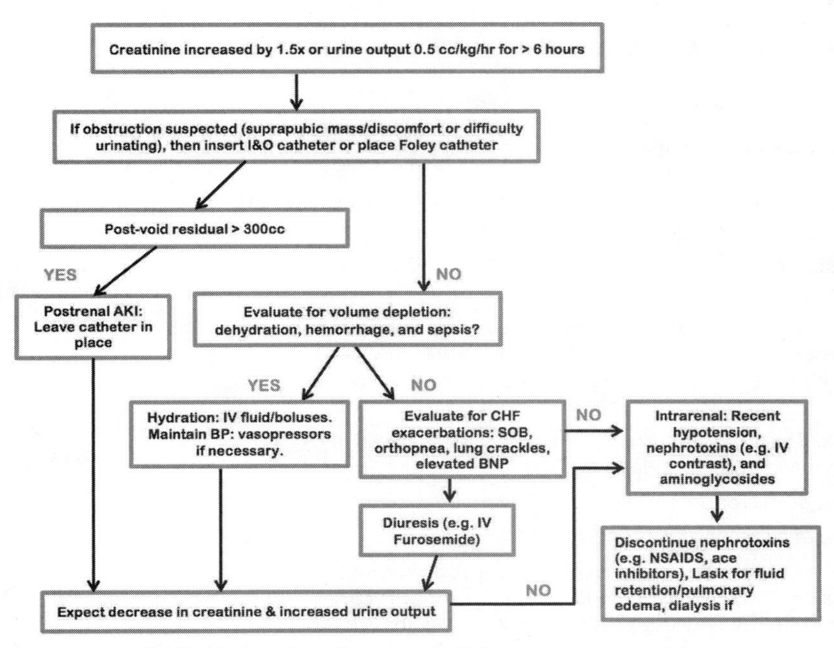

Collaborative Interventions (continued)

Supportive and Safety Care

Patients with acute renal failure, depending on the urgency and severity, are commonly cared for in the ICU. Extensive care is provided in the ICU and is not within the scope of this particular NovE-lesson; however, care of less critically ill patients typically includes:

- Monitor daily weight, intake, and output.
- Examine urine for amount, color, specific gravity, glucose, protein, blood, and sediment.
- Closely monitor serum creatinine, BUN, and electrolytes, particularly potassium.
- Continuously monitor EKG for any abnormalities that signal electrolyte imbalances, particularly hyperkalemia.
- Support nutritional therapy: protein-controlled diet. Restrict sodium, potassium, and phosphorus.
- Dialysis if necessary. Clinicians involved in peritoneal or continuous forms of dialysis require specialty preparation when the patient is dialyzed at the bedside. Patients receiving hemodialysis are typically transported for the procedure.
- Perform frequent assessments: mental status, oral mucus membranes, lung sounds, heart sounds, peripheral edema, skin turgor, bleeding from the dialysis access site or anticoagulation.
- Manage changing fluid and electrolyte imbalances to maintain hemodynamic stability.
- Monitor, clean, and protect temporary venous access sites, which commonly involve a non-tunneled catheter that can be dislodged.
- Prevent "never" events (e.g., catheter-related infections, deep vein thrombosis, pressure ulcers, urinary infections).
- Institute fall precautions and orthostatics when appropriate in patients with fluid and electrolyte imbalances, hemodynamic alterations (e.g., hypotensive).
- Provide mouth and skin care.
- Manage bowel function.
- Provide emotional support to the patient who is commonly experiencing a life-threatening condition. AKI has a high mortality rate, despite excellent intervention. Care often imposes pain and suffering from the invasive nature of many interventions, dietary restrictions, hemodynamic and electrolyte instability, and activity restrictions, to name a few. Collaborate with the health care provider if more intensive support from a psychiatrist is indicated.

Hyperkalemia

- Renal failure can produce high potassium (K+) levels through the inability of the kidneys to eliminate K+. Normal K+ is 5 g/dL. Levels >6 are associated with the development of fatal dysrhythmias.
- Call the Rapid Response Team if hyperkalemia is >6 mmol/L.
- Urgently obtain and evaluate a 12-lead EKG on patients with a K+ level >6 mmol/L (Alfonzo, et al., 2012).
- Continuously monitor heart rhythm for life-threatening EKG changes in patients with a K+ >6.5 mmol/L, or >6 mmol/L if the patient is acutely ill (Alfonzo, et al., 2012).
- **Immediate treatment consists of** a combination of the following to bring high potassium levels down and decrease the possibility of fatal dysrhythmias:
  - o Protect the heart: Administer calcium chloride or calcium gluconate to help stabilize the cardiac cell membranes and protect against dysrhythmias. Administer slowly over 5–10 minutes (Alfonzo, et al., 2012). Make certain the IV is intact, as tissue necrosis can occur if extravasation occurs.
  - o Shift K+ from serum into cells. This is only a temporary measure as the excess K+ content still remains in the body (Alfonzo, et al., 2012):
    - ■ Initiate a glucose/insulin bolus or infusion if K+ is >6.5 mmol/L.
    - ■ Consider a glucose/insulin bolus or infusion if K+ is >6 mmol/L.
  - o Do not recommend administration of an alkalizing agent, such as sodium bicarbonate, but it has been used in the past as a temporary maneuver to lower pH. Lowering pH causes a shift of K+ from the serum into the cells. Although this practice continues, there is no evidence to support its use.
  - o Nonpotassium sparing diuretics, such as furosemide (Lasix), can be used but may be slow to act.
  - o Shift K+ into intracellular space: Administer beta-agonist nebulizers (e.g., salbutamol), which can cause a temporary shift of K+ from the serum into the cells. Use as adjuvant rather than monotherapy, as it is not reliably effective (Alfonzo, et al., 2012).
  - o Remove K+ from the body: Calcium resonium has replaced the long-used Kayexalate (or sodium polystyrene sulfonate), which binds to K+ in the gut. These drugs are used to manage hyperkalemia by removing it via the GI system. It is administered either orally or in the form of a retention enema. It is not for emergency use as it is slow acting. Recent research suggests sodium polystyrene may not be as helpful as was thought. In addition, there is a rare incidence of colonic necrosis (Alfonzo, et al., 2012).
  - o Discontinuation of medications that can increase K+ levels, such as ACE inhibitors and K+ sparing diuretics (e.g., Aldactone), may be beneficial (Alfonzo, et al., 2012).
  - o Recheck serum K+ levels within a few hours to ensure that K+ level is decreasing (Alfonzo, et al., 2012).
  - o If the patient is not responsive to treatment or if K+ levels are very high (e.g., >6.5 mmol/L), dialysis is strongly considered. If higher, dialysis is required. Dialysis is commonly known as renal replacement therapy (RRT). Dialysis can be used to remove potassium and is the most effective technique available, particularly when cardiac function deteriorates (Alfonzo, et al., 2012).

Concept Check

5. **Which diet order is expected for a patient admitted with acute kidney injury?**

   A. NPO

   B. Clear liquids

   C. Full liquids

   D. Normal as tolerated

Answer question

Collaborative Interventions (continued)

Renal Replacement Therapy

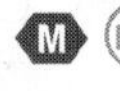 

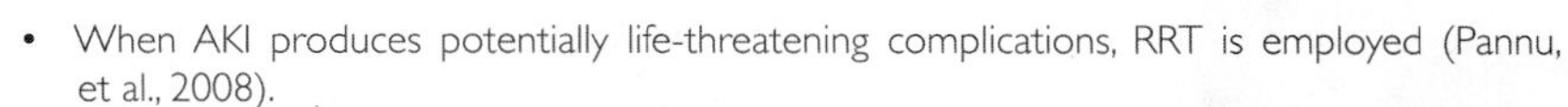

- When AKI produces potentially life-threatening complications, RRT is employed (Pannu, et al., 2008).

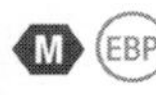

- The most common reasons to provide artificial support for the kidneys include (Pannu, et al., 2008):
  - o Refractory fluid overload or pulmonary edema not responsive to diuretics or inotropes
  - o Metabolic acidosis and hyperkalemia (refractory to medical therapy)
  - o Uremic complications such as pericarditis, encephalopathy, and bleeding (see diagram)
  - o Poisons that are dialyzable (e.g., toxic alcohols and salicylates)

Clinical Manifestations of Uremia

Neurologic	Metabolic	Cardiovascular
Apathy; lethargy Headache Insomnia Paresthesias Impaired cognition Gait impairments Seizure, ↓ LOC, Coma	Hyperkalemia Azotemia Hypocalcemia Hypermagnesia Hyperphosphatemia Acidosis Hyperlipidemia Hyperuricemia Malnutrition	Dysrhythmias Hypertension Coronary disease Heart failure Edema Pericarditis Pericardial effusion

Musculoskeletal Osteodystrophy Spontaneous fractures Bone pain	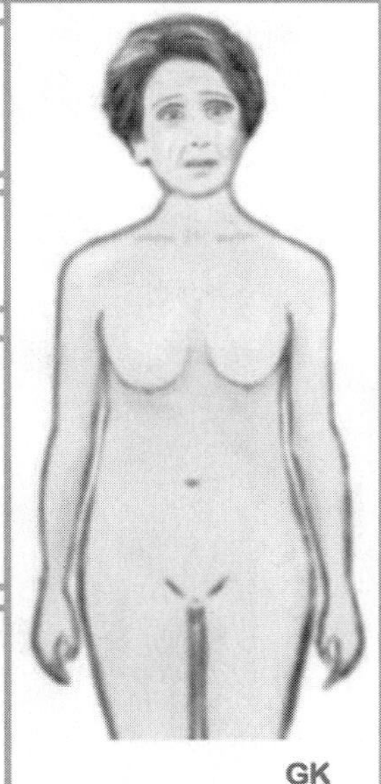	**Respiratory** Pleuritis Pulmonary edema Kussmaul's pattern
Endocrine Glucose intolerance Hyperparathyroidism		**Hematologic** Impaired coagulation Anemia
Urinary Hematuria Proteinuria Nocturia Fixed specific gravity Oliguria; anuria		**Gastrointestinal** Nausea & vomiting Abdominal pain Hiccups Anorexia Gastroenteritis Uremic fetor
Skin Dry skin; poor turgor Pruritis Uremic frost Pallor Uremic skin (yellow-green) Ecchymosis	GK	**Reproductive** Amenorrhea Spontaneous abortion Male impotence
		Immune ↓ Leukocytes Prone to infection

The table shows the types and extent of multisystem complications that can develop in patients with uremia. Patients can become very sick.

Source: Courtesy of George Kyriakdis/Santa Ana, CA

Types of RRT or Dialysis

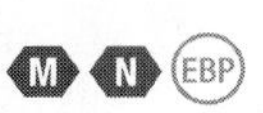

When less invasive interventions fail or cannot resolve the problems quickly, there are several different types of dialysis (or RRT) to remove metabolic wastes, toxins, and excess fluid and electrolytes. These include (Pannu, et al., 2008):

- Peritoneal dialysis: Dialysate is infused into the peritoneum to remove wastes and fluid.
- Intermittent hemodialysis: Blood is channeled into an external dialyzer that filters the wastes from the blood prior to reinfusion. This is the most effective and most commonly used RRT.

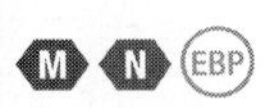

- Continuous RRT (CRRT): Blood is slowly but continuously filtered via several methods (e.g., diffusion, convection). CRRT is often a preferred mode in unstable patients (Kellum, et al., 2012; Pannu, et al., 2008).

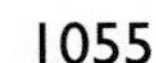

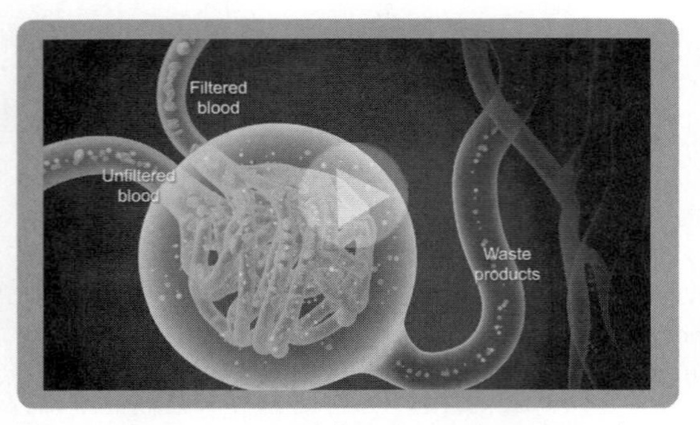

This animation reviews renal physiology and two types of renal replacement therapies to remove accumulated harmful wastes and excess fluid in acute kidney injury or renal failure. An overview introduces hemodialysis and peritoneal dialysis as methods to filter the blood.

Peritoneal Dialysis

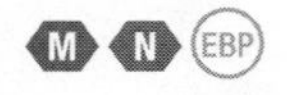

- Peritoneal dialysis (PD) is not widely used in adults in acute situations, as CRRT has greater benefit for most patients (Kellum, et al., 2012).

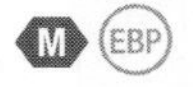

- PD is an effective treatment in the care of patients with renal failure (Kellum, et al., 2012).
- PD uses the peritoneum as a natural membrane for removal of solutes and excess fluid.

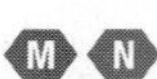
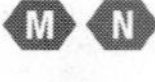

- PD requires a PD catheter to be surgically inserted. Ensure the site is clean, frequently inspected, and maintain a sterile dressing.

- Observe for complications, including catheter leakage, malfunction, and infection. These are not uncommon with PD.

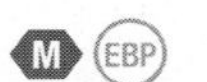

- Consider limitations of PD, which include (Kellum, et al., 2012):
  - o Low solute clearance
  - o Potential restriction of breathing due to dialysate expansion in peritoneal cavity limiting inspiration
  - o Contraindicated in patients after abdominal surgery or those with surgical drains

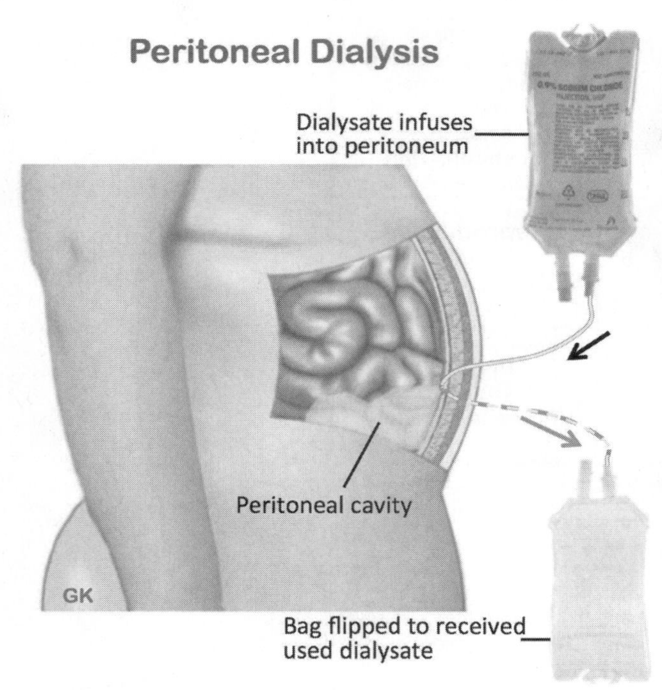

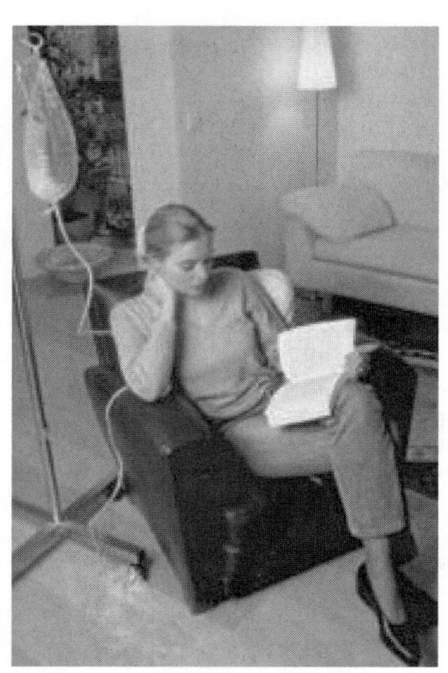

Patient receiving peritoneal dialysis at home.

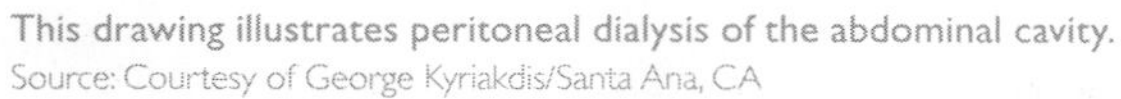

This drawing illustrates peritoneal dialysis of the abdominal cavity.

Source: Courtesy of George Kyriakdis/Santa Ana, CA

Collaborative Interventions (continued)

Hemodialysis

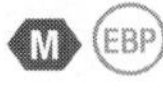

- By far, the most effective technique for renal replacement is hemodialysis (HD) (Kellum, et al., 2012).
- HD is commonly used in acute kidney injury.

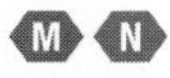

- Intermittent HD (IHD) is preferred when rapid removal of wastes or toxins and limited exposure to anticoagulation are needed. Availability and expertise of the staff are factors that determine RRT selection.
- IHD is becoming less common for inpatients due to the availability and preference for slower, continuous renal replacement techniques. However, HD remains common in outpatient care.

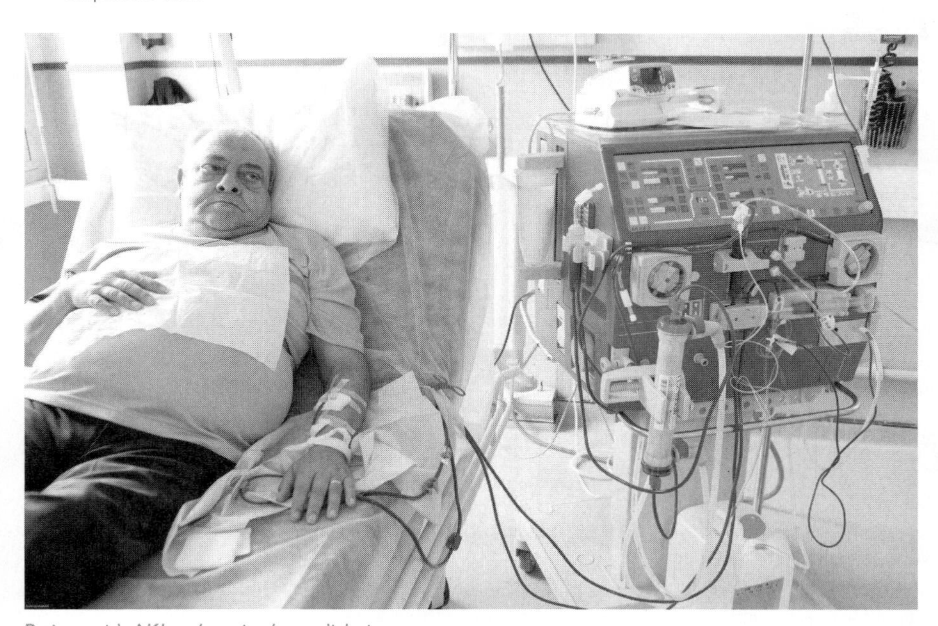

Patient with AKI undergoing hemodialysis.
Source: Phanie/RGB Ventures/SuperStock/Alamy

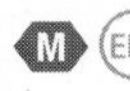

- Hemodialysis is intermittent and commonly performed for 3–6 hours per treatment. Although IHD is typically done three times per week, a suitable schedule is based on the patient's individual needs (Pannu, et al., 2008).
- HD involves diffusion of solutes (dissolved electrolytes) across a membrane to clear them from the blood. Solutes diffuse when there is a gradient (difference) between the blood and dialysate concentrations.
- Fluid is filtered by altering the hydrostatic pressure. Thus, a pressure gradient between the blood and dialysate causes fluid movement.

- In order to perform HD, vascular access needs to be created. This can be in the form of central venous access, or a surgically created access that allows for chronic access to the site.

A-V Fistula

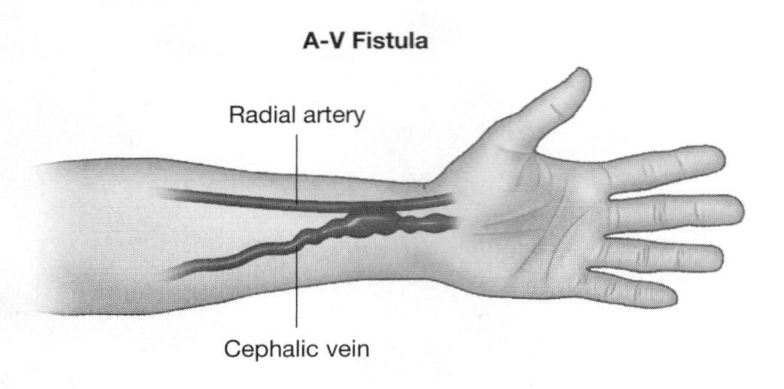

A-V Graft

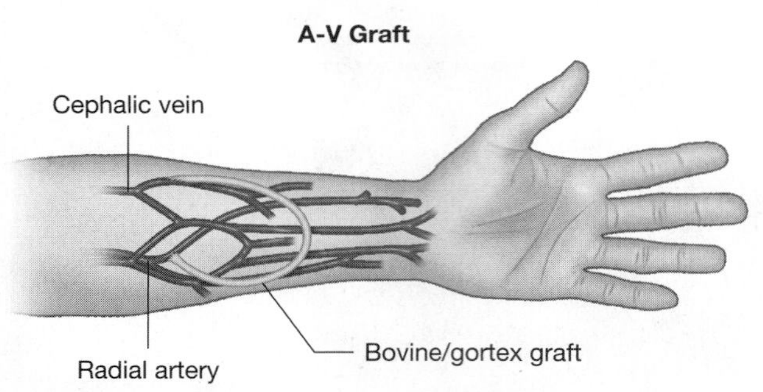

These anatomical illustrations depict both an arteriovenous (A-V) fistula and an A-V graft that are surgically formed in renal failure patients for long-term dialysis.

- During HD, blood is pumped and flows through an external filter that removes excess fluid and solutes (waste products).
- The filtered blood is then returned to the bloodstream.
- HD not only removes dangerously elevated electrolytes, such as potassium, but also aids in sodium control to improve hypertension management.
- M N During hospitalization, dialysis can be done at the bedside or the patient can be transported to a dialysis center. The patient's acuity is a determining factor in whether or not to dialyze at the bedside or to transport.

Continuous Dialysis

- CRRT is any continuous renal replacement therapy that extends over a 24-hour period.
- M EBP CRRT is recommended instead of intermittent hemodialysis (IHD) in patients who are hemodynamically unstable or have cerebral edema. Studies are inconclusive but the slower continuous removal of toxins and fluid should result in less instability, larger amounts of waste removal, and better removal of inflammatory mediators (Kellum, et al., 2012). Further, IHD may delay recovery from AKI.
- CRRT uses biocompatible dialyzer membranes in removal of wastes, which seem to have improved benefits.
- M N EBP CRRT includes a number of blood purification therapies. Blood may be purified with differing mechanisms of solute transport, various types of diffusion membrane, different dialysate solution, and variations in vascular access devices. For those who enter the specialty, evidence-based practices should guide care of the patients (Kellum, et al., 2012).
- Vascular access is temporary in AKI patients, unlike patients with chronic kidney disease who require long-term and permanent access via arteriovenous fistula or graft.
- M N EBP Priorities for vascular access using a dialysis catheter are based on expert opinion (Kellum, et al., 2012) and include:
  1. Right jugular vein is the primary site of choice.
  2. Femoral vein is the second choice
  3. Left jugular vein is the third choice.
  4. Subclavian vein on the dominant side is the fourth choice.
- CRRT is a slower renal replacement method than hemodialysis (HD), but it can exceed clearances provided by HD.

- The most commonly used continuous techniques are:
  - o Continuous venovenous hemofiltration: continuous removal of large and small wastes using solvent drag (convection). Convection occurs when wastes move from a higher **pressure** in the blood to lower filtrate pressure across a membrane.
  - o Continuous venovenous hemodialysis: continuous removal of small wastes using diffusion. Diffusion occurs when wastes move from a higher blood **concentration** to lower dialysate solution concentration across a membrane.
  - o Continuous venovenous hemodiafiltration: continuous removal of large and small wastes using both diffusion and convection.
  - o Slow continuous ultrafiltration: slowest removal of urea, does not require dialysate, and removes both large and small wastes using solvent drag (convection)
  - o Slow low-efficiency dialysis: alternative for slower fluid and toxin removal with reduced exposure time to anticoagulation risks. Uses a diffusion removal method but can be more expensive.

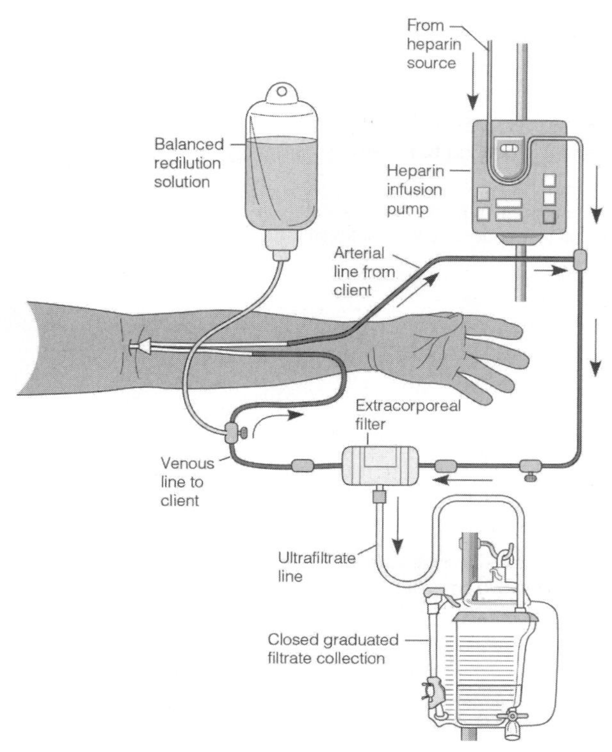

This diagram represents how continuous venovenous hemofiltration (CVVH) works.

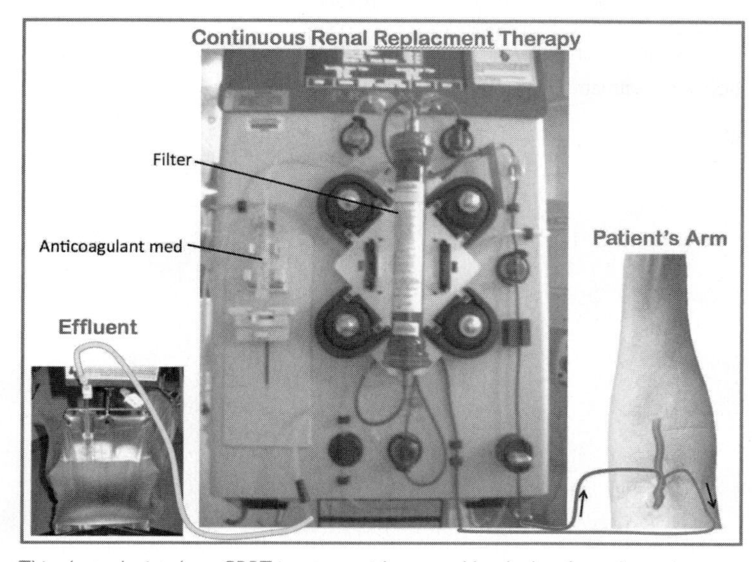

This photo depicts how CRRT is set up, with venous blood taken from the patient, filtered through the renal replacement system, and effluent being removed.

Collaborative Interventions (continued)

Prevention

There is little evidence-based practice regarding the prevention of AKI. However, given the understanding of pathophysiology of AKI and limitations in treatment, the following may be helpful:

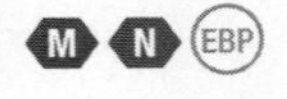

- Maintain adequate hydration. Administer IV normal saline to specifically prevent contrast-induced nephropathy. Normal saline should be administered at 1 mL/kg/hr, starting 12 hours before the procedure and continuing for 24 hours afterwards if the patient's condition can tolerate this rate (Kellum, et al., 2012; Tepel, Aspelin, & Lameire, 2006).

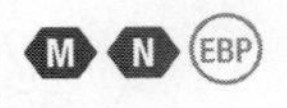

- Avoid depending on oral hydration alone to prevent contrast-induced AKI (Kellum, et al., 2012).
- Maintain hemodynamics (e.g., mean arterial pressure) for renal perfusion and good oxygenation, particularly when the patient is acutely ill or at high risk for AKI. Maintenance of adequate fluid volume is essential.

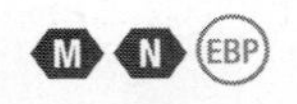

- Early identification of patients at risk is essential, especially for post-percutaneous coronary interventions: hypotension, heart failure, older than 75 years old, anemia, diabetes, renal disease, or intra-aortic balloon pump support (Pannu, et al., 2008).

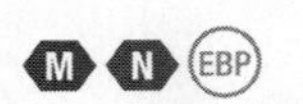

- Avoid nephrotoxins and monitor levels of nephrotoxic drugs (e.g., aminoglycosides, radioactive contrast, amphotericin B, vancomycin) when they are used (Kellum, et al., 2012).

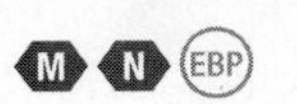

- Diuretics, fenoldopam, and dopamine do not help and should not be used to prevent AKI (Kellum, et al., 2012)

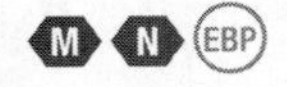

- Anticipate and investigate patients who are at risk for AKI in everyday practice. Collaborate with the health care provider to monitor creatinine and evaluate patients with (National Institute for Health and Care Excellence [NICE], 2013):
  - Heart failure
  - Chronic kidney disease, especially those with GFR <60 mL/min/1.73 m^2
  - Diabetes
  - Hypovolemia
  - Oliguria (urine output <0.5 mL/kg/hr)
  - Older than 65 years of age
  - Hepatic disease
  - Altered cognitive or neurologic status, which can lead to fluid deficit
  - Treatment with nephrotoxic medications (e.g., NSAIDs, diuretics, ACE inhibitors, angiotensin II receptor antagonists, aminoglycosides), particularly if hypovolemia occurred
  - Treatment with iodine contrast procedure
  - Urinary obstruction
  - Sepsis, severe sepsis, or septic shock
  - History of AKI

Patient Education

When caring for patients with complex illnesses, particularly those who require long-term and ongoing intervention, self-care, and education, clinicians require specialized and more in-depth preparation in that specialty. As an overview, education of patients with AKI commonly includes:

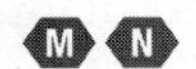

- Educate on the progression of AKI and anticipated treatments.

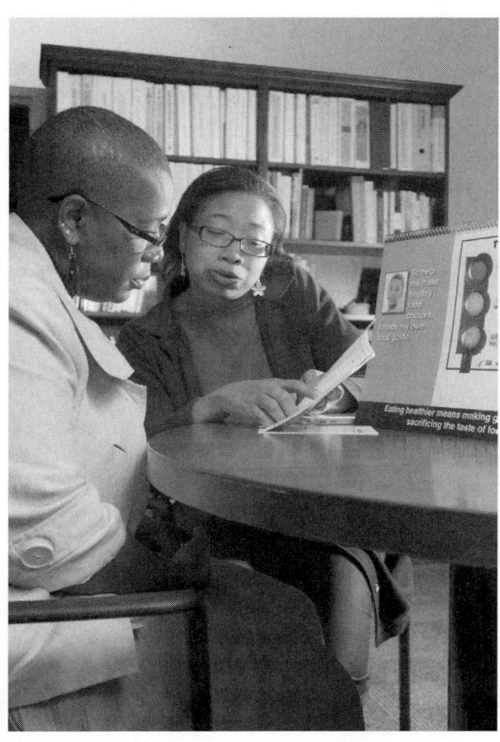

Educating the patient and family is key to preventing complications in these complex patients.

Source: Amanda Mills/Centers for Disease Control and Prevention

- Review signs, symptoms, and complications to report to the health care provider immediately (e.g., shortness of breath due to fluid overload, chest pain, muscle weakness that can signal electrolyte imbalances, fever, itching and/or rash, tachypnea, tachycardia, palpitations, confusion, dizziness, reduced urination, nausea or vomiting).
- Daily weights to provide early warning of water weight gain.
- Fluid and dietary modifications, which commonly include limiting sodium, phosphorus, and potassium intake. Fluid restrictions may be prescribed to patients who can benefit from suggestions as to how best allot fluid intake throughout the day.
- Activity modifications, such as pacing activities to balance with fatigue that is common. Resting more can prevent becoming overtired. Projects or tasks that cause fatigue can be broken into smaller tasks or delegated to others.
- Explain any procedures, including dialysis.
- Provide the patient and family with psychological support.
- Educate regarding advanced directives.
- Educate about disease, recognition of onset and prevention of recurrence of complications, medications, when to call the health care provider or 911, follow-up care, exercise and activity, smoking or substance cessation, weight management, and flu/pneumonia vaccines.
- Continue to carefully manage comorbid conditions, particularly diabetes, hypertension, hypercholesterolemia, and obesity, which can exacerbate kidney injury.
- Strongly encourage patients to adhere to lifestyle modifications and medical management because renal failure is a silent disease and can advance to the renal failure stage without clear warning. Follow-up care is the major method of tracking the disease's course.

Concept Check

6. What is the most effective and most commonly used form of renal replacement therapy?

A. Peritoneal dialysis

B. Intermittent dialysis

C. Continuous dialysis

D. Continuous venovenous hemodialysis

Answer question

Concept Check

7. Which intervention is of greatest value in preventing AKI?

A. Administration of diuretics

B. Administration of dopamine

C. Maintenance of mean arterial pressure

D. Monitoring serum creatinine

Answer question

Summary of Interventions

- Acute renal failure or acute kidney injury (AKI) is a common problem faced by hospitalized patients.
- Rapid recognition of AKI, by recognizing a rising creatinine level or a decreasing urine output, is a key nursing priority in order to prevent the deleterious effects of renal failure.
- Three types of AKI exist:
    - Prerenal: treated with IV fluids when caused by dehydration and diuretics, particularly in heart failure patients
    - Intrarenal: more difficult to correct, carries a higher mortality and may take several weeks to improve. Treatment usually consists of discontinuing nephrotoxic drugs. Treatment is otherwise supportive, attempting to alleviate: hyperkalemia, fluid retention, and acidosis. Dialysis may be necessary in severe conditions.
    - Postrenal: often due to an obstruction, which, if relieved, can correct this type of renal dysfunction

LO4:

Evaluation of Desired Collaborative Care Outcomes

Evaluation and reassessment should reveal attainment of previously established patient outcomes. In summary:

- The patient's mentation is clear, lungs are clear, skin turgor is elastic, and urine output balances with fluid intake.
- The patient is afebrile and has no findings associated with infection.
- The patient's weight is returning to desired or pre-illness level.
- The patient discusses activities that cause fatigue and works with the health care team to devise methods to alleviate that fatigue.
- The patient discusses anxiety-provoking situations and healthy coping mechanisms to address the same.
- The patient accurately describes the benefits of lifestyle changes and their impact on overall health.
- The patient discusses ways to avoid future episodes of AKI, including plans to actively participate in follow-up care.

References

Choudhury, D. (2010). Acute kidney injury: Current perspectives. *Postgrad Med, 122*(6), 29–40.

Dennen, P., Douglas, I., & Anderson, R. (2010). Acute kidney injury in the intensive care unit: An update and primer for the intensivist. *Crit Care Med, 38*(1), 261–275.

Dirkes, S. (2011). Acute kidney injury: Not just acute renal failure anymore? *Crit Care Nurs, 31*(1), 37–50. **www.aacn.org/WD/CETests/Media/C1113.pdf**

Kelso, L. A. (2012). Recognizing and preventing acute kidney injury. *Nuring 2014 Crit Care, 7*(2), 36–41.

Martin, R. (2010). Acute kidney injury: Advances in definition, pathophysiology, and diagnosis. *AACN Advanc Crit Care, 21*(4), 350–356.

Merhaut, S., & Trupp, R. J. (2010). Cardiorenal dysfunction. *AACN Advanced Crit Care, 21*(4), 357–364. **www.aacn.org/WD/CETESTS/Media/ACC2142.pdf**

Murphy, F., & Byrne, G. (2010). The role of the nurse in the management of acute kidney injury. *Brit J Nurs, 19*(3), 146–152. **www.austincc.edu/nursmods/rrc/rrc_lev4/rnsg_2432/documents/Nursesroleinthemanagementofacutekidneyinjury.pdf**

Ricci, Z., Cruz, D., & Ronco, C. (2008). The RIFLE criteria and mortality in acute kidney injury: A systematic review. *Kidney Int, 73*(5), 538–546. **www.nature.com/ki/journal/v73/n5/full/5002743a.html**

Richard, C. J. (2011). Preservation of vascular access for hemodialysis in acute care settings. *Crit Care Nurs Q, 34*(1), 76–83. doi: 10.1097/CNQ.0b013e3182048ca4.

Vrtis, M. C. (2013). Preventing and responding to acute kidney injury. *AJN Amer J Nurs, 113*(4), 38–47. **www.nursingcenter.com/lnc/cearticle?tid=1532495**

Yaklin, K. M. (2011). Acute kidney injury: An overview of pathophysiology and treatments. *Nephrol Nurs J, 8*(1), 13–18.

Clinical Practice Guidelines

Alfonzo, A., Soar, J., Nolan, J., et al. (2012). Treatment of acute hyperkalemia in adults. *The Renal Association, 2012: Guidelines.* **www.renal.org/docs/default-source/guidelines-resources/Treatment_of_Acute_Hyperkalaemia_in_Adults_-_FINAL_VERSION_JULY_2012.pdf?sfvrsn=0**

Fliser, D., Laville, M., Covic, A., et al. (2012). A European renal best practice (ERBP) position statement on the Kidney Disease Improving Global Outcomes (KDIGO) clinical practice guidelines on acute kidney injury: Part 1: definitions, conservative management and contrast-induced nephropathy. *Nephrol Dial Transplant, 27*, 4263–4272. **ndt.oxfordjournals.org/content/27/12/4263.full.pdf+html**

Kellum, J., Lameire, N., & the Kidney Disease: Improving Global Outcomes (KDIGO) Acute Kidney Injury Work Group. (2012). KDIGO clinical practice guideline for acute kidney injury. *Kidney Internationl Supp, 2*(1), 1–138. **www.kdigo.org/clinical_practice_guidelines/pdf/KDIGO AKI Guideline.pdf**

Lewington, A., & Kanagasundaram, S. (2011). *Clinical practice guidelines in acute kidney injury.* **www.renal.org/Clinical/GuidelinesSection/AcuteKidneyInjury.aspx**

Pannu, N., Klarenbach, S., Wiebe, N., et al. (2008). Renal replacement therapy in patients with acute renal failure: A systematic review. *JAMA, 299*(7), 793–805. **jama.jamanetwork.com/article.aspx?articleid=181491**

Tepel, M., Aspelin, P., Lameire, N. (2006). Contrast-induced nephropathy: A clinical and evidence-based approach. *Circulation, 113*, 1799–1806. **circ.ahajournals.org/content/113/14/1799.full.pdf+html**

Patient Education

National Institute for Health and Care Excellence (NICE). (2013). *Information for the public: Acute kidney injury: prevention, detection and management of acute kidney injury up to the point of renal replacement therapy, NICE clinical guideline 169.* **www.nice.org.uk/guidance/CG169/ifp/chapter/Acute-kidney-injury**

National Kidney Disease Education Program: Improving the Understanding, Detection, and Management of Kidney Disease. (2012). *Educate your patients: Kidney disease education lesson builder.* **nkdep.nih.gov/identify-manage/educate-patients.shtml**

Learning Outcomes for Chronic Kidney Disease

When you complete this lesson, you will be able to:

1. Recognize the clinical relevance of chronic kidney disease.
2. Consider the pathophysiology, etiology, risk factors, and clinical presentation of chronic kidney disease that determine the priority patient concerns.
3. Determine the most urgent and important nursing interventions and patient education required in caring for a patient with chronic kidney disease.
4. Evaluate attainment of desired collaborative care outcomes in patients with chronic kidney disease.

LO1:

What Is Chronic Kidney Disease?

- Chronic kidney disease (CKD), known in the past as chronic renal failure, is a progressive and irreversible reduction of kidney function due to loss of nephrons.

Chronic Kidney Disease

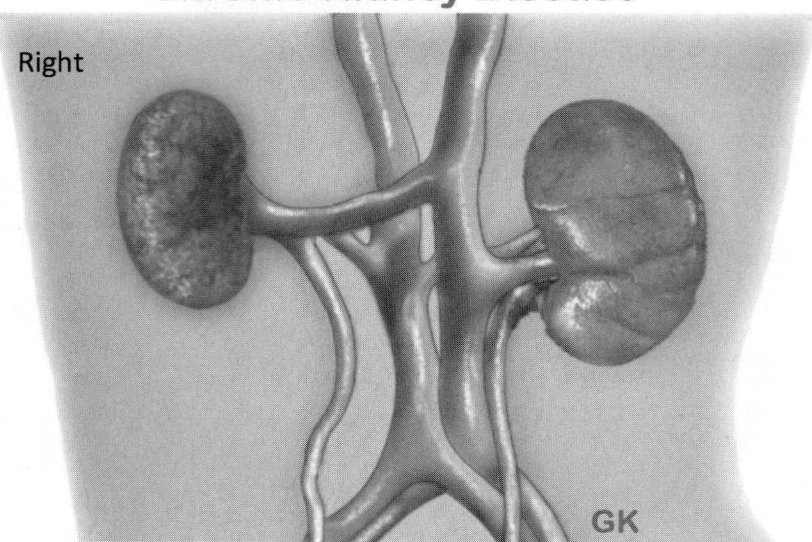

This image depicts a failing kidney (right) compared to a healthy one (left). The diseased kidney has a granular surface, is smaller, and has poor functioning.

Source: Courtesy of George Kyriakdis/Santa Ana, CA

- CKD may lead to end stage renal disease (ESRD), which could require dialysis or renal transplant.

LO1:

Clinical Relevance

- In the United States, the prevalence and incidence of kidney failure are rising, at very high costs (over $32 billion/year) for the continued poor outcomes.
- Twenty-six million American adults have CKD and millions of others are at increased risk.
- Kidney disease is the ninth leading cause of death in the United States.
- CKD is a major risk factor for heart disease.
- CKD affects people of all races. However, a higher incidence of CKD exists in African Americans, nearly four times greater than in Caucasians.

Renal Artery Stenosis with Kidney Failure

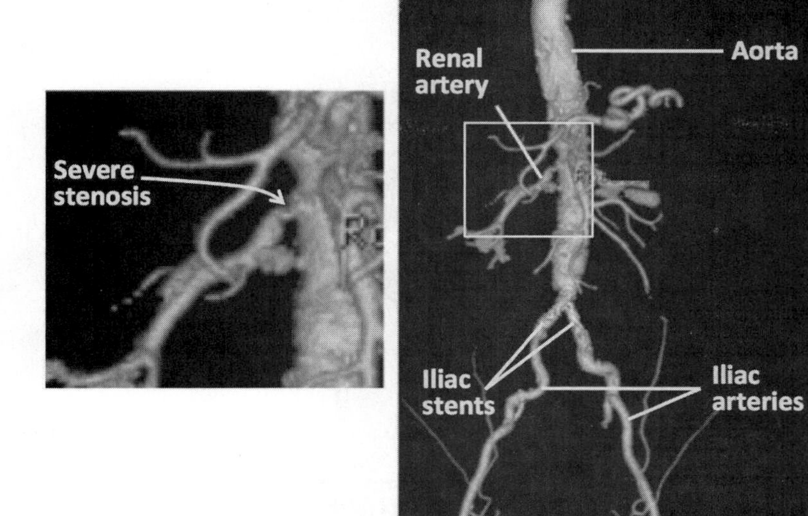

This 3D CT angiogram scan reveals severe renal stenosis (cutout), resulting in renal disease. Diffuse atherosclerotic disease also affects the iliac arteries, which required stenting.
Source: Courtesy of K. Kyriakdis

Concept Check

1. **What is true of kidney damage associated with chronic kidney disease?**
   A. It is reversible if treatment is started early.
   B. The damage may result in acute kidney injury.
   C. The damage is not curable.
   D. Damage is avoidable if good lifestyle choices are made.

Answer question

LO1:

Physiology of the Kidneys

- Blood perfuses the kidneys and is filtered in the nephron by the glomeruli.
- The filtered fluid, which normally contains no protein or albumin, passes through the renal tubules.
- Solutes are reabsorbed (e.g., Na+) and excreted (e.g., K+) in the tubules before the tubular fluid is excreted by the kidneys as urine.

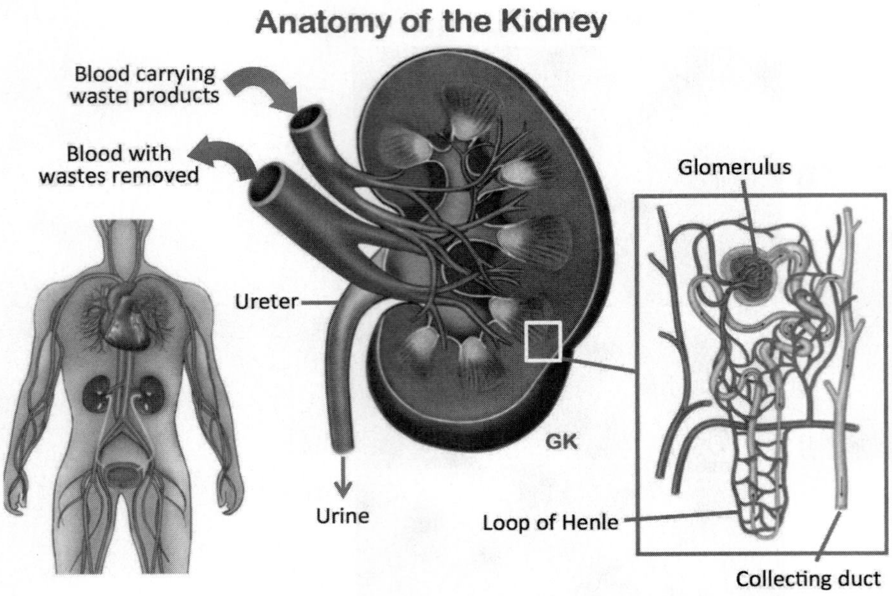

Anatomy of the Kidney

This diagram (left) illustrates the anatomy of the urinary system: the kidneys, ureters, and bladder. Arterial blood flowing into the kidney (middle) contains waste products while the blood flowing out has been filtered. The nephron or filtration structure (right) is responsible for removing wastes and excess fluid: collecting duct, ureter, loop of Henle, glomerulus, and renal tubule.
Source: Courtesy of George Kyriakdis/Santa Ana, CA

LO2:

Pathophysiology

- The loss of nephrons in CKD is at the center of all the clinical symptoms and prognosis for patients with this condition.
- Insults to the kidney result in nephron destruction. Some factors that can cause destruction of nephrons include recurrent infection, urinary obstruction, and autoimmune diseases affecting the kidney. These processes can result in glomerulosclerosis (scarring of the glomeruli) and tubulointerstitial fibrosis (scarring of the tubules and surrounding tissue). Factors that cause atherosclerosis are the most common cause of these conditions.

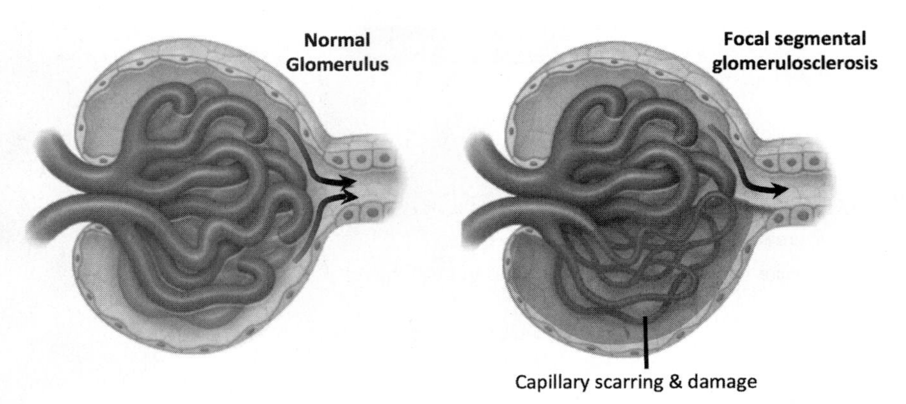

Left: A normal glomerulus filters the impurities out of the blood. Right: Focal segmental glomerulosclerosis (FSGS). In the damaged glomerulus, note the narrowing and distortion of the capillaries from sclerosis or scarring that limit filtration.

- Nephron injury occurs through the following two mechanisms:
  1. **Glomerulosclerosis:** Factors such as diabetes, smoking, and hypertension cause damage to the endothelial cells of the capillaries and arterioles of the kidneys.
     a. Endothelial damage causes the release of cytokines, which attract other inflammatory cells such as macrophages.
     b. Cytokines also cause a proliferation of smooth muscle cells, cell death, an increased permeability of the capillaries, and an increase in the production of collagen (fibrous tissue/scarring).
     c. These changes cause capillary dysfunction with leakage of albumin and, eventually, scarring and destruction of the glomeruli.

2. **Tubulointerstitial fibrosis:** The second mechanism for nephron injury has similar factors and processes that additionally affect the renal tubules.
    a. Albumin, glucose, and other substrates leak from the capillaries and trigger an inflammatory response of the cells within the tubules.
    b. Initially, dysfunction of the tubules occurs, with decreased ability to reabsorb water and sodium. The ability to excrete potassium, phosphorus, and acids is also diminished.
    c. Eventually there is scarring (fibrosis), atrophy, and destruction of the tubules and surrounding tissue.

- With destruction of the nephrons, a number of problems evolve:
    - Electrolyte abnormalities including hyperkalemia, hyperphosphatemia, and acidosis occur. Hyperkalemia can cause dangerous cardiac dysrhythmias. Hyperphosphatemia can cause the formation of calcium phosphate deposits in the blood vessels.
    - Uremia or the accumulation of serum toxins can cause confusion, coma, uremic encephalopathy, seizures, and peripheral neuropathy.
    - Anemia occurs when the creatinine is >2–3 mg/dL or when the blood urea nitrogen (BUN) is >60–80 mg/dL. Fibroblasts in the kidney produce a hormone called erythropoietin, which stimulates the bone marrow to produce red blood cells. High creatinine and BUN decrease renal erythropoietin, which causes bone marrow suppression. Anemia results.
    - Systemic inflammation may result in muscle wasting (sarcopenia). Cytokines produce an increase in muscle breakdown as well as a decrease in muscle development.
    - Cardiovascular disease is accelerated. This may be due, in part, to the systemic inflammation that occurs and the deposition of calcium in the blood vessels.

LO2:

Risk Factors

- African American, Native American, Hispanic/Latino, or Asian American
- Family history of kidney disease
- Diabetes
- Hypertension
- Heart disease
- Smoking
- Obesity
- Genetic mutation in uromodulin (the most prevalent urinary protein), the gene encoding uromodulin

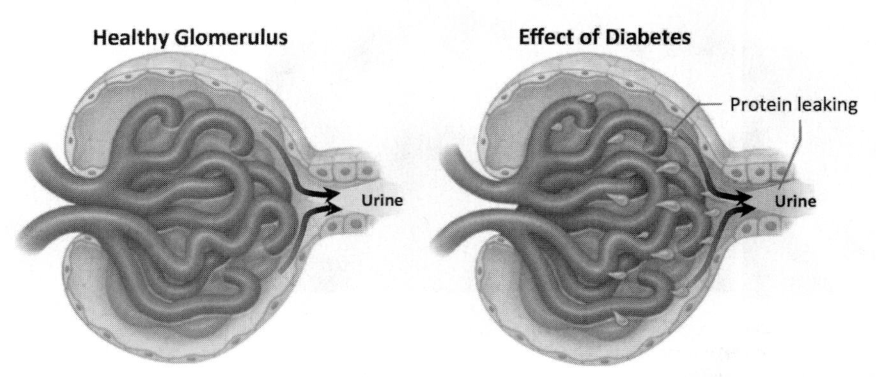

Diabetes places people at high risk for kidney disease because CKD can develop even when diabetes is controlled. This picture shows why early screening for protein in the urine may detect early stages.

Concept Check

2. Which electrolyte imbalance is the most common result of chronic kidney damage?
    A. Hyperkalemia
    B. Hypophosphatemia
    C. Hyponatremia
    D. Hypercalcemia

Answer question

LO2:

Causes

- **Hyperglycemia/diabetes**, particularly in Caucasians, Hispanics, and Native Americans
- **Hypertension**, particularly in African Americans
- Smoking
- Elevated LDL, triglycerides
- Diabetes and hypertension are the two most common causes of CKD and end stage kidney disease.

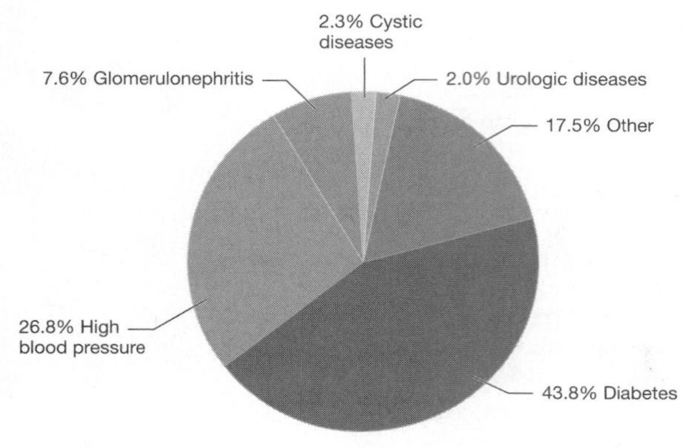

This graph reflects the most prevalent causes of kidney failure, which is the end stage of CKD. Diabetes is the most common cause of renal disease, followed by hypertension.

- Glomerulonephritis is an inflammation of the kidneys that results from either a systemic autoimmune response (e.g., lupus) or an autoimmune response that specifically targets the kidneys.
- Polycystic kidney disease is a hereditary disease that is characterized by the development of cysts in the kidneys. The cysts replace normal, functioning kidney tissue (see photo).

Polycystic Kidneys

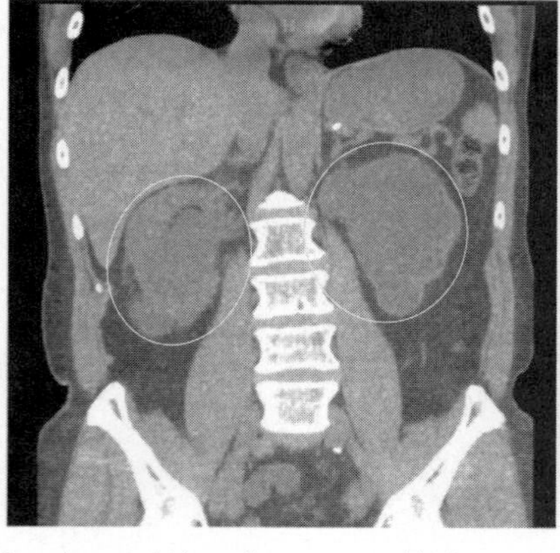

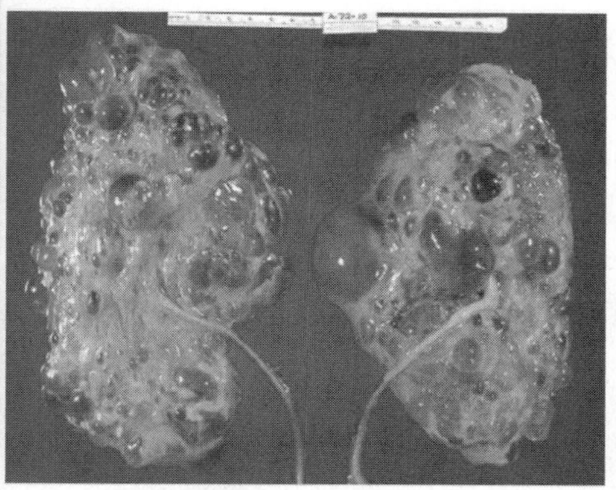

In polycystic kidney disease, normal kidney tissue is replaced by nonfunctioning, multiple fluid-filled cysts. The number of cysts results in massive enlargement of the kidneys. The CT scan (left) shows how enlarged and irregularly shaped the kidneys become (circled). The photo (right) reveals how the cysts destroy the normal tissue to cause kidney failure.

Sources: Courtesy of K. Kyriakidis & Centers for Disease Control and Prevention/Dr. Edwin P. Ewing, Jr.

- Recurrent kidney infections
- Chronic obstruction of urine flow (e.g., resulting from an enlarged prostate)

LO2:

Assessment Findings

- There may be no clinical symptoms with mild CKD.
- With moderate to severe CKD, symptoms from complications may include:
  - o Generalized malaise
  - o Listlessness
  - o Forgetfulness
  - o Loss of libido
  - o Pruritus
  - o Nausea, vomiting, anorexia
  - o A metallic taste
  - o Constipation
- Most patients have high blood pressure, which is exacerbated by volume overload.
- Pulse and respiratory rates can be rapid in the setting of anemia and metabolic acidosis.
- Patients with volume overload may develop peripheral edema or pulmonary edema, manifested by shortness of breath and tachypnea.
- Some patients, particularly those on dialysis, have hemoglobin levels that drop to very low values, yet can live normal lives.
  - o It is not uncommon to have a hemoglobin level <7 gm/dL in CKD.

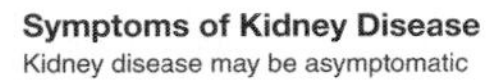
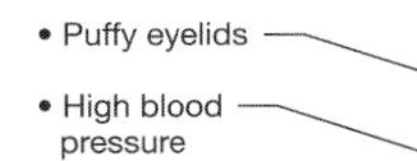

Symptoms of Kidney Disease
Kidney disease may be asymptomatic
• Puffy eyelids
• High blood pressure
• Loin pain
• Blood in urine/ tea color urine
• Frothy urine
• Cloudy urine
• Discomfort/ pain when passing urine
• Difficulty in passing urine
• Passing urine frequently
• Passing urine frequently at night
• Passing stone/sand with urine
• Swollen ankles
Symptoms of Kidney Failure
• Poor appetite, nausea, vomiting
• Tiredness
• Pale (anemia)
• Shortness of breath
• Drowsiness, coma, convulsion
Prevention of Kidney Disease
• Adequate water intake (8 cups per day) to maintain good urine volume
• Good personal hygiene, especially female to prevent urinary tract infection
• Balanced diet Avoid excessive salt and meat intake
• For patient with kidney stone, may need to avoid high intake of calcium
• Prevent complications from diabetes and high blood pressure. Good control of diabetes and blood pressure.
• Patient with kidney stones or urinary tract obstruction (large prostate) should seek early and adequate treatment.
• Be careful about taking drugs including pain killers and antibiotics.
• Early detection of kidney disease by routine examination of urine and blood test for kidney function.
• Early treatment of kidney disease

Concept Check

3. Which chronic kidney disease is hereditary?

A. Glomerulonephritis

B. Chronic obstructive disorder

C. Polycystic kidney disease

D. Lupus erythematosus

Answer question

LO2:

Diagnostics

Creatinine

- Serum creatinine measurement is an estimation of glomerular filtration rate (GFR) and is the most commonly used measure of renal function. Creatinine is a byproduct of muscle cells and is normally released in the course of muscle function.
- Creatinine production is determined by muscle mass. The higher the muscle mass, the higher the creatinine.
- Creatinine is released from the muscle cells at a relatively constant rate and is filtered through the glomerulus and not reabsorbed. The level is, therefore, a function of how fast it is produced (related to muscle mass) and how fast it is filtered (related to GFR and kidney function).
- The serum creatinine level must, therefore, always be interpreted with respect to the patient's weight, age, and sex, although in practice, this is often not done. Changes in serum creatinine reflect changes in kidney function and GFR.
- If creatinine of 1 mg/dL is baseline for a given patient with normal GFR, then:
  - o A creatinine of 2 mg/dL = 50% reduction in GFR
  - o A creatinine of 4 mg/dL = 70–85% reduction in GFR
  - o A creatinine of 8 mg/dL = 90–95% reduction in GFR
- The upper limit of the normal creatinine level can be as high as 1.6–1.9 mg/dL. What is normal for patients depends on their muscle mass. A creatinine of 1, therefore, could be abnormally high in a patient with low muscle mass (e.g., older adult women). Men generally have a higher muscle mass per kilogram of body weight and thus a higher serum creatinine level than women.
- Although GFR decreases by 1% per year after age 40, serum creatinine level generally remains stable because muscle mass usually decreases with age.

Glomerular Filtration Rate/Creatinine Clearance

- GFR (normal is >90 mL/hr) is an indicator of kidney function that measures the amount of fluid filtered by the kidneys.
- Creatinine clearance is used to approximate the GFR.
- Measuring creatinine clearance requires a 24-hour urine collection, which is not always convenient in a hospital setting.

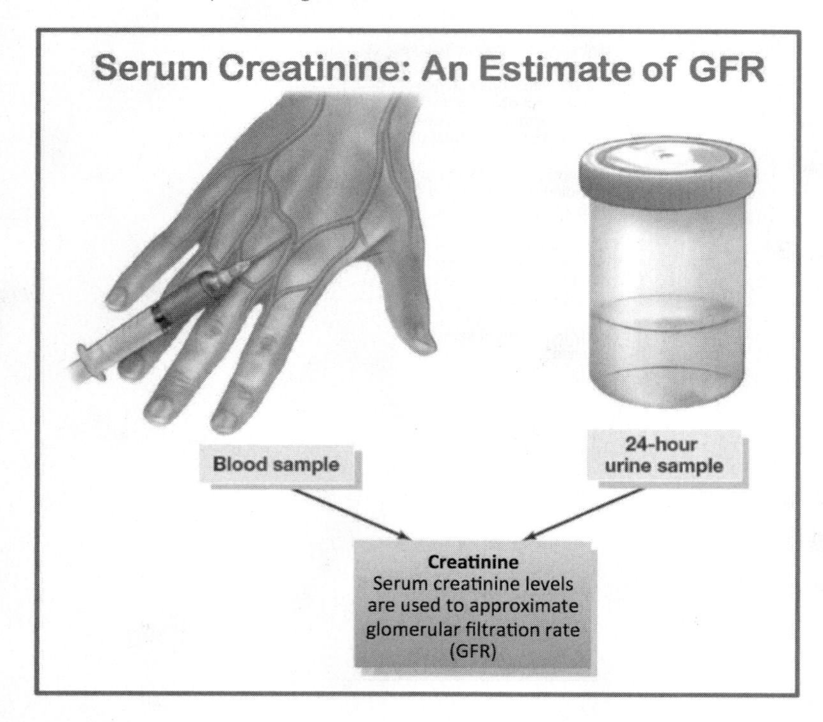

- However, there are a number of ways to estimate GFR based on serum creatinine, age, sex, and weight.
- Creatinine clearance can be estimated with the following formula:

$$\text{Creatinine clearance} = \frac{(140 - \text{age}) \times \text{weight (kg)} \times (0.85 \text{ if female})}{72 \times \text{serum creatinine (in mg/dL)}}$$

- These calculations are accurate only if creatinine is stable. If creatinine is increasing, these calculations underestimate the drop in GFR.

GFR

- Decreased GFR determines the stage of CKD.
- A decreased GFR is reflected in the creatinine clearance.
- The National Kidney Foundation's Kidney Disease Outcomes Quality Initiative (KDOQI) defines CKD as:
  - o Kidney damage or
  - o A decreased GFR of <60 mL/min/1.73 m^2 for 3 months or more.
- Early stages of CKD are often asymptomatic. Not until later stages do symptoms start to occur, at which time substantial renal damage has already occurred.

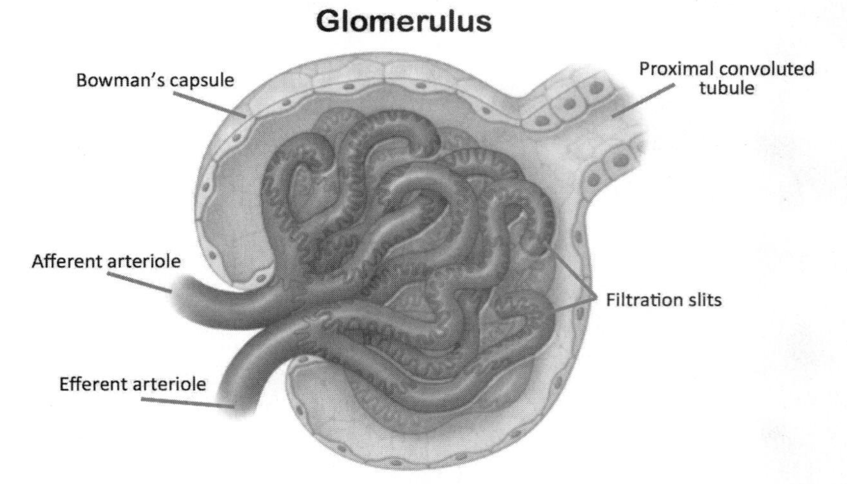

Each glomerulus is a cluster of blood capillaries surrounded by a Bowman's capsule. Blood enters the glomerulus and pressure forces fluid out of the blood through the filtration slits, creating a cell-free fluid that enters the renal tubule.

STAGE	GFR (CC/MIN)
Stage I	> 90
Stage II	60-89
Stage IIIa	45-59
Stage IIIb	30-44
Stage IV	15-29
Stage V	<15 or on dialysis

Stages of chronic kidney failure by GFR are listed.

Diagnostics (continued)

Blood Urea Nitrogen

- The urea concentration correlates poorly with the GFR.
- The reason for poor correlation is that the reabsorption of BUN along the tubule is a function of urine flow rate.
- With low urine flow rates of <30 mL/hour, urea clearance is as low as an estimated 30% of GFR.
- Under conditions of diuresis, with urine outputs >100 mL/hour, urea clearance can increase to 70–100% of GFR.
- In CKD, both BUN and creatinine are elevated.

Labs

- Albumin in the urine: Presence of albumin is usually a sign of kidney disease and can be used as a screening tool.

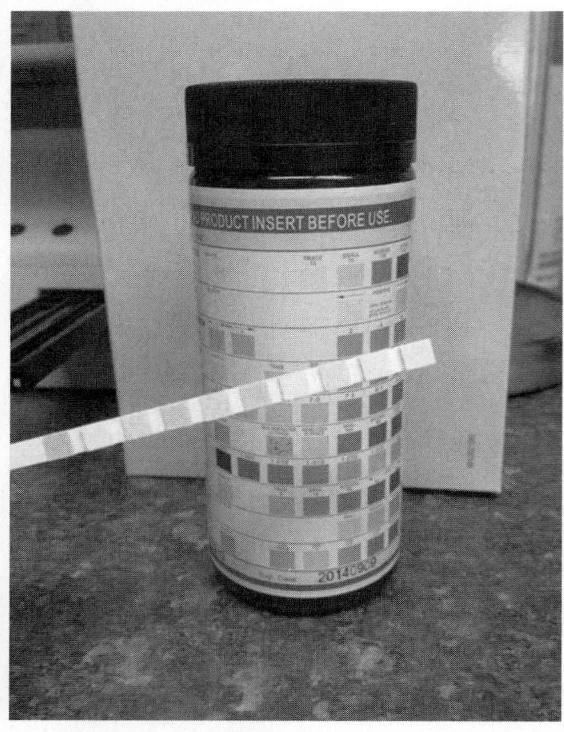

A simple urine screening test for albumin can signal kidney disease.

- Electrolytes: Patients with CKD commonly have electrolyte abnormalities, which may include a high potassium, low calcium, high phosphate, and low bicarbonate (a sign of acidosis).
- Hemoglobin and hematocrit: Anemia is a common problem in CKD. Because it develops slowly, patients' symptoms are not always apparent.

Ultrasound

- Renal ultrasound may show small kidneys with thinning of the renal cortex.
- Other abnormalities can also be diagnosed such as malignancy or polycystic kidney disease. Some of these diseases may show that the kidneys are enlarged.

Renal Cyst Noted on Ultrasound

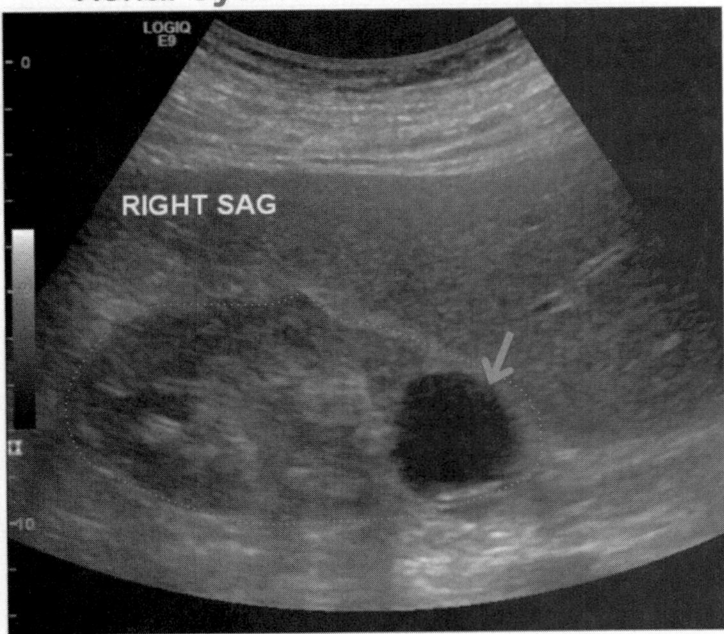

This photo is a longitudinal renal ultrasound scan of the kidney showing a large renal cyst (red arrow). The kidney is faintly outlined in a light blue dotted line.
Source: Courtesy of K. Kyriakdis

Concept Check

4. **What is the normal glomerular filtration rate (GFR)?**
   A. 40–45 mL/hr
   B. Less than 10 mL/hr
   C. 60 mL/hr
   D. Over 90 mL/hr

Answer question

Priority Patient Concerns and Desired Collaborative Care Outcomes

Prior to caring for patients with CKD, it is important to prioritize the patient's concerns that must guide the nursing care plan and interventions. Care for the patient is ordered and organized in accordance with the patient's priority and urgent needs. Desired collaborative care outcomes in patients with CKD typically include:

1. The patient will achieve and maintain normal fluid and electrolyte balance.
2. The patient will ingest sufficient calories to meet metabolic needs within the guidelines of dietary modifications.
3. The patient will be free of injury and participate in risk reduction assessment and prevention activities.
4. The patient will remain free of signs and symptoms of infection.
5. The patient will report reduction of fatigue and convey plans for fatigue management.
6. The patient will discuss use of healthy coping mechanisms that have helped manage anxiety.
7. The patient will verbalize understanding of procedures, maintenance of dialysis, and plan of care.
8. The patient will report pleasure in return to social interaction even if limited.

Considering these important care outcomes, prepare a list of the major 3–6 priority patient concerns or nursing diagnoses for patients with CKD. Be prepared to participate in a discussion of this list and/or to submit them as an assignment, as determined by your faculty. Resources you may find helpful in this assignment can include this lesson, the references, resources on nursing care plans, and standard nursing diagnoses manuals.

LO3:

Collaborative Interventions

Goals for CKD Management

Since there is no cure for CKD, the goals in managing CKD should focus on:

- Slowing the progression of the disease (Levin, et al., 2012)
- Preventing or managing diabetes, hypertension, cardiovascular disease, and other manageable causes that can either promote or exacerbate CKD and progression to ESRD (MacLeod, et al., 2008)
- Correcting the electrolyte abnormalities, volume overload, anemia that commonly results, and other complications of CKD (MacLeod, et al., 2008)
- Improving the patient's quality of life (Fox, et al., 2008)
- Educating the patient and family to improve adherence to the mutually determined medical regimen and modify lifestyle to slow progression of CKD

Evidence-Based Practices

CKD is a long-term, complex condition that requires multiple simultaneous interventions. In CKD patients, interventions are clinically prioritized based on the individual patient's needs with less emphasis on urgency unless there is significant deterioration or a complication. Currently, the following evidence-based practices (EBP) are recommended in the care of patients with CKD:

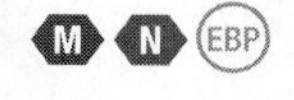

- Control hypertension: Evidence shows a reduction in the progression of CKD. The goal is to control blood pressure (BP) at <140/90 mmHg. Antihypertensive medications that are commonly used to control BP include (Levin, et al., 2012; MacLeod, et al., 2008):
    - o Angiotensin-converting enzyme (ACE) inhibitors (e.g., captopril), except in late stage CKD
    - o Angiotensin receptor blockers (ARBs) (e.g., losartan), except in late stage CKD
- Control hyperglycemia in diabetes with a target hemoglobin A1C <7%. Control slows kidney disease progression (see the Care of Patients with Diabetes NovE-lessons) (Levin, et al., 2012; MacLeod, et al., 2008).
- Administer lipid-lowering agents in hyperlipidemia to decrease cardiovascular events (e.g., myocardial infarction), which cause progression of CKD. However, the direct impact on renal disease progression is not as clear (MacLeod, et al., 2008).
- Urge smoking cessation. Smoking is associated with albuminuria and progression of renal disease. Smoking is also a risk factor for cardiovascular disease (MacLeod, et al., 2008).
- Encourage a healthy and controlled protein-energy diet. Dietary restriction of protein is controversial in patients with GFR >60 mL/min. Kidney Disease: Improving Global Outcomes (KDIGO) recommends controlling protein intake up to 0.8 g/kg/day in diabetics or patients with GFR <30 mL/min as they have a slower decline of GFR. In general, protein restrictions are not broadly recommended for CKD patients, but high protein intake is discouraged (ADA, 2010; MacLeod, et al., 2008).

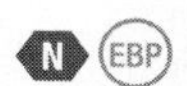

- Support patients, as needed, in making key decisions regarding the kinds of care and interventions they want (Registered Nurses' Association of Ontario [RNAO], 2009). Support can involve:
    - o Providing additional or clarifying information about their illness or condition
    - o Responding to questions about what to expect
    - o Assisting to prioritize issues of most importance in their care
    - o Intervening when the patient feels pressured by others to make decisions or feels alone
    - o Recognizing when the patient's ability to make decisions is impaired by physiologic or emotional stress (e.g., pain, fear, worry)
- Know key decisions that patients with CKD face (RNAO, 2009), which can include:
    - o How to manage the cost of many and expensive medications
    - o Whether or not to make lifestyle changes (e.g., quit smoking, alter dietary habits)
    - o Whether to adhere to medical regimen; how to modify it if needed
    - o Whether or not to pursue dialysis
    - o What kind of dialysis, if presented with options
    - o Whether to undergo renal transplant
    - o Whether to accept a kidney donated by a relative; how to talk to the donor
    - o Whether to pursue advanced directives and how
    - o When to transition to palliative care

- Carefully preserve and protect the veins in the patient's nondominant arm for vascular access, as many patients require dialysis. This is a critically important intervention (Fox, et al., 2008). Clinician must know and patients should be educated to protect vascular access:
  - o Blood may NOT be drawn from the nondominant arm or site protected for vascular access.
  - o IV lines may not be inserted in the nondominant arm. Central lines are preferable.
  - o Collaborate to consult a nephrologist early in the CKD illness.

Collaborative Interventions (continued)

Symptom Management

Patients with CKD predictably experience fluid, electrolyte, hematologic, and lifestyle alterations. The following recommendations guide observation for and management of the most common abnormalities. Based on a synthesis of the best evidence currently available, care of patients with CKD may further include:

Fluid and Electrolyte Abnormalities

- Sodium and fluid retention can result in both peripheral and pulmonary edema and can cause shortness of breath and hypoxemia. Maintain accurate intake and output records. The patient can monitor fluid retention by checking daily weights. For example, a gain of 1 kg over a short period of time indicates a gain of 1 L of fluid. Treatment includes (Levin, et al., 2012; MacLeod, et al., 2008):
  - o Sodium-restricted diet
  - o Diuretics
  - o Distribute the patient's fluid intake over 24 hours to avoid fluid overload
- Elevated potassium (K+) can cause cardiac dysrhythmias that may be fatal. It can be treated with:
  - o Low K+ diet
  - o Loop diuretics (e.g., furosemide, hydrochlorothiazide) (MacLeod, et al., 2008)
- Elevated phosphorus and calcium can cause calcifications in the tissue and blood vessels and can accelerate atherosclerosis. CKD reduces renal calcium reabsorption, which initiates a secondary hyperparathyroidism and, consequently, phosphorus and calcium are resorbed from the bone into the bloodstream. Treatment consists of:
  - o Medications that bind phosphate in the gut to prevent absorption
  - o Vitamin D (Fox, et al., 2008; MacLeod, et al., 2008)
- Acidosis can cause bone disease (osteoporosis) and muscle wasting. It affects insulin sensitivity and thyroid hormone secretion. Plasma bicarbonate (or CO_2) is a common lab test and indicates acidosis when low (<20 mEq/L). It occurs with a GFR <25 mL/hr and is treated with sodium bicarbonate or citrate, calcium acetate (PhosLo) or calcium carbonate (OsCal). Aluminum-based phosphate binders are currently rarely used (MacLeod, et al., 2008).

Anemia

Anemia develops early in most CKD patients and in virtually all patients by the late stages of CKD. In CKD, it results primarily from reduced erythropoietin production, but iron deficiency can also occur.

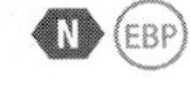

- Observe for anemia, which can cause symptoms of fatigue and shortness of breath (MacLeod, et al., 2008).
- It occurs with GFR <25 mL/hr.
- For safety, rule out bleeding as a priority (Fox, et al., 2008).
- Treat with IV or subQ injection recombinant erythropoietin, when decreased production is the cause (MacLeod, et al., 2008).
- Investigate and manage a hemoglobin level <11 g/dL. Iron deficiency can be a cause, which erythropoietin will not remedy (MacLeod, et al., 2008).
- Iron and folic acid supplements are given in anemia when iron or folate are low (see the Care of Patients with Anemia NovE-lesson).
- Consider and/or administer IV iron infusion if oral iron therapy is ineffective and depending on severity of the iron deficiency (McMurray, et al., 2012).
- Monitor patients for at least 60 minutes after IV iron infusion (McMurray, et al., 2012).

Activity Restrictions

- Patients are commonly more fatigued immediately following dialysis, particularly initially. They should be informed not to plan activities until the following day or late in the day or to rest between activities.
- Monitor patients for early warning signals of dialysis disequilibrium syndrome (DDS). DDS is a syndrome causing cerebral edema. Patients at highest risk are severely ill with confounding conditions (e.g., first dialysis, metabolic acidosis, head trauma, stroke, sepsis, meningitis) and are having either hemodialysis or continuous renal replacement therapy. DDS is currently rare since BUN is gradually reduced in dialysis, but this syndrome can be life threatening. Warning signs include: dizziness, confusion, headache, blurred vision, asterixis, restlessness, muscle cramps, and nausea. If suspected, collaborate with the health care provider to stop dialysis.
- Assess factors that contribute to fatigue, such as fluid and electrolyte imbalances, anemia, and depression (MacLeod, et al., 2008).
- Facilitate education with a **renal dietary consultant** who also understands the fluid restrictions (MacLeod, et al., 2008).

Manage Bowel Function

Patient must keep track of bowel movements. It is not unusual for patients to have constipation and fluid restrictions may exacerbate the problem. Work with the patient on dietary and lifestyle modifications (see the Care of Patients with GI Functional Disorders NovE-lesson regarding constipation) to prevent problems. Encourage the patient to convey problems as they may need stool softeners.

Concept Check

5. **Vitamin D is administered to treat which complication of CKD?**
   A. Elevated potassium
   B. Elevated phosphorus
   C. Acidosis
   D. Sodium and water retention

Answer question

Collaborative Interventions (continued)

Adjustment of Medications

It is important to keep in mind that CKD does not just affect the kidneys. It creates systemic changes that must be considered whenever any interventions are implemented. Due to drug interactions between multiple medications and the alterations that CKD itself creates with medications, consideration should be given to the following for potential adjustment:

- Medications and iodinized contrast used in procedures are cleared by the kidneys, the liver, or both. Consider how the severity of CKD can delay or preclude metabolism and clearance of drugs that can create toxicity.
- Particular medications and iodinized contrast that are primarily cleared by the kidneys need to be adjusted or discontinued. Those medications include:
  - o Metformin should not be used in patients with diabetes and CKD due to potentially fatal lactic acidosis (Fox, et al., 2008).
  - o ACE inhibitors, thiazide diuretics, and ARBs need to be replaced (and avoided) in patients in severe or advanced stages of CKD (Fox, et al., 2008).
- Vitamins, food supplements, and diet supplements should be discussed with the health care provider and/or pharmacist to ensure compatibility, needs, and avoidance of harm.
- Alka Seltzer or bicarbonate (e.g., baking soda) products for heartburn (MacLeod, et al., 2008)
- Phosphate preparations (e.g., phosphor soda) used for colonoscopy (Fox, et al., 2008)
- Phosphorus, aluminum, or magnesium containing medications such as antacids and laxatives (e.g., Milk of Magnesia, Amphojel, Mylanta, Fleet enema) to prevent elevated phosphorus (Fox, et al., 2008)
- Nonsteroidal anti-inflammatory drugs (NSAIDs) (e.g., ibuprofen, aspirin, naproxen, some cold or cough medicines) (Fox, et al., 2008)
- Herbal supplements or treatments (MacLeod, et al., 2008)
- Salt substitutes if they contain potassium (MacLeod, et al., 2008)
- Contrast dyes and nuclear tracers (e.g., gadolinium) used for diagnostic tests or scans, such as CT scans with contrast and angiography, can induce nephropathy (Fox, et al., 2008).
- Decongestants used to treat colds or flu

Additional Consultations

- Promote self-esteem as well as spiritual and emotional care. Refer to specialists in these areas when appropriate because of the tremendous lifestyle changes and decisions associated with end stage kidney disease.
- Consult psychiatric provider or social worker, clergy, and case manager as needed.

Dialysis

- Peritoneal or hemodialysis is needed when the GFR decreases to a point that electrolyte abnormalities, acidosis, uremia (accumulation of toxins), and volume overload cannot be controlled with medications. This usually occurs at GFR clearance of <10 mL/minute.
- Dialysis has a myriad of issues for the patient to become aware of and educated about. Chronic hemodialysis is a life-altering treatment because treatments are three times per week. Patients need to learn about the procedure, scheduling, symptoms that indicate a treatment is needed, and how to manage symptoms of CKD.
- Patients need to understand how thoroughly long-term hemodialysis affects their lives. While the treatment is lifesaving, it requires a major adjustment in their lives. Lifestyle modifications (e.g., stop smoking, limit alcohol, dietary changes, activity alterations) are discussed below when educating the patient.

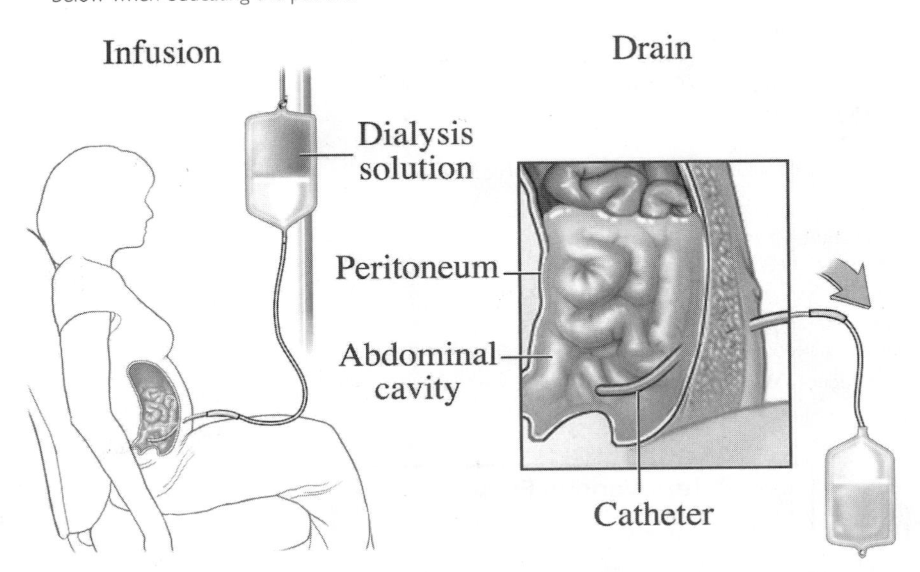

This drawing illustrates peritoneal dialysis using the abdominal cavity. Dialysis solution (dialysate) is infused into the abdomen where solutes are pulled into the fluid. The solution is then drained out of the abdomen, washing out toxins and excessive solutes.

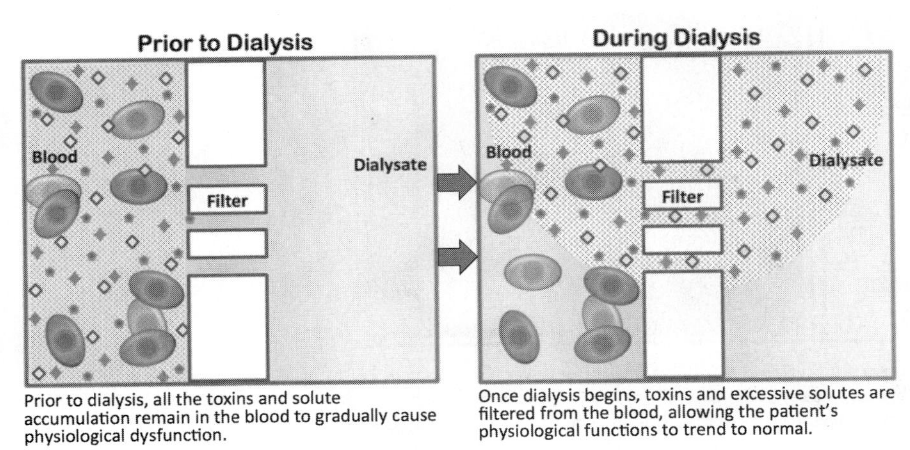

Prior to dialysis, all the toxins and solute accumulation remain in the blood to gradually cause physiological dysfunction.

Once dialysis begins, toxins and excessive solutes are filtered from the blood, allowing the patient's physiological functions to trend to normal.

Collaborative Interventions (continued)

Blood or Vascular Access

- When hemodialysis is necessary, blood access must be surgically prepared in advance.
- Three methods are used: arteriovenous (AV) fistula, synthetic AV graft using tubing, or, in emergent situations, access via a large vein. However, for long-term hemodialysis, the creation of an AV fistula is preferred for its durability, low complication rate, and good blood flow.
- AV fistulas involve anastomosing or surgically connecting an artery to a vein in the non-dominant arm. AV fistulas are preferable for long-term hemodialysis. In order to safely and repeatedly recannulate the fistula for dialysis, the venous wall must thicken or mature over time from the increased pressure and blood flow directly from the artery.

- Specific care and safety precautions that are imperative in the care of patients with an AV fistula or graft include:
  - o Avoid obtaining blood pressure measurements from the affected arm as compression can damage the fistula. Avoid any compression to the affected arm (or extremity).
  - o Do NOT allow venipunctures (e.g., lab work) or IV access from the affected arm. Ensure that the patient and family are educated and will act assertively to prevent venipunctures from the arm with the fistula.
  - o Routinely assess the circulation in the fistula and in the arm distal to the fistula. Palpate or auscultate for a bruit or thrill to ensure patency. Thrombosis of the fistula is a common complication and must be detected and managed early for intervention to be successful. Teach patient to assess circulation. Urgently notify the health care provider if thrombosis is suspected.
  - o Routinely assess circulation in the arm distal to the fistula as in a normal physical exam.
  - o Ensure meticulous sterile technique.
  - o Be attentive for any signs of infection at the fistula and needle insertion sites, unexpected enlargement of the fistula suggesting an aneurysm, or reduced blood flow suggesting thrombosis.
  - o Instruct the patient to avoid heavy lifting, carrying anything heavy, or allowing any type of compression on the fistula site, including sleeping with body weight on the affected arm.
  - o If edema occurs, elevate the arm to reduce dependent edema. Avoid using arm slings.
  - o Instruct about frequent, daily range-of-motion exercises.

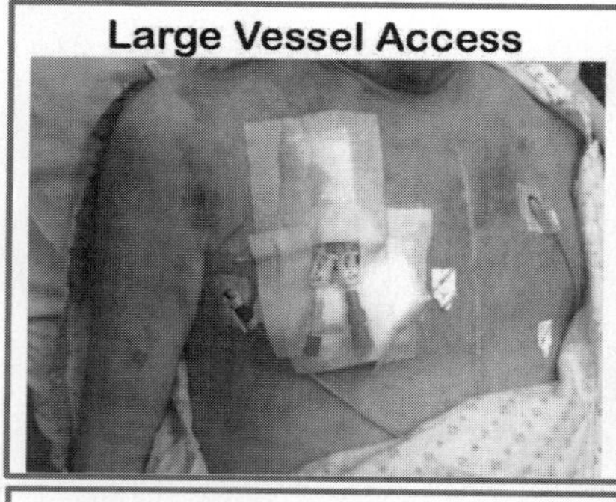

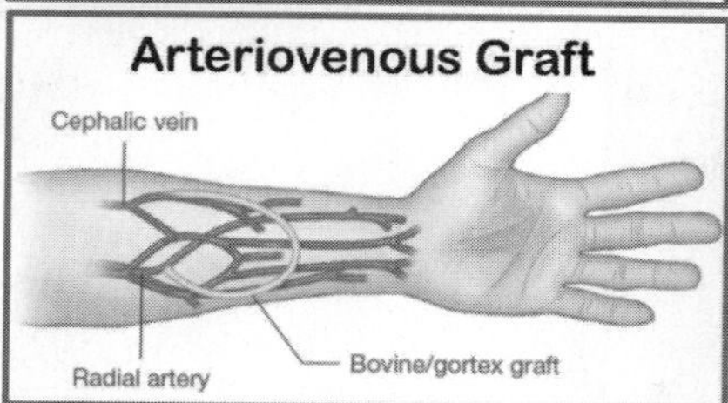

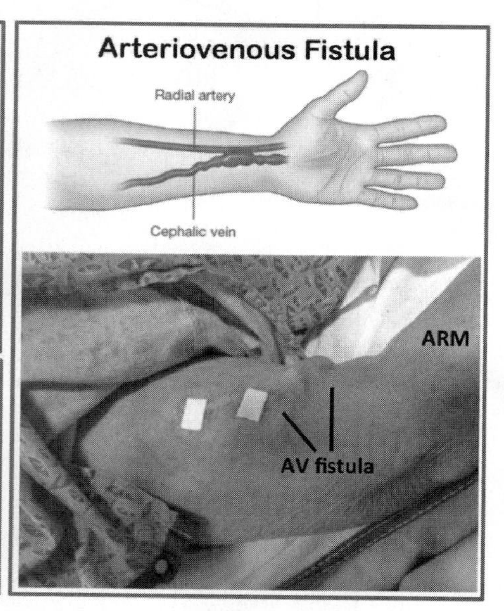

These images show the three vascular access methods for hemodialysis. Large vessel access is seen in a critically ill patient who has had cardiac bypass surgery in the past. The AV graft depicts how the bovine graft is an external access and avoids constant needle sticks in the patient's arm. For CKD patients, the AV fistula is common. The upper image shows the typical fistula created. The photo show that a fistula can be created in the upper arm if needed.

Source: Courtesy of K. Kyriakidis

Collaborative Interventions (continued)

Patient Education

Educate the patient and family regarding key issues:

- N — Underlying causes (and management) of CKD (diabetes and/or hypertension are the most common)
- N EBP — Urge vigilance about follow-up visits, as all patients with CKD are at higher risk for acute kidney injury and should be monitored for early warning signals (Levin, et al., 2012).
- M N EBP — Consult nutritionist or dietitian to best educate patients with renal failure, from early stage disease through all stages, including posttransplant patients (American Dietetic Association [ADA], 2010). Good and disease-appropriate nutrition can help the patient maintain good nutrition, impede disease progression, and delay the need for kidney transplantation (ADA, 2010).
- N EBP — Limit and plan sodium, potassium, phosphate, fat, and fluid intake, based on the patient's severity of CKD. Focus on a heart-healthy diet (Levin, et al., 2012).
- M N EBP — In the past, protein restriction was emphasized. However, current research does not generally support a protein-restricted diet, unless deemed necessary in specific instances (e.g., on dialysis, postrenal transplant). In the past, patients became malnourished and died of complications rather than their disease. Instead, a healthy diet is now recommended, with a controlled protein intake of approximately 0.8 gm/kg/day. Follow-up care should include evaluation for protein-energy malnutrition every 3–6 months (ADA, 2010; Levin, et al., 2013). Newer treatments trump the small benefit that restricted protein diets now contribute.
- M N EBP — Collaborate with nutritionist to increase controlled protein intake up to 0.9 gm/kg/day in patients with diabetic nephropathy and posttransplant (ADA, 2010).
- M N EBP — Collaborate with nutritionist to prepare the patient for energy intake of 25–35 kcal/kg/day (ADA, 2010).
- M N EBP — Avoid high or excessive protein intake (ADA, 2010).
- N — Avoid moderate to heavy use of alcohol. Consult the health care provider about alcohol use.
- N EBP — Encourage consulting the pharmacist before taking any over-the-counter drugs or protein supplements (Levin, et al., 2012).
- M N EBP — Consider monitoring and evaluating the patient's biochemical parameters (e.g., electrolytes, hematocrit, albumin) regularly to prevent or provide early detection of possible complications (ADA, 2010):
  - o Hypo- and hyperglycemia
  - o Inflammatory injury
  - o Fluid and/or electrolyte disturbances
  - o Hyperlipidemia
  - o Progression of kidney disease
  - o Protein-energy malnutrition
  - o Anemia
  - o Bone disorders
- N EBP — Collaborate with the health care provider and follow medical advice to manage comorbid conditions that can cause progression of CKD, particularly diabetes, hyperlipidemia, and hypertension (ADA, 2010).
- N — Immediately report signs, symptoms, and complications (fluid overload, weight gain >2 kg, injury, infection, mental status changes) to the health care provider.
- M N EBP — Encourage all patients with CKD to get the influenza vaccination (Levin, et al., 2012).
- M N EBP — Encourage patients at high risk for progression in their CKD to get hepatitis B and pneumonia vaccinations, unless contraindicated (Levin, et al., 2012).
- N EBP — Activity restrictions post-procedure. Otherwise, maintain as active a lifestyle as possible. Gradually increase activity when possible, as tolerated, to mitigate the catabolic effects on protein reserves (ADA, 2010).
- N EBP — Avoid herbal remedies as these may interact with the multiple medications prescribed (Levin, et al., 2012).
- N — Adjusting to the need for and schedule of frequent hemodialysis
- N — Family and psychological support, community resources
- M N — Dialysis procedure and precautions
- N — Community and online resources (National Kidney Foundation)
- M N — Advanced directives to concretize what the patient's preferences for care are and these are shared and known to care providers

Concept Check

6. What is the preferred access for hemodialysis?

A. Arteriovenous fistula

B. Synthetic AV graft

C. Subclavian vein

D. Femoral artery

Answer question

Education in Patients on Hemodialysis

Educate the patient and family regarding key issues:

- Compliance with medications and hemodialysis: Patients must typically take multiple medications, several times daily, for the rest of their lives.

- Hemodialysis typically requires travel to a dialysis center for treatment three times weekly, unless done at home. This regimen is challenging for any patient to comply with unless they understand the importance of the different components of their care.

- Lifestyle changes are paramount to long-term health and survival. Cardiovascular disease is a major contributor to mortality in CKD patients, so educate the patient for a heart-healthy lifestyle: healthy diet, smoking cessation, exercise, good management of comorbid conditions (e.g., diabetes, hypertension, obesity), and weight and stress management (see the Care of Patients with ACS NovE-lesson).

- Advanced directives: Some patients may not want to continue with such a regimen because of age, other underlying medical conditions, debility, or personal preferences.

LO1:

Renal Transplantation: Overview

- Renal transplantation is the transplant of a donated kidney into a patient with ESRD.
- Renal transplantation is recommended for patients with permanent renal failure (serum creatinine >8 mg/dL or GFR <10 mL/minute). It can provide a better quality of life and improved survival over prolonged dialysis.
- Patients usually live 10–15 years longer with a renal transplantation than they do on hemodialysis.
- Renal transplants are among the safest and most successful of all transplantations.
- Ideally, a patient with CKD receives a transplanted kidney rather than dialysis. However, the current shortage of kidney donors does not make this option realistic.
- Transplant recipients criteria must be met. Patients with advanced conditions that increase the risk of the procedure or preclude successful outcomes are poor transplant candidates.
- Kidney donors may be deceased or living. The most desirable donor is one with the closest tissue and blood type matches. Living related donors are commonly the best matches.
- Deceased donors are commonly gifted from patients who meet brain death criteria and who are additionally free of infective, malignant, or systemic disease that can affect the recipient (e.g., hepatitis, cancer, HIV).

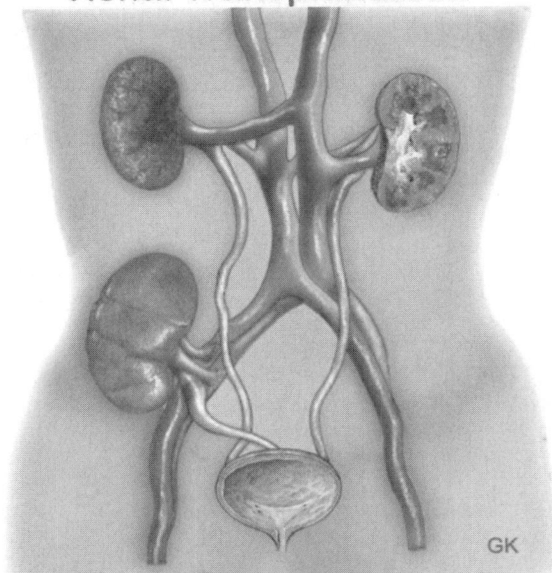

This image depicts the bilateral diseased and failing kidneys, leading to renal transplant.

Source: Courtesy of George Kyriakidis/Santa Ana, CA

Priority Patient Concerns and Desired Collaborative Care Outcomes: Renal Transplantation

Prior to caring for patients requiring renal transplantation, it is important to prioritize the patient's concerns that must guide the nursing care plan and interventions. Care for the patient is ordered and organized in accordance with the patient's priority and urgent needs. Desired collaborative care outcomes in patients requiring renal transplantation typically include:

1. The patient will report reduced anxiety from use of healthy coping mechanisms.
2. The patient will verbalize instructions for posttransplant medication, self-care, and follow-up requirements and will state signs and symptoms of rejection and complications.
3. The patient will discuss techniques to reduce exposure and harmful effects when inadequately protected from the environment.
4. The patient will discuss any feelings of distress regarding the donor that may arise.
5. The patient will identify ways that social interaction can be reestablished, even with necessary restrictions.

LO3:

Collaborative Interventions: Renal Transplantation

Care of a patient following transplant often requires intensive care with lifelong follow-up. Extensive specialty education and preparation are needed by clinicians who care for transplant patients. However, in addition to typical postoperative care for all surgical patients, the major interventions for renal transplant patients focus on:

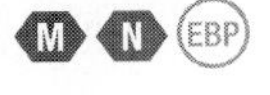

- Administer and maintain immunosuppressive (e.g., cyclosporine A, tacrolimus) medications (and combinations, if used) to prevent organ rejection (KDIGO Transplant Work Group, 2009).

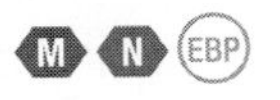

- Administer antiproliferative medications (e.g., mycophenolate, azathioprine, sirolimus) as prescribed to block acute cellular rejection. It is used concomitantly with immunosuppressants (KDIGO Transplant Work Group, 2009).

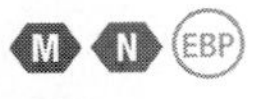

- Administer corticosteroids medications (e.g., methylprednisolone, prednisone) to prevent and/or treat organ rejection (KDIGO Transplant Work Group, 2009).

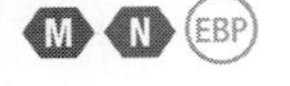

- Monitor closely for medications reaching target blood levels, for new signs of kidney injury, and for early warning signs of rejection, which include pain over transplant site, fever, edema, low urine output, tachycardia, and flu-like symptoms (KDIGO Transplant Work Group, 2009).

- Continue treatment of comorbid conditions (e.g., dyslipidemia, heart disease, diabetes), as in CKD, to prevent complications that can result in graft rejection or kidney injury (KDIGO Transplant Work Group, 2009).
- Control hypertension posttransplant to maintain the diastolic BP at <80 mmHg and systolic BP at <130 mmHg (KDIGO Transplant Work Group, 2009).
- Administer approved, inactivated vaccines (e.g., pneumonia) to all transplant patients (except hepatitis B), starting 6 months after transplant. Influenza vaccinations may be given under 6 months posttransplant (KDIGO Transplant Work Group, 2009).
- Adhere to meticulous infection control practices.
- Collaborate with patient to start early mobilization and self-care activities.
- Pain management
- Wound care
- Monitoring and early detection of potential complications, such as cancers, development of diabetes, mineral or bone disorders, neutropenia, anemia, hyperuricemia, and sexual or fertility dysfunction (KDIGO Transplant Work Group, 2009)
- Consult a pharmacist for more detailed information about multiple medications (e.g., best timing when to take the multiple medications with multiple doses, immunosuppressive medications and implications for sexual dysfunction).
- Address psychosocial aspects of transplantation. These can include pretransplant stress, role changes with the family, fear and anxiety, social and work related alterations, transplant outcomes, coping with donor death, body image changes, complex lifelong medical regimen, functional impairments, adjustment to new lifestyle, and depression. Collaborate with the health care provider if psychological consult is deemed necessary or helpful.

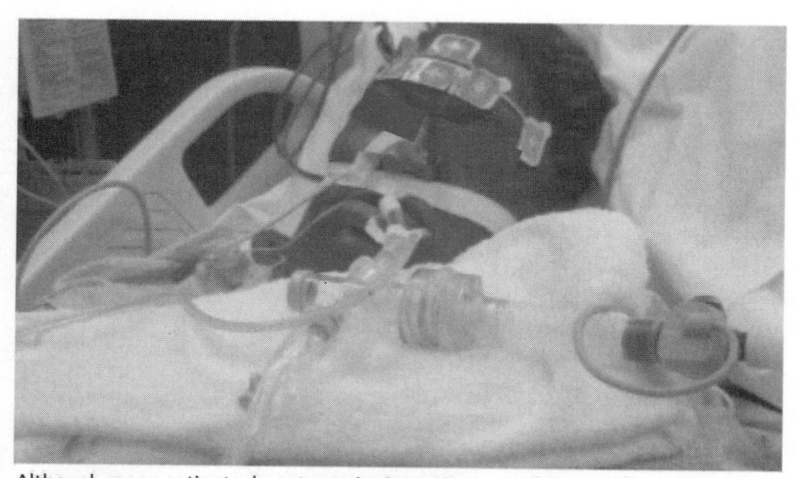

Although many patients do not require intensive care, this transplant patient had multiple comorbid conditions (e.g., hypertension, diabetes, morbid obesity) that complicated post-operative recovery.

Source: Copyright © 2014. NovEx Novice to Expert Learning, LLC.

Collaborative Interventions: Renal Transplantation (continued)

Patient Education

Education posttransplant is detailed and extensive. Proper preparation of the patient and family for discharge requires specialty education. In general, patient education for posttransplant patients should include:

- Adherence to treatment regimen. Observe for signs of nonadherence, provide early support, and collaborate with team about needed intervention (KDIGO Transplant Work Group, 2009).
- Cessation of smoking and any tobacco use (KDIGO Transplant Work Group, 2009)
- Weight management, particularly if obese (KDIGO Transplant Work Group, 2009)
- Detailed preparation about the multiple medications, their use in conjunction with medications for comorbid conditions, and the timing issues (e.g., with meals, what cannot be taken together)

- Early warning signs of infection when they may have a muted response due to immunosuppressive medications
- Consult a nutritionist for detailed instructions:
  - o New risk of infection to common organisms in raw or unwashed foods and nuts. Nutritionist can help with specific education for immunosuppressed patients
  - o Protein restrictions are no longer recommended and have been replaced with protein-controlled diets. Nutritionist can best guide patients with their individualized preferences (ADA, 2010).
- Be alert for early warning signs of rejection, which can include low-grade temperature elevation or fever, pain over transplant site, fever, edema, low urine output, tachycardia, aching joints, and flulike symptoms.
- Avoid exposure to pet wastes, soil, unchlorinated pools, and lakes to reduce the risk of infection to common organisms.
- Avoid exposure to individuals known to have infections and avoid public and crowded places during flu and cold seasons
- Early and progressive activity, exercise, self-care, and activities of daily living
- Follow a healthy lifestyle and proper diet (e.g., more fruits and vegetables) in addition to specific dietary instructions provided.
- Consider preparing and executing advanced directives.

Concept Check

7. Which information should be provided to a patient who has had renal transplantation?

A. Follow a protein restricted diet.

B. Reduce the amount of cooked vegetables eaten.

C. Early, progressive exercise is recommended.

D. Expect an occasional low-grade fever.

Answer question

Summary of Interventions: CKD

Collaborative interventions focus on:

- Slowing the progression of the disease and preventing cardiovascular disease. This includes controlling:
  - o Hyperglycemia
  - o Hypertension
  - o Smoking cessation
  - o Hyperlipidemia
- Correcting the electrolyte abnormalities, volume status, and anemia that can result
- Dialysis is often used in patients with ESRD to prolong life, but with significant trade-offs. For some patients, this requires major alterations in lifestyle and behaviors.
- Renal transplantation remains the best option for CKD, although not everyone with CKD is able to receive a transplant.
- Patient education is at the heart of a patient's long-term well-being, whether in CKD, ESRD, on dialysis, or postrenal transplantation.

LO4: Evaluation of Desired Collaborative Care Outcomes

Evaluation and reassessment should reveal attainment of previously established patient outcomes. In summary:

CKD

- The patient's fluid intake and output balance and electrolytes are within expected range.
- The patient's protein-related weight loss is minimal and there are limited findings of vitamin and mineral deficiencies.
- The patient remains injury free and discusses adoption of risk reduction modalities.
- The patient remains free of signs and symptoms of infection.
- The patient reports that fatigue is more manageable since using suggested techniques.
- The patient reports feeling less anxiety and more control over personal health.
- The patient accurately describes and discusses procedures, maintenance of dialysis, and plan of care.
- The patient reports returning to social interaction as capable and desired, without increasing risk of infection or fatigue.

Renal Transplantation

- Patient reports use of suggested healthy coping mechanisms and their effectiveness at reducing anxiety.
- The patient accurately describes posttransplant medication, self-care, and follow-up requirements and states signs and symptoms of rejection and complications.
- The patient describes techniques used to reduce exposure and potential harm from environmental threats to health, such as avoiding crowds and increasing healthy personal habits.
- The patient openly discusses or is gradually opening up to discussions about the donor and family and feelings associated with placement of nonself tissue within the body.
- The patient reports returning to enjoyable social activities, even if limited.

References

Avesani, C. M., Carrero, J. J., Axelsson, J., et al. (2006). Inflammation and wasting in chronic kidney disease: Partners in crime. *Kidney International, 70*, S8–S13. doi:10.1038/sj.ki.5001969 **www.nature.com/ki/journal/v70/n104s/full/5001969a.html**

Carrion, J. (2012). Vascular access devices for hemodialysis. *OR Nurse, 6*(1), 28–32.

Go, A. S., Chertow, G. M., Fan, D., et al. (2004). Chronic kidney disease and the risks of death, cardiovascular events, and hospitalization. *N Eng J Med, 351*, 1296–1305. doi: 10.1056/NEJMoa041031 **www.nejm.org/doi/full/10.1056/NEJMoa041031#t=article**

Kammerer, J., Garry, G., Hartigan, M., et. al. (2007). Adherence in patients on dialysis: Strategies for success. *Nephrol Nurs J, 34*(5), 479–486.

Kugler, C., Maeding, I., & Russell, C. (2011). Non-adherence in patients on chronic hemodialysis: An international comparison study. *J Nephrol, 24*(3), 366–375.

Nahas, M. E., & Bello, A. K. (2005). Chronic kidney disease: The global challenge. *Lancet, 365*(9456), 331–40.

Shankar, A., Klein, R., & Klein, B. (2006). The association among smoking, heavy drinking, and chronic kidney disease. *Amer J Epidemiol, 164*(3), 263–271. **aje.oxfordjournals.org/content/164/3/263.full**

Thomas-Hawkins, C., & Zazworsky, D. (2005). Self-management of chronic kidney disease. *AJN Amer J Nurs, 105*(10), 40–48. **www.nursingcenter.com/lnc/JournalArticle?Article_ID=604769&Journal_ID=54030&Issue_ID=604711&expiredce=1**

Wong, F. K. Y., Chow, S. K. Y., & Chan, T. M. F. (2010). Evaluation of a nurse-led disease management programme for chronic kidney disease: A randomized controlled trial. *International J Nurs Studies, 47*(3), 268–278. **www.journalofnursingstudies.com/article/S0020-7489%2809%2900234-X/abstract**

Clinical Practice Guidelines

American Dietetic Association. (2010). *Chronic kidney disease evidence-based nutrition practice guideline*. Chicago, IL: American Dietetic Association. **www.guideline.gov/content.aspx?id=23924**

Fox, H., Voleti, V., Khan, L., et al. (2008). A quick guide to evidence-based chronic kidney disease care for the primary care physician. *Postgraduate Medicine, 120*(2), 1–6. **fammed.buffalo.edu/unynet/files/Postgrad%20CKD%207-08.pdf.**

Kidney Disease: Improving Global Outcomes (KDIGO) Transplant Work Group. (2009). KDIGO clinical practice guideline for the care of kidney transplant recipients. *Am J Transplant, 9*(Suppl s3), S1–S155. **www.ncbi.nlm.nih.gov/pubmed/19845597**

Levin, A., Stevens, P. E., & Kidney Disease: Improving Global Outcomes (KDIGO) CKD Work Group. (2012). KDIGO 2012 clinical practice guideline for the evaluation and management of chronic kidney disease. *Kidney International Suppl, 3*(1), 1–163. **www.kdigo.org/clinical_practice_guidelines/pdf/CKD/KDIGO_2012_CKD_GL.pdf**

MacLeod, A., Ali, T., Allan, G., et al., & the Guideline Development Group. (2008). *Diagnosis and management of chronic kidney disease: A national clinical guideline 103*. Edinburgh: Scottish Intercollegiate Guidelines Network. **www.sign.ac.uk/pdf/sign103.pdf**

McMurray, J., Parfrey, P. S., & Kidney Disease: Improving Global Outcomes (KDIGO) Anemia Work Group. (2012). KDIGO 2012 clinical practice guideline for anemia in chronic kidney disease. *Kidney International Suppl, 2*(4), 279–335. **www.guideline.gov/content.aspx?id=38245&search=kdigo**

Registered Nurses' Association of Ontario (RNAO). (2009). *Decision support for adults living with chronic kidney disease*. Toronto, ON: Registered Nurses' Association of Ontario. **http://rnao.ca/sites/rnao-ca/files/Decision_Support_for_Adults_Living_with_Chronic_Kidney_Disease_1.pdf**

Patient Education

Berns, J. S. (2014). *Patient information: Chronic kidney disease (beyond the basics)*. **www.uptodate.com/contents/chronic-kidney-disease-the-basics?source=see_link**

National Institute for Health and Care Excellence (NICE). (2011). *Information for the public: Treating anaemia in people with chronic kidney disease, NICE clinical guideline 114*. **www.nice.org.uk/nicemedia/live/13329/52855/52855.pdf**

National Institute for Health and Care Excellence (NICE). (2008). *Information for the public: Identifying and treating long-term kidney problems (chronic kidney disease), NICE clinical guideline 73*. **www.nice.org.uk/nicemedia/live/12069/42120/42120.pdf**

Learning Outcomes for Glomerulonephritis

When you complete this lesson, you will be able to:

1. Recognize the clinical relevance of glomerulonephritis.
2. Consider the pathophysiology, etiology, risk factors, and clinical presentation of glomerulonephritis that determine the priority patient concerns.
3. Determine the most urgent and important nursing interventions and patient education required for a patient with glomerulonephritis.
4. Evaluate attainment of desired collaborative care outcomes for a patient with glomerulonephritis.

LO1:

What Is Glomerulonephritis?

- *Glomerulonephritis* is a term that encompasses several types of renal conditions that injure the glomeruli. Inflammation results and causes renal dysfunction. It is also referred to as nephritis.
- Glomerulonephritis can produce two syndromes: nephritic and nephrotic.
- Nephritic syndrome is characterized by hematuria, mild to moderate proteinuria, and one or more of the following: oliguria, edema, hypertension, and/or elevated serum creatinine.

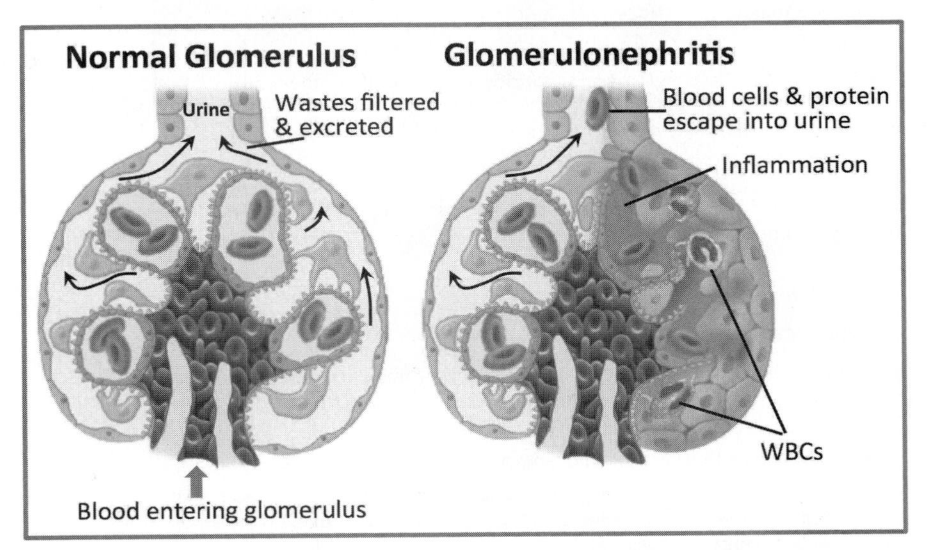

Glomerulonephritis is compared to a normally functioning glomerulus. The inflammation and dysfunction shown on the right can be due to one of many causes.

- Nephrotic syndrome is characterized by massive proteinuria (>3.5 g/day) and lipiduria, and often by hypoalbuminemia, hyperlipidemia, and generalized edema.
- In nephrotic syndrome, the capillary damage with increased glomerular permeability allows larger molecules to be filtered and excreted into the urine. It also results from a variety of diseases that damage the glomerulus, including those that cause glomerulonephritis. Causes of nephrotic syndrome, however, include diseases that may not involve inflammation of the glomeruli.
- **Syndromes are not diseases but are a collection of symptoms that appear together**. The purpose of separating nephrotic and nephritic syndromes is that the classification can help in determining possible causes and prognosis.
- Patients with glomerulonephritis may develop both nephritic and nephrotic syndrome, depending on where and how the glomerulus is affected. If both are present, a patient may have characteristics of one syndrome more than the other.
- Glomerulonephritis is a complex condition that results from immune system injury and is not yet clearly understood.

Concept Check

1. What is another name for glomerulonephritis?
   A. Urinary infection
   B. Nephrolithiasis
   C. Nephritis
   D. Interstitial fibrosis

Answer question

Nephritic Versus Nephrotic Syndromes

	Nephritic Syndrome	Nephrotic Syndrome
Proteinuria	++ (variable)	++++ (massive)
Edema	Mild	up to Severe
RBC's in urine	+++	+/-
HTN	+/-	No
Oliguria	Yes	No
Cellular inflammatory reaction	Yes	No
Hyperlipidemia/hyperlipiduria	No	Yes
Cause	Usually a type of glomerulonephritis	Glomerulonephritis as well as other causes

Characteristic findings that differentiate the nephritic from the nephrotic syndrome.

This table of key signs and symptoms is presented here because they define "what is" nephritic versus nephrotic syndromes.

LO1:

Clinical Relevance

- Glomerulonephritis may occur at any age but can be especially tragic in children who must deal with the renal damage for the rest of their lives with the prospect of failed or failing kidney function.
- It may complicate other life-threatening and disabling diseases.
- Renal compromise or failure presents a huge economic burden on the patient and on his or her family and, in the event dialysis or transplant becomes necessary, an expense borne by insurance or governmental agencies.
- Because of an impaired immune system and/or the deteriorated health status of the patient, other serious diseases and complications become much more prevalent. These patients thus require extensive care and incur tremendous suffering.
- The cost, nursing care, and support care required for these patients and for the increasing numbers of afflicted patients impose a burden on the health care delivery system and their families.
- Glomerulonephritis may strike an otherwise healthy and unsuspecting victim without warning.
- Onset of symptoms may not be noted by patient or family until the disease is far advanced.

LO2:

Pathophysiology

The pathophysiology in glomerulonephritis details the abnormal processes that occur in both nephritic and nephrotic syndromes, which are commonly overlapping and indistinguishable. Both syndromes are a constellation of symptoms, but nephrotic syndrome has some unique and differentiating pathophysiology, whether it develops in conjunction with nephritic syndrome or independent of it. The pathophysiologic description here details glomerulonephritis, which necessarily includes both syndromes as they evolve:

- Glomerulonephritis often results from the damage that large, circulating antigen–antibody complexes cause. These immune complexes form when antibodies are produced in response to particular antigens. Antigens bind to the antibodies, which are derived from a variety of sources. Antigens include:
  - Components of viruses or bacteria when infection is the cause (e.g., streptococcal glomerulonephritis)
  - Components of human cells when autoimmune diseases are the cause (e.g., systemic lupus)
  - Immune globulin IgA when IgA nephropathy is the cause
  - Components of the glomerulus itself

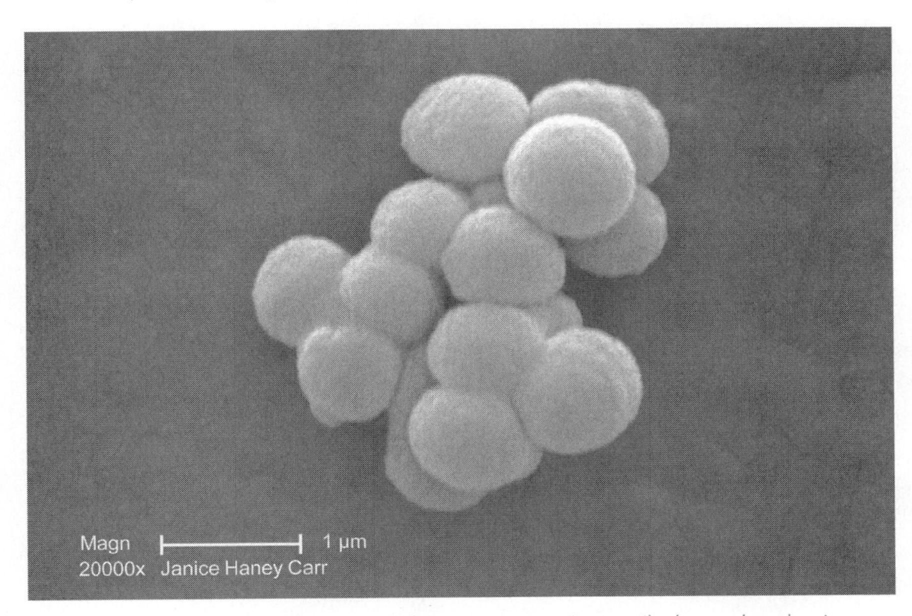

This photo shows *streptococcus* bacteria, which can set up an antigen–antibody complex when it invades. It is responsible as a causative agent in glomerulonephritis.
Source: Bette Jensen/Centers for Disease Control and Prevention

- Normally, the glomerulus filters the blood flowing into it. This filtration is driven by the pressure of blood flow into the glomerulus, which forces electrolytes, water, and toxins through the thin glomerular walls. Filtrate forms in the Bowman's capsule, which then drains into the renal tubules. As the filtrate passes through the different tubular segments, water and electrolytes can be reabsorbed.
- Glomerulonephritis results when the immune complexes from the various sources flow into the glomerulus and, during filtration, are deposited in and damage the capillary walls. The damage eventually moves outside the capillary into surrounding tissues.

Glomerulus with Immune Complex Deposits

Nephron

GK

Kidney

GK

Glomerulus

This photo shows where microscopic renal damage occurs, from kidney (left) to nephron to glomerulus (right). Immune complex deposits (bright green) in glomeruli that cause destruction are seen on microscopy with immunofluorescent staining.

Source: Courtesy of George Kyriakdis/Santa Ana, CA

- A normal glomerulus (see figure below) can be transformed into an inflamed one.
  - o The deposited immune complexes create "humps" in the capillaries and initiate inflammation by releasing cytokines. Cytokines signal an inflammatory response.
  - o As more inflammatory cells, such as macrophages and neutrophils are attracted, they release more cytokines.
  - o Other cells are stimulated to produce and deposit fibrous tissue.
  - o Both structural and glomerular changes ensue:
    - Obstruction of the capillary lumen
    - Leakage of RBCs and protein through the capillary wall as it swells and ruptures
    - Sodium and water retention
- The deposits of damaging immune complexes in the kidney are often the result of a systemic condition that affects multiple organs, such as the lungs, not the kidneys alone.
- Urine output may decrease.
- Excessive sodium and water retention may lead to hypertension.

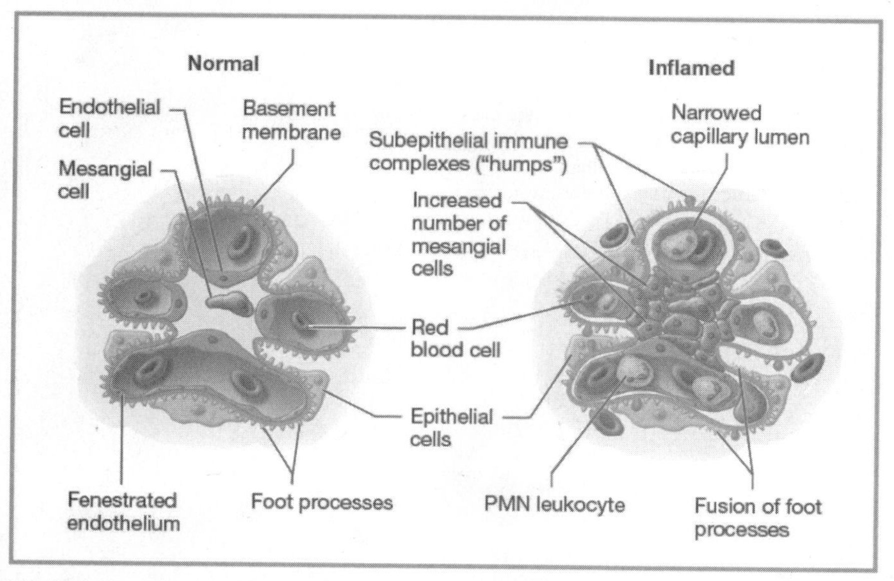

Left: Normal glomerulus. Right: The image shows how the deposited immune complexes set the inflammatory response in motion to initiate glomerulonephritis.

Nephrotic Syndrome

In glomerulonephritis, when protein leakage is extreme, additional and distinguishing pathophysiology develops to help identify it:

- If large amounts of protein leak from the capillaries, the patient may develop nephrotic syndrome.
- Loss of protein leads to low serum albumin levels.
- Albumin normally helps to hold fluid inside the intravascular space. When albumin is low in patients with nephrotic syndrome, fluid disproportionately moves into the extravascular space (edema).
- Fluid retention is exacerbated by the sodium and water retention that occurs in the glomeruli.
- Hypoalbuminemia is also thought to stimulate lipid production by the liver, leading to hyperlipidemia.
- Loss of other serum proteins needed for coagulation and immunity leads to a hypercoagulability and increased susceptibility to infection.
- Hypercoagulability puts these patients at increased risk for deep venous thrombosis (DVT), renal vein thrombosis, and pulmonary embolus.

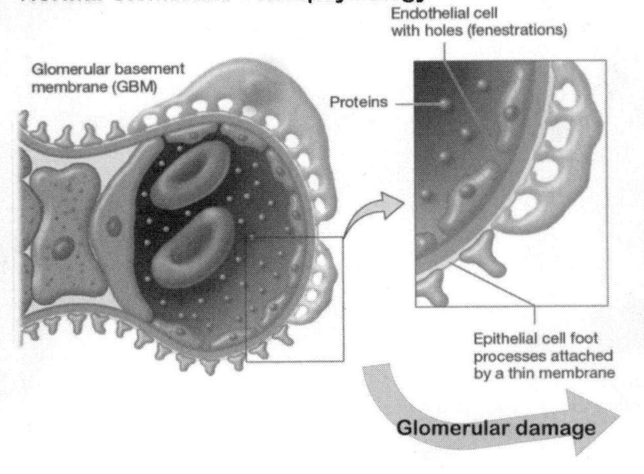

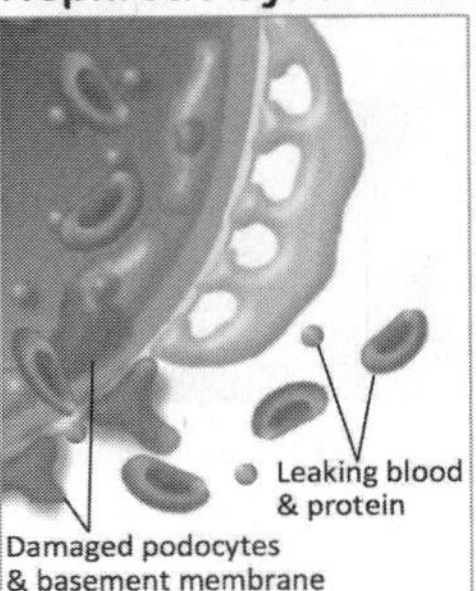

Drawn around the glomeruli are foot processes, which serve as barriers to keep protein and blood cells out of the urine. These are the endothelial cell, basement membrane, and epithelial cell (podocyte). The epithelial cell seems to be most important. Injury to these barriers causes protein and blood to leak into the urine.

Concept Check

2. **Which finding is associated with nephritic syndrome rather than nephrotic syndrome?**
   A. Massive proteinuria
   B. Hyperlipidemia
   C. Severe edema
   D. Oliguria

Answer question

LO2:

Risk Factors

- Streptococcal upper respiratory infections
- HIV
- Hepatitis B and C
- Systemic lupus erythematosus
- Diabetes mellitus
- Certain medications (e.g., NSAIDs)
- Cancer
- Addicting drugs, especially IV drugs, resulting in high risk for hepatitis B and C
- Genetic predisposition to certain subtypes
- "Unsafe" sex, resulting in high risk for hepatitis B and C

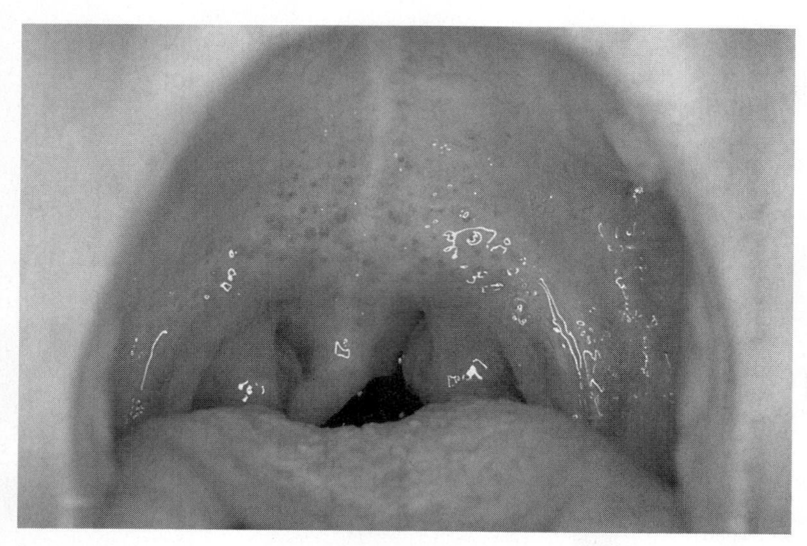

Streptococcus bacteria has infected the throat and caused oropharyngeal inflammation with petechial hemorrhages in the soft palate. This bacteria can enter the blood stream and result in glomerulonephritis, endocarditis, and/or sepsis.
Source: Dr. Heinz F. Eichenwald/Centers for Disease Control and Prevention

LO2:

Causes

Nephritic Syndrome

- Poststreptococcal glomerulonephritis: occurs weeks after pharyngitis
- IgA nephropathy: due to deposition of IgA complexes in the kidney; occurs within 1–2 days after upper respiratory tract infection (URTI)
- Crescentic glomerulonephritis
- Goodpasture's syndrome: Antiglomerular basement membrane (anti-GBM) antibodies are formed against basal membrane antigens; also affects the lung.
- Vasculitic disorders: Wegener's granulomatosis (affects lungs and upper airway), microscopic polyangiitis, Churg-Strauss vasculitis
- Membranoproliferative glomerulonephritis: secondary to systemic lupus erythematosus (SLE), hepatitis B and C
- Henoch-Schönlein purpura: systemic vasculitis—deposition of IgA in the skin and kidneys

Nephrotic Syndrome

- Minimal change glomerulonephritis is a common cause in which large amounts of protein are eliminated in the urine.
- Focal segmental glomerulosclerosis (FSGS) is the scarring of glomeruli in focal segments of the kidney.
- Membranous glomerulonephritis, which results from the buildup of damaging immune complexes
- Systemic lupus
- Hepatitis B and C
- HIV
- Diabetes mellitus
- Malignancy
- Medications (e.g., NSAIDs)

Concept Check

3. **What is the basic pathophysiologic mechanism associated with the development of glomerulonephritis?**
   A. Immune complex deposition
   B. Damage to vessels by hypotension
   C. Development of arteriosclerotic plaques
   D. Death of cells from apoptosis

Answer question

LO2:

Assessment Findings

- As many as half of patients may be asymptomatic when initially diagnosed.
- The onset and progression is variable and is usually associated with the type of glomerulonephritis.
- Onset of signs and symptoms may be acute with rapid progression to end stage renal disease.
- Onset may be acute with rapid resolution.
- Onset may be gradual with gradual progression over years (chronic glomerulonephritis).
- For details and to understand the relative significance of symptoms, see the Nephritic versus Nephrotic Syndromes table in the "What is Glomerulonephritis" section.
- Other signs and symptoms of glomerulonephritis may include fever and malaise.

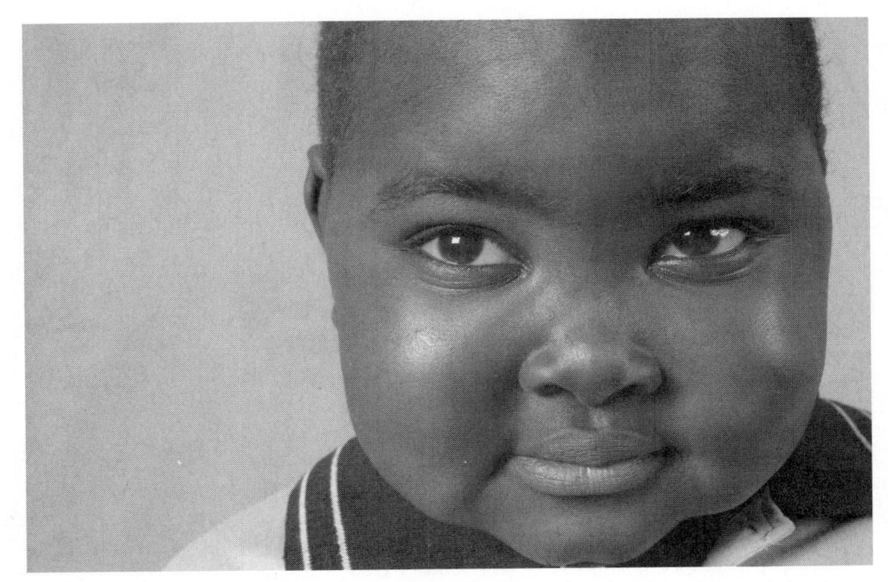

This 6-year-old boy suffers from nephrotic syndrome. His face is edematous from the protein loss. Although his generalized edema creates the appearance of being overweight, he suffers from muscle wasting. Hypertension and fatigue are additional manifestations.
Source: Medicimage/Alamy

Nephritic Syndrome

- Hematuria: Blood in the urine (rust or brown color, dark) suggests glomerular damage.
- Hypertension
- Decreased urine output
- Decreasing glomerular filtration rate
- Renal failure
- If advanced, can cause:
  - o Pruritus
  - o Lung edema with shortness of breath
  - o Encephalopathy

Nephrotic Syndrome

- Swelling (edema): facial, orbital, abdominal, lower extremities, and/or feet; tends to be worse than in glomerulonephritis
- Foamy urine (occurs because of large amounts of protein in the urine)
- Muscle wasting
- Patients are at increased risk for development of DVT and infections. DVT may present with leg swelling and pain.

Concept Check

4. Rusty-colored urine in a patient with nephritic syndrome suggests which complication?

A. Glomerular damage

B. Increased glomerular filtration rate

C. Protein in the urine

D. Increased risk of deep vein thrombosis

Answer question

LO2:

Diagnostics: Nephritic Versus Nephrotic Syndrome

Nephritic Syndrome

- Urinalysis: protein and RBCs. Examination of urine sediment shows red cell casts. Casts are cylindrical structures that are formed in the tubules. Casts with red cells in urine are suggestive of glomerular damage.
- Laboratory:
  - o May show electrolyte abnormalities (e.g., hyperkalemia or metabolic acidosis, elevated creatinine)
  - o Antiglomerular basement membrane antibody test to evaluate for Goodpasture's syndrome
  - o Antineutrophil cytoplasmic antibodies (ANCAs) to evaluate for Wegener's syndrome
  - o Antinuclear antibodies to evaluate for lupus

Nephrotic Syndrome

- Urinalysis: protein with 24-hour urine showing >3.5 grams, lipids (lipiduria)

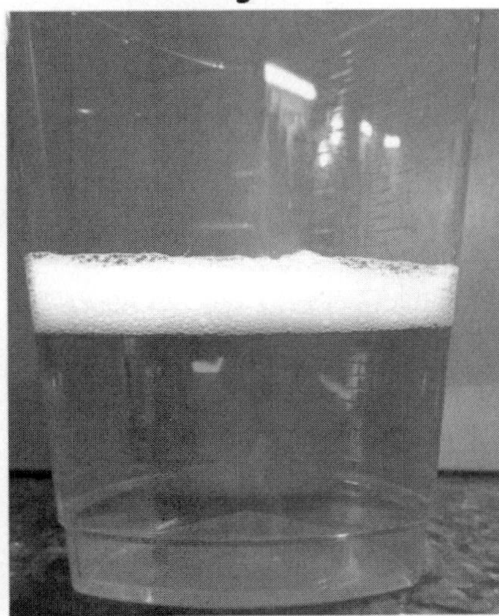

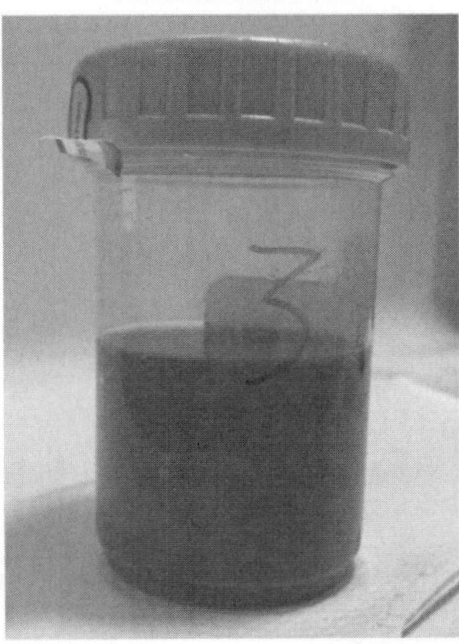

Foamy urine can suggest the presence of protein. Hematuria indicates the presences of blood. Nephrotic syndrome should be considered.
Source: Courtesy of K. Kyriakidis

- Laboratory:
  - o Elevated triglycerides and LDL
  - o Low albumin
  - o Possible high creatinine
- Imaging studies (e.g., ultrasound, CT scan, or MRI) rule out malignancy as a cause.

Both Syndromes

Biopsy: Examination of tissue is helpful in making a diagnosis in either syndrome. Tissue may show inflammation of the glomeruli and is examined for patterns of damage. In some types, only a section of glomeruli are affected. Other types may only have portions of each glomerulus affected (shown in photo, lower right). Tissue stains may also show different patterns.

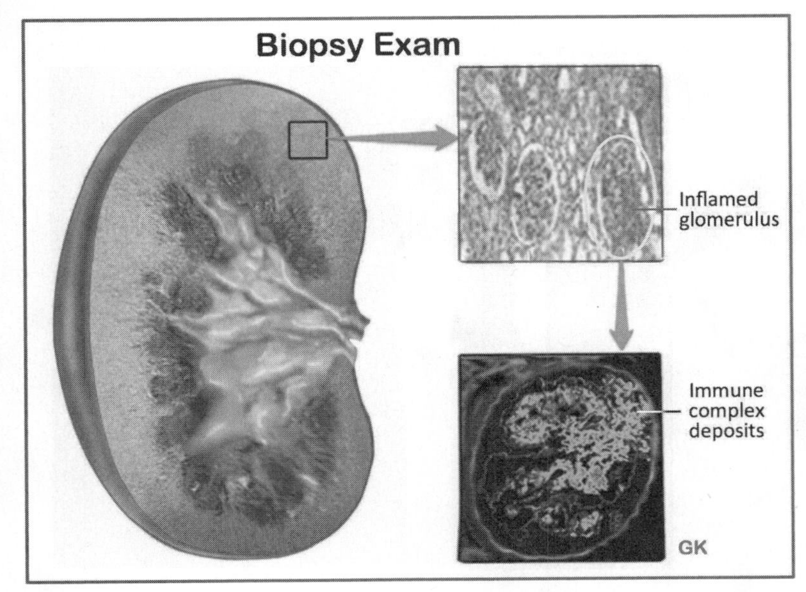

Source: Courtesy of George Kyriakdis/Santa Ana, CA

Priority Patient Concerns and Desired Collaborative Care Outcomes

Prior to caring for patients with glomerulonephritis, it is important to prioritize the patient's concerns that must guide the nursing care plan and interventions. Care for the patient is ordered and organized in accordance with the patient's priority and urgent needs. Desired collaborative care outcomes in patients with glomerulonephritis typically include:

1. The patient will evidence findings associated with balanced body fluids.
2. Patient will report pain has resolved or is reduced to tolerable level.
3. Patient's skin will return to an intact state, without edema or impairment.
4. Patient will remain infection free throughout course of illness and state understanding of preventive measures.
5. Patient will consume sufficient calories to support desired weight.
6. Patient will state understanding of disease process and treatment modalities.
7. Patient will be oriented to self and others, and demonstrate accurate interpretation of environment.

Considering these important care outcomes, prepare a list of the major 3–6 priority patient concerns or nursing diagnoses for patients with glomerulonephritis. Be prepared to participate in a discussion of this list and/or to submit them as an assignment, as determined by your faculty. Resources you may find helpful in this assignment can include this lesson, the references, resources on nursing care plans, and standard nursing diagnoses manuals.

LO3:

Collaborative Interventions

Goals of Treatment

- Care of patients with glomerulonephritis often calls for watching and waiting.
- If glomerulonephritis is rapidly progressive with increasing creatinine, treatment is aimed at decreasing the inflammation in the glomeruli.

Steroids

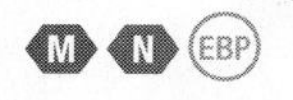

- Administer corticosteroid as the primary therapy for most of the inflammatory aspects in this disease (Cattran, et al., 2012):
  - o Prednisone
  - o Methylprednisolone

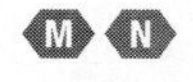

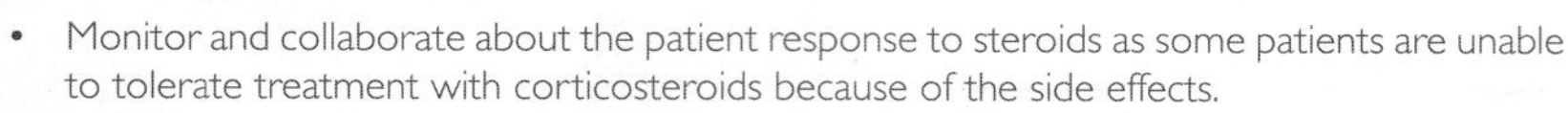

- Monitor and collaborate about the patient response to steroids as some patients are unable to tolerate treatment with corticosteroids because of the side effects.

- Use immunosuppressive drugs to also treat inflammation of the glomeruli. Some of these drugs are the same ones used for transplant patients and patients with autoimmune disorders. These drugs are used alone or in combination with corticosteroids (Cattran, et al., 2012).

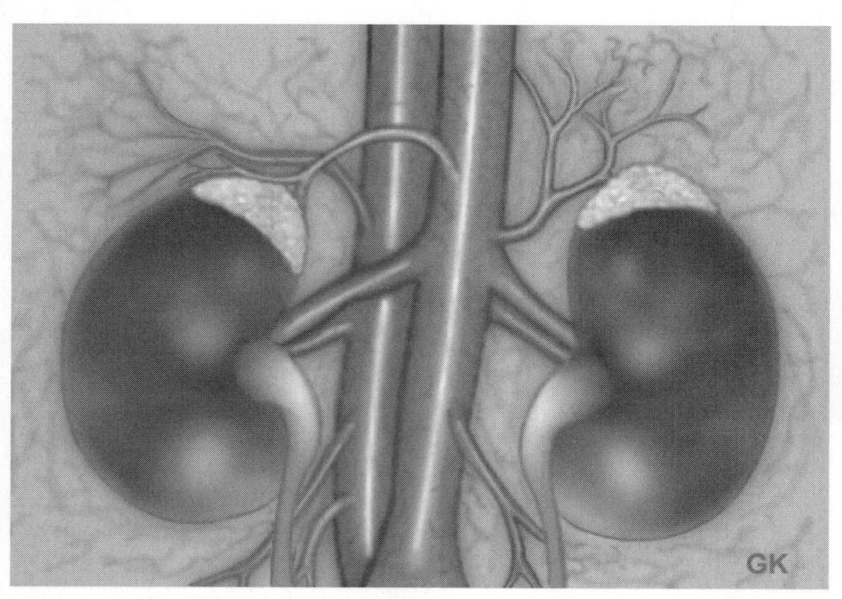

Nephrotic syndrome (NS) can be caused by a minimal change lesion (or lipoid nephrosis). Steroids as well as immunosuppressive medications like cyclosporine are successfully used with NS. These meds, however, are used with caution because of the high risk of toxicity.
Source: Courtesy of George Kyriakdis/Santa Ana, CA

Immune Treatments for Glomerulonephritis

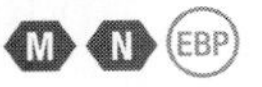

- Consider mycophenolate mofetil (CellCept) as an immune treatment (Cattran, et al., 2012):
  - o It is usually used for immunosuppression for transplant patients.
  - o There is some evidence for use in glomerulonephritis to limit the immune system response to inflammation.
  - o Use of this drug may allow steroids to be discontinued.

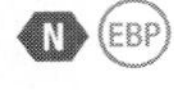

- Observe the patient's response to immunosuppressants, as systemic side effects are a possibility, including infections and certain types of cancers (e.g., lymphomas) (Cattran, et al., 2012).
- Consider plasmapheresis if glomerulonephritis is due to an immune disorder (Cattran, et al., 2012):
  - o Plasmapheresis is a plasma exchange process.
  - o The plasma portion of the blood is exchanged for IV fluids or donated plasma.
  - o The exchange removes antibodies and high concentrations of inflammatory-causing agents from the patient's blood.
  - o The patient's plasma is discarded.
  - o The aim of antibody and inflammatory agent removal is to mitigate the inflammatory response and reduce injury in the glomeruli.

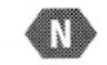

- Monitor the patient's hemodynamic stability during and after plasmapheresis (e.g., heart rate, blood pressure).

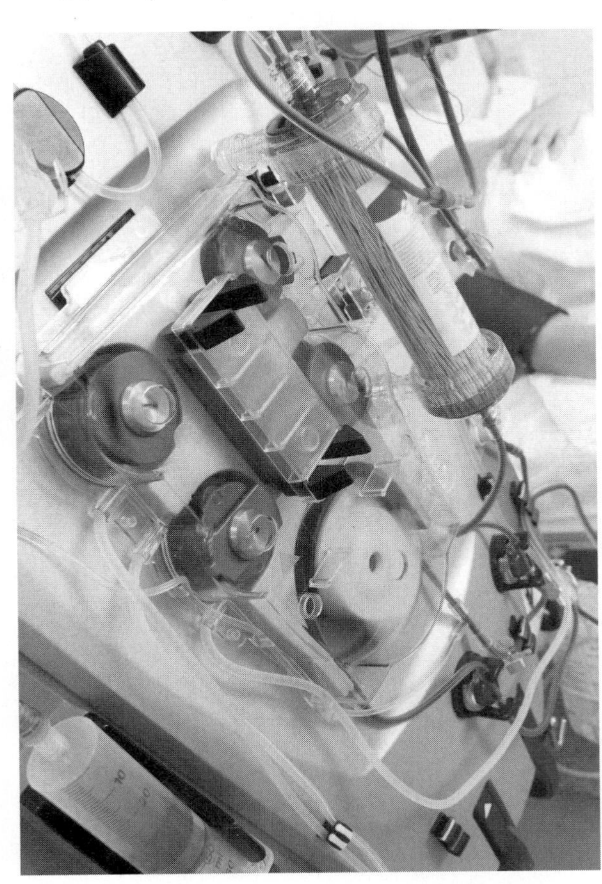

A patient is being treated with plasmapheresis. This procedure can be done at the bedside. This photo shows the major components of plasmapheresis treatment.
Source: beerkoff/Fotolia

Collaborative Interventions (continued)

Limiting Symptoms and Damage

Evidence-based interventions are aimed at treating or limiting the symptoms of glomerulonephritis as well as preventing or reducing damage to the kidneys. Care of the patient includes:

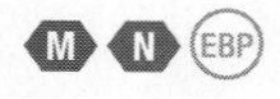

- Treatment for hypertension: Controlling hypertension is important to limit exacerbation of renal damage. Consider administering (Cattran, et al., 2012):
  - o Angiotensin-converting enzyme inhibitors (ACE inhibitor)
  - o Angiotensin receptor blockers

- Sodium restriction and diuretics are used to control or reduce edema (Cattran, et al., 2012).
- Consider treating hyperlipidemia using statins to prevent its damaging systemic effects.

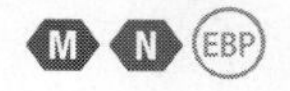

- Provide prophylaxis for DVT in hospitalized patients with nephrotic syndrome. They are at high risk for venous thromboembolic disease. Administer either subcutaneous low molecular weight heparin or unfractionated heparin for prophylaxis (Cattran, et al., 2012).

- Consider dialysis in patients with advanced kidney failure when the patient becomes poorly responsive to less invasive interventions.

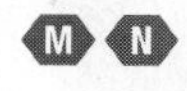

- When fluid restrictions are prescribed, a good rule of thumb for fluid allowance is 500–600 mL + the total urine output for the prior 24 hours.

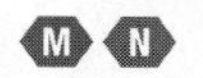

- Monitor for early warning signs and labs indicating hyperkalemia and hyperphosphatemia.

Concept Check

5. Which class of medications is the primary treatment for glomerulonephritis?

A. Antibiotics

B. Steroids

C. Diuretics

D. Antihypertensives

Answer question

Prevention

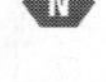

Many patients will ask if glomerulonephritis can be prevented. Clinicians need to be prepared to respond to patients and provide instructions about what they may do.

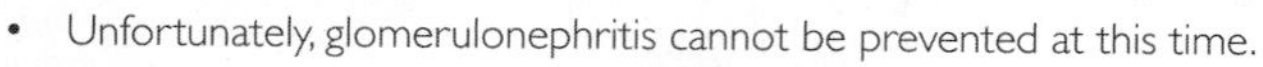

- Unfortunately, glomerulonephritis cannot be prevented at this time.

- Blood pressure control is one of the most important ways to avoid glomerulonephritis (Cattran, et al., 2012).
- Basic good personal hygiene and habits can help avoid risks of developing glomerulonephritis:
  - o Hand washing
  - o Completing an entire course of antibiotics
  - o Practicing safe sex
  - o Avoiding IV drugs is helpful in preventing viral infections such as HIV and hepatitis, which could lead to glomerulonephritis.

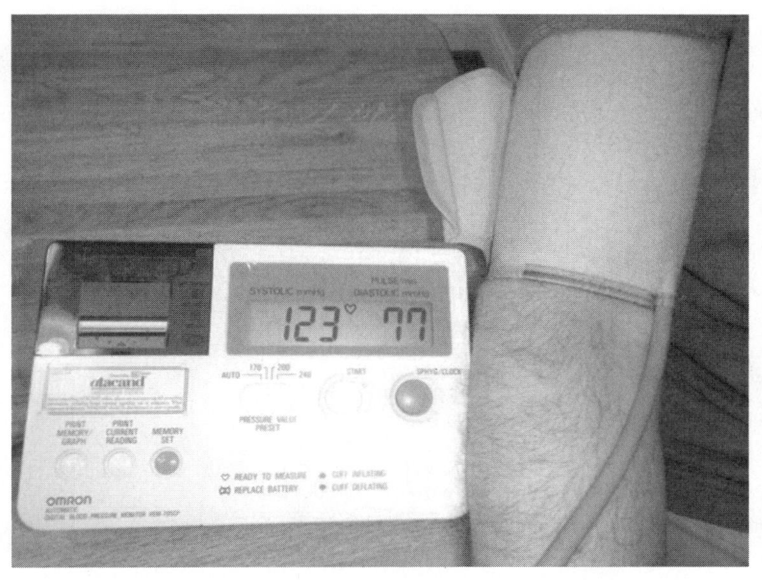

Research shows that blood pressure control is paramount in reducing the risk for glomerulonephritis, preventing further glomerular damage, and limiting progression into kidney failure.

Concept Check

6. In order to determine today's fluid restriction amount, which information should the nurse review?

A. Patient's weight

B. Total amount of oral fluids yesterday

C. Patient's basal metabolic rate

D. Amount of urine output for past 24 hours

Answer question

Comfort and Safety

- N Promote conservation of patient's energy during acute illness: Assist with activities of daily living, maintain a restful environment, and balance activity and rest.
- N Coordinate needed activities.
- N With recovery, promote activity as tolerated.
- N Anticipate that edema may cause shortness of breath and heart failure, limiting any activity. Plan minimal activity when edema limits ability.
- N Vigilant monitoring for infection and educating the patient to watch for infection are vital in these high-risk patients.
- N Promote methods to help the patient manage anxiety and fear related to the disease process and procedures (e.g., relaxation techniques, diversional activities, massage, exercise, and hobbies).
- N Observe for changes in mental functioning such as irritability, inability to read or to perform job-related functions, or other processes requiring concentration or changes in memory. Mental changes warn of increasing plasma levels of toxins that require evaluation.

Patient Education

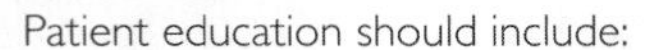

Patient education should include:

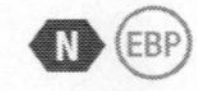

- Observation and reporting of side effects of corticosteroids (Cattran, et al., 2012):
  - o Weight gain
  - o Hyperglycemia
  - o Agitation
  - o Osteoporosis (destruction of bones)
  - o Easy bruising and thinning of the skin

- Purpose, desired effects, dosage, potential adverse side effects, and schedule of newly prescribed drugs

- Dietary or fluid restrictions

- Detection of fluid retention, measurement of weight and blood pressure

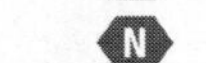

- When to notify the health care provider

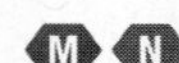

- Receiving pneumonia and influenza vaccinations, but no live vaccines (Sasaki, et al., 2009)
- If dialysis is necessary: scheduling, routines, access care, signs and symptoms of complications

Summary of Interventions

- Treatment usually consists of watchful waiting.
- When the disease is rapidly progressing, medications to decrease glomerular inflammation are used:
  - o Steroid therapy
  - o Antibiotics
- Symptom treatment consists of:
  - o Treatment of hypertension, commonly with angiotensin receptor blockers or ACE inhibitors, to prevent the progression of disease
  - o Sodium restriction and diuretics for edema
  - o Possible treatment of hyperlipidemia with statins
  - o DVT prophylaxis for hospitalized patients with nephrotic syndrome
- Patients who have developed end-stage renal disease require dialysis or kidney transplantation.

Concept Check

7. What lifestyle change is necessary for a patient with glomerulonephritis?

A. Increase exercise.

B. Liberal use of salt at meals

C. Get additional rest.

D. Avoidance of influenza vaccine

Answer question

LO4:

Evaluation of Desired Collaborative Care Outcomes

Evaluation and reassessment should reveal attainment of previously established patient outcomes. In summary:

- The patient has clear mentation, clear lungs, and elastic skin turgor, and urine output is balanced with fluid intake.
- Patient reports that pain is diminished to a level that does not interfere with activities of daily living.
- Patient's skin is intact.
- Patient has remained infection-free.
- Patient's weight remains within the desired range, and there is no evidence of muscle wasting or continued muscle wasting.
- Patient accurately discusses disease process and treatment plan.
- Patient is oriented to time, place, and self and demonstrates understanding of environmental input.

References

D'Agati, D., Kaskel, F., & Falk, R. J. (2011). Focal segmental glomerulosclerosis. *N Engl J Med, 365*(25), 2398–2411.

Lang, M. M., & Towers, C. (2001). Identifying poststreptococcal glomerulonephritis. *Nurse Pract, 26*(8), 34–49.

Lu, D. F., McCarthy, A. M., Lanning, L. D., et al. (2007). A descriptive study of individuals with membranoproliferative glomerulonephritis. *Nephrol Nurs J, 34*(3), 295–303.

Nasr, S. H., Fidler, M. E., Valeri, A. M., et al. (2011). Postinfectious glomerulonephritis in the elderly. *J Am Soc Nephrol, 22*(1), 187–195. doi: 10.1681/ASN.2010060611 **Jasn.asnjournals.org/content/22/1/187.full.pdf**

Nasr, S. H., Markowitz, G. S., Stokes, M. B., et al. (2008). Acute post infectious glomerulonephritis in the modern era: Experience with 86 adults and review of the literature. *Medicine* (Baltimore), *87*(1), 21–32.

Richardson, M. A. (2012). The many faces of minimal change nephrotic syndrome: An overview and case study. *Nephrol Nurs J, 39*(5), 365–375.

Clinical Practice Guidelines

Cattran, D., Feehally, J., et al. & Glomerulonephritis International Work Group, et al. (2012). Kidney Disease: Improving Global Outcomes (KDIGO) Clinical practice guideline for glomerulonephritis. *Kidney International Supplements, 2*(2), 139–241. **www.kdigo.org/clinical_practice_guidelines/pdf/KDIGO-GN-Guideline.pdf**

Sasaki, S., Yoshikawa, N., et al. (2009). Evidence-based practice guideline for the treatment of CKD. *Clin Exp Nephrol, 13*, 537–566. **www.jsn.or.jp/en/guideline/pdf/guideline2009.pdf**

Patient Education

Mayo Clinic Staff. (2014). *Nephrotic syndrome.* **www.mayoclinic.org/diseases-conditions/nephrotic-syndrome/basics/definition/con-20033385**

National Kidney Foundation. (2015). *Glomerulonephritis.* **www.kidney.org/atoz/content/glomerul.cfm**

Parmar, M. S. (2014). *Acute glomerulonephritis.* **emedicine.medscape.com/article/239278-overview**

STOP

Go to the online course and complete the NovE-Cases assigned by your instructor for this module.

Learning Outcomes for Diabetes Mellitus

When you complete this lesson, you will be able to:

1. Recognize the clinical relevance of diabetes mellitus.
2. Consider the pathophysiology, etiology, risk factors, and clinical presentation of diabetes mellitus that determine the priority patient concerns.
3. Determine the most urgent and important nursing interventions and patient education required in caring for a patient with diabetes mellitus.
4. Evaluate attainment of desired collaborative care outcomes for a patient with diabetes mellitus.

LO1:

What Is Diabetes?

Diabetes is an endocrine condition that results in hyperglycemia either from lack of insulin production or insulin resistance.

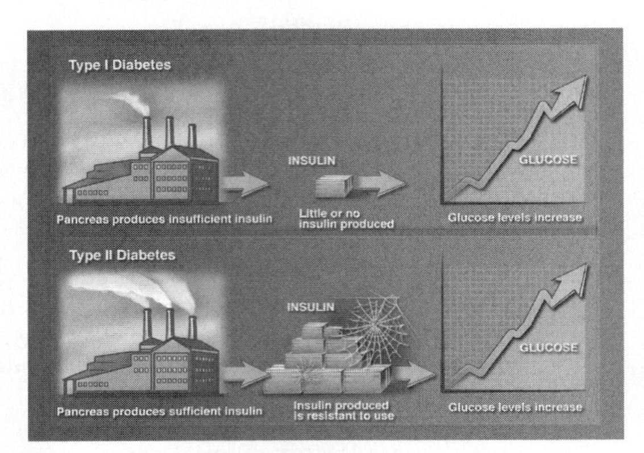

This illustration compares and contrasts diabetes type 1 with diabetes type 2. Insulin dependent, type 1 is shown first and is demonstrated by a factory (pancreas) that is putting out insufficient product (insulin). Type 2 is shown using a factory (pancreas) that puts out sufficient product (insulin) that simply is not utilized.

LO1:

Clinical Relevance

- Twenty-six million people (8.3% of the population) in the United States have diabetes mellitus. About 79 million have impaired glucose tolerance. The increased percentage in 50 years indicates that the disease is at an epidemic proportion.
- The total health care costs for diagnosed diabetes in 2012 was over $245 billion dollars.
- In 2007, diabetes was a contributing factor to 231,404 deaths. It is currently the seventh leading cause of death in the United States.
- The risk of stroke or heart disease in diabetics is two to four times greater than it is in the general population.
- Studies show that diabetes can be prevented or delayed by weight control and exercise.
- Complications of diabetes are debilitating and include heart disease, stroke, limb amputations, pain, blindness, and kidney failure. Complications can be decreased and sometimes avoided by proper education, treatment of hyperglycemia, and modification of risk factors.
- Patients admitted to the hospital for other conditions commonly have diabetes as a comorbid condition.
- Due to the prevalence of diabetes, all health care providers frequently care for patients with diabetes. Prior to diagnosis, 25% of diabetics already have complications.

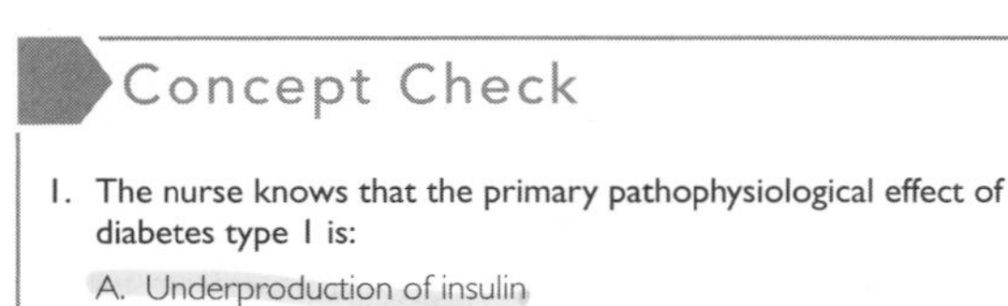

Concept Check

1. The nurse knows that the primary pathophysiological effect of diabetes type 1 is:
   A. Underproduction of insulin
   B. Overproduction of insulin
   C. Inability to use insulin
   D. Excess renal secretion of insulin

Answer question

LO2:

Pathophysiology

Type 1 Diabetes Mellitus

Type 1 diabetes mellitus is characterized by insulin deficiency or a deficiency in insulin production due to a loss of beta cells, which produce, store, and release insulin.

- Without insulin, the body cannot regulate blood glucose levels, and glucose, which is needed for energy production, cannot enter cells.
- With the body unable to regulate blood glucose levels, glucose accumulates in the blood and causes hyperglycemia.
- While the exact cause of type 1 diabetes is not known, it is postulated that it is caused by an abnormal autoimmune response against these insulin-producing cells.
- Viruses may stimulate this autoimmune response as well as cause direct infection and destruction of beta cells.

At the time of onset, most patients are otherwise healthy. The lack of insulin has three key physiologic effects:

- Decreased uptake of glucose by cells results in hyperglycemia.
- Glycogen gets converted to glucose in the liver (gluconeogenesis), also causes hyperglycemia.
- Fat cells release fatty acids, which are later converted to ketones by the liver. This process results in metabolic acidosis (diabetic ketoacidosis, or DKA). Diabetic ketoacidosis requires greater depth of understanding and is covered in a separate NovE-lesson.

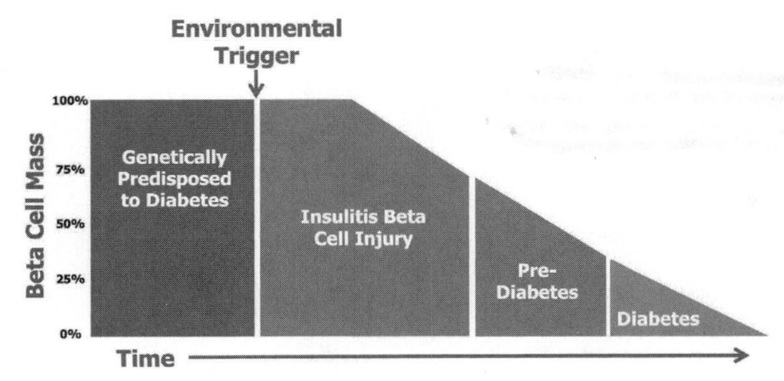

The natural history of type 1 diabetes is depicted in the diagram. Genetic factors may combine with environmental triggers to cause lymphocytes to infiltrate the pancreatic islets, destroy the beta cells, and create a lifelong dependency on exogenous insulin.
Source: Copyright © 2014, NovEx Novice to Expert Learning, LLC

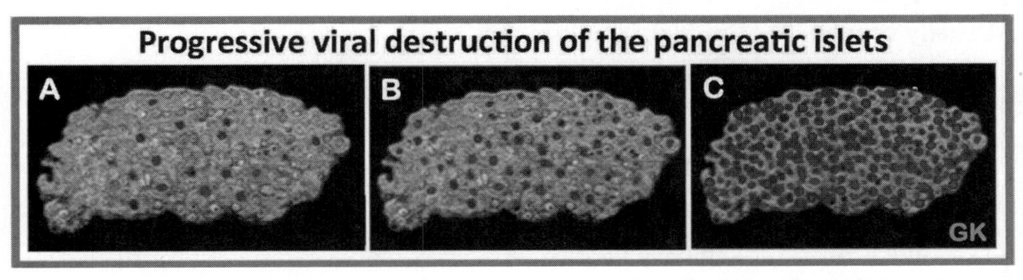

Source: Courtesy of George Kyriakidis/Santa Ana, CA

- The three microscopic fluorescent stains show beta cell–specific destruction in pancreatic islets (EMC mice) from a virus. Diabetes ensues:
  - o Uninfected control sample prior to viral destruction of beta cells
  - o Diffuse and significant beta cell destruction three days after viral infection
  - o Few beta cells remain 21 days after viral infection.
- Sections of the pancreas are stained with fluorescein-labeled anti-insulin.

Pathophysiology (continued)

Type 2 Diabetes Mellitus

Type 2 diabetes mellitus is primarily caused by insulin resistance. This is accompanied by a progressive dysfunction of insulin-secreting beta cells.

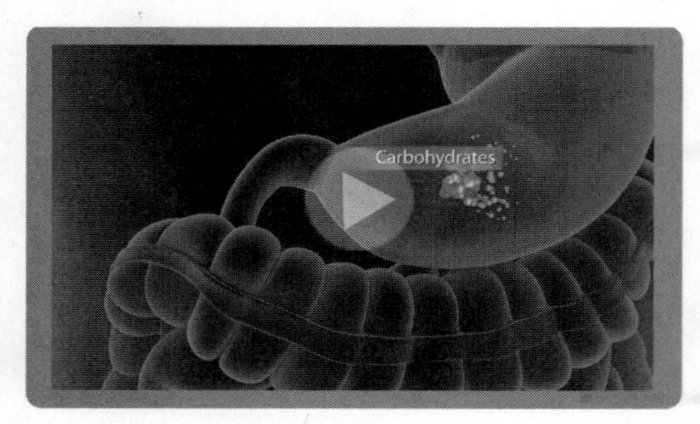

This animation shows type 2 diabetes, a condition in which the blood glucose level is too high. The animation shows the normal physiology of food absorption and insulin's mechanism of action. The pathology of type 2 diabetes is portrayed, including low insulin production, insulin resistance, hyperglycemia, and common symptoms. Acute complications are shown, including diabetic ketoacidosis, hyperosmolar hyperglycemic nonketotic syndrome, hypoglycemia (insulin shock), seizures, and diabetic coma. Chronic complications are displayed, including atherosclerosis, blindness, neuropathy, and renal failure. Multiple treatments are detailed at the end of the animation, including blood glucose monitoring, healthy eating, regular exercise, and medications.
Source:

- Normally, increased blood glucose after meals triggers an increase in insulin secretion by beta cells. Insulin then binds to insulin receptors on cells to allow glucose to enter.
- In patients with type 2 diabetes, these receptors are less sensitive to insulin (insulin resistance). Early in the course of type 2 diabetes, the insulin levels in the blood are higher than normal.
- Because of insulin resistance, patients with type 2 diabetes typically require daily doses of exogenous insulin that are much higher than physiologic levels (normal patient levels). This is in contrast to patients with type 1 diabetes who require daily dosing of insulin that are much closer to normal (a nondiabetic's normal insulin production level) in order to meet targeted glycemic goals.
- The mechanism that results in decreased insulin sensitivity is not clearly understood.
- However, insulin resistance has been linked to obesity and other metabolic conditions, such as polycystic ovarian syndrome.
- Hyperglycemia is toxic to beta cells, and eventually their destruction causes insulin levels to drop below normal in untreated patients. Type 2 diabetes, therefore, eventually becomes a problem of insulin resistance as well as insulin production.

Differences Between Type 1 and Type 2 Diabetes

	DM Type 1	DM Type II
Age at onset	Usually childhood	Usually adults
Presentation at onset	Usually sudden	Gradual, insidious
DKA	Common	Uncommon
Genetics	Yes	Yes
Weight	Normal	Commonly obese
Treatment	Requires insulin	Oral &/or insulin
Insulin requirements	Typically low	Typically high

DM = Diabetes mellitus
DKA = Diabetic ketoacidosis
Source:

Complications of Type 1 and Type 2 Diabetes

- Hyperglycemia, insulin resistance, and increased free fatty acids cause abnormalities in the function of vascular smooth muscle, endothelium (vascular cells lining the lumen), and platelets.
- The molecular changes that occur result in impairment of vascular relaxation and induce a propensity for clotting.
- Both small (microvascular) and large (macrovascular) arteries are affected. The progression of atherosclerosis that occurs is the main cause of complications and death in patients with diabetes.

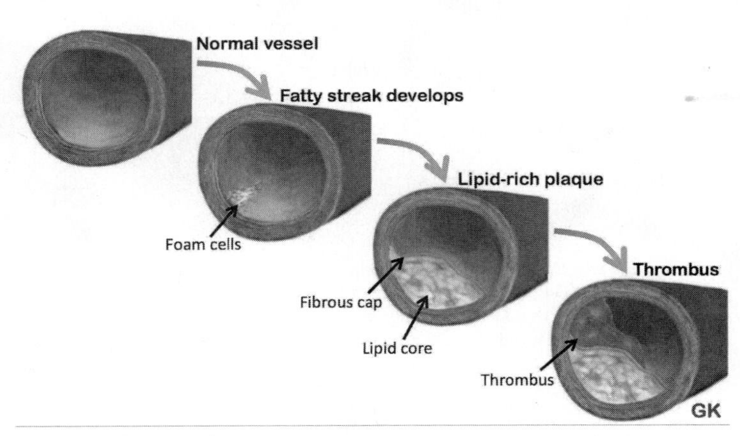

Diabetes is an especially significant secondary cause because patients tend to have an atherogenic combination of high triglycerides; high small, dense LDL fractions; and low HDLs (diabetic dyslipidemia, hypertriglyceridemic hyperapo B). Patients with type 2 diabetes are especially at risk. The combination may be a consequence of obesity and/or poor control of diabetes.

Source: Courtesy of George Kyriakidis/Santa Ana, CA

- Increased levels of stress are found in patients with diabetes (both types).
- The higher level of stress predisposes these patients to increased risk for infection, sepsis, and myocardial infarction.
- The result is the release of stress hormones (e.g., epinephrine, growth hormone, and cytokines), which have adverse effects on glucose levels, insulin production, and insulin sensitivity.
- Glucose control becomes more difficult under these circumstances.

Concept Check

2. **The nurse explains that coronary artery disease is associated with:**
   A. Primarily type 1 diabetes
   B. Primarily type 2 diabetes
   C. Both type 1 and type 2 diabetes
   D. Neither type 1 nor type 2 diabetes

Answer question

LO2:

Causes and Risk Factors

Type 1 Diabetes

- Family history of diabetes mellitus in a first-degree relative (parent or sibling)
- There are indications that certain genes may have increased risk.
- The farther from the equator a population lives, the greater the incidence of diabetes.
- Certain viruses (e.g., Epstein–Barr, mumps, Coxsackie) may initiate the destruction of pancreatic beta cells.
- Certain dietary factors may have influence:
  - o Excess nitrates in drinking water may increase risk.
  - o Omega-3 fatty acids may offer some protection.
  - o Low levels of vitamin D may increase risk.
  - o Preeclampsia or the mother's age being under 25 years may increase risk of diabetes in the baby.

Type 2 Diabetes

- Family history of diabetes mellitus in a first-degree relative.
- Ethnicity
  - o African Americans and Hispanics are at a much higher risk than Caucasians.
  - o Native Americans, Asian Americans, and Pacific Islanders are at a higher risk than Caucasians.
- History of gestational diabetes mellitus (develops during pregnancy)
- Metabolic syndrome—Insulin resistance, hypertension, dyslipidemia, and gout are often seen together. With one or more of these abnormalities, a patient is more likely to develop one or more of the remaining other traits (see photo).
- Previous hemoglobin A_{1c} greater than 5.7%, impaired glucose tolerance, or impaired fasting glucose
- Age of 45 years or more
- Obesity (body mass index of 25 kg/m^2 or higher)
- Abdominal obesity with a high waist–hip ratio
- Sedentary lifestyle
- Obstructive sleep apnea
- History of vascular disease
- Polycystic ovary syndrome

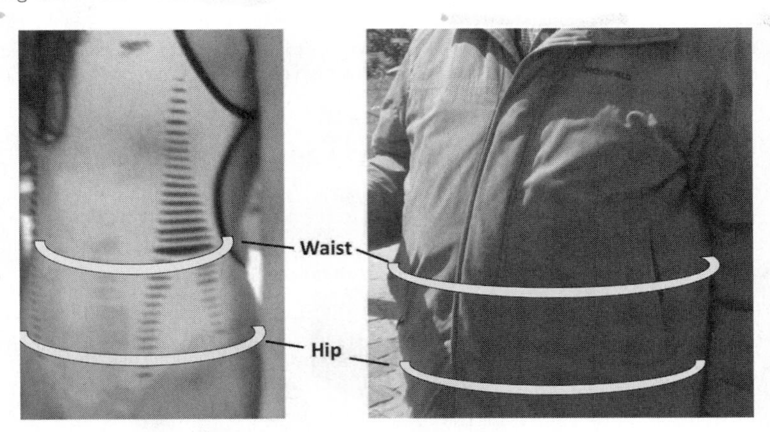

These photos compare the waist–hip measurement ratios. Left: The waist is measured at its narrowest point in a lean person, while the hips are measured at the widest point around the buttocks. Right: Measurement of an obese person with convex waist, it may be measured at about 1 inch above the navel. The hip is measured at its widest portion of the buttocks at left and at the great trochanters at right.

Source: Copyright © 2014, NovEx Novice to Expert Learning, LLC

LO2:

Assessment Findings: Type 1 and Type 2 Diabetes

Assessment findings related to hyperglycemia include:

- Polyuria and polydypsia due to osmotic diuresis
- Polyphagia (increased hunger)
- Weight loss
- Fatigue
- Blurred vision
- Changes in blood sugar levels cause fluid to move in or out of lenses of the eye, resulting in blurred vision.

Other symptoms related to complications of diabetes, such as:

- Foot numbness and pain due to neuropathy
- Visual loss due to retinopathy

Concept Check

3. The nurse would document polyphagia if the patient made which statement?

A. "I want to sleep all the time."

B. "I cannot get enough to eat."

C. "I urinate several times each day."

D. "I am always thirsty."

Answer question

LO2:

Diagnostics: Type 1 and Type 2 Diabetes

Glucose

- Glucose testing is usually performed by patients with a glucose meter. In the hospital, glucose can be quickly checked with point of care devices or be sent to the laboratory.
- Fasting plasma glucose (FPG) is defined as not eating for at least 8 hours.

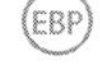

- The following table lists the criteria for diabetes (Handelsman, et al., 2011):

Results	Fasting Plasma Glucose
Normal	<100 mg/dL
Impaired	100 - 125 mg/dL
Diabetes	126 mg/dL **OR** random glucose ≥200mg/dL + symptoms

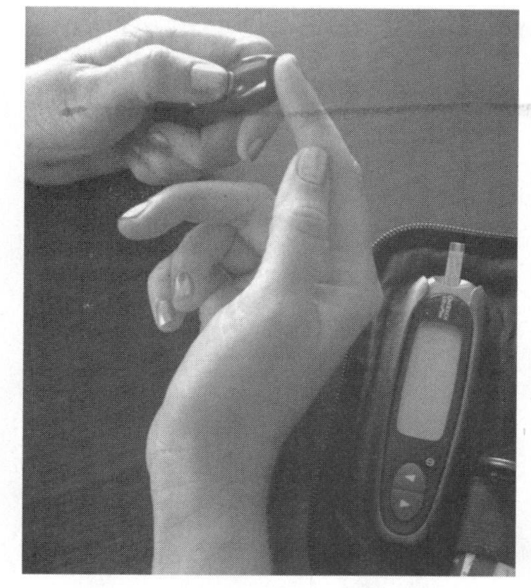

Caution: In some diabetics, blood glucose can dip dangerously low while sleeping. So, check blood glucose level at bedtime and upon waking. A snack before bed may help. For some, hormone fluctuations or dips in insulin levels may cause high readings in the morning. Regular monitoring is essential.

Glucose Tolerance

Oral glucose tolerance testing (OGTT) is primarily used for diagnosing diabetes. A standard dose (75 gm) of glucose is ingested, and two hours later, plasma glucose is measured.

- Two-hour plasma glucose values are shown in this table (Handelsman, et al., 2011):

Results	Oral Glucose Tolerance Test
Normal	<139 mg/dL
Impaired	140 - 199 mg/dL
Diabetes	≥200mg/dL

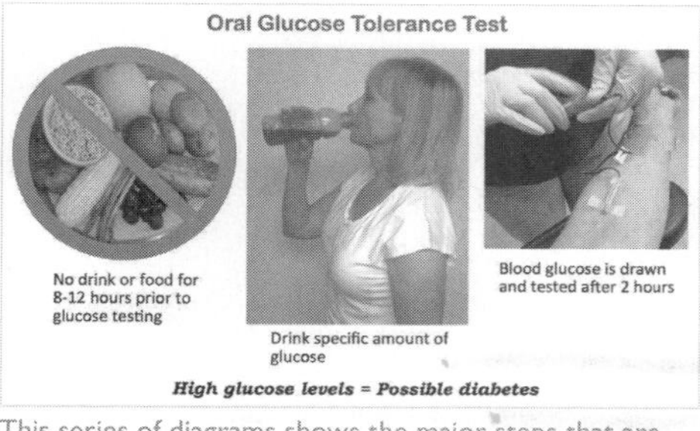

This series of diagrams shows the major steps that are required for patients in order to obtain an accurate oral glucose tolerance test. The NIH instructs patients to fast for 12 hours prior procedure. The patient drinks the glucose drink, and blood is tested two hours post-ingestion.

Hemoglobin A_{1c}

Hemoglobin A_{1c} (HbA_{1c}) levels reflect glucose levels over a period of 6–8 weeks. HbA_{1c} levels can be used to diagnose diabetes and guide therapy.

- Glucose binds to components of hemoglobin, including HbA_{1c}.
- HbA_{1c} levels reflect the serum glucose concentration over the life span of the RBCs. Higher levels reflect poorer glucose control.

Results	Hemoglobin A1C Tests
Normal	≤ 5.6%
Risk	5.7 – 6.0%
High Risk	6.0 - 6.5%
Diabetes	≥ 6.5%

- Target HbA_{1c} for diabetics is commonly ≤7.0. However, targets should be individualized.
- Lower targets decrease the likelihood of developing complications but increase the risk of hypoglycemia.

Diagnostics: Type 1 and Type 2 Diabetes (continued)

Urinalysis

- Urinalysis may show glucose when serum glucose is >180 mg/dL.
- Ketones on dipstick are an easy way to alert a patient about the onset of DKA.
- Protein /albumin is one of the earliest signs of diabetic nephropathy. Routine urine dipstick detects proteinuria of 300–500 mg/day.
- Urine WBCs (white blood cells), urine nitrite, and leukocyte esterase may indicate an infection, which can trigger worsening control of diabetes.

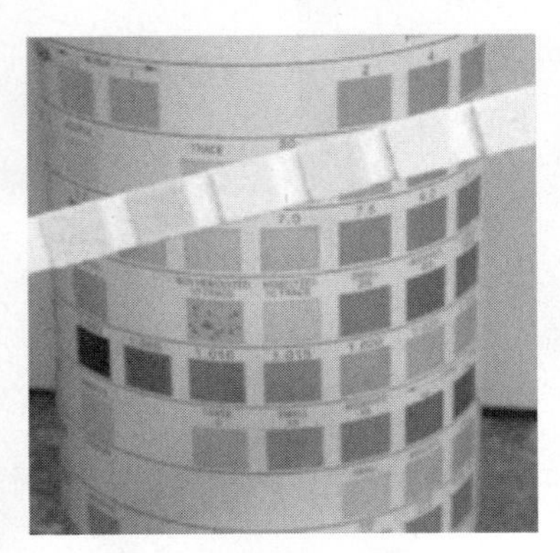

As part of many well visits, medical professionals typically perform a urine dipstick test, which can identify the existence and amounts of various elements in the body. Identifiable parameters include ions and metals, proteins and enzymes, blood cells, and various other parameters. Each section of a urine dipstick test reacts based on the existence and amount of the identified parameter.

Electrolytes

- Bicarbonate usually decreases in DKA.
- Serum creatinine may increase with diabetic nephropathy or dehydration (due to hyperglycemia).
- Other electrolyte abnormalities seen in diabetes can include hyperkalemia, hypokalemia, and hyponatremia. These may occur as a result of medications or kidney dysfunction.

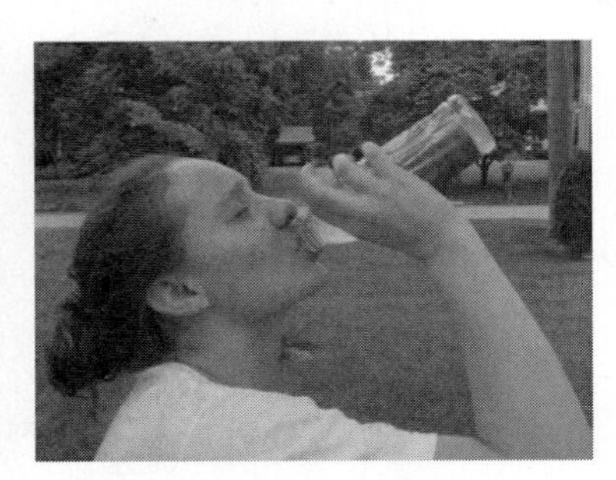

Electrolytes are crucial to the function of every cell in the body. This is why electrolytes are tightly regulated, and why the body expends considerable energy to maintain a constant balance between the various electrolytes. Under conditions where a disease such as diabetes upsets metabolic function, the body's electrolyte control system breaks down. Since the results of electrolyte imbalance can be severe, managing electrolytes is a major issue in diabetic care.

Concept Check

4. What does a hemoglobin A_{1C} of 6.3% indicate?

A. This is a normal level.

B. The patient is at risk for diabetes.

C. The patient is at a high risk for diabetes.

D. The patient is diabetic.

Answer question

Priority Patient Concerns and Desired Collaborative Care Outcomes

Prior to caring for patients with type 1 and type 2 diabetes mellitus, it is important to prioritize the patient's concerns that must guide the nursing care plan and interventions. Care for the patient is ordered and organized in accordance with the patient's priority and urgent needs. Desired collaborative care outcomes in patients with type 1 and type 2 diabetes mellitus typically include:

Diabetes Mellitus Type 1:

1. Patient will maintain HbA1c of <7% and blood glucose levels between 70–130 mg/dL (or per primary care provider recommendations).
2. Patient will remain infection-free.
3. Patient will make healthy dietary selections for meals.
4. Patient will demonstrate good glycemic control, risk factor identification, and improved nutritional and exercise management strategies for type 1 diabetes.

Diabetes Mellitus Type 2:

1. Patient will maintain blood glucose levels within prescribed range (typically 70–130 mg/dL).
2. Patient will state understanding of lifestyle choices and the association with type 2 diabetes.
3. Patient will collaborate with the health care team to determine ways to improve compliance with healthy lifestyle choices and prescribed medicine regimen.
4. Patient will demonstrate good sensory perception.
5. Patient will experience progressive reduction in fear and anger as coping with the medical diagnosis and lifestyle changes improve.

Considering these important care outcomes, prepare a list of the major 3–6 priority patient concerns or nursing diagnoses for patients with type 1 and type 2 diabetes mellitus. Be prepared to participate in a discussion of this list and/or to submit them as an assignment, as determined by your faculty. Resources you may find helpful in this assignment can include this lesson, the references, resources on nursing care plans, and standard nursing diagnoses manuals.

LO3:

Collaborative Interventions: Type 1 Diabetes

Goals in Diabetes Management

Clinical Practice Guidelines form the foundation for four goals of treatment in all diabetic patients (ADA, 2014; Handelsman, et al., 2011; Nathan, et al., 2009):

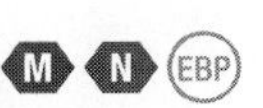

- Improving glycemic control is associated with decreased rates of complications including coronary artery disease, stroke, peripheral artery disease, retinopathy, nephropathy, and neuropathy. Intensive treatment has to be balanced with the risk of developing hypoglycemia. Glycemic control is achieved with:

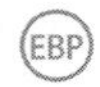

  - Weight loss and exercise: The American Diabetes Association (ADA) (2014) recommends 150 minutes per week of moderate exercise spread over 3 days of each week. Heart rate goal is 50–70% of maximum.
  - Pharmacologic therapy
    - Oral hypoglycemics (only in type 2 diabetics)
    - Insulin therapy

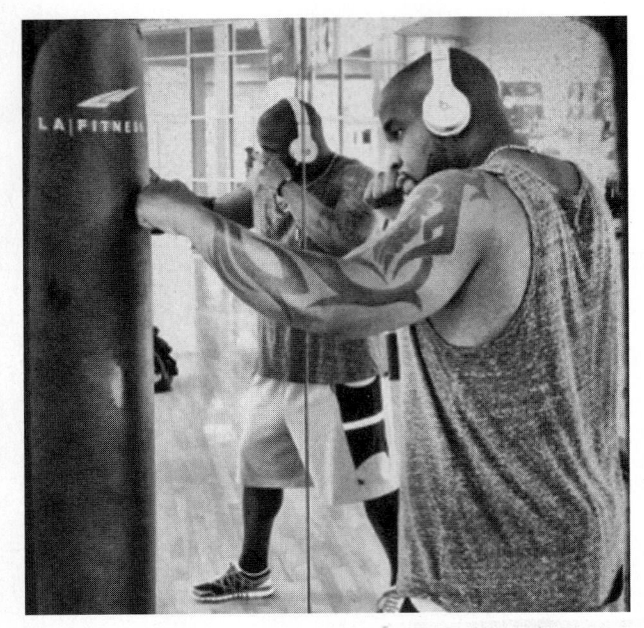

Exercise is safe—and highly recommended—for most people with type 2 diabetes, including those with complications. Along with diet and medication, exercise helps lower blood sugar and lose weight. However, the prospect of diving into a workout routine may be intimidating. Many newly diagnosed type 2 diabetics may not have exercised in years. If that's the case, start slow and work up.

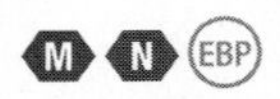

- Treating modifiable risk factors of atherosclerosis includes treatment of hypertension, dyslipidemia, smoking, obesity, and inactivity.

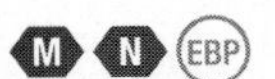

- Detection, prevention, and treatment of complications

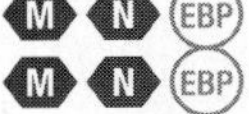

- Education of the family and patient on diabetes, preventing progression of the disease, and lifestyle changes.

LO3:

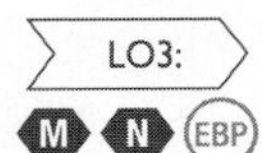

Collaborative Interventions: Type 2 Diabetes

This algorithm depicts the metabolic management of type 2 diabetes (Nathan, Buse, Davidson, et al., 2009). Check HbA_{1c} every 3 months until it is under 7% and then at least every 6 months. Interventions should be changed if HbA_{1c} is 7% or more. Except for glibenclamide (glyburide) or chlorpropamide (due to concerns regarding their safety), sulfonylureas can be used.

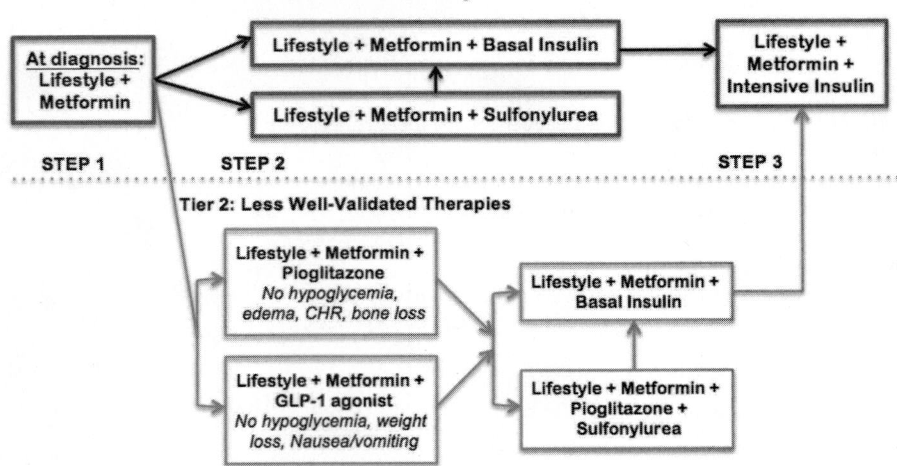

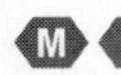 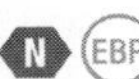

Oral Hypoglycemics

First-line medications

- Metformin decreases production of glucose by the liver.
- Sulfonylureas enhance insulin secretion by the pancreas.

Second-line medications

- Meglitinides stimulate insulin secretion.
- Thiazolidinediones increase the sensitivity of insulin receptors to insulin.
- DPP-IV inhibitors stimulate insulin secretion and inhibit glucagon secretion.
- Glucagon-like peptide agonists stimulate insulin production by the pancreas.
- Alpha-glucosidase inhibitors reduce the rate of digestion of complex sugars.

 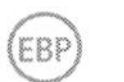 

Insulin

Initiation and adjustment of insulin regimens:

- Insulin regimens should be designed to take lifestyle and meal schedule into account. The algorithm can only provide basic guidelines for initiation and adjustment of insulin.
- Premixed insulins are not recommended during adjustment of doses; however, they can be used conveniently, usually before breakfast and/or dinner, if proportion of rapid- and intermediate-acting insulin is similar to the fixed proportions available.
- Treatment options for type 1 diabetes are presented in the animation.*

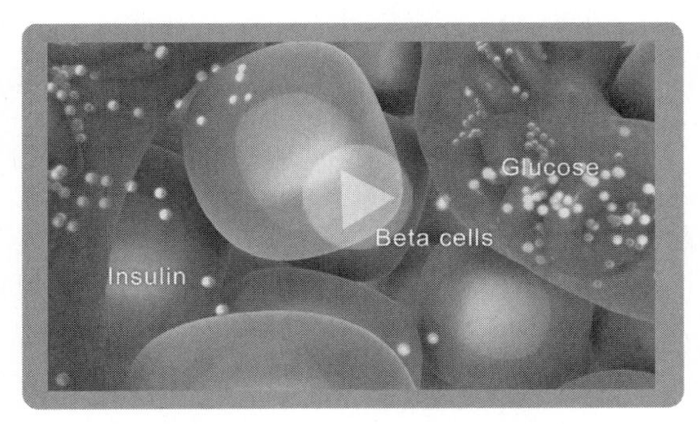

This animation explains the pathophysiology, causes, symptoms and treatment of type 1 diabetes. The condition of hyperglycemia is discussed as well as the goal of achieving a normal range. Treatment combinations of insulin replacement, blood glucose monitoring, a healthy diet, and exercise are explained.

*www.ncbi.nlm.nih.gov/pmc/articles/PMC2606813/.

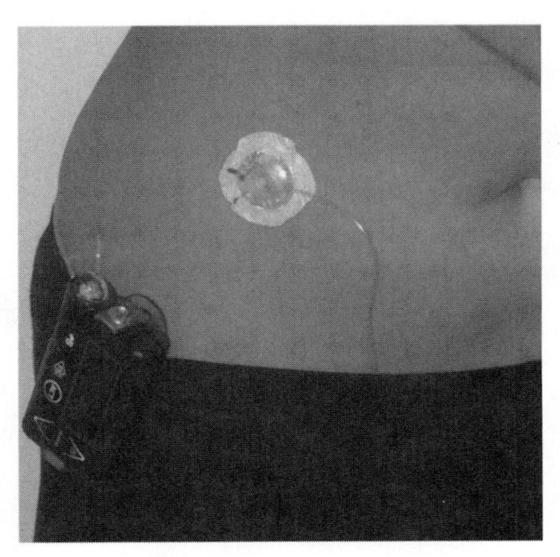

Insulin pumps are commonly used devices for controlling glucose levels in patients with type 1 diabetes.

Collaborative Interventions: Type 2 Diabetes (continued)

Complications

Management of diabetic complications has three key components:

- Prevention
- Screening: recognition of the complications early
- Treatment of the complication

The following section discusses the evidence-based practice recommendations by the American Diabetes Association, 2014; Handelsman, et al., 2011; Nathan, et al., 2009; and NICE, 2012.

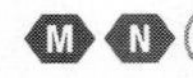

Atherosclerosis

Atherosclerotic diseases (CAD, PVD, stroke) are the leading cause of death in patients with diabetes mellitus.

Screening

Patients should be asked routinely about chest pain, shortness of breath with exertion, and symptoms of claudication. Patients with symptoms should be tested appropriately (e.g., stress test for chest pains).

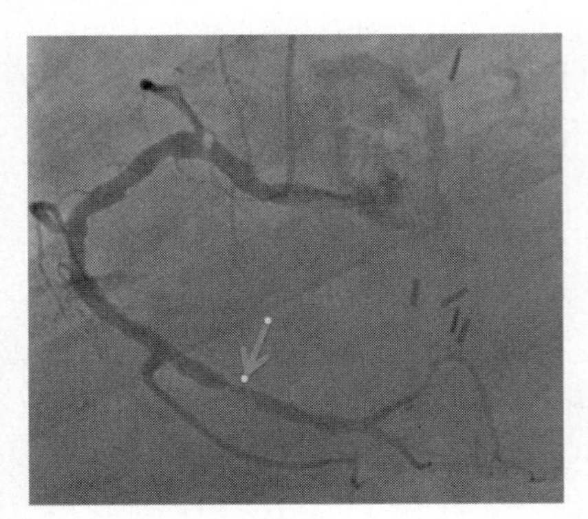

The narrowing of the silhouette of the right coronary artery (arrow) indicates an atherosclerotic lesion that has almost occluded the artery.
Source: Courtesy of K. Kyriakidis

Prevention

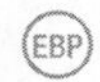

The American Association of Clinical Endocrinologists (Jellinger, et al., 2012) recommend the following evidence-based interventions to prevent or delay progression of atherosclerosis, which exacerbates diabetes:

- Glycemic control is essential.
- Lifestyle interventions include a healthy weight, exercise, and a heart-healthy diet. Moderate exercise for 150 minutes per week (heart rate goal of 50–70% of maximum) spread over 3 days of each week is recommended.
- Smoking cessation
- Treatment of hypertension includes goals of systolic BP <130 mmHg and diastolic BP <80 mmHg.
- Dyslipidemia treatment goals with aggressive lipid-modifying pharmacologic therapy for patients with diabetes and without apparent coronary artery disease include LDL of <100 mg/dL; patients with diabetes and/or with coronary artery disease should aim for LDL of <70 mg/dL (Brunzell, et al., 2008).
- Antiplatelet therapy (e.g., aspirin) in diabetic patients with high cardiovascular disease risk.

Treatment

Treatment of atherosclerotic diseases (e.g., coronary artery disease, peripheral vascular disease, and stroke) are complex. Patients should be started on aspirin or an antiplatelet agent.

Concept Check

5. What is the goal for systolic blood pressure in patients who have diabetes?
   A. <110 mmHg
   B. <120 mmHg
   C. <130 mmHg
   D. <140 mmHg

Answer question

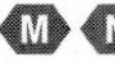 

Neuropathy

Damage to the nerves commonly occurs in people with diabetes. Damage can involve the peripheral nerves or the autonomic nerves.

- Peripheral neuropathy usually affects the feet first and is associated with pain and loss of sensation. Patients often describe the pain as a burning pain that is worse at night. Another common description is, "I feel like I'm walking with gravel in my shoes."
- When the autonomic system is affected, blood pressure may drop when standing suddenly. Involvement of the autonomic system may also cause gastrointestinal motility problems. Patients may have diarrhea and/or constipation. The stomach may empty slowly (gastroparesis), resulting in nausea, vomiting, and early satiety.

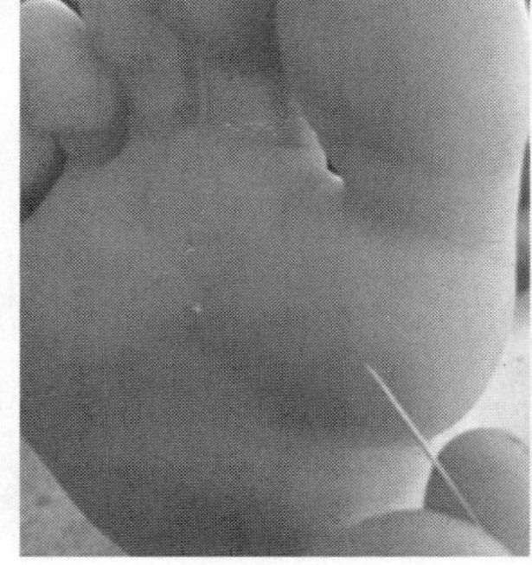
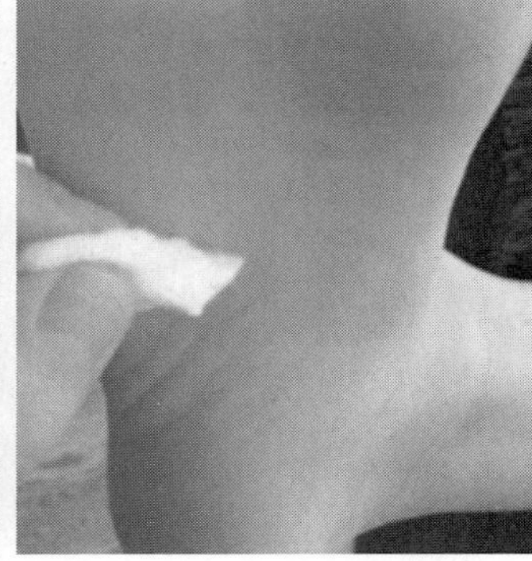

Although these are useful and time-honored techniques, the way that health care providers test sensation with a pin prick or cotton wool varies slightly. It is, therefore, difficult to have meaningful results when they are not standardized.

Screening

Patients should be queried about foot pain, foot numbness, and early satiety. Screening should take place yearly and can be done by checking with a pinprick, cotton wool, or tuning fork.

Prevention

Neuropathy prevention is mostly related to tight glycemic control.

Treatment

Pain is treated with various drugs, including tricyclics, antidepressants, gabapentin, and narcotics. Tricyclics and gabapentin usually do not offer immediate relief. This group of medications need to be taken over a period of time and on a regular basis to control pain.

  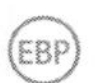

Diabetic Foot Problems

- Poor glucose control contributes to immune system dysfunction, increased incidence of infections, and slow wound healing. This is exacerbated by poor tissue perfusion from peripheral vascular disease.
- When patients develop foot infections, they often do not notice it early because of their lack of sensation due to neuropathy. The combination of lost sensation, a propensity for infections, poor perfusion, slow wound healing, and poor eyesight can be disastrous and may lead to amputation, sepsis, and death.
- Chronic leg ulcers from peripheral arterial disease and venous insufficiency, cellulitis, osteomyelitis, and gangrene are common problems.

Screening

During clinic visits or at hospital admission, the feet should always be examined thoroughly.

Prevention

Proper foot care that includes frequent foot checks, wearing well-fitting shoes, and proper nail care are essential.

Treatment

Infections are treated with antibiotics and debridement (if necessary). Revascularization can be required for severe peripheral vascular disease.

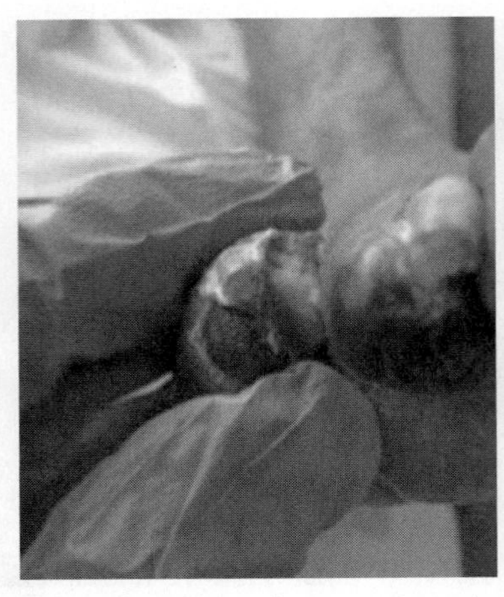
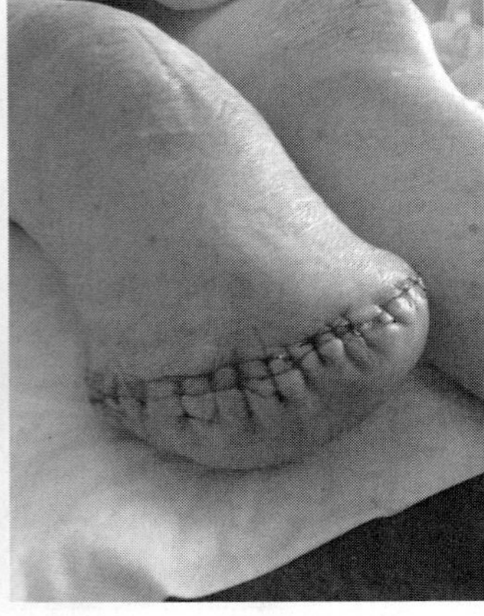

Diabetic foot ulcer involving several toes that has worsened to the point of necrosis and gangrene (left). The infection is extensive, involves the underlying bone and required amputation (right).
Sources: *(left)* Courtesy of R. Murphy; *(right)* Courtesy of K. Kyriakidis

Concept Check

6. Tight glycemic control helps to prevent the need for amputation in patients with diabetes by:

A. Decreasing immune response to pathogens

B. Encouraging shunting of blood to major organs

C. Promoting wound healing

D. Decreasing sensation to vulnerable areas

Answer question

Collaborative Interventions: Type 2 Diabetes (continued)

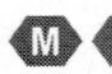

Nephropathy

Damage to the kidneys usually occurs over years and can progress to end stage renal disease.

Screening

- Urine albumin protein. Annual testing is recommended by the ADA. Leakage of urine protein is one of the earliest signs of diabetic nephropathy.
- Serum creatinine. Annual testing is recommended by the ADA.

Prevention

- Treat hypertension. Goals: systolic BP <130 mmHg and diastolic BP <80 mmHg
- Glycemic control

Treatment

ACE inhibitors, ARBs*, and some calcium channel blockers (e.g., verapamil, diltiazem) can reduce proteinuria.

*Angiotensin II receptor blockers

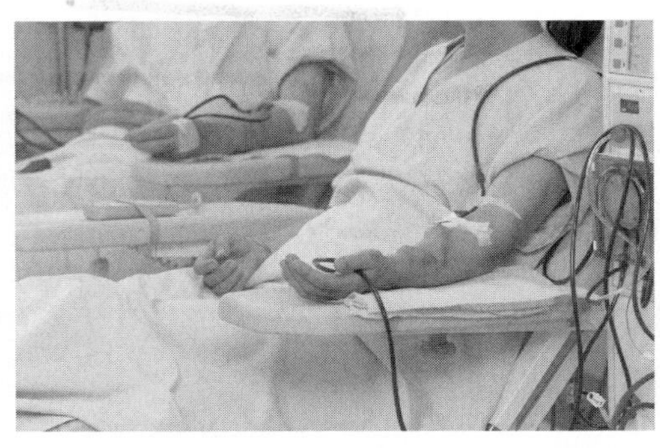

Kidney dialysis is very hard on the veins of the patient. Most patients need a shunt: a blood vessel especially strengthened to withstand the repeated connections to the dialysis machine. When the patient doesn't have an appropriate blood vessel, a plastic material is used. These plastic shunts do not last long, frequently becoming infected and inflamed.
Source: Picsfive/Shutterstock

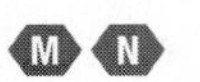
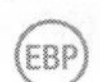

Diabetic Retinopathy

Diabetic retinopathy is one of the leading causes of blindness in the United States. Damage to the retina consists of:

- Macular edema, resulting from thickening of the macula from protein leakage
- Proliferation of blood vessels of the retina
- Hemorrhage and leakage of proteins
- Diabetic cataracts

Screening

A retinal eye exam on diagnosis of type 2 diabetes (within 5 years of diagnosis of type 1 diabetes) and every three years afterward if the exam is normal

Prevention

Glycemic control can prevent progression of diabetes and its harmful effects.

Treatment

- Laser photocoagulation for macular edema and hyperproliferative retinopathy
- Cataract surgery

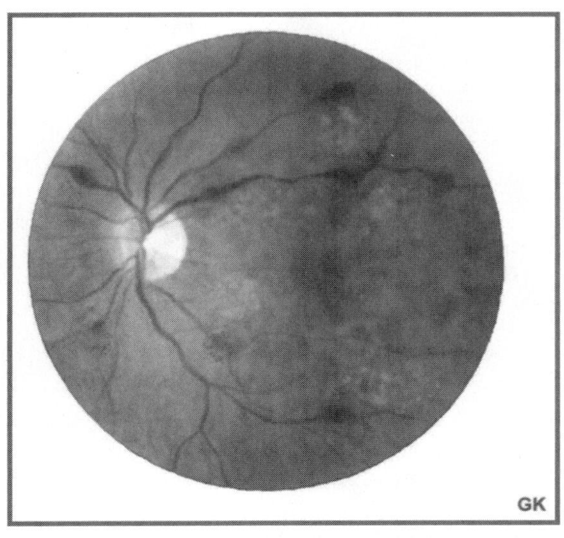

Red areas represent hemorrhages and the scattered yellowish areas are due to protein leakage. The optic nerve can be seen as the bright white spot to the lower left of center. The blood vessels are thickened.
Source: Courtesy of George Kyriakidis/Santa Ana, CA

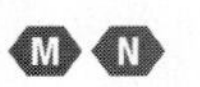

Male Erectile Dysfunction

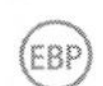

Male erectile dysfunction (ED) is the inability to achieve a penile erection and sustain it for sexual performance. Men with diabetes are commonly affected with ED 10–15 years sooner than nondiabetic men. This diabetic complication is often associated with poorly controlled hypertension, poor glucose control, unhealthy diet, obesity, and heavy tobacco use.

Screening

- During physical exams inquire about any problems with sexual performance.
- If ED is present, determine whether ED is organic or functional.

Prevention

- Glycemic control
- Manage hypertension to achieve goals: systolic BP <130 mmHg; diastolic BP <80 mmHg
- Regular exercise with weight management
- Healthy diabetic diet
- Smoking and substance abuse cessation
- Prevent other diabetic complications that lead to ED (e.g., neuropathy, atherosclerosis).

Treatment

Can include medication, penile injections, vacuum devices that aid achieving erection, prosthetic devices, or intraurethral suppositories.

Collaborative Interventions: Type 2 Diabetes (continued)

Emergencies (DKA and Hyperosmolar Coma)

Treatment of DKA and hyperosmolar coma require in-depth discussion of pathophysiology and care. Refer to the NovE-lesson on Diabetic Ketoacidosis and Hyperosmolar Hyperglycemic Crisis.

Patient Education

Educate patient and family about:

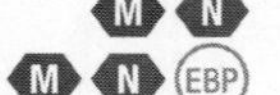

- Key evidence-based educational factors that help control diabetes and prevent the development of complications (ADA, 2014; Handelsman, et al., 2011; Nathan, et al., 2009; and NICE, 2012):
  - o Healthy diabetic-specific diet and counting carbs
  - o Regular exercise
  - o Proper use of prescribed medications*
  - o Blood glucose monitoring

*Please refer to the animation in the Collaborative Intervention: Insulin section.

- Seeking effective ways of coping with emotional stress, anxiety, and fear. Adverse effects of increased stress:
  - o Increases the risk of infection, sepsis, and myocardial infarction
  - o Impacts glucose levels, insulin production, and insulin sensitivity
  - o Makes glucose control more difficult

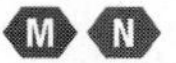
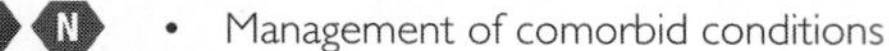

- Management of comorbid conditions

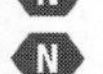

- Safety of wearing a medical alert

- Pneumonia and influenza vaccinations

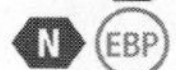

- Smoking cessation

- Ample patient education resources via the Centers for Disease Control and Prevention, National Institutes of Health, and national diabetes organizations

Begin education with your patient, but consult the diabetic educator or nurse specialist whenever possible.

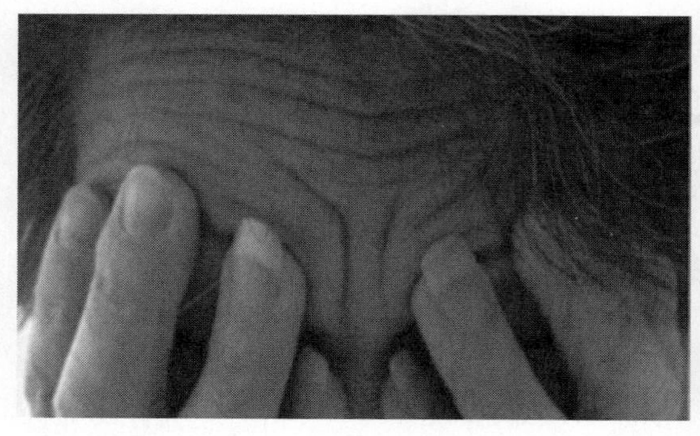

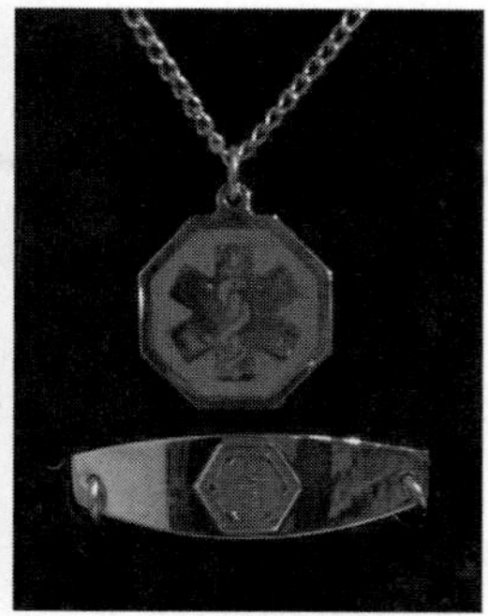

Left: Stress has adverse effects on the body, particularly in those with diabetes. Controlling stress or one's responses to stress can lower the risk of diabetes related problems and complications. Right: Wearing a medical alert bracelet or necklace can be life-saving to warn a rescuer of a life-threatening condition.
Source: *(both)* Copyright © 2014, NovEx Novice to Expert Learning, LLC

Overview of Diabetes Care

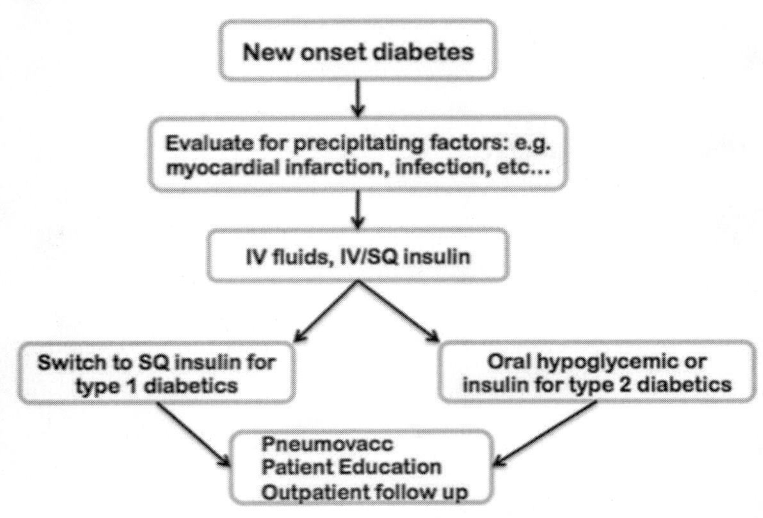

Summary of Interventions: Type 1 and Type 2 Diabetes

- Treatment of hyperglycemia includes:
  - Weight loss and exercise. The American Diabetes Association recommends 150 min/week of moderate exercise (heart rate goal is 50–70% of maximum) spread over 3 days of a week.
  - Pharmacologic therapy
    - Oral hypoglycemics (only in type 2 diabetics)
    - Insulin therapy is required for type 1 diabetics
- Treating modifiable risk factors of atherosclerosis includes treatment for hypertension, dyslipidemia, smoking, obesity, substance abuse, and inactivity.
- Detection, prevention, and treatment of complications—such as atherosclerosis, neuropathy, diabetic foot problems (including infections), retinopathy, erectile dysfunction, and DKA—are key to overall management.
- Education of the family and patient is essential for health maintenance.

Concept Check

7. The nurse identifies which effect of stress?

A. Decreases blood glucose

B. Decreases risk for sepsis

C. Increases risk for kidney stones

D. Changes insulin sensitivity

Answer question

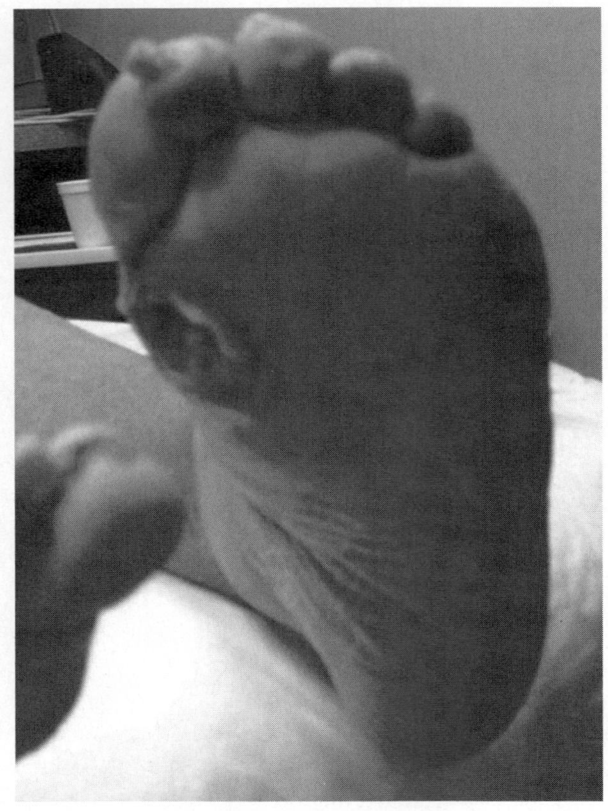

Detecting early warning signs of diabetic foot ulcers is critical for patients to prevent significant, slow-healing, and debilitating ulcers, as seen in this photo.
Source: Courtesy of K. Kyriakidis

LO4:

Evaluation of Desired Collaborative Care Outcomes

Evaluation and reassessment should reveal attainment of previously established patient outcomes. In summary:

Diabetes Mellitus Type 1:

- Patient's fasting and postprandial blood glucose measurements and hemoglobin A_{1c} levels are within the ranges expected.
- Patient is infection-free.
- Patient makes healthy dietary selections for meals.
- Patient is using knowledge to monitor and manage blood glucose, identify and understand risk factor modifications, improve nutritional intake, and begin exercise regimen.

Diabetes Mellitus Type 2:

- Patient's blood glucose levels are consistently within the prescribed range.
- Patient demonstrates healthy lifestyle changes.
- Patient reports improved compliance with lifestyle changes and taking medications as directed.
- Patient is not experiencing further, if any, diabetes-related changes in eyes, renal function, or peripheral blood flow.
- Patient discusses openly and without reservation the diagnosis and how she or he is coping.

References

2011 National Diabetes Fact Sheet. **www.cdc.gov/diabetes/pubs/pdf/ndfs_2011.pdf**

Aalaa, M., Malazy, O. T., Sanjari, M., et al. (2012). Nurses' role in diabetic foot prevention and care: A review. *J Diabetes & Metab Disorders, 11*, 24. doi: 10.1186/2251-6581-11-24.

American Diabetes Association. (2013). Standards of medical care in diabetes—2013. *Diabetes Care, 36*(Suppl 1), S11–S66. **http://care.diabetesjournals.org/content/36/Supplement_1/S11.full**

Brunzell, J. D., Davidson, M., Furberg, C. D., et al; American Diabetes Association; American College of Cardiology Foundation. (2008). Lipoprotein management in patients with cardiometabolic risk: consensus statement from the American Diabetes Association and the American College of Cardiology Foundation. *Diabetes Care, 31*, 811–822.

Creager, M. A., Lüscher, T. F., Cosentino, F., & Beckman, J. A. (2003). Review: Clinical cardiology: New frontiers diabetes and vascular disease, pathophysiology, clinical consequences, and medical therapy: Part I. *Circulation, 108*, 1527–1532.

Jellinger, P. S., Smith, D. A., Mehta, A. E., et al; AACE Task Force for Management of Dyslipidemia and Prevention of Atherosclerosis. (2012). American Association of Clinical Endocrinologists' guidelines for management of dyslipidemia and prevention of atherosclerosis. *Endo Practice, 18*(Suppl 1), 1–78. **www.aace.com/files/lipid-guidelines.pdf**

Kitabchi, A. E., Umpierrez, G. E., Miles, J. M, & Fisher, J. N. (2009). Hyperglycemic crisis in diabetes: Consensus statement by the American Diabetes Association. *Diabetes Care, 32*(7), 1335–1343. **http://care.diabetesjournals.org/content/32/7/1335.full.pdf+html**

Paterson, B. L., Thorne, S., & Dewis, M. (2007). Adapting to and managing diabetes. *J Nurs Scholarship*. doi: 10:1111/j.1547-5069.1998.tb01237.x

Clinical Practice Guidelines

American Diabetes Association. (2014). Executive summary: Standards of medical care in diabetes—2014. *Diabetes Care, 37*(Suppl 1), S5–S13. doi: 10.2337/dc14-S005

Handelsman, Y., Mechanick, J. I., Blonde, L., et al. (2011). American Association of Clinical Endocrinologists medical guidelines for clinical practices for developing a diabetes mellitus comprehensive care plan. *Endo Practice, 17*(Suppl 2), 1–53. **www.aace.com/files/dm-guidelines-ccp.pdf**

Nathan, D. M., Buse, J. B., Davidson, M. B., et al. (2009). Medical management of hyperglycemia in type 2 diabetes: A consensus algorithm for the initiation and adjustment of therapy. *Diabetes Care, 32*(1), 193–203. doi: 10:2337/dc08-9025

National Institute for Health and Clinical Excellence. (2012). Preventing type 2 diabetes—risk identification and interventions for individuals at high risk (PH38). London: NICE. **http://guidance.nice.org.uk/PH38**

Riethof, M., Flavin, P. L., Lindvall, B., et al., & Institute for Clinical Systems Improvement (ICSI). (2012). *Diagnosis and management of type 2 diabetes mellitus in adults*. Bloomington, MN: Institute for Clinical Systems Improvement. **www.guideline.gov/content.aspx?id=36905&search=diabetes**

Patient Education

American Association of Diabetes Educators. (2010). *Guidelines for the practice of diabetes education*. Chicago, IL: American Association of Diabetes Educators. **www.guideline.gov/content.aspx?id=24594&search=diabetes+mellitus**

Diabetes Care and Education: Patient Education Materials. **Dce.org/publications/education-handouts/**

Diabetes: Cleveland Clinic Health Information. **my.clevelandclinic.org/disorders/diabetes/endo_education.aspx**

Learning Outcomes for Hyperglycemic Crisis

When you complete this lesson, you will be able to:

1. Recognize the clinical relevance of hyperglycemic crisis.
2. Consider the pathophysiology, etiology, risk factors, and clinical presentation of hyperglycemic crisis that determine the priority patient concerns.
3. Determine the most urgent and important nursing interventions and patient education required in caring for a patient with hyperglycemic crisis.
4. Evaluate attainment of desired collaborative care outcomes for a patient with hyperglycemic crisis.

LO1:

What Is Hyperglycemic Crisis?

- Diabetic ketoacidosis (DKA) and hyperglycemic hyperosmolar state (HHS) are two conditions that are potentially life-threatening emergencies.
- Diabetic ketoacidosis is more common in type 1 diabetics. It is a combination of hyperglycemia, acidosis, and ketosis. DKA usually occurs in the setting of lack of insulin, which results in fatty acids being metabolized rather than glucose, and associated production of ketones.
- Hyperosmolar hyperglycemia occurs when blood sugar is >600 mg/dL (normal is <100 mg/dL) without evidence of ketoacidosis. It is a combination of hyperglycemia and hyperosmolarity with altered mental status. HHS is more common in type 2 diabetics.

LO1:

Clinical Relevance

DKA and HHS are **medical emergencies** that require prompt recognition and treatment with insulin and IV fluids.

- These conditions are often precipitated by other stressful or critical medical illnesses such as infection or myocardial infarction.
- Early recognition can be life saving.

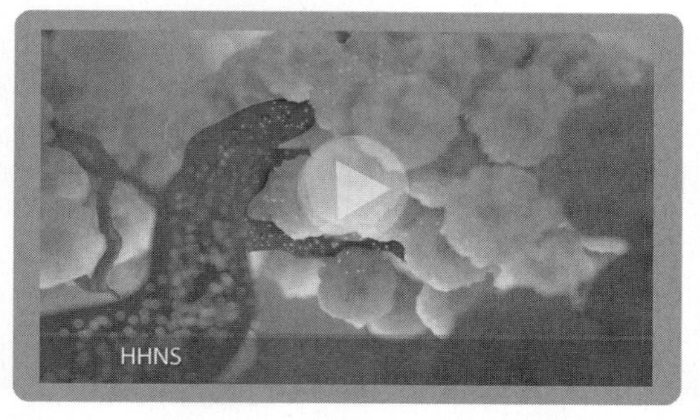

This animation explains the results of insulin resistance and its effect on the body. The buildup of glucose in the bloodstream results in a condition known as hyperglycemia and DKA.

Concept Check

1. Which patient is at the highest risk for development of HHS?
   A. 23-year-old patient with diabetes type 1
   B. 52-year-old patient with diabetes type 1
   C. 48-year-old patient with diabetes type 2
   D. A patient not diagnosed with either type of diabetes

Answer question

LO2:

Pathophysiology

Ketoacidosis

Hyperglycemic crisis usually occurs in the setting of an increase in counterregulatory hormones (e.g., cortisol, glucagon, growth hormone) and/or lack of insulin. Lack of insulin may be a result of noncompliance. An increase of counterregulatory hormones usually occurs during a stressful or critical medical illness (e.g., infection myocardial infarction). The lack of insulin and/or increase of counterregulatory hormones can have two major effects (see schematic).

- **Glycogenolysis.** Production of glucose (gluconeogenesis) by the liver is stimulated causing hyperglycemia.
- **Ketogenesis.** In DKA, metabolism shifts from carbohydrate to fat metabolism, similar to fasting states. Breakdown of stored fats into fatty acids and glycerol is an alternative source of energy. Fatty acids are then metabolized into ketoacids by the liver but produce a metabolic acidosis. The degree of acidosis depends on the rate of ketone production and excretion.

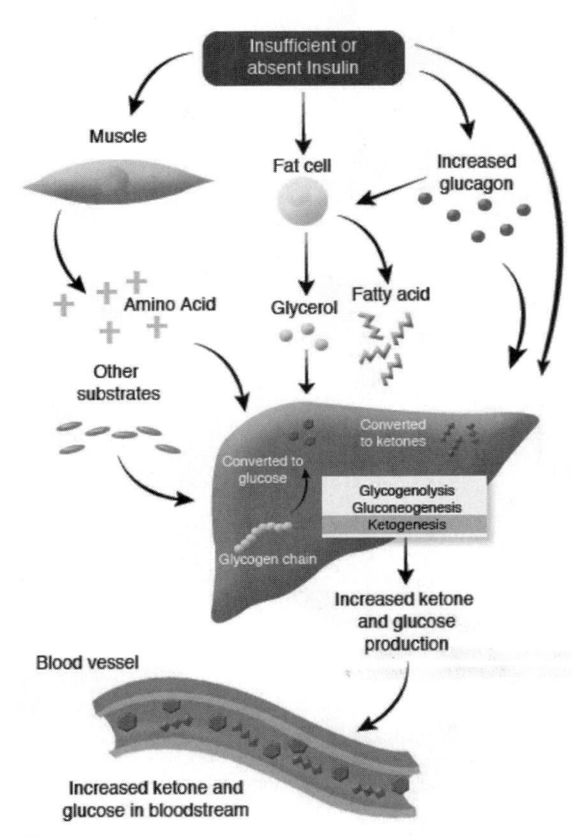

Diabetic ketoacidosis.

Pathophysiology (continued)

Effects of Hyperglycemia

- In hyperglycemia, the nephrons are unable to reabsorb all the glucose that was filtered.
- The unreabsorbed glucose draws potassium, sodium, and water into the tubules, and these are excreted in the urine. An osmotic diuresis occurs.
- This results in dehydration with loss of potassium and sodium.
- If the patient fails to drink due to low thirst or has limited volume replacement, hyperosmolarity develops along with hyperglycemia and mental changes (HHS).
- Although osmotic diuresis occurs with both DKA and HHS, the loss of intravascular volume is much more profound with HHS (approximately 9 L).

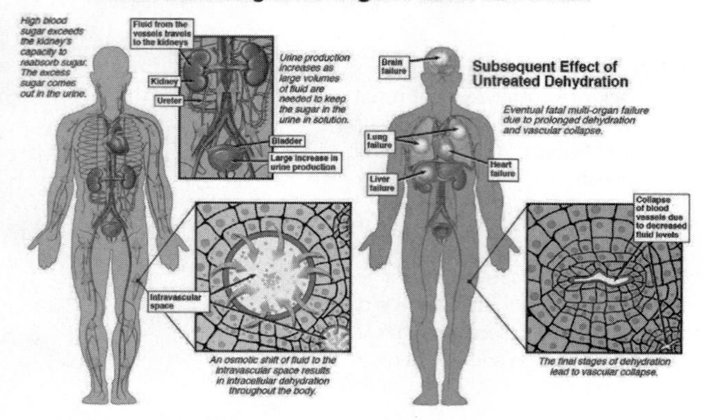

Failure to diagnose and treat nonketotic hyperglycemia with resulting multiorgan failure and death.

Basic Pathophysiology of Hyperglycemic Crises

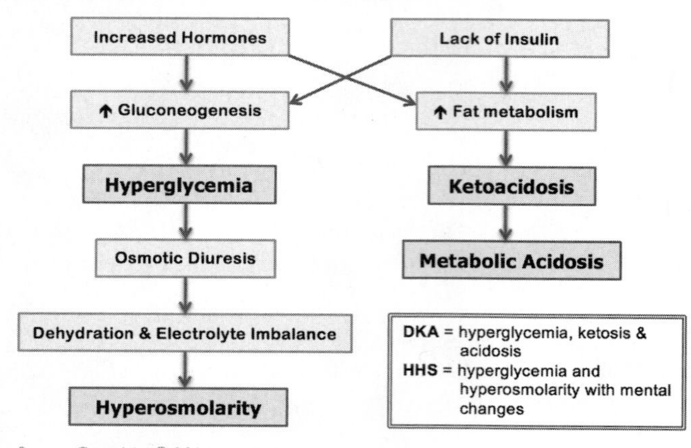

Effects on Potassium

- Even though potassium is lost with osmotic diuresis, serum potassium levels are usually normal to high. The serum potassium remains normal because the lack of insulin and metabolic acidosis (in DKA) shifts potassium out of cells and into the blood. However, the overall body potassium level is low.
- Once insulin treatment is initiated, serum potassium levels can drop precipitously (hypokalemia) because insulin causes a shift of potassium back into the cells. Further, correction of metabolic acidosis (in DKA) causes movement of potassium back into the cells, resulting in hypokalemia.
- When the needed fluids are replaced, the serum electrolytes are further diluted.

Causes

LO2:

DKA and HHS

- Most common: urinary tract infection, pneumonia, gastroenteritis
- Noncompliance with medication
- Acute medical illness
    - o Infection
    - o Myocardial infarction
    - o Pulmonary embolus
    - o Hepatic failure
    - o Renal failure
    - o Sepsis

Additional HHS

- Dehydration:
  - o Due to an illness that prevents adequate hydration or fluid intake
  - o Due to an illness that causes dehydration (vomiting, diarrhea)
- Substances that cause hyperglycemia or dehydration, or inhibit insulin (e.g., diuretics, beta blockers, calcium channel blockers, alcohol, cocaine)
- Noncompliance with oral hypoglycemic medications or insulin therapy

Concept Check

2. What is a common cause of HHS?

   A. Taking too much hypoglycemic medication

   B. Increased glucose intake

   C. Illness

   D. Drinking too much water

Answer question

LO2:

Assessment Findings

DKA

- Fatigue and weakness
- Polyuria, polydipsia
- Weight loss
- Nausea, vomiting
- Abdominal pain
- Fatigue
- Vital signs:
  - o Hyperventilation due to acidosis (Kussmaul)
  - o Hypotension
  - o Tachycardia due to dehydration
- Altered mental status
- Breath smells like acetone (nail polish remover)
- Decreased skin turgor
- Dry mucous membranes
- Evidence of skin infections
- Cardiac effects:
  - o Myocardial contractility is depressed.
  - o Arterial vasodilation
  - o Resistance to the effects of catecholamines (vasopressors may have a diminished effect)
  - o Vasoconstriction of pulmonary arteries

HHS

- Fatigue and weakness
- Polyuria, polydipsia
- Weight loss
- Vital signs:
  - o Tachycardia
  - o Hypotension
  - o Cardiovascular collapse, if hypotension is severe
- Hypothermia: poor prognostic factor
- Altered mental status
  - o Typically worse than in patients with DKA.
  - o Coma occurs in 20% of patients with HHS.
- Seizures
- Poor skin turgor
- Dry mucous membranes
- Renal failure

Common Characteristics of DKA vs. HHS

DKA	HHS
Typically younger patients	Typically older patients
Type 1 diabetes	Type 2 diabetes
Often undiagnosed diabetes	Uncontrolled diabetes for weeks
Develops rapidly (usually < 24 hours)	Develops over days.
Nausea, vomiting, abdominal pain	Usually no nausea, vomiting or abdominal pain
Hyperglycemia	Hyperglycemia, often over 600 mg/dL
Volume depletion, dehydration, polydipsia, polyuria	Volume depletion, dehydration, polyuria, hypotension, cardiovascular collapse
Altered mental status, lethargy, coma	Altered mental status, lethargy, coma, seizures
Underlying illness: infection, infarction, drugs (alcohol/cocaine), organ failure	Underlying illness: sepsis, stroke, MI, medication (diuretics, corticosteroids)
Kussmaul breathing – ketotic/acidotic breathing	No ketosis/acidotic breathing

LO2:

Diagnostics

*Note that "normal" lab values may vary from one reference to another. Many lab values are ranges rather than exact numbers. Recognizing meaningful abnormal values and following the patient's trend are the key points in "monitoring lab values."

DKA

- Hyperglycemia
  - o Blood glucose typically >250 mg/dL
- Ketosis
  - o Positive urine and plasma ketones
  - o Increased anion gap
- Dehydration
  - o Volume depletion: increased BUN/Cr ratio
  - o Increased creatinine (Cr)
- Acidosis
  - o Arterial pH ≤7.3
  - o Decreased bicarbonate level
- Electrolyte abnormalities (e.g., potassium, sodium, magnesium)

HHS

- Hyperglycemia
  - o Blood glucose level ≥600 mg/dL
  - o Often 800 or more to 1000 mg/dL
- No ketosis
  - o Absent-to-no ketones produced, so no acidosis present
  - o Anion gap normal
- Profound dehydration
  - o Serum osmolality ≥320 mOsm/kg
  - o Increased BUN/Cr ratio
  - o Increased creatinine
- No acidosis
  - o Serum pH >7.30
  - o Serum bicarbonate >18 mEq/L
  - o Anion gap normal
- Electrolyte abnormalities (e.g., potassium, sodium, magnesium)

Anion Gap

Positive ions − negative ions = anion gap OR
Sodium − [chloride + carbon dioxide (or bicarb)] = anion gap

- Example: 141 (sodium) − [116 (chloride) − 5 (carbon dioxide)] = anion gap of 20.

	2:39	4:25	6:25
Sodium			141
Potassium			5.6 H
Chloride			116 H
Carbon Dioxide			< 5 *L
BUN			14
Creatinine			0.77
Estimated GFR			>60
Glucose			298 H
Bedside Glucose	352 H	363 H	
Calcium			8.6
Troponin I			<0.1

- Average anion gap for a healthy adult is 8–12.
- The anion gap is nonspecific. It is increased when the number of unmeasured anions increases.
- The underlying condition must be identified and treated.
- Common causes of anion gap: lactic acidosis, ketoacidosis, presence of toxic substances such as aspirin or methanol

Concept Check

3. Which respiratory finding is common in DKA?
   A. Biot's
   B. Agonal
   C. Kussmaul's
   D. Eupneic

Answer question

Concept Check

4. Which arterial blood gas reading is expected in a patient diagnosed with HHS?
   A. 7.32
   B. 7.45
   C. 7.25
   D. 7.23

Answer question

Diagnostics (continued)

Labs:

- CBC: Leukocytosis may be present due to DKA or underlying infection.
- Complete metabolic panel (CMP): Serum sodium level usually is low. Increased BUN level is related to dehydration.
- Serum osmolality mildly elevated
- Serum acetone elevated in DKA
- UA (urinalysis): may indicate UTI, possibly ketones and elevated glucose
- **Arterial Blood Gases:** critical lab test to detect the presence and level of acidosis
- Blood cultures: needed when an infection is suspected
- Lactate: marker for tissue hypoxia/sepsis
- Cardiac markers (e.g., troponin): needed to identify evidence of myocardial infarction

EKG:

Look for abnormalities, infarction, or ischemia.

Imaging:

Perform if there is a problem suspected of precipitating DKA.

- CT chest: if pulmonary embolism is suspected
- CT abdomen: if infectious process or pancreatitis is suspected

Diagnostic Criteria: DKA and HHS

	HHS	DKA		
		Mild	Moderate	Severe
Blood glucose	>600 mg/dL	>250 mg/dL	>250 mg/dL	>250 mg/dL
Level of consciousness	Stupor or coma	Alert; oriented	Alert; drowsy	Stupor or coma
Arterial pH	>7.30	7.25–7.30	7.00–7.24	<7.00
Serum Ketones	Small	+	+	+
Urine Ketones	Small	+	+	+
Serum osmolality	>320 mOsm/kg	Variable	Variable	Variable
Serum bicarbonate	>18 mEq/L	15–18	10– <15	<10
Anion gap	Variable	>10	>12	>12

This table details the key criteria in diagnosing DKA and/or HHS. It further assists in making distinctions about the severity of the illness.

Source: Copyright © 2014, NovEx Novice to Expert Learning, LLC

Priority Patient Concerns and Desired Collaborative Care Outcomes

Prior to caring for patients with DKA and HHS, it is important to prioritize the patient's concerns that must guide the nursing care plan and interventions. Care for the patient is ordered and organized in accordance with the patient's priority and urgent needs. Desired collaborative care outcomes in patients with DKA and HHS typically include:

1. Patient will attain normovolemic state.
2. Patient will remain alert and oriented or return to pre-illness mental state.
3. Patient will demonstrate the ability to perform prescribed therapies to keep blood glucose within normal limits.
4. Patient will not experience severe or unresolved complications of disease process.
5. Patient's weight will progress toward desired level for height.

Considering these important care outcomes, prepare a list of the major 3–6 priority patient concerns or nursing diagnoses for patients with DKA and HHS. Be prepared to participate in a discussion of this list and/or to submit them as an assignment, as determined by your faculty. Resources you may find helpful in this assignment can include this lesson, the references, resources on nursing care plans, and standard nursing diagnoses manuals.

LO3:

Collaborative Interventions

Emergent Management of DKA and HHS

The most critical goal in the management of these two serious and often life-threatening conditions is the early recognition and treatment of the underlying illness. Management of DKA and HHS are similar. Four important therapies should be initiated simultaneously: rehydration, insulin, potassium, and correction of severe acidosis. The American Diabetes Association (ADA) provides evidence-based and consensus recommendations in the care of patients with DKA and HHS (2009):

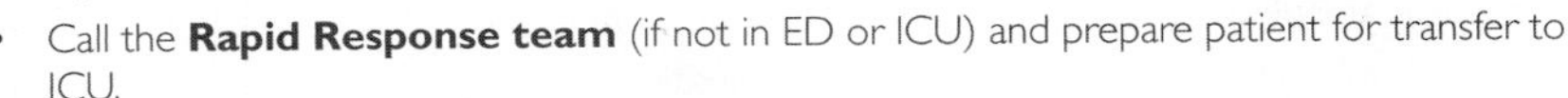

- Call the **Rapid Response team** (if not in ED or ICU) and prepare patient for transfer to ICU.

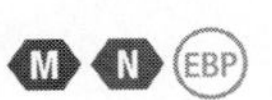

- **Fluid resuscitation:** Intravascular (IV) volume (**normal saline**) restoration to raise BP and glomerular perfusion. Several liters may be infused as boluses (e.g., 10–15 mL/kg/hr or 1.0 L/hr) initially, with caution in patients with heart failure.
    - o Start 2–3 IV access lines; one should be a central line.
    - o DKA patients may require 3–6 liters for resuscitation within the first 24 hours.
    - o HHS patients may require 8–10 liters for adequate resuscitation within the first 24 hours.

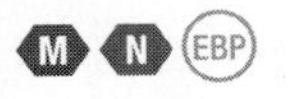

- **Correction of hyperglycemia: Continuous intravenous insulin** per hospital protocol (e.g., 0.1 units/kg/hr initially).

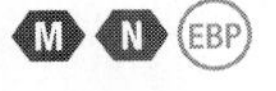

- Treat **electrolyte disturbances:**
    - o Potassium imbalances are the most serious and life-threatening electrolyte disturbances and must be treated immediately.
    - o In hypokalemia, infuse potassium without delay. Withhold insulin infusion until potassium is ≥3.3 mmol/L to prevent exacerbation of hypokalemia.
    - o Following rehydration and insulin infusion, the electrolytes shift between the intracellular, interstitial, and intravascular spaces, causing continued and sometimes opposite electrolyte imbalances. Prevention or correction of **hypokalemia**, **hyponatremia**, **hypophosphatemia**, and **hypomagnesia**.
    - o Cautious replacement in hypophosphatemia is indicated in anemia, respiratory depressions, and with cardiac failure.

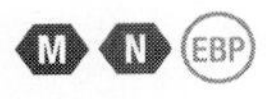

- Treat metabolic **acidosis/ketosis** with intravenous insulin. Do not use sodium bicarbonate unless pH <7.0.

M N
- **Antibiotics**, if indicated, should be started as soon as an infection is suspected and effectiveness of antibiotic(s) should be evaluated frequently.

M N
- **Monitor** serial electrolytes and arterial blood gases as indicated and bedside blood glucose hourly.

N
- Insert indicated devices and **continuously monitor:**
  - o Vital signs with bedside monitors (e.g., heart rate, blood pressure, respiratory rate, SpO_2)
  - o Cardiac rhythm, with continuous EKG monitor
  - o Physical exam, particularly neuro status. Cerebral edema signals a dire complication so early detection is critical.
  - o Intake and output: Urinary catheter is typically necessary.

M N
- Never event precautions are important:
  - o Use sequential compression device and anticoagulant to prevent venous thromboembolism.
  - o Regularly reposition the patient or employ rotational bed to prevent pressure ulcer development.
  - o Monitor for and prevent urinary catheter infection; remove catheter as soon as possible.
  - o Use sterile technique when handling central IV catheters and ensure proper dressing changes.
  - o Mobilize the patient at the earliest safe time.
  - o Institute fall precautions if patient has altered level of consciousness.
  - o Prevent air embolism when handling central IV access lines.

Collaborative Interventions (continued)

Transitioning from IV to Subcutaneous Insulin

As the patient stabilizes and his or her multiple abnormalties return to normal, care of the patient transitions. The transition period requires careful and gradual change to prevent recurrence of DKA and HHS (Kitabchi, et al., 2009):

M N
- A common error is to discontinue intravenous insulin when glucose returns to normal. Despite a normal glucose, acidosis may still be present. Insulin should be continued to allow removal of ketones by the body by reducing ketone production by the liver and adipose tissues and by increasing ketone utilization in the periphery.

M N
- Use American Diabetes Association (ADA) guidelines (Kitabchi, et al., 2009) for transitioning to subQ insulin once the patient is taking oral nutrition:
  - o Glucose <200 mg/dL in DKA or <250 mg/dL in HHS
  - o Anion gap ≤ 12 mEq/L in DKA
  - o Serum bicarbonate ≥ 15 mEq/L in DKA
  - o pH >7.30 in DKA
  - o Mental status returns to normal in HHS
  - o Osmolality returns to normal in HHS

M N
- The insulin transition should include a 1–2 hour overlap of IV and subQ doses.
- The above glucose, anion gap, bicarb, and pH parameters, along with return to normal mental status, signal the resolution of DKA or HHS.

N
- Once transferred to the medical-surgical unit, educate the patient about how to prevent DKA and HHS.

Concept Check

5. **Which patient usually requires the most intravenous fluid for resuscitation?**
   A. A patient with DKA
   B. A patient with HHS
   C. A patient whose HHS was caused by a myocardial infarction
   D. A patient whose DKA was caused by noncompliance with insulin therapy

Answer question

Concept Check

6. Which anion gap is normal for an adult?

A. 6

B. 10

C. 14

D. 16

Answer question

Concept Check

7. When is intravenous insulin discontinued in a patient being treated for HHS?

A. As soon as subcutaneous insulin is started

B. When the patient's blood glucose is <200 mg/dL

C. Once the patient is taking fluids orally

D. About an hour after the subcutaneous dosing is started

Answer question

Collaborative Interventions (continued)

Prevention

Prevention of DKA can improve if clinicians are attentive to the key patient exam findings that signal possible DKA and HHS. Whenever caring for a diabetic patient, the following should trigger concern, collaboration with team members, ongoing evaluation, and intervention as indicated:

- Illness in a diabetic that alters routine caloric intake or management of diabetes
- Loss of >5% of body weight within days (signaling an osmotic diuresis rather than actual loss of body weight)
- Tachypnea, with respiratory rate exceeding 30–35 breaths/minute
- Persistent hyperglycemia
- Altered level of consciousness requires urgent medical attention
- Persistent or uncontrolled fever
- Unresolving nausea and vomiting
- Educate the patient or review key points of sick-day management of diabetes, to include:
    - Use of short-acting insulin, not discontinuing insulin, or follow sick-day insulin therapy plan
    - Careful monitoring of blood glucose and urine ketones
    - Continued intake of calories and electrolytes. May be in the form of easily digestible liquids containing carbohydrates and salt.
    - Contact the health care provider to obtain any needed instructions, adjustments, and for follow-up.
    - Ongoing assessment and tracking of fever, weight loss, and oral intake
- Recognition and immediate intervention are critical in minimizing the hazards of DKA and HHS.

Summary of Interventions

DKA and HHS are serious complications of diabetes mellitus that require emergent hospitalization.

- Recognition and immediate intervention of the underlying illness
- Treatment focuses on the following:
  - o Intravenous hydration is critical.
  - o IV insulin is important for treatment of both hyperglycemia and ketoacidosis.
  - o Antibiotics are initiated if infection is suspected.
  - o Correction of electrolyte imbalances
  - o Correction of metabolic acidosis and ketosis
  - o Close monitoring of blood glucose and electrolytes guides treatment
  - o Close monitoring of vital signs and changes in the patient's physical findings are essential.
  - o Prevention involves education and early recognition.

LO4:

Evaluation of Desired Collaborative Care Outcomes

Evaluation and reassessment should reveal attainment of previously established patient outcomes. In summary:

- Patient's blood pressure is at pre-illness level, urine output is balanced with fluid intake, and there are no findings associated with hypovolemia.
- Patient is alert and oriented or is at pre-illness mental status.
- Patient accurately administers prescribed therapies and demonstrates techniques to keep blood glucose within normal limits.
- Patient's findings show illness and associated complications of disease process are resolving.
- Patient's BMI is improving toward desired level.

References

Clement, S., Braithwaite, S., Magee, M., et al. (2004). Management of diabetes and hyperglycemia in hospitals. *Diabetes Care, 27*(2), 553–591.

DeBeer, K., Michael, S., Thacker, M., et al. (2008). Diabetic ketoacidosis and hyperglycaemic hyperosmolar syndrome—Clinical guidelines. *Nurs Crit Care, 13*(1), 5–11.

Maletkovic, J., & Drexler, A. (2013). Diabetic ketoacidosis and hyperglycemic hyperosmolar state. *Endocrinology & Metabolism Clinics of North America, 42*(4), 677–695.

Savage, M., & Hilton, L. (2010). Managing diabetic ketoacidosis in adults: New national guidance from the Joint British Diabetes Societies. *J Diabetes Nurs, 14*(6), 220–225.

Tomky, D. (2005). Detection, prevention, and treatment of hypoglycemia in the hospital. *Diabetes Spectrum, 18*(1), 39–44.

Wall, R. (2013). Diabetic ketoacidosis and hyperosmolar hyperglycemia—A brief review. *Critical Care Alert, 21*(6), 41–45.

Clinical Practice Guidelines

American Diabetes Association. (2013). Standards of medical care in diabetes–2013. *Diabetes Care, 36*(Suppl. 1), S11–S66. doi:10:2337/dc13-S011

Kitabchi, A. E., Umpierrez, G. E., Miles, J. M., & Fisher, J. N. (2009). Hyperglycemic crisis in diabetes: Consensus statement by the American Diabetes Association. *Diabetes Care, 32*(7), 1335–1343. **http://care.diabetesjournals.org/content/32/7/1335.full.pdf+html**

Patient Education

American Diabetes Association. *Diabetes basics.* **www.diabetes.org/diabetes-basics/?loc=db-slabnav**

Hamdy, O. *Hypoglycemia.* **http://emedicine.medscape.com/article/122122-overview**

CARE OF PATIENTS WITH HYPERGLYCEMIA AND/OR HYPOGLYCEMIA DURING HOSPITALIZATION

Learning Outcomes for Hyperglycemia and Hypoglycemia

When you complete this lesson, you will be able to:

1. Recognize the clinical relevance of hyperglycemia and hypoglycemia during hospitalization.
2. Consider the pathophysiology, etiology, risk factors, and clinical presentation of hyperglycemia and hypoglycemia during hospitalization that determine the priority patient concerns.
3. Determine the most urgent and important nursing interventions and patient education required in caring for a patient with hyperglycemia or hypoglycemia during hospitalization.
4. Evaluate attainment of desired collaborative care outcomes for a patient with hyperglycemia or hypoglycemia during hospitalization.

LO1:

What Are Hyperglycemia and Hypoglycemia?

- Fasting blood sugar is a measure of blood glucose 8–12 hours after last eating. A normal result is <100 mg/dL.
- Random blood glucose measures glucose at any time. A normal result is <125 mg/dL. Glucose levels >125 mg/dL are defined as *hyperglycemia*.
- Hypoglycemia is a blood glucose level <70 mg/dL and associated with symptoms.
- Please refer to the Diabetes Mellitus Type 1 section to watch animations explaining hypoglycemia and hyperglycemina.

LO1:

Clinical Relevance

- Hyperglycemia and hypoglycemia are two of the most common problems encountered in hospitalized patients and can occur in diabetic and nondiabetic patients.
- Optimal control of blood glucose (i.e., avoiding hyper- and hypoglycemia) in the hospital is essential for the best possible outcome for patients.
- Patients with hyperglycemia in the hospital are at risk for adverse outcomes (e.g., higher rates of infection, higher mortality rates, longer hospital stays).
- Hypoglycemia is the most common adverse effect of intensive insulin therapy. It is also a common result of sliding scale insulin treatment, which is still widely used.
- Patients with type 1 diabetes who are receiving intensive care are at three times higher risk than patients without diabetes of experiencing hypoglycemia.
- Hypoglycemia can result in coma or death.

Concept Check

1. **What is the goal of glycemic control during hospitalization?**
   A. Keeping the patient slightly hypoglycemic
   B. Keeping the patient slightly hyperglycemic
   C. Avoiding both hypoglycemia and hyperglycemia
   D. The goal varies widely among patients.

Answer question

LO2:

Pathophysiology

Hyperglycemia During the Stress of Illness

- Normal glucose levels are usually maintained through a balance of insulin and stress hormones. Stress hormones counterbalance the effect of insulin, raising blood glucose. The hormones include glucagon, epinephrine, growth hormone, and cytokines.
- During hospitalization, surgery, critical illness, and infection can raise the levels of these hormones and cause hyperglycemia. Patients who were previously nondiabetic with normal glucose levels can develop hyperglycemia.
- Short periods of hyperglycemia result in abnormalities in the function of white blood cells and the immune system. These abnormalities are thought to impair wound healing and increase the risk of infection.
- Hyperglycemia also causes a large amount of glucose to enter the renal tubules. Normally, glucose is completely reabsorbed. However, when the ability of the nephrons to reabsorb glucose is overwhelmed (usually at a level of 180 mg/dL), the excess glucose is excreted in the urine, pulling water and electrolytes with it. This causes an increased urine output called osmotic diuresis. Osmotic diuresis can result in dehydration and/or electrolyte imbalances.

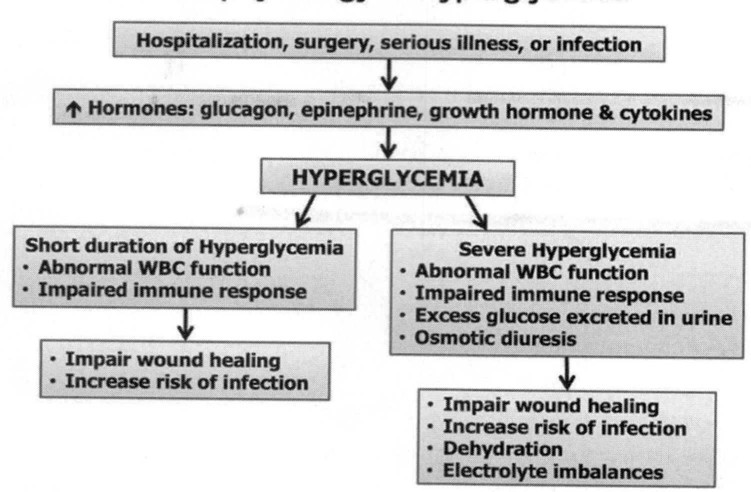

Source: Copyright © 2014, NovEx Novice to Expert Learning, LLC

Hypoglycemia During the Stress of Illness

- Hypoglycemia occurs when the plasma glucose concentrations fall too low.
- Hypoglycemia can occur in diabetic patients who may have taken their medications but were unable to eat, when the illness or its treatment interferes with normal medication action, breakdown, clearance, or when glucose production is impaired.
- Hypoglycemia is not a common problem for nondiabetic patients but may occur in patients who are not eating or those with critical illnesses involving sepsis or cardiac, renal, and hepatic failure. Glucose production can fail to keep pace with glucose utilization and cause the plasma glucose to fall too low.
- The brain is especially sensitive to even short periods of hypoglycemia. The brain does not store or manufacture glucose and is completely dependent on serum glucose levels to function. Although the brain is 2% of the body's total mass, it utilizes 25% of total glucose production. The brain, therefore, requires a steady supply of glucose to function properly. Hypoglycemia can mimic stroke-like symptoms and result in coma.

LO2:

Risk Factors

Hyperglycemia in Hospitalized Patients

- Surgery
- Infection
- Critical illness
- Sepsis
- Some medications
  - o Corticosteroid administration is a common cause.

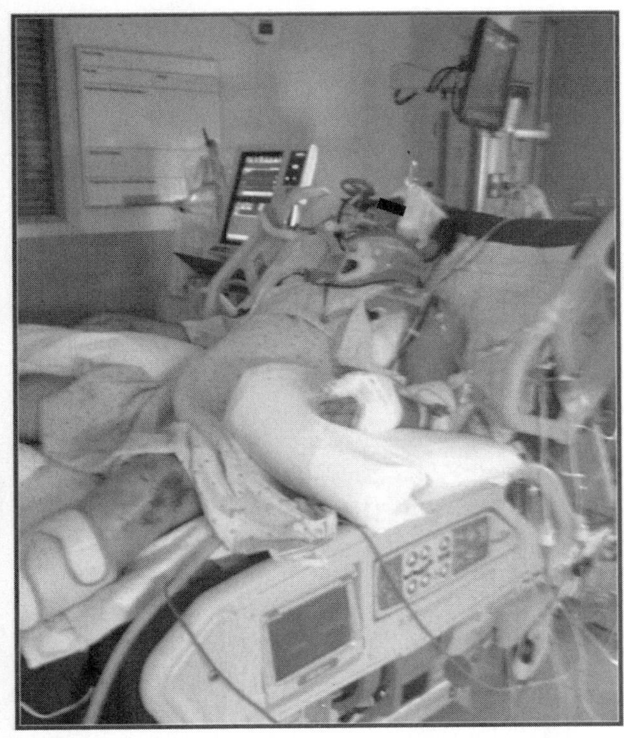

Patients who are critically ill, septic, or have cardiac, hepatic, or renal failure are at much higher risk for glycemic events. Glycemic events are linked to higher morbidity.

Hypoglycemia in Hospitalized Patients

- Sudden reduction of steroid dosage
- Renal failure or worsening kidney function
- Cardiac and hepatic failure
- Reduction of oral intake
- New NPO status or decreased PO intake
- Decrease in the rate of administration of dextrose IV infusion
- Interruption of enteral feeding or parenteral nutrition
- Premeal insulin given but meal not ingested
- Presence of an insulin pump

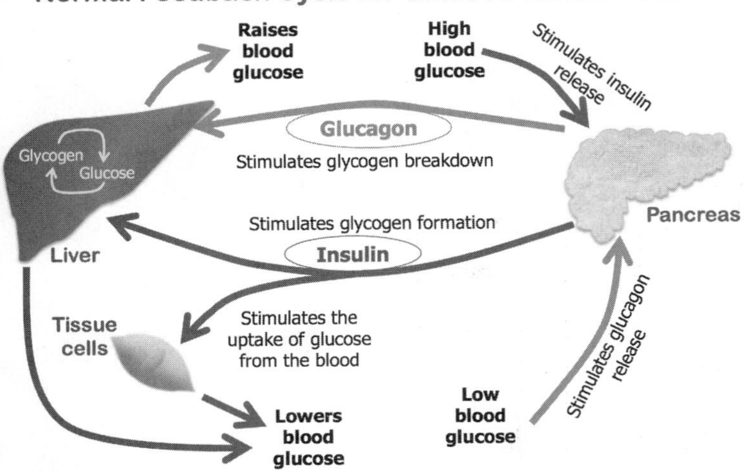

Risk factors for hypoglycemia can interfere with the glucose and insulin cycle above. Risk factors that predispose patients to hypoglycemic events include: cardiovascular disease, renal disorders, alcohol addiction, older age, gastroenteritis, poor nutritional state, and insulin overdose as a suicide method.

Concept Check

2. Which factor can cause hypoglycemia in a hospitalized patient?
   A. Inactivity
   B. Insulinoma
   C. Use of steroids
   D. Surgery

Answer question

LO2:

Causes

Hyperglycemia

- Patients with diabetes:
  - o Expired or insufficient insulin injection
  - o Improper injection of insulin
  - o Inactivity
  - o Inadequate dosage of oral medication
  - o Use of steroids
  - o Injury or surgery
  - o Severe emotional stress
- Certain hormones produced by the body to combat severe stress or illness can trigger hyperglycemia.

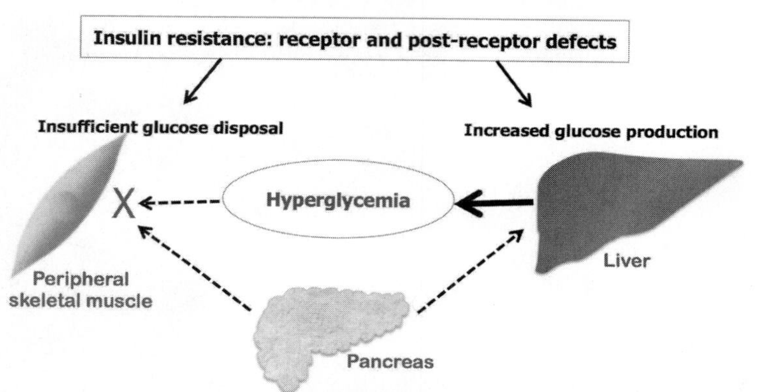

This graphic view depicts the causes of hyperglycemia in type 2 diabetes. Insulin fails to assist glucose to be used by muscle, yet the liver continues making glucose. In an attempt to secrete enough insulin to prevent hyperglycemia, the pancreas becomes exhausted from continual insulin production.

Hypoglycemia

- Diabetes with poor blood sugar regulation
- Drugs or medications (e.g., continued use of sliding scale insulin without regard for the patient's changing situation or caloric intake, medication or insulin errors)
- Excessive alcohol consumption
- Cortisol deficiency
- Some critical illnesses (e.g., sepsis)
- Malnourishment
- Insulinoma (a tumor of the pancreas)
- Reactive or postprandial hypoglycemia

LO2:

Assessment Findings

Hyperglycemia

Signs and symptoms usually do not occur until glucose levels are 250 mg/dL. They consist of:

- Headache
- Blurred vision
- Frequent urination
- Increased thirst
- Fatigue
- Weight loss
- Slow wound healing
- Thrush or genital itching
- More severe hyperglycemia with glucose >600:
    - o Confusion
    - o Coma

Hypoglycemia

- Early symptoms caused by adrenergic effects (epinephrine and glucagon release):
    - o Sweating and pallor
    - o Shakiness
    - o Headache
    - o Blurred vision
    - o Palpitations
    - o Hunger
    - o Anxiety or nervousness
    - o Dilated pupils
    - o Nausea/vomiting
- Neuroglycopenic effects resulting from reduced brain glucose:
    - o Irritability
    - o Dizziness
    - o Ataxia
    - o Seizures
    - o Combativeness
    - o Slurred speech
    - o Impaired judgment
    - o Emotional instability

These neurological manifestations are often mistaken for alcohol intoxication or stroke. Hypoglycemia should be considered in any patient who is confused or has a sudden decreased level of consciousness.

Concept Check

3. Which finding is usually not apparent until the patient's blood glucose level has exceeded 600 mg/dL?

A. Frequent urination

B. Fatigue

C. Confusion

D. Emotional instability

Answer question

LO2:

Diagnostics: Hyperglycemia and Hypoglycemia

- Electrolytes: Glucose may be high or low. Hyponatremia and hypokalemia may be associated with hyperglycemia. Anion gap and a low bicarbonate level may be present in diabetic ketoacidosis (DKA).
- Urinalysis may show evidence of ketones if DKA is developing.
- The Endocrine Society experts (Umpierrez, et al., 2012) recommend the following, although strong evidence is not yet available:
  - o Assess all patients with a diabetic history and make clear notation on the medical record.
  - o Use point of care (POC) testing of blood glucose (BG) for a minimum of 24–48 hours in patient with no diabetic history but with a BG >140 mg/dL. Treatment and continued monitoring is needed for persistently elevated BG.
  - o Point of contact: In stable inpatients, it is recommended that glucose be checked at bedtime and before meals.
  - o Use POC testing on normoglycemic patients, who are receiving therapies that can place them at higher risk for glycemic events, including parenteral or enteral nutrition, corticosteroids, and octreotides.
  - o Assess HbA1C in all inpatients who have diabetes or hyperglycemia (>140 mg/dL).

Priority Patient Concerns and Desired Collaborative Care Outcomes: Hyperglycemia and Hypoglycemia

Prior to caring for patients with hyperglycemia and hypoglycemia, it is important to prioritize the patient's concerns that must guide the nursing care plan and interventions. Care for the patient is ordered and organized in accordance with the patient's priority and urgent needs. Desired collaborative care outcomes in patients with hyperglycemia and hypoglycemia typically include:

1. Patient's blood glucose will return to desired level.
2. Patient will not experience delayed healing.
3. Patient will maintain desired electrolyte levels.
4. Patient will verbalize understanding of disease process and will use health management strategies.

Considering these important care outcomes, prepare a list of the major 3–6 priority patient concerns or nursing diagnoses for patients with hyperglycemia and hypoglycemia. Be prepared to participate in a discussion of this list and/or to submit them as an assignment, as determined by your faculty. Resources you may find helpful in this assignment can include this lesson, the references, resources on nursing care plans, and standard nursing diagnoses manuals.

LO3:

Collaborative Interventions

Hyperglycemia

Patients with hyperglycemia in the hospital are at risk for adverse outcomes (e.g., higher rates of infection). Intensive treatment, however, is not necessarily associated with decreased mortality because of the increased risk of hypoglycemia. Recommendations, therefore, are aimed at balancing the treatment of hyperglycemia and avoiding hypoglycemia. Regardless of the cause of hyperglycemia (i.e., diabetes, surgery, medications), optimal control needs to be achieved for the best outcome.

The following are recommendations by the American Association of Clinical Endocrinologists and American Diabetic Association or AACE/ADA (Moghissi, et al., 2009) and ADA (2013) for inpatient glycemic control.

Critically Ill Patients

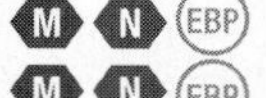

- Begin insulin therapy for persistent hyperglycemia (glucose level >180 mg/dL).

- The goal is to maintain **blood glucose (BG) level between 140–180 mg/dL**.
- Intravenous insulin infusion is the preferred method of treatment.

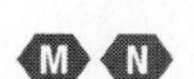

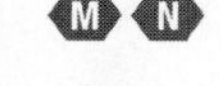

- Using a protocol that has proven effectiveness and a low occurrence of hypoglycemia is recommended.

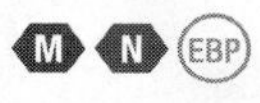

- Frequent glucose checks are necessary to prevent the occurrence of hypoglycemia and to achieve these goals.

Noncritically Ill Patients

In addition to the AACE/ADA recommendations, evidence-based recommendations also include those from the Endocrine Society (Umpierrez, et al., 2012) in the care of hospitalized patients who are not critically ill:

- The goal for glucose control, also called glycemic target, is strongly recommended by key authorities until sufficient evidence is available (Moghissi, et al, 2009; Umpierrez, et al, 2012). The glycemic target is **premeal BG <140 mg/dL and random BG <180 mg/dL**. Patients at high risk for hypoglycemia may need higher targets (e.g., <200 mg/dL), and patients who are more tightly controlled as outpatients may have lower blood glucose levels as targets.
- For patients on insulin therapy prior to hospitalization, continue to use a subcutaneous insulin schedule during hospitalization.
- Ideally, treatment should consist of subcutaneous administration of basal, nutritional, and correctional insulin. Basal insulin is administered around the clock with intermediate or long-acting insulin. Nutritional insulin is administered with meals using rapid-acting insulin. Correctional insulin is administered when glucose is elevated above the target range.

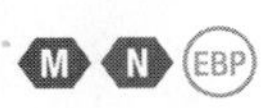

- Using only correctional insulin is often referred to as sliding scale insulin. It is not a good way to treat a patient in the long term because glucose is rarely in the target range and usually results in prolonged periods of both hyperglycemia and hypoglycemia.

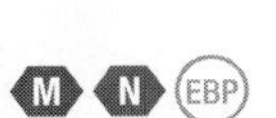

- Rapid- and long-acting insulin are combined to create a more normal pattern of insulin levels and better glucose control.

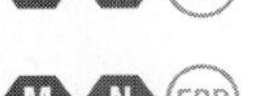

- Ongoing bedside POC testing of BG is recommended to guide glycemic management. BG measurements need to be coordinated with medications and nutritional intake.

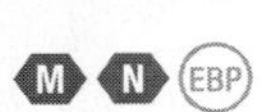

- Home oral diabetic medications may be continued in the hospital. However, oral diabetic medications should not be used to treat hyperglycemia that occurs in the hospital.

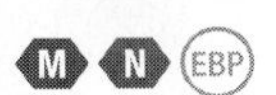

- Patients who require transition from continuous IV insulin to subcutaneous insulin, those receiving enteral or parenteral nutrition, those requiring perioperative BG control, and those with glucocorticoid-induced diabetes need condition-specific care. Consult a diabetic specialist to assist in guiding glycemic management in these patients.

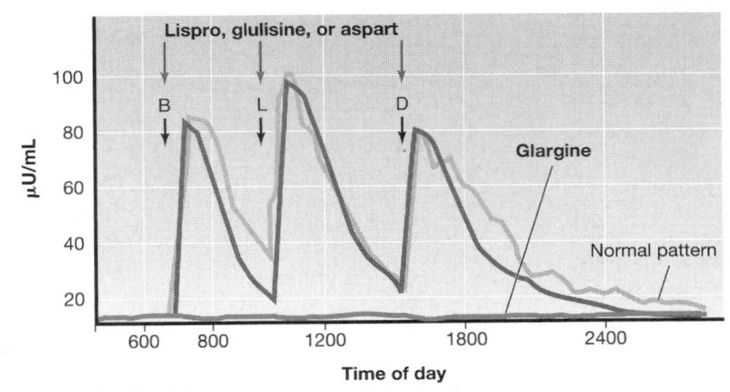

Graph: Type 1 Diabetes—Basal–Bolus Insulin Treatment with Insulin Analogues. Key points: Once-daily administration of long-acting glargine provides a steady supply of basal insulin. Mealtime administration of insulin lispro, glulisine, or aspart provides the meal-related bolus in insulin secretion.

Safety Issues

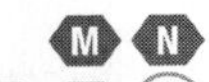

- Overtreatment and undertreatment of hyperglycemia is a major safety concern.

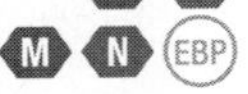

- In hospitalized patients who are eating a near-normal diet, guidelines recommend continuing the outpatient treatment regimen if BG is controlled, with a slight reduction if food intake is less than normal. If BG is not well controlled, insulin combinations are indicated.

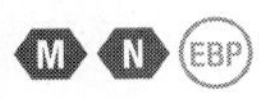

- In NPO patients, outpatient treatments should be discontinued and BG levels should guide combination insulin therapies (basal, prandial, and correction insulin).

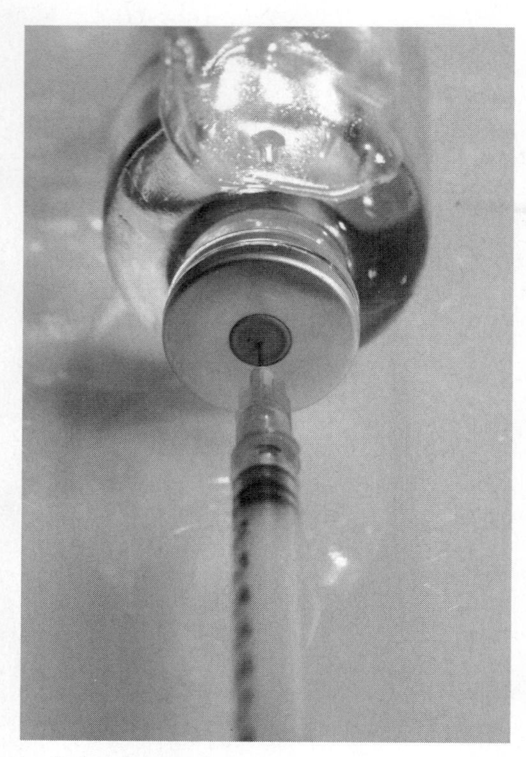

Insulin for administration.
Source: Luiscar74/Shutterstock

Concept Check

4. What is the high limit goal for blood glucose for patients who are critically ill?

A. 140 mg/dL

B. 160 mg/dL

C. 180 mg/dL

D. 200 mg/dL

Answer question

Concept Check

5. A hospitalized patient who takes oral medications to control diabetes type 2 has normal fasting blood glucose levels. What therapeutic changes does the nurse anticipate?

A. Discontinuation of oral medications

B. Changing therapy from oral medications to injectable insulin

C. Continuation of oral medications alone

D. Addition of injectable insulin to the oral medications

Answer question

Concept Check

6. What is the glycemic target in a critically ill patient?

A. 80–100 mg/dL

B. 100–110 mg/dL

C. 120–140 mg/dL

D. 140–180 mg/dL

Answer question

Collaborative Interventions (continued)

Hypoglycemia

Immediate Intervention

Evidence-based recommendations additionally include those from the Endocrine Society (Cryer, et al., 2009; Umpierrez, et al., 2012) and the ADA and Endocrine Society (Seaquist, et al., 2013). If low blood sugar (<70 mg/dL) is suspected, check for symptoms of hypoglycemia:

- A nurse-initiated protocol is needed to avoid and immediately treat hypoglycemia (BG <70 mg/dL).
- If patient is responsive and can safely swallow, obtain stat BG. Then, give a rapid-acting carbohydrate (e.g., hard candy, juice, cake frosting, oral glucose tablets or gel, or an equivalent concentrated glucose source.
- Patients who are on acarbose (Precose) or miglitol (Glyset) cannot rapidly digest carbohydrates, so only pure glucose (dextrose) is necessary to raise the blood glucose. Juices and table sugar will not help immediately. (See table below.)
- Obtain POC blood glucose and monitor response.
- Obtain IV access if possible and call the Rapid Response team.
- If the patient is on an insulin drip, stop the infusion, obtain a POC glucose, and give rescue medication if required (see table below).
- For less responsive patients, give an IV dextrose 50% (D50W) bolus. If there is no IV access, inject IM glucagon, obtain POC glucose, monitor response, and start IV.

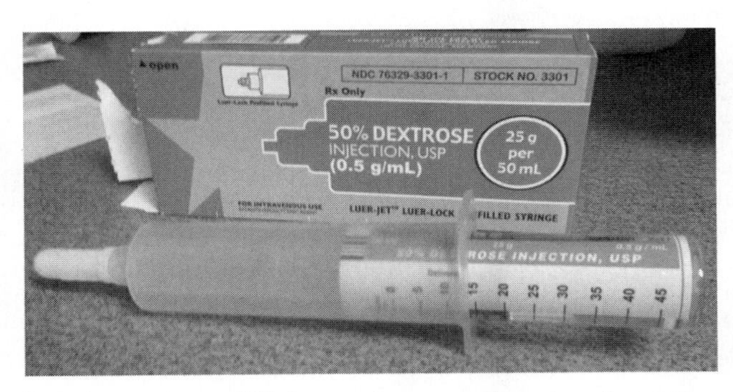

Pure glucose, given as 50% dextrose in emergent hypoglycemia, comes in a large 50cc syringe for IV bolus injection. Patients typically respond rapidly to this intervention.
Source: Courtesy of K. Kyriakidis

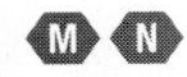

- For patients who are unconscious or obtunded, do not wait to get the POC glucose before treating suspected hypoglycemic event with D50W or glucagon.
- If initial recovery is achieved with simple glucose products, feed patient as soon as possible with a more complex meal (protein, fat, complex carbs) to sustain normal blood sugars.
- Blood glucose should be monitored every 1–2 hours until a steady glucose level is achieved.
- Assessment of oral intake, IV fluids, medications, and insulin dosing is performed to determine why the patient became hypoglycemic.

Safety Issues

When a patient exhibits signs and symptoms of hypoglycemia OR has blood glucose less than 70:	
Responsive patient and able to swallow **Mild-moderate hypoglycemia**	**Unresponsive patient or patient cannot swallow** **Severe hypoglycemia**
1. Stat blood glucose (BG), if not already obtained. 2. BG 49–69 mg/dL, treat with 15 grams of carbohydrate – Select one of the following: a. 4 ounces of fruit juice. If patient on Precose or Glyset, **DO NOT** give juice. b. 3 **glucose tablets**, followed by water c. 1 tube **Glucose gel** to buccal surface/side of mouth 3. BG less than 49 mg/dL, treat with 30 grams of carbohydrate (Select one of the following): a. 8 ounces of fruit juice. If patient on Precose or Glyset, **DO NOT** give juice. b. 6–8 **glucose tablets**, followed by water c. 2 tubes **Glucose gel** to buccal surface/side of mouth 4. If the BG is less than 40 prior to treatment: a. **Repeat test immediately (to confirm result)** b. Document a comment code in the meter c. Treat patient d. Dock meter as soon as possible e. Follow the Critical Value policy procedure 5. Repeat BG in 15 minutes. Repeat treatment if necessary. 6. If next mealtime is within 30 minutes, get tray as soon as possible. 7. If meal not scheduled in next 30 minutes, give snack with one carbohydrate (6 saltine crackers or 3 graham crackers) and one protein serving (8 ounces milk or peanut butter). 8. Repeat BG again in 60 minutes. 9. Notify physician as appropriate.	1. Stat blood glucose (BG), if not already obtained. 2. If the BG is less than 40 prior to treatment: a. **Repeat test immediately (to confirm result)** b. Document a comment code in the meter c. Treat patient d. Dock meter as soon as possible e. Follow the Critical Value policy procedure 3. If no IV access: a. Give **Glucagon IM** (Adult – 1 mg or Child – 0.5 mg for child weighing less than 20 kg.) (Obtain from Pharmacy). Administer immediately after reconstituting. b. Start IV or **D5W** at 100 ml/hour. c. Turn patient on side as vomiting is likely to occur. 4. If IV access, give **50% Dextrose** IV push (50 ml for adults, 25 ml for children under 20 kg). 5. If patient still not responsive in 5–10 minutes, repeat above steps. 6. When responsive, decrease IV rate to 50 ml/hour. 7. If **Glucagon** given, follow with a carbohydrate and protein snack when the patient is responsive. 8. Repeat BG in 15 minutes and at 60 minutes. 9. Notify physician of severe hypoglycemia and/or if **50% Dextrose** utilized.

This is an example of a hospital protocol for hypoglycemic patients.

Hypoglycemic treatment protocols should include:

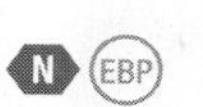

- Critical value reporting: Health care facilities should have an effective process for communication of blood glucose levels that are outside of set limits or a critical value.
- Actions to be taken in response to critical blood glucose levels should be defined and standardized.
- Policy should allow nurses to administer hypoglycemia rescue agents by following a standardized order set with minimal health care provider (HCP) oversight, but with appropriate HCP notification of event.
- Protocols are designed to prevent overtreatment that can cause hyperglycemia.

Prevention of Hypoglycemia

Clinical practice guidelines (Cryer, et al., 2009; Seaquist, et al., 2013) focus on recognition in patients who are unaware of hypoglycemia and reducing the risk and incidence:

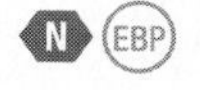

- BG monitoring:
  - Before meals and bedtime
  - At the onset of symptoms
  - During the night when indicated
  - Preprandial BG targets are 100–150 mg/dL.

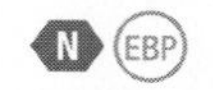

- Nutritional education:
  - Intake of adequate calories
  - Snacks between meals and at bedtime
  - Xanthine beverages (e.g., coffee, tea, chocolate) as tolerated

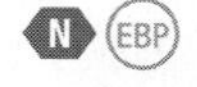

- Exercise:
  - Monitor BG before, during, and after exercise.
  - Snack before, during, and/or after exercise if BG <140 mg/dL.

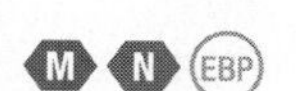

- Medication:
  - Adjust insulin or oral hypoglycemic medication when the patient is not eating or when tube feeding is on hold.
  - Combine rapid-acting insulins (e.g., aspart, lispro) to reduce the risk of hypoglycemia between meals.
  - Consider basal insulin to reduce the risk of nocturnal hypoglycemia.
  - Administer insulin in conjunction with meals, as needed.

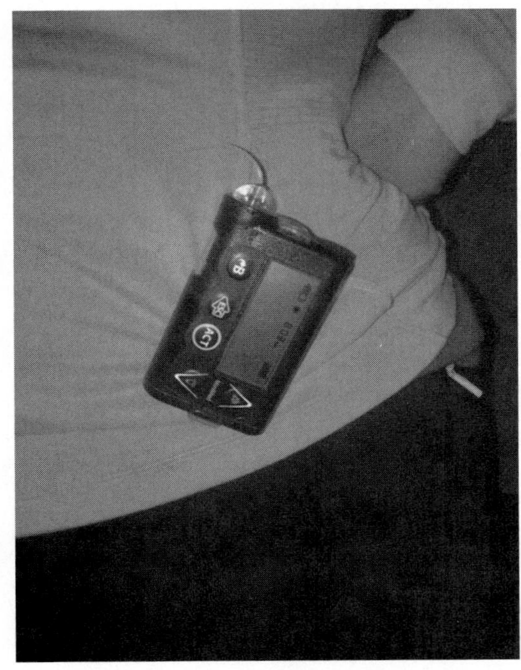

The insulin pump is used to automatically deliver basal insulin continuously, and bolus insulin at meal times by pressing the buttons. Before meals, a blood glucose value is entered into the pump to calculate the correction bolus to bring the blood glucose level back to the target value.
Source: Copyright © 2014, NovEx Novice to Expert Learning, LLC

Collaborative Interventions (continued)

Perioperative Considerations: Hyperglycemia and Hypoglycemia

- M N EBP For type 1 diabetic patients having surgery, continuous insulin infusion or basal with bolus insulins are recommended.
- M N EBP For type 2 diabetics on oral hypoglycemic drugs, medications should be held on the morning of surgery and resumed when the patient starts eating. Insulin therapy should be initiated if needed.
- M N EBP For patients on insulin, two different strategies may be used:
  1. Basal insulin can be continued at the home dose with initiation of dextrose-containing IV fluids.
  2. Basal insulin can be decreased to two thirds the dose.
- M N EBP Nutritional short-acting insulin should be discontinued and basal insulin is recommended postoperatively while the patient is NPO.
- M N EBP Basal bolus insulin is recommended in patients who are able to eat after surgery.
- Type 1 diabetics should never have basal insulin completely discontinued since this may result in DKA.

Patient Education and Discharge Planning: Hyperglycemia and Hypoglycemia

N
- Providers need to begin planning for discharge at the time of admission.

M N EBP
- Transitioning from inpatient to outpatient settings requires patient education and communication with the patients and their caregivers. Provide written instructions that summarize the verbal education and that are clearly understandable (Umpierrez, et al., 2012).

M N EBP
- Many patients come to the hospital with undiagnosed diabetes and require initial education.

M N EBP
- Consider raising glycemic target, and educate the patient, to avoid severe hypoglycemia in insulin-treated patients if a hypoglycemic event occurs.

M N EBP
- Collaborate with patient about potential need for bariatric surgery if the patient has a body mass index >35 kg/m^2 and type 2 diabetes.
- See NovE-lesson on Patient Education for Diabetes that includes:
  - o Diet and nutrition
  - o Medications
  - o Activity and exercise (ADA, 2013) N EBP
  - o Recognizing poorly controlled blood glucose
  - o Glucose monitoring
  - o Daily living issues
  - o Self-management

Concept Check

7. In general, what instruction should be provided to a patient who takes oral medications and is scheduled for elective surgery?

A. Discontinue oral medication 2 days before surgery.

B. Take oral medication with water prior to surgery.

C. Do not take oral medication on the morning of surgery.

D. Discontinue oral medication 1 week before surgery.

Answer question

Summary of Interventions

- Optimal control of blood glucose (i.e., avoiding hyperglycemia and hypoglycemia) in the hospital is essential for having the best possible outcomes for patients.

Hyperglycemia

- In ICU, the goal for the patient is to maintain blood **glucose levels between 140–180 mg/dL,** ideally with an IV infusion.
- For noncritical patients, the goal for glucose control is a **premeal BG <140 mg/dL and random BG <180 mg/dL**. Ideally, this is achieved with a combination of basal insulin and a nutritional bolus of insulin.

Hypoglycemia

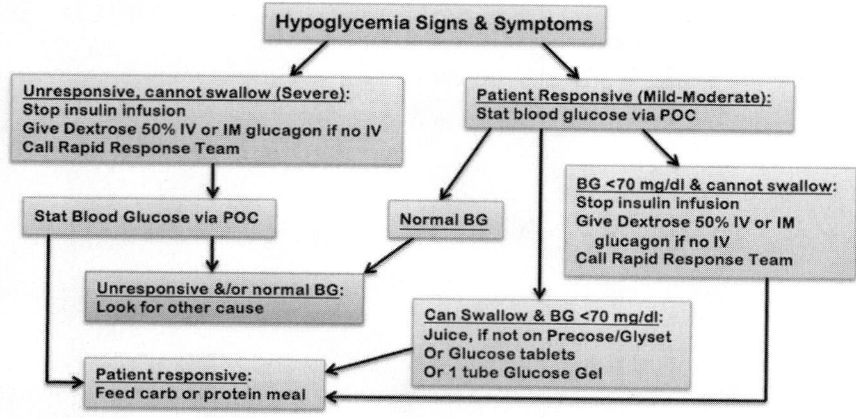

Hypoglycemia Signs & Symptoms
Unresponsive, cannot swallow (Severe):
Stop insulin infusion
Give Dextrose 50% IV or IM glucagon if no IV
Call Rapid Response Team
Patient Responsive (Mild-Moderate):
Stat blood glucose via POC
Stat Blood Glucose via POC
Normal BG
BG <70 mg/dl & cannot swallow:
Stop insulin infusion
Give Dextrose 50% IV or IM glucagon if no IV
Call Rapid Response Team
Unresponsive &/or normal BG:
Look for other cause
Can Swallow & BG <70 mg/dl:
Juice, if not on Precose/Glyset
Or Glucose tablets
Or 1 tube Glucose Gel
Patient responsive:
Feed carb or protein meal
BG = blood glucose
POC = Point of Care

Source: Copyright © 2014, NovEx Novice to Expert Learning, LLC

- Repeat treating with simple glucose if BG <70 mg/dL. Once initial recovery is achieved, feed patient as soon as possible with a more complex meal (protein, fat, complex carbs) to sustain normal blood sugars.
- Monitor patient's response using point of care (POC) glucose. Check at least hourly until glucose is stable.

LO4:

Evaluation of Desired Collaborative Care Outcomes: Hyperglycemia and Hypoglycemia

Evaluation and reassessment should reveal attainment of previously established patient outcomes. In summary:

- Patient's random blood glucose consistently measures between 70 and 125 mg/dL or at levels expected for the patient.
- Patient's recovery and healing are progressing at the expected rate, with wound specialist consultation as needed.
- Patient has no or only minor glucose-related changes in electrolyte levels.
- Patient accurately discusses blood glucose control treatment plan and demonstrates key strategies of control.

References

Harrison, R., Stalker, S., Henderson, R., & Lyerla, F. (2013). Use of a clinical decision support system to improve hypoglycemia management. *MEDSURG Nursing, 22*(4), 250–263.

Mompoint-Williams, D., Watts, P., & Appel, S. (2013). Detecting and treating hypoglycemia in patients with diabetes. *Nurse Practitioner, 38*(11), 11–14.

Pollock, F., & Funk, D. (2013). Acute diabetes management. *AACN Advanced Critical Care, 24*(3), 314–324.

Rutan, L., & Sommers, K. (2012). Hyperglycemia as a risk factor in the perioperative patient. *AORN, 95*(3), 352–364.

Tomky, D. (2005). Detection, prevention, and treatment of hypoglycemia in the hospital. *Diabetes Spectrum, 18*(1), 39–44.

Turchin, A., Matheny, M. E., Shubina, M., Scanlon, J. V., Greenwood, B., & Pendergrass, M. L.(2009). Hypoglycemia and clinical outcomes in patients with diabetes hospitalized in the general ward. *Diabetes Care, 32*(7), 1153–1157.

Wallace, C. (2012). Postoperative management of hypoglycemia. *Orthopaedic Nursing, 31*(6), 328–335.

Weant, K., Bailey, A., & Baker, S. (2013). Hyperglycemia in critical illness. *Advanced Emergency Nursing Journal, 35*(3), 209–216.

Clinical Practice Guidelines

American Diabetes Association. (2013). Standards of medical care in diabetes—2013. *Diabetes Care, 36*(suppl 1), S11–S66. doi:10:2337/dc13-S011

Cryer, P. E., Axelrod, L., Grossman, A. B., Heller, S. R., Montori, V. M., Seaquist, E. R., & Service, F. J. (2009). Evaluation and management of adult hypoglycemic disorders: An Endocrine Society Clinical Practice Guideline. *Journal of Clinical Endocrinology and Metabolism, 94*(3), 709–728. **www.endocrine.org/~/media/endosociety/Files/Publications/Clinical%20Practice%20Guidelines/FINAL-Standalone-Hypo-Guideline.pdf**

Moghissi, E. S., Korytkowski, M. T., DiNardo, M., Einhorn, D., Hellman, R., Hirsch, I. B., . . . , Umpierrez, G. E. (2009). American Association of Clinical Endocrinologists and American Diabetes Association consensus statement on inpatient glycemic control. *Diabetes Care, 32*(6), 1119–1131.

Seaquist, E. R., Anderson, J., Childs, B., Cryer, P., Dagogo-Jack, S., Fish, L., . . . , Vigersky, R. (2013). Hypoglycemia and diabetes: A report of a workgroup of the American Diabetes Association and the Endocrine Society. *Journal of Clinical Endocrinology and Metabolism, 98*(5), 1845–1859.

Umpierrez, G. E., Hellman, R., Korytkowski, M. T., Kosiborod, M., Maynard, G. A., Montori, V. M., . . . , Van den Berghe, G. (2012). Management of hyperglycemia in hospitalized patients in non-critical care setting: An Endocrine Society Clinical Practice Guideline. *Journal of Clinical Endocrinology and Metabolism, 97*(1), 16–38. **press.endocrine.org/doi/pdf/10.1210/jc.2011-2098**

Patient Education

Diabetes Education Online. (UCSF). (2015). *Hyperglycemic/hyperosmolar states.* **http://dtc.ucsf.edu/living-with-diabetes/complications/hyperglycemic-hyperosmolar-states/**

Diabetes Education Online. (UCSF). (2015). *Complications: Hypoglycemia.* **http://dtc.ucsf.edu/living-with-diabetes/complications/hypoglycemia/**

Mayo Clinic. (2013). *Hemoglobin A1c (HbA1c).* **www.mayoclinic.org/tests-procedures/a1c-test/basics/definition/prc-20012585**

Animation: **www.youtube.com/watch?v=jHRfDTqPzj4**

National Diabetes Information Clearinghouse (NDIC). (2012). *Hypoglycemia.* **http://diabetes.niddk.nih.gov/dm/pubs/hypoglycemia/#treatment**

Learning Outcomes for Insulin: Types and Administration

When you complete this lesson, you will be able to:

1. Discuss the similarities and differences among types and action profiles of insulin.
2. Recognize insulin administration precautions.
3. Distinguish what insulin combinations meet various patient needs.
4. Determine the important patient education and safety needs required when caring for a patient receiving insulin.

Insulin Types and Administration

This NovE-lesson teaches about:

- Insulin
  - Types of insulin
  - Insulin preparations, storage, and expiration
  - Insulin management
  - Action profiles and comparisons
  - Matching insulin action to patient needs
- Insulin administration
  - Insulin syringes
  - Injection sites
- Insulin precautions
  - Common errors: examples
  - Basal insulin
  - Pre-mixed insulin
  - High-alert medication
- Insulin administration
  - Approaches
  - Sliding scale
  - Basal + nutritional bolus combination
  - Glucose management programs
  - Carbohydrate counting
- Insulin needs during illness
- Collaborative interventions
  - Patient education and safety

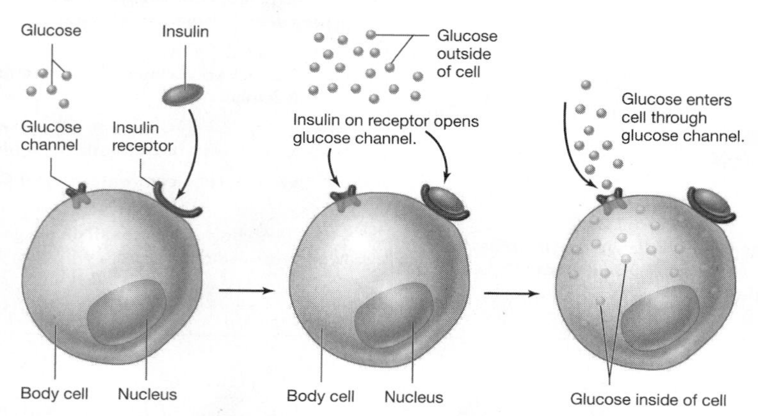

Insulin is key to unlocking a cell's glucose channel that allows glucose into the cell to be used as fuel. When glucose cannot enter, it remains locked out in the bloodstream, causing hyperglycemia.

LO1:

Insulin

Types of Insulin

- According to onset of action, there are currently four types of synthetic insulin: rapid-acting, short-acting or regular, intermediate-acting, and long-acting.
- Each type of insulin has a unique therapeutic:
  - o **Onset:** time when insulin begins lowering blood glucose
  - o **Peak:** time required to reach maximum therapeutic action
  - o **Duration:** length of effectiveness in lowering blood glucose
- Therapeutic glucose or glycemic control varies individually:
  - o Requires a combination of insulin types
  - o Variable number of daily injections
- Insulin is typically given subQ but is also infused IV, particularly in hospitalized patients.

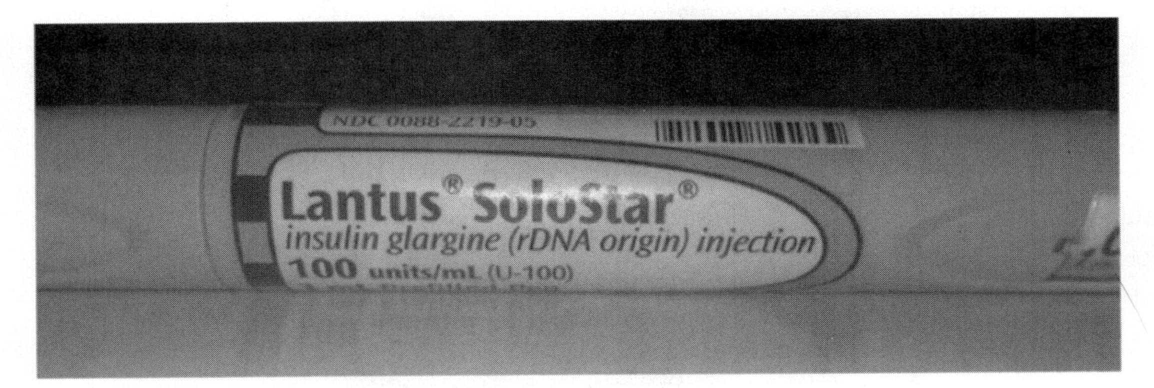

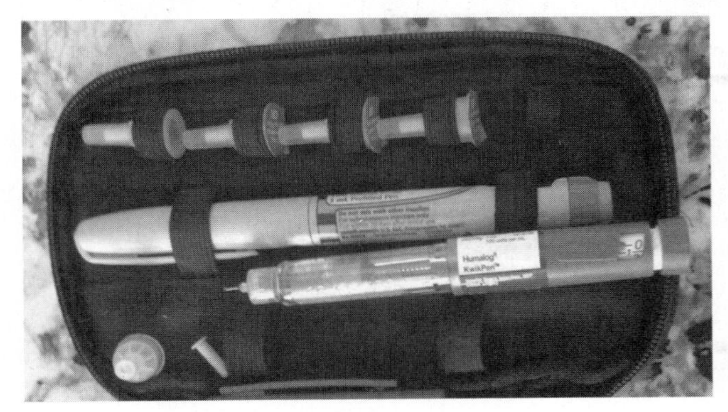

Types of insulin in prepared syringes.
Source: (*both*) Copyright © 2014, NovEx Novice to Expert Learning, LLC

Rapid-Acting Insulin—Humalog (lispro), Novolog (aspart), Apidra (glulisine)

- Onset is 15 minutes. Best given right before meals. Prior to administration of insulin, the food tray must be present and the patient must be willing and able to eat.
- Insulin availability mimics rise and fall in glucose that occurs with eating.
- Often combined with a daily long-acting insulin

Short-Acting, or "Regular," Insulin

- Also used around mealtime
- Takes longer to work than rapid-acting insulin: onset 30–45 minutes
- Peaks at about 2–3 hours
- Duration is 6–8 hours.

Intermediate-Acting Insulin—NPH (Humulin N, Novolin N), Lente

- Slower absorption due to substance that is added
- Cloudy in appearance
- Requires mixing before injection
- Later onset and longer duration than short-acting insulin

Long-Acting Insulin—Levemir (detemir), Lantus (glargine), Ultralente

- Typically have a small early peak, then a steady rate of absorption for most of the day. Often combined with fast-acting insulin for meal coverage.

LO2:

Insulin Preparations, Storage, and Expiration

- Follow the manufacturer's recommendations.
- As a general rule:
  - **Vials:**
    - Check expiration date and the date vials were first used or opened.
    - Whether refrigerated or not, the vial must be used within 28 days after first use.
    - Keep away from light and heat.
    - Do not freeze.
    - Discard if frozen or outdated.
  - **Cartridge system** (cartridges of insulin used to load the pen):
    - Do not refrigerate.
    - Discard after 28 days once used or opened.
    - Protect from heat and light.

Insulin (continued)

LO2:

Approach to Insulin Management

The four types of insulin are used to achieve good blood glucose control, whether the patient is eating intermittently or not at all.

The most current and effective approach to insulin management was recommended by the American Association of Clinical Endocrinologists and the American Diabetes Association (ADA) in the 2009 Consensus Statement.* The three-pronged approach involves these components:

1. **Basal insulin:** Ideally, basal insulin (e.g., glargine, detemir) is calculated to provide a constant, 24-hour, baseline level of insulin without peaks that suppress hepatic glucose release during fasting and/or between meals.
2. **Nutritional bolus or bolus insulin:** Bolus insulin prevents the postprandial glucose peaks that are predictable after each meal. Glucose from meals is converted into energy and prevents hyperglycemia. Rapid-acting insulins (e.g., aspart, glulisine, lispro) are commonly used because evidence shows that rapid-acting insulin provides better control over glucose peaks and potential hypoglycemia than regular insulin.
3. **Correctional insulin:** Patient sensitivity to insulin varies; so, although the "rules" for calculating insulin dosage *generally* work, adjustments are often needed for individuals. The correctional insulin is used to correct for the sensitivity factor. Rapid-acting insulins are the best choice in adjusting for these hyperglycemic glucose levels.

***Basal plus bolus insulin combinations** most accurately mimic normal physiologic insulin responses and provide the most effective glycemic control. Hence, they are strongly recommended as promoting the best outcomes.

Concept Check

1. Which dosage is calculated to provide a constant level of insulin?

   A. Basal
   B. Nutritional
   C. Bolus
   D. Correctional

Answer question

LO1: Insulin Action Profiles

Subcutaneous Administration

Insulin Preparations	Onset of Action	Peak	Duration	Uses
Aspart, Glulisine, Lispro	~ 15 minutes	1-2 hours	4-6 hours	Used to control the spike in blood sugar caused by meals. Typically used in combination with a long-acting insulin.
Human regular	30–60 minutes	2–4 hours	6–8 hours 6-10 hours	
Human NPH	2–4 hours	4–10 hours	12–20 hours	Intermediate-acting insulin that has a slower: onset of action, absorption rate, and longer duration. Can be used with basal insulin.
Levimir (Detemir)	2-3 hours	Flat	~ 14 hours	Long-acting insulin designed to be taken 1-2 times a day.
Glargine (Lantus)	2–4 hours	Flat	~ 24 hours	Long acting insulin designed to be taken once a day.

Concept Check

2. What is the onset of action of human NPH insulin?
   - A. 15 minutes
   - B. 30–45 minutes
   - C. 2–4 hours
   - D. 4–6 hours

Answer question

Concept Check

3. Which information on storage of insulin cartridges is correct?
   - A. Refrigerate.
   - B. May freeze if not opened
   - C. Discard 28 days after opening.
   - D. Keep in well-lit area.

Answer question

Insulin (continued)

LO1: **Insulin Action Comparisons**

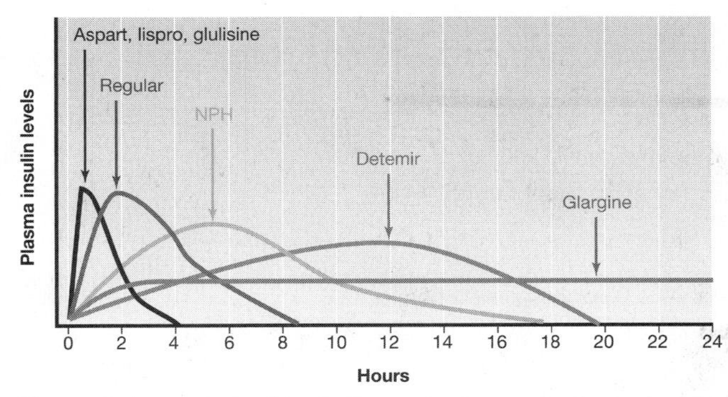

This graph depicts idealized insulin time-action (onset of action, peak, and duration) profiles after subcutaneous injection of insulin: aspart, lispro, glulisine, regular, NPH, detemir, and glargine.

LO3:

Match Insulin Action to Patient Needs

Many factors go into deciding which insulin regimen a person will use:

- Various people respond differently to each type of insulin.
- Each person's lifestyle affects how the body uses insulin.
- A variety of combinations may need to be tried before finding the best combination to control one's blood glucose.

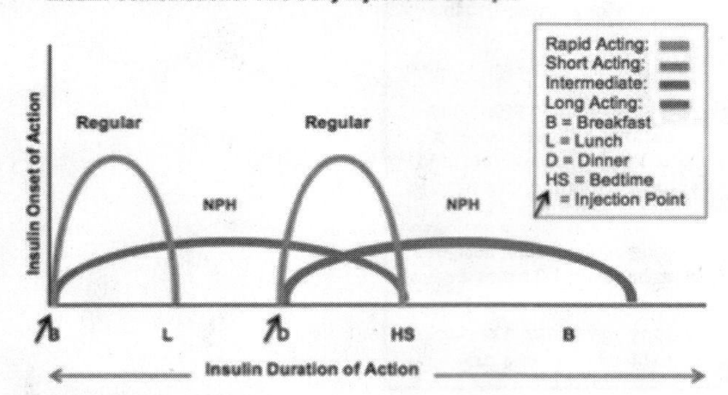

Source: Copyright © 2014, NovEx Novice to Expert Learning, LLC

- For instance (see graph above), one may need lower levels of insulin through the day except at breakfast and dinner. Therefore, two injections with both short- and intermediate-acting insulin may be given at the same time.
- However, other patients may need higher insulin levels during sleep (see below) when hormone levels can rise. Thus, delaying an intermediate dose until bedtime can help better meet this patient's physiological needs. The delay, however, creates the need for a third injection.
- These two examples provide ideas about how to assist the patient in adjusting insulin for optimal glucose control over 24 hours.

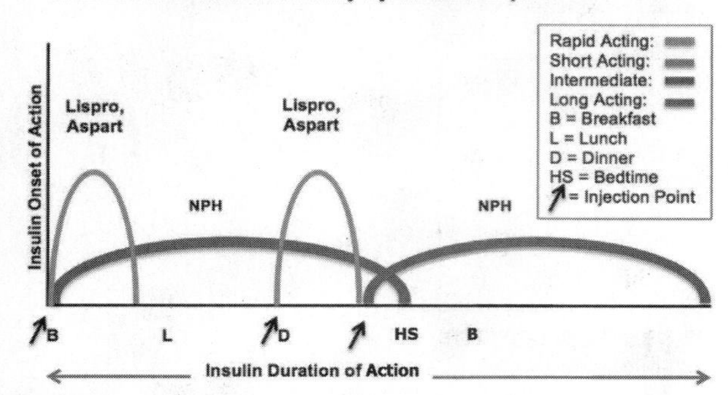

Source: Copyright © 2014, NovEx Novice to Expert Learning, LLC

LO2:

Insulin Administration

Insulin Syringes

- Insulin is dissolved in a liquid with the most common strength or concentration being 100 units of insulin per 1 milliliter (mL) of liquid.
- Insulin syringes in the United States will most likely have increments of U-100.
- These syringes may hold 1 mL or 0.5 mL, which equals 100 or 50 units of U-100 insulin respectively.
- Intravenous (IV) syringes have increments of 1 mL.
- IV syringes are frequently 3, 5, or 10 mL, which would hold 300, 500, or 1,000 units of insulin.
- ***Only insulin syringes should be used to give insulin.***

Correct

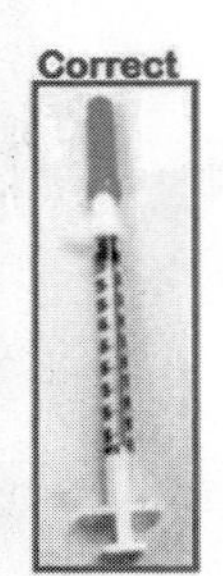

Incorrect

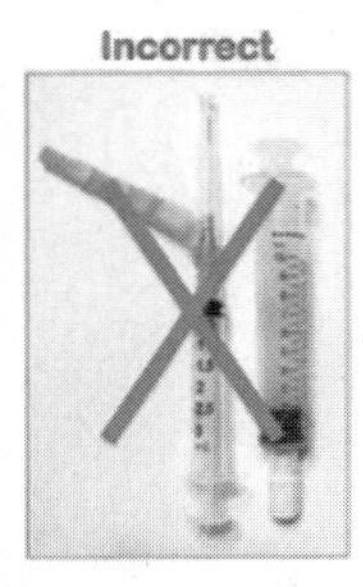

***Incorrect syringe selection and the resulting incorrect insulin dose can be harmful or fatal to the patient.**

Left: These are correct syringes to use for insulin administration. Right: Incorrect and dangerous syringes to avoid for insulin.

Concept Check

4. What is the most common kind of insulin syringe used in the United States?
   A. U-25
   B. U-50
   C. U-100
   D. U-200

Answer question

Insulin Administration (continued)

Insulin Injection Sites

- There are almost 70 easily accessible sites (shown in the chart) for rotation.
- The abdomen is commonly preferred because absorption is fastest while the arms are slower and the buttocks are slowest. The abdomen and arms are preferred for breakfast and lunch because of the rapid- or short-acting insulin used.
- This information is clinically useful. When insulin is needed to quickly act, use the abdomen. When long-acting insulin is given prior to sleep, the buttocks can be used.
- Insulin is more slowly absorbed when smoking and more rapidly absorbed after exercise when the skin temperature increases.

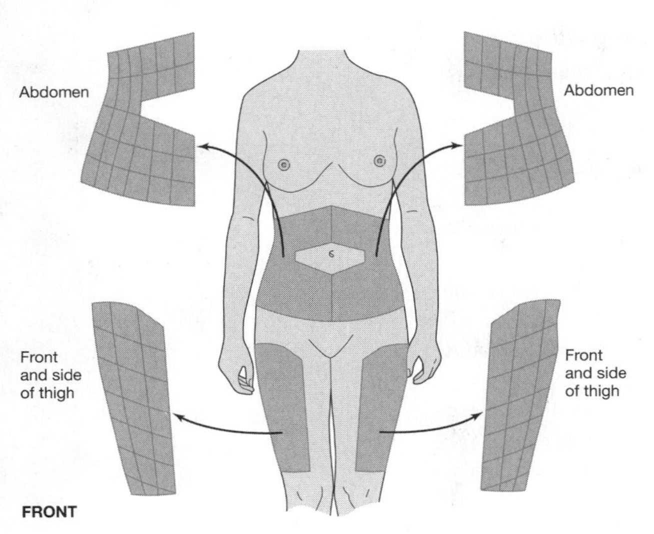

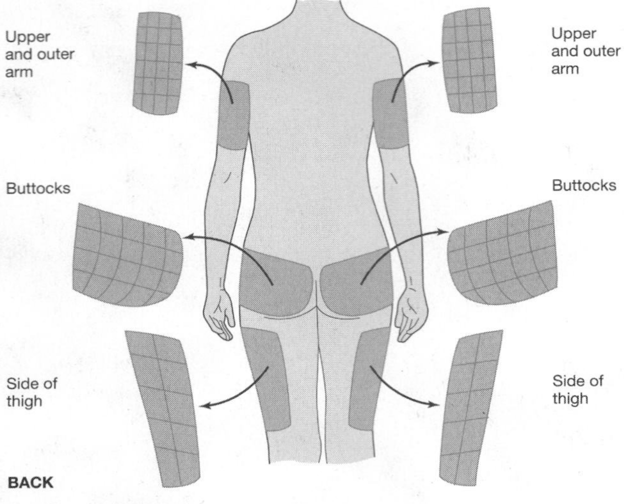

Sites for insulin injection.

- In the past, insulin injection sites were rotated to avoid the development of hard lumps and extra fat deposits. However, with the common use of human insulin, this recommendation is no longer current.
- Because insulin is absorbed at different rates with various sites, it is best to use the same region each day for specific meals to obtain a more predictable onset of action.

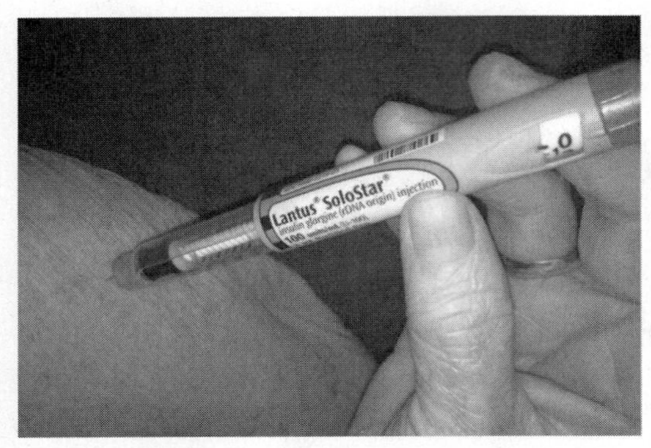

Injecting insulin.

LO2:

Insulin Precautions

Common Errors: Examples

Examples of incorrect insulin administration that can cause potential harm to your patient:

1. Administration of an ***intermediate***-acting insulin instead of a ***regular***, or ***short***-acting, insulin after meals can overdose the patient with insulin.
   - o The length of action of the ***intermediate*** insulin is 12–16 hours.
   - o Multiple doses during the day will cause the action times to overlap and cause hypoglycemia.
2. A sliding scale for dosing with ***regular*** insulin is ordered, and the blood glucose checks are performed every hour.
3. The blood glucose levels are elevated and, with every hourly reading, additional ***regular*** insulin is administered, causing an insulin overdose.
   - o The onset of action is 30–60 minutes, its peak is 2–4 hours, and duration of action for regular insulin is 6–8 hours.
   - o Hourly subcutaneous administration of regular insulin will cause the action times to overlap and cause hypoglycemia.
4. A type 1 diabetes patient is NPO for a test. The glargine insulin is held due to the patient's NPO status. The patient becomes **hyperglycemic**.
   - o Type 1 diabetics *require* a basal dose of insulin even when they are NPO.

Basal Insulin

Basal refers to the low level of insulin that is needed in the blood at all times.

- With type I diabetes, the pancreas does not make insulin, so when insulin doses are held, the body's cells are unable to utilize glucose for energy needs.
- This signals the body to break down stored glucose, which can lead to diabetic ketoacidosis (DKA).
- Unfortunately, without the basal insulin, the glucose cannot be utilized by the cells for energy.
- Often, a reduced dose (such as half the usual dose) of glargine could be administered, requiring the primary health care provider to give a one-time order.

Concept Check

5. Insulin is most quickly absorbed from which area?

A. Abdomen

B. Upper arm

C. Outer arm

D. Buttock

Answer question

LO1, 3:

Pre-Mixed Insulin

- Pre-mixed insulin is a combination of intermediate and regular insulin.
- It is usually used for non-ill persons and is often preferred in those with type 2 diabetes.
- It is difficult to adjust doses of pre-mixed insulin based on glucose readings. For those with type I diabetes, pre-mixed insulin is not recommended because they must adjust their pre-meal dosages frequently.
- Several combinations are available:
  - o 70/30 NPH/Regular Blend
  - o 50/50 NPH/Regular Blend
  - o 75/25 NPL/Humalog Blend

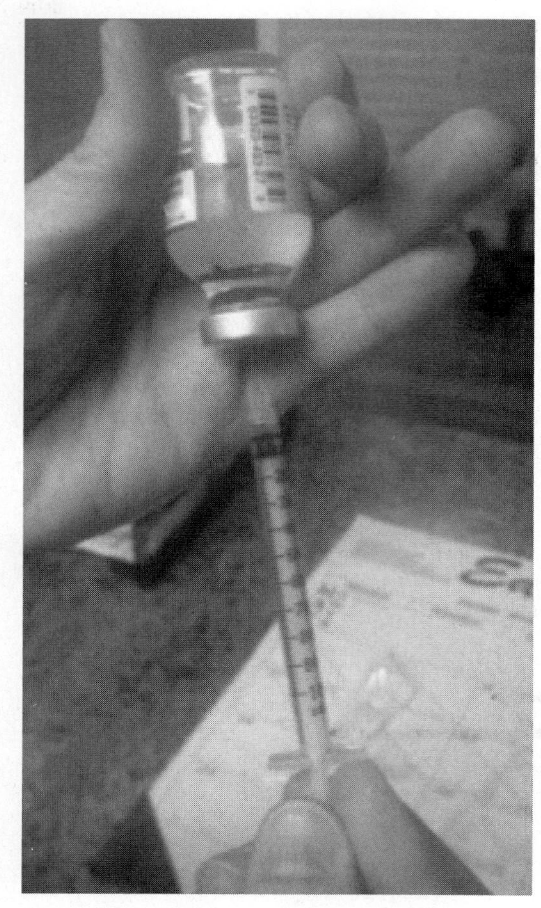

A study from Italy has found that older adult diabetic patients using self-mixed insulin commonly make errors in the measurement of their insulin. The researchers recommend using pre-mixed insulin to reduce difficulty and increase accuracy of insulin injections. The report of the study is published in *Diabetes Care*, November 1992.

LO2:

Insulin Precautions (continued)

Insulin Is a High-Alert Medication

- Medications that have the highest risk of causing harm if they are misused are called **high-alert medications**.
- In its hospital accreditation standards, The Joint Commission requires that hospitals have programs in place to reduce high-alert medication errors but leaves it up to each institution to determine how this should be accomplished.
- The Institute for Safe Medication Practices (ISMP) (1999) identified the drugs and situations that are most likely to cause harm. Insulin is among the top five medications known to have the highest risk of causing patient injury when improperly used.
- The Joint Commission recommends that insulin should be prepared by one nurse and then independently checked by a second nurse to ensure the proper dose, type, and amount of insulin that is correct for that particular dose.

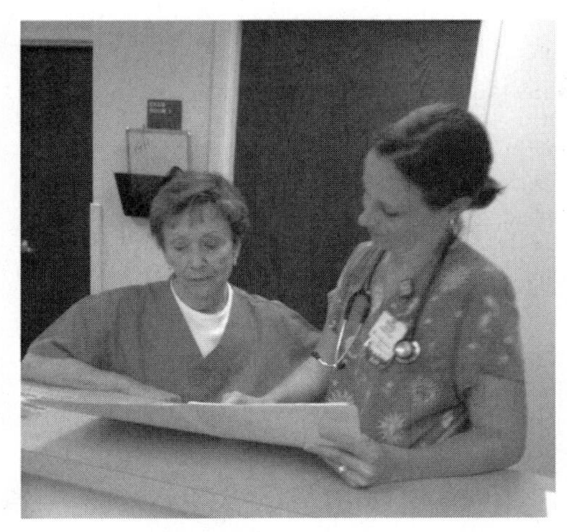

Many hospitals have created versions of a PINCH list to help nurses remember high-alert medications. **PINCH** stands for:

Patient-controlled analgesia, **P**otassium challenges, **I**nsulin drips, **N**arcotic drips, **C**hemotherapy, **H**eparin drips.

When a nurse administers a drug from this list, another nurse must double-check the order. Nurses must double-check the medication and the order at four different stages, including: when they hang the intravenous (IV) bag; when they change the IV bag; when the medication administration rate changes; and when the patient is transferred to another unit.

Source: Courtesy of R. Murphy

LO2:

Insulin Administration

Approaches

- **Sliding scale** is a term used to describe an "old" and traditional way to treat hyperglycemia. Examples are provided because, despite efforts to discourage the use of sliding scale insulin, it is still often used in current practice.
- **Basal + nutritional bolus combination** is a more physiologic way to approach glucose control as it targets prevention of hyperglycemia rather than treatment after it occurs. Basal insulin provides the constant 24-hour control, while bolus prevents predicted meal-related glucose elevations.
- **IV continuous** is a method that is usually used in a critical care setting.
- **Insulin pumps** are devices that provide a continuous subcutaneous insulin infusion and are worn by healthy individuals.
- **Carbohydrate counting** is a system that can be more precise in calculating the insulin needs of the person. This is usually used with healthy persons without cognitive impairments.

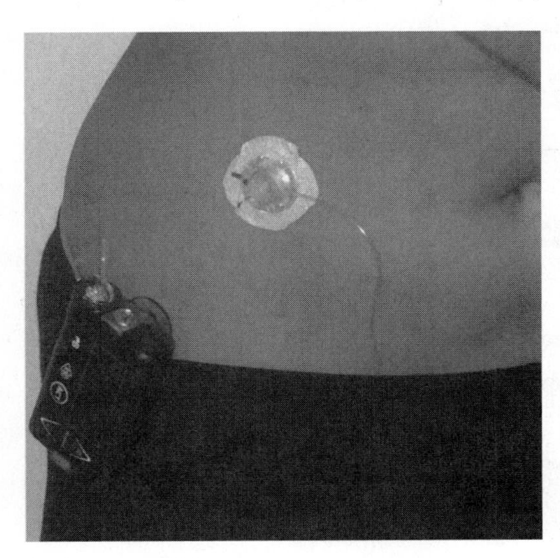

Insulin pump and infusion port.

Source: Copyright © 2014, NovEx Novice to Expert Learning, LLC

Sliding Scale Insulin (SSI) Approach

- Despite the ADA's discouragement and lack of research evidence, sliding scale insulin (SSI) is still used for glycemic control. SSI is a "reactive" rather than "proactive" approach to management, meaning that it treats hyperglycemia AFTER it occurs but does not help prevent its occurrence.
- The insulin dose is based on the blood glucose value when it is measured and is not based on the time when a meal arrives.
- This causes both **hypoglycemia** and **hyperglycemia**.
- If patients with type I DM are not given basal insulin, they are then predisposed to **dehydration** and **DKA**.
- Blood glucose levels can vary from 40 to 400, displaying a wide range.
- SSI continues to be used despite its ineffectiveness and potentially dangerous effects. Nurses have a role as change agents to improve patient care and safety.

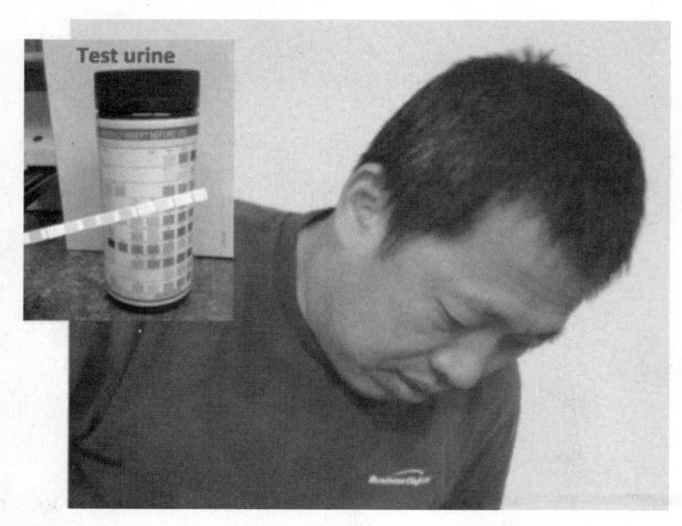

Ketoacidosis is a serious condition of glucose build-up in the blood and urine. A simple urine test can determine if high ketone levels are present. Life-saving treatment uses rapid replacement of fluids with a salt (saline) solution followed by low-dose insulin and potassium replacement.

Type of Insulin: ☐ Regular ☒ Novalog

Insulin Sliding Scale				Night (HS) Sliding Scale to prevent AM hypoglycemia	
Blood Sugar	Mild Thin, NPO, Elderly	Moderate Taking PO, Av Weight	Aggressive Steroids, infection, DM complications	Blood Sugar	Treatment
<70	Follow hypoglycemic flowchart				
70 – 150	No insulin	No insulin	No insulin	70 – 150	No insulin
151 – 200	2 units	3 units	4 units	151 – 200	No insulin
201 – 250	4 units	6 units	7 units	201 – 250	2 units
251 – 300	6 units	9 units	10 units	251 – 300	3 units
301 – 350	8 units	11 units	12 units	301 – 350	4 units
351 – 400	10 units	13 units	15 units	351 – 400	5 units
>400 call physician	12 units	15 units	17 units	>400	6 units and call physician

Signature: ______________ Date: ______________ Time: ______

Sliding scale insulin.
Source: Adapted with permission from Donna Schweitzer, RN, MSN, Bloomington, IL

Example 1: Blood glucose reading is **247** before lunch and you are using the Moderate sliding scale. You would administer **6 units** of Novalog insulin at this time. This does not address the amount of food eaten at this meal.
Example 2: If the reading at bedtime is **224**, then you administer **2 units** of Novalog insulin. The dose at night is often half of the daily dose to prevent night-time hypoglycemia.

Insulin Administration (continued)

LO2: Basal–Nutritional Bolus Insulin: Recommended Approach

- **Basal (long- or intermediate-acting)** insulin is slowly absorbed over 12 or 24 hours (depending on type given).
  - o It converts the glucose produced constantly (24 hours) by the liver into energy.
  - o It controls glucose production between meals and overnight.
  - o A constant level of insulin allows cells to take in glucose and function at all times.
- **Bolus doses with a rapid-acting insulin are given with meals.**
  - o It limits or prevents hyperglycemia after meals.
  - o The immediate rise and sharp peak at 1 hour post-meal is much like the normal physiologic activity of insulin and glucose. (See example below.)
- **Basal/bolus insulin** is currently the most effective evidence-based method of preventing glycemic events and complications.

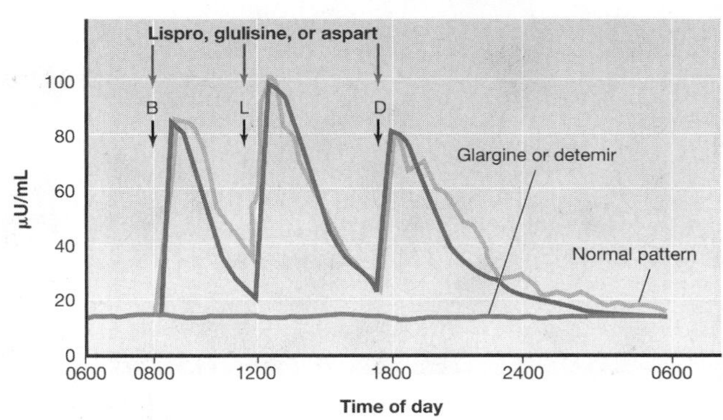

This is a current model of basal/bolus therapy. Either detemir or glargine are used as basal insulin, and then a premeal bolus is given; any one of the very rapid-acting insulin analogs (aspart, lispro, and glulisine) that closely mimics normal physiological response is much better. The peak is rapid and almost coincides with what happens with normal insulin secretion. It is a very good tool for meal control.

LO3: Glucose Management Programs

- Computer-based programs are available for hospitals to purchase.
- These programs take into account several biological factors that help determine the insulin rate.
- Management programs assist patients in targeting glucose range faster as well as preventing hypoglycemia.
- Reminds the nurse to obtain glucose reading

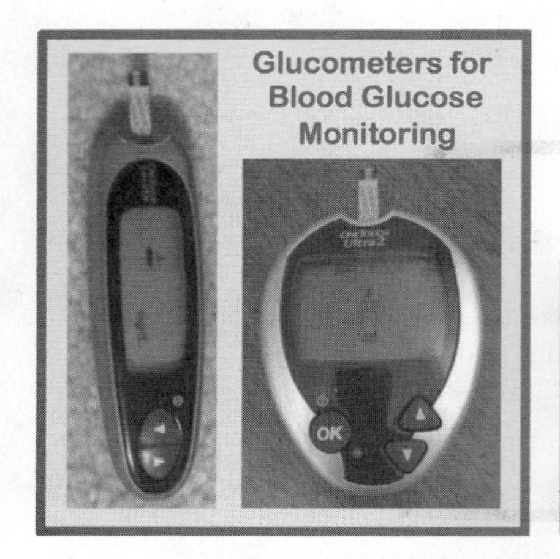

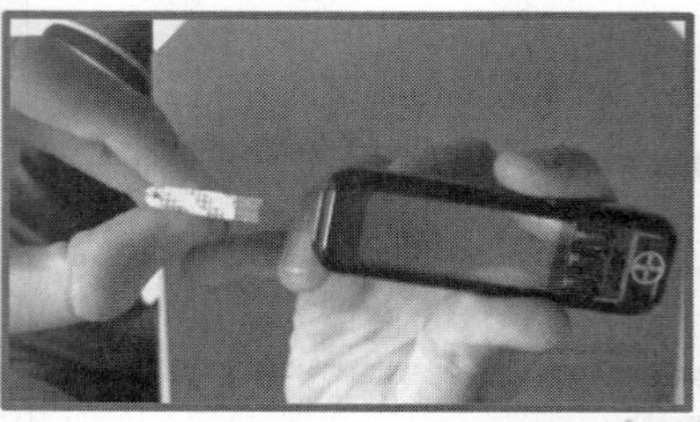
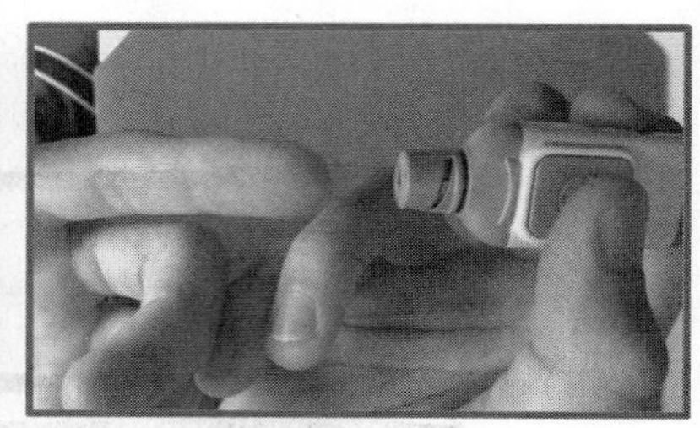
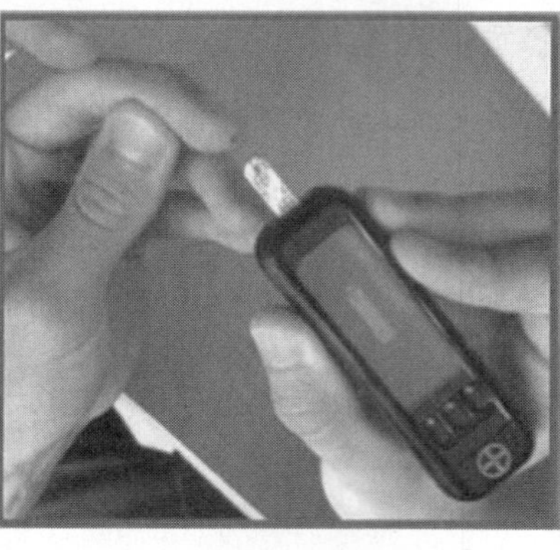
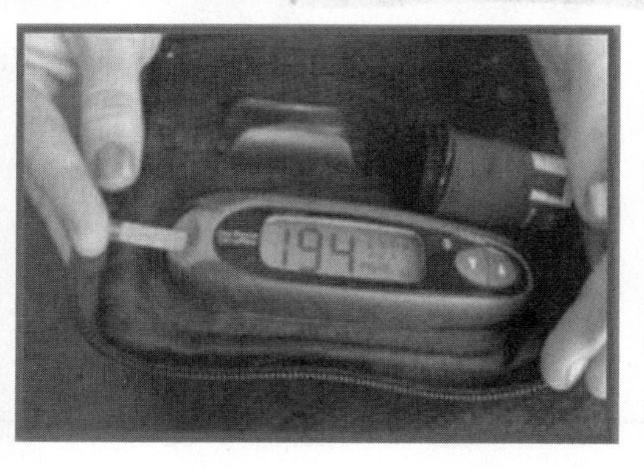

In patients with diabetes, blood glucose can be altered by many factors. So, it's important that they regularly monitor their glucose level. It is an essential daily habit in order to manage diabetes effectively and avert complications. Blood glucose monitoring requires a) a glucose meter, b) inserting a glucose test strip into the glucose meter, c) using a lancing device to prick the finger for blood, d) applying blood onto the test strip, and e) obtaining the glucose reading.

Concept Check

6. Which statement about sliding scale insulin administration is accurate?
   - A. It prevents hyperglycemia.
   - B. It is based on the time of meals.
   - C. It can cause both hyperglycemia and hypoglycemia.
   - D. Its use is supported by the ADA.

Answer question

Insulin Administration (continued)

LO3:

Carbohydrate Counting Approach

- Uses the carbohydrate content of the food to be eaten to determine mealtime insulin needs
- Carbohydrates are the macronutrient that have the most profound effect on blood glucose.
- Focuses on portion size
- The ADA recommends starting with 45–60 g per meal.

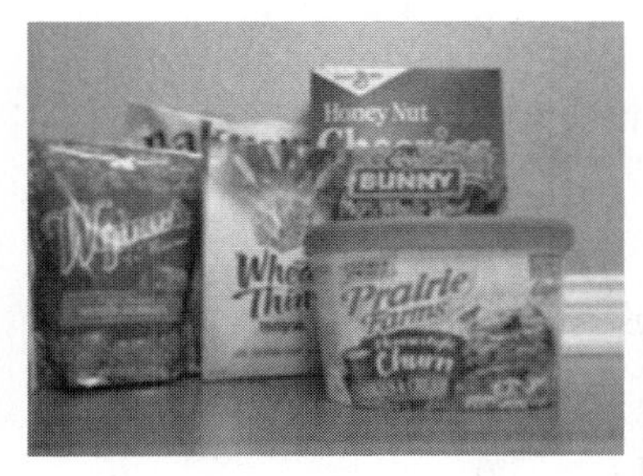

Starches contain carbohydrates and are in commonly consumed foods, like bread, cereal, rice, pasta, potatoes, crackers and corn. Starches are important energy sources. The body converts starches to glucose that can then be converted to energy. Other foods high in carbohydrates are seen in the photo. Food labels are a good source of information for carbohydrates counting.
Source: Copyright © 2014, NovEx Novice to Expert Learning, LLC

Calculating Carbohydrate/Insulin Ratio

15 Gm carb = 1 unit insulin

4 oz. juice	15 grams
½ cup oatmeal	15 grams
1 slice toast	15 grams
1 carton(1/2 pint) milk	15 grams
Total Carbohydrates	**60 gram**

Divide total carbohydrates (60) by insulin ratio (1:15)

60/15= 4 units rapid acting insulin for this meal's injection

Source: Copyright © 2014, NovEx Novice to Expert Learning, LLC

LO2:

Insulin Needs During Illness

- Blood glucose control becomes more difficult during illness or surgery.
- Type 1 diabetics ***continue to require insulin at all times, whether eating or not***. Basal, with sliding scale or bolus doses with meals, is strongly recommended.
- Close follow-up and communication with the physician is essential to manage glucose levels throughout illness and recovery.

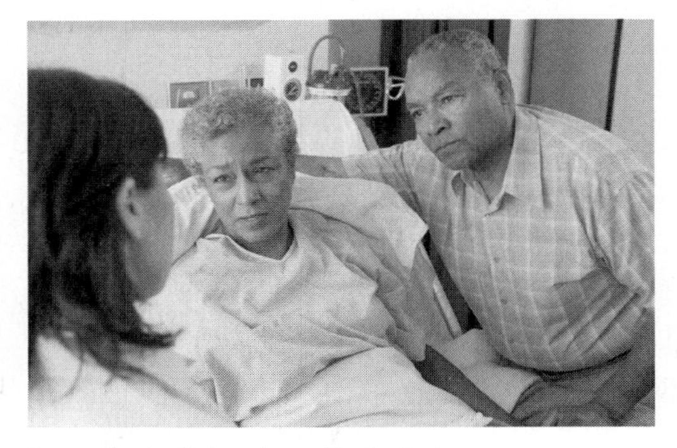

Source: Monkey Business Images/Shutterstock

LO4:

Collaborative Interventions

In this section, collaborative interventions include patients and their caregivers, when possible, as well as nurses and health care providers in order to provide patient safety and proper insulin administration:

- Mixing insulins: Draw up the clear insulin first, then the cloudy insulin (see photos).

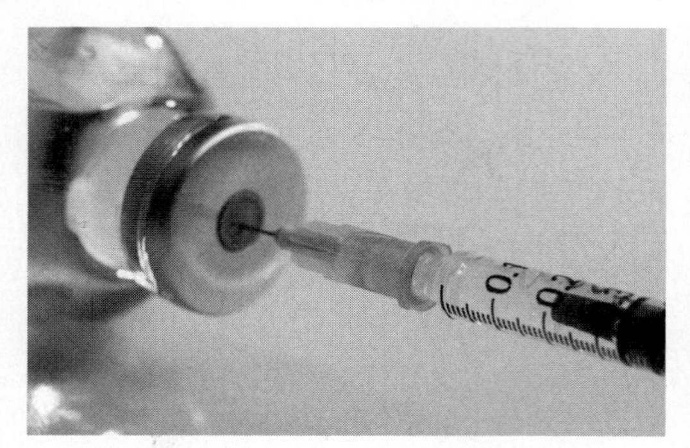
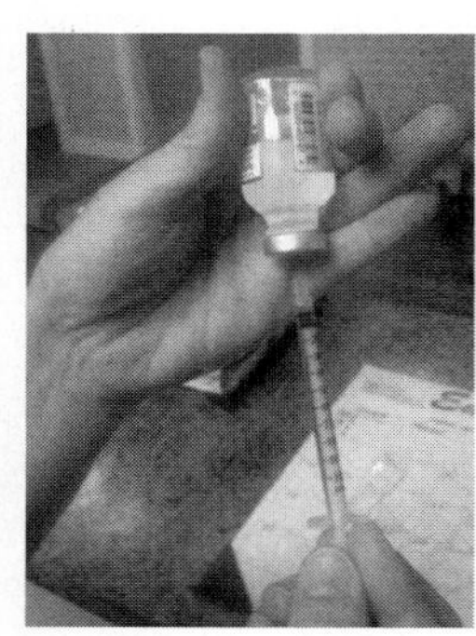

When mixing insulin for injection, draw up the clear (1), then the cloudy (2).
Sources: *(left)* Luiscar74/Shutterstock; *(right)* Courtesy of K. Kyriakidis

- High-alert medication and patient safety precautions (Joint Commission, 1999) to prevent accidental patient injury include:
  - o Strictly adhere to the hospital's medication check system that must include one nurse drawing up the correct dose and the second nurse validating the correct dose in the syringe.
  - o Do not store insulin and heparin together. The vials look very similar.
  - o When signing off on health care provider's insulin orders, ensure that "units" are spelled out. A simple "U" can be misinterpreted as a "0" and, for example, cause "4 units" to be misinterpreted as "40 units."
  - o Have a second nurse double check for the correct insulin concentration and infusion rates on an infusion pump.

- Actual procedure for injection:
  - o Wash hands.
  - o Inspect bottle (proper type of insulin, expiration date, stopper intact).
  - o Gently roll between hands.
  - o Cleanse skin with soap and water or alcohol pad.
  - o Pinch up the skin, push needle straight into the pinched-up skin at 90–45 degree angle.
  - o Push plunger all the way down, let go of pinched skin, leave needle in place for 5 seconds, and then remove.
  - o Dispose of single-use syringe safely!

- Assess patient's knowledge of and ability to perform insulin injections.

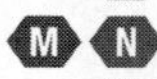

- Nutritional consult

- Diabetes educator consult

Collaborative Interventions (continued)

Patient Education and Safety

In addition to educating the patient and/or family about diabetes; recognition, prevention, and management of glycemic events; and early recognition of DKA and HHS, detailed education is needed regarding insulin to improve patient safety. Education should include:

- Evaluate and reinforce when the patient is given insulin at home (timing), which insulin is used, and in what doses.
- Teach or reinforce correct administration of insulin.
- Educate a reliable person to double-check dosages for patients who are newly insulin dependent.
- Review correct storage and care of insulin.
- Review signs and symptoms of hypoglycemia and hyperglycemia; review prevention.
- Review normal exercise patterns and meal plans.
- Review complications of insulin therapy (e.g., allergic reactions, lipodystrophy).

Concept Check

7. Which ratio is used in the carbohydrate counting method of glucose control?
   A. 15 g carbs/1 unit insulin
   B. 30 g carbs/1 unit insulin
   C. 2 units of insulin/45 g carbs
   D. 4 units of insulin/30 g carbs

Answer question

References

Cohen, M. R., & Kilo, C. M. (1999). High-alert medications: Safeguarding against errors. In M. R. Cohen (Ed.), *Medical errors*. Washington, DC: American Pharmaceutical Association.

Institute for Safe Medication Practices Medication Safety Alert. (2011). *Misadministration of IV insulin associated with dose measurement and hyperkalemia treatment.* **www.ismp.org/Newsletters/acutecare/articles/20110811.asp**

The Joint Commission Sentinal Event Alert. (1999). *High-alert medications and patient safety.* **www.jointcommission.org/assets/1/18/SEA_11.pdf**

Patient Education

American Diabetes Association. *Insulin basics.* **www.diabetes.org/living-with-diabetes/treatment-and-care/medication/insulin/insulin-basics.html**

Becton, Dickinson & Company. *Patient education.* **www.bd.com/us/diabetes/hcp/main.aspx?cat=3066&id=3120**

Fittante, A. (2011). *BD getting started fast food guide.* Franklin Lakes, NJ: Becton, Dickinson & Company. **www.bd.com/resource.aspx?IDX=23614**

Joslin Diabetes Center with Harvard Medical School. (2014). *How to improve the insulin injection experience.* **www.joslin.org/info/how_to_improve_the_insulin_injection_experience.html**

STOP

Go to the online course and complete the NovE-Cases assigned by your instructor for this module.

Learning Outcomes for Thyroid Disturbances

When you complete this lesson, you will be able to:

1. Recognize the clinical relevance of thyroid disturbances.
2. Consider the pathophysiology, etiology, risk factors, and clinical presentation of thyroid disturbance that determine the priority patient concerns.
3. Determine the most urgent and important nursing interventions and patient education required in caring for a patient with thyroid disturbance.
4. Evaluate attainment of desired collaborative care outcomes for a patient with thyroid disturbance.

LO1:

Thyroid Gland: Anatomy and Function

- The thyroid gland is located in the lower third of the anterior neck.
- The thyroid gland produces, stores, and releases into the circulation the thyroid hormones thyroxine (T4) and triiodothyronine (T3). T3 and T4 affect almost every cell in the body.
- Iodine is an essential element needed in order for the thyroid to produce hormones.
- Thyroid hormones regulate cell metabolism and affect oxygen consumption in almost every cell in the body.

Anatomy of the Thyroid Gland and Surrounding Anatomy

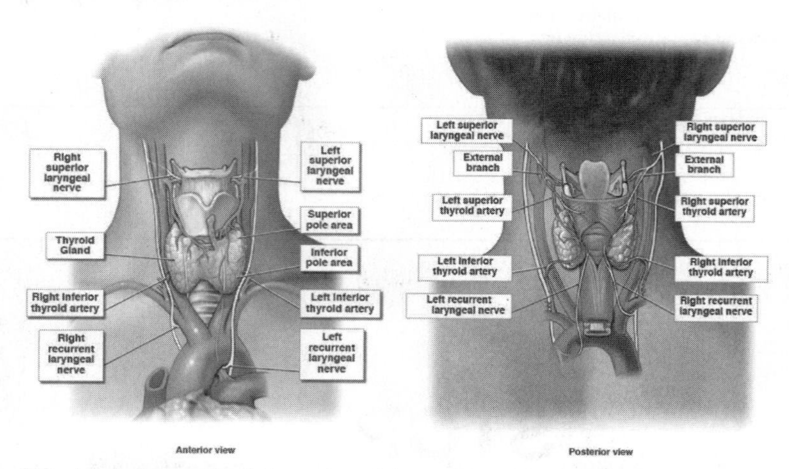

This picture shows a detailed overview of the anatomy of the thyroid gland and surrounding anatomy.

LO2:

Pathophysiology: Thyroid Disturbances

Thyroid hormones have an effect on multiple organ systems.

- Cell development
  - o The formation of proteins necessary for body function.
- Growth
  - o Thyroid hormones are essential for the healthy development of infants and children as well as continued healthy function through all stages of life.
- Metabolism
  - o Thyroid hormones regulate the metabolic activity of most tissues in the body.
- Specific body functions
  - o Cardiovascular system: Increases heart rate, contractility, and output.
  - o Central nervous system: mental function
  - o Reproductive system: necessary for normal reproduction

LO1:

What Are Thyroid Disturbances?

Thyroid disturbances commonly include:

- **Hyperthyroidism**, or excessive secretion of thyroid hormones, causes increased body metabolism.
- **Hypothyroidism**, or under secretion of thyroid hormones, causes decreased body metabolism.
- **Goiter** is an enlargement of the thyroid gland that can put pressure on surrounding structures.

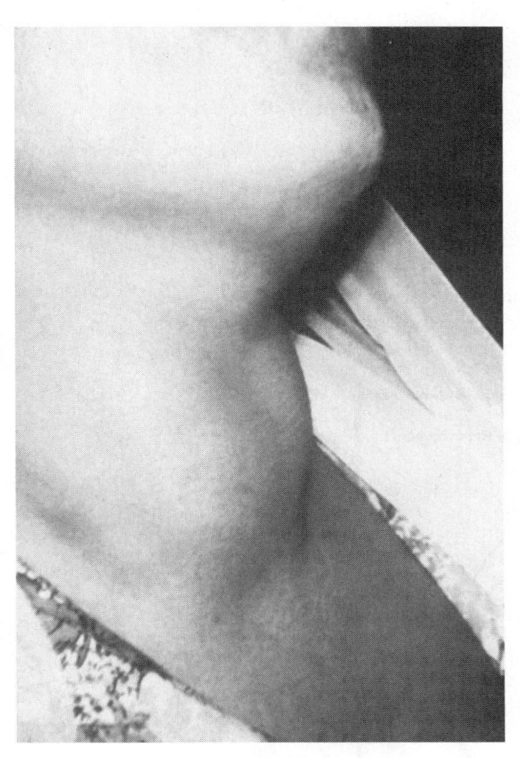

This photo displays a young woman with a very large goiter or enlarged thyroid gland, commonly found in hypothyroidism.
Source: Centers for Disease Control and Prevention

- **Nodules** are growths (fluid filled or solid) on the thyroid gland.
- **Cancer** of the thyroid is a common malignancy with an excellent long-term survival rate after treatment. There are several types of thyroid cancers. Papillary carcinomas comprise 80% of all thyroid cancers and often affect women between 20–55 years of age.

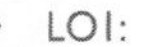

Clinical Relevance

- In the United States, approximately 10% of the population has hypothyroidism, while another 10% has an autoimmune form of thyroid disease, which may result in either hyperthyroidism or hypothyroidism.
- Almost 90% of people who reach their 80s have had a thyroid issue, primarily hypothyroidism.
- Thyroid cancer is the most common endocrine cancer, with fatalities 2:1 for men as compared to women.
- There are four types of thyroid cancer: papillary, follicular, anaplastic, and other. The majority are highly responsive to treatment and most (97.7%) are curable, depending on the stage at diagnosis.
- Most thyroid cancer occurs in women over 40 years of age.
- It is the sixth most common cause of cancer in women.
- Thyroid disease is one of the most common endocrine diseases.
- Thyroid disturbances may initially manifest with the new onset of many medical conditions, such as cardiac disease, making it important to assess thyroid function during the work-up of new onset of conditions.
- Hypothyroidism is often unrecognized. Therefore, many cases remain undiagnosed or misdiagnosed.

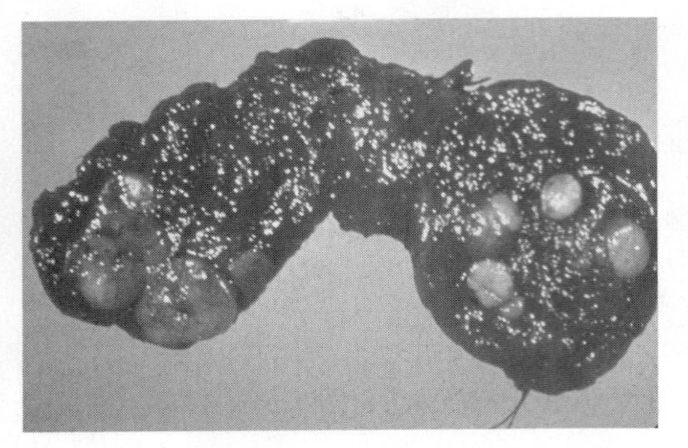

This photo reveals the severely invaded thyroid gland by cancer nodules.
Source: Dr. Jeffrey Norton/NCI Visuals Online

LO2:

Pathophysiology: Thyroid Regulation

The proper balance of thyroid hormones is controlled by the hypothalamus–pituitary–thyroid axis (see diagram). Synthesis and secretion of thyroid hormones also depend on the presence of adequate iodine and tyrosine, which are building blocks for thyroid hormones.

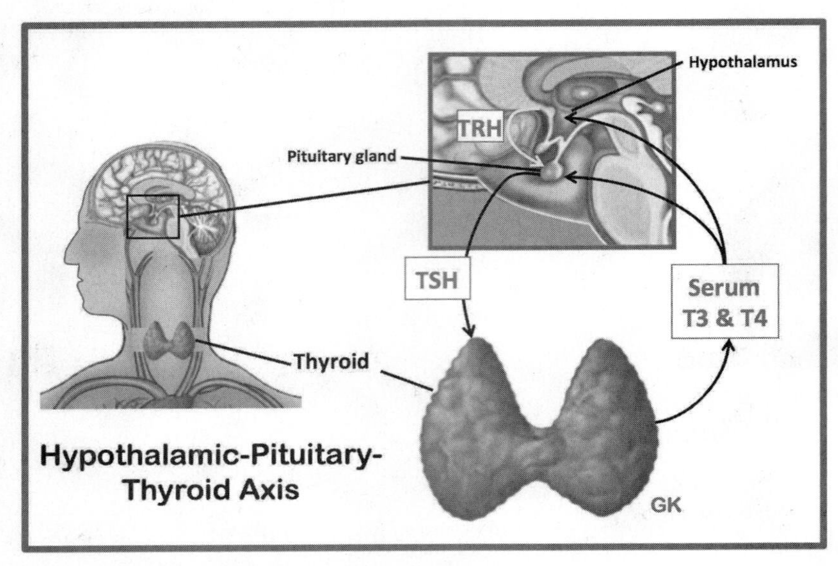

The normal hypothalamic-pituitary-thyroid axis.
Source: Courtesy of George Kyriakidis/Santa Ana, CA

- The hypothalamus produces thyrotropin-releasing hormone (TRH), which stimulates the pituitary gland to produce thyroid-stimulating hormone.
- Thyroid-stimulating hormone (TSH) in turn stimulates the thyroid to produce, and release T4 and T3 into the systemic circulation.
- Circulating T4 is converted into T3 (more active form of the hormone) by the liver, further increasing the circulating T3.
- Circulating hormones are taken up by cells affecting their metabolism. T4 can also be converted to more active form T3 by most cells.
- Both systemic T3 and T4 will inhibit release of TRH and TSH.

Thyroid Regulation Summary

- The amount of thyroid hormones T3 and T4 in the body is regulated by the pituitary gland and the hypothalamus. When the amount of thyroid hormones in the body decreases (see pictorial cycle):
    - o The pituitary releases TSH.
    - o The hypothalamus increases its production of TRH, which signals the pituitary to release more TSH.
- Both feedback loops cause the thyroid to release more T3 and T4.

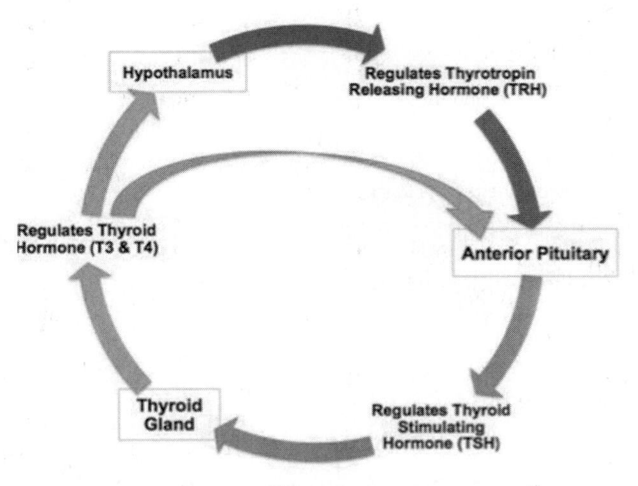

Thyroid regulation feedback loop.
Source: Copyright © 2014, NovEx Novice to Expert Learning, LLC

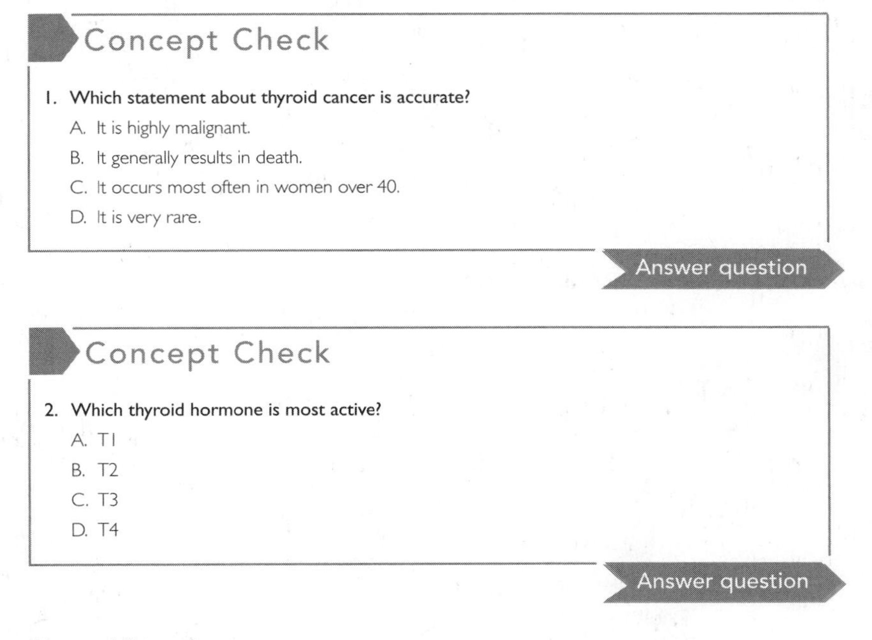
Concept Check

1. **Which statement about thyroid cancer is accurate?**
   A. It is highly malignant.
   B. It generally results in death.
   C. It occurs most often in women over 40.
   D. It is very rare.

Answer question

Concept Check

2. **Which thyroid hormone is most active?**
   A. T1
   B. T2
   C. T3
   D. T4

Answer question

Thyroid Disturbances

- **Hyperthyroidism** is the *overproduction* of thyroid hormone caused by overactive tissue in the thyroid gland. Since the thyroid controls the metabolic rate of cells in the body, this overproduction causes symptoms of *hypermetabolism*.
- **Hypothyroidism** is characterized by the *underproduction* of thyroid hormone, thus providing an insufficient supply to the body. This deficit downregulates the metabolism of cells, causing symptoms of *hypometabolism*.

LO2:

Risk Factors: Thyroid Disturbances

Conditions that can affect or disrupt the appropriate balance of thyroid hormones:

- Lack of iodine, which is essential in the production of thyroid hormones
- Pituitary tumors that result in decreased production of TSH
- Stimulation of the thyroid by antibodies causing overproduction of thyroid hormones
- Damage to the thyroid that can cause decreased production of thyroid hormones. Acute damage can also briefly cause release of stored thyroid hormones.

LO2:

Diagnostics: Thyroid Disturbances

*Note that "normal" lab values may vary from one reference to another. Many lab values are ranges rather than exact numbers. Recognizing meaningful abnormal values and following the patient's trend are the key points in "monitoring lab values."

- A combination of tests is needed to fully assess thyroid function.
- Each test, when run alone, will not give enough information to assess the thyroid function.
- Thyroid-stimulating hormone (TSH) is produced in the pituitary gland. TSH is released to stimulate the thyroid gland to produce T3 and T4. A normal value is 0.4 to 6 mU/L.
- Assessing the pituitary function by measuring TSH is necessary to develop a clear picture about the origin of an abnormality, which in turn can guide treatment.
- **T3** radioimmunoassay: Normal value is 75–195 ng/dL.
- **T4** radioimmunoassay: Normal is 4.5–11.2 ug/dL. This test measures *bound* and *unbound* T4 in the serum, which is not as helpful as a measurement of the free T4.
- **Free T4** (T4 not bound to protein): Normal is 0.7 to 2 ng/dL. This is a better measure of the T4 that is available for uptake by cells.

Interpreting Thyroid Tests

When the pathology is in the thyroid itself, the following patterns are seen in the serum levels of TSH and T3 and T4:

Thyroid Disorder	TSH	T3/T4
Hyperthyroidism	Low	High
Hypothyroidism	High	Low

Source: Copyright © 2014, NovEx Novice to Expert Learning, LLC

Other patterns are seen when the problem originates in the pituitary or hypothalamus.

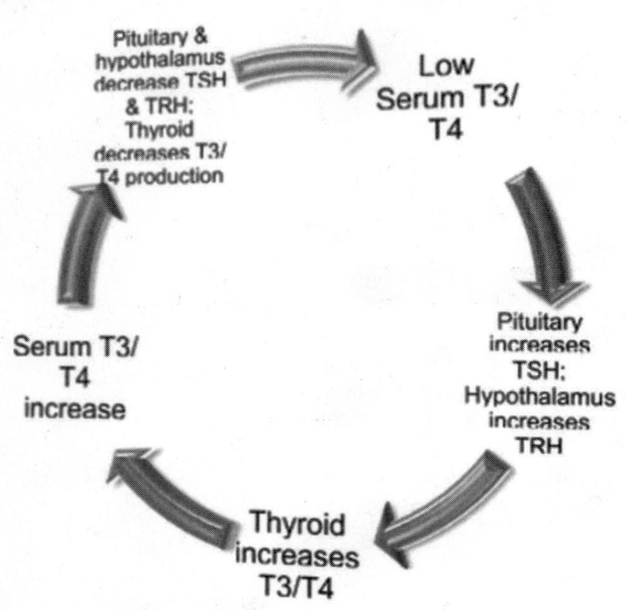

Thyroid Feedback Cycle. TSH = thyroid-stimulating hormone; TRH = thyrotropin-releasing hormone.
Source: Copyright © 2014, NovEx Novice to Expert Learning, LLC

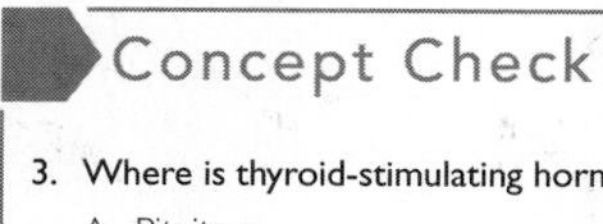

Concept Check

3. Where is thyroid-stimulating hormone (TSH) produced?
   A. Pituitary
   B. Hypothalamus
   C. Thyroid
   D. Parathyroid

Answer question

Diagnostics: Thyroid Disturbances (continued)

Thyroid Antibodies

- Autoimmune diseases occur when the body produces antibodies against tissues normally found in the body.
- **Hashimoto's thyroiditis and Graves' disease** are autoimmune diseases. Identifying the antibody can help determine the autoimmune thyroid disease as well as guide the treatment of the disease.
- **Hashimoto's disease:** Presence of **anti-thyroid peroxidase (anti-TPO)** and **anti-thyroglobulin (anti-Tg) antibodies** is a strong indicator. Definitive diagnosis is made by histological findings.
- **Graves' disease:** Presence of **thyroid-stimulating immunoglobulins (TSI)** is diagnostic.

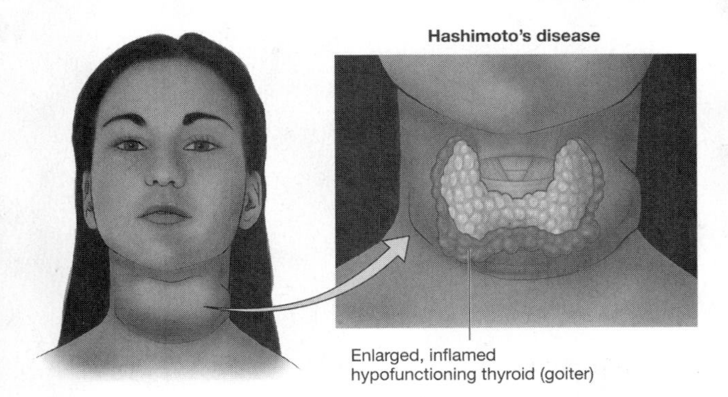

Hashimoto's disease is a chronic thyroiditis. It is a persistent inflammatory problem in the thyroid that develops slowly over time. It frequently causes hypothyroidism. The incidence is most common in middle-aged women.

Thyroid Assessment

Imaging

- **Radioactive iodine uptake:** The thyroid is the only area of the body that absorbs iodine.
  - o To test the thyroid function, a radioactive iodine liquid or pill is swallowed. The amount of iodine absorbed by the thyroid is measured and then compared to the dosage ingested.
  - o The measurements are usually obtained 6–24 hours after administering the iodine, using a device called a gamma probe.

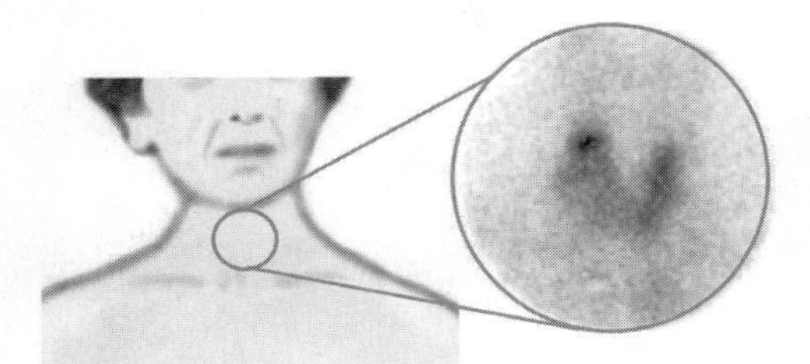

This diagram shows nuclear thyroid scan or radioactive iodine uptake test results. A normal thyroid uptake shows the outline of the entire thyroid gland. This image reveals prominent areas in the lower thyroid of decreased activity (reduced production of thyroid hormone) and corresponds with a large nodule in the patient's multinodular goiter.
Source: Courtesy of K. Kyriakidis

- **CT scan or ultrasound:** These noninvasive imaging tests can be used to look at the size and shape of the thyroid and the surrounding structures. Ultrasound is the most common imaging test utilized for thyroid disease. Nodules or cysts can be located for possible needle biopsy.

Biopsy

- Fine needle aspiration biopsy (FNAB): The biopsied tissue allows for a close exam of the thyroid cells and for the presence of cancer cells.

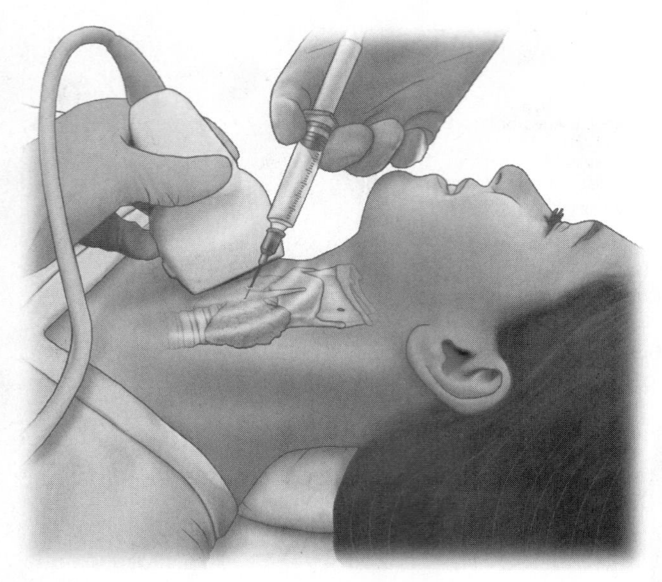

A very thin needle is used for aspiration biopsy. It is the most accurate test for evaluating thyroid nodules. Ultrasound can guide the needle biopsy of nodules so that nodular cells can be aspirated into the needle. The biopsied cells can then be examined by a cytologist.

Priority Patient Concerns and Desired Collaborative Care Outcomes: Thyroid Disturbances

Prior to caring for patients with thyroid disturbances, it is important to prioritize the patient's concerns that must guide the nursing care plan and interventions. Care for the patient is ordered and organized in accordance with the patient's priority and urgent needs. Desired collaborative care outcomes in patients with thyroid disturbances typically include:

1. Patient will demonstrate growing acceptance of current physical appearance and discuss rationale for their appearance.
2. Patient will maintain or return to desired body weight.
3. Patient will accurately discuss prescribed collaborative plan of care to improve symptoms.
4. Patient will report energy level adequate to maintain activities of daily living and periods of recuperative rest.

Considering these important care outcomes, prepare a list of the major 3-6 priority patient concerns or nursing diagnoses for patients with thyroid disturbances. Be prepared to participate in a discussion of this list and/or to submit them as an assignment, as determined by your faculty. Resources you may find helpful in this assignment can include this lesson, the references, resources on nursing care plans, and standard nursing diagnoses manuals.

LO2:

Hypothyroidism

Causes

- **Hashimoto's thyroiditis** is an autoimmune inflammation of the thyroid gland. The inflammation damages thyroid cells and makes them unable to produce T3 or T4.
  - o Hashimoto's thyroiditis is the most common cause of hypothyroidism in the United States in those over 6 years of age.
- Medical treatments to remove thyroid tissue such as surgery (removal when too little tissue remains to produce hormones) or radioablation (radioactive iodine therapy) of the thyroid is used to treat thyroid cancer.
- Lack of dietary iodine intake, not usually a problem in the United States, causes hypothyroidism and results in increased growth of thyroid tissue. Dietary iodine is needed to make T3 and T4.

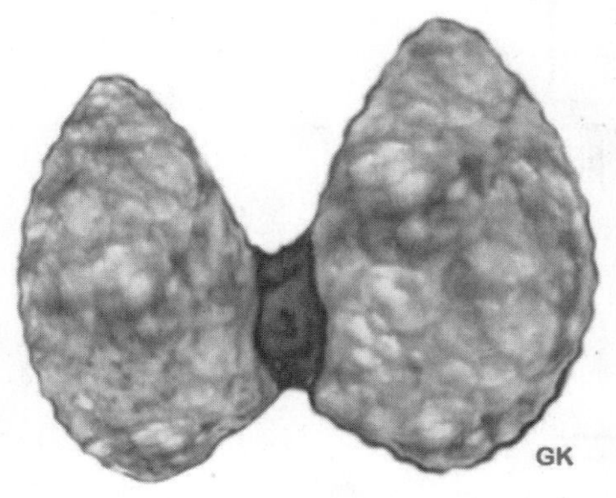

This photo shows the chronic lymphocytic inflammation seen in Hashimoto's thyroiditis. Note that the thyroid (both lobes) are invaded by the whitish nodular appearing tissue.
Source: Courtesy of George Kyriakidis/Santa Ana, CA

LO2:

Assessment Findings

Hypothyroidism is often overlooked by the patient because the onset of symptoms is usually gradual and slowly becomes increasingly apparent:

- Fatigue
- Weakness
- Weight gain or difficulty losing weight despite reduced food intake
- Coarse, dry hair and skin; hair loss
- Sensitivity to cold
- Muscle cramps and aches
- Constipation
- Depression
- Irritability
- Memory loss
- Abnormal menstrual cycles
- Decreased libido
- Slowed speech (severe cases)
- Jaundice (severe cases)
- Increase in tongue size (severe cases)

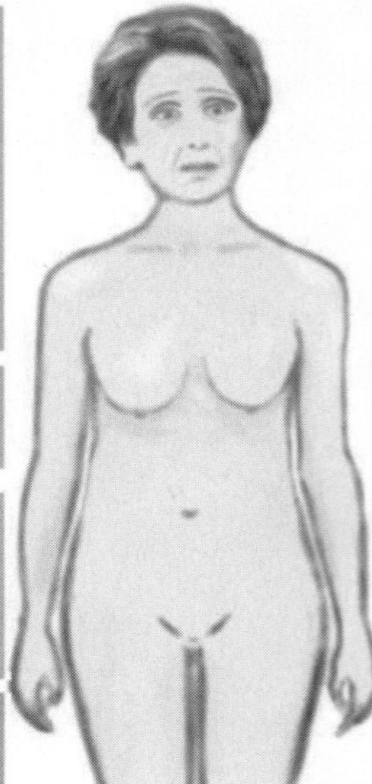

Effects of hypothyroidism on numerous organs.
Source: Courtesy of George Kyriakidis/Santa Ana, CA

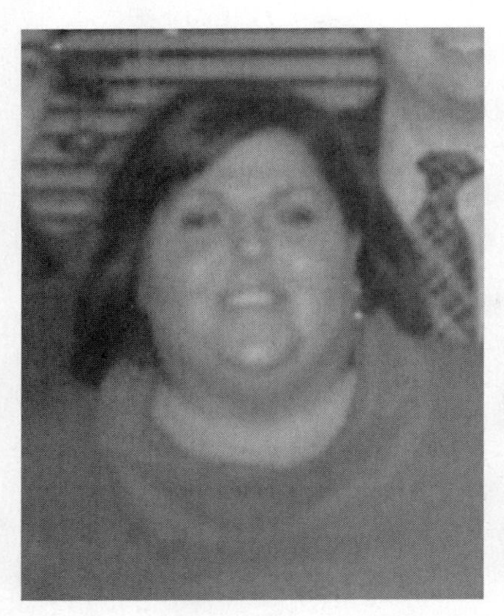

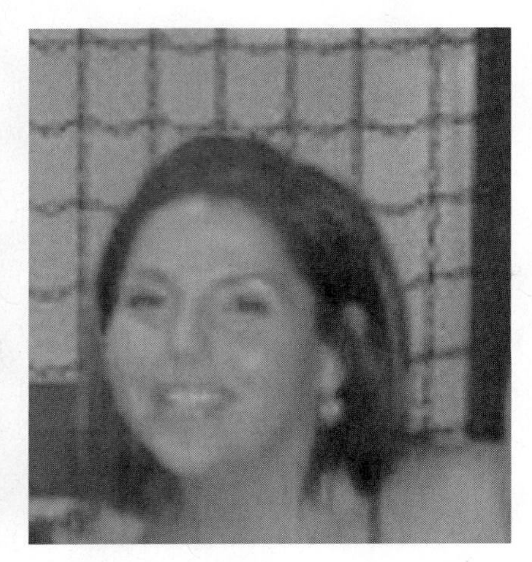

Before and after treatment of hypothyroidism.
Source: *(both)* Courtesy of R. Murphy

Concept Check

4. Which finding is associated with hypothyroidism?
   - A. Heat intolerance
   - B. Weight loss
   - C. Muscle weakness
   - D. Constipation

Answer question

Hypothyroidism (continued)

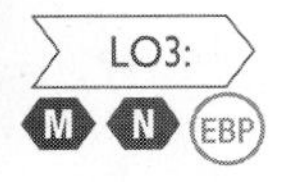

Collaborative Interventions

Hypothyroidism is usually a lifelong condition requiring lifelong treatment. Evidence-based practice recommendations (Garber, et al., 2012) include:

- The treatment of choice is synthetic thyroxine (T4), **levothyroxine**, an oral medication that is taken daily. Monotherapy is recommended.
- Doses may vary according to the individual patient's needs and level of thyroid function.
- Frequent blood test monitoring is usually needed at the beginning of treatment until the correct dose is identified.
- After finding the optimum dose, monitoring can usually be performed yearly.
- Iodine supplements and selenium should not be used to prevent or help manage hypothyroidism.

Supportive Care

Patients are commonly examined and diagnosed with hypothyroidism in an outpatient setting. Supportive care typically includes:

- Observe for early complications of hyperthyroidism in follow-up visits and educate the patient about the signs and symptoms.
- Educate patient regarding importance of medications and collaborate regarding a medication regimen.
- Teach patient about the lifelong requirement of thyroid replacement therapy.

Emergencies: Myxedema Coma

Myxedema coma or crisis is severe hypothyroidism and the cascade of metabolic problems that develop. Long-term and unrecognized or untreated hypothyroidism can lead to the life-threatening complication of myxedema coma.

- Myxedema coma arises from severe metabolic disorders: Hyponatremia, lactic acidosis, and hypoglycemia.
- Severe symptoms of hypothyroidism include hypothermia, severe hypotension that can progress to cardiovascular collapse, hypoventilation, bradycardia, decreased mental status, or coma.
- Infection, medication interactions, failure to take thyroid medications, and trauma are some conditions that precipitate this crisis.
- Treatments must be immediate and aggressive to prevent death. Evidence-based practice recommendations (Garber, et al., 2012) are highlighted:

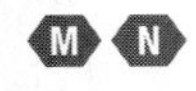

  o Transfer patient to ICU. Patient requires close monitoring and intervention, possibly mechanical ventilation.

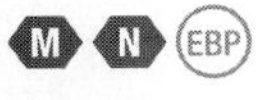

  o Administer thyroid hormones IV. Gastrointestinal absorption can be impaired. Combination T4 and T3 replacement therapy is recommended.

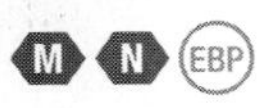

  o Give glucocorticoids unless adrenal insufficiency can be ruled out as a coexisting problem.

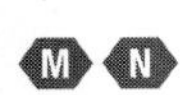

  o Identify and treat the cause as soon as possible (e.g., infection, trauma, failure to take prescribed medications, use of antidepressants).

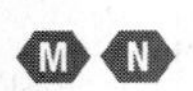

- Symptom Management and Comfort Care
  o Ensure good IV access for fluid (no hypotonic fluids), electrolyte, glucose, and medication administration.
  o Correct hypothermia using a warming blanket. Caution is warranted as rewarming can exacerbate the vasodilatation and consequently the hypotension.
  o Treat hypotension with fluid if volume depleted, with thyroid hormones if not severe, and by adding a vasopressor if severe, until T4 can correct the vascular problems.

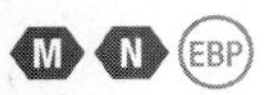

  o Use caution with opioids as these patients are hypersensitive to normal doses.
  o Closely monitor for early signs of complications, such as cardiac dysrhythmias, myocardial infarction, hemodynamic collapse, decreasing level of consciousness, increasing thyroid hormone levels.

LO2:

Hyperthyroidism

Causes

- **Graves' disease** is the most common cause of hyperthyroidism in the United States.
  - o It is an autoimmune disease caused by the production of antibodies that attach to the activating sites on the thyroid gland. This causes the gland to increase the production of T3 and T4.
  - o The thyroid gland becomes enlarged, creating a **goiter**.
  - o Graves' disease usually affects women in their 30s and 40s.
- Three common symptoms of Graves' disease are:
  - o Hypermetabolism
  - o Inflammation around the eyes causing swelling with occasional bulging of the eyes (exophthalmos) and blurred or double vision
  - o Pretibial myxedema or thickening of the lower leg skin and acropachy (swelling in hands and fingers)
- Toxic nodular goiter: nodule(s) that produce excess thyroid hormones
- Thyroiditis or inflammation of the thyroid gland
- Excess intake of thyroid hormones

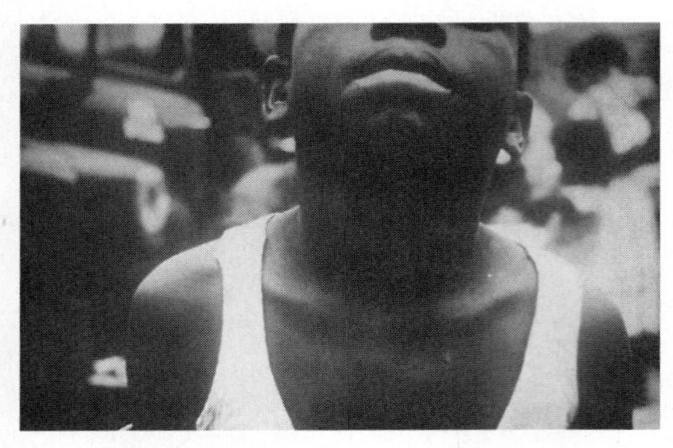

Goiter on the neck.
Source: Centers for Disease Control and Prevention

LO2:

Assessment Findings

Symptoms usually start out slowly and become increasingly apparent. Initially, the symptoms are commonly mistaken for nervousness due to stress:

- Palpitations or fast heart rate
- Heat intolerance
- Warm moist skin
- Nervousness
- Breathlessness
- Weight loss
- Increased bowel movements
- Light or absent menstrual periods
- Fatigue
- Insomnia
- Trembling hands
- Muscle weakness
- Hair loss
- Staring gaze
- Exopthalmos (primarily in Graves' disease)

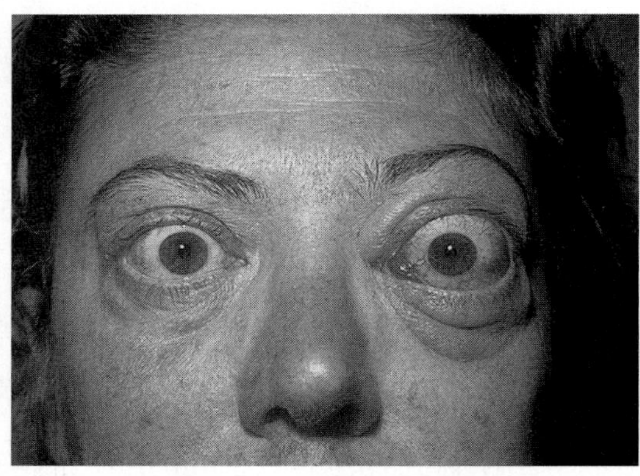

Patients with chronic or very acute hyperthroidism may develop exophthalmos or bulging of the eyes. Swelling of fat deposits and the muscles around the eyes cause the eyes to bulge outward.

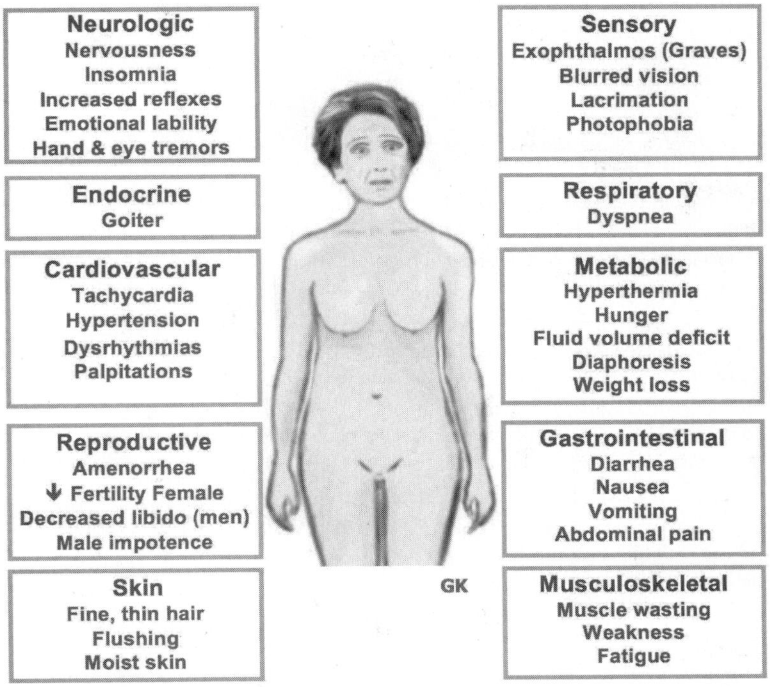

Neurologic
Nervousness
Insomnia
Increased reflexes
Emotional lability
Hand & eye tremors

Endocrine
Goiter

Cardiovascular
Tachycardia
Hypertension
Dysrhythmias
Palpitations

Reproductive
Amenorrhea
↓ Fertility Female
Decreased libido (men)
Male impotence

Skin
Fine, thin hair
Flushing
Moist skin

Sensory
Exophthalmos (Graves)
Blurred vision
Lacrimation
Photophobia

Respiratory
Dyspnea

Metabolic
Hyperthermia
Hunger
Fluid volume deficit
Diaphoresis
Weight loss

Gastrointestinal
Diarrhea
Nausea
Vomiting
Abdominal pain

Musculoskeletal
Muscle wasting
Weakness
Fatigue

GK

Effects of hyperthyroidism on numerous organs.
Source: Courtesy of George Kyriakidis/Santa Ana, CA

Hyperthyroidism (continued)

LO3:

Collaborative Interventions

The goal of treatment for hyperthyroidism is to diminish the amount of thyroid hormones being produced. Evidence-based practice guidelines from the American Association of Clinical Endocrinologists (Bahn, et al., 2011) recommend:

M N EBP

- **Beta blockers** (e.g., metoprolol, atenolol) are used to decrease the symptoms of hypermetabolism (e.g., palpitations, heat intolerance, nervousness, anxiety). Beta blockers do not affect the production of T3/ T4 but are used in acute situations to control symptoms until treatment to lower thyroid levels takes effect.

M N EBP

- **Thionamides** (e.g., propylthiouracil, methimazole)
  - o Can be taken to prevent the thyroid gland from making as much T3/T4
  - o Should be used in every patient who takes antithyroid therapy for Graves' disease
  - o Consider use prior to radioactive iodine in select patients.
  - o Pretreat patients going to surgery with methimazole to attain a euthyroid state.

M N EBP

- **Radioactive iodine** (RAI) can be used when a more permanent treatment is desired. Since the thyroid is the only area of the body that absorbs iodine, thyroid cells are killed by the radioactivity, resulting in less production of T3/T4.
  - o Administer sufficient radiation in a single dose to treat hyperthyroidism.
  - o Retreat with RAI if hyperthyroidism persists.

M N EBP

- **Surgical removal** of part or all of the thyroid gland can also permanently lower thyroid levels.
  - o Should have a total or near-total thyroidectomy if surgery is the primary intervention
  - o Should refer the patient to a high-volume thyroid surgeon
  - o Beta blockers and antithyroid medications should be weaned postoperatively.

Symptom Management and Comfort Care

After thyroidectomy, in addition to routine postoperative care, patient care commonly necessitates the following:

- Pain management is essential with analgesics.
- Elevate the head of bed to a semi-Fowler's position and use pillows to support the head and neck for comfort.
- Administer thyroid hormone replacement therapy, as prescribed, and give 1 hour prior to or 2 hours after meals to optimize absorption.
- Wound care and drain management are important to prevent infection and complications.
- Monitor for hypocalcemia or hypoparathyroidism (damage to parathyroid which lies in close proximity to thyroid).
- Monitor for digitalis toxicity, glycemic events, and/or bleeding times if the patient is on a digitalis preparation, insulin, and/or anticoagulants. Thyroid replacements can potentiate or alter digitalis, insulin, and anticoagulant effects.
- Observe for complications such as vocal cord injury, bleeding or hemorrhage, edema, respiratory distress, hypothyroidism, and laryngeal nerve damage.

Concept Check

5. Why are beta blockers given to patients with thyroid disturbances?

A. They decrease T3 production.

B. They increase T4 production.

C. They reduce the effects of hyperthyroidism.

D. They potentiate the action of other thyroid medications.

Answer question

Emergencies: Thyrotoxic Storm

Thyrotoxic (or thyroid) storm is a life-threatening but rare complication of thyrotoxicosis (too much thyroid hormone in the body).

- Hyperthyroidism (thyroid gland overproduces thyroid hormones) can cause thyroid storm. Excessive thyroid hormones cause the metabolic rate to rapidly rise. Without immediate and appropriate intervention, the mortality rate is high.
- The clinical manifestations overlap those of hyperthyroidism, but are more severe. Severe symptoms can include: high systolic but low diastolic blood pressure, tachycardia, extreme agitation, fevers up to 106°F, shock, delirium, jaundice, heart failure, coma, and death.
- It may be precipitated by trauma, infection, surgery (particularly thyroid surgery), severe thyrotoxicosis, noncompliance with therapies, and comorbid conditions.

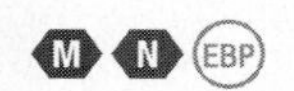

- Evidence-based treatment recommendations include (Bahn, et al., 2011):
    - o Transfer patient to ICU. They require close monitoring and intervention.
    - o Treat the precipitating factors.
    - o Initiate beta blockers immediately to control heart rate and reduce thyroid hormone synthesis.
    - o Give thionamides, preferably propylthiouracil (PTU) over methimazole, in severe situations to block thyroid hormone synthesis.
    - o Give iodine solution to prevent an increase in thyroid hormones that may be stored. Delay administration for 1–2 hours to prevent immediate synthesis of more thyroid hormones.
    - o Administer glucocorticoids (e.g., hydrocortisone) to replenish cortisol.

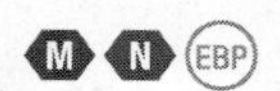

- Symptom Management and Comfort Care
    - o Secure IV access for fluid and electrolyte replacement and medication administration. Dextrose solutions may be needed to replace glycogen stores.
    - o Place NG tube as needed.
    - o Administer oxygen therapy, guided by SpO_2 and/or blood gases.
    - o Closely monitor vital signs, cardiac rhythm via EKG monitor, electrolytes, physical findings, patient responses, intake and output, bleeding times and blood counts, and early signs of deterioration (e.g., shock).
    - o Provide cooling blanket, antipyretics, or fan to reduce high fever while avoiding shivering. Use acetaminophen instead of aspirin or salicylates, which increase thyroid hormone circulating levels.
    - o Hemodynamic monitoring may be needed in severe situations.

Concept Check

6. The patient experiencing thyrotoxicosis would be best cared for in which area?

A. Intensive care unit

B. Home

C. Regular medical/surgical unit

D. Operating room

Answer question

LO2:

Thyroid Goiters

Causes

- **Hypothyroidism** is the most common cause of a goiter. When decreased production of thyroid hormones is detected through the pituitary-thyroid feedback loop, the pituitary gland increases production of TSH (thyroid-stimulating hormone) to stimulate the thyroid to make more T3 and T4. This stimulation will cause an increased growth of thyroid tissue.
- **Lack of dietary iodine intake** causes hypothyroidism and results in increased growth of thyroid tissue.
- Graves' disease causes the thyroid to enlarge, resulting in **hyperthyroidism**.
- A **nodule** or cancer growing in the thyroid creates enlargement of the gland.

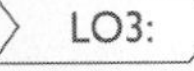

Collaborative Interventions

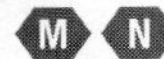

The primary intervention in patients with a goiter is to treat the underlying cause:

- Because goiters often develop due to hypothyroidism, a small dose of thyroid hormone (e.g., **levothyroxine**) may be used to reduce the amount of TSH that is produced by the pituitary gland.
- If thyroid diagnostics reveal hyperthyroidism as the cause of the goiter, a radioiodine uptake and scan should be completed to identify the cause of the hyperthyroidism.
- When a goiter is disfiguring, it may be surgically removed for cosmetic reasons.
- When a goiter is too large or it is pressing on or invading surrounding structures, surgical removal is preferred. Postoperative care is needed.

Total Thyroidectomy

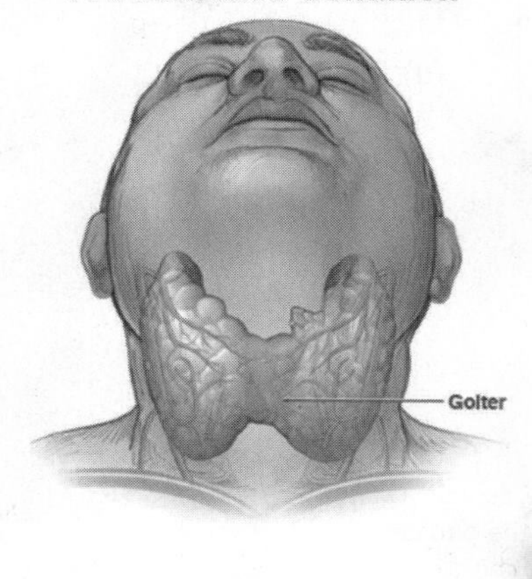

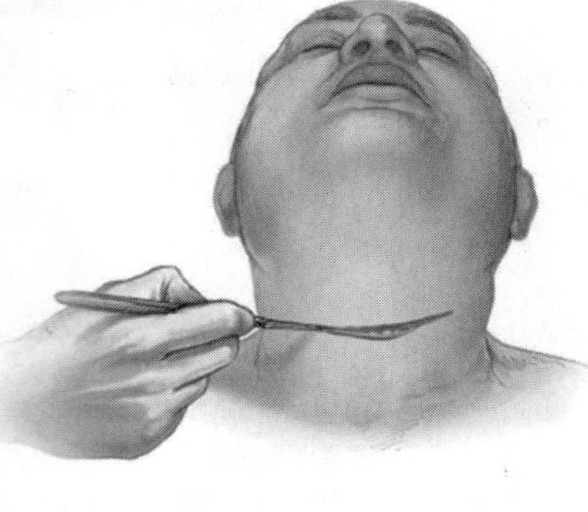

A. An incision is made in the neck.

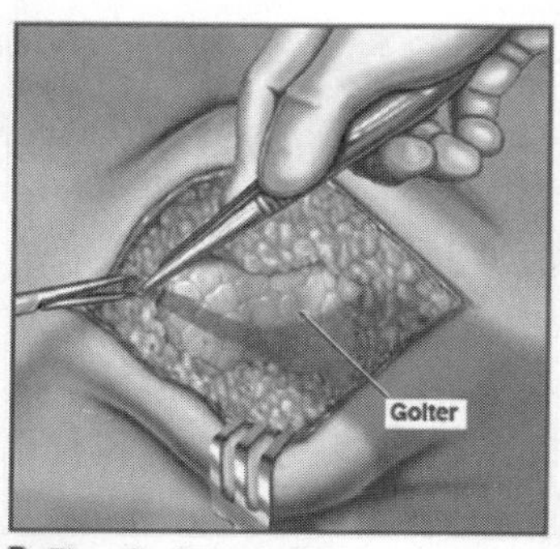

Goiter
B. The goiter is exposed.

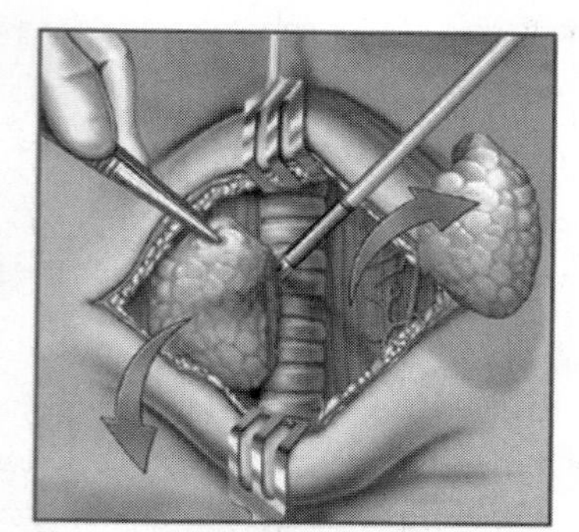

C. The left side of the goiter is removed, then the right side.

This illustration features the three major surgical steps involved in removing a goiter.
Source: © 2014 Nucleus Medical Media, All rights reserved

LO2:

Thyroid Nodules

Causes

- Nodules are abnormal growths of thyroid tissue.
- Thyroid nodules are common. At least 50% of people will develop one.
- Chances of developing a nodule increase with age.
- The majority are benign but a work-up is needed to assess if the nodule is:
  - o Cancerous
  - o Creating too much thyroid hormone
  - o Pressing on vital structures in the surrounding area
- Most nodules cause no symptoms.
- Depending on where it is located on the thyroid gland, the nodule may be seen as a lump on the neck.
- Rarely, it may cause difficulty in swallowing or hoarseness.

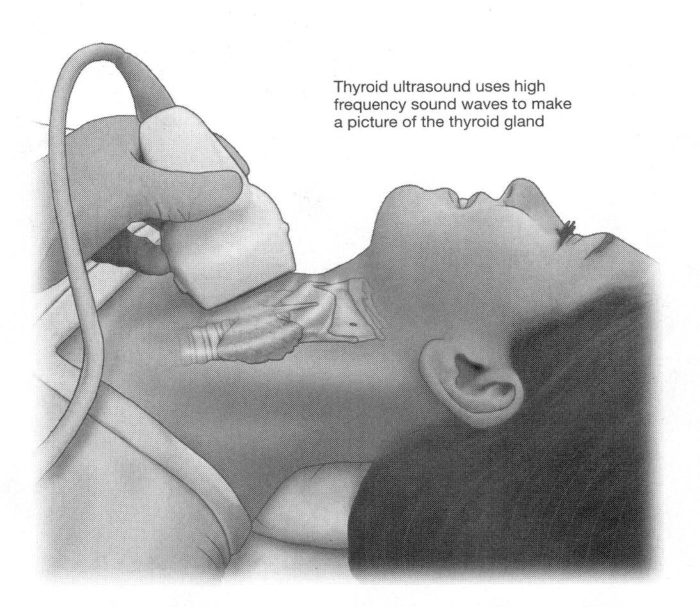
Thyroid ultrasound uses high
frequency sound waves to make
a picture of the thyroid gland

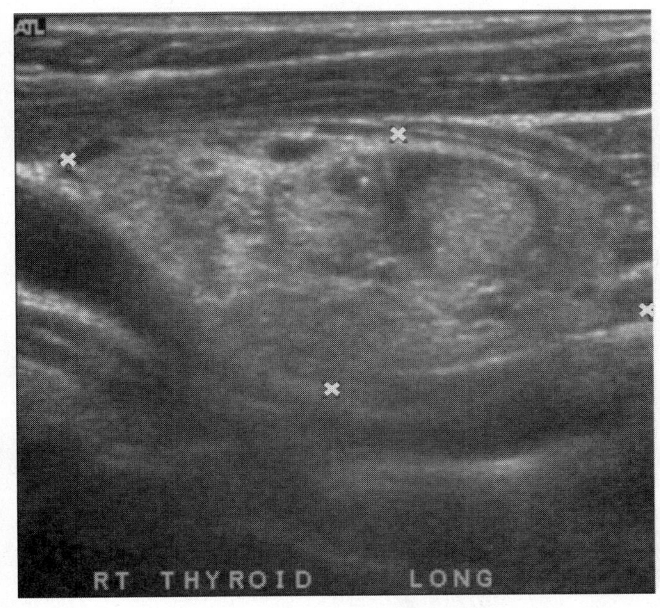
ATL
RT THYROID LONG

Upper: The thyroid ultrasound of the thyroid gland reveals the nodule palpated on exam. Lower: The largest nodule of several that were palpated in a multinodular goiter is shown above. The borders of the nodule are marked by the yellow Xs.

Source: (*lower*) Courtesy of K. Kyriakidis

LO3:

Collaborative Interventions

Evidence-based practice for the management of thyroid nodules are recommended by the American Thyroid Association, et al. (2014) and Gharib, et al. (2010):

- M N EBP After a **fine needle aspiration biopsy (FNAB)** procedure is performed, thyroidectomy is recommended for thyroid nodules indicating cancer, suspicious for cancer, or in high-risk patients. For benign or indeterminate cytology findings, the nodule can be observed over time for changes.
- M N EBP If a malignancy is found, surgery is the only way to remove the nodule and leave the remaining thyroid tissue unaffected.
- M N EBP If the FNAB shows a benign growth, the nodule may be monitored with examinations and serial ultrasounds.
- M EBP A repeat FNAB can be performed when a reassessment is needed.

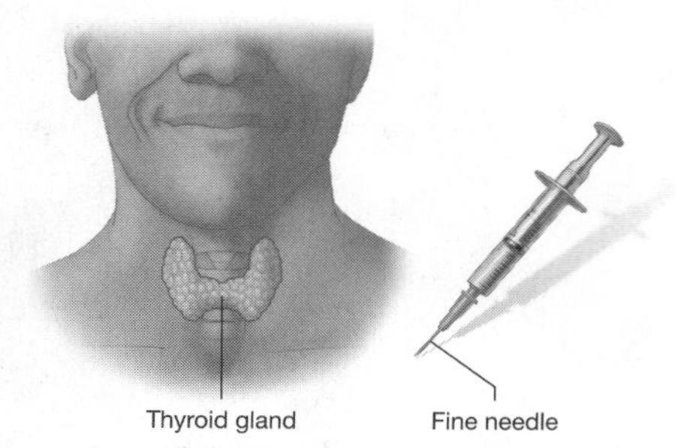

A fine needle biopsy is used if a cell sample from the thyroid gland is needed. A thin needle is inserted and a sample of cells and fluid are aspirated from the thyroid. The cells can then be examined to diagnose for potential thyroid disease or cancer.

LO2:

Thyroid Cancer

Causes

Malignant thyroid tumors:

- Commonly present as a painless, palpable, solitary nodule, often discovered during a routine exam.
- Firm, fixed nodules are more suggestive of malignancy.
- Rapid growth of a nodule is a highly suggestive sign.
- Symptoms may include hoarseness, dysphagia, and hemoptysis.
- The size of the tumor is related to survival. Tumors >4 cm are implicated in increased rate of recurrence and death.
- Malignancy is more commonly seen in those older than 60 and younger than 30 years old.
- Men have a 2:1 higher incidence of death from thyroid cancer than women.

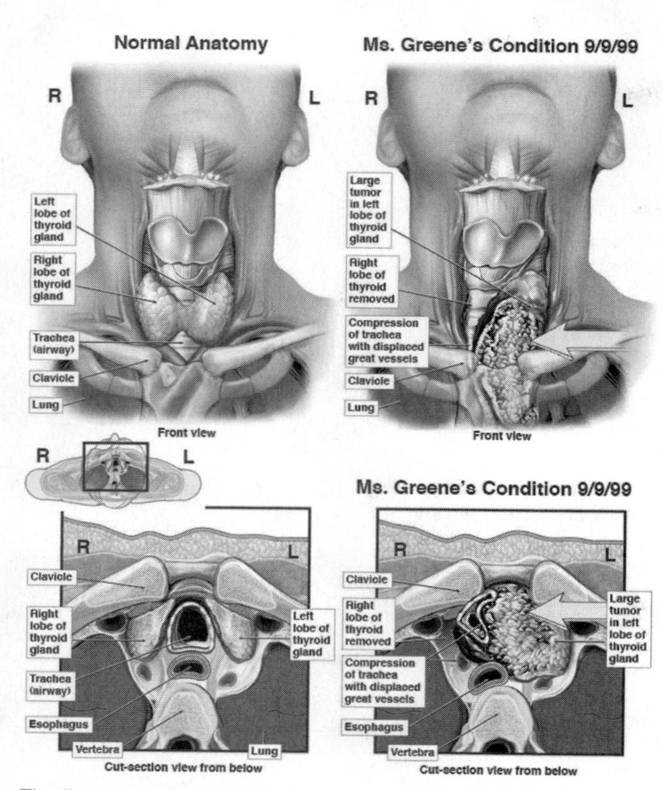

The illustrations depict a thyroid tumor with airway compression/occlusion.

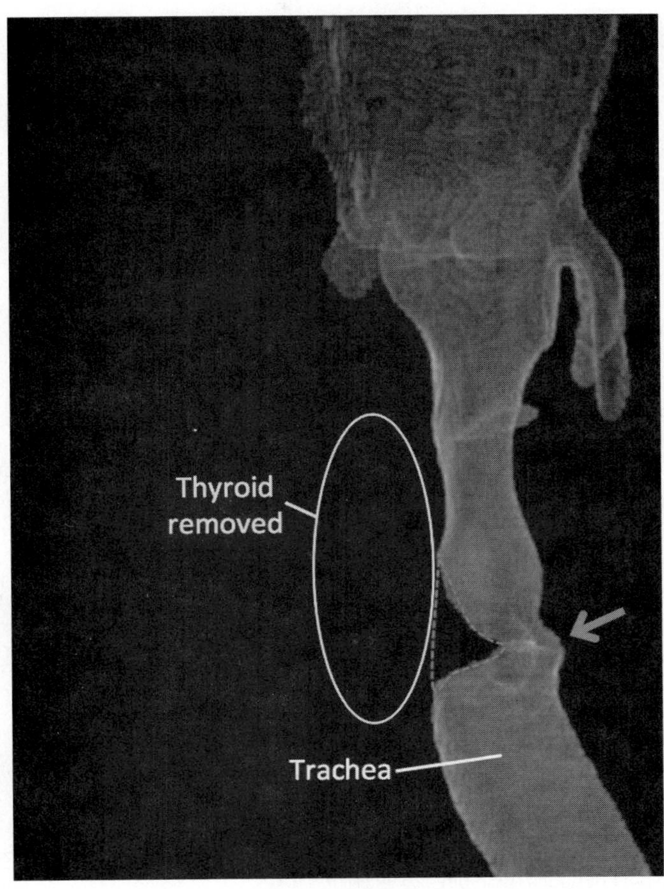

This 3D reconstruction of the trachea shows where the thyroid gland was located prior to removal due to cancer. The thyroid cancer is shown invading the trachea (red line) and is occluding the airway, causing about 40% obstruction. The red arrow points to the tracheal stenosis that results.
Source: Courtesy of K. Kyriakidis

LO3:

Collaborative Interventions

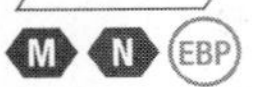

- **Surgical removal** of the cancerous area is the primary and most effective treatment (ATA, 2009):
  - o The surgery can be a partial or complete removal of the thyroid, depending on the size, stage, and location of the tumor.
  - o Postoperative care is detailed in Hyperthyroidism.

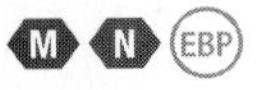

- **Radioactive iodine (RAI)** may be used after surgery to ablate any remaining thyroid tissue. In addition, ATA (2009) and Schlumberger, et al. (2012) showed that low doses were as effective as higher doses and had fewer adverse effects, except in patients with unifocal tumors <1 cm.

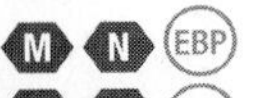

- **Levothyroxine suppression** may be used in moderate to high-risk patients (ATA, 2009).

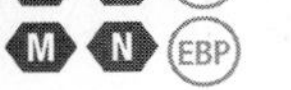

- **External radiation and chemotherapy** may be used if needed based on the type and extent of the malignancy (ATA, 2009).

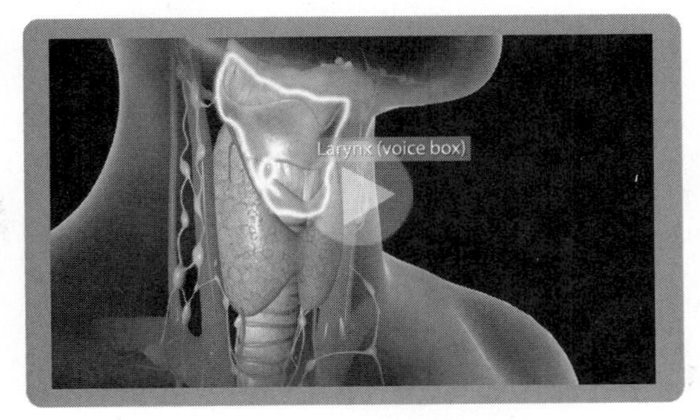

This animation reviews normal thyroid function to provide a good understanding of the four types of thyroid cancers. Treatments for the thyroid cancers are described and shown.
Source: © 2014 Nucleus Medical Media, All rights reserved

Patient Education: Thyroid Disturbances

- Education of patients and/or their families commonly needs to include the following:
  - N EBP Take medication daily on an empty stomach (Liwanpo & Hershman, 2009).
  - N EBP Avoid switching medications between brand names (Dong, et al., 1997).
  - N Never adjust the medication dosage without instruction from the health care provider.
  - N Dietary instructions such as a high-calorie diet for patients with hyperthyroidism and reducing iodine-rich foods in patients with hypothyroidism. Consult a dietician for specific guidance.
  - N EBP Instruct patient about interference with absorption of thyroid medications when taking supplements, like calcium- or aluminum-containing antacids, and iron tablets (Dong, et al., 1997). Supplements should not be taken within 4 hours of thyroid medication.
  - N Be aware and report signs and symptoms (detailed earlier) of hypothyroidism and hyperthyroidism, as treatment for one can cause the other.
  - N Always inform health care provider about any signs or symptoms, diagnostics, or treatments.
  - M N Educate for surgery (pre- and post-op), when indicated
  - N Instruct patients receiving radioactive iodine (RAI) treatments about bodily fluids and excretion precautions which contain RAI. Protect others from exposure to bodily fluids and double-flush the toilet during periods of treatment.
  - N Adhere to regular and essential follow-up appointments.
  - N Medical alert bracelets are suggested.
- M N Dosage adjustments may be needed:
  - As the patient ages
  - If thyroid disease worsens
  - Presence or new onset of comorbid conditions (e.g., heart failure, diabetes) can complicate thyroid function by causing drug interactions, which potentiate or hinder medication effects (e.g., with anticoagulant, digitalis preparation, insulin, oral hypoglycemics)
  - N EBP A high-fiber diet can interfere with absorption of thyroid medications (Dong, et al., 1997).
  - N EBP During pregnancy, consider the potential increased need for thyroxine (Mandel, et al., 1990).

Concept Check

7. What information is given to the patient prescribed thyroid replacement hormones?

A. Take your medication with milk.

B. Hold your medication on days you do not feel well.

C. Do not change brands of your medication.

D. If you are stressed, take an additional tablet each day.

Answer question

Summary of Interventions: Thyroid Disturbances

- **Hypothyroidism**
  - Synthetic thyroxine (T4), levothyroxine, an oral medication that is taken daily is the treatment of choice.
- **Hyperthyroidism**
  - Beta blockers are used in acute settings to control symptoms until treatment to lower thyroid levels takes effect.
  - Thionamides (i.e., propylthiouracil, methimazole) can be taken to suppress the thyroid gland from making as much T3 and T4.
  - Radioactive iodine or surgical removal of the thyroid can be used when a more permanent treatment is desired.

- Thyroid Cancer
  - o Surgery is the most effective treatment.
  - o Radioactive iodine is effective in ablating residual tissue.
  - o Levothyroxine suppression, external radiation, and chemotherapy may be used.
- Thyroid Goiter
  - o Treatment of the underlying hypothyroidism or hyperthyroidism
  - o Surgery if the goiter is invasive, obstructive, or disfiguring
- Thyroid Nodules
  - o After FNAB, thyroidectomy is recommended for malignancies or high risk.
- Patient Education

LO4:

Evaluation of Desired Collaborative Care Outcomes: Thyroid Disturbances

Evaluation and reassessment should reveal attainment of previously established patient outcomes. In summary:

- Patient demonstrates growing acceptance of body changes after understanding their origin.
- Patient's BMI is within normal range or is progressing toward normal.
- Patient demonstrates understanding of treatment regimen and is successfully managing disease at home.
- Patient reports resting well and having sufficient energy to complete daily activities.

References

Bray, D. (2014). Thyroid storm and the AACN synergy model. *RN Journal.* **Rnjournal.com/journal-of-nursing/thyroid-storm-and-the-aacn-synergy-model**

Brent, G. A. (2008). Clinical practice: Grave's disease. *N Engl J Med, 358*(24), 2594–2605.

Dahlen, R. (2002). Managing patients with acute thyrotoxicosis. *Crit Care Nurse, 22*(1), 62–69. **ccn.aacnjournals.org/content/22/1/62.long**

Kumrow, D., & Dahlen, R. (2002). Thyroidectomy: Understanding the potential for complications. *Medsurg Nursing, 11*(5), 228–235.

Nayak, B., & Burman, K. (2006). Thyrothoxicosis and thyroid storm. *Endocrinol Metab Clin North Am, 35*(4), 663.

Pearson, T. (2013). Hypothyroidism: Challenges when treating older adults. *J Gerontolog Nurs, 39*(1), 10–14.

Practice Guidelines

American Thyroid Association (ATA) Guidelines Taskforce on Thyroid Nodules and Differentiated Thyroid Cancer, Cooper, D. S., Doherty, G. M., et al. (2009). Revised American thyroid association management guidelines for patients with thyroid modules and differentiated thyroid cancer. *Thyroid, 19*(11), 1167–1214. doi: 10.1089/thy.2009.0110

Bahn, R. S., Burch, H. B., Cooper, D. S., et al. (2011). Hyperthyroidism and other causes of thyrotoxicosis: Management guidelines of the American thyroid association and American association of clinical endocrinologists. *Endocrine Practice, 17*(3), 456–520. **www.aace.com/files/hyperguidelinesapril2013.pdf**

Crawford, A., & Harris, H. (2014). Thyroid imbalances: Dealing with disorderly conduct. *Nursing 2014, 42*(11), 44–50. **www.nursingcenter.com/lnc/cearticle?tid=1440616**

Garber, J. R., Cobin, R. H., Gharib, H., et al. (2012). Clinical practice guidelines for hypothyroidism in adults: Cosponsored by the American association of clinical endocrinologists and the American thyroid association. *Thyroid, 22*(12), 1200–1235. doi: 10.1089/thy.2012.0205

Gharib, H., Papini, E., Paschke, R., et al. (2010). American Association of Clinical Endocrinologists, Associazione Medici Endocrinologi, and European Thyroid Association Medical guidelines for clinical practice for the diagnosis and management of thyroid nodules. *Endocr Pract, 12*(1), 63–102.

Schlumberger, M., Catargi, B., Borget, I., et al. (2012). Strategies of radioiodine ablation in patients with low-risk thyroid cancer. *N Engl J Med, 366*(18), 1663–1673. doi: 10.1056/NEJMoa1108586

Patient Education

American Thyroid Association. (2014). *ATA patient education.* **www.thyroid.org/patient-thyroid-information/ata-patient-education-web-brochures/**

American Thyroid Association. (2014). *Thyroid nodules.* **www.thyroid.org/patients/brochures/Nodules_brochure.pdf**

DHHS/NIH/NIDDK. (2014). *Hyperthyroidism.* **www.endocrine.niddk.nih.gov/pubs/hyperthyroidism/Hyperthyroidism_508.pdf**

DHHS/NIH/NIDDK. (2014). *Hypothyroidism.* **www.endocrine.niddk.nih.gov/pubs/hypothyroidism/Hypothyroidism_508.pdf**

Dong, B. J., Hauck, W. W., Gambertogloi, J. G., et al. (1997). Bioequivalence of generic and brand-name levothyroxine products in the treatment of hypothyroidism. *JAMA, 277*(15), 1205–1213. doi: 10.1001/jama.1997.03540390035032

Liwanpo, L., & Hershman, J. M. (2009). Conditions and drugs interfering with thyroxine absorption. *Clin Endocrinol Metab, 23*(6), 781–792. doi: 10.1016/j.beem.2009.06.006

Mandel, S. J., Larsen, R., Seely, E. W., & Brent, G. A. (1990). Increased need for thyroxine during pregnancy in women with primary hypothyroidism. *N Engl J Med, 323,* 91–96. doi: 10.1056/NEJM199007123230204

U.S. National Library of Medicine, NIH. (2014). *Thyroid diseases.* **www.nlm.nih.gov/medlineplus/thyroiddiseases.html**

Learning Outcomes for Adrenal Gland Disorders

When you complete this lesson, you will be able to:

1. Recognize the clinical relevance of adrenal gland disorders.
2. Consider the pathophysiology, etiology, risk factors, and clinical presentation of adrenal gland disorders that determine the priority patient concerns.
3. Determine the most urgent and important nursing interventions and patient education required in caring for a patient with adrenal gland disorder.
4. Evaluate attainment of desired collaborative care outcomes for a patient with adrenal gland disorder.

LO1:

What Are Adrenal Disorders?

Adrenal dysfunction occurs when the adrenal glands cannot perform their normal function. Causes of adrenal dysfunction include:

- Adrenal cortex disorders:
  - o **Adrenal insufficiency (AI) or Addison's disease** is a deficiency in adrenal cortical hormone production.
  - o **Adrenal hyperfunction:**
    - ■ **Excessive corticosteroid levels:** Cushing's syndrome
    - ■ **Excessive aldosterone levels:** Conn syndrome
- **Adrenal fatigue** is not a medical condition but is used in modern health publications.
- **Adrenal medulla tumors:** Adrenal neuroblastoma found in children

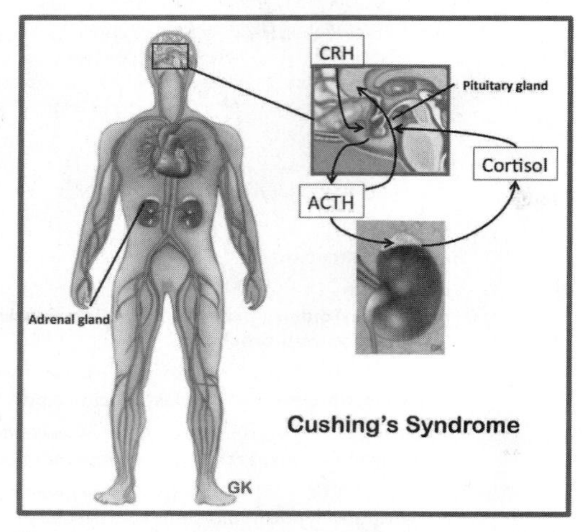

This diagram shows the organs and hormones involved in Cushing's syndrome. The pituitary gland, adrenal gland, cortisol, CRH from the hypothalamus, and ACTH are labeled.
Source: Courtesy of George Kyriakidis/Santa Ana, CA

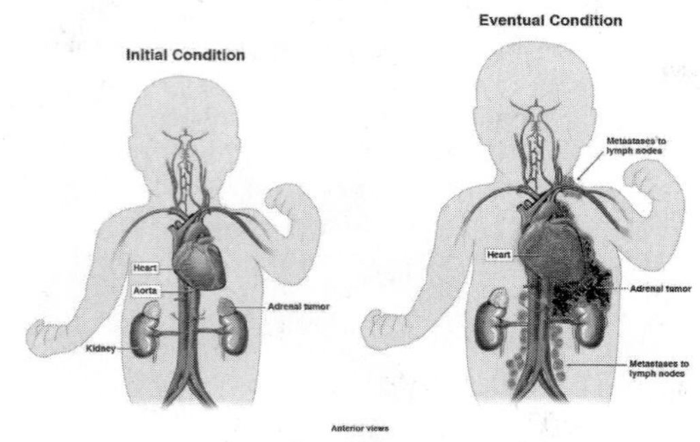

This illustration compares the left image, which shows an initial small tumor above the left kidney with an evolving image (right), which reveals a well-developed tumor that invades surrounding tissues.
Source: © 2014 Nucleus Medical Media. All rights reserved

LO1:

Clinical Relevance

- The adrenal glands play an important role in the body's metabolism.
- Acute adrenal insufficiency is a *medical emergency* that must be promptly identified and treated.
- Use of steroids, a common treatment for other conditions, can affect adrenal function.
- Long-term glucocorticoids usage is estimated at 1–3% of adults worldwide.

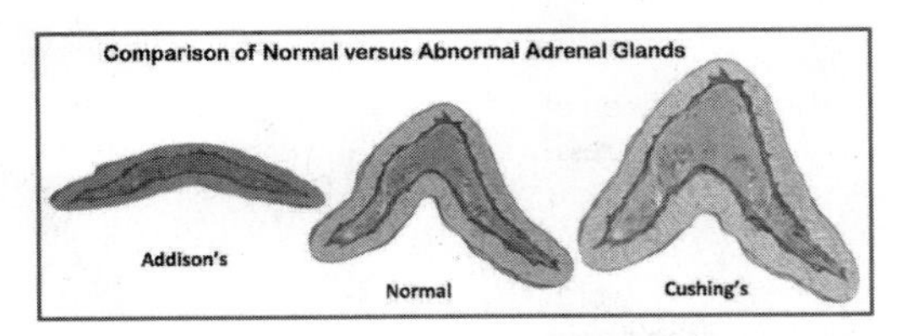

These pathology specimens show the differences between various adrenal diseases. The atrophied adrenal gland on the left reflects Addison's disease whereas the hypertrophied adrenal on the right reflects Cushing's disease. For comparison, the middle gland is normal.
Source: Courtesy of George Kyriakidis/Santa Ana, CA

Concept Check

1. Use of which medications has an adverse effect on the adrenal glands?
   A. Diuretics
   B. Steroids
   C. Vitamins
   D. Antibiotics

Answer question

LO2:

Pathophysiology

- Adrenal glands are located on top of each kidney.
- Each adrenal gland is made of two independent endocrine organs:
  - **Medulla:** The inner portion of the adrenal glands, the medulla, secretes the hormones epinephrine and norepinephrine. These alter blood pressure, heart rate, fight or flight, bronchodilation, and other key functions that are regulated by the sympathetic nervous system.
  - **Cortex:** The outer layer (cortex) secretes various hormones that include corticosteroids, male hormones (androgens), and mineralocorticoids, which regulate blood pressure along with sodium and potassium levels.

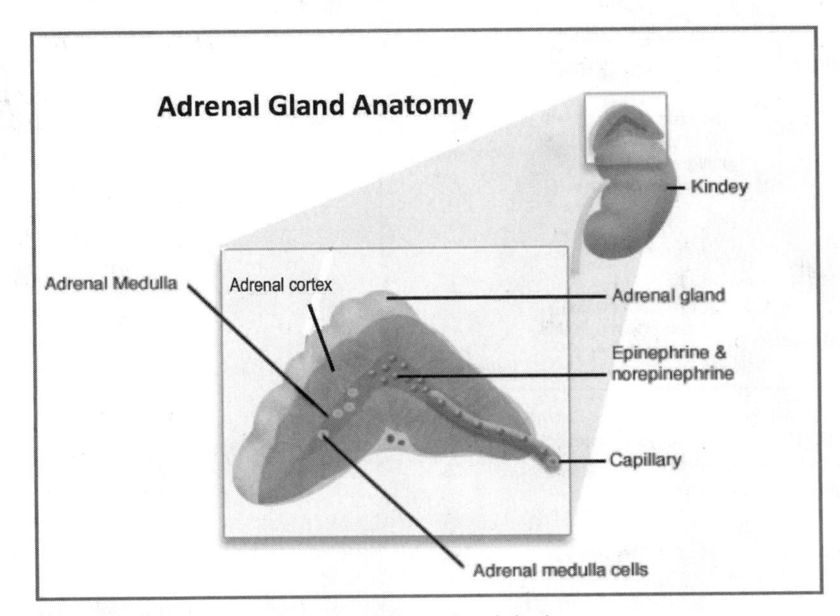

This exhibit depicts the normal anatomy of the adrenal glands.
Source: Copyright © 2014, NovEx Novice to Expert Learning, LLC

Adrenal Medulla

- The adrenal medulla is connected by preganglionic sympathetic fibers and is an extension of the sympathetic nervous system. The sympathetic nervous system is stimulated by stressors as well as by situations requiring extreme activity (e.g., exercise, perceived emergent or stressful situations).
- The medulla secretes hormones of *fight or flight*, epinephrine and norepinephrine, which help cope with physical and emotional stress. The principal cell responsible for secretion is called the chromaffin cell.
  - o **Epinephrine** increases heart rate and contractile force, facilitates blood flow to muscles and brain, causes smooth muscle relaxation, and helps convert glycogen to glucose in the liver (see picture of adrenal medulla).
  - o **Norepinephrine** increases heart rate and has strong vasoconstrictive effects that increase blood pressure.
- **Pheochromocytoma** is a rare tumor of the adrenals that results in excessive catecholamine (epinephrine and norepinephrine) secretion. Pheochromocytomas cause episodes of anxiety, sweating, palpitations, tachycardia, and hypertension. Surgery is the definitive treatment to remove the tumor; however, antihypertensive medications (alpha blockers, beta blockers, or calcium channel blockers) may be needed immediately to control hypertension.

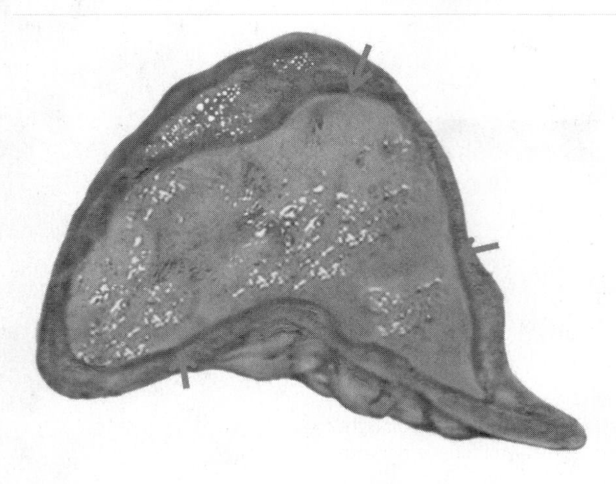

Pheochromocytoma (arrow) with small adrenal remnant (tail) to the right.
Source: Courtesy of George Kyriakidis/Santa Ana, CA

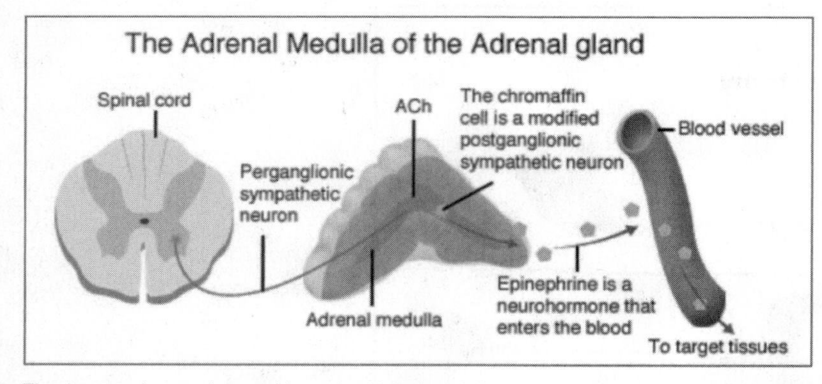

The diagram shows where and how the adrenal medulla secretes the hormones epinephrine and norepinephrine into the blood vessels. Thus, it functions as a neuroendocrine organ. Chromaffin cells, located in the medulla, produce the hormones.
Source: Copyright © 2014, NovEx Novice to Expert Learning, LLC

Pathophysiology (continued)

Adrenal Cortex

- The **adrenal cortex** secretes hormones called **corticosteroids** that affect metabolism:
  - o Maintenance of blood pressure
  - o Characteristics of men
- There are two main adrenocortical (made in the adrenal cortex) hormones:
  - o Glucocorticoids
  - o Mineralocorticoids
    - ■ Androgenic hormone is important but secreted in small amounts.

Adrenal Gland: Cortex & Medulla

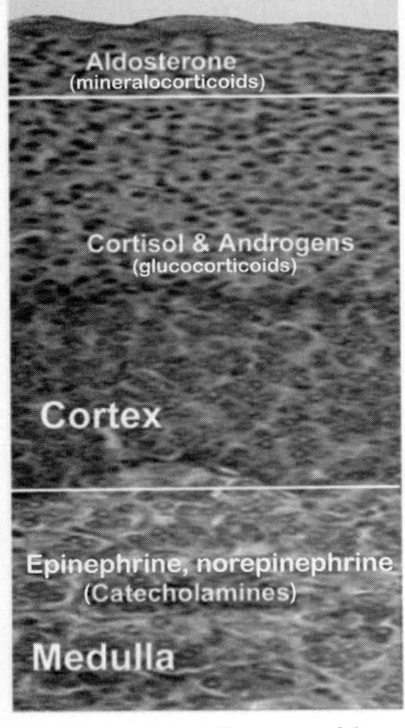

The adrenal gland is shown. The regions of the cortex that produce mineralocorticoids and glucocorticoids are labeled. The medulla, in the lower portion, secretes both epinephrine and norepinephrine.
Source: Courtesy of George Kyriakidis/Santa Ana, CA

Corticosteroids

- **Glucocorticoids (cortisol)** control the body's use of fats, proteins, and carbohydrates and help to maintain the tone of blood vessels. Physiologic stress such as severe sepsis, septic shock, or trauma usually results in an increase in cortisol levels but eventually can cause depletion of cortisol.
  - o **Adrenal insufficiency or Addison's disease** is a deficiency in adrenal cortical hormone production.
  - o **Cushing's syndrome** is an excessive and chronic production of corticosteroids.
- **Mineralocorticoid (aldosterone)** is a hormone that maintains blood volume and controls the amount of sodium retained and potassium secreted by the kidney. An aldosterone-producing adenoma or adrenal hyperplasia causes high levels of aldosterone (hyperaldosteronism) and can result in hypertension and hypokalemia.
- **Androgenic (androgen) hormone** has minimal effect on male characteristics. In women, androgen hormones promote sex characteristics and may be important for libido.

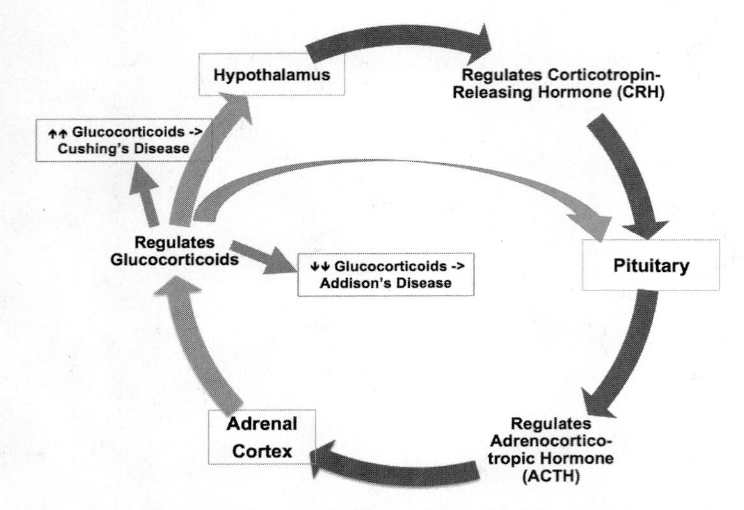

Hypothalamic-Pituitary-Adrenal Feedback System

Hypothalamus–Pituitary–Adrenal Axis

The adrenal glands are a part of the endocrine system and the hypothalamus–pituitary–adrenal (HPA) axis (see diagram).

- Stress triggers the release of corticotropin-releasing factor (CRF) from nerve cells in the hypothalamus.
- The CRF then stimulates the anterior pituitary gland to secrete adrenocorticotrophic hormone (ACTH).
- The ACTH stimulates the production of cortisol (glucocorticoid) and aldosterone in the adrenal cortex.
- Cortisol is then released into the bloodstream to respond to the body's stressors.
- Through a **negative feedback system**, an increase in cortisol signals:
    - The hypothalamus to stop releasing CRF, which consequently decreases the amount of ACTH and cortisol released into the bloodstream.
    - The pituitary directly to reduce the amount of ACTH.

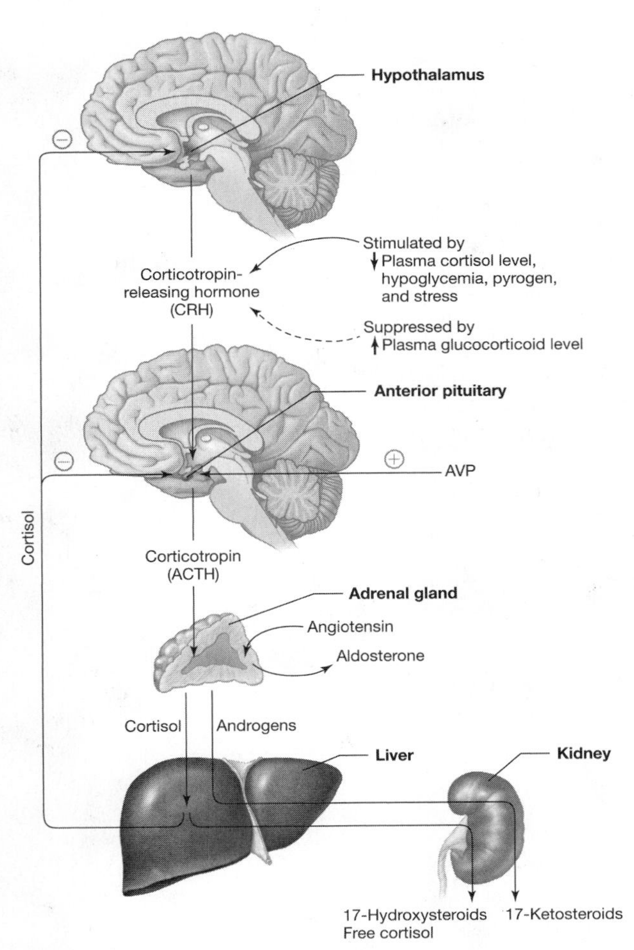

The diagram hints at the complexity of the endocrine system with many hormone-producing glands, including the adrenal glands. Many hormones influence the production and activity of others. The hormones shown here affect the brain, kidneys, and liver in addition to the heart, lungs, vascular system, and every organ system in the body. This diagram depicts the hypothalamus–pituitary–adrenal axis, which will be detailed later.

Concept Check

2. Which hormones are secreted from the adrenal medulla?
   - A. Catecholamines
   - B. Androgens
   - C. Cortiocosteroids
   - D. Mineralcorticoids

Answer question

Concept Check

3. What is the action of cortisol?
   - A. Helps maintain tone of blood vessels
   - B. Controls sodium retention by kidney
   - C. Affects female libido
   - D. Produces male secondary sexual characteristics

Answer question

Pathophysiology (continued)

Adrenal Insufficiency

Adrenal insufficiency (AI) can be classified as:

- Primary AI: Caused by diseases of the adrenal gland itself. Examples include infarction of the adrenal glands, HIV virus, hemorrhage, and autoimmune destruction of the adrenal.
- Secondary AI: Caused by interference with the pituitary releasing ACTH. This may be due to a pituitary tumor, trauma, or an infarction.
    - o Primary and secondary causes are relatively rare.
- Tertiary AI: Caused by the suppression of the hypothalamic–pituitary–adrenal function. A common cause of tertiary AI is from chronic and/or high dose glucocorticoid use. Glucocorticoid use is common for both endocrine and nonendocrine disorders. Long-term usage of glucocorticoids is estimated at 1–3% of adults worldwide.
    - o For those who have HPA suppression, high doses of glucocorticoids and/or chronic use can inhibit the production of CRH in the hypothalamus, ACTH in the pituitary, and/or cause adrenal atrophy.
    - o Adrenal suppression occurs when the inhibiting effects on HPA function continue after the glucocorticoids are stopped.
    - o High-dose glucocorticoid administration can render the adrenal glands unable to produce cortisol when glucocorticoids are abruptly halted. Slow tapering of glucocorticoids is recommended to allow the HPA function to recover.

Sudden loss of adrenal function causes a different response than a gradual loss:

- A sudden loss of adrenal function, as would occur with adrenal infarction or sudden withdrawal of corticosteroids, can result in hypotension and shock.
    - o These insults create an adrenal crisis.
    - o Acute AI is a medical emergency and must be promptly identified and treated.
- More gradual development of adrenal insufficiency usually has a more vague presentation. Lack of aldosterone may result in mild hypotension and hyperkalemia. Lack of cortisol can also cause hypoglycemia.

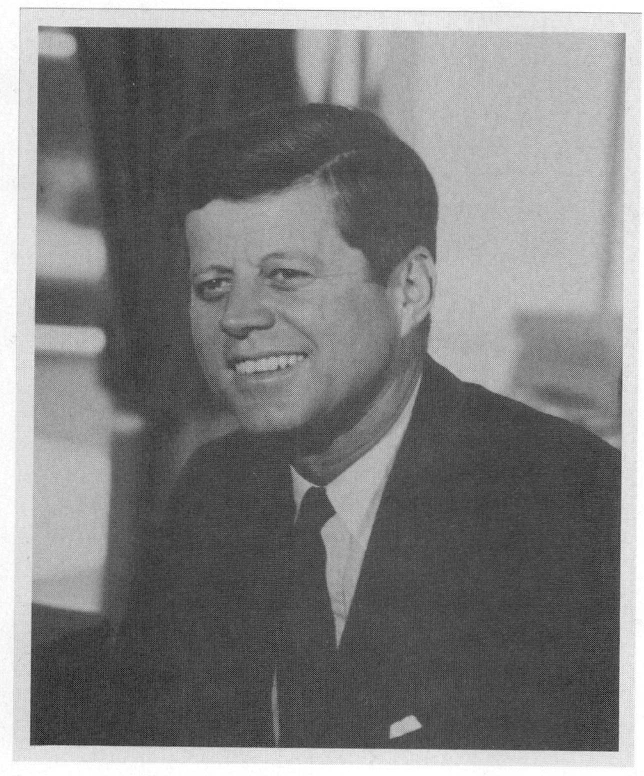

President John F. Kennedy was one of the best-known Addison's disease sufferers, and also possibly one of the first Addisonians to survive major surgery.
Source: National Archives and Records Administration

Concept Check

4. What is the most common cause of AI?

A. Adrenal infarction

B. Pituitary tumor

C. HIV

D. Long-term glucocorticoid use

Answer question

Risk Factors

Adrenal Insufficiency (Addison's)

Patients at highest risk for adrenal insufficiency are those with or having:

- Glucocorticoid use
- Cancer
- Adrenal surgery
- Autoimmune disease, such as lupus or type 1 diabetes
- Anticoagulant use
- Chronic infection (e.g., tuberculosis)

Corticosteroid Excess (Cushing's)

Patients at highest risk for corticosteroid excess are those with or having:

- Obesity
- Hypertension
- Type 2 diabetes
- Poorly controlled blood glucose levels

LO2:

Causes

Adrenal Insufficiency (Addison's)

Adrenal crisis (acute)

- Primary
  - o Bilateral hemorrhage (Waterhouse–Friderichsen syndrome)
  - o Bilateral adrenal infarction
- Secondary
  - o Pituitary infarction
- Tertiary
  - o Abrupt withdrawal of glucocorticoids
  - o Acute stress, such as infection or major surgery without an increase in corticosteroids

Chronic

- Primary
  - o Autoimmune destruction of adrenal tissue is the most common form of primary AI.
  - o Congenital adrenal hyperplasia
  - o Tuberculosis
  - o HIV infections
- Secondary
  - o Decreased release of ACTH from the pituitary due to tumors or hemorrhage
- Tertiary
  - o Decreased secretion of corticotropin-releasing hormone (CRH) by the hypothalamus

Corticosteroid Excess (Cushing's)

- Chronic administration of corticosteroids to treat immunologic and inflammatory disorders is, by far, the most common cause of this problem.
- Other rare causes include:
    - o Benign pituitary tumors (adenomas) produce excess ACTH (approximately 70% of cases).
    - o Adrenal masses (about 15% of cases)
    - o Ectopic ACTH syndrome (e.g., non-pituitary tumors that produce ACTH). These tumors commonly occur in the lungs or chest (approximately 15% of cases).

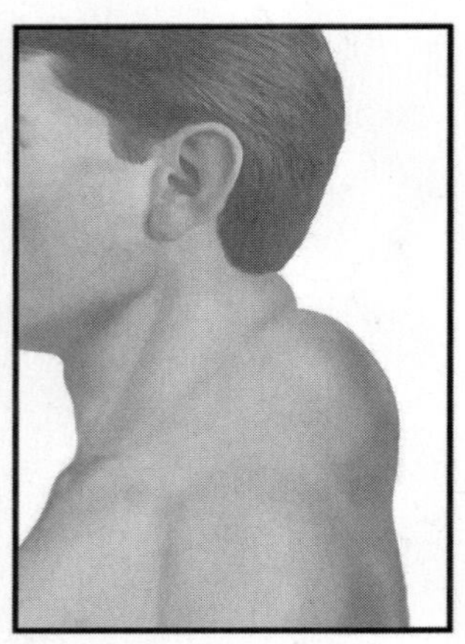

This diagram depicts the classic upper body obesity that affects people with Cushing's syndrome. Excessive fat around the neck is illustrated in a male figure.

LO2:

Assessment Findings

Adrenal Insufficiency (Addison's)

Adrenal Crisis

- **Shock due to circulatory collapse:** Decreased level of aldosterone allows large amount of sodium and water to be excreted through the kidneys.
- Anorexia, nausea, and vomiting
- **Abdominal pain**
- **Profound hypoglycemia:** Decreased levels of cortisol will decrease glucose production.
- **Weakness**, **fatigue**, lethargy
- Hyperkalemia
- Cardiac dysrhythmias
- Dizziness, confusion or coma

Chronic Adrenal Insufficiency

- Chronic malaise
- Fatigue, which worsens with activity
- Hyperpigmentation caused from excess melatonin production (hands, gums, face, neck, nails)
- Weight loss from anorexia, nausea, dehydration
- Muscle and joint pain
- Electrolyte imbalance due to lack of aldosterone that controls sodium and potassium excretion
    - o Hyponatremia and salt craving
    - o Hyperkalemia from sodium loss
- Azotemia: Elevated BUN (blood urea nitrogen) and creatinine

Corticosteroid Excess (Cushing's)

Clinical presentation of Cushing's:

- Weight gain
- Fatty deposits, mainly around the waist and abdomen, upper back, face and between the shoulders (buffalo hump)
- Arms and legs may remain thin
- Pink or purple stretch marks on the abdomen, thighs, breasts and arms
- Thinning fragile skin that bruises easily
- Acne
- Women may develop facial hair and have irregular menstrual periods.
- Moon facies
- Muscle weakness
- Skin ulcers (poor wound healing)

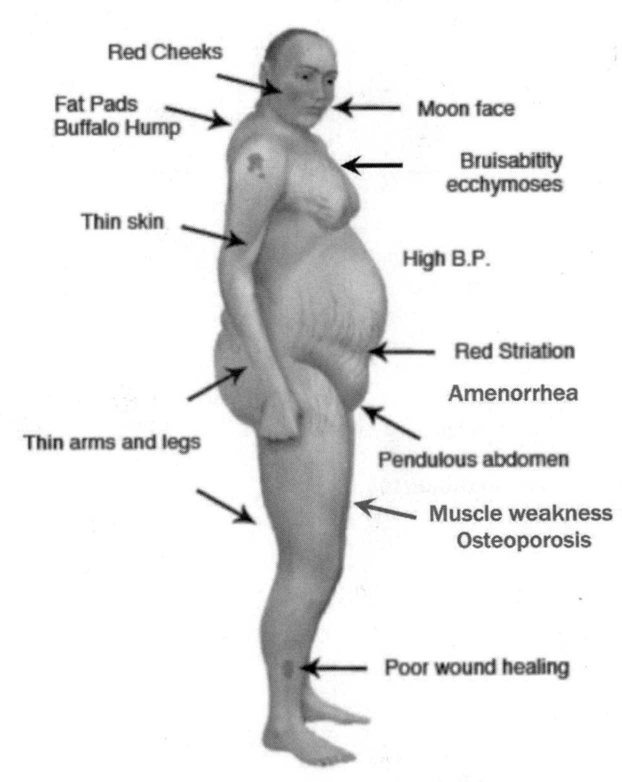

This diagram points out the major signs and symptoms noted on physical exam in a patient with Cushing's disease.

LO2:

Diagnostics

- Cortisol:
  - o A high level of cortisol is indicative of severe physiologic stress.
  - o A low level indicates an inability to respond to stress and adrenal insufficiency is likely.
  - o Both very high and very low levels of cortisol are associated with increased mortality from a critical illness.
  - o Cortisol levels can also be measured before and after synthetic ACTH is injected into the patient.
- ACTH level:
  - o A low ACTH in the setting of low cortisol indicates a pituitary problem.
- Electrolytes:
  - o A low glucose, low sodium, and high potassium may be a sign of adrenal insufficiency.
- Hyperglycemia may be present with corticosteroid excess.
- (EBP) CT scanning may be used to image the adrenal and can show evidence of hemorrhage, infarction, or malignancy (Funder, Carey, Fardella, et al., 2008).

Priority Patient Concerns and Desired Collaborative Care Outcomes

Prior to caring for patients with adrenal gland disorders, it is important to prioritize the patient's concerns that must guide the nursing care plan and interventions. Care for the patient is ordered and organized in accordance with the patient's priority and urgent needs. Desired collaborative care outcomes in patients with adrenal gland disorders typically include:

1. Patient will be able to perform activities of daily living without fatigue.
2. Patient will state acceptance of body appearance.
3. Patient will demonstrate ways to reduce stress and avoid infections.
4. Patient's skin will remain intact.
5. Patient will remain normovolemic.

Considering these important care outcomes, prepare a list of the major 3–6 priority patient concerns or nursing diagnoses for patients with adrenal gland disorders. Be prepared to participate in a discussion of this list and/or to submit them as an assignment, as determined by your faculty. Resources you may find helpful in this assignment can include this lesson, the references, resources on nursing care plans, and standard nursing diagnoses manuals.

LO3:

Collaborative Interventions: Adrenal Insufficiency or Addison's Disease

Acute adrenal insufficiency often presents with hypotension and hypoglycemia. Key treatment goals are to correct hypotension, reverse electrolyte imbalances, and correct cortisol deficit. Treatment recommendations (Marik, P. E., Pastores, S. M., Annane, D., 2008) involve:

M N
- **Aggressive IV fluid administration**, using large gauge IVs, is required to restore vascular fluid, raise blood pressure, and replace sodium. Start with 1–3 liters of 0.9% normal saline. If also hypoglycemia, use 5–10% dextrose in 0.9% normal saline. Avoid hypotonic saline!

M N
- **Vasopressors: Norepinephrine** is the vasopressor of choice for hypotension if refractory to fluid administration. Phenylephrine, dopamine, or epinephrine can be added.

M N
- Intravenous administration of **dexamethasone 4 mg or hydrocortisone 100 mg**. Taper (1–3 days) and change to oral route. Avoid dexamethasone in patients with septic shock or acute respiratory distress syndrome (ARDS).

M N
- Treat the cause, particularly an infectious cause.

M N
- **Treatment of hyperkalemia is crucial.** Give polystyrene sulfonates (Kayexalate, Kionex, or Resonium A) emergently, orally, or rectally.

M N
- Reverse additional electrolyte abnormalities: hyponatremia if persistent after isotonic saline and cortisol, hypercalcemia.

(The acute and poststabilization interventions and care are prioritized in the schematic.)

After stabilization, continued care includes:

M N EBP
- Acute and chronic adrenal insufficiency require glucocorticoid replacement, which may be given orally when patient is able to tolerate.

M N
- Continue isotonic or dextrose with isotonic saline for 24–48 hrs.

M N
- Determine precipitating cause of crisis and treat, particularly potential infection.

M N
- Diagnostics should be done to confirm adrenal insufficiency and type, if unknown.

M N
- Mineralocorticoid replacement: fludrocortisone daily.

M N
- Chronic adrenal insufficiency requires daily oral doses of glucocorticoid replacement.

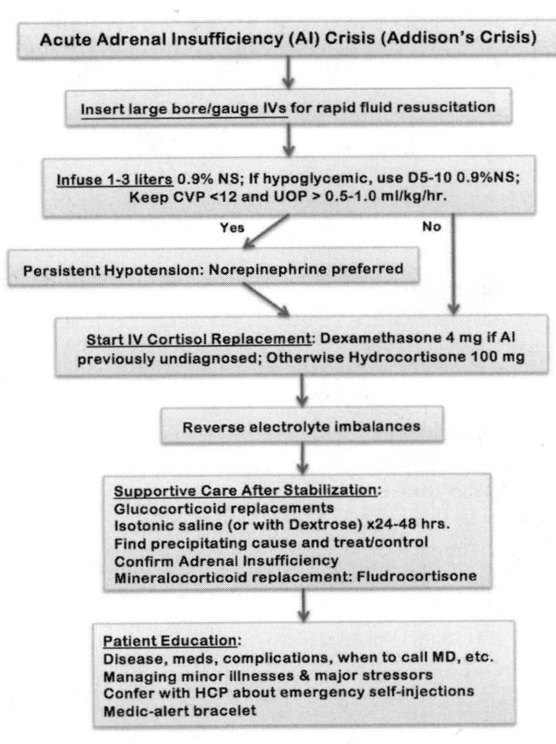
Acute Adrenal Insufficiency (AI) Crisis (Addison's Crisis)
Insert large bore/gauge IVs for rapid fluid resuscitation
Infuse 1-3 liters 0.9% NS; If hypoglycemic, use D5-10 0.9%NS;
Keep CVP <12 and UOP > 0.5-1.0 ml/kg/hr.
Yes
No
Persistent Hypotension: Norepinephrine preferred
Start IV Cortisol Replacement: Dexamethasone 4 mg if AI previously undiagnosed; Otherwise Hydrocortisone 100 mg
Reverse electrolyte imbalances
Supportive Care After Stabilization:
Glucocorticoid replacements
Isotonic saline (or with Dextrose) x24-48 hrs.
Find precipitating cause and treat/control
Confirm Adrenal Insufficiency
Mineralocorticoid replacement: Fludrocortisone
Patient Education:
Disease, meds, complications, when to call MD, etc.
Managing minor illnesses & major stressors
Confer with HCP about emergency self-injections
Medic-alert bracelet

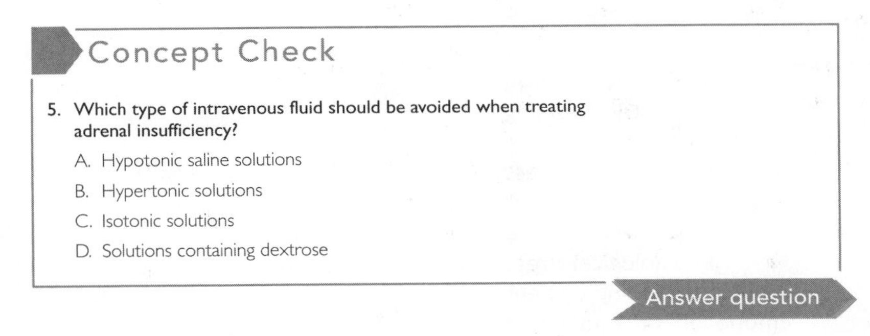

Concept Check

5. Which type of intravenous fluid should be avoided when treating adrenal insufficiency?
   A. Hypotonic saline solutions
   B. Hypertonic solutions
   C. Isotonic solutions
   D. Solutions containing dextrose

Answer question

Collaborative Interventions: Adrenal Insufficiency or Addison's Disease (continued)

Prevention: Hospitalized Patients at Risk for Adrenal Crisis

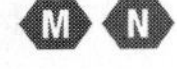

Patients who are under physiologic stress due to a medical illness or surgery normally require higher levels of corticosteroids to maintain proper metabolism and vessel tone. Normally, patients respond to the stressors by producing increased endogenous amounts of corticosteroids from their adrenal glands.

- However, some patients are unable to produce these essential higher levels due to known or unknown pituitary or adrenal problems. Patients who are unable to mount an adequate stress response may include those on chronic corticosteroid treatment for other illnesses. These patients require administration of supplemental corticosteroids to prevent adrenal crisis after surgery or during major or severe illness.
- **Recognizing the patients who are at risk for adrenal crisis is of great importance** when they undergo surgery or when they have an acute illness.
- Patients who are on corticosteroids because they have had pituitary surgery always need supplemental corticosteroids.
- Patients who are on prednisone of >20 mg daily for >3 weeks should be strongly considered for supplementation.
- Patients who are typically not at risk and do not require supplementation include those on:
  - o Prednisone <10 mg per day
  - o Alternate day dosing of corticosteroids
  - o Corticosteroids for <3 weeks
- Preventive doses for at risk surgical patients:

Type of Surgery	Steroid Supplementation at the Time of Surgery
Minor (e.g., hernia repair)	Hydrocortisone 25 mg IV on day of surgery
Moderate (e.g., joint replacement, open cholecystectomy)	Hydrocortisone 25 mg IV every 8 hours on day of surgery. Taper over 2 days.
Major (e.g., Cardiothoracic surgery, Trauma)	Hydrocortisone 50 mg IV every 8 hours on day of surgery. Taper over 2 days.

Patient Education: Adrenal Insufficiency

- Educate patients and the family to ensure that health care providers are aware of the adrenal problem and take extra precautions regarding prevention during major illness or surgery.
- Patients must routinely take prescribed glucocorticoids and inform health care provider when they are unable to tolerate oral intake.
- Educate patient on how to manage and prevent crisis during minor illness and major stressors by adjusting medications per health care provider (e.g., having self-injections of glucocorticoids, temporary increase in dosage).
- Educate all patients about their condition, precipitating factors, early recognition of complications, medications and side effects, when to call the health care provider or 911, and a medical alert bracelet.
- Educate the patient about complications, signs, symptoms of the opposite adrenal disorder resulting from treatment with medications, and healthy living habits.
- Stress management (e.g., exercise, yoga, meditation, guided imagery, music) can help normalize cortisol levels.

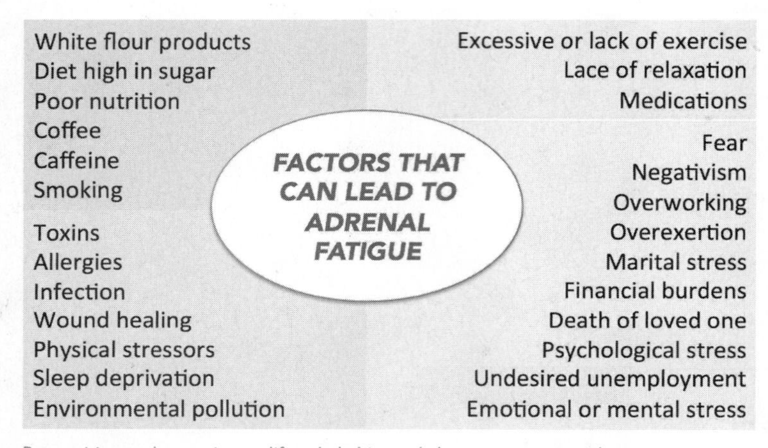

White flour products
Diet high in sugar
Poor nutrition
Coffee
Caffeine
Smoking
Toxins
Allergies
Infection
Wound healing
Physical stressors
Sleep deprivation
Environmental pollution
FACTORS THAT CAN LEAD TO ADRENAL FATIGUE
Excessive or lack of exercise
Lace of relaxation
Medications
Fear
Negativism
Overworking
Overexertion
Marital stress
Financial burdens
Death of loved one
Psychological stress
Undesired unemployment
Emotional or mental stress

Recognition and attention to lifestyle habits and changes are essential to maintaining healthy adrenal function and prevention of a crisis. The diagram points out many factors that can alter the need for or production of adrenal hormones.

Concept Check

6. Increased stress ___________ need for corticosteroids.
   A. Increases
   B. Decreases
   C. Eliminates
   D. Has no effect on

Answer question

LO3:

Collaborative Interventions: Corticosteroid Excess or Cushing's Syndrome

Care and treatment of the patient with Cushing's syndrome depends on the cause of the excessive cortisol levels:

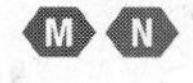

- The most common cause is excessive corticosteroid administration and should be suspected when patients are taking exogenous corticosteroids.
  - o If exogenous corticosteroids are the cause, ideally, the corticosteroid should gradually be withdrawn.

- However, withdrawal is not always possible in practice because the patients may require corticosteroids to treat their disease (e.g., lupus, inflammatory bowel disease, asthma).
- Occasionally, there are alternatives to treatment with corticosteroids with fewer side effects.
- A rare cause is a pituitary tumor and typically requires surgical removal (Biller, B. M., Grossman, A. B., Stewart, P. M., et al., 2008).

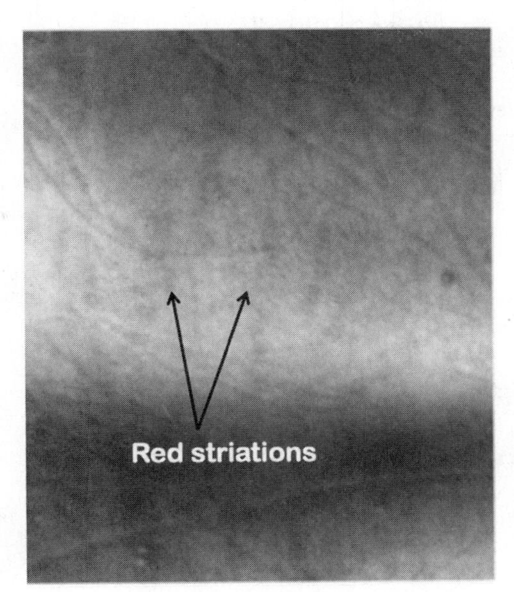

Cushing's syndrome is an often missed diagnosis but can reduce one's life span due to accompanying hypertension, osteoporosis, and diabetes in some. This photo shows a hallmark sign—the purple (or pink) stretch marks. Other hallmarks can include: fatty shoulder hump and moon face. Early recognition and treatment offer the patient the best opportunity for recovery.
Source: Courtesy of K. Kyriakidis

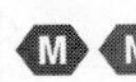

- Adrenalectomy is commonly the definitive intervention in primary hyperaldosteronism due to the high percentage of blood pressure and serum potassium levels of improvement (Funder, J. W., Carey, R. M., Fardella, C., et al., 2008).
  - o Both hypokalemia and hypertension should be managed closely preoperatively.
  - o Postoperative care specific to these patients includes: plasma aldosterone level, renin activity measurement, careful monitoring of potassium levels, discontinuation or reduction of antihypertensives, IV fluids with no potassium unless levels are low, moderately high sodium diet, and avoidance of the overuse of exogenous steroids.

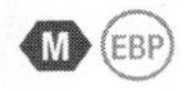

  - o In patients having laparoscopic adrenalectomy, the benefits of blood pressure normalization without medication far outweigh the risks of surgery.

Concept Check

7. How should discontinuation of long-term corticosteroids proceed?

A. Double dose for 2 days and then discontinue.

B. Taper doses over an extended period of time.

C. Switch doses to morning administration for 1 week before discontinuing.

D. Abruptly discontinue.

Answer question

Patient Education: Corticosteroid Excess

It is important to educate the patient and family prior to discharge about:

- The specific adrenal disorder
- Any prescribed medical and pharmacological interventions to ensure adequate understanding
- Interventions to prevent symptoms of adrenal disorders (e.g., skin breakdown, infections, hypertension)
- Signs and symptoms to assess for, such as stroke, how to prevent symptoms, and when to notify the health care provider
- Complications, signs, and symptoms of the opposite adrenal disorder resulting from treatment with medications

Summary of Interventions

- **Adrenal insufficiency** is treated with steroid supplementation.
- Adrenal insufficiency that develops abruptly can lead to adrenal crisis. Adrenal crisis is treated with:
  - o Corticosteroids
  - o Aggressive IV hydration, possibly vasopressors if hypotension is persistent
  - o Reverse electrolyte imbalances
- Preventing adrenal crisis perioperatively in patients on chronic high dose steroids can be avoided by starting a short supplement.
- **Corticosteroid excess** is usually treated with removal or reduction of corticosteroid treatment, if this is possible.

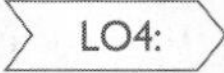

Evaluation of Desired Collaborative Care Outcomes

Evaluation and reassessment should reveal attainment of previously established patient outcomes. In summary:

- Patient reports being able to complete tasks of daily living without feeling exhausted.
- Patient identifies bodily changes due to disease process and reports the ability to cope with these changes.
- Patient discusses recognized stress factors, strategies to reduce them, and ways to prevent development of infection.
- Patient's skin is lesion free.
- Patient's blood pressure is within expected range, skin turgor is good, and urine output is balanced with fluid intake.

References

Coursin, D. B., & Connery, L. E. (2004). Assessment and therapy of selected endocrine disorders. *Anesthesiology Clinics of North America, 22*(1), 93–124.

Coursin, D., & Wood, K. (2002). Corticosteroid supplementation in adrenal insufficiency. *JAMA, 287*(2), 236–240.

Luken, K. (2007). Clinical manifestations and management of Addison's disease. *J Amer Academy Nurse Practitioners, 11*(4), 151–154.

Luliano, S., & Laws, E. R. (2013). Early recognition of Cushing's disease: A case study. *J Amer Assoc Nurse Practitioners, 25*(8), 402–406.

Grossman, A.B. (2010). Clinical review: The diagnosis and management of central hypoadrenalism. *J Clin Endocrinol Metab, 95*(11), 4855.

Nicholson, G., Burrin, J. M., & Hall, G. M. (1998). Perioperative steroid supplementation. *Anaesthesia, 53*, 1091–1104.

Clinical Practice Guidelines

Biller, B. M., Grossman, A. B., Stewart, P. M., et al. (2008). Treatment of adrenocorticotropin-dependent Cushing's syndrome: A consensus statement. *J Clin Endocrinol Metab, 93*, 2452.

Funder, J. W., Carey, R. M., Fardella, C., et al. (2008). Case detection, diagnosis, and treatment of patients with primary aldosteronism: An Endocrine Society's Clinical Guidelines. *J Clin Endocrinol & Metab, 93*(9), 3266–3281.

Marik, P. E., Pastores, S. M., Annane, D., et al., & American College of Critical Care Medicine. (2008). Recommendations for the diagnosis and management of corticosteroid insufficiency in critically ill adult patients: Consensus statements from an international task force by the American College of Critical Care Medicine. *Crit Care Med, 36*(6), 1937–1949.

Patient Education

Meyer, M. (2013). Addison's disease and Cushing's syndrome: The role of the nurse in patient education and interventions. *Mosby's Clinical Consult.* **www.nursingconsult.com/nursing/clinical-updates/full-text?clinical_update_id=199181**

Nieman, L., & Swearingen, B. (2013). *Cushing's syndrome and Cushing's disease: Your questions answered.* New York, NY: The Pituitary Society. **www.pituitarysociety.org**

Neiman, L. K. (2015). *Patient information: Adrenal insufficiency (Addison's disease).* **www.uptodate.com/contents/adrenal-insufficiency-addisons-disease-beyond-the-basics**

Nieman, L. K. (2015). *Patient information: Cushing's Syndrome.* **www.uptodate.com/contents/cushings-syndrome-beyond-the-basics?source=search_result&search=patient+information+cushing%27s&selectedTitle=2~150**

Learning Outcomes for Obesity

When you complete this lesson, you will be able to:

1. Recognize the clinical relevance of obesity.
2. Consider the pathophysiology, etiology, risk factors, and clinical presentation of obesity that determine the priority patient concerns.
3. Determine the most urgent and important nursing interventions and patient education required in caring for a patient with obesity.
4. Evaluate attainment of desired collaborative care outcomes for a patient with obesity.

LO1:

What Is Obesity?

- Obesity refers to the accumulation of excess body fat that leads to adverse health outcomes.
- Obesity is measured by the body mass index (BMI), which is a person's weight in kilograms divided by the height in meters.

BMI	Classification
< 18.5	Underweight
18.5–24.9	Normal weight
25.0–29.9	Overweight
30.0–34.9	Class I obesity
35.0–39.9	Class II obesity
≥ 40.0	Class III obesity

For adults 20 years of age or older.

LO1:

Clinical Relevance

Obesity is reaching epidemic proportions in the United States

- More than one-third of the adult population is obese.
- At least 2.8 million people die each year as a result of being overweight or obese.
- In 2008, medical costs associated with obesity were estimated at $147 billion by the Centers for Disease Control and Prevention (CDC).
- Obesity is increasing and is often referred to as the "obesity epidemic."
- Medical problems and mortality are increased in the obese population (see the following diagrams).

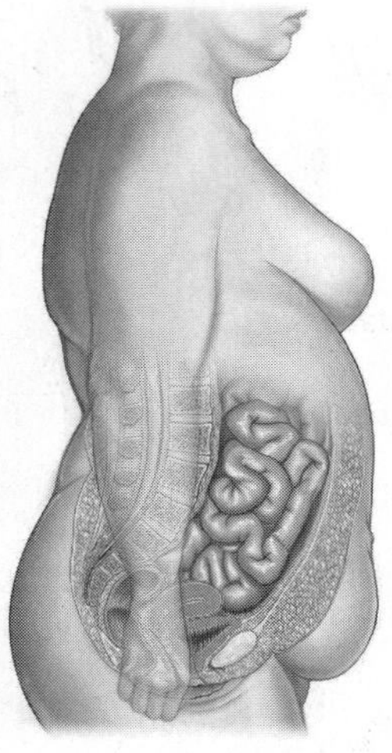

This illustration of an obese female shows the abdominal and pelvic cavities, particularly the small intestines.

Source: © 2014 Nucleus Medical Media, All rights reserved

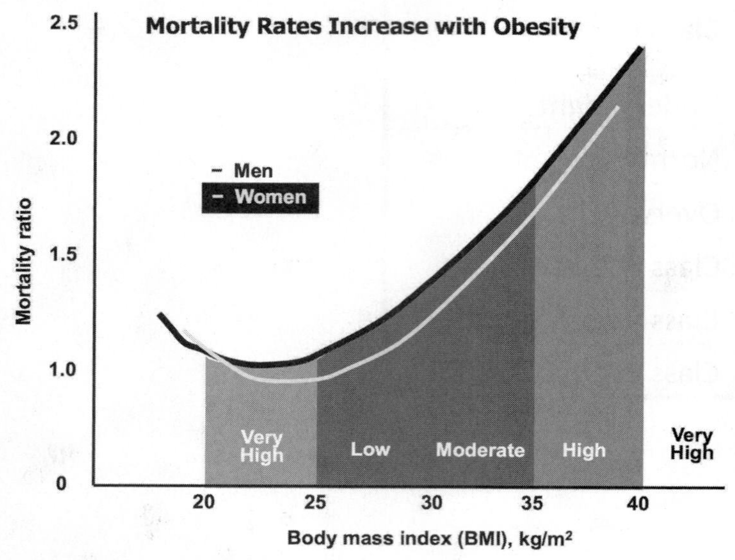

Mortality rate increases with obesity.

Source: Copyright © 2014, NovEx Novice to Expert Learning, LLC

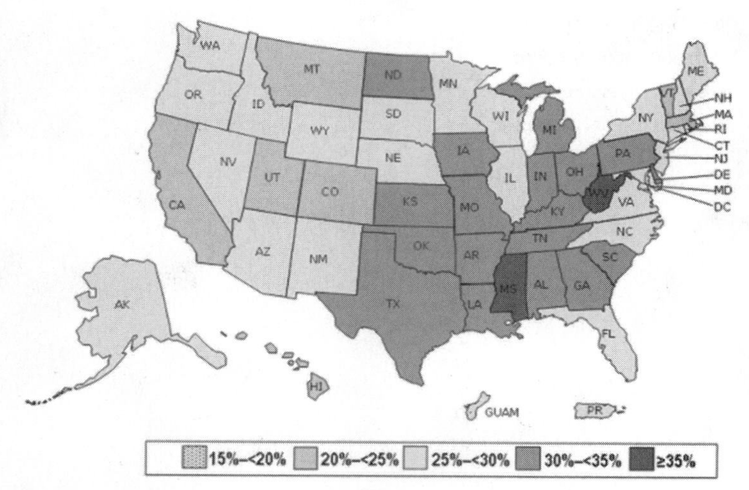

Obesity prevalent and increasing in United States. Percent of obese (BMI >30) in U.S. adults (2013).

Source: Centers for Disease Control and Prevention

LO2:

Pathophysiology

The primary cause of the majority of obesity is increased (caloric) food intake and decrease in physical activity.

- Hormonal influences may also play a role in the development of obesity, particularly leptin and its counterpart, ghrelin. The role that these hormones play in modulating appetite and fat storage have only been better understood recently and described. Research is ongoing.
- Overall, the pathophysiology represents interactions with a complex and incompletely understood hormonal system with environmental factors.

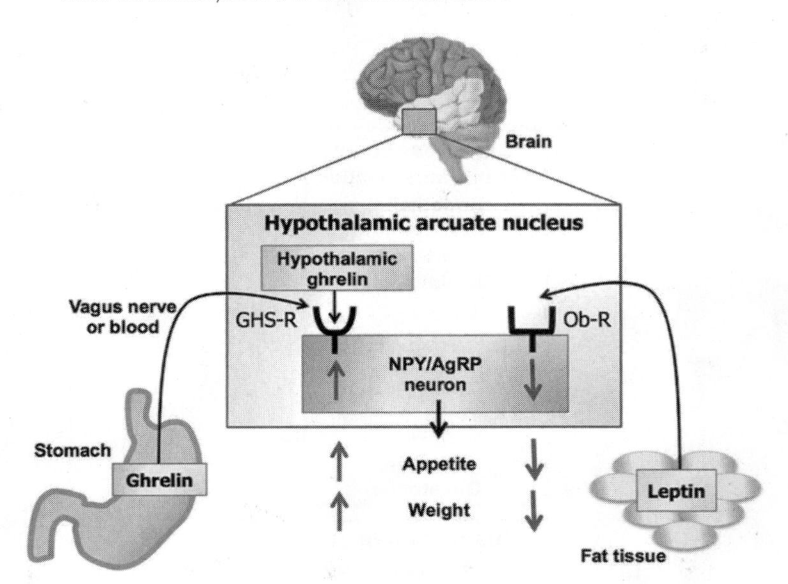

Leptin and ghrelin are key factors in appetite regulation and therefore affect body weight and fat. Hunger stimulates eating. Eating maintains or increases body weight. Both leptin and ghrelin are secreted by peripheral tissues, making them peripheral signals, but have central effects on the brain. *Leptin reduces hunger whereas ghrelin stimulates hunger. Normally, these hormones correlate to one's nutritional status and fat mass. The greater the fat mass, the more leptin produced. However, obesity unfortunately interferes with hormonal modulation.*

Metabolic Syndrome

- Metabolic syndrome describes central obesity (increased waist to hip ratio), associated with insulin resistance, hypertension, and dyslipidemia. There are slight differences in the definitions provided by the World Health Organization (WHO), the National Cholesterol Education Program, and other organizations.
- The development of insulin resistance depends on familial predisposition, weight gain, and lack of activity. Fat tissue is known to secrete hormones and cytokines that have significant metabolic effects on distant tissue. Increased visceral fat (fat around the internal organs) stores are associated with deleterious effects resulting in insulin resistance, hypertension, hyperlipidemia, and hyperglycemia or diabetes. All of these conditions predispose to the development of heart disease.
- The clinical usefulness of categorizing this as a syndrome is questionable because its treatment is basically directed at its components. However, treatment of insulin resistance, through weight loss and exercise, usually results in improvement in the rest of the components and conditions, including hypertension and hyperlipidemia.

Concept Check

1. **Which hormone is thought to decrease hunger?**
   A. Ghrelin
   B. Estrogen
   C. Testosterone
   D. Leptin

Answer question

Common Medical Consequences

- Diabetes
- Hypertension
- Hyperlipidemia
- Coronary artery disease
- Venous thromboembolic disease
- Gastro-esophageal reflux disease (GERD)
- Sleep apnea, respiratory insufficiency
- Osteoarthritis
- Increased risk of breast and colon cancer

Neuropsychosocial
Eating disturbance
Low self-esteem
Poor body image
Social isolation
Depression
Idiopathic intracranial hypertension

Respiratory
Sleep apnea
Asthma
Exercise intolerance

Endocrine
Type 2 diabetes
Menstrual disorder
Insulin resistance
Glucose intolerance
Precocious puberty
Polycystic ovarian syndrome

Hematology
Coagulopathy

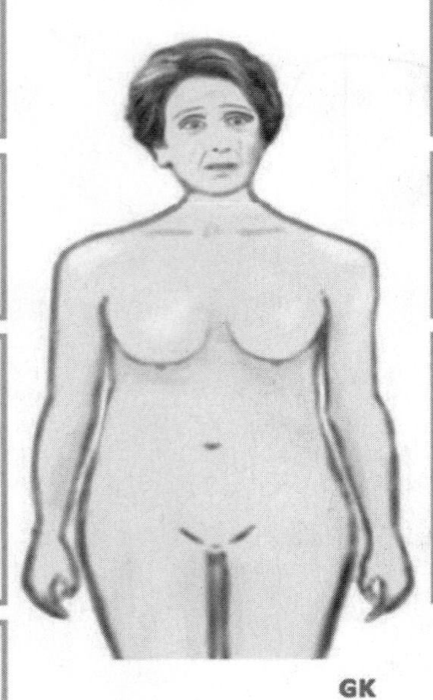

Cardiovascular
Chronic inflammation
Endothelial dysfunction
Hypertension
Dyslipidemia

Gastrointestinal
Gastro-esophageal reflux
Fatty liver
Gallstones

Musculoskeletal
Flat feet
Blount's disease
Sprained ankle
Fracture of forearm
Slipped capital femoral epiphysis

Source: Courtesy of George Kyriakidis/Santa Ana, CA

LO2:

Risk Factors and Causes

- Genetics
- Sedentary lifestyle
- Unhealthy diet or poor eating habits
- Smoking cessation
- Familial habits
- Particular medications
- Pregnancy
- Increasing age
- Medical conditions such as polycystic ovarian syndrome, Prader–Willi syndrome, diabetes or insulin resistance, and others.
- Lack of sleep
- Socioeconomic factors

LO2: Diagnostics

- Diagnosis of obesity and its severity is based upon measurement of the body mass index (BMI).
- Patients who are muscular may appear to be obese with this method:

BMI	Classification
Underweight	< 18.5
Normal weight	18.5–24.9
Overweight	25.0–29.9
Obesity	> 30.0

- **Waist to hip ratio** is a way of measuring visceral (abdominal) fat. Abdominal fat is more harmful. Waist to hip ratio is a stronger predictor of heart disease, diabetes, and mortality than BMI.
- The higher the waist to hip ratio, the greater the chance of developing complications of metabolic syndrome.
- Waist circumference is measured at the top of the iliac crest. This is usually the thinnest portion of the waist and is above the umbilicus. Hip circumference is measured around the widest portion. These measurements are taken after exhalation and with the patient relaxed. Obesity is defined by the WHO as waist/hip >0.95 for men and >0.8 for women.
- Alternatively, waist circumference alone can be used as a measure of risk. The AHA defines obesity as a circumference of >88 cm in women and >102 cm in men. If most of one's fat is around the waist (apple shaped) rather than at the hips (pear shaped), there is a higher risk for heart disease and type 2 diabetes. This risk increases with a waist size that is >35 inches for women or >40 inches for men.
- Other methods to measure body fat exist but are not convenient to use.

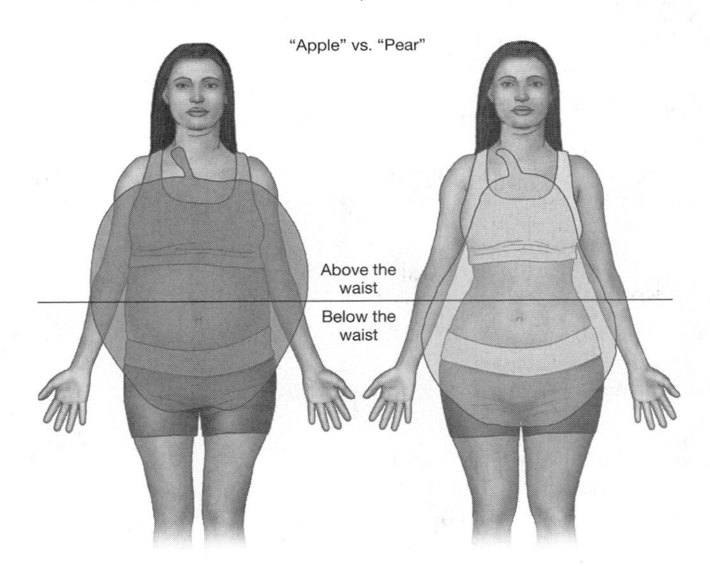

This picture compares a person with metabolic syndrome, or apple shape, with lower body, pear-shaped, obesity.

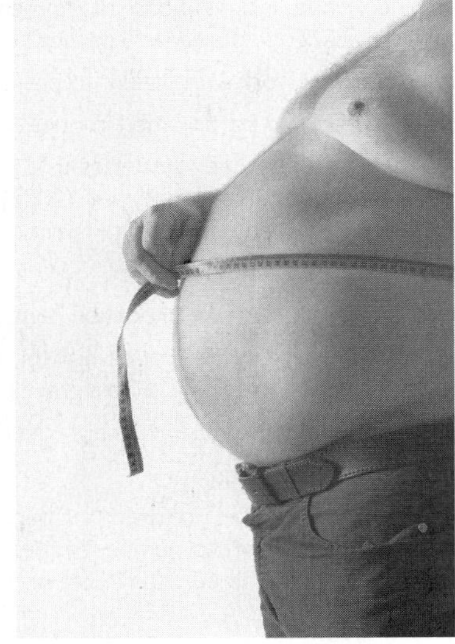

This photo shows the waist line of a person with metabolic syndrome who is at higher risk for multiple diseases.
Source: courtyardpix/Fotolia

Concept Check

2. Which finding is most significant for the development of heart disease?
   A. High BMI
   B. Low BMI
   C. High waist to hip ratio
   D. Low waist to hip ratio

Answer question

Priority Patient Concerns and Desired Collaborative Care Outcomes: Obesity

Prior to caring for patients who are obese, it is important to prioritize the patient's concerns that must guide the nursing care plan and interventions. Care for the patient is ordered and organized in accordance with the patient's priority and urgent needs. Desired collaborative care outcomes in patients who are obese typically include:

1. Patient will resume or gradually progress to return to ADL, self-care, and exercise.
2. Patient will eat a balanced diet.
3. Patient will demonstrate understanding that excess weight and poor nutrition increase risk for multiple disorders and will begin to modify risk factors.
4. Patient will exhibit positive or improved self-esteem.
5. Patient will accurately describe own body.

Considering these important care outcomes, prepare a list of the major 3–6 priority patient concerns or nursing diagnoses for patients who are obese. Be prepared to participate in a discussion of this list and/or to submit them as an assignment, as determined by your faculty. Resources you may find helpful in this assignment can include this lesson, the references, resources on nursing care plans, and standard nursing diagnoses manuals.

LO3:

Collaborative Interventions

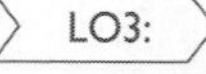

- Following medical evaluation, assess the patient's readiness for losing weight.

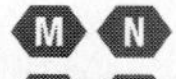

- If ready, continue interventions recommended by the American Gastroenterological Association (2002). If not ready to participate:
  - o Collaboratively work with patient to prevent further weight gain
  - o Identify barriers to participation in obesity therapy

Obesity therapy focuses on key strategies that are evidence-based and recommended by the American Gastroenterological Association (2002) and the Agency of Healthcare Research and Quality (2010). Aggressiveness of therapy guided by the patient's health risk:

- Dietary modifications should aim at:
  - o Reducing caloric intake with portion controlled servings
  - o Substituting energy-dense foods high in sugar and animal fat with low energy-dense foods (e.g., fruits, vegetables, whole grains)
  - o Limiting alcohol intake due to its high calories per gram
  - o Reducing fast-food intake

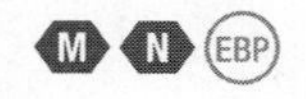

- Physical activity should be increased to a minimum of 30 minutes of cardiovascular exercise for 5 days per week. The total number of calories per week spent on exercise is the key. Eventually, increase exercise to 60–90 minutes of moderate-intensity exercise or 30–45 minute of vigorous exercise.

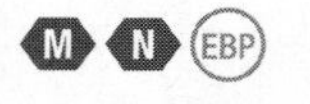

- Behavior modification and patient education improves the effectiveness and success of diet and exercise in weight loss.

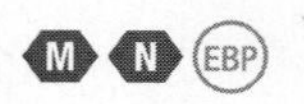

- Medications such as orlistat, lorcaserin, phentermine, and topiramate can modestly reduce weight. Drug therapy should only be given concurrently with the previously discussed interventions. Medication therapy needs to be monitored and discontinued when possible.

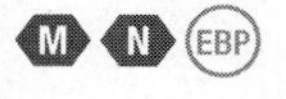

- Bariatric surgery should be considered if diet, exercise, and medications fail to help the patient attain a healthy body weight.

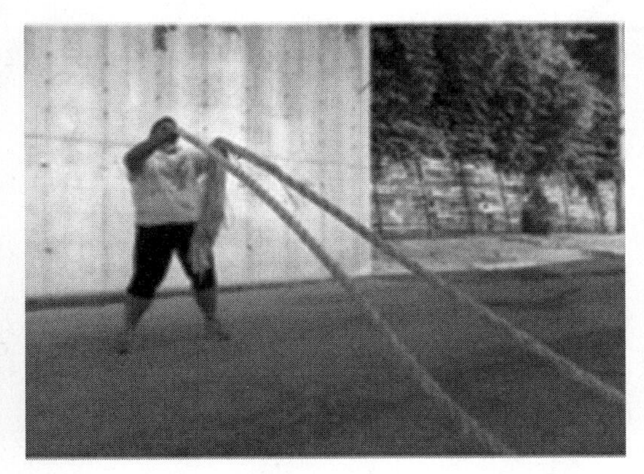

Source: Courtesy of R. Murphy

- Safety precautions are paramount when caring for obese patients:
  - o Whether admitted for obesity-related problems, bariatric surgery, or for another condition with obesity as a comorbid condition, obese patients must be carefully monitored and managed for skin problems and pressure ulcers. Carefully examine between skins folds in addition to normal sites (e.g., sacral area). Regularly reposition (every 2 hours) tubes and catheters to prevent them from burrowing into and disrupting the skin. Avoid excess moisture in skin folds that promote infections. Consult a wound specialist and dietician for wound-healing issues.
  - o Environmental factors that commonly pose risk, but require greater attention when assisting obese patients include wet or slippery floors, objects obstructing pathways, uneven flooring, small or difficult spaces in which to maneuver, poorly made or designed furnishings or baths, and uneven transfer surfaces.
  - o Be familiar with the patient's ability to cooperate and assist in weight-bearing activities prior to mobilizing the patient.
  - o Use assistive devices and team members to help mobilize the patient.
  - o A semi-Fowler's position may improve respiratory function. Obesity reduces expiratory reserve volume and functional residual capacity. Monitor for respiratory compromise, hypoventilation, and sleep apnea.
  - o During cardiac arrest, adequate CPR is difficult to assess without a Doppler to hear blood flow via the carotid arteries. Placement on a backboard presents a threat to both caregiver safety and to the patient's skin. Intubation should be performed by someone experienced or trained in situations where the landmarks are difficult to visualize.
  - o Medication administration can require taking the excess body fat into account. Intramuscular injections may require a longer length than the standard 1–1.5 inch needles.
  - o IV access may be a challenge and should be secured prior to a potential emergency.

Concept Check

3. What is the minimum amount of exercise an obese patient should get each week?

A. 30 minutes every day

B. At least 150 minutes each week

C. 15 minutes twice each day

D. 10 minutes three times each day

Answer question

Collaborative Interventions (continued)

Patient Education

Patient education for patients with obesity should include recommendations from the American Gastroenterological Association (2002).

- Educate about risk factor modification and treatment.
- Encourage a reduced calorie diet and portion control at every meal. Change grocery shopping to eliminate unhealthy choices and replace with nutritious options. Share the following sample grocery lists with patients.

Proteins	**Vegetables**	**Fruits** (low to medium in sugar)
Chicken breast	Broccoli	Lemon
Lean ground turkey	Asparagus	Lime
Lean ground beef	Lettuce (no Iceberg)	Rhubarb
Top sirloin steak (preferably grass fed)	Cauliflower	Raspberries
Wild game meat	Fresh green beans	Blackberries
Buffalo	Mushrooms	Cranberries
Swordfish	Peppers	Strawberries
Orange roughy fish	Onion	Papaya
Salmon	Peas	Blueberries
Tuna	Spinach	Watermelon
Trout	Kale	Papaya
Crab	Zucchini	Cantaloupe
Lobster	Cabbage	Honeydew
Shrimp	Artichokes	Plums
Egg whites or egg beaters (any sort of substitute)	Brussel sprouts	Oranges
Low fat cottage cheese	Cucumber	Kiwi
Tofu		
Veggie burgers		

Carbohydrates	**Good Fats**	**Fats to Avoid**
Baked potato	Avocados	Butter
Sweet potato	Sunflower seeds	Fried foods
Yams	Pumpkin seeds	Mayonnaise
Squash	Natural peanut butter	Sweets
Barley	Cold water fish	Whole-fat dairy
Beans (kidney, black, garbanzo)	Olives	Sugar-dense fruits and vegetables
Steamed brown rice	Low-fat cheese	Chips
Quinoa (high in protein)	Low-fat salad dressing	Fast foods
Steel cut oats	Low-sodium nuts	
Fat-free/low sugar yogurt	Flax seed oil	
Low-calorie popcorn (no butter)	Coconut oil	
	Grapeseed oil	
	Sunflower oil	
	Olive oil	

These lists provide a sample grocery shopping list of healthy, low calorie foods. It may be helpful to improve nutritional intake and/or better manage weight. One's health care provider or nutritionist may alter the list or provide further guidance.
Source: Copyright © 2014, NovEx Novice to Expert Learning, LLC

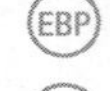

- Become active and/or exercise at least an hour each day of moderate-intensity exercise; however, exercise alone is not an effective strategy for weight loss.
- Employ behavior modification to accompany other weight loss strategies.

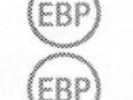

- Adhere to pharmacotherapy in conjunction with behavior modification to achieve effective results.

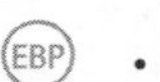

- Limit intake of sweetened or soda drinks.
- Eat most meals at home and limit restaurant and fast-food meals.

- Encourage regular self-weighing.

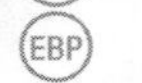

- Counsel on smoking cessation and educate about weight management interventions as patients who stop smoking are at risk for weight gain.

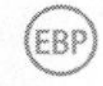

- Limit TV, computer, and video game time to <2 hours each day.
- Educate patient and family about disease process, medication use and side effects, recognition and avoidance of complications, management of comorbid conditions, smoking or drug cessation, follow-up care, and flu and pneumonia vaccines.

- Referral for physical therapist for individualized "exercise and activity" program

- Referral for nutrition consultation

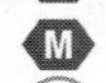

- Encourage individual or group support for psychological and/or behavioral support.

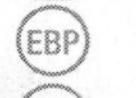

- Collaborate with health care providers to begin educating patients with BMI >40 kg/m^2 and those with severe obesity-related medical complication (e.g., heart failure, lipid disorders, arthritis, sleep apnea, diabetes, all causes of cancer, asthma, hypertension) about the benefits and effectiveness of bariatric surgery.

Priority Patient Concerns and Desired Collaborative Care Outcomes: Bariatric Surgery

Prior to caring for patients after bariatric surgery, it is important to prioritize the patient's concerns that must guide the nursing care plan and interventions. Care for the patient is ordered and organized in accordance with the patient's priority and urgent needs. Desired collaborative care outcomes in patients after bariatric surgery typically include:

1. Patient will maintain effective peripheral tissue perfusion without deep vein thrombosis.
2. Patient will maintain an effective breathing pattern without development of pulmonary emboli.
3. Patient's surgical recovery will not be delayed.
4. Patient will remain infection-free.
5. Patient will report that pain is at an acceptable level.

Considering these important care outcomes, prepare a list of the major 3–6 priority patient concerns or nursing diagnoses for patients after bariatric surgery. Be prepared to participate in a discussion of this list and/or to submit them as an assignment, as determined by your faculty. Resources you may find helpful in this assignment can include this lesson, the references, resources on nursing care plans, and standard nursing diagnoses manuals.

LO3:

Collaborative Interventions: Bariatric Surgery

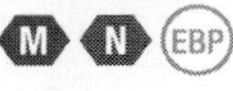

- Bariatric surgery is indicated for a BMI >40 and failure of nonsurgical treatments (American Gastroenterological Association, 2002).

- Surgery should be done in an accredited center with a multidisciplinary approach toward patient selection, education, and follow up.

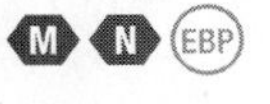

- Preoperatively, answer questions regarding surgery, offer reassurance, encourage smoking cessation for a minimum of 2 months prior, and establish baseline vital signs and physical exam (Mechanick, J. I., Youdim, A., Jones, D. B., et al., 2013).

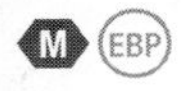

- Bariatric surgery can reverse medical problems associated with obesity such as diabetes, limited mobility from arthritis, hypertension, sleep apnea, and others, and therefore, influences the decision to recommend surgery (Mechanick, J. I., Youdim, A., Jones, D. B., et al., 2013).

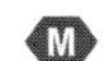

- Multiple surgical techniques have been developed that have two main mechanisms of action:
  - o Decreasing capacity of stomach with laparoscopic gastric banding
  - o Decreasing absorption area of small bowel by the Roux-en-Y-gastric bypass

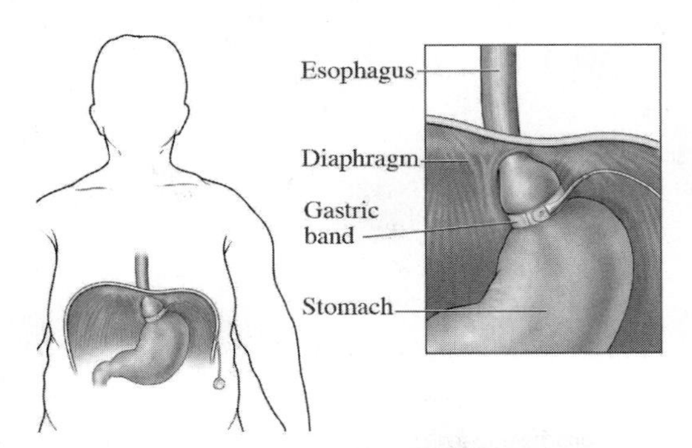

This diagram illustrates the surgical placement of a gastric band for treatment of obesity, known as Gastric Band Surgery. The diagram on the left shows the internal organs in relations to each other. A close-up view on the right depicts how the gastric band is placed around the upper portion of the stomach.

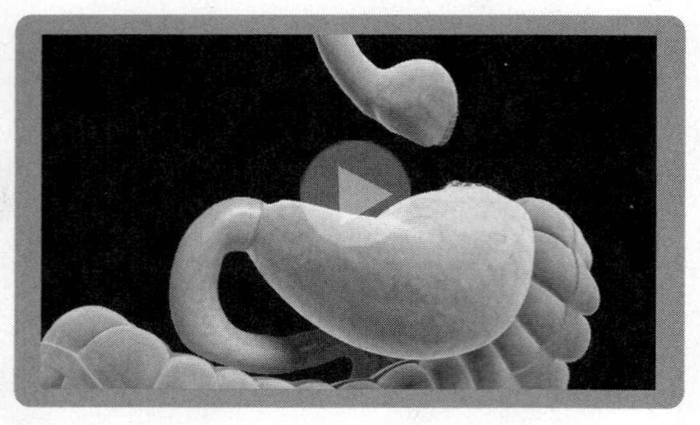

This animation demonstrates common surgical procedures used in bariatric surgery. Bariatric surgery is considered after less invasive weight reduction efforts and medications fail. It is performed on patients with a body mass index >40. If a serious medical condition, such as heart disease is exacerbated by obesity, patients with a BMI of ≥35 may receive surgery. Two types of bariatric surgery are shown: restrictive and malabsorptive. Gastric banding is a restrictive surgery while a biopancreatic diversion creates a malabsorptive result. Roux-en-Y, a gastric bypass, creates both restriction and malabsorption.

Concept Check

4. Which conditions are necessary prior to the patient being considered for bariatric surgery?

A. The patient must pledge to follow diet instructions.

B. The patient must have hypertension.

C. The patient must have failed nonsurgical weight management.

D. The patient must have diabetes mellitus.

Answer question

Collaborative Interventions: Bariatric Surgery (continued)

Postoperative Care of the Bariatric Patient

Postoperative care of the bariatric patient can require significant nursing care and includes evidence-based practice recommendations (Mechanick, J. I., Youdim, A., Jones, D. B., et al., 2013).

- Aggressive pulmonary toilet and monitoring:
  - M N o Auscultate lung sounds frequently as atelectasis can occur.
  - N o Have patient cough and deep breathe 10 times every hour.
  - N EBP o Use incentive spirometry to prevent respiratory infections.
  - M N EBP o Oxygen supplement as needed
  - N o Obese and morbidly obese patients are at high risk for hypoventilation syndrome and for obstructive sleep apnea. Monitor using capnography for rapid identification of respiratory complications.
- N Teach the patient to splint the wound when coughing to prevent dehiscence.
- M N EBP Mobilize the patient early to help prevent skin breakdown, respiratory complications, and promote circulation.
- M N EBP Administer prescribed anticoagulants (e.g., heparin or aspirin) and apply sequential compression devices and/or compression stockings to help prevent deep vein thrombosis.
- M N Order Big Boyz bed as indicated. These beds are considerably wider and built to accommodate the increased weight needed for patients.
- N Clinicians must take care to ensure sufficient help and/or appropriate use of equipment in moving the patient to avoid back injuries (see photo).

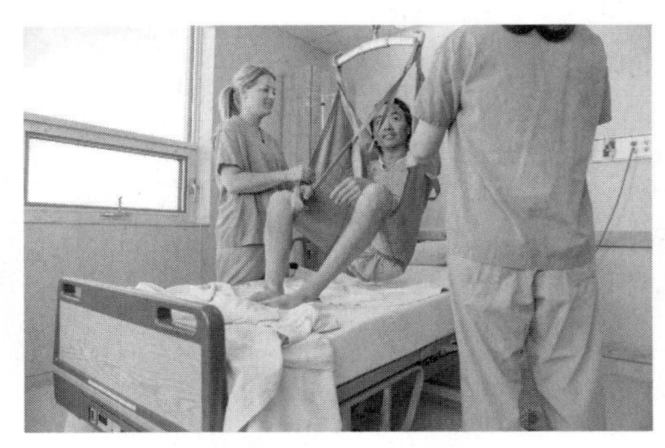

This photo shows the use of a lift to allow safe movement. It is particularly important to use for obese and bariatric patients.
Source: Tyler Olson/Fotolia

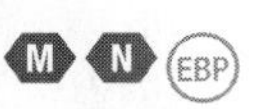

- Monitor for signs of anastomotic leak including respiratory distress, failure to wean from ventilator, and tachycardia over 120 beats/min sustained for more than 4 hours.
- Dietary and nutritional planning, guidance, and management should include:
  - o Clear liquids within 24 hours
  - o Staged progression of meals
  - o Nutrition counseling
  - o Nutritional supplements (e.g., minerals, iron, vitamins) when indicated

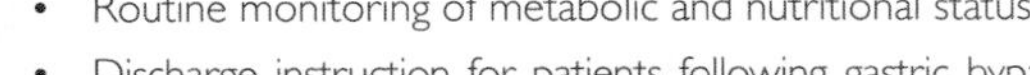

- Routine monitoring of metabolic and nutritional status
- Discharge instruction for patients following gastric bypass surgery should include education about dumping syndrome (undigested food is rapidly dumped by the stomach into the small intestines and creates nausea, cramping, and/or diarrhea) and ways to prevent it from occurring.
  - o More common in bypass surgery (not banding procedures), dumping syndrome can occur following meals and can cause loose stools.
  - o The nurse should educate the patient on eating solids and liquids at different times, eating very small frequent meals, and sitting up for 30–60 minutes following a meal to prevent the syndrome from occurring (see patient education).

Concept Check

5. Which patient is a candidate for bariatric surgery?

A. A healthy female whose BMI is 36

B. A healthy male whose BMI is 38

C. A female with heart disease whose BMI is 35

D. A male with hypertension whose BMI is 32

Answer question

Collaborative Interventions: Bariatric Surgery (continued)

Patient Education: Bariatric Surgery

Patient education for patients after bariatric surgery can vary among organizations and programs, but common issues for patients include:

M N
- Educate patient on ways to prevent dumping syndrome (avoid intake of solids without liquids, avoid lying down after meals, lie on left side).

N
- Eat small, frequent meals. Start by eating only three to five bites with a 20-minute pause prior to eating more. Eat slowly and chew food thoroughly.

N
- Avoid foods and activities that introduce air and gas (e.g., chewing gum, using straws, eating ice, drinking carbonated beverages), and eating sugar-dense foods (e.g., desserts, drinks, juices). (Follow your hospital's specific discharge instructions.)

M N
- Avoid or limit alcohol use. There is evidence of increased alcohol abuse and sensitivity following bariatric surgery.

M N
- Educate on standard for postoperative care, pain management, and wound management.

M N
- Reduced calorie diet. Reduce or avoid breads, raw fruits and vegetables, and unground meats.

M N
- Referral for physical therapy, dietitian, health care provider

N
- Educate patient and family about disease process, medication use and side effects, recognition and avoidance of complications, wound care, exercise, management of comorbid conditions, smoking and drug cessation, follow-up care, when to call the health care provider or 911, advanced directives, and flu and pneumonia vaccines.

M N
- Educate the patient about common complications and the need for ongoing follow-up care with health care provider related to electrolyte imbalances, metabolic panel, and persistent diarrhea and/or vomiting.

Concept Check

6. Which information should be included in dietary instruction for patients having bariatric surgery?

A. Initially, do not eat more than ½ cup of food at a time.

B. Drink sufficient fluids during meals.

C. Chew gum between meals to decrease hunger.

D. Avoid raw fruits and vegetables.

Answer question

Concept Check

7. Which position is most likely to increase the ability to breath in a patient who is obese?

A. Supine

B. Prone

C. High-Fowler's

D. Semi-Fowler's

Answer question

Summary of Interventions: Obesity

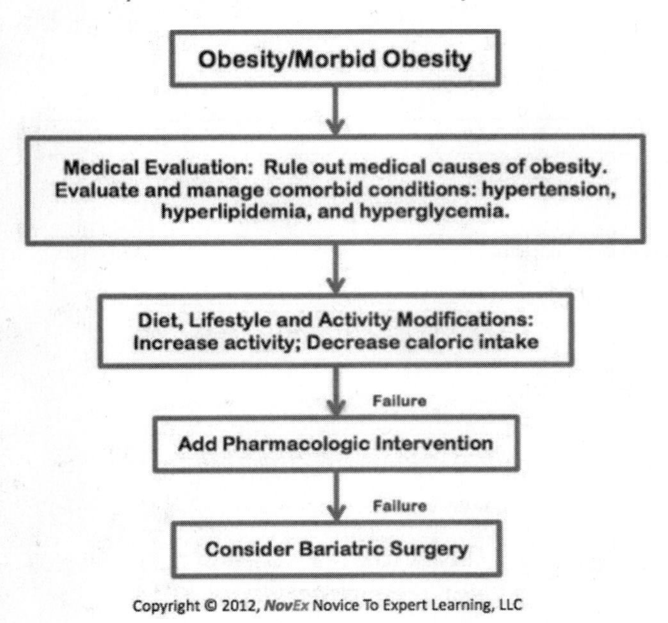

Source: Copyright © 2014, NovEx Novice to Expert Learning, LLC

Summary of Interventions: Bariatric Surgery

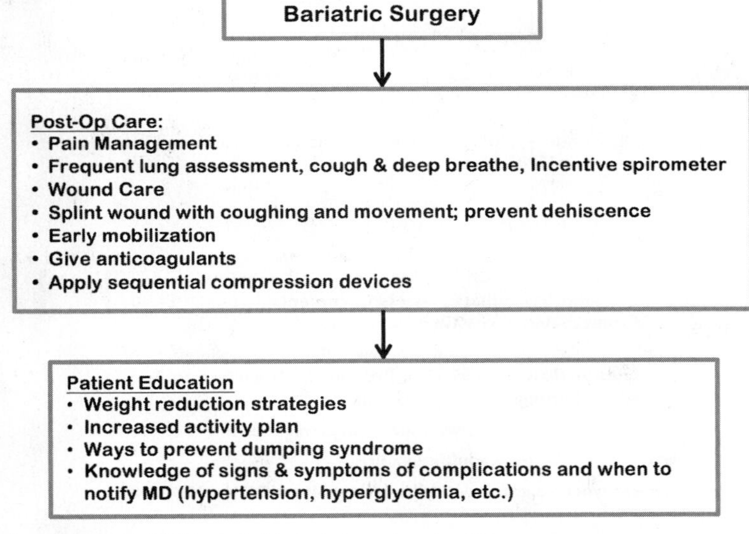

Source: Copyright © 2014, NovEx Novice to Expert Learning, LLC

LO4: Evaluation of Desired Collaborative Care Outcomes

Evaluation and reassessment should reveal attainment of previously established patient outcomes. In summary:

Obesity

- Patient reports progressive improvement in activity tolerance and participation in a daily exercise routine.
- Patient has increased percentage of diet based on lean meats, low-fat dairy, vegetables, and whole grains.
- Patient recognizes that food and exercise choices are significant factors in overall health.
- Patient reports feeling more confident and satisfied with self.
- Patient's description of body is based on reality.

Bariatric Surgery

- Patient has not developed deep vein thrombosis.
- Patient has not developed pulmonary embolism.
- Patient's surgical recovery is progressing at the expected or acceptable rate.
- Patient is infection-free.
- Patient reports that pain is diminished to an acceptable level.

References

Brown, J. (2012). *Managing obesity in adults. Nurs Times, 108* (48), 18–19. **www.nursingtimes.net/Journals/2012/11/22/v/x/f/121127-managing-obesity.pdf**

Burke, L. E., & Wang, J. (2011). Treatment strategies for overweight and obesity. *J Nurs Scholarship, 43*(4), 368–375. doi: 10.1111/j.1547-5069.2011.01424.x

Camden, S. G. (2009). Obesity: An emerging concern for patients and nurses. *OJIN: Online J Issues in Nursing, 14*(1). doi: 10.3912/OJIN.Vol14No1Man01

Goldie, C., & Brown, J. (2012). Managing obesity in primary care. *Nurs Times, 108, 14–16.* **www.nursingtimes.net/managing-obesity-in-primary-care/5039789.article**

McGinley, L. D. (2008). Best practices for safe patient handling of the morbidly obese patient. *Bariatric Nurs Surgical Patient Care, 3*(4), 255–260.

NHS National Institute for Health and Clinical Excellence. (2006). *Obesity: Guidance on the prevention, identification, assessment and management of overweight and obesity in adults and children: NICE clinical guideline 43.* National Collaborating Centre for Primary Care and the Centre for Public Health Excellence at NICE. London: NICE. **www.tinyurl.com/NICE-obesity**

World Health Organization. (2008). *Waist circumference and waist-hip ratio: Report of a WHO expert consultation.* Geneva, Switzerland: WHO Press. **whqlibdoc.who.int/publications/2011/9789241501491_eng.pdf**

Clinical Practice Guidelines

Agency of Healthcare Research and Quality. (2010). *Management of obesity: A national clinical guideline.* **www.guideline.gov/content.aspx?id=15597&search=obesity**

American Gastroenterological Association Clinical Practice Committee. (2002). American Gastroenterological Association medical position statement on obesity. *Gastroenterology, 123*(3), 879–881. **www.gastrojournal.org/article/S0016-5085(02)00179-8/fulltext**

Mechanick, J. I., Youdim, A., Jones, D. B., et al. (2013). Clinical practice guidelines for the perioperative nutritional, metabolic, and nonsurgical support of the bariatric surgery patient—2013 update: Cosponsored by American Association of Clinical Endocrinologists, the Obesity Society, and American Society for Metabolic & Bariatric Surgery. *EndocrPract, 19*(2), e1–e36. **www.guideline.gov/content.aspx?id=47785**

Patient Education

Hope Project. (Accessed 12/2013). *The health & obesity: Prevention & education project.* La Jolla, CA: The Hope Project. **cdhnfsite.wms.cdgsolutions.com/user-assets/Documents/PDF/HOPE%20Project%20Publicity%20Brochure.pdf**

Nutrition, Life Style by Poliquin website. **www.lifestylebypoliquin.com/Lifestyle/Nutrition/697/Eat_Protein_for_Breakfast_to_Stay_Alert_Throughout_the_Day.aspx**

Paleo Plan. (2013). *Recipes.* **www.paleoplan.com/recipes/**

www.cdc.gov/obesity/adult/index.html

www.mayoclinic.com/obesity/basics/definition/CON-20014834

Learning Outcomes for Pituitary Gland Disorders

When you complete this lesson, you will be able to:

1. Recognize the clinical relevance of pituitary gland disorders.
2. Consider the pathophysiology, etiology, risk factors, and clinical presentation of pituitary gland disorders that determine the priority patient concerns.
3. Determine the most urgent and important nursing interventions and patient education required in caring for a patient with pituitary gland disorders.
4. Evaluate attainment of desired collaborative care outcomes for a patient with pituitary gland disorders.

LO1:

What Are Pituitary Disorders?

- Pituitary dysfunction is anything that interferes with the normal function and hormone secretion of the pituitary gland (also known as the hypophysis).
- Tumors are the most common cause of pituitary dysfunction. Injuries may cause pituitary dysfunction, but most other causes are uncommon.
- Pituitary tumors may be benign or malignant (cancer). Pituitary carcinomas are malignant but extremely rare.
- Disorders caused by pituitary tumors generally fall into three categories:
  - o Tumor mass effects or tumors that grow and impinge upon the pituitary gland or surrounding brain tissue to cause dysfunction.
  - o **Hypopituitary** dysfunctions or hyposecretion, which include:
    - Benign pituitary adenomas: adenohypophyseal cells that are usually not cancer, grow slowly, and do not spread outside the pituitary gland. These are the most common cause of hypopituitarism.
    - Invasive pituitary adenomas: cells are not malignant and are slow growing, but they do spread. These are also benign.
  - o **Hyperpituitary** dysfunctions or hypersecretion, which include:
    - Prolactinomas: pituitary adenomas that result in an increased secretion of prolactin (most common in women of childbearing age)

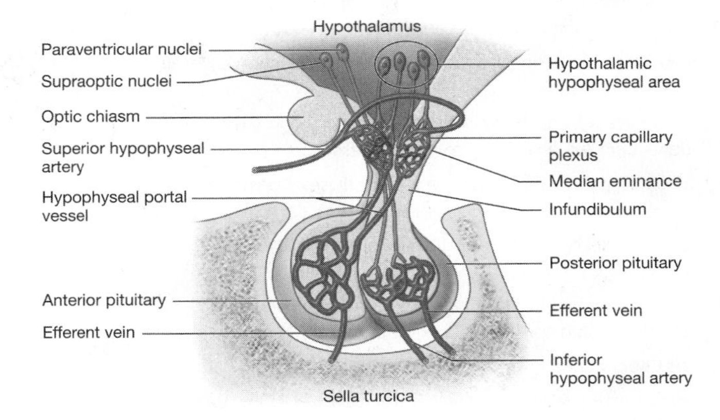

The location of the pituitary in close proximity to other vital structures in the brain allows pituitary tumors to affect many other functions.

Concept Check

1. What is the most common cause of pituitary dysfunction?
   A. Tumors
   B. Diabetes mellitus
   C. Congenital disorders
   D. Infection

Answer question

LO1:

Clinical Relevance

- Determining pituitary dysfunction is essential because of the important role of the pituitary on growth, metabolism, and normal functioning of the endocrine system.
- The pituitary also lies close to major blood vessels and nerves and can produce neurologic as well as hormonal symptoms.
- About 60 million people in the United States will develop a pituitary tumor.
- The mortality rate is low due to advanced medical and surgical management.
- Due to the proximity to the optic nerves, visual disturbance or loss of vision and other neurologic problems can result.
- One out of six individuals with pituitary tumors will develop symptoms, with the age of most common occurrence being between 30–40 years.

LO2:

Pathophysiology

The pituitary gland is a pea-sized gland that is located at the base of the brain. It has two lobes with different cellular structures and separate and distinct functions.

- The pituitary is often called the master endocrine gland due to its production of hormones that regulate the function of target endocrine glands.
- This regulatory gland influences cellular processes in the target glands (e.g., thyroid, adrenal) and throughout the body.
- Normal regulatory processes and the production and release of hormones are disrupted by pituitary tumors or uncommon genetic conditions. The pathophysiological consequences depend on the area of the pituitary gland that is affected. Hypersecretion or hyposecretion can adversely affect the normal functions, listed as follows.

The anterior lobe (adenohypophysis) secretes:

- Thyroid-stimulating hormone (TSH) or thyrotrophin: regulates the production of thyroid hormone by the thyroid gland, thereby regulating metabolism, growth, and activity by the nervous system
  - o Hyposecretion of TSH results in hypothyroidism (see the Care of Patients with Thyroid Disorders NovE-lesson)
- Growth hormone (GH) or somatotrophin: regulates muscle and bone mass, growth in children, well-being, fat distribution, and cartilage growth
  - o Hypersecretion of GH prior to puberty, before closure of the epiphyseal plates, can result in gigantism or extremely tall growth development.
  - o Hypersecretion of GH after puberty commonly results in acromegaly or a condition in which the forehead, maxilla, extremities, and tongue become enlarged.
- Adrenocorticotropic hormone (ACTH) or corticotropin: regulates cortisol production by the adrenal glands, blood glucose, and blood pressure
  - o Hypersecretion of ACTH creates excessive adrenal hormone release, resulting in Cushing syndrome (see the Care of Patients with Adrenal Disorders NovE-lesson)
- Prolactin (PRL) or lactotrophin: regulates milk production following childbirth, sex hormone levels, and fertility
- Luteininzing hormone (LH) or a gonadotrophin: regulates ovulation in females and testosterone production in males
- Follicle-stimulating hormone (FSH) or a gonadotrophin: helps regulate estrogen production by the ovaries and egg development in females and sperm production in males

The posterior lobe (neurohypophysis) secretes:

- Antidiuretic hormone (ADH) or vasopressin: regulates the body's water balance. ADH reduces water lost by the kidneys.
  - o Hypovolemia results in hyperosmolality, ADH is released and causes water reabsorption. Similarly, exogenous administration of ADH causes water to be reabsorbed by the kidneys.
  - o Conversely, hypoosmolality results in ADH suppression and a diuresis effect
  - o Abnormally, malignant tumors, head injury, pituitary surgery, or particular medications can cause overproduction of ADH. This condition is known as the syndrome of inappropriate ADH (SIADH). Excessive water retention (also called water intoxication) causes hyponatremia and other electrolyte imbalances.
- Hyposecretion of ADH causes diabetes insipidus (DI) or excessive loss of water in the urine (polyuria), which can be extreme. Dehydration and hypernatremia result. Infection, injury, tumor, and stroke are among potential causes of DI.
- Oxytocin: regulates milk flow during breastfeeding and increases uterine contractions during labor

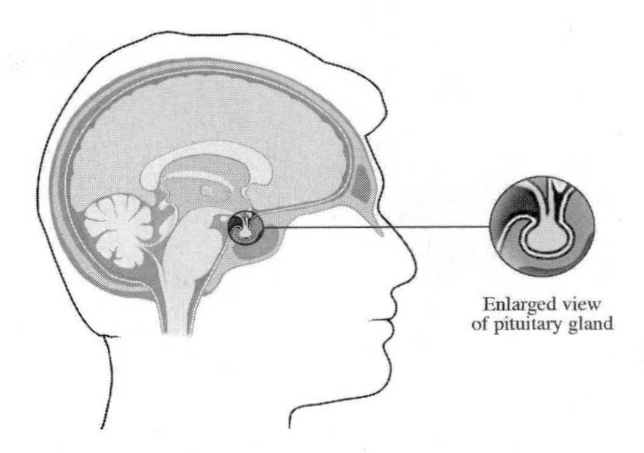

This image shows the pituitary gland, situated at the base of the brain.
Source: © 2014 Nucleus Medical Media, All rights reserved

Tumors

- Unless genetically inherited, pituitary dysfunction is generally caused by pituitary tumors. The pathophysiology of pituitary disorders stems from hyposecretion of hormones, hypersecretion, or mass effects.
- Tumor mass effects result from a tumor which presses upon the pituitary gland or upon brain tissue.
- Tumors may be functioning or secreting (meaning they make excessive amounts of one or more hormones), or nonfunctioning or nonsecreting (meaning they make no hormones). Most tumors are functioning.
- Tumors are classified as microadenomas (<1 cm) or macroadenomas (>1 cm). Some pituitary tumors can exist without producing symptoms.

Concept Check

2. Which lobe of the pituitary gland secretes growth hormone (GH)?

A. Posterior
B. Central
C. Lateral
D. Anterior

Answer question

LO2:

Risk Factors

Pituitary tumors are the most frequent cause of pituitary disorders; however, there is no known risk factor that predisposes a patient to tumors except in uncommon hereditary conditions. Therefore, there are no modifiable risk factors at the present.

LO2:

Causes

Hyperpituitarism

- Pituitary ademona (most common)
- Pituitary tumors
- Pituitary hyperplasia

Hypopituitarism

- Pituitary tumors (most common)
- Surgery to remove the pituitary gland
- Radiation therapy
- Trauma or head injury
- Infection
- Tumors near the pituitary
- Injury or infarction of the pituitary gland

LO2:

Assessment Findings

Symptoms of pituitary tumors are due to mass effect of the tumor on the pituitary gland with either overproduction or underproduction of hormones affecting target organs or other systems. Manifestations of tumors (malignant or benign) are identical and can include:

- Visual loss or disturbances
- Headaches
- Hair loss on the body
- Irregular and infrequent menstrual periods or no breast milk in women
- Facial hair loss, abnormal breast tissue growth, and impotence in men
- Reduced sex drive
- Slow sexual and growth development in children
- Other manifestations are related to interference with or additional production of hormones (hypopituitarism or hyperpituitarism)

Hypopituitarism

Symptoms Related to Pituitary Gland Deficiencies		
Pituitary Hormone Deficiency	**Target Gland**	**Symptoms**
ACTH (adrenocorticotropic hormone)	Adrenal	ACTH deficiency: weight loss, hypotension, chronic malaise, fatigue, nausea and vomiting, anorexia, hypoglycemia, depression
GH (growth hormone)	Many organs	GH deficiency: reduced muscle mass and strength, low exercise tolerance, fatigue, cold and heat sensitivity weight and fat gain, lower bone density, anxiety, depression
ADH (antidiuretic hormone)	Kidney	ADH deficiency: thirst, frequent urination
TSH (thyroid stimulating hormone)	Thyroid	TSH deficiency: weight gain, constipation, cold sensitivity, severe fatigue, malaise, muscle weakness, leg cramps, dry skin
Prolactin	Breast	Prolactin deficiency: loss of body hair, lack of milk production, fatigue
FSH & LH (follicle stimulating hormone and luteinizing hormone)	Gonads	FSH & LH deficiency: Men: hair loss, reduced libido, weakness, erectile dysfunction, infertility, headaches. Women: menstrual irregularity or amenorrhea, infertility

This table lists the pituitary hormone deficiencies, the organs they influence, and the symptoms that result.

Source: Copyright © 2014, NovEx Novice to Expert Learning, LLC

Hyperpituitarism

- Corticotrophin excess or Cushing's disease:
  - o Weight gain
  - o Moon face
  - o Red cheeks
  - o Muscle aches or myalgias
  - o "Buffalo" hump on back
  - o Malaise
  - o Easy bruising
  - o Poor wound healing
  - o Psychiatric manifestations
- Other effects can include hypertension or osteoporosis
- Growth hormone excess in adults: acromegaly (gigantism)
- Prolactin excess or hypogonadism
  - o Men: loss of sex drive, impotence
  - o Women: amenorrhea, infertility, excessive milk secretion

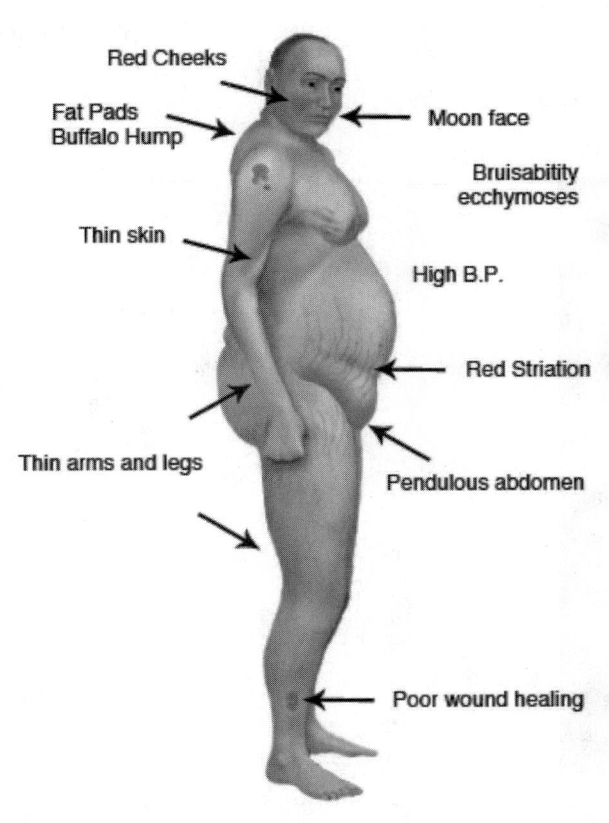

Symptoms in a patient with Cushing's disease.
Source: Copyright © 2014, NovEx Novice to Expert Learning, LLC

Concept Check

3. What is the reason for most visual disturbances associated with pituitary gland tumors?

A. Mass effect from the tumor
B. Increase of pituitary hormone
C. Decrease of pituitary hormone
D. Erosion of the retina

Answer question

Concept Check

4. Which lifestyle factor increases risk for pituitary tumors?

A. Smoking
B. High-fat diet
C. Sedentary lifestyle
D. There are no known risk factors.

Answer question

LO2:

Diagnostics

Pituitary Disorders

Labs:

- Serum prolactin levels
- Growth hormone levels
- Insulin-like growth hormone
- Glucose tolerance test
- 24-hour urine
- Dexamethasone suppression test
- Cortisol levels
- Thyroid hormone levels

EBP **Imaging** (Katznelson, et al., 2011):

- MRI of the brain is the preferred imaging study and provides better detail of the pituitary.
- CT scan is used if MRI is contraindicated (e.g., pacemaker).

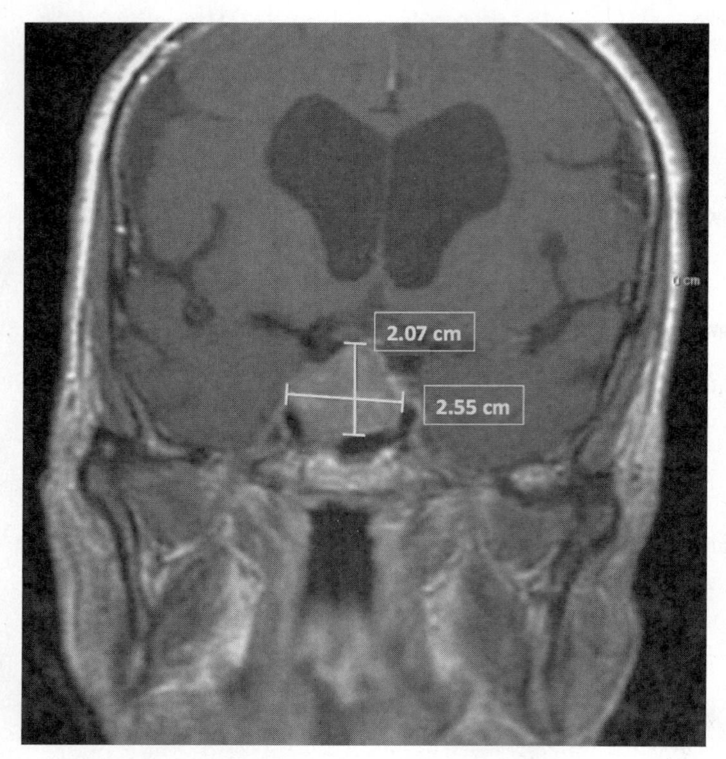

Brain MRI showing a 2.55 cm pituitary adenoma.
Source: Courtesy of K. Kyriakidis

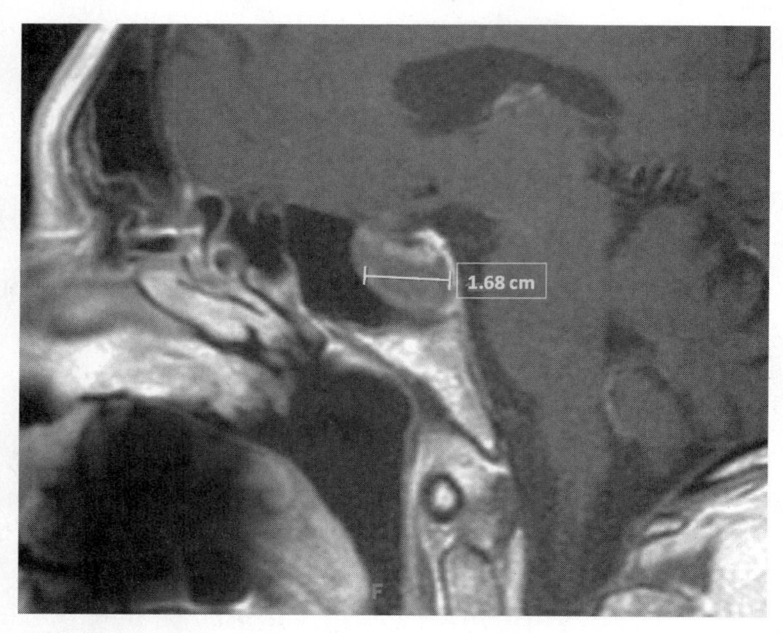

A 1.68 cm prolactinoma is seen on a brain MRI.
Source: Courtesy of K. Kyriakidis

Concept Check

5. **Thirst and frequent urination are findings associated with deficiency of which pituitary hormone?**
   A. ACTH
   B. ADH
   C. TSH
   D. FSH

Answer question

Concept Check

6. **Which finding is a manifestation of Cushing's disease?**
   A. Weight loss
   B. Malaise
   C. Pale skin
   D. Gaunt appearance of face

Answer question

Priority Patient Concerns and Desired Collaborative Care Outcomes

Prior to caring for patients with pituitary disorders, it is important to prioritize the patient's concerns that must guide the nursing care plan and interventions. Care for the patient is ordered and organized in accordance with the patient's priority and urgent needs. Desired collaborative care outcomes in patients with pituitary disorders typically include:

1. Patient will demonstrate growing acceptance of changes in body structures after understanding the causes.
2. Patient will demonstrate improved compliance with interventions to regulate hormones and improve pituitary functioning.
3. Patient will remain infection-free after surgery.
4. Fluid status will remain or return to expected range.
5. Patient will state return to or improvement in expected sexual patterns.

Considering these important care outcomes, prepare a list of the major 3–6 priority patient concerns or nursing diagnoses for patients with pituitary disorders. Be prepared to participate in a discussion of this list and/or to submit them as an assignment, as determined by your faculty. Resources you may find helpful in this assignment can include this lesson, the references, resources on nursing care plans, and standard nursing diagnoses manuals.

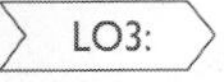

Collaborative Interventions

Medications

For many of the pituitary disorders, medication therapy is preferred to raise low hormone levels or to lower excessive hormone production. Drug combinations may be required:

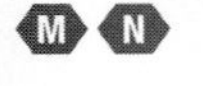

Hyperpituitarism

- Prolactinomas can be successfully treated with dopamine receptor agonists, such as bromocriptine and cabergoline.

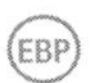

- Acromegaly can be treated with somatostatin analogues (SSAs), such as octreotide but surgery is recommended as the primary treatment with medication used as adjuvant therapy (Katznelson, et al., 2011.

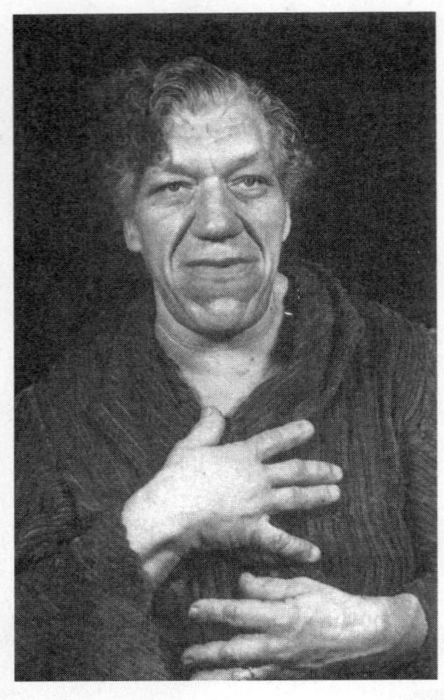

Patient with typical features of acromegaly or gigantism.

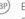

Hypopituitarism

- Hypothyroidism: Levothyroxine is commonly sufficient to manage this disorder.
- Adrenocoticosteroid deficiency: Cortisol is the treatment of choice.
- Hypogonadism:
  - o Male: Testosterone replacements can result in improvement.
  - o Female: Estrogen/progesterone replacements can alleviate problems.
- Growth hormone deficiency: Growth hormone replacement is needed.

Surgical Intervention

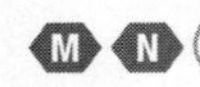

Evidence-based practices, recommended in the guidelines by the American Association of Clinical Endocrinologists (AACE) (2011) include:

- Microscopic transsphenoidal hypophysectomy surgery is the most common method used for pituitary tumor resection.
- Despite the surgical approach, it is the primary treatment for all patients with microadenomas, with select patients with macroadenomas, and with all patients with macroadenomas who also have mass effects caused by the tumor.
- The surgeon's experience and cure rates are linked to patient outcomes (mortality and morbidity).
- Adjuvant medical therapies are used in postoperative patients with persistent disease.
- Risks and benefits of medication, with any needed financial counseling, should be provided.
- Resection

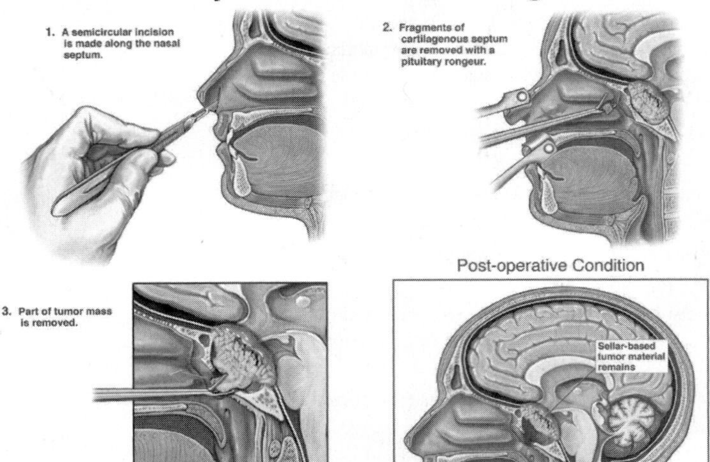
Invasive Pituitary Adenoma with Initial Surgical Excision
1. A semicircular incision is made along the nasal septum.
2. Fragments of cartilagenous septum are removed with a pituitary rongeur.
Post-operative Condition
3. Part of tumor mass is removed.
Sellar-based tumor material remains

This image is an illustration of trans-sphenoidalhypophysectomy surgery for a pituitary tumor.

Collaborative Interventions (continued)

Symptom Management and Comfort Care

- M N SIADH: Patients require multiple interventions in addition to primary treatment of the underlying cause. Care commonly involves:
    - o Fluid restriction to prevent exacerbation of water intoxication
    - o Treatment of hyponatremia (see the Fluid and Electrolyte NovE-lesson). IV fluids should be hypertonic saline to help alleviate the hyponatremia.
    - o Demeclocycline is an antibiotic but has the unusual property of promoting water excretion.
    - o Diuretics, particularly furosemide, can reduce water excretion.
- M N Diabetes insipidus: Extreme symptoms of dehydration and hypernatremia need to managed while treating the underlying cause. These typically include:
    - o Desmopressin (DDAVP) is used to replace ADH, increase water reabsorption, and is the treatment of choice. It can be administered orally, intranasally, intravenously, or subcutaneously.
    - o IV fluids should be hypotonic to help decrease the hypernatremia and treat dehydration.
    - o Force fluids orally if patient is able to take oral nutrition.
- Postoperative care includes routine care (e.g., wound care, infection precautions, early mobilization) but with particular attention to the following:
    - M N o Postoperative pain management is anticipated. Headache is common and may require narcotics.
    - M N o Nasal packing due to surgical approach is monitored for excessive bleeding. The nasal packing is removed within 2–3 days after surgery.
    - N o Incisional wound made under the lip for transnasal surgery requires mouth care at least every 4 hours. A humidified air mask may make breathing by mouth more comfortable.
    - N o Instruct the patient not to cough forcefully, blow nose, use incentive spirometer, or sneeze to prevent suture disruption.
    - N o Assess the patient frequently for new or worsening pituitary dysfunction (e.g., SIADH, cerebral salt waste syndrome, DI).
    - N o Monitor fluid intake and urine output.
    - M N o Monitor lab values for change: electrolytes, endocrine-related level, serum osmolality, urine specific gravity.
    - N o Monitor vital signs, hemodynamics and blood glucose. Frequently check neuro status for visual impairment, cerebral spinal fluid rhinorrhea, meningitis, or infection, subdural hematoma, and level of consciousness. Collaborate with the health care provider regarding severe headaches, light sensitivity, fever, rhinorrhea, epistaxis, and bleeding.
    - N o Attentiveness is needed to prevent never events as these patients often have urinary catheters, central lines, limited mobility, and venous stasis.

Patient Education

- Because pituitary dysfunction can cause significant physical changes, body image can be problematic for many of these patients. Assist patients to gain a realistic understanding about continued and/or unchanging physical alterations and provide support as needed. Inform patients if and which support groups are available.
- Early recognition and identification of symptoms of hyper- and hypopituitary disorders are important to prevent harmful effects of the disorders.
- Encourage collaborative interventions and educate the patient and family regarding diagnostic studies, medications, and possible surgical resection of the pituitary gland.
- Educate the patient about the disorder, signs and symptoms, medications, appropriate treatment strategies, and when to call their health care provider.
- Educate patient that potential moodiness, anxiety, depression, reduced sex drive, and/or nervousness can be hormone related. Encourage getting help as needed (e.g., support group, counselor, talk with HCP).
- Educate patients that some medications, particularly the somatostatin analogues (SSAs), can have serious adverse effects (Katznelson, et al., 2011).
- Educate diabetic patients that SSAs can inhibit insulin secretion and worsen glucose control (Katznelson, et al., 2011).

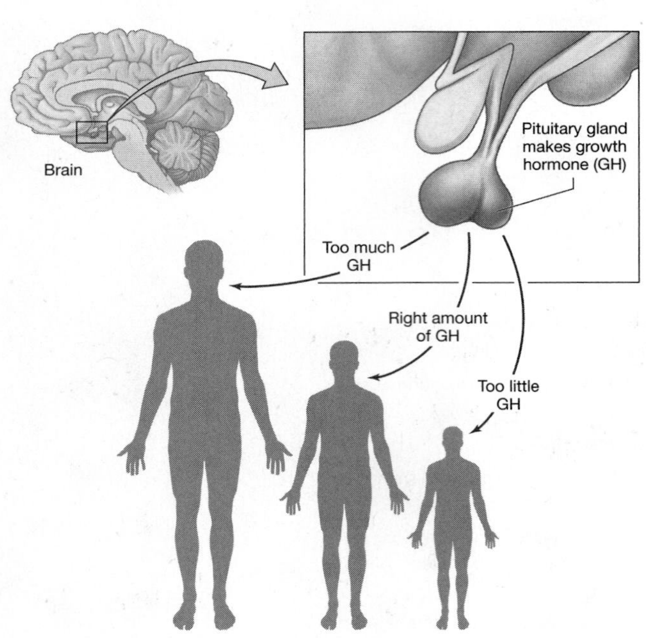

Growth hormone (GH), produced in the pituitary gland, exercises control over the body's growth rate and eventual size.

Concept Check

7. **Which intervention is appropriate for a patient with SIADH?**
   A. Discontinue diuretic.
   B. Restrict fluids.
   C. Administer D5W intravenous fluids.
   D. Give penicillin-based antibiotics.

Answer question

Summary of Interventions

- Pituitary tumors are treatable by resection.
- Some tumors can be managed with medication.
- Hypopituitary effects can be treated with hormone supplementation.
  - o Levothyoxine for hypothyroidism
  - o Cortisol for adrenocorticosteroid deficiency
  - o Growth hormone for growth hormone deficiency
  - o Testosterone or estrogen for hypogonadism

LO4:

Evaluation of Desired Collaborative Care Outcomes

Evaluation and reassessment should reveal attainment of previously established patient outcomes. In summary:

- Patient demonstrates increasing acceptance of physical changes and identifies those that can be modified by disease management.
- Patient accurately performs self-managed interventions in the treatment regimen and conveys a plan for self-management.
- Patient is infection-free.
- Patient is normotensive with expected skin turgor and fluid intake balances with urine output.
- Patient reports satisfactory or improving sexual function.

References

Crawford, A., & Harris, H. (2012). SIADH: Fluid out of balance. *Nursing 2012 .42*(9), 50–58.

John, C. A., & Day, M. W. (2012). Central neurogenic diabetes insipidus, syndrome of inappropriate secretion of antidiuretic hormone, and cerebral salt-wasting syndrome in traumatic brain injury. *Critical Care Nursing*, 32(2), e1–e7. doi:10.4037/ccn2012904

Skugor, M., & Hamrahian, A. H. (2014). *Pituitary disorders.* **www.clevelandclinicmeded.com/medicalpubs/diseasemanagement/endocrinology/pituitary-disorders/**

Yuan, W. (2013). Managing the patient with transsphenoidal pituitary tumor resection. *Journal of Neuroscience Nursing, 45*(2), 101–107. doi:10.1097/JNN.0b013e3182828e28l

Clinical Practice Guidelines

Freda, P. U., Beckers, A. M., Katznelson, L., et al., & Endocrine Society. (2011). Pituitary incidentaloma: an Endocrine Society clinical practice guideline. *Journal of Clinical Endocrinology and Metabolism, 96*(4), 894–904. **www.guideline.gov/content.aspx?id=34451&search=pituitary**

Katznelson, L., Atkinson, J. L., Cook, D. M., et al. (2011). American Association of Clinical Endocrinologists medical guidelines for clinical practice for the diagnosis and treatment of acromegaly—2011 update. *Endocrine Practice, 17*(Suppl. 4), 1–44.

Patient Education

Emory Pituitary Center. (2014). *Pituitary gland introduction.* **www.emoryhealthcare.org/pituitary/pituitary-gland.html**

Kattah, J. C. (2014). *Pituitary tumors.* **emedicine.medscape.com/article/1157189-overview#a0104**

Klibanski, A., & Tritos, N. (2013). *Pituitary disorders.* **www.hormone.org/diseases-and-conditions/pituitary/overview**

National Cancer Institute. (2014). *Pituitary tumors treatment.* **www.cancer.gov/cancertopics/pdq/treatment/pituitary/Patient**

Stanford Hospital & Clinics. (2014). *Diagnosis and treatment of acromegaly.* **neurosurgery.stanford.edu/pituitary/acromegaly.html**

STOP

Go to the online course and complete the NovE-Cases assigned by your instructor for this module.

Learning Outcomes for Osteoarthritis and Joint Replacement

When you complete this lesson, you will be able to:

1. Recognize the clinical relevance of osteoarthritis and joint replacement.
2. Consider the pathophysiology, etiology, risk factors, and clinical presentation of osteoarthritis and joint replacement that determine the priority patient concerns.
3. Determine the most urgent and important nursing interventions and patient education required in caring for a patient with osteoarthritis or joint replacement.
4. Evaluate attainment of desired collaborative care outcomes for a patient with osteoarthritis or joint replacement.

LO1:

What Is Osteoarthritis?

- Osteoarthritis (OA) describes degenerative abnormalities of joints that cause mechanical impairment in movement and symptoms.
- OA causes the loss of integrity in interarticular cartilage and often causes joint deformities.

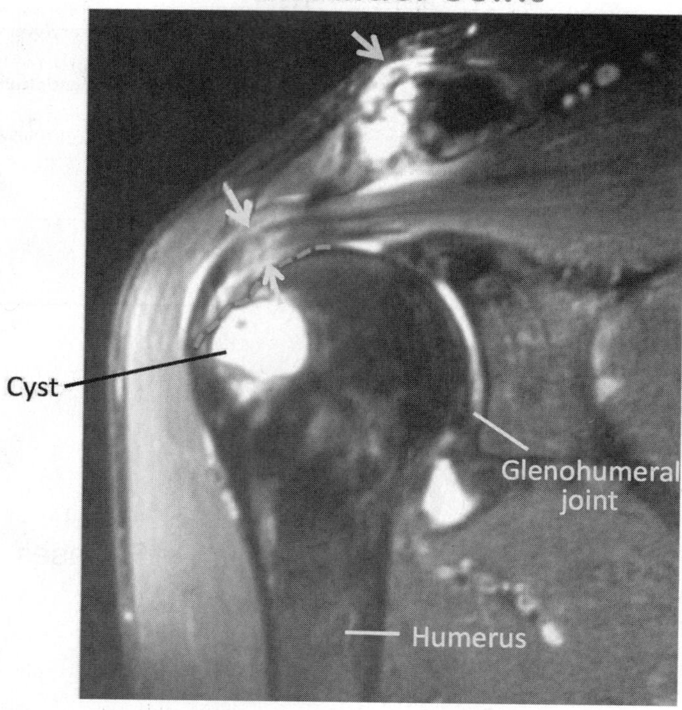

This CT scan reveals the extensive degenerative disease in the shoulder. Severe arthritic swelling (blue arrow) is causing impingement and tearing of the supraspinatus tendon (yellow arrows). When the arm is raised, the tendon is pinched (red dotted line), resulting in pain. The patient's pain is also related to the damage and loss of cartilage, with joint space narrowing in the glenohumeral joint. A large cyst is seen in the head of the humerus.
Source: Courtesy of William Stoddard/Fairbanks, AK

LO1:

Clinical Relevance

- OA is the most common form of arthritis.
- OA of the knee is one of the leading causes of mobility impairment.
- OA increases in prevalence with increasing age and body weight, two large demographics in the United States that are rapidly increasing in size each year.
- Over 600,000 knee replacements or arthroplasties are performed annually in the United States, and some experts in the field estimate that over 3 million will be performed each year by 2030.

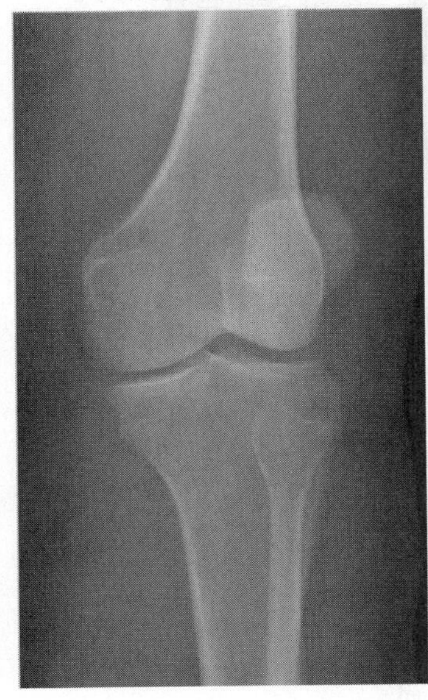

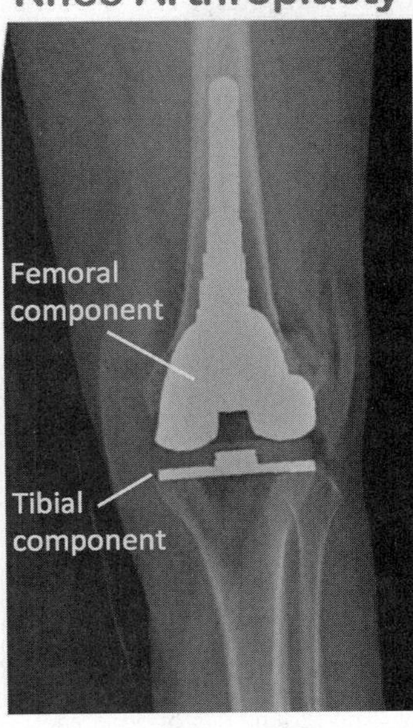

Comparison of a normal knee joint with a knee that has been surgically replaced. Note the prosthetic knee is implanted into the shaft of the upper bone in this particular patient.
Source: Courtesy of K. Kyriakidis

LO2:

Pathophysiology

- Cartilage is a unique tissue in that it has both compression and cushioning properties.
- Cartilage is located on the articular surface of the bones at joints and allows for smooth movement of the joints and "cushioning" of stresses.
- There is a continuous process of degradation and repair of cartilage tissue.
- Over time, an imbalance between these processes may cause cartilage, and therefore joint, deterioration.
- With the breakdown of cartilage, the body tries to repair the damage by forming bone spurs.

Healthy Joint

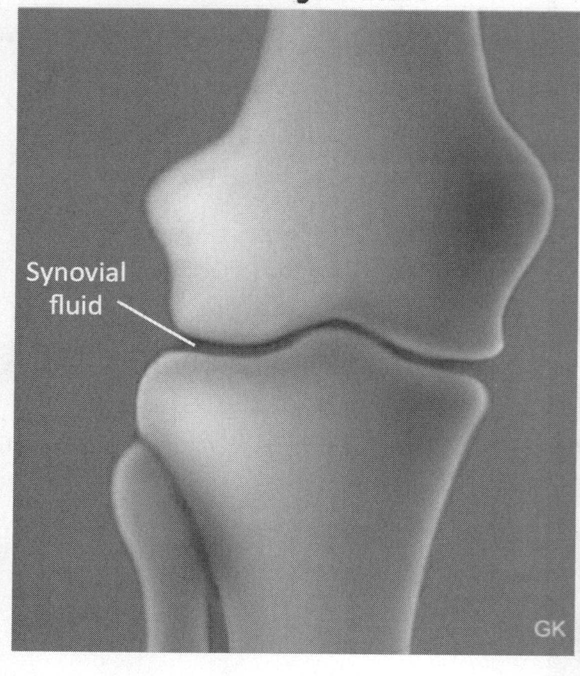

Early Osteoarthritis

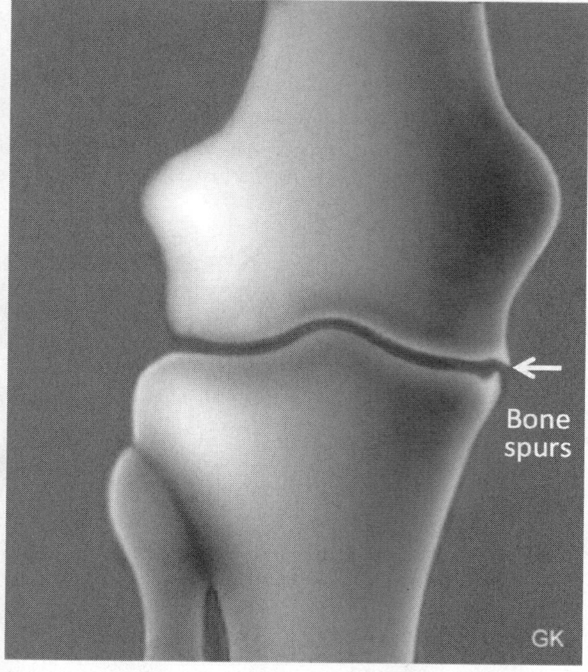

Left: Healthy joint. Right: In the development of early osteoarthritis, note the bone spurs that can arise near the outer joint as the body attempts to increase the bone area for weight bearing.

Source: *(both)* Courtesy of George Kyriakidis/Santa Ana, CA

- This imbalance is characterized by complex biochemical interactions involving inflammation, protein (and collagen) degradation, and cellular reactions.
- Over time, layers of cartilage break apart and wear away. The floating bits of bone and cartilage cause damage, stiffness, and pain.
- The joint loses normal motion and function over time.
- Progressive cartilage deterioration may cause abnormalities of the underlying bone such as osteophytes, sclerosis of the bone, and cysts in the bone beneath the damaged cartilage.

Moderate Osteoarthritis

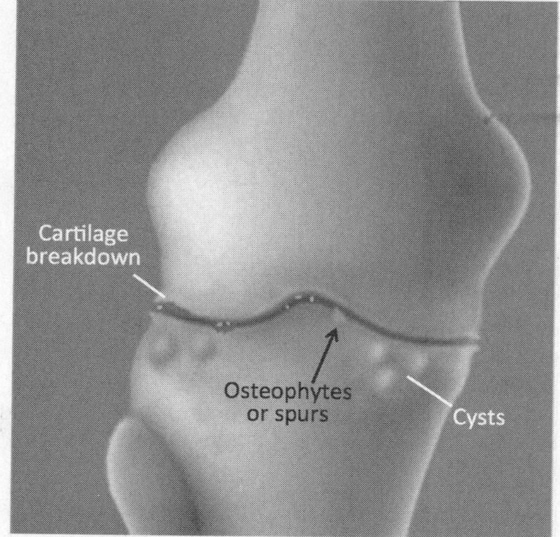

The image depicts moderate osteoarthritis where osteophytes are growing from the edges of the cartilage, cysts are forming, cartilage is starting to wear down, and bits of bone and cartilage are in the joint. All of these cause pain.

Severe Osteoarthritis

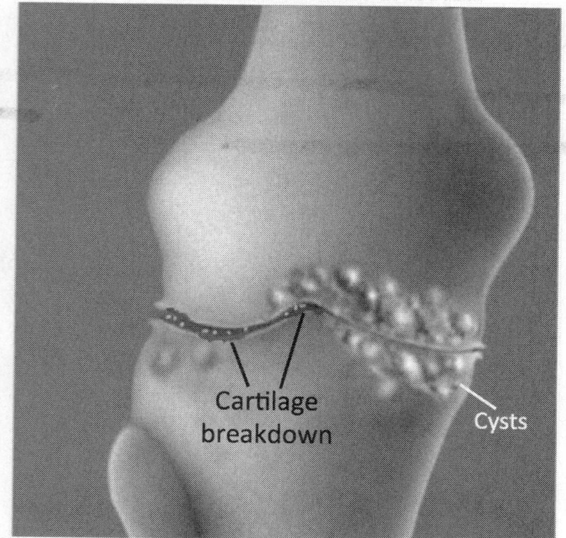

In severe osteoarthritis, note the cystic areas, revealing severely damaged cartilage, the worn cartilage, and bone fragments in the joint. Not shown is progressive bone on bone in the joint.

Source: *(both)* Courtesy of George Kyriakidis/Santa Ana, CA

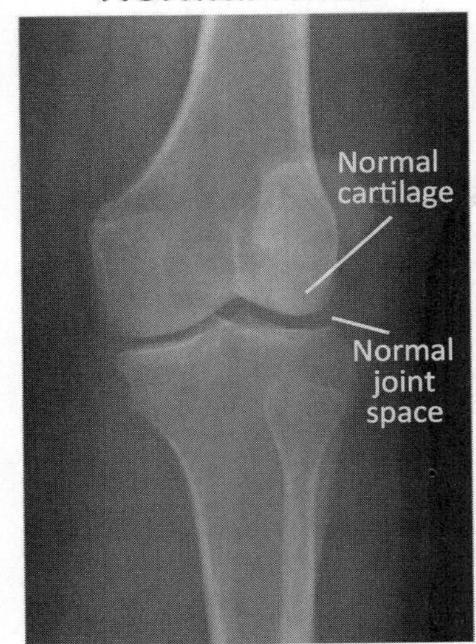

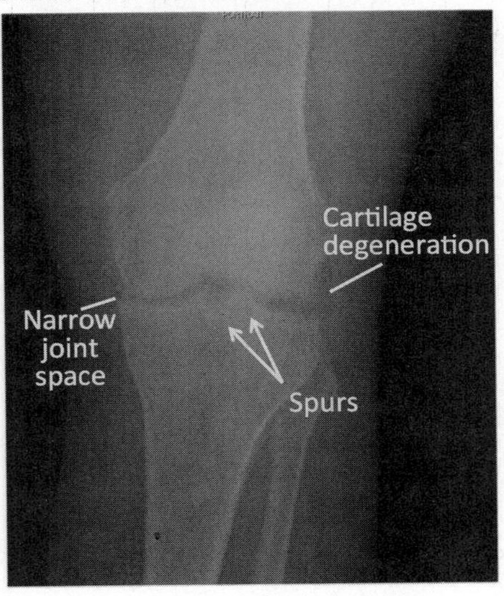

These *x*-rays show clear distinctions in the joints between normal and significant osteoarthritic changes. The osteoarthritic joint on the right has narrowing of the joint space between the tibia and the femur plus a bone spur that has formed. On the left, a normal knee joint has maintained a normal space between the bones, and no deterioration of the joint surfaces is seen.
Source: Courtesy of K. Kyriakidis

LO2:

Risk Factors and Causes

Factors that place patients at higher risk for developing or can result in osteoarthritis are:

- Increasing age, particularly over age 50
- Family history
- Previous trauma or injury to joint
- Increased weight (BMI)
- Congenital bone or joint abnormalities
- Joint injuries
- Gender: Women have higher prevalence.
- Sedentary lifestyle

Concept Check

1. **What is the basic pathophysiological process involved in the development of osteoarthritis?**
   A. Genetic alteration
   B. Degeneration
   C. Antigen deposition
   D. Hyperinflammation

Answer question

LO2:

Diagnostics

Clinical Exam

- In most situations, diagnosis of OA is clinically determined by medical history and examination.
- Osteoarthritis commonly occurs in the spine, hips, knees, and hands.

Areas Affected by Osteoarthritis

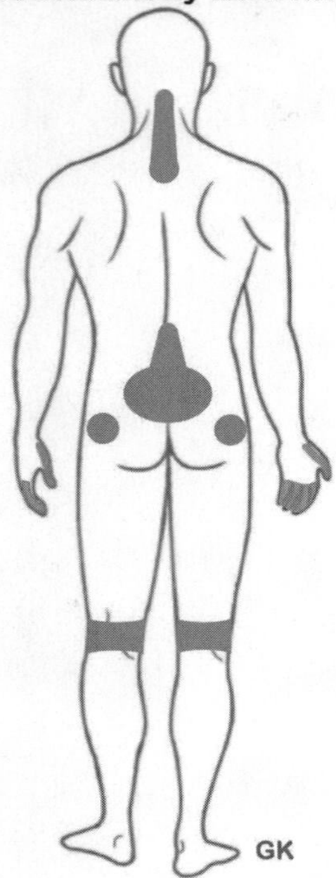

The sites on the human body most often affected by osteoarthritis are indicated by the blue areas on the body outline: hands (at the ends of fingers and thumb), spine (neck and lower back), knees, and hips.
Source: Courtesy of George Kyriakidis/Santa Ana, CA

- Joint pain and stiffness are the hallmark signs of OA, with impaired movement.
- Laboratory and x-ray tests are often used as adjunctive tests. Often, these tests help to rule out other causes of arthritis such as an inflammatory (rheumatoid) arthritis.
- Joint examination may show deformities, tenderness to palpation along the joint, and crepitus (creaking or crunching sound or feeling when the examiner moves joint through range of motion [ROM]).

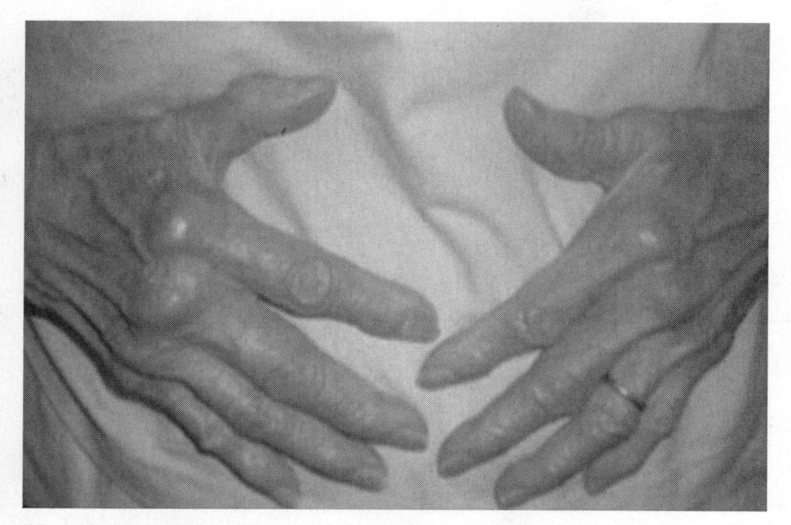

The obvious significant enlargement of the joints and ulnar deviation of the fingers due to joint deformities do not prevent this 88-year-old lady from doing needlework and other activities that require fine coordination of hand movement.
Source: Copyright © 2014, NovEx Novice to Expert Learning, LLC

Carpometacarpal Joint Collapse

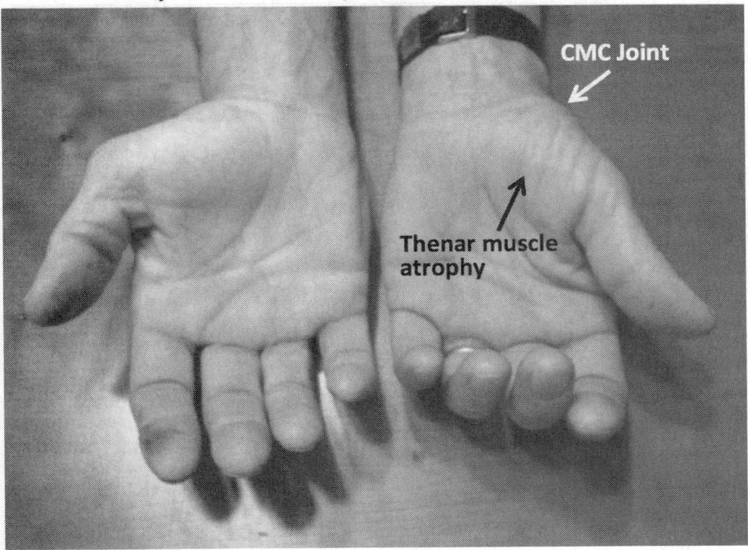

Clinical exam of this patient's left hand revealed severe pain in his carpometacarpal (CMC) joint. Thenar atrophy resulted from limited use of his hand due to pain.
Source: Courtesy of William Stoddard/Fairbanks, AK

Diagnostics (continued)

Laboratory

- Markers of inflammation in the body such as erythrocyte sedimentation rate (ESR) and C-reactive protein (CRP) are *not* elevated. Elevated values are seen with rheumatoid arthritis, lupus, and other inflammatory arthritides. In the past, osteoarthritis has been considered a noninflammatory arthritis, but recent evidence reveals that inflammation is associated with cytokines that are found in osteoarthritic joints. However, ESR and CRP are typically normal.
- Rheumatoid factor (RF) laboratory test is negative.
- Analysis of joint fluid, if performed, does not show inflammation.

Radiology

X-ray findings include:

- Joint space narrowing
- Bone spurs (osteophytes)
- Sclerosis of bone beneath cartilage
- Cysts in bone beneath cartilage
- Misalignment of the joint

Osteoarthritic Hand

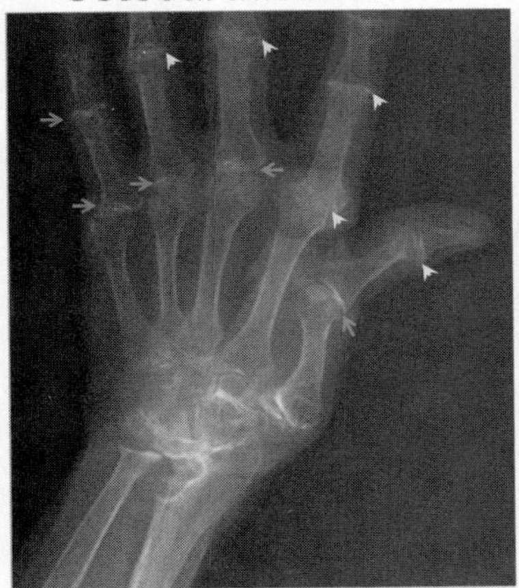

Diagnostic imaging revealed the extensive and erosive osteoarthritis of the finger joints (yellow arrows). There is little joint space in other joints (red arrows), with bone moving against bone, resulting in significant pain.

Spondylolisthesis of L5

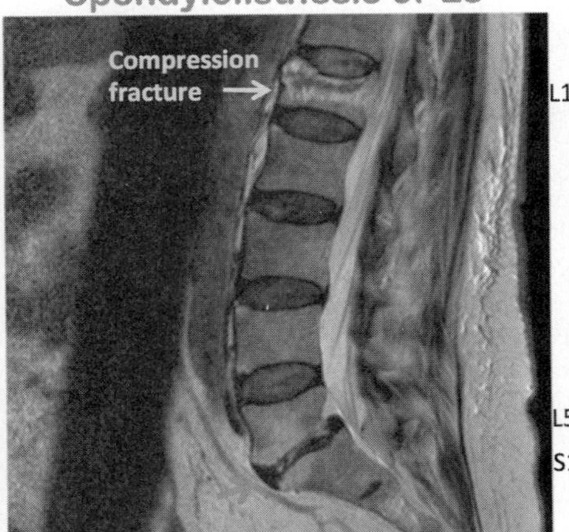

MRI of the lower spine, to diagnose the compression fracture at L1, revealed spondylolisthesis (osteoarthritis) at L5 on S1 with marked narrowing of the disc space (red arrow). Compare this joint space with the one above to appreciate the narrowing.

Source: Courtesy of K. Kyriakidis

Concept Check

2. Which laboratory result is common in osteoarthritis?

A. Elevated ESR

B. Positive RF

C. Inflammatory changes of joint fluid

D. Normal CRP

Answer question

Priority Patient Concerns and Desired Collaborative Care Outcomes

Prior to caring for patients with osteoarthritis, it is important to prioritize the patient's concerns that must guide the nursing care plan and interventions. Care for the patient is ordered and organized in accordance with the patient's priority and urgent needs. Desired collaborative care outcomes in patients with osteoarthritis typically include:

1. Patient will report that pain is absent or controlled enough not to interfere with activities of daily living (ADLs).
2. Patient will demonstrate increased mobility.
3. Patient will accurately discuss disease process and treatment modalities.
4. Patient will be free of DVT complications.
5. Patient will physically participate in daily activities, including ROM of all joints to perform self-care.

Considering these important care outcomes, prepare a list of the major 3–6 priority patient concerns or nursing diagnoses for patients with osteoarthritis. Be prepared to participate in a discussion of this list and/or to submit them as an assignment, as determined by your faculty. Resources you may find helpful in this assignment can include this lesson, the references, resources on nursing care plans, and standard nursing diagnoses manuals.

Concept Check

3. Which findings are common upon radiographic examination of osteoarthritic joints?

A. Joint space widening

B. Presence of osteophytes

C. Cysts throughout soft tissue

D. Softening of the bone beneath cartilage

Answer question

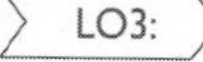

Collaborative Interventions

Care of osteoarthritis patients can often reduce pain and improve daily function. Care and education of the patient include:

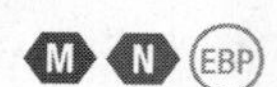

- Exercise is among the best interventions and focuses on strengthening, aerobics, ROM, balance, and agility (Jevsevar, et al., 2013). Performing activities of daily living is important, whether shopping, gardening, housework, cooking, walking, or other routine activities.

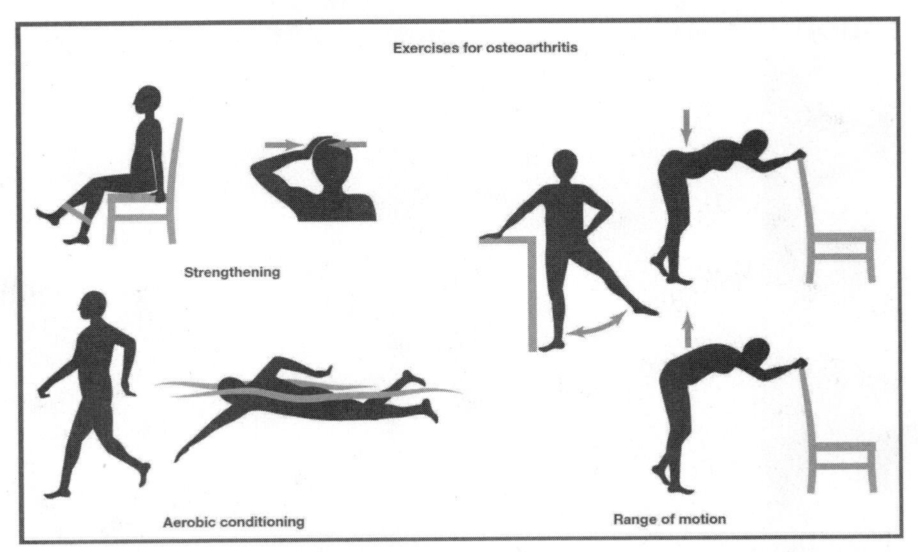

Numerous images display the kinds of exercises that may help patients with osteoarthritis.

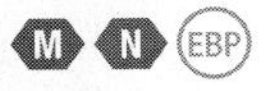

- Weight management to relieve stress on joints (Jevsevar, et al., 2013)
- Healthy diet

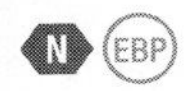

- Complementary therapies: heat and/or cold, massage, nerve stimulation, and acupuncture (Hochberg, et al., 2012)
  - o Heat is thought to stimulate the body's own healing power by improving circulation to the area and to reduce potential muscle spasms and stiffness. It can further alter the sensation of pain. Individuals may gain relief with either dry or wet methods of heat (e.g., heat lamp, warm soak, heating pad, and warm bath).
  - o Cold compresses may also be used to decrease edema and reduce spasms and therefore discomfort. The cold can offer a numbing effect for pain relief.
  - o Massage may be effective in relaxing muscle spasms around joints, alleviating stiffness, and enabling greater mobility with less pain.

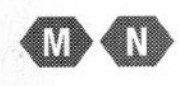

  - o Transcutaneous electrical nerve stimulation interferes with pain transmission by delivering a mild current through the skin. Pain relief, however, may be comparable to naproxen but is more costly.

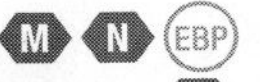

- Medications for pain relief (Jevsevar, et al., 2013)

- Surgery, if pain is unrelieved and debilitating

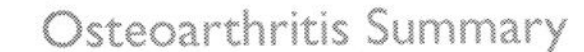

Osteoarthritis Summary

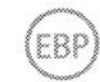

- As summarized in the image, treatment possibilities for osteoarthritis are rather limited at the present time. No drugs are currently known that prevent the progressive destruction of joints (Jevsevar, et al., 2013).

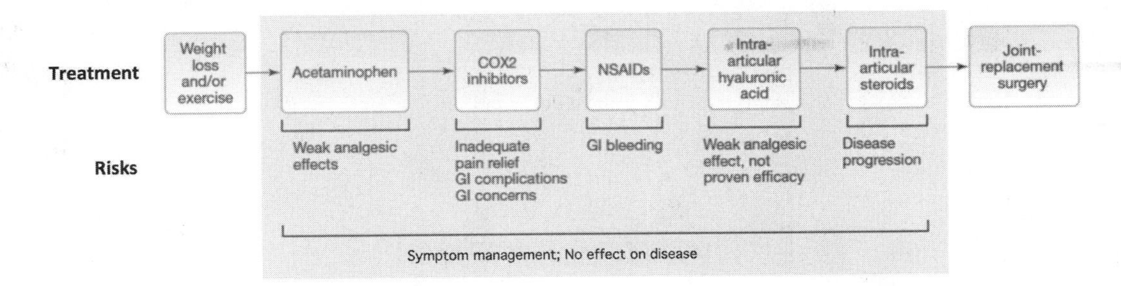

- Common sense measures, such as weight loss and physical exercise, offer little in the realm of prevention.

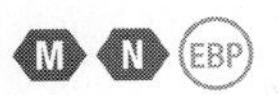

- For symptomatic relief, the choices progress as shown in the above figure, from analgesics and NSAIDs, to intra-articular injection of steroids or hyaluronic acid (Hochberg, et al., 2012). An injection of hyaluronic acid acts as a shock absorber and lubricant for the joint. It tends to be less effective in older patients and those with severe OA.

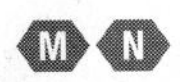

- Beyond these treatment modalities lies the ultimate option of joint replacement.

Hyaluronic Acid Injection

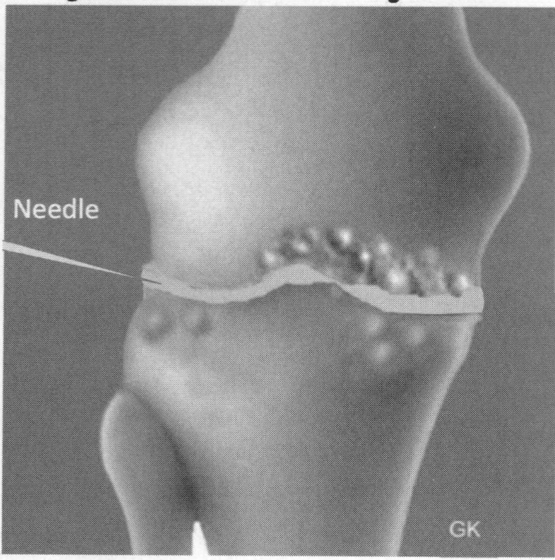

This photo depicts an injection of hyaluronic acid into the joint, providing a cushion and lubricant to reduce the bone-on-bone pain.

Source: Courtesy of George Kyriakidis/Santa Ana, CA

Concept Check

4. Which treatment is useful for osteoarthritis?

A. Cold to improve mobility

B. Cold to reduce swelling

C. Heat to increase immune response

D. Avoidance of heat or cold

Answer question

Collaborative Interventions (continued)

Joint Replacement

- When joint pain or dysfunction fails to respond to conservative measures such as NSAIDs and joint injections, a joint replacement is considered.
- Joint replacements can help with both pain and function.
- The most common joint replacements are of the knee and hip. However, other joints such as the shoulder and ankle can also be replaced.
- After hip and knee surgery, patients require similar treatment of pain with NSAIDs and narcotics, physical rehabilitation, and education.

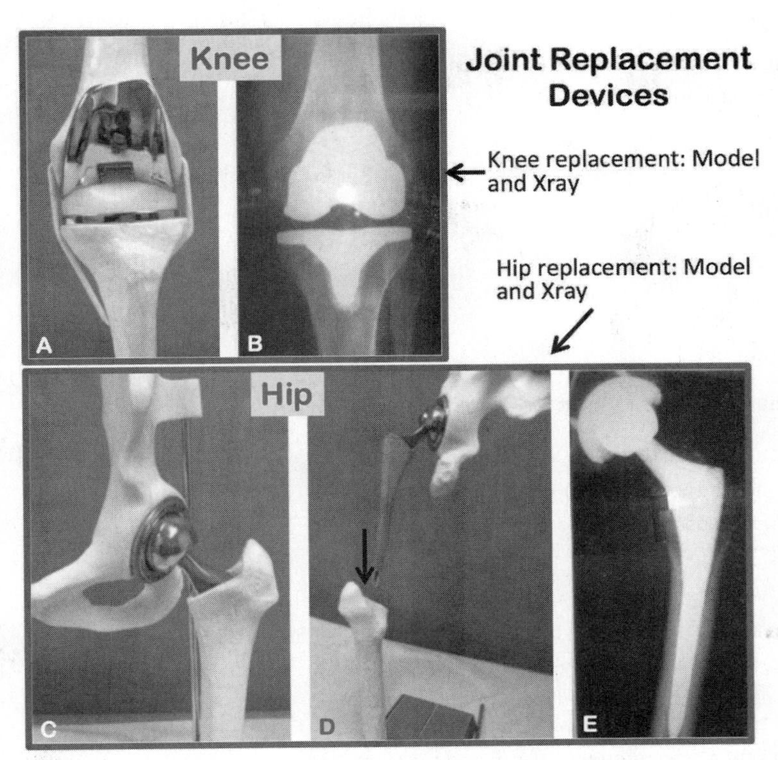

Knee and hip replacement devices are seen in photos A & C, showing how they are surgically positioned into a patient's boney joints. The metal replacements are cemented into the bone. As seen in D, the femoral hip portion is cemented deep into the femur. The end result can then be viewed on x-ray (photos B and E).
Source: Courtesy of K. Kyriakidis

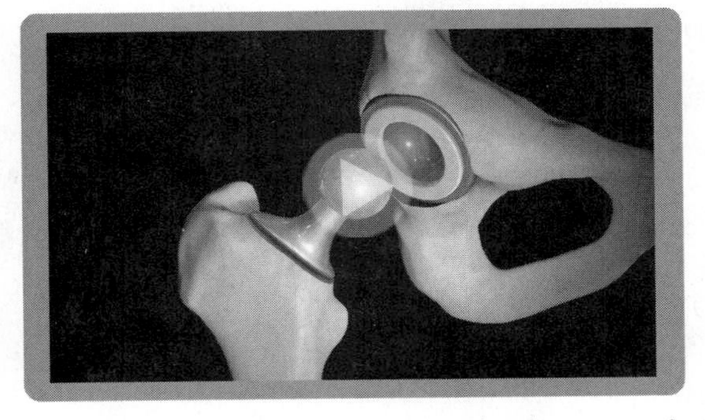

This is a similar video animation that describes the process of total hip replacement using minimally invasive surgery.
Source: © 2014 Nucleus Medical Media, All rights reserved

Preoperative Preparation and Care

Patients preparing for joint surgery require education to prepare well. To educate patients specific to joint replacement:

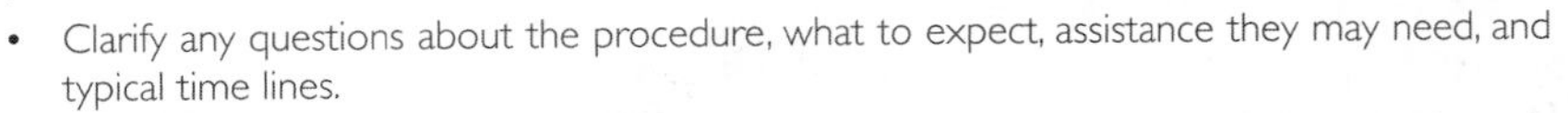

- Clarify any questions about the procedure, what to expect, assistance they may need, and typical time lines.

- Obtain a thorough history and exam of the patient's current ROM of affected joints for postop comparison.

- Review routine preop education to include:
  - o Pain control, commonly the use of a patient-controlled analgesia (PCA) pump
  - o Effective coughing, deep breathing, and use of incentive spirometry
  - o Early mobilization when appropriate
  - o Skin preparation
  - o Medications like antibiotics
  - o Advanced health care directives and bring a copy for the medical record
  - o Blood donation
  - o Nutrition
  - o Stop smoking
  - o Avoidance of drugs and alcohol use
- Instruct about expected postop activity restrictions. Educate about use of overbed trapeze to assist with movement and allow practice.
- Educate about postop joint exercises to strengthen muscles that stabilize and support the joint, avoid contractures, reduce muscle atrophy, and prevent DVT and pulmonary embolism.
- Discuss ways to prevent falls and improve safety upon returning home (see the Prevention: Fall Assessment section in the Care of Patients with Fractures NovE-lesson).

Postoperative Joint Replacement Care

- Provide comfort care and pain medications as ordered to control pain and discomfort.
- Administer IV fluids until adequate nutrition and medications can be taken orally.
- Provide wound care with careful, ongoing inspection of the wound (and drain) for signs of infection.
- Monitor vital signs and neurovascular checks (temperature, pulses, color, movement, sensation, and capillary refill) every 2–4 hours and taper as recovery progresses.
- Administer anticoagulants and antibiotics as indicated (Jacobs, et al., 2011).
- Use intermittent sequential compression device to help reduce the incidence of DVT (Jacobs, et al., 2011).
- Encourage early mobilization (Jacobs, et al., 2011). ROM exercises or continuous passive motion (CPM) device are needed until the patient is mobilized. Encourage use of assistive devices and techniques to avoid weight bearing on affected limb.
- Collaborate with the health care provider to consult physical therapy as early as indicated.
- Encourage adequate hydration.
- Administer stool softeners to reduce the incidence of constipation.
- Evaluate the need for and institute safety and fall precautions when caring for at-risk patients.

Concept Check

5. Which joint is most commonly replaced?

A. Hip
B. Shoulder
C. Ankle
D. Elbow

Answer question

Collaborative Interventions (continued)

Prevention of Complications

Joint replacements are associated with a number of complications. Prevention and treatment of the following complications are critical:

- "Never" events or complications that should never happen, including venous thromboembolism (Jacobs, et al., 2011).
- Indwelling urinary catheter should be removed as soon as possible to avoid catheter-associated urinary tract infection. Patients undergoing knee and hip replacements often have a catheter placed for surgery. Typically, they can have the catheter removed the same day.

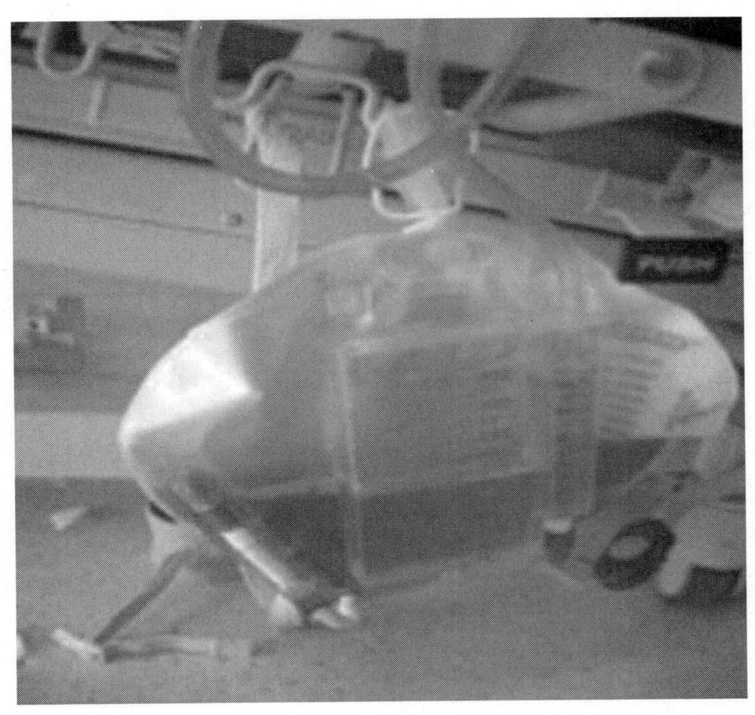

Indwelling urinary catheters are a leading cause of hospital-acquired infections. Evaluate them daily and remove as soon as feasible.
Source: Copyright © 2014, NovEx Novice to Expert Learning, LLC

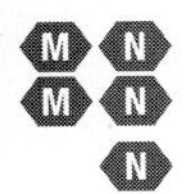

- Acute blood loss anemia
- Wound and joint infections
- Dislocation prevention
  - o All patients need to be educated on the limitation of ROM to prevent dislocation of their artificial joints.
  - o Depending on the dislocation and the joint, the patient is at risk for a return to surgery.
  - o The specific education is determined by the particular joint replaced (see the following Patient Education section).

Collaborative Interventions for Complications

Venous Thromboembolism

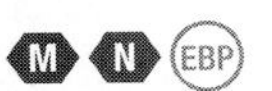

Patients having joint replacement are at increased risk for venous thromboembolism that can, potentially, be fatal. Prevention includes the use of anticoagulants for four weeks after surgery (Jacobs, et al., 2011):

- Low–molecular-weight heparin subcutaneously (Jacobs, et al., 2011)

Administering Subcutaneous Heparin

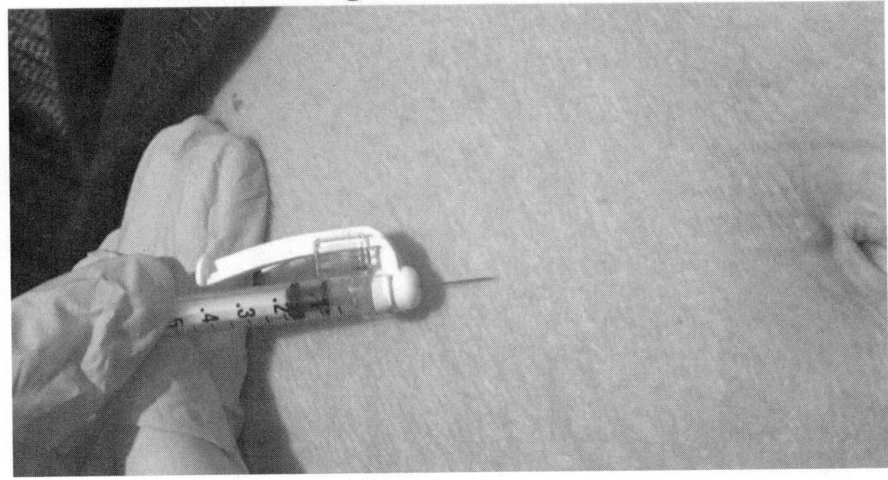

Unless contraindicated, anticoagulation is critical in orthopedic surgical patients.
Source: Courtesy of K. Kyriakidis

- Warfarin (Jacobs, et al., 2011)
- Factor Xa inhibitors (e.g., rivaroxaban) (Jacobs, et al., 2011)
- Factor IIa inhibitors (e.g., dabigatran) (Jacobs, et al., 2011)
- The above are often combined with mechanical compression devices (Jacobs, et al., 2011).
- Early mobilization (Jacobs, et al., 2011)
- Aspirin is sometimes used, but there is no evidence that it decreases thromboembolism in surgical patients.

Periprosthetic Joint Infections

- Joint infections usually occur as a result of contamination during surgery or hematogenous seeding by bacteria. All clinicians must remain vigilant about their own practices and those of others. A collaborative team climate better ensures open communication about potential issues and remedy.
- Treatment involves administering antibiotics and usually surgery.
- Surgery may consist of:
  - o Debridement consisting of removal of infected tissue and irrigation
  - o Removal of the joint followed by antibiotic treatment for 6 weeks followed by reimplantation of artificial joint
  - o Removal and replacement of joint at one time, followed by antibiotic treatment
- Prevention relies heavily on the surgeon's attentiveness to the comorbid conditions of the patient, to be especially vigilant with patients at high risk (e.g., rheumatoid arthritis, other systemic disease), to carefully select prophylactic antibiotics, and to remain vigilant postoperatively for characteristics of infection and identify the hematogenous source.
- Carefully evaluate the patient for evidence of infection prior to surgery in order to prevent hematogenous spread. Patients with evidence of infection may need to have surgery postponed (Sawyer, et al., 2012).
  - o Report fever immediately.
  - o Examine skin carefully for areas of erythema, skin breakdown, exudate (especially in patients with impaired sensation, e.g., diabetes) (Sawyer, et al., 2012).
  - o Monitor for and report symptoms of UTI, such as dysuria, frequency—check urinalysis.
- Provide prescribed prophylactic antibiotics, given at the beginning of anesthesia and every 8 hours for two doses (Sawyer, et al., 2012).
  - o IV cefazolin or
  - o IV vancomycin
- After surgery, evaluate surgical wounds for any evidence of infection or necrosis. Patients with wound infections should be treated promptly with antibiotics (Sawyer, et al., 2012).

Concept Check

6. **Which medication has the least evidence of effectiveness in preventing thromboembolism after joint replacement?**

A. Low-molecular-weight heparin

B. Aspirin

C. Factor Xa inhibitor

D. Factor IIa inhibitor

Answer question

Anemia

Blood loss during surgery is a common complication of joint replacements.

- Monitor patients who may become orthostatic, hypotensive, and tachycardic. Other symptoms may include weakness and shortness of breath.

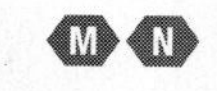

- Collaborate with the health care provider to quickly begin intravenous fluids for patients with orthostatic symptoms (lightheaded when standing, tachycardia, or hypotension).
- Consider transfusion in patients who remain symptomatic or with a hematocrit <21 (Carson, et al., 2012).

Collaborative Interventions (continued)

Patient Education

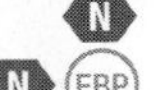

- Educate that pain may worsen for several weeks until edema diminishes.
- Instruct about the use of pain medications prior to experiencing significant pain (Sawyer, et al., 2012). Use as prescribed:
  - o Acetaminophen
  - o Nonsteroidal anti-inflammatory drugs (NSAIDs)
  - o Narcotics or analgesics
- Educate and have patient and/or caregiver repeat medications, dosages, frequency, and reason for use.
- Use ice (or frozen bag of peas) on the affected joint for 15 minutes to help relieve pain.
- After hip replacement, depending on the prosthesis, **hip precautions** are essential to prevent subluxation (partial) or total dislocation:
  - o Keep hip abducted and do not cross operated leg over other leg when sitting until otherwise instructed.
  - o Avoid walking pigeon-toed (internal rotation of hip).
  - o Avoid hip flexion past 90 degree angle when getting out of bed or chair.
  - o Do not lift knees above hips.
  - o Do not twist over surgical leg. Instead, pick feet up and step turn.
  - o Avoid low chairs and toilets that can cause bending at the waist more than 90 degrees. Use an elevated toilet seat and cushions on chairs.
  - o Avoid bending down to pick objects off the floor.
  - o Sleep on a firm mattress.
- Educate the patient to follow dressing changes as instructed by the health care provider. Be sure to keep it clean and dry. Report any redness, fever, odor, drainage, tenderness, or swelling at or around the incision.
- Continue ROM, muscle-strengthening, and aerobic exercises, as instructed by physical therapy prior to and following discharge. Alternatively, continue to participate in physical and/or occupational therapy sessions as prescribed.
- Evaluate and obtain assistive devices (e.g., raised toilet seat) as required. Educate the patient and caregiver on use of device (e.g., crutches, walker, cane) and observe patient's safe use prior to discharge.
- Remind the patient to stay hydrated, which can also reduce the chance of constipation.
- Avoid sitting for more than 45 minutes at a time. Change positions and walk to reduce complications like blood clots.
- Depending on the patient's progress, the nurse and/or physical therapy should prepare the patient for independence in ADLs by educating about how to:
  - o Get into and out of bed.
  - o Get into and out of the bath.
  - o Climb stairs.
  - o Get up and down safely with any assist device being used.
  - o Put on and take off pants or underwear.
  - o Put on and take off socks and shoes.
- Discuss home health care plan, as needed.
- Consult social worker if evaluation of work, home environment, or finances are of concern.
- Educate regarding disease condition, recognition and prevention of complications, medications, when to call health care provider, follow-up care, smoking cessation, alcohol moderation, weight management, and flu and pneumonia vaccinations.
- Avoid high-risk activities (e.g., running) and high-impact sports (e.g., downhill skiing) for the rest of patient's life to prevent fractures, prosthesis damage, and potential problems.
- Check with the health care provider and/or dentist about the latest recommendations for prophylactic antibiotic use prior to invasive procedures.

Summary of Interventions: Algorithm

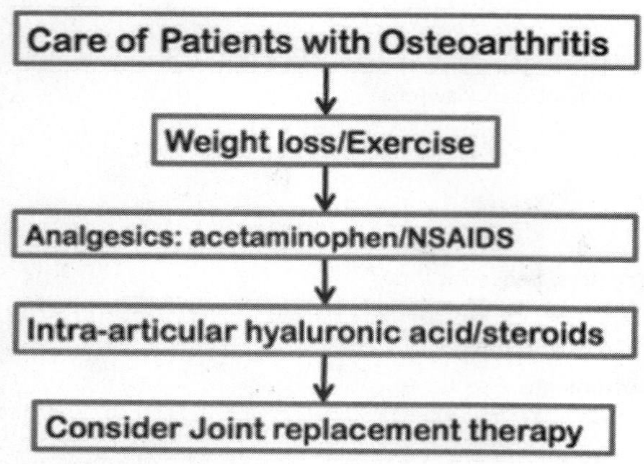

Source: Copyright © 2014, NovEx Novice to Expert Learning, LLC

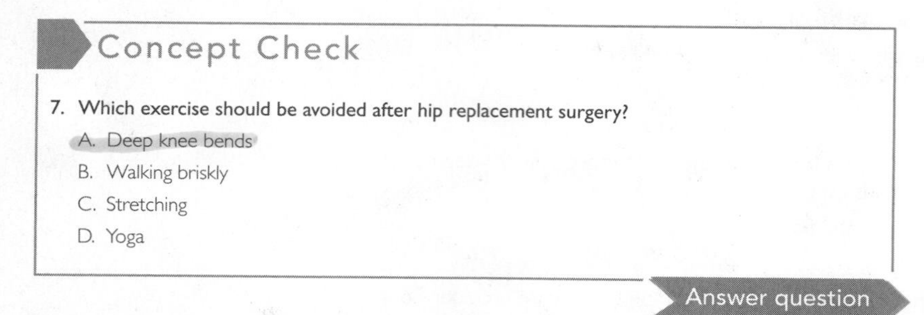

Concept Check

7. **Which exercise should be avoided after hip replacement surgery?**
   A. Deep knee bends
   B. Walking briskly
   C. Stretching
   D. Yoga

Answer question

LO4:

Evaluation of Desired Collaborative Care Outcomes

Evaluation and reassessment should reveal attainment of previously established patient outcomes. In summary:

- Patient reports that pain is diminished or is absent.
- Patient reports increased ability to comfortably participate in daily activities.
- Patient reports increased confidence in personal ability to effect symptom relief and to decrease effects of disease process.
- Patient has not experienced DVT.
- Patient reports improved joint mobility.

References

Carson, J. L., Terrin, M. L., Noveck, H., et al. (2011). Liberal or restrictive transfusion in high-risk patients after hip surgery. *The New England Journal of Medicine, 365*(26), 2453–2462. **www.nejm.org/doi/pdf/10.1056/NEJMoa1012452**

Davis, L. (2012). A new understanding of osteoarthritis. *The Clinical Advisor, 15*(4), 28–36.

Lucas, B. (2004). Nursing management issues in hip and knee replacement surgery. *British Journal of Nursing, 13*(13), 782–787. **smccd.edu/accounts/felixf/nurs232/nursingcareofhipreplacement.pdf**

Saufl, N., Owens, A., Kelly, I., et al. (2007). A multidisciplinary approach to total joint replacement. *Journal of Perianesthesia Nursing, 22*(3), 195–206. **dx.doi.org/10.1016/j.jopan.2007.03.007**

Shelton, L. R. (2013). A closer look at osteoarthritis. *The Nurse Practitioner, 38*(7), 30–36. **www.nursingcenter.com/lnc/CEArticle?an=00006205-201307000-00006&Journal_ID=54012&Issue_ID=1565784**

Sovani, S. & Grogan, S. P. (2013). Osteoarthritis: Detection, pathophysiology, and current/future treatment strategies. *Orthopedic Nursing, 32*(1), 25–36.

Wright, W. L. (2008). Management of mild-to-moderate osteoarthritis: Effective management by the nurse practitioner. *The Journal for Nurse Practitioner, 4*(1), 25–35. **www.npjournal.org/article/S1555-4155%2807%2900618-6/fulltext**

Clinical Practice Guidelines

Carson, J. L., Grossman, B. J., Kleinman, S., et al., & the Clinical Transfusion Medicine Committee of the AABB. (2012). Red blood cell transfusion: A clinical practice guideline from the AABB. *Annals of Internal Medicine, 157*(1), 49–58. doi: 10.7326/0003-4819-157-1-201206190-00429

Hochberg, M. C., Altman, R. D., April, K.T., et al. (2012). American College of Rheumatology 2012 recommendations for the use of nonpharmacologic and pharmacologic therapies in osteoarthritis of the hand, hip, and knee. *Arthritis Care & Research, 64*, 465–474. **onlinelibrary.wiley.com/enhanced/doi/10.1002/acr.21596**

Jacobs, J., Mont, M., Bozic, K., et al. (2011) Preventing venous thromboembolic disease in patients undergoing elective hip and knee arthroplasty. *The Journal of the American Academy of Orthopedic Surgeons, 19(12)*, 1–153. **www.aaos.org/Research/guidelines/VTE/VTE_full_guideline.pdf**

Jevsevar, D. S. (2013). Treatment of osteoarthritis of the knee, evidence-based guideline. *The Journal of the American Academy of Orthopedic Surgeons, 21*(9), 571–576. **www.aaos.org/Research/guidelines/TreatmentofOsteoarthritisoftheKneeGuideline.pdf**

Sawyer, M., Danielson, D., Dickson, E., et al. (2012). Perioperative Protocol. Health care protocol. *AHRQ National Guideline Clearinghouse*. **www.guideline.gov/content.aspx?id=48408&search=sawyer+danielson+dickson+2012**

Patient Education

Gecht-Silver, M. R., & Duncombe, A. M. (2015). Patient information: Arthritis and exercise. **www.uptodate.com/contents/arthritis-and-exercise-beyond-the-basics?source=search_result&search=arthritis+and+exercise&selectedTitle=1~150**

Kalunian, K. C. (2015). Patient information: Osteoarthritis symptoms and diagnosis—beyond the basics. **www.uptodate.com/contents/osteoarthritis-symptoms-and-diagnosis-beyond-the-basics**

National Association of Orthopaedic Nurses. (2009). *NAON patient education series: Total hip replacement.* Chicago, IL: NAON. (also in Spanish) **www.orthonurse.org/patienteducation**

National Association of Orthopaedic Nurses. (2009). *NAON patient education series: Total knee replacement.* Chicago, IL: NAON. (also in Spanish) **www.orthonurse.org/patienteducation**

National Institute of Arthritis and Musculoskeletal and Skin Diseases. (2013). *Osteoarthritis.* **www.niams.nih.gov/Health_Info/Osteoarthritis/**

Prouty, A., Cooper, M., Thomas, P. (2006). Multidisciplinary patient education for total joint replacement surgery patients. *Orthopaedic Nursing, 25*(4), 257–261.

CARE OF PATIENTS WITH FRACTURES: HIP, FEMUR, AND PELVIS

Learning Outcomes for Fractures

When you complete this lesson, you will be able to:

1. Recognize the clinical relevance of fractures.
2. Consider the pathophysiology, etiology, risk factors, and clinical presentation of fractures that determine the priority patient concerns.
3. Determine the most urgent and important nursing interventions and patient education required in caring for a patient with a fracture.
4. Evaluate attainment of desired collaborative care outcomes for a patient with a fracture.

LO1: What Are Hip and Femur Fractures?

- A fracture refers to a broken bone. Fractures result when the force exerted onto a bone exceeds the strength of the bone itself.
- The hip generally refers to the proximal end of the femur.
- Fractures of the hip are important clinically and can occur as a singular fracture or as a combination of fractures.
- Fractures usually result from trauma.
- The hip (femur) consists of structures that include:
  - o Proximal:
    - ■ Femoral head
    - ■ Femoral neck
    - ■ Greater trochanter
    - ■ Lesser trochanter
  - o Diaphysis or shaft
  - o Distal:
    - ■ Medial epicondyle
    - ■ Lateral epicondyle

Anatomy of the Hip Joint

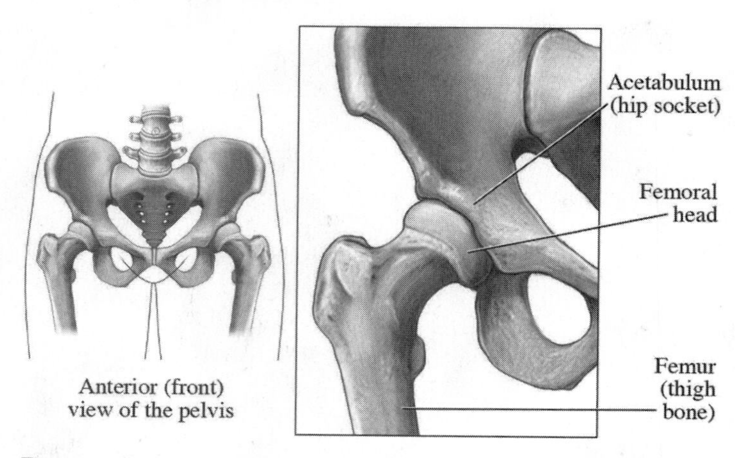

This image illustrates the pelvic anatomy with a closer look at the hip joint.

Femur: Anatomical & Xray Views

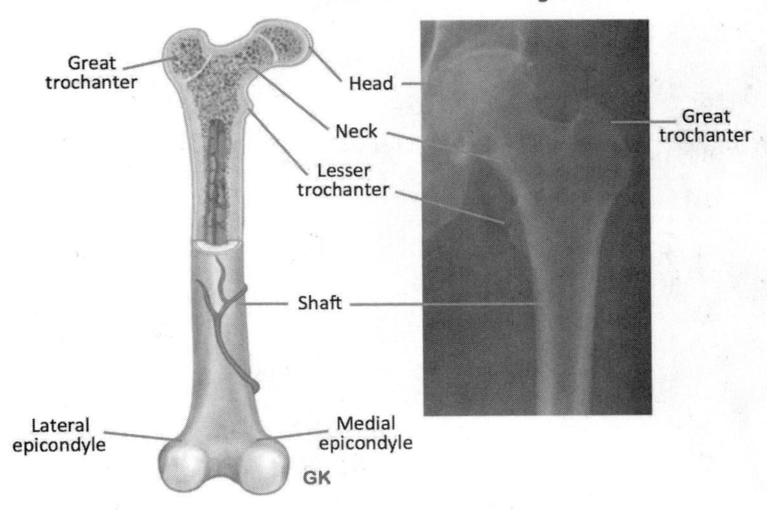

This image highlights the left femur.
Sources: Courtesy of George Kyriakidis/Santa Ana, CA, & K. Kyriakidis

LO1:

Clinical Relevance: Fractures

- Approximately 350,000 people break their hip every year in the United States. Two-thirds of those occur in people over 65 years of age.
- Incidence of hip fracture increases with age, with about half of hip fractures occurring in adults over 80 years of age.
- Over 95% of hip fractures result from falls, most commonly from falling sideways.
- Falls causing hip, femur, and pelvic fractures can be associated with another underlying disease process and/or associated injuries, such as osteoporosis, unsteady gait patterns, or pain with ambulation (related to arthritis, recent surgeries, sprains, leg fractures, or foot ulcers).
- Osteoporosis as an underlying disease is the leading cause of hip fracture.
- Mortality for hip fractures is about 12–37% within a year after the fracture.
- Between 25% and 75% of individuals who were independent before a fractured hip or femur are either unable to walk or unable to achieve previous levels of independence afterward.
- Delay in surgery may increase mortality from hip and femur fractures.
- Hip and femur fracture risk can double in stroke patients.
- Most pelvic fractures result from car, fall, and crush accidents.
- On average, people have about two fractures in their lifetime.

Concept Check

1. **Which structure is affected by a proximal femur fracture?**
   A. Medial epicondyle
   B. Femoral head
   C. Femoral diaphysis
   D. Lateral epicondyle

Answer question

LO2:

Pathophysiology: Fractures

- Hip and femur fractures are commonly the result of a traumatic event.
- With any traumatic injury, the mechanism of injury (MOI) is one component of the assessment in determining potential severity. Age, general physical health, and pre-existing medical conditions also factor into the assessment.
- MOI involves motion injuries, rapid deceleration forces forward and vertical, penetrating or blunt trauma, and compression or crush injuries.

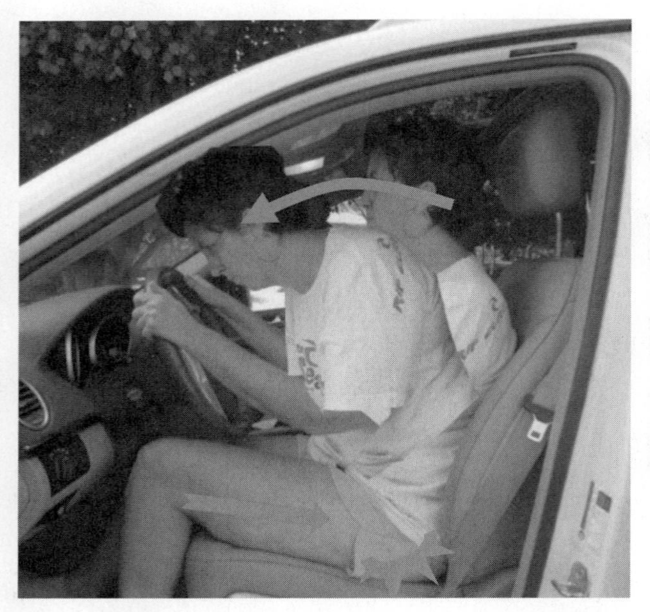

This image depicts how a hip is fractured from a motor vehicle accident.
Source: Courtesy of K. Kyriakidis

- If a patient has fallen, consider:
  - o Distance of the fall
  - o Body part that took the initial impact
  - o Type of surface the fall occurs on
  - o Age of the patient

Hip Fractures from Falls

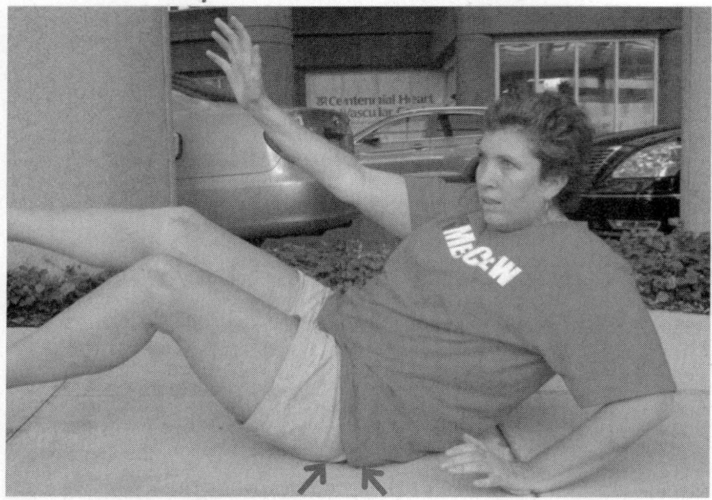

This image shows a common way that older patients sustain hip fractures.
Source: Courtesy of K. Kyriakidis

- Adults over 70 years of age are much more likely to sustain severe injuries and die from a ground-level or standing fall than younger patients.

Pathophysiology: Fractures (continued)

Femoral Shaft Fractures

- The femur is the largest and strongest bone of the body with an ample blood supply enclosed by protective, supportive tissues.

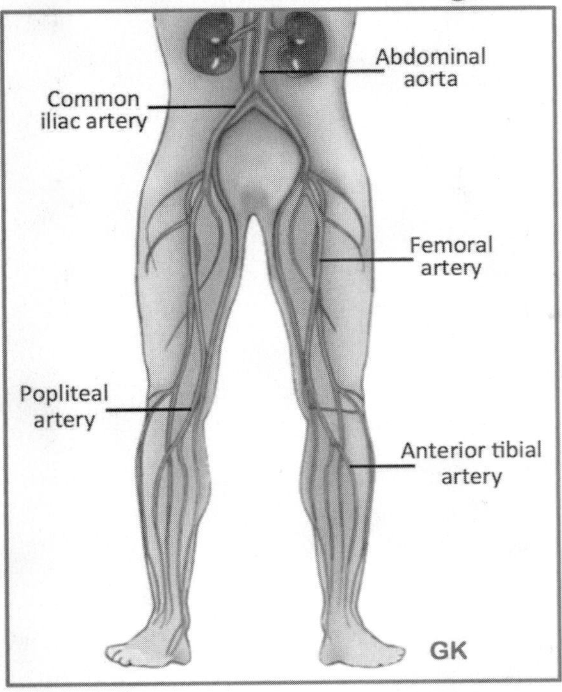

This image demonstrates the arterial circulation of the lower extremities.

Source: Courtesy of George Kyriakidis/Santa Ana, CA

- Substantial force is required to fracture the shaft of the femur in the absence of disease.
- Pathologic fractures, meaning fractures caused by an underlying disease process, such as a malignancy or osteoporosis, can occur with minimal force and result from weakening of the bone.

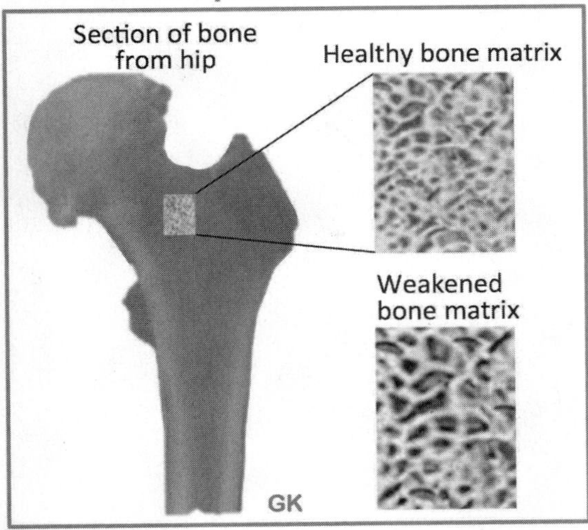

These images allow comparison of the effect of osteoporosis on bone.

Source: Courtesy of George Kyriakidis/Santa Ana, CA

Types

There are numerous types of femoral shaft fractures:

- Greenstick, spiral, oblique, or transverse (most common)
  - o Greenstick: Without actually breaking in two, the bone bends and/or cracks, making it an incomplete fracture. This is mostly seen in young children who have flexible and softer bones.
  - o Spiral: fractures that are caused by torque or twisting
  - o Transverse: The bone breaks at about a 90 degree angle. When bone breaks into two pieces, it is referred to as a simple fracture.
  - o Oblique: fractures that have a curved or sloping break in the bone. They appear to be diagonal.
  - o Type I fractures are often closed, meaning there is no break or puncture through the skin.
- Comminuted fractures are those where the bone breaks or fragments into multiple pieces or more than two. Comminuted fractures commonly cause displacement (displaced fracture) where the bone fragments move and no longer line up straight.
- Open or compound: fracture with broken bone protruding through the skin. The important distinction between an open versus closed fracture is that the bone is exposed to infection and the patient is therefore at risk for a deep bone infection.
- Femoral shaft fractures occur most commonly from a significant direct force to the femur or from an indirect force conducted from the knee.

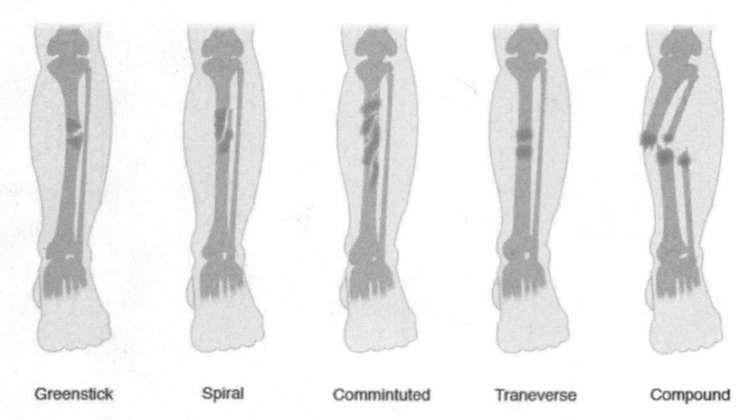

The images depict the most common types of bone fractures that patients experience.

Source: Copyright © 2014, NovEx Novice to Expert Learning, LLC

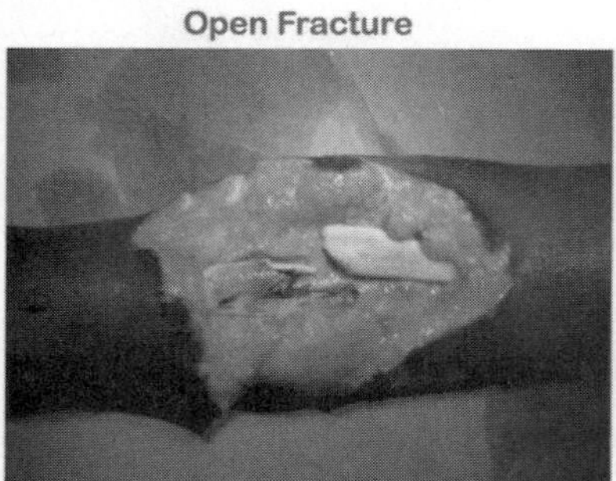

The photos shows an open fracture. Note that the wound appears to be a few weeks old. Courtesy of Wade Stoddard

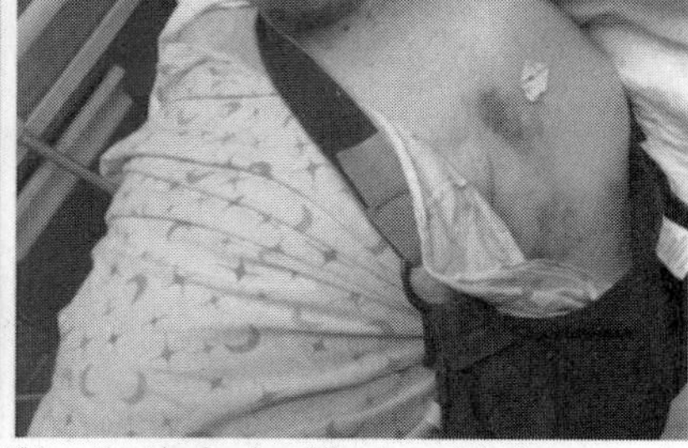

This patient had a closed fracture of the humerus a few weeks prior. Note the persistent bruising in the region surrounding the fracture. Courtesy of K. Kyriakidis

Name This Type of Fracture

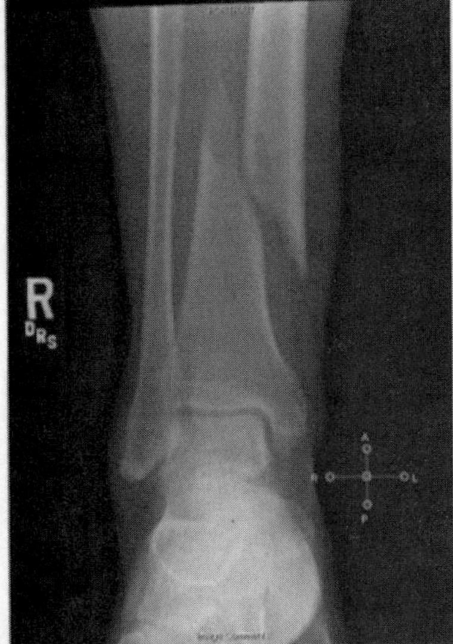

Carefully examine this tibial fracture. Can you determine the type(s) of fracture seen?

Answer: This fracture spirals from the back and downward toward the front and outer side, making it a spiral fracture. The bone is no longer aligned, making it a displaced fracture. It is also a closed fracture as there is no skin break.

Source: Courtesy of K. Kyriakidis

Pathophysiology: Fractures (continued)

Hip Fractures

There are several types of hip fractures:

- Intracapsular:
  - o Femoral head
  - o Femoral neck
  - o Intracapsular fractures have a higher rate of malunion, nonunion, or avascular necrosis of the femoral head.
- Extracapsular:
  - o Intertrochanteric
  - o Subtrochanteric

Types of Hip Fractures

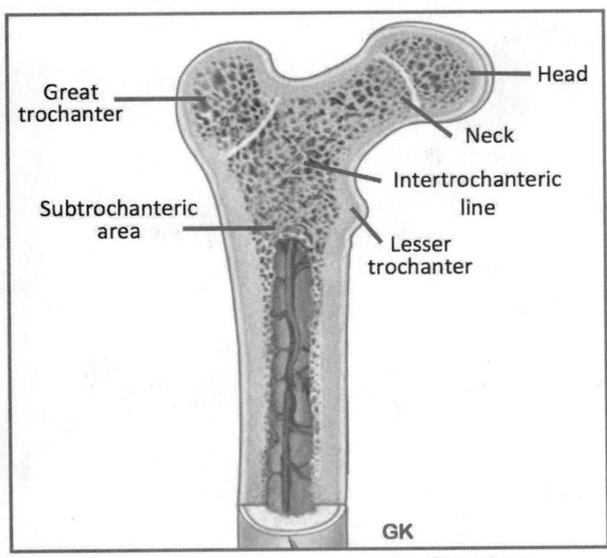

This image reflects common types of hip fractures.

Source: Courtesy of George Kyriakidis/Santa Ana, CA

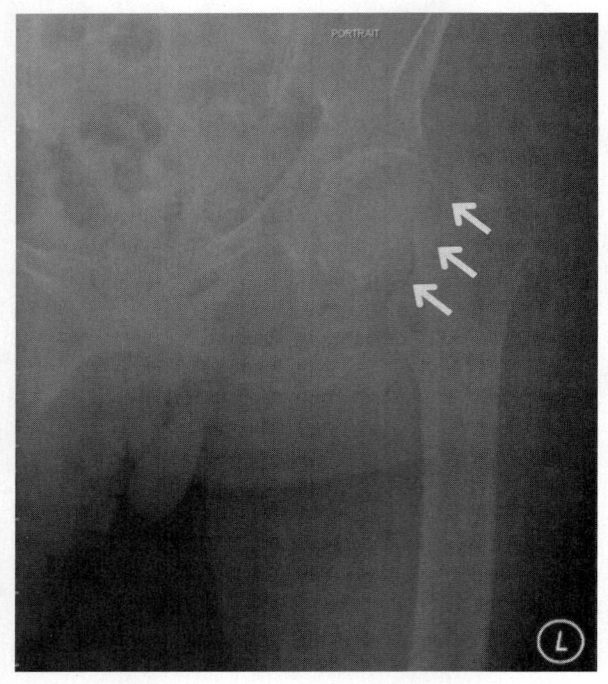

This CT scan reveals an intertrochanteric hip fracture. The damage is so severe that the whole femur neck is no longer visible on CT scan. Osteoporosis is notable in this patient.
Source: Courtesy of K. Kyriakidis

LO2:

Risk Factors: Hip and Femur Fractures

- Age: over 65 years
- Gender: About 80% are women.
- Heredity
- Polypharmacy, especially benzodiazepines and other psychoactive agents
- Previous hip fracture
- Tall stature
- Institutional living
- Neurologic impairment (e.g., history of stroke, depression)
- Decreasing bone mass (e.g., osteoporosis)
- Decreased mobility and/or gait disturbance
- Use of assistive devices for gait problems (e.g., walker or cane)
- Chronic medical conditions (e.g., asthma and hypertension)
- Visual impairment
- Self-perceived state of health, either fair or poor, with fear of falling

LO2:

Causes

Femur Fractures

- Trauma:
    - o High energy collision, most commonly motorcycle crashes or motor vehicle accidents, particularly in younger people
    - o Pedestrian hit by a car or vehicle
    - o Gunshot injury
- Falls from heights
- Low-force incident, such as a fall while standing, particularly in older adults or people with severe osteoporosis
- Physical abuse

Hip Fractures

The majority of hip fractures in adults are caused by:

- Trauma:
  - o Falls in older adults, mostly from a standing position
  - o Some from motor vehicle accidents
- Osteoporosis:
  - o Weakened bones

Older Woman After a Fall on Ice

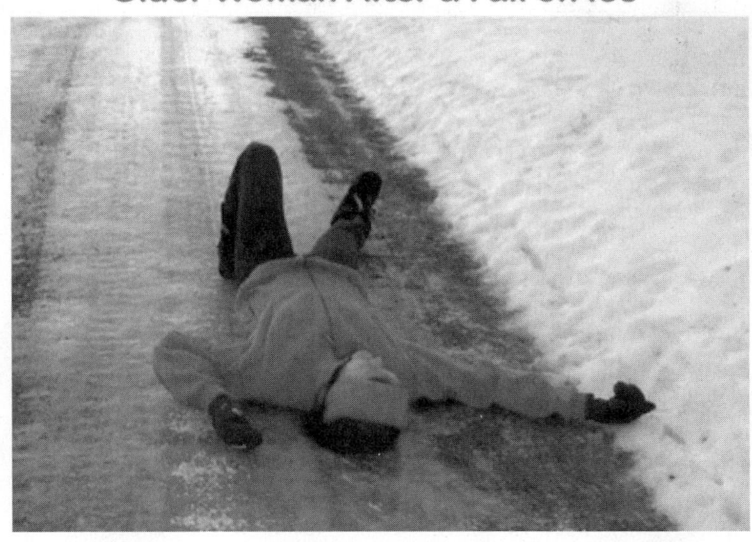

Older adults are at higher risk for falls, which is a common cause of hip fracture. Loose rugs, objects in the way, icy conditions, and poor lighting contribute to these falls.
Source: Courtesy of William Stoddard/Fairbanks, AK

LO2:

Assessment Findings: Fractures

- For the majority of patients with hip fractures, there is invariably a clear onset of the incident associated with some type of trauma or fall. This is followed by severe pain and inability to stand.
- The history and mechanism of injury is important for the health care provider to assess in questioning:
  - o How the fall occurred
  - o The height of the fall
  - o What surface the patient landed on
- It is important to determine the circumstances of the fall to discover an underlying problem.
- Many older patients have comorbidities that could contribute to a fall (e.g., heart disease, stroke).

Left Hip Hematoma & Fracture after a Fall

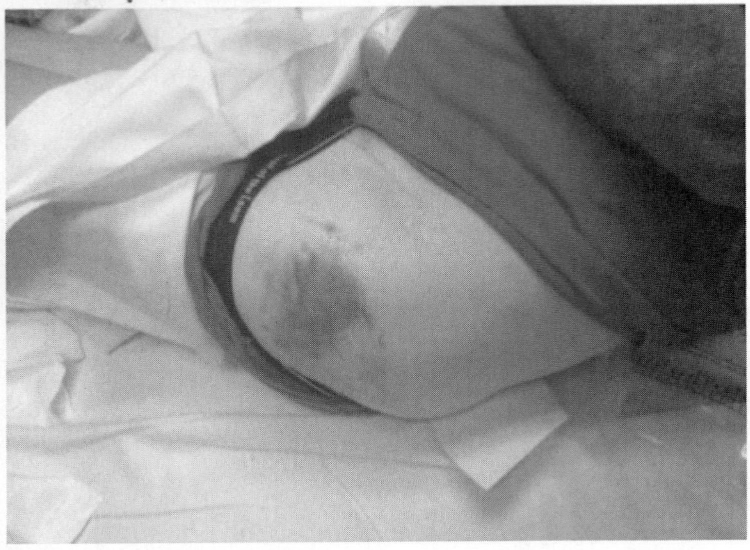

This photo shows the large hematoma with fracture on the patient's left hip after a fall.
Source: Courtesy of K. Kyriakidis

Concept Check

2. Which finding is a risk factor for hip or femur fracture?

A. Being a man
B. Being 50–64 years of age
C. Being tall
D. Taking calcium channel blockers

Answer question

Assessment Findings: Fractures (continued)

Hip and Femur Fractures

- The most common and notable signs and symptoms of hip or femur fracture include:
  - o Pain in hip, femur, or knee
  - o Limited range of motion or severe pain with passive movement
  - o Inability to stand or bear weight as usual
  - o Muscle spasms of the thigh
  - o Deformity of the extremity
  - o Hematoma at the fracture site
- Assess for associated injuries with history of fall, especially head or spinal trauma.
- Anatomical position of the affected extremity may provide information about the fracture:
  - o Femoral head fracture: 70% of patients with femoral head fractures and dislocations have other associated injuries.
  - o Femoral head dislocation:
    - ■ Posterior dislocation (most common): extremity adducted and internally rotated
    - ■ Anterior dislocation: extremity abducted and externally rotated

- Femoral neck: For partial or complete displacement, leg is shortened and externally rotated.
- Greater trochanteric fracture: Pain is noted with pressure, abduction, and extension, without deformity.
- Lesser trochanteric fracture: Pain is felt with flexion and internal rotation, without deformity or anatomical displacement.
- Intertrochanteric fracture: Extremity is shortened and externally rotated, with hip edema and ecchymosis, and pain with any movement.
- Subtrochanteric fracture: Proximal femur is flexed and externally rotated.
- Femoral shaft fracture:
  - Pain, swelling, and deformity at level of fracture of shaft are commonly seen.
  - Extremity may be shortened and crepitus present with movement.

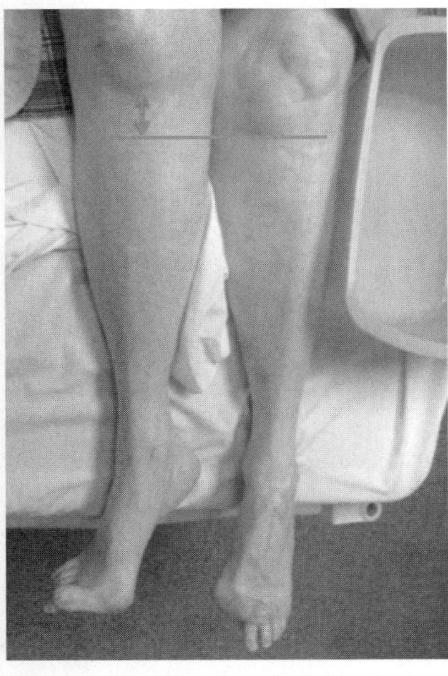

The photo shows a patient who is lying flat in bed. It reveals that her right leg is shortened and externally rotated. These are classic exam findings after an intertrochanteric hip fracture.
Source: Courtesy of K. Kyriakidis

  - Due to the extensive venous and arterial blood supply to the femur and musculature, careful, ongoing observation for an expanding hematoma, signs of shock, and/or neurovascular compromise distal to the injury is vital.

- Significant blood loss from hip and femur fractures can result in hypovolemic shock. Observe for tachycardia and hypotension.

Compartment Syndrome

- Compartment syndrome is an emergency and occurs when there is an increased pressure within a confined space.
- Compartment syndrome may occur with fractures because of associated bleeding and soft tissue edema.
- Bone, muscle, and blood vessels are confined by fascia and an increased pressure may lead to ischemia and necrosis of the tissue.
- Release of cytokines can cause a systemic inflammatory response. These patients usually require urgent surgery.
- Signs and symptoms that may indicate compartment syndrome include the 5 Ps:
  - Pain that is unrelenting and not relieved by narcotics
  - Paresthesias or numbness
  - Pulselessness
  - Pallor of the extremity
  - Paralysis of the affected limb. The affected limb may also be cold.

Compartment Syndrome?

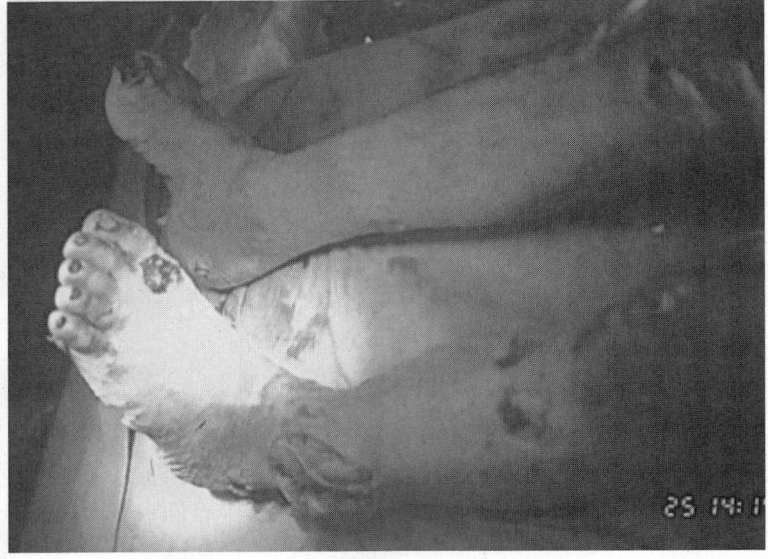

This patient suffered traumatic injury in Desert Storm. The obvious and extensive wounds require care. In addition, a clinician should be suspicious of the muscle and blood vessel damage with soft tissue edema in the left lower leg. The increased edema can be an early warning of developing compartment syndrome.
Source: Courtesy of William Stoddard/Fairbanks, AK

LO2:

Diagnostics: Hip and Femur Fractures

Imaging

- Standard x-rays
- CT scan can visualize some occult fractures not seen on standard x-rays.
- MRI can also detect subtle fractures and soft tissue abnormalities.

MRI: Right Femoral Neck Fracture

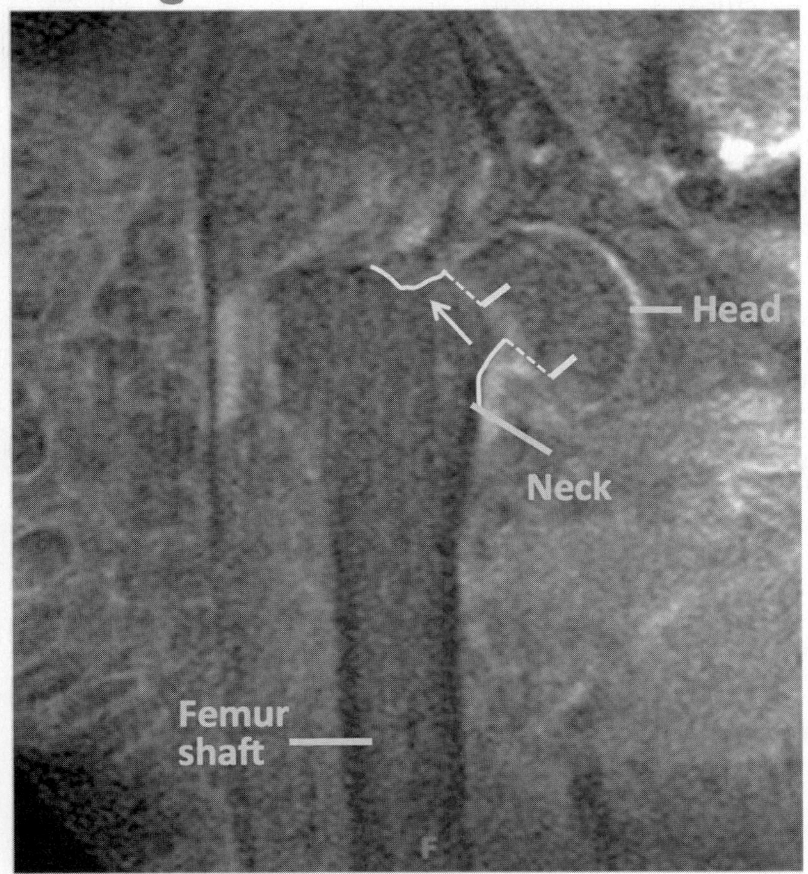

A right femoral neck fracture is seen in this MRI scan of the hip. The yellow lines should line up between the neck and head of the femur. However, the fracture resulted in a significant displacement. The head remains in the acetabular space. Edematous tissues are noted surrounding the hip.

Source: Courtesy of K. Kyriakidis

Electrocardiogram (EKG)

- Detection of dysrhythmias or ischemic change
- Cardiac and neurological workup if fall is result of dizziness or syncope, or if patient is at risk for cardiac event

Laboratory Results

- Complete blood count (CBC) as low hemoglobin and hematocrit can indicate anemia or blood loss.
- Elevated white blood cells (WBC) can indicate underlying infection.
- Comprehensive metabolic panel (CMP) can be obtained to observe for electrolyte imbalance and organ dysfunction.
- Urinalysis (UA) can indicate infection or renal failure.
- Type and cross match if blood loss is significant.
- Point-of-care cardiac enzymes identify cardiac problems.

Priority Patient Concerns and Desired Collaborative Care Outcomes: Hip and Femur Fractures

Prior to caring for patients with hip and femur fractures, it is important to prioritize the patient's concerns that must guide the nursing care plan and interventions. Care for the patient is ordered and organized in accordance with the patient's priority and urgent needs. Desired collaborative care outcomes in patients with hip and femur fractures typically include:

1. The patient will report pain is decreased to a tolerable level.
2. The patient will experience no findings associated with infection.
3. The patient will have normal capillary refill below the cast, distal extremity will be warm, and there will be no findings associated with neurological impairment.
4. The patient will remain injury free.
5. The patient will return to the amount of physical mobility expected, depending upon extent of injury.

Considering these important care outcomes, prepare a list of the major 3–6 priority patient concerns or nursing diagnoses for patients with hip and femur fractures. Be prepared to participate in a discussion of this list and/or to submit them as an assignment, as determined by your faculty. Resources you may find helpful in this assignment can include this lesson, the references, resources on nursing care plans, and standard nursing diagnoses manuals.

LO3:

Collaborative Interventions: Hip and Femur Fractures

Patients with hip and femur fractures experience pain, threat of infection, fluid demands, and possible oxygenation concerns. Care involves:

- **Fluids:**

  - o Observe for hypovolemia and treat with IV crystalloid bolus if indicated (NICE, 2011).
  - o Provide nothing by mouth (NPO) to restrict oral intake in anticipation of probable surgery.
- **Oxygen:**

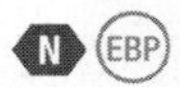

  - o Oxygen saturations should be monitored from emergency admission to 48 hours postoperative (Mak, et al., 2010).
  - o Supplemental oxygen to maintain SpO_2 >92%
- **Pain control:**

  - o Severe pain: provide parenteral or IV pain medications (e.g., opiates such as morphine, hydromorphone, or fentanyl) (NICE, 2011).
  - o Moderate pain: prefer ketorolac IM, if no contraindications
- **Antiemetics** (e.g., ondansetron, metoclopramide) for nausea or vomiting from pain or from opiates
- **Muscle relaxants** (e.g., lorazepam): IV meds for muscle spasms

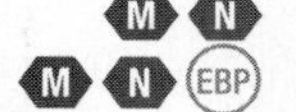

- **Prophylactic antibiotics** (e.g., cefazolin) at induction in surgery, especially for open fractures and tetanus toxoid if not up to date (Mak, et al., 2010)
- **Consults:**
  - o Orthopedic consult after x-ray results (NICE, 2011)

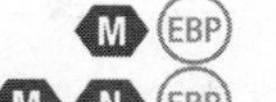

  - o Physical therapy postoperative consult can reduce complications (Mak, et al., 2010).
  - o Consider occupational therapy consult postoperatively (Mak, et al., 2010).
- **Immobilization:**
  - o Full spinal immobilization until spinal injury can be cleared
  - o Immobilize or avoid excess movement of injured extremity as sharp bone fragments can shear soft tissue structures and blood vessels.
- **Closely monitor:**
  - o Vital signs
  - o Ongoing neurovascular status distal to injury for compromise

- **Assessments:**

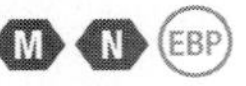
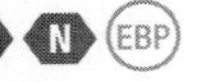

  - o Secondary assessment is crucial for other injuries, especially head trauma and spinal injuries (Mak, et al., 2010).
  - o **Consider comorbidities** present in the patient. Determine if the fall is recent or if the patient has been down for a period of time because injury can be complicated by rhabdomyolysis. Rhabdomyolysis, with muscle damage and release of tissue into the blood stream, can cause kidney damage and failure.
  - o Unexplained falls in older adults are often the result of an undiagnosed infection, e.g., urinary tract or pneumonia.
  - o Determine if the patient is on anticoagulant or antiplatelet therapy and observe for signs of increased bleeding.

Rhabdomyolysis

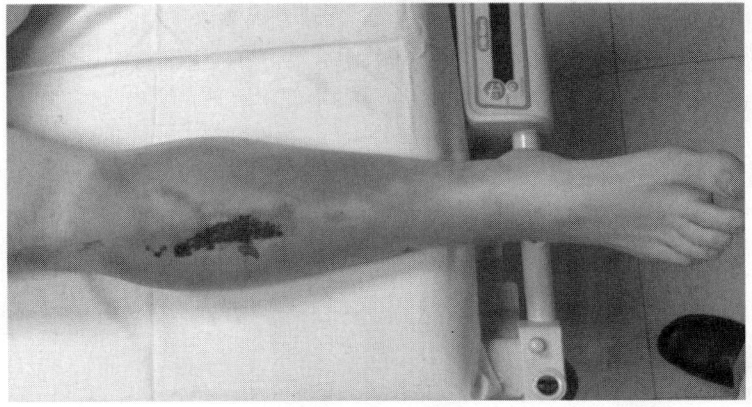

This patient developed rhabdomyolysis after falling and laying for hours without help. The ensuing muscle and tissue damage can be observed. The blackened elongated area on the shin is dried blood from an abrasion that was sustained in the fall.

Source: Courtesy of K. Kyriakidis

Concept Check

3. Which medication is commonly used to treat moderate pain associated with hip or femur fracture?
   - A. Oral NSAIDs
   - B. IV fentanyl
   - C. IM ondansetron
   - D. IM ketorolac

Answer question

Collaborative Interventions: Hip and Femur Fractures (continued)

Nonsurgical Intervention

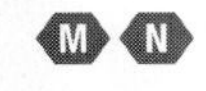

Hip reductions to treat dislocations are commonly performed in the operating room under general anesthesia, even though they are typically noninvasive. The degree of pain requires general anesthesia.

Surgical Intervention

- Most hip and femur fractures require surgical intervention for fixation and stabilization.

- Current guidelines recommend surgical intervention within 24 hours (Mak, et al., 2010).

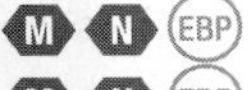

- Occasionally, surgery may be delayed in order to medically stabilize the patient and reduce operative risk (Mak, et al., 2010).

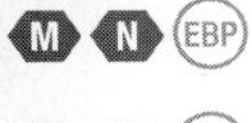

- Delays in surgical stabilization of fracture increase mortality rate (Mak, et al., 2010).

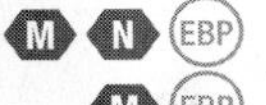

- Surgical interventions will depend on the type of fracture and the previous activity level of the patient (Mak, et al., 2010).

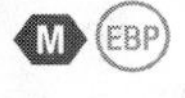

- The goal is to preserve the hip joint and restore function and mobility, and to decrease pain.

External Surgical Fixation

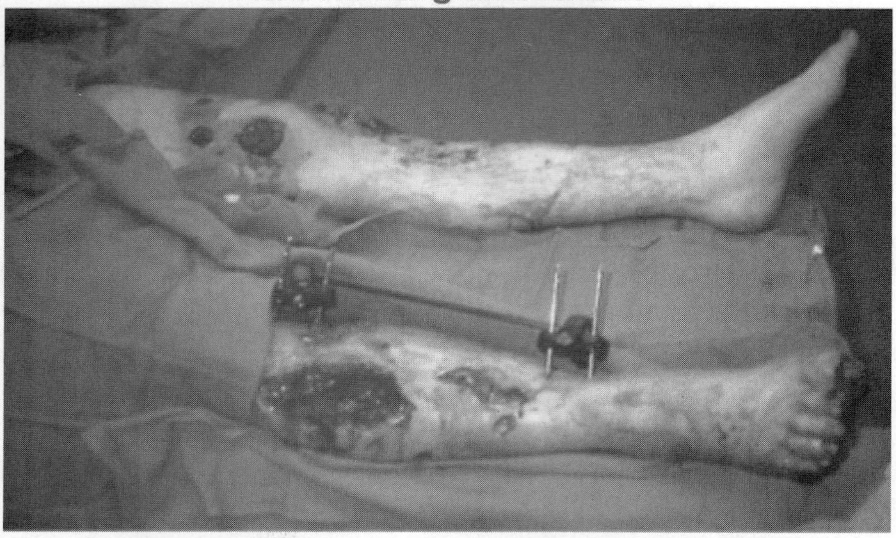

This photo was taken in a war zone and shows external fixation of a tibial fracture.

Source: Courtesy of William Stoddard/Fairbanks, AK

Internal Surgical Fixation

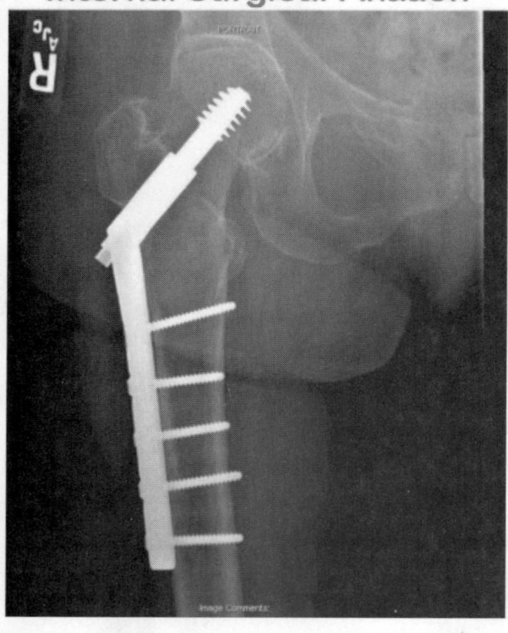

The x-ray shows the result of an internal fixation surgery on the hip where the metal and screws are clearly visible. This visual image provides a better understanding about why patients complain of aching at times.

Source: Courtesy of K. Kyriakidis

Right Hip Fracture with Hip Replacement Surgery

Post-fall Condition
Fracture through right femoral neck
R
Femoral head
A. An incision is made to expose the right hip and the femoral head is removed.
Prosthesis
B. The femur is reamed and a prosthesis is cemented in place.
Post-operative Condition
Prosthesis in place

From left to right: A severely fractured hip requires replacement. The middle image reveals the surgical procedure while the right image shows the metal hip device, inserted into the shaft of the femur, that is used to replace the femur head and neck. A better understanding about what a patient's surgery entails can inform the care provider about the pain, discomfort, and difficulties the patient may experience postoperatively.

Collaborative Interventions: Hip and Femur Fractures (continued)

Postoperative Care

Postoperative care should include:

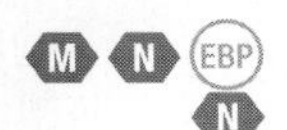

- Manage pain to achieve patient comfort and to improve mobility (Mak, et al., 2010).
- Observe for signs of wound or other infections (e.g., urinary, pulmonary, skin).

Normal Post-Surgical Wound

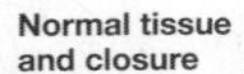

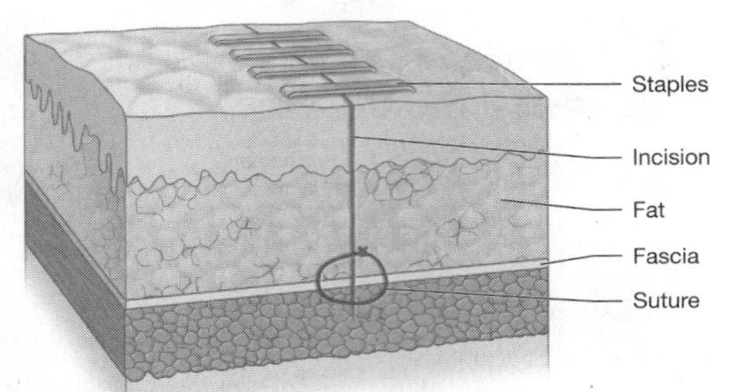

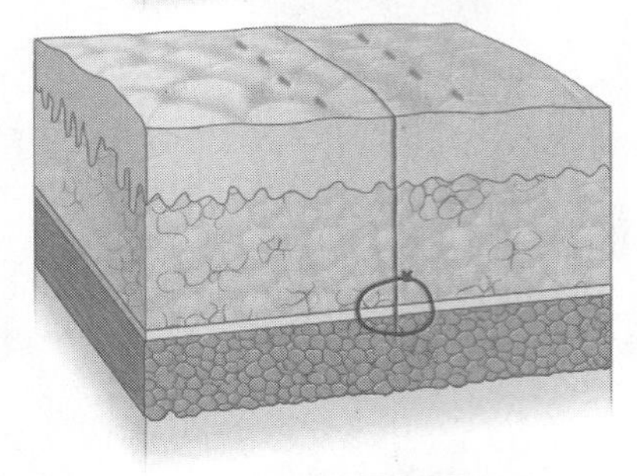

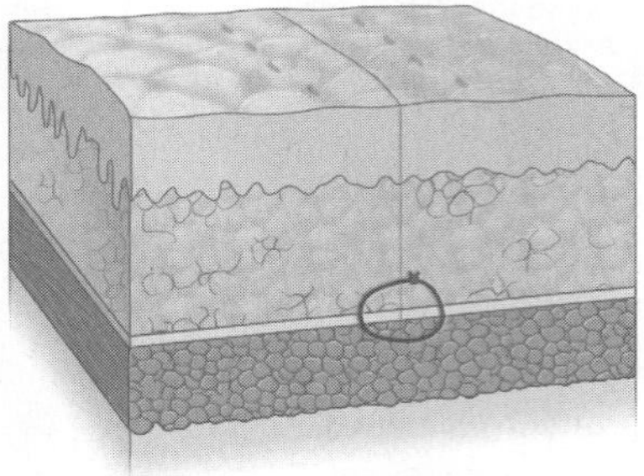

Observe the wound for normal healing postoperatively.

- Observe for postoperative bleeding.

- Maintain adequate fluid and nutritional intake in the postoperative period (Mak, et al., 2010) to support recovery and wound healing.
- Institute fall precautions per facility protocol.

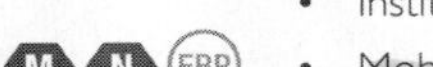

- Mobilize the patient early to improve healing and prevent multiple never events (e.g., DVT, pneumonia, pressure ulcers) (Mak, et al., 2010).

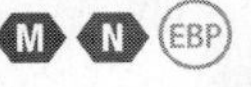

- Implement DVT prophylaxis in a majority of patients. A sequential pneumatic compression device is used for those who cannot take anticoagulants (Mak, et al., 2010).

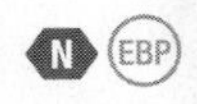

- Implement skin precautions to prevent pressure ulcers on bony prominences (Mak, et al., 2010).

- Be attentive to any potential pressure ulcer areas that may have been present prior to hospitalization by reviewing the admission assessment notes as a key reference point.

- Prevent other "never events" such as CAUTI, central line infections, air embolism, and others.

Collaborative Interventions: Hip and Femur Fractures (continued)

Prevention

Prevention of postoperative complications is key. Many interventions have been previously mentioned. A few more specific ones include:

Pressure Wounds

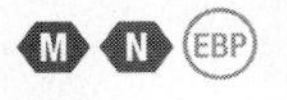

Pressure-relieving or alternating-pressure mattresses should be used on all fracture patients (Mak, et al., 2010).

Fall Assessment

- Risk for fall should be assessed on all patients presenting to the hospital and prior to discharge to identify those at risk. Each facility has a fall assessment scoring system to identify those at risk. Examples of patient function that are typically in an assessment tool for most facilities include:
  - o History of recent falls (past 3 months)
  - o Gait disturbance
  - o Balance problem
  - o Use of assist devices
  - o Medications: antiepileptics, benzodiazepines, diuretics, psychotropics, hypoglycemics
  - o Visual impairment
  - o Altered mental status
  - o Altered elimination
  - o Dizziness
  - o Men, but only slightly higher risk

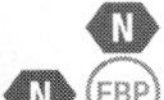

- Implement fall prevention strategies determined by the facility.
- When a patient is at risk for falls, patient education upon discharge should include avoidance of alcohol overuse, stop smoking, regular weight-bearing exercise, typical home environment changes, and need for assistance (e.g., removing scatter rugs, adding grab bars, replace glasses, wearing solid rubber-based shoes without heels, decluttering paths for movement, the patient's ability to climb steps without assistance, good lighting).

- For patients at high risk and who live alone, an alert system that they may activate should be considered. Older adults can sustain multiple injuries from a fall, including laying unattended for hours until someone finds them if they are unable to reach a phone to call for help.

Medications

Medications that may be considered are:

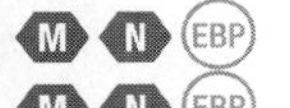

- Calcium supplements and bisphosphonates (Mak, et al., 2010)
- Supplemental vitamin D (Mak, et al., 2010)
- Parathyroid hormone and estrogen replacement may reduce bone loss and decrease the risk of fractures in those with osteoporosis.

Patients At Risk for Falls After Discharge

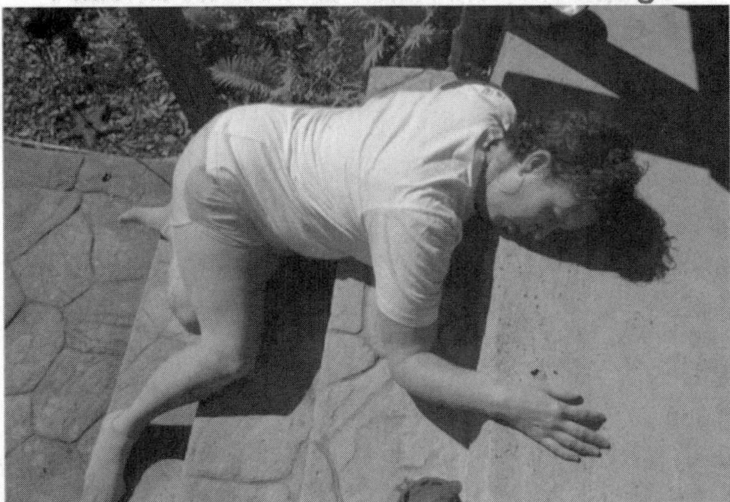

Patients should be educated with their caregivers to wait for assistance if stair climbing poses a fall risk. Many patients are fiercely independent so collaborating with the patient to explore other methods of assistance may be needed to support independent living.

Source: Courtesy of K. Kyriakidis

Intervention Summary: Hip and Femur Fractures

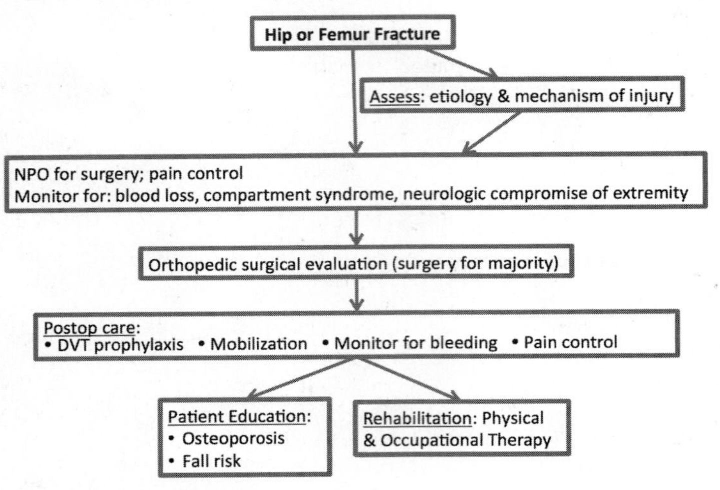

Hip or femur fracture algorithm.

LO1:

What Are Pelvic Fractures?

- The pelvis consists of a butterfly-shaped grouping of bones at the base of the spine, which include the pubis, ilium, and ischium.
- These bones form an anatomic ring with the sacrum.
- Pelvic fractures consist of 3% of all fractures, and over half are the result of minimal to moderate trauma.
- Pelvic fractures are associated with increased risk of pulmonary emboli.
- These bones are held in place by ligaments to form a girdle of bones.
- The pelvis forms one major ring in the center and two smaller rings that support and protect the bladder, intestines, and rectum.

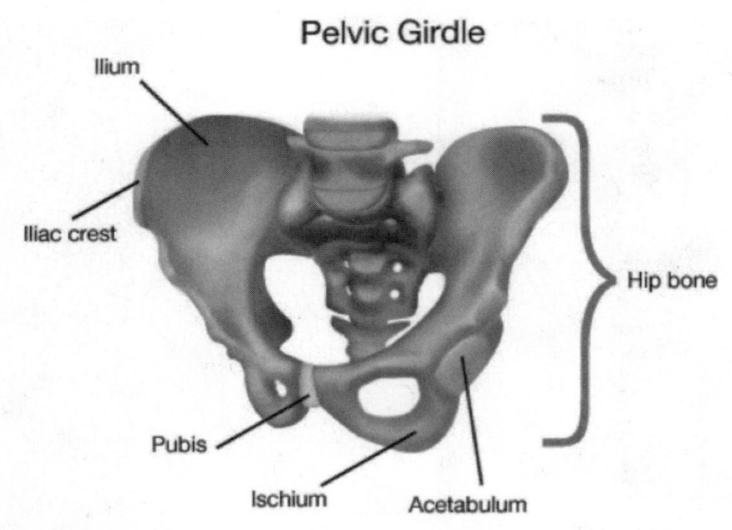

Normal pelvic anatomy.

Concept Check

4. What is true of pelvic fractures?
   A. Most result from substantial trauma.
   B. They increase risk for pulmonary emboli.
   C. Taking antiepileptic drugs increases risk.
   D. Alterations in elimination pattern increases risk.

Answer question

LO1:

Clinical Relevance: Pelvic Fractures

- Pelvic fractures are not common (3% of all fractures) and range widely from mild and stable to severe and unstable.
- Severe and unstable fractures are associated with severe traumatic events with other concurrent injuries.
- Over 50% of pelvic fractures occur as the result of a fall from standing, 95% of which are considered minor.
- Most fractures in older adults involve the pubic rami and do not disrupt the pelvic ring.
- Pre-existing bone disease, such as osteoporosis, enhances the likelihood of fractures from a fall.
- The pelvic bones contain and protect major blood vessels, organs, and nerves that can be compromised by pelvic fractures.

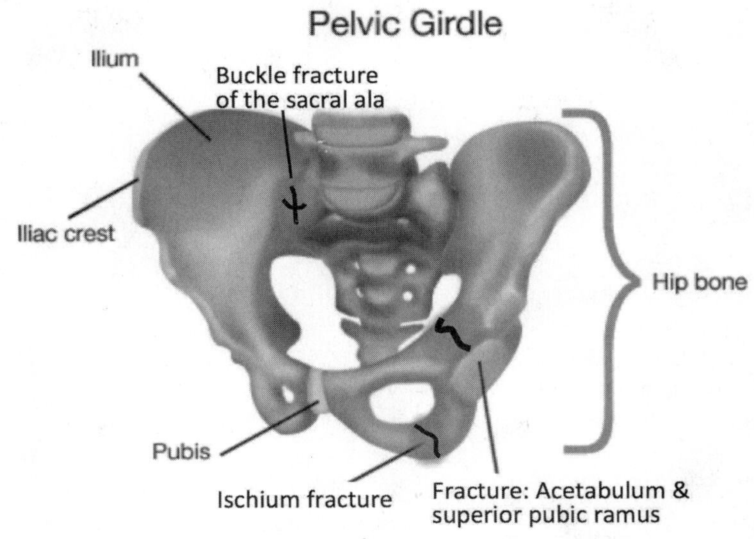

The image points out where most pelvic fractures tend to occur.

LO2:

Pathophysiology: Pelvic Fractures

- Like in hip and femur, pelvic fractures are commonly the result of a traumatic event.
- Similarly, the mechanism of injury (MOI) (e.g., age, general physical health, and pre-existing medical conditions) contribute to determining potential severity.
- **Stable** pelvic fracture: Pelvis has a singular fracture in the pelvic ring without displacement of bones and minimal bleeding.
- **Unstable** pelvic fracture: two or more fractures in the pelvic ring with moderate to severe bleeding
- Either fracture can be open, meaning that the skin has been broken, or closed, meaning that the skin is intact.
- Powerful dynamic forces are needed to produce multiple pelvic fractures.
- As a result, bleeding and damage to the extra-pelvic organs can occur.

Crush Injury of Pelvis

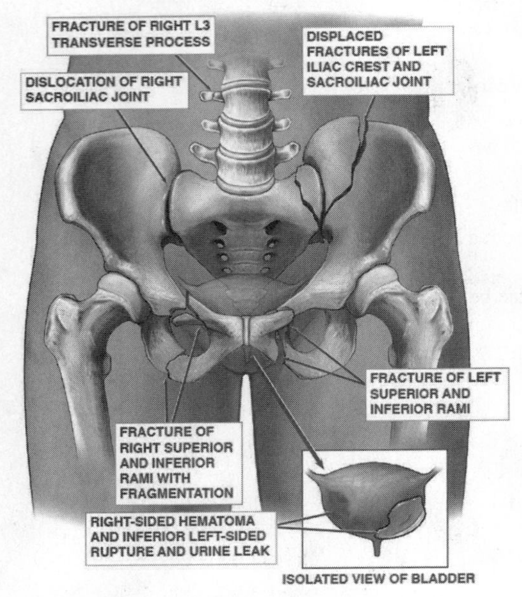

This anatomical image represents a severe unstable crush injury causing emergent surgery for organ repair.

Classification Systems for Pelvic Fractures

There are several classification systems for pelvic fractures. Title classification is one example:

- *Type A*: Sacroiliac complex is intact. Pelvic ring has a stable fracture. These do not require surgical intervention.
- *Type B*: Partial disruption of the posterior sacroiliac complex occurs due to internal or external rotation. These are considered unstable.
- *Type C*: Complete disruption of the posterior sacroiliac complex with vertical instability
  - o Type C results from significant force such as motor vehicle accident , fall from height, or severe crush injury.
  - o These are considered unstable.

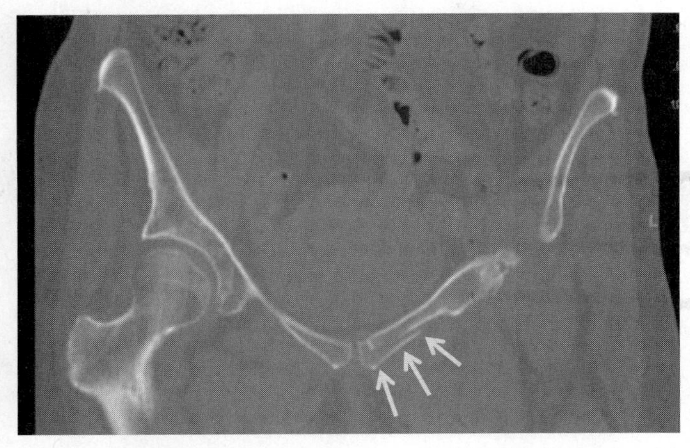

Pelvic fracture of the superior ramus on the patient's left side. This patient did not have a surgical repair and was deemed Type A fracture.

Source: Courtesy of K. Kyriakidis

LO2: Risk Factors: Pelvic Fractures

Risk factors for pelvic fracture are the same as those for hip and femur fracture:

- Age: over 65 year
- Gender: Approximately 80% are women.
- Heredity
- Polypharmacy, especially benzodiazepines and other psychoactive agents
- Previous hip fracture
- Tall stature
- Institutionalized living
- Neurologic impairment, such as history of stroke, and depression
- Decreasing bone mass (osteoporosis)
- Use of assistive devices for gait problems (e.g., walker or cane)
- Chronic medical conditions (e.g., asthma and hypertension)
- Decreased mobility or gait disturbance
- Visual impairment
- Self-perceived state of health, either fair or poor, and fear of falling

LO2: Causes: Pelvic Fractures

The majority of pelvic fractures in adults are caused by:

- Trauma:
  - o Falls in older adults, mostly from a standing position
  - o Some from motor vehicle accidents
- Osteoporosis:
  - o Weakened bones due to aging, postmenopause, calcium and vitamin D deficiencies, smoking, excessive alcohol consumption, and sedentary lifestyle

Displaced Pelvic Fracture

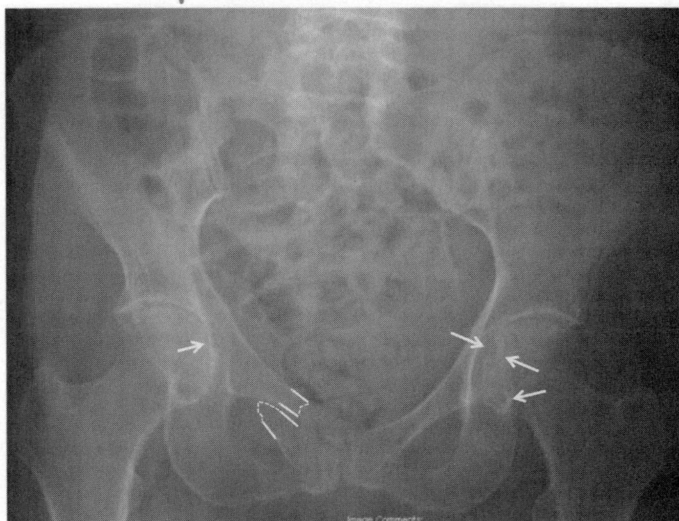

The Xray reveals a pelvic fracture from a car accident on the patient's right. The superior pubic ramus broke in two with the ends overlapping (yellow). Both femoral heads show degenerative changes or avascular necrosis (green arrows).

Source: Courtesy of K. Kyriakidis

LO2:

Assessment Findings: Pelvic Fractures

- History of trauma: Determine how the fall occurred, mechanism of injury, time of injury, general health of patient, and presence of comorbidities.
- Pain: particularly in the groin, hip, and lower back
- Abdominal pain
- Numbness and tingling in groin or legs
- Bleeding from vagina or urethra
- Difficulty urinating
- Unable to walk or stand
- Instability with hip adduction or motion can allude to a pelvic (specifically acetabular) fracture with or without hip fracture. A health care provider may find this on exam.

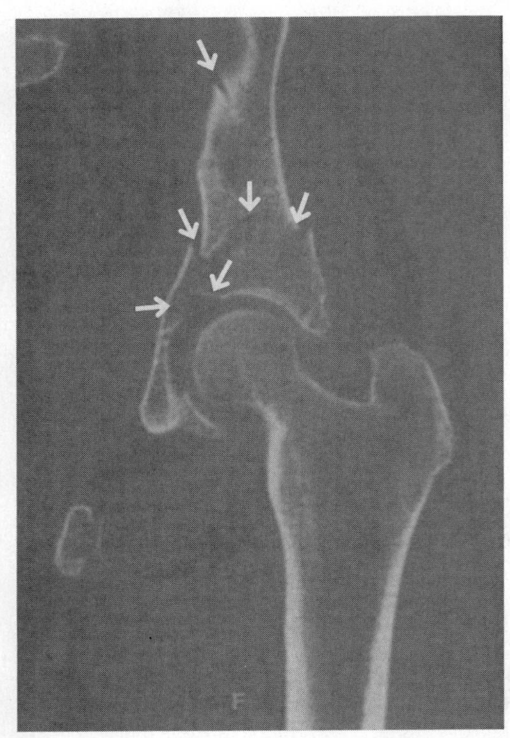

This CT scan of a hip joint reveals an acetabular fracture, just above and around the "socket" of the joint (arrows). Note the multiple fractured areas. This was caused by the force of the femoral head being forced into the pelvic structure.
Source: Courtesy of K. Kyriakidis

LO2:

Diagnostics: Pelvic Fractures

Imaging

- Standard x-rays
- CT scan to detect occult fractures not seen by x-rays
- MRI to detect subtle fractures and soft tissue abnormalities

EKG

Particularly observe for:

- Dysrhythmias
- Ischemic changes

Cardiac and Neurological Workup

If fall is result of dizziness or syncope or if at risk for cardiac event

Laboratory Results

- CBC: Low hemoglobin and hematocrit can indicate anemia or blood loss.
- WBC: Elevated WBC can indicate underlying infection.
- CMP (chemistry): Observe for electrolyte imbalance and organ dysfunction.
- Urinalysis (UA): Observe for signs of infection and renal failure.
- Type and cross match: if blood loss is significant or hemoglobin and hematocrit are low
- Point-of-care (POC): cardiac enzymes

Priority Patient Concerns and Desired Collaborative Care Outcomes: Pelvic Fractures

Prior to caring for patients with pelvic fractures, it is important to prioritize the patient's concerns that must guide the nursing care plan and interventions. Care for the patient is ordered and organized in accordance with the patient's priority and urgent needs. Desired collaborative care outcomes in patients with pelvic fractures typically include:

1. The patient will report pain is decreased to a tolerable level.
2. The patient will experience no findings associated with infection.
3. The patient will have normal capillary refill below the cast, distal extremity will be warm, and there will be no findings associated with neurological impairment.
4. The patient will remain injury free.
5. The patient will return to the amount of physical mobility expected, depending upon extent of injury.

Considering these important care outcomes, prepare a list of the major 3–6 priority patient concerns or nursing diagnoses for patients with pelvic fractures. Be prepared to participate in a discussion of this list and/or to submit them as an assignment, as determined by your faculty. Resources you may find helpful in this assignment can include this lesson, the references, resources on nursing care plans, and standard nursing diagnoses manuals.

LO3:

Collaborative Interventions: Pelvic Fractures

Immediate and Preoperative

Immobilization

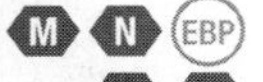

- After a fall or trauma, initially immobilize the affected area (Bhandari, et al., 2012).

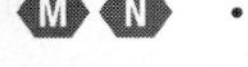

- Full spinal immobilization is necessary until spinal injury can be ruled out.

Fluids and Medications

- Observe and treat for tachycardia and/or hypovolemia, starting with crystalloid bolus and supplemental oxygen.
- Restrict oral intake—NPO initially.

Pain Control

- Collaborate with HCP to use parenteral pain medications with opiates (e.g., morphine, hydromorphone, fentanyl IV for severe pain, or ketorolac IM for moderate pain) if no contraindications as needed.

Assessments

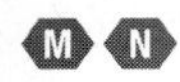

- Perform secondary assessment. This is crucial to identify concurrent injuries, especially head trauma and spinal injuries. Vital signs should be monitored closely.
- Observe perineal area for signs of bleeding, vaginal or urethral. Determine if patient has difficulty urinating or is unable to urinate.
- Monitor for shortness of breath or chest pain as pelvic fractures increase risk for pulmonary embolus.

Antiemetics

- May use medications (e.g., ondansetron, metoclopramide) for nausea and vomiting from pain or from opiates.

Anticoagulants

- Determine if patient is on anticoagulant or antiplatelet therapy for increased bleeding.

Infection and Antibiotics

- Collaborate on use of antibiotic (e.g., cefazolin) for open fractures or if internal organs have been damaged (e.g., bowel, bladder) or if infectious process is concurrently present.
- Avoid urinary catheter insertion until urethral injury has been ruled out or is unlikely by physical exam.

Tetanus Toxoid

- Administer tetanus toxoid when not up to date in patients with open fractures or wounds.

Consults

- Consider orthopedic consult after x-ray results for fracture treatment.
- Consider need for other specialist depending on internal organ damage (e.g., urologist, trauma surgeon).

Nonsurgical Intervention

- For minor, stable fractures, bed rest and pain medication (either with nonsteroidal medication or narcotics) are standard.
- Physical therapy is recommended with the use of assistive devices.
- Pelvic fractures can take 8–12 weeks to heal.

Surgical Intervention

- Initially, an external fixation device may be necessary in unstable patients (Bhandari, et al., 2012).
- A more permanent open reduction and internal fixation may be required.
- Repair of damaged organs and/or control of pelvic hemorrhage may be required.

Collaborative Interventions: Pelvic Fractures (continued)

Surgical or Nonsurgical Interventions

- Non–weight-bearing on the affected side for 8–12 weeks is recommended, depending on the injury.

Displaced Pelvic Fractures with Surgical Repair

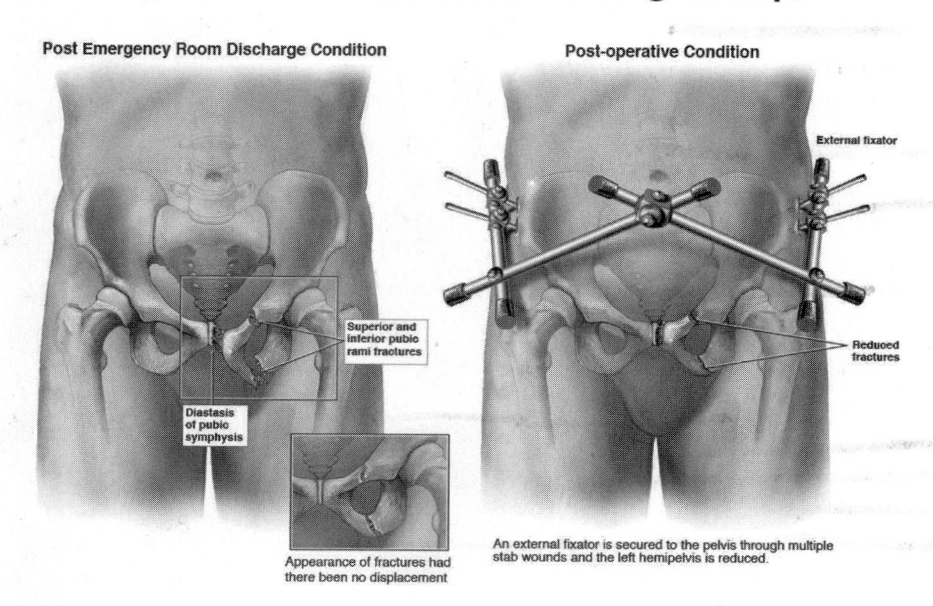

Complex Pelvic and Lumbar Spine Fractures and Pelvic Hematoma

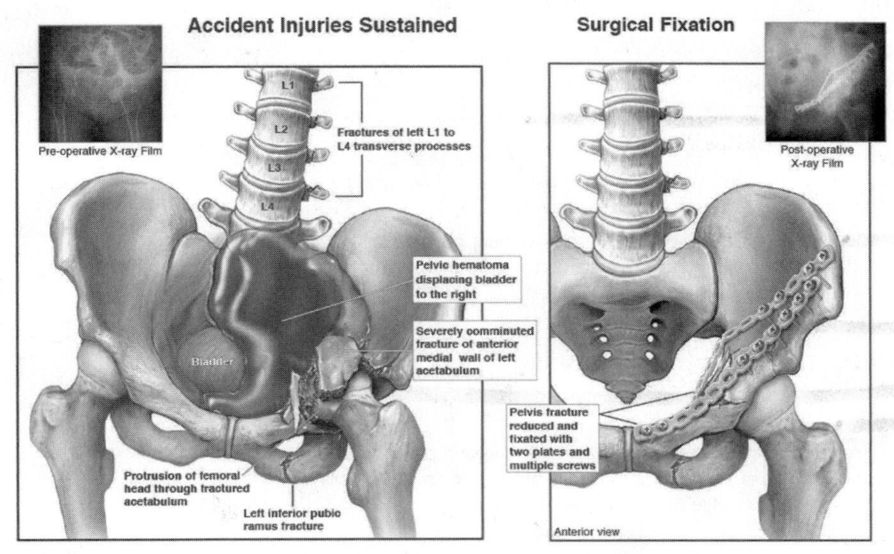

These four images provide examples of pelvic fractures (on the left) with different surgical repair fixations (on the right). The repair on the lower right required open reduction and evacuation of the large hematoma.

Concept Check

5. When is a urinary catheter placed in a patient suspected of having a pelvic fracture?
   - A. Immediately
   - B. Only in the absence of urethral damage
   - C. After radiographic evidence of fracture exists
   - D. Urinary catheters are not used in these patients.

Answer question

Postoperative Care

The goals of treatment are to restore the bony anatomy, prevent deformity, minimize discomfort, prevent complications, and to restore function and mobility.

N • Observe for complications: thromboembolism, wound or other infection (e.g., urinary, pulmonary, skin), bleeding, and malunion or nonunion.

N • Institute fall precautions per facility protocol.

N • Monitor closely for signs of blood loss and shock.

M N EBP • Monitor closely for neurovascular compromise in lower extremities (Bhandari, et al., 2012).

M N • Provide adequate nutrition and hydration.

M N EBP • Use prevention measures for DVT, such as a sequential compression device and subcutaneous heparin.

N EBP • Observe for formation of DVT or signs of pulmonary embolism (e.g., sudden shortness of breath and chest pain) (Bhandari, et al., 2012).

M N • Manage pain to make the patient comfortable and to encourage early mobilization when possible.

N • Implement skin precautions to prevent shear damage or pressure ulcers on bony prominences.

N • Document if pressure ulcers or wounds are present prior to hospitalization.

M N • Manage urethral injuries as directed by urologic consult. A suprapubic catheter may be in place due to urethral damage.

Collaborative Interventions: Pelvic Fractures (continued)

Prevention

Preventing pain, discomfort, and complications are central to the care of patient with fractures:

- **Pain prevention and management:**
  - o Because fractures are very painful, intervene to assess for pain and provide prescribed analgesics.
  - o Avoid constipation, which many narcotics can cause. Constipation should be avoided in pelvic fractures. Fluids, fiber, and stool softeners may be warranted.
  - o Immobilize the broken bone(s), which generally leads to improvement of pain. Cast, traction, and external fixation devices must be properly maintained by the nurse. Orthopedic procedures and protocols are often hospital and specialty specific.
  - o Maintain proper bone alignment and traction.
- **Prevention of infection:**
  - o Osteomyelitis is an infection of the bone and can occur following orthopedic injuries, especially in open wounds.
  - o Monitor for signs and symptoms of infection such as pain or changes in pain character, fever, redness, warmth, localized edema, tenderness (not only of fracture area), irritability, fatigue, nausea and/or vomiting, loss of range of motion, and elevated WBC counts.
  - o Urgently initiate ordered antibiotics when osteomyelitis or other infections are identified.
  - o Maintain clean, dry skin around traction entry points and external fixation devices. Nurses who care for orthopedic patients, like in any specialty, necessarily learn orthopedic specific nursing care and management of devices.

Prevention of Osteomyelitis

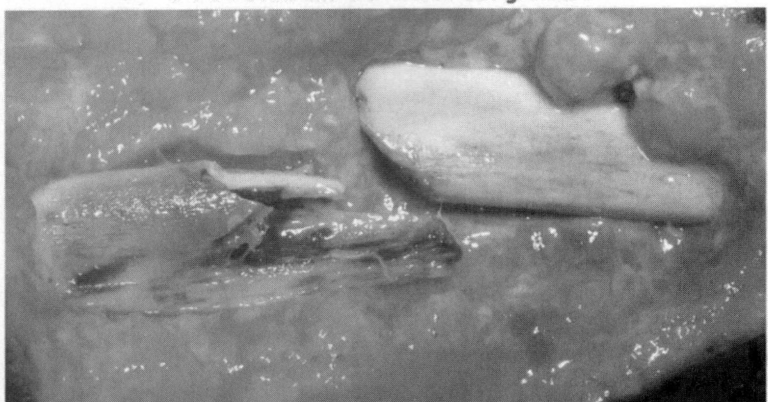

Patients following open orthopedic injuries, particularly where fractured bone is exposed for any extended time period, are at risk for osteomyelitis or infection. The wound above has been debrided and cleaned, but clinicians must remain vigilant for early warning signs of infection. Because osteomyelitis is commonly difficult to treat and can become chronic, prevention is key.

Source: Courtesy of Wade Stoddard

- **Restoration of mobility:**
  - o Encourage range of motion (ROM) exercises and ambulation as early as possible.
  - o Consult occupational therapy (OT) and/or physical therapy (Mak, et al., 2010).
  - o Educate on fall and trauma prevention.
- **Prevention of compartment syndrome:**
  - o Urgently notify the health care provider if suspicions arise about the development of compartment syndrome.
  - o Regularly perform neurovascular assessments and rapidly notify the health care provider of developing changes.
  - o Ensure properly fitting casts to help prevent compartment syndrome.
  - o Administer ordered anti-inflammatory medications when indicated.
  - o Monitor pressure compartments when indicated (Bhandari, et al., 2012).

- **Prevention of Pulmonary Embolism (PE) and DVT**
  - o Encourage early mobilization (Mak, et al., 2010).
  - o Initiate ROM above and below affected area.
  - o Consult PT, which can reduce morbidity and complications (Mak, et al., 2010).
  - o Administer ordered anticoagulants (Bhandari, et al., 2012).
  - o Use compression device to reduce the incidence of DVT (Bhandari, et al., 2012).
  - o Frequently perform pulmonary and oxygenation assessments and rapidly notify health care provider of concerning changes.

DVT Prevention

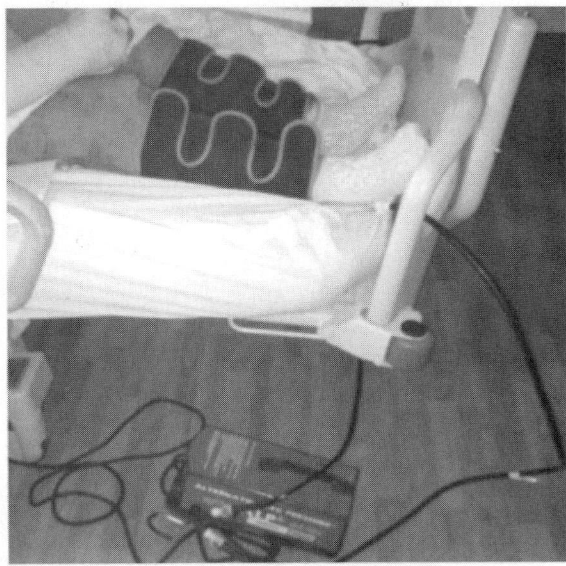

For less mobile patients, prevention of DVT is paramount. Sequential compression device use should be considered.

Collaborative Interventions: Pelvic Fractures (continued)

Patient Education and Discharge

- Typically, patients with pelvic fractures do not have casts. In atypical circumstances, if the patient is in a cast or traction:
  - o Encourage patient to wiggle toes or fingers when in cast or traction.
  - o Stress the need to keep cast clean and dry. Advise not to insert sharp objects inside the cast for scratching.
  - o Instruct patient to elevate the involved extremity and to apply cold (as prescribed) to help reduce swelling.
  - o Educate patient and family about the type, purpose, and maintenance of traction.
  - o Explain that a sensation of warmth within the cast is normal.
  - o Explain how to assess for compartment syndrome.
- Have the patient perform ROM exercises regularly.
- Teach to assess for numbness and tingling.
- Teach how to monitor the wound site and to care for the wound. Examine traction site every 4–6 hours.
- Follow up with physical therapist for rehabilitation.
- Follow up with occupational therapist if consulted.
- Educate the patient and family on how to prevent infections.
- Continue assessments for complications such as bleeding, DVT, PE, infection, and pneumonia.

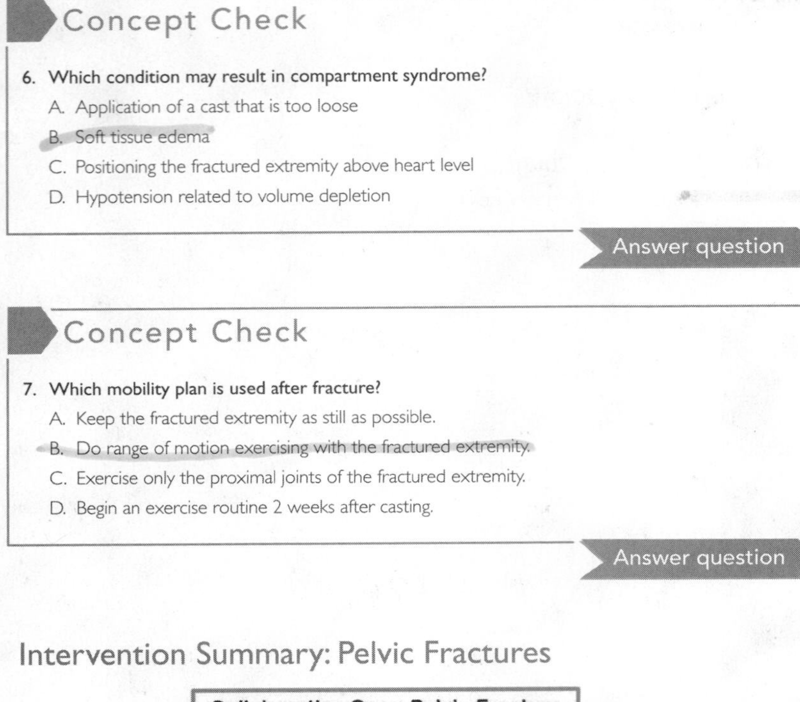

Concept Check

6. Which condition may result in compartment syndrome?
   A. Application of a cast that is too loose
   B. Soft tissue edema
   C. Positioning the fractured extremity above heart level
   D. Hypotension related to volume depletion

Answer question

Concept Check

7. Which mobility plan is used after fracture?
   A. Keep the fractured extremity as still as possible.
   B. Do range of motion exercising with the fractured extremity.
   C. Exercise only the proximal joints of the fractured extremity.
   D. Begin an exercise routine 2 weeks after casting.

Answer question

Intervention Summary: Pelvic Fractures

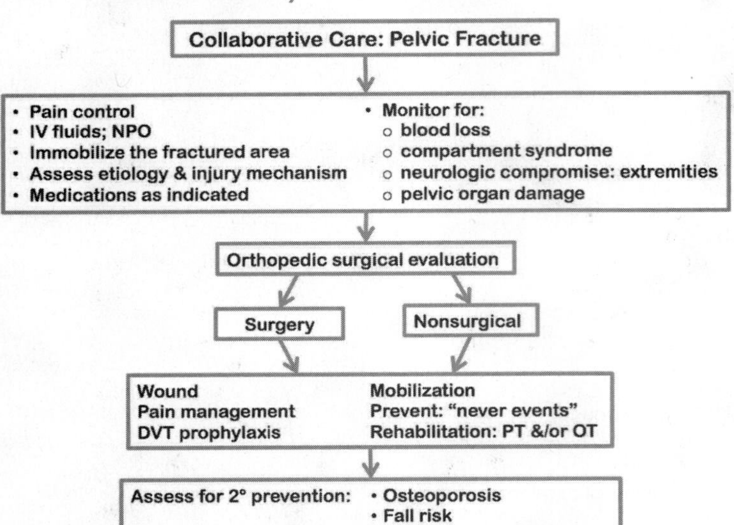

Summary of Interventions: Hip, Femur, and Pelvic Fractures

- Initial immobilization after a fall is necessary until other injuries can be ruled out. Stabilize the injured area.
- History is an important part of assessment of any patient with a fall complaint. Mechanism of injury, along with general health of the patient, and comorbidities are important in determining contributing factors to a fall.
- Assessment of other injuries and the circumstance of a fall is crucial in determining relevant factors of a fall and identifying other injuries.
- Hip and femur fracture can cause significant blood loss. Monitor for signs of hypovolemia, hemorrhage, and shock, with special attention to patients on anticoagulant therapy.
- Carefully and regularly assess to detect potential postoperative complications early and minimize them.
- Fall assessment should be performed on all patients to identify and minimize their risk.
- Altering modifiable risk factors can decrease the occurrence of falls.
- Use of supplemental calcium, estrogen, vitamin D, parathyroid hormone, and bisphosphonates can slow the progression of osteoporosis and susceptibility for fractures.

LO4:

Evaluation of Desired Collaborative Care Outcomes: Hip, Femur, and Pelvic Fractures

Evaluation and reassessment should reveal attainment of previously established patient outcomes. In summary:

- The patient reports that pain is controlled at a level that is tolerable.
- The patient has remained infection free.
- The patient has no findings associated with compartment syndrome.
- The patient has not fallen, any necessary prosthesis is intact, and no findings of DVT or PE are present.
- The patient has participated in physical therapy and has returned to the expected level of mobility.

References

Brauer, C. A., Coca-Perraillon, M., Cutler, D. M., et al. (2009). Incidence and mortality of hip fractures in the United States. *JAMA, 302*(14), 1573–1579.

Frakes, M. A., & Evans, T. (2004). Major pelvic fractures. *Critical Care Nurse, 24*(2), 18–30. **ccn.aacnjournals.org/content/24/2/18.full**

Frost, S. A., Nguyen, N. D., Black, D. A., et al. (2001). Risk factors for in-hospital post-hip fracture mortality. *Bone, 49*(3), 553–558.

Kobziff, L. (2006). Traumatic pelvic fractures. *Orthopaedic Nursing, 25*(4), 235–241. **www.nursingcenter.com/lnc/JournalArticle?Article_ID=659634&Journal_ID=403341&Issue_ID=659629&expiredce=1**

Maqbali, M. A. (2014). History and physical examination of hip injuries in elderly adults. *Orthopaedic Nursing, 33*(2), 86–92. **www.nursingcenter.com/lnc/CEArticle?an=00006416-201403000-00005&Journal_ID=403341&Issue_ID=2413893**

National Hospital Discharge Survey (NHDS). National Center for Health Statistics. (2010). **www.cdc.gov/nchs/data/databriefs/db182.htm**

Walker, J. (2011). Pelvic fractures: Classification and nursing management. *Nursing Standard, 26*(10), 49–57. **rcnpublishing.com/doi/pdfplus/10.7748/ns2011.11.26.10.49.c8816**

Clinical Practice Guidelines

Bhandari, M., et al. (2012). *Evidence-Based Orthopedics, First Edition.* **sgh.org.sa/Portals/0/Articles/Evidence-based%20Orthopedics.pdf**

National Institute for Health and Clinical Excellence. (2011). *Hip fracture: The management of hip fracture in adults.* CG124. London: NICE. **www.nice.org.uk/guidance/cg124/chapter/introduction**

Mak, J., Cameron, I. D., & March, L. M. (2010). Evidence-based guidelines for the management of hip fractures in older persons: An update. *The Medical Journal of Australia, 192*(1), 37–41. **www.mja.com.au/journal/2010/192/1/evidence-based-guidelines-management-hip-fractures-older-persons-update**

Patient Education

American Academy of Orthopaedic Surgeons. (2011). *Sports injury prevention for baby boomers.* **orthoinfo.org/topic.cfm?topic=A00178**

Cedars-Sinai. (2015). *Pelvic fracture.* **www.cedars-sinai.edu/Patients/Health-Conditions/Pelvic-Fracture.aspx**

Foster, K. W. (2015). *Hip fractures in adults.* **www.uptodate.com/contents/hip-fractures-in-adults**

Mechem, C. C. (2013). *Pelvic fracture in emergency medicine.* **emedicine.medscape.com/article/824856-overview**

University of Chicago Medicine. (2015). *Hip fracture.* **http://www.uchospitals.edu/specialties/orthopaedic-surgery/fractures/**

STOP

Go to the online course and complete the NovE-Cases assigned by your instructor for this module.

Learning Outcomes for Traumatic Brain Injury

When you complete this lesson, you will be able to:

1. Recognize the clinical relevance of traumatic brain injury.
2. Consider the pathophysiology, etiology, risk factors, and clinical presentation of traumatic brain injury that determine the priority patient concerns.
3. Determine the most urgent and important nursing interventions and patient education required in caring for a patient with traumatic brain injury.
4. Evaluate attainment of desired collaborative care outcomes for a patient with traumatic brain injury.

LO1:

What Is Traumatic Brain Injury?

- A traumatic brain injury (TBI) occurs when an individual sustains injury to the cranium or its contents.
- TBI occurs following motor vehicle accidents (MVA), falls, sports injuries, assaults, blast injuries, and other causes.
- The specific mechanisms that produce TBI include blunt (MVA or fall), penetrating (gun or knife), and blast (explosive devices).
- TBI is classified in a number of ways. It is defined in terms of primary and secondary injury as well as mild, moderate, or severe.

Traumatic Brain Injury from a Blast Wound and Shrapnel

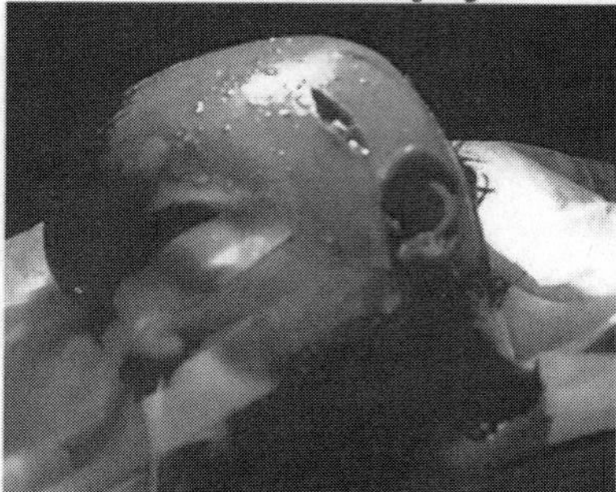

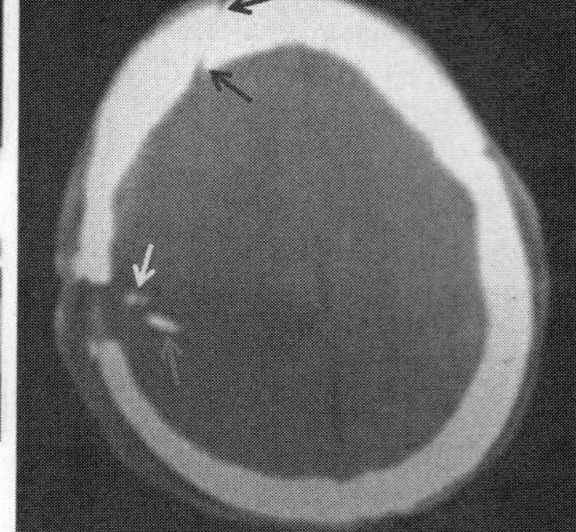

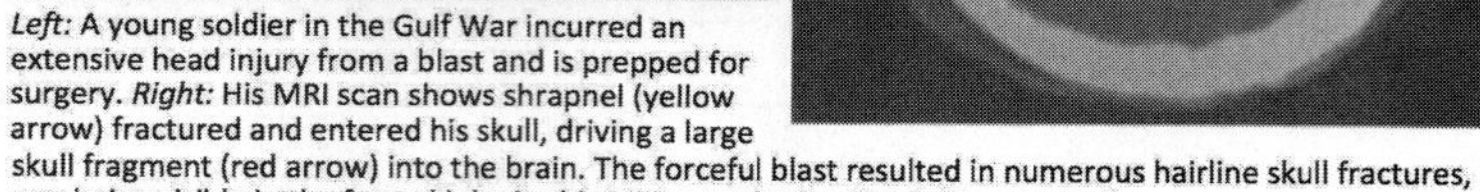

Left: **A young soldier in the Gulf War incurred an extensive head injury from a blast and is prepped for surgery.** ***Right:*** **His MRI scan shows shrapnel (yellow arrow) fractured and entered his skull, driving a large skull fragment (red arrow) into the brain. The forceful blast resulted in numerous hairline skull fractures, one being visible in the frontal lobe in this MRI over the forehead (blue arrows).**

Source: Courtesy of William Stoddard/Fairbanks, AK

- Concussions are also known as mild traumatic brain injuries that have a rapid onset but short duration.
- The nature of a concussion or mild TBI is more of a functional disturbance rather than a structural injury.

LO1:

Clinical Relevance

- There are 52,000 deaths and over 1,600,000 individuals treated in hospitals annually due to TBI (Centers for Disease Control and Prevention).
- Highest risk ages are birth to age 24.
- There were 45,000 military patients diagnosed with TBI between 2003 and 2007.
- Survivors of TBI usually face significant disabilities and complications that require ongoing medical care and rehabilitation.
- Patients over the age of 75 have the highest rate of TBI-related hospitalizations and death. Falls are the leading cause of TBI in this age group and often could have been prevented.
- Concussions account for approximately 80–90% of 1.4 million TBI patients' emergency visits, deaths, and hospitalizations yearly in the United States. Most of the 1.6–3.8 million TBIs occurring in sports and recreation are not treated in emergency rooms or hospitals.
- The economic impact is estimated at $60.4 billion in medical costs and lost productivity.

Head Injury from Impact

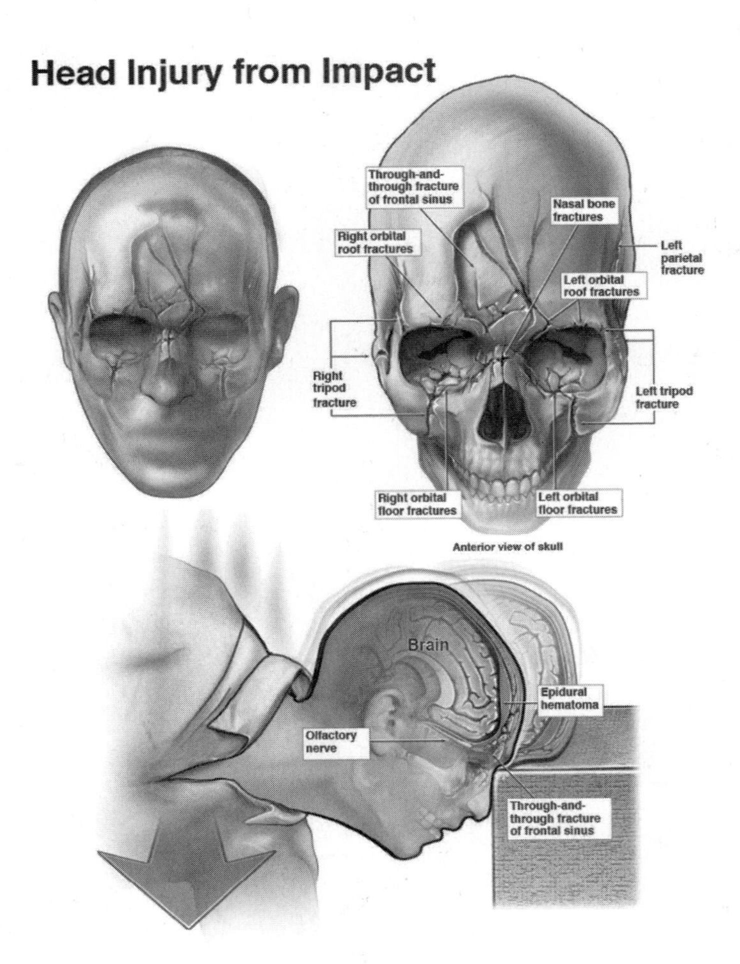

LO1:

Classification of TBI

Primary Brain Injury

- A primary brain injury occurs at the time of the traumatic event. It can result in:
  - o A fractured skull
  - o Torn blood vessels, sinuses, or dura
  - o Cranial nerve injuries
  - o Cellular changes due to the chemical response of the traumatic event
- Cerebral hypoperfusion or decreased blood flow to the brain typically occurs within the first 24 hours and is known as the hypoperfusion stage or phase 1.
- The primary injury can also produce direct injury to the brain.

Primary Brain Injury

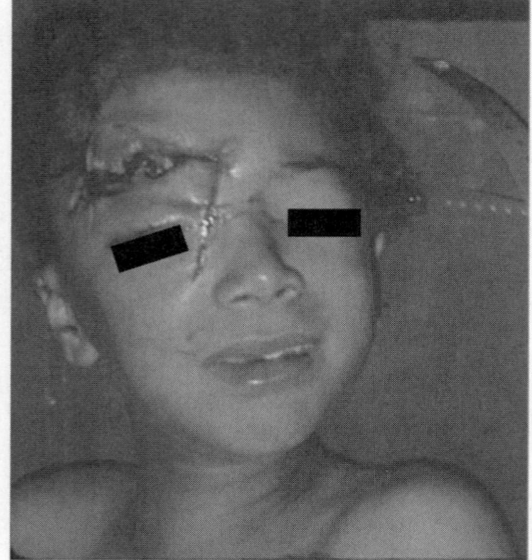

This child suffered an accidental primary brain injury with nasal, forehead (skull), and periorbital fractures. Depression of the skull complicated the injury and recovery.

Source: Courtesy of William Stoddard/Fairbanks, AK

Concept Check

1. What is the leading cause of TBI in patients over the age of 75?
   A. MVA
   B. Penetrating trauma
   C. Violence
   D. Falls

Answer question

Secondary Brain Injury

- Secondary injury to the brain is comprised of events that occur after the primary event that put the brain at risk for further injury.
- Causes of secondary injury include:
  - Hypotension
  - Hypoxia
  - Hyperthermia
  - Hypocapnia
  - Hypercapnia
  - Anemia

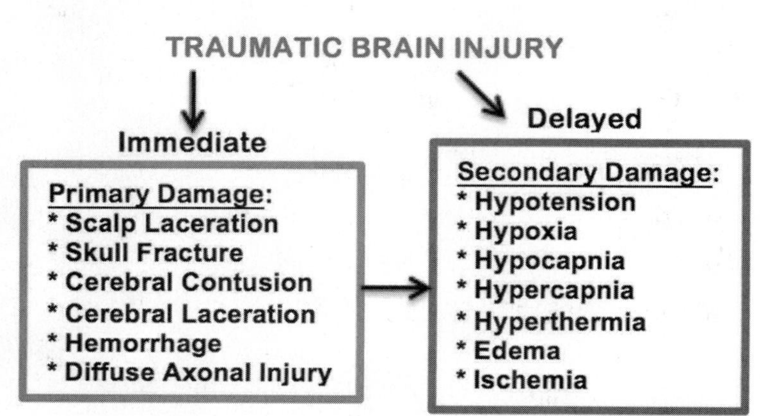

Source: Copyright © 2014, NovEx Novice to Expert Learning, LLC

- Changes in cerebral blood flow (CBF) to the brain during the first few weeks after the injury is another major cause of secondary brain cell injury.
- Phase 2 reflects cerebral hemodynamic changes that occur during the first three days following the brain injury:
  - From 24 hours up to 3–4 days, the brain is hyperemic, receiving more blood flow than required. Thus, phase 2 is called the hyperemic phase.
  - This excessive blood flow can lead to swelling and increased intracranial pressure (ICP), resulting in secondary injury to brain cells.
- Phase 3 occurs late in the first week and into the second week after TBI and results in lower CBF:
  - Vasospasm commonly occurs, so phase 3 is often referred to as the vasospasm phase.
  - Vasospasm can reduce cerebral blood flow and an increased risk for cerebral ischemia and further secondary cell injury or death.
- Primary and secondary injury can lead to cerebral edema, hemorrhages, and increased ICP. Left unchecked, the expanding contents in the cranial vault can lead to cerebral herniation and brain death. Medical personnel must be aware of the primary and secondary events and initiate steps to minimize their occurrence.

Secondary Brain Injury from Carotid Artery Hemorrhage

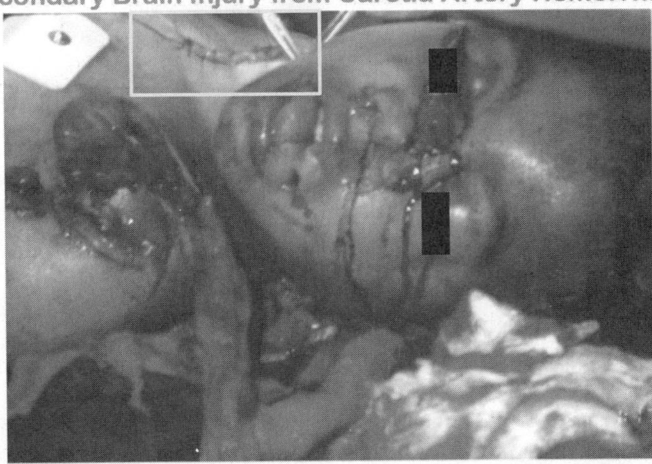

This young patient sustained a fatal brain injury secondary to hypoxia from carotid artery hemorrhage (yellow box). Despite successful surgery, she did not survive the prolonged hypoxia with consequent cerebral edema.

Source: Courtesy of William Stoddard/Fairbanks, AK

LO2:

Pathophysiology

Primary Brain Injuries

- The cranium's function is to protect the fragile brain. Trauma can result in fracture of the skull bones (see diagrams). Fractures can be linear or depressed, or occur in the bones at the base of the skull, known as basilar skull fractures.
- A linear fracture occurring in the temporal bone can lead to an epidural hematoma due to the location of the middle meningeal artery on the inside of the skull bones.
- Depressed skull fractures occur when the bone is broken and pushed inward, compressing and possibly bruising the brain. Depressed skull fractures require surgical intervention to lift the bone back into normal alignment.
- Basilar skull fractures occur in the base of the skull. If the anterior base is fractured, the patient can have bruising around the eyes with "raccoon eyes" type of appearance. Cerebrospinal fluid (CSF) may drain from the nose with associated loss of smell. A simple but positive test for glucose in the drainage strongly suggests CSF rather than nasal secretions. If the middle base is fractured, the patient can have fluid behind the tympanic membrane or leaking from the ear canal. If the posterior base of the skull is fractured, the patient may develop bruising behind the ear over the mastoid process.

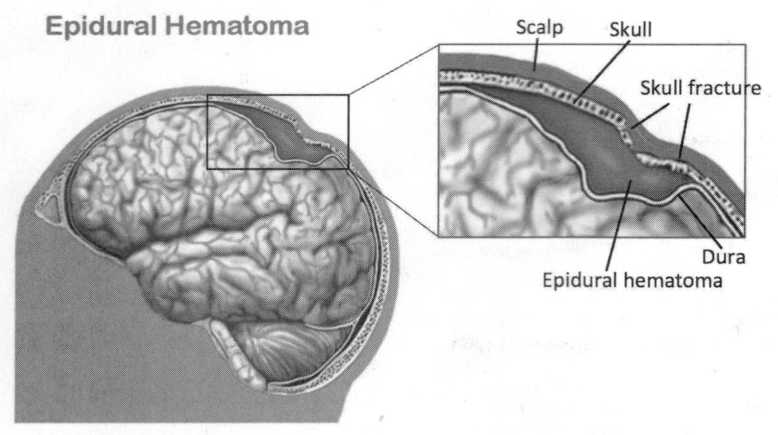

This illustrates a skull fracture resulting in an epidural hematoma. The bleeding within the cranial cavity places pressure on the frontal and parietal regions of the brain.
Source: Courtesy of George Kyriakidis/Santa Ana, CA

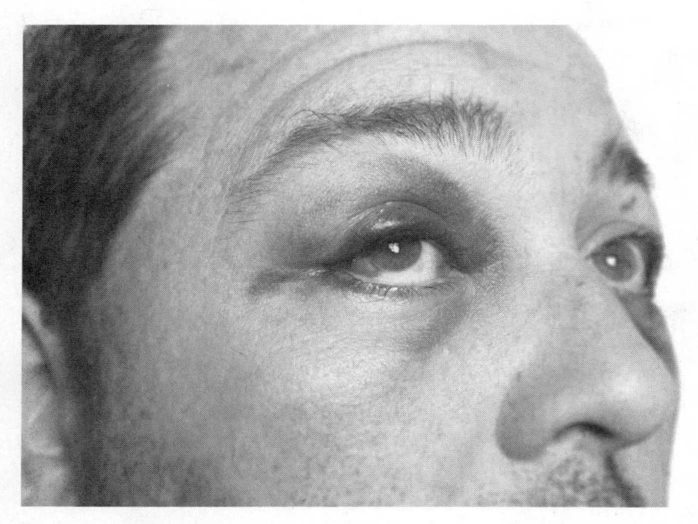

Basilar skull fracture with classic periorbital ecchymosis ("raccoon eyes"). Periorbital ecchymosis results from bleeding after a fracture in the anterior portion of the skull base. This finding may also be caused by facial fractures.
Source: tlorna/Fotolia

- If blood vessels or venous sinuses are broken in the cranium, the patient experiences bleeding inside the skull.
    - **Epidural hematomas** (see CT scan) occur when an artery on the outer surface of the dura is lacerated, causing arterial blood to rapidly accumulate in the space.

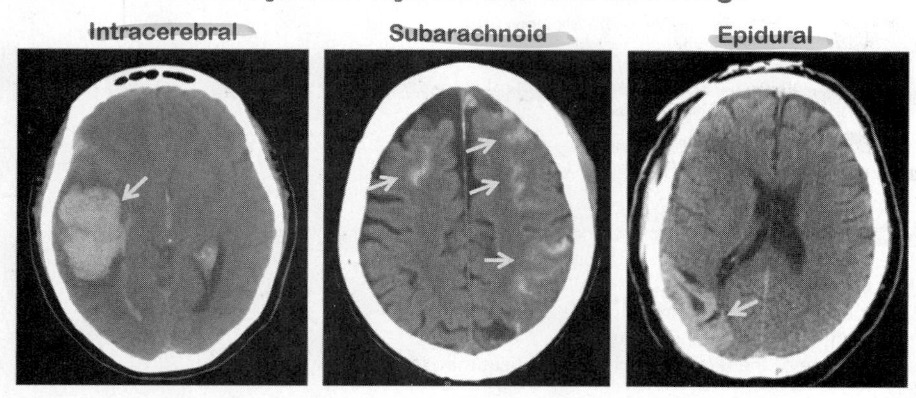

These CT scans show (left to right) a large intracerebral hemorrhage, diffuse subarachnoid hemorrhages, and a large epidural hematoma.
Source: Courtesy of K. Kyriadkis

- **Subdural hematomas** occur when bridging cortical veins that drain blood from the skull/meninges and brain break causing blood to accumulate in the space underneath the dura. Subdural hematomas can be acute, subacute, or chronic, meaning that the injury may manifest at the time of injury or may not present until days to weeks after the injury.
- **Intracerebral hematomas** result from bleeding within the brain tissue itself.
- **Subarachnoid hemorrhage** can occur following a traumatic event when small tears produce bleeding into the subarachnoid space.

- The brain and its coverings can be torn with trauma, which is known as shear injury. When the brain is injured, the injury produced is further classified as:
  - Focal: localized to one area
  - Diffuse: occurring over the entire brain

Concept Check

2. **Which term indicates that bleeding is occurring between the dura and the cranium?**

A. Epidural

B. Subdural

C. Intracerebral

D. Subarachnoid

Answer question

Pathophysiology (continued)

Diffuse Brain Injuries

- Diffuse brain injuries are the result of forces that stretch or shear the axons of the brain (white matter).
- The injury produced can be mild to severe and is often graded on a continuum. On the mild side of diffuse injury, where the axons are merely stretched, is cerebral concussion.

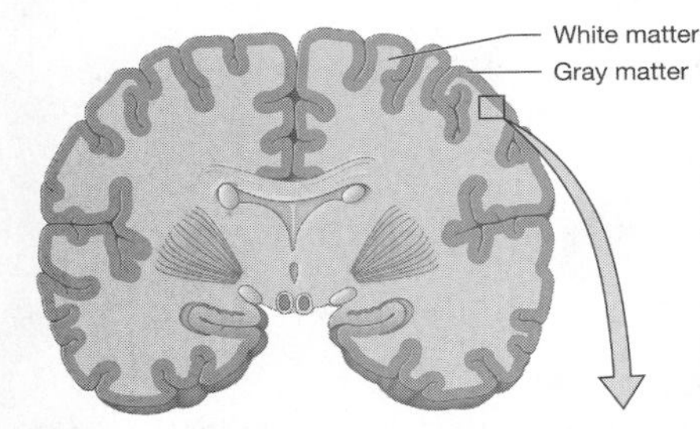

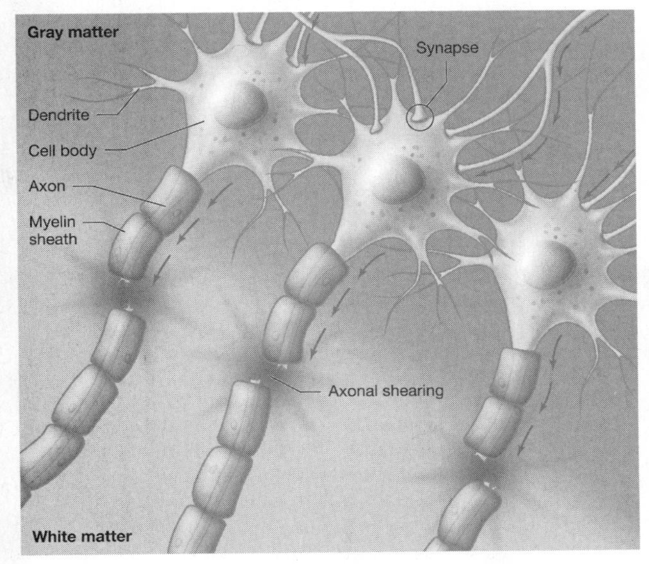

Diffuse axonal injury is depicted as shearing of the axons following an acceleration-deceleration injury. The lower picture shows how the axons are severed, at the junction of the white and gray matter, followed by death of the neurons.

- Defined as a loss of consciousness for less than 30 minutes, concussion causes patients to present with amnesia to the event that usually clears within 24 hours.
- Concussion patients in the acute phase rarely exhibit a motor or sensory deficit (inability to move or feel an arm or leg). Most TBIs are concussions. Specific interventions and care are presented later in this lesson.
- There are two types of concussions:
  - o Simple concussions gradually resolve within 7–10 days without neurologic complications.
  - o Complex concussions are recognized by symptoms that continue beyond 10 days and reappear with activity. Symptoms can include seizures, headache, confusion, altered level of consciousness, and cognitive impairment.
- Post-concussion syndrome may arise if the patient experiences headache, dizziness, problems with vision or hearing, insomnia, alcohol intolerance, irritability, and other minor symptoms (e.g., memory or concentration deficits) in less than 4 weeks post-concussion.
- Second impact syndrome is a condition that the patient can suffer if an athlete, for instance, already sustained a head injury (e.g., concussion) and incurs a second head injury. This second injury can prove devastating with diffuse cerebral edema that can cause headache, decreased consciousness, memory deficits, and confusion. Brain herniation and death can quickly follow. For this reason, patients are not released to play sports again without a physician determining the appropriate time period following evaluation.
- Diffuse axonal injury (DAI) is in the severe spectrum of diffuse injury, where the axons are sheared or severed. These patients present in coma and require full body systems support. Some DAI patients never wake up after injury.

Coup-Contrecoup

- An impact or blow to the skull can cause focal injury to the area of the brain that underlies the point of impact and can also produce injury to the opposite side of the brain (coup-contrecoup). The brain can be contused or bruised.
- The inferior and frontal/temporal lobes of the cerebral hemispheres are vulnerable to bruising due to their proximity to the base of the skull.
- When the brain becomes bruised, it can lead to further swelling. If the brain is contused in many areas, generalized cerebral swelling occurs, resulting in an increase in ICP.
- The 10 pairs of cranial nerves that originate in the brainstem/cerebellum area of the cranial vault can be damaged in the trauma. Injury or compression in this area can lead to multiple cranial nerve dysfunction.

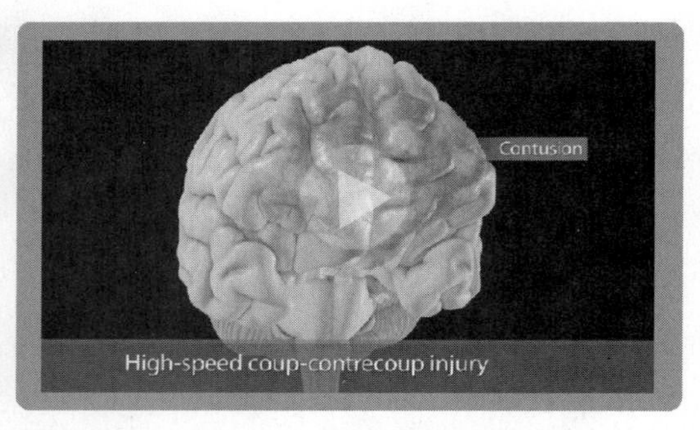

This animation depicts a closed head coup and contrecoup (or whiplash) injury resulting in TBI.

LO2: Risk Factors

- Males have a higher risk of hospitalization and three times higher risk of death from TBI as women.
- Older adults (age 65 or older)
- Young children (ages 0–14)

LO2:

Causes

Causes may vary and can result in a different severity of injury, but all result from a traumatic injury (e.g., blow, jolt, spinning, blast, penetration) to the head. The severity of injury is determined by factors such as the mechanism of injury, the nature of the impact, and its force.

- Falls, which account for about 40% of TBI injuries, especially in young children (ages 0–14) and older adults (age 65 or older)
- Blunt trauma injury is the second leading cause, predominantly in children when unintentionally being hit by an object.
- Contact sports, particularly boxing, football, soccer, baseball, basketball, lacrosse, hockey, or other high-impact sports
- Vehicle accidents that involve motorcycles, bikes, skateboards, cars, boats, and pedestrians are the third major cause of TBI.
- Assaults and violence account for approximately 20% of TBIs. Violence can include gunshot wounds, child abuse including shaking, penetrating wounds, and domestic abuse.
- Combat injuries from explosive blasts, shrapnel, or collision with objects due to a blast

LO2:

Assessment Findings

Assessment findings vary, depending on the severity of injury.

Mild TBI or Concussion

- Confusion, disorientation, amnesia, or dazed without loss of consciousness
- Loss of consciousness lasting a few seconds to minutes
- Headache
- Dizziness or imbalance
- Visual (blurred vision, diplopia), auditory (hard of hearing), or other sensory disturbances with taste, light, or smell
- Increased sleeping or drowsiness
- Insomnia
- Fatigue
- Nausea and/or vomiting
- Anxiety, mood disturbances, emotional lability, or depression
- Changes in memory, personality, or concentration
- Blank expression or dulled affect

Moderate-to-Severe TBI

- Loss of consciousness lasting minutes to hours. May be comatose.
- Seizures or convulsions
- Persistent and/or escalating headache
- Repeated episodes of nausea and vomiting
- Changes in pupil size in one or both eyes
- Inability to wake
- CSF drainage from ears or nose
- Loss of coordination or imbalance
- Numbness or weakness in digits
- Severe confusion or disorientation
- Agitation or combative behavior
- Slurring of speech

LO2:

Diagnostics

- Critical information includes:
  - Mechanism of injury
  - Condition of vehicle, bike, or helmet (if involved)
  - Glasgow Coma Scale (GCS) at the scene of the accident
  - Subsequent vital signs
  - Neurologic status
  - Interventions provided at the scene

Feature	Scale (responses)	Score
Eye opening	Spontaneous	4
	To verbal stimuli	3
	To pain	2
	No response	1
Verbal response	Oriented	5
	Confused	4
	Inappropriate words	3
	Incomprehensible speech	2
	No response	1
Best motor response	Obeys commands	6
	Moves to localized pain	5
	Flexion withdrawal from pain (normal)	4
	Abnormal flexion (decorticate)	3
	Abnormal extension (decerebrate)	2
	No response	1
Total Coma Score		3/15 – 15/15

Glasgow Coma Scale.

- A good history helps to establish a diagnosis and guides the team on priorities of care.
- Radiographic evaluation
  - o CT scan of the brain helps to determine the severity of the injury, mechanism of injury, and rule out potential bleeding.
  - o MRI may be informative in patients whose symptoms persist over 7 days.
- History and physical examination, combined with imaging studies, provide the diagnosis, as done with other neurologic disorders.
- Neuropsychological testing may be performed more commonly in professional sports, in cases of complex concussions, and in moderate-to-severe patients post-TBI.

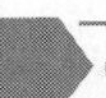

Concept Check

3. A patient who hit his forehead has both a frontal lobe and an occipital lobe contusion. What term is used to describe the occipital lobe injury?

A. Coup

B. Axonal

C. Shearing

D. Contrecoup

Answer question

Priority Patient Concerns and Desired Collaborative Care Outcomes

Prior to caring for patients with TBI, it is important to prioritize the patient's concerns that must guide the nursing care plan and interventions. Care for the patient is ordered and organized in accordance with the patient's priority and urgent needs. Desired collaborative care outcomes in patients with TBI typically include:

1. Patient will experience no hypoxia from decreased drive to breath.
2. Patient will return to pre-illness level of consciousness and alertness.
3. Patient, as much as possible, and family will express understanding of treatments and expected recovery.
4. Patient will maintain cerebral perfusion pressure (CPP) within desired range.
5. Patient's ICP will remain within desired range.

Considering these important care outcomes, prepare a list of the major 3–6 priority patient concerns or nursing diagnoses for patients with TBI. Be prepared to participate in a discussion of this list and/or to submit them as an assignment, as determined by your faculty. Resources you may find helpful in this assignment can include this lesson, the references, resources on nursing care plans, and standard nursing diagnoses manuals.

LO3:

Collaborative Interventions

The priorities in caring for patients with TBI are to completely and rapidly resuscitate the patient and to lessen the risk of secondary injury.

M N EBP
- Simultaneously assess airway, breathing, circulation and quantify the GCS. Stratification of level of injury and interventions are then triaged, which means that interventions are determined based on urgency of patient need (Badjatia, et al., 2007; Colorado Division of Workers' Compensation [CDWC], 2012).

M N EBP
- Obtain a history if the patient is alert. It is helpful to obtain an additional account of the history from a witness who can describe the circumstances if an incident occurred. Pay particular attention to information about the mechanism of injury, patient's level of consciousness at the scene, and period and duration of amnesia, when applicable (Vos, et al., 2012). History should include current medications, particularly aspirin, anticoagulants, antiplatelets, or any medication that increases the risk of bleeding or hemorrhage.

M N EBP
- Complete an urgent physical, neurologic, and surgical examination, when indicated (Vos, et al., 2012).

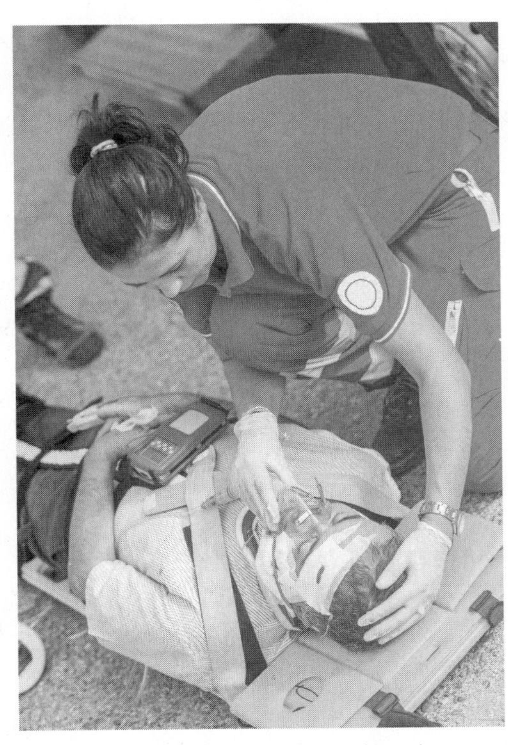

Patient with cervical spine collar on a backboard.
Source: william87/Fotolia

M N
- In patients with mild TBI, the neurologic exam should minimally include GCS, pupil size and reaction to light, and short-term memory.

M N EBP
- If hospitalized for mild to moderate TBI, initially check the patient every 30 minutes if the GCS is <15. If GCS is ≥ 15, check every 30 minutes for 2 hours, then every hour for 4 hours, and every 2 hours thereafter, if no abnormal findings arise (Vos, et al., 2012).

M N
- In the ED, continue spinal precautions that the prehospital care providers instituted (cervical spine collar and backboard).

M N EBP
- Hypoxia should be immediately addressed and corrected. Treat hypoxemia immediately to keep $SpO_2 > 92\%$ (Badjatia, et al., 2007). Cerebral oxygen saturation may be monitored along with ICP monitoring to assess cerebral oxygen delivery and guide treatment of increased ICP (American Association of Neuroscience Nurses [AANN], 2008; CDWC, 2012).

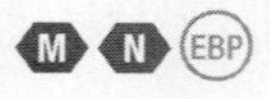

- Use endotracheal intubation if needed to maintain an adequate airway. Maintain normal $ETCO_2$ (End Tidal CO_2) between 35–40 mmHg to avoid hyperventilation, cerebral edema, and cerebral herniation (Badjatia, et al., 2007).

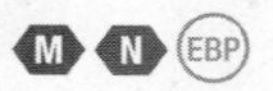

- Hypotension should be treated with volume resuscitation (normal saline) to establish adequate cerebral perfusion pressure (CPP >60 mmHg). Norepinephrine is suggested if a vasopressor is additionally needed (AANN, 2008; Badjatia, et al., 2007; CDWC, 2012).

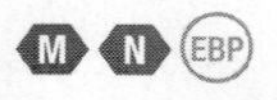

- Administer hyperosmolar medication (e.g., mannitol, hypertonic saline) if the patient's neurologic status deteriorates without hypotension or there are manifestations of transtentorial herniation (AANN, 2008; CDWC, 2012). Closely observe patient for possible pulmonary edema if hypertonic saline is administered, particularly in older or heart failure patients.

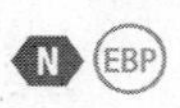

- Continuous monitoring for signs of low CPP or increased ICP (headache, somnolence, double vision, unequal pupils) is vital, and measurement of ICP is often performed for severe TBI (AANN, 2008; CDWC, 2012).

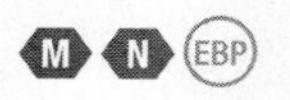

- Antiseizure (or anticonvulsant) medications are commonly provided early post-TBI to reduce risk of seizure. These anticonvulsants are often given for 1 week in patients with an intracerebral hemorrhage. Prevention of seizures can reduce complications due to seizures (AANN, 2008; CDWC, 2012).

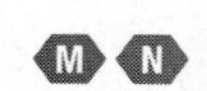

- Transport to the operating room may be required for evacuation of hematoma, as indicated, or for other injuries that are life-threatening.

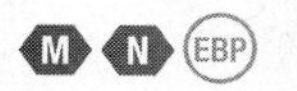

- If neurosurgical support is needed and not available, stabilize the patient and then transport expeditiously to a designated neurotrauma center (CDWC, 2012).

Collaborative Interventions (continued)

Minor, Moderate, and Severe Categories of TBI

TBI is categorized in terms of loss of consciousness (LOC), post-traumatic amnesia (PTA), and GCS on admission to the hospital.

Categories of Traumatic Brain Injuries

Category	Loss of Consciousness	Post-Traumatic Amnesia	Glasgow Coma Scale
Minor TBI	< 30 minutes	< 24 hours	13-15
Moderate TBI	30 min. to 24 hours	> 24 hours but < 7 days	9-12
Severe TBI	> 7 days	> 7 days	3-8

- Management of patients with severe TBI is complex. Each patient's individual needs are based on the severity of injury, presence of increased ICP, other organ/system involvement, functional neurologic assessment, age, presence of comorbidities, and overall premorbid health status.
- National consensus guidelines have been developed for minor TBI (i.e., American Academy of Neurology Guidelines for minor TBI) and severe TBI (i.e., Brain Trauma Foundation "Guidelines for Managing Severe TBI"). These guidelines serve as a basis for hospitals and practitioners to build hospital-based evidence relating to clinical guidelines and protocols for TBI.

Concept Check

4. What cerebral perfusion pressure is considered the minimum to be adequate?

A. 45 mmHg

B. 60 mmHg

C. 80 mmHg

D. 120 mmHg

Answer question

Collaborative Interventions (continued)

Minor TBI (GCS 13–15)

The patient with a minor TBI or concussion may or may not be admitted to the hospital (Vos, et al., 2012). Care of the patient commonly includes:

M N EBP
- Perform a neurologic exam. Patients with a normal neurologic exam, no substance involvement, no injuries or CSF leak, and/or a normal CT scan are commonly discharged to home (Vos, et al., 2012).

M N
- Administer acetaminophen to patients complaining of headache. When stable, prepare the patient for discharge. A cognitive screen is generally done prior to discharge to serve as a baseline.

N EBP
- Perform fall assessment and instruct the patient and family about fall precautions if warranted (Thompson & Mauk, 2011).

N
- If a seizure was associated with the injury, educate the patient and family about seizure precautions.

M N EBP
- Whether the patient is discharged home from the ED or admitted to the inpatient unit, provide discharge instructions to the patient and family to monitor the patient neurologically every 2–3 hours for the next 24 hours, even during night. Instruct them to ask simple questions to evaluate orientation (e.g., what is your name, what day is it, or where are you). Instruct the family to evaluate if the patient is acting appropriately. The patient should not drive for 24 hours (Thompson & Mauk, 2011; Vos, et al., 2012).

N EBP
- Give specific instructions to the patient and family for return to the hospital if the patient has any decline in neurologic status, worsening headache, seizures, confusion, incontinence, drowsiness and cannot be awakened, has repeated vomiting, exhibits irritable behavior, has unsteady gait, or has any unusual fluid (CSF) visibly leaking from the nose or ears (Thompson & Mauk, 2011; Vos, et al., 2012).

N EBP
- Tell the patient that sleep requirements are increased following concussion and that limiting stress is important (CDWC, 2012; Thompson & Mauk, 2011).

M N EBP
- Instruct the patient that return to work or school must be gradual in order to avoid undue cognitive or physical stress (Thompson & Mauk, 2011).

M N EBP
- Instruct the patient about the importance of avoiding alcohol, tobacco, and caffeine for a period of time after concussion (Thompson & Mauk, 2011).

M N EBP
- Instruct the patient to avoid contact sports for at least 1–2 weeks. Physician may follow the American Academy of Neurology guidelines to manage sports-related concussion. They are based on consensus opinion but there are no evidence-based guidelines at the current time (Bey & Ostick, 2009). Return to play is recommended only after assessment by health care professional is satisfactory (Thompson & Mauk, 2011).

M N EBP
- The patient should follow up with a health care provider who is familiar and experienced with minor head injury in order to receive the best guidance on resumption of normal activities. If the individual should experience signs or symptoms related to dysfunction that is cognitive, psychological, or physical, occurring even months after their injury, they should seek care with a physician specializing in TBI (CDWC, 2012; Vos, et al., 2012).
- Patients admitted to a medical–surgical unit typically have minor TBIs. Depending on the severity and type of injury, care can include:
  - M N — Care of any physical injuries
  - N EBP — Close neurological observation for any changes, particularly the patient's level of consciousness or post-concussion symptoms. Collaborate immediately with the health care provider if new or worsening symptoms evolve (CDWC, 2012).
  - M N EBP — Care and emotional comfort of the patient and family (CDWC, 2012) may, for example, involve fear of potential serious injury, inability to return to play, or restrictions that impact life demands.
  - N — Recruit counseling, pastoral, and/or social services in accordance with patient preferences.
  - M N EBP — Educate family about possible mood and memory changes (e.g., irritability) due to the TBI and on expected recovery, as determined by the type and severity of injury (CDWC, 2012).
  - M N EBP — Early mobilization when feasible helps prevent "never events" (CDWC, 2012).
  - N — Learn about the patient as a person prior to injury to assist in making good judgments about the evolving condition. TBI can cause a wide variety of alterations or impairments in the patient's emotional, physical, intellectual, and behavioral function. Early recognition is key to intervention.

Moderate TBI (GCS 9–12)

Patients presenting with a GCS of 9–12 fall into a category known as moderate head injury.

- This category is especially difficult to manage because there are no national consensus treatment guidelines for moderate TBI as there are in mild and severe TBI. Patients are generally not critical enough to require mechanical ventilation and aggressive blood pressure support.
- Provide close observation and monitoring of the neurologic status in moderate TBI patients who are usually admitted to the ICU. Patients at risk for deterioration include older adults and patients taking anticoagulants or platelet inhibitors. Due to the increased risk of bleeding, anticipate serial imaging with CT scans of the brain to monitor progression of the injury.
- Treat headache with acetaminophen as prescribed. The patient is usually given nothing to eat for a short period of time and then the diet is advanced slowly.
- Initiate DVT prophylaxis in these patients (AANN, 2008).
- Once stable, the patient is transferred to a medical–surgical unit for further monitoring and consultations with physical, occupational and speech therapists to determine if any functional deficits exist and whether recommendations for therapy are needed.

Collaborative Interventions (continued)

Severe TBI (GCS <9)

If the patient presents with a GCS of 3–8, the injury is considered severe. Continue care following initial lifesaving interventions:

- Immediately secure the airway with an endotracheal tube because the patient is not awake enough to protect the airway and clear secretions. Ensure the use of humidification.
- Continuously monitor vital signs, heart rhythm, SpO_2, and $ETCO_2$ if possible and as long as the patient is unstable or in critical condition. Treat hypoxia if PaO_2 <60 mmHg and/or SpO_2 <90% (Brain Trauma Foundation [BTF], 2007).
- Maintain hemodynamic stability, particularly systolic blood pressure (BP) ≥90 mmHg (AANN, 2008; BTF, 2007):
    - o Infuse fluids and/or vasopressor agents to achieve a cerebral perfusion pressure (CPP) between 50–70 mmHg. CPP equals mean arterial BP minus ICP. Avoid falling outside these parameters.
    - o Avoid aggressive interventions to maintain a CPP >70 mmHg due to the risk of pulmonary edema and adult respiratory distress syndrome.
    - o Norepinephrine is a preferred vasoactive medication.
    - o Avoid systemic hypotension, which compromises all body organs, including the brain.
- Secure IV access if not already done by EMT and administer fluids as prescribed.
- Anticipate and prepare for a CT scan within 15–30 minutes to evaluate the brain and skull radiographically. Other radiographic studies can be done to investigate other suspected injuries. Depending on the extent of brain injury, the neurosurgeon may perform a craniotomy for removal of blood clots, a craniectomy (temporary removal of a skull flap), and/or the insertion of an ICP monitor (Vos, et al., 2012).
- Continuous ICP and CPP monitoring is indicated for all patients with a GCS between 3–8 post-resuscitation, systolic blood pressure <90 mmHg, and/or radiographic evidence of injury (e.g., hematoma, edema, contusion, herniation, compression of basal cisterns) to inform collaborative interventions. ICP monitoring is also indicated in patients over age 40 and those with motor posturing. Following resuscitation and/or surgery, the severe TBI patient is admitted to the ICU (AANN, 2008; BTF, 2007; CDWC, 2012).
- Consider ventricular catheter or parenchymal ICP use over subdural, epidural, or subarachnoid monitors. The former are low cost and reliable. The latter tend to be less accurate (BTF, 2007).
- Maintain the ICP <20 mmHg unless the situation warrants a change in parameters. Clinical and CT scan data are used to substantiate the need for intervention (AANN, 2008; BTF, 2007):

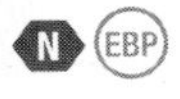

- o Raise the head of the bed to 30 degrees to reduce ICP and/or increase CPP (AANN, 2008).

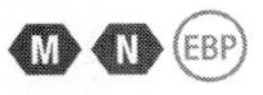

- o Do not use hyperventilation methods to reduce the ICP (AANN, 2008; BTF, 2007; CDWC, 2012).

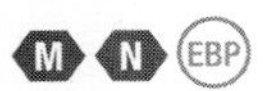

- o In accordance with hospital procedure, drain CSF to lower the ICP below 20 mmHg or parameters set by neurosurgeon and to raise CPP (AANN, 2008).

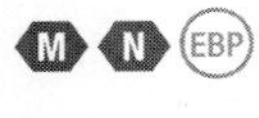

- o Administer sedation or analgesia, which can help prevent increased ICP (AANN, 2008). Propofol is the recommended sedative to control ICP in critically ill patients due to its rapid action, its short half-life, and the ability to provide windows without sedation for accurate neurologic assessment. Use caution with propofol as the drug can cause hypotension (BTF, 2007).

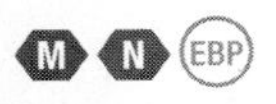

- o Administer prescribed mannitol to reduce ICP. Avoid hypotension when administering this medication (AANN, 2008; BFT, 2007).

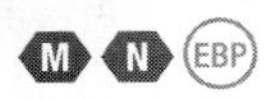

- o As soon as no spinal cord injury is confirmed, collaborate with the health care provider to remove or loosen cervical collar (AANN, 2008).

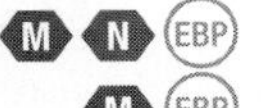

- o Control hyperthermia to prevent increased ICP (AANN, 2008).

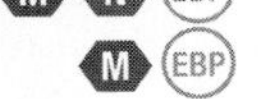

- o Inducing hypothermia is currently controversial but may be used by some health care providers to reduce ICP if intracranial hypertension is refractory (BTF, 2007).

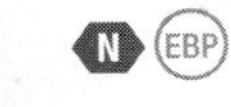

- Continuously monitor and manage hyperthermia which is associated with poor outcomes (CDWC, 2012).

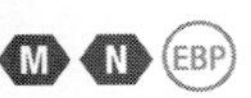

- Administer sedation and analgesia as needed, but attention to reassessment of neurologic status is imperative. Propofol is recommended, except at high doses (BTF, 2007; CDWC, 2012).

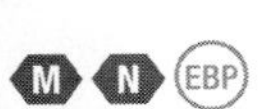

- Administer antiepileptic medications to reduce early, post-TBI seizures (within 7 days). Ensure hemodynamic stability prior to administration of barbiturates. Avoid prophylactic use of barbiturates to induce burst suppression EEG or to prevent late post-TBI seizures (AANN, 2008; BTF, 2007).

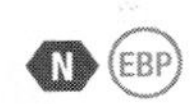

- Provide total nursing care for a patient who is immobile or limited in movement (CDWC, 2012).

Severe TBI Requiring Surgical Evacuation

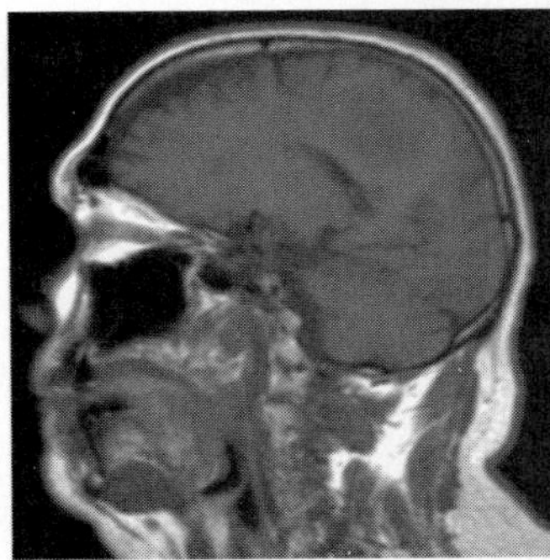

MRI scan shows severe traumatic brain injury requiring surgical evacuation. Large hemorrhagic area is enhanced in red.

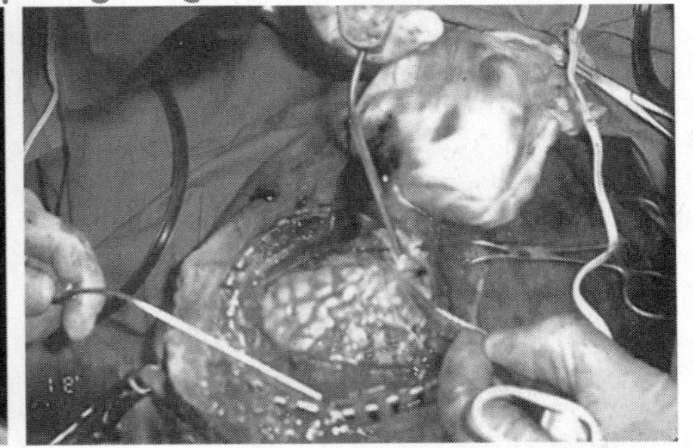

A surgical craniotomy is performed where a flap of the scalp is pulled back and a section of skull is removed to visualize and remove the hemorrhagic area. This quickly reduces pressure on the brain tissue.

Source: Courtesy of K. Kyriakidis & William Stoddard/Fairbanks, AK

Collaborative Interventions (continued)

Severe TBI (GCS <9) (continued)

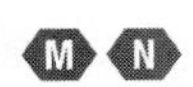

- Anticipate, observe for, and collaborate on autonomic storming, which is a result of sympathetic nervous system overactivity. Fever, diaphoresis, restlessness, hyperventilation, posturing, agitation, and tachycardia may manifest. Fever may falsely be understood as infection, resulting in an extensive and invasive infection work-up with treatment of antibiotics rather than treatment for autonomic storming.

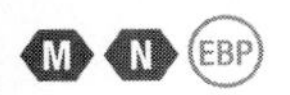

- Collaborate with the health care provider to initiate nutrition within 3 days post-TBI as metabolic demands greatly increase. Enteral or parenteral nutrition may be needed (AANN, 2008). Full caloric replacement should be attained by the seventh post-injury day. Early nutritional support reduces infection rate and overall complications. Patients with posturing and autonomic storming have even higher metabolic demands (BTF, 2007).

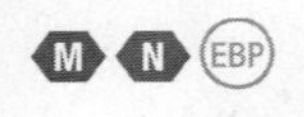

- Administer medications for DVT prophylaxis if the health care provider deems them safe, particularly in mechanically ventilated patients who are at much higher risk for DVT. If not safe due to the increased risk of intracranial bleed, initiate sequential compression devices for DVT prevention. When possible, both mechanical and pharmacologic prophylaxis are recommended (AANN, 2008; BTF, 2007).
- Administer prophylactic antibiotics in intubated patients to reduce the incidence of pneumonia. Consider early tracheostomy, particularly in patients who are expected to be mechanically ventilated for a prolonged time period. Extubate early whenever possible to reduce the risk of infection (BTF, 2007).
- Avoid the use of prophylactic antibiotics in patients with ventricular catheters for ICP monitoring. There is insufficient evidence to support antibiotic use (BTF, 2007).
- Manage and prevent hyperglycemic events by administering IV insulin per hospital protocol. Hyperglycemia aggravates hypoxic or injured brain tissues, expands the ischemic area, and worsens outcomes. Avoid the use of subcutaneous insulin, as it is potentially unsafe (AANN, 2008; BTF, 2007).
- Prevent all "never events" (e.g., pressure ulcers, catheter-related urinary tract infections, central line infection, and ventilator-related pneumonia) when at risk. Collaborate to discontinue all invasive lines as soon as not needed, mobilize as much as feasible, perform range-of-motion exercises, routinely reposition the patient, provide excellent mouth and perineal care, keep skin clean and dry, use vigilance to assure that everyone (including visitors) use excellent hand hygiene.
- Recommend a multidisciplinary team be coordinated to care for patients post-TBI as varied expertise is required to manage the physiological, functional, psychosocial, emotional, nutritional, occupational, educational, financial, and rehabilitation aspects of care. A case manager is often central in coordinating the team and the patient's care across settings and over time (CDWC, 2012).
- Avoid administering glucocorticosteroids as they have not proven useful and are not recommended. High doses are contraindicated and are associated with higher mortality (BTF, 2007; CDWC, 2012).
- Despite the potential physiological benefits of hyperbaric oxygen therapy, it is not recommended at this time and it can cause complications such as tension pneumothorax (CDWC, 2012).
- Once the team successfully controls the ICP and minimizes secondary injury, then medications and interventions are slowly titrated down and withdrawn. The patient is allowed to emerge from coma as much as possible.
- As the patient awakens, transference from ICU to a medical–surgical unit may occur. Assessments by physical therapy (PT), occupation therapy (OT), speech therapy (ST), and a physiatrist (physician of rehabilitation medicine) are done to determine the neurologic deficits caused by the injury and begin rehabilitation (CDWC, 2012). However, many patients may be transferred directly to a rehabilitation facility.
- Care and emotional comfort of the patient and family (CDWC, 2012) may, for example, involve life changes caused by serious injury, unexpected demands on the family, financial ramifications of a chronic injury, fear of death or prolonged coma, loss and grief, and personality changes. Preliminary research showed that agitation decreased in 73% of patients when caregivers engage the patient in individualized activities that align with the patient's abilities and interests (Waszynski, et al., 2013).
- Educate family about possible mood (e.g., aggression, irritability, argumentative), memory (e.g., disorganized, inattention, scattered), and personality (e.g., loss of inhibition, lack of impulse control) changes due to the TBI and on expected recovery, as determined by the type and severity of injury (CDWC, 2012).
- Following stabilization, the team determines discharge needs and proper patient placement for rehab. If the patient can actively participate in rehab 3 hours a day, then the patient may be considered a candidate for an acute rehabilitation unit. If the patient tolerates only 1–2 hours a day of therapy, then placement may be in a subacute rehabilitation unit. If the patient does not recover a participative level of functioning, then consideration for long-term care in a skilled nursing facility is needed (CDWC, 2012).

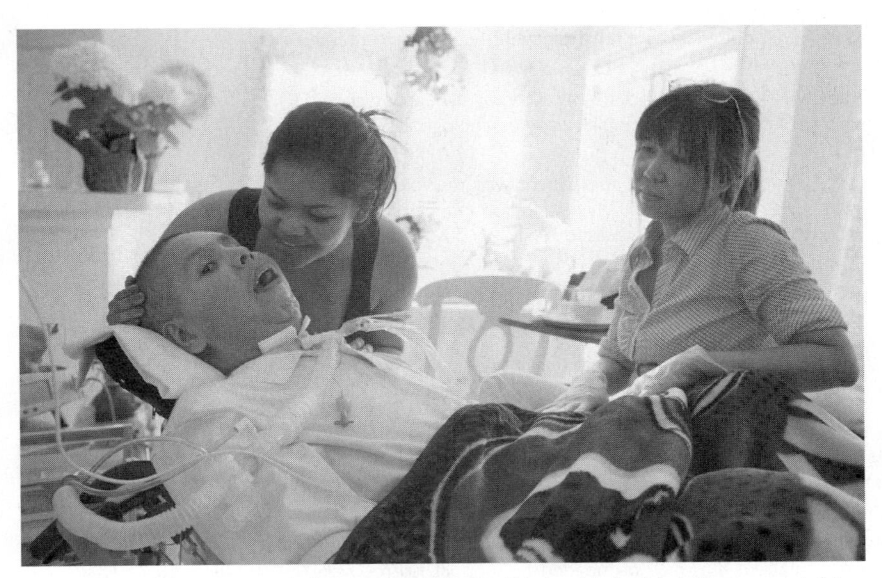

Joseph, 27, was injured when a bullet entered the back of his head in Baghdad. The traumatic injury left him paralyzed, brain-damaged, and blind. Joseph is awake and aware of his situation. Most patients with this severity of injury must be cared for in a skilled nursing facility; however, Joseph's family provides ICU-type care for him in their home, including mechanical ventilation and multiple other life supports. Joseph requires life-long constant care.

Source: Jacquelyn Martí/AP Images

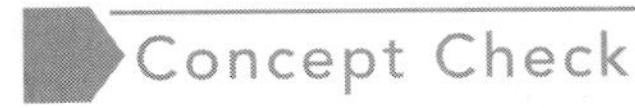

Concept Check

5. **Which findings are manifested during autonomic storming?**
   A. Hypoventilation
   B. Bradycardia
   C. Fever
   D. Somnolence

Answer question

Collaborative Interventions (continued)

TBI Post-ICU and Prior to Transfer to Rehab or Long-Term Care

As patients with moderate-to-severe TBIs recover and no longer need intensive care, even if they need extensive care, they often transfer to a medical–surgical unit while transitioning to rehab or skilled care. Depending on the patient's level of consciousness, care for these patients involves:

- Neurological observation for any changes, particularly the patient's level of consciousness (CDWC, 2012)
- Early, consistent mobilization and preventive measures to prevent "never events." TBI patients are at high risk for most never events (e.g., DVT, pneumonia, infection, falls), along with the hazards of immobility (muscle wasting, footdrop) (CDWC, 2012).
- Ensure nutritional support with airway protection, depending on the patient's ability to take oral nutrition (CDWC, 2012)
- Partial to total care may be needed, depending on the patient's abilities and the family's involvement.
- Care and emotional comfort of the family to learn to care for the patient and cope with unexpected life and role changes, demands, and stresses, such as, the patient's activities of daily living, bodily care, mobility, nutritional intake, personality changes, unemployment, rehabilitation, care of patient's and children, and cognitive and/or communication deficits, to name only a few (CDWC, 2012).
- Collaborate with the health care provider to recruit physical and speech therapy, counseling, social services and/or pastoral care, in accordance with patient's needs and preferences (CDWC, 2012).
- Speak to the patient and explain activities, whether the patient seems responsive or not. Encourage the family to interact with their loved one because hearing commonly remains intact.

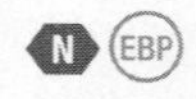

- Assist key family caregivers to learn daily, ongoing care for the patient (e.g., bathing, mouth care, safety, range of motion) (CDWC, 2012).

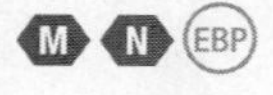

- Connect with behavioral therapy, which commonly includes a psychologist, neuropsychologist, and others to assist with recovery of the multiple cognitive and psychological issues that are expected (CDWC, 2012).

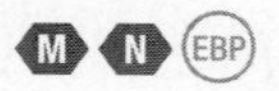

- Consider consulting cognitive rehab therapist to assist the patient with multiple potential deficits (e.g., working memory, impulse control, concentration, inhibition, interpersonal skills, cognitive efficiency) and learn compensatory cognitive skills for deficits (CDWC, 2012).

Patient and Family Support

Mild TBI

- Patients with a mild TBI or concussion require education that may include:

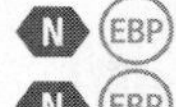

  - o Educate patient and family about fall precautions (Thompson & Mauk, 2011).

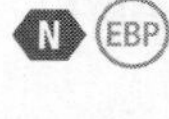

  - o Instruct about avoiding text messaging, activity on social media, video and computer games, and TV to provide cognitive rest. Schoolwork should be limited. Minimize activities that demand close attention or long periods of concentration. Increased cognitive activity delays recovery (Thompson & Mauk, 2011).

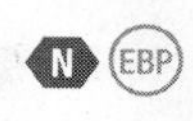

  - o Instruct about alerting teachers, coaches, employers, and others about the concussion incident and the short-term limitations that may be needed to support full recovery (Thompson & Mauk, 2011).

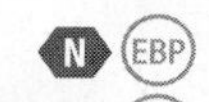

  - o Instruct about getting plenty of rest and sleep (Thompson & Mauk, 2011).

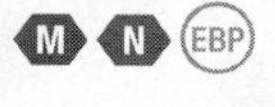

  - o Instruct about using acetaminophen or over-the-counter pain medications for relief of headache if not persistent past 7 days. Avoid frequent or daily use to prevent rebound headaches (Thompson & Mauk, 2011).

  - o Educate about avoiding the use of narcotics, particularly ones not prescribed for the patient, as they are central nervous system depressants and may mask evolving symptoms of more dangerous complications.

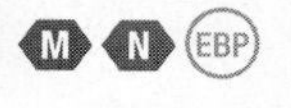

  - o Instruct about the aggregate effects of repeated mild TBI. A dangerous effect is that it can lead to eventual progressive cognitive impairment (Thompson & Mauk, 2011).

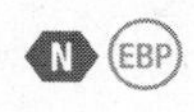

  - o Educate about post-concussive syndrome and its symptoms, which can include cognitive difficulties, headache, and dizziness that persist for weeks to months (Thompson & Mauk, 2011).

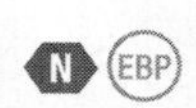

  - o Avoid caffeine, aspirin, alcohol, herbal supplements, or drugs, as they may exacerbate symptoms (Thompson & Mauk, 2011).

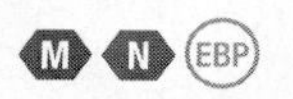

  - o Educate about second impact syndrome and urge the patient not to "return to play" until the health care provider recommends it is safe. A second concussion that occurs in close proximity to the first concussion and before symptoms of the first one have resolved can result in sudden fatal brain swelling (Thompson & Mauk, 2011).

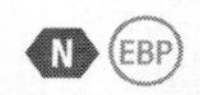

- Do not require a multidisciplinary team for treatment (CDWC, 2012).

Moderate-to-Severe TBI

The patient's and family's need for support (type and extent) are determined by the patient's severity of injury and possibilities for recovery. These are often determined by and may include:

- Most of these interventions are listed above in the moderate-to-severe interventions, as these must begin in rehabilitation, which can continue for months to years.
- Nurses commonly see patients in the most devastating stage post-TBI and rarely see patients years later, so they may be reluctant to offer what they think is false hope. But, following rehab, many TBI patients continue to gradually, possibly imperceptibly, recover for years (see Zach's photos).

Zach in His First Week of Rehab

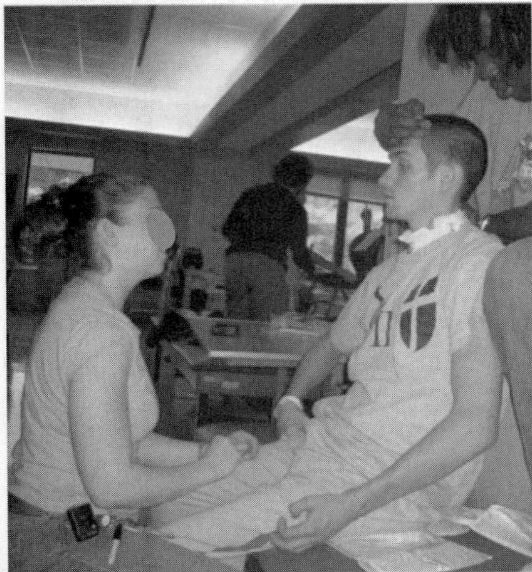

Zach, 25 years old, was struck by a car, which resulted in diffuse axonal shear damage. Zach was comatose for weeks and not expected to survive. Against the odds, this photo is Zach in a Rehab Center at 5 weeks post-TBI, not yet fully "awake".

Source: Courtesy of Zachary Phillips/Hendersonville, TN

Zach With Brother Jake After 4 Months in Rehab

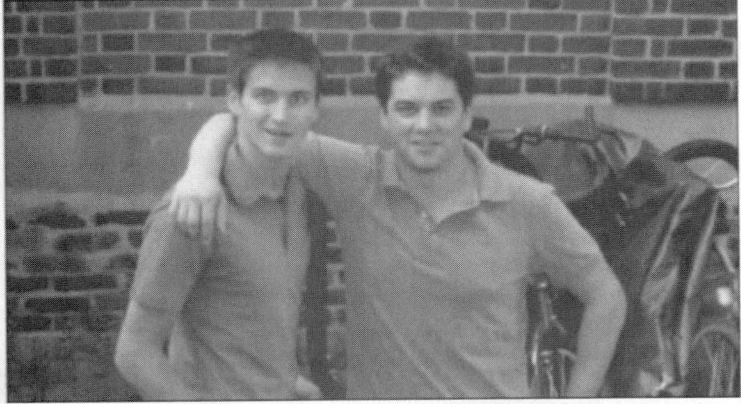

At 4 months post-TBI, Zach had fully evolved from his coma and graduated from wheelchair, to a walker, and then to a cane. He continued his rigorous daily exercise and rehabilitation to regain coordination, speech, and greater independence.

Source: Courtesy of Zachary Phillips/Hendersonville, TN

Zach at 6 Years Post Brain Injury

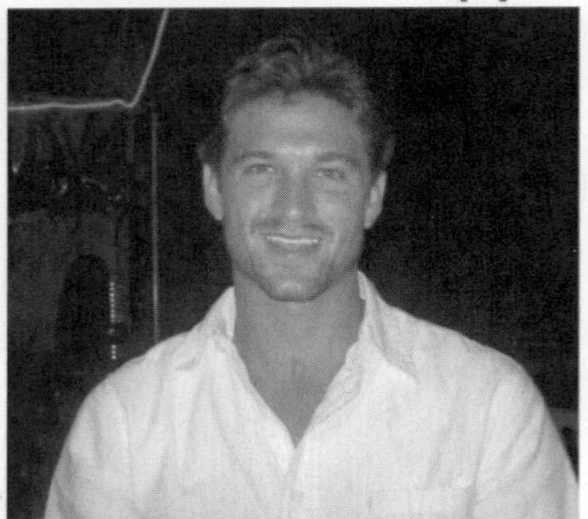

With hard work and a positive spirit, Zach reclaimed his independence and is an avid runner, cyclist, real estate agent, volunteer with TBI patients, and speaker for healthcare groups and students.

Source: Courtesy of Zachary Phillips/Hendersonville, TN

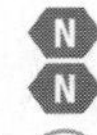

- o Offer as much positive reinforcement as is appropriate.
- o Support a family's hope in a realistic way.
- o Help reconnect the family with the patient as much as possible (CDWC, 2012)

Collaborative Interventions (continued)

Prevention

Education and awareness are the two main strategies for prevention.

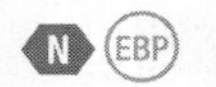

- Educate patients to wear a helmet when riding a bicycle, motorcycle, skiing, skating, skateboarding, horseback riding, and playing contact sports. Taking precautions can save lives and reduce devastating consequences (Thompson & Mauk, 2011).

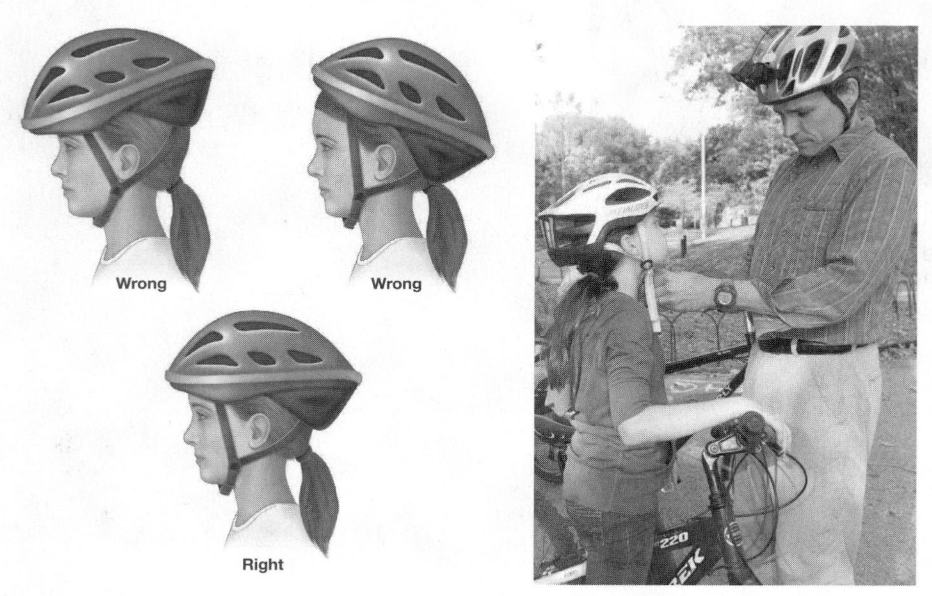

Left: This image displays the correct and incorrect ways of wearing a helmet for protection. Simple patient education can have life-changing results. Right: Adjusting a helmet to fit just right is primary in prevention and safety. An adult should ensure that a child's helmet fits properly.
Source: (*right*) CDC/Amanda Mills

- Headgear in sports should extend around the head and cover the ears to protect from player-to-player impacts. A helmet is needed in sports where head-to-head contact is likely (Thompson & Mauk, 2011).
- Wear a seatbelt and conform to child safety regulations (Thompson & Mauk, 2011).
- Do not drink and drive.
- Do not text while driving. Research suggests that texting is six times more dangerous than drinking.

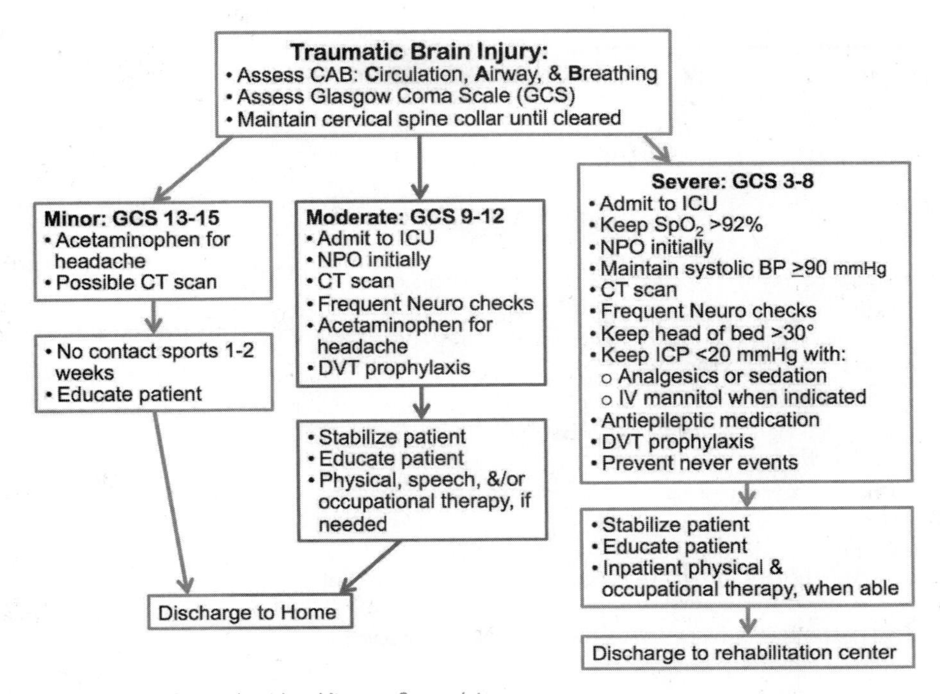

Traumatic Brain Injury algorithm: Minor to Severe Injury.

- Decrease the risk of falling in older adults:
  - o Avoid benzodiazepines, anticholinergics, and other medications that can increase the risk of falling (Thompson & Mauk, 2011).
  - o Use nonslip mats and avoid clutter in the home (Thompson & Mauk, 2011).
  - o Improve lighting in the home (Thompson & Mauk, 2011).
  - o Eye examinations to evaluate for cataracts or vision loss that may be correctable (Thompson & Mauk, 2011).
  - o Exercise regularly but not strenuously (Thompson & Mauk, 2011).
  - o Use safety aids (e.g., handrails).
- Restrict an athlete from return to play if signs of concussion persist such as headache, memory impairment, fatigue, dizziness, nausea, vomiting, insomnia, irritability, sense of being in a "fog," or alcohol intolerance. Adhere to physician instructions to delay return to play to prevent second impact injury (Thompson & Mauk, 2011).

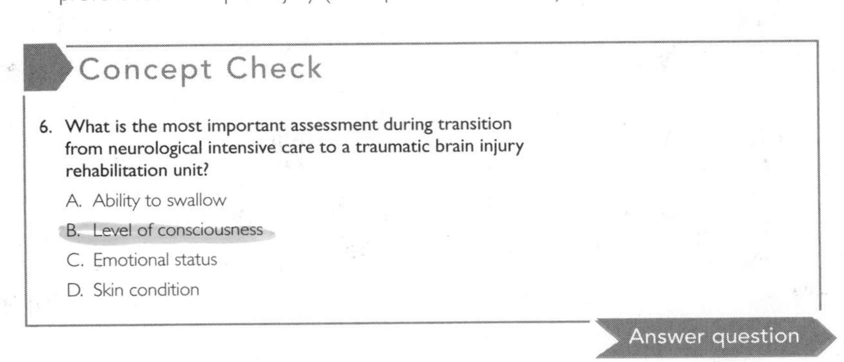

Concept Check

6. What is the most important assessment during transition from neurological intensive care to a traumatic brain injury rehabilitation unit?

A. Ability to swallow
B. Level of consciousness
C. Emotional status
D. Skin condition

Answer question

Concept Check

7. **Which finding is likely not associated with post-concussive syndrome?**

   A. Impaired short-term memory

   B. Dizziness upon standing

   C. Incontinence

   D. Headache

Answer question

Summary of Interventions

- As with all neurologic patients, close monitoring of the patient's progress is done to ensure the patient's needs are met.
- Specific interventions are determined by the severity of the injury and the patient's need for support and management through hospitalization.
- Individualization of care is imperative.
- Medical therapies focus upon reducing the extent of secondary brain injury with close attention to vital functions (primarily oxygenation and cerebral perfusion).
- Rehabilitation services and therapy are vital for the post-TBI patient as recovery occurs over months and years after injury.
- Gains in neurologic function can be made for years, so the patient and family should be encouraged to access the services needed to improve the quality of life for the individual with TBI.
- Educate for prevention. Brief moments of effort can prevent years to a lifetime of suffering and struggle.

LO4:

Evaluation of Desired Collaborative Care Outcomes

Evaluation and reassessment should reveal attainment of previously established patient outcomes. In summary:

- Patient's arterial blood gases have remained within expected range.
- Patient is at pre-illness level of alertness, wakefulness, and orientation to person, place and time.
- Patient, as much as possible, and family accurately discuss treatment modalities and expected level of recovery.
- Patient's CPP is >60 mmHg and has not appreciably deviated since admission.
- Patient's ICP has not exceeded desired level.

References

Bay, E. H., & Chartier, K. S. (2014). Chronic morbidities after traumatic brain injury: An update for the advanced practice nurse. *J Neuroscience Nursing, 46*(3), 142–152.

Bey, T., & Ostick, B. (2009). Second impact syndrome. *West J Emerg Med, 10*(1), 6–10. **www.ncbi.nlm.nih.gov/pmc/articles/PMC2672291/**

Blissitt, P. (2012). Controversies in the management of adults with severe traumatic brain injury. *AACN Advanced Critical Care, 23*(2), 188–203.

Centers for Disease Control and Prevention. (2014). *Injury prevention & control: Traumatic brain injury.* **www.cdc.gov/traumaticbraininjury/get_the_facts.html**

Dhandapani, M., Dhandapani, S., Agarwal, M., & Mahapatra, A. K. (2014). Pressure ulcer in patients with severe traumatic brain injury: Significant factors and association with neurological outcome. *J ClinNurs, 23*(7–8), 1114–1119. Doi: 10.1111/jocn.12396

Educational videos at **www.braininjury101.org**

Lump, D. (2014). Managing patients with severe traumatic brain injury. *Nursing 443*, 30–38. **journals.lww.com/ornursejournal/Fulltext/2013/05000/Managing_patients_with_severe_traumatic_brain.7.aspx**

Marshall, S., Bayley, M., & Berrigan, L. (2012). Clinical practice guidelines for mild traumatic brain injury and persistent symptoms. *Can Fam Physician, 58*(3), 257–267. **www.ncbi.nlm.nih.gov/pmc/articles/PMC3303645/**

Master, C. L., Balcer, L., & Collins, M. (2014). Concussion. *Ann Intern Med, 160*(3), ITC2-1-1.

Meier, C. (2013). Airway management in patients with brain injury. *Emerg Nurse, 21*(8), 18–23. doi: 10.7748/en2013.12.21.8.18.e1236

Moser, R. S., Schatz, P., & Jordan, B. D. (2005). Prolonged effects of concussion in high school athletes. *Neurosurgery, 57*(2), 300–306.

Rosario, E. R., Kaplan, S. E., Khonsari, S., & Patterson, D. (2014). Predicting and assessing fall risk in an acute inpatient rehabilitation facility. *Rehabil Nurs, 39*(2), 86–93. **onlinelibrary.wiley.com/doi/10.1002/rnj.114/full**

Tran, L.V. (2014). Understanding the pathophysiology of traumatic brain injury and the mechanisms of action of neuroprotective interventions. *J Trauma Nursing, 21*(1), 30–35.

Waszynski, C., Veronneau, P., Therrien, K., et al. (2013). Decreasing patient agitation using individualized therapeutic activities. *Amer J Nurs, 113*(10), 32–40. **www.mlanet.org/sites/default/files/education/pdf/ce500_articles.pdf**

Clinical Practice Guidelines

American Association of Neuroscience Nurses (AANN). (2008). *Nursing management of adults with severe traumatic brain injury*. Glenview, IL: Author. **www.guideline.gov/content.aspx?id=13576&search=traumatic+brain+injury**

Badjatia, N., Carney, N., Crocco, T. J., et al., & Brain Trauma Foundation. (2007). Guidelines for prehospital management of traumatic brain injury, 2nd edition. *Prehospital Emergency Care, 12*(1), S1–S53. **www.braintrauma.org/pdf/protected/Prehospital_Guidelines_2nd_Edition.pdf**

Brain Trauma Foundation (BTF). (2007). Guidelines for the management of severe traumatic brain injury, 3rd edition, a joint project of the Brain Trauma Foundation: Improving the outcome of brain trauma patients worldwide and American Association of Neurological Surgeons (AANS), Congress of Neurological Surgeons (CNS), and the AANS/CNS Joint Section on Neurotrauma and Critical Care. *J Neurotrauma, 24*(Suppl. 1), 1–116. **www.braintrauma.org/pdf/protected/Guidelines_Management_2007w_bookmarks.pdf**

Colorado Division of Workers' Compensation. (2012). *Traumatic brain injury medical treatment guidelines*. Denver, CO: Author. **www.guideline.gov/content.aspx?id=43752&search=severe+tbi#Section420**

Thompson, H. J., & Mauk, K. (2011). *Care of the patient with mild traumatic brain injury: AANN and ARN clinical practice guideline series.* **www.rehabnurse.org/uploads/files/cpgmtbi.pdf**

Vos, P., Alekseenko, Y., Battistin, L., et al. (2012). Mild traumatic brain injury. *AHRQ Guidelines, Eur J Neurol, 19*(2), 191–198. **www.guideline.gov/content.aspx?id=38468&search=minor+tbi**

Patient Education

American Association of Neurological Surgeons. (2011). *Patient information: Traumatic brain injury.* **www.aans.org/Patient%20Information/Conditions%20and%20Treatments/Traumatic%20Brain%20Injury.aspx**

Bowman, J. (2014). *Post-concussion syndrome.* **www.healthline.com/health/post-concussion-syndrome#Overview1**

Brainline.org. (2014). *About traumatic brain injury.* **www.brainline.org/landing_pages/TBI.html**

Centers for Disease Control and Prevention. (2015). *Heads up.* **www.cdc.gov/headsup/index.html**

Mayo Clinic Staff. (2014). *Concussion.* **www.mayoclinic.org/diseases-conditions/concussion/basics/definition/con-20019272**

Learning Outcomes for Spinal Cord Injury

When you complete this lesson, you will be able to:

1. Recognize the clinical relevance of spinal cord injury.
2. Consider the pathophysiology, etiology, risk factors, and clinical presentation of spinal cord injury that determine the priority patient concerns.
3. Determine the most urgent and important nursing interventions and patient education required in caring for a patient with spinal cord injury.
4. Evaluate attainment of desired collaborative care outcomes for a patient with spinal cord injury.

LO1:

What Is Spinal Cord Injury?

- When a traumatic event occurs to an individual, it can disrupt soft tissue surrounding the vertebral column, the ligaments holding the bones in place, the bones themselves, and the actual spinal cord.

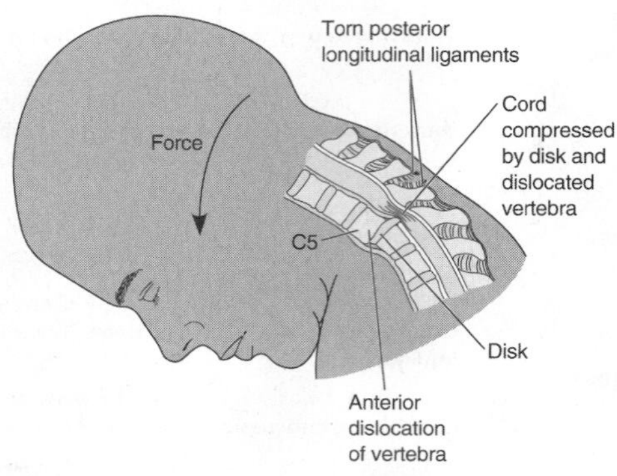

This medical illustration shows the head hyperflexion with a spinal fracture occurring at the C5 level. The C5/C6 disc is shown herniating anteriorly.

- Car accidents, interpersonal violence, falls and sports-related events are the leading cause of spine injury. Most injuries occur in the cervical spine with 30% of injuries occurring in the thoracic and lumbar regions.
- Specific mechanisms of injury include hyperextension, hyperflexion, rotation, compression, and penetration. Each produces the potential for localized trauma and injury to the vertebrae and spinal cord. The result is a primary and secondary injury.
- The primary injury causes a temporary or permanent loss of function in the spinal cord.
- The secondary injury includes the events (edema, hemorrhage, cellular changes) that occur following the initial injury that can reduce the blood flow to the spinal cord, creating further injury.
- Another significant type of spinal cord injury is nontraumatic. The main causes of this type are tumors, ischemia (spinal cord stroke), and spinal stenosis.

LO1:

Clinical Relevance

- Spinal cord injury (SCI) impacts over 10,000 persons in the United States each year. The injury can be devastating and drastically alter the quality of the individual's life. A previously independent individual can become dependent on others for activities of daily living if there is loss of significant motor function.
- Patients with spinal cord injuries frequently have medical complications such as pressure ulcers and recurrent urinary and pulmonary infections. These conditions often require recurring hospitalization and medical treatment.

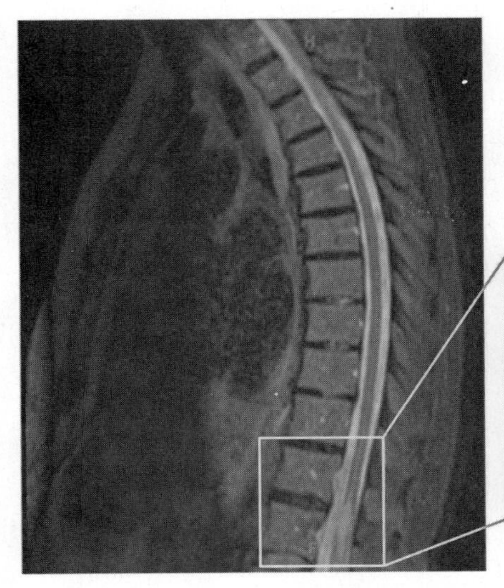

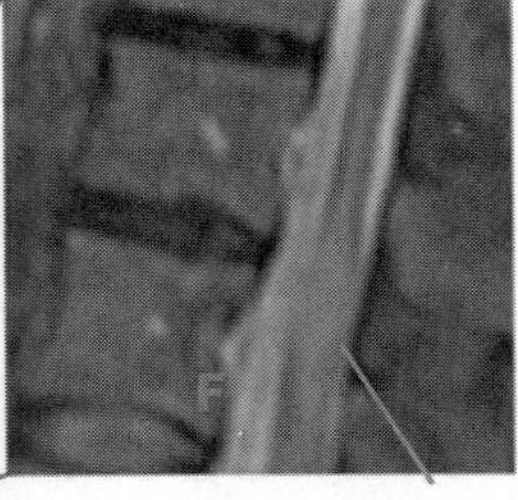

This MRI of the spine reveals a metastatic lesion from melanoma (cancer) invading the spinal cord. The patient developed an unexpected paraplegia. The magnified lesion on the spinal cord is highlighted in red for easy identification. The spinal cord damage resulted in an incontinent bladder, incontinent bowel, sexual dysfunction, and loss of motor function below the cancer.

Source: Courtesy of K. Kyriakidis

LO2:

Pathophysiology

- The very fragile spinal cord lies protected within the vertebral column. The 33 vertebrae and ligaments hold the spinal cord in place and, anatomically, protect it from harm.
- The spinal cord is a direct continuation of the medulla as it exits the brain and continues down to the bony level of the first or second lumbar vertebrae.
- When there is trauma to the back and neck, various types of injuries can be produced. The most minor is soft tissue injury. This type of injury is very common, especially when individuals are suddenly jolted in their motor vehicle (i.e., "whiplash").

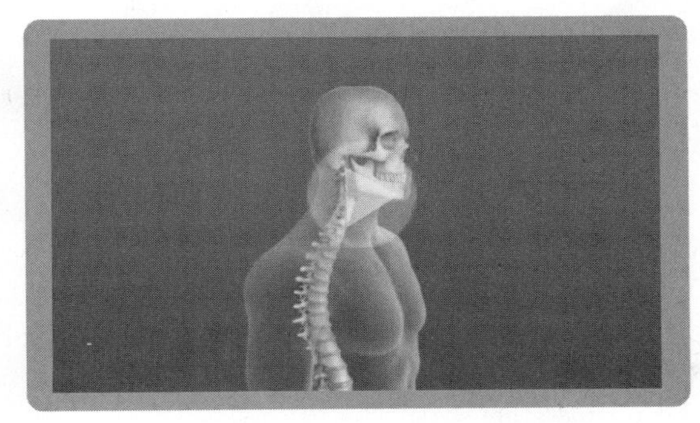

This animation depicts the anatomy of the cervical spine and intervertebral disc. Details include orientation of the cervical spine, movements of the cervical spine, and movement of intervertebral discs. A cross-section of the intervertebral disc and spinal cord highlights the nucleus pulposus, annulus fibrosus, spinal cord, dura mater, spinal root, and spinal nerve.

Source: © 2014 Nucleus Medical Media. All rights reserved

- Bone fractures may occur in the vertebral column. Simple breaks in the bone, compression or wedge fractures, and teardrop fractures can disrupt the bony alignment.
- If the ligaments holding the vertebrae in place are disrupted, the bones can shift out of alignment and compress the spinal cord itself. The specific location of a bone fracture is very important.
- Fractures of the first two cervical vertebrae can be life threatening by compressing the spinal cord, thus leading to immediate respiratory arrest.
- Fractures of the vertebrae can produce significant injury to the specific region of the spinal cord.

Spinal Cord Compression & Injury

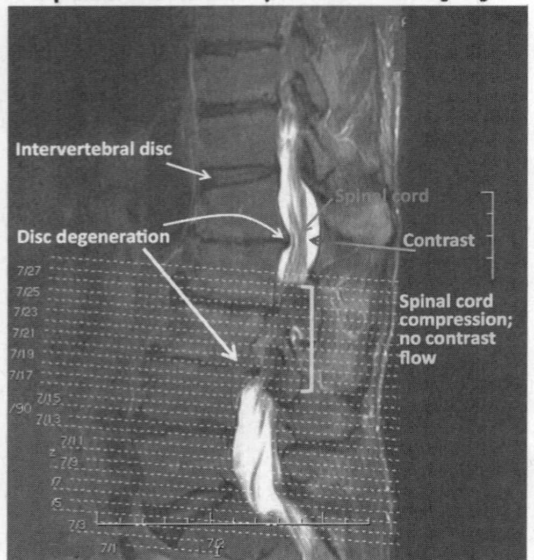

This MRI myelogram shows contrast surrounding the spinal cord except in the region of the yellow bracket where the cord is so compressed that no contrast is seen. It reveals why the patient has severe pain and limited function. Notice the collapsed intervertebral discs which cause the vertebral displacement.

Source: Courtesy of William Stoddard/Fairbanks, AK

Concept Check

1. The spinal cord is a direct continuation of which structure?
   A. Vertebrae
   B. Medulla
   C. Occipital lobe
   D. Disc

Answer question

Pathophysiology (continued)

Pathology and Types of Structures Injured

- Actual injury to the spinal cord itself is categorized by type of injury.
  - A **concussion** to the spine is a temporary loss of function.
  - A **contusion** is bruising in the spinal cord that causes hemorrhaging in the cord and edema.
  - A **laceration** of the cord cuts the actual cord leading to permanent damage.
- Bleeding around the spinal cord (epidural hematoma) can compress the cord and lead to reduced blood flow and cellular damage.
- In a similar manner, tumor growth adjacent to the spinal cord can cause compression. Specific blood vessels can become occluded or blocked causing a "stroke" to the spinal cord.
- Some injuries to the spine are considered complete, meaning there is a loss of motor and/or sensory function below the level of the lesion.
- Other injuries are classified as incomplete injuries.
  - One example is central cord syndrome, in which the patient has strong leg muscles and movement but weak arm muscles. This is due to damage to the neuronal tracts in the spinal cord that innervate the arms and sparing of the tracts that innervate the legs.
  - Another example is Brown–Séquard syndrome, which occurs following penetrating trauma and hemisection of the spinal cord. The patient loses motor and position sense, vibration, and touch on one side of the body, and a loss of pain and temperature sensation on the other side of the body.

Metastatic Cancer Invading the Spine With Loss of Function

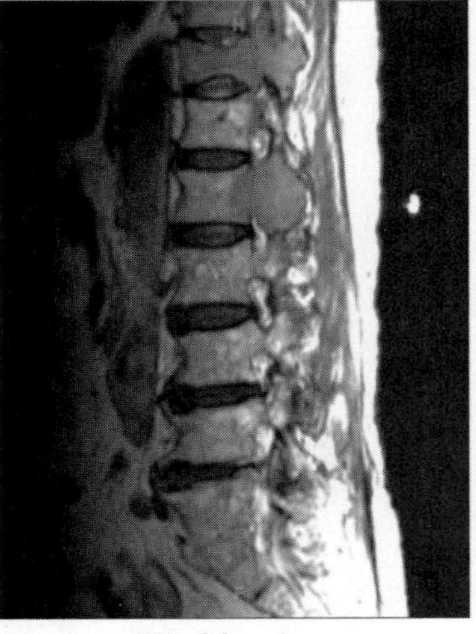

MRI of the spine

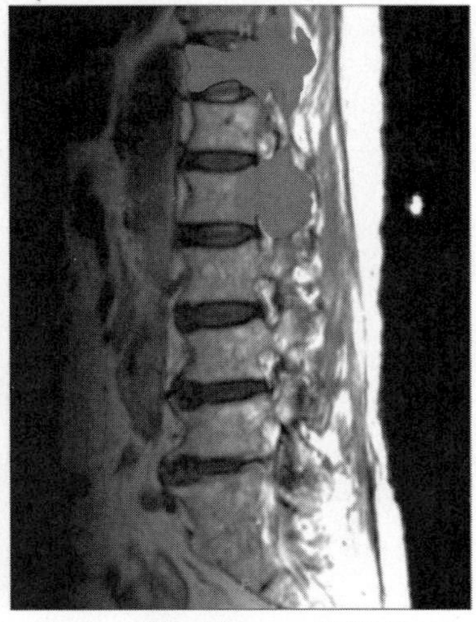

Identical MRI with cancer highlighted

The image on the left shows metastatic cancer invading the spine and causing SCI from compression and pathologic changes. On the right is an identical image with the tumor growths highlighted in red for easy recognition. The upper tumor has almost completely replaced the vertebra. Both vertebrae show cancerous growths intruding into the spinal cord.
Source: Courtesy of K. Kyriakidis

Pathology and Types of Structures Injured: SCI

C6-7 Disc Herniation with Spinal Cord Compression

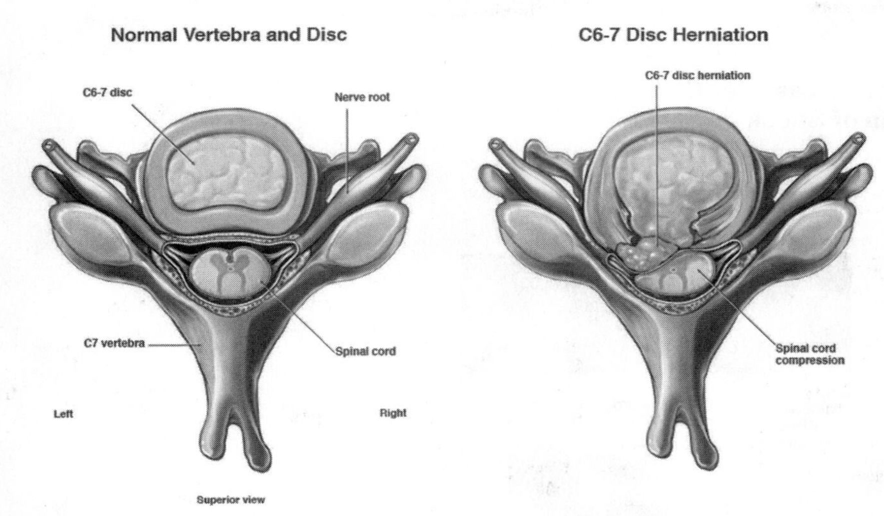

This illustration compares a normal disc with a herniated disc. The nucleus pulposus (central white matter) of the herniated disc is depicted protruding through the torn annulus fibrosus (pink) and compressing the spinal cord. Note the spinal cord compression points out why nerve damage occurs.
Source:

Injury to the Cord and Shock

When the spinal cord is injured, two types of shock occur with additional symptoms:

- The first is **spinal shock**. This is a temporary state where all motor, sensory, and reflex functions are lost. As spinal shock resolves, the patient's reflexes return, but motor function and sensation may not return.

Transected Spinal Cord

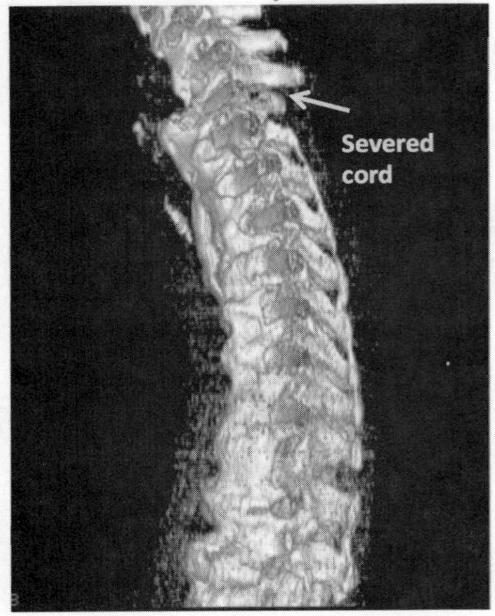

This CT scan reveals the devastating transection of the spinal cord (at T3) in this patient who then suffered neurogenic shock.

Source: Courtesy of K. Kyriakidis

- The second type of shock is **neurogenic shock**, which is an autonomic dysfunction that usually occurs in spinal cord injuries above the thoracic sixth level (T6). Due to loss of the sympathetic outflow in this region, the patient demonstrates hypotension, bradycardia, hypothermia, and loss of the ability to sweat below the level of the injury. Emergent intervention is needed.

Progressive Vasodilation to Vascular Collapse: Mechanism of Shock

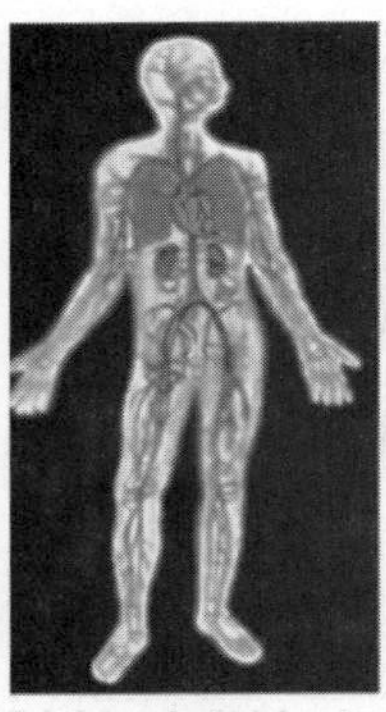

Arterial and arteriolar circulation

1. In this normal arteriole, a constant blood volume and flow sustain a constant blood pressure (BP).

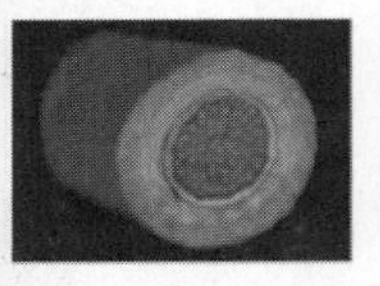

2. Early vasodilation occurs due to loss of sympathetic stimulation. Lumen widens as the wall thins. Without increased volume, BP begins to drop.

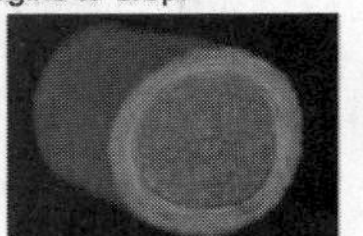

3. Autonomic dysfunction worsens, resulting in extreme vasodilation with a severe drop in BP, perfusion, and oxygenation.

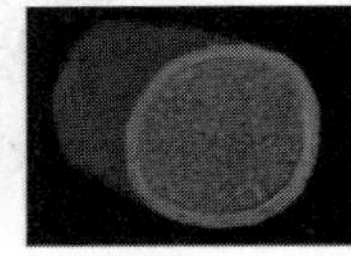

Note the changing vessel (1-4) diameter and muscle thinning as it expands. Blood flow gradually slows, becomes sluggish, and disseminated intravascular coagulation (microcoagulation) results.

4. As neurogenic shock ensues, circulatory collapse and blood clotting (DIC) result.

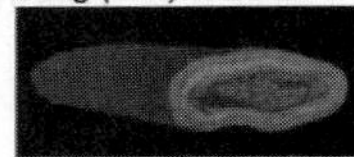

Source: Courtesy of George Kyriakidis/Santa Ana, CA

LO2:

Risk Factors

- Male gender: 80% of spinal cord injured victims from traumatic injuries are male.
- Age:
  - o Teens and young adults, age 15–30, have a significantly higher risk of SCI, particularly from motor vehicle crashes.
  - o Adults over 65 years of age have a higher risk of SCI, particularly from falls.
- Risky or unsafe activities, such as extreme sports or racing in a car
- Impact sports (e.g., football, soccer, diving)
- Drug or alcohol abuse
- Orthopedic conditions of the bone and joints, particularly osteoporosis or metastatic cancer

LO2:

Causes

- Sudden force injury (e.g., traumatic blow or motor vehicle crash)
- Stab wound
- Gunshot wound
- Hemorrhage or spinal "stroke"
- Cancer
- Inflammatory condition
- Arthritis
- Infectious organism
- Spinal degeneration of the disc or vertebrae

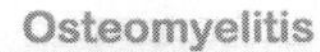

Osteomyelitis

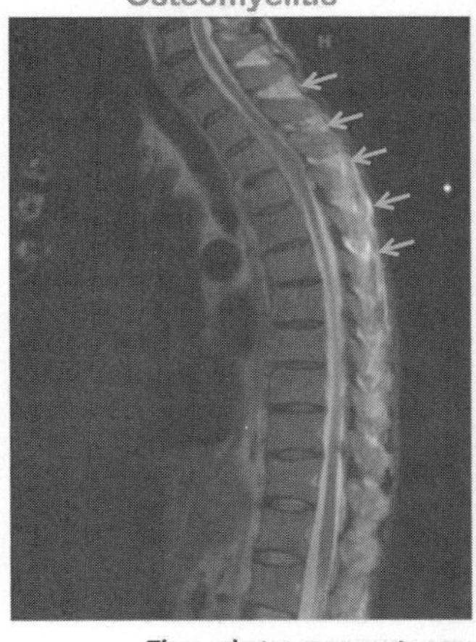

Metastatic Spinal Cancer

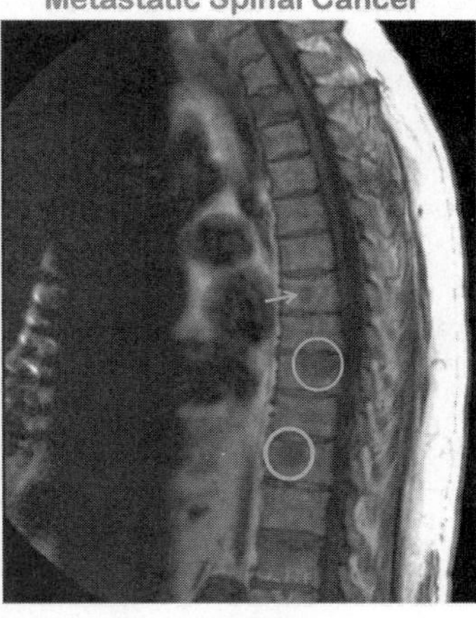

These photos represent some of the causes of spinal cord injury.

Source: Courtesy of K. Kyriakidis

Concept Check

2. The nurse recognizes which spinal cord level as the landmark for development of neurogenic shock?
   A. C1
   B. T3
   C. T6
   D. L1

Answer question

LO2:

Assessment Findings

Spinal Cord Innervation

Clinical findings following spinal cord injury are related to the level of the spinal cord injured. When injured, particularly in a complete injury where there is no longer any sensory or motor function at that level, the patient also loses all function controlled by spinal nerves below the level of injury.

- C1-4 innervates the phrenic nerve, which allows for movement of the diaphragm. Any injury to the upper cervical spine can paralyze the muscles required for breathing and result in apnea. As the most severe spinal cord injury, paralysis of the entire lower body (arms, legs, hands, feet, trunk) is expected. The highest cervical injuries may cause impaired speech and swallow.

- The cervical or neck region of the spinal cord controls deltoids (C5), biceps (C5-6), triceps (C7), wrist extensors (C6-7), finger flexion (C8), and finger extension (T1). Injury to the cervical spine can result in tetraplegia, more commonly known as quadriplegia, which can cause paralysis of all muscles and voluntary function below the neck. This typically involves loss of sensory and/or motor function of the hands, arms, legs, thoracic and abdominal regions, and the organs in the pelvis. Loss of motor function can be followed by hyperreflex activity, involuntary movement or twitching, and/or spastic movement, loss of bladder and bowel control, altered sexual function, pain or intense stinging or burning resulting from nerve damage, dyspnea, and inability to clear the airway. Loss of sensation or feeling to cold, heat, and touch, with numbness or tingling are expected.
- The thoracic region of the spinal cord innervates muscles of respiration (intercostal and abdominal muscles). Loss of function can affect the upper chest, back, abdomen, legs, and pelvic organs while preserving hand and arm function. This type of lower body paralysis is known as paraplegia.
- The lumbar and sacral regions of the spinal cord innervate the leg muscles.
- The lumbar region of the spinal cord controls hip flexion (L2), hip adductors (L2-4), hip abductors (L4-S1), quadriceps (L3-4), hamstrings (L4-5, S1), extension of the great toe (L5) and gastrocnemius (S1). Injury to the lumbar area may produce paraplegia due to loss of hip and leg movement. Loss of bowel and bladder control is expected.
- Injury to spinal nerve roots (the spinal cord ends in the lower thoracic spine) that branch off the lumbar and sacral region like a horse's tail may produce variable motor loss in the lower legs, absent Achilles reflex, radicular pain, and reflexive bowel and/or bladder function.
- Injury to the conus medullaris (bottom of the cord) can cause urinary retention, impotence, constipation, lax anal sphincter, saddle anesthesia, and minimal to no motor weakness.

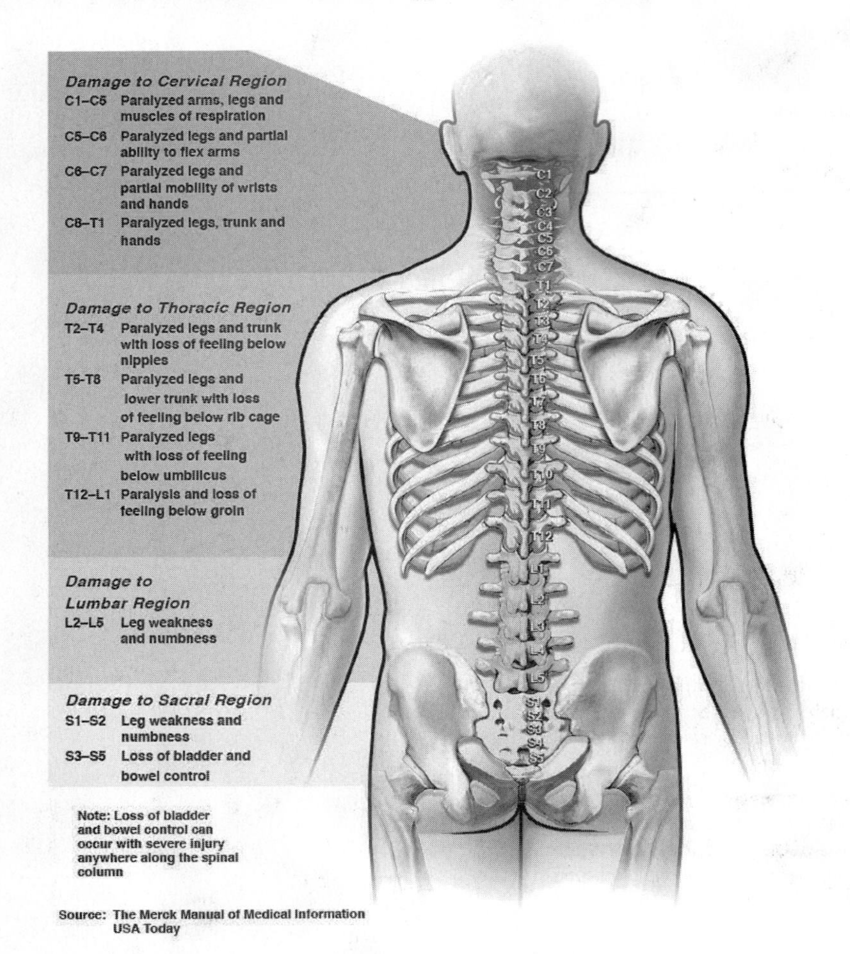
Effects of Nerve Damage along the Spinal Cord
Damage to Cervical Region
C1–C5 Paralyzed arms, legs and muscles of respiration
C5–C6 Paralyzed legs and partial ability to flex arms
C6–C7 Paralyzed legs and partial mobility of wrists and hands
C8–T1 Paralyzed legs, trunk and hands
Damage to Thoracic Region
T2–T4 Paralyzed legs and trunk with loss of feeling below nipples
T5-T8 Paralyzed legs and lower trunk with loss of feeling below rib cage
T9–T11 Paralyzed legs with loss of feeling below umbilicus
T12–L1 Paralysis and loss of feeling below groin
Damage to Lumbar Region
L2–L5 Leg weakness and numbness
Damage to Sacral Region
S1–S2 Leg weakness and numbness
S3–S5 Loss of bladder and bowel control
Note: Loss of bladder and bowel control can occur with severe injury anywhere along the spinal column
C1
C2
C3
C4
C5
C6
C7
T1
T2
T3
T4
T5
T6
T7
T8
T9
T10
T11
T12
L1
L2
L3
L4
L5
S1
S2
S3
S4
S5
Source: The Merck Manual of Medical Information
USA Today

This illustration portrays the effects of nerve damage along the spinal cord. It shows the spine, differentiating between the cervical, thoracic, lumbar, and sacral regions. Injuries that can result from damage to the spine at various levels are described.

General Assessment Findings

The clinical manifestations of spinal cord injury depend on the level of injury and any complicating factors. Symptoms further depend on whether the injury causes complete or incomplete loss of sensory and motor function to the affected regions. The major signs and symptoms can include:

- Neurologic: pain or intense stinging, areflexia (loss of reflexes), autonomic dysreflexia, loss of sensations, loss of temperature regulation resulting in hypo- or hyperthermia, neurogenic, or spinal shock
- Cardiovascular: hypovolemic shock, sudden severe hypertension, bradycardia, orthostatic hypotension, dysrhythmias, vascular/venous collapse, dependent edema
- Respiratory: apnea, difficulty breathing, decreased respiratory effort, decreased vital capacity, inability to clear secretions
- Musculoskeletal: loss of or weakness in movement—paraplegia, tetraplegia, variable paralysis, spasms, incoordination, muscle flaccidity
- Gastrointestinal: loss of bowel control/incontinence, paralytic ileus
- Urinary: neurogenic bladder, urinary incontinence, urinary retention

Concept Check

3. **Tetraplegia involves weakness or paralysis in which areas?**
   A. Upper extremities alone
   B. Lower extremities alone
   C. One side upper and lower extremity
   D. Both upper and lower extremities

Answer question

LO2:

Diagnostics

- Spinal cord injury is diagnosed by history and physical examination with emphasis on neurologic examination. Imaging studies are confirmatory and help delineate the etiology (see photo caption).
- Cervical spine films and computerized tomography (CT) and magnetic resonance imaging (MRI) scans are obtained to determine the extent of injury to the vertebral column, spinal cord, ligaments, and soft tissues.
- The American Spinal Injury Association (ASIA) has published an international standard for classifying spinal cord injuries that is widely used (ASIA scale) to guide rehabilitation and recovery planning. This scale uses sensory and motor functions at various points on the body.

Lumbar Spine: Identify the Problems

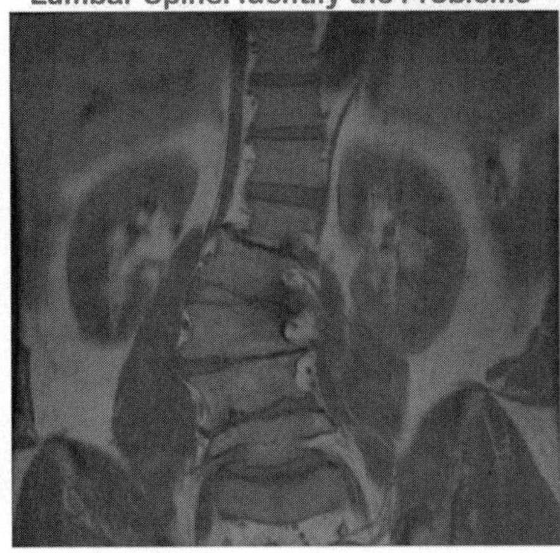

Answer: Collapsed Lumbar Spine

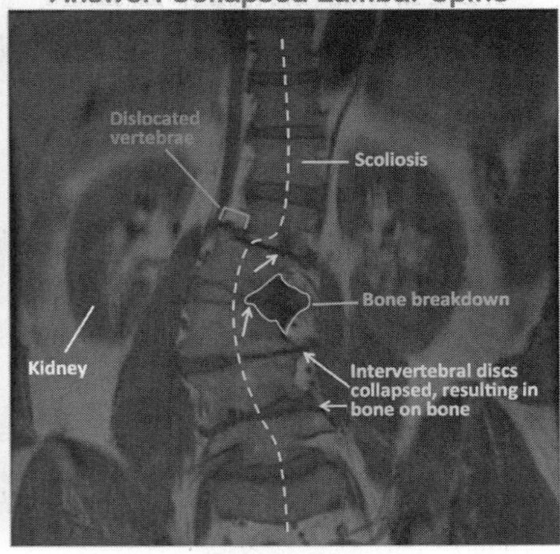

This patient is a very active outdoorsman who had a history of scoliosis and a back injury from a heavy object falling on his back in his youth. His back pain worsened over the years to the point when this MRI (left) was taken. Name four major problems seen. Right: This identical MRI points out the reasons for his back pain. Severe scoliosis (1) with multiple collapsed discs (2) led to pain from bone rubbing against bone. (3) Excruciating pain is compounded by the pressure placed on the spinal cord and pelvic nerves and the back spasms due to constant stretch on the ligaments. Note how severely offset the spinal column is (pink bracket), caused by the slipping and dislocation of the vertebrae (4) and is creating instability of the spinal column. Given the spinal instability, this patient is at risk for cord transection.

Source: Courtesy of William Stoddard/Fairbanks, AK

Priority Patient Concerns and Desired Collaborative Care Outcomes

Prior to caring for patients with spinal cord injury, it is important to prioritize the patient's concerns that must guide the nursing care plan and interventions. Care for the patient is ordered and organized in accordance with the patient's priority and urgent needs. Desired collaborative care outcomes in patients with a spinal cord injury typically include:

1. Patient will experience no further spinal injury.
2. Patient's respiratory status will be optimized using mechanical ventilation if necessary.
3. Patient will not experience damage from autonomic dysreflexia.
4. Patient's hemodynamic parameters will be maintained within desired limits.
5. Patient's skin will remain intact without decubitus ulcers.
6. Patient will discuss fearful feelings and report reduced fear after learning how ADLs are being managed.
7. Patient will report feeling more in control of personal health decisions.

Considering these important care outcomes, prepare a list of the major 3–6 priority patient concerns or nursing diagnoses for patients with spinal cord injury. Be prepared to participate in a discussion of this list and/or to submit them as an assignment, as determined by your faculty. Resources you may find helpful in this assignment can include this lesson, the references, resources on nursing care plans, and standard nursing diagnoses manuals.

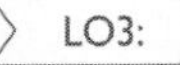

LO3:

Collaborative Interventions

Emergent Care

- When a spinal cord injury is suspected, **first responders** should:
  - EBP o Ensure that the spine is immobilized prior to moving the patient (Hadley, et al., 2013).
  - EBP o Place a cervical collar on patient and use a backboard to immobilize the spine to prevent any further injury (Hadley, et al., 2013).

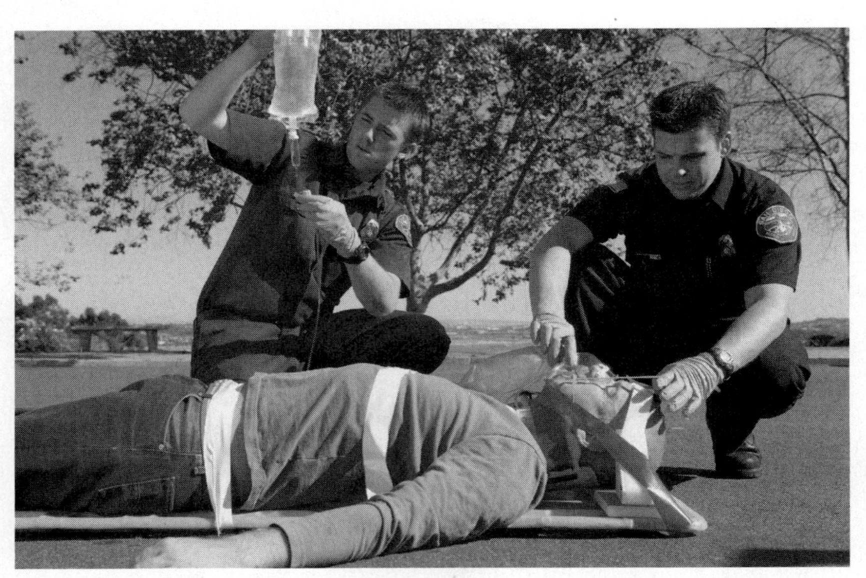

A pedestrian is shown with a possible neck injury. EMS workers are at the scene and have stabilized the man's neck with a neck brace to prevent further injury to the spinal cord.
Source: Juice Images/Fotolia

M N EBP
- Complete neurologic examinations must be performed:
  - o This is important because many SCI patients sustain a traumatic brain injury at the same time. A focused neurologic examination is conducted, noting motor movement in all muscle groups and the level of sensation. Not all SCI patients lose motor or sensory function (Gall, et al., 2008).
  - o Due to the complexity of the various levels of injury and their impact on vital functions, the patient must be repeatedly assessed (e.g., neuro check, Glasgow Coma Scale) to determine the impact on sensory and motor function. Note any pain that the patient complains of in the spine (Hadley, et al., 2013).
  - o SCI patients can break bones in the spine while initially remaining neurologically and functionally intact. Repeated assessments should be performed every 15–30 minutes, noting any change in level of function.
- The patient's airway and breathing are assessed to determine if they are able to maintain normal ventilation and oxygenation. If not, careful endotracheal intubation is done while maintaining perfect alignment of the cervical spine (Hadley, et al., 2013).
- Circulation is assessed by monitoring blood pressure (BP), pulse, and heart rhythm. Intravenous (IV) lines are started and fluid resuscitation follows if the patient is hypotensive (Hadley, et al., 2013).
- A mean arterial pressure (MAP) goal of 85–90 mmHg is desirable to support spinal perfusion (Aarabi, et al., 2013; Hadley, et al., 2013).
- Vasopressors like norepinephrine may be needed to maintain hemodynamic stability once volume resuscitation is completed (Aarabi, et al., 2013).
- An indwelling urinary catheter is placed in patients with a suspected spinal injury.
- Oral gastric tube placement may be necessary to decompress the stomach and to prevent regurgitation while lying flat on a backboard.
- The administration of high dose steroids (e.g., methylprednisolone) is controversial; however, there is no reliable evidence supporting a clinical benefit for SCI patients and it is not recommended. Some evidence suggests that it can do harm. Some physicians still administer high doses of steroids following SCI while other physicians avoid their use (Hurlbert, et al., 2013).
- Use of GM-1 ganglioside (or Sygen) is not recommended as there is no evidence to support its long-term benefit (Hurlbert, et al., 2013).
- Treatment of a spinal cord injury starts in the ED, as most patients incur SCI emergently or accidentally.

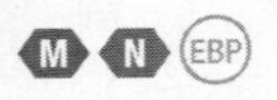

- The injured person is then admitted to the hospital, either the ICU or moved to a spinal cord injury treatment center, depending on the extent of injury (Aarabi, et al., 2013).
- Procedures are vital in treating spinal cord injuries:

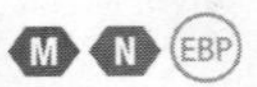

  1. Relief of pressure on the spine is accomplished using surgery or traction (a mechanical system of weights) (Fehlings, et al., 2012).
  2. Treatment to stabilize the spine is performed. Screws, metal plates, and other devices may be placed during surgery. In some cases, traction may be used instead (Fehlings, et al., 2012).
  3. Physicians who prescribe the steroid medication methylprednisolone administer it at this point. It is proposed to reduce swelling. If used, it is administered within 8 hours after injury for the purpose of helping to prevent nerve damage (Hurlbert, et al., 2013).

Concept Check

4. What is the most important goal of immediate care of a patient with a spinal cord injury?

A. Prevention of further spinal cord damage

B. Insertion of an endotracheal tube

C. Initiation of intravenous access

D. Assessment of level of injury

Answer question

Collaborative Interventions (continued)

Surgical Stabilization

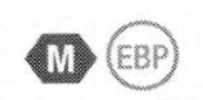

- Once the exact injury is isolated, the neurosurgeon or orthopedic surgeon determines how the spine must be immobilized and stabilized. If the patient requires surgery, the surgical procedure to stabilize the spine usually occurs within the first 24 hours, instead of leaving the patient immobilized on a firm type of bed with external traction devices (Aarabi, et al., 2013; Fehlings, et al., 2012).

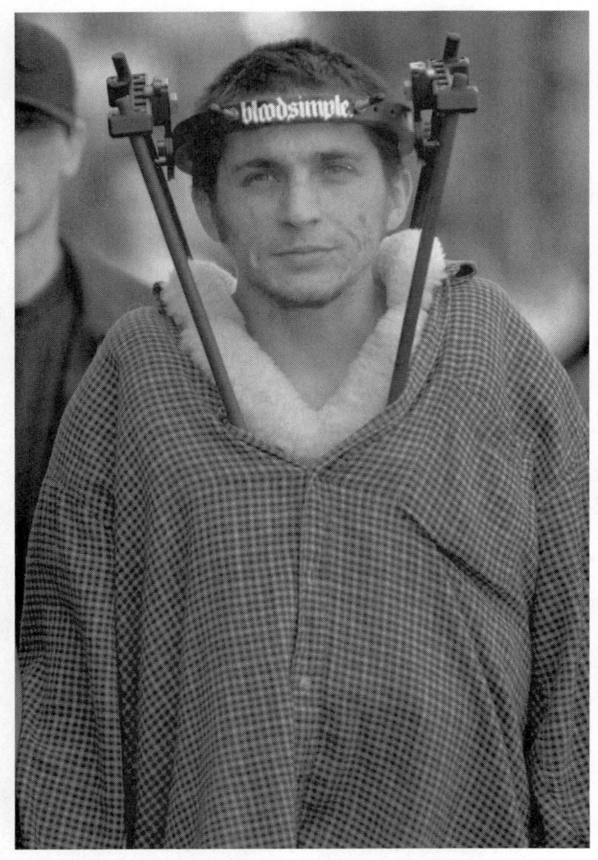

A "halo ring" or "crown" encircles and is fixed to the patient's head. This device is crucial for managing a variety of conditions that destabilize the cervical spine.

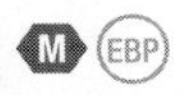

- Surgery may be necessary to alleviate compression on the spinal cord. Decompression is particularly important if it is focal and affects the anterior aspects (Aarabi, et al., 2013).

- If traction and/or spinal immobilization (e.g., halo apparatus) is needed, the patient may be on complete bed rest. A halo, for example, permits mobilization, is more comfortable, and reduces length of stay. Nursing care can involve:
    - o Ensure the pins are tight, secure, and cleaned twice daily.
    - o Ensure that traction is not too tight. Inspect the skin every 8 hours. Follow hospital-specific policy and procedure on skin and halo vest care.
    - o Log roll the patient employing three clinicians who secure the head, neck, shoulders, hips, and legs, and turn all simultaneously.
    - o Administer pain medication for headache or discomfort.
    - o Order a soft diet to avoid pain or discomfort from chewing.
    - o Maintain good body alignment.
    - o Provide routine care provided for all patients at bed rest.
    - o Prevent never events.
    - o Educate the patient to preferentially use eye movements rather than turning the head or neck. Educate loved ones to move to talk to patient to reduce the patient's need to turn to communicate.

Immediate and Intermediate Management

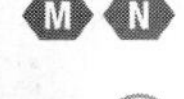

- SCI patients with neurologic deficits are usually admitted to the intensive care unit for management and close monitoring.

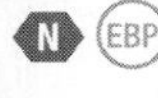

- Every body system can be impacted with SCI. Ensure the airway is supported and ventilatory support is provided as long as the patient's respiratory muscles are affected (Gall, et al., 2008).

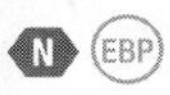

- The patient may have a depressed cough. The nurse may need to assist the patient with coughing by providing ideal body positioning and, at times, abdominal support (Gall, et al., 2008).

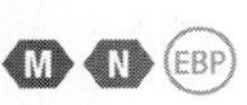

- BP management is important for the first 7 days, keeping the MAP >85 mmHg in order to ensure adequate perfusion of the spine. Pharmacological interventions may be required (Hadley, et al., 2013).

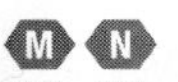

- H_2 blockers are administered to reduce the risk of gastric hemorrhage.

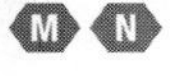

- Initial use of oral gastric or NG tubes provide gastric decompression until ready for enteral nutrition.

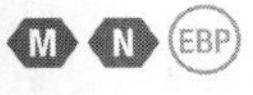

- Nutritional support is essential in spinal cord injured patients as they may experience a hypermetabolic state. Catabolic effects can result in increased loss of lean body mass (muscle), muscle atrophy, weight loss, and increased susceptibility to infection. Enteral nutrition, started within the first 48–72 hours after admission, is recommended, safe, and essential in most patients (American Dietetic Association [ADA], 2009; Dhall, et al., 2013).

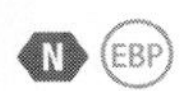

- If the patient has suffered motor paralysis, correct positioning of the extremities is important (Gall, et al., 2008). Postural alignment, whether turning patient or flat, includes:
    - o Observe a straight line from the nose to sternum to pubic symphysis to indicate spinal alignment.
    - o Ensure lateral alignment so that shoulders, hips, and legs show no signs of spinal rotation.
    - o Support the head and neck with pillows, pads or head blocks to maintain a midline position.
    - o Support limbs, hands, and feet to avoid contractures or hyperextension.

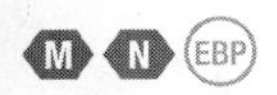

- It is imperative to prevent deep vein thrombosis with sequential compression devices and/or anticoagulation. Compression stockings continue to be used, but have not shown effectiveness in studies (Gall, et al., 2008).

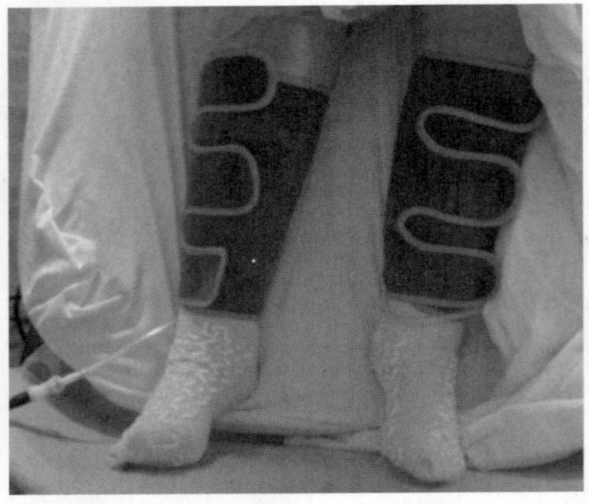

A sequential compression device provides pneumatic compression as an effective medical treatment to prevent deep vein thrombosis. The device is applied to a patient's legs. The air pump then repeatedly inflates and deflates to produce a pulsating pressure, thereby "massaging" the patient's legs.

Source: Courtesy of K. Kyriakidis

Collaborative Interventions (continued)

Prevention of Deep Vein Thrombosis and Pulmonary Embolism

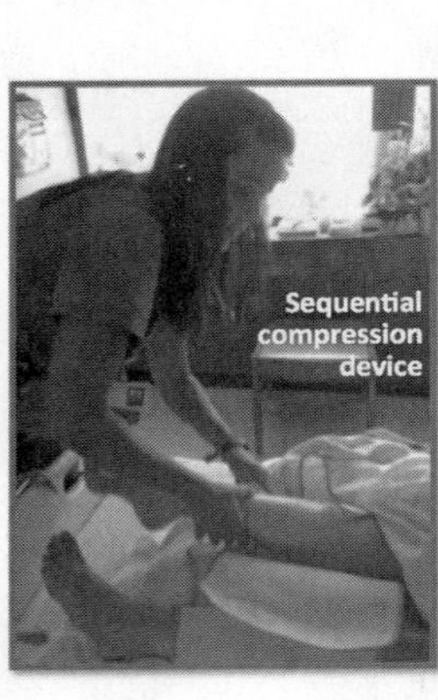

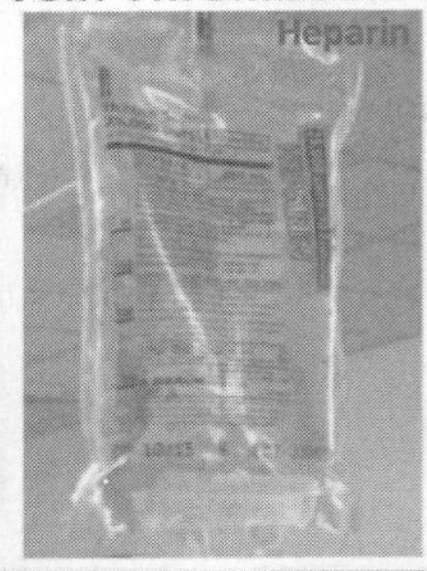

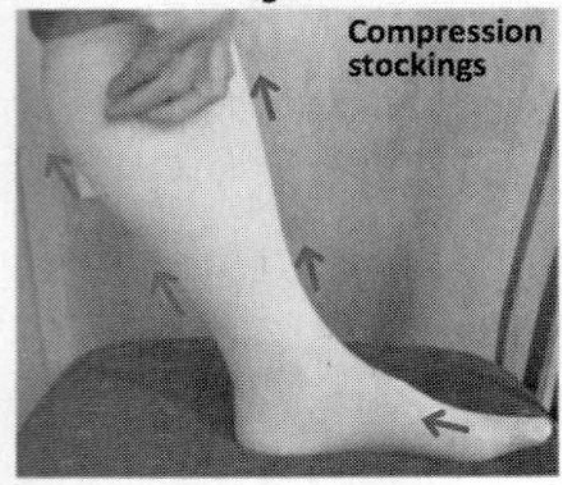

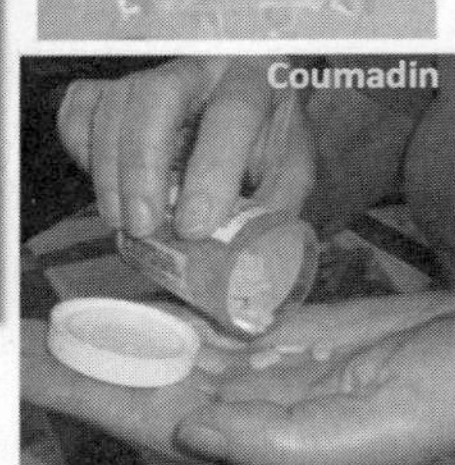

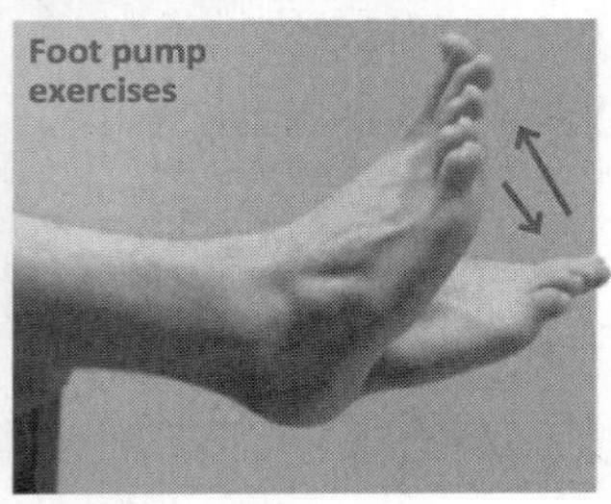

The images show five methods for preventing deep vein (venous) thrombosis (DVT) and life-threatening pulmonary embolism. The methods include sequential compression device, IV heparin, anticoagulant therapy medication (blood thinners, graduated compression stockings, and "foot pump" exercises). Early ambulation is one of the most critical methods.

Sources: Sequential compression device, Courtesy of Sarah Bateman/Nashville, TN; heparin, Courtesy of Sarah Dresen; coumadin, Courtesy of George Kyriakidis/Santa Ana, CA; compression stockings and foot pump, Copyright © 2014, NovEx Novice to Expert Learning, LLC

- Safety and supportive care should include:
  - o Care when moving patients to upright position to avert postural hypotension. Lower the patient's head immediately if dizziness is reported.
  - o Avoid moving the patient if postural hypotension develops; lower or lean the head of the chair back until dizziness dissipates.
  - o Monitor patient for early signs of any never events.
  - o Prevent bladder infections, urinary calculi, and promote good bowel function by ensuring adequate fluid intake.
  - o Remind and/or assist with range of motion exercises to prevent contractures in completely immobile patients.
  - o Anticipate potential for ileus soon after injury. Recognize early reduction or loss of bowel sounds and collaborate to intervene early.
  - o Bladder and bowel management are imperative for comfort and safety. Collaborate with team to develop a schedule for bladder and bowel training.

- Nurses must constantly monitor skin integrity and position the patient to prevent pressure ulcers on all pressure points, as some patients no longer have sensation. Rotation beds can be helpful.

M N EBP
- The indwelling urinary catheter should be removed as soon as possible. In and out catheterization is done as early as possible to begin bladder training. This also reduces the risk of urinary tract infections (Gall, et al., 2008).

M N EBP
- A bowel program is initiated with regular suppositories and stool softeners administered to help facilitate emptying. A daily routine should be established for bowel and bladder, focusing on timing (Gall, et al., 2008).

M N
- Pressure Relief Ankle Foot Orthosis (PRAFO) or similar boots are placed on the feet to prevent foot drop as SCI patients are at high risk.

N EBP
- Skin must be kept dry and intact. Frequent repositioning (with log roll) is needed to prevent skin breakdown (Gall, et al., 2008).

N EBP
- Exquisite nursing care and emotional and psychological support are central in the care of SCI patient and families. Excellent nursing care includes special attention targeted at prevention of complications (e.g., infections from wounds, catheters, invasive procedures; DVT; pneumonia; pressure ulcers; bowel impaction; hazards of immobility), early recognition and intervention of problems, mobilization to the extent possible in collaboration with physical therapy, and hygienic care, to name a few (Gall, et al., 2008).

M N EBP
- Early psychological support and consultation (Gall, et al., 2008).

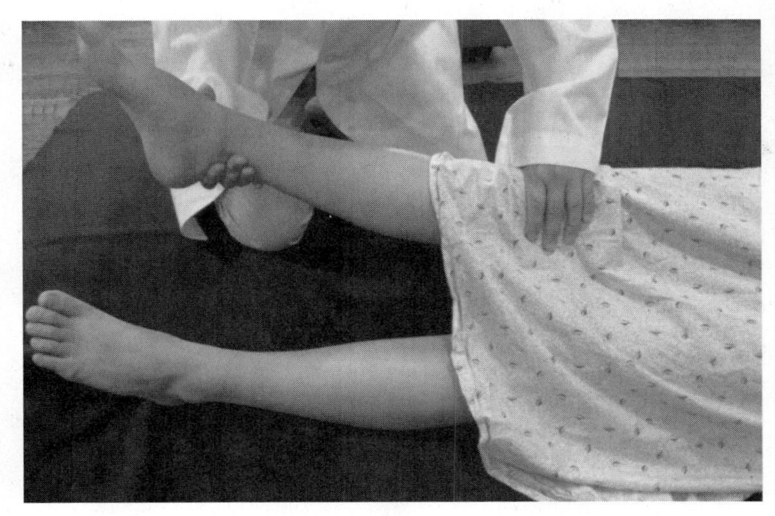

Physical therapy is commonly necessary for rehabilitation to assist patients with mobility after spinal cord injury.
Source: Courtesy of K. Kyriakidis

Concept Check

5. What is the MAP goal to ensure spinal perfusion during the first week post-injury?

A. 60 mmHg
B. 75 mmHg
C. 85 mmHg
D. 100 mmHg

Answer question

Collaborative Interventions (continued)

Psychological Support

M N EBP
- Psychological support to the patient and family is as important as any physical aspect of care (Gall, et al., 2008).

EBP
- The patient with paralysis often goes through the grieving process and may become depressed (Gall, et al., 2008).

M N EBP
- Consideration should be made to include antidepressants if depression is significant or prolonged (Gall, et al., 2008).

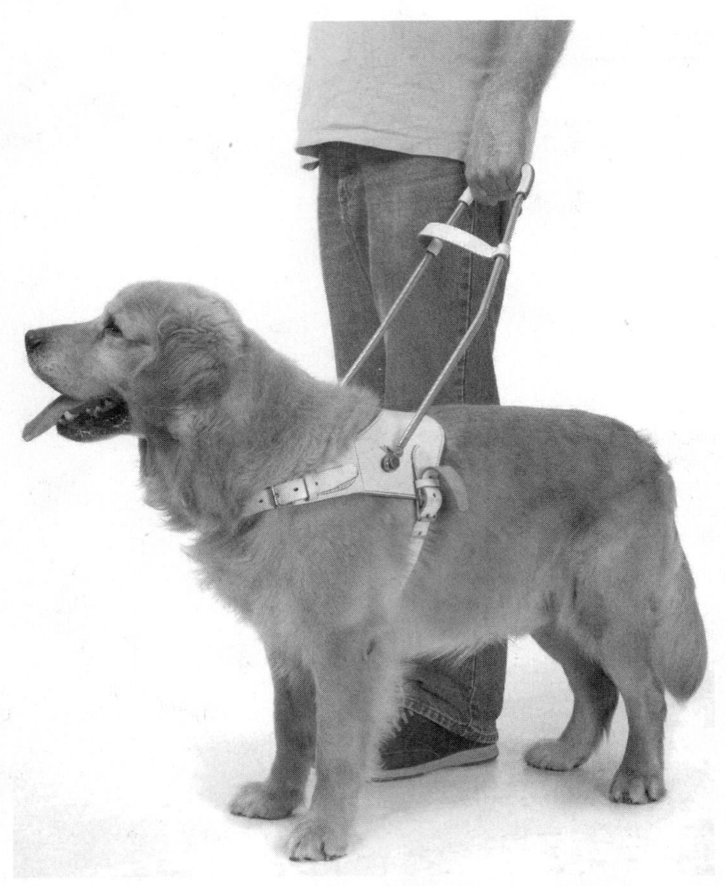

Service dogs can be a tremendous help to those who are disabled, particularly patients following spinal cord injury. Service dogs are specially trained to assist those living with physical disabilities and can assist people with severe depression. Tasks that the animals can perform include pulling a wheelchair or fetching dropped items as examples. Service dogs can also assist to break down social barriers.
Source: Jeroen van den Broek/Fotolia

Autonomic Hyperreflexia Danger

After the initial injury, SCI patients are at risk for the development of autonomic dysreflexia (AD) or hyperreflexia. AD refers to overactivation of the autonomic nervous system that results in a sudden onset of an excessively elevated blood pressure. Carefully monitor patients with lesions above T6 for early warning signs, as they are particularly susceptible in causing this syndrome. This neurologic emergency involves (Gall, et al., 2008):

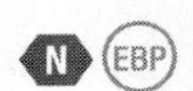

- A noxious stimulus below the level of injury should be suspected and removed if something triggers an extreme vasoconstriction (Gall, et al., 2008). Noxious stimuli can include:
  - o Urinary or rectal retention with distension
  - o Urinary tract infection
  - o Pressure ulcer
  - o Clothing that is too tight or irritating
  - o Sexual overstimulation
  - o Constipation
  - o Hemorrhoids, rectal infection, or inflammation
  - o Menstrual cramping or pain
  - o Labor and delivery
  - o Gastrointestinal infections or inflammation
  - o Bone fracture
  - o Sunburn
  - o Anything that causes the patient pain, irritation or discomfort can be a trigger

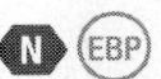

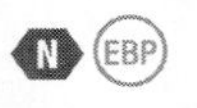

- Treat as a life-threatening complication if there is a distended bowel and/or bladder, pain, skin breakdown, or some other noxious stimulus below the level of injury that triggers AD (Gall, et al., 2008).

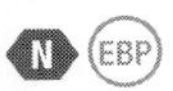

- Intervene quickly if the patient develops the acute onset of hypertension, throbbing headache, blurred vision, nasal congestion, nausea, diaphoresis, and bradycardia (Gall, et al., 2008). Left untreated, death, stroke, and/or seizures can occur.

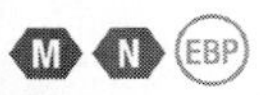

- The BP is excessively elevated and can be life threatening. It must be quickly lowered with IV medications. Removal of the cause is the cure for this disorder (e.g., emptying distended bladder) and can be lifesaving (Gall, et al., 2008)

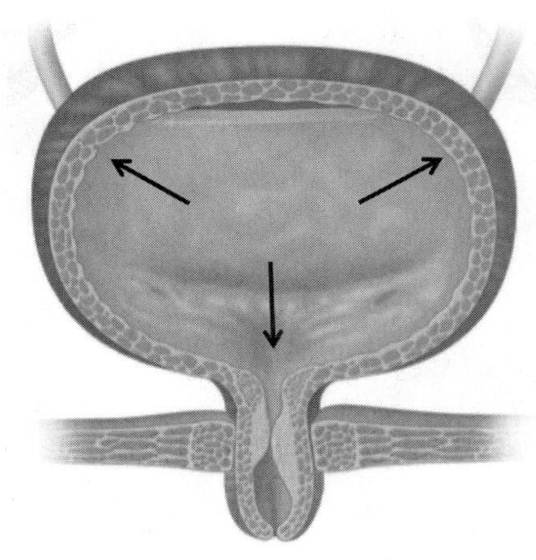

This image shows a full and distended bladder. In most people, a distended bladder poses no particular harm. However, in a patient with spinal cord injury, the distended bladder can initiate autonomic hyperreflexia, which can be life-threatening. While urinary catheterization should be avoided, it may be life-saving in this situation.

- Interventions first target treating the cause:
  - o As a priority, sit the patient up (and teach patient to sit) or elevate the head until BP returns to normal as this naturally helps orthostatically reduce the BP.
  - o Treat the cause, if known or strongly suspected. Talk with patient to gain understanding about related symptoms (e.g., last bladder and bowel emptying).
  - o Alleviate bladder distention immediately as it is a common cause (e.g., empty bladder, immediately insert intermittent catheter, change indwelling catheter if not draining) in about 85% of AD events.
  - o Check the BP every 3 minutes.
  - o Notify the health care provider immediately.
  - o If the BP does not trend down toward normal, remove tight clothing, check bowels or digitally stimulate to encourage emptying the bowel, and observe for any of the potential causes listed earlier to alleviate.
  - o If other interventions do not begin to lower the BP of >150 mmHg or if the BP is severely elevated, administer prescribed medication. A variety of antihypertensive medications are used and include nifedipine, captopril, nitrates, prazosin, and more.
- Never leave a patient with a history of AD alone because there may not be time to alert anyone once AD starts.

Collaborative Interventions (continued)

Chronic SCI Problems

There are many potential problems associated with SCI that may require intervention. Carefully monitor for the most prominent, including:

- Impaired gas exchange and/or ventilatory function
- Pressure ulcers (see animation)

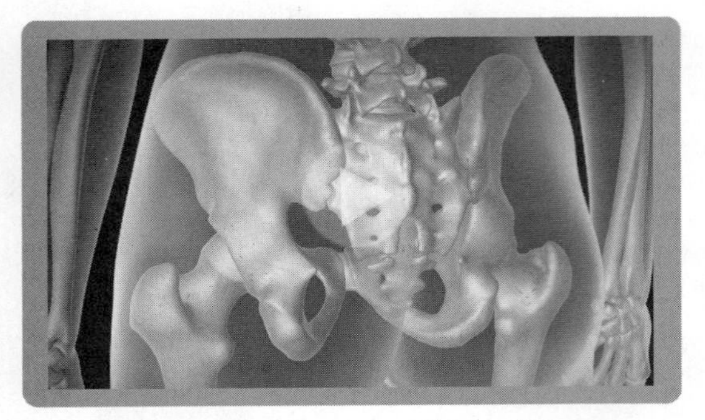

This animation provides an overview of how and where pressure sores or ulcers develop. Each of the four stages and their extent of damage are shown.

- Pneumonia
- Pulmonary embolism and/or DVT
- Orthostatic hypotension
- Altered thermoregulation
- Adynamic ileus
- Neurogenic bowel
- Alteration in genitourinary and/or GI system
- Recurrent urinary tract infections
- Sexual dysfunction
- Spasticity
- Contractures and immobility (see photo)

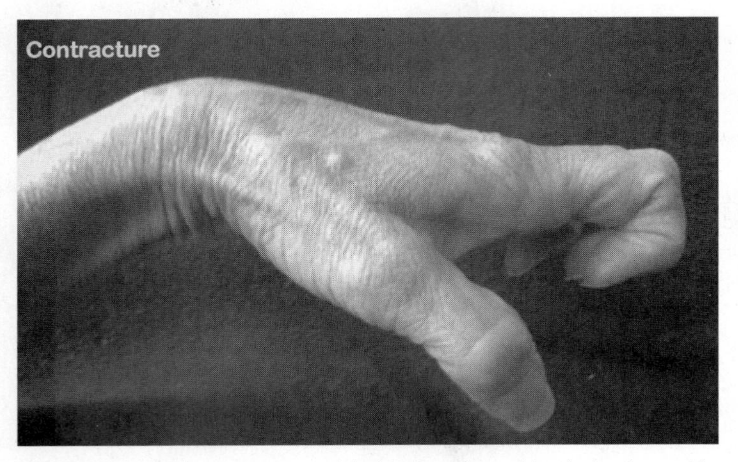

This photo depicts the contractures of the hand muscles, making the hand resemble a claw.

- Heterotopic ossification or formation of new bone in anatomically abnormal sites or tissues
- Grief and loss, altered coping, and body image

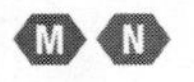
Interventions should be targeted at **prevention**, support, and to the actual problems as they arise.

Concept Check

6. Autonomic dysreflexia is uncommon below which level of spinal cord injury?

A. C2
B. T2
C. T4
D. T6

Answer question

Collaborative Interventions (continued)

Rehabilitation

To optimally improve the patient's outcomes, the patient must participate in all rehabilitation (rehab) services as early as possible.

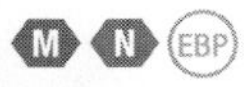

- Evaluation of nervous system function and dysfunction allows the team to plan the best possible rehabilitation for the patient (Gall, et al., 2008).
- The family or significant other should be given referrals to evaluate the various rehabilitation programs available in the area to optimize the patient's recovery (Gall, et al., 2008).

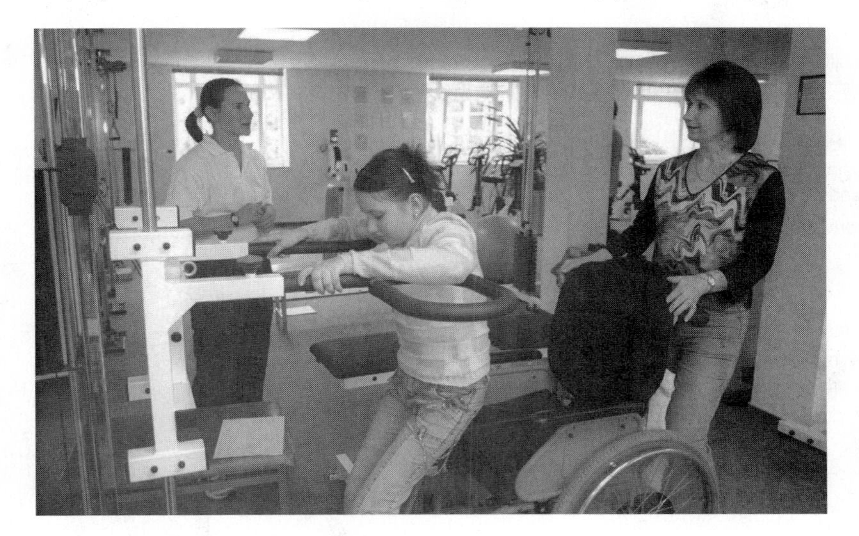

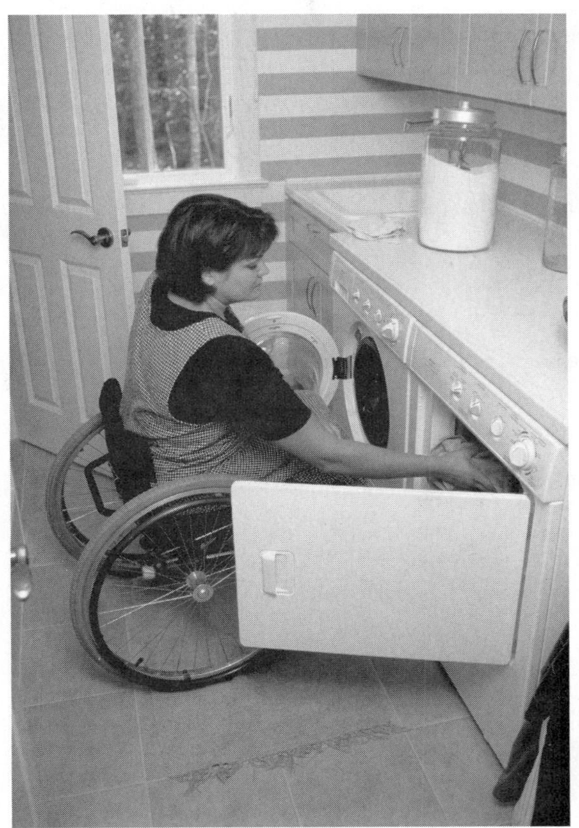

Innovative therapies are developing to involve patients in rehabilitation, exercise and activity at the earliest possible time, even before they can ambulate. Research is being conducted to learn about rehabilitation of the spinal cord injury and develop new treatments. Returning to activities of daily living is part of the rehabilitation process.

Source: (*upper*) Caro/Alamy; (*lower*) Richard Duncan, MRP, Sr. Proj. Mngr. North Carolina State University, The Center for Universal Design (CUD)/Centers for Disease Control and Prevention

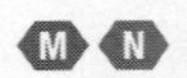

- Assist the patient and family as needed to consider a good match between the patient's needs and the rehab facility. Although the nurse may not assist with all factors to be considered, ensure that a knowledgeable and helpful professional discusses the following issues:
  - o Insurance coverage
  - o Services needed versus available
  - o Specialization in spinal cord injuries
  - o Affiliation with a medical center if needed for complications
  - o Cost of care
  - o Expertise and experience of the rehab team, which should minimally include a physiatrist (physician rehab specialist), specialty-prepared rehab nurses, physical therapist or physiotherapist, occupational therapist, social worker, psychologist, pastoral care, and patient and/or family educator.
  - o Clinicians with extensive knowledge about management of skin protection and healing, bladder and bowel training, autonomic dysreflexia, nutrition, spasticity, pain, sexuality, medications, and psychological and emotional responses to SCI and its consequences.
  - o Long-term care or link with secondary facility if needed
  - o Proximity to home
  - o Ability and staffing to individualize care
  - o Certified to take ventilator-dependent patients if applicable
  - o Link with reintegration programs into the community and/or peer support programs

- Patients commonly transfer to rehab prior to discharge home. The rehab team typically prepares the patient and family for discharge. Education depends on the severity of injury and may include:
  - o Care of the patient's bodily needs
  - o Assistance with activities of daily living
  - o Administration of medications
  - o Referrals to social services, home health, occupational therapist, nutritionist, physical therapist, community resources, and more
  - o Adaptation to assistive devices for mobility (e.g., wheelchair)
  - o Assistance with toileting and/or intermittent catheterization.

Collaborative Interventions (continued)

Collaborative Care

Patients with spinal cord injuries require extensive and comprehensive care that can only be provided by a team with complementary clinical expertise.

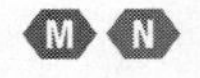

Collaborate to include the team members needed:

- Case manager
- Social worker
- Surgeon (possibly)
- Physical therapist
- Physiatrist and rehabilitation team
- Respiratory therapist
- Psychologist
- Speech therapist (possibly)
- Pastoral care (patient specific)
- Pharmacist
- Nutritionist
- Occupational therapist
- Home care
- Support and community resources (e.g., peer support, caregiver support)

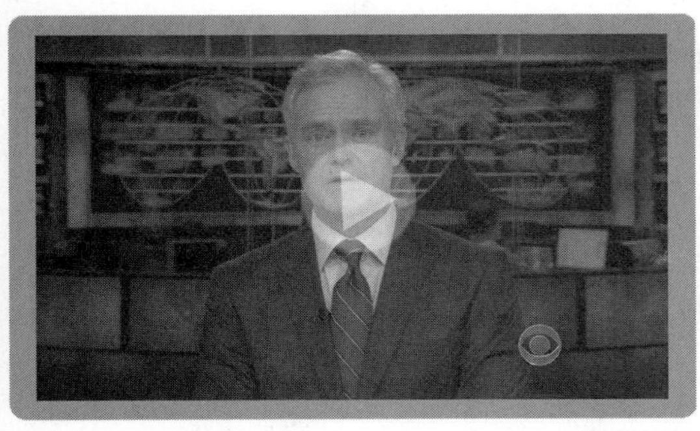

This is a video of a high school athlete who suffered from a life-changing spinal cord injury. The athlete and his mother discuss the resulting disability and hardships.
Source: CBS NEWS

Concept Check

7. When should referral to a rehabilitation program occur for a patient with a spinal cord injury?

A. As early as possible in the patient's recovery
B. As soon as the patient has made optimal physical recovery
C. After the patient has made successful transition from hospital to home
D. As soon as the patient is received in the ED post injury

Answer question

Summary of Interventions

- Stabilizing the patient's spine (collar or backboard) is a critical component of initial management.
- Respiratory, hemodynamic, and surgical stabilization are used as needed to manage acute spinal cord injury.
- Suspect and manage neurogenic shock if hypotension develops during the acute phase of spinal cord injury.
- To optimize the patient's outcome, participation in or transfer to rehabilitation is a critical intervention that should occur as early as the patient is stabilized.
- Attention to bowel and bladder function as well as skin integrity are important in both the acute and chronic phase of spinal cord injury.
- Autonomic hyperreflexia requires immediate elevation of the head and alleviation of the cause to lower the severe elevation in blood pressure caused by a noxious stimulus below the level of injury in a SCI patient.
- Prevention of the numerous hospital-acquired conditions is paramount (e.g., urinary and vascular catheter infections, pressure ulcers, DVT, wound infections, pneumonia).

LO4: Evaluation of Desired Collaborative Care Outcomes

Evaluation and reassessment should reveal attainment of previously established patient outcomes. In summary:

- Patient's spine is stabilized with no further spinal cord damage.
- Patient's respiratory status is at optimal condition allowed by level of injury.
- Patient accurately discusses risks and findings associated with autonomic dysreflexia and has not experienced permanent harm from it, if it occurred.
- Patient's hemodynamics are being maintained within desired limits.
- Patient's skin is intact without decubitus ulcers.
- Patient reports that fear has decreased as more is learned and experienced about managing the condition.
- Patient is an active participant in decision making regarding personal health.

References

Consortium for Spinal Cord Medicine. (2008). Early acute management in adults with spinal cord injury: A clinical practice guideline for health-care professionals. *Journal of Spinal Cord Medicine, 31*(4), 403–479. **www.ncbi.nlm.nih.gov/pmc/articles/PMC2582434/pdf/i1079-0268-31-4-408.pdf**

Krassioukov, A., Eng, J. J., Claxton, G., et al. (2010). Neurogenic bowel management after spinal cord injury: A systematic review of the evidence. *Spinal Cord, 48*(10), 718–733. **www.ncbi.nlm.nih.gov/pmc/articles/PMC3118252/pdf/nihms1767.pdf**

Krassioukov, A., Furlan, J. C., & Fehlings, M. G. (2003). Autonomic dysreflexia in acute spinal cord injury: An under-recognized clinical entity. *Journal of Neurotrauma, 20*(8), 707–716.

Rudyk, J., McKee, L., & Lamale, A. (2014). *Spinal cord injury.* **nursing.advanceweb.com/Continuing-Education/CE-Articles/Spinal-Cord-Injury-2.aspx**

Sarro, A., Anthony, T., Magtoto, R., & Mauceri, J. (2010). Developing a standard of care for halo vest and pin site care including the patient and family education: A collaborative approach among three greater Toronto area teaching hospitlas. *American Association of Neuroscience Nurses, 42*(3), 169–173.

Strever, T. (2014). Care of the patient with cervical spine injury. *OR Nurse 2014, 4*(4), 26–33. **www.nursingcenter.com/lnc/cearticle?tid=1037060**

Clinical Practice Guidelines

Aarabi, B., Hadley, M. N., Dhall, S. S., et al. (2013). Management of acute traumatic central cord syndrome (ATCCS). In Guidelines for the management of acute cervical spine and spinal cord injuries. *Neurosurgery, 72*(Suppl. 2), 195–204. Retrieved from **www.guideline.gov/content.aspx?id=44338&search=spinal+cord+injury+management**

American Dietetic Association. (2009). *Spinal cord injury. Evidence-based nutrition practice guideline.* Chicago, IL: Author. **www.andeal.org/search.cfm?keywords=spinal+cord+injury**

Dhall, S. S., Hadley, M. N., Aarabi, B., et al. (2013). Nutritional support after spinal cord injury. In Guidelines for the management of acute cervical spine and spinal cord injuries. *Neurosurgery, 72*(Suppl. 2), 255–259. **www.guideline.gov/content.aspx?id=44343&search=spinal+cord+injury+management**

Fehlings, M., Vaccaro, A., Wilson, J., et al. (2012). *Early versus delayed decompression for traumatic cervical spinal cord injury: Results of the surgical timing in acute spinal cord injury study (STASCIS).* **www.plosone.org/article/info%3Adoi%2F10.1371%2Fjournal.pone.0032037**

Gall, A., Turner-Stokes, L., & Guideline Development Group. (2008). Chronic spinal cord injury: Management of patients in acute hospital settings. *Royal College of Physicians.* **www.spinal.co.uk/userfiles/Professionals_Portal/RCP_SCI_Guidelines.pdf**

Hadley, M., Walters, B., Grabb, P., et al. (2013). Guidelines for the management of acute cervical spine and spinal cord injuries. *Neurosurgery, 72*(3), 1–259. **www.slideshare.net/INUB/guidelines-for-the-management-of-acute-cervical-spine-and-spinal-cord-injuries-neurosurgery-supplement-march-2013**

Hurlbert, R. J., Hadley, M. N., Walters, B. C., et al. (2013). Pharmacological therapy for acute spinal cord injury. In Guidelines for the management of acute cervical spine and spinal cord injuries. *Neurosurgery, 72* (Suppl. 2), 93–105. **www.guideline.gov/content.aspx?id=44291&search=spinal+cord+injury+management**

Patient Education

American Spinal Injury Association. (2014). *ASIA consumer guidelines for SCI rehabilitation.* **www.asia-spinalinjury.org/rehab/Consumer_Guidelines_SCI_Rehab_Draft_final_1.pdf**

Chin, L. S. (2014). *Spinal cord injuries.* **emedicine.medscape.com/article/793582-overview**

Consortium for Spinal Cord Medicine. (2008). Early Acute Management in Adults with Spinal Cord Injury: A Clinical Practice Guideline for Health-Care 2008. *Paralyzed Veterans of America.* **www.pva.org/site/apps/ka/ec/catalog.asp?c=ajIRK9NJLcJ2E&b=6423003&en=4nKxGFMfH3JGKPPiF2KDJLNsGhLIILMkFbKJIWNALrG&CategoryID=322146**

Mayo Clinic Staff. (2011). *Spinal cord injury.* **www.mayoclinic.com/health/spinal-cord-injury/DS00460/DSECTION=causes**

National Spinal Cord Injury Association. (2014). *Resource center: Ask us spinal cord central.* **www.sci-info-pages.com/factsheets.html**

Learning Outcomes for Neurological Inflammatory and Infectious Disorders

When you complete this lesson, you will be able to:

1. Recognize the clinical relevance of neurological inflammatory and infectious disorders.
2. Consider the pathophysiology, etiology, risk factors, and clinical presentation of neurological inflammatory and infectious disorders that determine the priority patient concerns.
3. Determine the most urgent and important nursing interventions and patient education required in caring for a patient with a neurological inflammatory or infectious disorder.
4. Evaluate attainment of desired collaborative care outcomes for a patient with a neurological inflammatory or infectious disorder.

LO1:

What Are Neurological Inflammatory and Infectious Disorders?

- Infection and inflammation in the central nervous system (CNS) can produce devastating results.
- When bacteria, viruses, or fungi infiltrate the CNS, they can spread infection and cause inflammation to the meninges, brain, spine (from brain to sacrum), and cranial nerves.
- The major infections of the CNS that are included in this lesson are meningitis, encephalitis, and Guillain-Barré Syndrome.

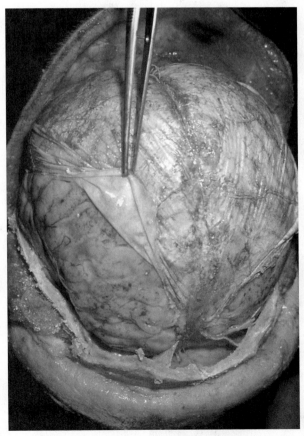

At autopsy, the patient's head was opened and revealed the purulent inflammation of leptomeninges beneath the dura that has been pulled back with hemostats. Note the purulent yellow, greenish gray exudate (pus) covering the brain. Also, the reddish specks are petechial hemorrhages caused by the bacterial infection.
Source: Centers for Disease Control and Prevention

LO1:

What Is Meningitis?

- Meningitis is an inflammation and infection of the membranes (known as meninges) covering the brain and the spinal cord.
- The meninges offer protection for the brain and spinal cord.
- Inflammation can cause edema that can trigger classic symptoms, including seizures.
- Of the pathogenic causes, bacteria are typically the most serious, life-threatening, and urgent.
- Some forms of meningitis are highly contagious.

LO1:

Clinical Relevance: Meningitis

- Recognizing meningitis is important because it can cause life-threatening conditions.
- Intervening with prompt treatment reduces morbidity and mortality in this potential emergency condition.
- Despite recovery from some types of meningitis, morbidity includes severe damage to organs and limbs in 20% of people.
- *Neisseria meningitidis* (epidemic meningitis or meningococcus) is contagious and can spread rapidly and extensively. It is important to be aware of appropriate isolation procedures and chemoprophylaxis (treating close contacts with antibiotics to prevent spreading of disease).

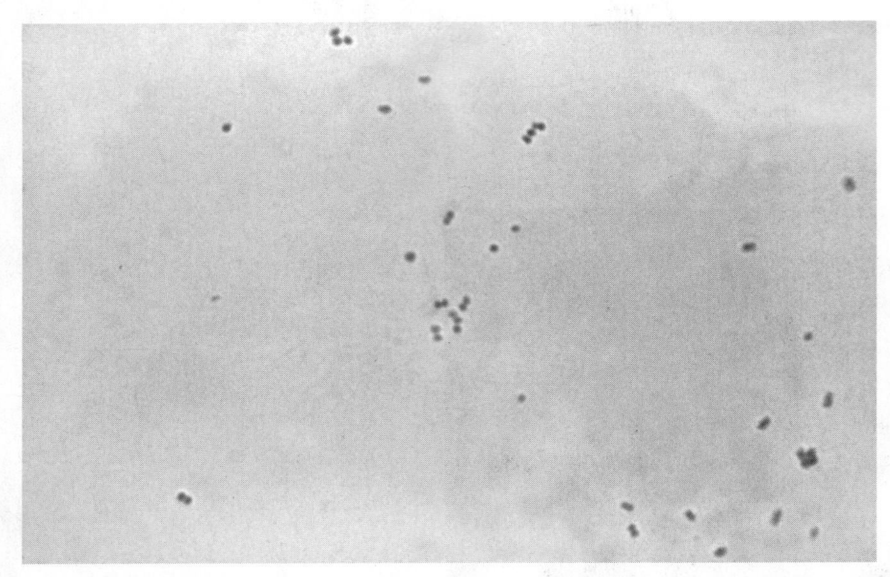

Meningitis may be caused by *Neisseria meningitidis* (meningococcus) bacterium. It is responsible for life-threatening sepsis and a major cause of childhood and adult death. This gram-negative bacteria appears upon gram staining.
Source: Centers for Disease Control and Prevention

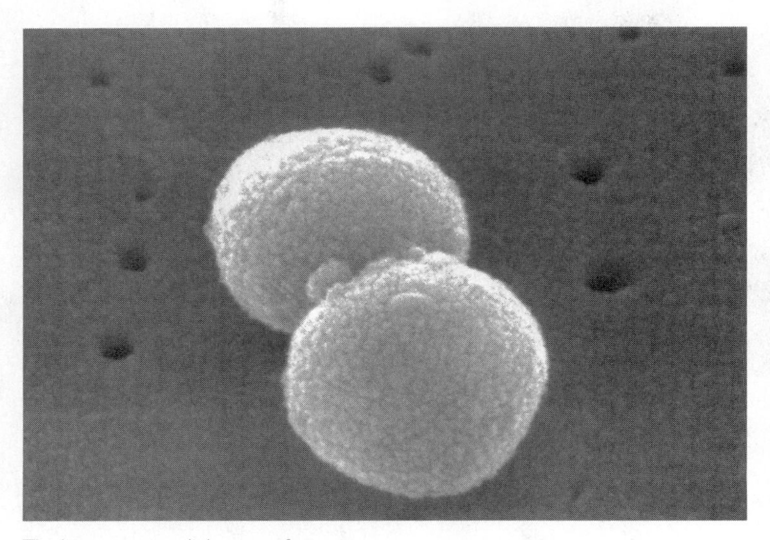

The bacterium is a diplococcus form.
Source: Dr. Richard Facklam/Janice Haney Carr/Centers for Disease Control and Prevention

- Approximately 4,100 patients with 500 deaths occur yearly in the United States while 1.2 million patients contract bacterial meningitis worldwide. Death occurs in 70% of patients with no treatment.
- Fungal meningitis is uncommon.
- Unlike other causes, viral meningitis is typically less severe and can resolve without treatment unless the patient is very young, very old, or has a weak immune system.

LO2:

Pathophysiology: Meningitis

- The pathogenesis of meningitis is that a pathogen (bacteria, virus, or fungus), typically, crosses the blood–brain barrier.
- The most common bacteria that cross the blood–brain barrier are *Streptococcus pneumoniae*, *Neisseria meningitides* (also known as meningococcal meningitis), and *Haemophilus influenzae*.

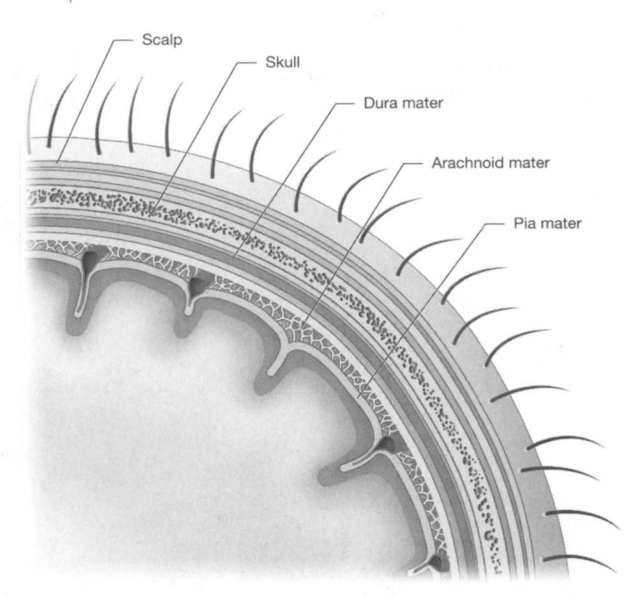

The drawing shows a section of the normal brain with the meningeal layers: dura mater, arachnoid mater, and pia mater. These layers encase the sensitive nerves and blood vessels covering the surface of the brain.

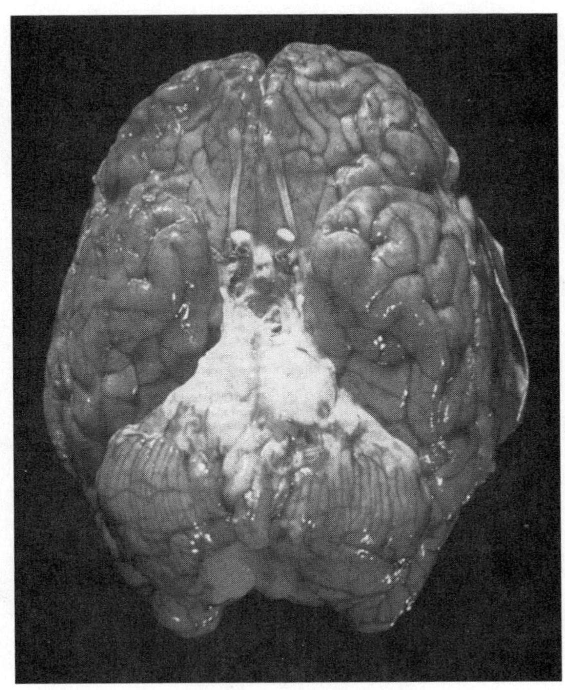

Bacterial meningitis is shown with the purulent and copious exudate. Note the dark burgundy blood vessels that reflect severe vascular congestion with venous thrombosis.
Source: Centers for Disease Control and Prevention

- The bacteria, virus, or fungus usually enter the CNS through open wounds, mucous membranes, infected tissue, or are introduced during a break in sterile technique during surgery (iatrogenic).
- Other means include open skull fractures, cerebrospinal fluid (CSF) leaks, sinusitis, otitis media, osteomyelitis, bloodborne (bacteremia), and septic emboli (e.g., from bacterial endocarditis).
- The pathogen then invades the subarachnoid space.
- When bacteria then enter the CNS (crossing through the blood–brain barrier), replication and infection commences.
- The pathogens activate the immune system. The complex immune reaction (e.g., increased white blood cells, cytokine release, complement) is initiated.
- The meninges become inflamed and cause the clinical signs and symptoms due to increased blood–brain barrier permeability with consequent edema, reduced cerebral blood flow with ischemia, white blood cells binding to capillaries with extravasation, and increased reactive oxygen species that cause cellular damage.
- The continued replication of bacteria with the accompanying immune response leads to cerebral edema, infarctions of the brain, hydrocephalus, and increased intracranial pressure (ICP).
- The patient's clinical presentation may differ, depending on the organism causing the meningitis.

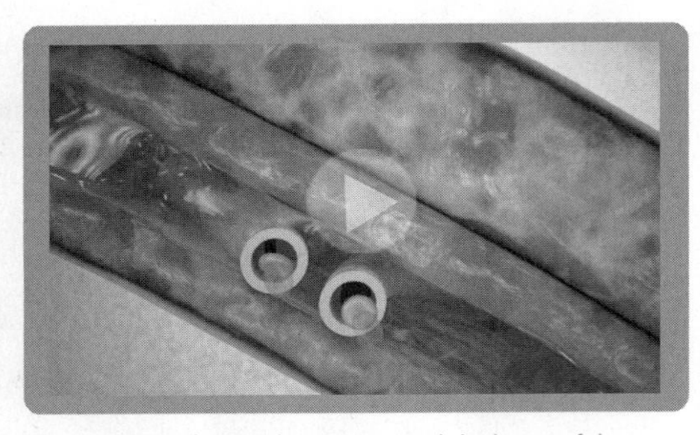

This animation depicts the anatomy and the layers of the meninges that cover the brain and spinal cord. It shows how viruses might spread, infect, and cause viral meningitis. The symptoms of viral meningitis between children and adults and treatments for the symptoms of viral meningitis are discussed.

LO2:

Risk Factors: Meningitis

- Age:
  - o Viral: young children
  - o Bacteria: 1.5–25 years old
  - o Older adults
- Crowded living conditions (e.g., college dorms, child care centers, military barracks) increase the risk of rapid spread.
- Defects in the immune system
- Infectious conditions adjacent to the CNS (e.g., sinusitis, otitis, mastoiditis)
- Bacteremia from conditions like endocarditis
- Trauma with head injury or skull fracture
- Post-splenectomy
- Recent neurosurgical interventions
- Pregnancy

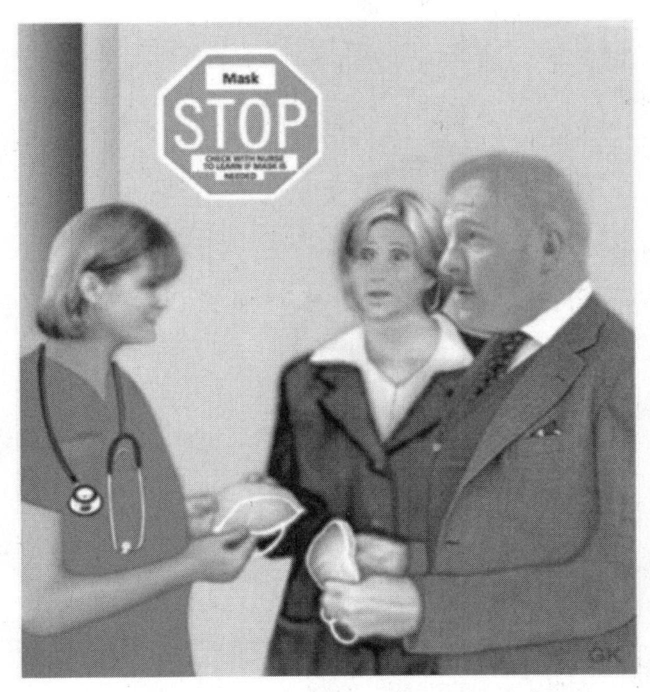

Infection control precautions should be implemented with all visitors for patients with or suspected of meningitis.
Source: Courtesy of George Kyriakidis/Santa Ana, CA

LO2:

Causes: Meningitis

- Bacteria that most frequently cause meningitis include *Neisseria meningitidis* (meningococcus), *Listeria*, *Haemophilus influenzae*, and *Streptococcus pneumoniae* (pneumococcus)
- Of the bacteria, *Neisseria* carries the highest mortality risk and is considered to be the most devastating to survivors.
- Viruses that most commonly cause meningitis include enterovirus, herpes simplex, and arboviruses (e.g., West Nile).
- The most common fungus to produce meningitis is *Cryptococcus neoformans*.
- Conditions that cause bacteremia (e.g., sinusitis, infective endocarditis)

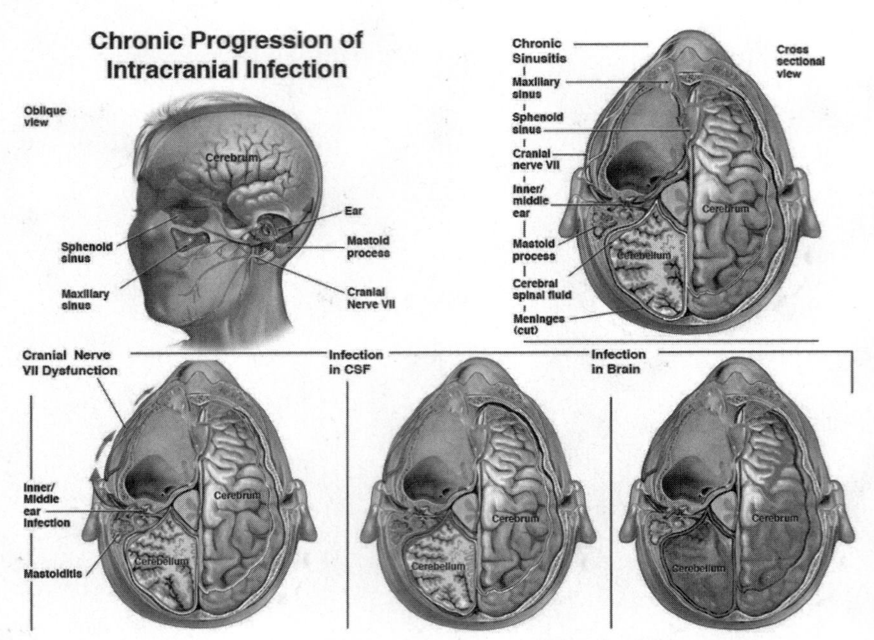

This exhibit features four views of the head and reveals the ear anatomy, the cerebellum and temporal lobes with surrounding meninges, sinuses, and mastoid regions. They illustrate how organisms can cause meningitis: Initial sinusitis with an arrow showing infection spreads from sinuses into inner ear. Arrows show the infection spreading into surrounding bone reflecting mastoiditis. Redness surrounding the meninges shows intracranial spread of infection and infection within the cerebrospinal fluid. Eventually, a massive colonization of the infection occurs around the brain.

Source:

- Nonpathogenic causes can include cancer, particular drugs (e.g., NSAIDs, methotrexate), inflammatory conditions (e.g., sarcoidosis), and physical injury.

Concept Check

1. **Which cause of meningitis has the highest mortality rate?**
   A. *Streptococcus pneumoniae*
   B. *Neisseria meningitides*
   C. *Haemophilus influenzae*
   D. Herpes simplex

Answer question

LO2:

Assessment Findings: Meningitis

- Patients with bacterial meningitis complain of a triad: headache, stiff neck, and photophobia. Most have general malaise but normal sensorium.
- Objective signs of meningitis include fever, nuchal rigidity (stiff neck), cranial nerve palsies, such as a III or VI nerve palsy, and changes in motor strength in severe cases.

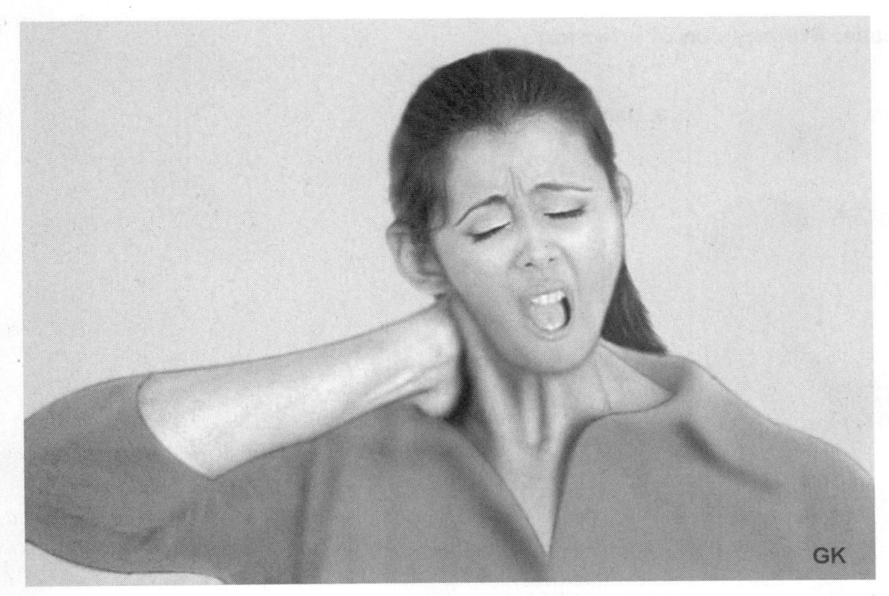

Nuchal rigidity or neck stiffness is seen in this child with meningitis.
Source: Courtesy of George Kyriakidis/Santa Ana, CA

- Findings that point more clearly to meningitis are combinations of:
  - o The triad above
  - o Non-blanching skin rash
  - o Altered mental status such as confusion, disorientation, and impaired memory
  - o Unusual skin color
  - o Positive Kernig's sign, which is inability to completely extend the leg when supine with thigh flexed toward abdomen
  - o Positive Brudzinski's sign, which is bending the head and neck forward causing flexion of the knees and hips
  - o Back rigidity
  - o Seizures
  - o Hypotension
  - o Shock
- General nonspecific findings include nausea, vomiting, tachycardia, lethargy, irritability, headache, loss of appetite, myalgia, chills, diarrhea, and dyspnea.
- In **meningococcal meningitis**, 50% of patients have a red or purple pinprick, non-blanching rash that progresses to purple blotches or purpura. The endotoxins released by the organisms damage the vessels and cause disseminated intravascular coagulation (DIC).
- Petechiae and purpura are primarily located on the trunk, lower extremities, mucous membranes, and conjunctiva. If the microvascular circulation is not ameliorated, tissue necrosis can ensue and gangrene can develop.
- **Viral meningitis** patients present with a milder clinical presentation. Besides general aches and malaise, the patient may have fever, headache, photophobia, and nausea and/or vomiting.
- **Fungal meningitis** patients complain of similar symptoms as those with the viral presentation.
- Meningitis can rapidly progress and produce systemic and devastating sequelae. Vasculitis is seen as petechiae and purpura, indicating DIC. Tissue necrosis can follow. As meningitis worsens, the brain and spinal tissues are damaged and can lead to death.

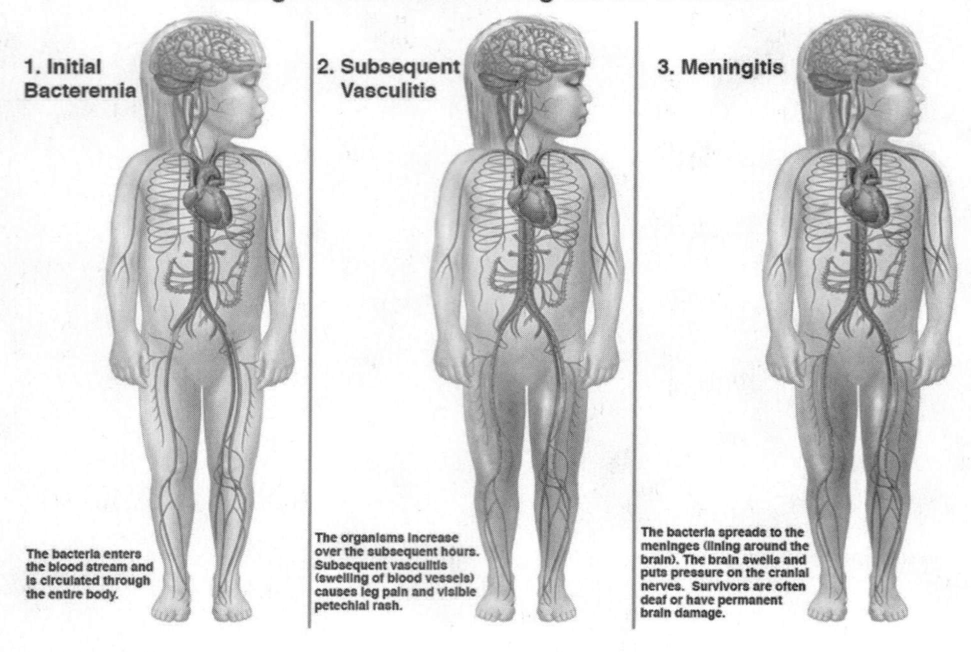

Meningococcal Disease: Progression of Infection
1. Initial Bacteremia
2. Subsequent Vasculitis
3. Meningitis
The bacteria enters the blood stream and is circulated through the entire body.
The organisms increase over the subsequent hours. Subsequent vasculitis (swelling of blood vessels) causes leg pain and visible petechial rash.
The bacteria spreads to the meninges (lining around the brain). The brain swells and puts pressure on the cranial nerves. Survivors are often deaf or have permanent brain damage.

Meningococcal disease: Progression of infection.
Source: © 2014 Nucleus Medical Media, All rights reserved

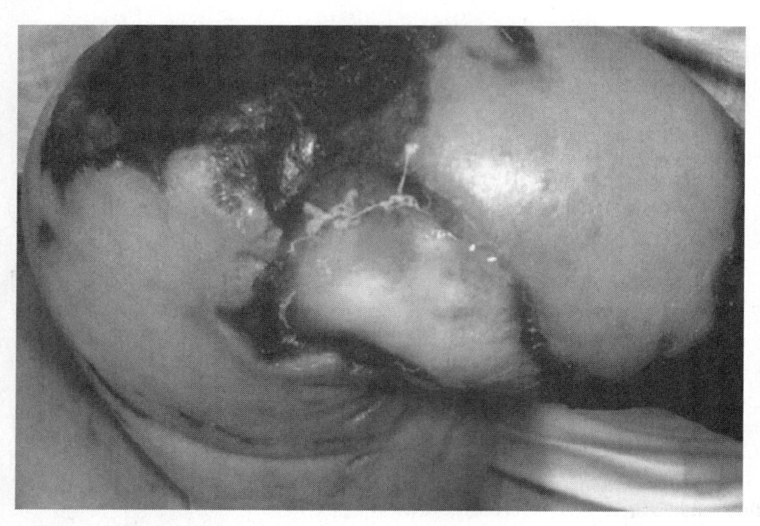

A patient with meningococcemia shows the devastating consequences of severe vasculitis. She developed DIC that resulted in widespread tissue necrosis, as seen here on the shoulder. This patient was unable to recover.
Source: Mr. Gust/Centers for Disease Control and Prevention

LO2:

Diagnostics: Meningitis

Cerebrospinal fluid (CSF) analysis combined with the clinical features and cultures provide the diagnosis of meningitis.

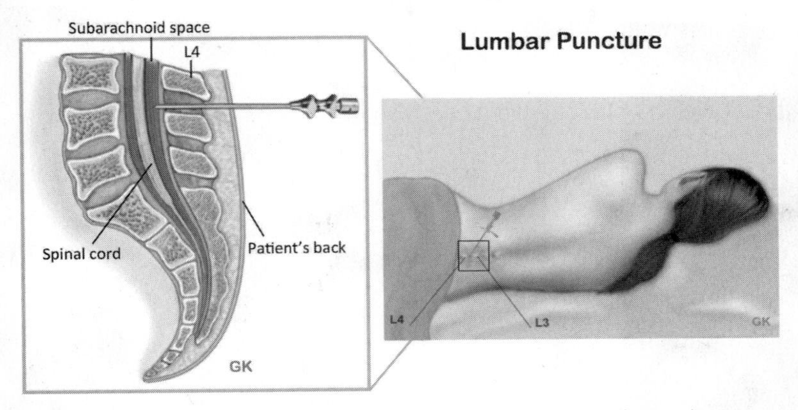

This image depicts a lumbar puncture that involves insertion of a needle into the spine in the subarachnoid space and the aspiration of CSF. The fluid can then be tested and cultured for infectious invaders.
Source: Courtesy of George Kyriakidis/Santa Ana, CA

Cerebrospinal Fluid

- After completing a physical assessment, the physician performs a lumbar puncture to evaluate the CSF.
- In normal CSF samples, white blood cells (WBCs) are rarely present (0–3 cells per mL).
- In bacterial meningitis, the CSF appears cloudy with 1,000–5,000 WBCs (primarily neutrophils), elevated protein, and a low CSF glucose level.
- In viral meningitis, the WBCs are 50–1,000 with fewer neutrophils, a protein count that is slightly elevated, and normal CSF glucose.
- Fungal meningitis has fewer WBCs with no neutrophils, slight elevation in protein, and low CSF glucose.

Comparison of Assessment Findings in Meningitis

Findings	Normal	Bacterial	Viral	Fungal
CSF sample	Clear	Cloudy	Clear	Clear/cloudy
WBCs (cell/mL)				
Lymphocyte	≤5	<100	<100	Few
Neutrophil	0	1,000–5,000	50–1,000	0
Protein (g/L)	<0.4	>1.0	0.4–1	0.4–1
Glucose (CSF:blood)	≥0.6	<0.4	≥0.6	<0.4

- CSF is sent to microbiology for gram stain and cultures to determine the specific organism.
- The CSF cultures for bacteria, virus, and fungus along with specialized tests, such as polymerase chain reaction (PCR) for *Neisseria meningitides* or other molecular diagnostic testing, can often identify the specific pathogen causing meningitis (see photo).

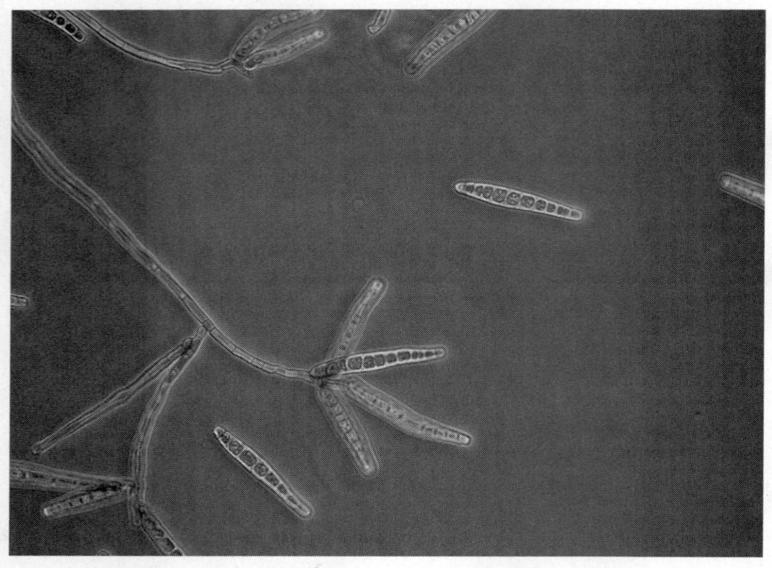

The fungus Exserohilum rostratum was cultured and responsible for the rare meningitis outbreak nationwide in Fall 2012.
Source: Centers for Disease Control and Prevention

Concept Check

2. The triad of symptoms associated with bacterial meningitis include headache, stiff neck, and what other finding?

A. Confusion

B. Loss of sense of smell

C. Pustular rash

D. Photophobia

Answer question

Priority Patient Concerns and Desired Collaborative Care Outcomes: Meningitis

Prior to caring for patients with meningitis, it is important to prioritize the patient's concerns that must guide the nursing care plan and interventions. Care for the patient is ordered and organized in accordance with the patient's priority and urgent needs. Desired collaborative care outcomes in patients with meningitis typically include:

1. Patient will be free from pain or experience a reduction in pain.
2. Patient will remain injury-free.
3. Patient's neurological condition will stabilize and improve with treatment.
4. Patient's mobility will not decline past baseline and will improve with treatment.
5. Patient's intracranial pressure will remain within desired range.

Considering these important care outcomes, prepare a list of the major 3–6 priority patient concerns or nursing diagnoses for patients with meningitis. Be prepared to participate in a discussion of this list and/or to submit them as an assignment, as determined by your faculty. Resources you may find helpful in this assignment can include this lesson, the references, resources on nursing care plans, and standard nursing diagnoses manuals.

LO3:

Collaborative Interventions: Meningitis

Priority Interventions: Antimicrobials

- Patients with meningitis can present with mild symptoms to life-threatening shock. In mild forms of meningitis, the patient may be alert and oriented with normal vital signs.

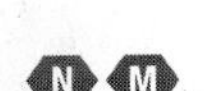

- Promptly see patients with possible meningitis in the emergency department (ED). Isolate them as a precautionary measure to contain the potential spread of the organism. Precautions recommended by the Centers for Disease Control and Prevention (CDC) include:
  - o In epidemic forms (*Neisseria meningitides*): Institute droplet precautions on admission and for 24 hours after administering antimicrobial agents. Also use masks and protect the face during intubation.
  - o In enteroviruses: Take contact precautions with infants and children.
  - o In *Mycobacterium tuberculosis*: Initiate airborne precautions if pulmonary infiltrates exist. Initiate airborne and contact precautions if infectious body fluids are draining.

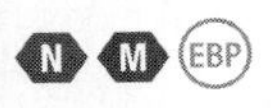

- Obtain blood cultures as quickly as possible so that antimicrobial therapy can be started (Tunkel, et al., 2004).

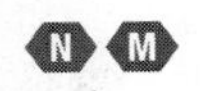

- Start IV fluids to ensure IV access for antibiotics, if hydrated, and to infuse fluids if patient is dehydrated and unable to drink.

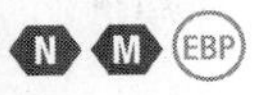

- **Initially treat for meningitis: It is of paramount importance to initiate IV antimicrobial therapy as soon as possible** (Tunkel, et al., 2004). Patients with meningitis are treated with antibiotics until bacterial meningitis is either ruled in or out because the consequences of delay can be severe or death.

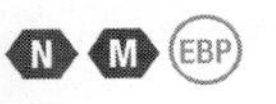

- **If bacterial meningitis, it is recommended that antibiotics be administered within 30 minutes of considering the diagnosis** (Tunkel, et al., 2004):
  - o Vancomycin and ceftriaxone gives broad spectrum coverage for *S. pneumoniae* and *N. meningitides*.
  - o Patients over 50 years of age are more likely to receive ampicillin, vancomycin, and rifampin as well as cefotaxime or ceftriaxone.
  - o Oral antibiotics are not recommended, as the concentration required to treat bacterial meningitis cannot be attained orally.

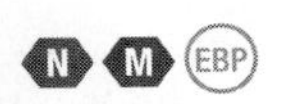

- If uncertain about meningitis, carefully examine and monitor until diagnostics can help confirm the condition. However, collaborate with the health care provider immediately to administer antibiotics if (Cloke, et al., 2010):
  - o A petechial rash begins to spread
  - o Purpura develop
  - o Findings pointing at bacterial meningitis or septicemia manifest
  - o The C-reactive protein or WBC counts (particularly neutrophils) are increased
- Steroids can also be used to treat bacterial meningitis:

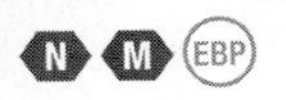

  - o Recommend administering dexamethasone (10 mg IV every 6 hours for 4 days [q6h × 4d]) 15–20 minutes prior to, or simultaneously with, first antibiotic infusion for suspected pneumococcal meningitis (Tunkel, et al., 2004).

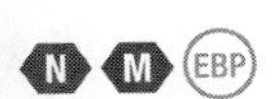

  - o Some physicians give steroids to all patients with bacterial meningitis, continue for 4 days, but discontinue if it is not bacterial meningitis; however, this approach is controversial. Benefit with other bacterial pathogens is unclear. Research suggests discontinuing steroids if the meningitis is other than pneumococcal meningitis (Tunkel, et al., 2004) as steroids are not benign.

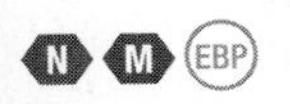

- If viral meningitis is suspected, administration of acyclovir may be indicated (usually for herpes simplex meningitis) (Steiner, et al., 2010).

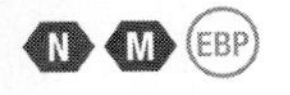

- If fungal meningitis is diagnosed, administer amphotericin B with or without flucytosine IV (Pappas, et al., 2009).

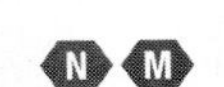

- Simultaneous with other interventions, collaborate with the public health department to control infection to protect the public. This action is required by law:
  - o All the patient's contacts are notified and treated if *Neisseria meningitidis* is the culprit organism.
  - o The source or problem is investigated if the infection is not clearly explainable.

Collaborative Interventions: Meningitis (continued)

Meningitis

Urgent administration of antibiotics is critical in patients with bacterial meningitis. Following or in conjunction with antibiotic administration, care of these patients require:

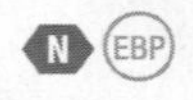

- Closely monitor and assess any patient suspected of having meningitis at least hourly (e.g., vital signs, level of consciousness, oxygen saturations, and capillary refill)(Cloke, et. al., 2010).

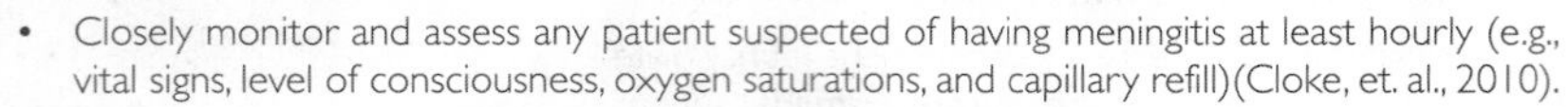

- Implement hospital's infection control precautions, depending on the cause of the meningitis.

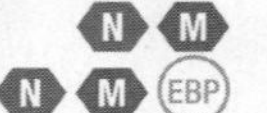

- Closely monitor the patient's neurological status for signs of increased ICP. If the patient has increased ICP, hydrocephalus should be suspected. The neurosurgeon may need to place a ventriculostomy ICP catheter in order to drain the CSF (Cloke, et al., 2010) and alleviate increased pressure on the brain.

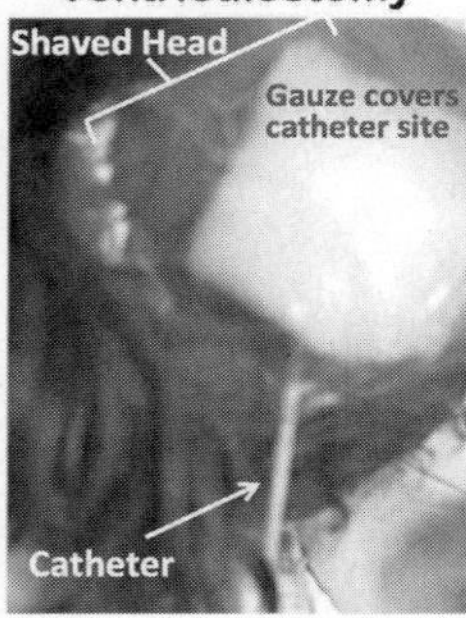

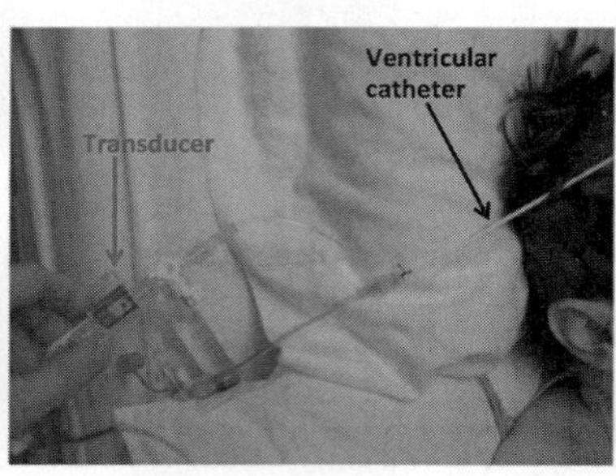

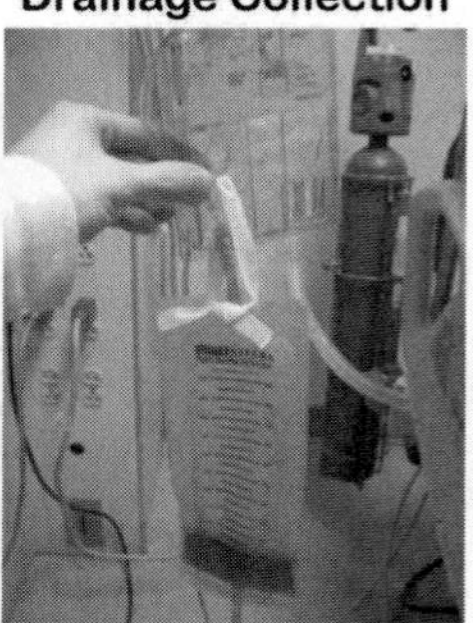

This series of images shows a ventriculostomy with pressure transducer (for monitoring and drainage) to alleviate the fluid buildup in the brain. From left to right, the illustrations show: a) ventricular catheter insertion site where the patient's hair was shaved, b) the pressure transducer system to monitor pressure, and c) the drainage system to collect the CSF to lower cerebral pressure.

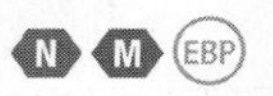
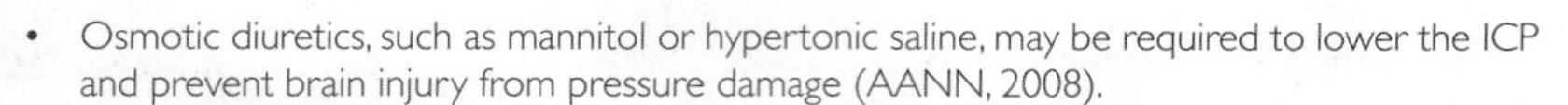

- Osmotic diuretics, such as mannitol or hypertonic saline, may be required to lower the ICP and prevent brain injury from pressure damage (AANN, 2008).

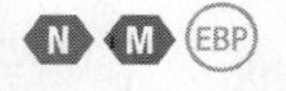

- Due to the increased risk of seizures, consider administering anticonvulsants in some patients with meningitis for a period of time (Cloke, et al., 2010).

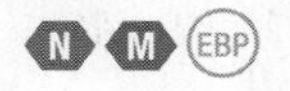

- Institute seizure precautions to ensure safety and protect the patient from injury (Cloke, et al., 2010).

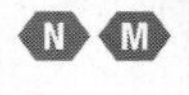

- Monitor for and treat fever and pain, such as headaches, with medication as prescribed. Fever may persist for 4–6 days or longer.
- Monitor for complications as the meningitis patient is at risk for problems such as disseminated intravascular coagulation, Waterhouse-Friderichsen syndrome (adrenal hemorrhage), or cerebral edema.
- In patients with severe meningitis and who are at risk for meningococcal septicemia, anticipate, monitor, and intervene if the following develop: acidosis, hypotension, hypoglycemia, hypokalemia, hypocalcemia, anemia, or coagulopathy.
- Avoid administration of activated protein C in patients with meningococcal septicemia.
- Prolonged hospitalization makes the patient with meningitis vulnerable to complications associated with immobility and multiple invasive therapies. Prevention of complications requires attentiveness. Implement all safety and preventive measures to avoid the multiple potential never events that include:
  - Ventilator-associated pneumonia
  - Catheter-associated urinary tract infection
  - Blood reaction from incompatibility
  - Intravenous catheter-related air embolism
  - Deep vein thrombosis (DVT) and pulmonary embolism
  - Glycemic events
  - Falls
  - Pressure ulcer
  - Wound site infection
  - Vascular catheter-associated infection

- Discuss and recommend the meningococcal vaccine, particularly for adolescents and young adults. The CDC recommends meningococcal vaccinations as an important preventative measure. College students and military persons, living in more crowded spaces like dorms or barracks, are at higher risk (Cloke, et al., 2010; Tunkel, et al., 2004).

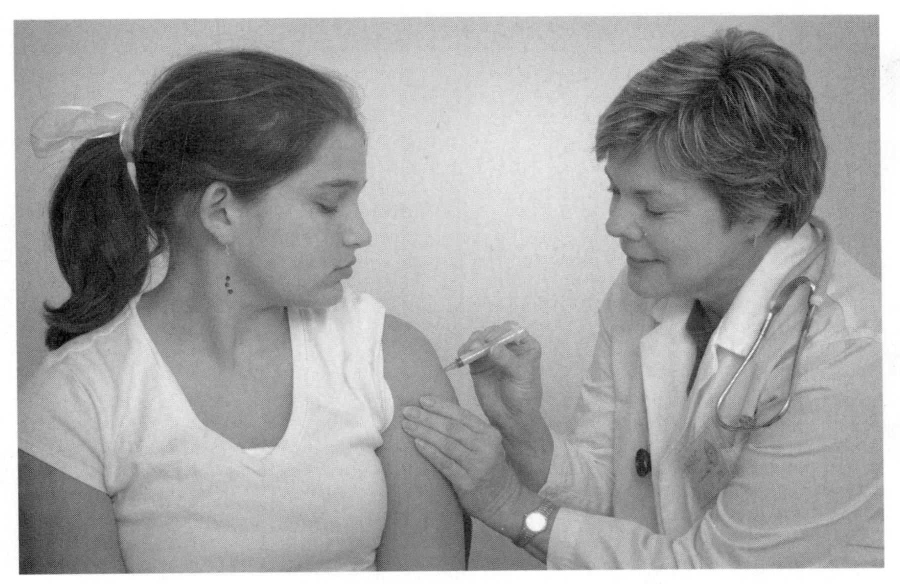

Vaccinations against meningococcal meningitis can help protect against a potentially deadly condition.
Source: Centers for Disease Control and Prevention/Judy Schmidt

N
- Comfort measures should be considered, depending on the patient's condition:
  - o Limit visitors and unnecessary stimulation if noise and stress make the patient uncomfortable.
  - o Maintain a quiet room if the patient experiences phonophobia (noise sensitivity) to reduce agitation and improve comfort.
  - o Maintain a dimly lit room if the patient experiences photophobia to reduce agitation and improve comfort.
  - o Cluster nursing interventions to minimize interrupted rest and reduce activity.
  - o Frequent linen changes may be needed if patient is very diaphoretic.
  - o Provide ongoing emotional support to patient and family. Recovery can be prolonged.

Collaborative Interventions: Meningitis (continued)

Shock Associated with Meningitis

N
- Vigilantly monitor for manifestations of shock (see the Shock NovE-lesson) and mobilize the team for urgent intervention if the patient shows early signs and symptoms of deterioration.

N EBP
- If the patient presents in shock with an altered level of consciousness and accompanying hypotension, call the Rapid Response Team and initiate a sepsis protocol (see the Sepsis NovE-lesson)(Cloke, et al., 2010). Care should be taken with fluid replacement so as not to overhydrate due to the risk of increased ICP and cerebral edema.

N M EBP
- Management of meningitis-associated shock is similar to other types of shock:
  - o Support perfusion: Fluids and vasopressors may be required (e.g., normal saline and norepinephrine).
  - o Protect the patient's oxygenation using intubation or BiPap, as indicated (Cloke, et al., 2010).

N M
- Provide or continue supportive care and medications such as antipyretics, analgesic agents, sedation agents, anticonvulsants, and antibiotics as needed.

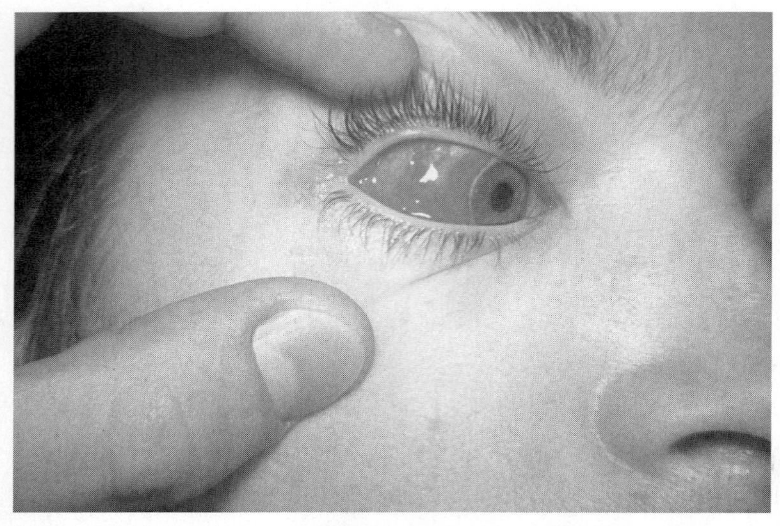

Subconjunctival hemorrahage.
Source: Centers for Disease Control and Prevention/Dr. Thomas F. Sellers/Emory University

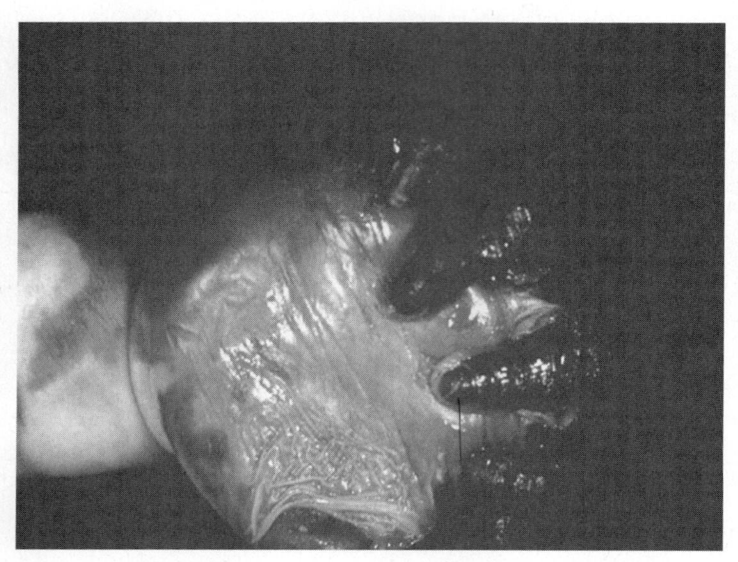

Acute meningococcemia is a severe, life-threatening illness marked by fever, vomiting, hypotension, meningitis, DIC, and other systemic symptoms. Classic dermatological findings are a stellate purpura with a central gunmetal gray color, which progresses into tissue necrosis, DIC, and gangrene (black), as seen here on the fingers of the hand.
Source: Mr. Gust/Centers for Disease Control and Prevention

Patient Education

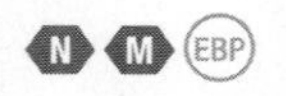

- Prior to discharge, discuss the patient's long-term needs, particularly neurological, orthopedic, psychological, social, renal, and/or cutaneous. Learning disabilities and seizures may result (Cloke, et al., 2010). Collaborate with team, particularly case manager, to link patient to needed resources.

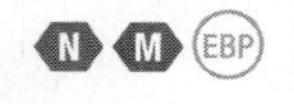

- Collaborate with the health care provider to have a formal audiological assessment done as significant-to-profound deafness is possible. Should ideally be completed prior to discharge (Cloke, et al., 2010).

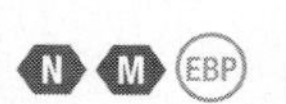

- Prior to infection, vaccinations provide the best protection in preventing bacterial meningitis (Cloke, et al., 2010; Tunkel, et al., 2004).

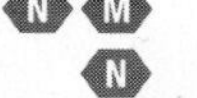

- After meningitis, immunizations against other causes of meningitis should be considered.

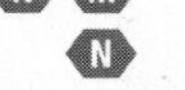

- Follow up with the health care provider after discharge.

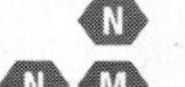

- Patients with viral meningitis, similar to the flu (viral in origin), typically recover in 7–10 days. Care for patients with viral meningitis include:
  - o Plenty of rest
  - o Increased fluid intake
  - o Good nutrition
  - o Acetaminophen or ibuprofen to treat fever, headache, and pain
  - o Monitoring for symptoms (e.g., irritability, fatigue, difficulty concentrating, uncoordinated movement, weakness, spasms) for gradual improvement within a week.

LO4:

Evaluation of Desired Collaborative Care Outcomes: Meningitis

Evaluation and reassessment should reveal attainment of previously established patient outcomes. In summary:

- Patient is calm and expresses decrease in pain level.
- Patient experiences no injury related to decreased sensory perception.
- Patient's neurological condition is back to baseline.
- Patient is returning to pre-illness level of mobility.
- Patient's intracranial pressure is within desired range.

LO1:

What Is Encephalitis?

- Encephalitis is an acute inflammation of the brain or brain parenchyma.
- Encephalitis differs from meningitis because meningitis is inflammation of the covering of the brain. However, some patients develop both.
- Patients develop a flu-like illness, but a severe headache can accompany it.
- Infectious encephalitis is caused by bacteria, virus, or fungus. The most common causative agent is viral.

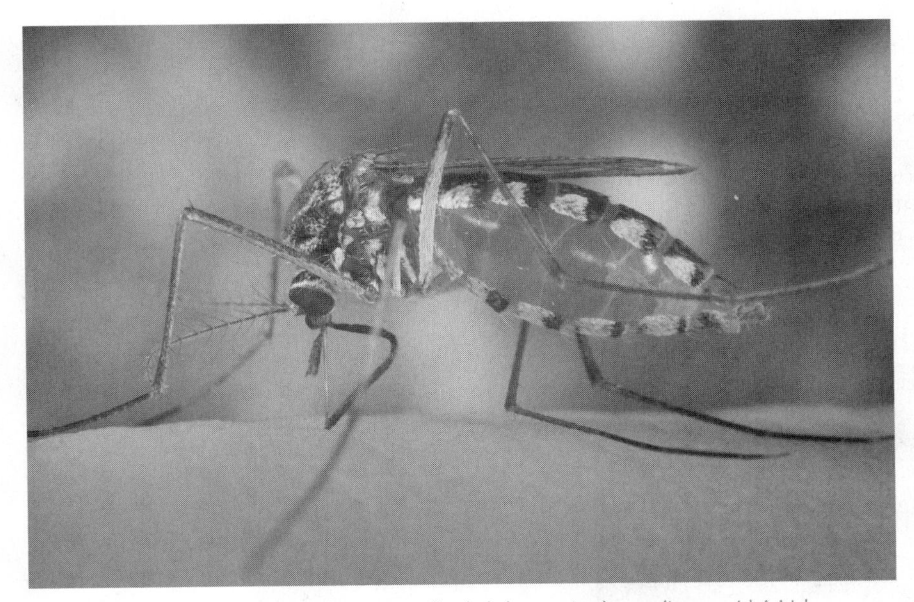

West Nile encephalitis is a potentially severe and/or lethal mosquito-borne disease with initial flu-like symptoms such as fever, nausea, vomiting, headache and diarrhea. Most have some neuro features of mild to severe encephalitis. Here, the red belly reveals blood that is visible through the translucent abdomen.

Source: Centers for Disease Control and Prevention/Frank Collins, PhD.

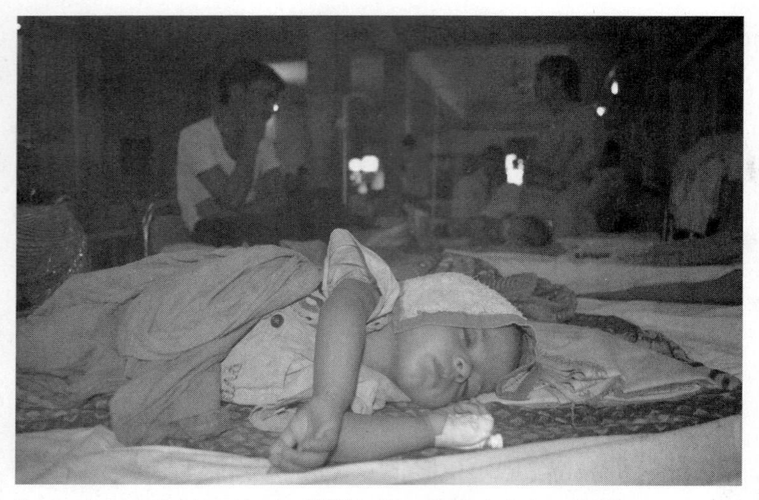

During the encephalitis epidemic of 2012 in Uttar Pradesh, India, a child has succumbed to encephalitis. Note the neck and body stiffness. The death toll rose into the hundreds after admitting over 2,500 patients to hospitals. The yearly monsoons bring encephalitis to all the surrounding regions. Children and the elderly are most affected.
Source: STRDEL/AFP/Getty Images

LO1:

Clinical Relevance: Encephalitis

- Encephalitis is a cause of seizures, coma, permanent brain damage, and death.
- Vectors (such as mosquitoes) are pervasive worldwide and spread organisms that can result in serious illness and possibly death. Control of vectors can reduce the incidence.
- The United States reports approximately 10,000–20,000 cases of encephalitis yearly. Approximately 50% of those patients remain undiagnosed.
- One of the major causes of encephalitis is herpes simplex virus. Early administration of the antiviral acyclovir (or antimicrobials for other invaders) can reduce morbidity and mortality.

Encephalitis with Unexpected Cyst

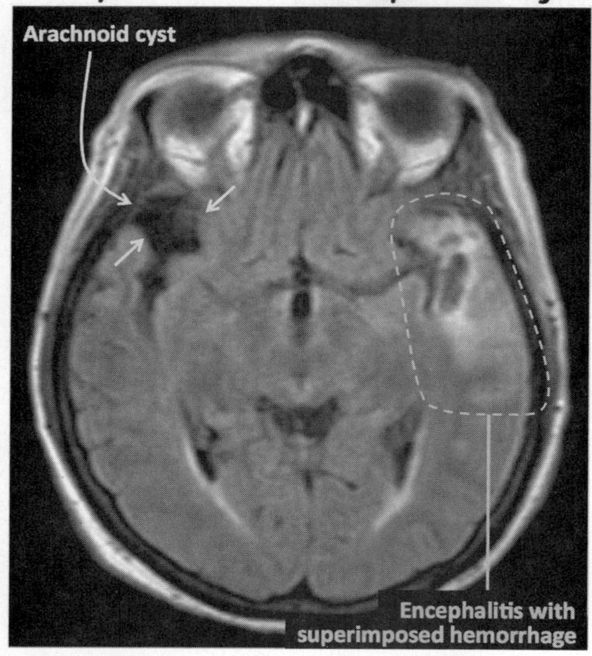

Encephalitis is important to recognize due to the severity and complications it may cause in the patient's condition. This MRI shows that encephalitis (right side of the brain) is complicated by hemorrhage. Note that an unexpected arachnoid cyst was revealed in the left side of the brain.
Source: Courtesy of K. Kyriakidis

LO2:

Pathophysiology: Encephalitis

- Viral encephalitis can originate from the respiratory system (concurrent illness such as mumps, measles, varicella), oral cavity (enterovirus and polio), oral/genital (herpes simplex), and bites from vectors such as animals carrying the rabies virus or mosquitoes carrying arboviruses.
- Since encephalitis is primarily caused by a virus, the transmission of a virus into the CNS is described:
  - o The virus enters the body and colonizes. Upon penetrating a cell, the virus transcribes and replicates the viral nucleic acid. It penetrates the CNS by entering through cerebral capillaries, choroid plexus, and/or along peripheral nerves.
  - o The virus attacks the susceptible neurons and causes cell lysis.
  - o The most common viruses are the herpes simplex virus and arboviruses (Saint Louis, Eastern or Western equine, or West Nile virus).

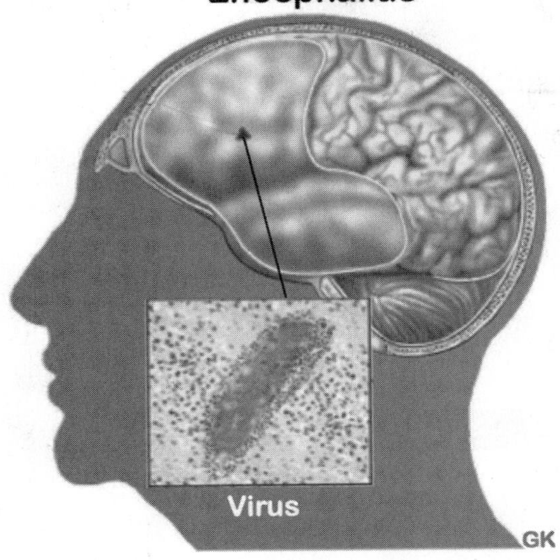

A virus is often a prevalent, rapidly erupting, serious, and potentially fatal cause of encephalitis. It occurs when the virus crosses into the parenchyma of the brain.
Source: Courtesy of George Kyriakidis/Santa Ana, CA

LO2:

Risk Factors and Causes: Encephalitis

- Travel to areas with endemic disease and mosquito activity (arboviruses including West Nile virus)
- Very young or old age
- Immunocompromised condition
- Most cases of encephalitis are sporadic without any specific risk factors.

Causes of Encephalitis

Causes	Transmission	
Herpes simplex virus	Person to person contact	
Human immunodeficiency virus (HIV)	Introduction of an infected person's bodily fluids or blood into that of another person	
Enteroviruses	Contact with bodily fluids	
Arboviruses	Bites from mosquito that are infected from animals (birds, squirrels)	
Animal-borne conditions	Bites from animals (dogs, cats) that are infected	

Concept Check

3. What is the most common causative agent of encephalitis?
   A. Bacteria
   B. Virus
   C. Fungus
   D. Prion

Answer question

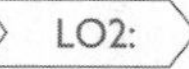

LO2: Assessment Findings: Encephalitis

- History and physical exam are important in the initial clinical diagnosis.
- Patients presenting with encephalitis usually complain of:
  - o Headache
  - o Confusion or altered cerebral function
  - o Fever
  - o Seizures
- In more severe cases, patients present with:
  - o Altered level of consciousness
  - o Personality changes such as aggressive or bizarre behavior
  - o Seizures
  - o Loss of sensation or movement
  - o Hallucinations
  - o Double vision
- An important distinction between encephalitis and meningitis is that patients with encephalitis show altered sensorium (confused state). That is not typically seen with meningitis.

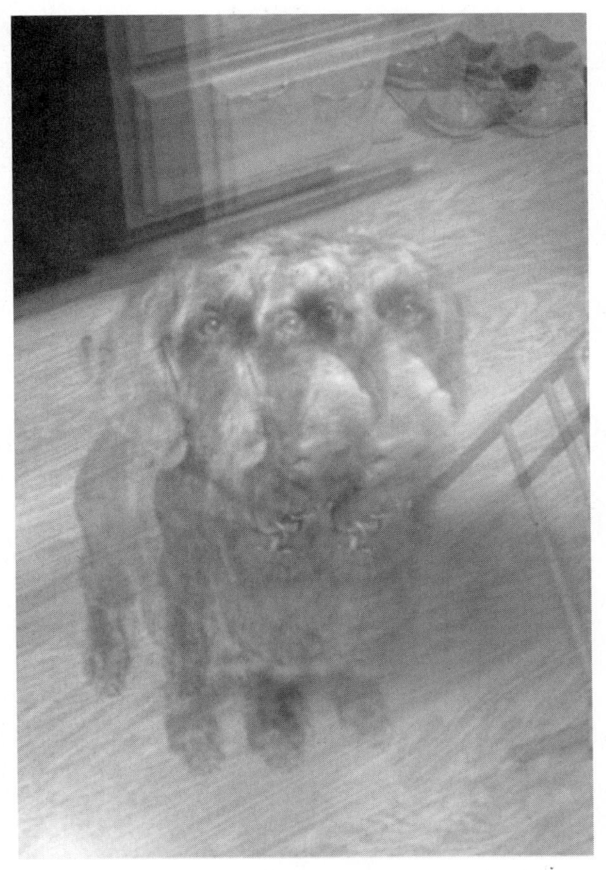

This patient, who was developing encephalitis, presented with headache, double vision, and confusion. Her history of recent and numerous mosquito bites in an area known for West Nile virus pointed to the likely diagnosis.
Source: Courtesy of Sarah E. Dresen

LO2:

Diagnostics: Encephalitis

- A brain CT or MRI scan, lumbar puncture (LP), and blood analysis with cultures are obtained to help diagnose the patient, along with the physical findings.
- CSF samples usually show an elevation in WBCs, with a lymphocytic predominance. CSF may also show elevated protein levels.
- CSF analysis can also provide diagnosis of pathogen through molecular genetic analysis (PCR) and cultures.
- Imaging of the brain is often performed. Some patients with encephalitis may have findings on imaging studies, particularly MRI (see photos).

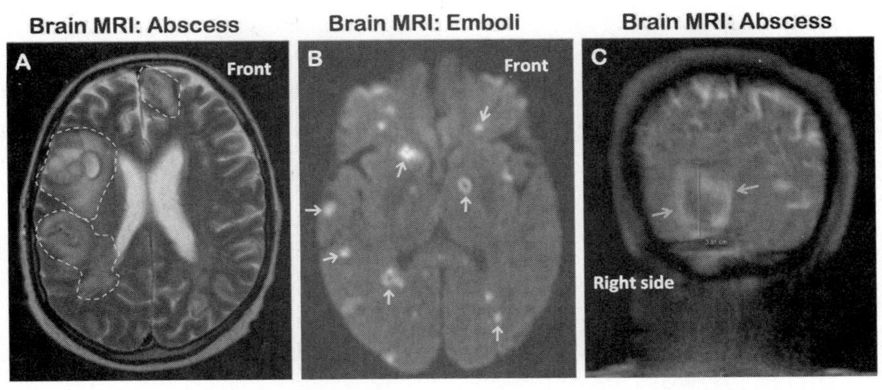

MRI brain scans assist to diagnose infected tissue. Examples are shown here: A) disseminated bacterial infection in a diabetic patient; B) multiple septic emboli in a patient with endocarditis, C) large brain abscess in a patient with meningitis.
Source: Courtesy of K. Kyriakidis

- In herpes encephalitis:
    - o LP results reveal an elevated opening CSF pressure plus lymphocytes, increased protein, and normal glucose.
    - o There is gyral enhancement with edema/hemorrhage of the inferior frontal and temporal lobes on CT or MRI of the brain.
    - o Blood is positive for HSV-1 antigen.
- If an arbovirus is the cause, expect:
    - o The ELISA serological assay for antiviral IgM (early rise)
    - o IgG (late) is positive
    - o West Nile virus reveals IgM capture of the ELISA antibody test.

Priority Patient Concerns and Desired Collaborative Care Outcomes: Encephalitis

Prior to caring for patients with encephalitis, it is important to prioritize the patient's concerns that must guide the nursing care plan and interventions. Care for the patient is ordered and organized in accordance with the patient's priority and urgent needs. Desired collaborative care outcomes in patients with encephalitis typically include:

1. Patient will remain injury-free.
2. Patient's intracranial pressure will remain within desired range.
3. Patient will remain alert and oriented.
4. Patient will participate in rehabilitation activities.

Considering these important care outcomes, prepare a list of the major 3–6 priority patient concerns or nursing diagnoses for patients with encephalitis. Be prepared to participate in a discussion of this list and/or to submit them as an assignment, as determined by your faculty. Resources you may find helpful in this assignment can include this lesson, the references, resources on nursing care plans, and standard nursing diagnoses manuals.

Concept Check

4. Which finding is characteristic of cerebral spinal fluid analysis in a patient with encephalitis?

A. Decreased white blood count
B. Increased lymphocytes
C. Decreased protein
D. Decreased red blood cell count

Answer question

Concept Check

5. A patient who has developed West Nile encephalitis has been exposed to what type of pathogen?

A. Herpes simplex
B. Varicella
C. Enterovirus
D. Arbovirus

Answer question

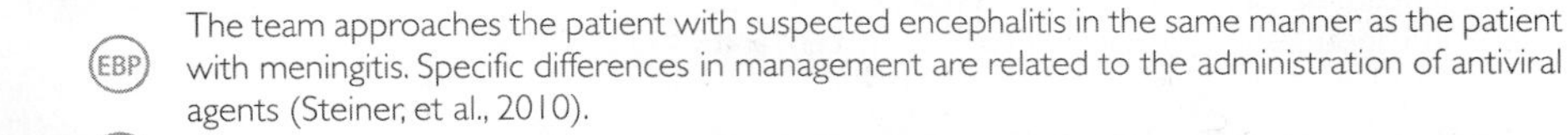

LO3: Collaborative Interventions: Encephalitis

The team approaches the patient with suspected encephalitis in the same manner as the patient with meningitis. Specific differences in management are related to the administration of antiviral agents (Steiner, et al., 2010).

- Administer acyclovir as the agent of choice for suspected herpes encephalitis. This medication is often started in patients with encephalitis while awaiting test results that may confirm the pathogen involved (Steiner, et al., 2010).
- Herpes encephalitis is currently the only virus that has a specific treatment. In all other forms of viral encephalitis, the primary therapies involve supporting the body systems.
- If the patient has been infected with an arbovirus, focus on symptom management with no specific antiviral agent to counter the arbovirus. Acyclovir may be started initially with encephalitis due to an arbovirus, but the management is typically related to supporting the body systems (see meningitis care).
- Anticipate and plan for recovery from encephalitis within a few weeks for mild cases.
- Administer IV fluids as needed if vomiting threatens to lead to dehydration. Avoid overhydration that can cause cerebral edema.
- Administer acetaminophen to manage fever, headache, and pain from neck stiffness.
- Implement seizure precautions as in meningitis. (See the Seizure NovE-lesson for safety and protection.)
- Administer antiepileptic medications if seizures occur. May be given prophylactically if meningeal edema is severe.
- Carefully monitor the patient to track changes and recognize the onset of any complications early.
- Ensure adequate rest and nutrition.
- If encephalitis is moderate to severe, prolonged hospitalization makes these patients vulnerable to complications associated with immobility (e.g., pressure ulcers, DVT) and multiple invasive therapies (e.g., vascular and urinary catheter-related infections, pneumonia if intubated). Prevention of never events requires excellent care, which includes implementing all safety and preventive measures. The multiple potential never events include:
    - Ventilator-associated pneumonia
    - Catheter-associated urinary tract infection
    - Intravenous catheter-related air embolism
    - Deep vein thrombosis and pulmonary embolism
    - Glycemic events
    - Falls
    - Pressure ulcer
    - Vascular catheter-associated infection
- Comfort measures should be considered, depending on the patient's condition:
    - Limit visitors and unnecessary stimulation if noise and stress make the patient uncomfortable.
    - Maintain a quiet room if the patient experiences phonophobia (noise sensitivity) to reduce agitation and improve comfort.
    - Maintain a dimly lit room if the patient experiences photophobia to reduce agitation and improve comfort.
    - Cluster nursing interventions to minimize interrupted rest and reduce activity.
    - Frequent linen changes may be needed if very diaphoretic.
    - Provide stool softener or mild laxative when needed to prevent constipation, straining during defecation, and the risk of increased ICP.
    - Provide ongoing emotional support to patient and family. Assist in reorienting the patient if delirious or confused. Recovery can be prolonged.

Patient and Family Education, Rehabilitation, and Discharge

- N More severe cases can result in significant neurological impairment that requires months or years of rehabilitation. Collaborate with the health care provider to ensure that patient and family obtain needed referrals.
- N M Collaborate to involve physical therapy, rehabilitation, case worker, nutritionist, and family as soon as possible for planning, prevention, and long-term care.
- N Chronic headache can occur after an acquired brain injury such as encephalitis. Educate families and the patient to seek follow-up medical care if chronic headache ensues.
- N Discuss cognitive impairments with the health care provider as consultations for cognitive rehabilitation and neuropsychology may be helpful.
- N Care of the patient mirrors that of patients with meningitis.
- N Educate patient to avoid alcohol, caffeine, and tobacco as these may aggravate the patient's condition.
- N M Educate regarding advanced directives.

LO4: Evaluation of Desired Collaborative Care Outcomes: Encephalitis

Evaluation and reassessment should reveal attainment of previously established patient outcomes. In summary:

- Patient has remained injury-free.
- Patient's intracranial pressure has remained within desired range.
- Patient is alert and oriented.
- Patient expresses willingness to participate in rehabilitation activities.

LO1: What Is Guillain-Barré Syndrome?

- Guillain-Barré Syndrome (GBS) is an acute, inflammatory, autoimmune disease that causes muscle weakness, sensory loss, and areflexia.
- It is considered an autoimmune disorder in which the body begins to attack itself.
- The attack occurs on the peripheral nervous system and results in demyelination of nerves (breakdown of the myelin covering the nerves). The result is an acute polyneuropathy.
- Due to the ensuing paralysis, Guillain-Barré is a medical emergency that requires immediate hospitalization.
- There is no cure for GBS, but most patients do eventually recover.

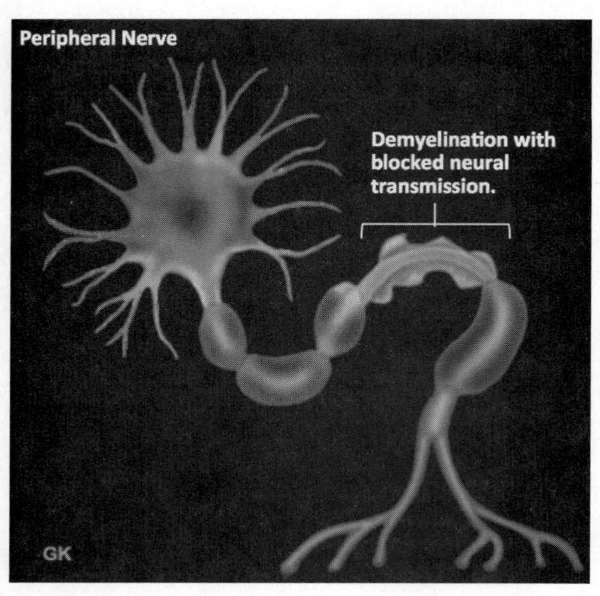

This image depicts the basic pathophysiology of peripheral nerve damage in patients with Guillain-Barré Syndrome.
Source: Courtesy of George Kyriakidis/Santa Ana, CA

LO1:

Clinical Relevance: Guillain-Barré Syndrome

- GBS can cause rapid muscular deterioration, may involve the respiratory system, and can cause respiratory failure.
- Muscle weakness can rapidly progress, so early recognition and intervention is lifesaving.
- Patients with GBS need to have respiratory function monitored closely, because approximately 30% require intubation and mechanical ventilation.
- When demyelination affects the vagus nerve, autonomic nervous system (cardiac and hemodynamic) dysfunction frequently occurs, endangering the patient's life with hyper- and hypotension and dysrhythmias.

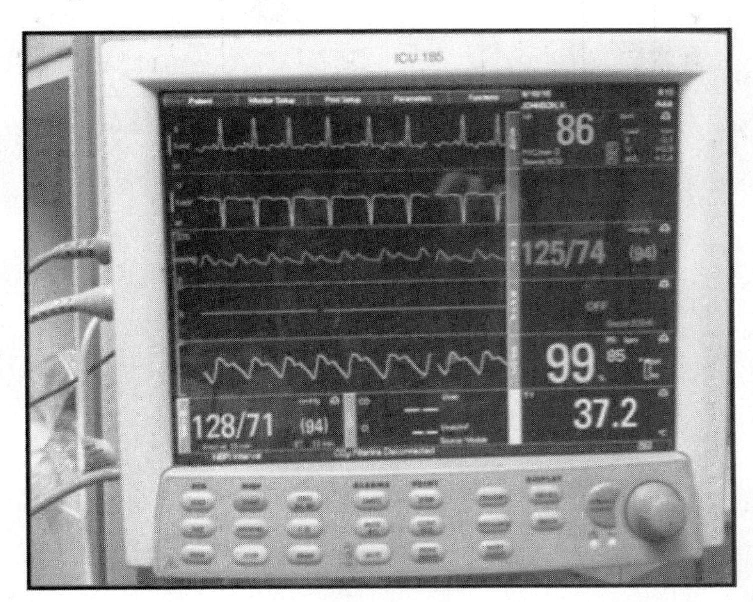

Patients with Guillain-Barré Syndrome require respiratory support with close monitoring for additional signs of deterioration. Guillain-Barré Syndrome can progressively lead to paralysis so close observation is required. Observe for life-threatening complications, such as dysrhythmias, hypotension, compromised respirations, and respiratory effort.

- Approximately 3,000–6,000 persons are afflicted by GBS yearly in the United States, whether they received a vaccine or not.

LO2:

Pathophysiology: Guillain-Barré Syndrome

- GBS is considered an autoimmune disorder in which the body fails to recognize and mistakenly begins to attack itself.
- The attack occurs on the peripheral nervous system and results in demyelination of nerves (breakdown of the myelin covering the nerves).
- Generally, 70% of the individuals diagnosed with Guillain-Barré have experienced a viral illness 2–3 weeks prior to the onset.
- Macrophages begin to attack the normal myelin, leading to demyelination.
- Impulses that normally travel quickly from nerve to nerve are slowed or stopped, creating the visible weakness seen in GBS.
- The majority of treated patients recover within approximately 40 days, as the Schwann cells that produce myelin escape damage.

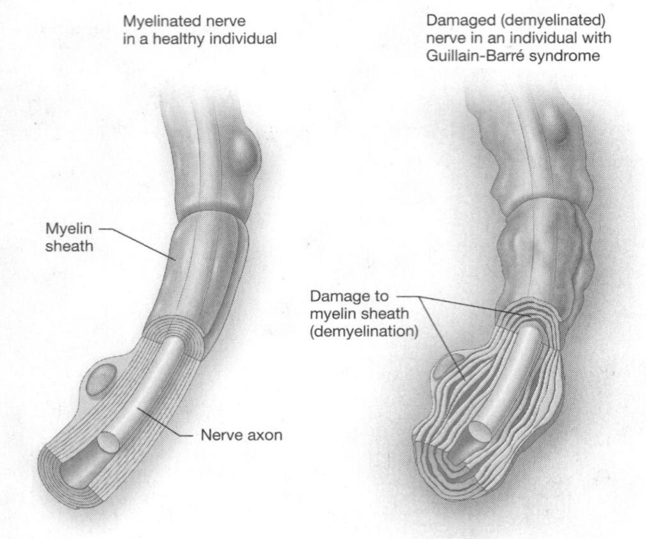

Guillain-Barré Syndrome is an uncommon condition in which the body's immune system attacks its nerves. Weakness and numbness of the extremities are early symptoms. These neurological losses may rapidly spread and cause total paralysis.

LO2: Risk Factors and Causes: Guillain-Barré Syndrome

- Infections, particularly *Campylobacter* (bacterial) and cytomegalovirus or CMV (viral), can trigger the autoimmune response against nerve-protecting myelin.
- Older adults are at higher risk as the incidence increases in the older population.
- There is a small but known risk in adults associated with the H1N1 vaccine, but there is no evidence that children are at any increased risk.

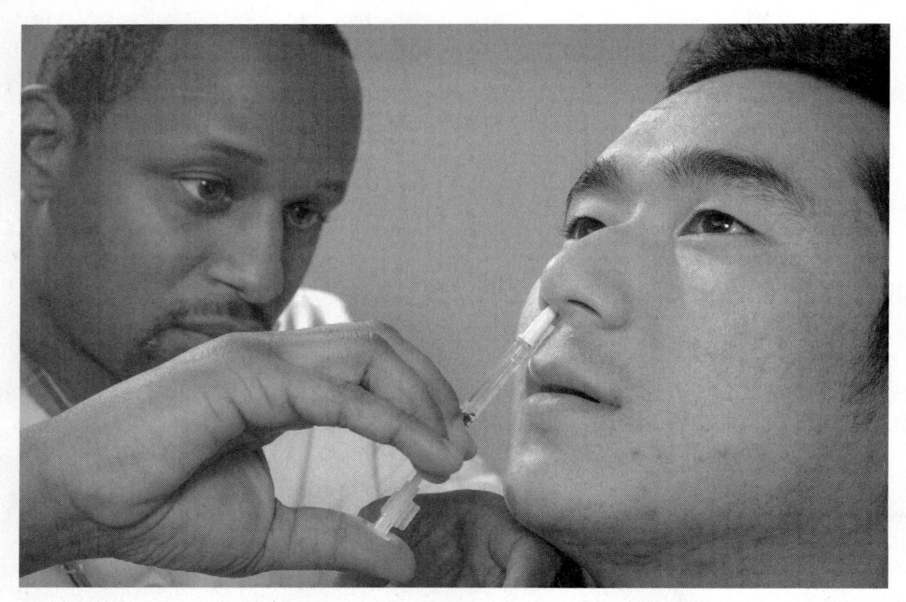

In 1976–1977, an unusually high rate of GBS was identified in the United States following the administration of inactivated 'swine' influenza A (H1N1) vaccines. In 2003, the Institute of Medicine (IOM) concluded that the evidence favored acceptance of a causal relationship between the 1976 swine influenza vaccines and GBS in adults.
Source: Centers for Disease Control and Prevention/Dr. Bill Atkinson

Concept Check

6. What causes the weakness associated with Guillain-Barré Syndrome?

A. Demyelination of peripheral nerves

B. Death of afferent central nerves

C. Decreased oxygenation of tissues at the synaptic junction

D. Accumulation of pus along nerve routes

Answer question

LO2:

Assessment Findings: Guillain-Barré Syndrome

- The person with Guillain-Barré develops a rapidly progressing weakness or numbness/tingling that commonly starts in the lower extremities and rapidly ascends. The primary symptom is ascending weakness.
- Variant forms can include descending GBS.
- In some patients, the weakness is limited to the lower extremities, but in others it can rapidly ascend and impact the diaphragm, which can impair normal breathing. Dyspnea, reduced tidal volume, and respiratory failure can occur.
- The numbness or sensory loss may or may not be present. Inappropriate nerve signals result in sensations like pain, crawling skin, and tingling.
- Individuals may lose their deep tendon reflexes.
- In some cases, loss of some of the cranial nerves that innervate the face or eyes can occur, causing facial weakness, speech difficulties, dysphagia, and related symptoms.
- Autonomic dysfunction with ileus, hypotension, hypertension, and/or cardiac dysrhythmias can occur.

LO2:

Diagnostics: Guillain-Barré Syndrome

- Diagnosis is made by combining clinical information (e.g., ascending paralysis) with diagnostic testing.
- Diagnosis of Guillain-Barré can be made by examining the CSF obtained via a lumbar puncture for increased protein.
- An electromyograph (EMG) is a nerve conduction study. EMG reveals slowing or impairment of the conduction of impulses.

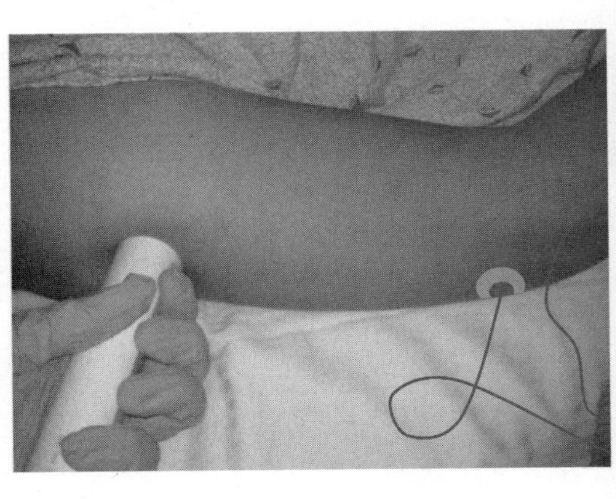

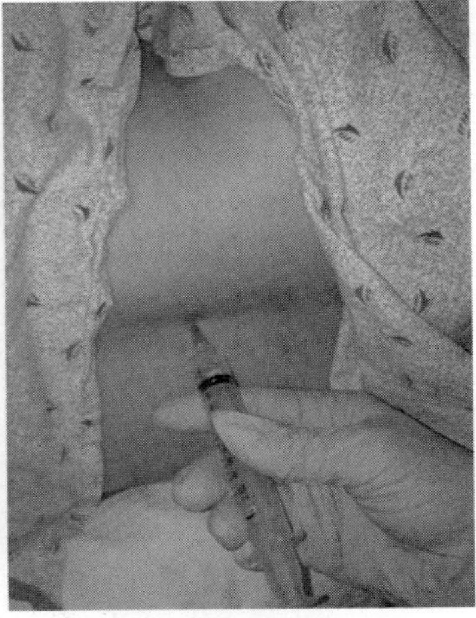

Left: The EMG test consists of two parts. The first part is called a nerve conduction study. Brief electrical shocks are delivered to the arm or leg to evaluate the peripheral nerve fibers by recording how well small electrical impulses travel through the nerve fibers. Injury or disease to the nerve or nerve fibers can impair this electrical transmission. Right: A lumbar puncture or spinal tap is performed to obtain cerebrospinal fluid to assist in diagnosis.

Source: *(both)* Copyright © 2014, NovEx Novice to Expert Learning, LLC

If interested in more detail about EMG, click: www.youtube.com/watch?v=k0uSpYd_lcs.

Priority Patient Concerns and Desired Collaborative Care Outcomes: Guillain-Barré Syndrome

Prior to caring for patients with Guillain-Barré, it is important to prioritize the patient's concerns that must guide the nursing care plan and interventions. Care for the patient is ordered and organized in accordance with the patient's priority and urgent needs. Desired collaborative care outcomes in patients with Guillain-Barré typically include:

1. Patient will have spontaneous ventilatory drive.
2. Patient will be able to clear airway.
3. Patient will maintain adequate mobility throughout disease process (either actively or passively according to disease progression).
4. Patient will state reduction in or freedom from fear.
5. Family will express understanding of the disease process and will state therapeutic ways of coping.

Considering these important care outcomes, prepare a list of the major 3–6 priority patient concerns or nursing diagnoses for patients with Guillain-Barré. Be prepared to participate in a discussion of this list and/or to submit them as an assignment, as determined by your faculty. Resources you may find helpful in this assignment can include this lesson, the references, resources on nursing care plans, and standard nursing diagnoses manuals.

LO3:

Collaborative Interventions: Guillain-Barré Syndrome

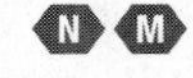

- Immediately triage patients with complaints of ascending weakness for admission to the hospital and provide supportive care, as in meningitis.

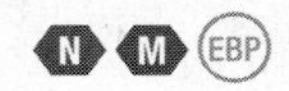

- Assess patient's vital signs, including blood pressure, heart rate, respirations, and temperature frequently. Obtain electrocardiogram in case autonomic dysfunction occurs and causes cardiac disturbances (Hughes, et al., 2005).
- Closely monitor respirations and oxygenation:

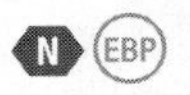

  - o Frequently assess airway and breathing to monitor for diaphragm involvement and neuromuscular respiratory failure (Hughes, et al., 2005), inability to clear secretions, risk of aspiration, and compromised gas exchange.

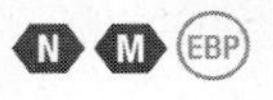

  - o In some instances, assess ventilatory parameters, including negative inspiratory force, tidal volume, and vital capacity, and measure every 8–12 hours to monitor diaphragm function (Hughes, et al., 2005).

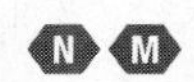

  - o If the patient's diaphragm becomes compromised, endotracheal intubation and ventilatory support is necessary.

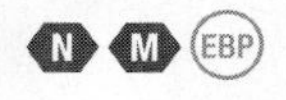

  - o Mechanical ventilation may be indicated for a short time or for weeks to months, depending on the progression of the disease (Hughes, et al., 2005). (Review endotracheal intubation in the Collaborative Interventions section of the Acute Lung Injury NovE-lesson).

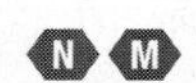

  - o Consider tracheostomy if the patient cannot be weaned from mechanical ventilation within 2–3 weeks.

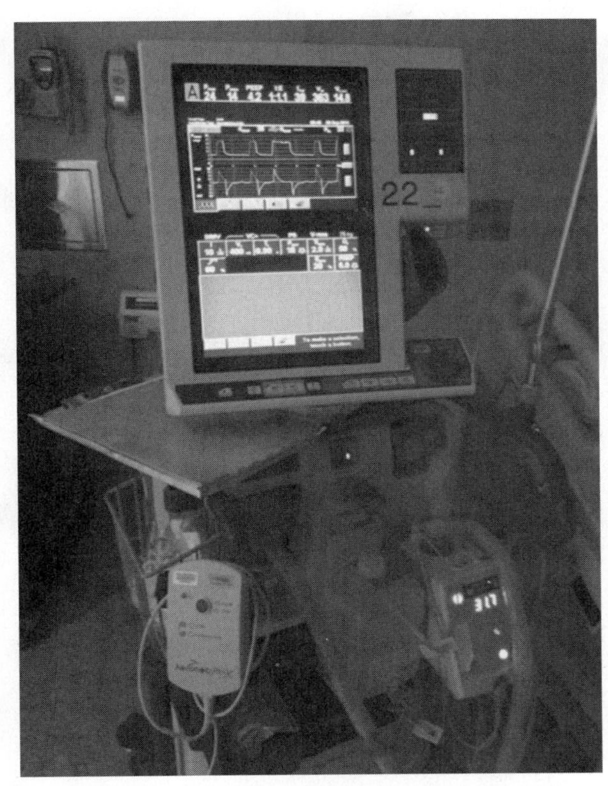

Some patients require life support during Guillain-Barré. Mechanical ventilation is a primary intervention. Nurses must be vigilant in recognizing when a patient has respiratory compromise to provide early rescue.
Source: Copyright © 2014, NovEx Novice to Expert Learning, LLC

- Monitor patients' cardiac rhythm and hemodynamics if autonomic disturbances arise. Patients with GBS can have life-threatening dysrhythmias and hyper- and hypotensive events.
- Conduct a neurological exam frequently. Assess for change in motor function of all extremities. Monitor patients for additional autonomic disturbances with complications that may include ileus, bronchial mucosa, and hyponatremia.
- Consider treatment for disease-causing antibodies:
  - If in the early stages of GBS, plasma exchange or plasmapheresis is recommended in an attempt to cleanse the blood or wash out antibodies causing the Guillain-Barré Syndrome (Patwa, et al., 2012).

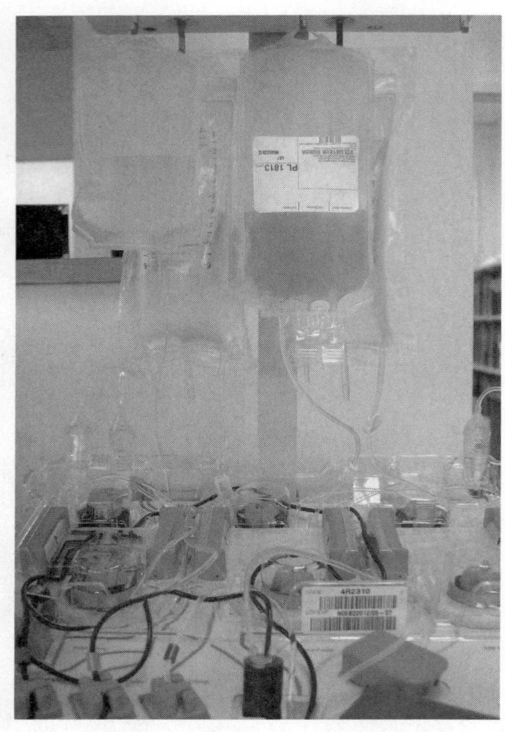

Blood plasma, containing the disease-causing antibodies, is seen collecting in the IV bag. Plasmapheresis is done to separate the plasma from the blood cells so that the plasma can be removed from the patient's body.
Source: Michelle Marsan/Shutterstock

- o Intravenous immunoglobulin (IVIG) is recommended as an alternative treatment with equal efficacy. IVIG contains antibodies from the donor, which help block the damage due to antibodies (Patwa, et al., 2012).
- o Evidence shows that there is no benefit to performing both plasmapheresis and IVIG together (Patwa, et al., 2012).
- o If patients receive IVIG, nurses should monitor for side effects, including anaphylaxis reactions such as chills, hypotension, and fluid shift. Monitoring of blood pressure, pulse, respirations, and temperature should be done frequently (Patwa, et al., 2012).

- Glucocorticoids have not been shown to be beneficial (Patwa, et al., 2012).

Collaborative Interventions: Guillain-Barré Syndrome (continued)

Symptom Management and Comfort Care

All body systems require support while the individual is hospitalized.

N M EBP
- Vigilantly manage the patient's pain. Acetaminophen and NSAIDs are first line choices but analgesic support (e.g., opioids) is imperative in many patients because individuals with Guillain-Barré often have significant neuropathic pain, especially in their feet (Hughes, et al., 2005).

N M
- Consider adjuvant therapy, which may be needed in conjunction with analgesics, such as tricyclic antidepressants, carbamazepine, gabapentin, tramadol, or mexiletine, to ameliorate neuropathic pain.

N M EBP
- Administer prophylactic anticoagulants (heparin) against deep vein thrombosis. Prophylaxis is imperative during immobility. If contraindicated, a sequential leg compression device should be used (Hughes, et al., 2005).

N
- Properly position and turn the patient frequently.

N M EBP
- Involve rehabilitation (rehab) specialists and occupational therapy early during hospitalization to assist the team in supporting mobility, cognition, and activities of daily living (Hughes, et al., 2005). Rehab should include good body and limb positioning, orthotics, nutrition, and posture with progressive resistive exercises.

N M EBP
- Collaborate with physical therapy for range of motion to the extremities to maintain flexibility and mobilization at the earliest possible time (Hughes, et al., 2005). However, care is needed to avoid overfatigue, which can impede recovery.

N EBP
- Prevent skin breakdown with good hygiene and skin care, which is especially important for patients who lose bladder and bowel control during this time (Hughes, et al., 2005).

N M
- Initiate enteral or parenteral nutrition within 24–48 hours. Recovery from this prolonged and debilitating illness can be complicated by under- or malnutrition.

N
- Assess bowel function daily to avoid or intervene early on ileus development. Avoid promotility medications that are contraindicated in patients with dysautonomia.

N M
- May need to consider urinary indwelling catheter for a limited period of time. Discontinue its use at the earliest possible time.

N
- Provide psychological support, which is imperative, as the patient will require long-term care.

N
- Educate patient and family regarding advanced directives and illness trajectory, and educate family in their role in caring for the patient.

N M
- As soon as the patient can participate in rehabilitation for 3 hours per day, expect transfer to an acute rehabilitation unit as a temporary measure, in preparation for transition home.

N
- Once the acute care period has passed, anticipate and plan with the health care provider for individuals who may require long-term care in a subacute rehabilitation unit or skilled nursing facility. Approval and bed space in other facilities can take time.

N M
- As in meningitis and encephalitis, due to long-term hospitalization that may be needed, implement safety and preventative care to avoid never events (details provided earlier).

N M
- Educate the patient that, after a year following recovery from GBS, immunizations are recommended as vaccinations are not a considerable risk factor associated with GBS.

Concept Check

7. The weakness that accompanies Guillain-Barré Syndrome typically begins in which region?

A. Hands

B. Face

C. Feet

D. Respiratory muscles

Answer question

Summary of Interventions: Guillain-Barré Syndrome

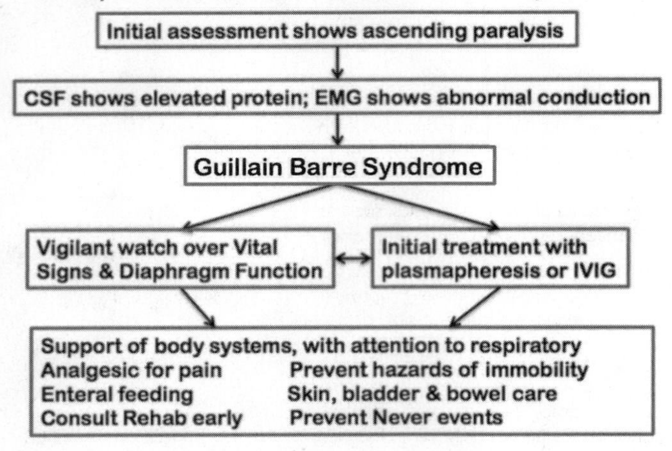

LO4:

Evaluation of Desired Collaborative Care Outcomes: Guillain-Barré Syndrome

Evaluation and reassessment should reveal attainment of previously established patient outcomes. In summary:

- Patient's spontaneous ventilatory drive has returned.
- Patient maintains a clear airway.
- Patient has returned to pre-illness mobility.
- Patient has stated reduction in or freedom from fear.
- Family has expressed understanding of the disease process and has stated therapeutic ways of coping.

Summary of Interventions: Neurological Infectious Disorders

- Individuals with meningitis, encephalitis, or Guillain-Barré Syndrome require immediate care by acute care hospitals.
- Some of these conditions are life-threatening and carry a high rate of mortality and morbidity.
- Antimicrobials are started immediately, if indicated.
- Supportive care (e.g., cardiac, hemodynamic, respiratory) is needed. Depending on duration of the illness, rehabilitation may be needed.
- Vigilance is needed to prevent any never events and any complications of immobility.
- Educate the patient and family about advanced directives.

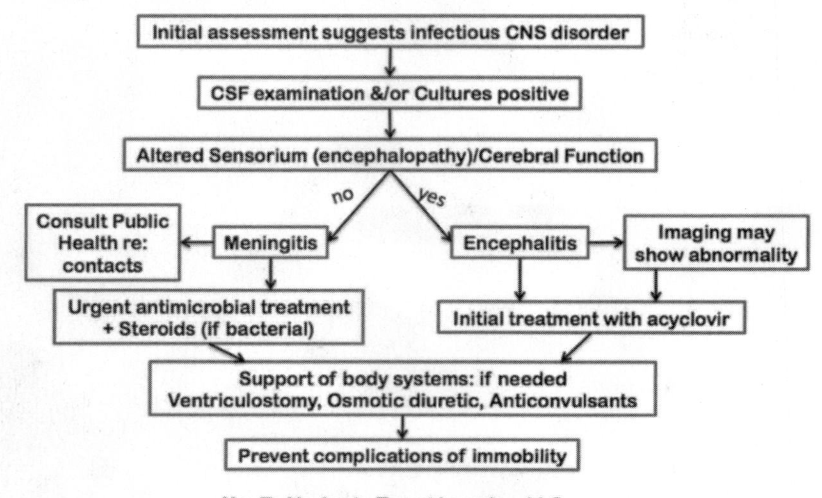

References

Bowyer, H. R., & Glover, M. (2010). Guillain-Barre syndrome management and treatment options for patients with moderate to severe progression. *J Neuroscience Nurs, 42*(5), 288–293.

Higginson, C. B., Maring, C., & Cook, A. (2010). Initial evaluation and management of bacterial meningitis in an emergent setting: A review. *AdvEmergNurs J, 32*(4), 301–313.

Matthews, C., Miller, L., & Mott, M. (2007). Getting ahead of acute meningitis and encephalitis. *Nursing 2014, 37*(11), 36–39. **www.nursingcenter.com/lnc/CEArticle?an=00152193-200711000-00035&Journal_ID=54016&Issue_ID=751243**

Siegel, J., Rhinehart, E., Jackson, M., et al., & the Healthcare Infection Control Practices Advisory Committee. (2007). *2007 guideline for isolation precautions: Preventing transmission of infectious agents in healthcare settings.* **www.cdc.gov/hicpac/2007IP/2007isolationPrecautions.html**

Stephens, D. S., Greenwood, B., & Brandtzaeg, P. (2007). Epidemic meningitis, meningococcaemia, and *Neisseria meningitides. Lancet. 369*(9580), 2196–2210.

Wisniewski, A. (2003). Combating infection: Closing in on clues to encephalitis. *Nursing 2014, 33*(4), 70–71.

Clinical Practice Guidelines

American Association of Neuroscience Nurses (AANN). (2008). *Nursing management of adults with severe traumatic brain injury.* Glenview, IL: Author. **www.guideline.gov/content.aspx?id=13576&search=traumatic+brain+injury**

Cloke, A., Guideline Development Group, et al. (2010, June). Bacterial meningitis and meningococcal septicaemia. *NICE Clinical Guideline, No. 102,* 45. **www.guideline.gov/content.aspx?id=23800#top**

Hughes, R., Wijdicks, E., Benson, E., et al. (2005). Supportive care for patients with Guillain-Barre Syndrome. *Arch Neurol, 62*(8), 1194–1198. **lib.ajaums.ac.ir/booklist/archives%20of%20neurology_Aug-8_26.pdf**

Pappas, P. G., Kauffman, C. A., Andes, D., et al. (2009). Clinical practice guideline for the management of candidiasis: 2009 update. *ClinInfec Dis, 48*(5), 503–535. **www.idsociety.org/uploadedFiles/IDSA/Guidelines-Patient_Care/PDF_Library/Candidiasis.pdf**

Patwa, H. S., Chaudhry, V., Katzberg, H., et al. (2012). Evidence-based guideline: Intravenous immunoglobulin in the treatment of neuromuscular disorders. *Neurology, 78*(13), 1009–1015. **www.neurology.org/content/78/13/1009.full**

Steiner, I., Budka, H., Chaudhuri, A., et al. (2010). Viral meningoencephalitis: A review of diagnostic methods and guidelines for management. *Eur J Neurol, 17*(8), 999–e57. **www.guideline.gov/content.aspx?id=24522&search=viral+meningitis**

Tunkel, A., Hartman, B., Kaplan, S., et al. (2004). Practice guidelines for the management of bacterial meningitis. *Clin Infect Dis,* 39(9), 1267–1284. **cid.oxfordjournals.org/content/39/9/1267.full#sec-5**

Patient Education

Centers for Disease Control and Prevention. (2014). *Arboviral encephalitides.* **www.cdc.gov/ncezid/dvbd/about.html**

Centers for Disease Control and Prevention. (2015). *Meningitis.* **www.cdc.gov/meningitis/index.html**

Harvard Medical School Patient Education Center. (2015). *Guillain-Barre syndrome.* **www.patienteducationcenter.org/articles/guillain-barre-syndrome/**

National Institute of Neurological Disorders and Stroke. (2015, April 17). *Meningitis and encephalitis fact sheet.* **www.ninds.nih.gov/disorders/encephalitis_meningitis/detail_encephalitis_meningitis.htm**

STOP

Go to the online course and complete the NovE-Cases assigned by your instructor for this module.

Learning Outcomes for Stroke

When you complete this lesson, you will be able to:

1. Recognize the clinical relevance of stroke.
2. Consider the pathophysiology, etiology, risk factors, and clinical presentation of stroke that determine the priority patient concerns.
3. Determine the most urgent and important nursing interventions and patient education required in caring for a patient with stroke.
4. Evaluate attainment of desired collaborative care outcomes for a patient with stroke.

LO1:

What Is Stroke?

- Stroke, the sudden development of focal neurologic deficits, occurs when arteries feeding the brain become blocked from the inside (known as ischemic stroke) or rupture causing blood to rapidly escape into the brain tissue or subarachnoid space (known as hemorrhagic stroke).
- Ischemic stroke accounts for 80–85% of all strokes whereas hemorrhagic stroke accounts for 15–20%.

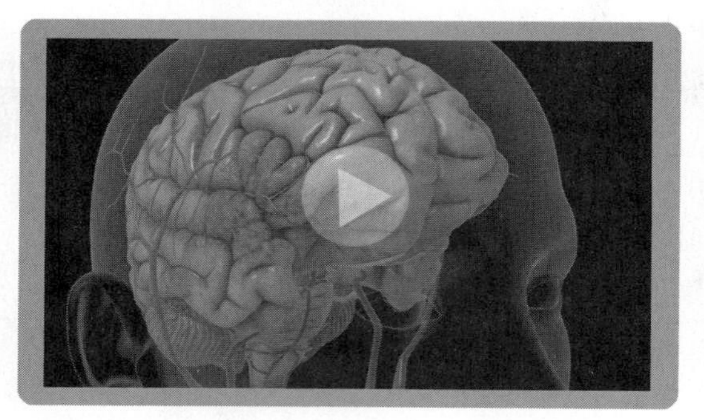

This animation gives a thorough explanation of stroke, covering anatomy and physiology, different types of stroke, and treatment.

Source: © 2014 Nucleus Medical Media, All rights reserved

LO1:

Clinical Relevance

- Stroke impacts over 795,000 people in the United States each year and is the third leading cause of death.
- Survivors of stroke often face considerable cognitive and physical disability. This may lead to recurrent hospitalizations for medical complications. Stroke is, therefore, a leading cause of chronic disability.
- Stroke is preventable! Modifying certain risk factors can lower the risk of stroke.

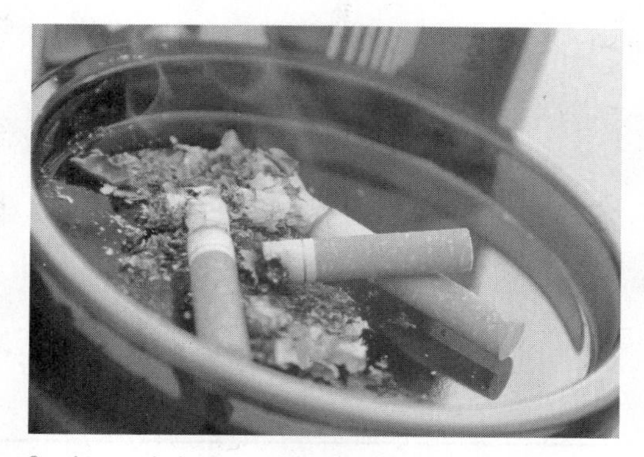

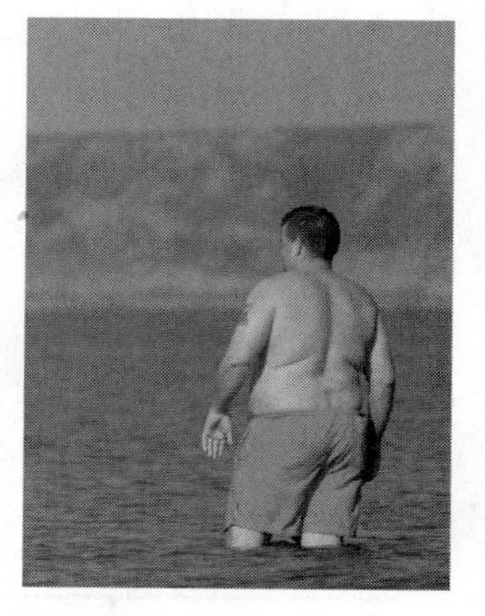

Smoking and obesity are clinically important risk factors. Behavior modification is central in prevention.

Sources: (*left*) Centers for Disease Control and Prevention; (*right*) Marilyn Barbone/Fotolia

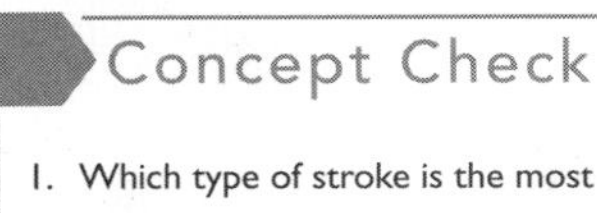
Concept Check

1. Which type of stroke is the most common?
   A. Hemorrhagic
   B. Subarachnoid
   C. Epidural
   D. Ischemic

Answer question

LO2:

Pathophysiology

- Because the understanding and care of a stroke patient depends, in part, on the etiology, it is important to differentiate between the two types.

Neurological Signs and Symptoms

Both types of stroke are discussed in this lesson.

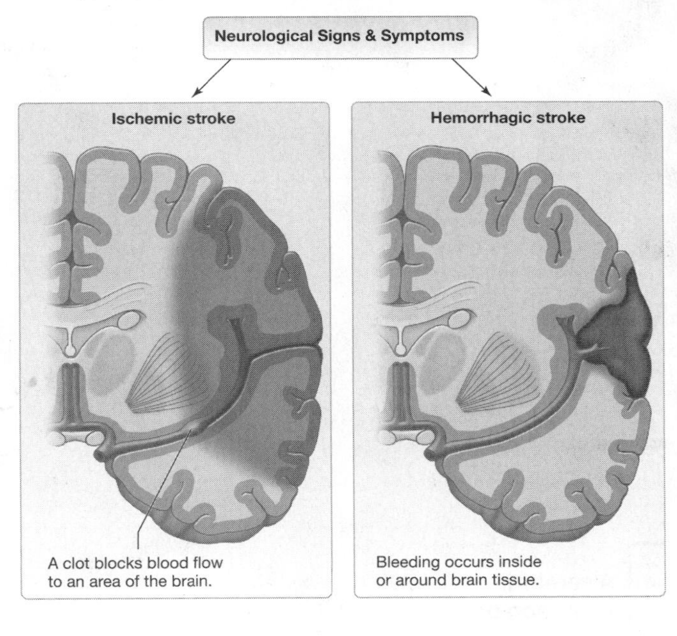
Neurological Signs & Symptoms
Ischemic stroke
Hemorrhagic stroke
A clot blocks blood flow to an area of the brain.
Bleeding occurs inside or around brain tissue.

LO1:

What Is Ischemic Stroke?

- Ischemic stroke (see photo) occurs due to blockage of an artery feeding the brain and is the most common type of stroke.
- The subtypes of ischemic stroke are thrombotic, embolic, lacunar, and cryptogenic (unknown cause).
  - o **Embolic stroke** occurs when an artery in the brain suddenly becomes blocked from a blood clot or some other material (i.e., vegetation from a heart valve) that travels up into the brain, lodges, and blocks an artery.

Bilateral Cerebellar Hemisphere Ischemia

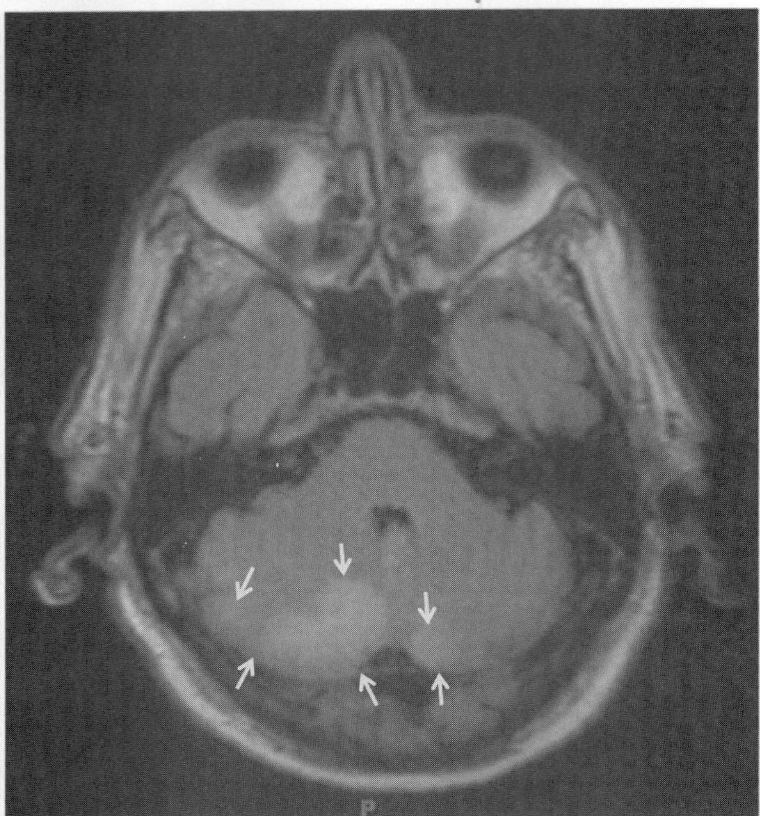

The MRI scan shows the image produced by an ischemic stroke and the damage (yellow arows) that can occur to surrounding tissue following an embolic event.
Source: Courtesy of K. Kyriakidis

- **Thrombotic stroke** occurs when an artery in the brain becomes narrow from atherosclerosis and a plaque ruptures. The sudden occlusion of one or more vessels usually occurs during periods of sleep.

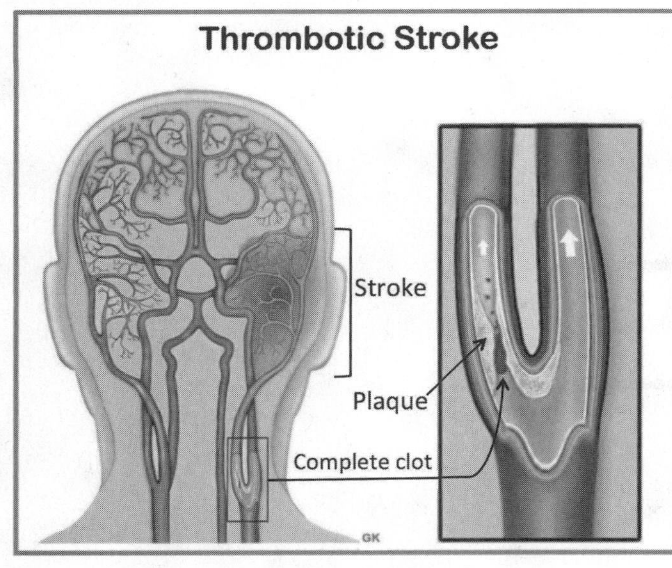

A cerebral infarction or stroke results from inadequate arterial perfusion with complete occlusion of the artery, commonly caused by an embolus or thrombus. Thrombi or emboli typically produce macroscopic areas of brain necrosis.

This image shows an artery blocked, or occluded, by a thrombus (stationary) plaque formation. As blood cells and other elements flow through the arterial lumen, the interior wall of the blood vessel (tunica intima) tears, allowing cholesterol deposits to form a plaque thrombus within the wall itself. Over time, the buildup can cause complete blockage of the artery, and tissue death beyond the site of the occlusion. This is a common cause of ischemic stroke.
Source: Courtesy of George Kyriakidis/Santa Ana, CA

- **Lacunar strokes** are blockages of the small cortical vessels of the brain. These very small infarcts can occur in multiple regions of the brain.
- **Cryptogenic stroke** is a large category that includes all the other causes for stroke. Too often when an individual has a stroke, the cause cannot be determined.

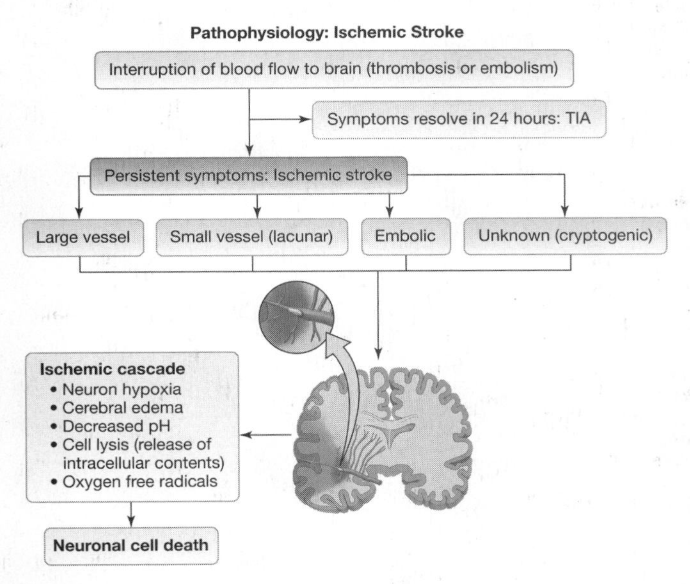

This schematic depicts the pathophysiology of ischemic stroke.

Transient Ischemic Attack

- A transient ischemic attack (TIA) occurs when stroke symptoms present but resolve in less than 24 hours. It is sometimes referred to as a mini-stroke.
- TIAs have the same origin as ischemic strokes.
- An interruption in blood flow to a portion of the brain causes temporary (often just for a few minutes) stroke symptoms, such as weakness or tingling in an arm or leg, difficulty speaking, temporary blurring or loss of vision, or affects one side of the body.
- TIAs do not cause brain damage, but they are important warning signs that a person is at risk for having a stroke.
- Patients experiencing a TIA should seek medical care right away to prevent a full stroke.

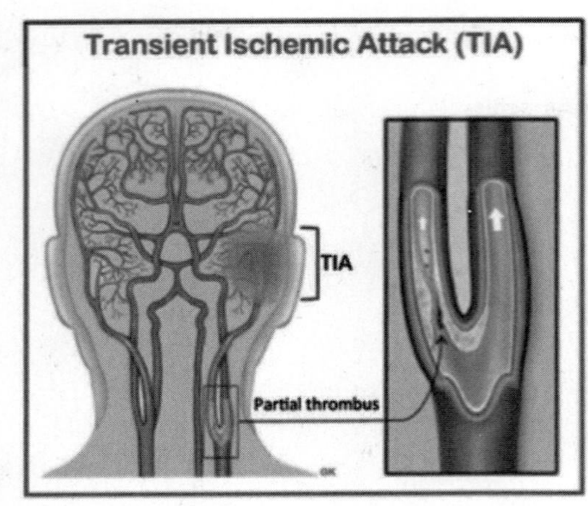

A TIA is a brief period when there is insufficient blood flow in an area of the brain. The lack of perfusion results in temporary but sudden loss of localized neurological function. Most TIAs resolve in <30 minutes.

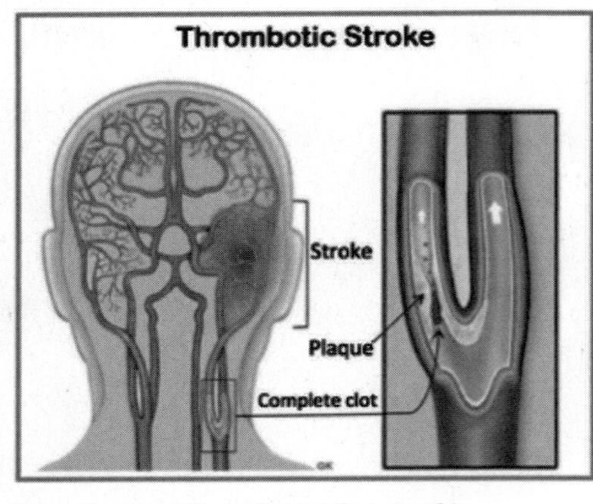

A cerebral infarction or stroke results from inadequate arterial perfusion with complete occlusion of the artery, commonly caused by an embolus or thrombus. Thrombi or emboli typically produce macroscopic areas of brain necrosis.

Source: Courtesy of George Kyriakidis/Santa Ana, CA

LO2:

Pathophysiology: Ischemic Stroke

- When part of the brain does not receive its blood supply, the brain cells become ischemic (see schematic) and the pathophysiologic mechanisms leading to cell death are triggered. The cells begin a process of cell death that starts within 30–60 minutes of the blockage.
- Collateral blood flow can potentially sustain the affected portion of the brain for a period of time, but if blood flow is not re-established in the blocked vessel, the brain cells will die within 6–8 hours from the start of the blockage.
- This TIME factor is important in trying to minimize brain damage in stroke. Because "TIME IS BRAIN," rapidly recognizing stroke symptoms and starting treatment are important factors in improving outcomes.

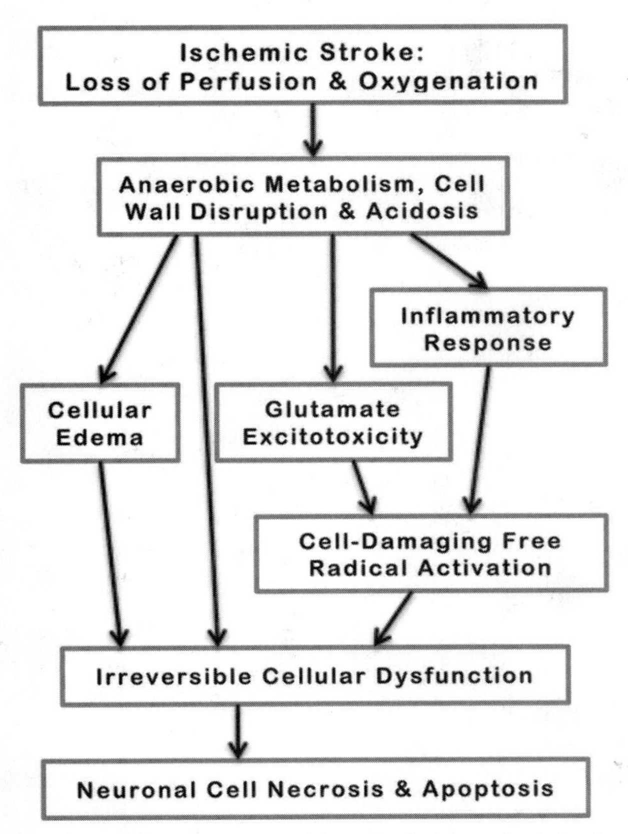

This schematic shows a summary of the pathophysiology of an ischemic stroke.
Source: Copyright © 2014, NovEx Novice to Expert Learning, LLC

- A key concept in stroke management is the ischemic penumbra. The penumbra is the area of brain surrounding the dead tissue, and it also suffers the effects of ischemia. The penumbra may be at risk for further damage or cell death. Ischemia leaves these cells "stunned" and they do not function properly.
- Usually after a stroke, blood pressure becomes elevated. This elevation in blood pressure helps to perfuse the penumbra and is the reason that blood pressure management after acute stroke (allowing blood pressure to increase) is important.
- As the cells are injured or die, they begin to swell (edema). When a large region of the brain swells, the subsequent widespread edema and pressure can impact the individual's level of consciousness. The patient can develop increased intracranial pressure (ICP). If the ICP becomes too high, the entire brain may undergo brain death. It is important to assess for increases in ICP so treatment can be initiated to lower it.

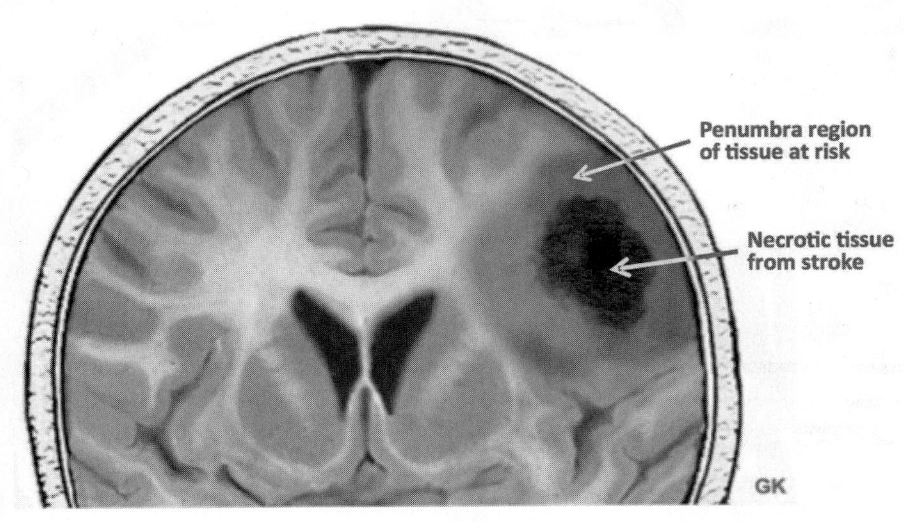

Note the extended amount of brain tissue at risk, as compared with the initial brain damage.
Source: Courtesy of George Kyriakidis/Santa Ana, CA

Cell Death

- When blood flow is not restored to a section of the brain, the cells go through a process of cell death. The cells that are injured or dying begin to swell (cerebral edema). When a large region of the brain swells, it can impact the individual's level of consciousness. The patient can develop increased ICP. After a large stroke, if the ICP increases too much, the entire brain may be secondarily injured from the effects of the edema and pressure, compressing the healthy tissue. Brain death may occur.
- It is important to assess for increases in ICP so treatment can be initiated as soon as possible to lower ICP.
- Two other factors can influence outcome in ischemic stroke:
  - o Poorly controlled blood glucose (>180 mg/dL)
  - o Elevations in body temperature >37°C
  - o Both can contribute to poorer outcomes and higher mortality.

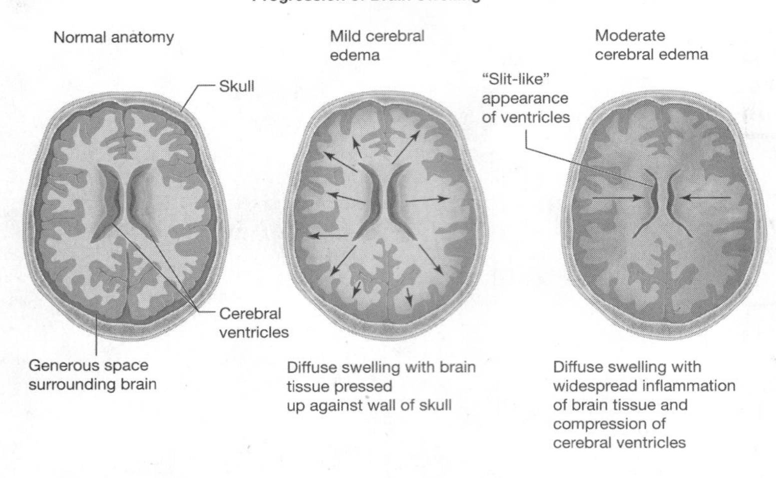

Pathological Evolution of a Stroke

Day 1

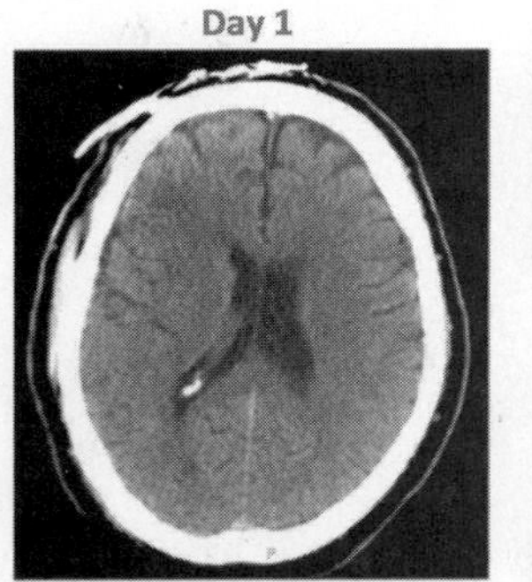

Initially, there is no sign in the CT scan of a stroke. The brain appears to be normal.

Day 3

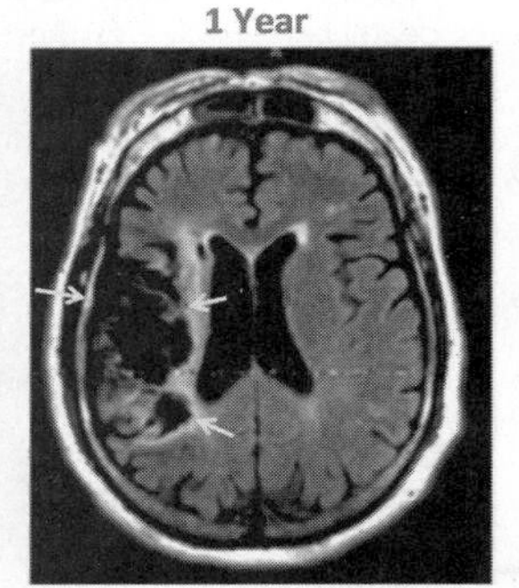

By Day 3, an acute large right middle cerebral artery infarction appears.

1 Year

At 1 year, extensive encephalomalacia (softening or loss of brain tissue) results from the stroke.

Source: Courtesy of K. Kyriakidis

LO2:

Risk Factors: Ischemic Stroke

Risk factors associated with stroke fall into two categories:

- Nonmodifiable risk factors include age, gender, heredity/family history, and race/ethnicity.
- Modifiable risk factors include hypertension, smoking, diabetes, cardiovascular disease, cardiac dysrhythmias such as atrial fibrillation, elevated cholesterol/lipids, carotid artery stenosis, hypercoagulable states, birth control pills, drug use, obesity, poor diet, and lack of physical activity.

LO2:

Causes: Ischemic Stroke

- Causes of ischemic stroke are extensive, but most common are:
  - o Atherosclerosis
  - o Vasoconstriction
  - o Aortic and cardioembolic disease
  - o Lipohyalinosis (lipid hyaline build up)
  - o Vascular occlusion
- A less typical but important cause is:
  - o Systemic hypoperfusion, often the result of cardiac arrest or lethal dysrhythmias. Hypoperfusion causes global rather than localized brain ischemia and damage.

Concept Check

2. What action protects the penumbra?

A. Allowing blood pressure to be higher than normal
B. Maintaining heart rate at lower than normal
C. Increasing blood glucose temporarily
D. Keeping the patient warmer than normal

Answer question

LO2:

Assessment Findings: Ischemic Stroke

- Individuals sustaining an ischemic stroke usually present with a focal deficit. Look for weakness or no movement in the face, arm, and/or leg on one side of the body.
- Numbness in the face, arm, or leg can occur. Patients with a blocked vessel in their dominant hemisphere, where their speech center is located, present with the inability to speak and/or understand the spoken word. This is called **aphasia**.

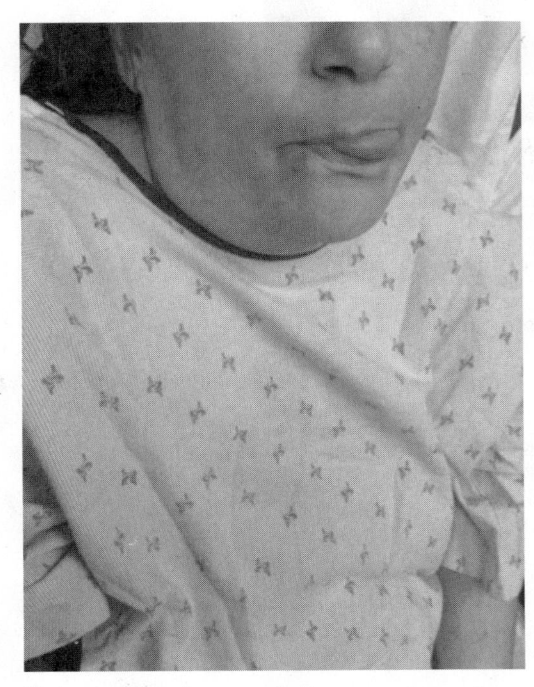

Notice the patient has control of her tongue from only one side. Difficulties with speech may accompany the loss of control.
Source: Courtesy of K. Kyriakidis

- Other findings for ischemic stroke are related to the specific vessel occluded. These include headache, visual loss (cortical blindness), loss of balance or dizziness, confusion, loss of coordination, and loss of spatial awareness or the ability to recognize one's own body parts or one side of the environment (often called unilateral neglect or extinction).
- Stroke patients may lose the ability to do math, read, write, and perform activities of daily living like brushing their teeth.
- It is important for the general public to be educated on stroke symptoms so the symptoms are recognized and the individual is rapidly transported to a hospital, particularly one with a certified stroke center.

LO2:

Diagnostics: Ischemic Stroke

- Diagnosis of ischemic stroke is based on clinical findings of a neurologic deficit that lasts 24 hours. Neurologic deficits that resolve within 24 hours are classified as TIA.

M N EBP

- Neurologic imaging (CT or MRI) is the most widely used test in diagnosis confirmation and classification of stroke subtype. CT scans can be performed quickly and are very good at differentiating a hemorrhagic stroke from an ischemic stroke. However, CT scans of the brain are often initially normal (Morgenstern, et al., 2010).

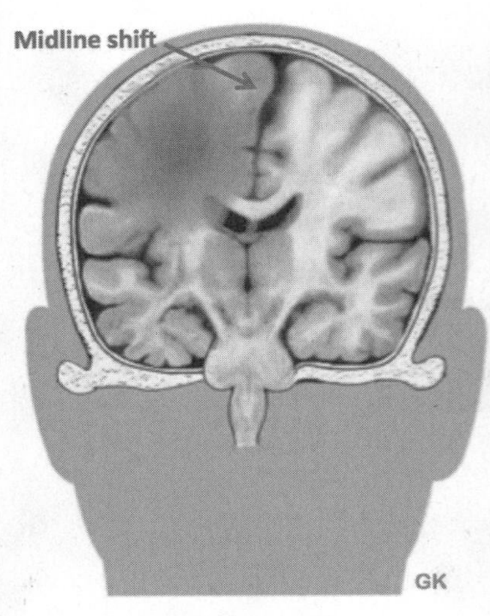

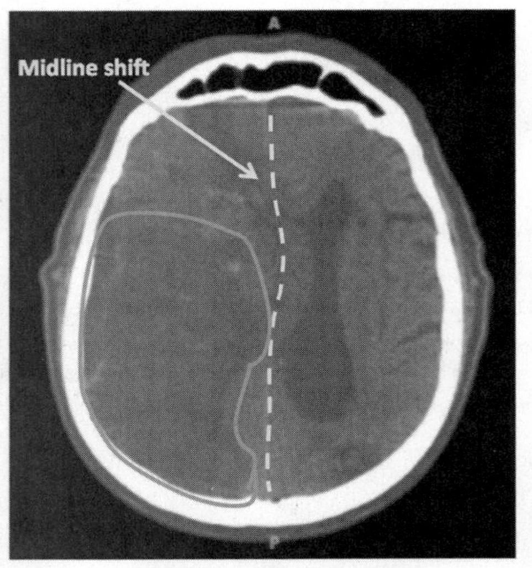

Vertical view

Horizontal view

Left: This image depicts the pathologic and anatomical changes due to a large hemispheric ischemic stroke with a midline shift from cerebral edema. Right: This CT scan reveals the same large ischemic stroke (blue circle) in a patient, with a subsequent midline shift from cerebral edema. The severity of the edema has compressed the adjacent ventricle.

Sources: Courtesy of George Kyriakidis, Santa Ana, CA, & K. Kyriakidis

- Glucose should be checked early on since hypoglycemia can present with symptoms similar to stroke.
- Cardiac monitoring is essential since it can detect atrial fibrillation, which is a common cause of embolic stroke.

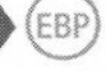

- MRI with contrast is more sensitive than CT at evaluating ischemic stroke, especially early on. See the CT and MRI images of the brain of a patient whose stroke symptoms started two hours earlier. The image on the left is a CT of the brain, and it appears normal. The MRI with contrast of the same brain shows the deficit clearly (Morgenstern, et al., 2010).

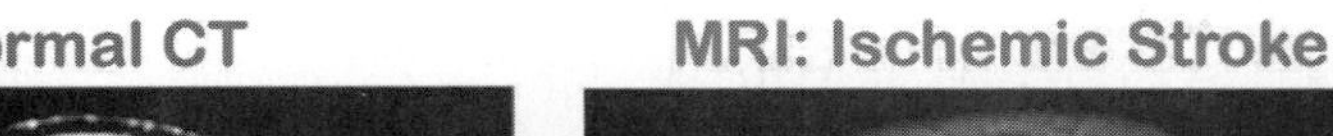

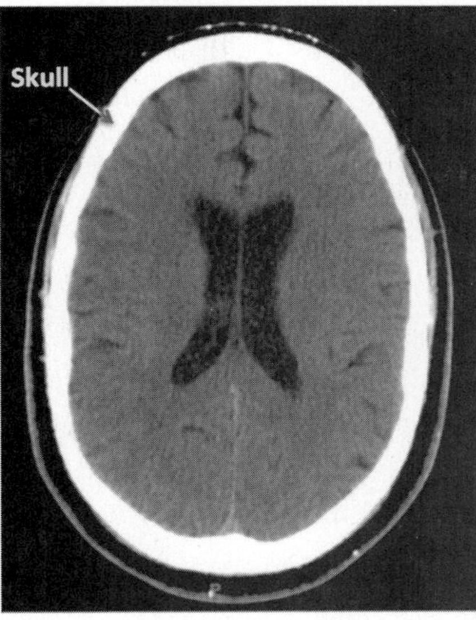

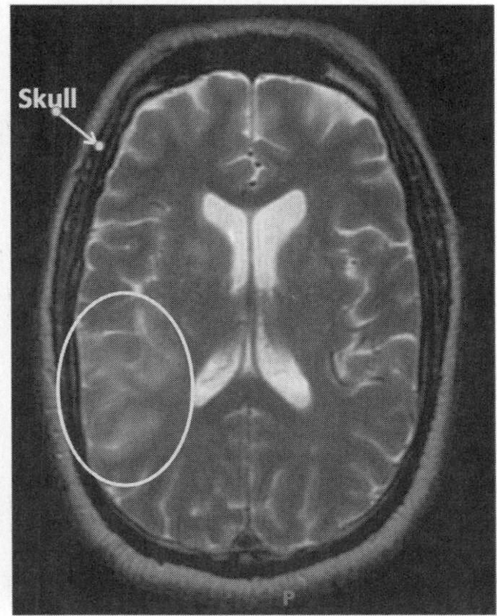

The CT brain scan on the left appears normal after a stroke. However, the MRI (right) of the same patient clearly shows the injured tissue (yellow circle).
Source: Courtesy of K. Kyriakidis

- Carotid and vertebral dopplers can determine presence of blockage in the carotid and vertebral arteries.
- MRI and CT angiography can help evaluate the above vessels as well as the intracranial vessels (Morgenstern, et al., 2010).
- Echocardiography can look for sources of blood clot that can embolize to the brain.

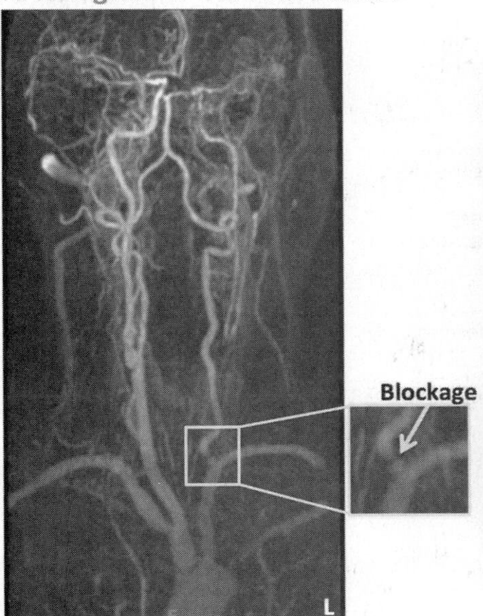

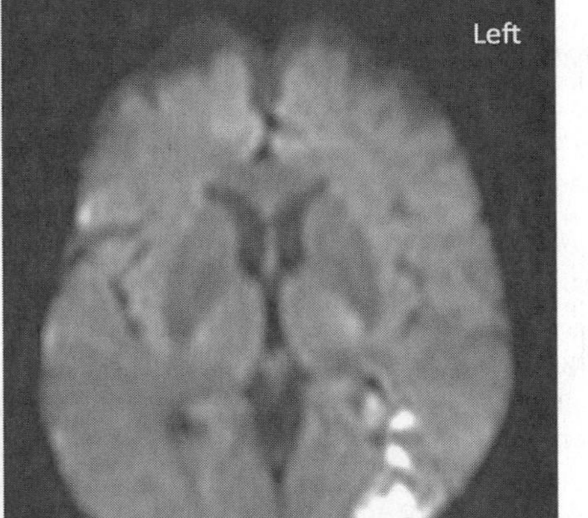

Left: The MR arteriogram of the carotid arteries shows the left common carotid is occluded at its origin. Blood flow is seen in the carotid beyond the blockage due to collateral blood flow and perfusion. Middle: This image is a close-up view of the blockage in the carotid artery. Right: The MRI shows the subsequent stroke on the patient's left side, caused by the carotid blockage.
Source: Courtesy of K. Kyriakidis

Priority Patient Concerns and Desired Collaborative Care Outcomes: Ischemic Stroke

Prior to caring for patients with ischemic stroke, it is important to prioritize the patient's concerns that must guide the nursing care plan and interventions. Care for the patient is ordered and organized in accordance with the patient's priority and urgent needs. Desired collaborative care outcomes in patients with ischemic stroke typically include:

1. Patient will state acceptance of body.
2. Patient will use effective alternative communication skills.
3. Patient will avoid falls.
4. Patient and family will use techniques to help stimulate and maintain the patient's memory.
5. Patient will not aspirate.
6. Patient and family will demonstrate effective coping mechanisms and realignment of roles.

Considering these important care outcomes, prepare a list of the major 3–6 priority patient concerns or nursing diagnoses for patients with ischemic stroke. Be prepared to participate in a discussion of this list and/or to submit them as an assignment, as determined by your faculty. Resources you may find helpful in this assignment can include this lesson, the references, resources on nursing care plans, and standard nursing diagnoses manuals.

Concept Check

3. **Stroke is diagnosed when neurological deficits last more than:**

   A. 1 hour

   B. 8 hours

   C. 12 hours

   D. 24 hours

Answer question

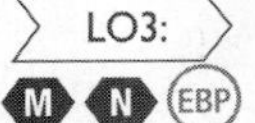

LO3:

Collaborative Interventions: Ischemic Stroke

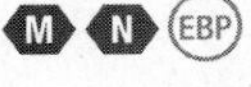

- Hospitals that have undergone intense training in stroke and built protocols for stroke management are best suited to care for the hyperacute stroke population (SIGN, 2010).

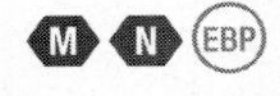

- Patients arriving via ambulance or brought in by their family must be rapidly assessed and triaged to a bed in the emergency department (ED). Delays in identification of stroke must be avoided (SIGN, 2010) as "time is brain." This saying means that about 1.9 million neurons are damaged and destroyed for every minute that a stroke goes untreated.

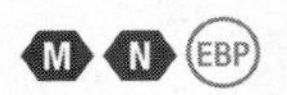

- The suspected stroke patient is brought to an acute ED bed where a stroke team quickly assesses the patient's airway, breathing, circulation, and stroke symptoms (SIGN, 2010).

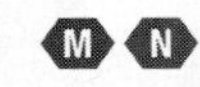

- One or more intravenous (IV) lines are placed, and blood samples are obtained for CBC, coagulation factors, and electrolytes. Infuse saline with no glucose solutions.

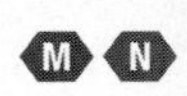

- Supplemental oxygen is started, as needed, if O_2 sats <92%. Continuous pulse oximetry monitoring is initiated.

- Continuous electrocardiogram (ECG) monitoring is needed.

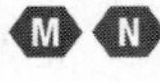

- A stat chest x-ray, 12-lead ECG, and CT scan of the brain are done within 25 minutes of arrival.

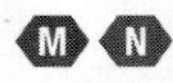

- Use central lines, NG tubes, urinary catheters, and arterial punctures with caution in the first 24 hours, particularly if thrombolytics are considered or used.

Initial Treatment in the ED

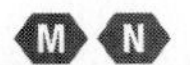

- Most stroke centers use the National Institutes of Health Stroke Scale (NIHSS) to quantify the severity of stroke (see form).
- An individual with no stroke symptoms on the NIHSS would score a 0.
  - o The highest score that can be obtained is 42.
- The level of stroke severity as measured by the NIHSS is:
  - o 0 = no stroke
  - o 1–4 = minor stroke
  - o 5–15 = moderate stroke
  - o 16–20 = moderate to severe stroke
  - o 21–42 = severe stroke

Category	Score/Description						
1a. Level of Consciousness (Alert, drowsy, etc.)	0 = Alert 1 = Drowsy 2 = Stuporous 3 = Coma						
1b. LOC Questions (Month, age)	0 = Answers both correctly 1 = Answers one correctly 2 = Incorrect						
1c. LOC Commands (Open/close eyes, make fist/let go)	0 = Obeys both correctly 1 = Obeys one correctly 2 = Incorrect						
2. Best Gaze (Eyes open - patient follows examiner's finger or face)	0 = Normal 1 = Partial gaze palsy 2 = Forced deviation						
3. Visual Fields (Introduce visual stimulus/threat to pt's visual field quadrants)	0 = No visual loss 1 = Partial Hemianopia 2 = Complete Hemianopia 3 = Bilateral Hemianopia (Blind)						
4. Facial Paresis (Show teeth, raise eyebrows and squeeze eyes shut)	0 = Normal 1 = Minor 2 = Partial 3 = Complete						
5a. Motor Arm - Left **5b. Motor Arm - Right** (Elevate arm to 90° if patient is sitting, 45° if supine)	0 = No drift 1 = Drift 2 = Can't resist gravity 3 = No effort against gravity 4 = No movement X = Untestable (Joint fusion or limb amp)	Left					
		Right					
6a. Motor Leg - Left **6b. Motor Leg - Right** (Elevate leg 30° with patient supine)	0 = No drift 1 = Drift 2 = Can't resist gravity 3 = No effort against gravity 4 = No movement X = Untestable (Joint fusion or limb amp)	Left					
		Right					
7. Limb Ataxia (Finger-nose, heel down shin)	0 = No ataxia 1 = Present in one limb 2 = Present in two limbs						
8. Sensory (Pin prick to face, arm, trunk, and leg - compare side to side)	0 = Normal 1 = Partial loss 2 = Severe loss						
9. Best Language (Name item, describe a picture and read sentences)	0 = No aphasia 1 = Mild to moderate aphasia 2 = Severe aphasia 3 = Mute						
10. Dysarthria (Evaluate speech clarity by patient repeating listed words)	0 = Normal articulation 1 = Mild to moderate slurring of words 2 = Near to unintelligible or worse X = Intubated or other physical barrier						
11. Extinction and Inattention (Use information from prior testing to identify neglect or double simultaneous stimuli testing)	0 = No neglect 1 = Partial neglect 2 = Complete neglect						
	TOTAL SCORE						

INITIAL	SIGNATURE	INITIAL	SIGNATURE	INITIAL	SIGNATURE

Collaborative Interventions: Ischemic Stroke (continued)

Thrombolytics

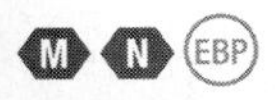

- The major intervention for ischemic stroke is the administration of tissue plasminogen activator (tPA), thrombolytic (Albers, et al., 2008).

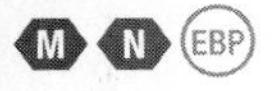

  - o This FDA-approved treatment must be given within 3–4½ hours of the start of the ischemic stroke (Albers, et al., 2008).

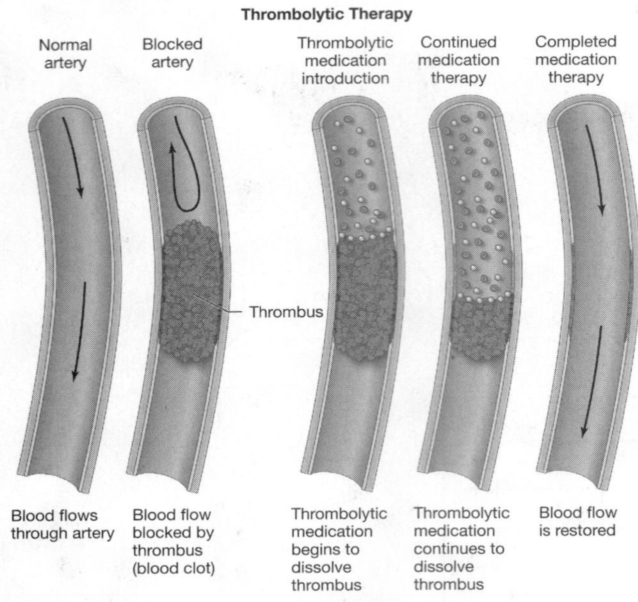

Thrombolytic Therapy
Normal artery
Blocked artery
Thrombolytic medication introduction
Continued medication therapy
Completed medication therapy
Thrombus
Blood flows through artery
Blood flow blocked by thrombus (blood clot)
Thrombolytic medication begins to dissolve thrombus
Thrombolytic medication continues to dissolve thrombus
Blood flow is restored

These five sections of an artery show: 1) normal anatomy with unobstructed blood flow; 2) large pretherapy thrombus causing complete blockage; 3) introduction of thrombolytic medication (small brightly colored dots) attacking the surface of the clot; 4) continued therapy breaking down and dissolving the clot; and 5) completion of therapy with a return to normal blood flow.

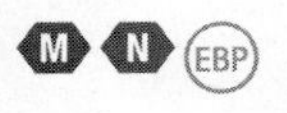

- The team must carefully review the patient's history (e.g., possible coagulopathy, meds like aspirin or warfarin), laboratory results (e.g., glucose, platelets, toxicology, and blood alcohol if suspicious), and CT scan of the brain to rule out any bleeding, and quantify the NIHSS score (Albers, et al., 2008).

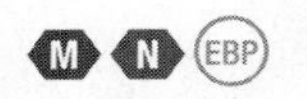

- Inclusion criteria for tPA include:
  - o Over 18 years of age (Albers, et al., 2008)
  - o NIHSS score ≥4
  - o CT scan of the brain showing no bleeding (Albers, et al., 2008)
- There are many contraindications to giving tPA, and studies have demonstrated only 3–12% of patients actually receive tPA for ischemic stroke.

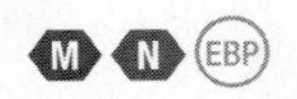

- Blood pressure needs to be lowered to <185/<110 prior to administration of tPA (Albers, et al., 2008). After thrombolytic therapy, maintain BP ≤180 mmHg systolic and ≤105 mmHg diastolic for at least 24 hours.
- Educate patients and families about the benefits, risks, and possible complications of thrombolytic therapy, particularly the risk of bleeding in patients who receive this therapy.
- Monitor the patient closely (neuro checks) for allergic reaction and intracranial hemorrhage after thrombolytic therapy for at least 24–36 hours when the risk of hemorrhage is the highest. Observe and report severe hypertension, onset of severe headache, changes in levels of consciousness, nausea, vomiting, or change in neurological responses. Stop thrombolytic infusion if in progress. Anticipate the need for STAT CT scan, lab work, and possible infusion of platelets.
- However, the majority of stroke patients are not eligible for thrombolytic therapy. The remaining patients benefit from specific supportive care with attention to prevention of acute complications (Albers, et al., 2008).

Treatment for Stroke

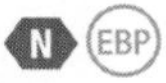

- It is imperative to keep the stroke patient NPO (nothing per mouth) until swallow screen is completed by the health care provider to determine if the patient is at increased risk for aspiration pneumonia (Adams, et al., 2007). Suspect swallowing difficulties if the patient:
  - o Chokes on own saliva
  - o Has garbled speech
  - o Lacks a swallow reflect
  - o Is drooling
  - o Shows facial muscular weakness
  - o Demonstrates gurgling in his/her voice
  - o Has a decreased level of consciousness (LOC)
  - o Has had a brainstem infarction, large hemispheric stroke, or multiple strokes

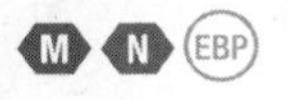

- If the patient cannot swallow safely, the speech pathologist or therapist must further evaluate the patient and recommend the specific type of diet and consistency of the food and fluids. If the patient is unsafe, then enteral or parenteral nutrition is started at some point (SIGN, 2010).

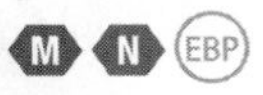

- Aspirin is the only effective antiplatelet drug in the treatment of acute stroke. Aspirin is administered orally if the patient can safely swallow or rectally if not (SIGN, 2010).

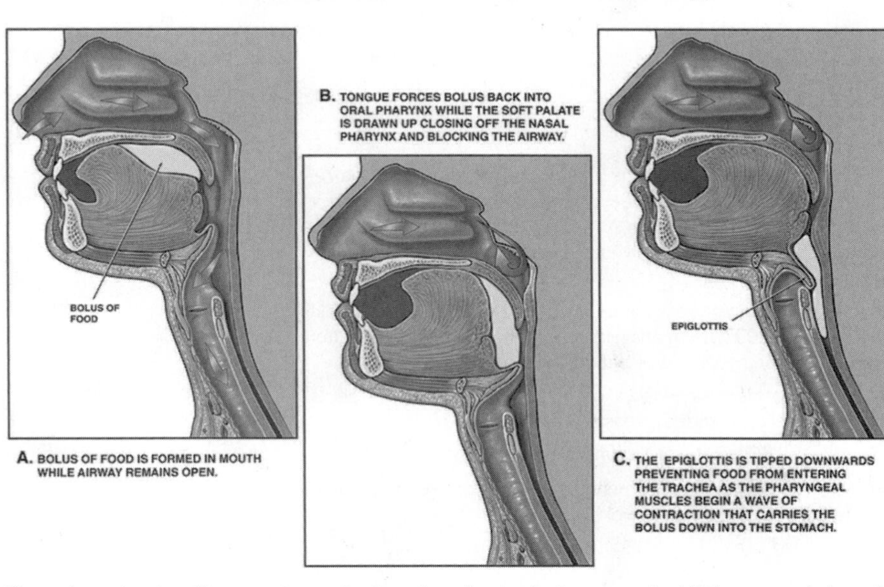
The Action of Swallowing
B. TONGUE FORCES BOLUS BACK INTO ORAL PHARYNX WHILE THE SOFT PALATE IS DRAWN UP CLOSING OFF THE NASAL PHARYNX AND BLOCKING THE AIRWAY.
BOLUS OF FOOD
EPIGLOTTIS
A. BOLUS OF FOOD IS FORMED IN MOUTH WHILE AIRWAY REMAINS OPEN.
C. THE EPIGLOTTIS IS TIPPED DOWNWARDS PREVENTING FOOD FROM ENTERING THE TRACHEA AS THE PHARYNGEAL MUSCLES BEGIN A WAVE OF CONTRACTION THAT CARRIES THE BOLUS DOWN INTO THE STOMACH.

These three drawings illustrate the mechanism of swallowing. It shows a sagittal (side cut away) view of the head and neck. In stroke patients, swallowing may be impaired and needs evaluation.

- Monitor patients closely for complications with neuro and BP checks every 15–30 minutes during the first 2–6 hours, followed by checks every 1–2 hours during the acute phase. Note that seizures are a potential complication that may occur early or late following stroke. Seizures can be life-threatening.

Collaborative Interventions: Ischemic Stroke (continued)

Blood Pressure Support

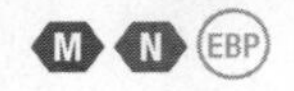

- A key goal in acute stroke management is perfusion of the ischemic penumbra, which can require higher pressures. Acute drops in blood pressure may cause further damage to this ischemic penumbra and, therefore, worsen the stroke and the patient's outcome (Adams, et al., 2007).

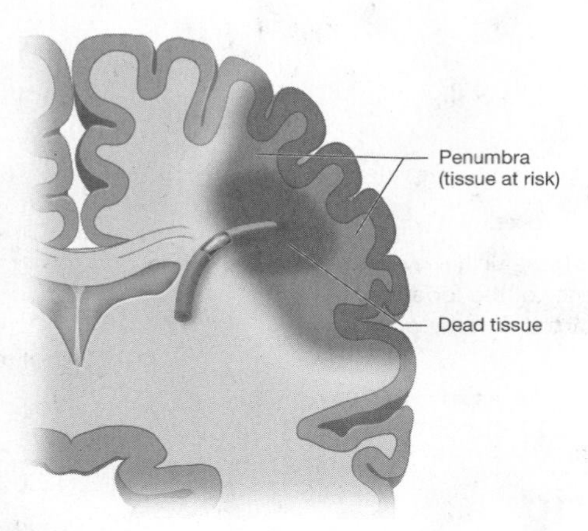

This image shows the large areas of brain tissue (penumbra) surrounding the initially damaged brain tissue. High perfusion pressures may be needed to prevent the penumbra from continued ischemia and consequently becoming part of the infarcted area.

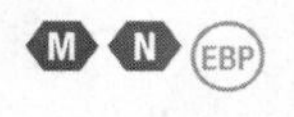

- Clinical hypotension takes on new meaning in the face of stroke. BP support may be required to maintain an adequate perfusion pressure. Collaborate with the team to maintain a **mean arterial pressure** (MAP) of 120–130 mmHg. A MAP in most non-stroke patients is 70–105 mmHg. Collaborate with team in patients who also have heart failure, coronary disease, and renal failure (Adams, et al., 2007).

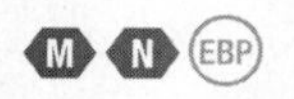

- Treatment of significantly elevated blood pressure is contraindicated unless the pressure exceeds 220/120 mm Hg (Adams, et al., 2007). BP management in patients immediately after stroke diverges from BP management in hypertensive patients without stroke.

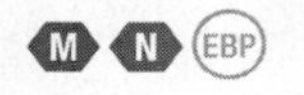

- If BP exceeds 220/120 mmHg and treatment is needed, short acting antihypertensive agents, such as labetalol or nicardipine, are recommended (Adams, et al., 2007).

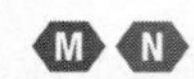

- If the patient does qualify for tPA, the BP treatment threshold is lowered.

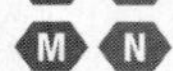

- After the acute phase of stroke, long-term BP management focuses on control and prevention of hypertension to reduce the risk of recurrent stroke.

Hospital Care

M N EBP
- Once admitted, oxygenation and ventilation are assessed for adequacy. The team watches the patient's ability to clear secretions from the airway (Adams, et al., 2007).

M N EBP
- The newly admitted patient undergoes frequent neurologic checks to monitor for neurologic decline secondary to cerebral edema (Adams, et al., 2007).

N EBP
- Vital signs are monitored closely to ensure the correct BP threshold is treated, depending on whether or not tPA was given. The stroke patient usually has continuous ECG (Adams, et al., 2007).

N EBP
- Monitor for dysrhythmias, which are not uncommon in the first 24 hours, particularly atrial fibrillation. Evaluate the patient's hemodynamic status if dysrhythmias are detected (Adams, et al., 2007).

M N EBP
- Glycemic control: Blood glucose levels should be carefully monitored and managed as a high priority in the first 24 hours.

M N EBP
  - o Administer insulin, in collaboration with the health care provider, when glucose exceeds 180 mg/dL. Hyperglycemia contributes to poorer outcomes and higher mortality and is common in two-thirds of all stroke patients. Maintain target glucose <140 mg/dL. Avoid glucose in IV solutions (Adams, et al., 2007).

M N EBP
  - o Administer glucose 50% as directed if hypoglycemia is detected. Hypoglycemia can exclude the patient from receiving thrombolytic therapy and can also lead to neurological abnormalities that mimic stroke (Adams, et al., 2007).

M N EBP
- Administer antipyretics (e.g., acetaminophen) and look for the source of infection (e.g., pneumonia, UTI) if fever >38°C develops (Adams, et al., 2007).

M N
- Monitor for intracranial edema with increased ICP, which may ensue as early as the first 24 hours in patients with large multilobar and cerebellar infarcts or as late as 3–4 days after middle cerebral artery (MCA)-related strokes. The goal is to detect and manage brain edema by reducing ICP to prevent brain herniation:

M N
  - o Observe for early warning signs such as altered level of consciousness, headache, and/or visual disturbances.

M N
  - o Late signs include pupillary abnormalities, respiratory pattern changes (e.g., Cheyne-Stokes if cerebral stroke, neurogenic hyperventilation if midbrain stroke, cluster if pons or medulla stroke, apneusis if pons stroke, or ataxia), BP changes like widening pulse pressure, and changes in heart rate like bradycardia.

M N EBP
  - o Monitor and collaboratively manage hyperthermia, hypoxemia, and hypercarbia (Adams, et al., 2007).

M N EBP
  - o Treatments to reduce increased ICP may include hyperventilation, drainage of cerebral spinal fluid (CSF), osmotics (e.g., furosemide, mannitol), and/or decompression via surgery. Reducing CO_2 concentrations by 5–10 mmHg using hyperventilation can lower ICP by as much as 25–30%. Hyperventilation is used short term with caution due to the potential for vasoconstriction that compromises brain perfusion. Use of mannitol requires close monitoring of the urine and serum osmolality (Adams, et al., 2007).

M N
  - o ICP monitoring and drainage should be done in the ICU setting and require meticulous care.

M N EBP
  - o Clinical practice guidelines strongly recommend avoiding the use of corticosteroids to treat increased ICP in patients with stroke (Adams, et al., 2007).

M N EBP
- Stroke patients are commonly at high risk for most of the **never events** (serious, preventable, costly events that should never happen). Prevention and safety are key. Care should include prophylaxis for deep vein thrombosis and pulmonary embolism, positioning (head of bed at 30 degrees) to prevent aspiration and pneumonia, falls and pressure ulcer prevention, meticulous care when using invasive monitoring and devices (particularly intubation and vascular and urinary catheters), and adequate range of motion to the arms and legs to avoid contractures (Adams, et al., 2007). Prevention is critical. Pulmonary embolism is responsible for 50% of deaths after stroke, as an example.

Collaborative Interventions: Ischemic Stroke (continued)

Supportive and Comfort Care

- Supportive care to prevent/reduce increased ICP should be discussed collaboratively with the team. Clinicians should:
  - M N EBP o Elevate the head of the bed 25–30 degrees except in patients with MCA stroke who have better outcomes with supine position. The risk of aspiration must be weighed against the potential benefits of the supine position (Summers, et al., 2009).
  - N o Provide good head and body alignment to reduce intrathoracic pressure and promote venous drainage.
  - M N o Provide good pain management.
  - N o Plan activities to avoid overtiring or overstimulating the patient.
  - N M EBP o Maintain normothermia as hyperthermia is associated with higher morbidity and mortality due to increased metabolic demands on the brain. Fever can, therefore, exacerbate ischemia and brain damage. Fever can be due to infection or can be neurogenic (Adams, et al., 2007).
- N Avoid fluid overload and dehydration in fluid management to improve outcomes.
- M N Depending on the location and extent of the stroke, electrolyte disturbances may be more prominent and require monitoring and management.
- M N Ensure adequate nutritional intake as soon as the swallowing assessment is completed. Nutrition should utilize the least invasive means that the patient can manage. Oral nutrition is best if the patient can swallow effectively. If not, enteral feedings are preferred over parenteral infusions to minimize infection risks. It is simpler, lowers costs, maintains intestinal mucosal function, and maintains normal digestion.
- M N Consult a dietitian for the best types of foods for intake, depending on the patient's nutritional feeding route, to determine the patient's caloric needs, and to adjust the caloric intake over time as needed.
- N Monitor weight every 3–7 days to evaluate nutritional support.
- N Reduce the risk of aspiration in patients on oral intake:
  - N o Sit the patient in high Fowler's position but preferably in a chair sitting up.
  - N o Have the patient sit for at least 30 minutes after meals.
  - N o Provide mouth care before and after meals. Mouth care before meals increases the production of saliva to facilitate swallowing. Mouth care after meals enables recognition of food pocketing in the mouth that can lead to aspiration.
  - N o Educate the patient and family that food is placed in the unaffected side of the mouth for eating.
  - N o Encourage the patient to take small frequent meals and take time to chew and swallow. Instruct the patient to do a chin-tuck when swallowing to reduce aspiration risk.
  - N o Ensure that food is in the patient's visual field and instruct the patient to scan the whole plate and tray if the patient has visual field loss.
  - N o Keep suctioning device near the patient during meals in case needed.
  - N o Avoid the use of straws to drink when lying in bed. This is a dangerous practice and increases the risk of aspiration.
  - N o Educate the family on all supportive and preventive care.
- Minimize the risk of infection, particularly pneumonia and urinary tract infections.
  - o About 35% of deaths in patients with strokes are due to pneumonia.
  - o Approximately 15–60% of stroke patients have urinary tract infections (UTI), and UTI is a predictor of poor outcomes. With altered sphincter control and use of indwelling urinary catheters, stroke patients are at high risk for UTI.
  - M N EBP o Avoid immobility, which leads to atelectasis and then pneumonia (Hinchey, et al., 2005). Evidence shows that this nurse-initiated intervention decreases the incidence of pneumonia.

- o Monitor airway and oxygenation along with structured swallowing assessments to reduce the incidence of pneumonia (Hinchey, et al., 2005). Evidence shows that nurse-initiated pulmonary toilet interventions decrease the incidence of pneumonia.
  - o Avoid the use of indwelling urinary catheters if at all possible and remove them as soon as indicated (Adams, et al., 2007). An indwelling catheter is not a good or appropriate solution to urinary incontinence, which occurs in 30–60% of patients after stroke (see the Urinary Incontinence NovE-lesson for detailed management and nursing care).
  - o Be alert, if the patient has an indwelling urinary catheter, for early signs of infection, which can include altered LOC along with typical signs of UTI (Adams, et al., 2007).
  - o Collaborate with HCP to administer antibiotic to treat real or suspected infection (Adams, et al., 2007).
- Reduce the risk of aspiration pneumonia in dysphagic patients, especially if they are "silent aspirators," by providing aggressive oral care to minimize bacterial counts if the patient is silently aspirating.
- Provide and collaborate with family and support services (e.g., clergy, psych team) to provide emotional and social support to prevent or manage possible depression and stress. Support may also be imperative for patients with communication, visual, cognitive, functional, and/or mobility problems.
- Be attentive to potential bowel dysfunction, which is common in stroke patients. Prevent constipation, the most common problem:
  - o Assess ongoing bowel function, hydration, and fluid intake.
  - o Become familiar with pre-stroke elimination pattern and work to restore the patient's normal pattern.
  - o Employ frequent mobility and hydration to avoid constipation. Make diet changes to improve fiber, fruits, and vegetables to enhance return to the patient's normal.
  - o Integrate stool softeners, suppositories, laxatives, and enemas if needed. These are *not* replacements for good nursing care to ensure that the patient moves their bowels at least every two days. The nurse must take responsibility for the patient's bowel care.
- Prevent morbidity due to immobility. Mobilizing patients is primarily a nursing responsibility, which can prevent contractures, atrophy, nerve-pressure palsy, and orthopedic complications. Ensure proper range of motion exercises (active if possible, passive if not) are performed in collaboration with physical therapy and correct positioning is used.
- Transfer the patient to rehabilitation at the earliest possible time to improve the patient's outcome.
- Avoid skin breakdown as patients with stroke are at high risk for problems.
  - o Assess the patient's skin frequently.
  - o Mobilize the patient early.
  - o Keep the patient clean if they have bladder or bowel incontinence, particularly in patients with diabetes, renal failure, and peripheral vascular disease.
  - o Use a risk-assessment tool to evaluate and predict the risk of pressure ulcer occurrence.
  - o Reposition the patient every 2 hours using appropriate techniques.
  - o Avoid friction involving the patient's skin, as friction can result in injury or tears.
  - o Use accepted skin care products but keep the patient's skin dry and clean.

Collaborative Interventions: Ischemic Stroke (continued)

Secondary Prevention

- Antiplatelet agents such as aspirin and clopidogrel are often used (Albers, et al., 2008).

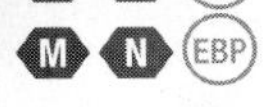

- Antithrombotic agents (warfarin, heparin) are also used depending on stroke etiology (Albers, et al., 2008).

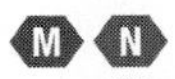

- Lipid-lowering agents (statins) are used after assessment of plasma lipid levels.
- Carotid endarterectomy (CEA) is a surgical procedure to remove the buildup of plaque in a carotid artery:
  - o Candidates for CEA include patients who sustain a mild stroke that is not debilitating and patients who have a TIA with carotid artery stenosis >50%.
  - o Patients who benefit from CEA include those in whom the location of the stenosis explains the symptoms. For example, a patient with transient right-sided weakness with 65% stenosis in the right carotid artery is not a good candidate for CEA as this patient should show left carotid stenosis.

- Stenting of the carotid artery is an alternative to CEA that is less invasive:
  - o Stenting consists of inserting a catheter, typically through the femoral artery, passing it through the aorta, and guiding it to the carotid artery with the help of x-ray (fluoroscopy) to locate the stenotic area.
  - o A stent is then placed in the area of stenosis to open the arterial lumen.
- Both CEA and stenting procedures are generally useful in reducing the incidence of future stroke, although stenting has more associated complications in patients who are older than 70. Complications of these procedures include infection, bleeding, myocardial infarction, and stroke (Brott, et al., 2004; Brott, et al., 2010; Rothwell, et al., 2004).
- Investigational methods: A number of investigational methods are being used in patients who are outside the normal window for administration of TPA in some centers. These include intra-arterial thrombolysis, mechanical clot disruption, and stenting of the occluded arteries.
- Primary prevention is focused on educating the patient and family members about the risks associated with stroke. Education should include taking antihypertensive and diabetic medications, warfarin for atrial fibrillation (when appropriate), and antiplatelet agents for cardiovascular and blood related disorders; disease process; recognition of complications; potential for seizure; when to call the health care provider; prevention of infections and the hazards of immobility. Educate the patient and family about modifiable risk factors by encouraging lifestyle changes, as indicated: Stop smoking, increase physical activity, promote healthy diet changes, manage weight, control cholesterol, and manage lipids. These changes are imperative to reduce the risk of future stroke.

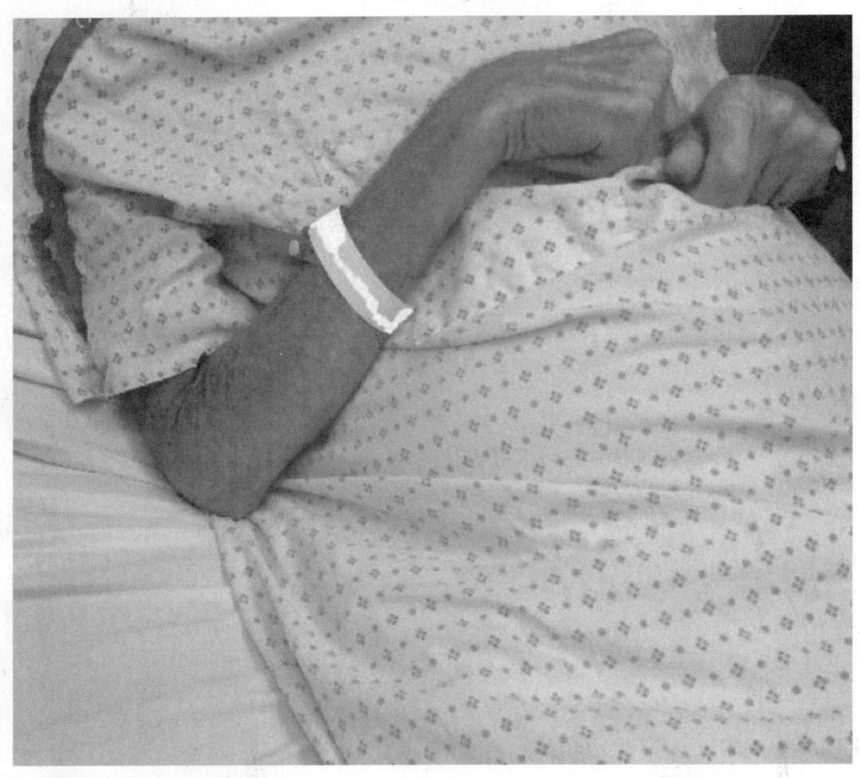

After stroke, this patent developed contractures of the arms. Preventing hazards of immobility that may follow stroke are imperative for the patient to maintain as much mobility and function as possible.

Source: Courtesy of K. Kyriakidis

Ischemic Versus TIA: Summary of Interventions

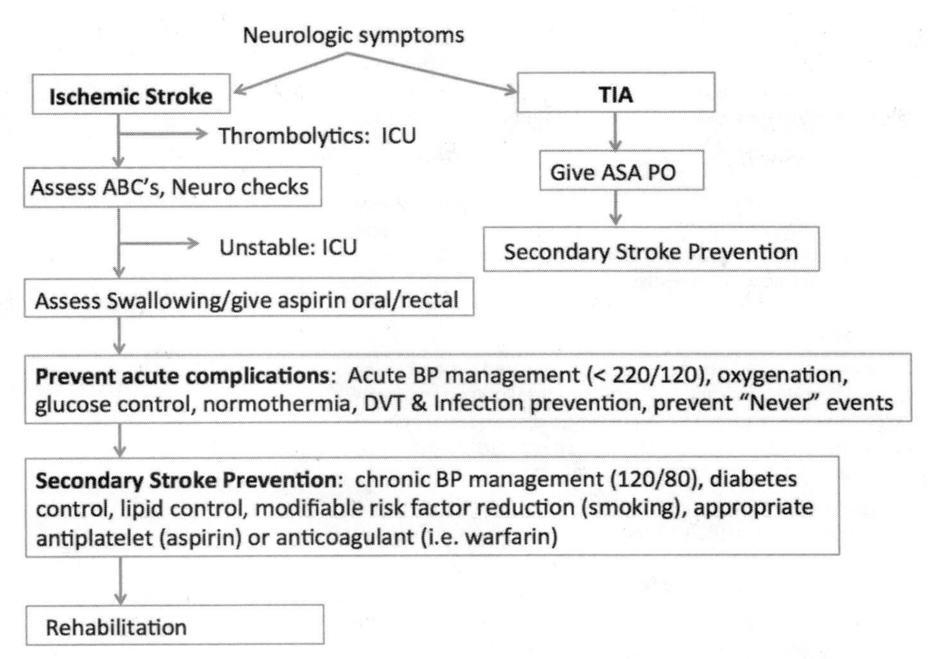

The schematic summarizes the care of patients with an ischemic stroke or transient ischemic attack.
Source: Copyright © 2014. NovEx Novice to Expert Learning, LLC

Collaborative Interventions: Ischemic Stroke (continued)

Impact of a Stroke

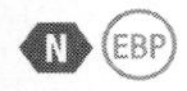

- Depending on the area of the brain impacted and severity of the stroke, patients can demonstrate varying loss of function, which can involve speech, movement, sensation, coordination, spatial awareness, and activities of daily living (refer to functional anatomy module). Individualization of nursing care should occur, and interventions geared toward maximizing the functions that are present (SIGN, 2010).

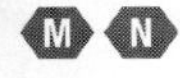

- Rehabilitation, as an inpatient and referral to an outpatient center, should begin as soon as the patient is stable and ready. Rehabilitation specialists are well prepared to assist patients to learn how to adapt to their acquired limitations and to acquire new skills in everyday living and work.

Dominant Hemisphere Stroke

- If the stroke occurs in the dominant hemisphere (usually the left hemisphere in the right-handed person), there can be a loss of speech or understanding speech.
- Commands may need to be given to the patient with visual cues. The speech pathologist may suggest strategies for the team to use to help patients communicate their needs to the staff.
- Patients can become very frustrated when they are unable to talk and express their wishes for care or communicate their immediate needs. Work with the patient to determine a good communication system.
- The dominant hemisphere stroke patient loses movement and possibly sensation in the opposite arm and/or leg. Care should be directed at correct positioning of the opposite arm/leg to ensure correct alignment and prevention of skin breakdown.
- Dominant hemisphere stroke patients may also lack initiation and need to be encouraged to engage in activities such as eating, bathing, and grooming. These patients may also undergo apraxia, which is the inability to perform planned motor acts.
- The ability to brush teeth or comb the hair are learned behaviors stored in the frontal lobe. The individual may be able to tell the health care provider that the toothbrush is for brushing teeth but they cannot put together the sequence of steps to accomplish the task.

Nondominant Hemisphere Stroke

- The patient sustaining a stroke in the nondominant hemisphere (usually the right hemisphere in right-handed people) can understand verbal commands and cues but usually neglects the left environment. Place the call light, phone, and urinal on the right side of the bed so the patient notices these items in the "side of the world they recognize." Expect the nondominant hemisphere stroke patient to have difficulty getting dressed since this function is found in the right parietal lobe.

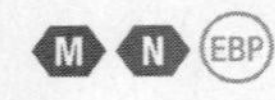

- Many stroke patients have visual field cuts or vision loss (SIGN, 2010). Approach the patient midline and move to the left side of the bed then the right side. Watch to see if the patient visually follows movement to the left or the right. If the patient does not follow to one side, then the health care team should approach the patient's midline and encourage him/her to learn to scan to the side the patient does not acknowledge or see.

Safety Factors for the Stroke Patient

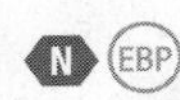

- Safety is important in the stroke patient since they are at risk for falls and other injuries. Physical therapy, occupational therapy, and speech therapy are consulted to assist in assessing the patient's deficits. Motor activity is increased after the patient is assessed, and needed caution is determined. Caution must be used when moving the patient into the sitting or standing position as well as ambulating (SIGN, 2010).

- Patients at higher safety-related risk are those with visual disturbances, altered LOC, cognitive deficits, balance and coordination disturbances, unilateral neglect, sensory deficits, affective disorders, swallowing deficits, motor dysfunctions, and abnormal posturing. Safety precautions need to accommodate to the patient's specific needs.

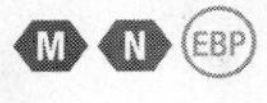

- Consultation with a physiatrist (health care provider specializing in rehabilitation medicine), usually on day 2 or 3, allows the team to plan the discharge needs and patient placement (home, acute rehabilitation, or skilled nursing facility) (SIGN, 2010).

- Patient education on secondary stroke prevention is absolutely vital prior to discharge. If the patient smokes, then smoking cessation counseling should be undertaken. Lastly, the health care provider determines the appropriate anticoagulation, antithrombotic, and/or statin medications to be taken at home after discharge (SIGN, 2010).

Concept Check

4. **What is the highest obtainable score on the NIH stroke scale?**

A. 20
B. 35
C. 42
D. 50

Answer question

LO1:

What Is Hemorrhagic Stroke?

- Hemorrhagic stroke is the rupture of an artery inside the brain. It accounts for 15–20% of all strokes, but it has the highest mortality risk. (Review the animation for hemorrhagic stroke in the "What is Stroke?" section.)

Subtypes

Subtypes of hemorrhagic stroke include intracerebral hemorrhage (ICH) and subarachnoid hemorrhage (SAH).

- ICH occurs when an artery or vein ruptures, causing blood to rapidly escape into the surrounding brain.
- SAH is further classified related to its mechanism. Aneurysmal SAH occurs following rupture of a brain aneurysm (abnormal weakness in the wall of the artery causing ballooning out of the artery). The blood rapidly escapes from the vessel into the subarachnoid space (SAS), ventricles, and/or surrounding brain tissue.
- Vascular malformations that rupture cause SAH as well as ICH. Aneurysms occur ten times more frequently than vascular malformations.

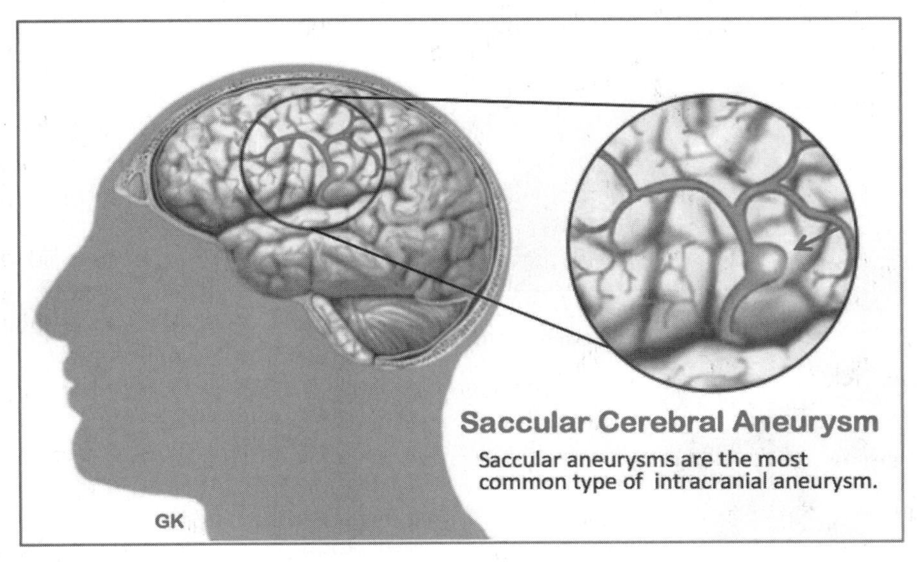

Saccular Cerebral Aneurysm
Saccular aneurysms are the most common type of intracranial aneurysm.
GK

Source: Courtesy of George Kyriakidis/Santa Ana, CA

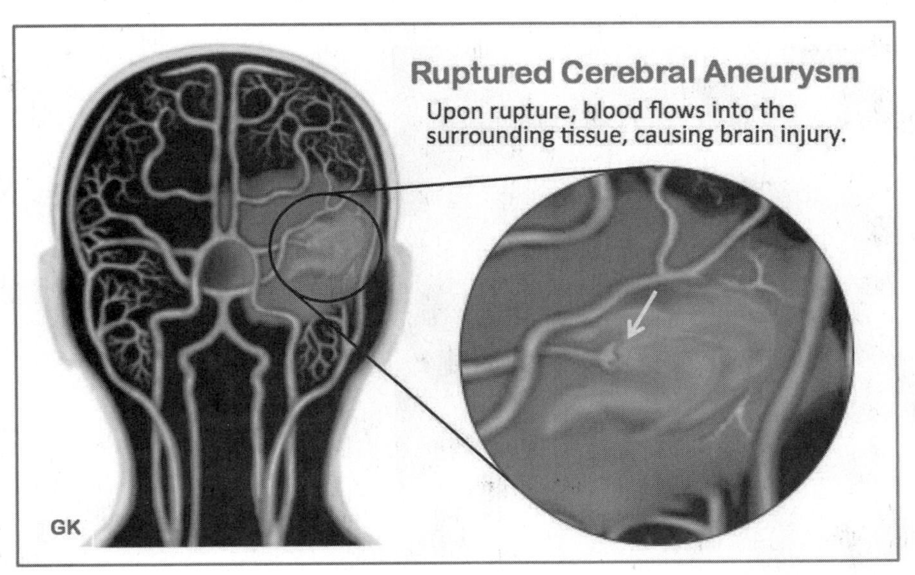

Ruptured Cerebral Aneurysm
Upon rupture, blood flows into the surrounding tissue, causing brain injury.
GK

Source: Courtesy of George Kyriakidis/Santa Ana, CA

LO1: Clinical Relevance: Hemorrhagic Stroke

- Hemorrhagic stroke requires prompt medical attention and has a high mortality rate.
- While it makes up 20% of all strokes, there are important differences from ischemic stroke in terms of treatment.

LO2: Pathophysiology: Hemorrhagic Stroke

- When ICH occurs, a hematoma forms at the site. Blood flow in the immediate area falls, and damage to local brain tissue occurs. Edema results from cell damage, causing the pressure inside the cranial vault to rise. Depending on the size of the hematoma, the pressure can produce minor (headache) to severe (coma) symptoms. There are also cellular changes over several days in the surrounding tissue where swelling occurs.
- Subdural and epidural hematomas are often caused by trauma to the head that disrupts blood vessels (see picture)

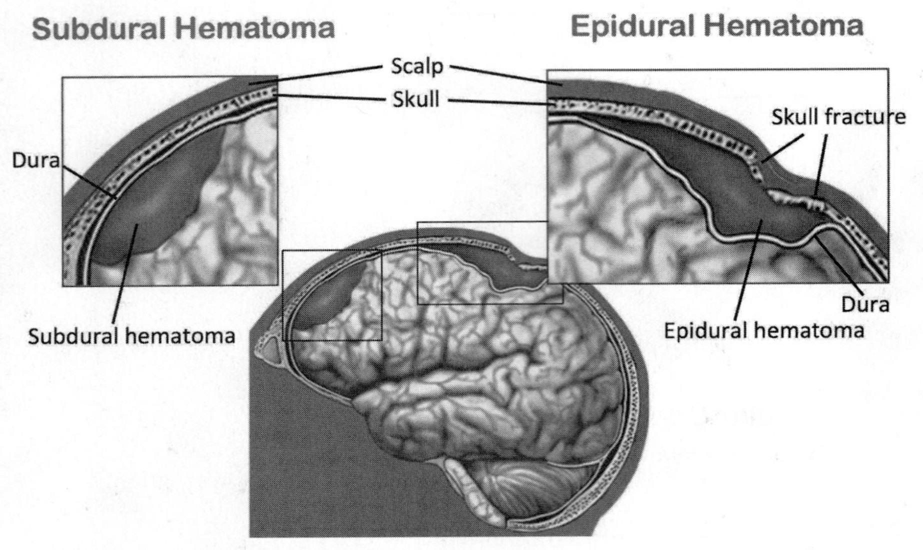

This picture compares an epidural with a subdural hematoma.
Source: Courtesy of George Kyriakidis/Santa Ana, CA

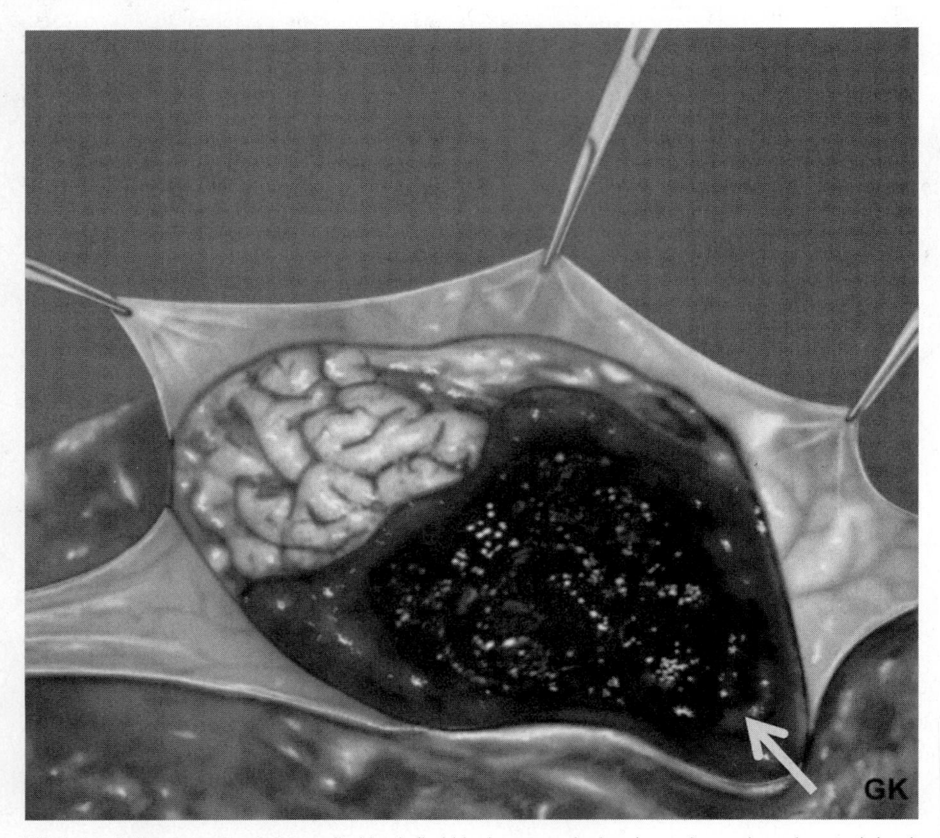

With the skull removed and dura pulled back (held by hemostats), the photo shows that a large subdural hematoma (dark red) lies under the dura and on the surface of the brain.
Source: Courtesy of George Kyriakidis/Santa Ana, CA

- In aneurysmal SAH, the ballooning of the artery usually occurs at bifurcations, where one artery comes off another artery. They come in different sizes and shapes (see picture).
- Aneurysms may be:
  - o Giant, which is defined as having a diameter >25 mm. Although giant aneurysms are much less common, they have a higher rate of rupture and clot formation within the aneurysm.
  - o Saccular with a rounded balloon appearing bulge. These are also called berry aneurysms and account for the majority of cerebral aneurysms.
  - o Fusiform in shape, which distend or dilate the entire circumference of the artery
  - o Dissecting, where the middle and outer layers of the vessel wall separate, dilate, and place the patient at risk for rupture and stroke
  - o Ruptured, which results in cerebral hemorrhage brain

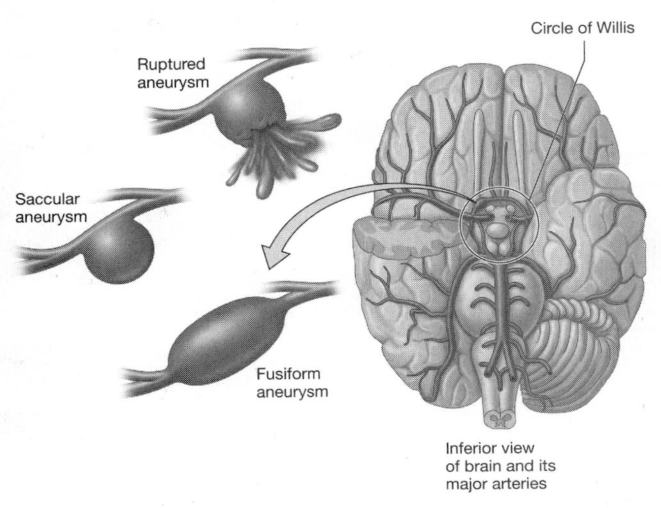

Several types of aneurysms that can lead to hemorrhagic stroke are illustrated.

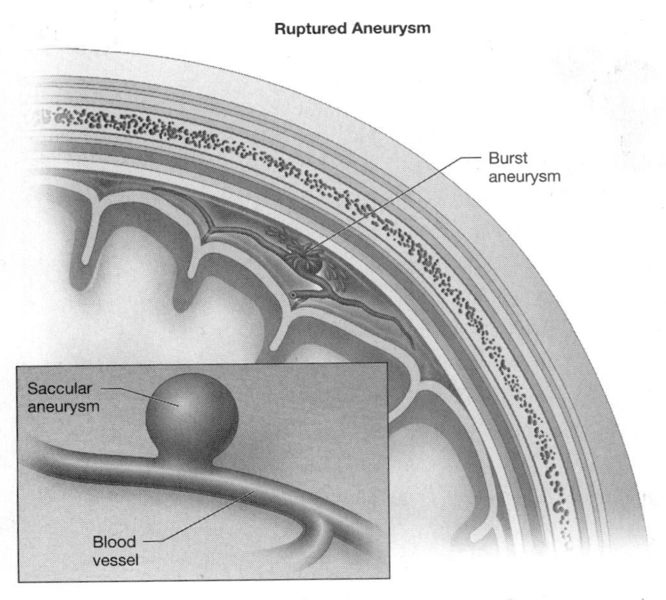

This picture shows the location of the aneurysm rupture (burst aneurysm) in the subarachnoid space.

- Usually the dome of the aneurysm ruptures, causing blood to rapidly escape the artery and enter the subarachnoid space, brain tissue, and/or ventricles. When an aneurysm ruptures, it can produce small or large amounts of blood. If large, it can lead to a sudden increase in ICP. Until the aneurysm is closed off with a surgical clip or coil, it can rebleed, leading to a high mortality. As a result of SAH, complications can develop, such as hydrocephalus (buildup of CSF in the brain because CSF reabsorption is slowed or blocked), hyponatremia and dehydration (loss of sodium and water due to the secretion of brain natriuretic hormone), and/or vasospasm (narrowing of the cerebral arteries in the brain from the free blood in the SAS). If left untreated, this can lead to inadequate blood flow through the artery or arteries to parts of the brain.

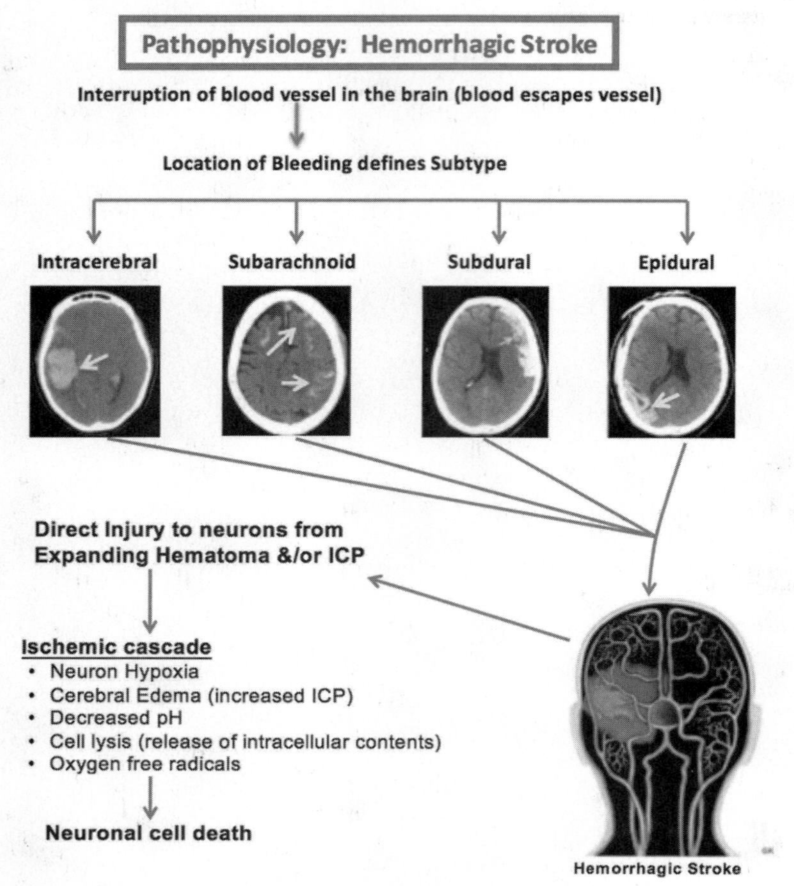

Sources: Courtesy of George Kyriakidis, Santa Ana, CA; K. Kyriakidis; & Copyright © 2014, NovEx Novice to Expert Learning, LLC

LO2:

Risk Factors and Causes: Hemorrhagic Stroke

Risk factor assessment and education are important to avoid the devastating effects of hemorrhagic stroke.

- Hypertension
- Diabetes
- Smoking
- Drug use (cocaine)
- Abnormalities of blood vessels (cerebral aneurysm, AVM)
- Use of anticoagulants (i.e., warfarin)
- Bleeding disorders
- Brain tumors
- Trauma

LO2:

Assessment Findings: Hemorrhagic Stroke

Common Assessment Findings

- Headache "worst of my life"
- Focal weakness of any body part, hemiparesis
- Coma
- Seizures
- Trouble speaking (aphasia)
- Loss of balance
- Visual changes or loss
- Double vision
- Changes in sensation of body parts
- Vomiting

Increased Intracranial Pressure

- **Increased ICP:** Patients presenting with ICH or SAH often demonstrate symptoms and signs of increased ICP.
- **Decreased level of consciousness (LOC):** If ICP increases, the patient's LOC becomes altered. Patients may present with syncope.
- **Inability to clear airway:** Airway compromise can occur if patients cannot clear secretions from their airway. The inability to protect the airway puts patients at greater risk for aspiration and pneumonia.
- **Hypercapnia:** In addition, as their LOC becomes more compromised, patients do not breathe deeply enough or fast enough, leading to increased carbon dioxide retention in their blood. The hypercapnia further worsens ICP due to the dilation it causes in the cerebral arteries.

Concept Check

5. Which condition is a complication of subarachnoid hemorrhage?

A. Hydrocephalus
B. Hypernatremia
C. Vascular dilation
D. Fluid overload

Answer question

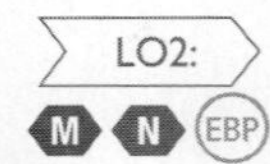

Diagnostics: Hemorrhagic Stroke

- Diagnosis of hemorrhagic stroke is based on history and clinical findings with confirmation using neurologic imaging (CT or MRI) (Morgenstern, et al., 2010).

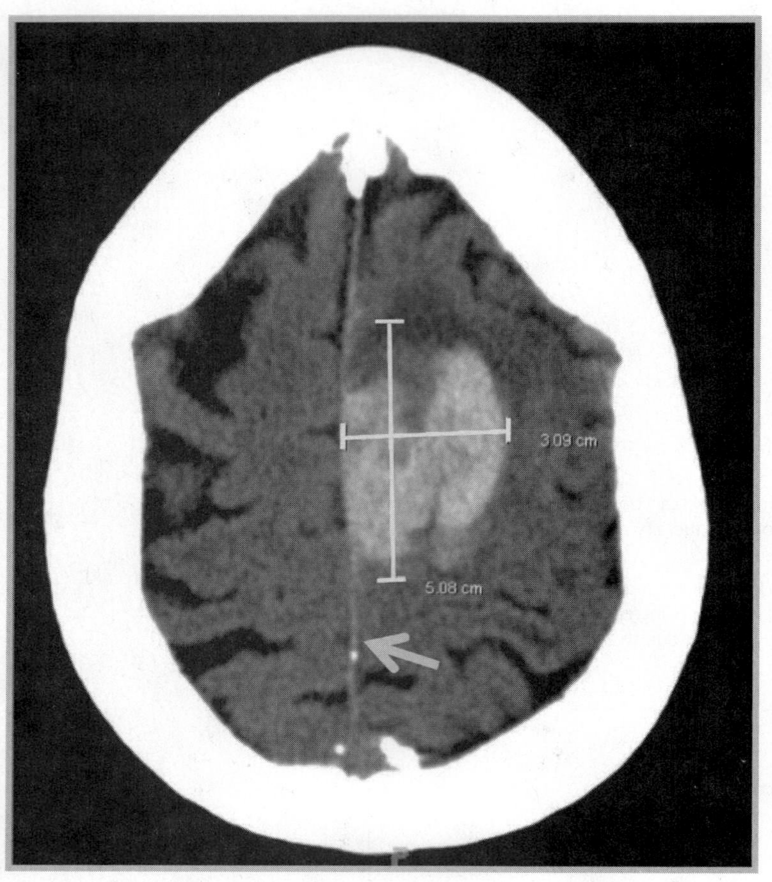

CT image showing a large intracerebral hemorrhage (bright white areas represent blood). Note the midline shift (arrow) of the brain from the hemorrhage and edema.
Source: Courtesy of K. Kyriakidis

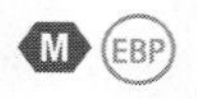

- CT scans are the most widely used tests in patients that present with stroke symptoms. CT scans can be performed quickly and are very good at differentiating a hemorrhagic stroke (right photo) from an ischemic stroke. However, CT scans of the brain are often initially normal (Morgenstern, et al., 2010).

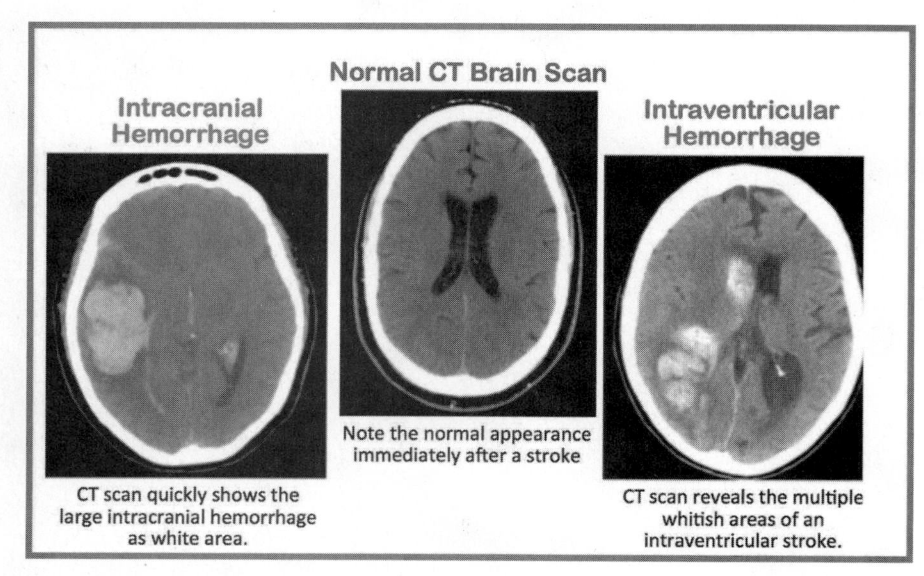

Source: Courtesy of K. Kyriakidis

Priority Patient Concerns and Desired Collaborative Care Outcomes: Hemorrhagic Stroke

Prior to caring for patients with hemorrhagic stroke, it is important to prioritize the patient's concerns that must guide the nursing care plan and interventions. Care for the patient is ordered and organized in accordance with the patient's priority and urgent needs. Desired collaborative care outcomes in patients with hemorrhagic stroke typically include:

1. Patient will report that pain is decreased.
2. Patient will exhibit no findings associated with increased intracranial pressure.
3. Patient's respirations will be regular and unlabored.
4. Patient's intracranial pressure will remain within desired range.
5. Patient will demonstrate reduction in confusion.

Considering these important care outcomes, prepare a list of the major 3–6 priority patient concerns or nursing diagnoses for patients with hemorrhagic stroke. Be prepared to participate in a discussion of this list and/or to submit them as an assignment, as determined by your faculty. Resources you may find helpful in this assignment can include this lesson, the references, resources on nursing care plans, and standard nursing diagnoses manuals.

Concept Check

6. Which finding is often associated with the presence of hemorrhagic stroke?

A. Atrial fibrillation

B. Sudden deafness

C. Inability to void

D. Headache

Answer question

LO3:

Collaborative Interventions: Hemorrhagic Stroke

Intracranial Hemorrhage

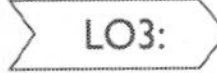

- Patients generally seek care in the ED if they sustain an ICH. The team determines the chief complaint and history. Frequent, repeated neurologic assessments are needed (Morgenstern, et al., 2010).
- Monitor and protect vital functions:

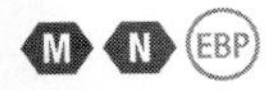

  - o First, assess the airway and breathing. If the patient's Glasgow Coma Score (GCS) is 3–8, intubation and mechanical ventilation are needed to support the airway. Monitor via pulse oximetry to ensure adequate oxygenation (SpO2 >92%).

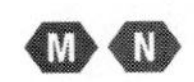

  - o Assess circulation by checking pulse and blood pressure. If the systolic BP is >150 mmHg, IV labetalol and/or nicardipine are used to lower SBP to 140 mmHg and reduce rebleeding risk. Continuously monitor the ECG for rate and rhythm (Morgenstern, et al., 2010).

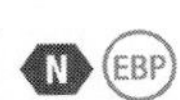

  - o Immediately start IV lines and administer normal saline.

  - o Obtain necessary labwork that includes CBC, electrolytes, blood glucose, and coagulation.

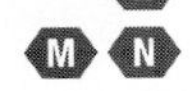

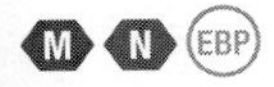

  - o Intervene immediately if there are signs of increased ICP. Raise the head of bed to 30 degrees and neck maintained midline. Mannitol or a hypertonic saline bolus may be used. Interventions such as sedation and analgesic medications are initiated as indicated for elevated ICP. Additional and more invasive interventions may be initiated upon transfer to the ICU if ICP remains elevated (Morgenstern, et al., 2010).

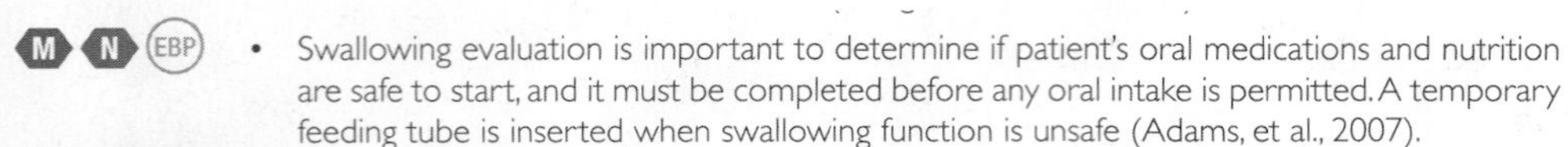

- Swallowing evaluation is important to determine if patient's oral medications and nutrition are safe to start, and it must be completed before any oral intake is permitted. A temporary feeding tube is inserted when swallowing function is unsafe (Adams, et al., 2007).

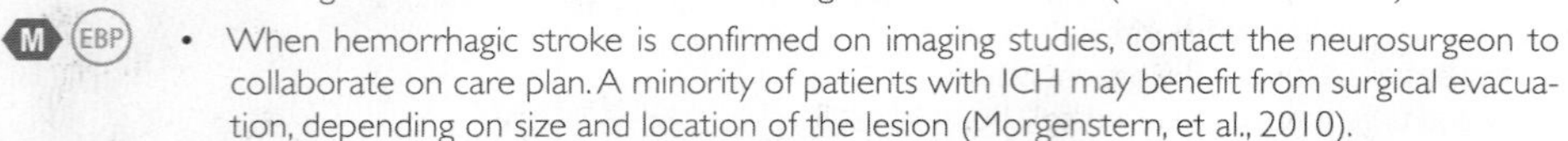

- When hemorrhagic stroke is confirmed on imaging studies, contact the neurosurgeon to collaborate on care plan. A minority of patients with ICH may benefit from surgical evacuation, depending on size and location of the lesion (Morgenstern, et al., 2010).

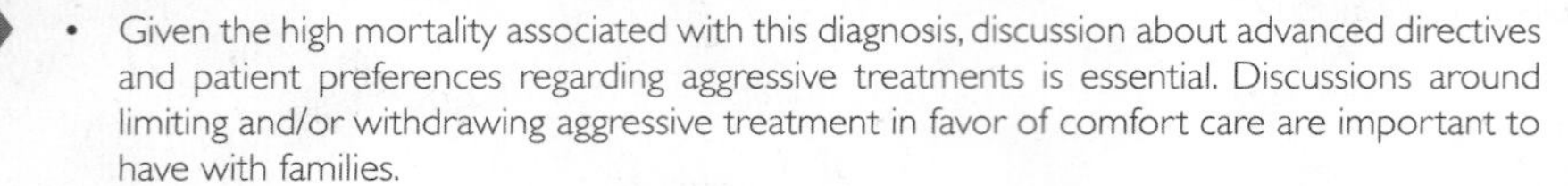

- Given the high mortality associated with this diagnosis, discussion about advanced directives and patient preferences regarding aggressive treatments is essential. Discussions around limiting and/or withdrawing aggressive treatment in favor of comfort care are important to have with families.
- When primary ICH occurs, the size and the location of the hemorrhage (i.e., dominant cerebral hemisphere where speech and major functions are located or nondominant cerebral hemisphere) are evaluated. This assessment along with the neurologic exam provides important information guiding prognosis, mobility, and overall level of disability.
- Major and immediate therapeutic interventions in the hospital concern:
  - o Reversing anticoagulation, blood thinners, and any coagulopathy (Morgenstern, et al., 2010)
  - o Treating elevated blood pressure (160/90 or higher); target MAP is 110 mmHg and target BP is 160/90
  - o Treating hyperglycemia and hypoglycemia to reduce adverse outcomes (Morgenstern, et al., 2010)
  - o Treating fever (Adams, et al., 2007)
- Additionally, prevent complications of immobility, including:
  - o Deep vein thrombosis (DVT) and pulmonary embolism using mechanical compression stockings (Morgenstern, et al., 2010)

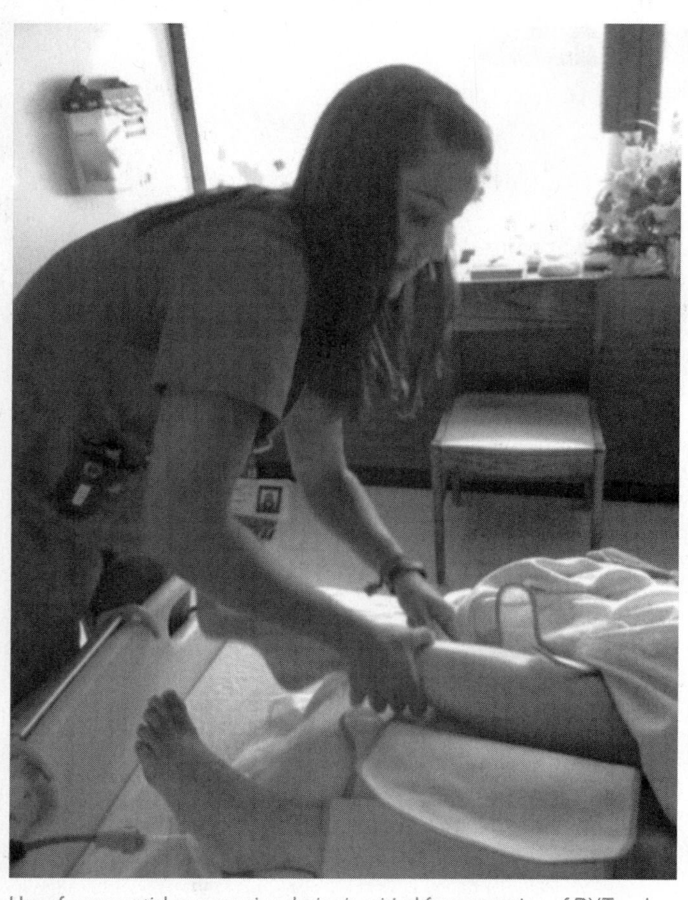

Use of a sequential compression device is critical for prevention of DVT and pulmonary embolism.
Source: Courtesy of Sarah Bateman/Nashville, TN

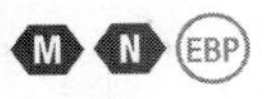

- o Infection with good hygiene and by removing catheters and invasive therapies as soon as appropriate (Adams, et al., 2007)

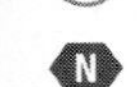

- o Skin breakdown and pressure wounds with early mobilization, repositioning, and physical therapy
- o Aspiration pneumonia by elevating the head of the bed to 30 degrees (Summers, et al., 2009)
- o Fall prevention by incorporating safety measures and patient/family education (SIGN, 2010)
- o Contractures using early and consistent range of motion exercises (Adams, et al., 2007)

- With small ICHs, patients are typically awake enough to protect their airway and adequately breathe. Frequently assess BP to prevent rebleeding. Neurologic checks continue every 1–2 hours to monitor for any neurologic changes. Attention to all body systems is important (Morgenstern, et al., 2010).

Collaborative Interventions: Hemorrhagic Stroke (continued)

Hospital, Supportive, Comfort, and Safety Care

Care of the hospitalized patient, supportive, comfort, and safety care of patients following hemorrhagic stroke are the same as the care for patients with ischemic stroke, unless specified in this section. The care is detailed earlier in this lesson, in the Collaborative Interventions in the Care of Patients with Ischemic Stroke section.

Aneurysm Treatment

- Treatment for the aneurysm can involve applying a clip or coiling to occlude a rupture or potential one.
  - o Clipping involves craniotomy and exposing the aneurysm before applying the clip onto the blood vessel.
  - o Coiling consists of inserting a catheter, typically through the femoral artery, and into the aorta. The catheter is then advanced into the brain with the help of x-ray (fluoroscopy) until it reaches the aneurysm. A platinum coil is then deployed that causes a clot to form in the aneurysm.

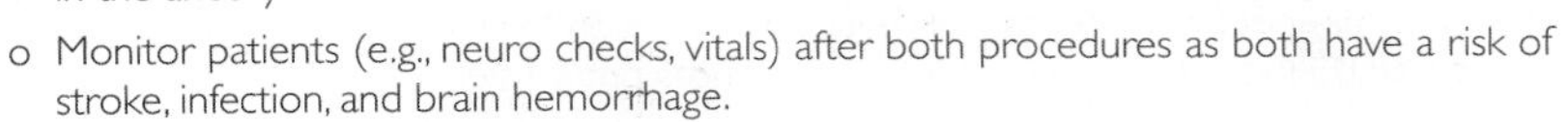

  - o Monitor patients (e.g., neuro checks, vitals) after both procedures as both have a risk of stroke, infection, and brain hemorrhage.

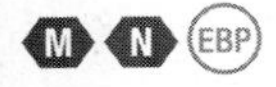

- If signs of hydrocephalus and/or increased ICP are present, collaborate with the HCP. An ICP ventriculostomy is commonly placed to drain off fluid (see picture). Draining cerebral spinal fluid (CSF) build up is a way to decrease the ICP. Usually the ventriculostomy is needed for 10–14 days. If CSF drainage is needed chronically (brain does not begin to reabsorb CSF), a permanent shunt can be placed inside the brain and drained into the peritoneum, called a ventriculoperitoneal shunt (American Association of Neuroscience Nurses [AANN], 2009).

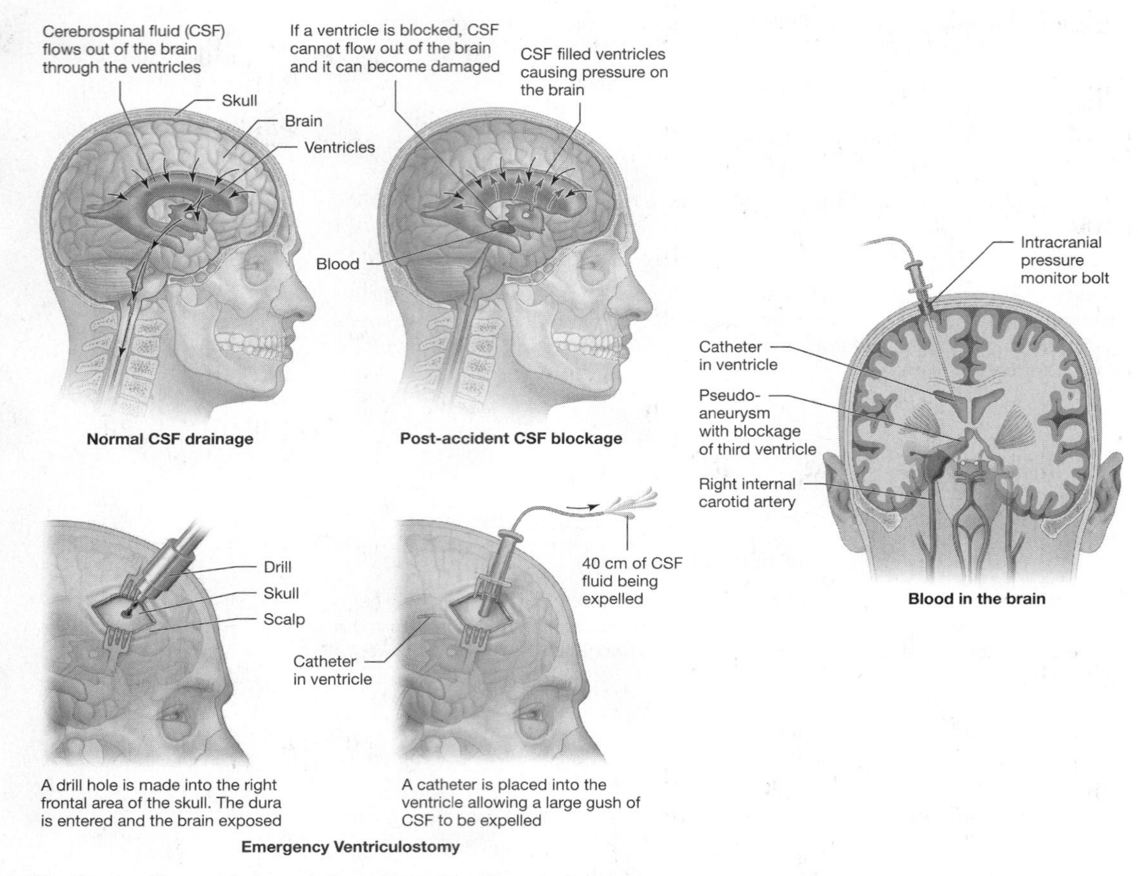

The drawings illustrate hydrocephalus and insertion of ventriculostomy.

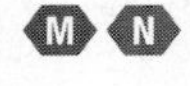

- Care of the aneurysmal SAH patient is similar to the patient with ICH. Depending on the severity of the bleed, the patient may or may not be on mechanical ventilation. Attention to management of all the body systems (see ICH) is similar. There are a few differences, primarily related to vasospasm.

Complications of Subarachnoid Hemorrhage (SAH)

Vasospasms

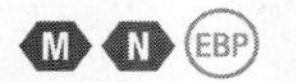

- The potential development of vasospasm requires continual reassessment for neurologic changes. Vasospasm is dangerous to the patient as it quickly leads to acute brain ischemia and damage (AANN, 2009).

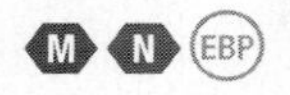

- Vasospasm is most likely to occur during days 4–14 after SAH bleed. In order to reduce the risk of vasospasm, all SAH patients are placed on nimodipine (calcium channel blocker) for 21 days (AANN, 2009).
- If the patient begins to demonstrate vasospasm as evidenced by a decline in neurologic function, increases in blood flow velocities on transcranial doppler (TCD ultrasound exam measures the speed of the blood in cerebral arteries), and/or CT angiogram, then:

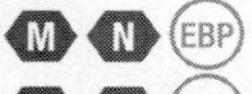

  o Infuse fluid to help dilate the arteries (AANN, 2009).

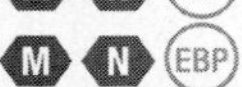

  o Increase BP artificially with vasopressor to counter the vasospasm (AANN, 2009).

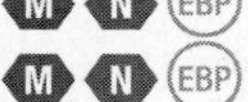

  o Consider initiating central venous pressure and/or invasive arterial line monitoring to guide the titration of vasoactive medications to raise the BP (AANN, 2009).

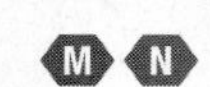

- If the patient's neurologic status worsens despite treatment, the neurosurgeon must be called immediately for further treatment.

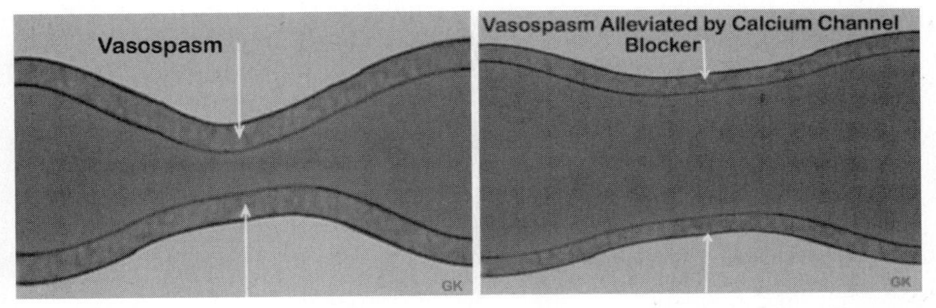

Left: This image shows vasospasm that may occur following subarachnoid hemorrhage. Right: After intra-arterial injection of nimodipine into the artery, the image demonstrates the treatment effect of increased diameter and improved perfusion of the vessels. The patient's clinical condition can rapidly improve after treatment.
Source: Courtesy of George Kyriakidis/Santa Ana, CA

Collaborative Interventions: Hemorrhagic Stroke (continued)

Subdural and Epidural Hematoma

- M These conditions are generally treated much like ICH. However, these patients typically benefit more from surgical evacuation of the hematoma.
- N Nursing care is directed at assessment of vital signs and body systems, support of the respiratory function, treatment of BP, delivery of nutrition, and monitoring and treating blood glucose levels.
- N As in all strokes described prior in detail, it is important to prevent the never events and the hazards of immobility, explained in detail earlier in this NovE-lesson.

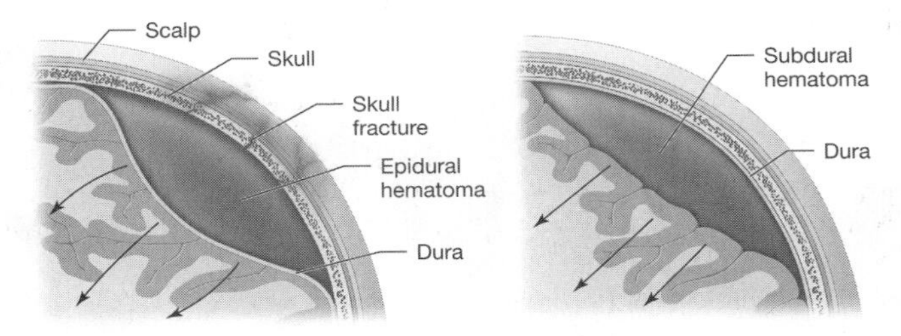

Note the different types and locations of hemorrhagic strokes. An epidural hematoma is depicted on the left and a subdural hematoma on the right.

Summary of Nursing and Medical Interventions

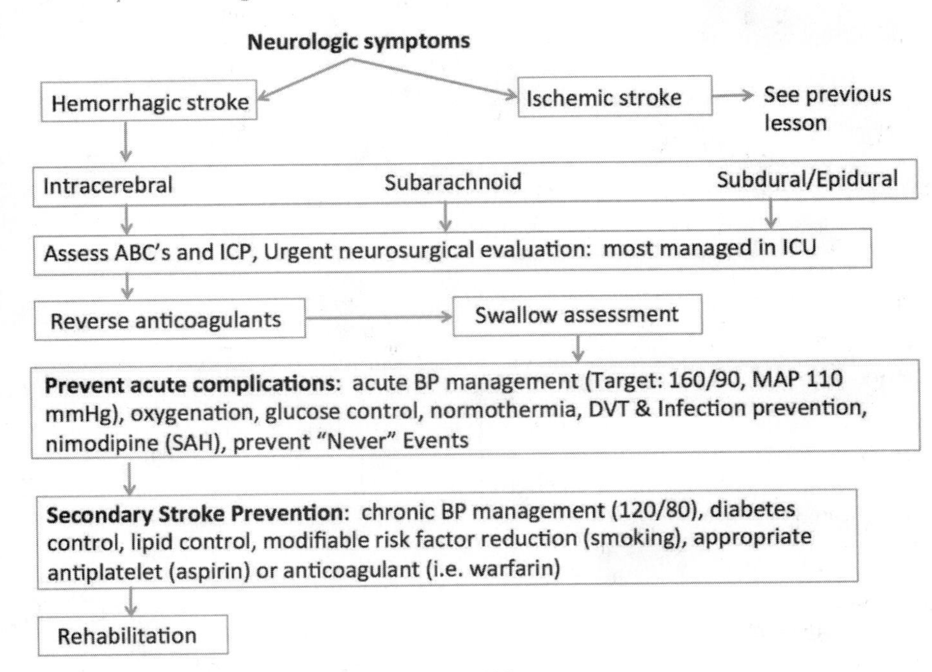

Source: Copyright © 2014, NovEx Novice to Expert Learning, LLC

Rehabilitation

- A collaborative team is essential to help assess and determine the patient's rehabilitation needs and possibilities. In addition to the patient, family, medical, nursing, and surgical teams, assessment and judgment is needed from physical therapists, occupational therapists, speech therapists, and social worker or case manager to determine the type and extent of the neurologic deficits for rehabilitation.
- To begin rehab, a mobility plan is developed. The patient increases activities, if able, from sitting up to standing and possibly ambulating with assistance. The ability to provide self-care (hygiene, dressing, eating, and other activities of daily living) is determined and a rehab plan is put into place.

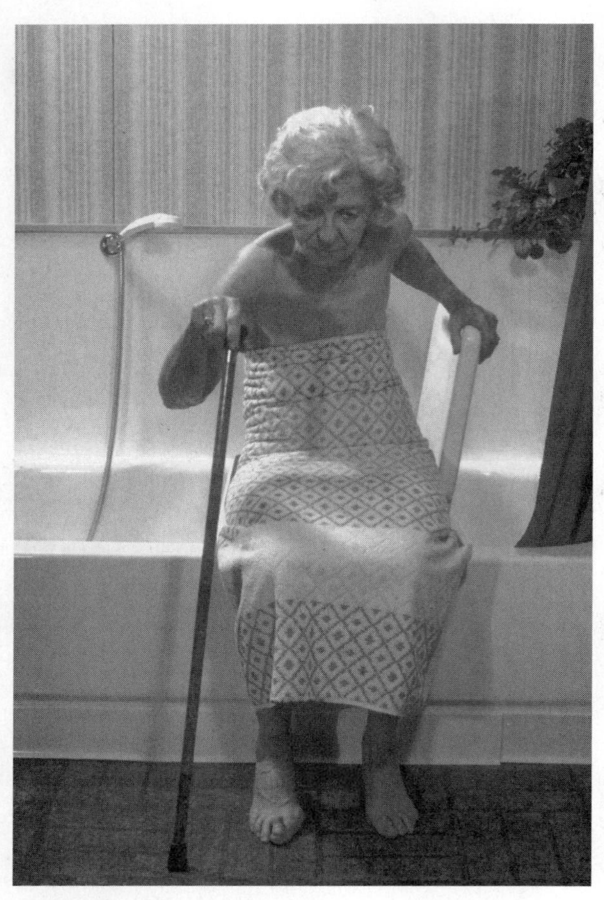

Patients and their caregivers must find ways to enable patients following stroke to regain greater independence in ADLs.
Source: CDC/Richard Duncan, MRP, Sr. Proj. Mngr, North Carolina State University, The Center for Universal Design (CUD)

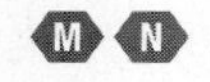

- Depending on the hemorrhage's impact on the individual, the discharge plan will vary. Patients may go home, may be transferred to an acute rehabilitation unit, or may be admitted to a skilled nursing facility.

Concept Check

7. Which patient typically benefits the most from a surgical procedure?

A. A patient with cerebral vasospasm
B. A patient with an epidural hematoma
C. A patient with a transient ischemic attack
D. A patient with a right parietal ischemic stroke

Answer question

Summary of Interventions: Ischemic and Hemorrhagic Strokes

- Stroke is a leading cause of death and disability in the United States.
- Determination of the stroke type (ischemic or hemorrhagic) is important in providing effective treatment.
- Provide support for vital functions.
- Thrombolytic therapy must be considered in all ischemic stroke patients when time of onset of symptoms to the time of treatment is <4.5 hours.
- Neurosurgical input and management is a key factor in providing the most appropriate care for hemorrhagic stroke.
- Patient and family education regarding general supportive care and rehabilitation with attention to prevention of acute complications is valuable for all stroke patients.

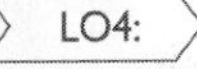

Evaluation of Desired Collaborative Care Outcomes

Evaluation and reassessment should reveal attainment of previously established patient outcomes. In summary:

Ischemic Stroke

- Patient expresses understanding of permanent body changes and demonstrates acceptance.
- Patient is able to communicate with caregivers.
- Patient has avoided falls.
- Patient has regained as much memory as possible, given the extent of stroke.
- Patient has avoided aspiration.
- The patient and family discuss how this stroke has changed their lives and how they are adapting to those changes.

Hemorrhagic Stroke

- Patient reports that headache has eased.
- Patient has no nausea or vomiting, heart rate and respiratory rate are within desired range, and mentation is clear.
- Patient's respirations are regular and unlabored.
- Patient's intracranial pressure remains within desired range.
- Patient demonstrates reduction in confusion.

References

Ischemic Stroke

Adams, H. P. (2009). Secondary prevention of atherothrombotic events after ischemic stroke. *Mayo Clinic proceedings, 84*(1), 43–51.

Adams, R. J., Albers, G., Alberts, M. J., et al. (2008). Update to the AHA/ASA recommendations for the prevention of stroke in patient with stroke and transient ischemic attack. *Stroke, 39*(5), 1647–1652.

Donnan, G. A., Fisher, M., Macleod, M., et al. (2008). Stroke. *Lancet, 371*(9624), 1612–1623.

Henkle, J. (2005). An update on transient ischemic attacks. *Journal of Neuroscience Nursing, 37*(5), 243–248.

Hinchey, J. A., Shephard, T., Furie, K., et al. (2005). Formal dysphagia screening protocols prevent pneumonia. *Stroke, 36*, 1972–1976.

Hinkle, J., & Guanci, M. M. (2007). Acute ischemic stroke review. *Journal of Neuroscience Nursing, 39*(5), 285–293, 310.

Mink, J., & Miller, J. (2011). Opening the window of opportunity for treating acute ischemic stroke. *Nursing, 41*(1), 24–32. doi: 10-1097/01. NURSE.0000391397.75203.54

Pugh, S., Mathiesen, C., Meighan, M., et al. (2009). Guide to the care of the hospitalized patient with ischemic stroke, 2nd edition. AANN Clinical practice guideline series. Glenview, IL: American Association of Neuroscience Nurses. **http://www.guideline.gov/content .aspx?id=13575**

Summers, D., Leonard, A., Wentworth, D., et al. on behalf of the AHA Council on Cardiovascular Nursing the Stroke Council. (2009). Comprehensive overview of nursing and interdisciplinary care of the acute ischemic stroke patient: A scientific statement from the American Heart Association. *Stroke, 40*(8), 2911–2944. doi: 10.1161/ STROKEAHA.109.192362.

Clinical Practice Guidelines

Adams, H. P. Jr, del Zoppo, G., Alberts, M. J., et al. (2007). Guidelines for the early management of adults with ischemic stroke: A guideline from the American Heart Association/American Stroke Association Stroke Council, Clinical Cardiology Council, Cardiovascular Radiology and Intervention Council, and the Atherosclerotic Peripheral Vascular Disease and Quality of Care Outcomes in Research Interdisciplinary Working Groups: The American Academy of Neurology affirms the value of this guideline as an educational tool for neurologists. *Stroke, 38*(5), 1655–1711 **stroke.ahajournals.org/content/38/5/1655 .full** and in *Circulation, 115*, e478–e534. **circ.ahajournals.org/ content/115/20/e478.full**

Albers, G. W., Amarenco, P., Easton, J. D., et al. (2008). Antithrombic and thrombolytic therapy for ischemic stroke: American College of Chest Physicians evidenced-based clinical practice guidelines (8th edition). *Chest, 133*(6_suppl), 630S–669S. **journal.publications.chestnet. org/article.aspx?articleid=1085940**

Brott, T. G., Brown, R. D. Jr, Meyer, F. B., et al. (2004). Carotid revascularization for prevention of stroke: Carotid endarterectomy and carotid artery stenting. *Mayo Clinic proceedings, 79*(9), 1197–1208.

Brott, T. G., Hobson, R. W. 2nd, Howard, G., et al., and CREST Investigators. (2010). Stenting versus endarterectomy for treatment of carotid-artery stenosis. *The New England Journal of Medicine, 363*(1), 11–23. **www.ncbi.nlm.nih.gov/pmc/articles/PMC2932446/**

Jauch, E. C., Saver, J. L., Adams, H. P., et al. and the American Heart Association Stroke Council, Council of Cardiovascular Nursing, Council on Peripheral Vascular Disease, and Council on Clinical Cardiology. (2013). AHA/ASA Guideline for the early management of patients with acute ischemic stroke: A guideline for healthcare professionals from the American Heart Association/American Stroke Association. *Stroke,* **stroke.ahajournals.org/content/ early/2013/01/31/STR.0b013e318284056a.full**

Morgenstern, L., Hemphill, J., Anderson, C., et al. and American Heart Association Stroke Council and Council on Cardiovascular Nursing. (2010). Guidelines for the management of spontaneous intracerebral hemorrhage: A guideline for healthcare professionals from the American Heart Association/American Stroke Association. *Stroke, 41*(9), 2108–2129. **stroke.ahajournals.org/content/41/9/2108.long**

Rothwell, P. M., Eliasziw, M., Gutnikov, S. A., et al. for the Carotid Endarterectomy Trialists Collaboration. (2004). Endarterectomy for symptomatic carotid stenosis in relation to clinical subgroups and timing of surgery. *Lancet, 363*(9413), 915–924. doi: dx.doi.org/10.1016/ S0140-6736(04)15785-1

Scottish Intercollegiate Guidelines Network (SIGN) (2010). Management of patients with stroke: Rehabilitation, prevention and management of complications, and discharge planning: A national clinical guideline. Edinburgh, Scotland: Scottish Intercollegiate Guidelines Network, SIGN publication; no. 118. **www.guideline.gov/content.aspx?id=23849**

Patient Education

Caplan, L. R. (2014). *Patient information: Ischemic stroke treatment.* **www .uptodate.com/contents/ischemic-stroke-treatment-beyond-the-basics**

Centers for Disease Control and Prevention. (2015). *Stroke patient education handouts.* **www.cdc.gov/stroke/materials_for_ patients.htm**

Hinkle, J., & Guanci, M. M. (2015). *Acute ischemic stroke review.* **www .medscape.com/viewarticle/567653**

Hinkle, J. (2015). *An update on transient ischemic attacks.* **www .medscape.com/viewarticle/514552**

Hemorrhagic Stroke

Arias, M., & Smith, L. N. (2007). Early mobilization of acute stroke patients. *Journal of Clinical Nursing, 16*(2), 282–288.

Liechty, J. A., & Heinzekehr, J. B. (2007). Caring for those without words: A perspective on aphasia. *Journal of Neuroscience Nursing, 39*(5), 316–318.

Mink, J., & Miller, J. (2011). Respond aggressively to hemorrhagic stroke. *Nursing, 2011, 41*(3), 36–42. doi: 10.097/01. NURSE.0000394077.52606.9b

Rank, W. (2013). Aneurysmal subarachnoid hemorrhage: Follow the guidelines. *Nursing, 43*(5), 42–50. doi: 10.1097/01. NURSE.000428692.56721.36

Clinical Practice Guidelines

American Association of Neuroscience Nurses. (2009). *AHRQ Guidelines: Care of the patient with aneurismal subarachnoid hemorrhage.* Glenview, IL: American Association of Neuroscience Nurses. **www .guideline.gov/content.aspx?id=34442**

Broderick, J., Connolly, S., Feldmann, E., et al. (2007). Guidelines for the management of spontaneous intracerebral hemorrhage in adults: 2007 update: A guideline from the American Heart Association/ American Stroke Association Stroke Council, High Blood Pressure Research Council, and the Quality of Care and Outcomes in Research Interdisciplinary Working Group. *Stroke, 38*(6), 2001–2023.

Connolly, E. S., Rabinstein, A. A., Carhuapoma, J. R., et al. (2012). AHA/ ASA Guidelines for the management of aneurysmal subarachnoid hemorrhage: A guideline for healthcare professionals from the American Heart Association/American Stroke Association. *Stroke, 43*(6), 1711–1737. **stroke.ahajournals.org/content/43/6/1711.full**

Patient Education

Caplan, L. R. (2014). Patient information: Hemorrhagic stroke treatment. **www.uptodate.com/contents/hemorrhagic-stroke-treatment-beyond-the-basics**

Liebeskind, D. S. (2015). Hemorrhagic stroke. **emedicine.medscape .com/article/1916662-overview**

Learning Outcomes for Brain Tumors

When you complete this lesson, you will be able to:

1. Recognize the clinical relevance of brain tumors.
2. Consider the pathophysiology, etiology, risk factors, and clinical presentation of brain tumors that determine the priority patient concerns.
3. Determine the most urgent and important nursing interventions and patient education required in caring for a patient with a brain tumor.
4. Evaluate attainment of desired collaborative care outcomes for a patient with a brain tumor.

LO1:

What Are Brain Tumors?

Brain tumors are a varied group of tumors that arise in the brain. They are generally classified as:

- **Primary** if the cell of origin lies within the brain
- **Metastatic** if the cell of origin lies outside the brain and migrates into the brain.

Tumors are further classified as:

- **Benign** if the cells are nonmalignant
- **Malignant** (cancer)

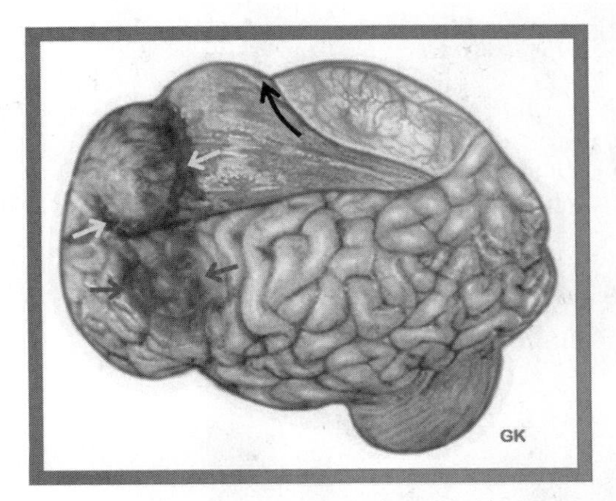

A meningioma (yellow arrows), which is peeled back with the dura, leaves an indented, compressed cerebral region (blue arrows) underneath.
Source: Courtesy of George Kyriakidis/Santa Ana, CA

LO1:

Clinical Relevance

- Primary malignant brain tumors account for about 2% of all cancers for adults.
- Approximately 50,000 primary malignant and benign brain tumors occur each year in the United States.
- People aged 50–79 have the highest incidence of brain tumors.
- Tumors metastasizing from another area of the body to the brain account for another 150,000 brain tumors annually in the United States.
- The lung, breast, skin, kidney, and gastrointestinal tract are the primary sites from which metastatic brain tumors originate.

LO2:

Pathophysiology

- Brain tumors can be benign or malignant:
  - o Benign tumors have cell structure that resembles normal tissue.
  - o Malignant tumors contain abnormal cells that undergo uncontrolled cell division.
  - o Malignant tumors tend to grow faster and can infiltrate the tissue around them.
  - o Both types of tumors can have harmful effects on the central nervous system.
- Local growth results in impingement of:
  - o Local brain tissue, including pituitary gland
  - o Blood vessels that can block blood flow and lead to ischemia
  - o Cranial nerves, causing functional impairment
  - o Brain ventricles that can prevent cerebrospinal fluid (CSF) flow, causing increased intra-cranial pressure (ICP)
  - o Meninges
- Local circulation is disrupted and may cause ischemia and necrosis of tissue.
- The location of the tumor determines what effects are seen. Examples are:
  - o A tumor in the left temporoparietal lobe may cause a right hemiparesis and right-sided loss of sensation.
  - o A tumor in the pituitary can press on the optic chiasm, causing vision loss.

CT Scan of Pituitary Mass

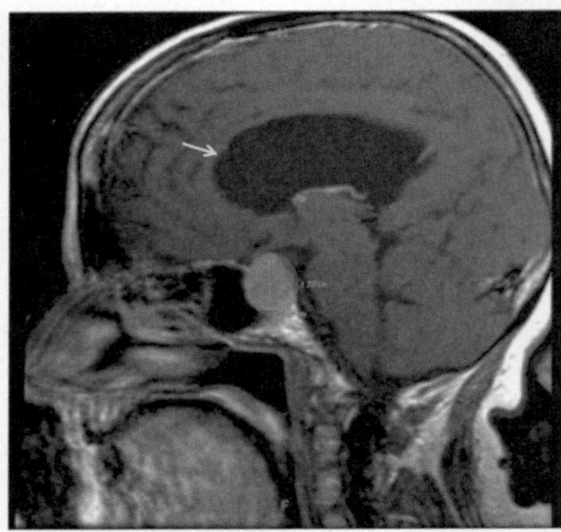

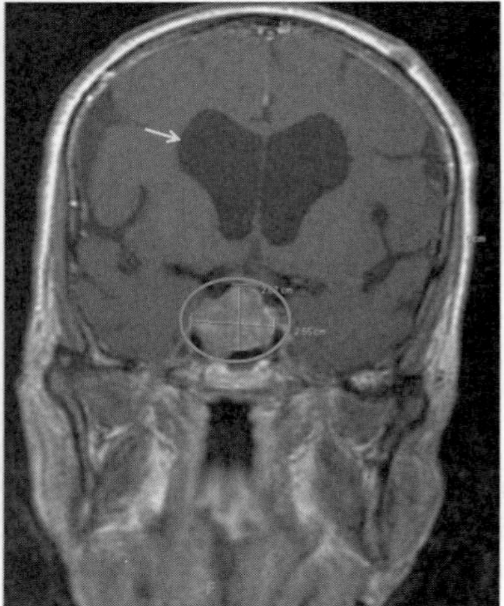

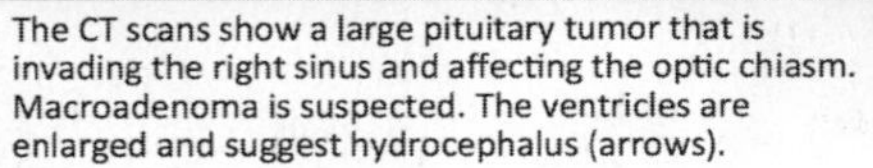

The CT scans show a large pituitary tumor that is invading the right sinus and affecting the optic chiasm. Macroadenoma is suspected. The ventricles are enlarged and suggest hydrocephalus (arrows).

Source: Courtesy of K. Kyriakidis

- ICP can result from any space-occupying lesion in the brain, since the space in the intracra-nial vault is fixed (see image).
- Edema often surrounds malignant tumors, worsening this problem.
- Edema occurs because the capillaries in malignant tumors are leaky.
- A tumor that is blocking the flow of CSF through the ventricles may result in accumulation of CSF and further increase the ICP (see image).

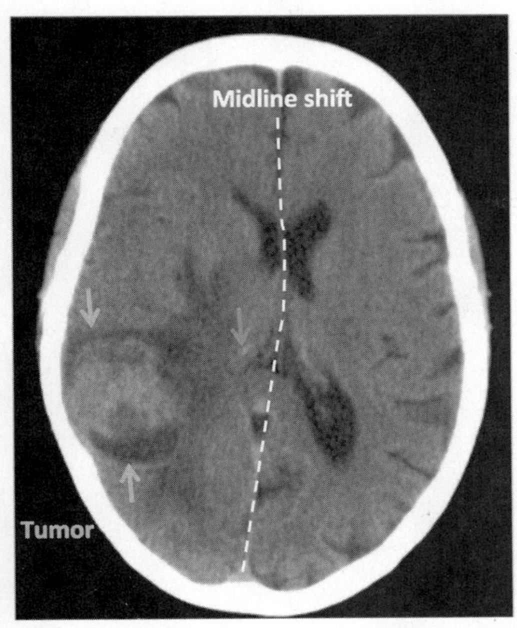

This CT scan shows a large tumor or glioblastoma (green arrows) that is pressing on and collapsing a ventricle (red arrow), thus blocking the flow of CSF through the ventricle in the cerebellum. The obstruction of flow results in accumulation of CSF fluid in the other ventricles and in increased intracranial pressure. The tumor with edema can be seen pressing the brain and causing a midline shift (white line).
Source: Courtesy of K. Kyriakidis

Concept Check

1. **Metastatic brain tumors most often arise from which tissue?**
   A. Lung
   B. Prostate
   C. Bone
   D. Muscle

Answer question

Pathophysiology (continued)

Seizures

- The pathophysiology of seizures caused by brain tumors is not clearly understood.
- Changes in pH, the balance of neurotransmitters (e.g., gliomas producing excessive amount of glutamate), and the cytokines released around the tumor may contribute to an environment that decreases the threshold for neurons to fire.
- During a seizure numerous neurons fire simultaneously. This activity may then spread to involve larger areas of the brain.

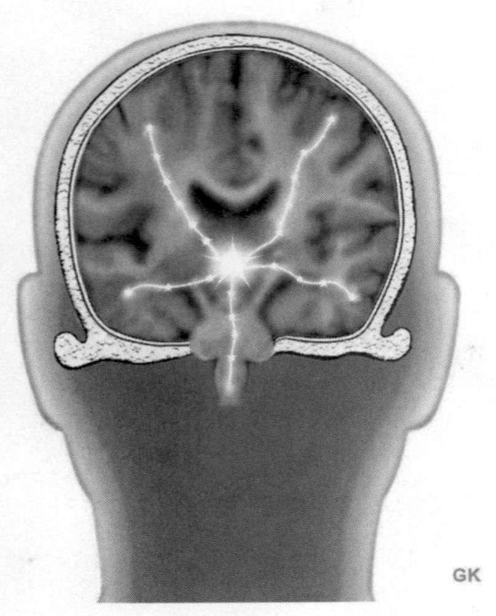

Headaches are commonly the earliest symptom of a brain tumor that patients have, but seizures make them seek medical care.
Source: Courtesy of George Kyriakidis/Santa Ana, CA

Types of Brain Tumors

Classification: Tumors can be categorized a number of ways:

- Benign or malignant
- Intrinsic (intra-axial) or extrinsic (extra-axial): Intrinsic tumors originate from glial cells while extrinsic tumors originate from the meninges, cranial nerves, and other tissues.
- Congenital tumors (e.g., hemangioblastoma and craniopharyngioma), which are present from birth
- Neuroendocrine tumors, which arise from the tissue in the pituitary gland and secrete hormones (e.g., adrenocorticotropic hormone or growth hormone)

Benign and Malignant Tumors

The classification of benign and malignant in brain tumors includes many factors other than the pathological appearance that influences the patient outcome.

- A **benign tumor** is typically slow-growing with distinct borders and rarely spreads. Removal is the treatment of choice if symptomatic, but these tumors can recur. If the benign tumor occurs in a vital area of the brain, the tumor, though benign, can have life-threatening or life-altering consequences.

Brain Tumor Sites Based on Type

Meningioma
Oligodendroglioma
Astrocytoma
Supratentorial ependymona
Pineal region tumor
Optic glioma
Medulloblastoma
Craniopharyngioma
Pituitary tumor
Cerebellar astrocytoma
Schwannomas
Brainstem glioma
Infratentorial ependymona
GK

There are many different types of brain tumors. They are usually categorized by the type of cell where the tumor originates, or by the area of the brain where they occur.
Source: Courtesy of George Kyriakidis/Santa Ana, CA

- A **malignant tumor** is typically invasive and rapid-growing and lacks distinct borders. These tumors often infiltrate (send roots) into adjacent tissue. Malignant tumors include:
  - o Glioblastoma
  - o Anaplastic astrocytoma
  - o Primary central nervous system (CNS) lymphoma
  - o Medulloblastoma
- Low-grade gliomas can be slow growing neoplasms (group of cells formed by abnormal proliferation). They often recur after treatment and can become malignant over time.
- A metastatic brain tumor originates from another part of the body (e.g., lungs, breast, colon, skin). Metastatic lesions are often multiple.

Pathophysiology (continued)

Intrinsic/Intra-Axial Tumors

The main intrinsic tumors classified by cellular origin are:

- **Astrocytomas** are diffusely infiltrating tumors and are subdivided into four grades:
  - o Grade I: Pilocystic astrocytoma
  - o Grade II: Diffuse astrocytoma
  - o Grade III: Anaplastic astrocytoma
  - o Grade IV: Glioblastoma multiforme
- **Oligodendroglial** tumors originate from white matter and usually occur in the frontal and parietal areas.
- **Ependymoma** tumors originate from cells inside the ventricles of the brain.
- **Embryonal** tumors may originate in fetal or embryonic tissues and develop in the brain following birth.
- **Pineal** tumors originate from pinocytes.
- **Medulloblastoma** tumors are malignant small cell tumors of the cerebellum and are usually seen in children under the age of 20.

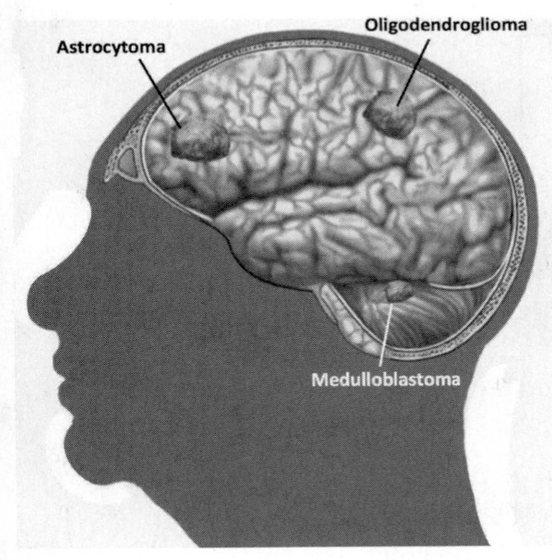

This image shows some of the types of brain tumors and their locations.
Source: Courtesy of George Kyriakidis/Santa Ana, CA

Concept Check

2. Which brain tumor is congenital?
   A. Glioblastoma
   B. Craniopharyngioma
   C. Meningeal
   D. Optic glioma

Answer question

Extrinsic/Extra-Axial Tumors

The main extrinsic tumors are classified by structural origin:

- **Schwannomas** are benign growths originating from Schwann cells of the nerve sheath. These tumors are not cancerous and instead push nerve fibers to the side. Because they commonly occur along cranial nerve VIII and affect balance and hearing, they are called acoustic neuroma, vestibular schwannoma, or acoustic neurilemoma.
- **Neurofibroma** is a benign tumor that grows on the peripheral nerve sheath.
- **Meningiomas** are slow growing, extra-axial tumors that come from the meninges and other structures.

LO2:

Risk Factors

- No definitive risk factor has been identified as the cause for the majority of brain tumors, but some associations have been made.
- Associated risk factors include:
    - o Race: more common in Caucasians
    - o Age: increases with age, usually over 50
    - o Gender: overall slightly more likely to occur in men
    - o Previous radiation exposure: ionizing radiation like that used to treat cancers or in the nuclear industry
    - o Vinyl chloride exposure
    - o Family history of brain tumors
    - o Immunosuppression therapy has the risk of developing central nervous system lymphomas.
- Exposure to environmental hazards, lifestyle habits, and genetics continue to be studied.

LO2:

Causes

- Unregulated cell growth underlies all brain tumors, the cause of which is a complex combination of genetic factors and environmental factors.

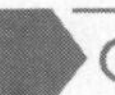

Concept Check

3. Which situation is a risk factor for the development of a brain tumor?

A. Being younger than 50 years of age

B. Female gender

C. Asian descent

D. History of immunosuppressant treatment

Answer question

LO2:

Assessment Findings

- When tumors grow in the CNS, they are confined to a closed space. As the tumors grow, they may cause an increase in ICP because the tissue immediately surrounding the tumor becomes edematous and compressed.
- There is increased vascular permeability to plasma, so vasogenic edema occurs.
- The tumors and edema produce symptomatology that is reflective of the location of the tumor, and individuals may complain of:
    - o Headache
    - o Mental status changes
    - o Visual problems such as blurred vision or loss of visual fields
- The individual with an expanding intracranial tumor may experience:
    - o Vomiting
    - o Altered level of consciousness
    - o Possible motor weakness

Focal or Regional Findings

- When the abnormal tumor growth infiltrates specific lobes or regions of the brain, the individual develops focal symptoms that reflect the impacted area:

Progression of Brain Swelling

Normal anatomy
Mild cerebral edema
Moderate cerebral edema
Skull
"Slit-like" appearance of ventricles
Cerebral ventricles
Generous space surrounding brain
Diffuse swelling with brain tissue pressed up against wall of skull
Diffuse swelling with widespread inflammation of brain tissue and compression of cerebral ventricles

This series shows cerebral comparisons as brain swelling progresses. The images (left to right): 1) Normal brain with fluid filled space surrounding it; 2) Mild cerebral edema with brain tissue pressing outward against the skull; 3) Moderate cerebral edema with further brain tissue swelling and inflammation, compressing the ventricles within the brain.

- o **Frontal lobe tumors** cause impaired affect, poor judgment, lack of insight, depression, apathy, motor weakness to the contralateral side, speech (expressive or comprehension), and abnormal behavior.
- o **Parietal lobe tumors** produce sensory disruptions with numbness occurring on the opposite side; neglect (person does not look to the other side of the body; right parietal tumor causes neglect to the left side and body); problems with reading, writing, math skills (left parietal); and inability to get dressed or draw (right parietal).

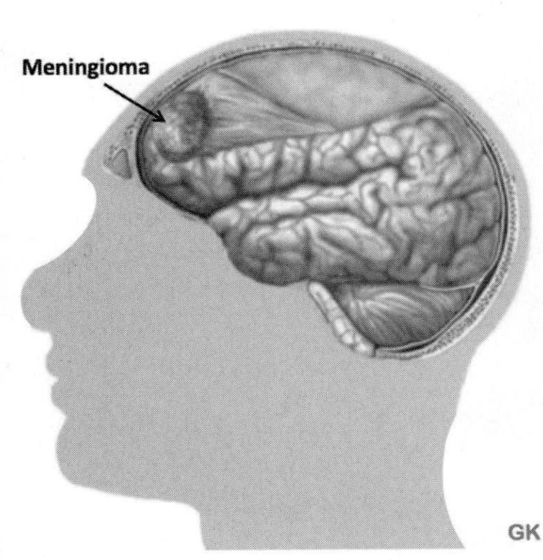

A large meningioma is shown in the frontal lobe, causing personality changes. Meningiomas, causing 30–40% of all brain tumors, are often benign.
Source: Courtesy of George Kyriakidis/Santa Ana, CA

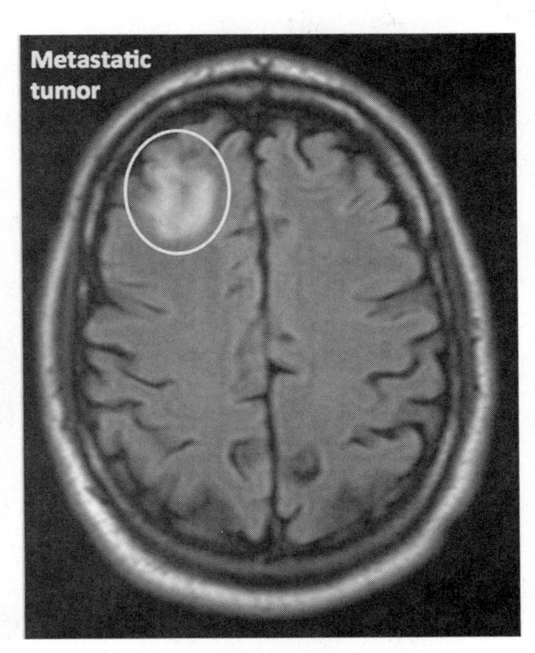

MRI image shows frontal lobe tumor surrounded by vasogenic edema. The family became concerned about the patient when he displayed speech, judgment, and behavioral changes.
Source: Courtesy of K. Kyriakidis

- o **Temporal lobe tumors** produce psychomotor seizures and receptive aphasia if on the left hemisphere.
- o **Occipital lobe tumors** can produce visual disturbances.
- o **Pituitary tumors** create visual field loss, Cushing's syndrome (ACTH secreting), or gigantism (GH secreting).
- o If tumors arise in the ventricles, they can cause **hydrocephalus**, the buildup of excessive CSF in the ventricles.
- o **Cerebellum tumors** produce problems with coordination and balance.
- **Brainstem tumors** create cranial nerve deficits, vomiting, and altered respirations.

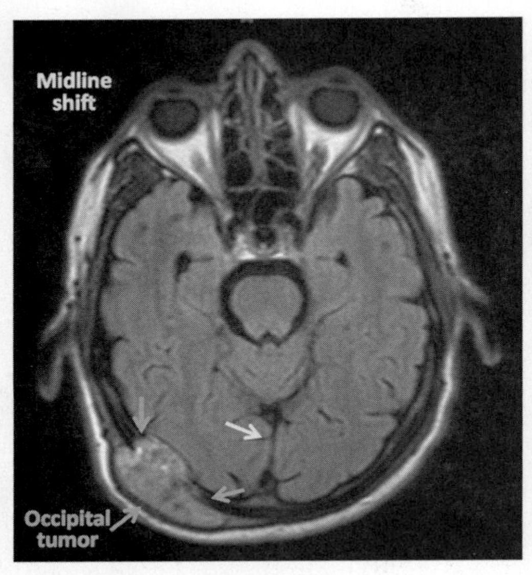

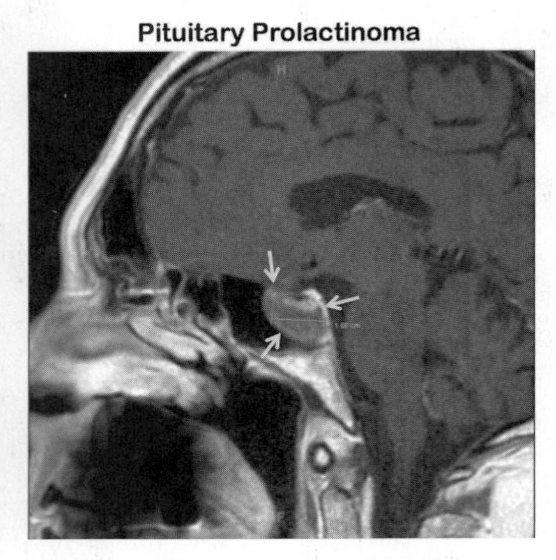

Left: This MRI scan shows a patient with a metastatic occipital tumor (back of the head). Notice that the tumor is causing the brain to shift to the opposite side. The increased intracranial pressure is likely responsible for the visual disturbances experienced by this patient. Right: This patient had a pituitary tumor, which impaired many of his key body functions, particularly hormonal and visual. The blue arrow shows the location and size of the pituitary tumor. Note that the tumor appears to have necrotic or cystic character in the lower portion.

Source: (*both*) Courtesy of K. Kyriakidis

Assessment Findings (continued)

Increased Intracranial Pressure

Tumors create increased ICP by displacing the normal structures inside the cranial vault. This effect produces signs and symptoms.

- **Early signs** of increased ICP include agitation, decreased level of consciousness, headache, nausea and vomiting.
- **Late signs** of increased ICP include hemiplegia, extensor/flexor posturing, and Cushing's triad (bradycardia, increased systolic blood pressure, widening pulse pressure).
- Some patients experience an acute seizure. This may be the first sign of a brain tumor.

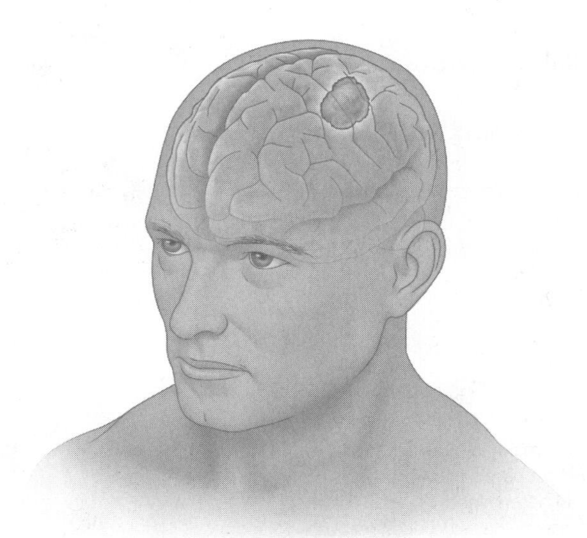

A brain tumor can be benign or malignant, primary, or secondary. Causes and risk factors include age, gender, family history, and exposure to chemicals. Symptoms range from headaches and leg and feet numbness to seizures. Treatment is dependant upon the type and location of the brain tumor. To learn more, click on www.medicinenet.com/neurology/focus.htm.

Concept Check

4. A brain tumor that causes receptive aphasia is most likely to be in which location?

A. Pituitary gland

B. Brainstem

C. Occipital lobe

D. Temporal lobe

Answer question

LO2:

Diagnostics

- History and physical assessment with neurologic imaging studies (CT or MRI) provide the diagnosis.
- Brain tumor type is determined after biopsy and review of tissue sample by a neuropathologist.

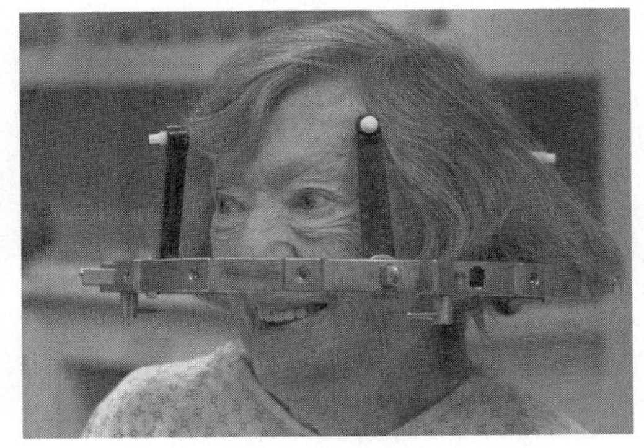

Stereotaxy is a minimally invasive method of obtaining tissue for biopsy, surgery, and other interventions. It involves a three-dimensional coordinates system to locate small targets inside the body and to perform an intervention on them (such as ablation [removal], implantation, radiosurgery [SRS], in addition to biopsy). The photo shows a patient in a stereotactic frame prior to a procedure.

Source: Susan Tripp Pollard/Contra Costa Times/ZUMA Press, Inc./Alamy

Priority Patient Concerns and Desired Collaborative Care Outcomes

Prior to caring for patients with brain tumors, it is important to prioritize the patient's concerns that must guide the nursing care plan and interventions. Care for the patient is ordered and organized in accordance with the patient's priority and urgent needs. Desired collaborative care outcomes in patients with brain tumors typically include:

1. The patient's intracranial pressure will remain within or not dangerously exceed desired range.
2. The patient will remain injury-free.
3. Patient will report that fear of unknown is minimized by teaching and support.
4. Patient will maintain or improve activity levels.
5. Patient and family will discuss losses associated with diagnosis and identify needs for support.

Considering these important care outcomes, prepare a list of the major 3–6 priority patient concerns or nursing diagnoses for patients with brain tumors. Be prepared to participate in a discussion of this list and/or to submit them as an assignment, as determined by your faculty. Resources you may find helpful in this assignment can include this lesson, the references, resources on nursing care plans, and standard nursing diagnoses manuals.

Concept Check

5. **Which finding is an early sign of increased intracranial pressure?**
   A. Agitation
   B. Hemiplegia
   C. Bradycardia
   D. Increased systolic blood pressure

Answer question

LO3:

Collaborative Interventions

Once a mass is identified, the patient is admitted to the appropriate unit relative to the stability of the patient. Those with significant signs of increased ICP are admitted to the intensive care unit.

Medications

M N EBP

- Benzodiazepines for rapid treatment of an active seizure (e.g., lorazepam, diazepam, midazolam) (National Institute for Health and Clinical Excellence [NICE], 2012)
- Anticonvulsants for seizure prevention and treatment of an active seizure (e.g., fosphenytoin, phenytoin); not indicated if no history of seizures (Mikkelsen, et al., 2010)
- IV steroids: Evidence shows that corticosteroids decrease cerebral edema (e.g., dexamethasone). Steroids may provide temporary increased ICP relief in brain metastases (Ryken, et al., 2010; Soffietti, et al., 2011).
- Hyperosmolar agents: Mannitol draws water out of the brain cells that is then excreted by the kidneys.
- H2 blockers to prevent gastrointestinal bleeding risk from steroid use (e.g., famotidine, cimetidine, ranitidine) (Kahrilas, et al., 2008).
- DVT prophylaxis (e.g., low-molecular-weight heparin) is recommended and effective. Preoperative use of venous thromboembolism prophylaxis is recommended (Finnish Medical Society Duodecim, 2010; Soffietti, et al., 2011).
- Analgesics (e.g., morphine, hydromorphone) are used carefully due to CNS depressant effects.

Monitoring

N

Patients with brain tumors should be closely monitored. This includes:

- Seizure precautions
- Vital signs and heart rhythm
- Frequent neurological assessments, particularly level of consciousness
- DVT development
- Analgesics: need and response

Psychological Support

- The diagnosis of a brain tumor is a devastating and life-altering event for the patient and family. Support and comfort are helpful as the patient adapts. Be attentive to how the patient and family tend to best cope with illness and support their individual beneficial coping mechanisms whenever possible (e.g., enabling them to take control, crying, anger, time alone, praying). Empathize with the devastating problem they are coping with rather than attempting to correct behaviors that can be difficult.
- Based on patient preferences, involve pastoral services or the patient's family minister for spiritual support.
- Provide alternative therapies (e.g., massage, relaxation, music therapy) as supportive care to patients according to patient preferences (NICE, 2012).
- Being attentive and providing caring practices are particularly comforting to families in distress and crisis. Knowing that the clinicians are watching out for and watching over their loved one can help lower their stress and distress levels.
- Educate about advanced directives.
- If the health care team and/or patient and family deem appropriate, discuss palliative care and hospice options as sources of supportive and comfort care.

Surgical Intervention

- Most common is open craniotomy with guided tumor debulking or removal (Kalkanis, et al., 2010).

Olfactory Groove Meningioma with Craniotomy and Surgical Excision

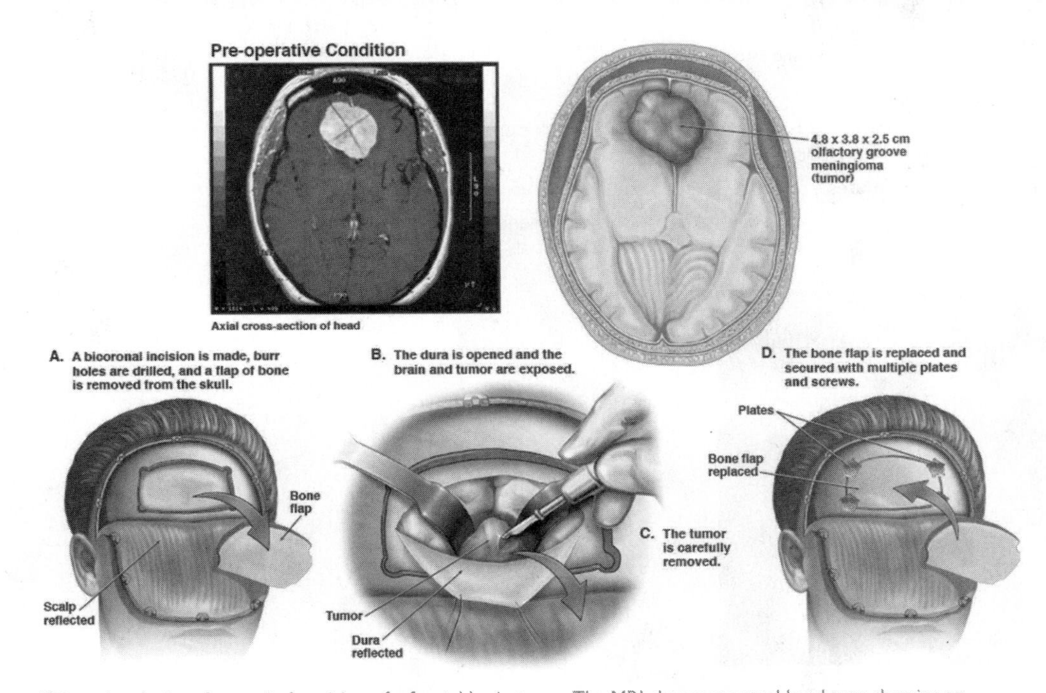

This series depicts the surgical excision of a frontal brain tumor. The MRI shows an actual head scan showing an olfactory groove meningioma (tumor) within the brain. The remaining images show multiple steps of the excision surgery, including the bicoronal incision, exposure and removal of the tumor, and replacement of the cranial bone flap using multiple plates and screws.

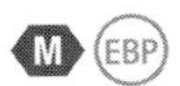

- Surgical removal of a single brain metastatic lesion may be considered (Soffietti, et al., 2011).

Collaborative Interventions (continued)

Radiation

- Radiation treatment uses radioactive energy to shrink and/or destroy cancer tissues. It can also assist in some patients to reduce advanced cancer-related symptoms.

- Radiation may be delivered using:
  - o Internal radiation or **brachytherapy**, which involves placing radioactive material (e.g., radioactive seeds) near or directly into a tumor, directing radiation at the tumor and sparing surrounding tissues. The targeted radiation can cause tumor shrinkage and death.

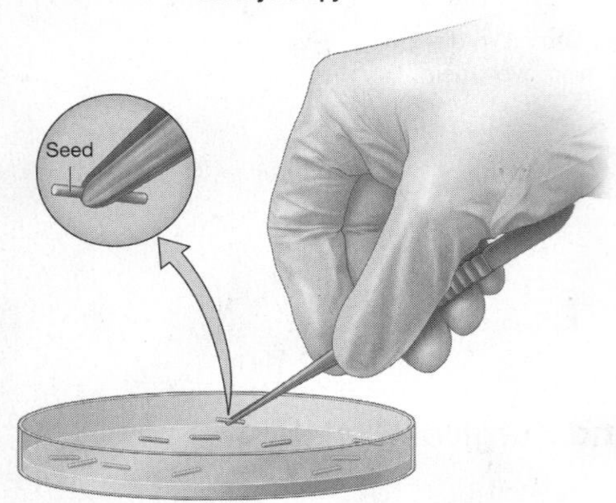

Brachytherapy involves implanting a radioactive seed into the tumors.

  - o Systemic radiation, which involves infusing or ingesting radioactive material that enters the bloodstream to destroy cancer cells.
  - o External beam radiation, which uses a beam of radiation targeted to cancer cells

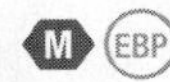

- Whole brain radiation therapy (WBRT) may be used as the sole treatment in newly diagnosed adults with single brain metastases in selected cancers (Gaspar, et al., 2010).

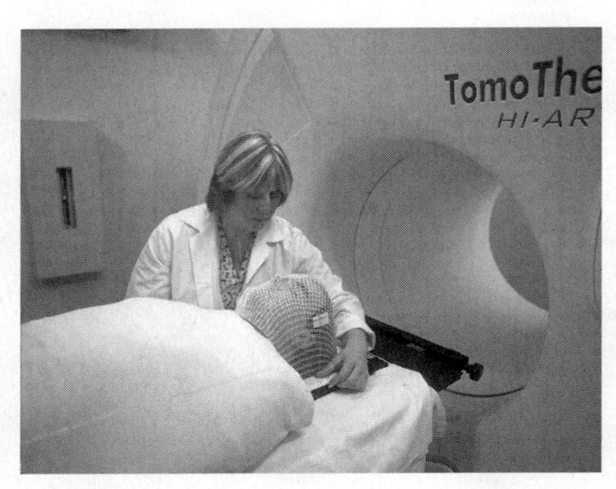

Patient receiving radiation therapy. Note the immobilizing head mesh (mask) to prevent patient movement and better ensure that the radiation is delivered to its intended focal point.

Source: National Cancer Institute

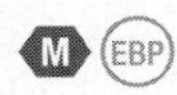

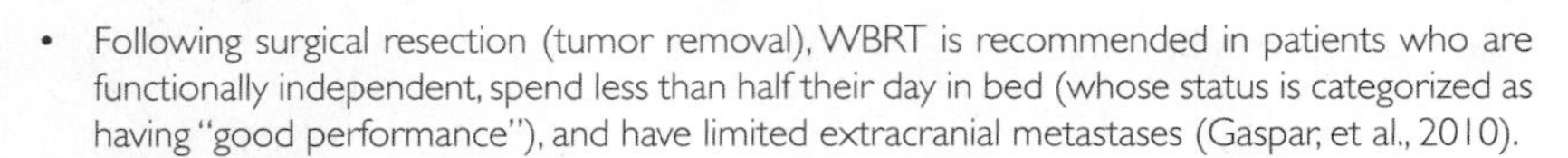

- Following surgical resection (tumor removal), WBRT is recommended in patients who are functionally independent, spend less than half their day in bed (whose status is categorized as having "good performance"), and have limited extracranial metastases (Gaspar, et al., 2010).

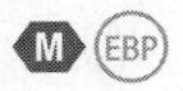

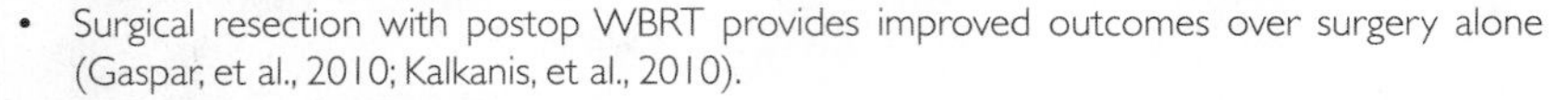

- Surgical resection with postop WBRT provides improved outcomes over surgery alone (Gaspar, et al., 2010; Kalkanis, et al., 2010).

- Radiation therapy may also involve the use of gamma knife radiosurgery in which approximately 200 narrow beams of radiation focus on the tumor with precision and destroy cancer cells without harm to tissues surrounding it. It is much safer than traditional surgery.

- Monitor for and instruct the patient that side effects are possible and may include nausea, vomiting, seizures, headache, loss of hair or hearing, skin alterations, memory and speech deficits, and extreme fatigue.

Chemotherapy

 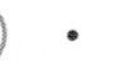

- Use of cytotoxic antineoplastic medications against cancer and some metastatic brain tumors that are chemosensitive (Soffietti, et al., 2011)

- Chemotherapy following WBRT for brain metastases is not recommended as it has shown no survival benefit (Mehta, et al., 2010).

Gene/Virus Therapy (experimental)

- Adenoviral vectors are used to target tumor cells for genetic change, chemosensitization, and more.

Collaborative Interventions (continued)

Postoperative Care

Depending on the type and extent of brain surgery, postoperative care can include:

- Neurological assessments:
  - o Should assess frequently and on an ongoing basis
  - o Include motor function, sensory, and level of consciousness checks.
  - o Routinely evaluate changes in level of consciousness. A decrease in level of consciousness could be due to:
    - Increasing intracranial pressure
    - Decrease in blood glucose level
    - Low sodium level
    - Excessive analgesics

- Implement seizure precautions.

- Monitor vital signs, including temperature, pulse, blood pressure, respirations, pulse oxygenation (SpO_2) and impairment in spontaneous movement.

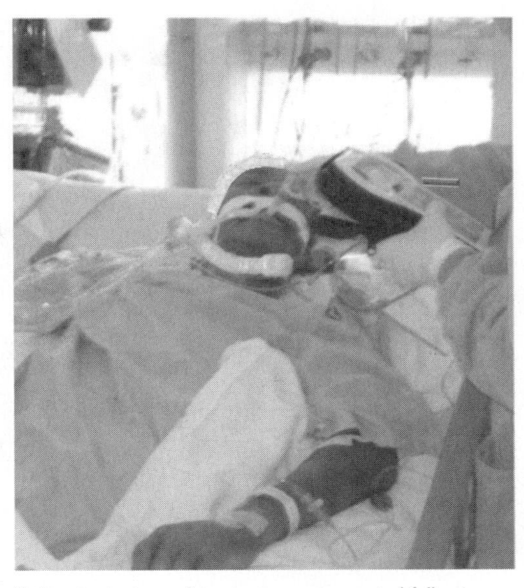

Patient in the immediate postoperative period following his brain tumor surgery.

Source: Copyright © 2014, NovEx Novice to Expert Learning, LLC

- Protect airway:
  - o If patient is intubated and on ventilator, follow weaning protocol as soon as possible.
  - o Prevent pneumonia using coughing, turning, and inspiratory spirometer.

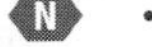

- Cardiac monitoring: Continuously observe for dysrhythmias (i.e., bradycardia, tachycardia).
- Wound and skin monitoring and care: Incision care and observation for infection, frequent turning and repositioning to prevent pressure sores
- May require management of drains or hemovacs

- Intake and output for pituitary tumors:
  - o Monitor closely for hormonal imbalances, most commonly antidiuretic hormone (ADH). Inappropriate ADH syndrome can result from injury by cancer or inflammation associated with a tumor.
  - o If too little ADH is secreted, the patient generates large amounts of urine and rapidly decompensates from hypovolemia.
  - o If the patient secretes an excessive amount of ADH, large amounts of water may be retained, causing volume overload and dramatically decreasing the serum sodium level.
  - o Strict intake and output tracking on these patients is imperative with appropriate fluid replacement as indicated.
  - o Patient should be NPO until fully awake and can swallow safely.
- Monitor ICP when ICP device is placed to manage intracranial pressure.
- Postoperative medications include administering prescribed:
  - o Steroids
  - o H_2 blockers
  - o Anticonvulsants
  - o Analgesic agents
- Prophylaxis against deep vein thrombosis (DVT) is vital as malignant brain tumors carry an increased risk of DVT (Soffietti, et al., 2011).
- Remove indwelling urinary catheter, central venous lines, and other invasive devices at the earliest possible time to prevent never events.
- Mobilize as soon as possible to prevent complications (e.g., DVT, pneumonia, skin breakdown) (RNAO, 2013).

Brain Surgery - Ventriculostomy and Placement of Intracranial Pressure (ICP) Monitor Bolt

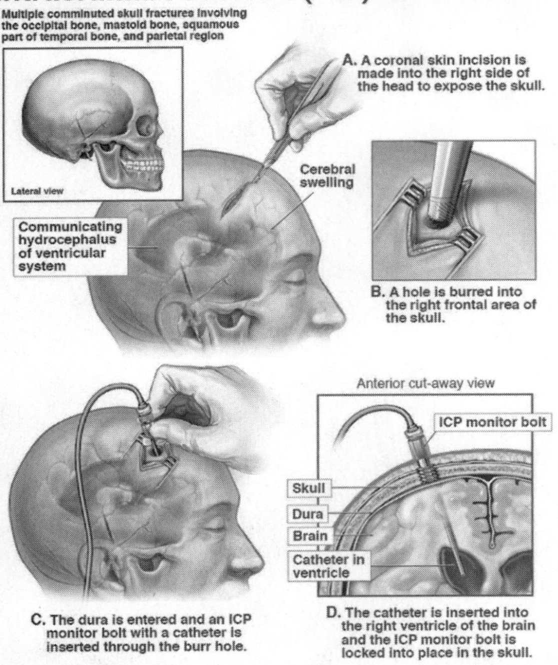

This series of medical illustrations shows the steps to place a ventriculostomy to monitor intracranial pressure: A. Incision into the scalp; B. Drilling into the frontal area of the skull; C. Dura opened and an intracranial pressure monitor bolt being inserted; D. Final position of the intracranial pressure monitor bolt with catheter tip residing deep in the ventricle of the brain to obtain the pressure reading.

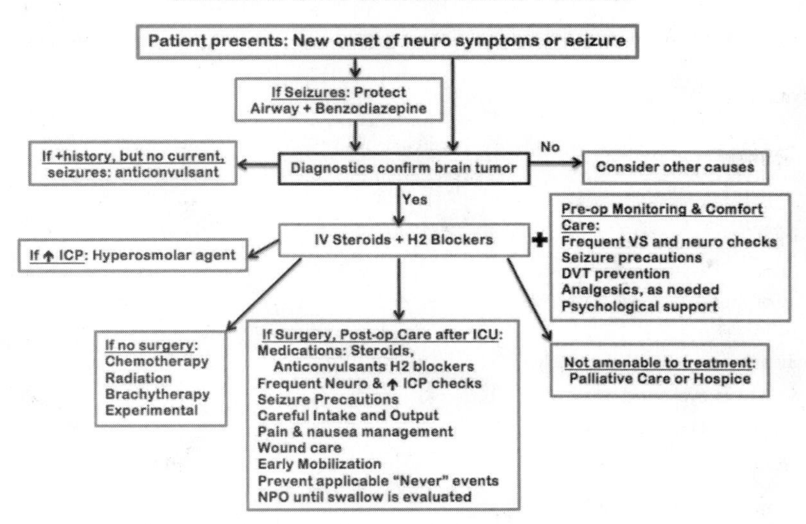

Source: Copyright © 2014, NovEx Novice to Expert Learning, LLC

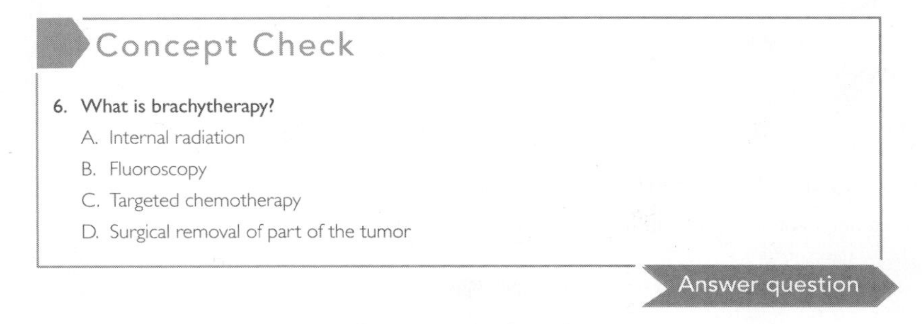

Concept Check

6. What is brachytherapy?
   - A. Internal radiation
   - B. Fluoroscopy
   - C. Targeted chemotherapy
   - D. Surgical removal of part of the tumor

Answer question

Collaborative Interventions (continued)

Patient Education

Educate the patient and family about:

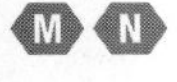

- What to expect, if possible. This is determined by the medical team unless the tumor is a frequent condition that the nurses see.
- Healthy diet and how to accommodate mouth blisters with certain therapies, such as chemotherapy (see the Care of Cancer Patients with Treatment Toxicities NovE-lesson)
- Medications, which may include steroids, anticonvulsants, H_2 blockers
- Seeking support for emotional upset and life changes depending on the degree of cognitive, behavioral, and functional impairments that evolve, if any
- Ongoing lifelong follow-up with CT and MRI, as recommended by the health care provider
- Rehabilitation: physical, speech, and/or occupational therapy, physiatrist
- Sources of support: National Cancer Institute, American Brain Tumor Association, American Cancer Society

Concept Check

7. Which long-term care provision is instituted for patients who have had brain surgery for tumor removal?
   - A. Daily administration of vitamin K
   - B. Seizure precautions
   - C. Strict bedrest
   - D. Management of indwelling urinary catheter

Answer question

Summary of Interventions

- **Histologic origin** and **location** of the tumor affect the specific interventions and overall prognosis.
- Medical treatments may include a combination of:
  - o Surgery
  - o Chemotherapy
  - o Brachytherapy
  - o Experimental therapies
  - o Palliative care or hospice
- Evidence-based practices support the use of steroids, benzodiazepines if seizures occur, anticonvulsants when appropriate, and H_2 blockers.
- Postoperative monitoring post-ICU continues to be essential, especially:
  - o Diligent intake and output; NPO until swallow is evaluated
  - o Seizure precautions; monitor for increasing intracranial pressure
  - o Wound care
  - o Pain and nausea management
  - o Early mobilization; prevent never events
  - o Educate the patient and family for discharge.
- Psychological support is important in the care of patients with a brain tumor because of possible life-threatening or life-altering effects.

LO4:

Evaluation of Desired Collaborative Care Outcomes

Evaluation and reassessment should reveal attainment of previously established patient outcomes. In summary:

- The patient's intracranial pressure is within desired range with no notable brain injury.
- The patient is injury free.
- The patient reports that education and support helped manage the feelings of fear.
- The patient remains active to the extent allowed by treatments and disease.
- The patient and family talk with one another about the patient's prognosis, make plans for the future, and make use of support as desired.

References

Armstrong, T. S., & Gilbert, M. R. (2000). Metastatic brain tumors: Diagnosis, treatment, and nursing interventions. *Clinical Journal of Oncology Nursing, 4*(5), 217–225. **www.ncbi.nlm.nih.gov/pubmed/11111453**

Bohan, E. M. (2013). Cognitive changes associated with central nervous system malignancies and treatment. *Seminars in Oncology Nursing, 29*(4), 238–247. doi:10.1016/j.soncn.2013.08.004

Cahill, J., & Armstrong, T. (2011). Caring for an adult with a malignant primary brain tumor. *Nursing 2014, 41*(6), 28–33. **journals.lww.com/nursing/Citation/2011/06000/Caring_for_an_adult_with_a_malignant_primary_brain.10.aspx**

Grant, R. (2004). Overview: Brain tumour diagnosis and management/Royal College of Physicians guidelines. *Journal of Neurology, Neurosurgery, and Psychiatry, 75*(Suppl. II), ii18–ii23. **jnnp.bmj.com/content/75/suppl_2/ii18.full.pdf+html**

McKinney, P. A. (2004). Brain tumours: Incidence, survival, and aetiology. *Journal of Neurology, Neurosurgery, and Psychiatry, 75*(Suppl. II), ii12–ii17. **jnnp.bmj.com/content/75/suppl_2/ii12.full**

Schaller, B., & Ruegg, S. J. (2003). Brain tumor and seizures: Pathophysiology and its implications for treatment revisited. *Epilepsia, 44*(9), 1223–1232. **onlinelibrary.wiley.com/doi/10.1046/j.1528-1157.2003.05203.x/full**

Tremont-Lukats, I. W., Ratilal, B. O., Armstrong, T., & Gilbert, M. R. (2008). Antiepileptic drugs for preventing seizures in people with brain tumors. *Cochrane Database of Systematic Reviews, 16*(2).

Clinical Practice Guidelines

Finnish Medical Society Duodecim. (2010). Prevention of venous thromboembolism. In *Evidence-based medical guidelines*. Helsinki, Finland: Wiley Interscience. John Wiley & Son. **www.guideline.gov/content.aspx?id=34957&search=dvt**

Gaspar, L. E., Mehta, M. P., Patchell, R. A., et al. (2010). The role of whole brain radiation therapy in the management of newly diagnosed brain metastases: A systematic review and evidence-based clinical practice guideline. *Journal of Neuro-Oncology, 96*(1), 17–32. **www.guideline.gov/content.aspx?id=25746&search=brain+tumor**

Kahrilas, P. J., Shaheen, M. J., & Vaezi, M. F. (2008). American Gastroenterological Association Institute technical review on the management of gastroesophageal reflux disease. *Gastroenterology, 135*(4), 1392–1413. **www.gastrojournal.org/article/S0016-5085(08)01605-3/fulltext#sec4.1**

Kalkanis, S. N., Kondziolka, D., Gaspar, L. E., et al. (2010). The role of surgical resection in the management of newly diagnosed brain metastases: A systematic review and evidence-based clinical practice guideline. *Journal of Neuro-Oncology, 96*(1), 33–43. **www.guideline.gov/content.aspx?id=25747&search=brain+tumor**

Mehta, M. P., Paleologos, N. A., Mikkelsen, T., et al. (2010). The role of chemotherapy in the management of newly diagnosed brain metastases: A systematic review and evidence-based clinical practice guideline. *Journal of Neuro-Oncology, 96*(1), 71–83. **www.guideline.gov/content.aspx?id=25749&search=brain+tumor**

Mikkelsen, R., Paleologos, N. A., Robinson, P. D., et al. (2010). The role of prophylactic anticonvulsants in the management of brain metastases: A systematic review and evidence-based clinical practice guideline. *Journal of Neuro-Oncology, 96*(1), 97–102. **www.guideline.gov/content.aspx?id=25751&search=seizure**

National Institute for Health and Clinical Excellence. (2012). *The epilepsies: The diagnosis and management of the epilepsies in adults and children in primary and secondary care* (Clinical guideline 137). London, UK: Author. **www.guideline.gov/content.aspx?id=36082&search=seizure**

Registered Nurses' Association of Ontario. (2013). *RNAO best practice guidelines*. **rnao.ca/sites/rnao-ca/files/Nursing_OS_and_BPGs_Phase_2_Oct._2013_0.pdf**

Ryken, T. C., McDermott, M., Robinson, P. D., et al. (2010). The role of steroids in the management of brain metastases: A systematic review and evidence-based clinical practice guideline. *Journal of Neuro-Oncology, 96*(1), 103–114. **www.guideline.gov/content.aspx?id=25752&search=brain+tumor**

Soffietti, R., Cornu, P., Delattre, J. Y., et al. (2011). Brain metastases. In N. E. Gilhus, M. P. Barnes, & M. Brainin (Eds.), *European handbook of neurological management* (2nd ed., pp. 437–446). Oxford: Blackwell-Wiley.

Patient Education

Bauman, G., & Macdonald, D. (2007). *"Benign" vs. "malignant" brain tumors.* **www.schulich.uwo.ca/oncology/education/undergraduate/docs/CNS.pdf**

Cancer Treatment Centers for America. (2014). *What is brachytherapy?* **www.brachytherapy.com/**

Huff, J. S. (2013). *Brain neoplasms.* **emedicine.medscape.com/article/779664-overview**

Mayo Clinic Staff. (2014). *Diseases and conditions: brain tumor.* **www.mayoclinic.org/diseases-conditions/brain-tumor/home/ovc-20117132**

Simon, H. (2013). *Brain tumors—primary.* **www.umm.edu/patiented/articles/who_gets_brain_tumors_000089_3.htm**

CARE OF PATIENTS WITH CHRONIC NEUROLOGIC CONDITIONS: DEMENTIA AND DELIRIUM

Learning Outcomes for Chronic Neurologic Conditions: Dementia and Delirium

When you complete this lesson, you will be able to:

1. Recognize the clinical relevance of dementia and delirium.
2. Consider the pathophysiology, etiology, risk factors, and clinical presentation of dementia and delirium that determine the priority patient concerns.
3. Determine the most urgent and important nursing interventions and patient education required in caring for a patient with dementia or delirium.
4. Evaluate attainment of desired collaborative care outcomes for a patient with dementia or delirium.

LO1:

Dementia and Delirium

- These common conditions affect the ability to think clearly, concentrate, solve problems, and remember. The diminished ability to perform these tasks is called cognitive decline.
- **Dementia** develops over the years and is irreversible.
- **Delirium** has a trigger such as a medication, intoxication, or an illness that causes a sudden decline. The degree of delirium fluctuates and usually improves after the trigger is removed.
- Patients who develop these conditions may no longer be able to care for themselves, and they can be challenging to care for by the family or health care providers.

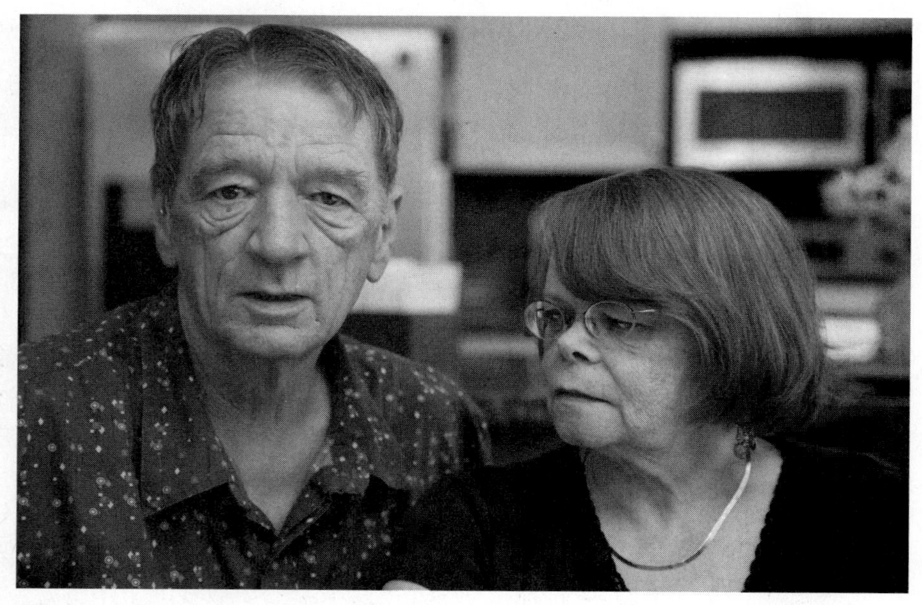

The decline in a loved one's mental capacities due to dementia is very difficult for loved ones to witness. As their intellectual abilities wane, family members often feel they are "losing" the person they love.
Source: Scott Griessel/Fotolia

LO1:

What Is Dementia?

- Dementia is a neurodegenerative syndrome that causes a progressive loss of cognitive function.
- Several types of conditions cause dementia, most of which show progressive decline of cognitive function over long periods of time (progression over years).

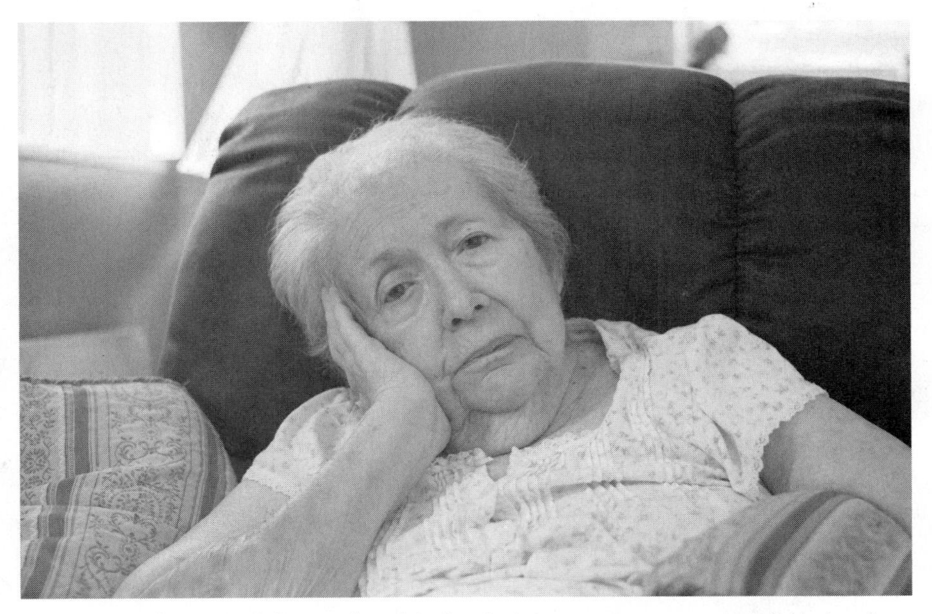

Dementia can affect any and all areas of cognitive functioning, so symptoms vary with individuals and depend upon the cause of the dementia. This photo reflects the confusion and memory loss that characterizes dementia.
Source: Fotoluminate LLC/Fotolia

LO1:

Clinical Relevance: Dementia

- One in eight to nine older (> age 65) adult Americans has Alzheimer's disease.
- With the aging of the population, dementia is increasingly more prevalent.
- Dementia is a leading cause of institutionalization of adults (nursing home placement).
- Direct cost of care for patients with dementia in the United States is $200 billion annually. This does not account for the cost of caregiver burden.

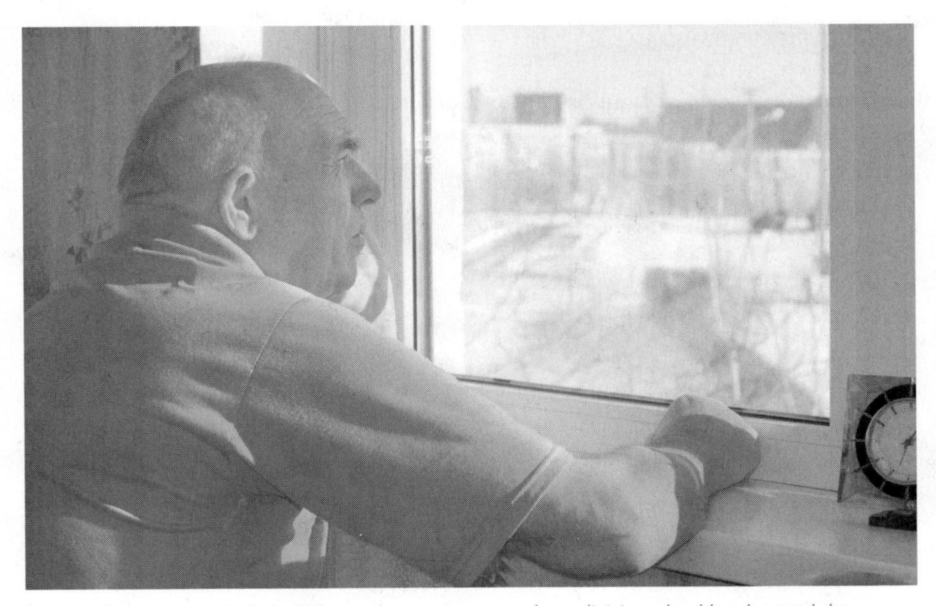

Because dementia, particularly Alzheimer's type, is so prevalent, clinicians should understand the implications in patients caring for themselves, taking medications, and living alone.
Source: Kolotype/Fotolia

Concept Check

1. **Which condition(s) is/are reversible?**
   A. Delirium
   B. Dementia
   C. Both delirium and dementia
   D. Neither delirium nor dementia

Answer question

LO2:

Pathophysiology: Dementia

- Numerous conditions cause dementia. Most dementias have neuron loss and brain atrophy, resulting in permanent cognitive dysfunction.
- Alzheimer's disease is the most common and is associated with over 50% of cases.
- Vascular dementia is another prominent cause. It is also known as multi-infarct dementia, where scattered cerebral infarctions are responsible for neuron loss and cognitive deficits.
- Lewy body dementia is associated with Parkinson's disease.
- Numerous other types of dementia are less common than those discussed (e.g., Creutzfeldt–Jakob, Huntington, HIV, traumatic brain injury, drug use).

Alzheimer's Disease

- Alzheimer's disease is a degenerative neurological disease.
- Abnormal protein deposits, called amyloid plaques, and neurofibrillary tangles are found in the brains of patients with Alzheimer's disease. How amyloid plaques are related to loss of neurons is not understood.
- Neurofibrillary tangles are masses of tangled, nonfunctional neurons.
- Loss of memory, especially short-term memory, is a characteristic of Alzheimer's disease and is likely due to the loss of neurons that produce acetylcholine, a neurotransmitter essential for new memory formation.
- The Alzheimer's Association provides an excellent tour of the brain with Alzheimer's at www.alz.org/braintour/alzheimers_changes.asp.

Normal Brain: Cortical Mass

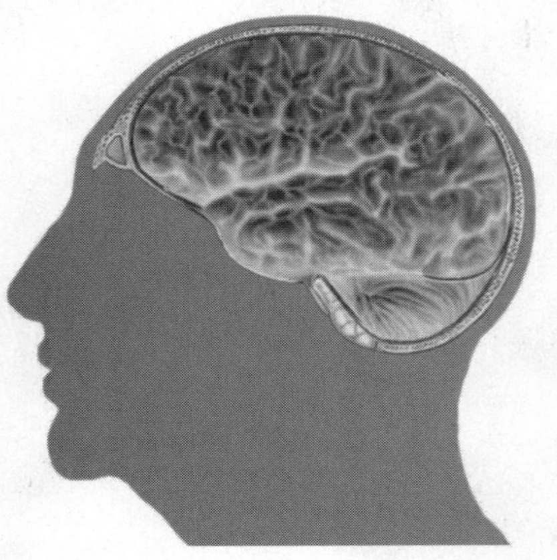

Alzheimer's: Loss of Cortical Mass

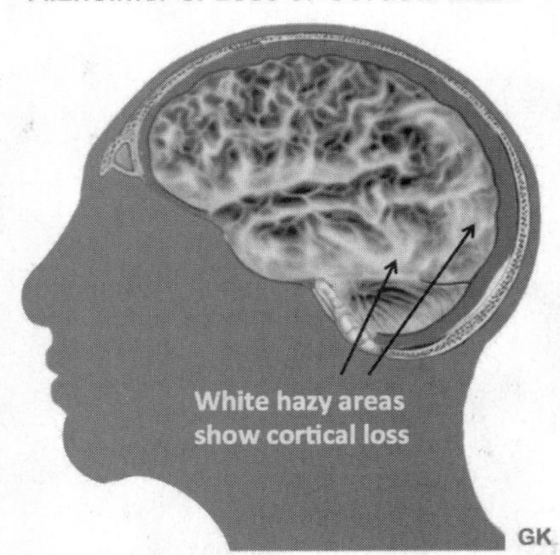
White hazy areas
show cortical loss
GK

This picture shows neural degeneration in people with Alzheimer's, but the concepts of brain atrophy/degeneration are the same, just not as widespread.
Source: Courtesy of George Kyriakidis/Santa Ana, CA

- Alzheimer's disease primarily affects the cortex of the brain by irreversibly damaging neurons and causing atrophy.
- The affected cerebral areas explain the cognitive deficits exhibited: decline in intelligence, forgetfulness, word-search problems, depression, wandering, hostility, personality alterations, and speech difficulties.

Areas of the Brain Most Affected by Alzheimer's Disease

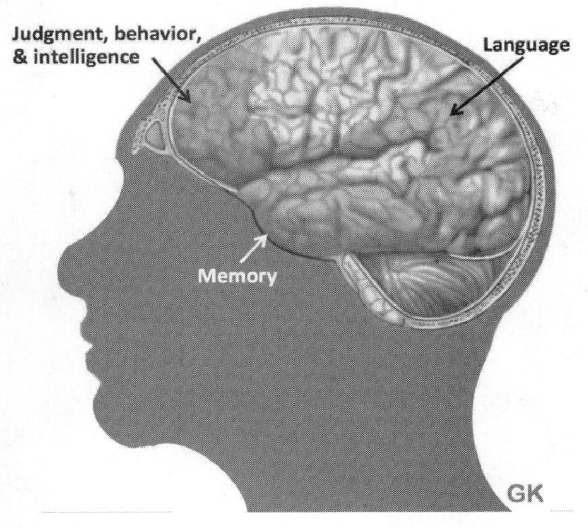

This illustration depicts color-coded regions of the brain indicating the areas of the cerebral cortex commonly affected by Alzheimer's disease: the frontal lobe governs intelligence, judgment, and social behavior while the temporal and parietal brain lobes govern memory and language.
Source: Courtesy of George Kyriakidis/Santa Ana, CA

Pathophysiology: Dementia (continued)

Vascular Dementia

- Dementia can develop over time from vascular disease.
- The development of atherosclerosis in the small vessels of the brain results in ischemia and multiple small strokes.
- These small strokes usually do not present with classical stroke symptoms (e.g., hemiparesis).
- Loss of neurons over time results in cognitive dysfunction.

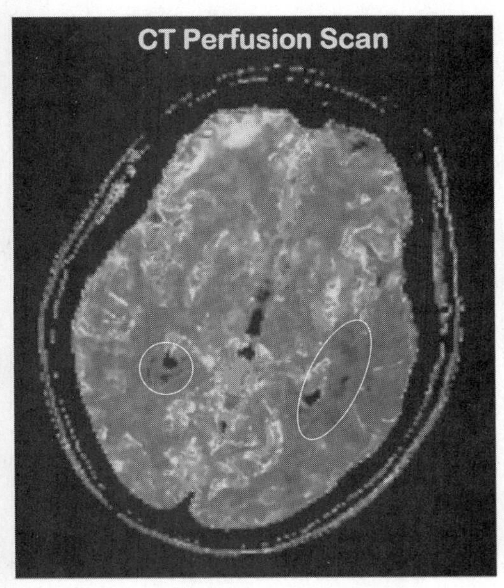

Red=high perfusion
Navy=low perfusion
Black=no perfusion

This CT perfusion scan reveals multiple ischemic (medium blue) and infarction (black & navy) areas throughout the brain. The white circled areas indicate cortical and subcortical infarctions in a vascular dementia patient.
Source: Courtesy of K. Kyriakidis

Lewy Body Dementia

- Patients with Lewy body type of dementia develop protein deposits in the brain called Lewy bodies.
- In this disorder, dopamine-generating neurons located in part of the midbrain are lost.

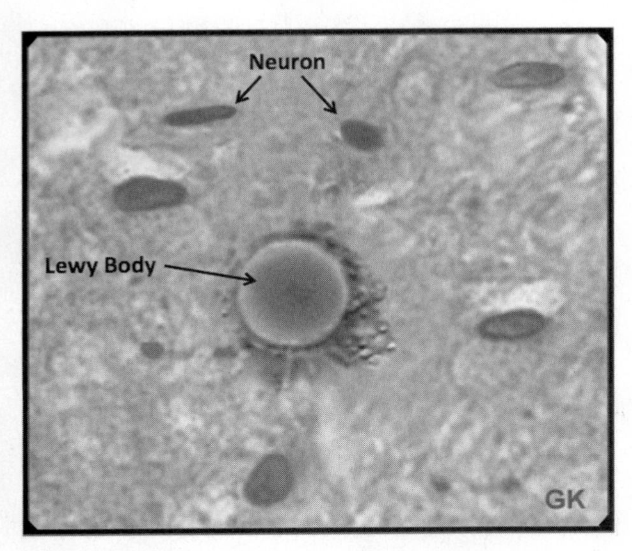

Lewy body dementia is one of the most common types of progressive dementia. Lewy body dementia usually occurs sporadically, in people with no known family history of the disease. However, rare familial cases have occasionally been reported. In Lewy body dementia, cells die in the brain's cortex (outer layer), and in a part of the mid-brain called the substantia nigra. Many of the remaining nerve cells in the substantia nigra contain abnormal structures called Lewy bodies that are the hallmark of the disease.
Source: Courtesy of George Kyriakidis/Santa Ana, CA

- As a result, patients may develop symptoms of Parkinson's disease characterized by:
  - Bradykinesia (slow movements)
  - Resting tremor ("pill rolling" tremor)
  - Rigidity
  - Slow gait with short steps
- Up to 30% of patients with Parkinson's disease develop dementia.

Concept Check

2. Patients with vascular dementia commonly experience which changes?

A. Motor impairment
B. Cognitive dysfunction
C. Sensory impairment
D. Bradykinesia

Answer question

LO2:

Risk Factors: Dementia

- Age is a primary risk factor.
- Vascular disease—a history of heart disease, stroke, or peripheral vascular disease
- Parkinson's disease
- Diabetes

Dementia: Risk Factors	
Age	Patients are at higher risk for vascular dementia, Alzheimer's disease and several other forms of dementia with advancing age.
Diabetes	Diabetes contributes to the development of both Alzheimer's and vascular dementia.
Atherosclerosis	This vascular problem reduces and can block cerebral perfusion and may result in stroke.
Genetics	Research shows that several genes place patients at higher risk for Alzheimer's dementia.
Alcohol Use & Smoking	Smoking is linked to higher risk of mental impairment and dementia and additionally increases the risk of atherosclerosis. Similarly, alcohol increases the risk of dementia.
Cholesterol	High low-density lipoprotein levels (bad cholesterol) increase the risk of vascular dementia.
Early Cognitive Impairment	Many, but not all, patients with cognitive deficits are at higher risk of dementia.
Down Syndrome	Research shows that patients with Down syndrome commonly develop Alzheimer's by middle age.
Plasma Homocysteine	A high level of homocysteine is a strong risk factor for both vascular and Alzheimer's dementia.

Researchers have identified several risk factors that affect the likelihood of developing one or more kinds of dementia. Some of these factors are modifiable, while others are not.

LO2

Causes: Dementia

Causes of dementia vary widely. Some types of dementia are irreversible while others are potentially reversible when the cause is successfully treated.

Progressive Causes

- Alzheimer's disease: most common cause in older adults
- Vascular disease: second most common cause
- Lewy body dementia
- Frontotemporal dementia
- Traumatic brain injury: from single incident (e.g., accident) or repetitive injury (e.g., football, boxing)
- Huntington's disease, which is inherited and results in nerve cell wasting
- HIV, which destroys brain tissue
- Creutzfeldt–Jakob disease, which may be inherited or acquired

Reversible Causes

- Infection: Lyme disease, meningitis, syphilis, encephalitis
- Nutritional abnormalities: thiamine deficiency, vitamin B-12 deficit
- Subdural hematoma
- Poisoning: Lead, pesticide
- Adverse reaction to medication
- Metabolic or endocrine disorder: hypothyroidism, hypernatremia, malabsorption of vitamin B-12, hypoglycemia
- Brain tumor
- Hypoxia: severe asthma, carbon monoxide poisoning, chronic lung disease
- Immune disorders: leukemia

LO2:

Assessment Findings: Dementia

- Generally, all dementias cause a gradual loss of cognitive function over time.
- Memory impairment is often a first sign. Other signs include language impairment, apathy, and loss of executive functioning (planning ability). The diagram that follows details the gradual loss.
- Sleep disturbances are common. Patients may sleep during the day and be awake at night.
- Wandering
- Eating disturbances occur frequently. Some patients with advanced dementia may stop eating altogether.
- Late stages of dementia tend to show severe cognitive impairment, dependence on caregivers, and neuropsychiatric symptoms.
- Dementia differs from delirium in that most common types of dementia cause a relentless progression of the disease that is not reversible.
- Psychosis often accompanies dementia. Parkinson's-related dementia and Lewy body dementia often produce hallucinations and Parkinsonian symptoms (e.g., bradykinesia and tremor).

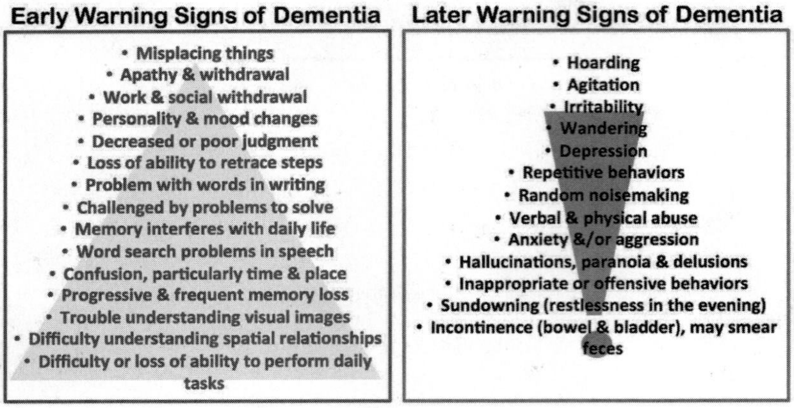

Early Warning Signs of Dementia

- Misplacing things
- Apathy & withdrawal
- Work & social withdrawal
- Personality & mood changes
- Decreased or poor judgment
- Loss of ability to retrace steps
- Problem with words in writing
- Challenged by problems to solve
- Memory interferes with daily life
- Word search problems in speech
- Confusion, particularly time & place
- Progressive & frequent memory loss
- Trouble understanding visual images
- Difficulty understanding spatial relationships
- Difficulty or loss of ability to perform daily tasks

Later Warning Signs of Dementia

- Hoarding
- Agitation
- Irritability
- Wandering
- Depression
- Repetitive behaviors
- Random noisemaking
- Verbal & physical abuse
- Anxiety &/or aggression
- Hallucinations, paranoia & delusions
- Inappropriate or offensive behaviors
- Sundowning (restlessness in the evening)
- Incontinence (bowel & bladder), may smear feces

Signs and symptoms of progressive decline in dementia.
Source: Copyright © 2014, NovEx Novice to Expert Learning, LLC

For the initial diagnosis, there are three things that the physician looks at:

- The medical symptoms
- Other physical conditions that might be responsible for similar symptoms
- The results of the MMSE memory test—Mini-Mental State Examination

LO2:

Diagnostics: Dementia

- The primary means of diagnosis is clinical assessment.
- Screening tools are available to assist in diagnosis, such as the Mini-Mental State Examination (MMSE). These can usually be completed in minutes.
- Formal neuropsychiatric testing may also be used to assist in diagnosis. This type of testing takes longer and may require more than 1 hour.
- Laboratory tests are often used to rule out reversible conditions (e.g., thyroid, electrolyte, infection, hypoxia, medications, vitamin, metal poisoning)
- CT and MRI scans are used to rule out reversible conditions in patients with dementia (e.g., inflammatory disease, tumor, abscess) (Sorbi, et al., 2012).

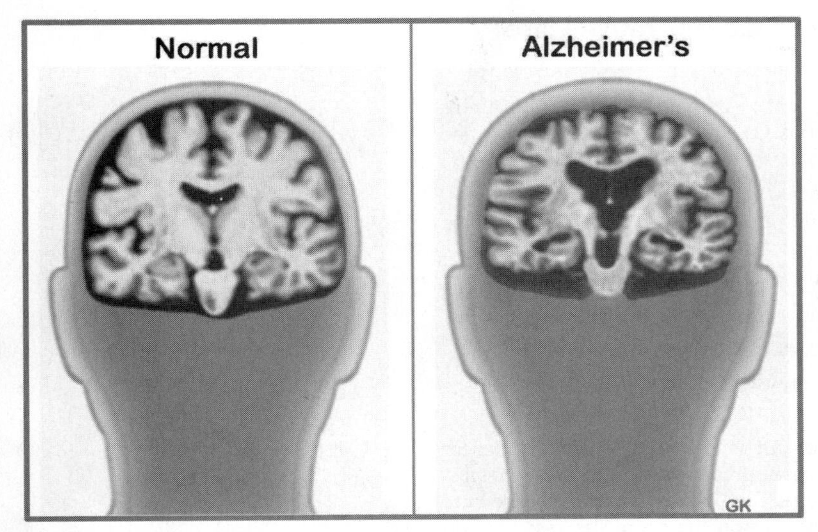

Alzheimer's disease leads to nerve cell death and tissue loss throughout the brain. As the disease progresses, brain tissue shrinks and the ventricles (chambers within the brain that contain cerebrospinal fluid) become larger. The damage disrupts communication between brain cells, crippling memory, speech, and comprehension.
Source: Courtesy of George Kyriakidis/Santa Ana, CA

Mini-Mental State Examination

- This is an example of the MMSE tool. It is simple to complete for patients without cognitive impairment.

Mini-Mental State Examination

Section	Question or Task	Maximum Score	Patient Score
Orientation	What is the date: year, season, date, day, month?	5	
	Where are we: country, county, town, hospital, floor?	5	
Registration	Name three objects for the patient to remember: 1 second to say each, then ask patient to recall all three. Repeat until the patient has learned all three. Count and record trials.	3	
	Ask patient to count backwards from 100 by 7s (93, 86, 79...): one point for each correct. Stop after 5 are correct. Alternatively spell "world" backwards.	5	
	Ask patient to name the 3 same objects you named above.	3	
Language	Show patient 2 objects and name them: (e.g., pencil, clock)	2	
	Repeat the following, "no ifs, ands, or buts"	1	
	Follow a 3-stage commend: "take a piece of paper in your right hand, fold it in half, and put it on the floor"	3	
	Read and obey the following: "close your eyes", "write a sentence," and "copy a design"	3	
Total Score		30	
Score Results:	< 17= severe dysfunction & severe dementia; 18-25=marked cognitive dysfunction and dementia; 26-28=borderline cognitive dysfunction; 29-30=normal		

A mini-mental status test is easy to administer. Scores of <26 may indicate the presence of dementia or delirium.
Source: Copyright © 2014, NovEx Novice to Expert Learning, LLC

Concept Check

3. Abnormal results on which examination best supports the diagnosis of Alzheimer's disease?
   A. Thyroid levels
   B. Electrolyte levels
   C. MRI
   D. Mini-Mental State Examination

Answer question

Priority Patient Concerns and Desired Collaborative Care Outcomes: Dementia

Prior to caring for patients with dementia, it is important to prioritize the patient's concerns that must guide the nursing care plan and interventions. Care for the patient is ordered and organized in accordance with the patient's priority and urgent needs. Desired collaborative care outcomes in patients with dementia typically include:

1. Patient and family will use strategies to help patient remain oriented to person, place, and time, as much as possible.
2. Patient and family will use strategies to help patient recognize surroundings and situations.
3. Family will demonstrate coping strategies that enable them to function within expectations.
4. Patient will provide or participate in part or all of activities of daily living (ADLs).
5. Caregiver and/or family members will discuss or demonstrate ways to prevent or reduce caregiver strain.

Considering these important care outcomes, prepare a list of the major 3–6 priority patient concerns or nursing diagnoses for patients with dementia. Be prepared to participate in a discussion of this list and/or to submit them as an assignment, as determined by your faculty. Resources you may find helpful in this assignment can include this lesson, the references, resources on nursing care plans, and standard nursing diagnoses manuals.

LO3:

Collaborative Interventions: Dementia

- There are no known cures, treatments, or lifestyle changes that are strongly recommended as preventing or delaying development of dementia (Parminder, et al., 2008; Sorbi, et al., 2012).
- Treatments may improve symptoms and functioning. Interventions include:

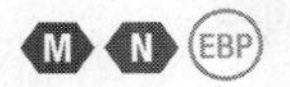

  - o Acetylcholinesterase inhibitors such as donepezil, galantamine, and rivastigmine have shown some efficacy in mild to moderate Alzheimer-related dementia for cognitive function and symptom management (Parminder, et al., 2008; Scottish Intercollegiate Guidelines Network [SIGN], 2006).
  - o Memantine, which blocks NMDA receptors, has also shown efficacy in moderate to severe Alzheimer (Parminder, et al., 2008).
  - o Memantine is ineffective in improving cognitive function in non-Alzheimer dementias (Sorbi, et al., 2012).
  - o Prevent delirium or confusion in the hospital by minimizing the use of medications that worsen confusion including benzodiazepines, narcotics, and anticholinergics (Fletcher, et al., 2012).
- Antipsychotics are used with caution to control adverse neuropsychiatric symptoms (e.g., agitation, aggression, mood and behavioral disorders, psychosis) of dementia but should not be used in patients with Lewy body dementia since it can worsen symptoms of Parkinson's disease (Fletcher, et al., 2012; SIGN, 2006; Sorbi, et al., 2012).
- Rule out other potentially reversible causes of cognitive impairment using diagnostic testing and history (Fletcher, et al., 2012).
- Treatments that are not recommended include (SIGN, 2006):
  - o Anti-inflammatories such as corticosteroids, hydroxychloroquine
  - o Estrogen
  - o Selegiline
  - o Anticonvulsants

Prevention of Delirium and Confusion

Evidence-based practices are included in the following preventive measures if the evidence and recommendation are both strong:

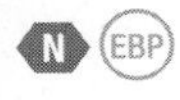

- Approach older adults with a high level of suspicion to improve early detection of onset of symptom (Registered Nurses' Association of Ontario [RNAO], 2012).

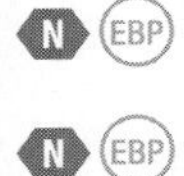

- Know and be alert to early recognition signs and symptoms that may be present and confound the presentation of other clinical conditions (RNAO, 2012).

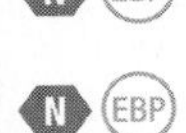

- Collaborate with the health care provider to use standardized tools to assess for cognitive changes (RNAO, 2012).

- Factor in the patient's physical disabilities or sensory alterations when assessing cognitive changes (RNAO, 2012).
- Collaborate with the health care provider and pharmacist about medications and advocate for those with the fewest adverse effects (RNAO, 2013).

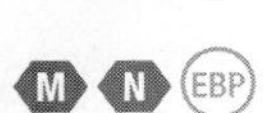

- Ensure early detection and treatment of dehydration, which can cause symptoms that mimic dementia and aggravate dementia (Fletcher, et al., 2012).

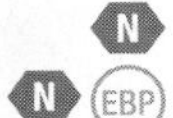

- Place patient's room near nurses' station for safety reasons and closer observation.

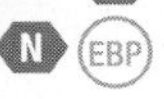

- Open visitation for familiar family members and caregivers who can help provide emotional care and comfort (Fletcher, et al., 2012).
- Discontinue invasive lines as soon as they are not necessary (e.g., IVs, NG tube, telemetry, and Foley catheters) to reduce stressful and unfamiliar challenges to patient.
- Improve and/or maintain orientation with the following:
    - o Family photos
    - o Windows with outside views

    - o Calendars and clocks large enough to see easily

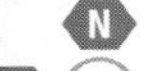

    - o Frequent reorientation to surroundings

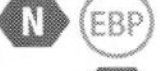

    - o Tranquil environment with periods of undisturbed rest (Fletcher, et al., 2012)

- If the patient has hearing aids or eyeglasses, they should be available and used during waking hours.

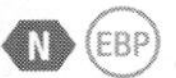

- Minimize disturbances at night, including noise and unnecessary interruptions (including vital signs if condition warrants). Educate family and caregivers for assistance (Fletcher, et al., 2012).

Collaborative Interventions: Dementia (continued)

Family and Caregiver Education and Support

Support and education for family and caregivers are necessary to reduce strain and optimize patient health. Education includes:

- Potentially increased need over time for caregiver support of patient: cognitive, activity, total care

- Prevent fecal and urinary incontinence since patients with dementia do not remember to toilet:
    - o Remind the patient to void or defecate regularly.
    - o Schedule fluid intake to avoid dehydration yet avoid incontinence during outings.
    - o Limit caffeine, which has diuretic effects.
    - o Work out a schedule with the patient that accommodates their routine voiding and defecating habits.
    - o Recommend incontinence products, which can be helpful.
    - o If incontinence is unusual for the patient, collaborate with the health care provider about potential urinary tract infection.
    - o Assist to reduce environmental barriers to hinder the patient's ability to use or get to the bathroom.

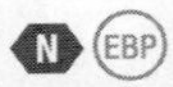

- Prevent falls: loose carpets, passageways, handrails, lighting (Fletcher, et al., 2012).

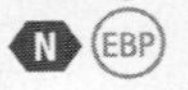

- Prevent safety hazards: wandering, burns, driving, ID bracelet (Fletcher, et al., 2012). Child-safe locks or items and install locks requiring keys are examples of reducing wandering.

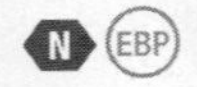

- Reduce anxiety and agitation: tranquil, low-stress and unhurried communications, environment, and meals (Fletcher, et al., 2012; SIGN, 2006). Reducing caffeine, junk food, and sugar in the diet can help reduce agitation.
- Involve the patient in activities that may slow the progression of dementia:

  - o Transition toward healthy lifestyle by maintaining a healthy diet, stop smoking and substance misuse, and managing weight within a healthy range.
  - o Manage comorbid conditions with the health care provider (e.g., diabetes, hypertension).

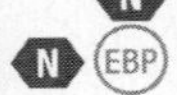

  - o Stay mentally stimulated and active with thinking activities, such as puzzles, word games, memory games, crossword puzzles (SIGN, 2006).

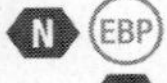

  - o Stay physically active and socially integrated with friends and family (SIGN, 2006).

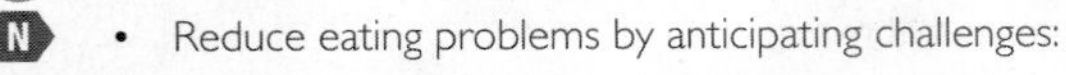

- Reduce eating problems by anticipating challenges:
  - o Difficulty handling utensils, change to a spoon or assist with cutting up food if needed
  - o Expect meals will get messier as getting food to the mouth becomes harder. An adult bib may be useful.
  - o Assist feeding the patient in later stages. Expect meals to take extended periods. May need to remind the patient to chew or swallow.
  - o Expect that foods may require being pureed, minced, or slurried as swallowing becomes less coordinated and/or the patient refuses to eat due to the constant challenge. Swallowing assessment may be needed.
  - o Expect that tube feedings may eventually become a safer method of eating when swallowing is ineffective and may become dangerous. Tube feedings are controversial and need to be discussed with the health care provider.

- Pick your priorities when everyday activities or care become a battle to determine which are necessary:

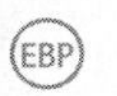

  - o Daily bath: full versus partial. Bathing involves being cold, vulnerable, and intruded upon, often by strangers. Using calm, gentle approaches with verbal support during bathing assisted caregivers in providing care (Hall, et al., 2013).
  - o Dressing: changing into clean clothes, appropriate dress, assistance dressing, purchasing clothes that make self-care easier (e.g., no zippers or shoe laces)
  - o Need to stop driving: Expect this to be extremely difficult as it takes away independence.
  - o Assist in managing finances (e.g., paying bills, handling money, spending money on items of value).
  - o Household cleaning and tasks
  - o Cooking or decisions about meals: may need assistance with decisions about what to eat or cook. Expect that cooking is likely to become a safety hazard.
  - o Using a telephone may become difficult. Later, the patient may not recognize a ringing phone. When they do answer, they are vulnerable to telemarketers.
  - o Be alert for depression as the patient's abilities decline and they recognize their growing limitations. Depression can complicate the patient's willingness or ability to participate in ADLs.

- Improving a patient's participation and defusing their resistance involves (Hall, et al., 2013):
  - o Offering choices
  - o Knowing the person and their individual preferences, including adapting to the patient's preferred schedule
  - o Providing time for privacy
  - o Providing a caregiver of the same gender whenever possible
  - o Providing simple, one step instructions to minimize stimuli
  - o Avoiding hurrying the patient through activities
  - o Encouraging the patient's participation in self-care whenever possible
  - o Using patience, gentleness, flexibility, sensitivity, creativity, and genuine engagement and interest in the person
  - o Using persuasion and avoid coercion while allowing the patient to remain in control
  - o Avoiding successive unpleasant tasks or activities
  - o Listening, being attentive to the patient's responses about their experiences (e.g., cold is cold), and responding by validating the patient's perceptions
- Enhance sleep and reduce problem behavior at night: Establish a calming night time ritual away from noise; leave a night light on to mitigate disorientation upon waking; limit caffeine and daytime napping; encourage exercise.
- Seek assistance and collaborate with the health care provider for more in-depth guidance when late stages of dementia ensue to consider how to best deal with potential issues if they present: wandering, violent behaviors of aggression toward caregivers, disorientation, hallucinations, communication, family or caregiver respite, safety.
- Refer to Alzheimer's caregiver centers, helplines, support groups, and resources.

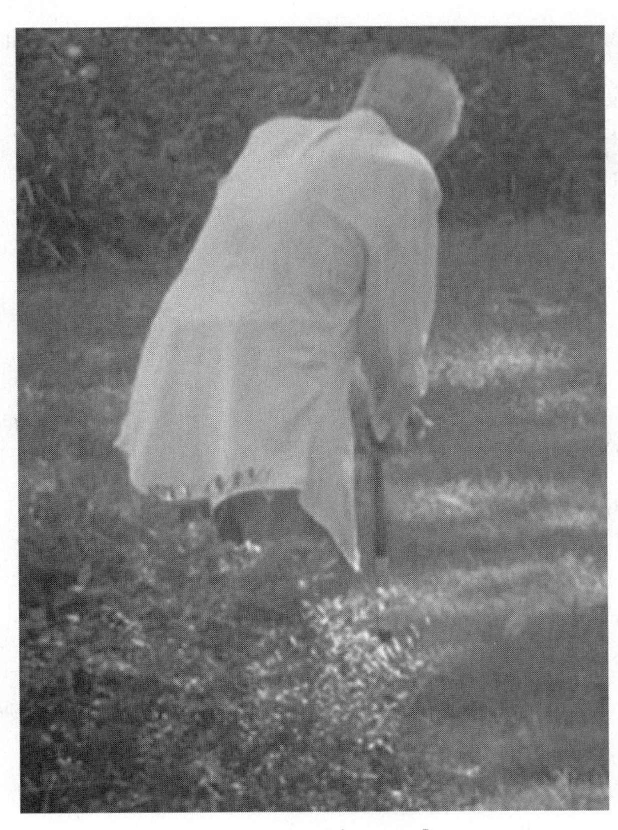

The need for total care evolves over the years. Support groups can help prepare caregivers for the social and life changes. Learning to cope with and support patients who wander (like this patient) and/or require 24 hours per day of care is commonly needed by family or caregivers.
Source: Courtesy of K. Kyriakidis

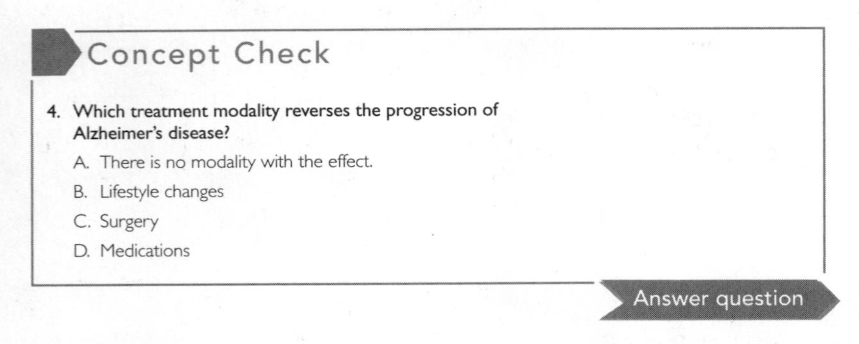

Concept Check
4. Which treatment modality reverses the progression of Alzheimer's disease?
A. There is no modality with the effect.
B. Lifestyle changes
C. Surgery
D. Medications
Answer question

Intervention Summary: Dementia

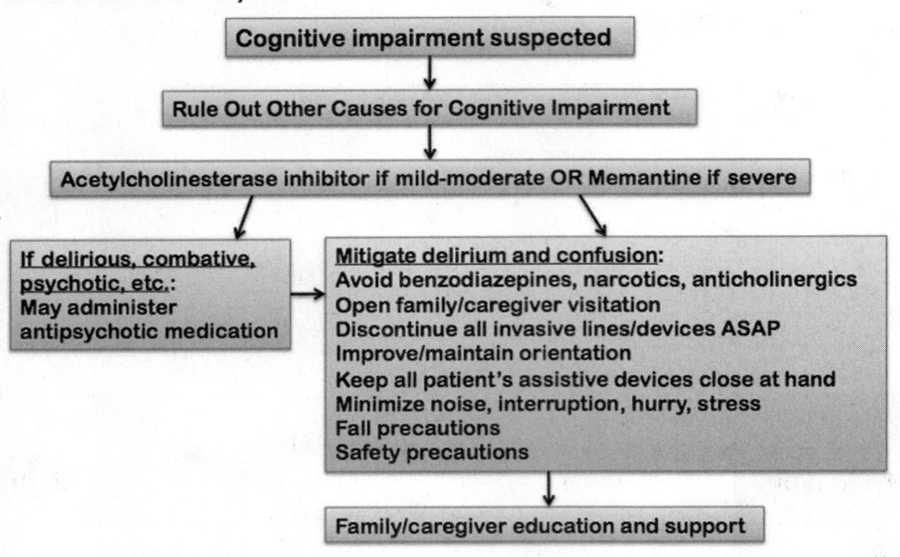

Summary of Interventions: Dementia

Dementias are a diverse group of conditions that cause progressive decline in cognitive functioning.

- Rule out other potentially reversible causes of cognitive impairment using diagnostic testing and history.
- Key interventions include the following:
  - o Some pharmacologic therapies exist that may help symptoms of the disease; however, there is no curative therapy.
  - o Preventing confusion and delirium in the hospital is a key intervention.
  - o Family and/or caregiver education and support is important.
  - o Driving is an issue that must be addressed when safety is compromised. It is very difficult for seniors to lose their independence.

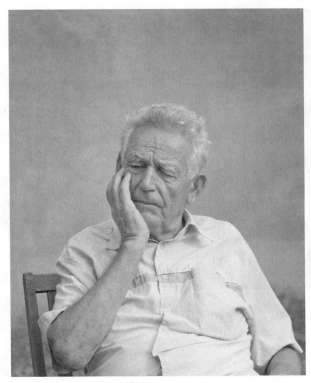

When seniors with dementia reach a state of significant confusion and memory loss, safety, particularly driving, can become a serious concern. Clinicians must confront the issue. Commonly, family consults the clinician with concerns first.
Source: Budimir Jevtic/Fotolia

LO4:

Evaluation of Desired Collaborative Care Outcomes: Dementia

Evaluation and reassessment should reveal attainment of previously established patient outcomes. In summary:

- Patient remains oriented to person, place, and time as long as possible given progressive nature of illness.
- Patient recognizes surroundings and situations as long as possible given progressive nature of illness.
- Family demonstrates findings associated with adequate coping within expected range.
- Patient retains the ability to help with self-feeding, dressing, hygiene, and social interaction for as long as possible given the progressive nature of the illness.
- Caregiver and family retain ability to provide care for patient while also caring for self.

LO1:

What Is Delirium?

- Delirium is an acute state of confusion that typically follows a fluctuating (agitated/combative versus somnolent/hypoactive) course.
- It is a clinical syndrome characterized by a change in cognitive functioning often with disorganized behavior and deficits in attention (inability to concentrate). It may involve visual and/or auditory hallucinations.
- Delirium is frightening and very upsetting for patients, particularly those who have hallucinations. Videos of patients sharing their experiences can be found on the Internet.

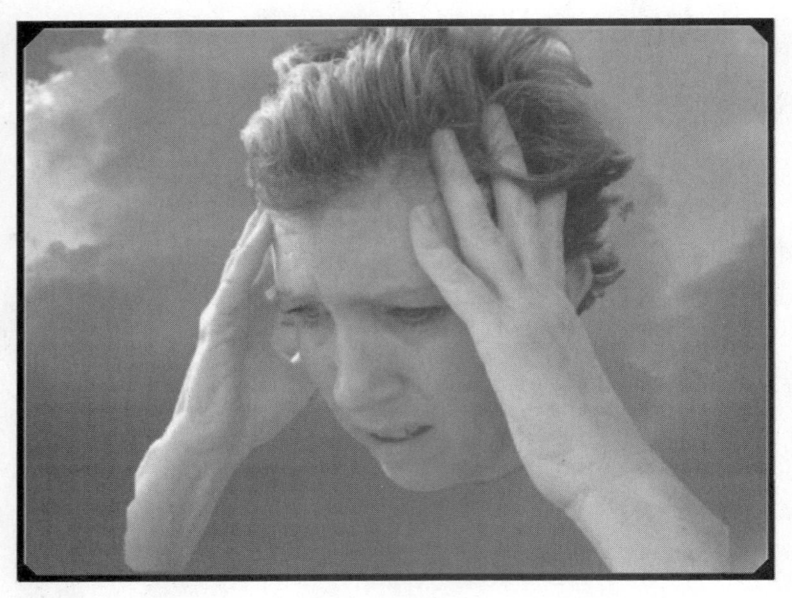

Onset of delirium can manifest as confusion and distress.
Source: Courtesy of K. Kyriakidis

LO1:

Clinical Relevance: Delirium

- Delirium is a common syndrome in hospitalized patients.
- As many as 30% of older adult patients in hospitals may experience delirium.
- More than 50% of ICU patients experience delirium.
- Delirium is associated with multiple complications, including suffering by patients, falls, prolonged hospitalization, and increased length of hospital stay.
- Prompt recognition and treatment can reduce patient suffering, complications, and reduce costs. Further, many patients continue to be frightened long after the experience.

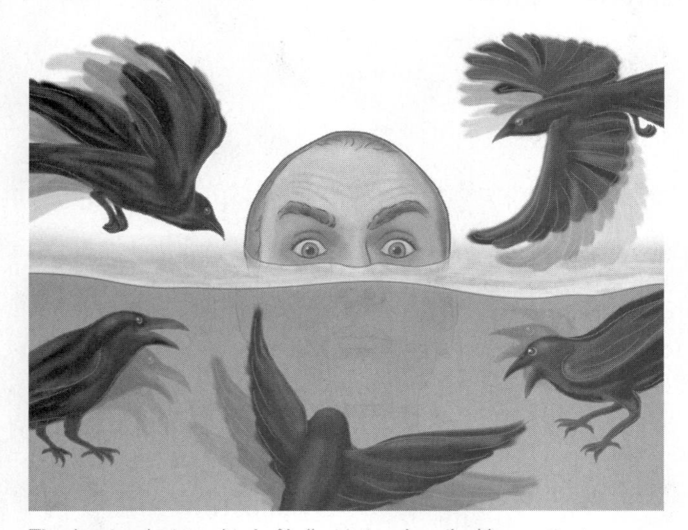

The drawing depicts a kind of hallucination described by a patient. Although older adults are at higher risk, anyone can develop delirium. Delirium may complicate the patient's condition and require more fiscal resources. Experts suggest that minor treatment changes in the patient's care may prevent delirium, reduce suffering, and limit costs in approximately 40% of affected patients.

LO2:

Pathophysiology: Delirium

- The pathophysiology of delirium is complex and poorly understood.
- A prominent theory is that neurotransmitters become imbalanced leading to a cognitive dysfunction.
- Another theory postulates that inflammatory mediators (cytokines) can disrupt neuronal function.

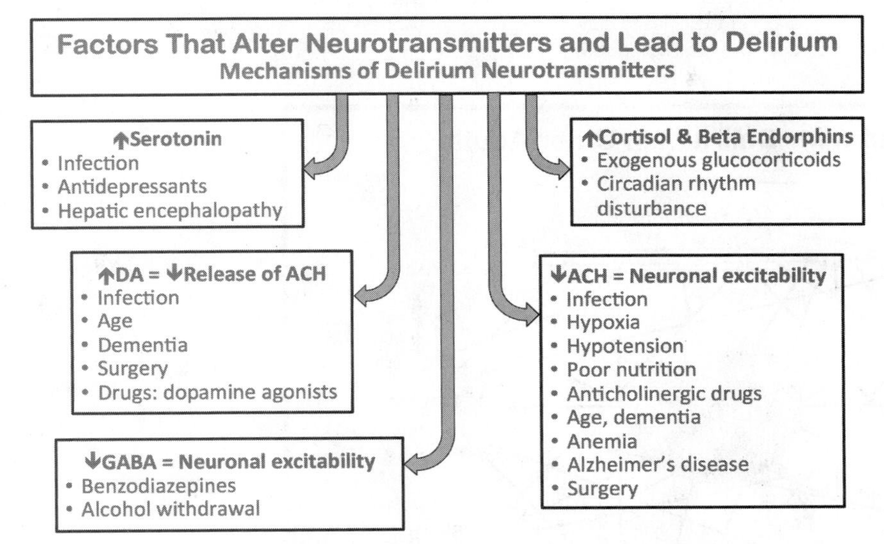

Factors That Alter Neurotransmitters and Lead to Delirium
Mechanisms of Delirium Neurotransmitters
↑Serotonin
• Infection
• Antidepressants
• Hepatic encephalopathy
↑Cortisol & Beta Endorphins
• Exogenous glucocorticoids
• Circadian rhythm disturbance
↑DA = ↓Release of ACH
• Infection
• Age
• Dementia
• Surgery
• Drugs: dopamine agonists
↓ACH = Neuronal excitability
• Infection
• Hypoxia
• Hypotension
• Poor nutrition
• Anticholinergic drugs
• Age, dementia
• Anemia
• Alzheimer's disease
• Surgery
↓GABA = Neuronal excitability
• Benzodiazepines
• Alcohol withdrawal

ACH=acetylcholine; DA=dopamine; GABA=gamma-aminobutyric acid

Source: Copyright © 2014, NovEx Novice to Expert Learning, LLC

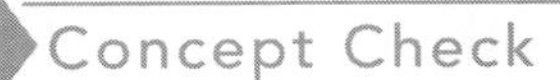

5. Which theory is postulated regarding the development of delirium?
   - A. Patients who experience delirium will likely go on to develop dementia later in life.
   - B. Delirium is caused by lack of attention to reorientation by busy medical staff.
   - C. Delirium results when insufficient cytokines are produced.
   - D. The cause of delirium may be an imbalance in neurotransmitters.

Answer question

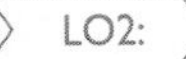

Risk Factors: Delirium

- Dementia
- Parkinson's
- Prior stroke
- Age older than 70
- Prior history of delirium

In older adults, delirium is one of five interrelated syndromes (see diagram for relationships). The other four are:

- Pressure ulcers
- Incontinence
- Falls
- Functional decline

These five interrelated syndromes share four risk factors:

- Older age
- Baseline cognitive deficiency
- Baseline functional impairment
- Compromised mobility

In older adults, even if one of the five syndromes is left unattended to and declines, the others inevitably follow. Notice that delirium is at the center, indicating that the older adult is at high risk of delirium if there is significant deterioration in their health status. Similarly, attentiveness and prevention of one of the conditions can decrease the likelihood of the others.

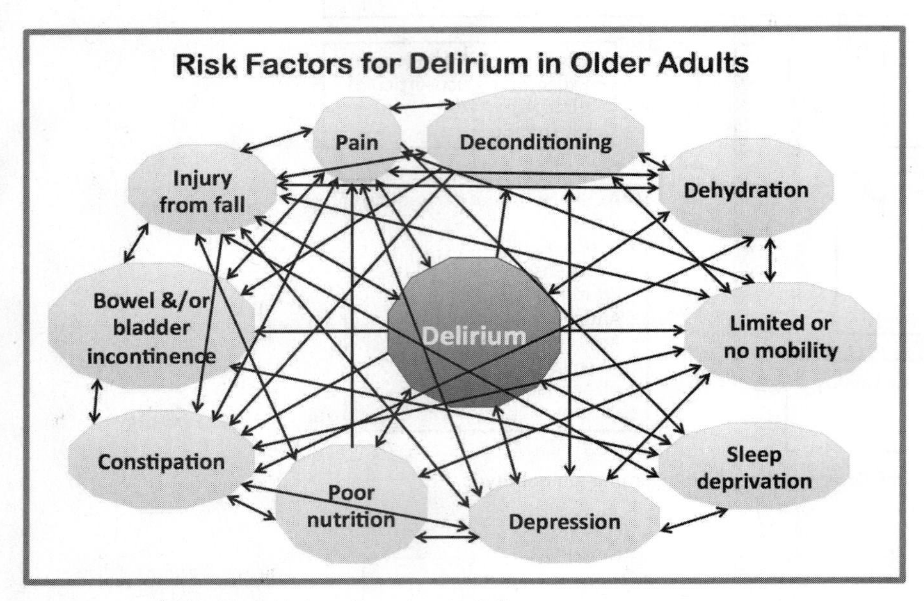

Source: Copyright © 2014, NovEx Novice to Expert Learning, LLC

LO2:

Causes: Delirium

- Recreational drugs and drug withdrawal (e.g., alcohol, narcotics, antihistamines) are a growing cause of "excited delirium," which is a more violent and extreme form of delirium.

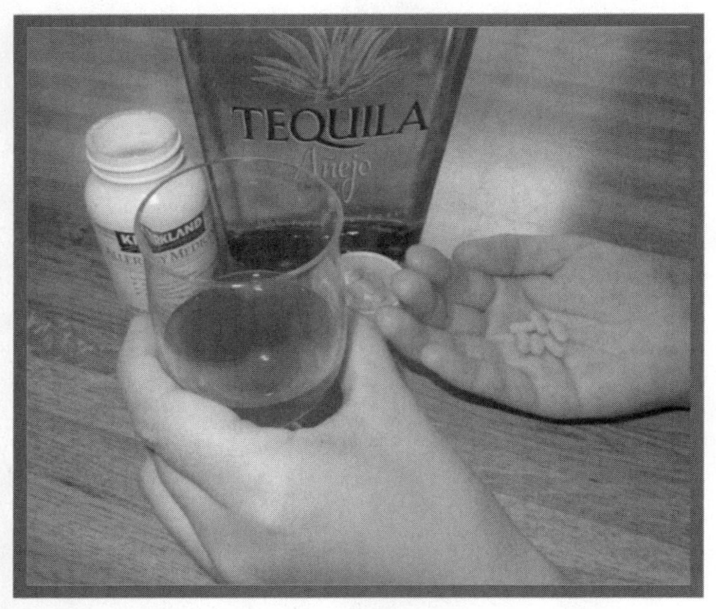

Violent delirium is an increasingly common emergency seen in young adults from mixing antihistamines and alcohol.
Source: Copyright © 2014, NovEx Novice to Expert Learning, LLC

- Critical illness, including sepsis
- Medications such as psychotropics, antihistamines, and muscle relaxers
- Hypoxemia, hypercapnia
- Electrolyte disorder (e.g., hyponatremia, hypercalcemia)
- Infections (febrile delirium)
- Liver failure
- Renal failure

Concept Check

6. **Which common, over-the-counter medication class may increase risk for the development of delirium?**
   A. Antihistamines
   B. Vitamin supplements
   C. Aspirin
   D. Mineral supplements

Answer question

LO2:

Assessment Findings: Delirium

- Delirium is a clinical diagnosis, based on assessment:
  - o There is sudden onset, developing over hours with a fluctuating course.
  - o There is a trigger (e.g., sepsis) (see Causes section).
  - o There is a disturbance in consciousness resulting in inattentiveness.
  - o Patient may be either hypoactive (e.g., somnolent, withdrawn) or hyperactive (e.g., agitated, restless). See diagram.
  - o Cognitive ability is decreased (confusion).

Assessing Consciousness: Linking Sedation and Delirium Monitoring

Step 1 Level of Consciousness: RASS

Scale	Label	Description
+4	COMBATIVE	Combative, violent, immediate danger to staff
+3	VERY AGITATED	Pulls to remove tubes or catheters; aggressive
+2	AGITATED	Frequent non-purposeful movement, fights ventilator
+1	RESTLESS	Anxious, apprehensive, movements not aggressive
0	ALERT & CALM	Spontaneously pays attention to caregiver
−1	DROWSY	Not fully alert, but has sustained awakening to voice (eye opening & contact >10 sec)
−2	LIGHT SEDATION	Briefly awakens to voice (eyes open & contact <10 sec)
−3	MODERATE SEDATION	Movement or eye opening to voice (no eye contact)

→ If RASS is ≥ −3 proceed to CAM-ICU (Is patient CAM-ICU positive or negative?)

Scale	Label	Description
−4	DEEP SEDATION	No response to voice, but movement or eye opening to physical stimulation
−5	UNAROUSEABLE	No response to voice or physical stimulation

→ If RASS is −4 or −5 → STOP (patient unconscious), RECHECK later

- There are multiple bedside evaluation tools to assist in diagnosis (Confusion Assessment Method for the ICU [CAM-ICU] scale).

Confusion Assessment Method for the ICU (CAM-ICU) Flowsheet

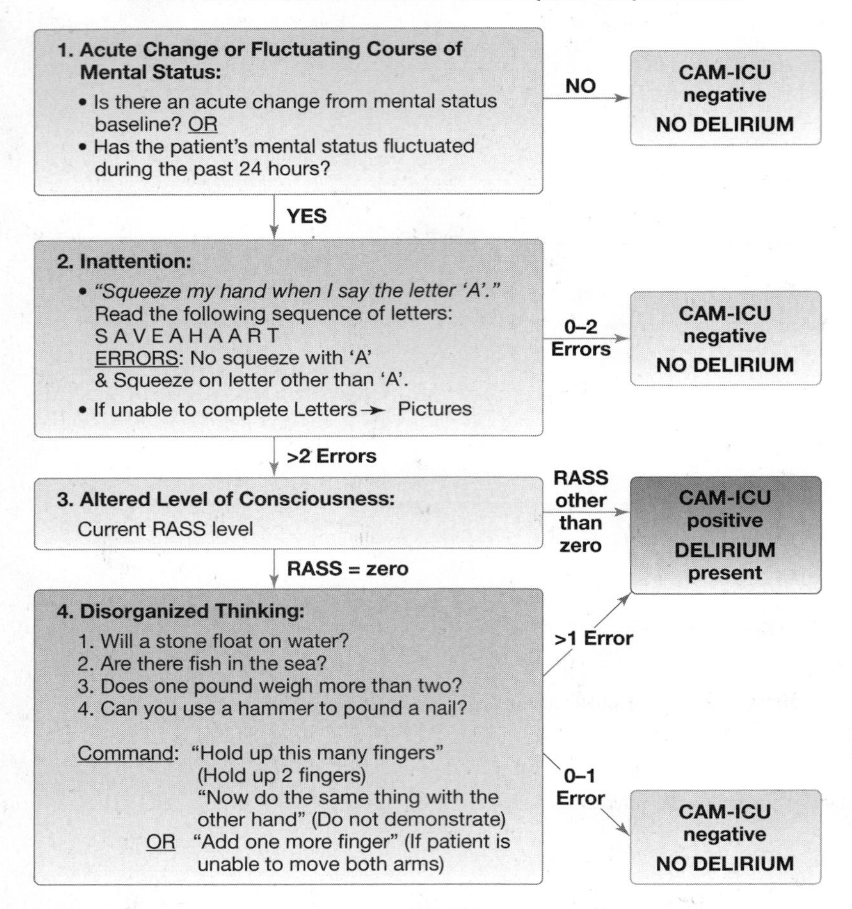

1. Acute Change or Fluctuating Course of Mental Status:
• Is there an acute change from mental status baseline? OR
• Has the patient's mental status fluctuated during the past 24 hours?
NO
CAM-ICU negative
NO DELIRIUM
YES
2. Inattention:
• "Squeeze my hand when I say the letter 'A'."
Read the following sequence of letters:
S A V E A H A A R T
ERRORS: No squeeze with 'A'
& Squeeze on letter other than 'A'.
• If unable to complete Letters → Pictures
0–2 Errors
CAM-ICU negative
NO DELIRIUM
>2 Errors
3. Altered Level of Consciousness:
Current RASS level
RASS other than zero
CAM-ICU positive
DELIRIUM present
RASS = zero
4. Disorganized Thinking:
1. Will a stone float on water?
2. Are there fish in the sea?
3. Does one pound weigh more than two?
4. Can you use a hammer to pound a nail?
Command: "Hold up this many fingers" (Hold up 2 fingers)
"Now do the same thing with the other hand" (Do not demonstrate)
OR "Add one more finger" (If patient is unable to move both arms)
>1 Error
0–1 Error
CAM-ICU negative
NO DELIRIUM

Differentiating Dementia, Delirium, and Depression

Dementia, delirium, and depression can occur simultaneously and confound the patient's care. It is important to differentiate which condition or conditions the patient is experiencing and manage them as well as possible to improve the patient's mental health.

	Dementia	Delirium	Depression
Onset	Usually slow, and insidious. Develops over years.	Acutely develops	Develops over months to years..
Progressive	Yes. Progressive over years.	Confusion fluctuates throughout the day	No
Mood	Normal	Normal	Depressed
Precipitating Cause	No. However, patients may suddenly get worse when there is a change in environment such as a move.	New medication, recreational drugs, alcohol, acute medical condition.	Social stressors such as loss of a spouse.

Priority Patient Concerns and Desired Collaborative Care Outcomes: Delirium

Prior to caring for patients with delirium, it is important to prioritize the patient's concerns that must guide the nursing care plan and interventions. Care for the patient is ordered and organized in accordance with the patient's priority and urgent needs. Desired collaborative care outcomes in patients with delirium typically include:

1. Patient will become reoriented to person, place, and time or will return to pre-delirium mental state.
2. Patient's memory will be restored, maintained, or improved compared to pre-delirium status.
3. Patient will experience prolonged periods of uninterrupted rest.
4. Patient will avoid injury.

Considering these important care outcomes, prepare a list of the major 3–6 priority patient concerns or nursing diagnoses for patients with delirium. Be prepared to participate in a discussion of this list and/or to submit them as an assignment, as determined by your faculty. Resources you may find helpful in this assignment can include this lesson, the references, resources on nursing care plans, and standard nursing diagnoses manuals.

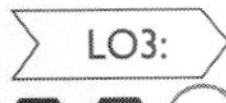

Collaborative Interventions: Delirium

M N EBP
- The primary focus is on treating underlying cause (e.g., medication adverse reaction, infection, sepsis, electrolyte imbalance) (Fletcher, et al., 2012; National Collaborating Centre for Acute and Chronic Conditions [NCCACC], 2010).

M N EBP
- Implement nonpharmacologic treatments as first-line therapies. Collaborate with team to (Fletcher, et al., 2012):
  - o Restore hydration.
  - o Alleviate pain.
  - o Encourage reassuring and trusted family members at bedside.
  - o Restore sleep and wake cycle.
  - o Remove unnecessary interventions (e.g., IVs, cardiac monitors) that can create disorientation.
  - o Provide reassurance, use calming techniques, and provide as tranquil an environment as possible.

N EBP
- Ensure safety and implement fall precautions (Fletcher, et al., 2012).

M N EBP
- Do not use physical restraints unless absolutely necessary as restraints can worsen the delirium (Fletcher, et al., 2012).

M N EBP
- Pharmacologic therapies such as low dose antipsychotics may be used if necessary. Avoid antipsychotic medications in patients with Lewy body-related dementia and Parkinson's disease (Fletcher, et al., 2012; NCCACC, 2010).

M N EBP
- Avoid drugs that may increase symptoms (e.g., narcotics, benzodiazepines, and sedatives) (Fletcher, et al., 2012; RNAO, 2010).

N EBP
- Collaborate with team to provide a therapeutic environment (RNAO, 2010; Tullman, et al., 2008):
  - o Encourage orientation and frequently reassure the patient (e.g., calendars, photos).
  - o Provide plenty of sleep and night time calming rituals.
  - o Reduce unnecessary sensory stimulation (e.g., lights, noise).
  - o Mobilize and exercise frequently.
  - o Communicate with simple, clear instructions.
  - o Minimize or remove as soon as feasible all invasive devices.
  - o Encourage familiar faces or loved ones to be at the bedside.
  - o Avoid psychotropic drugs until necessary.

N EBP
- Provide emotional, social, and psychological support to the patient and family (RNAO, 2010)

Prevention

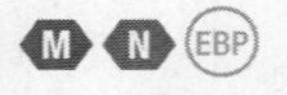

Early recognition of patients at high risk for delirium and prevention are key interventions (RNAO, 2010):

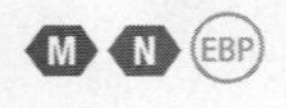

- Maintain a high level of suspicion and be alert at the time of admission to a hospital or long-term care facility of those at risk for delirium (e.g., over age 65, severely ill, cognitive impairment) (NCCACC, 2010).

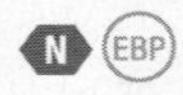

- Assess and monitor the following within hours of admission and then daily, if not more often when at high risk (NCCACC, 2010; RNAO, 2010; Tullmann, et al., 2008):
  - o Attention or how distractable
  - o Alertness
  - o Orientation
  - o Memory: may not remember current events or follow instructions
  - o Perceptual disturbances: may have illusions, auditory or visual hallucinations
  - o Thinking: difficulty organizing, slow responses, incoherent, illogical, rambling, topic hopping, garbled speech
  - o Physical function: agitation, level of mobility, appetite, sleep
  - o Social behavior: cooperative, withdrawn, moodiness, changes in communication

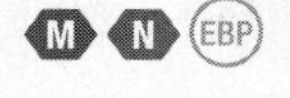

- Consult experienced professional in delirium (e.g., psych nurse specialist) to diagnose and manage the patient if delirium is present (NCCACC, 2010; RNAO, 2010).

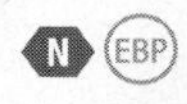

- Reduce or eliminate risk factors (e.g., medications causing adverse effects, infection, dehydration, pain, hypoxia) for delirium (Tullmann, et al., 2008).

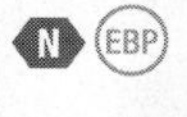

- Provide a therapeutic environment, which includes the interventions detailed previously (NCCACC, 2010; Tullmann, et al., 2008).

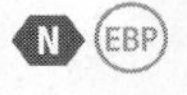

- Preserve what is familiar to the patient as much as possible, such as continuity of care provided by familiar team members, avoid transferring the patient between rooms or units (NCCACC, 2010).

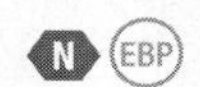

- Collaborate with the health care provider to correct or intervene in situations that can deteriorate and result in delirium (NCCACC, 2010):
  - o Correct dehydration.
  - o Prevent hypoxia.
  - o Provide good pain management.
  - o Recognize and treat infection. Avoid unnecessary invasive procedures or device use (e.g., indwelling urinary catheter, central line catheter).
  - o Manage constipation.
  - o Provide interventions to reduce further deterioration in mental status in patients who are cognitively impaired (e.g., lighting, clock, orient the patient, familiar persons).
  - o Mobilize the patient as much as possible and to the extent that the patient is capable.
  - o Encourage good nutritional intake. Collaborate with team if oral intake is inadequate.
  - o Attend to visual and auditory sensory deficits to ensure good communication and to meet patient needs.
  - o Provide needed rest and uninterrupted sleep whenever possible.

Summary of Interventions: Delirium

- Treat the underlying cause (e.g., discontinue any medications that may be causing or contributing to the delirium) as much as possible.
- Nonpharmacologic interventions are the first-line measures in management.
- When pharmacologic measures are needed, low dose antipsychotics (haloperidol) are preferred.

Concept Check

7. Which intervention is helpful in the treatment of delirium?

A. Use of restraints

B. Sedation with a benzodiazepine

C. Relaxing visiting hours

D. Enforcing complete bed rest

Answer question

LO4: Evaluation of Desired Collaborative Care Outcomes: Delirium

Evaluation and reassessment should reveal attainment of previously established patient outcomes. In summary:

- Patient is oriented to person, place, and time or is at pre-delirium mental state.
- Patient demonstrates memory at same level as pre-illness.
- Patient has prolonged periods of uninterrupted rest.
- Patient has no injuries.

References

Dementia

Andrews, J. (2013). Maintaining continence in people with dementia. *Nursing Times, 109*(27), 20–21. **www.nursingtimes.net/Journals/2013/07/05/o/e/m/100713-Maintaining-continence-in-people-with-dementia.pdf**

Bonner, A. (2014). When nurses lead. *J Gerontol Nurs, 2,* 1–5. doi: 10.3928/00989134-20140425-01

Davies, N., Maio, L., Rait, G., & Iliffe, S. (2014). Quality end-of-life care for dementia: What have family carers told us so far? A narrative synthesis. *Palliat Med.* **pmj.sagepub.com/content/early/2014/03/18/0269216314526766.full.pdf+html**

Konno, R., Kang, S., & Makimoto, K. (2014). A best-evidence review of intervention studies for minimizing resistance-to-care behaviours for older adults with dementia in nursing homes. *J Advanced Nurs.* doi: 10.1111/jan.12432

Mata, A. M. (2014). Breaking through the culture of fear in dementia care. *Brit J Nurs, 23*(7), 351.

Murray, A. (2014). The effect of dementia on patients, informal carers and nurses. *Nurs Older People, 26*(5), 27–31.

Clinical Practice Guidelines

Fletcher, K. (2012). Recognition and management of dementia. In: M. Boltz, E. Capezuti, T. Fulmer, & D. Zwicker (Eds.), *Evidence-based geriatric nursing protocols for best practice* (4th edition) (pp. 163–185). New York, NY: Springer Publishing Company. **www.guideline.gov/content.aspx?id=43921**

Hall, G. R., Gallagher, M., & Hoffmann-Snyder, C. (2013). *Bathing persons with dementia.* Iowa City, IA: University of Iowa College of Nursing, John A. Hartford Foundation Center of Geriatric Nursing Excellence.

Parminder, R., Pasqualina, S., Afisi, I., et al. (2008). Effectiveness of cholinesterase inhibitors and memantine for treating dementia: Evidence review for a clinical practice guideline. *Ann Intern Med, 148*(5), 379–397. **annals.org/article.aspx?articleid=739930**

Registered Nurses' Association of Ontario. (2012). *Best practice guidelines: Screening for delirium, dementia, and depression in the older adult.* **rnao.ca/sites/rnao-ca/files/storage/related/646_BPG_DDD_summary.pdf**

Registered Nurses' Association of Ontario. (2013). *Best practice guidelines: Caregiving strategies for older adults with delirium, dementia, and depression.* **rnao.ca/sites/rnao-ca/files/Caregiving_Strategies_for_Older_Adults_with_Delirium_Dementia_and_Depression.pdf**

Scottish Intercollegiate Guidelines Network (SIGN). (2006). *Management of patients with dementia. A national clinical guideline.* Edinburgh, Scotland: Scottish Intercollegiate Guidelines Network. **www.sign.ac.uk/pdf/sign86.pdf**

Sorbi, S., Hort, J., Erkinjuntti, T., et al., & European Federation of Neurological Societies (EFNS) Scientist Panel on Dementia and Cognitive Neurology. (2012). EFNS-ENS guidelines on the diagnosis and management of disorders associated with dementia. *Eur J Neurol, 19*(9), 1159–1179. **www.guideline.gov/content.aspx?id=38470&search=dementia**

Patient Education

Alzheimer's Association Alzheimer's and Dementia Caregiver Center. (2014). *Caregivers for Alzheimer's and dementia face special challenges.* **www.alz.org/care/**

Centers for Disease Control and Prevention. (2013). *Mental health: Dementia/Alzheimer's disease.* **www.cdc.gov/mentalhealth/basics/mental-illness/dementia.htm**

Family Caregiver Alliance National Center on Caregiving. (2004). *Caregiver's guide to understanding dementia behaviors.* **caregiver.org/caregivers-guide-understanding-dementia-behaviors**

Delirium

Carbone, M. K., & Gugliucci, M. R. (2014). Delirium and the family caregiver: The need for evidence-based education interventions. *Gerontologist.* doi: 10.1093/geron/gnu035

Chong, M. S., Chan, M., Tay, L., & Ding, Y.Y. (2014). Outcomes of an innovative model of acute delirium care: The geriatric monitoring unit (GMU). *Clin Interv Aging, 9,* 603–612. **www.ncbi.nlm.nih.gov/pmc/articles/PMC3986297/**

Inouye, S. K., Bogardus, S.T., Charpentier, P. A., et al. (1999). A Multicomponent Intervention to Prevent Delirium in Hospitalized Older Patients. *N Engl J Med, 340,* 669–676. doi: 10.1056/NEJM199903043400901

Morandi, A., Davis, D., Fick, D. M., et al. (2014). Delirium superimposed on dementia strongly predicts worse outcomes in older rehabilitation inpatients. *J Am Med Dir Assoc, 15*(5), 349–354. **www.ncbi.nlm.nih.gov/pmc/articles/PMC4004584/**

Patel, J., Baldwin, J., Bunting, P., & Laha, S. (2014). The effect of a multicomponent multidisciplinary bundle of interventions on sleep and delirium in medical and surgical intensive care patients. *Anaesthesia, 69*(6), 540–549. doi: 10.1111/anae.12638

Rompaey, V., Schuurmans, M. J., Shrotridge-Gaggett, L. M., et al. (2008). A comparison of the CAM-ICU and the NEECHAM Confusion Scale in intensive care delirium assessment: An observational study in non-intubated patients. *Crit Care, 12*(1): R16. **www.ncbi.nlm.nih.gov/pubmed/18282269**

Clinical Practice Guidelines

Fletcher, K. (2012). Recognition and management of dementia. In: M. Boltz, E. Capezuti, T. Fulmer, & D. Zwicker (Eds.), *Evidence-based geriatric nursing protocols for best practice* (4th edition) (pp. 163–185). New York, NY: Springer Publishing Company. **www.guideline.gov/content.aspx?id=43921**

National Collaborating Centre for Acute and Chronic Conditions. (2010). *Delirium: diagnosis, prevention and management. Clinical Guideline 103.* London, UK: National Institute for Health and Clinical Excellence (NICE).

Registered Nurses' Association of Ontario. (2010). *Best practice guidelines: Caregiving strategies for older adults with delirium, dementia, and depression 2010 supplement.* Toronto, Ontario: Registered Nurses' Association of Ontario. **rnao.ca/sites/rnao-ca/files/Caregiving_Strategies_for_Older_Adults_with_Delirium_Dementia_and_Depression.pdf**

Tullmann, D. F., Mion, L. C., Fletcher, K., et al. (2008). Delirium: Prevention, early recognition, and treatment. In: E. Capezuti, D. Zwicker, M. Mezey, T. Fulmer (Eds.), *Evidence-based geriatric nursing protocols for best practice* (3rd edition). New York, NY: Springer Publishing Company. **www.guideline.gov/content.aspx?id=43920**

Patient Education

Alagiakrishnan, K. (2014). *Delirium follow-up.* **Emedicine.medscape.com/article/288890-followup**

Francis, J., & Young, G. B. (2014). *Patient information: Delirium (beyond the basics).* **www.uptodate.com/contents/delirium-beyond-the-basics**

Mayo Clinic Staff. (2012). *Diseases and conditions: delirium.* **www.mayoclinic.org/diseases-conditions/delirium/basics/definition/con-20033982**

Learning Outcomes for Seizures

When you complete this lesson, you will be able to:

1. Recognize the clinical relevance of seizures.
2. Consider the pathophysiology, etiology, risk factors, and clinical presentation of seizures that determine the priority patient concerns.
3. Determine the most urgent and important nursing interventions and patient education required in caring for a patient with seizures.
4. Evaluate attainment of desired collaborative care outcomes for a patient with seizures.

LO1:

What Is a Seizure?

- A seizure (or convulsion) is an abnormal, synchronous firing of neurons in the brain.
- Seizures are classified as partial or generalized, depending upon the extent of the unregulated firing of neurons.
- Patients with recurrent or repeated seizures are diagnosed with epilepsy.

LO1:

Clinical Relevance

- Epilepsy and seizures affect nearly 3 million Americans of all ages with as much as 10% of the U.S. population suffering a seizure at some point in their life.
- The annual cost of seizures is approximately $17.6 billion in the United States in direct and indirect costs.
- Seizures are frightening for the patient and their families.
- Patients with seizures need first aid education for both themselves and their families and friends in order to protect the patient in the event of a seizure (see photo).
- Immediate response to seizures is often clouded by misdiagnosis. Seizures are sometimes mistaken for a cardiac arrest.
- Status epilepticus is a persistent seizure that can produce brain injury or death. Rapid and effective treatment is essential.

First Aid for Seizures

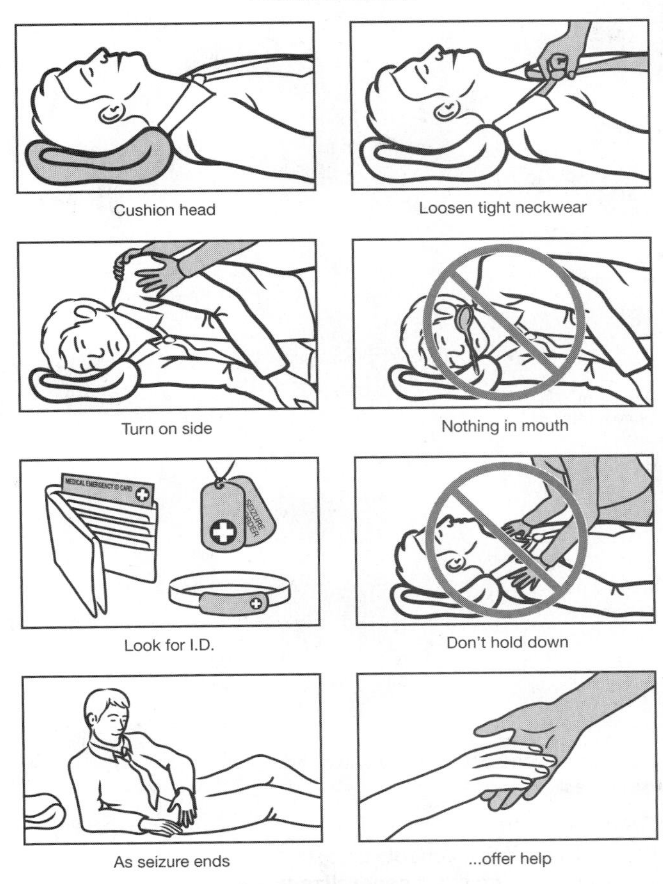
Cushion head
Loosen tight neckwear
Turn on side
Nothing in mouth
Look for I.D.
Don't hold down
As seizure ends
...offer help
If seizures are prolonged, call for help.

First aid involves a few simple steps that can help protect someone who is having a seizure. More detailed information is available through the Epilepsy Foundation.

LO2:

Pathophysiology

- The brain has 100 billion neurons with each neuron synapsing on average with 7,000 other neurons. Communication between neurons occurs through electrical impulses that propagate through the axons of a neuron.
- Neurotransmitter substances, released in the synapses, attach to receptors that can either activate or inhibit other neurons from firing. Some neurotransmitters are excitatory and others are inhibitory. This balance promotes orderly communication between neurons.
- An imbalance of these neurotransmitters can result in uninhibited firing of neurons that can spread to other parts of the brain.
- The balance among these neurotransmitters can be affected by numerous things, such as injury to brain tissue, electrolyte abnormalities, and drugs.

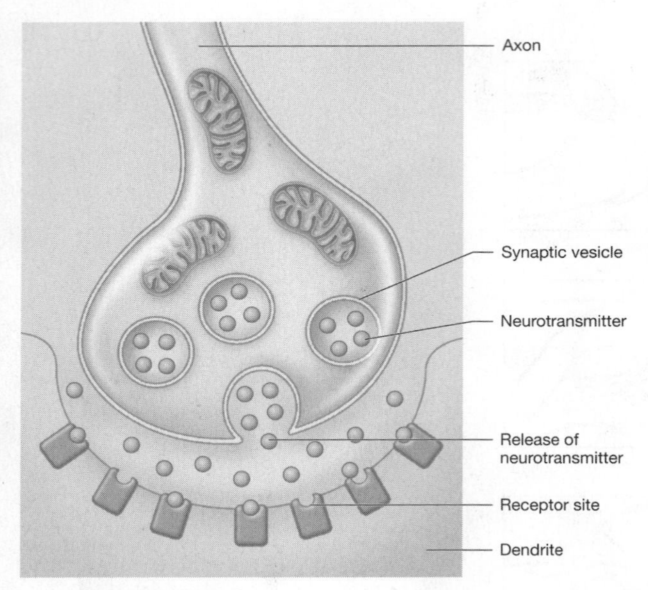

Our bodies synthesize (make) neurotransmitters. Some of the chemical building blocks for neurotransmitters, such as amino acids, come from the foods we eat. Neurons include places to store neurotransmitters. These storage areas, called vesicles, are located close to the ending of each axon. Neurons synthesize some neurotransmitters within the vesicle. Others neurotransmitters are synthesized in the body of the cell and shipped down to the vesicle.

- When only a part or one side of the brain is affected, uninhibited neuronal firing and the involuntary activity that ensues are called **partial seizures**.
- Symptoms that are manifested depend on the part of the brain involved.
- If the uninhibited firing spreads to involve the whole brain, areas that control consciousness are affected, and loss of consciousness usually occurs. These are called **generalized seizures**. There is also total loss of control over body movements.
- Seizures usually resolve after a few minutes. Persistent, uninhibited firing activity results in a prolonged seizure, called **status epilepticus**.

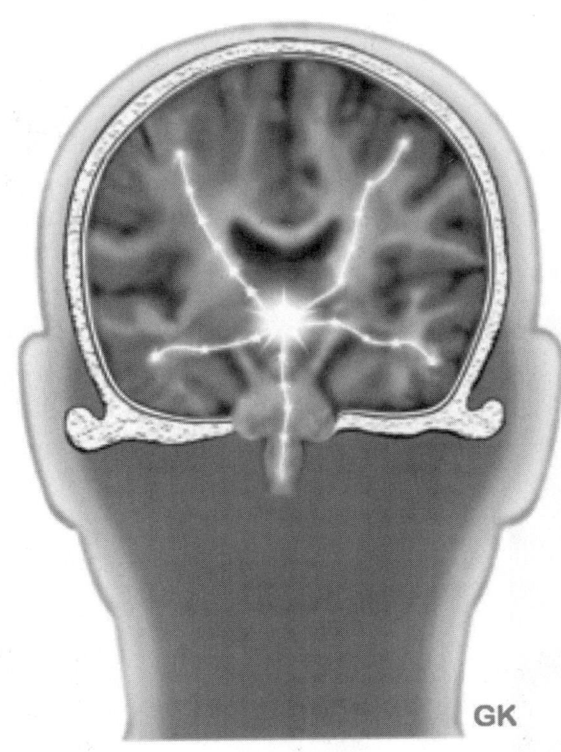

This image depicts the site of the seizure's origin. Note that in a generalized seizure, the abnormal electrical impulses are transmitted throughout the brain and, consequently, affect the whole body. If status epilepticus develops, it can be damaging and life threatening. Seizure activity that continues longer than 5 minutes can begin to damage neurons.

Source: Courtesy of George Kyriakidis/Santa Ana, CA

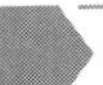

LO2:

Risk Factors and Causes

Causes and risk factors include:

- Electrolyte abnormalities (e.g., hyponatremia)
- Structural lesions of the brain (e.g., brain tumors)
- Central nervous system infections (e.g., meningitis, encephalitis)
- Stroke (e.g., hemorrhagic or ischemic)
- Intoxication or overdose of drugs (e.g., theophylline, tricyclic antidepressants)
- Withdrawal from drugs (e.g., alcohol, benzodiazepines)
- Idiopathic (e.g., epilepsy)
- Metabolic abnormities (e.g., hypoglycemia, hypoxia)

Concept Check

1. **Which type of seizure may be fatal?**
   A. General seizure
   B. Partial seizure
   C. Status epilepticus
   D. Convulsion

Answer question

LO2:

Assessment Findings

Early Warning of Impending Seizures

Some people who experience seizures experience a forewarning that they come to recognize:

- An **aura** is a sensation experienced before the onset of a seizure. This perception can be a smell, sound, or lights. The aura occurs while the patient is conscious. For many patients, an aura foretells of an imminent seizure.
- An aura may present as distorted sound or vision.
- The patient may experience the aura and/or seizure as very frightening.

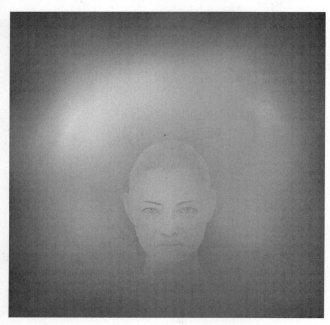

An artist captures what a patient describes as the aura she experiences. This is only one example.

Partial Seizures

Partial seizures occur in one specific region of the brain and may therefore present in various ways:

- Auras may be experienced.
- Motor signs such as eye or face twitching and hand jerking can occur. Sometimes individuals complain of an unusual taste in their mouth, hallucinate, or have a déjà vu experience.
- When partial seizures progress to involve consciousness, they are called **complex partial seizures**. These individuals demonstrate lip smacking, blinking, picking at clothes, and can also show bizarre behaviors such as wandering, running, or arm jerking. Patients with partial complex seizures usually do not remember the incident.
- Partial seizures can develop into generalized seizures that affect the entire brain.

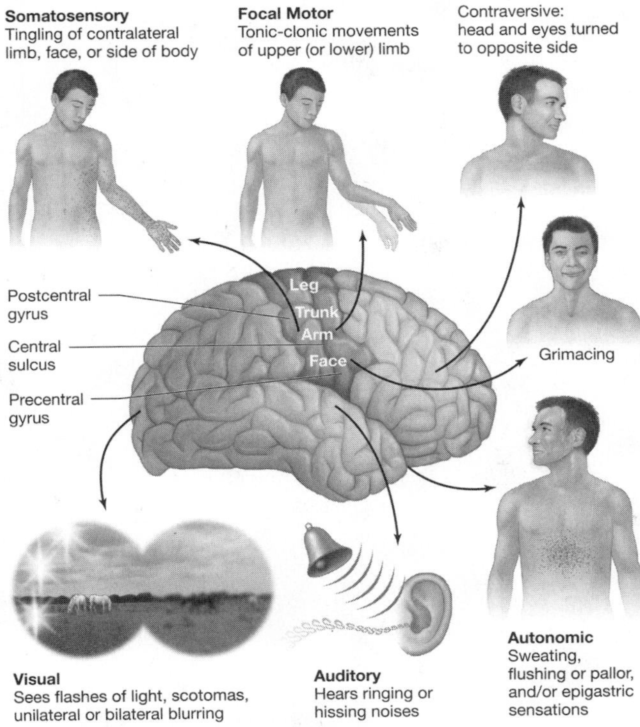

Partial seizures are the result of an abnormal paroxysmal discharge of cerebral neurons within a particular brain region, and they manifest focal symptoms and may progress to generalized seizures. Partial seizures are subdivided into simple partial seizures, in which there is no loss of consciousness, and complex partial seizures, which are always associated with loss of consciousness.

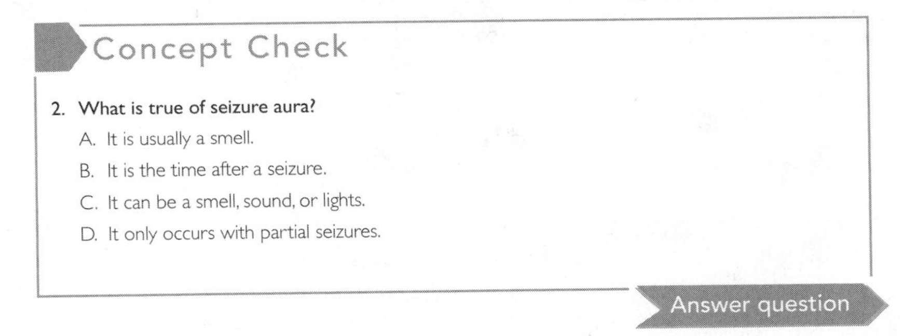

Concept Check

2. What is true of seizure aura?
   - A. It is usually a smell.
   - B. It is the time after a seizure.
   - C. It can be a smell, sound, or lights.
   - D. It only occurs with partial seizures.

Answer question

Assessment Findings (continued)

Generalized Seizures

- Generalized seizures affect both hemispheres of the brain. There are many different types of generalized seizures. Except for myoclonic seizures, there is a loss of consciousness.

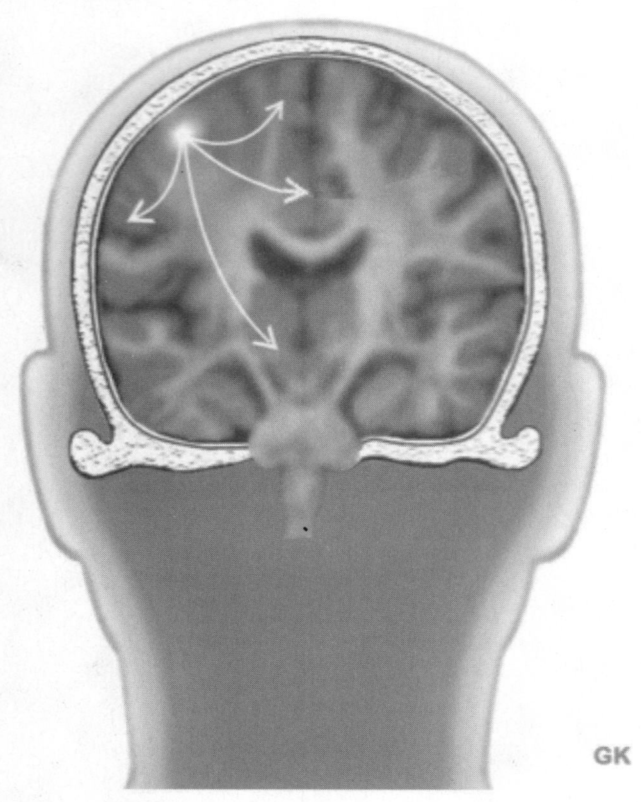

This image shows neuro stimulation from a partial seizure in which symptoms may manifest in part of the body. Partial seizures can become generalized to affect the additional areas of the brain.
Source: Courtesy of George Kyriakidis/Santa Ana, CA

Normal EEG | **Abnormal Epileptiform Interictals EEG**

Left: A normal EEG is shown above with the expected rhythmic activity. This should provide a general idea about how a normal EEG appears. ***Right***: This EEG reveals an abnormal epileptiform interictal pattern (circled in red) that can be seen between or after seizures. The ability to obtain an EEG during a seizure is difficult. However, detection of interictal epileptiform discharges is very informative about seizures.

Source: Courtesy of K. Kyriakidis

- **Absence seizures** are generalized seizures in which the individual has an impairment in responsiveness with little to no motor involvement and lasts <30 seconds.
- **Myoclonic generalized seizures** are sudden shock-like muscle contractions without impairment of consciousness.
- **Atonic generalized seizures** are drop attacks.The person simply drops to the ground with a loss of consciousness.
- **Tonic generalized seizures** are manifested by stiffening of the extensor muscles.
- **Clonic generalized seizures** are a sudden hypotonic episode followed by limb jerking.

- **Tonic–clonic seizures** (formally called **grand mal** and also known as **convulsions**) exhibit increased tone followed by rhythmic jerking of the body.

Tonic-Clonic or Grand Mal Seizure

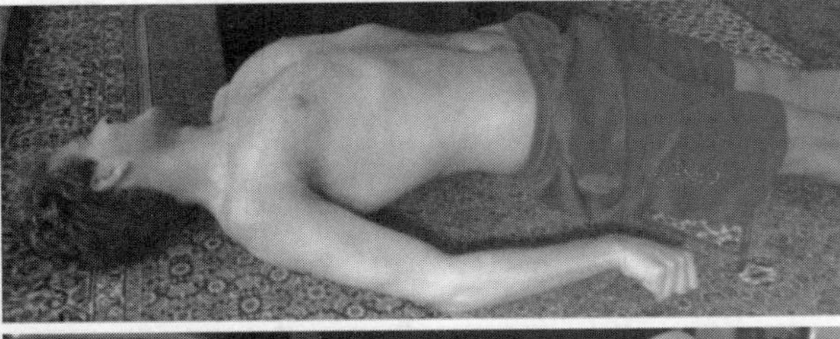

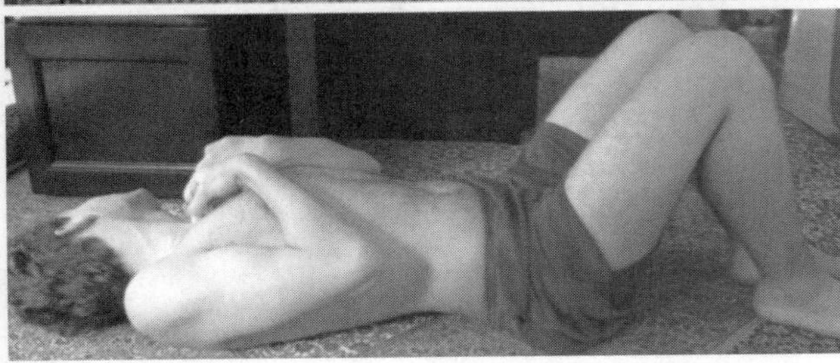

The illustrations depict involuntary movements commonly seen in grand mal or tonic–clonic seizures. A) Depicts tonic movement. B) Depicts clonic movement.

Source: Courtesy of K. Kyriakidis

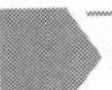

Concept Check

3. **How long does an absence seizure generally last?**
   A. Less than 30 seconds
   B. From 1 to 2 minutes
   C. No longer than 30 minutes
   D. Up to 45 minutes

Answer question

Postictal State

- Patients with either partial or generalized seizures usually have a period of confusion and weakness afterward that may last from minutes to hours.
- The patient may appear to be awake, but may not communicate or seem "present" for a temporary period.
- The patient may also have focal deficits such as a hemiparesis that may be mistaken for a stroke.

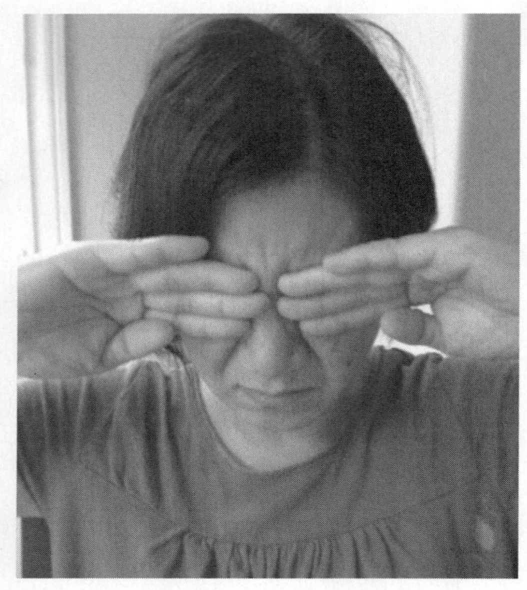

The postictal state refers to the period following a seizure. In addition to physical responses, a seizure can cause behavioral effects. Common behaviors after a seizure can last anywhere from a few seconds to a few days, and although frightening, they rarely cause long-term harm.
Source: Copyright © 2014, NovEx Novice to Expert Learning, LLC

LO2:

Diagnostics

- Obtain blood glucose via point of care (POC) device to evaluate for hypoglycemia.
- Laboratory tests may be ordered to identify the cause of seizures. These may include electrolytes and drug screen (e.g., low sodium, <120 mEq/L).
- If the patient has a history of seizures and is taking anticonvulsant medications, a drug level may be obtained to determine if the drug is in the therapeutic range.
- An electroencephalogram (EEG) may show an area of abnormal firing of the brain.
- A noncontrast computerized tomography (CT) or magnetic resonance imaging (MRI) of the brain may be ordered to determine if injury occurred during the seizure. These studies may also determine if there is any physical abnormality such as a brain tumor or vascular malformation that may have caused the seizure.
- Further tests, such as lumbar puncture, may be performed depending upon clinical circumstances (e.g., if CNS infections are a possibility).

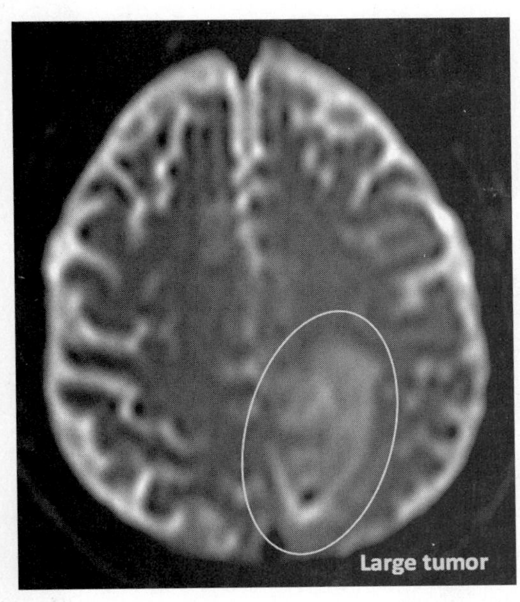

This MRI pictures the brain with a brain tumor in the right posterior region. The brain tumor is the most likely cause of the patient's seizures.
Source: Courtesy of K. Kyriakidis

Concept Check

4. What is the period immediately following a seizure called?

A. Postictal
B. Tonic
C. Absence
D. Myoclonic

Answer question

Priority Patient Concerns and Desired Collaborative Care Outcomes

Prior to caring for patients with seizures, it is important to prioritize the patient's concerns that must guide the nursing care plan and interventions. Care for the patient is ordered and organized in accordance with the patient's priority and urgent needs. Desired collaborative care outcomes in patients with seizures typically include:

1. Patient's airway will remain patent throughout seizure activity.
2. Patient will not experience injury during seizures.
3. Patient will state improved sense of power and describe measures to manage disease.
4. Patient will reorient to person, place, and time following seizures.
5. Patient will state a plan for using supportive measures to prevent social isolation (e.g., support groups, social work, counseling).

Considering these important care outcomes, prepare a list of the major 3–6 priority patient concerns or nursing diagnoses for patients with seizures. Be prepared to participate in a discussion of this list and/or to submit them as an assignment, as determined by your faculty. Resources you may find helpful in this assignment can include this lesson, the references, resources on nursing care plans, and standard nursing diagnoses manuals.

LO3:

Collaborative Interventions

- Call the Rapid Response Team if a seizure occurs.

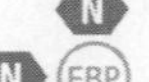

- Note the time the seizure starts, its progression, and its duration (Fisher, et al., 2009).
- Monitor and be prepared to manage cardiopulmonary functions. Administer CPR if the patient does not resume spontaneous respirations and/or pulse following seizure (National Institute of Health and Care Excellence [NICE], 2012).
- Note any precipitating or warning factors (e.g., aura). Carefully and completely describe these factors (Fisher, et al., 2009).
- Note the level of consciousness during and after the episode (e.g., unconscious, confused, dazed) (Fisher, et al., 2009).
- Identify and document the types of movement and the limbs involved during the seizure (ictus). May include twitching, jerking, stiffening, head turning, eye rolling or flickering, or deviation (Fisher, et al., 2009).

Safety Measures

Patients who are experiencing a seizure are at risk for accidental injury. Safety measures can help protect the patient and include:

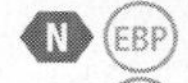

- Stay with the patient to keep him or her safe (Fisher, et al., 2009).
- Ensure that bedrail pads are placed to mitigate the risk for injury during a seizure (Seattle Children's Hospital [SCH], 2012).

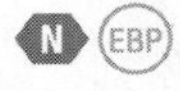

- When witnessing a seizure, attempt to assist the person to the ground (if not in bed) and turn the person onto a side (Fisher, et al., 2009).

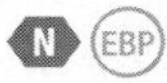

- Remove any objects in the environment that are near and can cause harm (Fisher, et al., 2009).

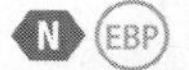

- Do not restrain the person who is seizing (Fisher, et al., 2009).
- Do not place anything or force any object into the person's mouth (Fisher, et al., 2009).
- If possible, place pillows under the head in order to reduce potential injury.

Support After the Seizure

- Once the seizure stops, quickly assess airway breathing and circulation (Fisher, et al., 2009).

- Apply supplemental oxygen and airway support while observing the level of consciousness (Fisher, et al., 2009).

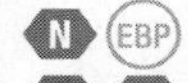

- Assess blood pressure and heart rate (SCH, 2012).
- Obtain blood glucose and basic metabolic panel (BMP) or electrolytes and/or kidney tests via POC.

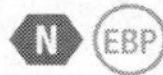

- During the post-seizure (known as postictal) period, observe the behavior and overall neurologic status. The patient may be temporarily weak, disoriented, or seem unable to speak (Fisher, et al., 2009).
- Examine the patient for any signs of injury or trauma.
- Note bleeding of the tongue or around the mouth.
- Assure the individual that he or she is safe (Fisher, et al., 2009).

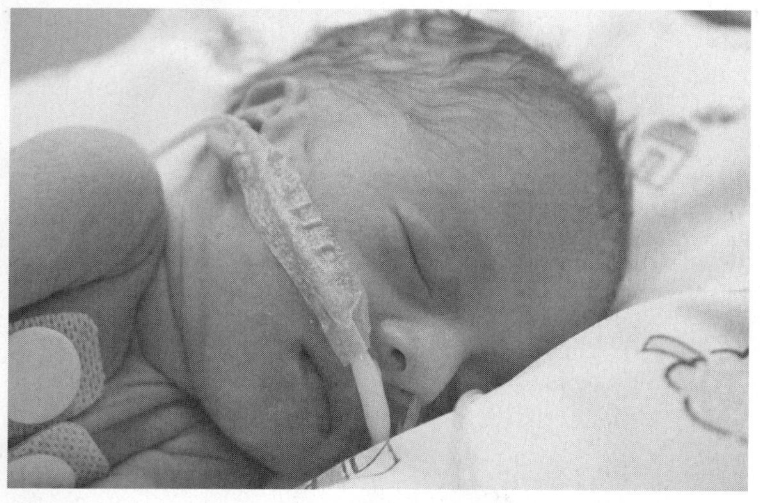

A peaceful moment in the ICU after 6 hours of on and off seizures on Halloween.
Source: Gert Vrey/Fotolia

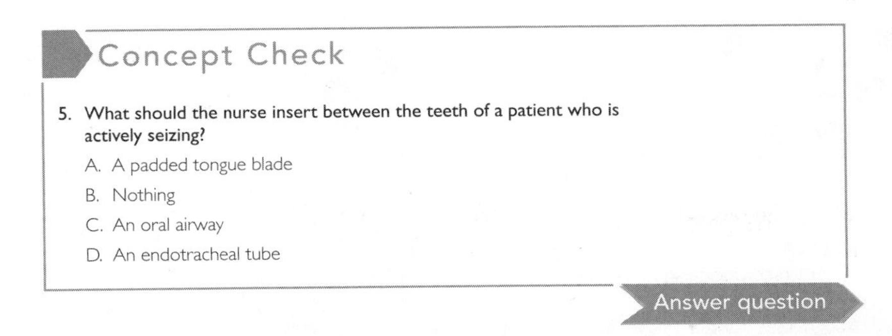

Concept Check

5. What should the nurse insert between the teeth of a patient who is actively seizing?

A. A padded tongue blade

B. Nothing

C. An oral airway

D. An endotracheal tube

Answer question

Collaborative Interventions (continued)

Medications Used in Seizures

Following diagnostic work-up, tests are interpreted to determine if the patient needs to be on anticonvulsant medication. A major goal of antiepileptic management is complete seizure control without adverse drug effects.

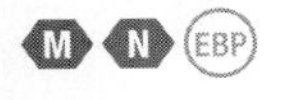

- First-time seizures may not require anticonvulsant treatment. However, if a second seizure occurs, anticonvulsant therapy is usually initiated (NICE, 2012).
- There are a number of different medications used to control seizures. Most commonly prescribed newer treatments include:
  - o Valproic acid (Depakote), 15–60 mg/kg/day. May not be used in women of childbearing age with first-time seizures (Glauser, et al., 2006; NICE, 2012).
  - o Levetiracetam (Keppra), 1000–3000 mg/day (Glauser, et al., 2006; NICE, 2012)
- Other commonly used drugs include:
  - o Phenobarbital, 60–250 mg/day. It is effective but has more side effects than other drugs (Glauser, et al., 2006).
  - o Phenytoin (Dilantin), 300–600 mg/day. It is effective. Side effects include gum hyperplasia (Glauser, et al., 2006).
  - o Carbamazepine (Tegretol), 600–1200 mg/day (Glauser, et al., 2006). Caution: Carbamazepine has the potential to exacerbate myoclonic seizures (NICE, 2012).
  - o Primidone (Mysoline), 25 mg three times/day (Glauser, et al., 2006).
  - o Lamotrigine (Lamictal), 100–300 mg/day (Glauser, et al., 2006). Caution: lamotrigine has the potential to exacerbate myoclonic seizures (NICE, 2012).
  - o Gabapentin (Neurontin), 900–3600 mg/day (Glauser, et al., 2006)
  - o Lacosamide (Vimpat), 10–400 mg/day
- In patients with absence or myoclonic seizures, avoid the use of carbamazepine, pregabalin, gabapentin, tiagabine, oxcarbazepine, vigabatrin, and phenytoin, which can exacerbate the seizure disorder (NICE, 2012).
- Be vigilant in monitoring for drug-related adverse effects (NICE, 2012).
- Surgical removal of a seizure focus may be considered in patients not responding to medications or other treatments (Fisher, et al., 2009).

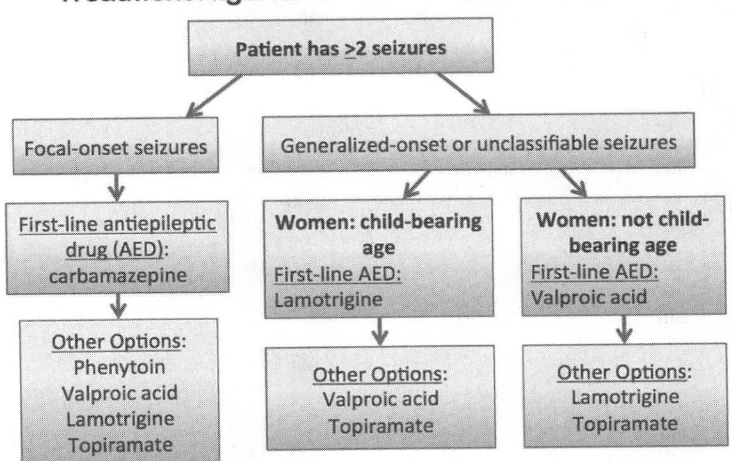

A suggested treatment algorithm. An AED is an antiepileptic drug.

Collaborative Interventions (continued)

Status Epilepticus

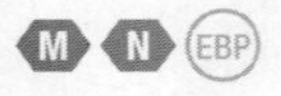

- In the individual with sustaining status epilepticus, the airway must be protected. Supplemental oxygen with bag, valve, and/or mask and pulse oximetry should be implemented (Fisher, et al., 2009).
- Consideration for endotracheal intubation should be considered if the seizure is prolonged.
- Ensure that the patient is safe and reduce the chance of injury by keeping the bedrails up and padding them around the patient (see photo) (Fisher, et al., 2009).

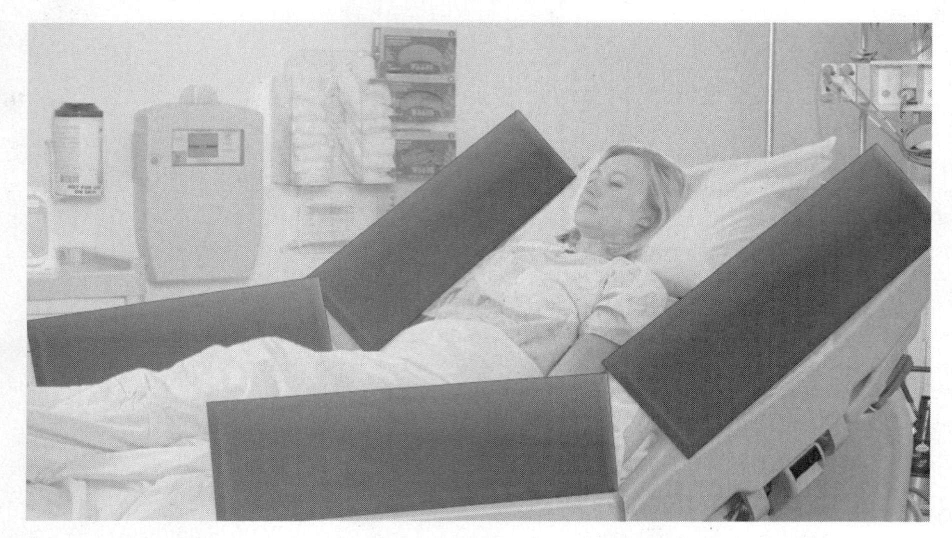

This image depicts the protective side rail pads used for safety when caring for patients with seizures.

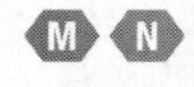

- After assessing blood pressure and heart rate, ensure IV access with two large bore IV catheters. Begin normal saline IV.
- Quickly check the blood glucose level and administer supplemental glucose if needed.
- Immediate medications to be administered include thiamine 100 mg and 50% dextrose if the bedside glucose is <70 mg/dL.
- Collaborate regarding need for lab tests, which may include blood cell count, metabolic panel, liver function tests, magnesium, calcium, phosphorus, ammonia, toxicology and alcohol, lactate, creatine phosphokinase (CPK), prolactin, and coagulation tests.
- In the event that the medication history is unknown, obtain blood levels of phenytoin, phenobarbital, primidone, carbamazepine, and valproic acid.

Immediate Treatment of Status Epilepticus

Immediately administer medications to stop the seizures. Collaboration with the health care provider is needed regarding type of seizure and medical history:

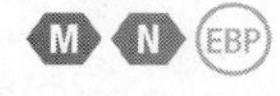

- IV lorazepam—administer 0.1 mg/kg at 2 mg/minute. Up to 8 mg can be given to a maximum of 0.3 mg/kg (SCH, 2012).
- An alternative is IV diazepam, 0.15 mg/kg at 5 mg/minute to a maximum of 10 mg.

If the seizure does not stop:

- Administer IV fosphenytoin, as ordered, 20 mg/kg at 150 mg/minute (phenytoin equivalent at a slower rate). If the patient is still seizing, administer an additional 5 mg/kg fosphenytoin IV, which may be followed with another 5 mg/kg to a total maximum of 30 mg/kg IV (SCH, 2012).

Alternatives:

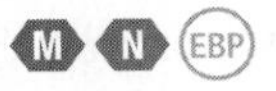

- IV phenobarbital—20 mg/kg at 50–100 mg/minute with additional 5–10 mg/kg if refractory. It may be given up to a maximum of 30 mg/kg with maintenance at 2–4 mg/kg/day (Fisher, et al., 2009).
- Divalproex sodium—25 mg/kg over 60 min × 1, then 10–15 mg/kg/day, divided every 6 hours
- Propofol—1–2 mg/kg × 1, then 1–15 mg/kg/hour IV drip
- IV midazolam—0.2 mg/kg × 1, then 0.75–10 mcg/kg/minute or 0.05–0.4 mg/kg/hour. *Note: Midazolam has never been tested officially for initial treatment of status epilepticus over lorazepam* (SCH, 2012).

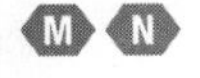

- Patients who are intubated and pharmacologically paralyzed will not show signs of tonic–clonic movements but may still be seizing. Avoid paralytic agents in patients with seizures.

Post-Status Epilepticus Seizure

- Reassess vital signs and include temperature. If the body temperature is elevated, initiate cooling measures immediately.
- A continuous EEG monitoring should be initiated as soon as possible to determine the extent of seizure activity and to indicate when the seizures stop. The individual with status epilepticus is managed in the ICU for the duration of the status. Assessment of neurologic status must be done on a regular basis.
- Once the seizures have halted, extensive diagnostic tests are done to determine if there is any permanent damage to the brain. Support of all major body systems is maintained while the patient is in the hospital.
- It is imperative that status epilepticus be halted as rapidly as possible in order to limit the damage to the brain. Individuals can sustain significant brain injury or even brain death if the seizure activity is prolonged.
- Recommend the approach to the long-term pharmacological treatment of patients with seizures to include (NICE, 2012):
  - If first-line monodrug therapy fails to effectively treat seizures, initiate a second monotherapy. Use caution and closely monitor during the pharmacologic transition. Taper the first drug slowly after second drug reaches adequate blood levels.
  - If the second drug is ineffective before tapering the first, collaborate with the health care provider about which to taper and then start another drug.
  - Recommend combination drug therapy if attempts at monodrug therapies fail.
- Avoid giving paralytic medications to patients with seizures because paralytics mask (hide) potential continued seizures (cerebral seizure activity) without any evident peripheral muscle movement. It can be dangerous for the patient to go untreated.

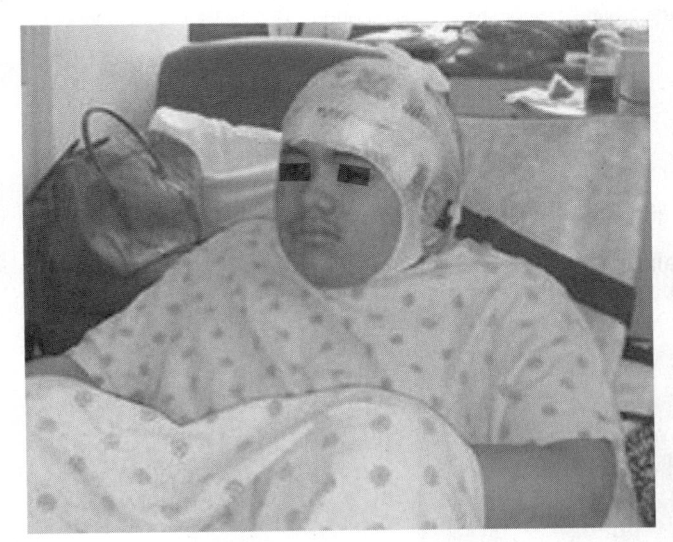

Young patient is prepared to have an EEG. He has numerous electrical probes on his head, which are covered by a stocking to hold them in place.
Source: Courtesy of K. Kyriakidis

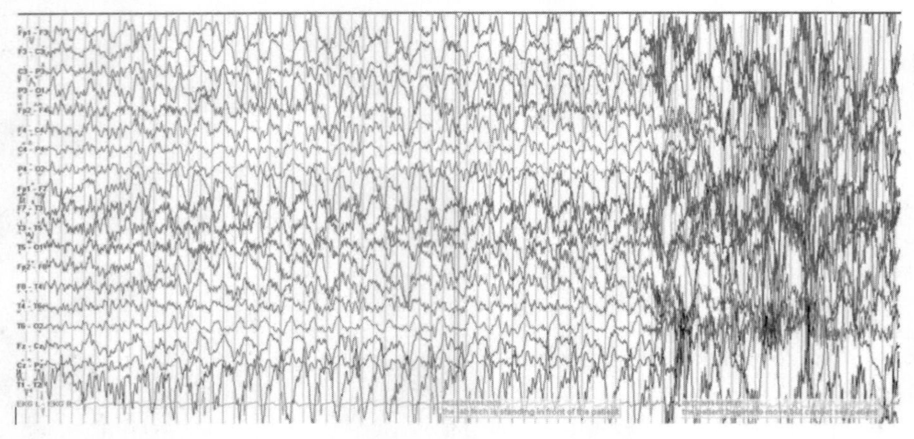

During an EEG, a generalized tonic-clonic or grand mal seizure occurred. The patient became unresponsive. Note the widespread outbreak of repetitive spike and polyspike complexes of high amplitude, seen to the right of the EEG.
Source: Courtesy of Dr. Colleen Vanderkolk

- Involve the epilepsy nurse specialist or comparable nurse on the team to ensure that the patient understands and gains access to the multiple health care and community resources needed to learn necessary information and support them over time (NICE, 2012).

Collaborative Interventions (continued)

Patient Education

The patient and family should be educated about seizure precautions to protect the patient and others. Patient should be aware of the following:

- Avoid bathing alone (showers are best) to protect the patient from accidental submersion underwater in case of a seizure.

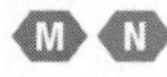

- Refrain from driving until receiving a physician's release. State laws vary but all prohibit driving for a period of time, on average 6–12 months, after a seizure until the patient is stabilized and adherent to medication regimen.

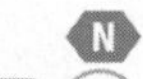

- Avoid use of any equipment that can cause harm to self or others if a seizure occurred.

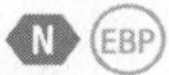

- Actions to take if the individual has a seizure (Fisher, et al., 2009):
  - o Stay calm and time the seizure. Look for seizure ID bracelet.
  - o Loosen tight-fitting clothing around the neck.
  - o Ensure that the patient is safe. Help patient to the ground if he or she is falling or about to fall.
  - o Support the head with a cushion or by gently holding both sides. Move nearby objects to prevent striking the patient.
  - o Place pillows around the patient to protect him or her from injury.
  - o Do not try to open mouth or put objects in the mouth. Do not give food or drink.
  - o Do not restrain his or her involuntary movements as this can result in injury.

Recovery Position Post-Seizure

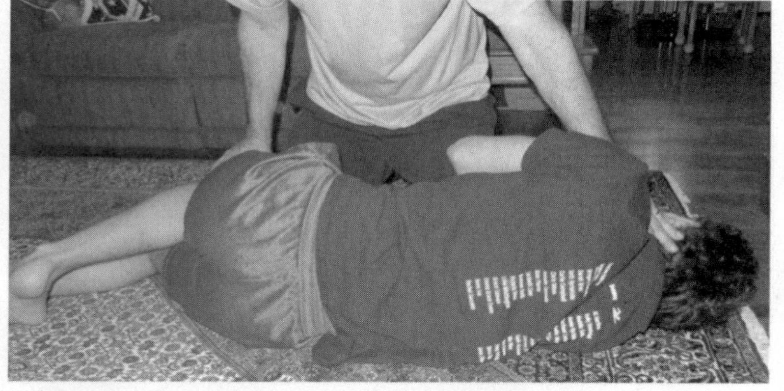

In the recovery phase post-seizure, support that patient's head, keep the patient's head to the side to prevent aspiration, and keep the patient turned off his or her back.

Source: Courtesy of K. Kyriakidis

- o Turn the patient onto a side to prevent aspiration.
  - o Call EMS or 911 for help if the seizure lasts over 5 minutes, results in injury, produces physical distress, patient is pregnant, fails to return to consciousness, or there is concern.
- After a seizure, family or friends can offer support until the patient is fully aware and oriented again. Care during the postictal period may include:
  - o Reassure the person that he or she is safe without restraining. Be supportive and reassuring.
  - o Give the patient time to recover fully from being dazed, tired, and weak. With recovery, the patient begins to know who and where he or she is.
  - o Observe for injuries, particularly in the mouth.
- Safety is the main issue addressed in patient and family education. The National Seizure Disorders Foundation and the Epilepsy Foundation are two excellent sources that families and friends may be referred to for simple and clear education.
- Educate the patient to avoid and be aware of possible triggers: dietary deficiencies (e.g., low calcium or magnesium), low blood glucose, fatigue, stress, anger and other strong emotions, loud music, flashing lights, sleep deprivation, alcohol and drugs (of special concern), fever, intense exercise, excessive caffeine, dehydration, menstrual periods, and certain medications for other conditions.

Signs & Symptoms: Postictal State

- ✓ Confusion, amnesia
- ✓ Drowsiness
- ✓ Hypertension
- ✓ Headache, migraine
- ✓ Nausea
- ✓ Muscle soreness
- ✓ Sore cheek or tongue

This table lists major manifestations that patients commonly experience after a seizure, during the postictal period.

- Educate patients who smoke that they risk starting a fire if they have a seizure while smoking.

- Educate the patient that many of the drugs prescribed for seizure control require that a specific level be achieved in the blood. Low levels may be ineffective, and high levels may be associated with toxic side effects (Fisher, et al., 2009). Patients need to have routine blood levels tested.
- Educate young women and women of childbearing age that special precautions are needed and they should routinely see their health care provider if pregnant or pregnancy is anticipated (Fisher, et al., 2009).
- Prior to discharge, it is imperative to educate the patient and family about their medication administration, side effects, specific dietary restrictions, and other medication considerations (Fisher, et al., 2009).
- A subset of patients who have not responded well to antiepileptic drugs may respond to dietary manipulation with the introduction of a ketogenic diet to control seizures. Consult a nutritionist to assist with this type of diet as it is high in fats and low in carbohydrates. Excessive fats result in increased ketones which have effectively controlled seizures in some when anticonvulsants have been ineffective (Fisher, et al., 2009)
- Encourage patient to verbalize frustrations, feelings of stigma, fear, social isolation, anger, or any concerns so that help and support may be offered (Fisher, et al., 2009).
- Introduce the patient to the multiple health care and community resources available. Support groups can be very helpful in learning to live comfortably and safely with the potential of seizures, in most situations. Resources include: Epilepsy Foundation of America and American Epilepsy Society.

Concept Check

6. What is characteristic of a ketogenic diet?

A. It includes additional carbohydrates.
B. It is low sodium.
C. It is high fat.
D. It emphasizes meal timing.

Answer question

Summary of Interventions

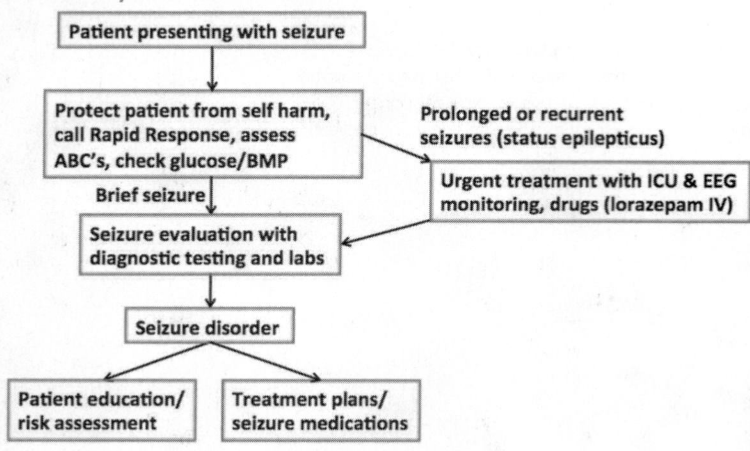

LO4:

Evaluation of Desired Collaborative Care Outcomes

Evaluation and reassessment should reveal attainment of previously established patient outcomes. In summary:

- Patient's airway was not compromised during seizure activity.
- Patient remains injury free.
- Patient reports feeling more empowered to manage illness.
- Patient is able to state person, place, and time following seizures.
- Patient reports attendance at support groups, social activities, and/or other preferred methods of support.

Concept Check

7. What is the priority goal for a patient with status epilepticus?

A. Protect the patient from injury to extremities.
B. Stop the seizure.
C. Determine seizure trigger.
D. Intubate the patient.

Answer question

References

Balamurugan, E., Aggarwal, M., Lamba, A., Dang, N., & Tripathi, M. (2013). Perceived trigger factors of seizures in persons with epilepsy. *Seizure European Journal Epilepsy, 22*(9), 743–747.

Devinsky, O. (2004). Effects of seizures on autonomic and cardiovascular function. *Epilepsy Currents, 4*(2), 43–46. **www.ncbi.nlm.nih.gov/pmc/articles/PMC531654/**

Miller, W. R. (2014). Patient-centered outcomes in older adults with epilepsy. *Seizure.* **www.ncbi.nlm.nih.gov/pubmed/24838071**

Reddig, R.T., Nixdorf, K. E., & Jensen, M. B. (2011). The prophylactic use of an antiepileptic drug in intracerebral hemorrhage. *Clinical Neurology and Neurosurgery, 113*(10), 895–897. **www.ncbi.nlm.nih.gov/pubmed/21824722**

Clinical Practice Guidelines

Fisher, R., & Long, L. (2009). *Care of the patient with seizures* AANN Clinical Practice Guideline Series, Revised 2009. **www.aann.org/pdf/cpg/aannseizures.pdf**

Glauser, T., Ben-Menachem, E., Bourgeois, B., et al. (2006). ILAE treatment guidelines: Evidence-based analysis of antiepileptic drug efficacy and effectiveness as initial monotherapy for epileptic seizures and syndromes. *Epilepsia, 47*(7), 1094–1120. **staging.ilae.org/Visitors/Documents/Guidelines.pdf**

National Institute of Health and Care Excellence. (2012). *The epilepsies: The diagnosis and management of the epilepsies in adults and children in primary and secondary care* (NICE clinical guideline 137). **guidance.nice.org.uk/cg137**

Patient Education

Epilepsy Foundation of America. (2005). *Ketogenic diet.* **www.epilepsy.com/learn/treating-seizures-and-epilepsy/dietary-therapies/ketogenic-diet**

Epilepsy Foundation of America. (2007). *Epilepsy.* **www.epilepsy.com/learn/about-epilepsy-basics#**

National Seizure Disorders Foundation. *Seizure First Aid – A Real Life Saver.* **nationalseizuredisordersfoundation.org/seizure-first-aid/**

Seattle Children's Hospital & Research Foundation. (2013). *Seizure acute management: Emergency department version 1.2.* **www.google.com/url?sa=t&rct=j&q=&esrc=s&source=web&cd=1&ved=0CCQQFjAA&url=http%3A%2F%2Fwww.seattlechildrens.org%2Fpdf%2Fseizure-acute-management-pathway.pdf&ei=fzu7U-OeLqbfsATszoD4Aw&usg=AFQjCNHkWaJz5czHqLC9vYLSYqCjL3SmMQ&bvm=bv.70138588,d.cWc**

U.S. National Library of Medicine. (2012). *Epilepsy.* **www.ncbi.nlm.nih.gov/pubmedhealth/PMH0001714/**

STOP

Go to the online course and complete the NovE-Cases assigned by your instructor for this module.